ARCHIVES OF GENERAL PSYCHIATRY

JANUARY 1994

LIFETIME AND 12-MONTH PREVALENCE OF *DSM-III-R* PSYCHIATRIC DISORDERS IN THE UNITED STATES: RESULTS FROM THE NATIONAL COMORBIDITY SURVEY
R. C. Kessler et al

SUICIDALITY AND 5-HYDROXYINDOLEACETIC ACID CONCENTRATION ASSOCIATED WITH A TRYPTOPHAN HYDROXYLASE POLYMORPHISM
D. A. Nielsen et al

CSF BIOCHEMISTRIES, GLUCOSE METABOLISM, AND DIURNAL ACTIVITY RHYTHMS IN ALCOHOLIC, VIOLENT OFFENDERS, FIRE SETTERS, AND HEALTHY VOLUNTEERS
M. Virkkunen et al

PERSONALITY PROFILES AND STATE AGGRESSIVENESS IN FINNISH ALCOHOLIC, VIOLENT OFFENDERS, FIRE SETTERS, AND HEALTHY VOLUNTEERS
M. Virkkunen et al

WHO NEUROPSYCHIATRIC AIDS STUDY, CROSS-SECTIONAL PHASE:
I. STUDY DESIGN AND PSYCHIATRIC FINDINGS
II. NEUROPSYCHOLOGICAL AND NEUROLOGICAL FINDINGS
M. Maj et al

REGIONAL CEREBRAL BLOOD FLOW MEASURED DURING SYMPTOM PROVOCATION IN OBSESSIVE-COMPULSIVE DISORDER USING OXYGEN 15–LABELED CARBON DIOXIDE AND POSITRON EMISSION TOMOGRAPHY
S. L. Rauch et al

American Medical Association
Physicians dedicated to the health of America

New dosing guidelines optimize relapse control for Larry

Establish a safe, effective oral haloperidol dose

How Much?	**Initial month's dose is 10 to 15 times patient's daily oral dose[3]** ■ Elderly ■ Debilitated ■ Stabilized on oral doses <10 mg/day	**Initial month's dose is 20 times patient's daily oral dose[3]** ■ Maintained on oral doses >10 mg/day ■ Tolerant to oral medication ■ At risk for relapse
	Supplementation with oral haloperidol can be used during periods of dose adjustments	
How Often?	■ Once a month ■ Since first injection should not exceed 100 mg, the balance of the first month's dosage can be administered 3 to 7 days later	
How High?	■ Total monthly dose should not exceed 450 mg ■ Maximum volume per injection site should not exceed 3 mL	
Maintenance	■ 10 to 15 times daily oral dose depending on clinical response	■ 10 to 15 times daily oral dose depending on clinical response ■ If 20 times the daily oral dose is used, monthly dose should be reduced based on clinical response (by approximately 25% of the original dose, each month for 2 months) until appropriate maintenance dose is reached[4]

■ In a recent multicenter trial, a 200-mg monthly maintenance dose of HALDOL Decanoate provided the most consistent relapse prevention when compared to lower decanoate doses of 25 mg, 50 mg, and 100 mg. In this study, patients had a lower rate of extrapyramidal side effects on all dosage levels of depot therapy than at the start of the study when most patients were on oral medication.[5]

HALDOL® Decanoate 50 / HALDOL® Decanoate 100
(haloperidol) **(haloperidol)**

For IM Injection Only

Brief Summary

The following is a brief summary only. Before prescribing, see complete prescribing information in HALDOL and HALDOL Decanoate product labeling.

CONTRAINDICATIONS: Since the pharmacologic and clinical actions of HALDOL Decanoate 50 and HALDOL Decanoate 100 are attributed to HALDOL haloperidol as the active medication, CONTRAINDICATIONS, WARNINGS, and additional information are those of HALDOL, modified to reflect the prolonged action. HALDOL is contraindicated in severe toxic central nervous system depression or comatose states from any cause and in individuals who are hypersensitive to this drug or have Parkinson's disease.

WARNINGS: ***Tardive Dyskinesia:*** Tardive dyskinesia, a syndrome consisting of potentially irreversible, involuntary, dyskinetic movements may develop in patients treated with antipsychotic drugs. Although the prevalence of the syndrome appears to be highest among the elderly, especially elderly women, it is impossible to rely upon prevalence estimates to predict, at the inception of antipsychotic treatment, which patients are likely to develop the syndrome. Whether antipsychotic drug products differ in their potential to cause tardive dyskinesia is unknown. Both the risk of developing tardive dyskinesia and the likelihood that it will become irreversible are believed to increase as the duration of treatment and the total cumulative dose of antipsychotic drugs administered to the patient increase. However, the syndrome can develop, although much less commonly, after relatively brief treatment periods at low doses. There is no known treatment for established cases of tardive dyskinesia, although the syndrome may remit, partially or completely, if antipsychotic treatment is withdrawn. Antipsychotic treatment, itself, however, may suppress (or partially suppress) the signs and symptoms of the syndrome and thereby may possibly mask the underlying process. The effect that symptomatic suppression has upon the long-term course of the syndrome is unknown. Given these considerations, antipsychotic drugs should be prescribed in a manner that is most likely to minimize the occurrence of tardive dyskinesia. Chronic antipsychotic treatment should generally be reserved for patients who suffer from a chronic illness that 1) is known to respond to antipsychotic drugs, and 2) for whom alternative, equally effective, but potentially less harmful treatments are **not** available or appropriate. In patients who do require chronic treatment, the smallest dose and the shortest duration of treatment producing a satisfactory clinical response should be sought. The need for continued treatment should be reassessed periodically. If signs and symptoms of tardive dyskinesia appear in a patient on antipsychotics, drug discontinuation should be considered. However, some patients may require treatment despite the presence of the syndrome. (For further information about the description of tardive dyskinesia and its clinical detection, please refer to ***ADVERSE REACTIONS***.)

Neuroleptic Malignant Syndrome (NMS): A potentially fatal symptom complex sometimes referred to as Neuroleptic Malignant Syndrome (NMS) has been reported in association with antipsychotic drugs. Clinical manifestations of NMS are hyperpyrexia, muscle rigidity, altered mental status (including catatonic signs) and evidence of autonomic instability (irregular pulse or blood pressure, tachycardia, diaphoresis, and cardiac dysrhythmias). Additional signs may include elevated creatine phosphokinase, myoglobinuria (rhabdomyolysis) and acute renal failure. The diagnostic evaluation of patients with this syndrome is complicated. In arriving at a diagnosis, it is important to identify cases where the clinical presentation includes both serious medical illness (e.g., pneumonia, systemic infection, etc.) and untreated or inadequately treated extrapyramidal signs and symptoms (EPS). Other important considerations in the differential diagnosis include central anticholinergic toxicity, heat stroke, drug fever and primary central nervous system (CNS) pathology. The management of NMS should include 1) immediate discontinuation of antipsychotic drugs and other drugs not essential to concurrent therapy, 2) intensive symptomatic treatment and medical monitoring, and 3) treatment of any concomitant serious medical problems for which specific treatments are available. There is no general agreement about specific pharmacological treatment regimens for uncomplicated NMS. If a patient requires antipsychotic drug treatment after recovery from NMS, the potential reintroduction of drug therapy should be carefully considered. The patient should be carefully monitored, since recurrences of NMS have been reported. Hyperpyrexia and heat stroke, not associated with the above symptom complex, have also been reported with HALDOL.

Usage in Pregnancy: (see ***PRECAUTIONS - Usage in Pregnancy***)

Combined Use With Lithium: (see ***PRECAUTIONS-Drug Interactions***)

General: Bronchopneumonia, sometimes fatal, has followed use of antipsychotic drugs, including haloperidol. Prompt remedial therapy should be instituted if dehydration, hemoconcentration or reduced pulmonary ventilation occur, especially in the elderly. Decreased serum cholesterol and/or cutaneous and ocular changes have been reported with chemically-related drugs, although not with haloperidol. See ***PRECAUTIONS - Information for Patients*** for information on mental and/or physical abilities and on concomitant use with other substances.

PRECAUTIONS: Administer cautiously to patients: (1) with severe cardiovascular disorders, due to the possibility of transient hypotension and/or precipitation of anginal pain (if a vasopressor is required, epinephrine should not be used since HALDOL may block its vasopressor activity and paradoxical further lowering of blood pressure may occur; metaraminol, phenylephrine or norepinephrine should be used); (2) receiving anticonvulsant medications, with a history of seizures, or with EEG abnormalities, because HALDOL may lower the convulsive threshold. If indicated, adequate anticonvulsant therapy should be concomitantly maintained; (3) with known allergies or a history of allergic reactions to drugs; (4) receiving anticoagulants, since an isolated instance of interference occurred with the effects of one anticoagulant (phenindione). Concomitant antiparkinson medication, if required, may have to be continued after HALDOL is discontinued because of different excretion rates; if both are discontinued simultaneously, extrapyramidal symptoms may occur. Intraocular pressure may increase when anticholinergic drugs, including antiparkinson drugs, are administered concomitantly with HALDOL. When HALDOL is used for mania in bipolar disorders, there may be a rapid mood swing to depression. Severe neurotoxicity may occur in patients with thyrotoxicosis receiving antipsychotic medication, including HALDOL.

Information for Patients: Mental and/or physical abilities required for hazardous tasks or driving may be impaired. Alcohol should be avoided due to possible additive effects and hypotension.

Drug Interactions: Patients receiving lithium plus haloperidol should be monitored closely for early evidence of neurological toxicity and treatment discontinued promptly if such signs appear. As with other antipsychotic agents, it should be noted that HALDOL may be capable of potentiating CNS depressants such as anesthetics, opiates, and alcohol.

Carcinogenesis, Mutagenesis and Impairment of Fertility: No mutagenic potential of haloperidol was found in the Ames Salmonella microsomal activation assay. Negative or inconsistent positive findings have been obtained in *in vitro* and *in vivo* studies of effects of haloperidol on chromosome structure and number. The available cytogenetic evidence is considered too inconsistent to be conclusive at this time. Carcinogenicity studies using oral haloperidol were conducted in Wistar rats (dosed at up to 5 mg/kg daily for 24 months) and in Albino Swiss mice (dosed at up to 5 mg/kg daily for 18 months). In the rat study survival was less than optimal in all dose groups, reducing the number of rats at risk for developing tumors. However, although a relatively greater number of rats survived to the end of the study in high dose male and female groups, these animals did not have a greater incidence of tumors than control animals. Therefore, although not optimal, this study does suggest the absence of a haloperidol related increase in the incidence of neoplasia in rats at doses up to 20 times the usual daily human dose for chronic or resistant patients. In female mice at 5 and 20 times the highest initial daily dose for chronic or resistant patients, there was a statistically significant increase in mammary gland neoplasia and total tumor incidence; at 20 times the same daily dose there was a statistically significant increase in pituitary gland neoplasia. In male mice, no statistically significant differences in incidences of total tumors or specific tumor types were noted. Antipsychotic drugs elevate prolactin levels; the elevation persists during chronic administration. Tissue culture experiments indicate that approximately one-third of human breast cancers are prolactin dependent *in vitro*, a factor of potential importance if the prescription of these drugs is contemplated in a patient with a previously detected breast cancer. Although disturbances such as galactorrhea, amenorrhea, gynecomastia, and impotence have been reported, the clinical significance of elevated serum prolactin levels is unknown for most patients. An increase in mammary neoplasms has been found in rodents after chronic administration of antipsychotic drugs. Neither clinical studies nor epidemiologic studies conducted to date, however, have shown an association between chronic administration of these drugs and mammary tumorigenesis: the available evidence is considered too limited to be conclusive at this time.

Usage in Pregnancy: Pregnancy Category C. Safe use in pregnancy or in women likely to become pregnant has not been established; use only if benefit clearly justifies potential hazards to the fetus.

Nursing Mothers: Infants should not be nursed during drug treatment.

Pediatric Use: Controlled trials to establish the safety and effectiveness of intramuscular administration in children have not been conducted.

ADVERSE REACTIONS: Adverse reactions following the administration of HALDOL Decanoate 50 or HALDOL Decanoate 100 are those of HALDOL haloperidol. Since vast experience has accumulated with HALDOL, the adverse reactions are reported for that compound as well as for haloperidol decanoate. As with all injectable medications, local tissue reactions have been reported with haloperidol decanoate.

CNS Effects: Extrapyramidal Symptoms (EPS) — EPS during the administration of HALDOL (haloperidol) have been reported frequently, often during the first few days of treatment. EPS can be categorized generally as Parkinson-like symptoms, akathisia, or dystonia (including opisthotonos and oculogyric crisis). While all can occur at relatively low doses, they occur more frequently and with greater severity at higher doses. The symptoms may be controlled with dose reductions or administration of antiparkinson drugs such as benztropine mesylate USP or trihexyphenidyl hydrochloride USP. It should be noted that persistent EPS have been reported; the drug may have to be discontinued in such cases. ***Withdrawal Emergent Neurological Signs*** — Abrupt discontinuation of short-term anti-psychotic therapy is generally uneventful. However, some patients on maintenance treatment experience transient dyskinetic signs after abrupt withdrawal. In certain cases these are indistinguishable from "Tardive Dyskinesia" except for duration. It is unknown whether gradual withdrawal will reduce the occurrence of these signs, but until further evidence is available HALDOL should be gradually withdrawn. ***Tardive Dyskinesia*** — As with all antipsychotic agents HALDOL has been associated with persistent dyskinesias. Tardive dyskinesia, a syndrome consisting of potentially irreversible, involuntary, dyskinetic movements, may appear in some patients on long-term therapy or may occur after drug therapy has been discontinued. The risk appears to be greater in elderly patients on high-dose therapy, especially females. The symptoms are persistent and in some patients appear irreversible. The syndrome is characterized by rhythmical involuntary movements of tongue, face, mouth or jaw (e.g., protrusion of tongue, puffing of cheeks, puckering of mouth, chewing movements). Sometimes these may be accompanied by involuntary movements of extremities and the trunk. There is no known effective treatment for tardive dyskinesia; antiparkinson agents usually do not alleviate the symptoms of this syndrome. It is suggested that all antipsychotic agents be discontinued if these symptoms appear. Should it be necessary to reinstitute treatment, or increase the dosage of the agent, or switch to a different antipsychotic agent, this syndrome may be masked. It has been reported that fine vermicular movement of the tongue may be an early sign of tardive dyskinesia and if the medication is stopped at that time the full syndrome may not develop. ***Tardive Dystonia*** — Tardive dystonia, not associated with the above syndrome, has also been reported. Tardive dystonia is characterized by delayed onset of choreic or dystonic movements, is often persistent, and has the potential of becoming irreversible. ***Other CNS Effects*** — Insomnia, restlessness, anxiety, euphoria, agitation, drowsiness, depression, lethargy, headache, confusion, vertigo, grand mal seizures, and exacerbation of psychotic symptoms including hallucinations, and catatonic-like behavioral states which may be responsive to drug withdrawal and/or treatment with anticholinergic drugs.

Body as a Whole: Neuroleptic malignant syndrome (NMS), hyperpyrexia and heat stroke have been reported with HALDOL. (See ***WARNINGS*** for further information concerning NMS.)

Cardiovascular Effects: Tachycardia, hypotension, hypertension and ECG changes, including prolongation of the Q-T interval and ECG pattern changes compatible with the polymorphous configuration of torsades de pointes.

Hematologic Effects: Reports of mild, usually transient leukopenia and leukocytosis, minimal decreases in red blood cell counts, anemia, or a tendency toward lymphomonocytosis; agranulocytosis rarely reported and only in association with other medication.

Liver Effects: Impaired liver function and/or jaundice.

Dermatologic Reactions: Maculopapular and acneiform reactions, isolated cases of photosensitivity, loss of hair.

Endocrine Disorders: Lactation, breast engorgement, mastalgia, menstrual irregularities, gynecomastia, impotence, increased libido, hyperglycemia, hypoglycemia and hyponatremia.

Gastrointestinal Effects: Anorexia, constipation, diarrhea, hypersalivation, dyspepsia, nausea and vomiting.

Autonomic Reactions: Dry mouth, blurred vision, urinary retention, diaphoresis, and priapism.

Respiratory Effects: Laryngospasm, bronchospasm and increased depth of respiration.

Special Senses: Cataracts, retinopathy and visual disturbances.

Other: Cases of sudden and unexpected death have been reported in association with the administration of HALDOL. The nature of the evidence makes it impossible to determine definitively what role, if any, HALDOL played in the outcome of the reported cases. The possibility that HALDOL caused death cannot, of course, be excluded, but it is to be kept in mind that sudden and unexpected death may occur in psychotic patients when they go untreated or when they are treated with other antipsychotic drugs.

Postmarketing Events: Hyperammonemia has been reported in a 5½ year old child with citrullinemia, an inherited disorder of ammonia excretion, following treatment with HALDOL.

IMPORTANT: Full directions for use should be read before HALDOL or HALDOL Decanoate products are administered or prescribed.

For information on symptoms and treatment of overdosage, see full prescribing information.

The short-acting HALDOL injectable form is intended only for acutely agitated psychotic patients with moderately severe to very severe symptoms.

10/13/92

References: 1. American Psychiatric Association Highlights: Selecting patients for depot neuroleptic therapy. *Relapse*. 1991;1(3):5,6. 2. Youssef HA. A five-year follow-up study of chronic schizophrenics and other psychotics treated in the community: depot haloperidol decanoate versus other neuroleptics. *Adv Ther*. 1989;6(4):186-195. 3. HALDOL® Decanoate Package Insert. McNeil Pharmaceutical. Spring House, PA 19477. Revised 10/13/92. 4. Ereshefsky L, Toney G, Lyman RC, Saklad SR, Anderson CB, Richards AL. Haloperidol decanoate: an effective dosing strategy. Presented at the American Psychiatric Association 144th Annual Meeting. May 1991; New Orleans, La. 5. Davis JM, Kane JM, Marder SR, et al. Dose response of prophylactic antipsychotics. *J Clin Psychiatry*. 1993;54(suppl 3):24-30.

ARCHIVES OF GENERAL PSYCHIATRY

VOL 51 NO. 1, JAN 1994

Original Articles

Lifetime and 12-Month Prevalence of *DSM-III-R* Psychiatric Disorders in the United States: Results From the National Comorbidity Survey 8
Ronald C. Kessler, PhD; Katherine A. McGonagle, PhD; Shanyang Zhao, PhD; Christopher B. Nelson, MPH; Michael Hughes, PhD; Suzann Eshleman, MA; Hans-Ulrich Wittchen, PhD; Kenneth S. Kendler, MD

CSF Biochemistries, Glucose Metabolism, and Diurnal Activity Rhythms in Alcoholic, Violent Offenders, Fire Setters, and Healthy Volunteers 20
Matti Virkkunen, MD; Robert Rawlings, MS; Riitta Tokola, MD; Russell E. Poland, PhD; Alessandro Guidotti, MD; Charles Nemeroff, MD, PhD; Garth Bissette, PhD; Konstantine Kalogeras, MD; Sirkka-Liisa Karonen, PhD; Markku Linnoila, MD, PhD

Personality Profiles and State Aggressiveness in Finnish Alcoholic, Violent Offenders, Fire Setters, and Healthy Volunteers 28
Matti Virkkunen, MD; Eila Kallio, PhD; Robert Rawlings, MS; Riitta Tokola, MD; Russell E. Poland, PhD; Alessandro Guidotti, MD; Charles Nemeroff, MD, PhD; Garth Bissette, PhD; Konstantine Kalogeras, MD; Sirkka-Liisa Karonen, PhD; Markku Linnoila, MD, PhD

Suicidality and 5-Hydroxyindoleacetic Acid Concentration Associated With a Tryptophan Hydroxylase Polymorphism 34
David A. Nielsen, PhD; David Goldman, MD; Matti Virkkunen, MD; Riitta Tokola, MD; Robert Rawlings, MS; Markku Linnoila, MD, PhD

American Medical Association

Physicians dedicated to the health of America

WHO Neuropsychiatric AIDS Study, Cross-sectional Phase I: Study Design and Psychiatric Findings 39
Mario Maj, MD, PhD; Robert Janssen, MD; Fabrizio Starace, MD; Michael Zaudig, MD; Paul Satz, PhD; Bhirom Sughondhabirom, MD; Mesu'A-Kabwa Luabeya, MD; Rolf Riedel, MD; David Ndetei, MD; Helena M. Calil, MD, PhD; Eric G. Bing, MD; Michael St. Louis, MD; Norman Sartorius, MD, PhD

WHO Neuropsychiatric AIDS Study, Cross-sectional Phase II: Neuropsychological and Neurological Findings 51
Mario Maj, MD, PhD; Paul Satz, PhD; Robert Janssen, MD; Michael Zaudig, MD; Fabrizio Starace, MD; Lou D'Elia, PhD; Bhirom Sughondhabirom, MD; Mahamoudi Mussa, MD; Dieter Naber, MD; David Ndetei, MD; George Schulte, MD; Norman Sartorius, MD, PhD

Regional Cerebral Blood Flow Measured During Symptom Provocation in Obsessive-Compulsive Disorder Using Oxygen 15–Labeled Carbon Dioxide and Positron Emission Tomography 62
Scott L. Rauch, MD; Michael A. Jenike, MD; Nathaniel M. Alpert, PhD; Lee Baer, PhD; Hans C. R. Breiter, MD; Cary R. Savage, PhD; Alan J. Fischman, MD, PhD

Letters to the Editor

Violence in the Severely Mentally Ill 71
Martin A. Weiler, MD

In Reply 71
Sheilagh Hodgins, PhD

Are Stress Hormones and Serotonin Related to Aggression in Primates? 72
Victor I. Reus, MD

In Reply 73
J. Dee Higley, PhD; Patrick T. Mehlman, PhD; David Taub, PhD; Stephen J. Suomi, PhD; Sue B. Higley; James M. Vickers, DVM; Markku Linnoila, PhD, MD

Cingulotomy in a Case of Concomitant Obsessive-Compulsive Disorder and Tourette's Syndrome 73
Lee Baer, PhD; Scott L. Rauch, MD; Michael A. Jenike, MD; N. H. Cassem, MD; H. Thomas Ballantine, MD; Peter A. Manzo; Robert L. Martuza, MD

Departments

Instructions for Authors 6

Classified Advertising 75

ARCHIVES OF GENERAL PSYCHIATRY

MANUSCRIPT CRITERIA AND INFORMATION

Mail manuscripts to the Assistant to Chief Editor, Grayson S. Norquist, MD, *Archives of General Psychiatry,* UCLA Neuropsychiatric Institute, 760 Westwood Plaza, Los Angeles, CA 90024. Telephone: (213) 206-0226. Manuscripts are received with the understanding that they are not under simultaneous consideration by another publication. Accepted manuscripts become the permanent property of the ARCHIVES. They may not be republished without permission from the publisher (AMA).

Editing. Copyediting follows AMA style and requires corresponding author approval. The authors are responsible for all statements made in their work, including changes made by the copy editor and authorized by the corresponding author.

Reprints. Forms for ordering are included with the edited typescript sent for approval. Reprints are shipped 6 to 8 weeks after publication.

Cover Letter

- In the cover letter, designate one author as correspondent and provide a complete address and telephone number.
- For a manuscript to be reviewed, considered, or edited, the following statement must be signed by *all* authors:

"I have been sufficiently involved in this work to take public responsibility for its validity and final presentation as an original publication. I can provide documentation of my work upon reasonable request and I have fulfilled the obligations for full disclosure and authorship as described by *Archives of General Psychiatry*. . . ." This signed statement must conclude with *one* of the two following sentences: "Accordingly, I hereby transfer, assign, or otherwise convey all copyright ownership to the AMA in the event such work is published by the AMA." [OR] "No copyright ownership can be transferred since this work was produced in the course of my official duties as a US government officer or employee."

Manuscript Preparation[1,2]

- Submit an original double-spaced typescript and 3 copies.
- **Manuscripts will not be returned after the review process.** If authors want them, they *must* request this on submission, **providing a self-addressed, postage-paid envelope.**
- Type—double-spaced throughout (including references) —on one side only of $8\frac{1}{2} \times 11$-in white bond paper. If a word processor is used, do not justify right-hand margins. Use a letter-quality printer.
- Titles should not exceed 42 characters per line, including punctuation and spaces. Title page needs full names, academic affiliations, addresses to which reprint requests should be sent, and, if the paper was presented at a meeting, the organization, place, and date of presentation.
- Include a structured abstract of 135 words or less, stating in defined sections, the Background, Methods, Results, and Conclusions.
- Use Système International (SI) measurements throughout the manuscript.
- Use generic names of drugs, unless the specific trade name is directly relevant to the discussion.
- Do not use abbreviations in the title or abstract. Limit their use in the text.
- *Do not use footnotes or appendixes.* Such materials should either be incorporated into the text or offered to interested readers on request.
- Include name and affiliation of statistical reviewer, if appropriate.
- Acknowledge fully any material taken from other publications, and submit written permission from the owner to reprint in any language or form without limitation.

Tables. Double-space on separate sheets of $8\frac{1}{2} \times 11$-in white bond paper. Title all tables and number them in the order of

ARCHIVES OF GENERAL PSYCHIATRY

VOL 51 NO. 2, FEB 1994

Original Articles

Dose-Response Study of N,N-Dimethyltryptamine in Humans: I. Neuroendocrine, Autonomic, and Cardiovascular Effects 85
Rick J. Strassman, MD, Clifford R. Qualls, PhD

Dose-Response Study of N,N-Dimethyltryptamine in Humans: II. Subjective Effects and Preliminary Results of a New Rating Scale 98
Rick J. Strassman, MD; Clifford R. Qualls, PhD; Eberhard H. Uhlenhuth, MD; Robert Kellner, MD, PhD

Maintenance Imipramine Therapy for Secondary Depression in Schizophrenia: A Controlled Trial 109
Samuel G. Siris, MD; Paul C. Bermanzohn, MD; Susan E. Mason, PhD; Mitchell A. Shuwall, PhD

Striatal D_2 Dopamine Receptor Characteristics in Neuroleptic-Naive Schizophrenic Patients Studied With Positron Emission Tomography 116
Jarmo Hietala, MD; Erkka Syvälahti, MD; Klaus Vuorio, MD; Kjell Någren, PhD; Pertti Lehikoinen, PhD; Ulla Ruotsalainen, MSc; Viljo Räkköläinen, MD; Ville Lehtinen, MD; Uno Wegelius, MD

Neuropsychological Deficits in Neuroleptic Naive Patients With First-Episode Schizophrenia 124
Andrew J. Saykin, PsyD; Derri L. Shtasel, MD; Raquel E. Gur, MD, PhD; D. Brian Kester, MS; Lyn H. Mozley, MS; Paul Stafiniak, MS; Ruben C. Gur, PhD

American Medical Association
Physicians dedicated to the health of America

All articles published, including editorials, letters, and book reviews, represent the opinions of the authors and do not reflect the policy of the American Medical Association, the Editorial Board, or the institution with which the author is affiliated, unless this is clearly specified.

Plasma Homovanillic Acid Levels in First-Episode Schizophrenia: Psychopathology and Treatment Response 132
Amy R. Koreen, MD; Jeffrey Lieberman, MD; Jose Alvir, DrPH; David Mayerhoff, MD; Antony Loebel, MD; Miranda Chakos, MD; Farooq Amin, MD; Thomas Cooper, MA

News and Views

Assessing the Validity of an Animal Model of Deficient Sensorimotor Gating in Schizophrenic Patients 139
Neal R. Swerdlow, MD, PhD; David L. Braff, MD; Navid Taaid, MA; Mark A. Geyer, PhD

Letters to the Editor

Clinical Response to Clozapine in Patients With Schizophrenia 159
David Pickar, MD; Robert E. Litman, MD; Walter W. Hong, MD; Tom P. Su, MD; Ellen M. Weissman, MD; John K. Hsiao, MD; William Z. Potter, MD, PhD

The Relation of Parenthood to Suicide 160
David C. Clark, PhD, Jan Fawcett, MD

In Reply 160
Georg Høyer, MD, PhD, Eiliv Lund, MD, PhD

Departments

Classified Advertising 162

Instructions for Authors—See January 1994 Issue, page 6.

ARCHIVES OF GENERAL PSYCHIATRY

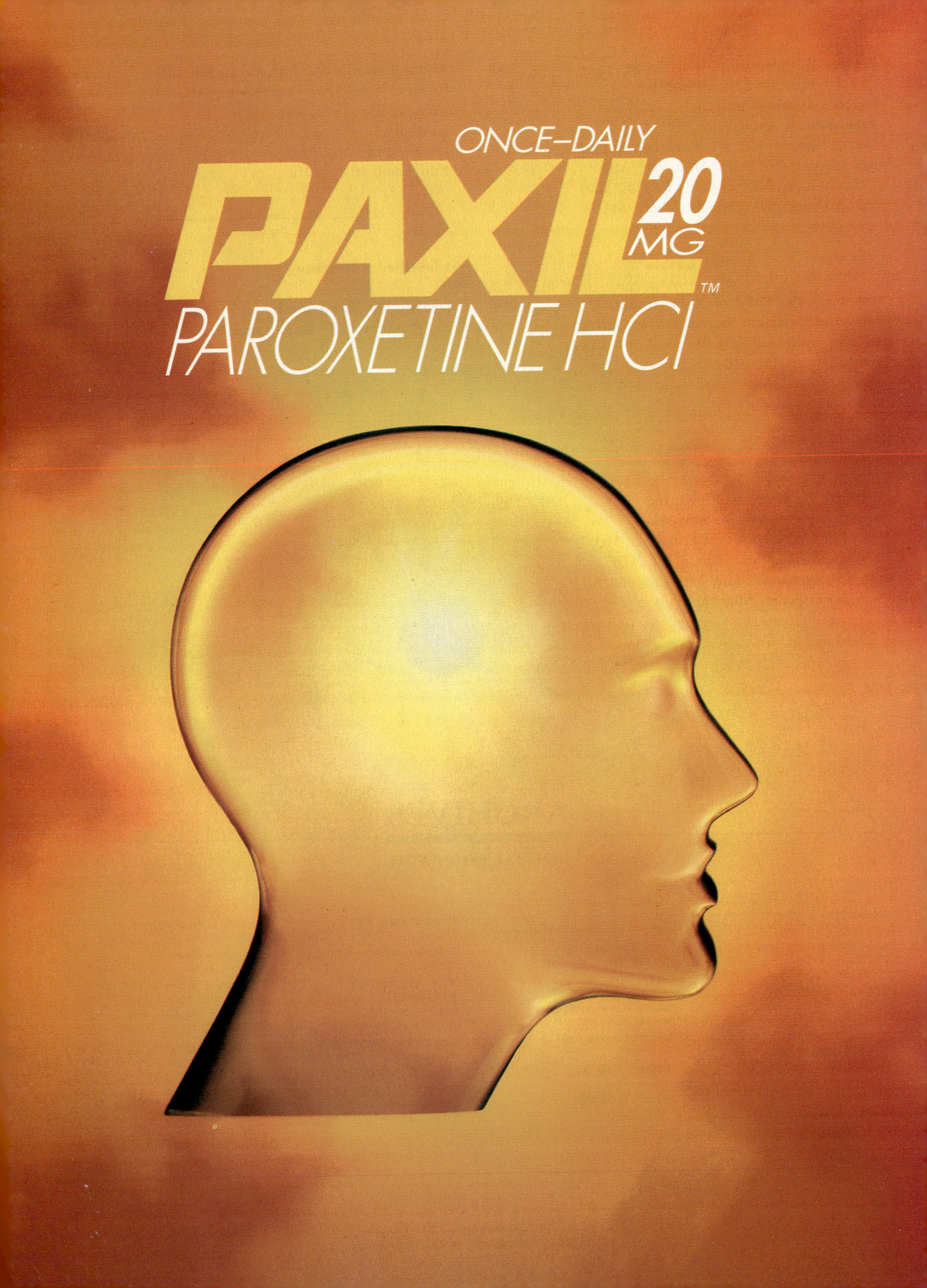
ONCE–DAILY
PAXIL 20 MG™
PAROXETINE HCl

ARCHIVES OF GENERAL PSYCHIATRY

VOL 51 NO. 3, MAR 1994

Editorial

The Third Editor of the ARCHIVES—Jack D. Barchas, MD 173
Michael D. Springer, George D. Lundberg, MD

Original Articles

Psychotherapy and Pharmacotherapy for Ambulatory Cocaine Abusers 177
Kathleen M. Carroll, PhD; Bruce J. Rounsaville, MD; Lynn T. Gordon, RN, MPA; Charla Nich, MS; Peter Jatlow, MD; Roseann M. Bisighini; Frank H. Gawin, MD

Increased Pressure for Rapid Eye Movement Sleep at Time of Hospital Admission Predicts Relapse in Nondepressed Patients With Primary Alcoholism at 3-Month Follow-up 189
J. Christian Gillin, MD; Tom L. Smith, PhD; Michael Irwin, MD; Nelson Butters, PhD; Anna Demodena; Marc Schuckit, MD

Subanesthetic Effects of the Noncompetitive NMDA Antagonist, Ketamine, in Humans: Psychotomimetic, Perceptual, Cognitive, and Neuroendocrine Responses 199
John H. Krystal, MD; Laurence P. Karper, MD; John P. Seibyl, MD; Glenna K. Freeman; Richard Delaney, PhD; J. Douglas Bremner, MD; George R. Heninger, MD; Malcolm B. Bowers, Jr, MD; Dennis S. Charney, MD

American Medical Association
Physicians dedicated to the health of America

All articles published, including editorials, letters, and book reviews, represent the opinions of the authors and do not reflect the policy of the American Medical Association, the Editorial Board, or the institution with which the author is affiliated, unless this is clearly specified.

The International Personality Disorder Examination: The World Health Organization/Alcohol, Drug Abuse, and Mental Health Administration International Pilot Study of Personality Disorders 215
Armand W. Loranger, PhD; Norman Sartorius, MD, PhD; Antonio Andreoli, MD; Peter Berger, MD; Peter Buchheim, MD; S. M. Channabasavanna, MD; Bina Coid, PhD; Alv Dahl, MD; Rene F. W. Diekstra, PhD; Brian Ferguson, MD; Lawrence B. Jacobsberg, MD, PhD; W. Mombour, MD; Charles Pull, MD; Yutaka Ono, MD; Darrel A. Regier, MD

Perspectives

Diagnosing Personality Disorders: A Review of Issues and Research Methods 225
Mark Zimmerman, MD

Letters to the Editor

Psychoneuroimmunology and Human Immunodeficiency Virus Type 1 Infection Revisited 246
Karl Goodkin, MD, PhD; C. L. Mulder, MD; Nancy T. Blaney, PhD; Gail Ironson, MD, PhD; Mahendra Kumar, PhD; Mary Ann Fletcher, PhD

In Reply 247
Samuel Perry, MD, Judith Rabkin, PhD

Pindolol Induces a Rapid Improvement of Depressed Patients Treated With Serotonin Reuptake Inhibitors 248
Francesc Artigas, PhD; Victor Perez, MD; Enric Alvarez, MD

The Diagnostic Interview Schedule and Anorexia Nervosa in Hong Kong 251
Sing Lee, MRCPsych

Departments

Classified Advertising 253

Instructions for Authors—See January 1994 issue, page 6.

Beginning April 1, 1994, manuscripts should be sent to:

Jack D. Barchas, MD
Editor, Archives of General Psychiatry
Department of Psychiatry
Cornell Medical Center
525 E 68th St
New York, NY 10021

ARCHIVES OF GENERAL PSYCHIATRY

The First in a New Chemical Class of Non-benzodiazepine Sleep Agents

AMBIEN™

(ZOLPIDEM TARTRATE) C IV

5-MG & 10-MG TABLETS

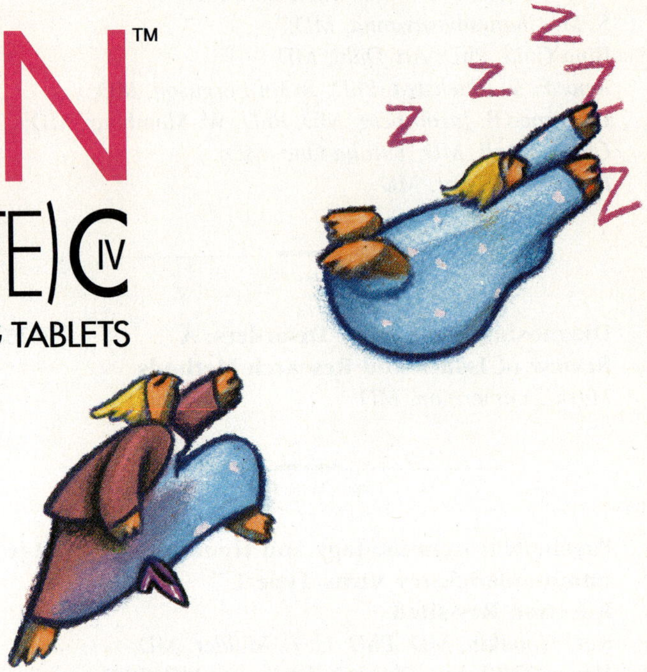

- AMBIEN—an imidazopyridine, chemically unrelated to benzodiazepines or any other sleep agent
- Extensive clinical experience—over 500 million doses prescribed throughout Europe[1]

With AMBIEN, Patients Fall Asleep Fast and Get a Full Night's Sleep

AMBIEN Generally Preserves Normal Sleep Physiology[2-5]

Mean Percentage of Time in Each Sleep Stage[2]

	Stage 1	Stage 2	Stages 3&4	REM
AMBIEN	8.8%	56.5%	16.1%	18.6%
Natural Sleep	8.8%	56.7%	14.3%	20.5%

No statistically significant difference from natural sleep (at baseline) for all sleep stages, in a double-blind, controlled study of 12 healthy volunteers.[2] The clinical significance is unknown.

With AMBIEN, Patients Awaken Refreshed and Alert

- A short half-life — mean 2.5 hours, with no active metabolites
- No evidence of significant daytime sedation or psychomotor impairment[1,2,5,6]

Although AMBIEN is generally not associated with next-day effects, until your patients know how they will react to this sleep agent, they should not engage in activities requiring mental alertness or motor coordination after taking AMBIEN (eg, driving or operating hazardous machinery). Potential impairment of the performance of such activities may occur the day following ingestion of AMBIEN

SEARLE

Please see references and brief summary of prescribing information on last page of this advertisement.

ARCHIVES OF GENERAL PSYCHIATRY

VOL 51 NO. 4, APR 1994

Original Articles

Schizophrenia and Temporal Lobe Epilepsy: A Neuropsychological Analysis 265
James M. Gold, PhD; Bruce P. Hermann, PhD; Christopher Randolph, PhD; Alan R. Wyler, MD; Terry E. Goldberg, PhD; Daniel R. Weinberger, MD

Cannabis Abuse and the Course of Recent-Onset Schizophrenic Disorders 273
Don H. Linszen, MD, PhD; Peter M. Dingemans, PhD; Marie E. Lenior, MA

Fluphenazine vs Placebo Supplementation for Prodromal Signs of Relapse in Schizophrenia 280
Stephen R. Marder, MD; William C. Wirshing, MD; Theodore Van Putten, MD; Jim Mintz, PhD; Joanne McKenzie, RN; Kathleen Johnston-Cronk, MS; Malca Lebell, PhD; Robert P. Liberman, MD

Analysis of the D_4 Dopamine Receptor Gene Variant in an Italian Schizophrenia Kindred 288
Fabio Macciardi, MD, PhD; Arturas Petronis, MD, PhD; Hubert H. M. Van Tol, PhD; Cecilia Marino, MD; M. Cristina Cavallini, MD; Enrico Smeraldi, MD; James L. Kennedy, MD

Epidemiology of Nonaffective Acute Remitting Psychosis vs Schizophrenia: Sex and Sociocultural Setting 294
Ezra Susser, MD, DrPH; Joseph Wanderling, MA

Haloperidol Addition in Fluvoxamine-Refractory Obsessive Compulsive Disorder: A Double-blind, Placebo-Controlled Study in Patients With and Without Tics 302
Christopher J. McDougle, MD; Wayne K. Goodman, MD; James F. Leckman, MD; Nicole C. Lee, MSNC; George R. Heninger, MD; Lawrence H. Price, MD

American Medical Association
Physicians dedicated to the health of America

All articles published, including editorials, letters, and book reviews, represent the opinions of the authors and do not reflect the policy of the American Medical Association, the Editorial Board, or the institution with which the author is affiliated, unless this is clearly specified.

ARCHIVES
OF
GENERAL PSYCHIATRY

The ARCHIVES OF GENERAL PSYCHIATRY is a member of the consortium of AMA journals listed below. The ARCHIVES reaches more than 27 500 readers in 85 countries each month. The complete text of all AMA journals is available on the MEDIS database from Mead Data Central, Dayton, Ohio.

The Journal of the American Medical Association (JAMA)
Archives of Dermatology
Archives of Family Medicine
Archives of General Psychiatry
Archives of Internal Medicine
Archives of Neurology
Archives of Ophthalmology
Archives of Otolaryngology—Head & Neck Surgery
Archives of Pathology & Laboratory Medicine
Archives of Pediatrics & Adolescent Medicine
Archives of Surgery

The ARCHIVES OF GENERAL PSYCHIATRY (ISSN 0003-990x) is published monthly by the American Medical Association, 515 N State St, Chicago, IL 60610, and is an official publication of the Association. Second-class postage rates paid at Chicago and at additional mailing office. GST registration number: R126 255 556. Canada Post International Publications Mail (Canadian Distribution) Sales Agreement No. 318633.

Printed in the USA.

SUBSCRIPTION RATES—The subscription rates for the ARCHIVES OF GENERAL PSYCHIATRY are as follows: $90 for 1 year, $163 for 2 years in the United States and US possessions; other countries, 1 year, $125; 2 years, $233 for expedited air delivery. (Rates for subscriptions for delivery to Japan or South Korea are available through exclusive agents—contact the publisher.) Special rates for residents and medical students in the United States and US possessions are available. Address inquiries to: Subscriber Services Center, American Medical Association, 515 N State St, Chicago, IL 60610. Phone: (800) 262-2350. Fax: (312) 464-5831. For mailing addresses outside the US and US possessions, see Foreign Subscription Information.

CHANGE OF ADDRESS—POSTMASTER, send all address changes to Subscriber Services, American Medical Association, 515 N State St, Chicago, IL 60610. Please notify us of address change at least 6 weeks in advance to ensure uninterrupted service. Include both old and new addresses, a recent mailing label, and new ZIP code. For mailing addresses outside the US and US possessions, see Foreign Subscription Information.

SUBSCRIBER SERVICES—For information about subscribing to any of the AMA publications, change of address, missing issues, or purchasing back issues, please contact Subscriber Services, American Medical Association, 515 N State St, Chicago, IL 60610, or call (312) 670-SUBS (670-7827) between 8:30 AM and 4:30 PM CST. For mailing addresses outside the US and US possessions, see Foreign Subscription Information.

FOREIGN SUBSCRIPTION INFORMATION—Subscriptions outside the United States and US possessions are served according to geographic region. Please address correspondence to the following three offices based on delivery address: 1) For delivery in North America, Central America and South America, contact Subscriber Services, AMA, 515 N State St, Chicago, IL 60610, phone: 1-312-760-7827, fax: 1-312-464-5831; 2) For delivery in the United Kingdom, contact Professional & Scientific Publications, BMA House, Tavistock Square, London WC1H 9JR, England, phone: 44-071-383-6270, fax: 44-071-383-6402; 3) For delivery in all other countries, contact JAMA & Archives Reader Services Centre, Karl-Mand-Strasse 2, D-56070 Koblenz, Germany, phone: 49-261-80706-53, fax: 49-261-80706-54.

REPRINTS—Authors place their reprint order at the time the edited typescript is reviewed and should allow 4 to 6 weeks for delivery following publication. Requests for individual reprints should be sent directly to the author at the address shown in the article.

For bulk reprint orders for commercial distribution, please contact Mark Kuhns, 600 Third Ave, New York, NY 10016, phone (212) 867-6640, fax (212) 953-2497. For reprint orders in limited quantities for educational distribution, please contact Rita Houston, 515 N State St, Chicago, IL 60610, phone (312) 464-2512, fax (312) 464-5835.

PERMISSIONS—Contact Laslo Hunyady, Permissions Assistant, 515 N State St, Chicago, IL 60610, phone (312) 464-2513.

ADVERTISING PRINCIPLES—Each advertisement in this issue has been reviewed and complies with the principles governing advertising in AMA scientific publications. A copy of these principles is available on request. The appearance of advertising in AMA publications is not an AMA guarantee or endorsement of the product or the claims made for the product by the manufacturer.

Tryptophan Depletion in Patients With Obsessive-Compulsive Disorder Who Respond to Serotonin Reuptake Inhibitors 309
Linda C. Barr, MD; Wayne K. Goodman, MD; Christopher J. McDougle, MD; Pedro L. Delgado, MD; George R. Heninger, MD; Dennis S. Charney, MD; Lawrence H. Price, MD

Familial Correlates of Reduced Central Serotonergic System Function in Patients With Personality Disorders 318
Emil F. Coccaro, MD; Jeremy M. Silverman, PhD; Howard M. Klar, MD; Thomas B. Horvath, MD; Larry J. Siever, MD

Incidence of Dementia in a Population Older Than 75 Years in the United Kingdom 325
Eugene S. Paykel, MD, FRCP, FRCPsych; Carol Brayne, MSc, MD, MRCP, MFPHM; Felicia A. Huppert, PhD; Caroline Gill, MSc; Claire Barkley, MB, ChB, MRCPsych; Eric Gehlhaar, MB, MRCPsych, DGM; Lynn Beardsall, PhD; Deborah M. Girling, MA, MB, BChir, MRCPsych; Penelope Pollitt, PhD; Daniel O'Connor, MD, FRANZCPsych

Letters to the Editor

Schizophrenia After Prenatal Exposure to the Dutch Hunger Winter of 1944-1945 333
Peter Jones, MD

In Reply 333
Ezra Susser, MD, DrPH, Shang P. Lin, PhD

Age of Onset in Familial Schizophrenia 334
Lynn E. DeLisi, MD; Nick Bass, MD; Angela Boccio, MS; Gail Shields, MD; Carla Morganti, MD; Antonio Vita, MD

Naltrexone and Alcohol Dependence: Some Methodological Issues 335
Chittaranjan Andrade, MD, N. Sanjay Kumar Rao, MBBS

In Reply 335
Joseph R. Volpicelli, MD, PhD; Arthur I. Alterman, PhD; Charles P. O'Brien, MD, PhD

Departments

Classified Advertising 337

Instructions for Authors— See January 1994 Issue, page 6.

Beginning April 1, 1994, manuscripts should be sent to:

Jack D. Barchas, MD
Editor, Archives of General Psychiatry
Department of Psychiatry
Cornell Medical Center
525 E 68th St, Box 171
New York, NY 10021

ARCHIVES OF GENERAL PSYCHIATRY

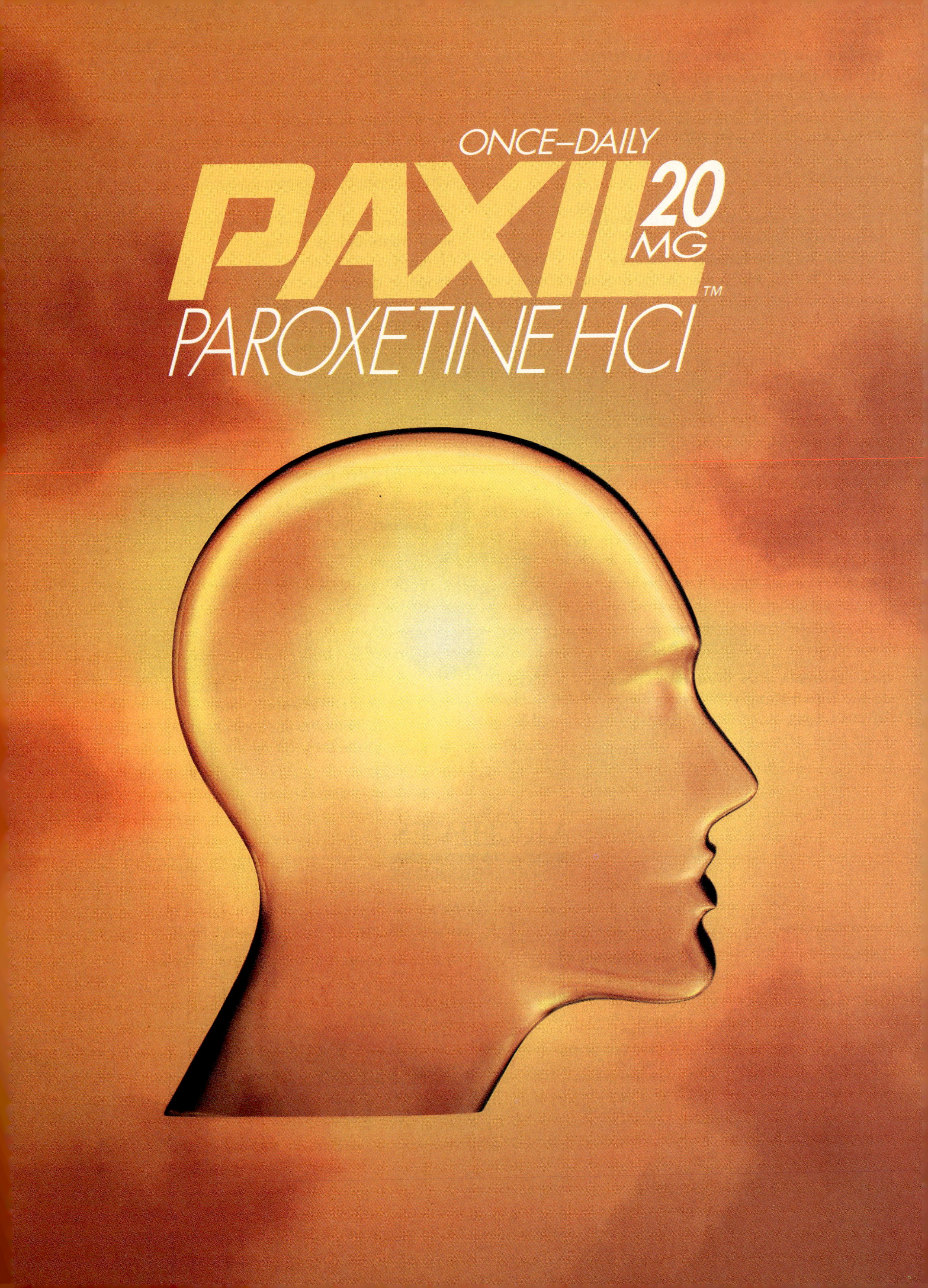
ONCE–DAILY
PAXIL 20 MG
™
PAROXETINE HCl

ARCHIVES
OF
GENERAL PSYCHIATRY

VOL 51 NO. 5, MAY 1994

News and Views

Standardized Assessment for Panic Disorder Research: A Conference Report 346
M. Katherine Shear, MD, Jack D. Maser, PhD

Original Articles

***DSM-III-R* Generalized Anxiety Disorder in the National Comorbidity Survey** 355
Hans-Ulrich Wittchen, PhD; Shanyang Zhao, PhD; Ronald C. Kessler, PhD; William W. Eaton, PhD

Childhood-Onset Dysthymic Disorder: Clinical Features and Prospective Naturalistic Outcome 365
Maria Kovacs, PhD; Hagop S. Akiskal, MD; Constantine Gatsonis, PhD; Phoebe L. Parrone, MS

Psychiatric and Medical Effects of Anabolic-Androgenic Steroid Use: A Controlled Study of 160 Athletes 375
Harrison G. Pope, Jr, MD, David L. Katz, MD, JD

Psychiatric Disorders in Relatives of Probands With Panic Disorder and/or Major Depression 383
Risë B. Goldstein, PhD, MPH; Myrna M. Weissman, PhD; Phillip B. Adams, PhD; Ewald Horwath, MD; Jennifer D. Lish, PhD; Dennis Charney, MD; Scott W. Woods, MD; Christina Sobin, PhD; Priya J. Wickramaratne, PhD

Cognitive Behavioral Treatment Compared With Nonprescriptive Treatment of Panic Disorder 395
M. Katherine Shear, MD; Paul A. Pilkonis, PhD; Marylene Cloitre, PhD; Andrew C. Leon, PhD

American Medical Association
Physicians dedicated to the health of America

All articles published, including editorials, letters, and book reviews, represent the opinions of the authors and do not reflect the policy of the American Medical Association, the Editorial Board, or the institution with which the author is affiliated, unless this is clearly specified.

James S. Todd, MD
Executive Vice President

Kenneth E. Monroe
Deputy Executive Vice President

Larry E. Joyce
Senior Vice President

George D. Lundberg, MD
Editor-in-Chief, Scientific Publications

Robert L. Kennett
Vice President, Publishing

Nawin Gupta, PhD
Director, Publishing Operations Division

Cheryl Iverson
Director, Editorial Processing Division

Michael D. Springer
Associate Publisher

John P. Cahill
Manager, Advertising Sales

Geoffrey A. Flick
Manager, Marketing Services

Advertising Offices: East: Phillip B. Altamore, Donald M. Blatherwick, John L. Reeves, 600 Third Ave, Suite 3700, New York, NY 10016 (212) 867-6640. **Diagnostics/Devices:** M. J. Mrvica Associates, 155 S White Horse Pike, Berlin, NJ 08009; (609) 768-9360. **Midwest/Far West:** Peter L. Payerli, 515 N State St, Chicago, IL 60610 (312) 464-2551.

ARCHIVES OF GENERAL PSYCHIATRY

The ARCHIVES OF GENERAL PSYCHIATRY is a member of the consortium of AMA journals listed below. The ARCHIVES reaches more than 27 500 readers in 85 countries each month. The complete text of all AMA journals is available on the MEDIS database from Mead Data Central, Dayton, Ohio.

The Journal of the American Medical Association (JAMA)
Archives of Dermatology
Archives of Family Medicine
Archives of General Psychiatry
Archives of Internal Medicine
Archives of Neurology
Archives of Ophthalmology
Archives of Otolaryngology—Head & Neck Surgery
Archives of Pathology & Laboratory Medicine
Archives of Pediatrics & Adolescent Medicine
Archives of Surgery

The ARCHIVES OF GENERAL PSYCHIATRY (ISSN 0003-990x) is published monthly by the American Medical Association, 515 N State St, Chicago, IL 60610, and is an official publication of the Association. Second-class postage rates paid at Chicago and at additional mailing office. GST registration number: R126 255 556. Canada Post International Publications Mail (Canadian Distribution) Sales Agreement No. 318633.

Printed in the USA.

SUBSCRIPTION RATES—The subscription rates for the ARCHIVES OF GENERAL PSYCHIATRY are as follows: $90 for 1 year, $163 for 2 years in the United States and US possessions; other countries, 1 year, $125; 2 years, $233 for expedited air delivery. (Rates for subscriptions for delivery to Japan or South Korea are available through exclusive agents—contact the publisher.) Special rates for residents and medical students in the United States and US possessions are available. Address inquiries to: Subscriber Services Center, American Medical Association, 515 N State St, Chicago, IL 60610. Phone: (800) 262-2350. Fax: (312) 464-5831. For mailing addresses outside the US and US possessions, see Foreign Subscription Information.

CHANGE OF ADDRESS—POSTMASTER, send all address changes to Subscriber Services, American Medical Association, 515 N State St, Chicago, IL 60610. Please notify us of address change at least 6 weeks in advance to ensure uninterrupted service. Include both old and new addresses, a recent mailing label, and new ZIP code. For mailing addresses outside the US and US possessions, see Foreign Subscription Information.

SUBSCRIBER SERVICES—For information about subscribing to any of the AMA publications, change of address, missing issues, or purchasing back issues, please contact Subscriber Services, American Medical Association, 515 N State St, Chicago, IL 60610, or call (312) 670-SUBS (670-7827) between 8:30 AM and 4:30 PM CST. For mailing addresses outside the US and US possessions, see Foreign Subscription Information.

FOREIGN SUBSCRIPTION INFORMATION—Subscriptions outside the United States and US possessions are served according to geographic region. Please address correspondence to the following three offices based on delivery address: 1) For delivery in North America, Central America and South America, contact Subscriber Services, AMA, 515 N State St, Chicago, IL 60610, phone: 1-312-760-7827, fax: 1-312-464-5831; 2) For delivery in the United Kingdom, contact Professional & Scientific Publications, BMA House, Tavistock Square, London WC1H 9JR, England, phone: 44-071-383-6270, fax: 44-071-383-6402; 3) For delivery in all other countries, contact JAMA & Archives Reader Services Centre, Karl-Mand-Strasse 2, D-56070 Koblenz, Germany, phone: 49-261-80706-53, fax: 49-261-80706-54.

REPRINTS—Authors place their reprint order at the time the edited typescript is reviewed and should allow 4 to 6 weeks for delivery following publication. Requests for individual reprints should be sent directly to the author at the address shown in the article.

For bulk reprint orders for commercial distribution, please contact Mark Kuhns, 600 Third Ave, New York, NY 10016, phone (212) 867-6640, fax (212) 953-2497. For reprint orders in limited quantities for educational distribution, please contact Rita Houston, 515 N State St, Chicago, IL 60610, phone (312) 464-2512, fax (312) 464-5835.

PERMISSIONS—Contact Laslo Hunyady, Permissions Assistant, 515 N State St, Chicago, IL 60610, phone (312) 464-2513.

ADVERTISING PRINCIPLES—Each advertisement in this issue has been reviewed and complies with the principles governing advertising in AMA scientific publications. A copy of these principles is available on request. The appearance of advertising in AMA publications is not an AMA guarantee or endorsement of the product or the claims made for the product by the manufacturer.

The Time Course of Nonchronic Major Depressive Disorder: Uniformity Across Episodes and Samples 405
William Coryell, MD; Hagop S. Akiskal, MD; Andrew C. Leon, PhD; George Winokur, MD; John D. Maser, MD; Timothy I. Mueller, MD; Martin B. Keller, MD; for the National Institute of Mental Health Collaborative Program on the Psychobiology of Depression—Clinical Studies

Sympathetic Nervous System Activity in Major Depression: Basal and Desipramine-Induced Alterations in Plasma Norepinephrine Kinetics 411
Richard C. Veith, MD; Nancy Lewis, RN; Oscar A. Linares, MD; Robert F. Barnes, MD; Murray A. Raskind, MD; Enrique C. Villacres, MD; M. Michele Murburg, MD; E. Alexandra Ashleigh, MD; Sonia Castillo, PhD; Elaine R. Peskind, MD; Marcella Pascualy, MD; Jeffrey B. Halter, MD

Letters to the Editor

No Evidence of a Schizophrenia Locus in a Second Pseudoautosomal Region 427
Zhe Wu Wang, MD; Donald W. Black, MD; Nancy Andreasen, MD, PhD; Raymond R. Crowe, MD

Lower-Dose Therapy With Traditional Neuroleptics in Chronically Hospitalized Schizophrenic Patients 427
Robert C. Smith, MD, PhD

Correction and Amplification 429
Hector R. Bird, MD

Alcohol Dependence May Be the Missing Link Between Posttraumatic Stress Disorder and Panic 429
Eve J. Wiseman, MD

In Reply 430
John H. Krystal, MD; Steven M. Southwick, MD; Dennis S. Charney, MD

Familial Obsessive-Compulsive Disorder Presenting as Pathological Jealousy Successfully Treated With Fluoxetine 430
Simon Wright, MB, ChB, MRCPsych

Biologic Theories of Sexual Orientation 431
Nathaniel McConaghy, DSc, MD

Theories of Sexual Orientation: A Reappraisal 432
Douglas Berger, MD; Hiroyuki Suematsu, MD; Yutaka Ono, MD

In Reply 432
William Byne, MD, PhD, Bruce Parsons, MD, PhD

Departments

Correction 422

Classified Advertising 430

Instructions for Authors—
See January 1994 issue, page 6.

ARCHIVES
OF
GENERAL PSYCHIATRY

ARCHIVES OF GENERAL PSYCHIATRY

VOL 51 NO. 6, JUNE 1994

Original Articles

Mental Illness in the Biological and Adoptive Relatives of Schizophrenic Adoptees: Replication of the Copenhagen Study in the Rest of Denmark 442
Seymour S. Kety, MD; Paul H. Wender, MD; Bjørn Jacobsen, MD; Loring J. Ingraham, PhD; Lennart Jansson, MD; Britta Faber, MD; Dennis K. Kinney, PhD

Independent Diagnoses of Adoptees and Relatives As Defined by *DSM-III* in the Provincial and National Samples of the Danish Adoption Study of Schizophrenia 456
Kenneth S. Kendler, MD; Alan M. Gruenberg, MD; Dennis K. Kinney, PhD

Neuropsychological Deficits in Schizophrenics: Relationship to Age, Chronicity, and Dementia 469
Robert Heaton, PhD; Jane S. Paulsen, PhD; Lou Ann McAdams, PhD; Julie Kuck, MA; Sidney Zisook, MD; David Braff, MD; M. Jackuelyn Harris, MD; Dilip V. Jeste, MD

Myelination of a Key Relay Zone in the Hippocampal Formation Occurs in the Human Brain During Childhood, Adolescence, and Adulthood 477
Francine M. Benes, MD, PhD; Mary Turtle; Yusuf Khan; Peter Farol

American Medical Association

Physicians dedicated to the health of America

The Panicogenic Effects of Cholecystokinin-Tetrapeptide Are Antagonized by L-365,260, a Central Cholecystokinin Receptor Antagonist, in Patients With Panic Disorder 486
Jacques Bradwejn, MD, FRCPC; Diana Koszycki, MA; Anne Couëtoux du Tertre, MD; Harold van Megen, MD; Johan den Boer, MD; Herman Westenberg, PhD; Lawrence Annable, DipStat

Increased Density of Guanine Nucleotide–Binding Proteins in the Postmortem Brains of Heroin Addicts 494
Pablo V. Escriba, PhD; Magdalena Sastre, PhD; Jesús A. García-Sevilla, MD

Letters to the Editor

Lithium Prophylaxis in American Patients With Unipolar Disorder 502
Mogens Schou, MD

In Reply 502
Mitchell S. Nobler, MD, Harold A. Sackeim, PhD

Maintenance Therapy in Depression 503
Gary J. Barnes, FRANZCP, Quentin Jones

In Reply 504
Ellen Frank, PhD, David J. Kupfer, MD

Klein's Suffocation Theory of Panic 505
Steven Taylor, PhD, S. Rachman, PhD

In Reply 506
Donald F. Klein, MD

Departments

Classified Advertising 508

Instructions for Authors—See January 1994 issue, page 6.

ARCHIVES OF GENERAL PSYCHIATRY

ARCHIVES
OF
GENERAL PSYCHIATRY

VOL 51 NO. 7, JULY 1994

Letters to the Editor

The Prevalence of Schizophrenia in Ireland 513
E. Fuller Torrey, MD

In Reply 513
Dermot Walsh, MB, FRCPI,
Kenneth S. Kendler, MD

Neural Circuits in Schizophrenia 515
Robert W. McCarley, MD;
Martha E. Shenton, PhD;
Brian F. O'Donnell, PhD;
Paul G. Nestor, PhD

In Reply 516
William T. Carpenter, Jr, MD;
Robert W. Buchanan, MD;
Brian Kirkpatrick, MD;
Carol Tamminga, MD;
Frank Wood, PhD

Original Articles

Life Events and the Research Diagnostic Criteria Endogenous Subtype: A Confirmation of the Distinction Using the Bedford College Methods 519
Ellen Frank, PhD;
Barbara Anderson, MS;
Charles F. Reynolds III, MD;
Angela Ritenour; David J. Kupfer, MD

Life Events and Endogenous Depression: A Puzzle Reexamined 525
George William Brown, PhD;
Tirril Olivia Harris, MA;
Cathy Hepworth, MPhil

American Medical Association
Physicians dedicated to the health of America

A Controlled Prospective Study of *DSM-III* Adjustment Disorder in Childhood: Short-term Prognosis and Long-term Predictive Validity 535
Maria Kovacs, PhD; Constantine Gatsonis, PhD; Myrna Pollock, MSW; Phoebe Lucy Parrone, MS

Minor Depression in a Cohort of Young Adults in Israel 542
Andrew E. Skodol, MD; Sharon Schwartz, PhD; Bruce P. Dohrenwend, PhD; Itzhak Levav, MD; Patrick E. Shrout, PhD

Impaired Autonomic Nervous System Habituation in Those at Genetic Risk for Schizophrenia 552
J. Meggin Hollister, MA; Sarnoff A. Mednick, PhD, DrMed; Patricia Brennan, PhD; Tyrone D. Cannon, PhD

A Multicenter Investigation of Fixed-Dose Fluoxetine in the Treatment of Obsessive-compulsive Disorder 559
Gary D. Tollefson, MD, PhD; Alvin H. Rampey, Jr, PhD; Janet H. Potvin, PhD; Michael A. Jenike, MD; A. John Rush, MD; Roberto A. Dominguez, MD; Lorrin M. Koran, MD; M. Katherine Shear, MD; Wayne Goodman, MD; Laura A. Genduso, PharmD

Incentives Improve Outcome in Outpatient Behavioral Treatment of Cocaine Dependence 568
Stephen T. Higgins, PhD; Alan J. Budney, PhD; Warren K. Bickel, PhD; Florian E. Foerg; Robert Donham, MA; Gary J. Badger, MS

Patterns of Risk in First-Degree Relatives of Patients With Alzheimer's Disease 577
Jeremy M. Silverman, PhD; Ge Li, MD, PhD; Michele L. Zaccario; Christopher J. Smith; James Schmeidler, PhD; Richard C. Mohs, PhD; Kenneth L. Davis, MD

Departments

Classified Advertising 587

Instructions for Authors—
See January 1994 issue, page 6.

ARCHIVES
OF
GENERAL PSYCHIATRY

ARCHIVES
OF
GENERAL PSYCHIATRY

VOL 51 NO. 8, AUGUST 1994

News and Views

Interpersonal Psychotherapy: Current Status 599
Myrna M. Weissman, PhD, John C. Markowitz, MD

Original Articles

High-Dose Selegiline in Treatment-Resistant Older Depressive Patients 607
Trey Sunderland, MD; Robert M. Cohen, MD, PhD; Susan Molchan, MD; Brian A. Lawlor, MD; Alan M. Mellow, MD, PhD; Paul A. Newhouse, MD; Pierre N. Tariot, MD; Edward A. Mueller, MD; Dennis L. Murphy, MD

The 24-Hour Profiles of Cortisol, Prolactin, and Growth Hormone Secretion in Mania 616
Paul Linkowski, MD, PhD; Myriam Kerkhofs, PhD; Anne Van Onderbergen, MD; Philippe Hubain, MD; Georges Copinschi, MD, PhD; Mireille L'Hermite-Balériaux, MS; Raoul Leclercq, MD; Michele Brasseur, MD; Julien Mendlewicz, MD, PhD; Eve Van Cauter, PhD

Carbamazepine Increases Cerebrospinal Fluid Thyrotropin-Releasing Hormone Levels in Affectively Ill Patients 625
Lauren B. Marangell, MD; Mark S. George, MD; Garth Bissette, PhD; Peggy Pazzaglia, MD; Teresa Huggins, PhD; Robert M. Post, MD

American Medical Association
Physicians dedicated to the health of America

James S. Todd, MD
Executive Vice President
Kenneth E. Monroe
Deputy Executive Vice President
Larry E. Joyce
Senior Vice President
George D. Lundberg, MD
Editor-in-Chief, Scientific Publications
Robert L. Kennett
Vice President, Publishing
Nawin Gupta, PhD
Director, Publishing Operations Division
Cheryl Iverson
Director, Editorial Processing Division

Michael D. Springer
Associate Publisher
John P. Cahill
Manager, Advertising Sales
Geoffrey A. Flick
Manager, Marketing Services

Advertising Offices: East: Phillip B. Altamore, Donald M. Blatherwick, John L. Reeves, 600 Third Ave, Suite 3700, New York, NY 10016 (212) 867-6640. **Diagnostics/Devices:** M. J. Mrvica Associates, 155 S White Horse Pike, Berlin, NJ 08009; (609) 768-9360. **Midwest/Far West:** Peter L. Payerli, 515 N State St, Chicago, IL 60610 (312) 464-2551.

Elevation of Serum Free Triiodothyronine, Total Triiodothyronine, Thyroxine-Binding Globulin, and Total Thyroxine Levels in Combat-Related Posttraumatic Stress Disorder 629
John Mason, MD; Steven Southwick, MD; Rachel Yehuda, PhD; Sheila Wang, PhD; Sherry Riney; Douglas Bremner, MD; David Johnson, PhD; Hadar Lubin, MD; Dudley Blake, PhD; Gang Zhou; Fred Gusman, MSW; Dennis Charney, MD

Risk Factors for Spontaneous Dyskinesia in Schizophrenia 643
Wayne S. Fenton, MD; Richard Jed Wyatt, MD; Thomas H. McGlashan, MD

Neuropsychological Functioning in Siblings Discordant for Schizophrenia and Healthy Volunteers 651
Tyrone D. Cannon, PhD; Lisa Eyler Zorrilla, MA; Derri Shtasel, MD; Raquel E. Gur, MD, PhD; Ruben C. Gur, PhD; Elysa J. Marco; Paul Moberg, PhD; R. Arlen Price, PhD

Letters to the Editor

Retrocallosal White Matter Abnormalities in Patients With Obsessive-compulsive Disorder 663
Hans C. Breiter, MD; Pauline A. Filipek, MD; David N. Kennedy, PhD; Lee Baer, PhD; Dawn A. Pitcher; Michael J. Olivares; Perry F. Renshaw, MD, PhD; Verne S. Caviness, Jr, MD, DPhil; Michael A. Jenike, MD

Mania Induced by Citalopram 664
Christian Bryois, MD, François Ferrero, MD

Arachidonic Acid: A Common Link in the Biology of Schizophrenia? 665
M. Peet, MB, FRCPsych; J. D. E. Laugharne, MD, MRCPsych; D. F. Horrobin, DPhil; G. P. Reynolds, PhD

Interactions of Serotonin Reuptake Inhibitors With Tricyclic Antidepressants 666
Anand P. Popli, MD; Ross J. Baldessarini, MD; Jonathan O. Cole, MD

Departments

Instructions for Authors 594

Call for Papers 641

Classified Advertising 668

ARCHIVES OF GENERAL PSYCHIATRY

MANUSCRIPT CRITERIA AND INFORMATION

Submit manuscripts to Jack D. Barchas, MD, Editor, ***Archives of General Psychiatry,* Cornell Medical Center, Dept of Psychiatry, Box 171, 525 E 68th St, New York, NY 10021.** Manuscripts are received with the understanding that they are not under simultaneous consideration by another publication, have not been published previously, and have the approval of each author. Accepted manuscripts become the permanent property of the ARCHIVES. They may not be republished without permission from the publisher (AMA).

Editing. Copyediting follows AMA style and requires corresponding author approval. The authors are responsible for all statements made in their work, including changes made by the copy editor and authorized by the corresponding author.

Reprints. Forms for ordering are included with the edited typescript sent for approval. Reprints are shipped 6 to 8 weeks after publication.

Cover Letter

- In the cover letter, designate one author as correspondent and provide a complete address and telephone and fax numbers.

- For a manuscript to be reviewed, considered, or edited, the following statement must be signed by *all* authors:

"I have been sufficiently involved in this work to take public responsibility for its validity and final presentation as an original publication. I can and will provide documentation of my work upon reasonable request and I have fulfilled the obligations for full disclosure and authorship as described by *Archives of General Psychiatry*. . . ." This signed statement must conclude with *one* of the two following sentences: "Accordingly, I hereby transfer, assign, or otherwise convey all copyright ownership to the AMA in the event such work is published by the AMA." [OR] "No copyright ownership can be transferred since this work was produced in the course of my official duties as a US government officer or employee."

Manuscript Preparation[1,2]

- Submit an original double-spaced typescript and 7 copies.
- **Manuscripts will not be returned after the review process.** Unpublished manuscripts will be destroyed.
- Type—double-spaced throughout (including references)—on one side only of 8½ × 11-in white bond paper. Number all pages. Do not justify right-hand margins. Use a printer of at least letter quality.
- Titles cannot exceed 200 characters, including punctuation and spaces, and should be as brief as possible.
- The title page should list full names, degrees, academic affiliations and their locations, and the name and address to whom reprint requests should be sent. If the paper was presented at a meeting, include the organization, place, and date of presentation. Acknowledgment of grant or drug company support should also be made on this page. Include a word count of the text, excluding abstract, references, and tables.

- Include a structured abstract of 135 words or less that states in defined sections the Background, Methods, Results, and Conclusions.

- Use Système International (SI) measurements throughout the manuscript.

- Use generic names of drugs, unless the specific trade name is directly relevant to the study design or discussion.

- Do not use abbreviations in the title or abstract. Limit their use in the text.

- *Do not use footnotes or appendixes.* Such materials should either be incorporated into the text or offered to interested readers on request.

- Include a statistical analysis section under *Methods* that fully describes the application of each statistical procedure used. If a test is used that is not commonly presented in the ARCHIVES, briefly describe its purpose and how it is to be interpreted. Results should report the test statistic (eg, χ^2, F or t value), degrees of freedom, and P value. Measures of central tendency (eg, means) should be accompanied by measures of variability (eg, standard deviations). In the cover letter, state the name of your statistical consultant, if appropriate.

- Acknowledge fully any material taken from other publications, and submit written permission from the owner to reprint in any language or form without limitation.

Tables. Double-space on separate sheets of 8½ × 11-in white bond paper. Title each one and number them in the order of their citation in the text. If a table must be continued, repeat the title on a second sheet, followed by "(cont)." Any explanatory notes to be printed with the table must be typed single-spaced beneath the table.

Figures. Once manuscripts are accepted, two sets of professionally prepared, high-contrast glossy prints (preferably in a proportion of 5 × 7 in) are required. If full-color figures are necessary, the ARCHIVES may pay part of the expense with the balance to be borne by the author.

- Number figures according to their order in the text. Type the figure number, proper orientation (eg, top), name of the senior author, and an abbreviated title on a gummed label; affix it to the back of the print.

- Double-space legends (maximum length, 40 words) on a separate sheet of 8½ × 11-in paper.

References. Number references in the order they are mentioned in the text; do *not* alphabetize. In text, tables, and legends, identify references with superscript arabic numbers. In listing ref-

ARCHIVES OF GENERAL PSYCHIATRY

VOL 51 NO. 9, SEPTEMBER 1994

Original Articles

Reduction of Cerebral Blood Flow in Older Depressed Patients 677
Ira M. Lesser, MD; Ismael Mena, MD; Kyle B. Boone, PhD; Bruce L. Miller, MD; C. Mark Mehringer, MD; Marcy Wohl, RN

Mood-Lowering Effect of Tryptophan Depletion: Enhanced Susceptibility in Young Men at Genetic Risk for Major Affective Disorders 687
Chawki Benkelfat, MD; Mark A. Ellenbogen; Peggy Dean, RN; Roberta M. Palmour, PhD; Simon N. Young, PhD

Increased Evening Activation of the Hypothalamic-Pituitary-Adrenal Axis in Depressed Patients 701
Elizabeth A. Young, MD; Roger F. Haskett, MD; Leon Grunhaus, MD; Atul Pande, MD; Virginia Murphy Weinberg, RN; Stanley J. Watson, MD, PhD; Huda Akil, PhD

Suicide and Mortality Patterns in Anxiety Neurosis and Depressive Neurosis 708
Christer Allgulander, MD

American Medical Association
Physicians dedicated to the health of America

Noradrenergic Dysregulation During Discontinuation of Cocaine Use in Addicts 713
Christopher J. McDougle, MD; Jed E. Black, MD; Robert T. Malison, MD; Ralf C. Zimmermann, MD; Thomas R. Kosten, MD; George R. Heninger, MD; Lawrence H. Price, MD

Buspirone Treatment of Anxious Alcoholics: A Placebo-Controlled Trial 720
Henry R. Kranzler, MD; Joseph A. Burleson, PhD; Frances K. Del Boca, PhD; Thomas F. Babor, PhD; Patricia Korner, RN; Joseph Brown, PhD; Michael J. Bohn, MD

Predicting Early Onset of Male Antisocial Behavior From Preschool Behavior 732
Richard E. Tremblay, PhD; Robert O. Pihl, PhD; Frank Vitaro, PhD; Patricia L. Dobkin, PhD

Untreated Anxiety Among Adult Primary Care Patients in a Health Maintenance Organization 740
Sheila K. Fifer, PhD; Susan D. Mathias, MPH; Donald L. Patrick, PhD, MSPH; Peter D. Mazonson, MD, MBA; Deborah P. Lubeck, PhD; Don P. Buesching, PhD

Departments

Instructions for Authors 675

Call for Papers 697

Classified Advertising 751

ARCHIVES OF GENERAL PSYCHIATRY

ARCHIVES OF GENERAL PSYCHIATRY

VOL 51 NO. 10, OCTOBER 1994

News and Views

Effects of the Menstrual Cycle on Dependent Variables in Mood Disorder Research **761**
Ellen Leibenluft, MD; Patricia L. Fiero, MA; David R. Rubinow, MD

Original Articles

Elevated Cerebrospinal Fluid Levels of Oxytocin in Obsessive-compulsive Disorder: Comparison With Tourette's Syndrome and Healthy Controls **782**
James F. Leckman, MD; Wayne K. Goodman, MD; William G. North, PhD; Phillip B. Chappell, MD; Lawrence H. Price, MD; David L. Pauls, PhD; George M. Anderson, PhD; Mark A. Riddle, MD; Maureen McSwiggan-Hardin, MSN; Christopher J. McDougle, MD; Linda C. Barr, MD; Donald J. Cohen, MD

Changes in Cerebrospinal Fluid Neurochemistry During Treatment of Obsessive-compulsive Disorder With Clomipramine **794**
Margaret Altemus, MD; Susan E. Swedo, MD; Henrietta L. Leonard, MD; Dan Richter; David R. Rubinow, MD; William Z. Potter, MD; Judith L. Rapoport, MD

Neuropsychological Impairments in Deficit vs Nondeficit Forms of Schizophrenia **804**
Robert W. Buchanan, MD; Milton E. Strauss, PhD; Brian Kirkpatrick, MD; Constanze Holstein, MS; Alan Breier, MD; William T. Carpenter, Jr, MD

American Medical Association

Physicians dedicated to the health of America

All articles published, including editorials, letters, and book reviews, represent the opinions of the authors and do not reflect the policy of the American Medical Association, the Editorial Board, or the institution with which the author is affiliated, unless this is clearly specified.

Autonomic Abnormalities in Schizophrenia: State or Trait Indicators? 813
Michael E. Dawson, PhD; Keith H. Nuechterlein, PhD; Anne M. Schell, PhD; Michael Gitlin, MD; Joseph Ventura, MA

Awareness of Illness in Schizophrenia and Schizoaffective and Mood Disorders 826
Xavier F. Amador, PhD; Michael Flaum, MD; Nancy C. Andreasen, MD, PhD; David H. Strauss, MD; Scott A. Yale, MSW; Scott C. Clark, MD; Jack M. Gorman, MD

Letters to the Editor

Genetic and Environmental Influences of Twins in Posttraumatic Stress 838
Scott Lurie, MD, Pleas Geyer, MD

In Reply 838
William R. True, PhD, MPH; John Rice, PhD; Andrew C. Heath, DPhil

Departments

Instructions for Authors 759

Call for Papers 839

Classified Advertising 840

ARCHIVES OF GENERAL PSYCHIATRY

ARCHIVES OF GENERAL PSYCHIATRY

VOL 51 NO. 11, NOVEMBER 1994

News and Views

Diagnostic Interview for Genetic Studies: Rationale, Unique Features, and Training 849
John I. Nurnberger, Jr, MD, PhD; Mary C. Blehar, PhD; Charles A. Kaufmann, MD; Carolyn York-Cooler; Sylvia G. Simpson, MD; Jill Harkavy-Friedman, PhD; Joanne B. Severe, MS; Dolores Malaspina, MD; Theodore Reich, MD; and collaborators from the NIMH Genetics Initiative

Comment

The Diagnostic Interview for Genetic Studies 863
Allen Frances, MD

Original Articles

Serotonin and the Neurobiology of Depression: Effects of Tryptophan Depletion 865
Pedro L. Delgado, MD; Lawrence H. Price, MD; Helen L. Miller, MD; Ronald M. Salomon, MD; George K. Aghajanian, MD; George R. Heninger, MD; Dennis S. Charney, MD

Dose-Response Studies With Protirelin 875
James C. Garbutt, MD; James P. Mayo, MD; Karley Y. Little, MD; Gregory M. Gillette, MD; George A. Mason, PhD; Bess Dew, RN; Arthur J. Prange, Jr, MD

American Medical Association
Physicians dedicated to the health of America

All articles published, including editorials, letters, and book reviews, represent the opinions of the authors and do not reflect the policy of the American Medical Association, the Editorial Board, or the institution with which the author is affiliated, unless this is clearly specified.

Regional Cerebral Blood Flow in Mood Disorders, III: Treatment and Clinical Response 884
Mitchell S. Nobler, MD; Harold A. Sackeim, PhD; Isak Prohovnik, PhD; James R. Moeller, PhD; Sukdeb Mukherjee, MD; David B. Schnur, MD; Joan Prudic, MD; D. P. Devanand, MD

Specificity of Ethanollike Effects Elicited by Serotonergic and Noradrenergic Mechanisms 898
John H. Krystal, MD; Elizabeth Webb; Ned Cooney, PhD; Henry R. Kranzler, MD; Dennis S. Charney, MD

Allelic Variation in the D_4 Dopamine Receptor (DRD4) Gene Does Not Predict Response to Clozapine 912
Peter A. Rao, MD; David Pickar, MD; Pablo V. Gejman, MD; Anca Ram, MD; Elliot S. Gershon, MD; Joel Gelernter, MD

Hypochondriasis and Panic Disorder: Boundary and Overlap 918
Arthur J. Barsky, MD; Maria C. Barnett, MPH; Paul D. Cleary, PhD

Letters to the Editor

The Effect of Diagnostic Hierarchy in Genetic Epidemiological Studies of Psychiatric Disorders 926
Marc-André Roy, MD, Kenneth S. Kendler, MD

In Reply 927
Priya Wickramaratne, PhD, Myrna M. Weissman, PhD

Brain Atrophy or Dystrophy in Schizophrenia: When Did It Happen? 927
Janice R. Stevens, MD

Departments

Instructions for Authors 847

Correction 864

Classified Advertising 928

ARCHIVES OF GENERAL PSYCHIATRY

ARCHIVES OF GENERAL PSYCHIATRY

VOL 51 NO. 12, DECEMBER 1994

Original Articles

Backward Masking in Schizophrenia and Mania: I. Specifying a Mechanism 939
Michael Foster Green, PhD; Keith H. Nuechterlein, PhD; Jim Mintz, PhD

Backward Masking in Schizophrenia and Mania: II. Specifying the Visual Channels 945
Michael Foster Green, PhD; Keith H. Nuechterlein, PhD; Jim Mintz, PhD

Comment

Parsing Cognition: The Power of Psychology Paradigms 952
Philip S. Holzman, PhD

Original Articles

Developmental Brain Abnormalities in the Offspring of Schizophrenic Mothers: II. Structural Brain Characteristics of Schizophrenia and Schizotypal Personality Disorder 955
Tyrone D. Cannon, PhD; Sarnoff A. Mednick, PhD, DrMed; Josef Parnas, MD; Fini Schulsinger, MD; Johannes Praestholm, MD; Aage Vestergaard, MD

Clinical Characteristics and Predisposing Factors in Acute Drug-Induced Akathisia 963
Perminder Sachdev, MD, PhD, FRANZCP, Jane Kruk, BSc(Hons)

The Boundary of Social Phobia: Exploring the Threshold 975
Jonathan R. T. Davidson, MD; Dana C. Hughes, RN, PhD; Linda K. George, PhD; Dan G. Blazer, MD, PhD

American Medical Association
Physicians dedicated to the health of America

All articles published, including editorials, letters, and book reviews, represent the opinions of the authors and do not reflect the policy of the American Medical Association, the Editorial Board, or the institution with which the author is affiliated, unless this is clearly specified.

Birth Complications Combined With Early Maternal Rejection at Age 1 Year Predispose to Violent Crime at Age 18 Years 984
Adrian Raine, DPhil; Patricia Brennan, PhD; Sarnoff A. Mednick, PhD

One-Year Follow-up of Psychotherapy and Pharmacotherapy for Cocaine Dependence: Delayed Emergence of Psychotherapy Effects 989
Kathleen M. Carroll, PhD; Bruce J. Rounsaville, MD; Charla Nich, MS; Lynn T. Gordon, RN, MPA; Philip W. Wirtz, PhD; Frank Gawin, MD

Editorial

Some Issues for the New Director of NIMH 998
Jack D. Barchas, MD, Peter M. Marzuk, MD

Letters to the Editor

Clinical Action of Remoxipride 1001
Robert Conley, MD; Carol A. Tamminga, MD, James An Nguyen, MD

All Prepaid Health Care Systems Are Not Equal 1002
Abby L. Wasserman, MD

In Reply 1002
Kenneth B. Wells, MD, MPH, Roland Sturm, PhD

Serotinin$_{2A}$ Receptors in Schizophrenia: Relation to Suicide 1003
Herbert Y. Meltzer, MD

In Reply 1003
Marc Laruelle, MD; Anissa Abi-Dargham, MD; Manuel F. Casanova, MD; Daniel R. Weinberger, MD; Joel E. Kleinman, MD, PhD

Effects of Alterations in Plasma Tryptophan Levels on Aggressive Feelings 1004
Anthony J. Cleare, MBBS, Alyson J. Bond, PhD

In Memoriam

Mary Catherine Neidigh Freedman 1005

Departments

Reviewers List 933

Instructions for Authors 937

Index to Volume 51 1007

Classified Advertising 1020

ARCHIVES OF GENERAL PSYCHIATRY

their citation in the text. If a table must be continued, repeat the title on a second sheet, followed by "(cont)." Any explanatory notes to be printed with the table must be typed single-spaced beneath the table.

Figures. For accepted manuscripts, two sets of professionally prepared, high-contrast glossy prints (preferably in a proportion of 5 × 7 in) are required. If full-color figures are necessary, the ARCHIVES may pay part of the expense with the balance to be borne by the author.

- Number figures according to their order in the text. Type the figure number, name of the senior author, and an abbreviated title on a gummed label; affix it to the back of the print.

- Double-space legends (maximum length, 40 words) on a separate sheet of 8½ × 11-in paper.

References. Number references in the order they are mentioned in the text; do *not* alphabetize. In text, tables, and legends, identify references with superscript arabic numbers. In listing references, follow AMA style, abbreviating names of journals according to *Index Medicus*. *NOTE:* List all authors and/or editors.

Examples:

1. DuBois RN, Lazenby AJ, Yardley JH, Hendrix TR, Bayless TM, Giardiello FM. Lymphocytic enterocolitis in patients with 'refractory sprue.' *JAMA*. 1989;262:935-937.

2. Ritchie JM, Greene NM. Local anesthetics. In: Gilman AG, Goodman LS, Rall TW, Murad F, eds. *The Pharmacological Basis of Therapeutics*. 7th ed. New York, NY: Macmillan Publishing Co Inc; 1985:309-310.

Informed Consent. State that informed consent for human investigation was obtained. Do not use real names or initials. Authors must ensure that patient confidentiality is in no way breached.

Obligations for Full Disclosure and Authorship[3,4]

The collegiality of reliable science communications entails full, open exchange of information about a report and its history. The cover letter with the submission should fully inform the editor. Authors' identification of special circumstances, vested interests, or sources of bias that might be deemed to affect the integrity of the reported information is requisite for the review process. The same obligations apply to referees. The review process and all communications to the Chief Editor must observe the custom of strict confidentiality. If authors have any questions about their involvement, disclosures, or possible duplicative material, or other special circumstances relevant to the integrity of the scientific communication, the editor will gladly confer confidentially with them.

Readers, in turn, should be provided sufficient data to arrive at their own informed assessments of the report's integrity. They can usually be informed of the history, divisions of labor, or special circumstances of a report within the published text and with the identification of affiliations and full acknowledgments of aid, advice, and support.[4]

Authorship does not claim expertise in every aspect of the work. It does mean that each author within his or her own limits has exerted sufficient reasonable effort to vouch for the validity of the entire work and to bear public accountability for maintaining the integrity of the scientific information communicated. Each author must have had enough substantial involvement in generating and formulating the published product to bear such accountability.

Letters

The purpose is to provide significant news or clarification of general interest. **Author(s) receive only a brief acknowledgment of acceptance or rejection.** The Chief Editor reserves the right to edit the material prior to publication.

Letters intended for publication *must* follow manuscript preparation guidelines (eg, double-spaced, copyright transfer). They generally should not exceed 750 words. Illustrative material is not usually accepted; brief tables may occasionally be considered.

References

1. Iverson CI, Dan BB, Glitman P, et al. *American Medical Association Manual of Style.* 8th ed. Baltimore, Md: Williams & Wilkins; 1988.

2. International Committee of Medical Journal Editors. Uniform requirements for manuscripts submitted to biomedical journals. *Ann Intern Med.* 1988;108:258-265.

3. Freedman DX. The meaning of full disclosure. *Arch Gen Psychiatry.* 1988;45:689-691.

4. Freedman DX. Megamultiple authorship. *Arch Gen Psychiatry.* 1982;39:351.

Checklist

____ (1) Cover letter including all information deemed necessary for the editor's review.

____ (2) Statement on copyright and authorial responsibility, signed by *all* authors.

____ (3) Corresponding author identified and telephone number and address provided.

____ (4) Original manuscript (including structured abstract, references, legends, tables, and figures) plus 3 copies.

____ (5) Right-hand margin unjustified.

____ (6) Copies of publications considered to be helpful for the review process or that bear on any possible overlap of published data.

____ (7) Self-addressed, postage-paid envelope for return of manuscripts (if desired).

Lifetime and 12-Month Prevalence of *DSM-III-R* Psychiatric Disorders in the United States

Results From the National Comorbidity Survey

Ronald C. Kessler, PhD; Katherine A. McGonagle, PhD; Shanyang Zhao, PhD; Christopher B. Nelson, MPH; Michael Hughes, PhD; Suzann Eshleman, MA; Hans-Ulrich Wittchen, PhD; Kenneth S. Kendler, MD

Background: This study presents estimates of lifetime and 12-month prevalence of 14 *DSM-III-R* psychiatric disorders from the National Comorbidity Survey, the first survey to administer a structured psychiatric interview to a national probability sample in the United States.

Methods: The *DSM-III-R* psychiatric disorders among persons aged 15 to 54 years in the noninstitutionalized civilian population of the United States were assessed with data collected by lay interviewers using a revised version of the Composite International Diagnostic Interview.

Results: Nearly 50% of respondents reported at least one lifetime disorder, and close to 30% reported at least one 12-month disorder. The most common disorders were major depressive episode, alcohol dependence, social phobia, and simple phobia. More than half of all lifetime disorders occurred in the 14% of the population who had a history of three or more comorbid disorders. These highly comorbid people also included the vast majority of people with severe disorders. Less than 40% of those with a lifetime disorder had ever received professional treatment, and less than 20% of those with a recent disorder had been in treatment during the past 12 months. Consistent with previous risk factor research, it was found that women had elevated rates of affective disorders and anxiety disorders, that men had elevated rates of substance use disorders and antisocial personality disorder, and that most disorders declined with age and with higher socioeconomic status.

Conclusions: The prevalence of psychiatric disorders is greater than previously thought to be the case. Furthermore, this morbidity is more highly concentrated than previously recognized in roughly one sixth of the population who have a history of three or more comorbid disorders. This suggests that the causes and consequences of high comorbidity should be the focus of research attention. The majority of people with psychiatric disorders fail to obtain professional treatment. Even among people with a lifetime history of three or more comorbid disorders, the proportion who ever obtain specialty sector mental health treatment is less than 50%. These results argue for the importance of more outreach and more research on barriers to professional help-seeking.

(Arch Gen Psych. 1994;51:8-19)

From the Institute for Social Research (Drs Kessler, McGonagle, and Zhao, Mr Nelson, and Ms Eshleman) and Department of Sociology (Dr Kessler), The University of Michigan, Ann Arbor; the Virginia Polytechnic Institute and State University, Blacksburg (Dr Hughes); the Max Planck Institution of Psychiatry, Munich, Germany (Dr Wittchen); and the Departments of Psychiatry (Dr Kendler) and Human Genetics (Dr Kendler), Medical College of Virginia/ Virginia Commonwealth University, Richmond.

THIS REPORT presents data on the lifetime and 12-month prevalence of 14 *DSM-III-R* psychiatric disorders assessed in the National Comorbidity Survey (NCS). The NCS is a congressionally mandated survey designed to study the comorbidity of substance use disorders and nonsubstance psychiatric disorders in the United States. The NCS is the first survey to administer a structured psychiatric interview to a representative national sample in the United States. The need for such a survey was noted 15 years ago in the report of the President's Commission on Mental Health and Illness.[1] It was impossible to undertake such a survey at that time, though, due to the absence of a structured research diagnostic interview capable of generating reliable psychiatric diagnoses in general population samples. Recognizing this need, the National Institute of Mental Health, Bethesda, Md, funded the development of the Diagnostic Interview Schedule (DIS),[2] a research diagnostic interview that can be administered by trained interviewers who are not clinicians. The DIS was first used

See Methods on next page

METHODS

SAMPLE

The NCS is based on a stratified, multistage area probability sample of persons aged 15 to 54 years in the noninstitutionalized civilian population in the 48 coterminous states. The inclusion of respondents aged as young as 15 years, compared with the 18-year-old lower age limit found in most general population surveys, was based on an interest in minimizing recall bias of early-onset disorders. The exclusion of respondents aged older than 54 years was based on evidence from the ECA Study that active comorbidity between substance use disorders and nonsubstance psychiatric disorders is much lower among persons aged older than 54 years than among those aged 54 years and younger. The NCS also includes a supplemental sample of students living in campus group housing. The survey was administered by the staff of the Survey Research Center at the University of Michigan (UM), Ann Arbor, between September 14, 1990, and February 6, 1992. The response rate was 82.6%. Cooperation in listed households did not differ markedly by age or sex, the only two listing variables available for all selected respondents. A total of 8098 respondents participated in the survey. Based on previous evidence that survey nonrespondents have higher rates of psychiatric disorder than respondents,[11,12] a supplemental nonresponse survey was carried out in parallel with the main survey. In this supplemental survey, a random sample of initial nonrespondents was offered a financial incentive to complete a short form of the diagnostic interview. Elevated rates of both lifetime and current psychiatric disorders were found among these initial nonrespondents. A nonresponse adjustment weight was constructed for the main survey data to compensate for this systematic nonresponse. A second weight was used to adjust for variation in probabilities of selection both within and between households. A third weight was used to adjust the data to approximate the national population distributions of the cross-classification of age, sex, race/ethnicity, marital status, education, living arrangements, region, and urbanicity as defined by the 1989 US National Health Interview Survey.[13] A comparison of weighted and unweighted NCS data with national distributions on a range of demographic variables is presented in **Table 1**.

DIAGNOSTIC ASSESSMENT

The psychiatric diagnoses reported below are based on the *DSM-III-R*.[6] The diagnostic interview used to generate these diagnoses is a modified version of the Composite International Diagnostic Interview (CIDI),[14] a state-of-the-art structured diagnostic interview based on the DIS and designed to be used by trained interviewers who are not clinicians.[15] We deleted diagnoses known to have low prevalence in population-based surveys, such as somatization disorder. We also deleted the Folstein-McHugh Mini-Mental State Examination, which is included in the full CIDI, based on pilot test results showing that respondents in the 15- to 54-year-old age range only rarely have high error scores and that those with high error scores in this age range disproportionately come from the foreign-born and the poorly educated population groups. Our modifications of the remaining sections of the CIDI included adding commitment and motivation probes for recall of lifetime episodes, and including clarifying probes for CIDI questions found in pilot work to be unclear or confusing to respondents.

The *DSM-III-R* diagnoses included in the core NCS include major depression, mania, dysthymia, panic disorder, agoraphobia, social phobia, simple phobia, generalized anxiety disorder, alcohol abuse, alcohol dependence, drug abuse, drug dependence, antisocial personality disorder (ASPD), and nonaffective psychosis (NAP). Twelve-month diagnoses of substance use disorders were made in the subsample of respondents who qualified for the lifetime diagnosis and who reported at least one *DSM-III-R* symptom in the 12 months prior to the interview. Nonaffective psychosis is a summary category made up of schizophrenia, schizophreniform disorder, schizoaffective disorder, delusional disorder, and atypical psychosis. We also constructed a summary category for 12-month "severe" disorder, defined as (1) 12-month mania or NAP, (2) lifetime mania or NAP with 12-month treatment or role impairment, or (3) 12-month depression or panic disorder with severe impairment (hospitalization or use of antipsychotic medication).

World Health Organization field trials of the CIDI have documented good interrater reliability,[16,17] test-retest reliability,[18,19] and validity of almost all diagnoses.[20-26] The exception is acute psychotic disorder, which has been shown to be diagnosed with low reliability and validity in structured interviews like the CIDI.[27,28] Based on this evidence, the NCS included clinical reinterviews with respondents who reported any evidence of psychotic symptoms. These reinterviews were administered by experienced clinicians using an adapted version of the Structured Clinical Interview for *DSM-III-R*,[29] an instrument with demonstrated reliability in the diagnosis of schizophrenia.[30] The NCS diagnoses of schizophrenia and other nonaffective psychotic disorders (NAPs) are based on these clinical reinterviews rather than on the UM-CIDI interviews.

INTERVIEWERS AND INTERVIEWER TRAINING

As noted above, the NCS was carried out by the field staff of the Survey Research Center at the UM. The 158 interviewers who participated in the NCS had an average of 5 years of prior interviewing experience with the Survey Research Center. In addition, the NCS interviewers went through a 7-day study-specific training program in the use of the UM-CIDI. Fieldwork was closely monitored throughout the entire data collection period. Three field quality control procedures are worth noting. First, completed interviews were edited by one of 18 regional supervisors before they were returned to the national field office. This al-

Continued on next page

lowed rapid detection of missing data and unclear responses. Incomplete interviews were returned to the interviewer, who recontacted the respondent to obtain the missing information. Second, a random sample of respondents was recontacted by the field supervisors to verify the accuracy of interviewer performance. Third, the field edits were checked at the national field office as soon as interviews were received. This provided a second check on interviewer performance as well as a check on the accuracy of the supervisor's editing. Supervisors were contacted whenever errors were found, and the interview was sent back to the field for resolution.

ANALYSIS PROCEDURES

As a result of the complex sample design and weighting, special software was required to estimate SEs. Standard errors of proportions were estimated by using the Taylor series linearization method.[31] The PSRATIO program in the OSIRIS software package[32] was used to make these calculations. Standard errors of odds ratios (ORs) were estimated by using the method of Balanced Repeated Replication in 44 design-based balanced subsamples.[33,34] The LOGISTIC program in the SAS software package[35] was used to make these calculations.

in the Epidemiologic Catchment Area (ECA) Study, a landmark study that interviewed more than 20 000 respondents in a series of five community epidemiologic surveys. The ECA Study has been the main source of data in the United States on the prevalence of psychiatric disorders and utilization of services for these disorders for the past decade.[3-5]

The NCS was designed to take the next step beyond the ECA Study. Three main advances are noteworthy. First, the NCS diagnoses are based on *DSM-III-R*[6] rather than *DSM-III*[7] criteria. Questions are also included in the interview that allow some comparisons with *DSM-IV*[8] and with the *International Classification of Diseases (ICD-10)* Diagnostic Criteria for Research.[9] Second, while the ECA Study was designed primarily as a prevalence and incidence study, the NCS was designed to be a risk factor study as well. As a result, the NCS interview contains a much more comprehensive risk factor battery than the ECA Study, including family history Research Diagnostic Criteria[10] assessments of parental psychopathology, questions about childhood family adversity, measures of social networks and support, and information about stressful life events and difficulties. Third, while the goals of the ECA Study to include institutional respondents and clinical reappraisals made it necessary to carry out the ECA Study in a small number of local samples, our different goals made it possible to carry out the NCS in a national sample. As a result, we are able to study regional variations in specific psychiatric disorders and urban-rural differences in unmet need for services as well as to provide the first nationally representative data that can be used in the current debate about health care policy in the United States.

RESULTS

THE PREVALENCE OF PSYCHIATRIC DISORDERS

The results in **Table 2** show UM-CIDI/*DSM-III-R* prevalence estimates of the 14 lifetime and 12-month disorders assessed in the core NCS interview. Lifetime prevalence is the proportion of the sample who *ever* experienced a disorder, while 12-month prevalence is the proportion who experienced the disorder at some time in the 12 months before the interview. The prevalence estimates in Table 2 are presented without exclusions for *DSM-III-R* hierarchy rules. Standard errors are reported in parentheses.

The most common psychiatric disorders were major depression and alcohol dependence. More than 17% of respondents had a history of major depressive episode (MDE) in their lifetime, and more than 10% had an episode in the past 12 months. More than 14% of respondents had a lifetime history of alcohol dependence, and more than 7% continued to be dependent in the past 12 months. The next most common disorders were social and simple phobias, with lifetime prevalences of 13% and 11%, respectively, and 12-month prevalences close to 8% and 9%, respectively. As a group, substance use disorders and anxiety disorders were somewhat more prevalent than affective disorders. Approximately one in every four respondents reported a lifetime history of at least one substance use disorder, and a similar number reported a lifetime history of at least one anxiety disorder. Approximately one in every five respondents reported a lifetime history of at least one affective disorder. Anxiety disorders, as a group, are considerably more likely to occur in the 12 months before the interview (17%) than either substance use disorders (11%) or affective disorders (11%), suggesting that anxiety disorders are more chronic than either substance use disorders or affective disorders. The prevalence of other NCS disorders was quite low. Antisocial personality disorder, which was only assessed on a lifetime basis, was reported by more than 3% of respondents, while schizophrenia and other NAPs were found among only 0.7% of respondents. It is important to remember that the diagnosis of NAP was based on clinical reinterviews using the Structured Clinical Interview for *DSM-III-R* diagnosis rather than on the lay CIDI interviews. The prevalence estimates for NAP based on the UM-CIDI were considerably higher but were found to have low validity when judged in comparison with the clinical reappraisals (K.S.K., William Eaton, PhD, Janie Abelson, MSW, R.C.K., oral communication, September 1992).

As shown in the last row of Table 2, 48% of the sample reported a lifetime history of at least one UM-CIDI/*DSM-*

Table 1. Characteristics of NCS Respondents Compared With Those of the Total US Population*

	US Population†	% NCS Weighted	% NCS Unweighted
Sex			
M	49.1	49.5	47.5
F	50.9	50.5	52.5
Race			
W	75.0	75.3	75.1
B	11.9	11.5	12.5
Hispanic	8.6	9.7	9.1
Other	4.5	3.5	3.3
Education, y			
0-11	22.5	22.3	18.2
12	36.8	37.4	33.1
13-15	21.2	21.7	26.3
≥16	19.5	18.6	22.4
Marital status			
Married/cohabitation	59.8	62.9	54.4
Separated/widowed/divorced	10.1	10.0	15.5
Never married	30.1	27.1	30.1
Region			
Northeast	20.0	20.2	19.2
Midwest	24.6	23.8	25.6
South	33.7	36.4	35.6
West	21.7	19.6	19.6
Age, y			
15-24	25.5	24.7	21.8
25-34	30.8	30.1	32.4
35-44	25.9	27.1	27.7
45-54	17.8	18.1	18.1
Urbanicity			
Large MSAs	71.2	67.8	68.9
Small MSAs	8.1	7.5	6.5
Not MSAs	20.7	24.7	24.6
Total N	65 244‡	8098	8098

**NCS indicates National Comorbidity Survey; large MSAs, counties in the US Bureau of the Census–defined metropolitan statistical areas with 250 000 or more residents; small MSAs, counties in MSAs containing less than 250 000 residents; and not MSAs, counties that are not in MSAs.*

†The US population characteristics are based on results from the 1989 US National Health Interview Survey.

‡There were 65 244 household members in the sample households interviewed as part of the 1989 US National Health Interview Survey.

III-R disorder, and 29% had one or more disorders in the 12 months before the interview. While there is no meaningful sex difference in these overall prevalences, there are sex differences in the prevalences of specific disorders. Consistent with previous research,[36-40] men are much more likely to have substance use disorders and ASPD than women, while women are much more likely to have affective disorders (with the exception of mania, for which there is no sex difference) and anxiety disorders than men. The data also show, consistent with a trend found in the ECA Study,[41] that women in the household population are somewhat more likely to have NAP than men, although this sex difference is not statistically significant ($P>.05$).

A final observation about the results in Table 2 is that the sum of the individual prevalence estimates across the 14 disorders consistently exceeds the prevalence of having any disorder. This means that there is considerable comorbidity among these disorders. For example, while the 48% lifetime prevalence in the total sample means that 48 of every 100 respondents in the sample reported a lifetime history of at least one disorder, a summation of lifetime prevalence estimates for the separate disorders shows that these 48 individuals reported a total of 102 lifetime disorders (2.1 per person). As demonstrated in the next section of the article, this comorbidity is quite important for understanding the distribution of psychiatric disorders in the United States.

THE IMPORTANCE OF COMORBIDITY

It is beyond the scope of this article to delve into the many different types of comorbidity that exist in the NCS. Nevertheless, the aggregate results in **Table 3** document that these patterns are very important in understanding the distribution of psychiatric disorders among persons aged 15 to 54 years in the United States and provide an empirical rationale for more detailed examination of particular types of comorbidity in future analyses. The four rows of Table 3 represent the number of lifetime disorders reported by respondents. As shown in the first column, 52% of respondents never had any UM-CIDI/*DSM-III-R* disorder, 21% had one, 13% had two, and 14% had three or more disorders. Only 21% of all the lifetime disorders occurred in respondents with a lifetime history of just one disorder. This means that the *vast majority* of lifetime disorders in this sample (79%) were comorbid disorders. Furthermore, an even greater proportion of 12-month disorders occurred in respondents with a lifetime history of comorbidity. It is particularly striking that close to six (59%) of every 10 12-month disorders and nearly nine (89%) of 10 severe 12-month disorders occurred in the 14% of the sample with a lifetime history of three or more disorders. These results show that while a history of some psychiatric disorder is quite common among persons aged 15 to 54 years in the United States, the major burden of psychiatric disorder in this sector of our society is concentrated in a group of highly comorbid people who constitute about one sixth of the population. The more detailed disaggregation and investigation of these people is a major focus of the NCS.

UTILIZATION OF SERVICES

Although previous national surveys have asked about utilization of professional services for emotional problems,[42,43] no national survey until now has included a diagnostic assessment that could be used to define unmet need. This was done in the NCS by assessing both lifetime and recent

Table 2. Lifetime and 12-Month Prevalence of UM-CIDI/*DSM-III-R* Disorders*

	Male				Female				Total			
	Lifetime		12 mo		Lifetime		12 mo		Lifetime		12 mo	
Disorders	%	SE	%	SE	%	SE	%	SE	%	SE	%	SE
Affective disorders												
Major depressive episode	12.7	0.9	7.7	0.8	21.3	0.9	12.9	0.8	17.1	0.7	10.3	0.6
Manic episode	1.6	0.3	1.4	0.3	1.7	0.3	1.3	0.3	1.6	0.3	1.3	0.2
Dysthymia	4.8	0.4	2.1	0.3	8.0	0.6	3.0	0.4	6.4	0.4	2.5	0.2
Any affective disorder	14.7	0.8	8.5	0.8	23.9	0.9	14.1	0.9	19.3	0.7	11.3	0.7
Anxiety disorders												
Panic disorder	2.0	0.3	1.3	0.3	5.0	1.4	3.2	0.4	3.5	0.3	2.3	0.3
Agoraphobia without panic disorder	3.5	0.4	1.7	0.3	7.0	0.6	3.8	0.4	5.3	0.4	2.8	0.3
Social phobia	11.1	0.8	6.6	0.4	15.5	1.0	9.1	0.7	13.3	0.7	7.9	0.4
Simple phobia	6.7	0.5	4.4	0.5	15.7	1.1	13.2	0.9	11.3	0.6	8.8	0.5
Generalized anxiety disorder	3.6	0.5	2.0	0.3	6.6	0.5	4.3	0.4	5.1	0.3	3.1	0.3
Any anxiety disorder	19.2	0.9	11.8	0.6	30.5	1.2	22.6	0.1	24.9	0.8	17.2	0.7
Substance use disorders												
Alcohol abuse without dependence	12.5	0.8	3.4	0.4	6.4	0.6	1.6	0.2	9.4	0.5	2.5	0.2
Alcohol dependence	20.1	1.0	10.7	0.9	8.2	0.7	3.7	0.4	14.1	0.7	7.2	0.5
Drug abuse without dependence	5.4	0.5	1.3	0.2	3.5	0.4	0.3	0.1	4.4	0.3	0.8	0.1
Drug dependence	9.2	0.7	3.8	0.4	5.9	0.5	1.9	0.3	7.5	0.4	2.8	0.3
Any substance abuse/dependence	35.4	1.2	16.1	0.7	17.9	1.1	6.6	0.4	26.6	1.0	11.3	0.5
Other disorders												
Antisocial personality	5.8	0.6	...	...	1.2	0.3	...	...	3.5	0.3	...	...
Nonaffective psychosis†	0.6	0.1	0.5	0.1	0.8	0.2	0.6	0.2	0.7	0.1	0.5	0.1
Any NCS disorder	48.7	0.2	27.7	0.9	47.3	1.5	31.2	1.3	48.0	1.1	29.5	1.0

**UM-CIDI indicates University of Michigan Composite International Diagnostic Interview; NCS, National Comorbidity Survey.*
†Nonaffective psychosis includes schizophrenia, schizophreniform disorder, schizoaffective disorder, delusional disorder, and atypical psychosis.

utilization of services from a wide variety of professionals in a number of different treatment settings. Summary results (**Table 4**) show that only four of every 10 respondents with a lifetime history of at least one UM-CIDI/*DSM-III-R* disorder ever obtained professional help for their disorders, only one in four obtained treatment in the mental health specialty sector, and about one in 12 were treated in substance abuse facilities. While nearly six in 10 persons who have a lifetime history of three or more disorders ever received professional treatment, only four in 10 of these highly comorbid people were treated in the mental health specialty sector, and about one in seven received treatment in substance abuse facilities. Among respondents with a 12-month disorder, only one in five obtained any professional help in the past year, one in nine obtained treatment in the mental health specialty sector, and one in 25 were treated in substance abuse facilities. Only about one third of persons with three or more disorders in the past year received any professional treatment in the past year, slightly more than one in five were treated in the mental health service sector, and about one in 12 received treatment in substance abuse facilities. These national patterns are broadly consistent with those from the five-site ECA sample,[5,44] in showing that the vast majority of people with recent disorders have not had recent treatment.

DEMOGRAPHIC CORRELATES OF DISORDER

Bivariate risk factor associations are reported for groupings of disorders in **Table 5** (lifetime) and **Table 6** (12 months). Based on findings in Table 3 that the majority of both lifetime and 12-month disorders, and the vast majority of severe disorders, occurred in people with a history of three or more disorders, we also included three or more disorders as an outcome variable in Tables 5 and 6. Associations are shown in the form of ORs with 95% confidence intervals (CIs). As noted above, these CIs are based on complex variance estimation techniques that adjust for the weighting and clustering of the sample data.

Sex

As mentioned previously in the discussion of Table 2, the NCS data are consistent with those of previous epidemiologic studies, in finding that women have higher prevalences than men of affective disorders (with the exception of mania, for which there is no sex difference), anxiety disorders, and NAP, and that men have higher rates than women of substance use disorders and ASPD. Furthermore, we find that women have higher prevalences than men of both lifetime and 12-month comorbidity of three or more disorders.

Table 3. The Concentration of Lifetime and 12-Month Disorders Among Persons With Lifetime Comorbidity

No. of Lifetime Disorders	Proportion of Sample		Proportion of Lifetime Disorders		Proportion of 12-mo Disorders		Proportion of Respondents With Severe 12-mo Disorders*	
	%	SE	%	SE	%	SE	%	SE
0	52.0	1.1	...	...	...	...	...	...
1	21.0	0.6	20.6	0.6	17.4	0.8	2.6	1.7
2	13.0	0.5	25.5	1.0	23.1	1.0	7.9	2.1
≥3	14.0	0.7	53.9	2.7	58.9	1.8	89.5	2.8

**Severe 12-month disorders include active mania, nonaffective psychosis, or active disorders of other types that either required hospitalization or created severe role impairment.*

Age

In the absence of an extremely young age at onset, cohort effects, differential mortality, selection bias associated with age, and age-related differences in willingness to report symptoms, one would expect to find increasing lifetime prevalence of all disorders with age. However, the results in Table 5 show quite a different pattern, with the highest prevalences generally in the group aged 25 to 34 years and declining prevalences at later ages. This pattern is broadly consistent with the results of recent epidemiologic surveys,[36,45] in documenting increasing psychopathology in more recent cohorts. The pattern is even more pronounced in Table 6, where it is shown that 12-month disorders are consistently most prevalent in the youngest cohort (age range, 15 to 24 years) and generally decline monotonically with age.

Race

While the NCS results concerning sex and age are consistent with those of previous epidemiologic studies, this is less true for the results concerning race. Blacks in the NCS have significantly lower prevalences of affective disorders, substance use disorders, and lifetime comorbidity than whites. There are no disorders where either lifetime or active prevalence is significantly higher among blacks than whites. More detailed analyses (results available from the first author [R.C.K.]) show that these effects cannot be explained by controlling for income and education. The lower prevalence of affective disorders is consistent with, but more pronounced than, the ECA finding of a slightly lower rate in the 30- to 64-year-old age range among blacks than whites.[46] The lower prevalence of substance use disorders among blacks is consistent with the ECA finding of higher prevalence of drug and alcohol abuse and dependence among young whites compared with that among young blacks.[47,48] Our failure to find black-white differences in anxiety disorders (or, in more detailed analyses not reported here, in panic disorder, simple phobia, or agoraphobia) is consistent with the ECA finding that blacks and whites have similar prevalences of panic disorder[49] but inconsistent with the ECA finding that blacks have nearly twice the lifetime prevalence of simple phobia and agoraphobia.[50]

Hispanics in the NCS have significantly higher prevalences of current affective disorders and active comorbidity than non-Hispanic whites. There are no disorders where either lifetime or active prevalence is significantly lower among Hispanics than among non-Hispanic whites. The higher rate of affective disorders is inconsistent with that of the ECA Study, which found higher lifetime rates among whites and no race difference in active prevalence.[46] The failure to find a white vs Hispanic difference in anxiety disorders is inconsistent with the ECA finding that Hispanics have significantly lower lifetime rates of panic.[50] Furthermore, the NCS does not replicate the ECA finding that Hispanics have elevated rates of alcohol use disorders compared with whites.[47]

Socioeconomic Status

Consistent with previous research,[3,37,51-54] rates of almost all disorders decline monotonically with income and education. The ORs in Tables 5 and 6 comparing the lowest with highest income groups are significant in all equations. The coefficients comparing the middle vs highest income groups are significant in predicting anxiety disorders, ASPD, and comorbidity. The ORs for education are somewhat more variable, but the general pattern is still one of decline in the ORs from the lowest to highest education groups. One noteworthy exception is that lifetime substance use disorder is significantly higher in the *middle* education subsamples than among those with either the lowest or highest education. The significant ORs for both income and education are consistently larger in predicting 12-month than lifetime prevalence, which means that socioeconomic status is associated not only with onset but also with course of disorder. It is unclear from these data, though, whether this is due to causal influence or to drift. Finally, there is a consistent tendency for socioeconomic status to be more powerfully related to anxiety disorders than to affective disorders, suggesting indirectly that the resources associated with socioeconomic status are more protective against the onset and/or exacerbation of worries and fears than of sadness. We are un-

Table 4. Lifetime and 12-Month Utilization of Professional Services*

	No Disorder	Any Disorder	≥3 Disorders
Lifetime			
Any professional†			
%	15.3	42.0	58.8
SE	1.3	1.1	1.8
Mental health specialty‡			
%	8.1	26.2	41.0
SE	1.2	1.1	2.1
Substance abuse facility§			
%	0.3	8.4	14.8
SE	0.2	0.7	1.5
12 mo			
Any professional			
%	7.0	20.9	34.2
SE	0.7	1.1	3.0
Mental health specialty			
%	2.7	11.5	22.5
SE	0.6	0.8	2.6
Substance abuse facility			
%	0.1	4.0	8.6
SE	0.04	0.7	2.5

**Top part of Table 4 relates to lifetime disorders/utilization; bottom part, 12-month disorders/utilization.*

†Any professional indicates hospitalization or outpatient treatment by a mental health specialist, physician, social worker, counselor, nurse, or other health professional, including treatment in a substance abuse facility.

‡Mental health specialty indicates hospitalization or outpatient treatment by a psychiatrist or psychologist or treatment in a substance abuse facility.

§Substance abuse facility indicates hospitalization for drug or alcohol problems or treatment in a drug or alcohol outpatient clinic or drop-in center or program for people with emotional problems with alcohol or drug abuse.

aware of any previous research on this issue, although this consistent pattern in our data suggests that this might be a fruitful area for future investigation.

Urbanicity

Urbanicity is examined here at the county level by distinguishing major metropolitan counties (major metropolitan areas), urbanized counties that are not in major metropolitan areas (other urban areas), and rural counties (rural). It is important to note that significant within-county differences in the prevalence of some disorders has been found in previous research.[55] Within-county comparisons will be made in later analyses of the NCS, but these comparisons cannot yet be carried out because of current incompleteness in the NCS geocoding, pending release of final matching information from the 1990 census.

As seen in Tables 5 and 6, the effects of urbanicity at the county level are generally not significant. The single exception is that residents of major metropolitan counties are more likely than residents of rural counties to have comorbidity in the 12 months before the interview (OR=1.44). The coefficient that compares residents of other urbanized counties with residents of rural counties on the same outcome is very similar in magnitude (OR=1.41) and significant at the .06 level, which means that it is the low rate of comorbidity in rural America rather than a high rate in major metropolitan counties that underlies this pattern. This one significant coefficient could have occurred by chance in 22 different comparisons (two urbanicity coefficients for each of 11 outcomes), although there is a general trend in the data for rural residents to have the lowest levels of disorder (in 10 of the 11 outcomes in Tables 5 and 6).

Region

There are a number of significant regional differences in lifetime prevalence. Substance use disorders, ASPD, and comorbidity are all highest in the West. Anxiety disorders are highest in the Northeast. Virtually all disorders are lowest in the South. None of these patterns, however, is replicated in parallel analyses of 12-month disorders, implying that region is associated in different ways with onset and course.

COMMENT

LIMITATIONS

Two data collection limitations need to be noted. First, the NCS is a cross-sectional survey that relies entirely on retrospective reports to assess the prevalence of lifetime disorders. Commitment and memory probes were used to minimize recall problems, but we recognize that whatever success we had in this regard was only partial. Long-term longitudinal data collection is needed to evaluate the magnitude of recall failure and to adjust for its effects on prevalence estimates. Second, even in cases where respondents describe recent disorders, our diagnostic assessment is based on only a single structured interview administered by nonclinicians. This is a practical necessity in a survey as large and geographically dispersed as the NCS. Yet, it is important to recognize that we pay a price for this ease of implementation in reduced diagnostic precision, which could have been improved if it had been possible to use clinical interviewers, to carry out multiple interviews, and to use ancillary information from informants and institutional records. The fact that these things were not done means that the prevalences reported here should be interpreted as estimates rather than as definite diagnoses.

PREVALENCE

The NCS results show that psychiatric disorders are more prevalent than previous research would lead us to believe. Close to half of all respondents report a lifetime history of at least one UM-CIDI/*DSM-III-R* disorder. One fifth of re-

Table 5. Demographic Correlates of Lifetime Psychiatric Disorders*

	Any Affective Disorder		Any Anxiety Disorder		Any Substance Use Disorder		ASPD†		Any Disorder		≥3 Disorders	
	OR	95% CI	OR	95% CI	OR	95% CI	OR	95% CI	OR	95% CI	OR	95% CI
Sex												
M	1.00	...	1.00	...	1.00	...	5.16‡	2.90-9.20	1.00	...	1.00	...
F	1.82‡	1.56-2.12	1.85‡	1.58-2.16	0.40‡	0.34-0.46	1.00	...	0.95	0.83-1.08	1.24‡	1.02-1.50
Age, y												
15-24	0.85	0.65-1.11	1.13	0.90-1.43	1.36‡	1.01-1.83	2.56‡	1.52-4.30	1.15	0.92-1.43	1.18	0.88-1.58
25-34	0.97	0.77-1.22	1.13	0.90-1.42	1.99‡	1.53-2.57	1.83‡	1.08-3.12	1.36‡	1.12-1.65	1.47‡	1.07-2.02
35-44	1.06	0.81-1.38	1.05	0.83-1.34	1.58‡	1.25-1.99	1.01	0.50-2.03	1.20	0.99-1.46	1.19	0.87-1.62
45-54	1.00	...	1.00	...	1.00	...	1.00	...	1.00	...	1.00	...
Race												
W	1.00	...	1.00	...	1.00	...	1.00	...	1.00	...	1.00	...
B	0.63‡	0.46-0.87	0.77	0.58-1.01	0.35‡	0.27-0.46	0.89	0.56-1.41	0.50‡	0.41-0.60	0.67‡	0.45-0.98
Hispanic	0.96	0.72-1.27	0.90	0.71-1.15	0.80	0.62-1.03	1.43	0.92-2.23	0.86	0.69-1.06	0.99	0.73-1.35
Income, $												
0-19 000	1.56‡	1.23-1.98	2.00‡	1.66-2.41	1.27‡	1.05-1.54	2.98‡	1.71-5.20	1.49‡	1.25-1.78	2.46‡	1.87-3.24
20 000-34 000	1.19	0.89-1.60	1.52‡	1.21-1.90	1.06	0.80-1.41	2.16‡	1.15-4.06	1.21	0.95-1.53	1.71‡	1.20-2.43
35 000-69 000	1.16	0.88-1.51	1.48‡	1.16-1.90	1.06	0.83-1.36	1.59	0.82-3.10	1.21	0.97-1.49	1.55‡	1.12-2.15
≥70 000	1.00	...	1.00	...	1.00	...	1.00	...	1.00	...	1.00	...
Education, y												
0-11	0.98	0.80-1.20	1.86‡	1.53-2.26	0.99	0.77-1.27	14.13‡	6.05-32.99	1.17	0.96-1.42	2.15‡	1.60-2.90
12	1.00	0.82-1.24	1.76‡	1.42-2.20	1.25‡	1.05-1.48	4.29‡	2.07-8.90	1.25‡	1.07-1.46	2.09‡	1.52-2.86
13-15	1.05	0.89-1.25	1.44‡	1.15-1.79	1.20‡	1.01-1.43	3.32‡	1.43-7.72	1.21‡	1.04-1.40	1.73‡	1.25-2.39
≥16	1.00	...	1.00	...	1.00	...	1.00	...	1.00	...	1.00	...
Urbanicity												
Major metropolitan	1.26	0.91-1.76	0.98	0.76-1.26	1.09	0.82-1.45	1.27	0.80-1.99	1.10	0.83-1.47	1.20	0.86-1.68
Other urban	1.20	0.85-1.71	1.00	0.74-1.35	1.10	0.80-1.51	0.98	0.61-1.58	1.09	0.78-1.53	1.18	0.80-1.73
Rural	1.00	...	1.00	...	1.00	...	1.00	...	1.00	...	1.00	...
Region												
Midwest	1.06	0.85-1.33	1.17	0.93-1.46	1.21	0.96-1.54	1.34	0.89-2.00	1.19	0.94-1.49	1.00	0.76-1.33
Northeast	1.00	0.76-1.30	1.29‡	1.07-1.56	1.33‡	1.04-1.69	1.49	0.83-2.69	1.25‡	1.03-1.52	1.35	0.98-1.85
West	1.32	1.00-1.74	1.15	0.87-1.52	1.57‡	1.15-2.14	2.40‡	1.49-3.85	1.38‡	1.05-1.81	1.43‡	1.03-1.98
South	1.00	...	1.00	...	1.00	...	1.00	...	1.00	...	1.00	...

*ASPD indicates antisocial personality disorder; OR, odds ratio; and CI, confidence interval.
†Results concerning ASPD exclude respondents aged 15 to 17 years because the diagnosis requires that the respondent be at least 18 years of age.
‡$P<.05$ (two tailed).

spondents have a lifetime history of an affective disorder, one fourth have a history of an anxiety disorder, and one fourth have a history of a substance use disorder. A 12-month prevalence of at least one disorder is nearly 30% in the sample as a whole, with more respondents reporting a 12-month anxiety disorder (17.2%) than either affective disorders (11.3%) or a substance use disorder (11.3%). The high ratio of a 12-month to lifetime anxiety disorder prevalence suggests indirectly that they are more chronic than either affective disorders or substance use disorders.

The fact that the NCS prevalence estimates are higher than in previous epidemiologic surveys could be due, at least in part, to secular trends. A number of methodologic factors could also be involved, including the fact that the NCS is based on a national sample, concentrates on a younger age range than previous surveys, uses a correction weight to adjust for nonresponse bias, and reports *DSM-III-R* diagnoses while earlier epidemiologic surveys used the *DSM-III* diagnostic system. Any attempt to compare prevalence estimates in the NCS with those in earlier surveys needs to grapple with the implications of all these issues.

It is also important to recognize that while the diagnostic instrument used in the NCS is very similar to the diagnostic instrument used in the ECA Study and other recent epidemiologic studies (the DIS), there are differences in wording and depth of probing that could have important effects on prevalence estimates. For example, the UM-CIDI assesses phobias by presenting the respondent with three separate lists containing a total of 20 prototypic feared objects and situations (six for social phobia, nine for simple phobia, and five for agoraphobia), while the version of the DIS used in the ECA Study combined all these objects and situations into a single list containing a total of only 15 items. The assessment of social phobia, in par-

Table 6. Demographic Correlates of 12-Month Psychiatric Disorders*

	Any Affective Disorder		Any Anxiety Disorder		Any Substance Use Disorder		Any Disorder		≥3 Disorders	
	OR	95% CI	OR	95% CI	OR	95% CI	OR	95% CI	OR	95% CI
Sex										
M	1.00	...	1.00	...	1.00	...	1.00	...	1.00	...
F	1.76†	1.43-2.18	2.19†	1.88-2.55	0.37†	0.31-0.43	1.18†	1.07-1.31	1.55†	1.15-2.10
Age, y										
15-24	1.67†	1.14-2.44	1.40†	1.09-1.80	3.65†	2.29-5.84	2.06†	1.66-2.56	2.08†	1.17-3.70
25-34	1.32	0.89-1.96	1.13	0.85-1.51	2.65†	1.72-4.06	1.51†	1.20-1.88	1.66	0.88-3.16
35-44	1.35	0.93-1.96	0.98	0.76-1.26	2.00†	1.31-3.05	1.24	0.98-1.56	1.36	0.75-2.49
45-54	1.00	...	1.00	...	1.00	...	1.00	...	1.00	...
Race										
W	1.00	...	1.00	...	1.00	...	1.00	...	1.00	...
B	0.78	0.54-1.14	0.90	0.65-1.26	0.47†	0.35-0.64	0.70†	0.55-0.90	1.04	0.53-2.06
Hispanic	1.38†	1.02-1.86	1.17	0.93-1.49	1.04	0.74-1.46	1.11	0.91-1.35	1.86†	1.23-2.82
Income, $										
0-19 000	1.73†	1.29-2.32	2.12†	1.63-2.77	1.92†	1.36-2.71	1.92†	1.54-2.39	3.36†	1.95-5.79
20 000-34 000	1.13	0.80-1.59	1.56†	1.18-2.06	1.12	0.79-1.60	1.24	0.97-1.57	2.10†	1.16-3.83
35 000-69 000	1.01	0.75-1.37	1.50†	1.15-1.97	1.11	0.75-1.64	1.20	0.93-1.55	1.66†	1.02-2.73
≥70 000	1.00	...	1.00	...	1.00	...	1.00	...	1.00	...
Education, y										
0-11	1.79†	1.31-2.43	2.82†	2.26-3.51	2.10†	1.56-2.84	2.33†	1.91-2.84	3.76†	2.45-5.76
12	1.38†	1.00-1.89	2.10†	1.66-2.67	1.80†	1.40-2.32	1.79†	1.46-2.21	2.54†	1.70-3.78
13-15	1.37†	1.02-1.84	1.60†	1.19-2.15	1.70†	1.20-2.42	1.58†	1.28-1.96	2.06†	1.18-3.59
≥16	1.00	...	1.00	...	1.00	...	1.00	...	1.00	...
Urbanicity										
Major metropolitan	1.21	0.76-1.92	1.04	0.77-1.41	1.09	0.79-1.50	1.05	0.75-1.47	1.44†	1.00-2.08
Other urban	1.11	0.69-1.79	1.18	0.85-1.63	1.12	0.77-1.64	1.11	0.78-1.60	1.41	0.97-2.04
Rural	1.00	...	1.00	...	1.00	...	1.00	...	1.00	...
Region										
Midwest	0.84	0.63-1.13	1.07	0.81-1.41	1.22	0.97-1.53	1.04	0.80-1.34	0.79	0.56-1.11
Northeast	0.87	0.62-1.21	1.24	0.99-1.57	1.30	0.98-1.72	1.09	0.85-1.39	1.08	0.74-1.59
West	0.98	0.59-1.64	1.12	0.86-1.47	1.13	0.86-1.48	1.02	0.77-1.33	1.07	0.61-1.88
South	1.00	...	1.00	...	1.00	...	1.00	...	1.00	...

*OR indicates odds ratio; CI, confidence interval.
†P<.05 (two tailed).

ticular, is more thorough in the UM-CIDI than in the DIS, and this may explain why the NCS estimate of the prevalence of social phobia is much higher than the ECA estimate.

A final methodologic factor of importance in accounting for the comparatively higher NCS prevalence estimates is that the NCS included more sensitive probes for lifetime recall than did earlier epidemiologic surveys. Two aspects of this probing are noteworthy. First, based on the results of pilot tests that showed that respondents underreport stem questions once they recognize that positive responses will lead to more detailed questions, we included diagnostic stem questions for a number of disorders in a life review section that was administered before probing any positive stem responses. Second, this life review section used probes to stimulate motivation for lifetime recall in an effort to aid memory search. Based on these refinements, NCS respondents reported more positive responses to virtually all stem questions than ECA respondents. This, in turn, led to higher prevalence estimates.

The higher prevalence in the NCS compared with that in the ECA Study is particularly pronounced for MDE (lifetime prevalence of 17.1% in the NCS compared with 6.3% in the ECA Study). We suspect that this is due, at least in part, to the fact that failure to recall lifetime episodes of MDE is greater than for other disorders and that our refinements to aid recall had a more powerful effect on estimates of MDE than other disorders. This cannot explain the fact, though, that 12-month prevalence of MDE is much higher in the NCS than in the ECA Study. A factor relevant to this difference is that the NCS used three separate stem questions for MDE concerning periods of feeling "sad, blue, or depressed," feeling "down in the dumps or gloomy," and "losing interest in most things like work, hobbies, or things you usually like to do for fun." The ECA Study, in comparison, used only one stem question that combined the content of our first and third questions. It is noteworthy that the estimated prevalence of MDE in the NCS is quite similar to the estimates in previous epidemiologic studies that used clinical interviews like the Schedule for Affective Disorders and Schizophrenia and the Structured Clinical Interview for *DSM-III-R*.[56-58] The fact that our refinements did not lead to overreporting is indicated by the fact that blind clinical reappraisals of the UM-CIDI diagnosis of MDE in a random subsample of NCS respondents using the Structured Clinical Interview for *DSM-III-R*[29] as the validation standard yielded a positive predictive value of 0.70 (±0.10), a rate that compares favorably with that of similar investigations of the ECA diagnostic classification of MDE.[2,27,28]

COMORBIDITY

One important accomplishment of the ECA Study was that it documented that comorbidity among psychiatric disorders is quite high in the general population. More than 60% of the ECA respondents with at least one lifetime disorder had two or more disorders.[3] The ECA respondents with comorbidity were also found to have higher utilization of services.[59] It was also found that mental disorders are associated with substance abuse prevalence and specialty sector treatment.[60] The NCS was designed to build on these results and to provide more fine-grained data about the prevalence, causes, and consequences of psychiatric comorbidity. We have taken a first step in that direction in the present report. We find that 56% of NCS respondents with a history of at least one disorder had two or more disorders. We also find that the majority of lifetime disorders and an even greater percentage of 12-month disorders occur in the roughly one sixth of the population with a lifetime history of three or more disorders. The fact that this segment of the population accounts for a higher percentage of 12-month disorders than lifetime disorders means that comorbidity is, in general, associated with a more serious course of illness, a result consistent with the findings of clinical investigations.[61-65] Future analyses of the NCS data will disaggregate this overall pattern to investigate the possibility that the effect of comorbidity on course can be further specified as due to particular primary disorders, secondary disorders, or primary-secondary combinations and whether these effects are specified by age at onset, family history, and other individual differences.

UTILIZATION OF SERVICES

Our findings regarding utilization of services are broadly consistent with those of previous research,[5,43,44] in showing that the majority of people with psychiatric disorders receive no professional treatment and that fewer yet receive treatment in the mental health specialty sector. Although more likely than others to obtain treatment, we also found that fewer than half of people with three or more lifetime comorbid disorders ever obtained mental health specialty sector treatment.

It is noteworthy that the ECA estimate of the percentage of people with a disorder who received any professional treatment during the past 12 months is roughly 25% higher than the NCS estimate.[5] This finding, coupled with the fact that the NCS finds a considerably higher 12-month prevalence of disorder than the ECA Study, means that the NCS finds considerably more unmet need for mental health services than the ECA Study. More detailed analyses are planned to investigate this difference and to determine how much of it is due to time trends, to the fact that the ECA Study was based on a largely urbanized population where access to professional services is greater than in the rest of the population, or to other reasons.

RISK FACTORS

For the most part, the risk factor results reported above are consistent with previous investigations in finding more affective disorders and anxiety disorders among women, more substance use disorders and ASPD among men, and declining rates of most disorders with age and higher socioeconomic status. The other risk factor results are more provisional, though, due to the fact that they either fail to replicate previous research (in the case of the results regarding race) or are new results (in the cases of urbanicity and region). It is important to remember, in this regard, that we examined close to 200 separate coefficients in the risk factor analysis. It is quite likely that some of the significant results in this large set are due to chance. Future analyses of the NCS need to examine these risk factor results in more detail to determine whether they are stable. Perhaps the most interesting of these results concerns the fact that respondents living in rural areas have a 40% lower odds of 12-month comorbidity of three or more disorders than their urban counterparts. This association is much more powerful than the associations of urbanicity with the prevalence of individual disorders, which means that while rural Americans are no more likely to suffer from a psychiatric disorder, their disorders are more likely to be "pure" than comorbid. If this result is stable, it has important implications for the provision of services to the rural mentally ill, where medical care is more likely to come from the general medical sector than from the specialty mental health sector. Comorbidity is recognized as a major complication that impedes the ability of the general medical sector to provide effective care.[63] The fact that 1-year comorbidity of three or more disorders is lowest in rural areas means that the magnitude of this complication is considerably less than expected from our total population estimate.

Another intriguing aspect of the results regarding low prevalence of disorder in rural counties is that this is true despite the fact that rural Americans are exposed to much greater financial adversity than their urban counterparts.[66] The same can be said for the low prevalence of affective and substance use disorders among blacks compared with that among whites, patterns that exist despite the fact that blacks have much lower aggregate levels of both income and education than whites.[66] Future analyses of the NCS data will explore these patterns in more depth with the expectation that some as yet unknown resources protect rural people and blacks from the adverse psychiatric effects that we would otherwise expect to be associated with their stressful lives.

Accepted for publication August 16, 1993.

The National Comorbidity Survey (NCS) is a collaborative epidemiologic investigation of the prevalence, causes, and consequences of psychiatric morbidity and comorbidity in the United States. The NCS is supported by the US Alcohol, Drug Abuse, and Mental Health Administration, Rockville, Md (grants MH46376 and MH49098), with supplemental support from the W. T. Grant Foundation, New York, NY (grant 90135190). Preparation of this report was also supported by a Research Scientist Development Award to Dr Kessler (grant MH00507). Ronald C. Kessler, PhD, is the principal investigator. Collaborating NCS sites and investigators are as follows: The Addiction Research Foundation, Toronto, Ontario (Robin Room, PhD); Duke University Medical Center, Durham, NC (Dan Blazer, MD, and Marvin Swartz, MD); The Johns Hopkins University, Baltimore, Md (James Anthony, PhD, William Eaton, PhD, and Philip Leaf, PhD); the Max Planck Institute of Psychiatry, Munich, Germany (Hans-Ulrich Wittchen, PhD); the Medical College of Virginia, Richmond (Kenneth Kendler, MD); The University of Michigan, Ann Arbor (Lloyd Johnston, PhD, and Ronald Kessler, PhD); the National Institute of Mental Health, Bethesda, Md (Darrell Kirch, MD, and Darrel Regier, MD); New York (NY) University (Patrick Shrout, PhD); State University of New York, Stony Brook (Evelyn Bromet, PhD); The University of Toronto (Ontario) (R. Jay Turner, PhD); and Washington University School of Medicine, St Louis, Mo (Linda Cottler, PhD). A complete list of NCS publications can be obtained from the NCS Study Coordinator, Room 1006, Institute for Social Research, The University of Michigan, Box 1248, Ann Arbor, MI 48106-1248.

The authors appreciate the detailed comments provided by Naomi Breslau, PhD, Evelyn Bromet, PhD, William Eaton, PhD, Lee Robins, PhD, Frank Sullivan, PhD, and Myrna Weissman, PhD, and the anonymous journal reviewers.

Reprints not available.

REFERENCES

1. The President's Commission on Mental Health and Illness, eds. *Report to the President From the President's Commission on Mental Health, Volume I.* Washington, DC: US Government Printing Office; 1978. Stock No. 040-000-00390-8.
2. Robins LN, Helzer JE, Croughan JL, Ratcliff KS. National Institute of Mental Health Diagnostic Interview Schedule: its history, characteristics and validity. *Arch Gen Psychiatry.* 1981;38:381-389.
3. Robins LN, Locke BZ, Regier DA. An overview of psychiatric disorders in America. In: Robins LN, Regier DA, eds. *Psychiatric Disorders in America: The Epidemiologic Catchment Area Study.* New York, NY: Free Press; 1991:328-366.
4. Bourdon KH, Rae DA, Locke BZ, Narrow WE, Regier DA. Estimating the prevalence of mental disorders in U.S. adults from the Epidemiologic Catchment Area Study. *Public Health Rep.* 1992;107:663-668.
5. Regier DA, Narrow WE, Rae DS, Manderscheid RW, Locke BZ, Goodwin FK. The de Facto US Mental and Addictive Disorders Service System: Epidemiologic Catchment Area prospective 1-year prevalence rates of disorders and services. *Arch Gen Psychiatry.* 1993;50:85-94.
6. American Psychiatric Association. *Diagnostic and Statistical Manual of Mental Disorders, Revised Third Edition.* Washington, DC: American Psychiatric Association; 1987.
7. American Psychiatric Association. *Diagnostic and Statistical Manual of Mental Disorders, Third Edition.* Washington, DC: American Psychiatric Association; 1980.
8. Task Force on *DSM-IV*: American Psychiatric Association. *Diagnostic and Statistical Manual of Mental Disorders, Fourth Edition Draft Criteria.* Washington, DC: American Psychiatric Association; March 1993.
9. World Health Organization. Mental health and behavioral disorders (including disorders of psychological development). In: *International Classification of Diseases—10th Revision.* Geneva, Switzerland: World Health Organization; 1991: chap 5. Diagnostic Criteria for Research, Draft for Field Trials.
10. Endicott J, Andreasen N, Spitzer RL. *Family History Research Diagnostic Criteria.* New York, NY: Biometrics Research, New York State Psychiatric Institute; 1978.
11. Allgulander C. Psychoactive drug use in a general population sample, Sweden: correlates with perceived health, psychiatric diagnoses, and mortality in an automated record-linkage study. *Am J Public Health.* 1989;79:1006-1010.
12. Eaton WW, Anthony JC, Tepper S, Dryman A. Psychopathology and attrition in the Epidemiologic Catchment Area Study. *Am J Epidemiol.* 1992;135:1051-1059.
13. US Department of Health and Human Services. *National Health Interview Survey: 1989 (Computer File).* Hyattsville, Md: National Center for Health Statistics; 1992.
14. World Health Organization. *Composite International Diagnostic Interview (CIDI), Version 1.0.* Geneva, Switzerland: World Health Organization; 1990.
15. Robins LN, Wing J, Wittchen H-U, Helzer JE. The Composite International Diagnostic Interview: an epidemiologic instrument suitable for use in conjunction with different diagnostic systems and in different cultures. *Arch Gen Psychiatry.* 1988;45:1069-1077.
16. Wittchen H-U, Robins LN, Cottler LB, Sartorius N, Burke JD, Regier DA, and Participants in the Multicentre WHO/ADAMHA Field Trials. Cross-cultural feasibility, reliability and sources of variance in the Composite International Diagnostic Interview (CIDI). *Br J Psychiatry.* 1991;159:645-653.
17. Cottler LB, Robins LN, Grant BF, Blaine J, Towle LH, Wittchen H-U, Sartorius N, and Participants in the WHO/ADAMHA Field Trials. The CIDI-core substance abuse and dependence questions: cross-cultural and nosological issues. *Br J Psychiatry.* 1991;159:653-658.
18. Semler G, von Cranach M, Wittchen H-U, eds. Comparison between the Composite International Diagnostic Interview and the Present State Examination. Report to the WHO/ADAMHA Task Force on Instrument Development; February 1987; Geneva, Switzerland.
19. Wacker HR, Battegay R, Mullejans R, Schlosser C. Using the CIDI-C in the general population. In: Stefanis CN, Rabavilas AD, Soldatos CR, eds. *Psychiatry: A World Perspective.* Amsterdam, the Netherlands: Elsevier Science Publishers; 1990:138-143.
20. Semler G, ed. *Reliabilitat und Validitat des Composite International Diagnostic Interview: Inaugural-Dissertation zur Erlangung des akademischen Grades eines Doktors der Philosophie.* Mannheim, Germany: Universitat Mannheim; 1989.
21. Spengler P, Wittchen H-U. Procedural validity of standardized symptom questions for the assessment of psychotic symptoms: a comparison of the CIDI with two clinical methods. *Compr Psychiatry.* 1989;29:309-322.
22. Janca A, Robins LN, Cottler LB, Early TS. Clinical observation of CIDI assessments: an analysis of the CIDI field trials—wave II at the St. Louis site. *Br J Psychiatry.* 1992;160:815-818.
23. Leitmeyer P, ed. *Zur Symptomerfassung mit dem standarisierten Interview CIDI-C in der Allgemeinpraxis: Inaugural Dissertation zur Erlangung des medizinischen Doktorgrades fur klinische Medizin.* Mannheim, Germany: Universitat Mannheim; 1990.
24. Farmer AE, Katz R, McGuffin P, Bebbington P. A comparison between the Present State Examination and the Composite International Diagnostic Interview. *Arch Gen Psychiatry.* 1987;44:1064-1068.
25. Farmer AE, Jenkins PL, Katz R, Ryder L. Comparison of CATEGO-derived *ICD-8* and *DSM-III* classifications using the Composite International Diagnostic Interview in severely ill subjects. *Br J Psychiatry.* 1991;158:177-182.
26. Wittchen H-U, Burke JD, Semler G, Pfister H. Recall and dating of psychiatric

symptoms: test-retest reliability of time-related symptom questions in a standardized psychiatric interview. *Arch Gen Psychiatry.* 1989;46:437-443.
27. Anthony JC, Folstein M, Romanoski AJ, von Korff MR, Nestadt GR, Chahal R, Merchant A, Brown CH, Shapiro S, Kramer M, Gruenberg EM. Comparison of the lay Diagnostic Interview Schedule and a standardized psychiatric diagnosis: experience in eastern Baltimore. *Arch Gen Psychiatry.* 1985;42:667-675.
28. Helzer JE, Robins LN, McEvoy LT, Spitznagel E. A comparison of clinical and Diagnostic Interview Schedule diagnoses. *Arch Gen Psychiatry.* 1985;42:657-666.
29. Spitzer RL, Williams JBW, Gibbon M, First MB. The structured clinical interview for *DSM-III-R* (SCID), I: history, rationale, and description. *Arch Gen Psychiatry.* 1992;49:624-629.
30. Williams JBW, Gibbon M, First MB, Spitzer RL, Davies M, Borus J, Howes MJ, Kane J, Harrison GP Jr, Rounsaville B, Wittchen H-U. The structured clinical interview for *DSM-III-R* (SCID), II: multisite test-retest reliability. *Arch Gen Psychiatry.* 1992;49:630-636.
31. Woodruff RS, Causey BD. Computerized method for approximating the variance of a complicated estimate. *J Am Stat Assoc.* 1976;71:315-321.
32. University of Michigan. *OSIRIS VII.* Ann Arbor, Mich: Institute for Social Research, The University of Michigan; 1981.
33. Kish L, Frankel MR. Balanced repeated replications for standard errors. *J Am Stat Assoc.* 1970;65:1071-1094.
34. Koch GG, Leneshow S. An application of multivariate analysis to complex sample survey data. *J Am Stat Assoc.* 1972;67:780-782.
35. SAS Institute. *SAS 6.03.* Cary, NC: SAS Institute; 1988.
36. Robins LN, Regier DA, eds. *Psychiatric Disorders in America: The Epidemiologic Catchment Area Study.* New York, NY: Free Press; 1991.
37. Canino GJ, Bird HR, Shrout PE, Rubio-Stipec M, Bravo M, Martinez R, Sesman M, Guevara L. The prevalence of specific psychiatric disorders in Puerto Rico. *Arch Gen Psychiatry.* 1987;44:727-735.
38. Hwu H-G, Yeh EK, Chang LY. Prevalence of psychiatric disorders in Taiwan defined by the Chinese Diagnostic Interview Schedule. *Acta Psychiatr Scand.* 1989;79:136-147.
39. Wells JE, Bushnell JA, Hornblow AR, Joyce PR, Oakley-Browne MA. Christchurch Psychiatric Epidemiology Study, I: methodology and lifetime prevalence for specific psychiatric disorders. *Aust N Z J Psychiatry.* 1989;23:315-326.
40. Wittchen H-U, Essau CA, von Zerssen D, Krieg JC, Zaudig M. Lifetime and six-month prevalence of mental disorders in the Munich follow-up study. *Eur Arch Psychiatry Clin Neurosci.* 1992;241:247-258.
41. Keith SJ, Regier DA, Rae DS. Schizophrenic disorders. In: Regier DA, Robins LN, eds. *Psychiatric Disorders in America: The Epidemiologic Catchment Area Study.* New York, NY: Free Press; 1991:33-52.
42. Gurin G, Veroff J, Feld SC. *Americans View Their Mental Health.* New York, NY: Basic Books Inc Publishers; 1960.
43. Veroff J, Kulka RA, Douvan E. *Mental Health in America: Patterns of Help-Seeking From 1957 to 1976.* New York, NY: Basic Books Inc Publishers; 1981.
44. Shapiro S, Skinner EA, Kessler LG, von Korff M, German PS, Tischler GL, Leaf PJ, Benham L, Cottler L, Regier DA. Utilization of health and mental health services: three Epidemiological Catchment Area sites. *Arch Gen Psychiatry.* 1984;41:971-978.
45. Cross-National Collaborative Group. The changing rate of major depression. *JAMA.* 1992;268:3098-3105.
46. Weissman MM, Bruce ML, Leaf PJ, Florio LP, Holzer C III. Affective disorders. In: Robins LN, Regier DA, eds. *Psychiatric Disorders in America: The Epidemiologic Catchment Area Study.* New York, NY: Free Press; 1991:53-80.
47. Helzer JE, Burnam A, McEvoy LT. Alcohol abuse and dependence. In: Robins LN, Regier DA, eds. *Psychiatric Disorders in America: The Epidemiologic Catchment Area Study.* New York, NY: Free Press; 1991:81-115.
48. Anthony JC, Helzer JE. Syndromes of drug abuse and dependence. In: Robins LN, Regier DA, eds. *Psychiatric Disorders in America: The Epidemiologic Catchment Area Study.* New York, NY: Free Press; 1991:116-154.
49. Horwath E, Johnson J, Hornig CD. Epidemiology of panic disorder in African-Americans. *Am J Psychiatry.* 1993;150:465-469.
50. Eaton WW, Dryman A, Weissman MM. Panic and phobia. In: Robins LN, Regier DA, eds. *Psychiatric Disorders in America: The Epidemiologic Catchment Area Study.* New York, NY: Free Press; 1991:155-179.
51. Bruce ML, Takeuchi DT, Leaf PJ. Poverty and psychiatric status: longitudinal evidence from the New Haven Epidemiologic Catchment Area Study. *Arch Gen Psychiatry.* 1991;48:470-474.
52. Holzer CE, Shea B, Swanson JW, Leaf PJ, Myers JK, George L, Weissman MM, Bednarski P. The increased risk for specific psychiatric disorders among persons of low socioeconomic status. *Am J Psychiatry.* 1986;6:259-271.
53. Stansfeld SA, Marmot MG. Social class and minor psychiatric disorder in British civil servants: a validated screening survey using the General Health Questionnaire. *Psychol Med.* 1992;22:739-749.
54. Myers JK. Social factors related to psychiatric disorders. *Soc Psychiatry Psychiatr Epidemiol.* 1984;19:53-61.
55. Robins LN, Helzer JE, Weissman MM, Orvaschel H, Gruenberg E, Burke JD Jr, Regier DA. Lifetime prevalence of specific psychiatric disorders in three sites. *Arch Gen Psychiatry.* 1984;41:949-958.
56. Boyd JH, Weissman MM. Epidemiology of affective disorders: a reexamination and future directions. *Arch Gen Psychiatry.* 1981;38:1039-1046.
57. Kendler KS, Neale MC, Kessler RC, Heath AC, Eaves LJ. A population-based twin study of major depression in women. *Arch Gen Psychiatry.* 1992;49:257-266.
58. Weissman MM, Myers JK, Harding PS. Psychiatric disorders in a U.S. urban community: 1975-1976. *Am J Psychiatry.* 1978;135:459-462.
59. Helzer JE, Pryzbeck TR. The co-occurrence of alcoholism with other psychiatric disorders in the general population and its impact on treatment. *J Stud Alcohol.* 1988;49:219-224.
60. Regier DA, Farmer ME, Rae DS, Locke BZ, Keith SJ, Judd LL, Goodwin FK. Comorbidity of mental disorders with alcohol and other drug abuse: results from the Epidemiologic Catchment Area (ECA) Study. *JAMA.* 1990;264:2511-2518.
61. Bukstein OG, Brent DA, Kaminer Y. Comorbidity of substance abuse and other psychiatric disorders in adolescents. *Am J Psychiatry.* 1989;146:1131-1141.
62. Hesselbrock MN, Meyer RE, Keener JJ. Psychopathology in hospitalized alcoholics. *Arch Gen Psychiatry.* 1985;42:1050-1055.
63. Kessler RC, McGonagle KA, Carnelley KB, Nelson CB, Farmer MA, Regier DA. Comorbidity of mental disorders and substance use disorders: a review and agenda for future research. In: Leaf P, ed. *Research in Community and Mental Health.* Greenwich, Conn: JAI Press Inc. In press.
64. Marlatt GA, Gordon JR. Determinants of relapse: implications for the maintenance of behavioral change. In: Davidson P, Davidson S, eds. *Behavioral Medicine: Changing Health and Lifestyles.* New York, NY: Brunner/Mazel Inc; 1980.
65. Vaillant GE. Natural history of male psychological health VIII: antecedents of alcoholism and 'orality.' *Am J Psychiatry.* 1980;137:181-186.
66. Rosenblatt PC. *Farming Is in Our Blood: Farm Families in Economic Crisis.* Ames: Iowa State University Press; 1990.

CSF Biochemistries, Glucose Metabolism, and Diurnal Activity Rhythms in Alcoholic, Violent Offenders, Fire Setters, and Healthy Volunteers

Matti Virkkunen, MD; Robert Rawlings, MS; Riitta Tokola, MD; Russell E. Poland, PhD; Alessandro Guidotti, MD; Charles Nemeroff, MD, PhD; Garth Bissette, PhD; Konstantine Kalogeras, MD; Sirkka-Liisa Karonen, PhD; Markku Linnoila, MD, PhD

Background: There is an extensive literature describing a central serotonin deficit in alcoholic, impulsive, violent offenders and fire setters. In the present study, we investigated biochemical concomitants of impulsivity and aggressiveness, and the physiological consequences of reduced central serotonin turnover.

Methods: Forty-three impulsive and 15 nonimpulsive alcoholic offenders and 21 healthy volunteers were studied in the forensic psychiatry ward of a university psychiatric department. The subjects underwent lumbar punctures and oral glucose and aspartame challenges, and their diurnal activity rhythm was measured with physical activity monitors. Discriminant function analyses were used to investigate psychophysiological and biochemical concomitants of aggressive and impulsive behaviors.

Results: Alcoholic, impulsive offenders with antisocial personality disorder had low mean cerebrospinal fluid (CSF) 5-hydroxyindoleacetic acid (5-HIAA) and corticotropin levels and high mean CSF testosterone concentrations. Compared with healthy volunteers, they showed increased physical activity during the daytime. Alcoholic, impulsive offenders with intermittent explosive disorder had a low mean CSF 5-HIAA concentration and blood glucose nadir after an oral glucose challenge, and desynchronized diurnal activity rhythm. Healthy volunteers had mean CSF 5-HIAA concentrations that were intermediate between those of alcoholic, impulsive and nonimpulsive offenders. Alcoholic, nonimpulsive offenders had a significantly higher mean CSF 5-HIAA concentration than all the other groups, including healthy volunteers.

Conclusions: In the present sample, a low CSF 5-HIAA concentration was primarily associated with impulsivity and high CSF testosterone concentration, with aggressiveness or interpersonal violence.

(Arch Gen Psychiatry. 1994;51:20-27)

From the Departments of Psychiatry (Drs Virkkunen and Tokola) and Clinical Chemistry (Dr Karonen), University of Helsinki (Finland); Laboratory of Clinical Studies, Division of Intramural Clinical and Biological Research, NIAAA, Bethesda, Md (Mr Rawlings and Dr Linnoila); Division of Biological Psychiatry, Harbor–UCLA Medical Center, Torrance (Dr Poland); Fidia-Georgetown Neuroscience Institute, Washington, DC (Dr Guidotti); Department of Psychiatry, Emory University, Atlanta, Ga (Dr Nemeroff); Department of Psychiatry, Duke University Medical Center, Durham, NC (Dr Bissette); and Clinical Neuroendocrinology Branch, Intramural Research Program, NIMH, Bethesda (Dr Kalogeras).

A LOW concentration of 5-hydroxyindoleacetic acid (5-HIAA) in cerebrospinal fluid (CSF) has been associated with an increased risk of suicide attempts, unprovoked interpersonal violence, and early-onset alcoholism in men. These findings have been among the most replicated in modern biological psychiatry.[1]

In a series of studies, we observed that compared with Finnish alcoholic, nonimpulsive violent offenders and American healthy volunteers, Finnish alcoholic, impulsive violent offenders and fire setters have relatively low CSF 5-HIAA concentrations.[2,3] They also have low blood glucose nadirs during oral glucose tolerance tests and sleep irregularly in the forensic psychiatry ward.[4] Based on these observations, we have postulated that in alcoholic, impulsive violent offenders, deficient central serotonin turnover is conducive to disturbances of diurnal activity rhythm and glucose metabolism.[5] The neuroanatomical substrate whose dysfunction, secondary to reduced central serotonin turnover, could explain the constellation of our psychobiological findings is the suprachiasmatic nucleus. It receives a serotonergic input from the dorsal and median raphe nuclei[6] and functions as an endogenous circadian pacemaker[7] and also as a regulator of glucose metabolism.[8]

In follow-up and family history studies on offenders, we found a low CSF 5-HIAA concentration and propensity to low blood glucose concentrations to be predictive of recidi-

See Materials and Methods on next page

MATERIALS AND METHODS

SUBJECTS AND PROCEDURES

All subjects gave written informed consent and the study protocol was approved by the Department of Psychiatry and Helsinki University Central Hospital Institutional Review Boards in Finland. An ad hoc prisoner representative of the Helsinki University Central Hospital Review Board evaluated the protocol. In the United States, the protocol was approved by the National Institute of Mental Health Institutional Review Board and the Office for Protection from Research Risks.

Healthy volunteers were recruited through advertisements in the press. They were paid for their participation. Prospective subjects were asked to participate in a psychobiological study elucidating biochemical, behavioral, and genetic correlates of violent behavior under the influence of alcohol. The advertisement further defined that the volunteers had to be free of current or past drinking problems and mental disorders. After recruitment, the volunteers underwent a psychiatric interview and a physical examination and gave a venous blood sample to establish normal blood count, liver enzymes, and serum creatinine concentration. They were asked to follow a low monoamine and caffeine-free diet, not to use any alcohol or medicines for a week prior to admission, and to stay as inpatients in the research ward for 3 days and 3 nights. Only volunteers free of a lifetime and family history of major mental disorders, alcohol dependence, and substance abuse in their first-degree relatives were included in the sample.

On the first full day after a night on the ward, patients underwent a lumbar puncture between 8 and 9 AM. On the next 2 days they underwent double-blinded, random order, oral glucose or aspartame tests starting at 8 AM. Throughout their stay, the volunteers wore physical activity monitors on their left wrist.

Alcoholic, violent offenders and impulsive fire setters were ordered to undergo forensic psychiatric examinations by their trial judges. They spent an average of 1 month being drug-free and on the low monoamine diet in the research ward. The offenders were asked to volunteer and were explained the procedures by a physician not involved in the study. In addition to routine blood tests similar to those administered to the healthy volunteers, γ-glutamyltransferase levels in the 48 hours prior to the start of the study were measured to ascertain alcohol abstinence. The offenders wore the physical activity monitors on their left wrist continuously for 10 days and nights. Following lumbar punctures, they underwent double-blinded, random order, oral glucose and aspartame tests on two consecutive days.

PSYCHIATRIC DIAGNOSES, FAMILY HISTORY, AND CHARACTERISTICS OF THE CRIME

All subjects, including the volunteers, were administered the Schedule of Affective Disorders and Schizophrenia–Lifetime Version test,[14] a structured family history questionnaire,[11] and underwent a clinical interview by one of us (M.V.) to derive lifetime *DSM-III-R*[15] diagnoses and to elicit a family history of psychiatric and substance abuse disorders, alcoholism, and attempted or completed suicide. To maintain reasonable continuity with diagnostic practices in our previous studies, intermittent explosive disorder was diagnosed according to *DSM-III*[16] criteria, which, unlike *DSM-III-R*, permits diagnosis when the behavior is exhibited under the influence of alcohol. The psychiatrist knew the criminal history of the offenders by the time of the interview but was blind to the results of the biochemical and diurnal activity rhythm analyses.

As in our previous studies, the alcoholic offenders were divided in impulsive and nonimpulsive groups by the forensic research psychiatrist (M.V.) based on the characteristics of the index crime described in the police report. (A crime was termed *impulsive* when the victim was previously unknown to the offender, when no provocation or only verbal altercation preceded the attack, no premeditation could be documented, and no economic motivation such as robbery or burglary was evident. Impulsive fire setting excluded setting fires for insurance fraud. Nonimpulsive crimes were all clearly premeditated.)[2,3] The alcoholic, impulsive offender group was further subdivided into groups with antisocial personality or intermittent explosive disorder. This was done to examine whether these two clinically distinct disorders are psychobiologically different as well. Ten subjects in the alcoholic, impulsive offender group were fire setters.

BIOCHEMICAL VARIABLES

All biochemical variables were quantified by investigators who were blind to the clinical characteristics of the subjects.

Monoamine Metabolites

The CSF samples were obtained by a neurologist (R.T.) at 8 AM after bed rest for 1 night with only water permitted after 8 PM. The samples were collected into a large polypropylene tube on wet ice. After the first 12 mL had been drawn, the tube was capped, inverted, and the CSF sample was aliquoted into 1-mL tubes on dry ice. The samples were stored in a freezer at −80°C and shipped via air freight on dry ice from Helsinki to Bethesda, Md, where homovanillic acid (HVA), 5-HIAA, and MHPG concentrations were measured with a liquid chromatographic procedure using electrochemical detection.[17]

Neuropeptides and Hormones

Cerebrospinal fluid concentrations of DBI,[18] CRH,[19] AVP,[20] corticotropin,[21] and free testosterone[22] were measured with separate radioimmunoassays.

Oral Glucose and Aspartame Tolerance Test

At 8 AM, after a 12-hour overnight fast, the subjects consumed 1 g/kg of body weight (4 mL/kg) of glucose solution or an identical volume of an aspartame solution of indistinguishable sweetness (Leiras, Turku, Finland). Fifteen-milliliter blood samples were drawn from an antecubital vein into an

Continued on next page

aprotinin-containing test tube (12.5 mIU/mL, Antagosan Behringwerke, Marburg, Germany) before and 15, 30, 60, 90, 120, 180, 240 and 300 minutes after the administration of the liquid. For the first 2 hours of the test, the subjects rested in bed. Thereafter, they were allowed to move in the ward, but resting was encouraged. Blood glucose concentration was measured with an enzymatic assay.[3] Glucagon was quantified immediately after the samples were thawed with a double antibody separation radioimmunoassay (Diagnostic Products Corporation, Los Angeles, Calif). Insulin was quantified in antibody-coated test tubes (Coat-A-Count, Diagnostic Products Corporation). Between-assay variation for insulin was 4.6% at 215 pmol/L and for glucagon, 5.1% at 44.8 ng/L. All samples were assayed in duplicate. When results of duplicate determinations showed discrepancies of more than 5%, the samples were reanalyzed.

PHYSICAL ACTIVITY MONITORING

The activity monitors are small watch-size devices with a movement sensor, as well as clock and memory functions that permit continuous recording of activity for a period of 10 days.[23] The data were decoded and stored on an Apple Macintosh computer (Apple Computers, Cupertino, Calif).

DATA ANALYSES

All analyses were computed using the BMDP statistical package.[24] Parametric and nonparametric analyses of variance, correlation coefficients, and post hoc *t* tests were used for comparisons of individual means when appropriate. Bonferroni-correction was used for multiple comparisons within each analysis of variance. Two-tailed probabilities were applied except when clearly dimensional a priori hypotheses were tested as stated in the introduction. Because of the large number of correlational analyses, only results with a probability value of less than .01 were included. Preliminary analyses revealed no differences between the various groups in mean weight, height, or baseline glucose, insulin, and glucagon concentrations. Also age, weight, height, or season of collection did not contribute significantly to the variation of any of the psychobiological variables in the present sample. Therefore, these variables were not statistically adjusted in any of the analyses reported below. All results are expressed as means and SDs.

To directly examine biochemical concomitants of impulsiveness, a stepwise linear discriminant analysis was computed on the CSF biochemical variables for the alcoholic, impulsive-nonimpulsive offender grouping including the fire setters. A similar analysis was conducted on the alcoholic offender–healthy volunteer grouping after excluding the fire setters to investigate biochemical concomitants of aggressiveness or violent behavior. The prior probabilities used were .5 and .5, respectively, and the jackknife was used for estimation of error rates.

Oversampling of alcoholic offenders for the glucose and aspartame tolerance tests and the diurnal activity rhythm monitoring and technical difficulties with lumbar punctures and certain assays led to unequal sample sizes in various comparisons. The sample sizes are, therefore, included in all Figures and Tables.

vist violent criminality after release from prison.[9] Suicide attempts and completed suicides are primarily associated with low 5-HIAA and 3-methoxy-4-hydroxyphenylglycol (MHPG) concentrations in the CSF.[10] Moreover, alcoholic sons of alcoholic fathers, who have been convicted of violent crimes, have the lowest CSF 5-HIAA concentrations.[11] This latter finding suggests that there may exist a familial trait associated with early-onset alcohol abuse, impulsive and violent criminality, and low CSF 5-HIAA concentration. We have also observed that alcoholic, impulsive and nonimpulsive offenders have mean free testosterone concentrations in CSF that are similar,[12] but alcoholic, impulsive offenders have low urinary free cortisol outputs.[13]

In the present study, we attempt to differentiate biochemical concomitants of impulsivity vs aggressiveness or violent behavior. Thus, we investigated age- and sex-matched Finnish healthy volunteers as inpatients in the same psychiatry department as the alcoholic, violent offenders. Furthermore, we examined relationships between symptoms of the putative functional deficits of the suprachiasmatic nucleus and CSF 5-HIAA concentrations. The a priori hypotheses explored are as follows: (1) low CSF 5-HIAA concentration is associated with impulsivity of the index crime, a history of suicide attempts, a disturbance of diurnal activity rhythms, and abnormalities of glucose metabolism; (2) free testosterone concentration in CSF is correlated with aggressiveness or violent behavior rather than impulsiveness; (3) concentrations of the anxiety and adrenocortical stress response-associated neuropeptides, diazepam-binding inhibitor (DBI), corticotropin-releasing hormone (CRH), arginine vasopressin (AVP), and corticotropin in CSF are low in impulsive violent offenders.

RESULTS

DEMOGRAPHIC CHARACTERISTICS AND PSYCHIATRIC DIAGNOSES

Heights, weights, ages, and lifetime *DSM-III-R* diagnoses are indicated in **Table 1**.

BIOCHEMICAL VARIABLES

All γ-glutamyltransferase analyses yielded results that were within the normal range.

CSF Monoamine Metabolite Concentrations

Mean CSF 5-HIAA concentration was significantly lower among the alcoholic, impulsive than among the alcoholic, nonimpulsive offenders. The alcoholic, nonimpul-

Table 1. Demographic Characteristics and Lifetime Psychiatric Diagnoses Among Alcoholic Offenders and Healthy Volunteers

	Impulsive Offenders			
Characteristics	Antisocial Personality Disorder (n=23)	Intermittent Explosive Disorder (n=20)	Nonimpulsive Offenders (n=15)	Control Subjects (n=21)
Mean (±SD) height, cm	179.2±4.5	179.6±5.2	179.3±6.0	179.9±6.5
Mean (±SD) weight, kg	73.5±8.4	79.6±11.4	78.1±12.3	81.8±13.8
Mean (±SD) age, y	26.1±6.2	35.4±10.5	30.2±7.7	27.9±9.1
Conduct disorder	0	0	1	0
Borderline personality disorder	23	17	4	0
Dysthymia	7	8	6	0
Major depressive disorder	0	4	4	0
Passive-aggressive personality disorder	0	1	6	0
Schizoid personality disorder	0	1	1	0
Narcissistic personality disorder	1	1	0	0
Dependent personality disorder	0	1	4	0

Table 2. Mean 24-Hour Physical Activity Monitor Counts*

Area Under the Curve										
ASP	IED	NI	HV	ANOVA	ASP-IED	ASP-NI	ASP-HV	IED-NI	IED-HV	NI-HV
129.6	120.4	103.8	75.3	...	...	...	...	...	...	...
45.6	66.3	54.9	41.7	.0181	...	...	...†	...	...	...
21	16	15	16	...	...	...	...	...	...	...

**ASP indicates antisocial personality disorder; IED, intermittent explosive disorder; NI, nonimpulsive offenders; HV, healthy volunteers; and ANOVA, analysis of variance.*

†*P*<.005 *with the Bonferroni corrected two-tailed test.*

sive offenders had significantly higher mean CSF 5-HIAA concentrations than did the healthy volunteers. Among the alcoholic, impulsive offenders, subjects with antisocial personality and intermittent explosive disorder had similar mean CSF 5-HIAA concentrations (**Figure 1**). Of the alcoholic, violent offenders, 25 had made a suicide attempt. Their mean CSF 5-HIAA concentration was lower than that of the nonattempting offenders (58.8±25.2 vs 68.5±24.7 nmol/L; $P<.05$, one-tailed probability).

In the discriminant analysis on the impulsive-nonimpulsive grouping of the alcoholic offenders, the only variable selected with an overall correct jackknife classification rate of 78% was CSF 5-HIAA concentration. Mean CSF HVA and MHPG concentrations did not differ between any of the groups in the post hoc comparisons, even though analysis of variance showed a significant overall difference at the $P<.05$ level for HVA (**Figure 2**).

CSF Free Testosterone Concentration

Alcoholic, impulsive offenders with antisocial personality disorder had higher mean CSF testosterone concentrations than did healthy volunteers (**Figure 3**). In the discriminant analysis on the alcoholic, violent offenders–healthy volunteers grouping, the first variable entered was free testosterone concentration in CSF followed by 5-HIAA and MHPG concentrations in CSF. The overall correct jackknife classification based on CSF free testosterone concentration was 60%. This was improved to 64% by adding the effects of the CSF 5-HIAA and MHPG concentrations.

CSF Peptide Concentrations

Mean CSF corticotropin concentration was significantly lower among alcoholic, impulsive offenders with antisocial personality disorder than among healthy volunteers (**Figure 4**). Among the alcoholic offenders, suicide attempters had significantly lower mean CSF corticotropin concentrations than did nonattempters (5±1 pmol/L [n=22] vs 6±2 pmol/L [n=38]; $P<.008$). There were no significant differences among any of the groups in mean DBI, CRH, and AVP concentrations in CSF (data on file).

Correlational Analyses

Cerebrospinal fluid concentration of 5-HIAA correlated positively with CSF HVA concentration (r=.68; n=67; $P<.01$). Testosterone levels in CSF correlated negatively with AVP concentration in CSF (r=−.45; n=37; $P<.01$), and CSF corticotropin concentration correlated positively with that of AVP (r=.46; n=38; $P<.01$).

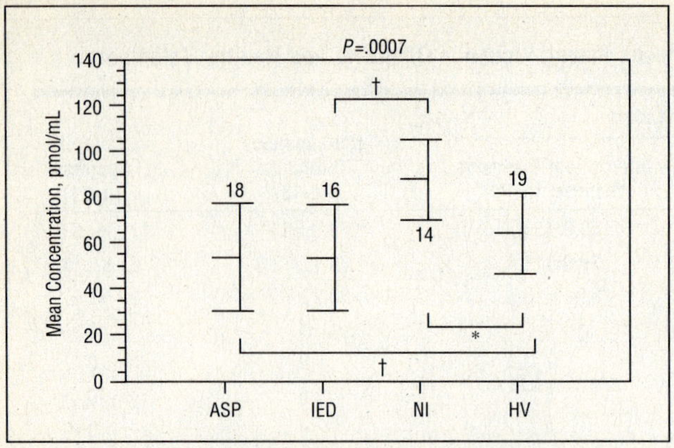

Figure 1. *Mean cerebrospinal fluid 5-hydroxyindoleacetic acid concentrations. ASP indicates antisocial personality disorder; IED, intermittent explosive disorder; NI, nonimpulsive offenders; HV, healthy volunteers; asterisk,* P<.05*; and dagger,* P<.01.

Oral Glucose and Aspartame Tolerance Tests

Alcoholic, impulsive offenders with intermittent explosive disorder had significantly lower mean blood glucose nadir during the glucose tolerance test than did healthy volunteers (**Figure 5**). Plasma insulin and glucagon concentrations did not differ significantly between the groups at any point during the oral glucose tolerance test (data on file). There were no significant differences between groups in any of the biochemical variables at any point during the aspartame tolerance test.

PHYSICAL ACTIVITY MONITORING

Alcoholic, impulsive offenders with antisocial personality disorder had significantly higher mean total 10 day-night activity counts than did healthy volunteers. Alcoholic, impulsive offenders with intermittent explosive disorder had indistinguishable day and night activity counts in a striking difference from the other groups (**Figure 6**).

COMMENT

PSYCHIATRIC DIAGNOSES AND CLASSIFICATION OF THE CRIMES

The main apparent difference between our earlier studies and the current one is that all except two of the alcoholic offenders met the criteria for *DSM-III-R* diagnosis of alcohol dependence rather than alcohol abuse. This is because the *DSM-III-R* criteria for alcohol dependence include a number of subjects who were previously defined as abusers according to *DSM-III* classification.[25] To avoid bias, the psychiatrist was blind to the results of all biochemical, physiological, and psychological tests at the time of making the diagnoses. The main weakness of the present design was that the diagnoses were made by the forensic research psychiatrist (M.V.) who was familiar with the crimes and the backgrounds of the alcoholic offenders and aware of who

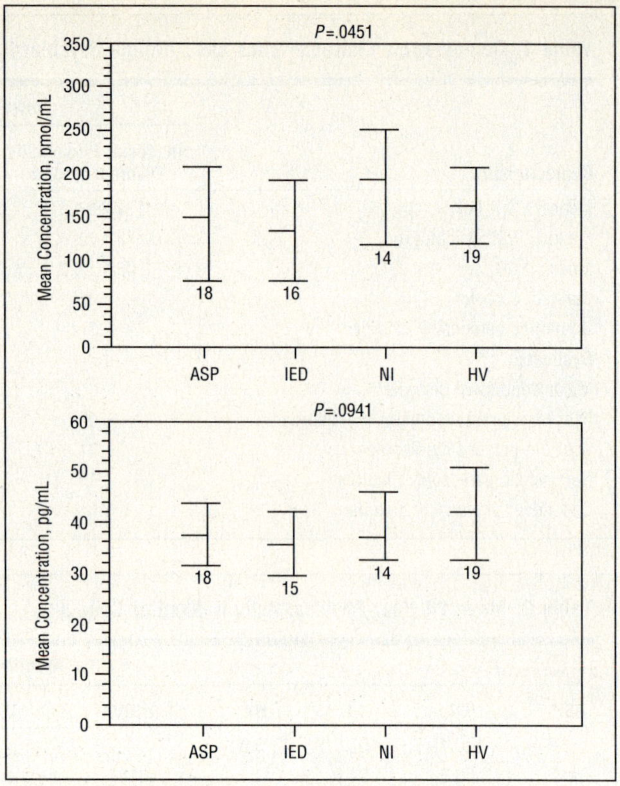

Figure 2. *Mean cerebrospinal fluid homovanillic acid (top) and 3-methoxy-4-hydroxyphenylglycol (bottom) concentrations. ASP indicates antisocial personality disorder; IED, intermittent explosive disorder; NI, nonimpulsive offenders; and HV, healthy volunteers.*

was an offender and who a healthy volunteer. To partially remedy the situation, the Schedule of Affective Disorder and Schizophrenia interview[14] was used as a source of structured information to bolster the reliability of the diagnostic data.

DIURNAL ACTIVITY RHYTHMS

The present results demonstrate that alcoholic, impulsive violent offenders with intermittent explosive disorder exhibit a profound diurnal activity rhythm disturbance. In rodents, intact serotonergic input to the suprachiasmatic nucleus facilitates entrainment of the circadian activity rhythm by light.[26] If the same principle holds for humans, the disturbed diurnal activity rhythm observed in these offenders may also be secondary to deficient central serotonergic neurotransmission. On the other hand, roughly one half of alcoholic, impulsive offenders with antisocial personality disorder exhibited a clear activity difference between the day and night times despite an equally low mean CSF 5-HIAA concentration. Compared with healthy volunteers, however, they showed increased mean total 24-hour activity counts throughout the monitoring period. This finding is commensurate with the history of attention deficit disorder and hyperactivity in many of the alcoholic offenders with antisocial personality disorder,[4] since this disorder has been reported to be associated with increased diurnal physical activity.[27]

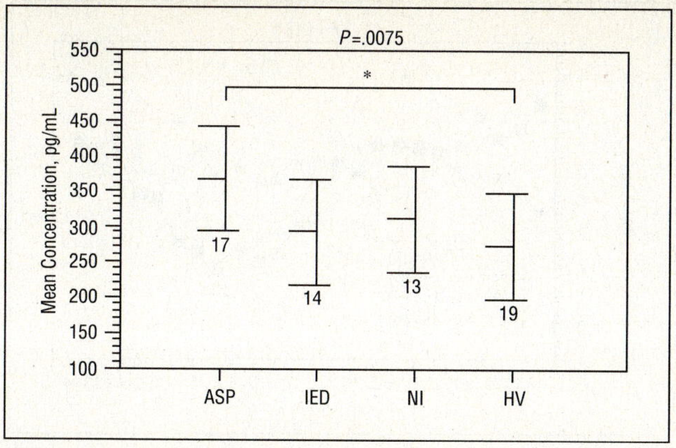

Figure 3. *Mean cerebrospinal fluid testosterone concentrations. ASP indicates antisocial personality disorder; IED, intermittent explosive disorder; NI, nonimpulsive offenders; HV, healthy volunteers; and asterisk,* $P<.01$.

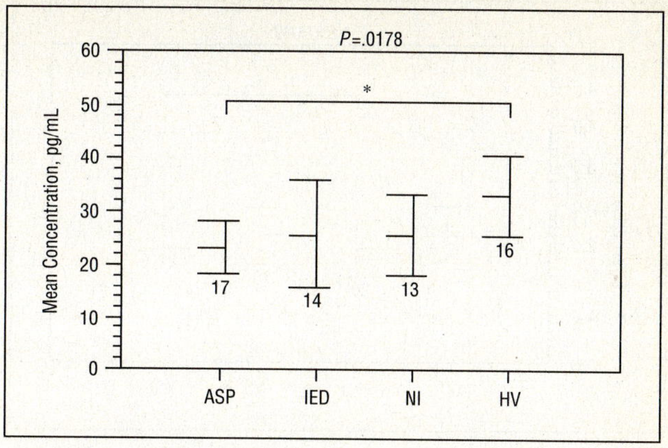

Figure 4. *Mean cerebrospinal fluid corticotropin concentrations. ASP indicates antisocial personality disorder; IED, intermittent explosive disorder; NI, nonimpulsive offenders; HV, healthy volunteers; and asterisk,* $P<.05$.

GLUCOSE METABOLISM

In accordance with the previous findings of Virkkunen,[28] mean blood glucose nadir was significantly lower in the alcoholic, impulsive violent offenders with intermittent explosive disorder than in the healthy volunteers. There was, however, no difference between the alcoholic impulsive and nonimpulsive offenders on this variable. Thus, the low blood glucose nadir was not correlated to CSF 5-HIAA concentration across the different groups of offenders. The difference between the intermittent explosive offenders and healthy volunteers could be either secondary to alcohol dependence or due to differences in time during which the two groups were on the low monoamine diet prior to the glucose challenge. No differences between the groups were found in glucagon and insulin concentrations at any point during the oral glucose tolerance test. The appropriate investigation of glucose metabolism in these subjects requires further study using the technique of euglycemic insulin clamp.

CSF 5-HIAA CONCENTRATION

Compared with previous results using American healthy volunteers,[3] the Finnish healthy volunteers with no family history of alcoholism or major depression in their first-degree relatives had relatively low CSF 5-HIAA concentrations. This may be partially owing to the inability to admit Finnish volunteers between early May and early September and the fact that the American healthy volunteers, who were primarily college students, were studied during their summer vacations between June and September when the CSF 5-HIAA concentration reaches its seasonal peak.[29] Thus, the CSF 5-HIAA concentrations among the American healthy volunteers probably represent an overestimate and those among the Finnish healthy volunteers an underestimate of the real mean value. Sampling of additional volunteers during all four seasons is needed to permit a truly adequate comparison between volunteers and violent offenders. In our previous studies, alcoholics, different from healthy volunteers, showed a lack of seasonal variation in CSF 5-HIAA and HVA concentrations.[30] In accordance with this observation, we again did not find any seasonal variation in CSF monoamine metabolite concentrations in the alcoholic offenders despite adequate sampling during all four seasons. The present results replicate our earlier observation[2] of a low mean CSF 5-HIAA concentration in alcoholic offenders with a history of a suicide attempt compared with alcoholic offenders without such a history.

In animal and human studies, indexes of reduced central serotonin turnover have been associated with the inability to tolerate delay and impaired impulse control.[31] A postmortem human study found that 5-HIAA concentration in the prefrontal cortex, but not in other brain regions, correlated positively with 5-HIAA concentration in CSF.[32] This apparent anatomic-neurochemical relationship is intriguing, because of the postulated role of the prefrontal cortex in impulse control.[33] Direct behavioral observation in concert with functional brain imaging and CSF studies will be necessary to support or refute the hypothesized relationships between reduced frontal serotonin turnover, low CSF 5-HIAA concentration, and impaired impulse control in humans.

CSF HVA AND MHPG CONCENTRATIONS

Differences in the mean CSF HVA concentrations between the groups had a similar profile but were relatively smaller than differences in mean CSF 5-HIAA concentrations. As expected, CSF 5-HIAA and HVA concentrations were highly correlated with each other. As we proposed previously,[34] and as supported by the results of the discriminant analysis, the small differences between the groups in mean CSF HVA concentrations are probably secondary to the differences in mean CSF 5-HIAA concentrations. Consequently, frontal dopamine turnover as partially reflected by CSF HVA concentration[34-36] may be less important for impulse control than frontal serotonin turnover.

Of the CSF monoamine metabolites, MHPG showed the lowest correlations with behavioral measures used in the present study. In general, we have been unable to consistently relate static measures of noradrenergic functions to

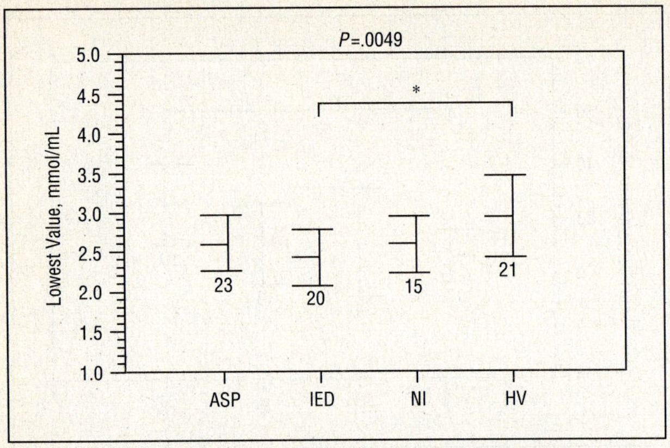

Figure 5. *Blood glucose nadir using the glucose tolerance test during the first 5 hours following an oral (1 g/kg of body weight) glucose challenge. ASP indicates antisocial personality disorder; IED, intermittent explosive disorder; NI, nonimpulsive offenders; HV, healthy volunteers; and asterisk,* P<.01.

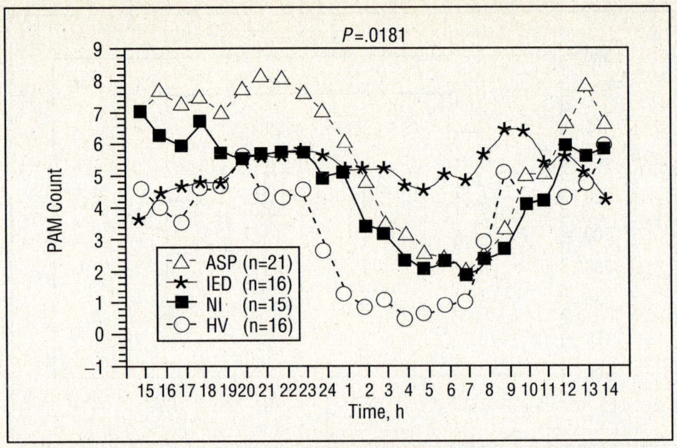

Figure 6. *Mean hourly physical activity monitoring (PAM) counts. ASP indicates antisocial personality disorder; IED, intermittent explosive disorder; NI, nonimpulsive offenders; and HV, healthy volunteers.*

trait measures of impulsivity and aggressiveness,[37] even though we earlier found an association between a history of attempted suicide and low CSF MHPG concentration in Finnish offenders.[10] Recent studies on rhesus monkeys in the wild and neuroendocrine studies in humans have found, however, that increased noradrenergic reactivity may be associated with state measures of aggressiveness and irritability.[38,39]

CSF FREE TESTOSTERONE CONCENTRATION

Mean CSF free testosterone concentration was higher in alcoholic, impulsive offenders with antisocial personality disorder than in healthy volunteers. The high CSF testosterone concentrations could be the result of a lack of inhibition of luteinizing hormone–releasing hormone and luteinizing hormone outputs by circulating cortisol.[40] Thus, the earlier report of low urinary free cortisol outputs in alcoholic, impulsive violent offenders[14] could explain the high CSF testosterone concentrations observed in the current similar group of subjects. In support of this reasoning, Mason et al[41] reported a negative correlation between repeatedly measured plasma testosterone concentrations and urinary free cortisol output in depressed and schizophrenic men.

The literature concerning testosterone levels and human aggressiveness was comprehensively reviewed.[42] According to this review, despite a host of apparently conflicting reports, the following findings are relatively strong: (1) plasma free or saliva testosterone correlates better with aggressiveness than plasma total testosterone concentration; (2) a repetitive pattern of aggressive behaviors that starts early in life is often associated with elevated testosterone concentrations; (3) a pattern of repetitive aggressiveness under the influence of alcohol is associated with elevated testosterone concentrations.

We elected to quantify CSF free testosterone concentrations because this pool of the hormone is directly available to the central nervous system neurons and relatively free of the fluctuations characteristic of plasma testosterone concentration that are due to the pulsatile pattern of excretion of the hormone. Our findings are in general agreement with conclusions based on the above-mentioned review on testosterone and human aggression. Moreover, the results of the discriminant analyses support the notion that the rate of central serotonin turnover is positively correlated with impulse control, and central availability of testosterone with outward directed aggressiveness.[43,44]

CSF DBI, CRH, AVP, AND CORTICOTROPIN CONCENTRATIONS

Alcoholic offenders with antisocial personality disorder had CSF DBI, CRH, and AVP concentrations similar to those in the healthy volunteers but relatively low CSF corticotropin concentrations. At the level of the pituitary, CRH and AVP act synergistically to facilitate the release of corticotropin.[45] Earlier studies showing strong positive correlations in normal volunteers between CSF concentrations of CRH and corticotropin[21,46] and between those of AVP and corticotropin,[46] the latter also replicated in the present sample, support the notion that such a relationship may also exist in the brain.

A large number of animal studies on corticotropin and learning have found that this neuropeptide facilitates consolidation of memory.[47] We speculate that the low mean CSF corticotropin concentration in the alcoholic offenders with antisocial personality disorder may be concordant with the often stated clinical observation that such patients exhibit difficulties with learning from experience. On the other hand, the meaning of the low mean CSF corticotropin concentration among alcoholic offenders who had attempted suicide remains obscure.

In conclusion, among alcoholic, violent offenders and fire setters, low CSF 5-HIAA concentration seems to be associated with impaired impulse control. Alcoholic offenders with intermittent explosive disorder had low blood glucose nadirs after an oral glucose administration and striking diurnal activity rhythm dysregulation. Alcoholic offenders with antisocial personality disorder had high CSF free testosterone and low corticotropin concentrations and showed increased diurnal physical activity. Concentration of free testosterone in CSF may be associated with outward directed aggressiveness, and that of corticotropin may be associated with learning from experience. Interrelationships between serotonin and glucose metabolism dysregulation need further study to elucidate the basic physiologic mechanisms involved.

Accepted for publication August 4, 1993.

This study was supported in part by Research Scientist Development Award MH 00534 from the National Institute of Mental Health, Bethesda, Md (Dr Poland).

We are grateful to Michael Eckardt, PhD, David Goldman, MD, David Pickar, MD, and William Z. Potter, MD, PhD, for their constructive criticism of the article.

Reprint requests to National Institute on Alcohol Abuse and Alcoholism, Bldg 10, Room 3C103, Bethesda, MD 20892 (Dr Linnoila).

REFERENCES

1. Roy A, Virkkunen M, Linnoila M. Serotonin in suicide, violence, and alcoholism. In: Coccaro E, Murphy D, eds. *Serotonin in Major Psychiatric Disorders.* Washington, DC: American Psychiatric Association; 1991:187-208.
2. Linnoila M, Virkkunen M, Scheinin M, Nuutila A, Rimon R, Goodwin FK. Low cerebrospinal fluid 5-hydroxyindoleacetic acid concentration differentiates impulsive from nonimpulsive violent behavior. *Life Sci.* 1983;33:2609-2614.
3. Virkkunen M, Nuutila A, Goodwin FK, Linnoila M. Cerebrospinal fluid monoamine metabolites in male arsonists. *Arch Gen Psychiatry.* 1987;44:241-247.
4. Roy A, Virkkunen M, Guthrie S, Linnoila M. Indices of serotonin and glucose metabolism in violent offenders, arsonists and alcoholics. In: Mann JJ, Stanley M, eds. *Psychobiology of Suicidal Behavior.* New York, NY: New York Academy of Science; 1986:202-220.
5. Linnoila M, Virkkunen M, Roy A. Biochemical aspects of aggression in man. In: Bunney WE Jr, Costa E, Potkin SG, eds. *Clinical Neuropharmacology.* New York, NY: Raven Press; 1986;(suppl 1):377-379.
6. Palkovits M, Saavedra JM, Jacobovits DM, Kizer JS, Zaborsky L, Brownstein MJ. Serotonergic innervation of the forebrain: effects of lesions on serotonin and tryptophan hydroxylase levels. *Brain Res.* 1977;130:121-134.
7. Moore RY, Eichler VB. Loss of a circadian adrenal corticosterone rhythm following suprachiasmatic lesions in the rat. *Brain Res.* 1972;42:201-206.
8. Yamamoto H, Nagai K, Nagakava H. Additional evidence that the suprachiasmatic nucleus is the center for regulation of insulin secretion and glucose homeostasis. *Brain Res.* 1984;304:237-241.
9. Virkkunen M, DeJong J, Bartko J, Goodwin FK, Linnoila M. Relationship of psychobiological variables to recidivism in violent offenders and impulsive fire setters: a follow-up study. *Arch Gen Psychiatry.* 1989;46:600-603.
10. Virkkunen M, DeJong J, Bartko J, Linnoila M. Psychobiological concomitants of history of suicide attempts among violent offenders and impulsive fire setters. *Arch Gen Psychiatry.* 1989;46:604-606.
11. Linnoila M, DeJong J, Virkkunen M. Family history of alcoholism in violent offenders and impulsive fire setters. *Arch Gen Psychiatry.* 1989;46:679-681.
12. Roy A, Virkkunen M, Guthrie S, Poland R, Linnoila M. Monoamines, glucose metabolism, suicidal and aggressive behaviors. *Psychopharmacol Bull.* 1986; 22:661-665.
13. Virkkunen M. Urinary free cortisol secretion in habitually violent offenders. *Acta Psychiatr Scand.* 1985;72:40-44.
14. Spitzer R, Endicott J. *Schedule of Affective Disorders and Schizophrenia—Lifetime Version.* Third Edition. New York, NY: New York State Psychiatric Institute; 1978.
15. American Psychiatric Association, Committee on Nomenclature and Statistics. *Diagnostic and Statistical Manual of Mental Disorders, Revised Third Edition.* Washington, DC: American Psychiatric Association; 1987.
16. American Psychiatric Association, Committee on Nomenclature and Statistics. *Diagnostic and Statistical Manual of Mental Disorders, Third Edition.* Washington, DC: American Psychiatric Association; 1980.
17. Scheinin M, Chang W-H, Kirk K, Linnoila M. Simultaneous determination of 3-methoxy-4-hydroxyphenylglycol, 5-hydroxyindoleacetic acid, and homovanillic acid in cerebrospinal fluid with high performance liquid chromatography using electrochemical detection. *Anal Biochem.* 1983;131:246-253.
18. Barbaccia M, Costa E, Ferrero P, Guidotti A, Roy A, Sunderland T, Pickar D, Paul S, Goodwin FK. Diazepam binding inhibitor: a brain neuropeptide present in human spinal fluid: studies in depression, schizophrenia and Alzheimer's disease. *Arch Gen Psychiatry.* 1986;43:1143-1147.
19. Smith MA, Bissette G, Slotkin TA, Kwight DL, Nemeroff CB. Release of corticotropin releasing factor from rat brain regions in vitro. *Endocrinology.* 1986;118:1997-2001.
20. Altemus M, Pigott T, Kalogeras KT, Demitrack M, Dubbert B, Murphy DL, Gold PW. Abnormalities in the regulation of vasopressin and corticotropin releasing factor secretion in obsessive compulsive disorder. *Arch Gen Psychiatry.* 1992;49:9-20.
21. Kling MA, Roy A, Doran AR, Calabrese JR, Rubinow DR, Whitfield HJ Jr, May C, Post RM, Chrousos GP, Gold PW. Cerebrospinal fluid immunoreactive corticotropin-releasing hormone and adrenocorticotropin secretion in Cushing's disease and major depression: potential clinical implications. *J Clin Endocrinol Metab.* 1991;72:260-271.
22. Rahe RH, Karson S, Howard NS Jr, Rubin RT, Poland RE. Psychological and physiological assessments on American Hostages freed from captivity in Iran. *Psychosom Med.* 1990;52:1-16.
23. Wehr TA, Wirz-Justice A, Goodwin FK, Breitmeir J, Craig C. 48 hour sleep-wake cycles in manic-depressive illness: naturalistic observations and sleep deprivation experiments. *Arch Gen Psychiatry.* 1982;39:559-565.
24. *BMDP Statistical Software Manual.* Los Angeles: University of California Press; 1990.
25. Cotter LB, Helzer JE, Mager D, Spitznagel EM, Compton WM. Agreement between *DSM-III* and *-III-R* substance use disorders. *Drug Alcohol Depend.* 1991;29:17-25.
26. Morin LP, Blanchard J. Depletion of brain serotonin by 5, 7-DHT modifies hamster circadian rhythm response to light. *Brain Res.* 1991;566:173-185.
27. Porrino LJ, Rapoport JL, Behar D, Sceery W, Ismond DR, Bunney WE Jr. A naturalistic assessment of motor activity of hyperactive boys. *Arch Gen Psychiatry.* 1983;40:681-687.
28. Virkkunen M. Reactive hypoglycemic tendency among habitually violent offenders. *Nutr Rev.* 1986;44(suppl):94-103.
29. Brewerton RD, Berrettini WH, Nurnberger JI, Linnoila M. Analysis of seasonal fluctuations of CSF monoamine metabolites and neuropeptides in normal controls: findings with 5-HIAA and HVA. *Psychiatry Res.* 1988;23:257-265.
30. Roy A, Adinoff B, Linnoila M. Cerebrospinal fluid variables among alcoholics lack seasonal variation. *Acta Psychiatr Scand.* 1991;24:187-194.
31. Soubrie P. Reconciling the role of central serotonin neurons in human and animal behavior. *Behav Brain Sci.* 1986;9:319-364.
32. Stanley M, Traskman-Benz L, Dorovini-Zis K. Correlations between aminergic metabolites simultaneously obtained from human CSF and brain. *Life Sci.* 1985; 37:1279-1286.
33. Miller LA. Impulsivity, risk-taking, and the ability to synthesize fragmented information after frontal lobectomy. *Neuropsychologia.* 1992;30:69-79.
34. Agren H, Mefford IN, Rudorfer MV, Linnoila M, Potter WZ. Interacting neurotransmitter systems: a non-experimental approach to the 5-HIAA–HVA correlation in human CSF. *Psychiatry Res.* 1986;20:175-193.
35. Ellsworth JD, Leahy DJ, Roth RH Jr, Redmond D Jr. Homovanillic acid concentration in brain, CSF and plasma as indicators of central dopamine function in primates. *J Neural Transm.* 1987;68:51-62.
36. Weinberger D, Berman KF, Illowsky BP. Physiological dysfunction of dorsolateral prefrontal cortex in schizophrenia. *Arch Gen Psychiatry.* 1988;45:609-615.
37. Roy A, Pickar D, DeJong J, Karoum F, Linnoila M. Suicidal behavior in depression: relationship to noradrenergic function. *Biol Psychiatry.* 1989;25:341-350.
38. Higley JD, Mehlman PT, Taub DM, Higley SB, Suomi SJ, Vickers D, Linnoila M. Cerebrospinal fluid monoamine and adrenal correlates of aggression in free-ranging rhesus monkeys. *Arch Gen Psychiatry.* 1992;49:436-441.
39. Coccaro EF, Lawrence T, Trestman R, Gabriel S, Klar HM, Siever LJ. Growth hormone responses to intravenous clonidine challenge correlate with behavior irritability in psychiatric patients and healthy volunteers. *Psychiatry Res.* 1991;39:129-139.
40. Steiger A, von Bardeleben V, Wiedeman K, Holsboer F. Sleep EEG and nocturnal secretion of testosterone and cortisol in patients with major endogenous depression during acute phase and after remission. *J Psychiatr Res.* 1991;25:169-177.
41. Mason JW, Giller EL, Kosten TR. Serum testosterone differences between patients with schizophrenia and those with affective disorder. *Biol Psychiatry.* 1988;23:357-366.
42. Archer J. The influence of testosterone on human aggression. *Br J Psychol.* 1991;82:1-28.
43. Ehrenkranz J, Bliss E, Sheard MH. Plasma testosterone: correlation with aggressive behavior and social dominance in man. *Psychosom Med.* 1976;36:469-475.
44. Dabbs JM Jr, Frady RL, Carr TS, Besh NF. Saliva testosterone and criminal violence in young adult prison inmates. *Psychosom Med.* 1987;49:174-182.
45. Sapolsky RM, Plotsky PM. Hypercortisolism and its possible neural bases. *Biol Psychiatry.* 1990;27:937-952.
46. Berrettini WH, Nurnberger JI Jr, Zerbe RL, Gold PW, Chrousos GP, Tomai T. CSF neuropeptides in euthymic bipolar patients and controls. *Br J Psychiatry.* 1987;150:208-212.
47. De Wied D, Jolles J. Neuropeptides derived from proopiocortin: behavioral, physiological and neurochemical effects. *Physiol Rev.* 1982;62:976-1059.

ORIGINAL ARTICLE

Personality Profiles and State Aggressiveness in Finnish Alcoholic, Violent Offenders, Fire Setters, and Healthy Volunteers

Matti Virkkunen, MD; Eila Kallio, PhD; Robert Rawlings, MS; Riitta Tokola, MD; Russell E. Poland, PhD; Alessandro Guidotti, MD; Charles Nemeroff, MD, PhD; Garth Bissette, PhD; Konstantine Kalogeras, MD; Sirkka-Liisa Karonen, PhD; Markku Linnoila, MD, PhD

Background: Based on clinical observations in a series of studies on Finnish alcoholic, violent offenders, we asserted that the impulsive offenders represented an extreme group of type 2 alcoholics. We also observed that these subjects were vulnerable to hypoglycemia after the administration of oral glucose load. Furthermore, we believe that while being hypoglycemic, the impulsive offenders are particularly irritable and aggressive. In the present study, we addressed these issues by studying psychological trait and state variables in a new group of violent offenders and fire setters, and age- and sex-matched healthy volunteers.

Methods: Fifty-eight alcoholic, violent offenders and impulsive fire setters and 21 healthy volunteers were administered the Karolinska scales of personality and the Rosenzweig picture frustration test after an oral aspartame and glucose challenge.

Results: The psychological test results and the criminal histories of the offenders, together with biochemical measurements, suggest that a low 5-hydroxyindoleacetic acid concentration in cerebrospinal fluid in the alcoholic offenders is associated with irritability and impaired impulse control, and a high free testosterone concentration in cerebrospinal fluid is associated with increased aggressiveness, monotony avoidance, sensation seeking, suspiciousness, and reduced socialization.

Conclusion: Finnish alcoholic, impulsive offenders have personality profiles characteristic of Scandinavian early-onset male alcoholics with antisocial traits, who have been also referred to as type 2 alcoholics.

(Arch Gen Psychiatry. 1994;51:28-33)

From the Departments of Psychiatry (Drs Virkkunen, Kallio, and Tokola) and Clinical Chemistry (Dr Karonen), University of Helsinki (Finland); Laboratory of Clinical Studies, Division of Intramural Clinical and Biological Research, National Institute on Alcohol Abuse and Alcoholism, Bethesda, Md (Mr Rawlings and Dr Linnoila); Division of Biological Psychiatry, Department of Psychiatry, Harbor–UCLA Medical Center, Torrance, Calif (Dr Poland); Fidia-Georgetown Neuroscience Institute, Washington, DC (Dr Guidotti); Department of Psychiatry, Emory University, Atlanta, Ga (Dr Nemeroff); Department of Psychiatry, Duke University Medical Center, Durham, NC (Dr Bissette); and Clinical Neuroendocrinology Branch, Intramural Research Program, National Institute of Mental Health, Bethesda (Dr Kalogeras).

TO STUDY psychobiological concomitants of disorders of impulse control, we investigated a total of 101 alcoholic, violent offenders, 33 fire setters and 27 healthy volunteers during the past 12 years. We observed that among alcoholic criminal offenders, impulsive violent behavior and fire setting are associated with low concentrations of the main serotonin metabolite 5-hydroxyindoleacetic acid (5-HIAA) in the cerebrospinal fluid (CSF).[1-3] Equally violent alcoholic offenders who premeditate on their crimes have normal to high CSF 5-HIAA concentrations.[1,3] Compared with healthy volunteers, all alcoholic violent offenders had relatively high CSF free testosterone concentrations and low blood glucose nadirs after an oral glucose administration.[3] Furthermore, alcoholic, impulsive offenders with antisocial personality disorder had low CSF corticotropin concentrations combined with low CSF 5-HIAA and testosterone concentrations.[3]

In our studies, the distinction between impulsive and nonimpulsive criminality is based on the police reports. This categorization, even though it yields highly reproducible results[1-3] is decided by the forensic research psychiatrist (M.V.), who also makes the psychiatric diagnoses according to *DSM-III* and *DSM-III-R* criteria.[3] The information concerning the criminal histories of the offenders may unduly influence the diagnoses made by the psychiatrist. Therefore, we wanted to investigate, and if necessary partially remedy,

See Materials and Methods on next page

MATERIALS AND METHODS

Subjects, procedures, and diagnostic and family history workups and biochemical analyses are detailed elsewhere.[3]

PSYCHOLOGICAL TESTING

All tests were scored without knowledge of the subjects' diagnoses, conditions, or results of the biochemical analyses. The Wechsler Adult Intelligence Scale[13] and the Minnesota Multiphasic Personality Inventory[14] were administered to all offenders as an integral part of the forensic psychiatric examination. Due to time constraints, the Wechsler Adult Intelligence Scale and Minnesota Multiphasic Personality Inventory were not administered to the healthy volunteers.

Karolinska Scales of Personality

The KSP has 135 questions grouped in 15 scales measuring psychic anxiety, somatic anxiety, muscular tension, psychasthenia, inhibition of aggression, detachment, impulsiveness, monotony avoidance, socialization, indirect aggression, verbal aggression, irritability, suspicion, guilt, and social desirability. The scales have been normalized for the Swedish population, and they are thought to measure relatively stable personality traits. The scales have been statistically grouped into three factors. Factor 1 contains scales quantifying impulsivity, psychopathy, sensation seeking, and socialization; factor 2 comprises scales related to aspects of anxiety; factor 3 is derived from the Buss-Durkee hostility inventory and measures aggressiveness.[15]

Rosenzweig Picture Frustration Test

This is a structured projective procedure that gauges responses to 24 cartoon pictures depicting conflict situations in everyday life.[11] There is a blank caption box above the person on the right in each picture. The subject is instructed to imagine himself as this person and asked to write the first thought elicited by the picture in the box. Direction of aggression and reaction type bias scores are assigned to each response. Direction of aggression is scored as extrapunitiveness (directed to the environment); intropunitiveness (directed to oneself); and impunitiveness (aggression avoided). Type of reaction is scored as obstacle dominance (frustration), ego defense (dominated by the ego of the subject), and need-persistence (solving the problem).

DATA ANALYSES

All analyses were computed using the BMDP statistical package.[16] Parametric and nonparametric analyses of variance, correlation coefficients, and post hoc *t* tests for comparisons of individual means were computed when appropriate. Bonferroni's correction was used for multiple comparisons. Two-tailed probabilities were applied throughout. Preliminary analyses revealed no differences among the various groups in mean weight, height, or baseline glucose, insulin, and glucagon concentrations. Also age, weight, height, or season did not contribute significantly to the variation of any of the psychobiological variables in the present sample. Therefore, these variables were not statistically adjusted in any of the analyses reported below.

this potential weakness in our studies. For this purpose, we chose the Karolinska scales of personality (KSP), a personality inventory based on constructs derived from theories of biological bases of temperament dimensions underlying certain psychiatric disorders.[4] The KSP has been standardized and extensively used in Scandinavian countries in studies on depression,[5] personality disorders,[6] alcoholism,[7] and chronic pain.[8] Thus the KSP affords the opportunity to compare the personality profiles of our subjects with those of independently diagnosed patient groups with similar psychiatric diagnoses. Moreover, the biochemical measurements enable us to test the theoretical assumptions concerning biological bases of dimensions of personality used in constructing the KSP.[4]

In a review article on serotonin and impulse control,[9] we pointed out that similar to a low CSF 5-HIAA concentration, many of the alcoholic impulsive offenders also have low blood glucose nadirs after an oral glucose administration. Moreover, we had postulated, as a part of our proposed model to explain psychobiological concomitants of impulsivity,[10] that it is during such episodes of low blood glucose levels caused by inebriation that these alcoholic impulsive offenders are most likely to exhibit unprovoked, interpersonally violent behavior or set fires impulsively. To test this hypothesis, we chose the Rosenzweig[11] picture frustration test to measure impulsive aggressiveness after an oral glucose administration. The choice was influenced by a report describing a strong negative correlation between the outward-directed aggression score on the Rosenzweig test and blood glucose nadir in healthy volunteers after an oral administration of glucose.[12]

RESULTS

DEMOGRAPHIC CHARACTERISTICS AND PSYCHIATRIC DIAGNOSES

Ages, heights, weights, *DSM-III-R*[17] and *DSM-III*[18] diagnoses, IQs, and characteristics of the index crime are indicated in Tables 1 and 2 of the accompanying article.[3]

Mean Scores on the Karolinska Scales of Personality (KSP) and Minnesota Multiphasic Personality Inventory (MMPI)*

	Mean (±SD) Score										
Scale	ASP (n=23)	IED (n=20)	NI (n=15)	HV (n=21)	ANOVA	ASP-IED	ASP-NI	ASP-HV	IED-NI	IED-HV	NI-HV
					KSP						
Psychic anxiety	25.3±5.9	26.5±7.4	25.1±6.2	19.4±4.3	.0014	...	...	$P<.01$	...	$P<.01$	$P<.05$
Somatic anxiety	27.1±6.6	25.4±7.9	23.5±5.6	16.2±4.4	...	...	...	$P<.01$	...	$P<.01$	$P<.01$
Muscular tension	23.6±6.6	22.3±7.5	21.2±5.6	15.0±3.5	.0001	...	...	$P<.01$	...	$P<.01$	$P<.05$
Detachment	25.4±5.2	25.0±4.4	24.1±5.2	19.9±5.4	.0020	...	...	$P<.01$	...	$P<.05$	...
Monotony avoidance	28.1±5.4	23.2±5.4	24.8±5.5	25.0±2.5	.0120	$P<.01$	...	...	...	...	...
Indirect aggression	13.7±2.6	13.8±3.0	11.4±2.8	9.8±3.3	...	...	...	$P<.01$	...	$P<.01$	...
Suspicion	13.1±2.4	12.7±3.0	10.9±2.7	9.4±2.6	.0001	...	...	$P<.1$	...	$P<.01$	...
					MMPI						
Psychopathic deviate	28.8±4.4	26.6±6.0	23.5±7.0	...	.0263	...	$P<.05$	...	...	...	...

**ASP indicates antisocial personality disorder; IED, intermittent explosive disorder; NI, nonimpulsive offenders; HV, healthy volunteers; and ANOVA, analysis of variance.* P *values are based on Bonferroni's correction applied to compensate for the numbers of post hoc comparisons.*

The alcoholic offenders were divided into impulsive and nonimpulsive groups based on the characteristics of the index crime as in our previous studies. (A crime was termed *impulsive* when the victim was previously unknown to the offender, when no provocation or only verbal altercation preceded the attack, no premeditation could be documented, and no economic motivation such as robbery or burglary was evident. Impulsive fire setting excluded setting fires for insurance fraud.[1,2]) There were 10 fire setters in the impulsive offender group. The data on the alcoholic, impulsive offenders were further divided according to their *DSM-III* (intermittent explosive disorder) and *DSM-III-R* Axis 2 diagnoses.

BIOCHEMICAL ANALYSES AND PHYSICAL ACTIVITY MONITORING

Results of these variables are reported in the accompanying article.[3]

PSYCHOLOGICAL TESTING

Alcoholic offenders with antisocial personality disorder had significantly lower ($P<.5$) mean full-scale IQs (95.8±13.0) than did alcoholic offenders with intermittent explosive disorder (109.4±13.4). The mean IQ of the alcoholic, nonimpulsive offenders was 98.6±20.1.

Minnesota Multiphasic Personality Inventory

Mean psychopathic deviate score was higher for all alcoholic, impulsive offenders, especially alcoholic offenders with antisocial personality disorder, than for alcoholic, nonimpulsive offenders (**Table**).

Karolinska Scales of Personality

Mean impulsiveness, and impulsiveness and monotony avoidance scores were significantly higher and socialization scores significantly lower among alcoholic offenders with antisocial personality disorder than in any other group of subjects (**Figure 1**). Alcoholic offenders with either antisocial personality or intermittent explosive disorder had significantly higher mean irritability scores than did healthy volunteers (Figure 1). Mean verbal aggression score for alcoholic offenders with antisocial personality disorder was significantly higher than for alcoholic, nonimpulsive offenders and healthy volunteers (Figure 1). All groups of alcoholic offenders had higher mean psychasthenia scores than did healthy volunteers (Figure 1). Mean socialization scores were lowest among alcoholic offenders with antisocial personality disorder, followed by alcoholic offenders with intermittent explosive disorder, alcoholic nonimpulsive offenders, and healthy volunteers. Differences between mean socialization scores were statistically significant for groups other than alcoholic offenders with intermittent explosive disorder and alcoholic nonimpulsive offenders (Figure 1). All groups of alcoholic offenders had higher mean psychic and somatic anxiety and muscular tension scores than did healthy volunteers (Table). Alcoholic offenders with antisocial personality and intermittent explosive disorder had significantly higher mean detachment, indirect aggression, and suspicion scores than did healthy volunteers (Table). Alcoholic offenders with antisocial personality disorder had significantly higher monotony avoidance scores than did alcoholic offenders with intermittent explosive disorder (Table).

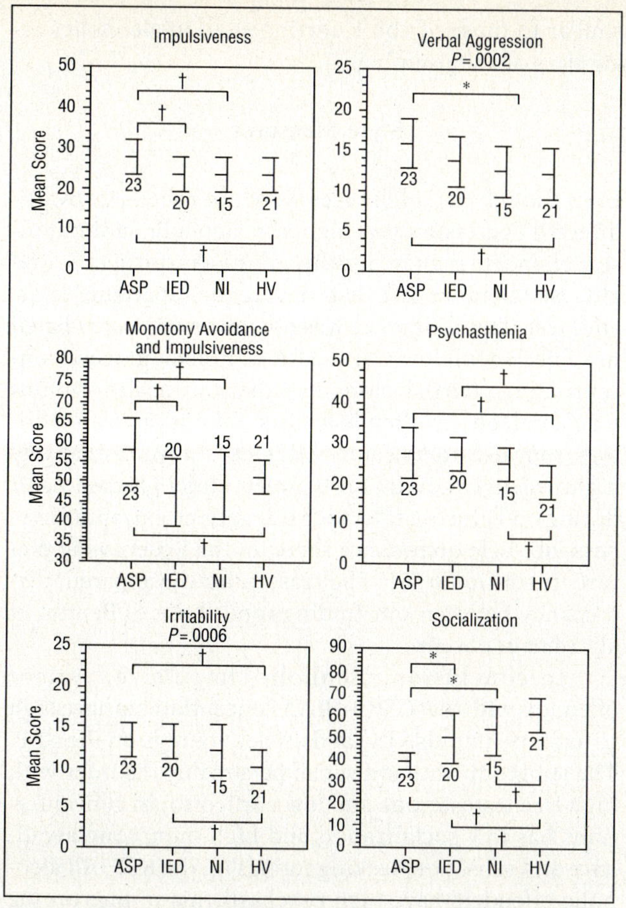

Figure 1. *Mean scores on the Karolinska scales of personality postulated a priori to differ between the groups. ASP indicates antisocial personality disorder; IED, intermittent explosive disorder; NI, alcoholic, nonimpulsive offenders; HV, healthy volunteers; asterisk,* P<.05, *using the corrected Bonferroni test for the number of post hoc comparisions; and dagger,* P<.01.

State Measures

Alcoholic nonimpulsive offenders had a significantly larger difference in the mean Rosenzweig extrapunitiveness–obstacle dominance scores between the glucose and the aspartame tolerance tests than did the healthy volunteers with higher scores during the glucose tolerance test (**Figure 2**). There were no other significant differences in any of the total or change scores on any of the dimensions of the Rosenzweig test.

CORRELATIONAL ANALYSES

Concentration of 5-HIAA in CSF correlated positively with the KSP inhibition of aggression score (r=.28; n=67; P<.01). Testosterone concentration in CSF correlated negatively with the KSP socialization score (r=−.41; n=63; P<.01) and positively with the suspicion score (r=.33; n=63; P<.01).

Concentration of diazepam-binding inhibitor in CSF correlated positively with the KSP psychasthenia score (r=.35; n=62; P<.01) and negatively with monotony avoidance score (r=−.43; n=62; P<.01) and monotony avoidance and impulsivity scores (r=−.29; n=62; P<.01).

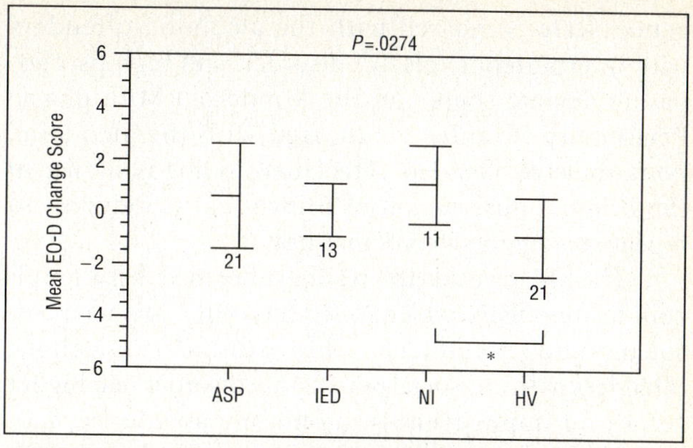

Figure 2. *Mean change scores related to glucose and aspartame administration on the extrapunitiveness–obstacle dominance (EO-D) dimension of Rosenzweig picture frustration test. ASP indicates antisocial personality disorder; IED, intermittent explosive disorder; NI, alcoholic, nonimpulsive offenders; HV, healthy volunteers; and asterisk,* P<.05, *using the corrected Bonferroni test for the number of post hoc comparisons.*

Concentration of corticotropin in CSF correlated positively with the KSP socialization score (r=.41; n=60; P<.01) and negatively with the psychic anxiety score (r=−.28; n=60; P<.01), the somatic anxiety score (r=−.34; n=60; P<.01), the indirect aggression score (r=−.28; n=60; P<.01), and the irritability score (r=−.43; n=60; P<.01).

COMMENT

CORRELATIONAL ANALYSES

The correlations between CSF 5-HIAA and testosterone concentrations and scores on the subscales of the KSP support the inference that central serotonin turnover is associated with impulse control and CSF free testosterone concentration is associated with aggressiveness. Furthermore, the positive correlation between CSF testosterone concentrations and the suspicion scores may parallel the original observation of Wilson et al[19] that administration of methyltestosterone to depressed men produces paranoid reactions.

The overall correlations between the diazepam-binding inhibitor concentration in CSF and scores on the subscales of the KSP support the suggestion that diazepam-binding inhibitor is an anxiogenic peptide.[20] Moreover, the correlations between CSF corticotropin concentrations and scores on the subscales of the KSP are congruent with findings in animal studies on behavioral effects after central administration of corticotropin.[21]

PSYCHOLOGICAL TESTS

Trait Measures

Alcoholic offenders with antisocial personality disorder had low IQs based on the Wechsler Adult Intelligence Scale compared with the alcoholic offenders with intermittent explosive disorder, and high psychopathic deviate scores on the Minnesota Multiphasic Personality Inventory compared with the alcoholic, nonimpulsive offenders. The latter finding is similar to the original observation of Brown and Goodwin[22] in repeatedly aggressive US marines.

The KSP revealed interesting differences between alcoholic, impulsive violent offenders with antisocial personality and intermittent explosive disorders. Alcoholic offenders with antisocial personality disorder had higher scores on impulsiveness, monotony avoidance, monotony avoidance and impulsiveness, and a lower score on socialization than did alcoholic offenders with intermittent explosive disorder. These findings support the notion that these two groups should remain diagnostically separate as suggested by previous psychobiological findings.[23]

The personality profiles of the alcoholic, impulsive violent offenders in the present study are similar to those found by von Knorring et al[7] in early-onset male alcoholics with low platelet monoamine oxidase (MAO) activity. Platelet MAO activity shows a similar inverse correlation to CSF 5-HIAA concentration with impulsive, aggressive, and antisocial traits.[24] Concentration of 5-HIAA in CSF correlates positively but relatively weakly with platelet MAO activity,[25] which has been suggested to be an "indirect indicator of the capacity of the central serotonin system."[26] In humans, platelet MAO activity is not correlated with brain MAO activity[27] but in nonhuman primates, platelet MAO,[28] and in mice,[29] brain MAO activity, may be reduced by testosterone. Thus, if biochemical correlates of impulsivity and aggressiveness are not studied separately and the population under study includes subjects with both characteristics, spurious low positive correlations may be found between platelet MAO and CSF 5-HIAA concentration. The present findings corroborate our earlier suggestions that the alcoholic, impulsive, violent offenders whom we have investigated may be a subgroup of type 2 or early-onset, antisocial male alcoholics.[7,30]

Interestingly, alcoholic, impulsive offenders who met the diagnostic criteria for antisocial personality disorder and intermittent explosive disorder and had low CSF 5-HIAA concentrations had high scores on the KSP anxiety-related scales. This finding supports the suggestion by Apter et al[31] that low CSF 5-HIAA concentration is associated with both impaired impulse control and increased anxiety. Unpublished findings in peer-reared rhesus monkeys (D. Higley, PhD, S. Suomi, PhD, M.L., unpublished data, November 1992) also show anxiety and impulsive aggressiveness coexisting in parentally neglected nonhuman primates with low CSF 5-HIAA concentrations. Psychasthenia ratings were, however, elevated among all alcoholic offenders regardless of CSF monoamine or hormone concentrations. This finding is similar to those of von Knorring et al[7] in alcoholics regardless of subgrouping.

State Measures

Even though the differences were not robust, outward-directed aggression was higher in alcoholic, nonimpulsive offenders than in healthy volunteers during the oral glucose tolerance test than during the aspartame tolerance test. This difference was not, however, exacerbated in subjects with low CSF 5-HIAA or blood glucose concentrations. Furthermore, in either our healthy volunteers or alcoholic offenders we could not replicate findings from an earlier healthy volunteer study of a relatively high negative correlation between blood glucose nadir during oral glucose tolerance test and the extrapunitiveness–obstacle dominance score on the Rosenzweig picture frustration test.[12] The reasons for the apparent discrepancy between our findings and those of Benton et al[12] remain obscure.

In conclusion, alcoholic, impulsive, violent offenders with low CSF 5-HIAA concentrations have high irritability, impulsivity, and anxiety ratings on the KSP. The subgroup with antisocial personality disorder with high free testosterone and low corticotropin concentrations has low socialization and high monotony avoidance and sensation-seeking ratings on the KSP. All alcoholic offenders have high psychasthenia ratings on the KSP. We could not replicate an earlier finding of a high negative correlation between blood glucose nadir after an oral glucose challenge and outward-directed aggression rating on the Rosenzweig picture frustration test.

Accepted for publication August 4, 1993.

This study was supported in part by Research Scientist Development Award MH 00534 from the the National Institute of Mental Health, Bethesda, Md (Dr Poland).

We are grateful to Michael Eckardt, PhD, David Goldman, MD, David Pickar, MD, and William Z. Potter, MD, PhD, for their constructive criticism of the article.

Reprint requests to National Institute on Alcohol Abuse and Alcoholism, Bldg 10, Room 3C103, Bethesda, MD 20892 (Dr Linnoila).

REFERENCES

1. Linnoila M, Virkkunen M, Scheinin M, Nuutila A, Rimon R, Goodwin FK. Low cerebrospinal fluid 5-hydroxyindoleacetic acid concentration differentiates impulsive from nonimpulsive violent behavior. *Life Sci.* 1983;33:2609-2614.
2. Virkkunen M, Nuutila A, Goodwin FK, Linnoila M. Cerebrospinal fluid monoamine metabolites in male arsonists. *Arch Gen Psychiatry.* 1987;44:241-247.
3. Virkkunen M, Rawlings R, Tokola R, Poland RE, Guidotti A, Nemeroff C, Bissette G, Kalogeras K, Karonen SL, Linnoila M. CSF biochemistries, glucose metabolism, and diurnal activity rhythms in alcoholic, violent offenders, fire setters, and healthy volunteers. *Arch Gen Psychiatry.* 1994;51:20-27.
4. Schalling D, Asberg M, Edman G, Oreland L. Markers for vulnerability to psy-

chopathology: temperament traits associated with platelet MAO activity. *Acta Psychiatr Scand.* 1987;76:172-182.
5. Perris C, Eiseman M, von Knorring L, Oreland L, Perris H. Personality traits and monomine oxidase activity in platelets in depressed patients. *Neuropsychobiology.* 1984;12:201-205.
6. von Knorring L, Oreland L, von Knorring A-L. Personality traits and platelet MAO activity in alcohol and drug abusing teenage boys. *Acta Psychiatr Scand.* 1987;75:305-314.
7. von Knorring L, von Knorring A-L, Smigan L, Lindberg U, Edholm M. Personality traits in subtypes of alcoholics. *J Stud Alcohol.* 1987;48:523-527.
8. von Knorring L, Almay BGL, Johansson F. Personality traits in patients with idopathic pain disorder. *Acta Psychiatr Scand.* 1987;76:490-498.
9. Roy A, Virkkunen M, Guthrie S, Linnoila M. Indices of serotonin and glucose metabolism in violent offenders, arsonists and alcoholics. In: Mann JJ, Stanley M, eds. *Psychobiology of Suicidal Behavior.* New York, NY: New York Academy of Science; 1986:202-220.
10. Linnoila M, Virkkunen M, Roy A. Biochemical aspects of aggression in man. In: Bunney WE Jr, Costa E, Potkin SG, eds. *Clinical Neuropharmacology.* New York, NY: Raven Press; 1986;(suppl 1):377-379.
11. Rosenzweig S. The current status of the Rosenzweig picture frustration study as a measure of aggression in personality. In: Brain PF, Benton D, eds. *Multidisciplinary Approaches to Aggression Research.* Amsterdam, the Netherlands: Elsevier Science Publishers; 1981:113-115.
12. Benton D, Kumari N, Brain PF. Mild hypoglycemia and questionnaire measures of aggression. *Biol Psychol.* 1982;14:129-135.
13. Wechsler D. *The Measurement of Adult Intelligence.* 3rd ed. Baltimore, Md; Williams & Williams; 1950.
14. Dahlstrom WM, Welch GS. *MMPI Handbook: A Guide to Use in Clinical Practice Research.* Minneapolis: University of Minnesota Press; 1960.
15. Buss AH. *The Psychology of Aggression.* New York, NY: John Wiley & Sons Inc; 1961.
16. *BMDP Statistical Software Manual.* Los Angeles: University of California Press; 1990.
17. American Psychiatric Association, Committee on Nomenclature and Statistics. *Diagnostic and Statistical Manual of Mental Disorders, Revised Third Edition.* Washington, DC: American Psychiatric Association; 1987.
18. American Psychiatric Association, Committee on Nomenclature and Statistics. *Diagnostic and Statistical Manual of Mental Disorders, Third Edition.* Washington, DC: American Psychiatric Association; 1980.
19. Wilson IC, Prange AJ, Lara PP. Methyltestosterone and imipramine in men: conversion of depression to paranoid reaction. *Am J Psychiatry* 1974;131:21-24.
20. Barbaccia M, Costa E, Ferrero P, Guidotti A, Roy A, Sunderland T, Pickar D, Paul S, Goodwin FK. Diazepam binding inhibitor: a brain neuropeptide present in human spinal fluid—studies in depression, schizophrenia and Alzheimer's disease. *Arch Gen Psychiatry.* 1986;43:1143-1147.
21. De Wied D, Jolles J. Neuropeptides derived from proopiocortin: behavioral, physiological and neurochemical effects. *Physiol Rev.* 1982;62:976-1059.
22. Brown GL, Goodwin FK. Diagnostic, clinical and personality characteristics of aggressive men with low CSF 5-HIAA. *Clin Neuropharmacol.* 1984;7:756-757.
23. Virkkunen M. Insulin secretion during the glucose tolerance test among habitually violent and impulsive offenders. *Aggres Behav.* 1986;12:303-310.
24. Klinteberg af B, Schalling D, Edman G, Oreland L, Asberg M. Personality correlates of platelet monoamine oxidase (MAO) activity in female and male subjects. *Neuropsychobiology.* 1987;18:89-96.
25. Oreland L, Wiberg A, Asberg M, Traskman L, Sjostrand L, Thoren P. Platelet MAO activity and monoamine metabolites in cerebrospinal fluid in depressed and suicidal patients and in healthy controls. *Psychiatry Res.* 1981;4:21-33.
26. Oreland L, Shaskan EG. Monomine oxidase activity as a biological marker. *Trends Pharmacol Sci.* 1983;4:21-33.
27. Young W, Laws E, Sharbrough F, Weinshilbonm RM. Human monoamine oxidase, lade of brain and platelet correlation. *Arch Gen Psychiatry.* 1986;43:604-609.
28. Redmond E, Baulu J, Murphy D, Loriaux L, Ziegler M, Lake R. The effects of testosterone on plasma and platelet monoamine oxidase (MAO) and plasma dopamine beta hydroxylase (DBH) activity in the male rhesus monkey. *Psychosom Med.* 1976;38:315-326.
29. Hoff KM. Interactions of testosterone with monoamine oxidase in mouse brain maturation. *Gen Pharmacol.* 1977;8:55-57.
30. Virkkunen M, Linnoila M. Serotonin in early onset, male alcoholics with violent behavior. *Ann Med.* 1990;22:327-331.
31. Apter A, von Pragg H, Plutchik R, Sevy S, Korn M, Brown SL. Interrelationships among anxiety, aggression, impulsivity, and mood: a serotonergically linked cluster? *Psychiatry Res.* 1990;32:191-199.

Suicidality and 5-Hydroxyindoleacetic Acid Concentration Associated With a Tryptophan Hydroxylase Polymorphism

David A. Nielsen, PhD; David Goldman, MD; Matti Virkkunen, MD; Riitta Tokola, MD; Robert Rawlings, MS; Markku Linnoila, MD, PhD

Background: To examine whether the tryptophan hydroxylase (TPH) gene, which codes for the rate-limiting enzyme in the biosynthesis of serotonin, may be a factor influencing serotonin turnover and behaviors controlled by serotonin.

Methods: Using a polymerase chain reaction–based method, TPH genotype was determined in DNA samples from 56 impulsive and 14 nonimpulsive, alcoholic, violent offenders and 20 healthy volunteers.

Results: In the behaviorally extreme impulsive group, we observed a significant association between TPH genotype and cerebrospinal fluid 5-hydroxyindoleacetic acid (5-HIAA) concentration. No association of TPH genotype with impulsive behavior was detected. The polymorphism was also associated with a history of suicide attempts in all violent offenders, independent of impulsivity status and cerebrospinal fluid 5-HIAA concentration.

Conclusion: In some individuals, a genetic variant of the TPH gene may influence 5-HIAA concentration in the cerebrospinal fluid and predisposition to suicidal behavior.

(Arch Gen Psychiatry. 1994;51:34-38)

FAMILY AND twin studies have implicated genetic contributions in certain kinds of antisocial[1] and suicidal behaviors,[2,3] alcoholism,[4-6] and several personality variables.[7] Alcoholism and antisocial and suicidal behaviors are strongly interrelated, often coexisting in patients and their blood relatives. These disorders are clinically heterogeneous and are likely to be causally complex. However, based on concentrations of cerebrospinal fluid (CSF) 5-hydroxyindoleacetic acid (5-HIAA), the principal metabolite of the neurotransmitter serotonin, it may be possible to identify a more homogeneous group of patients with a deficit of brain serotonin metabolism. For example, in alcoholic violent offenders, only the impulsive subgroup commonly has low CSF 5-HIAA concentrations.[8] Nonimpulsive alcoholics who otherwise manifest the same behaviors may not differ from controls.[9] Decreased serotonin turnover, as indicated by low CSF 5-HIAA concentrations, is postulated to be associated with anxiety-related intolerance to delay and deficient impulse control[10] and is associated with behaviors such as suicidality,[2,3,11-15] impulsive violence,[8,16,17] depression,[18,19] and alcoholism.[20]

Individuals with low CSF 5-HIAA concentrations may have alterations in genes controlling serotonin synthesis and metabolism. Although CSF 5-HIAA concentration is a partially heritable trait in rhesus monkeys,[21] the genetic factors determining individual differences in serotonin biosynthesis and catabolism are essentially unknown. Many of the genes potentially important in controlling serotonin metabolism have been cloned, including tryptophan hydroxylase (TPH),[22,23] aromatic L-amino acid decarboxylase,[24] serotonin transporter,[25,26] several serotonin receptors,[27] and mono-

From the Laboratories of Neurogenetics (Dr Nielsen and Dr Goldman) and Clinical Studies (Dr Linnoila and Mr Rawlings), Division of Intramural Clinical and Biological Research, National Institute on Alcohol Abuse and Alcoholism, Bethesda, Md, and the Department of Psychiatry, University of Helsinki (Finland) (Drs Virkkunen and Tokola).

See Subjects and Methods on next page

SUBJECTS AND METHODS

SUBJECTS AND PSYCHIATRIC DIAGNOSIS

The sample consisted of violent offenders and arsonists and control subjects, who were healthy volunteers with no mental disorders. All were offspring of Finnish Caucasian parents. The general characteristics of these subjects have been described.[33] The violent offenders and arsonists were classified as impulsive (n=56) or nonimpulsive (n=14) based on their crimes. Impulsive crimes were unpremeditated and unprovoked, whereas nonimpulsive crimes were clearly premeditated.[33] The mean ($\pm$SEM) ages of these groups were as follows: impulsive violent offenders, 30$\pm$1 years; nonimpulsive violent offenders, 31$\pm$2 years; and healthy volunteers, 33$\pm$2 years. Subjects were interviewed and diagnosed by a psychiatrist (M.V.) using *DSM-III* criteria.[34] All subjects were evaluated for a history of suicide attempts. The history was considered to be positive only when medical records documenting a severe attempt were available, a relative or partner endorsed the history, or there were scars corroborating the history. Of the impulsive group, 28 had antisocial personality disorder, 27 had intermittent explosive disorder, and one 17-year-old subject had conduct disorder. All offenders met criteria for alcohol abuse or dependence. Written informed consent was obtained after the nature, risks, and hazards of the study were explained.

GENETIC AND BIOCHEMICAL VARIABLES

Tryptophan hydroxylase genotype analysis and quantification of CSF 5-HIAA concentrations were made by investigators who were unaware of the clinical history of the subjects.

TPH Genotype Analysis

Tryptophan hydroxylase genotype was determined by single-strand polymorphism analysis.[29,35] Briefly, DNA isolated from Epstein-Barr virus immortalized lymphoblastoma cell lines was amplified using polymerase chain reaction with the primers HTHSSCP4, 5′-TTCAGATCCCTTCTATACCCCA-GAG-3′ and HTHSSCP5, 5′-GGACATGACCTAAGAGT-TCATGGCA-3′. These primers are specific to the boundaries of the intron corresponding to intron 7 of the mouse TPH gene.[22] The resulting phosphorus 32–labeled fragment was digested with *Hae* III, denatured with 90% formamide and 9.5 mmol/L of sodium hydroxide at 100°C for 2 minutes, electrophoresed through a nondenaturing 5% polyacrylamide gel, and visualized by autoradiography.

CSF 5-HIAA Concentration

Cerebrospinal fluid samples were obtained by lumbar puncture between 8 and 9 AM after overnight bedrest. Concentration of 5-HIAA in the first 12 mL of CSF drawn was measured with high-performance liquid chromatography using electrochemical detection.[32]

amine oxidases A and B.[28] All could play a role in modulating serotonin-dependent behaviors.

We previously identified a polymorphism in the human TPH gene using the single-strand conformational polymorphism method.[29] This polymorphic site is located in the intron corresponding to intron 7 of the mouse TPH gene. Using this polymorphism, TPH was genetically mapped to the short arm of chromosome 11 in close proximity to tyrosine hydroxylase. Two alleles, referred to as U and L, are abundant in Caucasian subjects, with the rarer U allele present at a frequency of 0.40.

Tryptophan hydroxylase catalyzes the oxygenation of tryptophan to 5-hydroxytryptophan, which is decarboxylated to serotonin. Monoamine oxidases A and B deaminate serotonin to 5-hydroxyindoleacetaldehyde, whose oxidation product is 5-HIAA. The concentration of serotonin in the frontal cortex is positively correlated with lumbar CSF 5-HIAA concentration.[30] Because the hydroxylation of tryptophan can be rate-limiting in serotonin biosynthesis,[31] we hypothesized that TPH genotype could be different in individuals with a low CSF 5-HIAA concentration and might be associated with behaviors controlled by serotonin. To test this hypothesis, we determined TPH genotype,[29] CSF 5-HIAA concentration,[32] and history of suicide attempts in a behaviorally extreme and genetically relatively homogeneous population of Finnish alcoholics.

RESULTS

A population association between TPH genotype and CSF 5-HIAA concentration is shown in **Figure 1** and **Table 1**. The frequency of the rarer TPH allele (U) in the total population was 0.41, not significantly different from the frequency in the impulsive (0.44) and nonimpulsive (0.39) offenders or control subjects (0.35). However, the impulsive offenders showed a highly significant relationship between CSF 5-HIAA concentration and TPH genotype (P=.0036) (Figure 1, left, and Table 1). Impulsive offenders with the UU genotype had the highest CSF 5-HIAA concentration (76$\pm$9 nmol/L) while the LL group had the lowest (45$\pm$4 nmol/L). Impulsive offenders with the UL genotype also had low CSF 5-HIAA concentrations (46$\pm$5 nmol/L). No association was observed between TPH genotype and CSF 5-HIAA concentration in the nonimpulsive offenders or control subjects (Table 1).

A significant association of TPH genotype with a history of suicide attempts was observed in all violent offend-

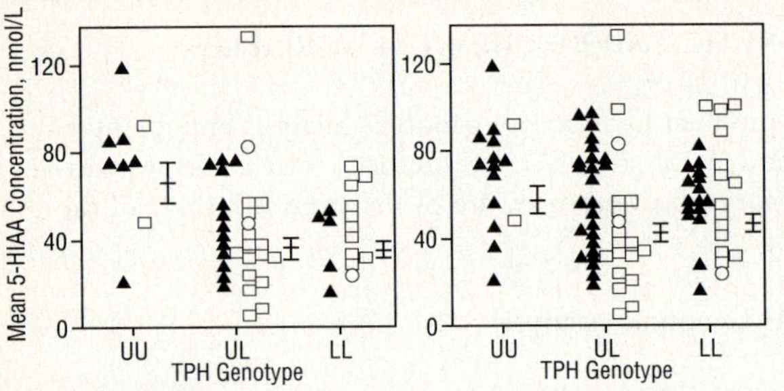

Figure 1. *Relationship between tryptophan hydroxylase (TPH) genotype, mean (±SEM) 5-hydroxyindoleacetic acid (5-HIAA) concentration, and history of suicide attempts. The 5-HIAA concentrations of the subjects are plotted against their TPH genotypes for impulsive subjects (left) and all subjects (right). Triangles represent subjects who had never attempted suicide; squares, suicide attempters; and circles, those who had committed suicide.*

Table 1. Population Association Between Tryptophan Hydroxylase Genotype and 5-Hydroxyindoleacetic Acid (5-HIAA) Concentration

	Mean 5-HIAA Concentration, nmol/L*		
Variable	Impulsive	Nonimpulsive	Control
Genotype†			
UU	76±9 (9)	69±13 (3)	56±11 (3)
UL	46±5 (31)	86±8 (5)	63±9 (8)
LL	45±4 (16)	89±6 (6)	65±3 (9)
P‡	.0036	NS	NS
5-HIAA concentration§	50±3 (56)	83±5 (14)	63±4 (20)
Frequency of UU	0.16	0.21	0.15
U allele frequency	0.44	0.39	0.35

*Mean concentrations were determined as described by Scheinin et al.[32] Numbers in parentheses are numbers of subjects.

†Tryptophan hydroxylase genotype was determined as described by Nielsen et al.[29]

‡Probabilities for the association of 5-HIAA to genotype were calculated with one-way analyses of variance. NS indicates not significant.

§Frequency of attempted suicide is presented as the frequency of subjects attempting suicide with the ratio of suicide attempters to total subjects in parentheses.

ers without respect to impulsivity (**Table 2**). The frequency of the U allele was 0.32 in individuals who had attempted suicide and 0.54 in those who had not. Only two (6%) of 36 suicide attempters had the UU genotype compared with 10 (29%) of 34 who had never attempted suicide. A significant association was observed between attempted suicide and TPH genotype ($P=.016$). A similar association was observed between TPH genotype and a history of multiple suicide attempts in the violent offenders (**Figure 2**). A history of multiple suicide attempts was most prevalent in subjects with the LL genotype, and to a lesser extent with the UL genotype, indicating an association between the L allele and repetitive suicidal behavior.

No association was observed between TPH genotype and primary psychiatric diagnosis of the subjects as shown in **Table 3**. The frequencies of the TPH genotypes in offenders with antisocial personality disorder, intermittent explosive disorder, and nonimpulsive violent offenders and control groups were not significantly different.

COMMENT

This study demonstrates that TPH genotype is associated with CSF 5-HIAA concentration in impulsive alcoholic violent offenders. To our knowledge, this is the first report to implicate a specific gene in the predisposition to a behavior (suicidality) postulated to be regulated by serotonin. Tryptophan hydroxylase genotype was associated with a history of suicidal behavior in the alcoholic violent offenders. However, TPH genotype was not associated with impulsivity or psychiatric diagnosis. The low turnover of serotonin as indicated by low CSF 5-HIAA concentrations in impulsive, alcoholic, violent offenders with at least one TPH L allele may reflect a reduced capacity to hydroxylate tryptophan to 5-hydroxytryptophan in the biosynthesis of serotonin. Since the TPH polymorphism is located in an intron of the gene, it may alter the processing of the TPH pre–messenger RNA (mRNA), but, more likely, it is not functionally significant. The association would then indicate the existence of a genetically linked mutation elsewhere in the TPH gene that alters enzyme activity. This could occur through a variety of mechanisms including a difference in gene transcription, mRNA processing, mRNA stability, enzymatic activity, or enzyme stability. Although highly unlikely, the associations may also be due to linkage disequilibrium of the TPH polymorphism with a second, nearby gene involved in the regulation of CSF 5-HIAA concentration and suicidal behavior.

This Finnish population is an advantageous group to search for a behavioral association to serotonergic genetic markers. The Finns are genetically more homogeneous than many other populations, such as American Caucasians, and in Finland one in 4000 individuals commit suicide each year, the third highest incidence rate among industrialized nations.[36] In addition, many of the subjects in this study had very low concentrations of CSF 5-HIAA.

The association may be strong only for impulsive offenders as they are phenotypically more extreme and are more likely to carry a linked mutation in the TPH gene. Other possibilities include the relatively small number of subjects in the nonimpulsive offender and control groups or genetic/environmental interactions. That is, the impulsive offenders, all of whom were also alcoholic, may be more phenotypically extreme in serotonin function either due to unknown environmental interactions or concomitant disturbances in other genes influencing the synthesis and metabolism of serotonin. Such postulated abnormalities would permit TPH to function as the primary regulator of serotonin turnover. However, since the as-

Table 2. Population Association Between Tryptophan Hydroxylase Genotype and History of Suicide Attempts

	History of Suicide Attempts					
	Impulsive		Nonimpulsive		All Violent Offenders	
Variable	With, No. (%)	Without, No.	With, No. (%)	Without, No.	With, No. (%)	Without No.
Genotype*						
UU	2 (22)	7	0 (0)	3	2 (17)	10
UL	18 (58)	13	1 (20)	4	19 (53)	17
LL	11 (69)	5	4 (67)	2	15 (65)	7
P†	.072		.095		.016	
Total	**31**	**25**	**5**	**9**	**36**	**34**
U allele frequency	0.54	0.35	0.56	0.10	0.54	0.32

**Genotype was determined as described by Nielsen et al.[29]*
†Probabilities were calculated with the Pearson χ^2 test.

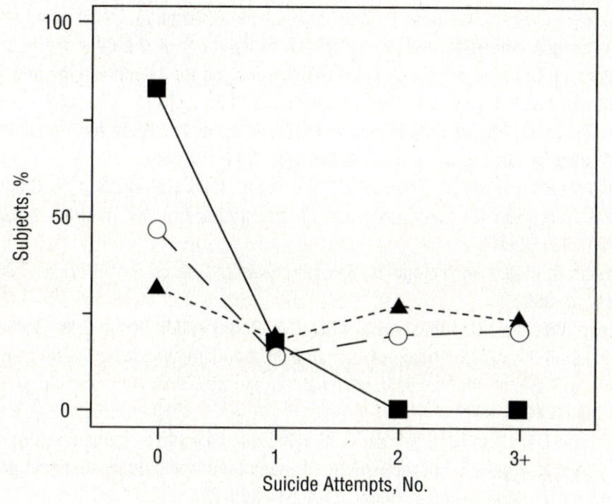

Figure 2. *Relationship between tryptophan hydroxylase genotype and lifetime history of multiple suicide attempts. For each genotype, the fraction of subjects having each genotype (UU, squares; UL, circles; LL, triangles) is plotted against the number of suicide attempts they have made in their lives.*

Table 3. Population Association Between Tryptophan Hydroxylase Genotype and Psychiatric Diagnosis*

	No. of Subjects			
	Impulsive†			
Variable	Antisocial Personality Disorder	Intermittent Explosive Disorder	Nonimpulsive	Control
Genotype†				
UU	4	4	3	3
UL	16	15	5	8
LL	8	8	6	9
Total	**28**	**27**	**14**	**20**
Frequency of UU	0.14	0.15	0.21	0.15
U allele frequency	0.43	0.43	0.39	0.35

**Psychiatric diagnoses were made as described in "Subjects and Methods." One 17-year-old subject with conduct disorder had a UU genotype.*
†Genotype was determined as described by Nielsen et al.[29]

sociations of TPH genotype with CSF 5-HIAA concentration and suicidal behavior was observed in alcoholics, alcohol or alcohol abuse may be a necessary component in the association with CSF 5-HIAA and suicidal behavior.

It is highly unlikely that the associations are due to genetic admixture or ethnic stratification in suicidal and nonsuicidal subjects or in those with low and high CSF 5-HIAA concentrations. Tryptophan hydroxylase allele frequency has been determined in two additional Caucasian populations. In 72 unrelated Caucasian individuals (Centre d'Etude du Polymorphisme Humaine parents), the U allele frequency was 0.40[29] and in 39 Caucasian Swedes, the U allele frequency was 0.41 (D.A.N., L. Traskman-Bendz, MD, H. Erikson, MD, D.G., unpublished results, 1993). By comparison, the U allele frequency was 0.41 in the Caucasian Finns studied herein. Contingency table analysis of the distribution of TPH genotypes also showed no statistically significant interpopulation difference (χ^2=.89; *df*=4; *P*=.93).

It is interesting that almost all offenders who attempted suicide (34 of 36) had either the LL or UL genotype, independent of CSF 5-HIAA concentration. Therefore, the presence of the L allele was associated with an increased risk of suicide attempts. Because CSF 5-HIAA concentration correlates with suicidal behavior in some populations,[11-15] the relationship of suicidality to TPH genotype was expected. This correlation suggests a more complex relationship in which TPH genotype plays a larger role. However, TPH genotype did not have an association with the psychiatric diagnoses of the subjects.

A genetic link between TPH and serotonin turnover may yield valuable insights into the inheritance of several other neuropsychiatric diseases. For example, abnormal serotonin metabolism has been implicated in Tourette's syndrome and autism, both of which have a genetic component.[37] It may be possible that TPH participates either directly or indirectly in the development of these diseases.

These findings, detected in a population of impulsive offenders, need to be confirmed in additional population samples, by genetic linkage in families or definitively, by identification of a functional variant of the human TPH gene. Previously, Abbar et al[38] found no association between two unspecified TPH polymorphisms and suicidal behavior in an unspecified group of psychiatric patients. Relating TPH genotype to behavior and CSF 5-HIAA concentrations among groups of high-risk patients could eventually lead to an improved ability to identify individuals who are predisposed to suicidal behavior and facilitate implementation of preventative measures.

Accepted for publication September 2, 1993.

Reprint requests to National Institute on Alcohol Abuse and Alcoholism, 9000 Rockville Pike, Bldg 10, Room 3C102, Bethesda, MD 20892 (Dr Nielsen).

REFERENCES

1. Crowe RR. An adoption study of antisocial personality. *Arch Gen Psychiatry.* 1974;31:785-791.
2. Roy A, Segal NL, Centerwall BS, Robinette CD. Suicide in twins. *Arch Gen Psychiatry.* 1991;48:29-32.
3. Rosenthal N, Davenport Y, Cowdry RW, Webster MH, Goodwin FK. Monoamine metabolites in cerebrospinal fluid of depressive subgroups. *Psychiatry Res.* 1980;3:113-119.
4. Cloninger CR, Bohman M, Sigvardsson S. Inheritance of alcohol abuse: cross-fostering analysis of adopted men. *Arch Gen Psychiatry.* 1981;38:861-868.
5. Bohman M, Cloninger CR, von Knorring AL, Sigvardsson S. An adoption study of somatoform disorders, III: cross-fostering analysis and genetic relationship to alcoholism and criminality. *Arch Gen Psychiatry.* 1984;41:872-878.
6. Linnoila M, DeJong J, Virkkunen M. Family history of alcoholism in violent offenders and impulsive fire setters. *Arch Gen Psychiatry.* 1989;46:613-616.
7. Loehlin JC. Partitioning environmental and genetic contributions to behavioral development. *Am Psychol.* 1989;44:1285-1292.
8. Linnoila M, Virkkunen M, Scheinin M, Nuutila A, Rimon R, Goodwin FK. Low cerebrospinal fluid 5-hydroxyindoleacetic acid concentration differentiates impulsive from nonimpulsive violent behavior. *Life Sci.* 1983;33:2609-2614.
9. Limson R, Goldman D, Roy A, Lanparski D, Ravitz B, Adinoff B, Linnoila M. Personality and cerebrospinal fluid monoamine metabolites in alcoholics and controls. *Arch Gen Psychiatry.* 1991;48:437-441.
10. Soubrie P. Reconciling the role of central serotonin neurons in human and animal behavior. *Behav Brain Sci.* 1986;9:319-364.
11. Asberg M, Traskman L, Thoren P. 5-HIAA in the cerebrospinal fluid. *Arch Gen Psychiatry.* 1976;33:1193-1197.
12. Roy A, Virkkunen M, Linnoila M. Serotonin in suicide, violence, and alcoholism. In: Coccaro E, Murphy D, eds. *Serotonin in Major Psychiatric Disorders.* Washington, DC: American Psychiatric Association; 1991:187-208.
13. Virkkunen M, De Jong J, Bartko J, Linnoila M. Psychobiological concomitants of history of suicide attempts among violent offenders and impulsive fire setters. *Arch Gen Psychiatry.* 1989;46:604-606.
14. Roy A, Agren H, Pickar D, Linnoila M, Doran AR, Cutler NR, Paul SM. Reduced CSF concentrations of homovanillic acid and homovanillic acid to 5-hydroxyindoleacetic acid ratios in depressed patients: relationship to suicidal behavior and dexamethasone nonsuppression. *Am J Psychiatry.* 1986;143:1539-1545.
15. Roy A, DeJong J, Linnoila M. Cerebrospinal fluid monoamine metabolites and suicidal behavior in depressed patients. *Arch Gen Psychiatry.* 1989;46:609-612.
16. Brown GL, Ballenger JC, Minichiello MD, Goodwin FK. Human aggression and its relationship to cerebrospinal fluid 5-hydroxyindoleacetic acid, 3-methoxy-4-hydroxyphenylglycol, and homovanillic acid. In: Sandler M, ed. *Psychopharmacology of Aggression.* New York, NY: Raven Press; 1979;31-148.
17. Roy A, Adinoff B, Linnoila M. Acting out hostility in normal volunteers: negative correlation with levels of 5-HIAA in cerebrospinal fluid. *Psychiatric Res.* 1988; 24:187-194.
18. van Praag HM, Korf J. Endogenous depressions with and without disturbances in the 5-hydroxytryptamine metabolism: a biochemical classification? *Psychopharmacology (Berl).* 1971;19:148-152.
19. Asberg M, Thoren P, Traskman L, Bertilsson L, Ringberger V. Serotonin depression: a biochemical subgroup within the affective disorders? *Science.* 1976; 191:478-480.
20. Ballenger JC, Goodwin FK, Major LF, Brown GL. Alcohol and central serotonin metabolism in man. *Arch Gen Psychiatry.* 1979;36:224-227.
21. Higley D, Thompson WT, Champoux M, Goldman D, Hasert MF, Kraemer GW, Scanlan JM, Suomi SJ, Linnoila M. Paternal and maternal genetic and environmental contributions to cerebrospinal fluid monoamine metabolites in Rhesus monkeys (*Macaca mulatta*). *Arch Gen Psychiatry.* 1993;50:615-623.
22. Stoll J, Goldman D. Isolation and structural characterization of the murine tryptophan hydroxylase gene. *J Neurosci Res.* 1991;28:457-465.
23. Boularand S, Darmon MC, Ganem Y, Launay J-M, Mallet J. Complete coding sequence of human tryptophan hydroxylase. *Nucl Acids Res.* 1990;18:4257.
24. Sumi-Ichinose C, Ichinose H, Takahashi E, Hori T, Nagatsu T. Molecular cloning of genomic DNA and chromosomal assignment of the gene for human aromatic L-amino acid decarboxylase, the enzyme for catecholamine and serotonin biosynthesis. *Biochemistry.* 1992;31:2229-2238.
25. Hoffman BJ, Mezey E, Brownstein MJ. Cloning of the serotonin transporter affected by antidepressants. *Science.* 1991;254:579-580.
26. Blakely RD, Berson HE, Fremeau RT, Caron MG, Peek MM, Bradley CC. Cloning and expression of a functional serotonin transporter from the rat brain. *Nature.* 1991;354:66-70.
27. Julius D. Molecular biology of serotonin receptors. *Annu Rev Neurosci.* 1991; 14:335-360.
28. Bach AW, Lan NC, Johnson DL, Abell CW, Bemenek ME, Kwan S-W, Seeburg PH, Shih JC. cDNA cloning of human liver monoamine oxidase A and B: molecular basis of differences in enzymatic properties. *Proc Natl Acad Sci U S A.* 1988;85:4934-4938.
29. Nielsen DA, Dean M, Goldman D. Genetic mapping of the human tryptophan hydroxylase gene on chromosome 11 using an intronic conformational polymorphism. *Am J Human Genet.* 1992;51:1366-1371.
30. Stanley M, Traskman-Bendz L, Dorovini-Zis K. Correlations between aminergic metabolites simultaneously obtained from human CSF and brain. *Life Sci.* 1985; 37:1279-1286.
31. Cooper JR, Melcer I. The enzymatic oxidation of tryptophan to 5-hydroxytryptophan in the biosynthesis of serotonin. *J Pharmacol Exp Ther.* 1961;132:265-268.
32. Scheinin M, Chang W-H, Kirk KL, Linnoila M. Simultaneous determination of 3-methoxy-4-hydroxyphenylglycol, 5-hydroxyindoleacetic acid and homovanillic acid in cerebrospinal fluid with high-performance liquid chromatography using electrochemical detection. *Anal Biochem.* 1983;131:246-253.
33. Virkkunen M, Rawlings R, Tokola R, Kallio E, Poland RE, Guidotti A, Nemeroff C, Bissette G, Kalogeras K, Karonen S-L, Linnoila M. CSF biochemistries, glucose metabolism, and diurnal activity rhythms in alcoholic, violent offenders, fire setters, and healthy volunteers. *Arch Gen Psychiatry.* 1994;51:20-27.
34. American Psychiatric Association, Committee on Nomenclature and Statistics. *Diagnostic and Statistical Manual of Mental Disorders.* Washington, DC: American Psychiatric Association; 1980.
35. Orita M, Suzuki Y, Sekiya T, Hayashi K. Rapid and sensitive detection of point mutations and DNA polymorphisms using the polymerase chain reaction. *Genomics.* 1989;5:874-879.
36. Lester D. The availability of firearms and use of firearms for suicide: a study of 20 countries. *Acta Psychiatr Scand.* 1990;81:146-14738.
37. Comings DE, Comings BG. Clinical and genetic relationships between autism-pervasive developmental disorder and Tourette syndrome: a study of 19 cases. *Am J Med Genet.* 1991;39:180-191.
38. Abbar M, Amadeo S, Malafosse A, Shenk L, Mallet J, Castelnau D. An association study between suicidal behavior and tryptophan hydroxylase markers. *Clin Pharmacol.* 1992;15(suppl 1):299.

WHO Neuropsychiatric AIDS Study, Cross-sectional Phase I

Study Design and Psychiatric Findings

Mario Maj, MD, PhD; Robert Janssen, MD; Fabrizio Starace, MD; Michael Zaudig, MD; Paul Satz, PhD; Bhirom Sughondhabirom, MD; Mesu'A-Kabwa Luabeya, MD; Rolf Riedel, MD; David Ndetei, MD; Helena M. Calil, MD, PhD; Eric G. Bing, MD; Michael St. Louis, MD; Norman Sartorius, MD, PhD

Background: Most available studies on the psychiatric, neuropsychological, and neurological complications of HIV-1 infection and AIDS have been conducted in Western countries, on samples of well-educated, mostly white, homosexual men. Concerns about generalizability of the results of those investigations prompted the WHO to implement the cross-cultural venture called WHO Neuropsychiatric AIDS study.

Methods: This project aims to assess the prevalence and natural history of HIV-1–associated psychiatric, neuropsychological, and neurological abnormalities in representative subject samples enrolled in the five geographic areas predominantly affected by the HIV-1 epidemic. Assessment is made by a data collection instrument including six modules. The intercenter and intracenter reliability in the use of each module has been formally evaluated. The study consists of a cross-sectional phase and a longitudinal follow-up.

Results: The cross-sectional phase was completed in five centers. This paper reports on the results of psychiatric assessment, which revealed a significantly higher prevalence of current mental disorders in symptomatic seropositive persons compared with seronegative controls among intravenous drug users in Bangkok and homosexuals/bisexuals in São Paulo. The mean global score on the Montgomery-Asberg Depression Rating Scale was significantly higher in symptomatic seropositive individuals than in matched seronegative controls in all centers.

Conclusions: These results suggest that the significance of the psychopathological complications of symptomatic HIV-1 infection may have been underestimated by previous studies conducted on self-selected samples of well-educated, middle-class, mostly white, homosexual men.

(Arch Gen Psychiatry. 1994;51:39-49)

From the Division of Mental Health and Global Programme on AIDS World Health Organization, Geneva, Switzerland (Drs Maj, Starace, and Sartorius); the Department of Psychiatry I, University of Naples, Italy (Drs Maj and Starace); the Division of HIV/AIDS, Centers for Disease Control and Prevention, Atlanta, Ga (Drs Janssen and St. Louis); the Max-Planck Institute for Psychiatry, Munich, Germany (Dr Zaudig); the Neuropsychiatric Institute, UCLA, Los Angeles, Calif (Drs Satz and Bing); the Department of Psychiatry, Chulalongkorn University, Bangkok, Thailand (Dr Sughondhabirom); the Centre of Neuropsychopathology, University of Kinshasa (Zaire), (Dr Luabeya); the Projet SIDA, Kinshasa, Zaire (Drs Luabeya and St. Louis); the Department of Psychiatry, University of Munich (Germany), (Dr Riedel); the Department of Psychiatry, University of Nairobi (Kenya), (Dr Ndetei); and the Department of Psychobiology, Escola Paulista de Medicina, São Paulo, Brazil (Dr Calil).

According to recent worldwide estimates by the World Health Organization (WHO), Geneva, Switzerland,[1] 85% of adults infected with the human immunodeficiency virus type 1 (HIV-1) live outside Western industrialized countries, over 75% of HIV-1 infections in adults have been transmitted through heterosexual intercourse, and more than 45% of HIV-1–infected subjects are women. Despite this, the overwhelming majority of the available studies assessing the prevalence and the natural history of the psychiatric, neuropsychological, and neurological complications of HIV-1 infection have been conducted in Western Europe or in North America on samples of well-educated, mostly white, homosexual men.

Focusing on psychiatric research, to our knowledge, the only three published investigations that evaluated the prevalence of HIV-1–associated mental disorders by using structured diagnostic interviews and operational diagnostic criteria were all carried out in the United States. The first of these studies[2] examined, by using the Diagnostic Interview Schedule[3] and the *DSM-III* diagnostic criteria,[4] a sample of 56 well-educated, middle-class homosexual men (all but one white) who were subdivided into four small groups (patients with acquired immunodeficiency syndrome [AIDS], patients with AIDS-related complex, asymptomatic or mildly symptomatic HIV-1–seropositive subjects, and HIV-1–seronegative controls). The second study[5] assessed, by the Struc-

See Subjects and Methods on next page

SUBJECTS AND METHODS

PARTICIPATING CENTERS

The cross-sectional phase of the WHO Neuropsychiatric AIDS Study has been completed in five centers: Chulalongkorn University, Bangkok, Thailand; Mama Yemo Hospital/Projet SIDA, Kinshasa, Zaire; University of Munich (Germany); Kenyatta Hospital, Nairobi, Kenya; and Emilio Ribas Hospital, São Paulo, Brazil. Data collection is ongoing in a sixth center (UCLA, Los Angeles, Calif).

The above-mentioned centers were selected in the five geographic areas that are predominantly affected by the HIV-1 epidemic (sub-Saharan Africa, North America, Latin America, western Europe, and Southeast Asia). Since sub-Saharan Africa accounted, as to the late 1980s, for about 60% of all HIV-1 infections,[10] we selected two centers in that area and one center in each of the others.

The criteria used for the selection of the centers were the following: (1) history of successful collaboration with the WHO; (2) availability of at least one outpatient unit (either a general medical clinic or a clinic for infectious diseases, excluding HIV-1 clinics) attended by both HIV-1–seropositive and HIV-1–seronegative persons; (3) comparability, with respect to sex ratio and distribution of HIV-1 at-risk groups, between the HIV-1–seropositive cases ascertained at the above-mentioned unit(s) during the last month and the whole population of HIV-1–seropositive subjects living in the relevant geographic area (as described by the WHO[10]); (4) availability of a laboratory unit able to perform HIV-1 serological tests (both enzyme-linked immunosorbent assay and Western blot), of a microbiology unit, and of a neuroradiology unit with a functioning computed tomography scanner; (5) availability of neuropsychiatric staff with previous research experience, including at least one professional trained in neuropsychological testing (in the São Paulo center, the trained personnel were partially supplied by the Escola Paulista de Medicina); and (6) ability to provide counseling for HIV-1–seropositive persons. The protocol of the study was approved by human subject review committees both at WHO headquarters and at each participating center.

SUBJECTS

Three samples of subjects were recruited in each center: (1) asymptomatic HIV-1–seropositive persons (groups II and III according to the Centers for Disease Control and Prevention [CDC[11]], Atlanta, Ga); (2) symptomatic HIV-1–seropositive persons (CDC group IV); and (3) HIV-1–seronegative controls matched to seropositive persons by sex, age (±5 years), education (±3 years), and HIV-1 at-risk group.

A total of 955 subjects (186 in Bangkok, 205 in Kinshasa, 183 in Munich, 203 in Nairobi, and 178 in São Paulo) completed the cross-sectional evaluation. Subjects who were enrolled but who dropped out before the assessment was completed were three (1.6%) in Bangkok, 12 (5.5%) in Kinshasa, two (1.1%) in Munich, 15 (6.9%) in Nairobi, and 15 (7.8%) in São Paulo. In the three centers where the attrition rate exceeded 5%, dropouts did not differ significantly from the other subjects with respect to any sociodemographic variable.

STUDY DESIGN

Subject recruitment took place between October 1990 and August 1991. Every third subject who was attending the selected outpatient medical unit(s) and who was aged older than 18 years, able to count from one to 25 in his or her native language, and able to read a series of 10 numbers was asked to participate by one of the physicians in charge of the unit(s). After signing an informed consent form, the subject was provisionally enrolled, received pretest counseling, and had blood drawn for HIV-1 serological tests. Two weeks later, at a return visit, test results and posttest counseling were provided. The HIV-1–seropositive persons and the HIV-1–seronegative individuals who were suitable for matching were definitively enrolled. In all these subjects, a second blood sample was drawn (for CD4 and CD8 counts and for the VDRL [test]), and the sociodemographic and medical modules of the data collection instrument were administered. The remaining modules of the instrument were applied 1 month later. The HIV-1 serostatus of recruited subjects was unknown to the examiners who performed

tured Clinical Interview for *DSM-III-R*[6] and the *DSM-III-R* diagnostic criteria,[7] a sample of 154 well-educated, middle-class, predominantly white homosexual/bisexual men who were all physically asymptomatic (HIV-1–seropositive and HIV-1–seronegative subjects who were evaluated before serological testing, plus subjects who were known to be HIV-1 seropositive). The third investigation[8] evaluated, by using the Structured Clinical Interview for *DSM-III-R* and the *DSM-III-R* criteria, 208 well-educated, middle-class, predominantly white homosexual men who were subdivided into HIV-1–seropositive subjects (asymptomatic, mildly symptomatic, or with AIDS-related complex) and HIV-1–seronegative controls.

Each of the above-mentioned studies found a high lifetime prevalence of mental disorders (in particular, of major depression) in all serogroups, and each found a lack of significant differences between HIV-1–sero-positive subjects and HIV-1–seronegative controls with respect to the prevalence of either lifetime or current mental disorders. The most recent study[8] found low rates of current depressive and anxiety disorders in both HIV-1–seropositive and HIV-1–seronegative subjects, concluding that HIV-1 infection per se is not associated with an increased risk of psychiatric "syndromal" disorders, although the frequency of mood changes (feeling sad, worried, or anxious) may be increased.

Despite the methodological strengths of those three

cognitive/neuropsychological, psychiatric, and neurological assessments. Confidentiality was strictly maintained: forms that linked personal identifiers and data were available only to the principal investigator of each center, and these forms were kept in a locked file.

DATA COLLECTION INSTRUMENT

The data collection instrument included six modules: (1) sociodemographic survey, (2) cognitive/neuropsychological assessment, (3) psychiatric assessment, (4) neurological assessment, (5) medical assessment, and (6) laboratory tests. The sociodemographic survey collected information on sex, age, education level, present work status, language, and HIV-1 at-risk group (if any). The psychiatric module is described below in this article, whereas the cognitive/neuropsychological and neurological modules are presented in the accompanying article.[9] The medical assessment included (1) a physical examination and a questionnaire on subjective symptoms (collecting information sufficient for staging of HIV-1 infection according to the CDC) and (2) a general medical history (collecting information on past and recent medical diseases, use of prescribed medications, alcohol and drug abuse, and time at first diagnosis of HIV-1 infection or AIDS). The laboratory test module collected the results of HIV-1 serological tests, CD4 and CD8 counts, VDRL, and specific diagnostic tests, as appropriate.

PSYCHIATRIC ASSESSMENT

The module used for psychiatric assessment included (1) the sections for psychotic, affective, and anxiety disorders of the Composite International Diagnostic Interview,[12] a structured interview that incorporates algorithms for psychiatric diagnosis according to the *International Classification of Diseases, 10th Revision*[13] (*ICD-10*), and *DSM-III-R*[7]; (2) the 18-item version[14] of the Brief Psychiatric Rating Scale[15] (BPRS); and (3) the Montgomery-Asberg Depression Rating Scale[16] (MADRS). We preferred the MADRS to the Hamilton Rating Scale for Depression[17] because the former is less loaded with somatic items that may generate equivocal results in HIV-1–infected subjects.[18] We did not find a rating scale for anxiety with the same characteristics, so we did not use any specific scale for anxiety symptoms.

The training of the psychiatrists of the participating centers in the use of the above-mentioned instruments took place in Atlanta in November and December 1989. All the researchers received formal training in the use of the Composite International Diagnostic Interview, according to the training manual developed by the WHO.[19] Moreover, they were trained in the administration of the two rating scales by the discussion of a series of live and videotaped examinations of HIV-1–seropositive subjects presenting with psychiatric symptoms or signs.

After the training, the intracenter and intercenter reliability in the use of the two rating scales was evaluated by the joint independent assessment of a further series of live and videotaped psychiatric interviews. The satisfactory results of this assessment have been reported in a previous article.[20]

ANALYSIS OF PSYCHIATRIC DATA

The asymptomatic and symptomatic HIV-1–seropositive subjects assessed in each center were compared separately with HIV-1–seronegative controls with respect to the prevalence of individual current (ie, past month) and lifetime (not including current) psychiatric diagnoses according to *ICD-10* and *DSM-III-R*, with the mean scores on the individual items of the BPRS and the MADRS, and with the mean global scores on the same scales. Comparisons were made by using the Scheffé test for continuous measures and the χ^2 test (with a Bonferroni correction for multiple testing) for categorical measures. Within each center, the effect of the interaction sex×serogroup on the global score of each rating scale was assessed by two-way analysis of variance. The same analysis was performed in Munich (the only center where all the main groups at risk for HIV-1 infection were substantially represented) to test the effect on the above-mentioned global scores of the interaction risk group×serogroup (subjects belonging to more than one at-risk group were excluded from the analysis). Within each center and each serogroup, correlations between global scores on rating scales and the CD4 count were explored by the Pearson coefficient.

investigations, it is obvious that their results cannot be generalized to the broad population of persons with HIV-1 infection. Not only were the subject samples not representative of that population from the sociodemographic viewpoint, but in two of the studies[5,8] they were recruited by newspaper advertisements and talks to specific community groups, whereas in the other one[2] the recruitment methods were not specified. Moreover, only one of the studies[2] covered all the stages of HIV-1 infection, and with very small sample sizes.

Concerns about the generalizability of the currently available information on the psychiatric, as well as the neuropsychological and the neurological, complications of HIV-1 infection have prompted the implementation of the WHO Neuropsychiatric AIDS Study. This is a research project that aims to assess the prevalence and the natural history of the above-mentioned complications in the five geographic areas that are predominantly affected by the HIV-1 epidemic (sub-Saharan Africa, North America, Latin America, western Europe, and Southeast Asia), in subject samples representing the broad population of HIV-1–infected persons living in those areas with respect to sex ratio and distribution of HIV-1 at-risk groups.

The study consists of a cross-sectional phase and a longitudinal follow-up. Herein, we report on the cross-sectional phase, describing the study design and the results of the psychiatric evaluation in the present report,

Table 1. Sociodemographic Characteristics of Subjects Evaluated in European, American, African, and Asian Centers*

	Munich, Germany			São Paulo, Brazil		
	HIV-1– (n=67)	A/HIV-1+ (n=42)	S/HIV-1+ (n=74)	HIV-1– (n=77)	A/HIV-1+ (n=55)	S/HIV-1+ (n=46)
Sex, % M	80.6	85.7	89.2	70.1	70.9	80.4
Age, y†	32.6±6.7	32.1±6.2	35.7±7.4	29.7±7.5	28.5±7.4	34.2±7.5
Education, y†	13.6±3.5	12.1±3.9	12.6±3.9	9.0±3.3	7.9±3.5	9.5±4.9
HIV-1 at-risk group (if any), %‡						
Homosexuals/bisexuals	22.4	21.4	29.7	45.4	50.9	58.7
IV drug users	10.4	16.7	14.9	7.8	10.9	10.9
Blood recipients	22.4	28.6	32.4	0	1.8	4.4

*HIV-1 indicates human immunodeficiency virus type 1; HIV-1–, HIV type 1–seronegative subjects; A/HIV-1+, asymptomatic HIV type 1–seropositive subjects; S/HIV-1+, symptomatic HIV type 1–seropositive subjects; and IV, intravenous.

†Data are given as mean±SD.

‡Some subjects belonging to two at-risk groups are counted twice.

Table 2. Background Medical and Immunological Information on Subjects Evaluated in European, American, African, and Asian Centers*

	Munich, Germany			São Paulo, Brazil		
	HIV-1– (n=67)	A/HIV-1+ (n=42)	S/HIV-1+ (n=74)	HIV-1– (n=77)	A/HIV-1+ (n=55)	S/HIV-1+ (n=46)
Medical history, %						
History of head traumas†	0	0	0	1.3	1.9	4.7
History of malaria†	0	0	0	0	0	2.2
History of syphilis†	1.5	7.1	8.1	0	9.1	8.7
Current alcohol abuse, %†	0	0	0	2.6	1.9	2.2
Current use of opiates, amphetamines, or nonprescribed sedatives, %	1.5	2.4	2.7	1.3	1.8	2.2
Current use of prescribed medications, %						
Zidovudine	0	2.4	47.3‡	0	0	4.3
Antidepressants	0	0	0	3.9	1.8	2.2
Antipsychotics	0	2.4	0	2.6	1.8	0
Anxiolytics	0	0	0	3.9	3.6	2.2
Immunological measures, mean±SD						
CD4 count, $\times 10^9$/L	1.08±0.23	0.62±0.16	0.20±0.16§	0.83±0.21	0.50±0.22	0.35±0.37§
CD4/CD8 ratio	1.8±0.5	0.8±0.4	0.5±1.9§	1.4±0.3	0.9±0.3	0.7±0.6§

*HIV-1 indicates human immunodeficiency virus type 1; HIV-1–, HIV type 1–seronegative subjects; A/HIV-1+, asymptomatic HIV type 1–seropositive subjects; and S/HIV-1+, symptomatic HIV type 1–seropositive subjects.

†See text for definitions.

‡Significant overall intracenter differences among serogroups: $P<.001$ (by χ^2 test).

§Significant overall intracenter differences among serogroups: $P<.0001$ (by analysis of variance).

||Significant overall intracenter differences among serogroups: $P<.001$ (by analysis of variance).

and the neuropsychological and neurological findings in an accompanying article.[9]

RESULTS

SOCIODEMOGRAPHIC AND MEDICAL CHARACTERISTICS OF THE SAMPLE

The sociodemographic characteristics of the subjects evaluated in the five centers are summarized in **Table 1**. There was no significant intracenter difference among the three serogroups, as expected on the basis of the study design. The samples collected in the centers were obviously different as to sex ratio and mean education level, whereas they were very similar with respect to mean age. Homosexuals/bisexuals, intravenous (IV) drug users, and blood recipients were almost absent in the African centers, whereas they were all substantially represented in Munich. Homosexuals/bisexuals were the predominant group in São Paulo, while the sample assessed in Bangkok was almost completely composed of IV drug users.

Kinshasa, Zaire			Nairobi, Kenya			Bangkok, Thailand		
HIV-1– (n=85)	A/HIV-1+ (n=52)	S/HIV-1+ (n=68)	HIV-1– (n=65)	A/HIV-1+ (n=66)	S/HIV-1+ (n=72)	HIV-1– (n=59)	A/HIV-1+ (n=89)	S/HIV-1+ (n=38)
56.5	63.5	51.5	75.4	63.6	66.7	88.1	86.4	86.8
33.9±7.8	32.3±7.6	33.8±7.6	30.0±8.6	30.7±8.6	33.2±9.6	31.4±6.3	28.4±6.8	30.7±6.9
10.8±2.4	9.6±2.4	9.9±2.7	8.2±2.6	7.1±3.9	7.1±3.6	8.6±3.4	8.4±3.5	8.8±4.2
1.2	3.8	0	3.0	0	4.2	5.3	7.9	7.9
0	0	0	1.5	0	1.4	81.4	75.3	73.7
4.7	1.9	5.9	1.5	6.1	6.9	0	3.4	2.7

Kinshasa, Zaire			Nairobi, Kenya			Bangkok, Thailand		
HIV-1– (n=85)	A/HIV-1+ (n=52)	S/HIV-1+ (n=68)	HIV-1– (n=68)	A/HIV-1+ (n=66)	S/HIV-1+ (n=72)	HIV-1– (n=59)	A/HIV-1+ (n=89)	S/HIV-1+ (n=38)
0	0	0	0	3.0	2.8	8.5	9.0	7.9
97.6	96.2	98.5	72.3	84.8	91.5	3.4	1.1	2.7
1.2	0	0	12.5	19.7	20.0	1.7	1.1	10.5
1.2	0	0	1.5	1.5	6.9	0	0	0
0	0	0	1.5	7.6	5.6	81.4	75.3	73.7
0	0	0	0	0	3.2	0	0	7.9
0	1.9	0	0	0	1.4	1.7	2.2	0
0	1.9	0	0	0	0	1.7	0	0
16.7	17.3	33.8	0	1.5	2.9	43.9	26.1	40.0
1.15±0.37	0.55±0.27	0.28±0.27§	0.86±0.43	0.58±0.34	0.38±0.71‖	1.00±0.41	0.64±0.41	0.46±0.35‖
1.2±0.6	0.3±0.2	0.2±0.2§	1.1±0.4	0.5±0.4	0.4±1.0§	1.1±0.5	0.6±0.3	0.5±0.3‖

These sociodemographic characteristics are consistent, as expected on the basis of the study design, with those of the whole population of HIV-1–seropositive persons living in the relevant geographic areas (as reported by the WHO[10]), with the only exception the high proportion of blood recipients in Munich (due to the specific interest in problems of HIV-1–infected hemophiliacs of some research groups at the University of Munich, which prompted many subjects belonging to this at-risk group to refer to that center).

The percentage of patients fulfilling CDC criteria for AIDS, within the group of symptomatic HIV-1–seropositive subjects, was 40.5% in Munich, 41.3% in São Paulo, 36.8% in Kinshasa, 41.7% in Nairobi, and 26.3% in Bangkok. There were three cases of central nervous system opportunistic infections in Munich (all of them of cerebral toxoplasmosis), four in São Paulo (two of cerebral toxoplasmosis and two of cryptococcal meningitis), two in Kinshasa (both of cryptococcal meningitis), and none in Nairobi and Bangkok.

As shown in **Table 2**, a history of head traumas causing loss of consciousness and requiring hospital-

Table 3. Prevalence of Current Mental Disorders in Subjects Evaluated in European, American, African, and Asian Centers*

	Munich, Germany			São Paulo, Brazil		
	HIV-1− (n=67)	A/HIV-1+ (n=42)	S/HIV-1+ (n=74)	HIV-1− (n=77)	A/HIV-1+ (n=55)	S/HIV-1+ (n=46)
ICD-10 diagnosis, %						
Acute schizophrenialike psychotic disorder	0	0	0	0	0	2.2
Depressive episode	0	4.8	4.0	7.8	10.9	19.6
Dysthymia	1.5	0	2.7	1.3	1.8	2.2
Generalized anxiety disorder	0	0	0	0	1.8	2.2
Any mental disorder†	1.5	4.8	6.7	9.1	14.7	26.2‡
DSM-III-R diagnosis, %						
Schizophreniform disorder	0	0	0	0	0	2.2
Major depressive episode	0	4.8	4.0	7.8	10.9	17.4
Dysthymia	0	0	2.7	1.3	0	2.2
Generalized anxiety disorder	0	0	0	0	1.8	2.2
Any mental disorder†	0	4.8	6.7	9.1	12.7	24.0‡

**HIV-1 indicates human immunodeficiency virus type 1; HIV-1−, HIV type 1–seronegative subjects; A/HIV-1+, asymptomatic HIV type 1–seropositive subjects; S/H symptomatic HIV type 1–seropositive subjects; and* ICD-10, International Classification of Diseases, 10th Revision.

†*Among those covered by the sections for psychotic, affective, and anxiety disorders of the Composite International Diagnostic Interview.*

‡*Significant differences (symptomatic seropositive vs seronegative subjects):* $P<.05$.

§*Significant differences (symptomatic seropositive vs seronegative subjects):* $P<.01$.

Table 4. Prevalence of Lifetime (Excluding Current) Mental Disorders in Subjects Evaluated in European, American, African, and Asian Ce

	Munich, Germany			São Paulo, Brazil		
	HIV-1− (n=67)	A/HIV-1+ (n=42)	S/HIV-1+ (n=74)	HIV-1− (n=77)	A/HIV-1+ (n=55)	S/HIV-1+ (n=46)
ICD-10 diagnosis, %						
Schizophrenia	0	0	0	0	0	0
Acute schizophrenialike psychotic disorder	0	0	0	0	1.8	2.2
Bipolar affective disorder	0	0	0	0	0	0
Depressive episode/recurrent depressive disorder	3.0	4.8	5.4	19.5	21.8	26.1
Dysthymia	1.5	0	2.7	1.3	1.8	2.2
Panic disorder	0	0	0	0	0	0
Generalized anxiety disorder	1.5	2.4	1.3	3.9	5.4	6.5
Any mental disorder†	6.0	7.2	9.4	24.7	30.8	37.0
DSM-III-R diagnosis, %						
Schizophrenia	0	0	0	0	0	0
Schizophreniform disorder	0	0	0	0	1.8	2.2
Bipolar disorder	0	0	0	0	0	0
Major depression	1.5	4.8	5.4	15.6	18.2	21.7
Dysthymia	0	0	2.7	1.3	0	2.2
Panic disorder	0	0	0	0	0	0
Generalized anxiety disorder	1.5	2.4	1.3	3.9	5.4	6.5
Any mental disorder†	3.0	7.2	9.4	20.8	25.4	32.6

**HIV-1 indicates human immunodeficiency virus type 1; HIV-1−, HIV-1 type 1–seronegative subjects; A/HIV-1+, asymptomatic HIV type 1–seropositive subjects; S symptomatic HIV type 1–seropositive subjects; and* ICD-10, International Classification of Diseases, 10th Revision.

†*Among those covered by the sections for psychotic, affective, and anxiety disorders of the Composite International Diagnostic Interview.*

ization was absent or rare in all the centers (with the partial exception of Bangkok), as was current alcohol abuse (defined as the consumption of at least five alcoholic beverages per day during the last month). A previous diagnosis of malaria (made by a physician) was very frequent in the African centers (actually, almost all subjects recruited in Kinshasa had suffered from this disease). A previous diagnosis of syphilis (made by a physician) was more common in HIV-1–seropositive subjects than in HIV-1–seronegative per-

Kinshasa, Zaire			Nairobi, Kenya			Bangkok, Thailand		
HIV-1− (n=85)	A/HIV-1+ (n=52)	S/HIV-1+ (n=68)	HIV-1− (n=65)	A/HIV-1+ (n=66)	S/HIV-1+ (n=72)	HIV-1− (n=59)	A/HIV-1+ (n=89)	S/HIV-1+ (n=38)
0	0	0	0	0	0	0	0	0
0	0	4.4	0	3.0	5.5	3.4	10.1	21.0‡
1.2	0	0	0	1.5	0	0	1.1	0
0	1.9	1.5	0	0	1.4	0	0	2.6
1.2	1.9	5.9	0	4.5	7.1	3.4	11.2	23.6§
0	0	0	0	0	0	0	0	0
0	0	4.4	0	3.0	5.5	1.7	9.0	18.4§
1.2	0	0	0	1.5	0	0	0	0
0	1.9	1.5	0	0	1.4	0	0	0
1.2	1.9	5.9	0	4.5	6.9	1.7	9.0	18.4‡

Kinshasa, Zaire			Nairobi, Kenya			Bangkok, Thailand		
HIV-1− (n=85)	A/HIV-1+ (n=52)	S/HIV-1+ (n=68)	HIV-1− (n=65)	A/HIV-1+ (n=66)	S/HIV-1+ (n=72)	HIV-1− (n=59)	A/HIV-1+ (n=89)	S/HIV-1+ (n=38)
0	0	0	0	0	0	0	1.1	0
0	0	0	0	0	0	0	0	2.6
0	0	0	0	0	0	0	0	2.6
2.3	3.8	7.3	4.6	7.5	11.1	16.9	22.5	26.3
1.2	0	0	0	1.5	0	0	1.1	0
1.2	1.9	1.5	0	0	0	0	0	0
0	1.9	1.5	1.5	1.5	1.4	0	0	2.6
4.7	7.6	10.3	6.1	10.5	12.5	16.9	24.7	34.1
0	0	0	0	0	0	0	0	0
0	0	0	0	0	0	0	0	2.6
0	0	0	0	0	0	0	0	2.6
2.3	3.8	7.3	4.6	6.1	9.7	13.6	21.3	23.7
1.2	0	0	0	1.5	0	0	0	0
1.2	1.9	1.5	0	0	0	0	0	0
0	1.9	1.5	1.5	1.5	1.4	0	0	0
4.7	7.6	10.3	6.1	9.1	11.1	13.6	21.3	28.9

sons in four of five centers, but the difference was never statistically significant.

About half of symptomatic HIV-1–seropositive subjects recruited in Munich were receiving treatment with zidovudine at the time of the assessment, whereas this drug was rarely used in the other centers. Prescribed psychotropic medications were taken by very few subjects (with the only exception benzodiazepines, used by a substantial proportion of individuals in Bangkok and Kinshasa, mainly at low doses, for the management of sleep disturbances).

Table 5. Mean Scores on the MADRS in Subjects Evaluated in European, American, African, and Asian Centers*

	Munich, Germany			São Paulo, Brazil		
	HIV-1– (n=67)	A/HIV-1+ (n=42)	S/HIV-1+ (n=74)	HIV-1– (n=77)	A/HIV-1+ (n=55)	S/HIV-1+ (n=46)
Apparent sadness	0.3±0.6	0.5±0.6	1.3±1.0†	0.7±1.0	0.9±1.1	1.6±1.3‡
Reported sadness	0.4±0.6	0.7±1.0	1.6±1.4†	0.9±1.3	1.0±1.2	1.5±1.4
Inner tension	0.4±0.5	0.5±0.7	0.8±0.9	0.9±1.2	1.1±1.1	1.4±1.2
Reduced sleep	0.6±0.8	0.7±1.0	1.3±1.4†	0.7±1.4	0.8±1.4	1.7±1.7‡
Reduced appetite	0.3±0.3	0.4±0.6	0.9±1.0†	0.5±1.0	0.7±1.0	1.6±1.7†
Concentration difficulties	0.4±0.5	0.5±0.7	1.1±1.3†	1.0±1.4	1.0±1.2	1.6±1.6‡
Lassitude	0.3±0.3	0.4±0.5	0.9±0.9†	0.7±1.1	0.6±1.1	1.7±1.4†
Inability to feel	0.3±0.1	0.5±0.4	1.2±0.9†	0.7±1.2	0.9±1.1	1.3±1.5‡
Pessimistic thoughts	0.2±0.4	0.3±0.9	0.7±1.1‡	0.8±1.3	1.0±1.5	1.6±1.7‡
Suicidal thoughts	0.1±0.1	0.2±0.7	0.6±0.9‡	0.2±0.7	0.6±1.2	0.8±1.2‡
Global score	3.0±4.1	4.1±5.9	10.3±7.7†	7.8±9.1	8.7±9.6	14.9±10.3†

**MADRS indicates Montgomery-Asberg Depression Rating Scale; HIV, human immunodeficiency virus; HIV-1–, HIV type 1–seronegative subjects; A/HIV-1+, asymptomatic HIV type 1–seropositive subjects; S/HIV-1+, symptomatic HIV type 1–seropositive subjects. All values are mean±SD.*

†Significant differences (symptomatic seropositive vs seronegative subjects): P<.01.

‡Significant differences (symptomatic seropositive vs seronegative subjects): P<.05.

Finally, the expected intracenter differences among serogroups were found with respect to immunological measures (Table 2).

PSYCHIATRIC FINDINGS

The overall prevalence of current mental disorders was significantly higher in symptomatic (but not in asymptomatic) HIV-1–seropositive subjects, compared with seronegative controls, in Bangkok and São Paulo. This difference remained significant when the analysis was restricted to IV drug users in the former center (21.4% vs 2.1%, $P<.01$) and to homosexuals/bisexuals in the latter (33.3% vs 5.7%, $P<.01$). Within the other three sites, the difference between symptomatic seropositive and seronegative persons only approached statistical significance (**Table 3**).

The only individual diagnoses for which the current prevalence was significantly increased in symptomatic seropositive subjects compared with controls were those of *ICD-10* depressive episode and *DSM-III-R* major depression in the Bangkok center. This increase remained significant when the analysis was restricted to the group of IV drug users (17.8% vs 2.1%, $P<.05$). No diagnosis had an increased current prevalence in asymptomatic seropositive persons in any center (Table 3).

The overall prevalence of lifetime mental disorders was not significantly increased in either symptomatic or asymptomatic HIV-1–seropositive subjects, compared with controls, in any center. No individual diagnosis had an increased lifetime prevalence in either group of seropositive subjects. Bangkok and São Paulo were the centers with the highest rates of lifetime mental disorders in all serogroups, mainly due to the high prevalence of major depression (**Table 4**). More precisely, the highest prevalence of lifetime mental disorders was found in IV drug users assessed in Bangkok (20.8% among seronegative subjects, 28.3% among asymptomatic seropositive persons, and 35.7% among symptomatic seropositive subjects) and in homosexuals/bisexuals evaluated in São Paulo (17.1% in seronegative subjects, 21.4% in asymptomatic seropositive individuals, and 29.6% in symptomatic seropositive subjects).

No significant sex difference was observed in any center and within any serogroup with respect to the overall prevalence of either current or lifetime mental disorders.

Symptomatic HIV-1–seropositive subjects had consistently higher mean scores on the MADRS compared with those of seronegative controls: of 50 item comparisons in the five centers, 44 showed a significant difference between the two groups, and the mean global score was always significantly increased in the former. Only two significant differences on individual items (both in Bangkok) were observed between physically asymptomatic HIV-1–seropositive subjects and controls (**Table 5**). The mean MADRS global score was significantly higher in women than in men among symptomatic HIV-1–seropositive subjects who were assessed in Kinshasa ($P<.05$) and in Munich ($P<.001$). No significant sex difference in this respect was found among either HIV-1–seronegative or asymptomatic HIV-1–seropositive persons in any center. The effect of the sex×serogroup interaction on the MADRS global score was found to be significant in Munich ($F=10.6$, $df=2$, $P<.0001$). In this center, the effect of the interaction risk group×serogroup did not reach statistical significance. The correlation between the MADRS global score and the CD4 count was significant only in symptomatic seropositive subjects assessed in Kinshasa and Munich ($P<.01$).

Kinshasa, Zaire			Nairobi, Kenya			Bangkok, Thailand		
HIV-1− (n=85)	A/HIV-1+ (n=52)	S/HIV-1+ (n=68)	HIV-1− (n=65)	A/HIV-1+ (n=66)	S/HIV-1+ (n=72)	HIV-1− (n=59)	A/HIV-1+ (n=89)	S/HIV-1+ (n=38)
0.3±0.8	0.5±1.3	1.3±1.5†	0.3±0.8	0.7±1.2	1.5±1.7†	0.3±0.8	1.4±1.1‡	2.1±1.4†
0.5±1.2	0.9±1.5	1.9±1.7†	0.3±1.0	0.7±1.5	1.5±1.6†	0.5±0.9	1.3±1.2‡	2.1±1.5†
0.1±0.3	0.1±0.5	0.3±0.8	0.2±0.8	0.3±0.9	0.8±1.3‡	0.5±1.0	0.5±1.0	1.1±1.3‡
0.2±1.0	0.1±0.5	0.9±1.7‡	0.6±1.5	1.1±1.8	1.9±2.1†	0.7±1.4	0.8±1.3	2.9±1.9†
0.5±1.5	0.5±1.4	1.8±2.1†	0.3±1.0	0.8±1.6	1.7±2.0†	0.3±0.8	0.7±1.2	1.5±1.7†
0.2±0.7	0.3±1.0	1.2±1.7†	0.3±1.1	0.3±0.9	1.2±1.7†	0.5±1.0	0.4±0.9	0.6±1.1
0.2±0.9	0.6±1.4	1.7±1.8†	0.3±1.0	0.6±1.3	1.5±1.8†	0.5±1.0	0.5±1.1	0.8±1.3
0.2±0.9	0.4±1.3	1.1±1.7†	0.4±1.0	0.5±1.2	1.2±1.7†	0.2±0.6	0.2±0.7	0.5±1.2
0.1±0.7	0.5±1.2	0.7±1.3‡	0.2±0.8	0.3±1.0	1.2±1.6†	0.2±0.8	0.5±1.0	1.5±1.2‡
0.1±0.6	0.3±0.9	0.3±0.9‡	0.2±0.7	0.1±0.4	0.7±1.2‡	0.4±0.9	0.4±1.0	1.2±1.7‡
2.4±4.9	4.3±7.7	11.5±10.7†	3.3±7.9	5.5±9.0	10.1±13.4†	4.1±6.8	6.8±6.9	13.3±9.9†

The mean BPRS global score and the mean scores on the BPRS items "somatic concern," "anxiety," and "depressed mood" were significantly increased in symptomatic but not in asymptomatic HIV-1–seropositive subjects, compared with those in seronegative controls, in all the centers (data available on request). In the Munich center, the mean BPRS global score was significantly higher in women than in men among symptomatic HIV-1–seropositive subjects ($P<.05$), and the effect of the interaction sex×serogroup was significant ($F=3.4$, $df=2$, $P<.05$). The effect of the interaction risk group×serogroup was not significant.

COMMENT

STUDY DESIGN

To our knowledge, the WHO Neuropsychiatric AIDS Study is the first investigation focusing on the psychiatric, neuropsychological, and neurological complications of HIV-1 infection that presents simultaneously the following characteristics: (1) being carried out in all the geographic areas significantly affected by the HIV-1 epidemic, (2) being conducted on subject samples that represent the broad population of HIV-1–infected persons living in the abovementioned areas with respect to sex ratio and distribution of HIV-1 at-risk groups, and (3) using standardized assessment instruments with high intercenter reliability.

Contrary to many previous investigations carried out in this research field, the WHO study did not rely on advertisements or contacts with specific communities for subject recruitment. Subjects were consecutively recruited from outpatient units to which they had referred for medical advice. This recruitment modality, besides being by far the most feasible in developing countries, is, in our opinion, less prejudicial to the representativeness of enrolled samples than self-selection (especially when the latter mostly involves people belonging to community organizations who are likely to be less vulnerable to psychiatric problems[8]). Of course, a limitation involved in the recruitment procedure adopted in the present study is the exclusion of the most severe cases of AIDS, which are unlikely to be seen in outpatient units.

HIV-1–seronegative controls were recruited from the same clinics where HIV-1–seropositive persons were enrolled. This ensured comparability of the groups with respect to socioeconomic background, medical history, and at-risk behaviors, and it helped to maintain the blindness of the investigators to the subjects' serostatus (blindness is obviously very difficult to preserve when probands and controls are recruited from different sources).

Very few exclusion criteria were adopted in the study. We only excluded subjects who were lacking in the minimum arithmetic skills necessary to perform neuropsychological tests and those who were aged younger than 18 years (to simplify consent procedures). Illiteracy, current alcohol or drug abuse, a history of head injury requiring hospitalization, or a history of other infectious diseases possibly affecting the central nervous system were not exclusion criteria. Indeed, some of the abovementioned conditions (illiteracy, drug abuse, or a history of other infectious diseases possibly affecting the central nervous system) were too frequent in some of our centers to be excluded without impairing the representativeness of the collected samples, whereas some others (alcohol abuse, history of head injury requiring hospitalization) were so rare as to be easily controlled for in statistical analysis.

The assessment of each subject took place in three sessions. This was necessary to (1) avoid overrecruitment of HIV-1–seronegative individuals (in the second session, after disclosure of HIV-1 serostatus, only HIV-1–seronegative subjects suitable for matching to already recruited HIV-1–seropositive persons were definitively enrolled) and (2) introduce an interval between notification of test results and psychiatric assessment.

PSYCHIATRIC FINDINGS

The results of the psychiatric assessment carried out in the present cross-sectional phase of the WHO Neuropsychiatric AIDS Study diverge in part from those obtained in the three previous investigations[2,5,8] that adopted a structured diagnostic interview and operational diagnostic criteria. The main discrepancy concerns the overall prevalence of current mental disorders that was significantly increased in symptomatic HIV-1–seropositive persons, compared with seronegative controls, in two of five centers in the present study, whereas it did not differ significantly between HIV-1–seropositive and HIV-1–seronegative subjects in the three investigations mentioned above. This discordance is probably in part explained by the different recruitment procedures that were adopted: in two of the previous studies mentioned above,[5,8] the assessed subjects were volunteers, mostly involved in formal or informal support groups (thus representing a self-selected sample of persons whose vulnerability to psychiatric problems was likely to be reduced[8]), whereas in our investigation subjects were consecutively enrolled from outpatient medical units. Differences in the time lapse occurring between notification of serostatus and psychiatric assessment may also have been of importance (see below). Furthermore, it is important to stress that the comparison between our data and those obtained in the three studies mentioned above[2,5,8] is hampered by the fact that in the second of those investigations[5] all the assessed seropositive subjects were asymptomatic, whereas in the third,[8] data concerning symptomatic and asymptomatic seropositive subjects were pooled.

THE CURRENTLY predominant view[2,5,8,21] that some behaviors at risk for HIV-1 infection are associated with high rates of psychiatric syndromes, independent from the occurrence of the infection, was supported by the findings from the present study, which found the highest overall prevalence of lifetime mental disorders within all serogroups among IV drug users assessed in Bangkok and homosexuals/bisexuals evaluated in São Paulo. We also observed, however, that within the last two subject samples, the prevalence of current mental disorders was significantly increased in symptomatic HIV-1–seropositive persons compared with HIV-1–seronegative controls. Unfortunately, we could not perform a systematic comparison of risk groups within each of the centers because in most of them, some of the groups were insufficiently represented. Moreover, due to the lack of information for most subjects about the length of infection before enrollment, we could not assess what proportion of HIV-1–associated psychiatric syndromes was a reactivation of mental disorders whose onset preceded the occurrence of the infection.

We made an attempt to evaluate, in our subject samples, the prevalence of adjustment disorders, but we finally gave up the effort, for the following reasons: (1) the Composite International Diagnostic Interview, in its original validated version, does not include specific questions for those disorders, and it does not incorporate algorithms for the relevant diagnosis according to either *ICD-10* or *DSM-III-R;* and (2) it is extremely difficult, in HIV-1–seropositive subjects, to distinguish adjustment disorders from "physiological" stress reactions. Actually, the present formulation of the diagnostic criteria for adjustment disorders, in both *ICD-10* and *DSM-III-R,* is such that any subsyndromal constellation of depressive or anxiety symptoms or signs, if associated with an obvious stressor such as HIV-1 infection or disease, may justify such a diagnosis.

The other major discrepancy between the results of our study and those of the most recent of the American investigations mentioned above[8] concerns the prevalence of depressive symptoms and signs in HIV-1–seropositive subjects. In our symptomatic seropositive subjects, the significant increase of the MADRS global score was a consistent finding across the centers, whereas in the previous study mentioned above, the mean global score on the Hamilton Rating Scale for Depression was not significantly increased in seropositive subjects compared with seronegative persons. The following explanations of this inconsistency can be proposed: (1) the different structure of the adopted rating scales; (2) the fact that the sample of seropositive subjects described by Williams et al[8] actually included both symptomatic and asymptomatic subjects (although the former represented 60.5% of the sample); (3) the above-mentioned differences in the recruitment procedures; and (4) the different time lapse occurring in the two studies between notification of serostatus and psychiatric assessment (in the study by Williams et al,[8] 90% of subjects had been aware of their serostatus for at least 3 months before the evaluation, whereas in our investigation, most subjects—85.9% in Kinshasa, 77.9% in Nairobi, 51.1% in Bangkok, 48.3% in São Paulo, and 34.4% in Munich—did not know their serostatus at the time of study entry, so that the interval between notification and psychiatric assessment was 1 month).

The significant effect of the interaction sex×serogroup on the MADRS global score in Munich is an intriguing finding, which, however, should be verified by investigations specifically focusing on sex differences in the psychological impact of HIV-1 infection.

On the whole, the results of the psychiatric evaluation performed within the cross-sectional phase of the WHO Neuropsychiatric AIDS Study suggest that the significance of the psychopathological complications of symptomatic HIV-1 infection may have been underestimated by previous studies carried out on self-selected samples of well-educated, middle-class, mostly white homosexual men. Depressive symptoms and signs and even a syndromal diagnosis of major depression are probably not a rare occurrence in CDC group IV subjects. Moreover, the fact that only two of our 22 subjects who fulfilled *DSM-III-R* criteria for major depression were receiving antidepressant treatment at the time of the assessment indicates that this syndrome frequently goes unnoticed and untreated. This is a finding on which clinicians dealing with HIV-1–seropositive persons should probably reflect.

Accepted for publication December 29, 1992.

The authors are indebted to Josè Esparza, MD, David Heymann, MD, Susan Holck, MD, and Roy Widdus, MD, Global Programme on AIDS, World Health Organization, Geneva, Switzerland, for their help and advice. Moreover, they would like to thank Constantin Gatsonis, PhD, Harvard University, Boston, Mass, and Justin McArthur, MD, The Johns Hopkins University, Baltimore, Md, for their collaboration in setting up the design of the study, and Hans-Ulrich Wittchen, PhD, Max-Planck Institute, Munich, Germany, for his help in training the researchers in the use of the Composite International Diagnostic Interview. The study was carried out in the centers with the help of the following researchers (besides those mentioned among the authors of the accompanying article): N. Karnjanathanalers, MD, S. Piyasirisilp, MD, T. Hemachudha, MD, J. Suttipan, MD, P. Worakul, MD, N. Suwanwela, MD, M. Harnvanich, MD, P. Phanuphak, MD, and A. Sughondhabirom, MD, Bangkok, Thailand; J. Perriens, MD, Y. Mukadi, MD, K. Tshala, MD, and I. Lebughe, MD, Kinshasa, Zaire; H. Hippius, MD, and C. Perro, MD, Munich, Germany; R. N. Kang'ethe, MD, M. B. Sebit, MD, J. M. Mburu, MD, P. A. Kigamwa, MD, and M. G. Lukwago, MD, Nairobi, Kenya; and C. A. Bolcato, PhD, J. Valença, MD, H. H. Campos, PhD, N. M. Oliveira, MD, G. Filelini, MD, and J. Suleiman, MD, São Paulo, Brazil.

Reprint requests to Division of Mental Health, World Health Organization, 1211 Geneva 27, Switzerland (Dr Maj).

REFERENCES

1. Global Programme on AIDS. *Current and Future Dimensions of the HIV/AIDS Pandemic: A Capsule Summary (January 1992).* Geneva, Switzerland: World Health Organization; 1992.
2. Atkinson JH, Grant I, Kennedy CJ, Richman DD, Spector SA, McCutchan JA. Prevalence of psychiatric disorders among men infected with human immunodeficiency virus: a controlled study. *Arch Gen Psychiatry.* 1988;45:859-864.
3. Robins LN, Helzer JE, Croughan J, Williams JVW, Spitzer RL. *NIMH Diagnostic Interview Schedule: Version III (May 1981).* Rockville, Md: National Institute of Mental Health; 1981.
4. American Psychiatric Association. *Diagnostic and Statistical Manual of Mental Disorders, Third Edition.* Washington, DC: American Psychiatric Association; 1980.
5. Perry S, Jacobsberg LB, Fishman B, Frances A, Bobo J, Kaplan Jacobsberg B. Psychiatric diagnosis before serological testing for the human immunodeficiency virus. *Am J Psychiatry.* 1990;147:89-93.
6. Spitzer RL, Williams JVW, Gibbon M, First MB. *Structured Clinical Interview for* DSM-III-R *(SCID).* New York, NY: New York State Psychiatric Institute; 1987.
7. American Psychiatric Association. *Diagnostic and Statistical Manual of Mental Disorders, Revised Third Edition.* Washington, DC: American Psychiatric Association; 1987.
8. Williams JVW, Rabkin JG, Remien RH, Gorman JM, Ehrhardt AA. Multidisciplinary baseline assessment of homosexual men with and without human immunodeficiency virus infection, II: standardized clinical assessment of current and lifetime psychopathology. *Arch Gen Psychiatry.* 1991;48:124-130.
9. Maj M, Satz P, Janssen R, Zaudig M, Starace F, D'Elia L, Sughondhabirom B, Mussa M, Naber D, Ndetei D, Schulte G, Sartorius N. WHO Neuropsychiatric AIDS Study, cross-sectional phase II: neuropsychological and neurological findings. *Arch Gen Psychiatry.* 1993;51:51-61.
10. Global Programme on AIDS. *Current and Future Dimensions of the HIV/AIDS Pandemic: A Capsule Summary (September 1990).* Geneva, Switzerland: World Health Organization; 1990.
11. Centers for Diseases Control. CDC classification system for HIV infection and revised case definition for AIDS. *MMWR Morb Mortal Wkly Rep.* 1986;35:334-339.
12. World Health Organization. *Composite International Diagnostic Interview (CIDI).* Geneva, Switzerland: World Health Organization; 1987.
13. World Health Organization. *The ICD-10 Classification of Mental and Behavioural Disorders: Clinical Descriptions and Diagnostic Guidelines.* Geneva, Switzerland: World Health Organization; 1992.
14. Hedlund JL, Vieweg BW. The Brief Psychiatric Rating Scale (BPRS): a comprehensive review. *J Operational Psychiatry.* 1980;11:48-65.
15. Overall JE, Gorham DR. The Brief Psychiatric Rating Scale. *Psychol Rep.* 1962; 10:799-812.
16. Montgomery S, Asberg M. A new depression scale designed to be sensitive to change. *Br J Psychiatry.* 1979;134:382-389.
17. Hamilton M. A rating scale for depression. *J Neurol Neurosurg Psychiatry.* 1960;23:56-62.
18. Harker JO, Satz P, Jones FD-L, Verma RC, Gan MP, Mathisen G, Poer HL, Cherninsky A. Measurement of depression and neuropsychological impairment in HIV-1 infection. *J Clin Exp Neuropsychol.* In press.
19. World Health Organization. *Composite International Diagnostic Interview (CIDI) Training Manual (Draft).* Geneva, Switzerland: World Health Organization; 1989.
20. Maj M, Janssen R, Satz P, Zaudig M, Starace F, Boor D, Sughondhabirom B, Bing E, Luabeya M, Ndetei D, Riedel R, Schulte G, Sartorius N. The World Health Organization's cross-cultural study on neuropsychiatric aspects of infection with the human immunodeficiency virus 1 (HIV-1): preparation and pilot phase. *Br J Psychiatry.* 1991;159:351-356.
21. Holland JCB, Tross S. The psychosocial and neuropsychiatric sequelae of the acquired immunodeficiency syndrome and related disorders. *Ann Intern Med.* 1985;103:760-764.

ORIGINAL ARTICLE

WHO Neuropsychiatric AIDS Study, Cross-sectional Phase II

Neuropsychological and Neurological Findings

Mario Maj, MD, PhD; Paul Satz, PhD; Robert Janssen, MD; Michael Zaudig, MD; Fabrizio Starace, MD; Lou D'Elia, PhD; Bhirom Sughondhabirom, MD; Mahamoudi Mussa, MD; Dieter Naber, MD; David Ndetei, MD; George Schulte, MD; Norman Sartorius, MD, PhD

Background: The neuropsychological and neurological complications of HIV-1 infection and AIDS were explored within the cross-sectional phase of the WHO Neuropsychiatric AIDS Study. Special attention was devoted to the controversial issue of the prevalence and clinical significance of subtle cognitive deficits in asymptomatic seropositive subjects.

Methods: A neuropsychological test battery validated for cross-cultural use, a structured interview for the diagnosis of dementia, a rating scale of functioning in daily living activities, and a neurological module were administered to representative samples of seropositive subjects and to matched seronegative controls living in the five geographic areas predominantly affected by the HIV-1 epidemic. Data are available for five centers.

Results: The prevalence of global neuropsychological impairment was significantly increased in asymptomatic seropositive subjects compared with controls in only two centers. A significant effect of education on neuropsychological performance was observed among asymptomatic seropositive individuals. In the two African centers, low-education, but not high-education, asymptomatic seropositive persons had an impaired performance. The frequency of impaired functioning in daily living activities and of neurologic abnormalities was higher in symptomatic, but not in asymptomatic, seropositive subjects compared with controls in all centers.

Conclusions: These data suggest that the risk of subtle cognitive deficits may be increased in asymptomatic stages of HIV-1 infection. However, these deficits are not associated with neurologic changes and do not seem to affect subjects' social functioning.

(Arch Gen Psychiatry. 1994;51:51-61)

From the Division of Mental Health and Global Programme on AIDS, World Health Organization, Geneva, Switzerland (Drs Maj, Starace, and Sartorius); the Department of Psychiatry I, University of Naples (Italy) (Drs Maj and Starace); the Neuropsychiatric Institute, UCLA, Los Angeles, Calif (Drs Satz and D'Elia); the Division of HIV/AIDS, Centers for Disease Control and Prevention, Atlanta, Ga (Dr Janssen); the Max-Planck Institute for Psychiatry, Munich, Germany (Dr Zaudig); the Department of Psychiatry, Chulalongkorn University, Bangkok, Thailand (Dr Sughondhabirom); the Centre of Neuropsychopathology, University of Kinshasa, and the Projet SIDA, Kinshasa, Zaire (Dr Mussa); the Department of Psychiatry, University of Munich (Germany) (Dr Naber); the Department of Psychiatry, University of Nairobi (Kenya) (Dr Ndetei); and the Emilio Ribas Hospital, São Paulo, Brazil (Dr Schulte).

SEVERAL GAPS still exist in the currently available knowledge of the neuropsychological complications of the infection produced by the human immunodeficiency virus type 1 (HIV-1).

A first controversial issue is whether subtle cognitive changes occur in a significant proportion of physically asymptomatic HIV-1–seropositive persons; in fact, although many studies[1-5] did not find any significant difference in the performance on neuropsychological tests between these subjects and matched HIV-1–seronegative controls, several others[6-10] found significant differences on measures of attention, concentration, information-processing speed, and verbal memory. The clinical significance of these possible early mild abnormalities as predictors of the future development of dementia also remains open to research; currently available evidence[11,12] suggests that HIV-1–associated cognitive dysfunction may remain stable for years, and it may even improve spontaneously in some cases,[13] but further well-designed long-term follow-up investigations, carried out on samples representative of the broad population of HIV-1–infected individuals, are clearly needed. Another set of unresolved issues concerns the relationships between HIV-1–associated cognitive impairment and the immunological, medical, neurological, and psychopathological aspects of the infection: divergent findings have been reported, for instance, concerning the correlation between neuropsychological performance and CD4

See Subjects and Methods on next page

SUBJECTS AND METHODS

SUBJECTS

The subject samples evaluated in the cross-sectional phase of the WHO Neuropsychiatric AIDS Study and the modalities of their enrollment are described in an accompanying article.[26]

COGNITIVE/NEUROPSYCHOLOGICAL ASSESSMENT

The module used for cognitive/neuropsychological assessment included (1) a brief questionnaire on subjective complaints concerning cognitive functioning (with specific items for memory, concentration, speech, and thinking); (2) a battery of neuropsychological tests (see below); (3) an adapted structured interview for the objective evaluation of cognitive performance (SIDAM[27]), which incorporates algorithms for the diagnosis of dementia according to the *International Classification of Diseases, 10th Revision (ICD-10)*[28] and *DSM-III-R*[29]; and (4) a rating scale of performance in activities of daily living (ADL), which collects information from the subject and a key informant and provides individual scores for 17 items corresponding to different ADLs, plus a global rating of disability.

The neuropsychological battery included the following tests: the Timed Gait; the Block Design subtest of the Escala de Inteligencia Wechsler para Adultos (EIWA), ie, the Spanish version of the Wechsler Adult Intelligence Scale[30]; the Digit Symbol subtest of the EIWA; the Grooved Pegboard, dominant and nondominant[31]; the Verbal Fluency Test, animals and first names[32]; the Trail Making A[33]; the WHO/UCLA Auditory Verbal Learning Test; the Color Trails 1 and 2; and the WHO/UCLA Picture Memory and Interference Test (for the last four tests, see below). The functional domains assessed by this battery are as follows: (1) motor speed/fine motor control (Timed Gait, Color Trails 1 and 2, EIWA Block Design and Digit Symbol, Grooved Pegboard, and Trail Making A); (2) sustained attention (Color Trails 1 and 2 and Trail Making A); (3) selective attention (Color Trails 2 and EIWA Digit Symbol); (4) cognitive flexibility (Color Trails 2 and EIWA Digit Symbol); (5) perceptual-motor analysis (EIWA Block Design); (6) verbal memory (WHO/UCLA Auditory Verbal Learning Test); (7) visual memory (WHO/UCLA Picture Memory and Interference Test); and (8) verbal fluency (Verbal Fluency Test, animals and first names).

The tests included in the neuropsychological battery were selected by an international committee of experts on the basis of the following criteria: (1) ability to tap the functional domains that have been claimed to be affected in symptomatic HIV-1 infection, (2) sensitivity to mild degrees of cognitive or motor dysfunction, (3) suitability for large-scale administration, and (4) suitability for use in a cross-cultural context. At the time of its first meeting (July 1989), the committee pointed out that no available test of either verbal or visual memory fulfilled all the above criteria and that the Trail Making B, which is a standard in HIV-1 research, was not suitable for cross-cultural use, due to the presence of letters and written instructions. It was decided, therefore, to develop three new tests (one of verbal memory, one of visual memory, and one replacing the Trail Making B). These tests (the WHO/UCLA Auditory Verbal Learning Test, the WHO/UCLA Picture Memory and Interference Test, and the Color Trails) were validated by a prepilot study.[34]

The WHO/UCLA Auditory Verbal Learning Test is similar to the Rey Auditory Verbal Learning Test,[35] in that it is a list-learning task. However, all of its items have been carefully selected (from categories such as parts of the body, tools, household objects, and common transportation vehicles) to be familiar to a variety of cultures.

The Color Trails 1 and 2 have been developed following the idea of the Trail Making A and B. However, to minimize cultural bias, no letters or written instructions are used in them. Both tests consist of several numbered circles colored in vivid pink or yellow: in Color Trails 1, each number is represented by only one color, whereas in Color Trails 2, each number is printed twice—once in a pink and once in a yellow circle. In Color Trails 1, the subject is instructed to draw a line between the numbered circles one after the other, following the number sequence. In Color Trails 2, the subject must maintain the sequence of numbers and alternate between pink and yellow.

The WHO/UCLA Picture Memory and Interference is a completely new test, based on a large series of line drawings representing a variety of objects familiar to most cultures. The test is presented visually with verbal instructions. It consists of four sections called Books. In Book 1, the subject is presented with a series of 20 drawings (targets) printed on 3×5-in cards. He or she is instructed to remember the target drawings. Immediately after, he or she is presented with 50 more drawings and asked to indicate, by saying yes or no, whether he or she saw each of the cards in the target group. The recognition set includes 20 original targets and 30 distractors. In Book 2, the subject is presented with 20 new targets that he or she is again instructed to remember, followed by a 50-item recognition trial. He or she is asked to identify with a yes response only those cards that were targets in Book 2. Among the 50 recognition items, there are 20 targets from Book 2, 10 new distractors, 10 old distractors from Book 1, and 10 old targets from Book 1 that now serve as distractors. In Book 3, the subject is once again presented with 20 new targets that are to be memorized, and then with another 50-item recognition trial. Again, he or she is instructed to respond with a yes only to those items that were targets in the most recent book. Among the 50 recognition items, there are now 20 targets from Book 3, 10 new distractors, five old distractors from Book 1, five old distractors from Book 2, five old targets from Book 1 that are now distractors, and five old targets from Book 2 that are now distractors. In Book 4, the subject is presented with 15 items that appeared as targets in the preceding books, and is instructed to indicate whether the item was originally seen as a target in Book 1, 2, or 3.

The researchers involved in neuropsychological assessment in all the centers were trained in the use of the test battery by means of a workshop held in Nairobi, Kenya, in March 1990. Further details on this training, as well as on the tests composing the battery, can be found in a previous article.[22]

The SIDAM was adapted for use in a cross-cultural context by amending some items (a copy of this international version is available on request from WHO headquarters). The high intercenter and intracenter reliability in the use of this instrument is reported in the above-mentioned preliminary article.[22]

The ADL rating scale was constructed ex novo with items appropriate to a cross-cultural context. Its suitability and acceptability were proved by the pilot investigation preceding the present cross-sectional phase of the WHO Neuropsychiatric AIDS Study.[22]

NEUROLOGICAL ASSESSMENT

The module used for neurological assessment included the following parts: (1) a screening neurological examination (including 11 sections: level of consciousness, cranial nerves, antisaccadic eye movements, muscle strength, coordination, involuntary movements, reflexes, sensory, Romberg test, gait, and other abnormalities); (2) a detailed neurological examination (including six sections: cranial nerves, involuntary movements, tone, motor, coordination, and sensory); (3) a neurological history; and (4) a neurological summary. A manual of instructions was produced that is available on request from WHO headquarters. Neurological diagnoses were made according to the operational criteria proposed by the WHO[16] and by the American Academy of Neurology (AAN), Minneapolis, Minn.[36] The training of the researchers and the intercenter and intracenter reliability data are reported in the above-mentioned preliminary article.[22]

ANALYSIS OF COGNITIVE/ NEUROPSYCHOLOGICAL DATA

The asymptomatic and symptomatic HIV-1–seropositive subjects evaluated in each center were compared separately with the HIV-1–seronegative controls with respect to the prevalence of impairment on individual neuropsychological tests and of global neuropsychological impairment. Impairment on each test was defined as a performance 2 or more SDs worse than the mean of the seronegative group. Global impairment was defined as an impaired performance on at least three of 10 tests (impairment on one or both Grooved Pegboard tests or on one or both Verbal Fluency tests was counted as one impaired test). A comparison with regard to the prevalence of global neuropsychological impairment was also performed between high-education and low-education asymptomatic and symptomatic HIV-1–seropositive subjects and the corresponding subgroups of HIV-1–seronegative controls: high-education subjects were those whose number of years of education was higher than the 25th percentile of the frequency distribution in the entire sample recruited in that center. All the above comparisons were made by using the χ^2 test or the Fisher's Exact Test, as appropriate. A Bonferroni correction for multiple testing was made. In comparing the prevalence of global neuropsychological impairment in each seropositive group with that of seronegative controls in each center, the possible confounding effect of depressive symptoms was evaluated by calculating the odds ratios (ORs) in the two subgroups obtained by stratifying for the global score on the Montgomery-Asberg Depression Rating Scale (MADRS[37]) (cutoff=19/20) and by applying Woolf's test for OR heterogeneity.[38]

A stepwise logistic regression analysis[39] was performed separately in asymptomatic and symptomatic HIV-1–seropositive subjects (of all centers lumped together) by using global neuropsychological performance as the dependent variable, whereas independent variables were center, sex, age, education (years of schooling), history of head traumas (causing loss of consciousness and requiring hospitalization), current use of anxiolytics, history of malaria, history of syphilis, CD4 count, current and lifetime psychiatric diagnosis (according to either *ICD-10* or *DSM-III-R*), and presence of prominent depressive symptoms (ie, a score of at least 20 on the MADRS). Treatment with zidovudine and current use of opiates were not included because they overlapped almost completely with the "center" variable. The same logistic regression analysis was also performed in HIV-1–seronegative and asymptomatic HIV-1–seropositive subjects of all the centers by using global neuropsychological performance as the dependent variable and all the above-mentioned parameters plus HIV-1 serostatus as independent variables. In all logistic regression analyses, the adjusted ORs with 95% confidence intervals (CIs) were calculated for all dichotomous independent variables that entered the models. Correlations of neuropsychological test scores with the CD4 count and MADRS global score were explored in each seropositive group by the Pearson coefficient.

The asymptomatic and symptomatic HIV-1–seropositive individuals evaluated in each center were compared separately with HIV-1–seronegative controls with respect to the prevalence of subjective cognitive complaints, the mean total score on the ADL rating scale, and the prevalence of a diagnosis of dementia according to *ICD-10* and *DSM-III-R*. Comparisons were made by using the Scheffé test for continuous measures and the χ^2 test (with the Bonferroni correction for multiple testing) for categorical measures. Associations between the occurrence of at least one subjective cognitive complaint, on the one hand, and the presence of global neuropsychological impairment and of prominent depressive symptoms, on the other, were assessed in each serogroup by the χ^2 test.

Continued on next page

ANALYSIS OF NEUROLOGICAL DATA

The asymptomatic and symptomatic HIV-1–seropositive subjects assessed in each center were compared separately with HIV-1–seronegative controls with respect to the prevalence of impairment on individual sections of the neurological examination and the prevalence of current neurological diagnoses according to WHO and AAN criteria. Comparisons were made by using the Scheffé test for continuous measures and the χ^2 test (with the Bonferroni correction for multiple testing) for categorical measures.

The χ^2 test was used to assess, in each serogroup, associations between the occurrence of impairment on each section of the neurological examination, on the one hand, and the presence of global neuropsychological impairment, of prominent depressive symptoms, and of any *ICD-10* or *DSM-III-R* psychiatric diagnosis, on the other. The Scheffé test was applied in each seropositive group to compare neurologically impaired vs nonimpaired subjects with respect to the mean CD4 count and mean total score on the ADL rating scale.

count,[2,5] or the impact of depression on cognitive functioning,[14,15] in HIV-1–seropositive individuals. Finally, although several estimates of the prevalence of HIV-1–associated dementia have been produced,[16] they are hampered by the very rare utilization of structured diagnostic interviews and operational diagnostic criteria.

A more general limitation of research concerning HIV-1–associated cognitive impairment is that available studies have been almost exclusively conducted on samples of well-educated, mostly white, homosexual men in Western industrialized areas. Reports from developing countries, in this research field, are very few, and the findings from these reports are inconsistent. For example, concerning the prevalence of dementia among patients with acquired immunodeficiency syndrome (AIDS) in sub-Saharan Africa, figures as high as 54%[17] and as low as 3.2%[18] can be found in the literature. These findings hardly can be compared with each other and with those obtained in Western countries, owing to huge differences in population-sampling procedures and assessment methods.[19]

And yet, there are reasons to suspect that interregional differences in the prevalence and the natural history of HIV-1–associated neuropsychological changes do exist. It is possible that subtle cognitive deficits become apparent earlier in HIV-1–infected subjects living in some developing countries because their "cerebral reserve" (ie, redundancy of cerebral networks) may be reduced by organic or psychosocial factors (eg, malnutrition, other infectious diseases affecting the central nervous system, and lack of social and educational stimulation).[20-23] On the other hand, progression to severe cognitive impairment may be prevented, in the same contexts, by early death due to wasting syndrome or opportunistic infections, so

Table 1. Prevalence of Impairment on Individual NP Tests in Subjects Evaluated in European, American, African, and Asian Centers*

	Munich, Germany			São Paulo, Brazil		
Test, % Impaired	HIV-1– (n=67)	A/HIV-1+ (n=42)	S/HIV-1+ (n=74)	HIV-1– (n=77)	A/HIV-1+ (n=55)	S/HIV-1+ (n=46)
Timed Gait	3.0	0	0	3.9	1.8	15.2
Auditory Verbal Learning (trials 1-5)	1.5	16.7†	28.4‡	0	5.5	19.6§
Color Trails 1	4.5	4.8	13.5	2.6	7.3	15.2‖
Color Trails 2	3.0	4.8	20.3†	3.9	0	8.7
EIWA Block Design	3.0	7.1	9.5	1.3	5.5	4.3
EIWA Digit Symbol	1.5	2.4	16.2†	1.3	3.6	4.3
Grooved Pegboard, D	6.0	2.4	10.8	5.2	5.5	10.9
Grooved Pegboard, ND	6.0	2.4	23.0†	3.9	1.8	8.7
Trail Making A	4.5	4.8	10.8	6.5	3.6	6.5
Verbal Fluency, animals	0	7.1	21.6§	0	3.6	6.5
Verbal Fluency, first names	1.5	4.8	18.9§	3.9	3.6	2.2
Picture Memory and Interference (all books)	3.0	9.5	24.3§	5.2	14.5	6.5

**NP indicates neuropsychological; HIV-1, human immunodeficiency virus type 1; HIV-1–, HIV type 1–seronegative subjects; A/HIV-1+, asymptomatic HIV type 1–seropositive subjects; S/HIV-1+, symptomatic HIV type 1–seropositive subjects; EIWA, Escala de Inteligencia Wechsler para Adultos; D, dominant; and ND, nondominant.*

†Significant intracenter differences (asymptomatic or symptomatic seropositive vs seronegative subjects): $P<.01$.

‡Significant intracenter differences (asymptomatic or symptomatic seropositive vs seronegative subjects): $P<.0001$.

§Significant intracenter differences (asymptomatic or symptomatic seropositive vs seronegative subjects): $P<.001$.

‖Significant intracenter differences (asymptomatic or symptomatic seropositive vs seronegative subjects): $P<.05$.

that the prevalence of the dementia syndrome may be found to be lower than in Western countries.[24]

The very rare utilization of standardized assessment and diagnostic instruments and the shortage of studies conducted in developing countries are also evident in the literature on neurological complications of HIV-1 infection. This insufficiency of reliable empirical data has generated contrasting views, such as the one expressed in the World Health Organization (WHO) Bangui clinical definition of AIDS[25] (according to which neurological impairment is just a "minor" manifestation of HIV-1 infection in Africa) and that contained in a recent article by Howlett et al[17] (according to which "neurological disorders are among the main clinical features of AIDS and HIV disease in Africa").

Within the cross-sectional phase of the WHO Neuropsychiatric AIDS Study, we assessed the prevalence of HIV-1–associated neuropsychological and neurological abnormalities in representative samples of HIV-1–seropositive subjects living in the five geographic areas predominantly affected by the HIV-1 epidemic. Herein, we report the results of this assessment.

RESULTS

NEUROPSYCHOLOGICAL FINDINGS

As asymptomatic HIV-1–seropositive subjects were compared with HIV-1–seronegative controls with respect to the prevalence of impairment on individual neuropsychological tests, only a few significant differences were observed. On the contrary, symptomatic HIV-1–seropositive individuals differed significantly from controls on numerous neuropsychological measures (their performance was significantly worse on Timed Gait, Color Trails 2, EIWA Digit Symbol, Trail Making A, and Verbal Fluency, animals, in three centers) (**Table 1**).

The prevalence of global neuropsychological impairment was significantly higher in symptomatic HIV-1–seropositive subjects than in controls in all the centers. A similar significant difference was found between asymptomatic HIV-1–seropositive subjects and HIV-1–seronegative individuals in São Paulo, Brazil, and Kinshasa, Zaire, but not in the other centers. In Kinshasa and in Nairobi, the prevalence of global neuropsychological impairment was significantly higher in low-education, but not in high-education, asymptomatic HIV-1–seropositive subjects compared with the corresponding subgroups of HIV-1–seronegative individuals (**Table 2**). Woolf's test for OR heterogeneity provided no evidence of multiplicative interaction between HIV-1 seropositivity and MADRS global score in any of the above comparisons.

On stepwise logistic regression analysis, performed separately in asymptomatic and symptomatic seropositive subjects, the following variables entered the model: education in the former group (improvement $\chi^2=17.9$, $df=1$, $P<.00001$; 81.7% of subjects correctly classified; OR=6.49 [CI, 2.46 to 7.12]); age (improvement $\chi^2=14.0$, $df=1$, $P<.001$); lifetime psychiatric diagnosis (improvement $\chi^2=10.2$, $df=1$, $P<.01$); center (improvement $\chi^2=12.8$, $df=4$, $P<.05$); depressive symptoms (improvement $\chi^2=7.1$,

Kinshasa, Zaire			Nairobi, Kenya			Bangkok, Thailand		
HIV-1– (n=85)	A/HIV-1+ (n=52)	S/HIV-1+ (n=68)	HIV-1– (n=65)	A/HIV-1+ (n=66)	S/HIV-1+ (n=72)	HIV-1– (n=59)	A/HIV-1+ (n=89)	S/HIV-1+ (n=38)
4.7	5.8	29.4‡	4.6	6.0	22.2†	3.4	12.4	57.9‡
2.4	0	10.3	0	6.0	6.9	5.1	3.4	10.5
3.5	7.7	16.2†	7.7	9.0	12.5	3.4	5.6	13.2
4.7	7.7	17.6†	7.7	9.0	20.8	3.4	12.4	23.7†
3.5	13.5‖	19.1†	4.6	9.0	13.9	10.2	12.4	15.8
2.4	3.8	14.7†	4.6	10.4	22.2†	6.8	4.5	7.9
2.4	5.8	16.2†	1.5	0	5.6	0	14.6†	18.4†
5.9	3.8	17.6‖	1.5	0	2.8	6.8	6.7	7.9
3.5	7.7	16.2†	6.2	7.5	15.3†	3.4	6.7	18.4‖
1.2	0	1.5	1.5	7.5	12.5‖	1.7	5.6	23.7†
3.5	3.8	8.8	0	0	2.8	0	5.6	18.4†
2.4	0	5.9	3.1	3.0	6.9	5.1	2.2	5.3

Table 2. Prevalence of Global NP Impairment by Education in Subjects Evaluated in European, American, African, and Asian Centers*

	Munich, Germany			São Paulo, Brazil		
	HIV-1−	A/HIV-1+	S/HIV-1+	HIV-1−	A/HIV-1+	S/HIV-1+
Low-education subjects, % impaired	5.0	11.8	31.0†	0	20.0	28.6
High-education subjects, % impaired	2.1	4.0	22.2‡	0	2.9	6.3
Total sample, % impaired	3.0	7.1	25.7§	0	9.1†	13.0‡

**NP indicates neuropsychological; HIV-1, human immunodeficiency virus type 1; HIV-1−, HIV type 1–seronegative subjects; A/HIV-1+, asymptomatic HIV type 1–seropositive subjects; and S/HIV-1+, symptomatic HIV type 1–seropositive subjects.*

†Significant intracenter differences (asymptomatic or symptomatic seropositive vs seronegative subjects): P<.05.

‡Significant intracenter differences (asymptomatic or symptomatic seropositive vs seronegative subjects): P<.01.

§Significant intracenter differences (asymptomatic or symptomatic seropositive vs seronegative subjects): P<.001.

df=1, *P*<.01); and sex (improvement χ^2=5.0, *df*=1, *P*<.05) in the latter group (83.2% of subjects correctly classified in the final model; OR=3.33 [CI, 1.40 to 7.85] for lifetime psychiatric diagnosis, and OR=2.89 [CI, 1.20 to 6.96] for depressive symptoms). On the stepwise logistic regression analysis performed in seronegative and asymptomatic seropositive subjects, the variables entering the model were education (improvement χ^2=17.0, *df*=1, *P*<.00001) and HIV-1 serostatus (improvement χ^2=10.2, *df*=1, *P*<.01) (95.1% of subjects correctly classified in the final model; OR=3.81 [CI, 1.79 to 8.85] for education, and OR=3.66 [CI, 1.52 to 8.85] for serostatus). When the education×serostatus interaction was run as an independent variable, it entered the model with an improvement χ^2 of 31.7 (*df*=1, *P*<.00001; 95.1% of subjects correctly classified; OR=8.58 [CI, 4.01 to 18.36]).

Only a few significant correlations between neuropsychological test scores and the CD4 count were observed among either asymptomatic or symptomatic HIV-1–seropositive persons. The most frequently involved tests were Color Trails 1 (*P*<.01 among asymptomatic subjects in Nairobi; *P*<.05 among both asymptomatic and symptomatic persons in Munich, Germany) and Color Trails 2 (*P*<.01 among asymptomatic subjects in Munich; *P*<.05 among symptomatic individuals in Munich and Kinshasa).

Table 3. Performance in ADLs of Subjects Evaluated in the Five Centers*

	Total Score on ADL Rating Scale, Mean±SD†		
Center	HIV-1−	A/HIV-1+	S/HIV-1+
Munich, Germany	34.3±1.3	35.2±3.1	39.7±8.7‡
São Paulo, Brazil	35.4±6.5	35.6±7.2	40.1±8.4‡
Kinshasa, Zaire	34.2±2.0	35.0±4.1	40.2±14.7‡
Nairobi, Kenya	34.2±4.2	34.6±2.5	39.2±10.1‡
Bangkok, Thailand	35.0±2.3	36.1±4.6	45.5±11.5‡

**ADLs indicates activities of daily living; HIV-1, human immunodeficiency virus type 1; HIV-1−, HIV type 1–seronegative subjects; A/HIV-1+, asymptomatic HIV type 1–seropositive subjects; and S/HIV-1+, symptomatic HIV type 1–seropositive subjects.*

†Higher scores indicate worse performance.

‡Significant intracenter differences (symptomatic seropositive vs seronegative subjects): P<.05.

Significant correlations between neuropsychological test scores and the MADRS global score were more frequent, especially in symptomatic seropositive subjects. The most frequently involved tests were Color Trails 1 (*P*<.01 among both asymptomatic and symptomatic subjects in Munich and symptomatic persons in São Paulo; *P*<.05 among symptomatic subjects in Nairobi and Bangkok, Thailand), EIWA Digit Symbol (*P*<.01 among asymptomatic individuals in Bangkok; *P*<.05 among both asymptomatic and symptomatic subjects in Munich and among symptomatic persons in Bangkok), and Grooved Pegboard, dominant (*P*<.001 among asymptomatic subjects in Munich; *P*<.01 among symptomatic individuals in Munich and Kinshasa; and *P*<.05 among asymptomatic subjects in Nairobi).

The proportion of symptomatic seropositive subjects presenting at least one subjective cognitive complaint was significantly higher than that of seronegative persons in all the centers (12.2% vs 0%, *P*<.01 in Munich; 17.4% vs 3.9%, *P*<.05 in São Paulo; 21.8% vs 1.2%, *P*<.01 in Kinshasa; 15.3% vs 3.1%, *P*<.05 in Nairobi; and 15.8% vs 3.4%, *P*<.05 in Bangkok). A similar difference between asymptomatic seropositive subjects and controls was detected only in Kinshasa (9.6% vs 1.2%, *P*<.05). The most frequent subjective complaints in symptomatic seropositive subjects were those concerning memory disturbances, concentration problems, and slowness of thinking (the prevalence of each of these complaints was significantly higher in these subjects than in seronegative controls in three of five centers). There was no significant difference between asymptomatic seropositive subjects and controls with respect to the prevalence of individual subjective complaints.

The presence of at least one subjective cognitive complaint was significantly associated with global neuropsychological impairment in symptomatic seropositive subjects assessed in Munich (*P*<.01) and São Paulo (*P*<.001), whereas no significant association was found in asymptomatic seropositive subjects in any center. The association between the occurrence of at least one subjective cognitive complaint and the presence of prominent depressive symptoms was significant in asymptomatic seropositive subjects enrolled in Munich (*P*<.01), Kinshasa (*P*<.001), and Nairobi (*P*<.05), and in symptomatic seropositive individuals assessed in Kinshasa (*P*<.01) and Nairobi (*P*<.05).

Kinshasa, Zaire			Nairobi, Kenya			Bangkok, Thailand		
HIV-1–	A/HIV-1+	S/HIV-1+	HIV-1–	A/HIV-1+	S/HIV-1+	HIV-1–	A/HIV-1+	S/HIV-1+
0	25.0†	19.0	0	22.7†	25.0†	0	5.7	22.1
1.4	2.8	19.1‡	5.1	0	10.4	2.4	3.7	16.0
1.2	9.6†	19.1§	4.6	7.5	15.3†	1.7	4.5	18.4†

The mean total score on the ADL rating scale was significantly higher in symptomatic HIV-1–seropositive subjects than in controls in all the centers, and it was consistently not increased in asymptomatic HIV-1–seropositive subjects (**Table 3**). Actually, none of the 17 items of the ADL rating scale explored in the five centers showed any significant difference between asymptomatic HIV-1–seropositive and HIV-1–seronegative individuals.

No case of dementia according to either *ICD-10* or *DSM-III-R* was detected in HIV-1–seronegative and asymptomatic HIV-1–seropositive persons in any of the centers. The prevalence of the syndrome in symptomatic HIV-1–seropositive patients ranged from 5.4% to 6.9% according to *ICD-10* criteria and from 4.4% to 6.5% according to *DSM-III-R* criteria in all the centers except Bangkok, where no case of dementia was diagnosed (**Table 4**).

NEUROLOGICAL FINDINGS

The prevalence of neurological impairment was significantly higher in symptomatic (but not in asymptomatic) HIV-1–seropositive individuals, compared with seronegative controls, in all the centers. The most frequently involved items of the neurological examination were frontal release signs (significant difference between symptomatic seropositive subjects and controls in all the centers), antisaccadic eye movements (significant differences in three centers), and muscle strength (same as antisaccadic eye movements). Of 65 item comparisons in the five centers, no one showed a significant difference between asymptomatic seropositive subjects and controls (**Table 5**).

Predominantly sensory neuropathy was the most common neurological diagnosis in symptomatic HIV-1–seropositive subjects, and it occurred in one physically asymptomatic HIV-1–seropositive subject, both in São Paulo and in Bangkok. Inflammatory polyneuropathy was the other diagnosis sporadically made (one case in Munich) in the asymptomatic seropositive group. Myopathy was very rare also in symptomatic seropositive subjects (one case in Munich and one case in Bangkok), as was acute inflammatory demyelinating polyradiculoneuropathy diagnosed according to AAN criteria (one case each in Munich, Kinshasa, and Nairobi) (**Table 6**). No neurological diagnosis was made in HIV-1–seronegative subjects.

In all the centers, impairment on each section of neurological examination was not significantly associated, in any serogroup, either with the presence of prominent depressive symptoms or with any *ICD-10* or *DSM-III-R* psychiatric diagnosis, whereas several associations were found between the occurrence of individual abnormal neurological items and the presence of global neuropsychological impairment in symptomatic (but not in asymptomatic) seropositive subjects (**Table 7**). As neurologically impaired symptomatic seropositive subjects were compared with nonimpaired ones, the former had a significantly decreased mean CD4 count in Munich and Nairobi and a significantly increased mean total score on the ADL rating scale (that is, a worse performance in ADLs) in Munich and Kinshasa. No significant

Table 4. Prevalence of Dementia According to *ICD-10* and *DSM-III-R* Criteria in Subjects Evaluated in the Five Centers*

	ICD-10 Diagnosis of Dementia, %			*DSM-III-R* Diagnosis of Dementia, %		
Center	HIV-1–	A/HIV-1+	S/HIV-1+	HIV-1–	A/HIV-1+	S/HIV-1+
Munich, Germany	0	0	5.4	0	0	5.4
São Paulo, Brazil	0	0	6.5	0	0	6.5
Kinshasa, Zaire	0	0	5.9	0	0	4.4
Nairobi, Kenya	0	0	6.9	0	0	5.5
Bangkok, Thailand	0	0	0	0	0	0

*ICD-10 *indicates* International Classification of Diseases, 10th Revision*; HIV-1, human immunodeficiency virus type 1; HIV-1–, HIV type 1–seronegative subjects; A/HIV-1+, asymptomatic HIV type 1–seropositive subjects; and S/HIV-1+, symptomatic HIV type 1–seropositive subjects.*

Table 5. Findings on Neurological Examination in Subjects Evaluated in European, American, African, and Asian Centers*

Results of Neurological Examination	Munich, Germany HIV-1– (n=67)	Munich, Germany A/HIV-1+ (n=42)	Munich, Germany S/HIV-1+ (n=74)	São Paulo, Brazil HIV-1– (n=77)	São Paulo, Brazil A/HIV-1+ (n=55)	São Paulo, Brazil S/HIV-1+ (n=46)
Normal, %	94.0	92.9	51.4†	89.6	83.6	45.7†
Abnormal, %						
Level of consciousness	0	2.4	0	0	0	2.2
Cranial nerves	1.5	0	5.4	0	0	2.2
Antisaccadic eye movements	4.5	2.4	20.3‡	9.1	16.4	41.3†
Muscle strength	0	4.8	14.9‡	0	3.6	8.7§
Coordination	0	0	10.8§	0	0	10.9§
Involuntary movements	0	0	1.4	0	0	4.3
Reflexes	0	0	14.9‡	7.7	9.1	21.7
Frontal release signs	0	0	13.5‡	0	0	8.7§
Sensation	0	0	9.5§	0	0	6.5
Romberg test	0	2.4	8.1§	0	0	0
Gait	0	0	18.9‖	0	0	6.5
Tone	0	2.4	10.8§	0	0	2.2
Atrophy	0	2.4	4.1	0	0	8.7§

**HIV-1 indicates human immunodeficiency virus type 1; HIV-1–, HIV type 1–seronegative subjects; A/HIV-1+, asymptomatic HIV type 1–seropositive subjects; and S/HIV-1+, symptomatic HIV type 1–seropositive subjects.*

†*Significant differences (symptomatic seropositive vs seronegative subjects):* $P<.0001$.

‡*Significant differences (symptomatic seropositive vs seronegative subjects):* $P<.01$.

§*Significant differences (symptomatic seropositive vs seronegative subjects):* $P<.05$.

‖*Significant differences (symptomatic seropositive vs seronegative subjects):* $P<.001$.

difference with respect to the mean CD4 count and mean total score on the ADL rating scale was found between neurologically impaired and nonimpaired asymptomatic seropositive subjects.

COMMENT

The results of the cross-sectional phase of the WHO Neuropsychiatric AIDS Study confirm that the symptomatic stages of HIV-1 infection are characterized by a significant impairment of cognitive functions. This finding holds in outpatient samples, excluding the most severe cases of AIDS. Fine motor control, sustained and selective attention, cognitive flexibility, and verbal memory are the most frequently affected functional domains, and the pattern of impairment does not seem to differ in the various geographical contexts. Cognitive impairment is associated with a significant worsening of the performance in daily living activities.

Findings concerning physically asymptomatic HIV-1–seropositive subjects are more ambiguous. Of 60 test comparisons performed in the five centers, only three showed a significant difference between asymptomatic seropositive and seronegative subjects. Nevertheless, the prevalence of global neuropsychological impairment was significantly higher in asymptomatic HIV-1–seropositive persons than in controls in two centers, and HIV-1 serostatus was one of the variables affecting global neuropsychological performance in the stepwise logistic regression analysis performed for seronegative and asymptomatic seropositive subjects of all the centers. Anyway, it is important to stress that the performance in daily living activities of asymptomatic seropositive subjects was not significantly impaired in any center.

The "cerebral reserve" theory is partially supported by the data collected. Within two centers in developing countries (Kinshasa and São Paulo), the prevalence of neuropsychological impairment was significantly higher in asymptomatic HIV-1–seropositive subjects than in HIV-1–seronegative controls, and also the corresponding Nairobi data approached statistical significance. Moreover, low-education, but not high-education, asymptomatic seropositive persons had an impaired neuropsychological performance in the two African sites, and a significant effect of the education level on the prevalence of the impairment in asymptomatic seropositive subjects of all the centers was detected by the stepwise logistic regression analysis. This last finding confirms the preliminary evidence obtained in the Multicenter AIDS Cohort Study.[40] Inadequate educational stimulation may in itself be a factor affecting "cerebral reserve" (by limiting the development of efficient synaptic connections between neurons), but a low-education level may also be seen as an indicator of a socioenvironmental situation where other factors reducing the redundancy of cerebral networks (such as other infectious diseases and malnutrition) are at work.

Cognitive impairment was not found to be significantly related to immunological status: in fact, only very few correlations were observed between neuropsychological test scores and the CD4 count, either in asymptomatic or in symptomatic HIV-1–seropositive subjects, and no significant effect of the CD4 count on global neuropsychological performance was revealed by the stepwise logistic regression analysis. However, the question of the relationship between

Kinshasa, Zaire			Nairobi, Kenya			Bangkok, Thailand		
HIV-1– (n=85)	A/HIV-1+ (n=52)	S/HIV-1+ (n=68)	HIV-1– (n=65)	A/HIV-1+ (n=66)	S/HIV-1+ (n=72)	HIV-1– (n=59)	A/HIV-1+ (n=89)	S/HIV-1+ (n=38)
82.4	76.9	58.8‡	84.6	78.8	59.7‡	67.8	63.3	34.2‡
0	0	2.9	0	0	0	0	0	0
0	0	0	0	0	1.4	5.1	2.2	5.3
10.6	17.3	25.0§	18.5	22.4	30.6	8.5	9.0	21.0
0	0	4.4	0	0	1.4	1.7	3.4	21.0‡
0	0	2.9	0	0	1.4	0	0	2.6
0	0	0	0	0	1.4	1.7	0	2.6
4.7	5.8	10.3	3.1	1.5	9.7	22.0	23.6	34.2
1.2	7.7	11.8§	0	0	9.7§	18.6	23.6	44.7†
0	0	2.9	0	0	2.8	0	0	2.6
0	0	2.9	0	0	2.8	0	0	2.6
0	0	4.4	0	0	1.4	0	0	2.6
0	0	1.5	0	0	0	0	0	0
0	0	0	0	0	0	1.7	2.2	10.5

cognitive and immunological decline will be more appropriately addressed by the follow-up phase of the present investigation.

Our findings indicate that the presence of prominent depressive symptoms is significantly associated with the occurrence of subjective cognitive complaints, especially in asymptomatic seropositive subjects. On the other hand, subjective cognitive complaints of asymptomatic seropositive persons do not correlate significantly to the objective neuropsychological performance (in line with findings from a previous report by van Gorp et al[41]). It is essential, therefore, that any definition of HIV-1–associated "mild cognitive impairment" require an objective test validation: the operational diagnostic criteria

Table 6. Prevalence of Neurological Diagnoses in Seropositive Subjects Evaluated in the Five Centers*

	Munich, Germany		São Paulo, Brazil		Kinshasa, Zaire		Nairobi, Kenya		Bangkok, Thailand	
	A/HIV-1+ (n=42)	S/HIV-1+ (n=74)	A/HIV-1+ (n=55)	S/HIV-1+ (n=46)	A/HIV-1+ (n=52)	S/HIV-1+ (n=68)	A/HIV-1+ (n=66)	S/HIV-1+ (n=72)	A/HIV-1+ (n=89)	S/HIV-1+ (n=38)
Diagnosis according to WHO criteria, %										
Myelopathy	0	5.4	0	2.8	0	1.7	0	3.3	0	2.7
Inflammatory polyneuropathy	2.4	5.4	0	6.5	0	1.7	0	3.3	0	0
Predominantly sensory neuropathy	0	8.1	2.0	6.5	0	1.7	0	8.3	1.2	5.4
Myopathy	0	1.3	0	0	0	0	0	0	0	2.7
Diagnosis according to AAN criteria, %										
Myelopathy	0	5.4	0	2.8	0	1.7	0	3.3	0	2.7
Acute inflammatory demyelinating polyradiculoneuropathy	0	1.3	0	0	0	1.7	0	1.6	0	0
Predominantly sensory neuropathy	0	8.1	2.0	6.5	0	1.7	0	8.3	1.2	5.4
Myopathy	0	1.3	0	0	0	0	0	0	0	2.7

**HIV-1 indicates human immunodeficiency virus type 1; A/HIV-1+, asymptomatic HIV type 1–seropositive subjects; S/HIV-1+, symptomatic HIV type 1–seropositive subjects; WHO, World Health Organization (Geneva, Switzerland); and AAN, American Academy of Neurology (Minneapolis, Minn). No neurological diagnosis was made in HIV type 1–seronegative subjects.*

Table 7. Significant Associations Between Impairment on Individual Sections of Neurological Examination and Global NP Impairment in Symptomatic Seropositive Subjects Evaluated in the Five Centers*

Sections of Neurological Examination	S/HIV-1+, *P*				
	MU	SP	KI	NA	BG
Level of consciousness	...	...	...	...	...
Cranial nerves	...	...	...	...	...
Antisaccadic eye movements	...	...	<.01	...	...
Muscle strength	...	...	<.01	...	...
Coordination	<.01	...	...	...	...
Involuntary movements	...	...	...	...	...
Reflexes	...	...	...	...	...
Frontal release signs	...	<.05	<.01	...	...
Sensation	<.001	...	<.01	...	...
Romberg test	...	...	...	...	...
Gait	...	...	...	...	...
Tone	...	...	...	...	...
Atrophy	...	<.01	...	...	...

**NP indicates neuropsychological; HIV-1, human immunodeficiency virus type 1; S/HIV-1+, symptomatic HIV type 1–seropositive subjects; MU, Munich, Germany; SP, São Paulo, Brazil; KI, Kinshasa, Zaire; NA, Nairobi, Kenya; and BG, Bangkok, Thailand.*

recently produced by the WHO[42] and by the AAN[36] for HIV-1–associated minor cognitive/motor disorder may be a first step in this direction.

The results of the present study show that the prevalence of dementia in the symptomatic stages of HIV-1 infection is almost the same in developed and in developing countries, with the exception of Thailand (where the explosion of the epidemic has been more recent, and most HIV-1 cases are not likely to have reached an advanced stage). The nonincreased prevalence of dementia in sub-Saharan Africa is not in contradiction to the possible earlier onset of HIV-1–related cognitive impairment: the more rapid progression of the infection, in fact, may cause the death of several subjects before they are able to reach the most severe stages of cognitive deterioration[24] (although this hypothesis needs to be substantiated by a long-term follow-up study).

It is important to emphasize that what we assessed in the present investigation is the prevalence of the dementia syndrome according to *ICD-10* and *DSM-III-R*, which does not necessarily correspond to that of the "AIDS dementia complex"[43] (since this last entity is defined also by the presence of motor symptoms and signs and is diagnosed by the exclusion of the etiological role of opportunistic infections). We preferred, in fact, to rely on a "syndromic" diagnosis that can be made by using a standard algorithm based on a structured interview.

The results of the present cross-sectional phase of the WHO study confirm that neurological impairment is a frequent occurrence in the symptomatic stages of HIV-1 infection, and that frontal release signs, impaired antisaccadic eye movements, and muscle weakness are the most frequent neurological abnormalities. As expected, the prevalence of neurological signs was the highest among all serogroups in the Bangkok center, where most subjects were intravenous drug users. We were able to confirm the significant association reported by Stern et al[10] between neurological and neuropsychological impairment only in symptomatic HIV-1–seropositive subjects, and in part of the centers, whereas no association was found in asymptomatic seropositive subjects in any center.

To our knowledge, our study was the first to adopt operational diagnostic criteria for HIV-1–associated neurological disorders (it is important to note, in this connection, the 100% consistency between the WHO and the AAN diagnoses of myelopathy, predominantly sensory neuropathy, and myopathy). The pattern of neurological disorders was very similar across the centers, including the two African sites, which may suggest a reconsideration of the WHO Bangui clinical definition of AIDS (that regards neurological impairment as only a "minor" manifestation of HIV-1 infection in Africa). The occurrence of a case of inflammatory polyneuropathy in an otherwise asymptomatic HIV-1–seropositive subject is not surprising, since it is known that this condition may be the first manifestation of HIV-1 infection.[44] Less expected, and of greater interest, is the occurrence, among asymptomatic seropositive subjects, of two cases of predominantly sensory neuropathy, a disorder that is regarded as rare in Centers of Disease Control and Prevention groups II and III.[16]

The cross-sectional phase of the WHO study will now be followed by a longitudinal one. This will approach the key issues of the evolution of HIV-1–associated cognitive impairment and of the relationship between this evolution and the immunological, medical, neurological, and psychopathological aspects of the infection. Moreover, it will verify the existence of a continuity between mild cognitive abnormalities that possibly occur in the asymptomatic phases of the infection and the subsequent development of dementia.

Accepted for publication December 29, 1992.

The authors are indebted to Alex Chervinsky, PhD, Neuropsychiatric Institute, UCLA, Los Angeles, Calif, and Andrew J. Saykin, PsyD, University of Pennsylvania, Philadelphia, for their participation in the development of the module for cognitive/neuropsychological assessment; to Eric N. Miller, PhD, and Wilfred G. van Gorp, PhD, Neuropsychiatric Institute, UCLA, for their help in training the researchers in the use of neuropsychological tests; and to Darwin Boor, MD, Department of Neurology, Emory University, Atlanta, Ga, for his help in developing the module for neurological assessment and in training the researchers in the use of this module. The committee that selected the neuropsychological tests included the following experts: Paul Satz, PhD, UCLA (Chairman); François Boller, PhD, Institut National de la Santé et de la Recherche Médicale (INSERM), Paris, France; Ron R. Hijman, PhD, State University, Utrecht, the Netherlands; Elly Katabira, MD, Mekerere University, Kampala, Uganda; Stephen

H. Koslow, MD, National Institute of Mental Health, Rockville, Md; David Ndetei, MD, University of Nairobi, Kenya; Andrew J. Saykin, PsyD, University of Pennsylvania; John Sidtis, PhD, University of Minnesota, Minneapolis; Thiravat Hemachudha, MD, Chulalongkorn University, Bangkok, Thailand; and Michael Zaudig, MD, Max-Planck Institute, Munich, Germany.

Reprint requests to Division of Mental Health, World Health Organization, 1211 Geneva 27, Switzerland (Dr Maj).

REFERENCES

1. Tross S, Price RW, Navia B, Thaler HT, Gold J, Hirsch DA, Sidtis JJ. Neuropsychological characterization of the AIDS dementia complex: a preliminary report. *AIDS.* 1988;2:81-88.
2. Goethe KE, Mitchell JF, Marshall DW, Prey RN, Cahill WT, Leger GD, Hoy LJ, Boswell RN. Neuropsychological and neurological function of human immunodeficiency virus seropositive asymptomatic individuals. *Arch Neurol.* 1989;46:129-133.
3. Janssen RS, Saykin AJ, Cannon L, Campbell J, Pinsky PF, Hessol NA, O'Malley TM, Lifson AR, Doll LS, Rutherford GW, Kaplan JE. Neurologic and neuropsychologic manifestations of human immunodeficiency virus (HIV-1) infection: association with AIDS-related complex but not asymptomatic HIV-1 infection. *Ann Neurol.* 1989;26:592-600.
4. Koralnik IJ, Beumanoir A, Hausler R, Kohler A, Delacoux R, Hirschel B. A controlled study of early neurologic abnormalities in men with asymptomatic human immunodeficiency virus infection. *N Engl J Med.* 1990;323:864-870.
5. Miller EN, Selnes OA, McArthur JC, Satz P, Pecker JT, Cohen BA, Sheridan K, Machado AN, van Gorp WG, Visscher B. Neuropsychological performance in HIV-1-infected homosexual men: the Multicenter AIDS Cohort Study (MACS). *Neurology.* 1990;40:197-203.
6. Grant I, Atkinson JH, Hesselink JR, Kennedy CJ, Richman DD, Spector SA, McCutchan JA. Evidence for early central nervous system involvement in acquired immunodeficiency syndrome (AIDS) and other human immunodeficiency virus (HIV) infections: studies with neuropsychological testing and magnetic resonance imaging. *Ann Intern Med.* 1987;107:828-836.
7. Poutianen E, Livainen M, Elovaara I, Valle S-L, Lahdervirta J. Cognitive changes as early signs of HIV infection. *Acta Neurol Scand.* 1988;78:49-52.
8. McKegney FP, O'Dowd MA, Feiner C, Selwyn P, Drucker E, Friedland GH. A prospective comparison of neuropsychologic function in HIV-seropositive and seronegative methadone-maintained patients. *AIDS.* 1990;4:565-569.
9. Wilkie FL, Eisdorfer C, Morgan R, Loewenstein DA, Szapocznik J. Cognition in early HIV infection. *Arch Neurol.* 1990;47:433-440.
10. Stern Y, Marder K, Dell K, Chen J, Dooneief G, Goldstein S, Mindry D, Richards M, Sano M, Williams J, Gorman J, Ehrhardt A, Mayeux R. Multidisciplinary baseline assessment of homosexual men with and without human immunodeficiency virus infection, III: neurologic and neuropsychological findings. *Arch Gen Psychiatry.* 1991;48:131-138.
11. Selnes OA, Miller EN, McArthur JC, Gordon B, Munoz A, Sheridan K, Fox R, Saah AJ. HIV-1 infection: no evidence of cognitive decline during the asymptomatic stages. *Neurology.* 1990;40:204-208.
12. Riccio M, Pugh K, Catalan J, Jadresic D, Baldweg D, Hawkins D. Neuropsychological findings in CDC group II gay men: one year follow-up of the St. Stephen's cohort study. In: Abstracts of the Seventh International Conference on AIDS; June 16-21, 1991; Florence, Italy. Abstract M.B. 2058.
13. Temoshok L, Drexler M, Canick JP, Sweet DM, Hollander H. Neuropsychological change on longitudinal assessment: prevalence and patterns in HIV spectrum disorders. In: Abstracts of the Fifth International Conference on AIDS; June 4-9, 1989; Montreal, Quebec. Abstract W.B.O. 44.
14. Naber D, Riedel R, Perro C, Schick U, Vieler T, Binder J, Einhaupl K. Neuropsychological deficits in HIV-infected patients: relationship to depression. *Biol Psychiatry.* 1991;29:176S.
15. Lunn S, Skydsbjerg M, Schulsinger K, Parnas J, Pedersen C, Mathiesen L. A preliminary report on the neuropsychologic sequelae of human immunodeficiency virus. *Arch Gen Psychiatry.* 1991;48:139-142.
16. World Health Organization. *Report of the Second Consultation on the Neuropsychiatric Aspects of HIV-1 Infection, Geneva, January 11-13, 1990.* Geneva, Switzerland: World Health Organization; 1990.
17. Howlett WP, Nkya WM, Mmuni KA, Missalek WR. Neurological disorders in AIDS and HIV disease in the northern zone of Tanzania. *AIDS.* 1989;3:289-296.
18. Belec L, Martin PMV, Vohito MD, Gresenguet G, Tabo A, Georges AJ. Low prevalence of neuropsychiatric clinical manifestations in central African patients with acquired immune deficiency syndrome. *Trans R Soc Trop Med Hyg.* 1989;83:844-846.
19. Maj M. Organic mental disorders in HIV-1 infection. *AIDS.* 1990;4:831-840.
20. Grady CL, Haxby JV, Horwitz B, Sundaram M, Berg G, Shapiro M, Friedland RP, Rapoport SI. Longitudinal study of the early neuropsychological and cerebral metabolic changes in dementia of the Alzheimer type. *J Clin Exp Neuropsychol.* 1988;10:576-596.
21. Perry S, Belsky-Barr D, Barr WB, Jacobsberg L. Neuropsychological function in physically asymptomatic, HIV-seropositive men. *J Neuropsychiatry.* 1989;1:286-302.
22. Maj M, Janssen R, Satz P, Zaudig M, Starace F, Boor D, Sughondhabirom B, Bing E, Luabeya M, Ndetei D, Riedel R, Schulte G, Sartorius N. The World Health Organization's cross-cultural study on neuropsychiatric aspects of infection with the human immunodeficiency virus 1 (HIV-1): preparation and pilot phase. *Br J Psychiatry.* 1991;159:351-356.
23. Satz P. Threshold theory: brain reserve capacity and symptom onset after brain injury. *Neuropsychology.* In press.
24. Perriens JH, Mussa M, Luabeya M, Kayembe K, Kapita B, Brown C, Piot P, Janssen R. Neurological complications of HIV-1-seropositive internal medicine inpatients in Kinshasa, Zaire. *J Acquir Immune Defic Syndr.* 1992;5:333-340.
25. World Health Organization. Acquired immunodeficiency syndrome (AIDS): provisional WHO clinical case definition for AIDS. *Wkly Epidemiol Rec.* 1986;61:72-73.
26. Maj M, Janssen R, Starace F, Zaudig M, Satz P, Sughondhabirom B, Luabeya M, Riedel R, Ndetei D, Calil HM, Bing EG, St. Louis M, Sartorius N. WHO Neuropsychiatric AIDS Study, cross-sectional phase I: study design and psychiatric findings. *Arch Gen Psychiatry.* 1993;51:39-49.
27. Zaudig M, Mittelhammer J, Hiller W, Pauls A, Thora C, Morinigo A, Mombour W. SIDAM: a structured interview for the diagnosis of dementia of the Alzheimer type, multi-infarct dementia and dementias of other ethiology according to *ICD-10* and *DSM-III-R. Psychol Med.* 1991;21:225-236.
28. World Health Organization. *The* ICD-10 *Classification of Mental and Behavioural Disorders: Clinical Description and Diagnostic Guidelines.* Geneva, Switzerland: World Health Organization; 1992.
29. American Psychiatric Association. *Diagnostic and Statistical Manual of Mental Disorders, Revised Third Edition.* Washington, DC: American Psychiatric Association; 1987.
30. Wechsler D; Green RF, Martinez JN, adaptation-eds. *Manual para la Escala de Inteligencia Wechsler para Adultos.* Cleveland, Ohio: The Psychological Corp; 1968.
31. Matthews CG, Klove J. *Instruction Manual for Adult Neuropsychology Test Battery.* Madison: University of Wisconsin Medical School; 1964.
32. Benton AL, Hamsher K. *Multilingual Aphasia Examination.* Iowa City: University of Iowa; 1977.
33. Reitan RM, Wolfson D. *The Halstead-Reitan Neuropsychological Test Battery: Theory and Clinical Interpretation.* Tucson, Ariz: Neuropsychology Press; 1985.
34. Maj M, D'Elia L, Satz P, Janssen R, Zaudig M, Uchiyama C, Starace F, Galderisi S, Chervinsky A. Evaluation of three new neuropsychological tests designed to minimize cultural bias in the assessment of HIV-1-seropositive persons: a WHO study. *Arch Clin Neuropsychol.* 1993;8:123-135.
35. Rey A. *L'examen clinique en psychologie.* Paris: Presses Universitaires de France; 1964.
36. American Academy of Neurology AIDS Task Force. Nomenclature and research case definitions for the neurological manifestations of human immunodeficiency virus type-1 infection. *Neurology.* 1991;41:778-785.
37. Montgomery S, Asberg M. A new depression scale designed to be sensitive to change. *Br J Psychiatry.* 1979;134:382-389.
38. Woolf B. On estimating the relation between blood group and disease. *Ann Hum Genet.* 1955:19:251-253.
39. Norusis MJ. *SPSS/PC+ Advanced Statistics.* Chicago, Ill: SPSS Inc; 1988.
40. Satz P, Morgenstern H, Miller EN, Selnes OA, McArthur JC, Cohen BA, Wesch J, Becker JT, Jacobson L, D'Elia LF, van Gorp W, Visscher B. Low education as a possible risk factor for early cognitive abnormalities in HIV-1: new findings from the Multicenter AIDS Cohort Study (MACS). *AIDS.* In press.
41. van Gorp W, Satz P, Hinkin C, Selnes OA, Miller EN, McArthur JC, Cohen BA, Paz D. Metacognition in HIV-1 seropositive asymptomatic individuals: self-ratings versus objective neuropsychological performance. *J Clin Exp Neuropsychol.* 1991;13:812-819.
42. Maj M, Starace F, Sartorius N. *Mental Disorders in HIV-1 Infection and AIDS.* Bern, Switzerland: Hans Huber Publishers; 1993.
43. Price RW, Brew B, Sidtis J, Rosenblum M, Scheck AC, Cleary P. The brain in AIDS: central nervous system HIV-1 infection and AIDS dementia complex. *Science.* 1988;239:586-592.
44. Berger JR, Moskowitz L, Fischl M, Kelley RE. Neurologic disease as the presenting manifestation of AIDS. *South Med J.* 1987;80:683-686.

Regional Cerebral Blood Flow Measured During Symptom Provocation in Obsessive-Compulsive Disorder Using Oxygen 15–Labeled Carbon Dioxide and Positron Emission Tomography

Scott L. Rauch, MD; Michael A. Jenike, MD; Nathaniel M. Alpert, PhD; Lee Baer, PhD; Hans C. R. Breiter, MD; Cary R. Savage, PhD; Alan J. Fischman, MD, PhD

Background: The study was designed to determine the mediating neuroanatomy of obsessive-compulsive disorder (OCD).

Methods: The short half-life tracer oxygen 15–labeled carbon dioxide was used to allow for repeated positron emission tomographic determinations of regional cerebral blood flow on each of eight patients with OCD during a resting and a provoked (symptomatic) state.

Results: Individually tailored provocative stimuli were successful in provoking OCD symptoms, in comparison with paired innocuous stimuli, as measured by self-report on OCD analogue scales (P=.002). Omnibus subtraction images demonstrated a statistically significant increase in relative regional cerebral blood flow during the OCD symptomatic state vs the resting state in right caudate nucleus (P<.006), left anterior cingulate cortex (P<.045), and bilateral orbitofrontal cortex (P<.008); increases in the left thalamus approached but did not reach statistical significance (P=.07).

Conclusions: These findings are consistent with results of previous functional neuroimaging studies and contemporary neurocircuitry models of OCD. The data further implicate orbitofrontal cortex, caudate nucleus, and anterior cigulate cortex in the pathophysiology of OCD and in mediating OCD symptoms.

(Arch Gen Psychiatry. 1994;51:62-70)

Despite dramatic advances in the pharmacologic and behavioral treatment of patients with obsessive-compulsive disorder (OCD), there remains much to be learned about its pathophysiology.[1-6] With the current availability of high-resolution functional imaging techniques, such as positron emission tomography (PET), single-photon-emission computed tomography, and echoplanar magnetic resonance imaging, there is now an opportunity to study the mediating neuroanatomy of OCD in ways never before possible.

A number of investigators have used PET[7-14] and single-photon-emission computed tomography[15,16] to compare patients with OCD and control subjects in an effort to characterize group differences. While there has been considerable agreement among investigators' results, this approach has led to some inconsistent and conflicting findings.[17] It is likely that there is much between-subject variation as well as intraindividual variation due to the presence or absence of OCD symptoms at the time of imaging. Moreover, such paradigms do not distinguish between functional brain characteristics dependent on a symptomatic state vs OCD trait. Finally, the techniques of anatomic localization and statistical analysis previously used may contribute to false-negative as well as false-positive results.

One previous functional imaging study was designed to investigate blood flow changes associated with an OCD symptomatic state. Using a xenon 133 gas inhalation technique, Zohar et al[18] studied 10 patients with OCD who had washing compulsions. When each patient lis-

From the Departments of Psychiatry (Drs Rauch, Jenike, Baer, Breiter, and Savage) and Radiology (Drs Rauch, Alpert, Breiter, and Fischman) and Division of Nuclear Medicine/Positron Emission Tomography Laboratory (Drs Rauch, Alpert, and Fischman), Massachusetts General Hospital and Harvard Medical School, Boston.

See Patients and Methods on next page

PATIENTS AND METHODS

PATIENTS

Inclusion criteria were the elements of the *DSM-III-R* diagnosis of OCD[19] (as determined by clinical interview). In addition to *DSM-III-R* criteria, all patients had been ill for at least 1 year, were at least 18 years of age, and were right-handed. Exclusion criteria were the presence of major medical illness or other major psychiatric disorder (eg, schizophrenia, eating disorder, generalized anxiety disorder, major depression [current], or bipolar disorder). All patients had been free of all psychoactive drugs for at least 2 weeks before the study.

Subjects were recruited from our OCD Clinic and Research Unit patient population. All subjects underwent a full psychiatric and medical evaluation, including two diagnostic interviews. Additional historical data were obtained when available.

All studies were performed with the approval of the Subcommittee on Human Studies of the Massachusetts General Hospital, Boston. Informed consent was obtained from each patient.

The study population was composed of eight subjects, five men and three women with a mean (±SE) age at study of 36.1±2.0 years (range, 27 to 44 years); age at onset of OCD of 18.1±2.1 years (range, 10 to 28 years); duration of illness at study of 18.1±2.9 years (range, 3 to 29 years); and severity of illness, as measured by Yale-Brown Obsessive-Compulsive Scale, of 24.4±3.4 (range, 11 to 33). As subjects were scanned in both resting and provoked states, they served as their own controls.

OCD SYMPTOM PROVOCATION PARADIGM

After an initial habituation phase, patients with OCD underwent PET scanning twice in a resting state, while responding to an innocuous control stimulus, and twice again in a provoked state, while responding to a provocative stimulus that was tailored to induce each patient's symptoms. In all cases, the subjects participated in the process of identifying an appropriately provocative stimulus, so as to ensure sufficient but not overwhelming provocation of symptoms (**Table 1**). A balanced-order paradigm intended to control for order effects was deemed impractical. Pilot experience revealed that, once provoked, subjects remained symptomatic for up to several hours, precluding a paradigm dependent on prompt return to a resting state.

Ten-point analogue scales based on self-reporting were used to quantify the severity of each subject's anxiety (Anxiety Analogue Scale [AAS]) and OCD symptoms (OCD Analogue Scale [OCDAS]) during an initial habituation period as well as during each scanning period. A response of 10 was equated with the most severe symptoms ever previously experienced by the subject; 0 was equated with complete absence of symptoms. These scales provided clinical measures by which to gauge the magnitude of each subject's response to the different stimuli (innocuous vs provocative).

After being fully situated in the scanner, each subject was allowed to habituate, during which time analogue scale scores were obtained every 3 minutes. Completion of habituation was operationalized as both AAS and OCDAS scores remaining constant for two consecutive measurement periods.

After habituation, each subject proceeded to the resting phase of the paradigm. For each of two resting scans, the subject was exposed to an innocuous stimulus matched to his or her individualized provocative stimulus in terms of primary sensory stimulation. For example, the subject was shown a "clean" glove, and it was identified as such. This glove was then placed on the patient's left arm and remained there for approximately 2 minutes, throughout the acquisition phase for the first resting scan. Immediately after placement of the stimulus, the subject was instructed to close his or her eyes and to allow his or her thoughts to focus on the stimulus. Once the eyes were closed, PET acquisition commenced. At the end of each scan, the glove was removed and the subject was asked to indicate the severity of his or her anxiety and OCD symptoms on the corresponding scales. This procedure was repeated to achieve a complete set of data for each of two resting scans for each subject.

Next, the procedure was repeated for two provoked scans, during which the subject was exposed to an individualized provocative stimulus (eg, a "contaminated" glove) in place of the innocuous stimulus. In all conditions, the scans were performed with low background noise and lighting, with eyes closed and ears open.

PET FACILITIES AND PROCEDURES

A 15-slice whole-body tomograph (Scanditronix PC4096, General Electric, Milwaukee, Wis) was used in its stationary mode to acquire the PET data used in this study. A detailed report on the physical properties and reconstruction software have been published elsewhere.[20] The slice geometry consisted of contiguous slices with center-to-center distance of 6.5 mm (axial field equal to 97.5 mm) and axial resolution of 6.0 mm full width half maximum. Image reconstruction was performed with a measured attenuation correction and a Hanning-weighted reconstruction filter set to yield 8.0-mm in-plane spatial resolution (full width half maximum). Additional corrections were made in the reconstruction process to account for scattered radiation, random coincidences, and counting losses due to dead time in the camera electronics.

SUBJECT POSITIONING

A head immobilization apparatus including a custom-molded thermoplastic face mask (True Scan, Annapolis, Md) was used to minimize head motion. Within the PET scanner, the head was aligned, relative to the canthomeatal line,

Continued on next page

by means of the horizontal and vertical projected laser lines whose position was known with respect to the slice positions of the scanner. Once the head immobilization apparatus was in place, the patient was fitted with nasal cannulas and an overlying face mask, attached to radiolabeled gas inflow and vacuum, respectively.

IMAGE ACQUISITION

Before emission scanning, several transmission measurements were made with an orbiting pin source. Each PET data acquistion run consisted of 20 measurements, the first three with 10-second duration each and the remaining 17 with 5-second duration each. Subjects began inhaling $^{15}O-CO_2$ gas 30 seconds after initiation of the scan and finished 60 seconds later. Scans 4 through 15 were summed after reconstruction to form images of relative blood flow.

The subjects were studied during a 1-minute period in which they continuously inhaled tracer quantities of $^{15}O-CO_2$ while breathing room air. The concentration of the delivered gas was 2960 MBq/L with a flow rate of 2 L/min, further diluted by free mixture with room air within the face mask, resulting in a rapidly rising count rate in the brain, reaching terminal count rates of 100 000 to 200 000 events per second. Previous work in our laboratory (unpublished data, 1991) with the use of radial artery cannulation demonstrated that the integrated counts during inhalation periods up to 90 seconds are a linear function over the flow range 0 to 130 mL/min per 100 g. Therefore, for data to be produced with units of flow relative to whole brain, no arterialized blood, and thus no arterial line, was necessary.

IMAGE TRANSFORMATION

The scan data were pooled, by slice over all runs, to form images of higher statistical quality. Whole-slice tracings for each slice across conditions were compared within subjects to rule out detectable intrascan or interscan head movement. In this study, no data required correction or exclusion on that basis.

The pooled images were examined visually, and the coordinates of midline structures across all slices were recorded and used in a least-squares fitting procedure to estimate the parameters of the midsagittal plane. Transverse section images of all the emission and transmission scans were resliced parasagittally at 5.1-mm intervals.

The brain surface of a 10.2-mm parasagittal slice was manually outlined at the 50% threshold level (nominal). Surface data missing from the parasagittal emission slice were filled in from the more complete sagittal transmission images when necessary.

Parameters for the transformation of PET data to the coordinate system of Talairach and Szikla[21] and Talairach and Tournoux[22] were obtained by deforming the 10-mm sagittal plane from the Talairach and Szikla brain atlas[21] until a best least-squares match was obtained. This nonlinear fitting procedure allowed us to estimate directly the location of the frontal pole, occipital pole, vertex, anterior and posterior commissures, and the tilt angle. The equation of the midsagittal plane and the location of the landmarks listed above are sufficient to compute the Talairach transformation, including three magnifications along the anterior commissure–posterior commissure (AC-PC) line and one vertical magnification. Quality of the fitting procedure was judged both by the SEs of the parameters and by visual comparison of the manually drawn brain surface and the fit to the atlas contour.

With the use of the transformation parameters determined above, PET image sets were transformed to the three-dimensional space defined by Talairach and Szikla.[21] A second quality-control step was then performed by projecting a computerized version of the Talairach and Szikla atlas[21] onto the transformed PET data, with a digitized Talairach mapping program. This allowed visual confirmation of the transformation by comparison of the outlines of structures in the atlas and key features in the PET images.

IMAGE NORMALIZATION, SUBTRACTION, AND STATISTICAL ANALYSES

The mean concentration in each run was obtained as an area-weighted sum of the concentration of each slice and adjusted to a nominal value of 50 mL/min per 100 g. The data were then rescaled and smoothed with a two-dimensional gaussian filter 20 mm in width (full width half maximum).[23] These images were pooled over all subjects for each scanning condition, and pairwise subtractions were performed (within subject and between conditions) to yield images of mean difference, SD, number of data points contributing to each pixel (N), and t statistic, as well as omnibus subraction images (OSIs; with values in z score units). The data were processed as described by Friston et al[23] to produce OSIs, which are images of standardized normal deviates.

The basic approach for statistical analysis and hypothesis testing was adapted from Friston et al,[23] allowing computation of a pixel threshold depending on image smoothness and the number of pixels in the region of interest (ROI) corresponding to the hypothesis to be tested. In this manner, the threshold for statistical significance was adjusted appropriately for multiple comparisons (ie, many pixels). Image smoothness was measured as described by Friston et al[23] and found to be 14.2 mm.

Once the transformations of the PET data were performed, the data expressed in stereotaxic space, and OSIs created, two different types of analyses were performed: (1) ROI analyses were performed on the PET data with region boundaries generated by the mapping program to test our a priori hypotheses, and (2) post hoc review of the OSIs was performed for the whole brain in search of additional regions of statistically significant activation. In both types of analyses, OSIs of provoked minus relaxed conditions were used.

Table 1. Challenge Stimulus, Symptom Provoked, and Resulting Change in OCD and Anxiety Score After Provocation for Each Subject*

	Challenge Stimulus			OCD Score		Anxiety Score	
Patient	Innocuous	Provocative	Provoked Symptom	Rest	Provocation	Rest	Provocation
1	Mental image of wristwatch	Mental image of unlocked door	Checking obsessions	1.5	3.5	3.0	5.0
2†	Photo of pet dog	Photo of serial killer	Violent obsessions	2.0	9.0	4.0	6.0
3†	Clean rubber glove	Rubber glove contaminated in trash can	Contamination obsessions	0	3.0	1.0	4.0
4	Clean dollar bill	Dollar bill thought to be involved in purchase of illegal drugs	Contamination obsessions	0.5	5.0	0	5.0
5	Clean rubber glove and image of clean glove	Clean glove and image of touching floor at home	Contamination obsessions	1.0	2.5	1.0	1.0
6	Clean rubber glove	Rubber glove contaminated by touching floor	Contamination obsessions	1.0	6.5	2.0	5.5
7	Clean rubber glove	Rubber glove contaminated in toilet	Contamination obsessions	3.0	5.5	3.0	4.5
8†	Clean towel	Towel contaminated by touching after defecating	Contamination obsessions	1.0	10.0	1.0	10.0
Mean	...	...	...	1.25	5.63‡	1.88	5.13§
SE	...	...	...	0.33	0.97	0.48	0.88

*OCD indicates obsessive-compulsive disorder.
†OCD and anxiety scores were based on a single scan for these patients. For all other patients, score represents mean of two scans.
‡Increase in OCD Analogue Scale score significant by dependent $t(7)=4.68$, $P=.002$.
§Increase in Anxiety Analogue Scale score significant by dependent $t(7)=3.25$, $P=.012$.

tened to an audiotape of a situation specific to his or her individual contamination fears, cerebral blood flow (CBF) significantly increased as compared with a relaxed state. When the patients actually touched the feared contaminant (ie, in vivo exposure), CBF was significantly decreased in virtually all cortical areas. With the ^{133}Xe technique, it was impossible for the investigators to tell where the cortical blood flow had been shunted. One hypothesis they entertained was that blood was being shunted away from the cortex to subcortical areas, such as the caudate nuclei, or to the orbital gyri, areas that have been found to have high metabolic activity in some PET studies. The results of the xenon study indicated that the obsessional state of the patient at the time of imaging may have strong effects on the pattern of CBF and may be a source of intraindividual variation.

In the present study, by using oxygen 15–labeled carbon dioxide, a highly diffusible tracer radiopharmaceutical with a 2-minute half-life, we studied CBF patterns in both a resting state and a few minutes later in a provoked obsessional state. In this manner, OCD symptomatic state–dependent characteristics could be identified, and each patient could serve as his or her own control. Furthermore, by using PET, the advantages of higher spatial resolution and visualization of subcortical structures were exploited.

We sought to test the following hypotheses: that in comparison with the resting state, provocation of OCD symptoms would result in increased regional CBF (rCBF) in (1) orbitofrontal cortex, (2) caudate nuclei, (3) anterior cingulate cortex, and (4) thalamus. These hypotheses were based in part on previous functional neuroimaging studies in OCD and were also in keeping with the most current pathophysiologic models of OCD.[4,13]

RESULTS

The study yielded usable data in the form of 13 scans in each condition from the eight subjects studied. For three subjects, data from one scan in each condition, rather than two, were generated because of technical difficulties (N=2) and a subject's discomfort from lying flat for the necessary scanning time (N=1).

CLINICAL INDEXES

For all eight subjects, the provocative stimuli caused increased OCD symptoms, as measured by the OCDAS, as compared with the innocuous stimuli (Table 1). Mean (±SE) OCDAS scores were 1.25±0.33 for the resting condition and 5.63±0.97 for the provoked condition, representing a mean increase in OCDAS of 4.38 with provocation. The increase in OCDAS scores associated with provocation was statistically significant ($t[7]=4.68$, $P=.002$). Mean AAS scores were 1.88±0.48 for the resting condition and 5.13±0.88 for the provoked condition, representing a mean increase in AAS of 3.25 with provocation. The increase in AAS scores associated with provocation was also statistically significant ($t[7]=3.25$, $P=.012$). Moreover, the correlations between OCDAS and AAS scores were statistically significant for both the resting ($r=.77$, $P=.026$) and provoked ($r=.85$, $P=.007$) conditions.

OMNIBUS SUBTRACTION IMAGES

Pertinent omnibus subtraction images (OSIs) are shown in **Figure 1** and **Figure 2**. They are presented in two different ways to illustrate optimally both the important find-

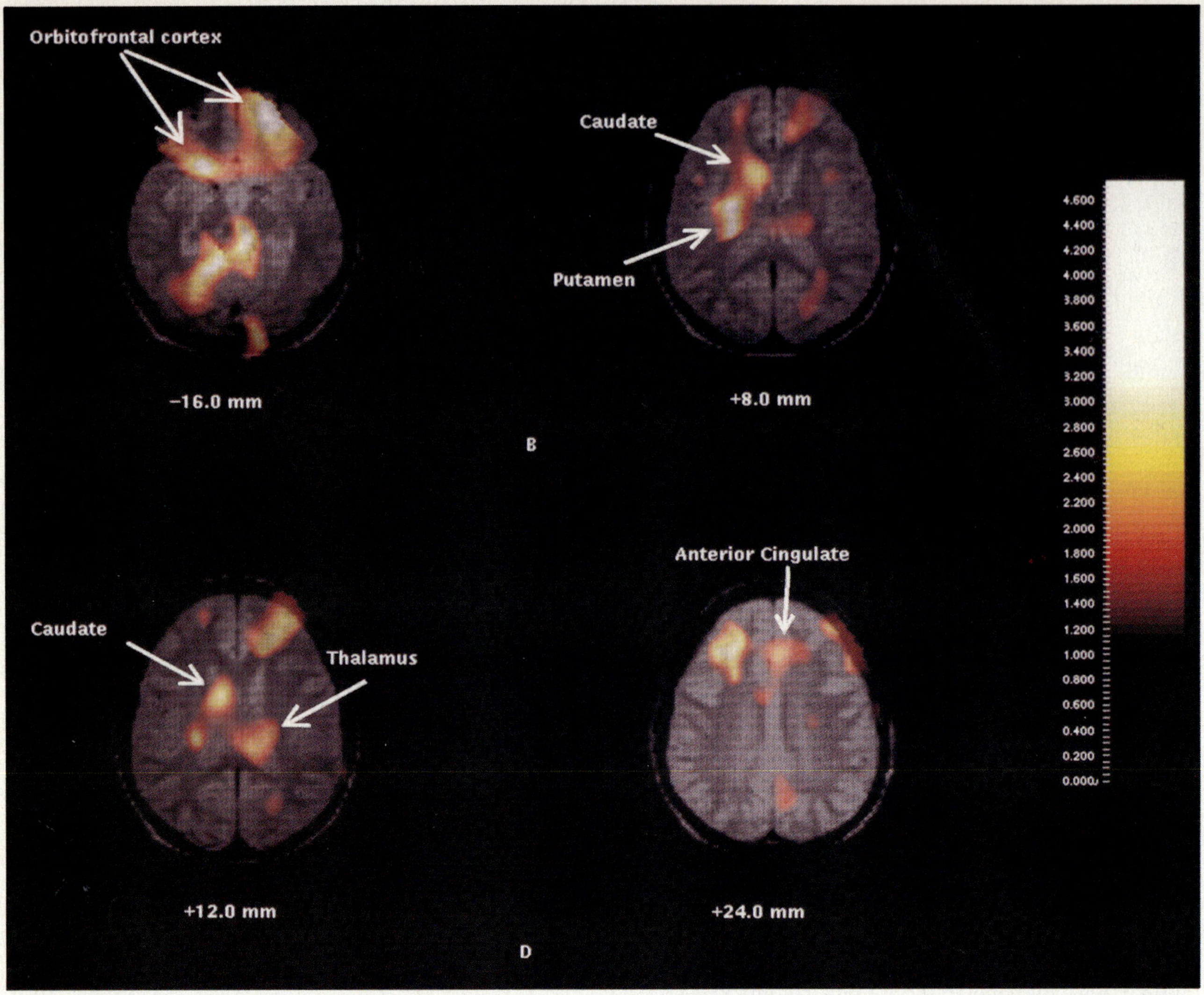

Figure 1. *Positron emission tomographic omnibus subtraction images of provoked minus resting conditions for all subjects (N=8; 13 scans per condition) displayed with a "hot iron" scale in units of z score, superimposed over a normal magnetic resonance image transformed to Talairach space, for the purpose of anatomic reference. All images are transverse sections parallel to the anterior commissure–posterior commissure plane, shown in conventional neuroimaging orientation (top=anterior, bottom=posterior, right=left, and left=right). Each transverse section is labeled with its z coordinate, denoting its position with respect to the anterior commissure–posterior commissure line (superior >0). Activation is found within regions of interest corresponding to a priori hypotheses. A shows orbitofrontal cortex bilaterally (P<.008); B and C, right caudate nucleus (P<.006); C, left thalamus (P=.07); and D, anterior cingulate cortex (P<.045). Other areas of substantial activation include (B) right putamen and left (C) and right (D) middle frontal cortex (not labeled).*

ings and the method used. In Figure 1, OSIs are superimposed over a normal magnetic resonance image, which has been transformed to Talairach space, to serve as an anatomic reference for the reader. In Figure 2, the OSIs are displayed with superimposed ROIs (white dashed lines) from the digitized atlas generated by the mapping program.

The ROIs corresponding to the a priori hypotheses were systematically inspected. Maximum pixel values with units in terms of *z* scores were identified within the boundaries of each ROI. These values were compared with significance thresholds reflecting an a priori criterion of $P<.05$ for one-tailed *t* tests and dependent on the number of pixels for each respective ROI (**Table 2**).

In the case of orbitofrontal cortex, for the horizontal slice 16 mm inferior to the AC-PC line, the OSI maximum pixel value within the ROI was 3.50, with one centroid of activation located in right posterior orbitofrontal cortex and another in left anterior orbitofrontal cortex. The number of pixels for orbitofrontal cortex was 414, resulting in a significance threshold ($P<.05$) of greater than 2.85. Thus, the 3.50 value reflected a probability value of $P<.008$. In the case of caudate nucleus, for the horizontal slice 8 mm superior to the AC-PC line, the OSI maximum pixel value within the ROI was 2.53 (right caudate only). The number of pixels for the caudate nuclei was 36 (18×2, since no hypothesis was made regarding laterality), resulting in a significance threshold ($P<.05$) of greater than 1.50. Thus, the 2.53 value reflected a probability value of $P<.006$. In the case of anterior cingulate cortex, for the horizontal slice 24 mm superior to the AC-PC line, the OSI maximum pixel value within the ROI was 2.24 (left of midline only). The number of pixels for

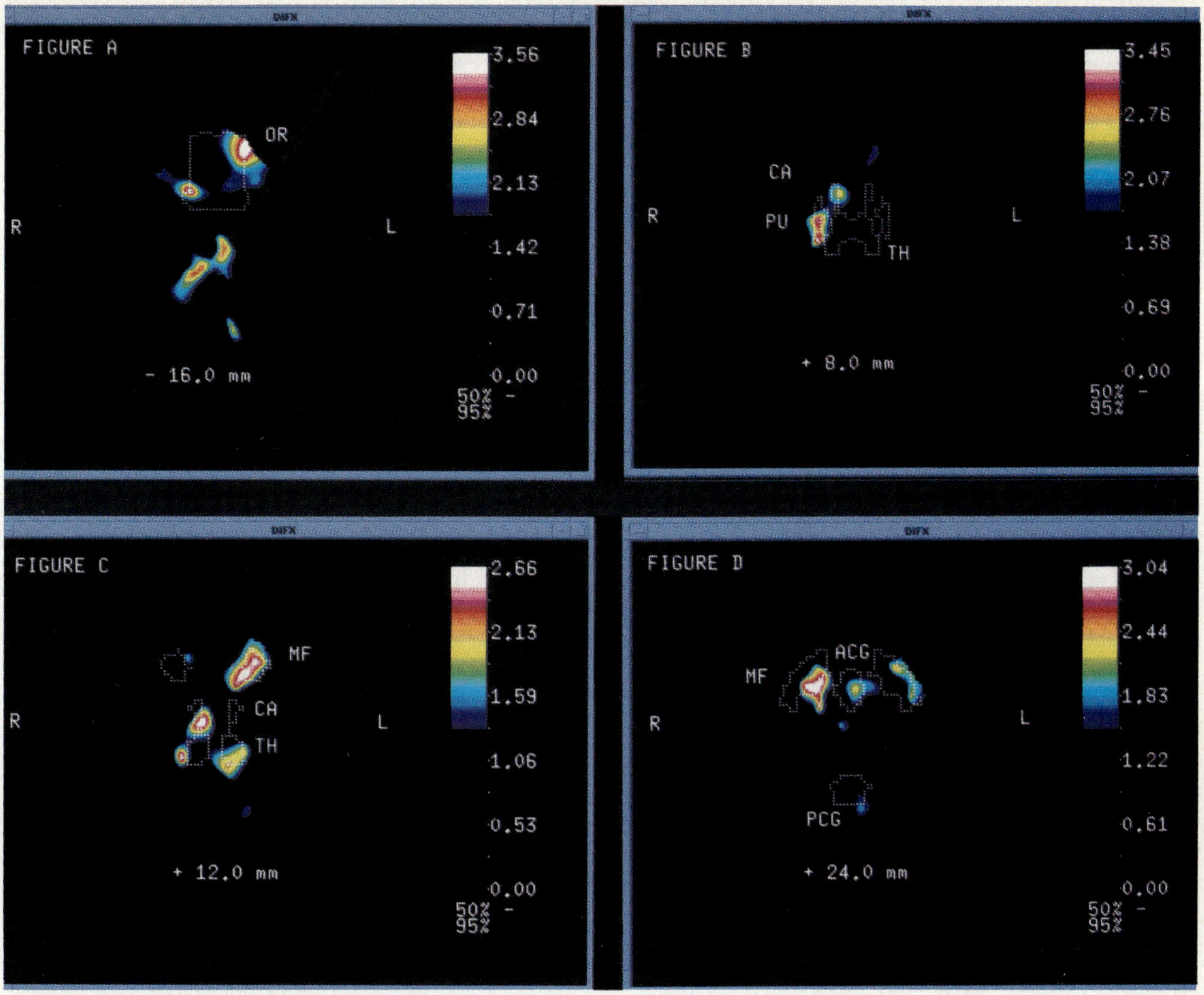

Figure 2. *Positron emission tomographic omnibus subtraction images of provoked minus resting conditions for all subjects (N=8; 13 scans per condition) displayed with a Sokoloff color scale in units of z score. White dashed outlines reflecting the boundaries of brain regions of interest as defined via a digitized version of the Talairach and Szikla[21] atlas are superimposed for anatomic reference. All images are transverse sections parallel to the anterior commissure–posterior commissure plane, shown in conventional neuroimaging orientation (top=anterior, bottom=posterior, right=left, and left=right). Each transverse section is labeled with its z coordinate, denoting its position with respect to the anterior commissure–posterior commissure line (superior >0). Activation is demonstrated within regions of interest corrresponding to a priori hypotheses. A shows orbitofrontal cortex bilaterally (P<.008); B and C, right caudate nucleus (P<.006); C, left thalamus (P=.07); and D, anterior cingulate cortex (P<.045). Other areas of marked activation include right putamen (B) and left (C) and right (D) middle frontal cortex. ACG indicates anterior cingulate cortex; CA, caudate nucleus; MF, middle frontal cortex; OR, orbitofrontal cortex; PCG, posterior cingulate cortex; PU, putamen; and TH, thalamus.*

the anterior cingulate cortex was 95, resulting in a significance threshold (*P*<.05) of greater than 2.20. Thus, the 2.24 value reflected a probability value of *P*<.045. In the case of thalamus, for the horizontal slice 12 mm superior to the AC-PC line, the OSI maximum pixel value within the ROI was 2.07 (left thalamus only). The number of pixels for the thalamus was 114 (57×2), resulting in a significance threshold (*P*<.05) of greater than 2.25. Thus, the 2.07 value did not achieve statistical significance based on the a priori criterion, but it did approach significance, reflected by a probability value of *P*=.07.

Post hoc inspection of all sections of the OSIs revealed several areas of high maximum pixel values indicative of substantial relative activation. Owing to the post hoc nature of these analyses, however, the threshold for significance (at *P*<.05) was adjusted for multiple comparisons to reflect that the ROI was essentially the whole brain. Therefore, corresponding pixel numbers for each slice were in excess of 2000. Consequently, thresholds for significance required maximum pixel values on the order of greater than 3.5. No structures were identified that met this stringent criterion. Still, a few structures did approach significance and contained maximum pixel values that would, in some cases, have achieved significance had a priori hypotheses pertaining to them been made. It is worth mentioning these structures, as future studies might test the hypothesis that they are activated by this paradigm. Specifically, the regions of subthreshold activation were left angular gyrus (maximum pixel value, 2.70), left visual association cortex (maxi-

Table 2. Regions of Interest With A Priori Hypothesis of Significant Increase With Provocation of Obsessions

Region of Interest	No. of Pixels*	Significance Threshold†	Actual Maximum Pixels‡	P§	Maximum Pixel Coordinates‖
Orbitofrontal cortex	414	2.85	3.50	.008	21.04, 51.89, −16.0 (left); −19.76, 18.74, −16.0 (right)
Caudate	36	1.50	2.53	.006	−9.56, 14.91, 8.0
Anterior cingulate	95	2.20	2.24	.045	4.46, 32.76, 24.0
Thalamus	114	2.25	2.07	.070	13.39, −27.6, 12.0

*Values represent the number of pixels within the region of interest for the slice examined.

†Values represent the z score threshold corresponding to P=.05, based on the number of pixels in the region of interest and the degree of smoothness in these images (Friston et al[23]).

‡Values represent the actual maximum pixel value (in z score units) within the region of interest from the omnibus subtraction image.

§Based on one-tailed t tests, with the a priori threshold for significance established at P<.05.

‖Coordinates defining the location of the maximum pixel values within each region of interest from the omnibus subtraction images in Talairach space[22] are expressed as "x, y, z"; x>0 is left of the midsagittal plane, y>0 is anterior to the anterior commissure, and z>0 is superior to the anterior commissure–posterior commissure line.

mum pixel value, 2.17), bilateral middle frontal cortex (maximum pixel value, 3.04), middle cingulate cortex (maximum pixel value, 2.36), right putamen (maximum pixel value, 3.14), and frontal eye fields (maximum pixel value, 3.13).

Finally, correlation analyses using the Pearson product-moment statistic were performed for OCDAS and AAS scores with rCBF at four sites of significant activation (ie, right posterior and left anterior orbitofrontal cortex, right caudate nucleus, and left anterior cingulate). Circular ROIs of fixed radius (21 to 26 pixels in area) were positioned around the centroid of maximal statistical activation, and mean rCBF values within each targeted ROI were determined. For the provoked state, only rCBF within left anterior orbitofrontal cortex was significantly correlated with OCDAS score ($r[7]=.74$, $P<.04$), and no correlations approached statistical significance for AAS score (all $P>.10$). Of note, this analysis was repeated for provoked-relaxed differences in analogue scores and rCBF values. This maneuver yielded only a significant *negative* correlation between right posterior orbitofrontal cortex and OCDAS ($r[7]=-.83$, $P<.01$), and again no correlations approaching significance for AAS score. No adjustments were made for multiple comparisons for these analyses (total, eight for OCDAS and eight for AAS).

COMMENT

Insel[17] recently published a thorough review of the considerable literature regarding functional neuroimaging studies and OCD. Positron emission tomographic studies comparing patients with OCD with controls[7-9] have consistently shown increased glucose metabolism in the orbitofrontal cortex, but with variability as to laterality, as well as inconsistent caudate and anterior cingulate abnormalities. Single-photon-emission computed tomographic studies using the ligand technetium Tc 99m hexamethylpropyleneamine oxime to compare patients with OCD and normal subjects have yielded similarly inconsistent findings.[15,16]

Examining changes associated with treatment, Benkelfat et al[11] reported that the left caudate–gray matter metabolic ratios decreased with improvement in nondepressed patients with OCD treated with clomipramine. Most recently, Baxter et al[13] reported on the results of two groups of nine patients with OCD who underwent fludeoxyglucose F 18 PET scans before and after treatment with fluoxetine or behavioral therapy. Responders to either treatment showed lowered metabolism in the head of the right caudate–ipsilateral hemisphere in comparison with pretreatment values, after successful treatment; no such differences were exhibited by treatment nonresponders or controls. Concurrently, Swedo et al[14] reported on a PET study of 13 subjects receiving a variety of pharmacotherapies for OCD. They found a decrease in whole-brain normalized right orbitofrontal metabolism that correlated with symptom improvement.

Thus, it has been reproducibly demonstrated that patients with OCD have increased glucose metabolism in orbitofrontal cortex and caudate nuclei in comparison with controls, and that normalization of metabolism in those structures is associated with posttreatment symptom improvement. The orbitofrontal cortex, cingulate cortex, and caudate nuclei are part of a circuit, also including the thalamus, that may be involved in the regulation of both consciously perceived emotional concerns and repetitive behaviors.[1,4,5] It is important to note that Baxter et al[13] showed interregional correlations between these structures, both before and after treatment, in patients with OCD, which have not been seen for normal subjects or unipolar depressed subjects.[24] Therefore, taken together, there is much evidence to support a role for this circuit in a neurobiologic model of OCD.[4-6,13,17]

Still, no previous PET studies had looked at differences between a resting and an obsessional state in the same patient during a brief period in an effort to determine how inconsistencies among studies may be due to variations in the mental state of obsessional patients at the time of the PET scans. Nor had any group used such a PET paradigm to investigate the mediating functional neuranatomy of OCD symptoms.

In the present study, invoking a within-subject symptom provocation paradigm, we found statistically significant activation in right caudate nucleus, left anterior cingulate cortex, and bilateral orbitofrontal cortex in the provoked (symptomatic) vs resting condition. Activation in the left thalamus approached, but did not achieve, the threshold for statistical significance. These findings, to some extent, represent a replication and extension of the findings reported by Zohar et al[18] using the more limited xenon technique. More importantly, the findings confirmed a priori hypotheses consonant with current pathophysiologic models of OCD.[4,13] Specifically, this pattern of activation supports the model of a frontostriatothalamofrontal loop in mediating OCD symptoms. Activation of cingulate cortex is likewise consistent with its prominent role within the Papez circuit[25] and limbic system, perhaps mediating anxiety in a less specific manner.

The correlation analyses performed between analogue scale scores and rCBF lack adequate power to be conclusive. Still, the finding that the analogue scale, OCDAS, is positively correlated with rCBF in left anterior orbitofrontal cortex for the provoked state and negatively correlated with rCBF in right posterior orbitofrontal cortex for provoked minus resting data suggest that these two regions may play opposing roles in mediating and suppressing OCD symptoms respectively. This could account for much of the variability in laterality of orbitofrontal findings in past studies where subjects were scanned in "neutral" states and intersubject comparisons were required. Interpretation of lateralized findings in this study is mitigated, however, by the lateralized nature of stimulus presentation. The absence of significant correlation between AAS and rCBF for the ROIs examined fails to inform as to which structures are responsible for mediating anxiety nonspecifically.

Post hoc OSI analyses of the provoked minus resting data revealed activations of comparable magnitude in several other structures. Because of the post hoc nature of these analyses, however, appropriate adjustment of the threshold for statistical significance in the face of multiple comparisons caused these differences to fall short of statistical significance. Nonetheless, it is important to attempt replication of these findings and to explore further the meaning of activation in these stuctures if the findings are reproducible. For instance, the notion that ongoing obsessions might be associated with activation of structures thought to mediate visual (areas 18 and 19) and language (angular gyrus) association functions is quite plausible and intuitively appealing.

Limitations of the present study include the small number of subjects and their heterogeneity with regard to OCD symptoms. Subjects with contamination fears are overrepresented in this sample. In the future, study populations could be composed of patients with pure OCD symptom subtypes. Replication with larger numbers could also provide sufficient power to test questions pertaining to interregion as well as symptom severity by regional activation correlations.

This study also suffers from limitations intrinsic to the methods and technologies used. The technique of signal normalization to whole brain does not allow for detection of changes in whole-brain CBF. Moreover, localization of change in rCBF is constrained by the spatial resolution of PET. Head movement cannot be absolutely prevented, and there are limitations in the sensitivity for its detection and correction. Together with the technique of stereotaxic transformation, these must be acknowledged as potential sources of error in terms of precise anatomic localization. Coupled with the statistical approach of Friston et al,[23] these factors contribute to the risk of type II errors. Still, the advantages of this technique remain: the capability to sum data across subjects, and superior power for identifying locations of differential activation, by avoiding dependence on large, arbitrary, or anatomically restrictive ROIs (regions of interest).

Finally, no control group was studied to allow identification of the rCBF profile associated with the nonspecific anxious state. Although this study serves to identify the mediating anatomy of OCD symptoms, it is important to distinguish which, if any, of those changes are attributable to anxiety in a nonspecific sense. Toward that end, future studies must determine the mediating anatomy of the anxious state for subjects with other anxiety disorders as well as normal controls.

Mountz et al[26] used an analogous PET paradigm to study simple phobics, in which exposure to provocative stimuli (ie, small animals) produced significant differences in anxiety and physiologic measurements between "resting" and "provoked" scans. Absolute global CBF and rCBF were significantly lower during provoked scans than during resting scans. However, when apppropriate normalizations were performed, no global or regional CBF differences among scans achieved statistical significance. Application of the techniques used in our study to the replication of their experiment might provide superior power and more revealing results.

In summary, the present study used the tracer $^{15}O-CO_2$ to allow repeated PET determinations of rCBF on each of a group of patients with OCD during a resting as well as a provoked state. Findings included a relative increase in rCBF during the OCD symptomatic state vs the resting state in right caudate nucleus, left anterior cingulate cortex, and bilateral orbitofrontal cortex. Activation in the left thalamus approached, but did not reach, statistical significance. These findings are consistent with results of previous neuroimaging studies, as well as contemporary theories of the pathophysiology of OCD. The OCDAS scores were positively correlated with activation of left anterior orbitofrontal cortex and negatively correlated with activation of right posterior orbitofrontal cortex, which suggests lateralized opposing influences on OCD symptoms. Unexpected regions of activation, although of substantial magnitude, in lieu of a priori hypotheses, did not achieve statistical significance. These regions, including the left angular gyrus and visual association cortex, should be further investigated. Future studies should seek to replicate these findings and to delineate the mediating anatomy of the nonspecific anxious state. There is also a need to develop alternative activation paradigms that herald diagnostic or prognostic value in the evaluation of OCD and that may allow for parallel study of related disorders.

Accepted for publication February 25, 1993.

This work was supported in part by a CIBA-Geigy Unrestricted Postdoctoral Fellowship Fund and by grant 5T32CA09362-11 from the National Cancer Institute, Bethesda, Md.

We wish to thank Dmitry Berdichevsky, MS, Avis Loring, RT(N), Peter Manzo, and Steve Weise for their technical assistance.

Reprint requests to OCD Unit, Ninth Floor, Massachusetts General Hospital—East, 149 13th St, Charlestown, MA 02129 (Dr Rauch).

REFERENCES

1. Jenike M. Obsessive-compulsive disorder: a question of a neurologic lesion. *Compr Psychiatry.* 1984;25:298-304.
2. Schwartz JM, Baxter LR, Mazziotta JC, Gerner RH, Phelps ME. The differential diagnosis of depression: relevance of positron emission tomography studies of cerebral glucose metabolism to the bipolar-unipolar dichotomy. *JAMA.* 1987; 258:1368-1374.
3. Jenike MA, Baer L, Minichiello WE, eds. *Obsessive Compulsive Disorder: Theory and Management.* 2nd ed. Chicago, Ill: Year Book Medical Publishers; 1990.
4. Modell J, Mountz J, Curtis G, Greden J. Neurophysiologic dysfunction in basal ganglia/limbic striatal and thalamocortical circuits as a pathogenetic mechanism of obsessive-compulsive disorder. *J Neuropsychiatry.* 1989;1:27-36.
5. Baxter LR, Schwartz JM, Guze BH, Bergman K, Szuba MP. Neuroimaging in obsessive-compulsive disorder: seeking the mediating neuroanatomy. In: Jenike MA, Baer L, Minichiello WE, eds. *Obsessive Compulsive Disorder: Theory and Management.* 2nd ed. Chicago, Ill: Year Book Medical Publishers; 1990:167-188.
6. Rauch SL, Jenike MA. Neurobiological models of obsessive compulsive disorder. *Psychosomatics.* 1993;34:20-32.
7. Baxter LR Jr, Phelps JM, Mazziotta JC, Guze BH, Schwartz JM. Local cerebral glucose metabolic rates in obsessive-compulsive disorder: a comparison with rates in unipolar depression and normal controls. *Arch Gen Psychiatry.* 1987; 44:211-218.
8. Baxter L, Schwartz J, Mazziotta J, Phelps ME, Pahl JJ, Buze BE, Fairbanks L. Cerebral glucose metabolic rates in nondrepressed patients with obsessive-compulsive disorder. *Am J Psychiatry.* 1988;145:1560-1563.
9. Nordahl TE, Benkelfat C, Semple W, Gross M, King AC, Cohen RM. Cerebral glucose metabolic rates in obsessive-compulsive disorder. *Neuropsychopharmacology.* 1989;2:23-28.
10. Swedo SE, Schapiro MB, Gady CL, Cheslow DL, Leonard HL, Kumar A, Friedland R, Rapoport SI, Rapoport JL. Cerebral glucose metabolism in childhood-onset obsessive-compulsive disorder. *Arch Gen Psychiatry.* 1989;46:518-523.
11. Benkelfat C, Nordahl TE, Semple WE, King AC, Murphy DL, Cohen RM. Local cerebral glucose metabolic rates in obsessive-compulsive disorder: patients treated with clomipramine. *Arch Gen Psychiatry.* 1990;47:840-848.
12. Sawle GV, Hymas NF, Lees AJ, Frackowiak RSJ. Obsessional slowness: functional studies with positron emission tomography. *Brain.* 1991;114:2191-2202.
13. Baxter LR Jr, Schwartz JM, Bergman KS, Szuba MP, Guze BH, Mazziotta JC, Alazraki A, Selin CE, Ferng H-K, Munford P, Phelps ME. Caudate glucose metabolic rate changes with both drug and behavior therapy for obsessive-compulsive disorder. *Arch Gen Psychiatry.* 1992;49:681-689.
14. Swedo SE, Pietrini P, Leonard HL, Schapiro MB, Rettew DC, Goldberger EL, Rapoport SI, Rapoport JL, Grady CL. Cerebral glucose metabolism in childhood-onset obsessive-compulsive disorder: revisualization during pharmacotherapy. *Arch Gen Psychiatry.* 1992;49:690-694.
15. Machlin S, Harris G, Pearslon G, Hoehn-Saric R, Jeffery P, Camargo E. Elevated medial-frontal cerebral blood flow in obsessive-compulsive patients: a SPECT study. *Am J Psychiatry.* 1991;148:1240-1242.
16. Rubin RT, Villanueva-Meyer J, Anath J, Trajmar PG, Mena I. Regional xenon 133 cerebral blood flow and cerebral technetium Tc 99m-HMPAO uptake in unmedicated patients with obsessive-compulsive disorder and matched normal control subjects: determination by high-resolution single-photon emission computed tomography. *Arch Gen Psychiatry.* 1992;49:695-702.
17. Insel TR. Toward a neuroanatomy of obsessive-compulsive disorder. *Arch Gen Psychiatry.* 1992;49:739-744.
18. Zohar J, Insel T, Berman K, Foa E, Hill J, Weinberger D. Anxiety and cerebral blood flow during behavioral challenge: dissociation of central from peripheral and subjective measures. *Arch Gen Psychiatry.* 1989;46:505-510.
19. American Psychiatric Association, Committee on Nomenclature and Statistics. *Diagnostic and Statistical Manual of Mental Disorders, Revised Third Edition.* Washington, DC: American Psychiatric Association; 1987.
20. Kops ER, Herzog H, Schmid A, Holte S, Feinendegen LE. Performance characteristics of an eight-ring whole body PET scanner. *J Comput Assist Tomogr.* 1990;14:437-445.
21. Talairach J, Szikla Z. *Atlas of Stereotactic Anatomy of the Telencephalon.* Paris, France: Masson et Cie; 1967.
22. Talairach J, Tournoux P. *Co-Planar Stereotaxic Atlas of the Human Brain.* New York, NY: Thieme Medical Publishers Inc; 1988.
23. Friston K, Frith C, Liddle P, Franckowiak R. Comparing functional (PET) images: the assessment of significant change. *J Cerebral Blood Flow Metab.* 1991; 11:690-699.
24. Baxter LR. Neuroimaging studies of obsessive compulsive disorder. *Psychiatr Clin North Am.* 1992;15:871-884.
25. Papez JW. Proposed mechanism of emotion. *Arch Neurol Psychiatry.* 1937; 38:725-743.
26. Mountz J, Modell J, Wilson M, Curtis G, Lee M, Schmaltz S, Kuhl D. Positron emission tomographic evaluation of cerebral blood flow during state anxiety in simple phobia. *Arch Gen Psychiatry.* 1989;46:501.

Violence in the Severely Mentally Ill

The article by Hodgins[1] in the June 1992 issue of the ARCHIVES is important because it appears to contradict the notion that patients with major mental illness are no more likely than the general population to commit violent and nonviolent crime. Hodgins reported that men and women with severe mental illness were 2.5 and 5.0 times more likely than the general population to be convicted of crime, respectively, and concluded that "the findings raise fundamental questions about these disorders, their etiology, and their treatment." The problem with this conclusion is that 49% of men and 43% of women with major mental disorders also had a diagnosis of substance abuse or dependence. Given that men and women with substance-abuse problems alone were 20 and 32 times more likely to be convicted, respectively, it could be concluded that the tendency to commit crime may be a function of substance abuse or dependence and not of major mental illness. The author should have separated subjects with major mental illness who were not substance abusers to assess the contribution of mental illness alone. If the substance abusers are removed from this group, it is plausible that the rate of crime will be lower than in the general population. I hope the author presents these data in the reply as should have been done in the original article.

Martin A. Weiler, MD
Creighton-Nebraska Department of Psychiatry
2205 S 10th St
Omaha, NE 68108

1. Hodgins S. Mental disorder, intellectual deficiency, and crime: evidence from a birth cohort. *Arch Gen Psychiatry.* 1992;49:476-483.

In reply

Unraveling the relationships between major mental disorders, substance abuse and dependence, and criminality is not easy because existing data suggest that they are rather complex. Assuming that they are linear and causal, as does Weiler, oversimplifies the problem and thereby limits the type of explanatory models that will be developed and the statistical analyses that can be performed.[1]

There is now good evidence to suggest that among persons who develop schizophrenia, major depression, and bipolar disorder, rates of substance abuse and dependence are elevated compared with rates in persons without disorders.[2-4(chap 9)] *As well, persons with major mental disorders are at increased risk for personality disorders*[4 (chap 12),5] *(S.H., J. Toupin, PhD, and L. Tremblay, PhD, unpublished data, 1991). Is the increased vulnerability for substance abuse related to the major disorder, to the personality disorder, or to both, or is it independent of the two? Is criminality related to the major disorder, the personality disorder, alcohol- and drug-use disorders, any combination of these disorders, or to none of them?*

Existing data suggest at least four hypotheses regarding the relations between the major disorders, substance abuse, and criminality. The first hypothesis proposes that substance abuse is one aspect of antisocial behavior, as has been noted among adolescent boys who are developing bipolar disorder.[6,7] *Alternatively, substance abuse may be one manifestation of an antisocial personality disorder, which has been found to be prevalent among offenders with major mental disorders.*[8,9] *A third hypothesis suggests that substance abuse may be an attempt by adolescents to cope with the development of anxiety and other symptoms, as in the first stages of schizophrenia.*[10] *A fourth hypothesis is that substance abuse has nothing to do with the criminality, as in the case of a patient who behaves violently, not while intoxicated but rather in response to hallucinations. These hypotheses are not mutually exclusive, and they could all be correct, applying to different subgroups of patients, or they could all be wrong. However, to my knowledge, they have not yet been tested.*

As was previously reported,[11] *in the Swedish cohort (unlike what Weiler understood), 49% of the male* offenders *with a major mental disorder (not of the men with a major mental disorder) and 43% of the female* offenders *with a major mental disorder (not of the female subjects with a major mental disorder) had secondary diagnoses of substance-use (alcohol and other drugs) disorders. Another 20% of the male offenders with major mental disorders and another 19% of the female offenders with major mental disorders were substance abusers in childhood but had no adult diagnoses of substance-use disorders.*[12] *The finding that about half the offenders with major disorders did not have additional diagnoses of substance-use disorders concurs with results from the studies of unbiased samples of homicide offenders. In these investigations,*[13-15] *despite the fact that populations of homicide offenders were assessed by a psychiatrist and, more often than not, by more than one psychiatrist, about half of those with major disorders did not receive additional diagnoses relating to substance abuse.*

Before jumping to any conclusions, consider the following facts. First, the study reported was a record study and involved "treated" cases as opposed to "true" cases of major disorders and of substance-use disorders. Second, among both the men and the women with major disorders, there is less criminality than among the men and the women with substance-use disorders. Third, as was reported previously,[11,12] more of the children who eventually developed major mental disorders and became criminal, compared with those who only developed major mental disorders, had been identified by child welfare authorities as substance abusers. Fourth, the prevalence of substance-use disorders is higher among the subjects with major mental disorders than among the other subjects. In fact, 32.9% of the men with major mental disorders and 10.0% of the women with major mental disorders had additional diagnoses of substance-use disorders. The prevalence is high given that these were file diagnoses made during a period when little or no attention was paid to concurrent disorders. Fifth, among the male subjects who had no substance-abuse problems in childhood or adulthood, 31.9% of those with major disorders and 26.2% of those with no disorder had at least one registration for crime. Among the women who had no substance-abuse problems in childhood or adulthood, 9.1% of those with major mental disorders and 4.1% of those with no disorder had at least one registration for a crime. Finally, taking into account only adult diagnoses, a similar picture emerges. Among the male subjects who had no diagnoses of substance-use disorders, 29.4% of those without disorders and 36.4% of those with major disorders had at least one registration for crime. Among the women with no substance-use disorders, 4.9% of those without disorders and 8.5% of those with major disorders had at least one registration for crime.

Sheilagh Hodgins, PhD
Department of Psychology
Universite de Montreal
CP 6128, Suc A
Montreal, Quebec H3C 3J7

1. Magnusson D, Bergman L. A pattern approach to the study of pathways from childhood to adulthood. In: Robins LN, Rutter M, eds. *Straight and Devious Pathways From Childhood to Adulthood.* Cambridge, England: Cambridge University Press; 1990:101-115.
2. Regier DA, Farmer ME, Rae DS, Locke BZ, Keith SJ, Judd LL, Goodwin FK. Comorbity of mental disorders with alcohol and other drug abuse: results from the Epidemiologic Catchment Area (ECA) Study. *JAMA.* 1990;264:2511-2518.
3. Mueser KT, Yarnold PR, Levinson DF, Singh H, Bellack AS, Keey K, Morrison RL, Yadalam KG. Prevalence of substance abuse in schizophrenia: demographic and clinical correlates. *Schizophr Bull.* 1990;16:31-56.
4. Goodwin FK, Jamison KR. *Manic Depressive Illness.* New York, NY: Oxford University Press; 1990:chap 9, chap 12.
5. Leveillee S. *Le Support Social Chez les Schizophrenes Dans la Communaute.* Montreal, Quebec: Universite de Montreal; 1993. Doctoral thesis.
6. Carlson G, Strober M. Affective disorders in adolescence. *Psychiatr Clin North Am.* 1979;2:511-526.
7. Bowden CL, Sarabia F. Diagnosing manic depressive illness in adolescents. *Compr Psychiatry.* 1980;21:263-269.
8. Cote G, Hodgins S. Co-occurring mental disorders among criminal offenders. *Bull Am Acad Psychiatry Law.* 1990;18:271-281.
9. Abrams KM, Teplin LA. Co-occurring disorders among mentally ill jail detainees: implications for public policy. *Am Psychol.* 1991;46:1036-1045.
10. Bukstein OG, Brest DA, Kaminer Y. Co-morbidity of substance abuse and other psychiatric disorders in adolescents. *Am J Psychiatry.* 1989;146:1131-1141.
11. Hodgins S. Mental disorder, intellectual deficiency, and crime. *Arch Gen Psychiatry.* 1992;49:476-483.
12. Hodgins S. The criminality of mentally disordered persons. In: Hodgins S, ed. *Mental Disorder and Crime.* Newbury Park, Calif: Sage Publications; 1993: 3-21.
13. Lindquist P. Criminal homicide in northern Sweden. *Int J Law Psychiatry.* 1989;8:19-37.
14. Gottlieb P, Gabrielsen G, Kramp P. Psychotic homicides in Copenhagen from 1959 to 1983. *Acta Psychiatr Scand.* 1987;76:285-292.
15. Beaudoin MN, Hodgins S. Homicide, schizophrenia and substance abuse or dependency. *Can J Psychiatry.* In press.

Are Stress Hormones and Serotonin Related to Aggression in Primates?

In both the abstract and "Comment" section of their recent report, Higley et al[1] state that plasma cortisol concentrations and "stress hormones" (plural emphasized) were positively correlated with a measurement of aggression. It is not clear what this is based on, since the correlation between plasma cortisol and aggression ratings in Table 2 of their article is essentially zero. If this is not a typographical error, it puts into question the authors' claim of a relationship between increased stress, serotonin, and aggression in their animal population, as does the absence of significant intercorrelations between 5-hydroxyindoleacetic acid (5-HIAA) levels in the cerebrospinal fluid (CSF) and the other stress measures identified, ie, CSF norepinephrine and plasma corticotropin.

Although it is in support of other work, the conclusion that the findings indicate that excessive aggression is related to diminished CSF 5-HIAA concentrations in nonhuman primates also seems overstated, in view of the graphic presentation of data. This correlation seems critically dependent on one subject, who had both the highest measure of aggressivity and the lowest CSF 5-HIAA value. Although it is impossible to be completely certain without examining the raw values, it appears that the second, fourth, and fifth most aggressive primates had CSF 5-HIAA values above the mean, and that approximately 11 of 16 monkeys at or above the mean for aggressivity had 5-HIAA values that were at or above the mean as well. This is not compelling support for the primary hypothesis that *interindividual* differences in aggressivity ratings are correlated negatively with CSF 5-HIAA levels as a trait. While the biological characteristics of the most aggressive primate seem worthy of continued study, the data presented do not indicate that broader statements about the relationship between 5-HIAA concentrations and excessive aggression in primate society as a whole are warranted.

Victor I. Reus, MD
Department of Psychiatry
University of California
School of Medicine
Langley Porter Hospital
401 Parnassus Ave
Box F-0984
San Francisco, CA 94143-0984

1. Higley JD, Mehlman PT, Higley SB, Suomi SJ, Linnoila M, Vickers JH. Cerebrospinal fluid monoamine and adrenal correlates of aggression in free-ranging rhesus monkeys. *Arch Gen Psychiatry.* 1992;49:436-441.

In reply

Dr Reus criticizes as "overstated" and "critically dependent on one subject" our reporting of a significant relationship between CSF 5-HIAA concentrations and aggression. We note that even when the single subject in question is dropped from the analysis, the results remain statistically significant (r=.46, P<.05). *While our study is the first, to our knowledge, to correlate interindividual differences in CSF 5-HIAA with aggression in nonhuman primates, our primary hypothesis of a negative correlation between aggression and CSF 5-HIAA was based on other cited studies of nonhuman primates, showing that increasing or decreasing serotonin activity pharmacologically produces the decrease or increase in aggression, respectively.*

In a follow-up study of these subjects, we extended this initial finding. We reported at the meeting of the American Society of Primatology[1] *that when direct behavioral observations of these animals are collected, they are more impulsive and engage in aggressive acts with a high likelihood of personal injury. As we stated in the report, we believe that these results are a promising beginning for developing a primate model "assessing the role of serotonin in the acquisition of social competence and the appropriate expression of aggression." This is by no means an overstatement of our findings.*

Dr Reus also notes that "in both the abstract and 'Comment' section of the report, [we] state that plasma cortisol concentrations and stress hormones are correlated with a measurement of aggression." Plasma cortisol is not, however, cited in the "Comment" section of the article. Leaving the word cortisol in the abstract was an unfortunate error on our part. It should have been deleted from the abstract where it remained from an early version of the manuscript presented at the 1991 meeting of the American Society of Primatology that included preliminary findings using a subset of the subjects. Our conclusions were not based on results from the cortisol analyses. Because cortisol was not mentioned or considered in the "Comment" section of the article, this error does not affect the interpretation or overall conclusions of our study.

Finally, the lack of intercorrelations between different stress measures and CSF 5-HIAA is not surprising. Because different hormones and neurotransmitters change differentially over time, intercorrelations are expected to be significant only if the various measures are collected at the appropriate time points. For example, while corticotropin is the major controlling factor of cortisol release, the correlation between corticotropin and cortisol was not significant. Indeed, in a master's thesis on rhesus monkeys from our laboratory, Scanlan[2] *showed that the timing of the peak plasma corticotropin and cortisol concentrations is different, with corticotropin peaks preceding cortisol peaks by over an hour. Nor do all stress measures respond uniformly to the same stressor, as illustrated repeatedly by Lang*[3,4] *in a phenomenon that he appropriately calls "Fear is Not a Lump." It is hoped that the roles that different stress hormones and neurotransmitters play in serotonin-mediated aggression will become clear as we continue our study of aggression in nonhuman primates.*

J. Dee Higley, PhD
Laboratory of Clinical Studies
National Institute of Alcohol Abuse and Alcoholism
National Institutes of Health
Animal Center Bldg 112, PO Box 289
Poolesville, MD 20837
Patrick T. Mehlman, PhD
David Taub, PhD
Laboratory Animal Breeders and Services
Yemassee, SC
Stephen J. Suomi, PhD
Sue B. Higley
Laboratory of Comparative Ethology
National Institute of Child Health and Human Development
Bethesda, Md
James M. Vickers, DVM
Pathobiology and Primatology Laboratory
Food and Drug Administration
Bethesda, Md
Markku Linnoila, PhD, MD
Office of the Scientific Director
National Institute of Alcohol Abuse and Alcoholism
Bethesda, Md

1. Mehlman PT, Higley JD, Faucher I, Corr J, Taub DM, Dodson A, Lilly A, Linnoila M, Suomi S. CNS 5-HIAA and aggression in free-ranging adolescent rhesus males. *Am J Primatol.* 1992;27:46-47.
2. Scanlan JM. *Adrenocortical and Behavioral Responses to Acute Novel and Stressful Conditions: The Influence of Gonadal Status, Time Course of Response, Age, and Motor Activity.* Madison: University of Wisconsin; 1984. Thesis.
3. Lang PJ. Fear reduction and fear behavior: problems in treating a construct. In: Shlien JM, ed. *Research in Psychotherapy.* Washington, DC: American Psychological Association; 1968:90-103.
4. Lang PJ. The cognitive psychophysiology of emotion: fear and anxiety. In: Tuma AH, Maser J, eds. *Anxiety and the Anxiety Disorders.* Hillsdale, NJ: Lawrence Erlbaum Associates Pub: 1985:131-170.

Cingulotomy in a Case of Concomitant Obsessive-Compulsive Disorder and Tourette's Syndrome

We recently reported on the extensive uncontrolled experience at Massachusetts General Hospital (MGH), Boston, suggesting the possible efficacy of cingulotomy for treating obsessive-compulsive disorder (OCD).[1] Recent evidence suggests a familial link between OCD and Tourette's syndrome (TS),[2] yet there is only one previous report regarding the effects of cingulotomy on the symptoms of TS (in two patients at MGH who underwent surgery to treat concomitant severe OCD).[3]

We now report the case of a man who had concomitant OCD and TS. He underwent two separate bilateral radiofrequency cingulotomies via burr holes, first in December 1989, and again in June 1991, to reduce his OCD symptoms. This patient's experience is instructive because his OCD symptoms appear to have improved following these cingulotomies, while his tics were unchanged or worse.

Report of a Case. A 35-year-old man had been followed up in our OCD clinic between 1987 and 1988 and was diagnosed as having OCD (onset at 5 years of age of a wide variety of counting, repeating, and touching rituals, along with urges to blurt out obscenities) and associated TS (numerous motor and vocal tics numbering in the hundreds per day since 5 years of age). For additional evaluation we referred him to a neurology clinic specializing in TS, where he was diagnosed as having TS associated with idiopathic OCD. The patient reported that he was easily able to discriminate his OCD symptoms from his TS symptoms based on his subjective sensations leading to compulsions or tics. He failed to respond to behavior therapy and medications (including adequate trials of clomipramine hydrochloride, fluoxetine hydrochloride, haloperidol, pimozide, and clonidine hydrochloride).

At the time of his first surgical procedure, while taking fluoxetine hydrochloride (60 mg/d), he was assessed by Structured Clinical Interview for *DSM-III-R* as meeting Axis I criteria for OCD, current major depression superimposed on dysthymia, and substance (alprazolam) and alcohol abuse (the patient reported that alcohol was the only substance that helped control his tics). Assessment by Structured Interview for *DSM-III-R* Personality—Revised yielded Axis II diagnoses of borderline, histrionic, and mixed personality disorders. At this time his score on the Yale-Brown Obsessive Compulsive Scale (YBOCS) was 26 (with compulsions occurring over 8 hours per day), and on the Beck Depression Inventory (BDI) was 28.

Three months after the first operation, while still receiving the same medication, he reported a decrease in urges to touch and break things, with a YBOCS score of 12 (compulsions still occurring over 8 hours a day, but with no obsessions), and BDI score of 15. On Clinical Global Improvement (CGI) scale, the patient rated his OCD, depression, and anxiety as all "slightly better," and his tics as "slightly worse" (with reported emergence of a new vocal tic). Sixteen months after cingulotomy, again still receiving the same medication, his YBOCS score had increased to 21 (with reemergence of a number of obsessions) and BDI score was 27. Compared with the baseline on the CGI scale, OCD was "not improved," his depression and anxiety were "slightly better," and tics were "not improved."

When he returned 18 months after surgery for evaluation prior to a second cingulotomy, his YBOCS score was 22 (with compulsions occupying 8 hours per day and obsessions 3 to 8 hours per day), and BDI score was 10. Compared with baseline on the CGI scale, he reported his depression and anxiety were "much improved," but his OCD and tics were again rated as "not improved."

Nine months after the second operation, the patient reported that both obsessions and compulsions were occurring less than 1 hour per day, and YBOCS score was 11 and BDI score was 5. Compared with the baseline on CGI, he rated his OCD and anxiety as "much improved," depression as "very much improved," and tics as "minimally worse." At the most recent assessment, 13 months after the second operation, YBOCS score remained at 11 (obsessions and compulsions both occurring less than 1 hour per day), and on the CGI scale, OCD and anxiety continued to be rated as "much improved," depression "very much improved," and tics as "minimally worse."

Comment. While no conclusions can be drawn from this single case, it appears that, although cingulotomy may have produced improvement in this patient's previously treatment-resistant obsessions and compulsions, his case provides no evidence that the two cingulotomies had any beneficial effect on his tics. This finding is consistent with the only previous report in the literature,[3] and suggests that, based on these three cases, cingulotomy alone does not appear to be an effective treatment for TS and associated tics.

Lee Baer, PhD
Scott L. Rauch, MD
Michael A. Jenike, MD
N. H. Cassem, MD
H. Thomas Ballantine, MD
Peter A. Manzo
Department of Psychiatry
Massachusetts General Hospital-East
Building 149
13th St, Floor 9
Charlestown, MA 02129
Robert L. Martuza, MD
Washington, DC

1. Jenike MA, Baer L, Ballantine HT, Martuza RL, Tynes S, Giriunas I, Buttolph ML, Cassem NH. Cingulotomy for refractory obsessive-compulsive disorder: a long-term follow-up of 33 patients. *Arch Gen Psychiatry.* 1991;48:548-555.
2. Pauls DL, Towbin KE, Leckman JF, Zahner GEP, Cohen DJ. Gilles de la Tourette's syndrome and obsessive-compulsive disorder: evidence supporting a genetic relationship. *Arch Gen Psychiatry.* 1986;43:1180-1182.
3. Kurlan R, Kersun J, Ballantine HT, Caine ED. Neurosurgical treatment of severe obsessive-compulsive disorder associated with Tourette's syndrome. *Mov Disord.* 1990;5:152-155.

ORIGINAL ARTICLE

Dose-Response Study of N,N-Dimethyltryptamine in Humans

I. Neuroendocrine, Autonomic, and Cardiovascular Effects

Rick J. Strassman, MD, Clifford R. Qualls, PhD

Background: To begin applying basic neuropharmacological hypotheses of hallucinogenic drug actions to humans, we generated dose-response data for intravenously administered dimethyltryptamine fumarate's (DMT) neuroendocrine, cardiovascular, autonomic, and subjective effects in a group of experienced hallucinogen users.

Methods: Dimethyltryptamine, an endogenous mammalian hallucinogen and drug of abuse, was administered intravenously at 0.05, 0.1, 0.2, and 0.4 mg/kg to 11 experienced hallucinogen users, in a double-blind, saline placebo–controlled, randomized design. Treatments were separated by at least 1 week.

Results: Peak DMT blood levels and subjective effects were seen within 2 minutes after drug administration, and were negligible at 30 minutes. Dimethyltryptamine dose dependently elevated blood pressure, heart rate, pupil diameter, and rectal temperature, in addition to elevating blood concentrations of β-endorphin, corticotropin, cortisol, and prolactin. Growth hormone blood levels rose equally in response to all doses of DMT, and melatonin levels were unaffected. Threshold doses for significant effects relative to placebo were also hallucinogenic (0.2 mg/kg and higher). Subjects with five or more exposures to 3,4-methylenedioxymethamphetamine demonstrated less robust pupil diameter effects than those with two or fewer exposures.

Conclusions: Dimethyltryptamine can be administered safely to experienced hallucinogen users and dose-response data generated for several measures hypothesized under serotonergic modulatory control. Additional studies characterizing the specific mechanisms mediating DMT's biological effects may prove useful in psychopharmacological investigations of drug-induced and endogenous alterations in brain function.

(Arch Gen Psychiatry. 1994;51:85-97)

HALLUCINOGENIC drugs reliably induce a unique constellation of subjective effects in humans. They elicit perceptual illusions and hallucinations, primarily visual but often auditory. Mood effects range from euphoria to panic to bland indifference. Somatic effects include dissociation, relaxation, or tension.[1] "Classic" hallucinogens include phenethylamines (eg, mescaline), indolealkylamines (eg, psilocybin and dimethyltryptamine [DMT]), and the lysergamides (eg, lysergic acid diethylamide [LSD]).[2]

These unique compounds were the focus of intensive clinical research in the 1950s and 1960s. The discovery of LSD may arguably have been as important to the development of a "biological" psychiatry as was the contemporaneous discovery of chlorpromazine. Hallucinogens' use in clinical research was associated with acceptable risks when subjects, both psychiatric patients and normal controls, were carefully screened, prepared, and followed up.[3] Clinical research with hallucinogens, however, became increasingly difficult with their widespread abuse by young adults. Highly publicized "adverse reactions" to hallucinogens, primarily LSD,[4] resulted in their placement into the restrictive schedule I of the Controlled

From the Departments of Psychiatry (Dr Strassman) and Medicine (Dr Qualls), School of Medicine, and the Department of Mathematics and Statistics (Dr Qualls), University of New Mexico, Albuquerque.

See Subjects and Methods on next page

SUBJECTS AND METHODS

The protocol was approved by the Scientific Advisory Committee of the General Clinical Research Center (GCRC) and the Human Research Review Committee of the University of New Mexico School of Medicine, Albuquerque, the New Mexico State Pharmacy Board, the US Drug Enforcement Administration, and the US Food and Drug Administration.[23] Witnessed written informed consent was obtained from all subjects. Confidentiality and anonymity were maintained throughout the study.

SUBJECTS

We recruited only experienced hallucinogen users. All subjects but one were recruited by word of mouth; this last subject responded to an announcement sent to a graduate student training office at a local university.

Subjects were initially interviewed by one of us (R.J.S.) to screen for medical and/or psychiatric conditions and assess level of experience with, and ability to manage dysphoric reactions to, hallucinogenic drugs. Subjects were dropped from further consideration if they were taking any medications long-term, had a history of psychosis not secondary to drugs or fever, or had a chronic medical disorder.

Prospective subjects then received a Structured Clinical Interview for *DSM-III-R* (SCID-R), Outpatient Version,[24] administered by a trained psychiatric research nurse. First-degree relatives' psychiatric histories were obtained during the SCID-R. Diagnoses were confirmed by discussion with two research psychiatrists. We then performed a medical history, physical examination, and laboratory screening tests (including a complete blood count with differential cell count, 24-item chemistry panel, thyroid functions [including thyrotropin], urinalysis, and electrocardiogram).

The demographic characteristics of our subjects are given in the **Table**. Subject 11 was dropped after receiving the nonblind (0.04- and-0.4-mg/kg) doses and the 0.05-, 0.1-, and 0.2-mg/kg doses because he had a major depressive episode precipitated by multiple personal stressors that appeared unrelated to his participation in the study. He responded to desipramine hydrochloride. The average (±SEM) age (excluding subject 11) was 41.5±1.5 years. The group was high functioning, with only one subject not being a professional or student in a professional training program. There was a high incidence of prior major depression in the group. Only one subject was suffering any current Axis I disorder; this was an adjustment disorder resulting from an impending divorce. There also was a high incidence of first-degree relatives suffering from depression and/or alcohol abuse. The number of exposures to hallucinogens ranged from six to "hundreds." Two subjects described a history of cocaine dependence/abuse, currently in remission; the remainder had little or no exposure to cocaine or amphetamines. Not all subjects had used marijuana equally, although all had some experience with it.

METHYLENEDIOXYMETHAMPHETAMINE USE

Of interest was the breakdown of subjects by amount of methylenedioxymethamphetamine (MDMA, "Ecstasy") use. All but two had used MDMA at least once. Six of the 11 subjects had used MDMA five or more times; five had used it twice or less. Methylenedioxymethamphetamine is a mammalian serotonergic neurotoxin[25] with equivocal long-term effects on human neuroendocrine and/or behavioral function.[26] Thus, we were interested in assessing differential effects of the serotonergic agonist, DMT, in these two groups of users. For the sake of approximating equal cell sizes, we described the six former subjects as having had high exposure and the latter five as having had low or no exposure.

DRUG

Dimethyltryptamine fumarate was prepared by David E. Nichols, PhD, Purdue University, West Lafayette, Ind. Purity, determined by gas chromatography–mass spectrometry and high-performance liquid chromatography, was greater than 99.9%. It was prepared for clinical administration by the Inpatient Pharmacy of the University of New Mexico Hospital in vials containing 40 mg/mL. Sterility and pyrogenicity testing revealed no abnormalities in a representative sample of vials. The dimethyltryptamine fumarate solution was drawn into a sterile tuberculin syringe at the appropriate dose and diluted with sterile saline to 1.0 mL before administration.

PROCEDURES

Nonblind Drug Administration

First, all subjects received nonblind administrations of 0.04 and 0.4 mg/kg of intravenous (IV) dimethyltryptamine fumarate in the GCRC, usually on consecutive days. Previous work[22] had demonstrated no tolerance to the cardiovascular and subjective effects of a full IM dose of DMT given twice daily for 5 consecutive days. Thus, we did not believe tolerance to DMT's effects would occur at this interval. We decided to administer the drug IV rather than IM as had been reported previously.[16] This was because of our initial dose-finding studies using a subject with experience smoking DMT free base, the usual form and route of administration by recreational users.[27] The onset and intensity of effect of 1.0 mg/kg of IM dimethyltryptamine fumarate was described by this subject as significantly less rapidly developing and hallucinogenic than his previous experience with the smoked drug. Further dose-finding studies with him and another experienced DMT smoker established that 0.4 mg/kg of IV dimethyltryptamine fumarate produced a "rush" and hallucinogenic effect comparable with those seen with a "full dose" of smoked free base.

The nonblind days served several purposes. They allowed us to assess the cardiovascular and subjective effects of a subclinical and fully hallucinogenic dose of dimethyltryptamine in a novel and potentially anxiety-provoking setting. These days also provided the research team and subjects an opportunity to become acquainted and familiar with each other in the research center setting without the extensive blood drawing and use of the rectal thermistor that could exaggerate any potentially paranoid reactions. Subjects also were able to "calibrate" themselves to what to expect regarding minimal and maximal effects of the drug, one of the purposes of the double-blind study being whether they could distinguish among incremental doses of DMT. Finally, these nonblind days provided subjects with the opportunity to drop out of the study before we had collected extensive data on them.

Subjects were admitted to the GCRC by 9 AM after having fasted since midnight. An IV line was inserted into a forearm vein and kept patent with heparinized saline. Subjects were allowed to relax for 30 minutes before the drug was given. Dimethyltryptamine was infused over 30 seconds and flushed with 5 mL of sterile saline over the next 15 seconds. Blood pressure and heart rate (HR) were taken with an automatic cuff several times before and frequently during the 30 minutes following drug administration. The research team (a registered nurse and psychiatrist) sat quietly on either side of the subject, attentive to verbal and nonverbal cues, but did not offer any direction or advice unless absolutely necessary during the first several minutes, the time of the peak effect of the drug. Sublingual nitroglycerin, and IV diphenhydramine and diazepam, were available at the bedside for sustained hypertension, allergic reactions, or excessive anxiety, respectively. As drug effects resolved, discussion focused on the nature of the subject's experiences. After subjects ate a snack or meal, they were discharged home.

No subject withdrew voluntarily after the nonblind days. One subject was withdrawn because of a marked diastolic blood pressure response (to >105 mm Hg) to the 0.04-mg/kg dose.

Double-blind, Placebo-Controlled, Randomized Drug Administration

A computer-generated randomization sequence was coded and kept by the Inpatient Pharmacy of the University of New Mexico Hospital. Subjects were admitted by 9 AM to a dimly lit (<100 lux) room on the GCRC. Two IV lines were started: a small-gauge metal needle in one arm for drug administration, and a large-gauge, three-holed plastic angiocatheter for blood withdrawal. A reusable rectal thermistor probe (YS-400, Yellow Springs Instruments, Yellow Springs, Ohio), configured to a physiological monitor (Vita-Log PMS-8, CPS Inc, Palo Alto, Calif), was inserted. The monitor sampled rectal temperature every minute, and the thermistor probe has an accuracy of ±0.03°C. Blood pressure and HR (vital signs), and pupil diameter (measured by placing a card with black circles differing by 1-mm increments juxtaposed 10 to 15 cm from the subject's eyes), were taken at 30, 15, and 2 minutes before drug administration. Blood samples for corticotropin, β-endorphin, prolactin, GH, cortisol, and melatonin levels were drawn 30 and 2 minutes before drug administration. Drug and saline flush were administered over 45 seconds, and time 0 was when the saline flush was completed. Doses were 0.05, 0.1, 0.2, and 0.4 mg/kg of dimethyltryptamine fumarate and sterile saline placebo. Blood samples were drawn, and pupil diameter and vital signs measured 2, 5, 10, 15, 30, and 60 minutes after drug administration. Study sessions occurred at an interval of at least 1 week and took place from January to September 1991. The one woman subject was studied during the early follicular phase of her cycle. A negative serum pregnancy test drawn the night before her study days was always available before drug administration.

ASSAYS

Dimethyltryptamine (free base) blood levels were assayed using the gas chromatography–mass spectrometry technique of Walker et al.[28] Limit of detectability was 1 ng/mL. Corticotropin and β-endorphin levels were assayed by immunoradiometric assays (Nichols Diagnostic Laboratories, San Juan Capistrano, Calif), and lower limits of detectability were 0.2 and 2.2 pmol/L, respectively. Limits of detectability for cortisol, GH, and prolactin radioimmunoassays (all from Diagnostic Products, Los Angeles, Calif) were 6 nmol/L, 1 μg/L, and 1 μg/L, respectively. Growth hormone and prolactin values below 1 μg/L were entered as 0.9 μg/L. The melatonin radioimmunoassay[29] limit of detectability was 5 pmol/L. All assays were performed in duplicate.

STATISTICS

Variable values are given as mean±SEM. All analyses were performed using PC SAS Version 6.03 (Cary, NC). Several derived variables were computed for analyses. Baseline values for blood pressure, HR, and pupil diameter were derived by averaging the three values obtained before drug administration (ie, −30, −15, and −2 minutes). Baseline temperature was computed by averaging values for 5 minutes immediately preceding drug administration. Hormone baseline values were computed by averaging results from the −30- and −2-minute samples. Maximum rise above baseline is indicated ΔMax; ΔAUC represents the area under the curve above baseline, calculated by the trapezoidal rule.

Our primary statistical tool was the univariate analysis of variance (ANOVA) with repeated measures, with dose as the repeated factor. Pairwise comparisons, when the overall F value generated a $P<.05$, were performed using the "contrast" statement in the general linear models procedure in SAS. To assess a possible modulatory role of methylenedioxymethamphetamine exposure on dimethyltryptamine's effects on a particular variable, we performed a two-way univariate repeated-measures ANOVA using MDMA history as the independent variable.

Continued on next page

MISSING DATA

We did not analyze blood hormone level results for the one female subject in the group because her veins collapsed at some point for almost every session, and her blood data were incomplete. However, we did analyze her autonomic and cardiovascular responses.

Pupil diameter was difficult to measure consistently, as subjects varied widely in their ability and/or desire to open their eyes during acute drug intoxication. Thus, these measurements were obtained at the subjects' discretion. Additionally, several subjects had technically poor rectal temperature tracings because of difficulties with probe placement, and these data could not be used. Two subjects had unsatisfactory temperature data for the 0.05- and 0.2-mg/kg sessions; one had no 0.1-mg/kg session data; and one had no temperature data from his placebo session. Finally, one subject refused the rectal thermistor probe, and no temperature data were collected from him. As SAS cannot perform repeated-measures ANOVA on subjects with missing data, we used a less robust one-way ANOVA for the temperature and pupil diameter data, with dose as the independent variable. Fisher's Least Significant Difference Test for pairwise comparisons was performed if the overall F value generated a significance of $P<.05$. To assess the effect of DMT exposure on MDMA's effects on pupil diameter and rectal temperature, we performed a two-way ANOVA with dose and MDMA history as independent factors.

Substances Act. Human studies with these drugs effectively ended in the mid-1970s. Despite legal restrictions and severe penalties for manufacture, possession, and distribution of hallucinogens, their use among college students has held relatively steady over the past 20 years.[5]

Basic research into the mechanisms of action of hallucinogens continued, however, and contributed to recent advances in serotonin (5-HT) receptor pharmacology.[6] Recent behavioral, in vivo, and ligand binding data suggest agonist or partial agonist effects at the 5-HT_2, 5-HT_{1A}, and 5-HT_{1C} receptors.[7-10] Dopaminergic[11] and noradrenergic[12] effects have been described but not studied recently.

Hallucinogenic drugs have diffuse and relatively well-documented biological effects, presumably related to their serotoninergic properties. Growth hormone (GH), prolactin, β-endorphin, corticotropin, and cortisol levels are all affected by serotonergic stimuli.[13] Consistent with the presumed serotonergic properties of the classic hallucinogens, levels of several of these hormones increase with their administration. For example, human prolactin blood levels rise in response to dimethyltryptamine,[14] and rat plasma corticoid levels are stimulated by LSD.[15] Cardiovascular variables, core temperature, and pupillary diameter also are affected by serotonergic hallucinogens. Examples of these effects include DMT's hypertensive and mydriatic,[16] LSD's pyretogenic and mydriatic,[17,18] and psilocybin's hypertensive and tachycardic[19] properties.

Dimethyltryptamine is a short-acting hallucinogen, first discovered in hallucinogenic Amazonian snuffs.[20] It was later synthesized and determined to be active by parenteral (intramuscular [IM]) administration only.[16] Its discovery in human body fluids prompted a flurry of investigations into its possible biosynthesis in man and its role as a putative endogenous psychotogen.[21] Difficulties distinguishing peripheral levels of DMT between normal controls and patients with endogenous psychoses led to a loss of interest in the function of this hallucinogenic tryptamine.[22]

It has been impossible to test in humans hypotheses of hallucinogen mechanisms of action developed from basic research. Systematic psychopharmacological investigations are the necessary interface bridging recent neuropharmacological findings to human effects. Dose-response investigations applying current psychiatric research methods to assess hallucinogens' effects can generate data providing the bases for more experimental studies, such as selective blockade with receptor subtype antagonists.

Several properties recommend DMT as an appropriate drug with which to renew such investigations. Its short duration minimizes prolonged dysphoric reactions in the potentially stressful environment of a modern clinical research center. The lack of a widespread "folklore" concerning its effects provides less bias and expectations from subjects. Finally, DMT's role in human brain function has yet to be explicated in normal and pathological states. That is, understanding effects and mechanisms of action of DMT may shed light on the etiology and treatment of endogenous hallucinatory conditions.

We have performed a dose-response study of the neuroendocrine, cardiovascular, autonomic, and subjective effects of dimethyltryptamine fumarate using a double-blind, placebo-controlled, randomized design. This article focuses on biological data generated by this study.

RESULTS

The major findings of this study are the following: (1) Intravenous dimethyltryptamine fumarate was fully hallucinogenic in doses of 0.2 and 0.4 mg/kg. Effects were felt nearly instantaneously, peaked within 2 minutes after injection, and resolved within 20 to 30 minutes. The time course of DMT blood levels matched the march of subjective effects. (2) Multiple biological variables rose dose dependently in response to DMT. The time course of elevations in blood levels of pro-opiomelanocortin

Demographic Characteristics of Subjects*

Subject No./ Age, y/Sex	Occupation	Axis I Diagnoses	Marital Status	Family Psychiatric History	Times Used: Marijuana	Cocaine, Amphetamines	Hallucinogens	Methylene dioxymethamphetamine
1/45/M	Construction worker	None	Divorced ×2, married	None	10-20	0	10-20	10
2/39/F	Psychologist	None	Divorced ×2, married	Father, depression, chronic; eating disorder?; mother, "hysterical"	100s	50-100	>50	75-100
3/38/M	Physician	Major depression, resolved; cannabis dependence, partial remission	Divorced ×1	Father, depression (taking amitriptyline hydrochloride)	1000s	3	50	1
4/45/M	Psychologist	Adjustment disorder, depressed	Divorced ×3	Brother, adjustment disorder, mixed	>400	15	30	10-15
5/34/M	Graduate student	Alcohol dependence, in remission; cannabis abuse, in remission	Never married	Brother, major depression	1000s	20-25	20-30	1
6/37/M	Resident physician	Major depression, resolved	Never married	None	1000s	15-20	50-60	0
7/42/M	City administrator	None	Divorced ×1, married	None	100s	<10	>100	5-10
8/36/M	Drug dealer	Cannabis dependence, in remission; cocaine dependence, in remission; stimulant abuse, in remission	Divorced ×1, married	Father, alcohol abuse	1000s	100s	>200	5-10
9/46/M	Owner of large business	Adjustment disorder, depressed, resolved; alcohol abuse, in remission	Divorced ×1	Mother, alcohol abuse; father, alcohol abuse	100s	50-100	6	0
10/45/M	Restaurant manager, writer	Cocaine dependence, in remission; alcohol abuse, in remission; major depression, resolved; depressive disorder, NOS, resolved	Divorced ×3	Father, alcohol abuse	100s	100	>100	10-12
11/38/M	Physician	Prolonged (18-mo) grief reaction vs major depression, resolved	Divorced ×2	Mother, major depression; father, alcohol abuse	50	3	75-100	8
12/50/M	Counselor	None	Divorced ×2, married	Alcohol abuse	100s	15-20	10	2

**NOS indicates not otherwise specified. Subject 11 suffered a major depression during the study and was withdrawn before completing it. His data are included for illustrative purposes.*

(POMC) peptides (corticotropin and β-endorphin), HR, blood pressure, and pupil diameter paralleled subjective effects and DMT blood concentrations. Elevations of prolactin and cortisol blood levels lagged 5 to 10 minutes behind these changes. Core temperature and GH effects did not begin until the first set of perturbations had almost resolved (15 to 30 minutes) and may not have peaked by 60 minutes after DMT administration.

DMT BLOOD LEVELS

There was no measurable DMT in blood samples before drug administration or after saline placebo administration for any subject except for subject 4. He had measurable DMT levels at one point before active drug administration and twice after placebo injection. His low levels in these circumstances are consistent with endogenous levels in a study of normal volunteers using a similar assay.[30] However, he regularly took "Chinese herbs" and "homeopathic tinctures" as tonics, unlike any of our other subjects.

Plasma levels of DMT peaked at the first blood draw, 2 minutes after the injection was completed, closely corresponding to peak psychological effects. Generally, a doubling of dose resulted in a doubling of ΔMax values. These data are displayed in **Figure 1**. As previously de-

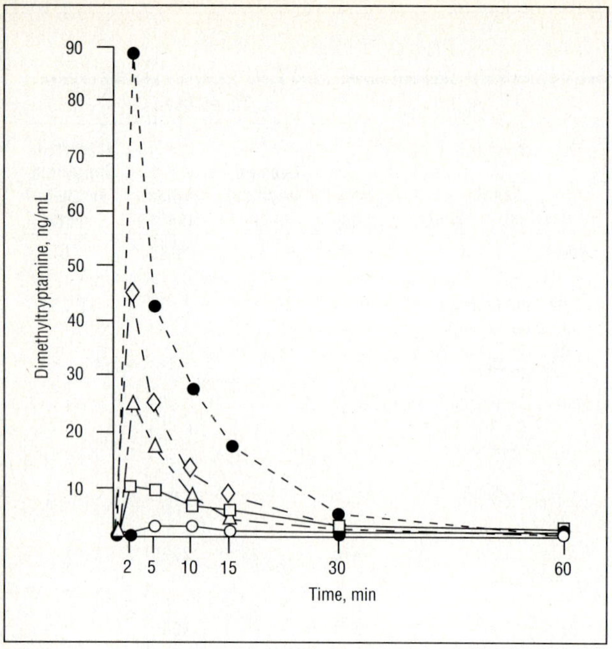

Figure 1. *Mean dimethyltryptamine (free base) values in 10 subjects after four doses of intravenous dimethyltryptamine fumarate (0.05 mg/kg [squares], 0.1 mg/kg [triangles], 0.2 mg/kg [diamonds], and 0.4 mg/kg [closed circles]) and saline placebo (open circles).*

scribed,[31] DMT levels varied widely among subjects, peak values ranging from 32 to 204 ng/mL after the 0.4-mg/kg injection.

BASELINE EFFECTS

There were no differences among baseline values for any biological variable among the five treatment conditions.

NEUROENDOCRINE EFFECTS
POMC PEPTIDES

The ΔAUC and ΔMax for both corticotropin and β-endorphin rose dose dependently in response to dimethyltryptamine fumarate, with the 0.4-mg/kg dose's effects being statistically greater than all other doses for both of these variables. The effects of placebo and the 0.05- and 0.1-mg/kg doses could not be separated statistically. Of interest was the stimulation of corticotropin and β-endorphin levels by saline placebo. This has the appearance of a conditioned response to placebo injection in all these subjects who had previously received the somewhat anxiety-provoking 0.4-mg/kg dose nonblind. These data are displayed graphically in **Figure 2** (corticotropin) and **Figure 3** (β-endorphin).

Prolactin

The ΔMax and ΔAUC for prolactin demonstrated a significant dose-dependent stimulatory effect of dimethyltryptamine fumarate. The 0.4-mg/kg dose raised both of these variables significantly more than placebo and the 0.05- and 0.1-mg/kg doses. The effects of 0.4 and 0.2 mg/kg on ΔMax prolactin could not be distinguished from each other, although the 0.4-mg/kg dose's effects on ΔAUC were significantly greater than those of 0.2 mg/kg. The effects of 0.2, 0.1, and 0.05 mg/kg of dimethyltryptamine fumarate and of placebo on ΔAUC were not statistically separable. These data are graphically presented in **Figure 4**. Note that prolactin effects were slightly delayed relative to the POMC peptides.

Cortisol

The ΔAUC and ΔMax for cortisol both demonstrated dose-dependent stimulatory effects of dimethyltryptamine fumarate. The 0.4-mg/kg dose raised these two variables more than all other doses. The effects of 0.4 mg/kg on ΔAUC for cortisol could not be statistically distinguished from the effects of 0.2 mg/kg, however. Neither could the 0.4-mg/kg dose's effects on ΔMax for cortisol be separated statistically from 0.2 and 0.05 mg/kg. Effects of the 0.05-, 0.1-, and 0.2-mg/kg doses on ΔAUC and ΔMax were not statistically different, although their effects were numerically greater than those of saline. These data are graphically presented in **Figure 5**.

Growth Hormone

There was a trend for DMT to produce a rise in ΔAUC for GH. The ΔMax for GH rose in response to DMT administration. Although all doses of DMT raised GH lev-

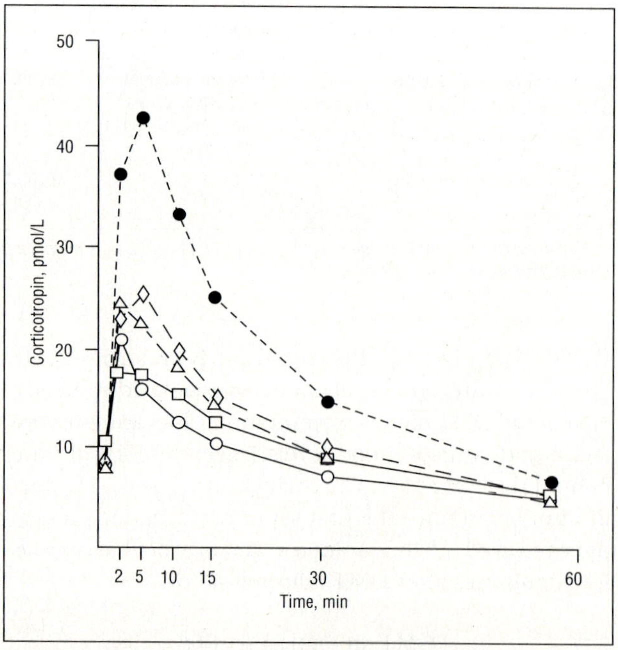

Figure 2. *Mean blood corticotropin values in 10 subjects after four doses of intravenous dimethyltryptamine fumarate (0.05 mg/kg [squares], 0.1 mg/kg [triangles], 0.2 mg/kg [diamonds], and 0.4 mg/kg [closed circles]) and saline placebo (open circles).*

els relative to saline placebo, effects of different doses could not be distinguished from each other. These data are graphically displayed in **Figure 6**. Note the delay in GH effects relative to the other neuroendocrine results.

Melatonin

We only assayed six subjects' blood samples for melatonin from their 0.4-mg/kg sessions. Utilizing one-sample *t* tests, there was no effect of 0.4 mg/kg of dimethyltryptamine fumarate on either ΔMax or ΔAUC for melatonin (data not given), so the remaining samples were not assayed.

AUTONOMIC EFFECTS

Rectal Temperature

The ΔMax and ΔAUC for temperature demonstrated a significant effect of dimethyltryptamine fumarate. For ΔAUC, the 0.4-mg/kg dose's effects were greater than those of 0.1 and 0.05 mg/kg and saline, but could not be distinguished from those of 0.2 mg/kg. The effects of 0.2, 0.1, and 0.05 mg/kg of drug and of saline could not be statistically separated. For ΔMax in temperature, the 0.4- and 0.2-mg/kg doses' effects were greater than those produced by 0.1 or 0.05 mg/kg or placebo. The ΔMax effects of 0.4 and 0.2 mg/kg could not be statistically separated from each other; neither could the effects of the three latter treatments be separated. These data are graphically displayed in **Figure 7**, where the delayed effect relative to other variables can be seen.

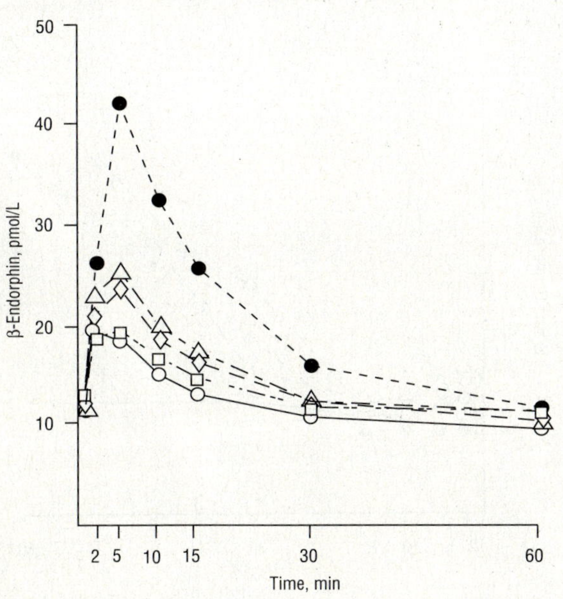

Figure 3. *Mean blood β-endorphin values in 10 subjects after four doses of intravenous dimethyltryptamine fumarate (0.05 mg/kg [squares], 0.1 mg/kg [triangles], 0.2 mg/kg [diamonds], and 0.4 mg/kg [closed circles]) and saline placebo (open circles).*

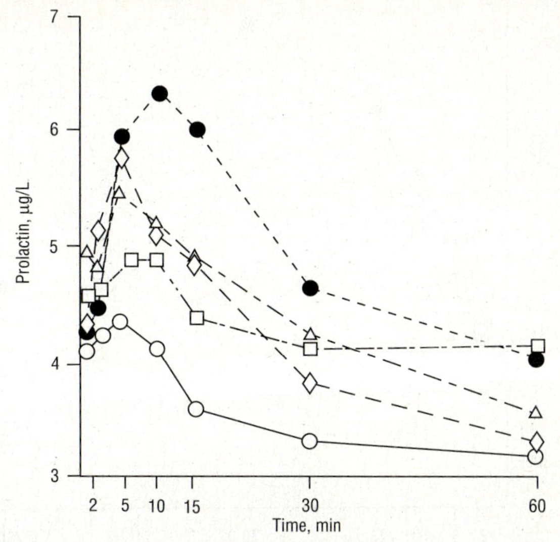

Figure 4. *Mean blood prolactin values in 10 subjects after four doses of intravenous dimethyltryptamine fumarate (0.05 mg/kg [squares], 0.1 mg/kg [triangles], 0.2 mg/kg [diamonds], and 0.4 mg/kg [closed circles]) and saline placebo (open circles).*

Pupil Diameter

As discussed in the "Procedures" section, our data for pupil diameter contained the most missing points and should be interpreted cautiously. Missing values made a calculation of ΔAUC pupil diameter impossible for the more disruptive 0.2- and 0.4-mg/kg doses. Furthermore, these data were analyzed using ANOVA without repeated measures, a less robust analytic tool.

The ΔMax pupil diameter demonstrated significant effects of DMT. The 0.4-mg/kg dose increased pupil diameter more than all other treatments. Effects of placebo and 0.05, 0.1, and 0.2 mg/kg could not be distinguished from each other. These data are displayed graphically in **Figure 8**.

CARDIOVASCULAR EFFECTS

Dimethyltryptamine dose dependently elevated ΔMax and ΔAUC values for both HR and mean arterial blood pressure (MAP). For ΔMax HR, effects of 0.4 and 0.2 mg/kg were significantly greater than those of 0.1 and 0.05 mg/kg and saline; these latter three treatments' effects were not distinguishable from each other. Neither were the effects of 0.4 and 0.2 mg/kg separable from each other. Effects on ΔAUC HR were less clearly separable by dose but followed the same pattern.

The 0.4-mg/kg dimethyltryptamine fumarate dose raised ΔAUC MAP significantly more than 0.1 and 0.05 mg/kg and saline. These latter three treatments' effects could not be distinguished from each other. Neither were the

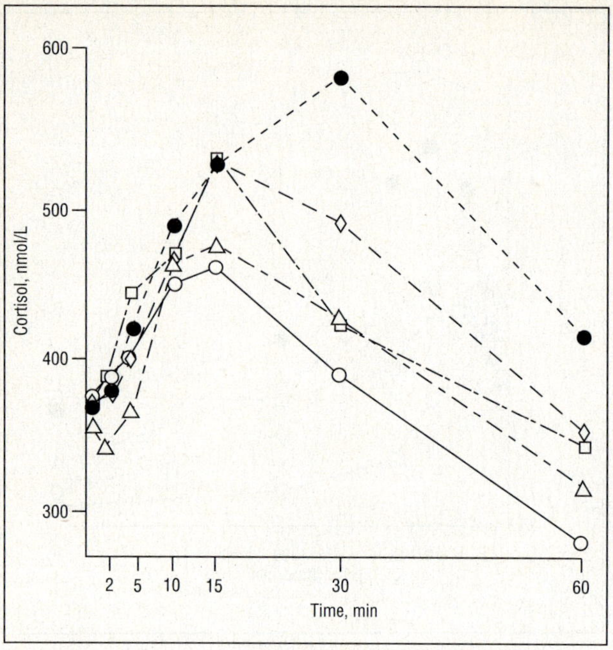

Figure 5. *Mean blood cortisol values in 10 subjects after four doses of intravenous dimethyltryptamine fumarate (0.05 mg/kg [squares], 0.1 mg/kg [triangles], 0.2 mg/kg [diamonds], and 0.4 mg/kg [closed circles]) and saline placebo (open circles).*

effects of 0.2 and 0.4 mg/kg statistically separable. The 0.4- and 0.2-mg/kg doses caused significantly greater elevations of ΔMax MAP than 0.1 and 0.05 mg/kg and saline; the two former doses' effects could not be distinguished from each other. These data are graphically displayed in **Figure 9** (HR) and **Figure 10** (MAP).

MDMA EFFECTS

For all of the biological variables under investigation, only ΔMax pupil diameter values were smaller across all doses of DMT in the high-exposure compared with the low- or no-exposure MDMA group (high exposure, 0.6±0.2 mm; low or no exposure, 1.5±0.2 mm; F=11.3, *P*=.002).

SUBJECTIVE EFFECTS

A detailed description of subjective effects, and the development of and preliminary data generated by our new rating scale, the Hallucinogen Rating Scale (HRS), are presented in a companion article.[32] Briefly, subjects felt the onset of effects before the 45-second infusion was completed. Peak hallucinogenic effects (with 0.2 and 0.4 mg/kg) occurred usually by the first blood draw and vital signs check, at 2 minutes after injection, a useful temporal reference point for subjects. Subjects remained moderately intoxicated for another 10 to 20 minutes. They felt relatively normal at 20 to 30 minutes after injection. Several described a relaxed, "at ease" feeling for an additional 30 minutes.

All subjects but one experienced visual hallucinatory phenomena at 0.2 and 0.4 mg/kg of dimethyltryptamine fumarate. Brief, poorly formed auditory hallucinations were experienced by most subjects. Somatic effects consisted of an intense rush, felt throughout the body or specifically in the head, and bodily dissociation, usually associated with a transient anxious or fearful emotional reaction. Cognitive effects were not particularly profound; rather, an "observing ego" was maintained, alert and attentive to the perceptual and somatic effects of the drug. The 0.2-mg/kg dose's perceptual perturbations, rush, and disorganizing effects were less intense than for 0.4 mg/kg, and 0.2 mg/kg was the dose preferred by many subjects. The 0.1-mg/kg dose of dimethyltryptamine fumarate produced hallucinatory phenomena in only one subject (the woman in the study). Somatic effects predominated, and many subjects disliked this dose the most. The 0.05-mg/kg dose was mistaken for placebo by several subjects. If effects were noted, they were usually somatic, with a warm, relaxed, and "floating" bodily sensation.

COMMENT

We safely administered graded doses of IV DMT, an endogenous hallucinogen and schedule I drug of abuse, to a group of experienced hallucinogen users. Dose-dependent responses were observed for several neuroendocrine, cardiovascular, and autonomic variables in a randomized, double-blind, saline placebo–controlled design. Peak psychological effects paralleled the time course of DMT blood levels, which appeared, peaked, and fell rapidly. Blood levels of the POMC peptides, corticotropin and β-endorphin, closely followed the course of DMT

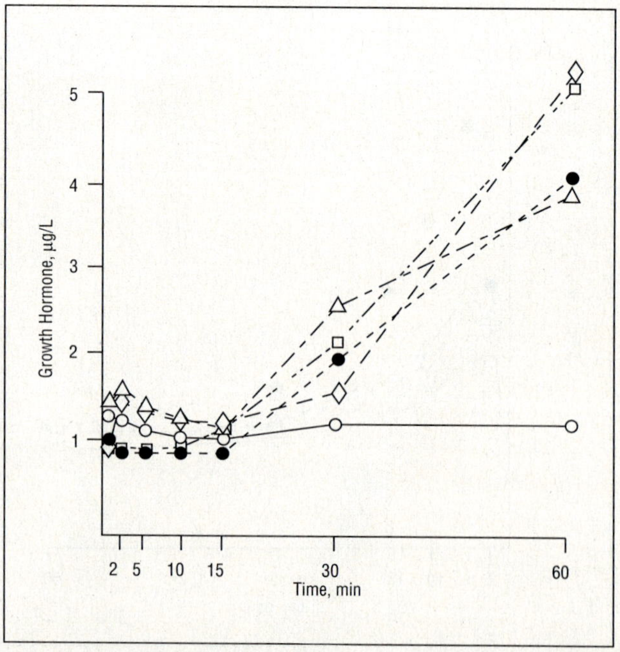

Figure 6. *Mean blood growth hormone values in 10 subjects after four doses of intravenous dimethyltryptamine fumarate (0.05 mg/kg [squares], 0.1 mg/kg [triangles], 0.2 mg/kg [diamonds], and 0.4 mg/kg [closed circles]) and saline placebo (open circles).*

levels and hallucinogenic effects, as did pupil diameter and cardiovascular responses. Cortisol and prolactin levels rose in a dose-dependent fashion and followed the first group of variables' course by 5 to 10 minutes. Core temperature and GH stimulation were most delayed, although GH effects were not separable by dose. Stimulation of daytime melatonin levels was not seen.

The threshold for significant biological effects of dimethyltryptamine relative to placebo was also that for its hallucinogenic properties: 0.2 mg/kg and higher. The 0.4-mg/kg dose of IV dimethyltryptamine fumarate produced blood levels and psychological effects comparable with those seen with administration of more than twice higher doses of IM dimethyltryptamine hydrochloride or creatine sulfate.[31] However, the IV route generated a more rapid onset (nearly instantaneous) and offset for these effects than the IM route.

Dimethyltryptamine, found in Amazonian hallucinogenic plant mixtures and human body fluids, meets electrophysiological,[33] pharmacological,[34] and behavioral[35] criteria for hallucinogenicity in lower animals. It had been used safely in humans in this country and Europe.[14,16,31] Its short duration of action was believed capable of providing a discrete, more manageable hallucinogenic state in a clinical research setting than might the 8- to 12-hour effects of lysergic acid diethylamide.

Hallucinogenic drugs are serotonergic agonists or partial agonists, in addition to having adrenergic and dopaminergic properties. The 5-HT receptor subtypes of interest include the $5\text{-}HT_{2/1C}$ and $5\text{-}HT_{1A}$.[36,37] We therefore chose our measured variables because they are believed regulated or modulated to a significant degree by serotonergic neurotransmission. These variables included multiple neuroendocrine markers, blood pressure, HR, rectal temperature, and pupil diameter. As DMT has nearly equal affinities for both the $5\text{-}HT_2$ and $5\text{-}HT_{1A}$ subtypes,[34] many of the effects to be discussed may devolve from activation of either; however, functional interactions in humans also have been described[38] and may be important.

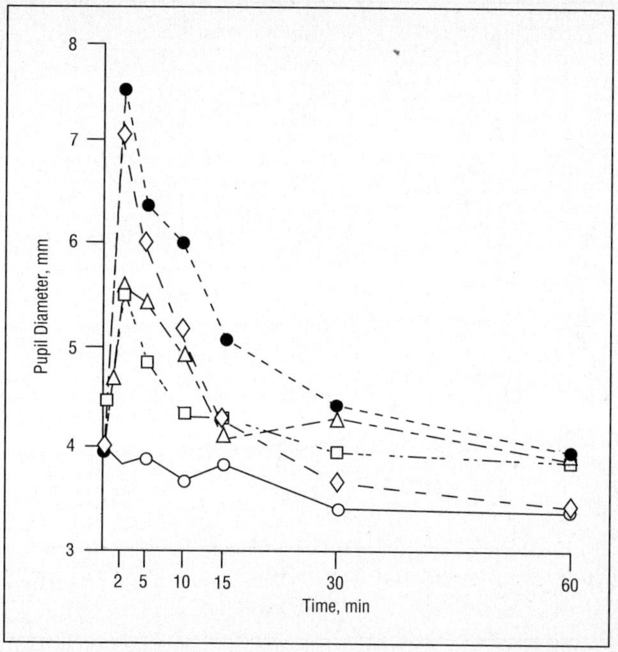

Figure 8. *Mean pupil diameter values in 11 subjects after four doses of intravenous dimethyltryptamine fumarate (0.05 mg/kg [squares], 0.1 mg/kg [triangles], 0.2 mg/kg [diamonds], and 0.4 mg/kg [closed circles]) and saline placebo (open circles).*

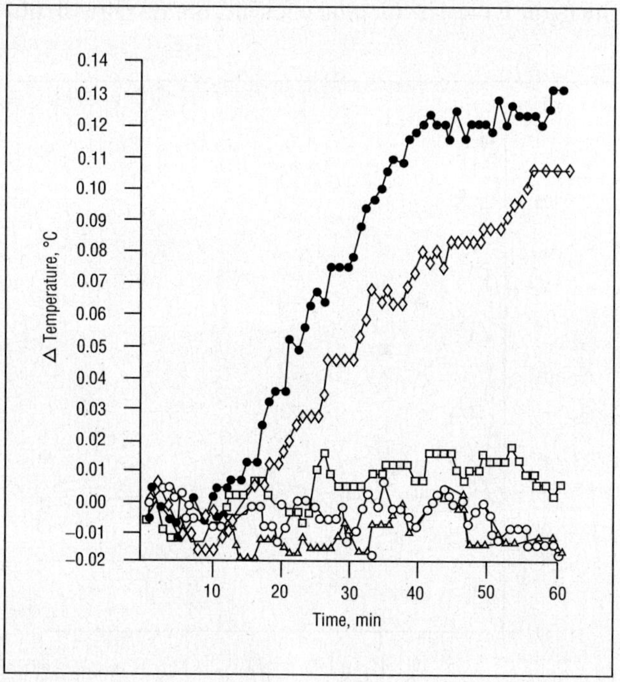

Figure 7. *Mean rectal temperature values relative to baseline temperature in 10 subjects after four doses of intravenous dimethyltryptamine fumarate (0.05 mg/kg [squares], 0.1 mg/kg [triangles], 0.2 mg/kg [diamonds], and 0.4 mg/kg [closed circles]) and saline placebo (open circles). Baseline temperature values were calculated by averaging the values of the 5 minutes immediately preceding dimethyltryptamine administration.*

Levels of the POMC peptide hormones, corticotropin and β-endorphin, both rose dose dependently in our subjects. They rose quite quickly, peak values being seen at 5 minutes after injection. With doses of 0.1 mg/kg and higher, ΔAUC and ΔMax values for these two hormones were nearly identical, confirming their corelease.[39] These rises in β-endorphin and corticotropin extend human[40,41] data demonstrating serotonergic stimulatory effects. Either $5\text{-}HT_{1A}$[42] or $5\text{-}HT_2$[43] subtypes may be involved.

Prolactin levels rose in our subjects in a dose-dependent manner, confirming and extending the data of Meltzer et al,[14] wherein cyproheptadine inconsistently blocked DMT's stimulatory effect. Multiple experimental procedures[44-47] have suggested a stimulatory effect of serotonergic neurotransmission on prolactin levels. Subtype delineation is not clearly understood, but both $5\text{-}HT_{1A}$[48] and $5\text{-}HT_2$[49] receptors appear involved.

Cortisol levels rose dose dependently in our subjects, consistent with the robust elevation of corticotropin described above, and with earlier human data.[14] Se-

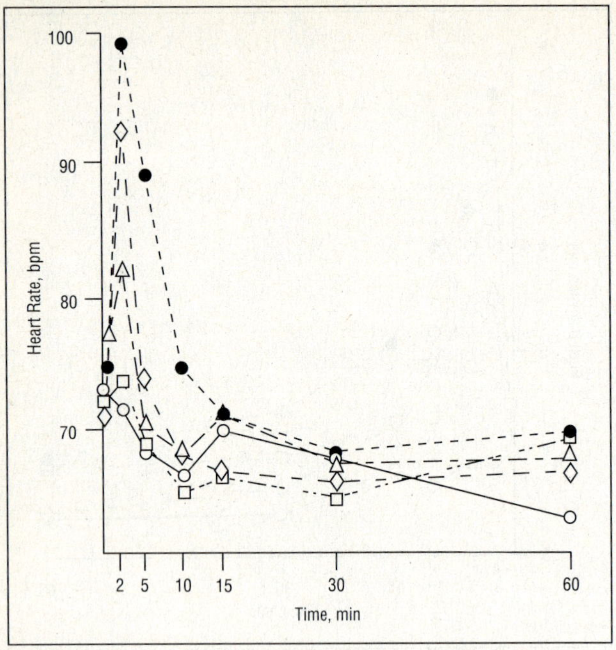

Figure 9. *Mean heart rate values (in beats per minute [bpm]) in 11 subjects after four doses of intravenous dimethyltryptamine fumarate (0.05 mg/kg [squares], 0.1 mg/kg [triangles], 0.2 mg/kg [diamonds], and 0.4 mg/kg [closed circles]) and saline placebo (open circles).*

rotonin receptor activation stimulates peripheral cortisol levels, most likely via corticotropin release,[50] with relevant subtypes having been discussed previously. The cortisol effects in our subjects did not provide as useful a differentiation among doses as the POMC hormones.

Hallucinogen-induced hyperthermia in humans[51] may occur by means of central[52] and/or peripheral[53] 5-HT_2 activation. Dimethyltryptamine's hyperthermic effects are probably mediated by the 5-HT_2 subtype, as 5-HT_{1A} agonists are hypothermic in man.[42] The delayed time course of the temperature rise seen with DMT is of interest and may reflect more complex homeostatic mechanisms controlling this variable than those with a more rapid time course.

Previous human studies have described variable effects of longer-acting hallucinogenic drugs on cardiovascular variables, including hypotension and hypertension, and tachycardia and bradycardia.[54] Dimethyltryptamine's excitatory cardiovascular properties confirm and extend previous human data[55] and suggest 5-HT_2 agonism. The 5-HT_2 agonists usually elicit a rise in blood pressure, without reliable increases in HR.[56,57] In contrast, 5-HT_{1A} agonists generally produce a drop in blood pressure, again without consistent HR effects.[58]

Dimethyltryptamine resembles other classic hallucinogens in its mydriatic properties[59]; this pupillary dilatation may be 5-HT_2 mediated.[60] As the pupillary diameter data were both the least reliably measured (ie, we did not use automated equipment, which also could have measured more dynamic features of pupillary function) and contained the most missing values, they must be considered preliminary.

We found no dose dependency of DMT's stimulation of blood GH levels. Meltzer et al[14] demonstrated a cyproheptadine-sensitive stimulatory effect of one DMT dose on peripheral GH levels in humans. Perhaps if we had continued drawing samples for 2 hours, as did Meltzer et al, we might have found better separation of effects by dose.

Subjective effects of IV dimethyltryptamine were consistent with previous reports of parenterally administered DMT[16,31,61] and were marked by perceptual, dissociative, affective, and cognitive alterations typical of the classic hallucinogens. Onset from the IV route was nearly instantaneous, rather than taking several minutes to develop, and effects were shorter than previously published IM data. However, this time course is quite similar to reports of DMT smoked free base.[27] The three subjects in the group with experience smoking DMT free base all volunteered that the IV route was somewhat more rapid and intense in onset and effects than smoking the compound. In this regard, DMT is actively transported across the blood-brain barrier in the rat.[62] A more detailed account of these effects and their quantification by a new rating scale are described in a companion article.[32]

Dimethyltryptamine, as a putative directly acting 5-HT agonist in humans, can be most appropriately compared with 6-chloro-2-(1-piperazinyl) pyrazine (MK-212) and *m*-chlorophenylpiperazine (*m*-CPP), although only *m*-CPP has been given intravenously to humans. Neither drug produces the typical hallucinogenic syndrome in normal sub-

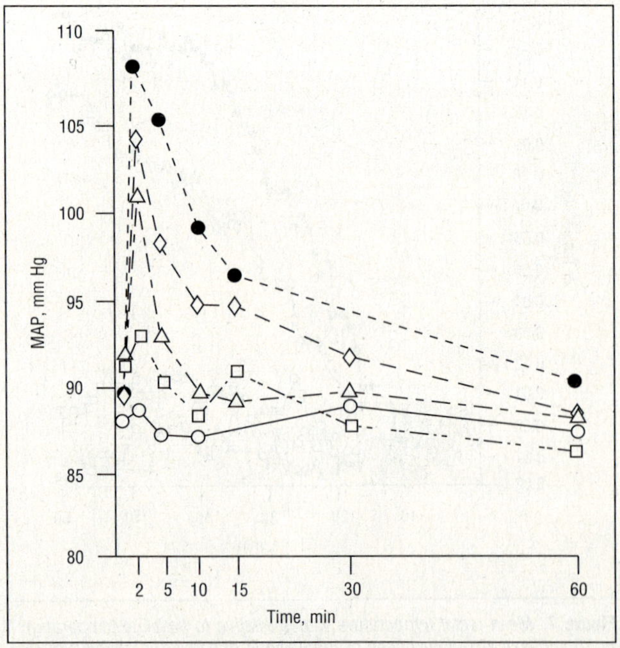

Figure 10. *Mean arterial blood pressure (MAP) values in 11 subjects after four doses of intravenous dimethyltryptamine fumarate (0.05 mg/kg [squares], 0.1 mg/kg [triangles], 0.2 mg/kg [diamonds], and 0.4 mg/kg [closed circles]) and saline placebo (open circles).*

jects; however, behavioral effects may be more disruptive in psychiatric samples.[63,64] Both *m*-CPP and MK-212 have complex effects at multiple 5-HT receptor subtypes, in addition to effects on other neurotransmitters.[65]

Intravenous *m*-CPP's biological effects are similar to those of DMT. Cortisol and GH stimulation is comparable in magnitude to DMT's, but the prolactin response to DMT is smaller.[66] Similarly, GH responses are delayed relative to those of prolactin and cortisol. Hyperthermic effects of IV *m*-CPP also are relatively delayed and are greater than those seen with DMT.[67] However, temperature data were collected longer for IV *m*-CPP than for DMT, and we may have missed a rise of similar magnitude. Behaviorally, IV *m*-CPP's peak effects occur somewhat later than those of DMT,[67] perhaps related to DMT's previously mentioned active transport into the brain.

Orally administered MK-212 elevates prolactin and cortisol (but not GH) blood levels,[64] blood pressure, and body temperature.[68] As MK-212 has never been given intravenously to humans, a comparison of the temporal sequence of its effects with IV DMT or *m*-CPP is not possible.

The only biological effect demonstrated in subjects with a greater cumulative exposure to the serotonergic neurotoxin MDMA relative to the group with less exposure was a decreased pupillary response to all doses of DMT. This is opposite to what might be expected based on augmented behavioral effects of hallucinogens in amine-depleted[69] or denervated[70] animals. We are unable to explain this finding, except to note that our pupil diameter data were the least complete and objectively measured, and were analyzed by ANOVA without repeated measures.

We erroneously hypothesized that daytime melatonin levels might be elevated secondary to DMT administration, based on the presence of 5-HT_2 receptors on pineal tissue[71] and stimulation by DMT of a requisite enzyme for melatonin synthesis.[72] However, the lack of a stimulatory effect of DMT on melatonin is relevant regarding the specificity of our neuroendocrine results. Previous work[73] showed that melatonin levels doubled after a "stressful" long-distance race, although β-endorphin levels rose to only half those noted in the present DMT study. These two sets of data make it unlikely that a "stress" effect (ie, purely sympathetic activation) drove our neuroendocrine variables; if so, either melatonin levels would have risen or β-endorphin effects would have been much greater.

CAVEATS

Our sample of subjects had a heavy loading of personal (50%) and family (67%) histories of affective disorder and/or alcohol abuse, both of which may be associated with abnormalities in serotonergic responsivity.[74,75] Thus, the data generated from this study may not be generalizable to strictly "normal" subjects. In addition, nine of 11 subjects had been divorced, there being a total of 17 divorces in this group. Although not specifically assessed, this high rate of divorce may imply a certain degree of impulsivity within our subjects, another condition in which serotonergic abnormalities have been described.[76]

One subject's blood pressure response to a screening, nonblind dose of 0.04 mg/kg caused him to be withdrawn from further participation. After completing this study, while screening additional subjects for subsequent protocols, another subject with a history of borderline essential hypertension (currently asymptomatic) also had a robust diastolic response to 0.05 mg/kg of dimethyltryptamine fumarate and was withdrawn from further sessions. Thus, we recommend that subjects with a history of hypertension, even though currently asymptomatic, not be considered for IV DMT studies. In addition, all prospective subjects must first be screened with the low, minimally psychoactive 0.05-mg/kg dose; diastolic blood pressure responses to more than 100 mm Hg contraindicate exposure to higher doses of DMT.

CONCLUSION

Human data are necessary to begin bridging basic neuropharmacological and clinical psychopharmacological concepts of hallucinogenic drugs' effects and mechanisms of action.[77] Using careful screening and preparation of subjects, attentive yet unobtrusive supervision of the acute drug intoxication, and follow-up, DMT was safely administered to a group of experienced hallucinogen users and normative dose-response data generated. The most salient biological variables, based on our data, seem to be corticotropin, prolactin, core temperature, blood pressure, HR, and pupil diameter. Pupil diameter studies, if performed, would benefit from the use of automated equipment.

We believe the importance of these data derive from at least two perspectives. The first is that of understanding effects and mechanisms of action of these intriguing drugs. Many of DMT's biological effects in psychiatrically healthy hallucinogen users are now much better characterized. The properties of other classic and nonclassic hallucinogens (such as 1-(2,5-dimethoxy-4-methylphenyl)-2-aminopropane (DOM) now can be assessed for their degree(s) of similarity. In addition, although serotonergic mechanisms are believed primary in mediating hallucinogens' effects, these data can help validate this hypothesis by performing human studies using selective 5-HT receptor subtype antagonists. Experiments also can be designed to assess the relative contributions of noradrenergic and dopaminergic neurotransmission.

Second, DMT might be considered an additional serotonergic probe of neuroendocrine and behavioral variables in research attempting to characterize neurotransmission in normal volunteers and psychiatrically ill subjects with presumed serotonergic abnormalities. Although the hallucinogenic effects of DMT are not separable from its threshold effects (relative to placebo) on the multiple biological factors presented herein, these effects, if judiciously managed, should not present insurmountable difficulties. *m*CPP, for example, increases several patient populations' symptoms but remains a valuable tool for human serotonergic studies. However, it must be emphasized that until DMT's effects are mechanistically characterized in normal subjects, there would not be sufficient data to conclude that altered responses to DMT necessarily implicated altered 5-HT function.

Accepted for publication November 4, 1992.

This investigation was supported by grant RO3-DAO6524 from the National Institute on Drug Abuse, Rockville, Md; the Scottish Rite Foundation for Schizophrenia Research, NMJ, Lexington, Mass; grant RR00997-13 from the National Institutes of Health General Clinical Research Center, Rockville; the Scott Rogers Fund of the University of New Mexico, Albuquerque; and University of New Mexico Department of Psychiatry research funds.

We thank David E. Nichols, PhD, for synthesis of the dimethyltryptamine fumarate used in this study; Cynthia Geist, RN, and the nursing staff of the GCRC, 5E, University of New Mexico Hospital, for nursing support; Katy Zownir-Brazis, RN, for performing the SCID-R interviews; E. Jonathan Lisansky, MD, for assistance in diagnosis; Joy McLeod, Alberta Bland, and Susan Lee for laboratory assistance; David S. Schade, MD, for development of the dimethyltryptamine assay; and Richard Dorin, MD, and Russel Reiter, PhD, for assistance in performing assays.

Reprint requests to Department of Psychiatry, University of New Mexico, 2400 Tucker Ave NE, Albuquerque, NM 87131-5326 (Dr Strassman).

REFERENCES

1. Freedman DX. On the use and abuse of LSD. *Arch Gen Psychiatry.* 1968;18:330-347.
2. Nichols D, Oberlender R, McKenna D. Stereochemical aspects of hallucinogenesis. In: Watson R, ed. *Biochemistry and Physiology of Substance Abuse, III.* Boca Raton, Fla: CRC Press Inc; 1991:1-39.
3. Cohen S. Lysergic acid diethylamide: side effects and complications. *J Nerv Ment Dis.* 1960;130:30-40.
4. Strassman R. Adverse reactions to psychedelic drugs: a review of the literature. *J Nerv Ment Dis.* 1984;172:577-595.
5. Pope H Jr, Ionescu-Pioggia M, Aizley H, Varma D. Drug use and life style among college undergraduates in 1989: a comparison with 1969 and 1978. *Am J Psychiatry.* 1990;147:998-1001.
6. Peroutka S, Snyder S. Multiple serotonin receptors: differential binding of [3H]5-hydroxytryptamine, [3H]lysergic acid diethylamide and [3H]spiroperidol. *Mol Pharmacol.* 1979;16:687-690.
7. Glennon R, Titeler M, McKenney J. Evidence for 5-HT_2 involvement in the mechanism of action of hallucinogenic agents. *Life Sci.* 1985;35:2505-2511.
8. Spencer D Jr, Glaser T, Traber J. Serotonin receptor subtype mediation of the interoceptive discriminative stimuli induced by 5-methoxy-N,N-dimethyltryptamine. *Psychopharmacology.* 1987;93:158-166.
9. Yagaloff K, Hartig P. ^{125}I-lysergic acid diethylamide binds to a novel serotonergic site on rat choroid plexus epithelial cells. *J Neurosci.* 1985;5:3178-3183.
10. Buckholtz N, Zhou D, Freedman DX, Potter W. Lysergic acid diethylamide (LSD) administration selectively downregulates $serotonin_2$ receptors in rat brain. *Neuropsychopharmacology.* 1990;3:137-148.
11. Ahn H, Makman M. Interaction of LSD and other hallucinogens with dopamine-sensitive adenylate cyclase in primate brain: regional differences. *Brain Res.* 1979;162:77-88.
12. Horita A, Hamilton A. Lysergic acid diethylamide: dissociation of its behavioral and hyperthermic effects by DL-alpha-methyl-p-tyrosine. *Science.* 1969;164:78-79.
13. Van de Kar L. Neuroendocrine pharmacology of serotonergic (5-HT) neurons. *Ann Rev Pharmacol Toxicol.* 1991;31:289-320.
14. Meltzer H, Wiita B, Tricou B, Simonovic M, Fang V. Effects of serotonin precursors and serotonin agonists on plasma hormone levels. In: Ho B, Schoolar J, Usdin E, eds. *Serotonin in Biological Psychiatry.* New York, NY: Raven Press; 1980:117-139.
15. Halaris A, Freedman DX, Fang V. Plasma corticoids and brain tryptophan after acute and tolerance dosage of LSD. *Life Sci.* 1976;17:1467-1472.
16. Sai-Halasz A, Brunecker G, Szara S. Dimethyltryptamine: ein neues Psychoticum. *Psychiatr Neurol.* 1958;135:285-301.
17. Horita A, Dille J. The pyretogenic effect of lysergic acid diethylamide. *Science.* 1954;120:1110-1111.
18. Greiner T, Burch N, Edelberg R. Psychopathology and psychophysiology of minimal LSD-25 dosage: a preliminary dosage-response spectrum. *Arch Neurol Psychiatry.* 1958;79:208-210.
19. Isbell H. Comparison of the reactions induced by psilocybin and LSD-25 in man. *Psychopharmacologia.* 1959;1:29-38.
20. Fish M, Johnson N, Horning E. Piptadenia alkaloids: indole bases of *P. peregrina* (L.) Benth. and related species. *J Am Chem Soc.* 1955;77:5892-5895.
21. Barker S, Monti J, Christian S. N,N-dimethyltryptamine: an endogenous hallucinogen. *Int Rev Neurobiol.* 1981;22:83-110.
22. Gillin J, Kaplan J, Stillman R, Wyatt R. The psychedelic model of schizophrenia: the case of N,N-dimethyltryptamine. *Am J Psychiatry.* 1976;133:203-208.
23. Strassman R. Human hallucinogenic drug research in the United States: a present-day case history and review of the process. *J Psychoactive Drug.* 1991;23:29-38.
24. Spitzer R, Williams J, Gibbon M. *Structured Clinical Interview of* DSM-III-R: *Outpatient Version.* New York, NY: Biometric Research Dept, New York State Psychiatric Institute; 1987.
25. McKenna D, Peroutka S. Neurochemistry and neurotoxicity of 3,4-methylenedioxymethamphetamine (MDMA, 'Ecstasy'). *J Neurochem.* 1990;54:14-22.
26. Price L, Ricaurte G, Krystal J, Heninger G. Neuroendocrine and mood responses to intravenous L-tryptophan in 3,4-methylenedioxymethamphetamine (MDMA) users. *Arch Gen Psychiatry.* 1989;46:20-22.
27. Stafford P. *Psychedelics Encyclopedia.* Rev ed. Boston, Mass: Houghton Mifflin Co; 1982:308-331.
28. Walker R, Mandel L, Kleinman J, Gillin J, Wyatt R, VandenHeuvel W. Improved selective ion monitoring mass-spectrometric assay for the determination of N,N-dimethyltryptamine in human blood utilizing capillary column gas chromatography. *J Chromatogr.* 1979;162:539-546.
29. Webley G, Mehl H, Willey K. Validation of a sensitive direct assay for melatonin for investigation of circadian rhythms in different species. *J Endocrinol.* 1985;106:387-394.
30. Angrist B, Gershon S, Sathananthan, Walker R, Lopez-Ramos B, Mandel L, VandenHeuvel W. Dimethyltryptamine levels in blood of schizophrenic patients and control subjects. *Psychopharmacology.* 1976;47:29-32.
31. Kaplan J, Mandel L, Stillman R, Walker R, VandenHeuvel W, Gillin J, Wyatt R. Blood and urine levels of N,N-dimethyltryptamine following administration of psychoactive doses to human subjects. *Psychopharmacologia.* 1974;38:239-245.
32. Strassman RJ, Qualls CR, Uhlenhuth EH, Kellner R. Dose-response study of N,N-dimethyltryptamine in humans, II: subjective effects and preliminary results of a new rating scale. *Arch Gen Psychiatry.* 1994;51:98-108.
33. Aghajanian G, Foote W, Sheard M. Action of psychotogenic drugs on single midbrain raphe neurons. *J Pharmacol Exp Ther.* 1970;171:178-187.
34. Deliganis A, Pierce P, Peroutka S. Differential interactions of dimethyltryptamine (DMT) with 5-HT_{1A} and 5-HT_2 receptors. *Biochem Pharmacol.* 1991;41:1739-1744.
35. Jenner P, Marsden C, Thanki C. Behavioral changes induced by N,N-dimethyltryptamine in rodents. *Br J Pharmacol.* 1980;69:69-80.
36. Pierce P, Peroutka S. Hallucinogenic drug interactions with neurotransmitter

receptor binding sites in human cortex. *Psychopharmacology.* 1989;97:118-122.
37. Sanders-Bush E, Breeding M. Choroid plexus epithelial cells in primary culture: a model of $5HT_{1C}$ receptor activation by hallucinogenic drugs. *Psychopharmacology.* 1991;105:340-346.
38. Charig E, Anderson I, Robinson J, Nutt D, Cowen P. L-tryptophan and prolactin release: evidence for interaction between $5\text{-}HT_1$ and $5\text{-}HT_2$ receptors. *Hum Psychopharmacol.* 1986;1:93-97.
39. Vale W, Spiess J, Rivier C, Rivier J. Characterization of a 41-residue ovine hypothalamic peptide that stimulates secretion of corticotropin and β-endorphin. *Science.* 1981;213:1394-1396.
40. Lewis D, Sherman B. Serotonergic regulation of adrenocorticotropin secretion in man. *J Clin Endocrinol Metab.* 1984;58:458-462.
41. Petraglia F, Facchinetti F, Martignoni E, Nappi G, Volpe A, Genazzani A. Serotonergic agonists increase plasma levels of β-endorphin and β-lipotropin in humans. *J Clin Endocrinol Metab.* 1984;59:1138-1142.
42. Anderson I, Cowen P, Grahame-Smith D. The effects of gepirone on neuroendocrine function and temperature in humans. *Psychopharmacology.* 1990;100:498-503.
43. Calogero A, Bernardini R, Margioris A, Bagdy G, Gallucci W, Munson P, Tamarkin L, Tomai T, Brady L, Gold P, Chrousos G. Effects of serotonergic agonists and antagonists on corticotropin-releasing hormone secretion by explanted rat hypothalami. *Peptides.* 1989;10:189-200.
44. Kato Y, Nakai Y, Imura H, Chichara K, Ohgo S. Effect of 5-hydroxytryptophan (5-HTP) on plasma prolactin levels in man. *J Clin Endocrinol Metab.* 1974;38:695-697.
45. Asnis G, Eisenberg J, van Praag H, Lemus C, Friedman J, Miller A. The neuroendocrine response to fenfluramine in depressives and normal controls. *Biol Psychiatry.* 1988;24:117-120.
46. Demisch L, Neubauer M. Stimulation of human prolactin secretion by mescaline. *Psychopharmacology.* 1979;64:361-363.
47. Aloi J, Insel T, Mueller E, Murphy D. Neuroendocrine and behavioral effects of *m*CPP in rhesus monkeys. *Life Sci.* 1984;34:1325-1331.
48. Smith C, Ware C, Cowen P. Pindolol decreases prolactin and growth hormone responses to intravenous L-tryptophan. *Psychopharmacology.* 1991;103:140-142.
49. Van de Kar L, Lorens S, Urban J, Bethea C. Effect of selective serotonin (5-HT) agonists and $5\text{-}HT_2$ antagonists on prolactin secretion. *Neuropharmacology.* 1989;28:299-305.
50. Calogero A, Bagdy G, Szemeredi K, Tartaglia M, Gold P, Chrousos G. Mechanisms of serotonin receptor agonist-induced activation of the hypothalamic-pituitary-adrenal axis in the rat. *Endocrinology.* 1990;126:1888-1894.
51. Snyder SH, Faillace L, Hollister L. 2,5-Dimethoxy-4-methyl-amphetamine (STP): a new hallucinogenic drug. *Science.* 1967;158:669-670.
52. Won S, Lin M. 5-Hydroxytryptamine receptors in the hypothalamus mediate thermoregulatory responses in rabbits. *Naunyn Schmiedebergs Arch Pharmacol.* 1988;338:256-261.
53. Cohen M, Fuller T, Wiley S. Evidence for $5\text{-}HT_2$ receptors mediating contraction in vascular smooth muscle. *J Pharmacol Exp Ther.* 1981;21:421-425.
54. Denber H, Merlis S. Studies on mescaline, VI: therapeutic aspects of the mescaline-chlorpromazine combination. *J Nerv Ment Dis.* 1955;122:463-469.
55. Turner W, Merlis S. Effect of some indolealkylamines on man. *Arch Neurol Psychiatry.* 1959;81:121-129.
56. Dabire H, Chaouche-Teyara K, Cherqui C, Fournier B, Laubie M, Schmitt H. Characterization of DOI, a putative $5\text{-}HT_2$ receptor agonist in the rat. *Eur J Pharmacol.* 1989;168:369-374.
57. Rittenhouse P, Bakkum E, Van de Kar L. Evidence that the serotonin agonist, DOI, increases renin secretion and blood pressure through both central and peripheral $5\text{-}HT_2$ receptors. *J Pharmacol Exp Ther.* 1991;259:58-65.
58. Dreteler G, Wouters W, Saxena P. Systemic and regional hemodynamic effects of the putative $5\text{-}HT_{1A}$ receptor agonist flesinoxan in the cat. *J Cardiovasc Pharmacol.* 1989;14:770-776.
59. Klee G, Bertino J, Weintraub W, Callaway E III. The influence of varying dosage on the effects of lysergic acid diethylamide (LSD-25) in humans. *J Nerv Ment Dis.* 1961;132:404-409.
60. Millson D, Haworth S, Rushton A, Wilkinson D, Hobson S, Harry J. The effects of a $5\text{-}HT_2$ antagonist (ICI 169,369) on changes in waking EEG, pupillary responses and state of arousal in human volunteers. *Br J Clin Pharmacol.* 1991;32:447-454.
61. Rosenberg D, Isbell H, Miner E. Comparison of placebo, *N*-dimethyltryptamine, and 6-hydroxy-*N*-dimethyltryptamine in man. *Psychopharmacology.* 1963;4:39-42.
62. Yanai K, Ido T, Ishiwata K, Hatazawa J, Takahashi T, Iwata R, Matsuzawa T. In vivo kinetics and displacement study of a carbon-11-labeled hallucinogen, *N,N*-[^{11}C]dimethyltryptamine. *Eur J Nucl Med.* 1986;12:141-146.
63. Seibyl J, Krystal J, Price L, Woods W, Heninger G, Charney D. 5-HT function in the biochemical and behavioral responses to *m*CPP in healthy subjects and schizophrenics. *Soc Neurosci Abstr.* 1989;15:1236.
64. Lowy M, Meltzer H. Stimulation of serum cortisol and prolactin secretion in humans by MK-212, a centrally active serotonin agonist. *Biol Psychiatry.* 1988;23:818-828.
65. Murphy D, Lesch K, Aulakh C, Pigott T. Serotonin-selective arylpiperazines with neuroendocrine, behavioral, temperature and cardiovascular effects in humans. *Pharmacol Rev.* 1991;43:527-552.
66. Charney D, Goodman W, Price L, Woods W, Rasmussen S, Heninger G. Serotonin function in obsessive-compulsive disorder. *Arch Gen Psychiatry.* 1988;45:177-185.
67. Murphy D, Mueller E, Hill J, Tolliver T, Jacobsen F. Comparative anxiogenic, neuroendocrine and other physiologic effects of *m*-chlorophenylpiperazine given intravenously and orally to healthy volunteers. *Psychopharmacology.* 1989;98:275-283.
68. Lee H, Bastani B, Friedman L, Ramirez L, Meltzer H. Effect of the serotonin agonist, MK-212, on body temperature in schizophrenia. *Biol Psychiatry.* 1992;31:460-470.
69. Appel JB, Freedman DX. Chemically-induced alterations in the behavioral effects of LSD-25. *Biochem Pharmacol.* 1964;13:861-869.
70. Nisbet AF, Marsden CA. Increased behavioural response to 5-methoxy-N,N-dimethyltryptamine but not to RU-24969 after intraventricular 5,7-dihydroxytryptamine administration. *Eur J Pharmacol.* 1984;104:177-180.
71. Ebadi M, Govitrapong P. Neural pathways and neurotransmitters affecting melatonin synthesis. *J Neural Transm.* 1986;21(suppl):125-158.
72. Hartley R, Smith J. The activation of pineal hydroxy-indole-O-methyl-transferase by psychotomimetic drugs. *J Pharm Pharmacol.* 1973;25:751-752.
73. Strassman R, Appenzeller O, Lewy A, Qualls C, Peake G. Increase in plasma melatonin, β-endorphin, and cortisol after a 28.5-mile mountain race: relationship to performance and lack of effect of naltrexone. *J Clin Endocrinol Metab.* 1989;69:540-545.
74. Price L, Charney D, Delgado P, Heninger G. Serotonin function and depression: neuroendocrine and mood responses to intravenous L-tryptophan in depressed patients and healthy comparison subjects. *Am J Psychiatry.* 1991;148:1518-1525.
75. Lee M, Meltzer H. Neuroendocrine responses to serotonergic agents in alcoholics. *Biol Psychiatry.* 1991;30:1017-1030.
76. Fishbein D, Lozovsky D, Jaffe J. Impulsivity, aggression, and neuroendocrine responses to serotonergic stimulation in substance abusers. *Biol Psychiatry.* 1989;25:1049-1066.
77. Freedman DX. Hallucinogenic drug research: if so, so what? *Pharmacol Biochem Behav.* 1986;24:407-415.

ORIGINAL ARTICLE

Dose-Response Study of N,N-Dimethyltryptamine in Humans

II. Subjective Effects and Preliminary Results of a New Rating Scale

Rick J. Strassman, MD; Clifford R. Qualls, PhD; Eberhard H. Uhlenhuth, MD; Robert Kellner, MD, PhD†

Background: Validation of animal models of hallucinogenic drugs' subjective effects requires human data. Previous human studies used varied groups of subjects and assessment methods. Rating scales for hallucinogen effects emphasized psychodynamic principles or the drugs' dysphoric properties. We describe the subjective effects of graded doses of N,N-dimethyltryptamine (DMT), an endogenous hallucinogen and drug of abuse, in a group of experienced hallucinogen users. We also present preliminary data from a new rating scale for these effects.

Methods: Twelve highly motivated volunteers received two doses (0.04 and 0.4 mg/kg) of intravenous (IV) dimethyltryptamine fumarate "nonblind," before entering a double-blind, saline placebo-controlled, randomized study using four doses of IV DMT. Subjects were carefully interviewed after resolution of drug effects, providing thorough and systematic descriptions of DMT's effects. They also were administered a new instrument, the Hallucinogen Rating Scale (HRS). The HRS was drafted from interviews obtained from an independent sample of 19 experienced DMT users, and modified during early stages of the study.

Results: Psychological effects of IV DMT began almost immediately after administration, peaked at 90 to 120 seconds, and were almost completely resolved by 30 minutes. This time course paralleled DMT blood levels previously described. Hallucinogenic effects were seen after 0.2 and 0.4 mg/kg of dimethyltryptamine fumarate, and included a rapidly moving, brightly colored visual display of images. Auditory effects were less common. "Loss of control," associated with a brief, but overwhelming "rush," led to a dissociated state, where euphoria alternated or coexisted with anxiety. These effects completly replaced subjects' previously ongoing mental experience and were more vivid and compelling than dreams or waking awareness. Lower doses, 0.1 and 0.05 mg/kg, were primarily affective and somaesthetic, while 0.1 mg/kg elicited the least desirable effects. Clustering of HRS items, using either a clinical, mental status method or principal components factor analysis provided better resolution of dose effects than did the biological variables described previously.

Conclusions: These clinical and preliminary quantitative data provide bases for further psychopharmacologic characterization of DMT's properties in humans. They also may be used to compare the effects of other agents affecting relevant brain receptors in volunteer and psychiatric populations.

(Arch Gen Psychiatry. 1994;51:98-108)

THE "CLASSICAL" hallucinogens include lysergic acid diethylamide (LSD), psilocybin, and mescaline. Above threshold doses, they reliably elicit a unique constellation of perceptual, emotional, cognitive, interoceptive, and volitional effects, in a usually clear sensorium.[1] Although other drugs might cause similar symptoms (eg, subanesthetic doses of the dissociative anesthetics ketamine hydrochloride and phencyclidine hydrochloride (PCP); amphetamines; marijuana; and anticholinergic deliriants), they can be differentiated clinically from the classical hallucinogens. For example, hallucinogens do not produce general anesthesia at high doses as do PCP or ketamine.

Despite limited cogent human psychopharmacologic studies for many years, basic neuropharmacologic work regarding hallucinogens' effects and mechanisms of action continued. Attention has

From the Department of Psychiatry (Drs Strassman, Uhlenhuth, and Kellner) and General Clinical Research Center (Dr Qualls), University of New Mexico School of Medicine, and the Department of Mathematics and Statistics (Dr Qualls), University of New Mexico, Albuquerque.
†Dr Kellner died November 15, 1992.

See Subjects, Materials, and Methods on next page

SUBJECTS, MATERIALS, AND METHODS

A detailed description of the recruitment, screening, assessment, and characterization of the 12 experienced hallucinogen users who participated in this study was presented previously.[14] Briefly, subjects were recruited by "word-of-mouth," and those with current Axis I disorders (except for one subject with an Adjustment Disorder), ongoing medical illness, or long-term medication use were excluded from participation. The number of previous exposures to hallucinogens ranged from six to "hundreds."

One of the 12 subjects was withdrawn halfway through the study because a recurrence of major depression developed that was associated with the onset of several stressors. He was treated with and responded to desipramine hydrochloride. Thus, the data described in this article are from 11 subjects (one woman and 10 men).

Six of the 11 subjects had used 3,4-methylenedioxymethamphetamine (MDMA, "Ecstasy") five or more times; five had taken it twice or less. 3,4-methylenedioxymethamphetamine is a mammalian serotonergic neurotoxin[16] with equivocal long-term effects in humans.[17] To approximate equal cell sizes to assess differential responses to the "serotonergic probe" DMT, we described the six former subjects as "high exposure" and the latter five as "low-no exposure."

DRUG ADMINISTRATION

Witnessed written informed consent was obtained. The method of, and rationale for, intravenous (IV) (rather than intramuscular) DMT administration were described in detail in the preceding article. All subjects received, on separate days, low (0.04 mg/kg) and high (0.4 mg/kg) doses of dimethyltryptamine fumarate, nonblind, in the inpatient unit of the General Clinical Research Center of the University of New Mexico Hospital, Albuquerque. The DMT was infused over 30 seconds and the IV tube was flushed with sterile saline for an additional 15 seconds.

Because the effects of DMT were so brief, we (R.J.S. and a research nurse) did not attempt to question or interview subjects during the acute intoxication, allowing them an unimpeded opportunity to observe the onset, plateau, and resolution of effects. Conversation focused on the effects of the injection once subjects were able and willing to begin talking. Other issues were discussed at the subject's discretion, but we emphasized descriptive rather than exploratory or therapeutic themes. The HRS was given 30 minutes postinfusion, after the single IV line was removed.

A similar format was used in the double-blind, saline placebo-controlled, randomized phase of the study. Furthermore, a rectal temperature probe was placed 30 minutes before drug administration, as was an additional forearm catheter for blood sampling until 60 minutes after injection. The HRS was administered after the last blood sample was drawn, and the probe and IV lines were removed. Double-blind treatments were 0.05, 0.1, 0.2, and 0.4 mg/kg of dimethyltryptamine fumarate, and sterile saline. Sessions were separated by at least 1 week for men, and at least 1 month for the only woman, who always was studied during the early follicular phase of her menstrual cycle.

HALLUCINOGEN RATING SCALE

The details of the development, drafting, modification, scoring, and analysis of the HRS are described in an "Appendix" available on request from the authors. Briefly, 19 experienced hallucinogen users, who had also used DMT, were interviewed, providing a thorough description of the effects of smoked DMT free base, its usual form of "street" use.[18] In drafting the HRS, we attempted to include effects of DMT common to other hallucinogens, as well as those believed unique to DMT. The version finally used for the double-blind study contained 126 individual items. When filling out the HRS, subjects were asked to recall their experiences from the immediately preceding session. Almost all questions were scored 0 to 4: 0, "not at all"; 1, "slightly"; 2, "moderately"; 3, "quite a bit"; and 4, "extremely."

STATISTICS

Statistical procedures were performed using PC-SAS Version 6 (SAS, Cary, NC). Two-tailed $P<.05$ were considered significant.

In screening for dose effects, a one-way analysis of variance (ANOVA) with the factor *dose*, without repeated measures (because SAS discards observations with even one missing value in its repeated measures procedure), was performed for each question. All questions were retained for further analyses if they demonstrated a dose-related response at $P<.05$.

Two methods were used to place HRS items into groups. The first was a clinical mental status method, choosing six conceptually coherent "clusters." These were as follows: (1) *Somaesthesia*—interoceptive, visceral, and cutaneous/tactile effects; (2) *Affect*—emotional/affective responses; (3) *Perception*—visual, auditory, gustatory, and olfactory experiences; (4) *Cognition*—alterations in thought processes or content; (5) *Volition*—a change in capacity to willfully interact with themselves, the environment, or certain aspects of the experience; and (6) *Intensity*—strength of the various aspects of the experience.

In addition, we obtained factors using a principal components factor analysis with a variance maximum (VARIMAX) rotation. The number of factors was set at six, to correspond to the number of clinical clusters.

The major analysis was a one-way ANOVA with repeated measures, with factor *dose* repeated, performed on the values for each set of clusters and factors. To assess whether extent of prior MDMA use affected these quantified subjective responses to DMT, a two-way repeated measures ANOVA, with repeated factor *dose* and class variable *MDMA history*, was performed.

focused on their serotonergic[2] in addition to dopaminergic[3] and noradrenergic[4] properties. Current research emphasizes the agonist or partial agonist properties of hallucinogens at serotonin (5-HT) receptors, specifically the 5-HT_2,[5,6] 5-HT_{1A},[7] and 5-HT_{1C}[8] subtypes.

N,N-dimethyltryptamine (DMT) is a prototypical indole hallucinogen, originally discovered in plants,[9] but later found in lower animals[10] and humans,[11] with well-characterized and relatively typical neuropharmacologic[12] and behavioral[13] properties. Its short duration of action, relative obscurity, history of safe use in clinical research, and unknown function in humans joined to make it an attractive candidate with which to begin a reexamination of human hallucinogenic drug effects.

Hallucinogens, as psychopharmacologic agents, can be characterized at multiple levels. Interfacing the animal and human "biological" data is possible by applying the relevant methodology to the clinical research setting. Thus, the neuroendocrine, cardiovascular, and autonomic (pupil diameter and rectal temperature) effects of graded doses of DMT, in 11 experienced hallucinogen users, were described in the preceding article.[14] However, the generalizability of animal to human data is more problematic when behavioral effects are addressed.[15]

The older human literature described a broad spectrum of effects of hallucinogens, using many different methods of data collection and a variety of experimental subjects. Our approach to assessing subjective effects of DMT was to study individuals who had repeatedly used hallucinogens. We believed that experienced users would be capable of carefully observing and describing subjective effects of DMT and less prone to development of acute adverse reactions to this short-acting, highly disruptive compound in the stressful setting of a modern clinical research center. We also thought it desirable to allow subjects, as much as possible, to use their (or a comparable cohort's) own words to describe the effects of DMT. Thus, to quantify the effects of DMT, we developed a rating scale based on descriptions of the psychological properties of DMT and other hallucinogens from similarly experienced hallucinogen users. We hoped this might provide an important "resonance" between our subjects' experiences and the words and phrases used by this independent sample.

This article describes the psychological properties of different doses of DMT using descriptions of effects clustered by a clinical, mental status method. It also presents our initial attempt to quantify these effects using a newly developed rating scale, the Hallucinogen Rating Scale (HRS).

RESULTS

The main findings were that 0.2 and 0.4 mg/kg IV dimethyltryptamine fumarate elicited the nearly instantaneous onset of visual hallucinatory phenomena, bodily dissociation, and extreme shifts in mood, which totally replaced subjects' previously ongoing mental experiences. Auditory effects were noted in about half the subjects. Effects resolved quickly; the time course paralleled DMT blood levels described previously. Lower doses, 0.05 and 0.1 mg/kg, were not hallucinogenic; emotional and somaesthetic effects predominated. Analyses of preliminary HRS data suggest its ability to quantify and statistically distinguish dose effects.

In this section, we emphasize effects of the highest, 0.4 mg/kg, hallucinogenic dose. Effects are presented by clinical cluster, to demonstrate the heuristic value of such grouping.

0.4-MG/KG DOSE

Subjects were almost uniformly overwhelmed at the intensity and speed of onset of this dose given for the first time nonblind. All subjects described an intense, rapidly developing, and usually transiently anxiety-provoking "rush" throughout their body and "mind." This developed before the 45-second infusion was completed. The rush, compared with a "freight train" by several subjects, immediately and completely disrupted normal mental function, replacing it with hallucinogenic effects. This rush progressed rapidly to a state wherein most subjects lost awareness of their bodies, and many were not cognizant of being in the hospital or participating in an experiment for the first minute or two of the experience. The three subjects who had smoked DMT free base agreed IV effects were more overwhelming and rapid in onset.

PERCEPTION

Visual imagery predominated in all subjects. At this dose, there was little difference between what was "seen" with eyes opened or closed. Examples of this phenomena included the following comments. "I tried closing my eyes but I saw the same things with my eyes closed as I did with them open." "[The visions were so real] I had to open my eyes to reorient. When I did, the visions were overlaid on top of you. I closed my eyes and then that removed the interference with what I had been seeing." Visual imagery included concrete, formed, more or less recognizable visual images. These were both familiar and novel, such as "a fantastic bird," "a tree of life and knowledge," "a ballroom with crystal chandeliers," human and "alien" figures (such as "a little round creature with one big eye and one small eye, on nearly invisible feet"), "the inside of a computer's boards," "ducts," "DNA double helices," "a pulsating diaphragm," "a spinning golden disc," "a huge fly eye bouncing in front of my face," tunnels, and stairways. Many subjects described kaleidoscopic geometric patterns that were not obviously representational; for example, "beautiful, colorful pink cobwebs; an elongation of light;" "tremendously intricate tiny geometric colors, like being 1 inch from a color TV." Subjects described the colors as brighter, more intense, and deeply saturated than those seen in normal awareness or dreams: "It was like the blue of a desert sky, but on another planet.

The colors were 10 to 100 times more saturated." Foreground-background distinctions were merged in these visions: "As far as I could see, all the way to the visual 'horizon,' there were hundreds of forms of beautiful women. Then, they became superimposed onto a [pastoral] scene that one might sketch. The figures made it a three-dimensional or four-dimensional scene."

As EFFECTS resolved, subjects would open eyes and note that the visual field was overlaid by geometric patterns, with undulating movement and intensification of colors of external objects. Several described a curious "decomposition" of external visual perceptual continuity that altered their ability to process normally what they saw. For example, one subject said, "I looked up and saw how mechanical and essentially soul-less you were. Your movements were not your own, they were no longer smooth and coordinated." There was also an enhancement of depth perception, most subjects referring to the room, and particularly a door in the room, as being "much more three-dimensional."

Auditory effects were noted in about half the subjects. They were not formed (eg, music or voices) but were usually high-pitched, "whining/whirring," "chattering," "crinkling/crunching," or at times comical, such as the "boing, sproing" sounds heard in cartoons. They were heard at the onset of effects, simultaneous with the rush and resolved just as quickly. Some subjects' auditory acuity seemed enhanced: "I was hyperaware of all the sounds you were making in the room; settling in your chair, the blood drawing equipment, the blood pressure cuff inflating." For others, outside auditory stimulation receded far from awareness. One subject said, "I was just totally overwhelmed. If there were noises next door, I couldn't hear them, they didn't matter."

SOMAESTHESIA

These effects were typical of a highly stimulatory "fear response." Several commented on their "breath catching in the throat," or the "wind being knocked out of me" at the onset of effects. Many described a transient heaviness in the chest, a sense of constriction and pressure. One subject said, "I was worried that the vibration would blow my head up. The colors and vibration were so intense, I thought I would pop. I didn't think I would stay in my skin." Another said, "There's that feeling of the dip in the road, swinging on a swing, your stomach sinks. The flushes run through you, your legs twitch." One subject exclaimed, before the infusion was complete, "Here we go!" This rush often progressed to a sense of detachment or dissociation from the body. The loss of awareness of physical experience coincided with the most intense display of hallucinatory images. Comments such as "I no longer had a body"; "I thought I had died"; "My body dissolved; I was pure consciousness"; "I sensed you hovering over me trying to resuscitate me as if I had just come into an emergency room" were typical.

Some male subjects described a sexual effect of the highest dose: a hot and pleasurable sensation developing in the genital area. No one experienced orgasm or ejaculated. Some subjects described a sense of "flying," "falling," a decrease in sense of bodily weight, or rapid movement. Sensations of hot, cold, and alternations between the two were common.

AFFECT

Subjects initially were anxious as the rush developed. However, they quickly settled into the experience within 15 to 30 seconds after injection. Many subjects, perhaps due to their experienced nature, were able to dissociate their emotional responses from the physical fear response. For example, "I felt the familiar body reaction, the fear, but there was no emotional response on my part. I didn't panic"; or "I tried to get myself worked up over what I was seeing, but I just wasn't able to respond emotionally."

Most described the high dose as exciting, euphoric, and highly positively charged. "I feel great, like I had a revelation or something." These qualities were often associated with the visual hallucinatory display: "The bird and I just flew. Wings! Aaaah! It was slow, majestic, grand, slow and lovely. So much beauty! So much richness!" It was not unusual for subjects to describe extremely different emotional reactions alternating with each other, or existing simultaneously, such as fear and euphoria, anxiety and relaxation.

COGNITION

Subjects found the high dose to be compellingly novel and unusual, if not somewhat disorienting. For example, "It was so alien. You immediately try to associate something familiar to it, but you can't." Another commented, "Things are coming into focus. I'm feeling human again. I had no idea what was going on. I was in the middle of the galaxy and there was no one to help me. For a second, I needed help. It just happened so fast."

However, subjects also found they were able to maintain, after some initial confusion, a watchful, observing ego. They almost uniformly remarked at how qualitatively unchanged their thinking processes were (although many described a speeding up of these processes). For example, "My intellect wasn't altered at all. I was just alert to what was unfolding during the experience"; "My mind was definitely at a different place, but it was commenting on the state as it was going on along"; "As I started to come down a little, I got journalistic. I became an observer."

Reality testing was affected inasmuch as subjects were often unaware of the experimental setting, so absorbing were the phenomena. For example, in response to a nurse describing a dream of hers at the end of a subject's double-blind 0.4-mg/kg session, he said, "What you are describing was a dream. This is real. It's totally unexpected, quite constant, and objective." Despite this subject's claim, many others remarked on the degree of similarity between dreams and their experiences at this dose. "This was a dream, not a hallucination. Dreams have story lines such as I experienced today; hallucinations do not."

Some subjects emerged from the intoxication with new perspectives on their personal and/or professional lives. One said, "It changed me. My self-concept seemed small, stupid and insignificant after what I saw and felt. It's made me admit that I can take more responsibility; I can do more in areas I never thought I could. It's so unnatural and bizarre you have to find your own source of strength to navigate in it." Another "saw clearly how the personal self and consciousness are just slowed down and less refined versions of 'pure consciousness.' "

Others, however, found the cognitive effects less sanguine, noting an unpleasant discrepancy between their observation of everyday reality and their apperception of it. For example, "Everything looked right but just a little off. It was as if the room were designed to make me feel uneasy. The wall colors were malevolent; the clock looked all right, but weirdly so, not quite right, as if it were just starting to move every time I glanced at it. It was like a New Age horror film, because things didn't really *look* that different." Another said, "It didn't feel like my normal mode of thinking. You know how schizophrenics talk about different meanings to things? A leaf on the ground takes on new meaning, and they get into it in a big way? That kind of thing."

Some found these effects emotionally unsettling, their intellectual and emotional bases for everyday experience having been severely disrupted. Parts of subsequent drug sessions were sometimes spent "working through" responses to previous high dose(s).

Many subjects referred to a sense of an "other intelligence" present within the hallucinatory state. This was usually described as "supra-intelligent," but "emotionally detached." " 'They' were aware of me, but not particularly concerned. It was like what a parent would feel looking into a playpen at his 1-year-old laying there"; or "It was business as usual for them, there was a lot to do." Others had a clear view of "alien beings": "The 'elves' were prankish and ornery in their nature. There were four of them by the highway; they totally commanded the scene—it was their territory. They were about my height and held up placards, showing me all this incredibly beautiful, complex, swirling geometric stuff."

VOLITION

Almost every subject found the high dose to cause an almost complete loss of control. They felt quite regressed, more or less completely helpless, and unable to function either physically or psychologically in a normal manner. For example, "I'm glad you two were on both sides of me. It was reassuring. I don't know what I would have done if I were alone in that state"; "The blood pressure cuff was sort of refreshing, reminding me I was being looked after, that I had a body. I had to remember to breathe"; "I knew enough to open my eyes to get reoriented"; "I felt like an infant."

Subjects were not capable of affecting willfully the progression of effects during the earliest stages. For example, one said, "I tried telling myself to let go, but even that thought was swept aside in the rush of effects." Several described being "forced" to attend to certain aspects of the experience, by the "other intelligences." For example, "There was a sense of *being told*: 'Look at this, look at that, pay attention!' I tried to let go, which helped"; "One of the elves made it impossible for me to move. There was no issue of control; they were totally in control. They wanted me to look here and there. That was all I could do"; "I wanted to focus to the left, but something was forcing me to view the hallucinations to the right."

INTENSITY

Many subjects described a wavelike pattern of intensity levels with this dose. For example, "There would be alternating an awareness, or consciousness, of the scene at hand. Then there would come another wave, like the ocean, knocking me over." Many subjects, including those with experience smoking DMT, said they had been "higher than ever before" with this dose of DMT.

The first, nonblind, high dose usually was more anxiety ridden (particularly for the first 30 seconds after injection) than the subsequent high dose. That is, subjects were prepared to "lose control" after having been in that state previously. Their understanding that the drug experience was essentially safe, that they "would live" and not "lose their minds" was strengthened by having had the high dose before. Finally, their confidence in the research team to unobtrusively support their regressed state grew as their participation in the study progressed.

0.2-MG/KG DOSE

This was the threshold dose for hallucinogenic effects. Nearly all subjects had some visual hallucinations, but auditory ones were less common. Some found this to be their "dose of choice," being less frightening than the 0.4-mg/kg dose, but generating enough perceptual and affective responses to be interesting, novel, and pleasurable. The rush was difficult to distinguish, at the onset, from the 0.4-mg/kg dose, but it soon became apparent that the intensity of the experience would be less than the highest dose.

0.1-MG/KG DOSE

This dose was least enjoyed by subjects. They felt the somaesthetic sensations of excitation and the "drive to discharge" more striking than the perceptual or affective changes. They were "physically" expecting a hallucinogenic effect, but were left only with uncomfortable physical tension. One

Table 1. Clinical Clusters: Responses to DMT and Placebo*

Factor	Saline	Dose, mg/kg 0.05	0.1	0.2	0.4	F	P
Intensity	0.25±0.12 (E)	0.98±0.18 (D)	1.47±0.18 (C)	2.18±0.23 (B)	2.94±0.15 (A)	38.71	.0001
Somaesthesia	0.12±0.06 (D)	0.51±0.11 (C)	0.81±0.14 (B)	1.19±0.19 (AB)	1.50±0.20 (A)	27.52	.0001
Affect	0.36±0.09 (D)	0.81±0.13 (C)	0.92±0.09 (C)	1.41±0.22 (B)	1.81±0.19 (A)	28.10	.0001
Perception	0.13±0.07 (C)	0.45±0.10 (C)	0.88±0.19 (C)	1.61±0.18 (B)	2.19±0.11 (A)	34.60	.0001
Cognition	0.14±0.08 (E)	0.51±0.14 (D)	0.66±0.15 (C)	1.29±0.26 (B)	1.78±0.28 (A)	25.97	.0001
Volition	0.32±0.07 (D)	0.74±0.10 (C)	1.04±0.16 (B)	1.41±0.14 (B)	1.89±0.16 (A)	22.55	.0001

*DMT indicates N,N-dimethyltryptamine fumarate. Summary of clinical cluster values in response to four doses of intravenous DMT and saline placebo in 11 subjects. Values are mean ±SEM. P is the P value corresponding to the overall F statistic obtained by repeated measures analysis of variance. Means in a given row with the same letter are not significantly different by repeated measures tests of contrast (α=.05).

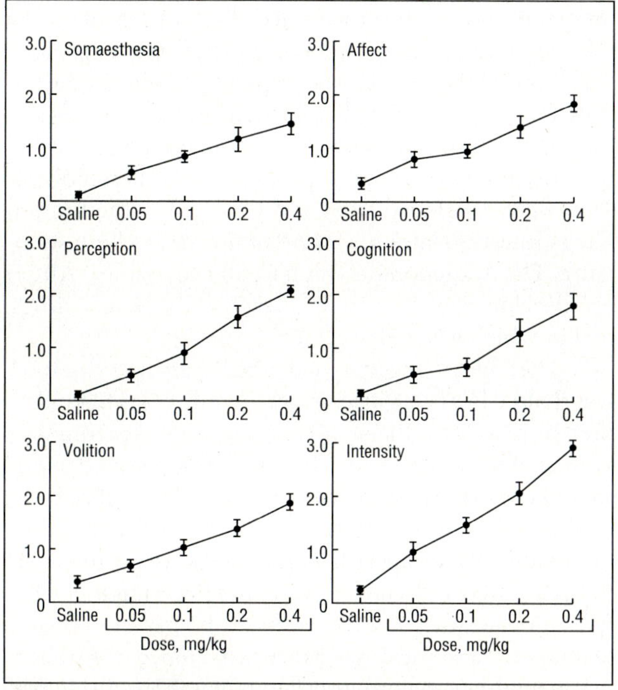

Mean (±SEM) raw values for the six clinical clusters derived from the Hallucinogen Rating Scale, in 11 subjects, after four doses of intravenous N,N-dimethyltryptamine (DMT) and saline placebo.

subject remarked, "You'll never sell this dose. It had all of the physical effects without any of the mental ones." Another said, "My body feels like pepper tastes."

0.05-MG/KG DOSE

Several subjects mistook this dose for placebo. Those who were able to distinguish it from saline remarked on its relaxing, comforting, and "warm" physical effects. One former heroin user likened it to the "soft cotton batting" of IV heroin. There were no perceptual (auditory or visual) effects at this dose.

Subjects were relatively consistent in their styles of reacting to all doses of DMT. That is, those who began speaking early did so after receiving all doses; those who preferred a longer period of silence with eyes closed did so after receiving all doses, too. Many, even if they were able to speak early on, chose to remain silent with eyes closed so as to be able to follow carefully the progression of effects.

HALLUCINOGEN RATING SCALE

Seventy-five of 126 questions demonstrated a significant effect of *dose* by a one-way ANOVA. All but one of these 75 ("What dose do you think you received today?") were included in computations choosing factors and clusters and in assessing the effects of *dose* on these groups of questions. Tables containing questions grouped by clinical cluster and principal components factor are contained in the Appendix available from the authors on request.

The results of a one-way ANOVA with repeated measures on mean raw scores for each cluster, with repeated factor *dose*, are presented in **Table 1** and graphically displayed in the **Figure**. Five of the six clusters discriminated between placebo and the lowest dose of DMT (0.05 mg/kg). Two clusters, Intensity and Cognition, discriminated among all doses.

The hallucinogenic "break point," between 0.2 and 0.1 mg/kg, was statistically separable for four clusters: Intensity, Affect, Perception, and Cognition. Volition, Perception, Affect, and Intensity demonstrated significant differences between 0.4 and 0.2 mg/kg.

Three of the six principal components factors discriminated between placebo and 0.05 mg/kg of dimethyltryptamine fumarate, whereas two factors discriminated among all five doses. However, they were better able to discriminate between the hallucinogenic 0.2-mg/kg and nonhallucinogenic 0.1-mg/kg dimethyltryptamine fumarate doses (six of six, compared with four of six clinical clusters). **Table 2** displays these results.

Table 2. Principal Components Factors: Responses to DMT and Placebo*

Factor	Saline	Dose, mg/kg 0.05	0.1	0.2	0.4	F	*P*
F1	0.38±0.15 (D)	1.02±0.20 (C)	1.10±0.15 (C)	1.60±0.24 (B)	2.28±0.23 (A)	23.89	.0001
F2	0.14±0.06 (E)	0.66±0.12 (D)	1.22±0.24 (C)	2.17±0.26 (B)	2.54±0.18 (A)	51.51	.0001
F3	0.18±0.05 (D)	0.37±0.10 (D)	0.58±0.13 (C)	1.05±0.21 (B)	1.41±0.24 (A)	12.62	.0001
F4	0.23±0.10 (D)	0.64±0.13 (CD)	0.81±0.09 (C)	1.30±0.18 (B)	1.97±0.16 (A)	30.23	.0001
F5	0.20±0.08 (E)	0.51±0.10 (D)	1.01±0.14 (C)	1.33±0.14 (B)	1.69±0.17 (A)	33.37	.0001
F6	0.19±0.06 (D)	0.47±0.12 (D)	0.70±0.15 (C)	1.18±0.19 (B)	1.51±0.19 (A)	22.95	.0001

**DMT indicates N,N-dimethyltryptamine fumarate. Summary of principal component factor values in response to four doses of intravenous DMT and saline placebo in 11 subjects. Values are mean±SEM.* P *is the* P *value corresponding to the overall F statistic obtained by repeated measures analysis of variance. Means in a given row with the same letter are not significantly different by repeated measures tests of contrast (α=.05).*

A two-way repeated measures ANOVA, with repeated factor *dose* and class variable *MDMA history*, demonstrated no effect of degree of prior MDMA exposure on either set of item groupings, across all doses.

TECHNICAL COMMENT ON ASSESSMENT OF SUBJECTIVE EFFECTS

Human studies assessing the psychological and subjective effects of hallucinogens used many approaches. Complicating these different observational and data collecting models were issues regarding the (1) subject sample and (2) purpose of drug administration. As no drug's effects are as responsive to environmental cues as are the effects of hallucinogens,[19-21] "set" and "setting" issues should be considered when interpreting these data.[22] Set refers to the psychophysiologic state and the expectations of the subject; setting refers to the physical environment and experimenters' expectations within which sessions occur.

Clinical observations by skilled clinicians were among the first attempts to describe a general pattern of the effects of hallucinogens in humans. These observations used behavioral-descriptive[23,24] and psychodynamic[25,26] perspectives, providing colorful and provocative descriptions. However, it was difficult to transfer these observational techniques from one research center to another. Attempts were made to quantify some of these psychological effects,[27] but similar problems arose attempting to generalize scores on, for example, "echolalia" or "regression to infancy" from study to study.

A parallel course of research applied previously validated psychological instruments to the hallucinogenic drug state. These included, for example, the Minnesota Multiphasic Personality Inventory (MMPI),[28] Rorschach,[29] Weschler intelligence tests,[30] and the Clyde Mood Scale,[31] and provided comparisons between hallucinogen effects and previously characterized psychopathologic syndromes. Additionally, these studies quantified effects of these drugs on relatively well-characterized psychological functions. However, none of these tests were originally developed specifically for quantification of hallucinogenic drug effects.

Three rating scales were used most frequently to quantify the psychological properties of hallucinogens. Two were developed specifically for LSD—the Linton-Langs questionnaire and the Abramson et al questionnaire. The Addiction Research Center Inventory (ARCI) was developed to assess the characteristics of several drugs, one of which was LSD.

The Linton-Langs questionnaire,[32,33] developed in 1962, was drafted by reviewing current literature on LSD and on the psychoanalytic theory of consciousness. A preliminary version of the scale was administered to the researchers and their colleagues who took LSD; the scale was modified based on their experiences. Experimental subjects had no previous hallucinogen experience, and they were not told what drug they were to receive or what the effects might be. The questionnaire was administered by members of the research team. Four "empirical" scales were developed from the experimental data, factoring questions that showed a high degree of correlation. For example, Scale "A" contained items related to "impaired control or attention," "loss of inhibition," "elation," and "subjective feeling of having developed new powers of insight." This scale was used by other investigators and for other hallucinogens.[34]

The Abramson et al questionnaire,[35] developed in 1955, was drafted by reviewing the literature on LSD. It was administered to subjects, volunteer "non-psychotic" adults, by a member of the research team. Subjects received saline placebo or one of two doses of LSD. Sessions took place in groups, known to affect an individual's response to LSD, relative to taking it alone.[36] Only five of 47 questions could distinguish between "high dose" LSD (usually 100 μg) and placebo. Emphasis was on somatic and perceptual symptoms such as dizziness, unsteadiness, sweating, paresthesias, blurred vision, "inner trembling," and weakness. Groups of questions were clustered in an a priori manner among "physiological," "perceptual," and "cognitive" categories. This scale was used at the Addiction Research Center, Lexington, Ky,[37] where several questions were included in the development of the ARCI.

The most commonly used rating scale for drug effects is the ARCI,[38] a 550-item, true-false test, developed in 1958. Subjects whose responses were used in drafting the ARCI were detoxified opiate addicts serving prison terms for violations of narcotics laws. Subjects' responses on sentence completion tasks under multiple conditions were used in drafting this scale as were some MMPI and other rating scale items.[39] Treatment conditions of these prisoner-subjects in the initial ARCI study included no-drug, saline placebo, two doses of LSD, and several other psychoactive drugs. Five "Group Variability" scales[40] were derived, characterizing common properties of a particular drug or drugs. These scales ultimately were used to describe novel compounds as, for example, more or less "morphine-like" or "LSD-like," rather than having effects on perception or cognition per se. The LSD scale contained items related to symptoms of anxiety, tension, depersonalization, and changes in perception and sensation (the "dysphoria" items). Regarding dose effects, little difference was noted between 1 and 1.5 μg/kg of LSD in non-LSD scales, whereas higher scores on the LSD scale were noted with the latter dose. A short, early version of the ARCI was used to assess two doses of DMT,[41] demonstrating less positive responses after the lower dose. The ARCI also was used to characterize the effects of the phenethylamine hallucinogen 2,5-dimethoxy-4-methamphetamine (DOM).[42]

OUR DESCRIPTION of subjective effects of DMT used reports obtained by experienced hallucinogen users who were well prepared for the effects of the drug. In addition, these subjects (and those whose descriptions provided the initial data for development of the HRS) found hallucinogens highly desirable. Thus, our sample differed from those used to characterize hallucinogens' effects in previous studies, and the experimental expectations were such that the entire gamut of effects could be reasonably assumed covered by our methodology. We believe the clustering of symptoms, as reflected by items on the HRS, provides a clinically useful manner of capturing some of the subtleties of DMT's effects. However, qualitative effects on clusters were not quantified in this preliminary report of the HRS. That is, affect was measured only relative to the multiple treatment conditions, and we did not parse affective changes into qualitative categories, such as "euphoria," dysphoria, or "anxiety." However, further refinement of scoring the HRS may provide these data.

The HRS was designed to assess the effects of hallucinogens, but our data concern only DMT, an unusually fast and short-acting compound. Additional testing of its ability to similarly characterize other hallucinogens is necessary. Validating the DMT-derived factors/clusters with an independent sample of DMT studies also is important.

COMMENT

We describe the subjective effects of multiple doses of the short-acting, endogenous hallucinogen, DMT in 11 experienced hallucinogen users, in a double-blind, placebo-controlled, randomized design. We also present preliminary data suggesting the utility of a new instrument, the HRS, to quantify DMT's effects.

The effects of DMT were nearly instantaneous in onset, paralleling blood levels of DMT, described in the preceding article.[14] Our subjects' descriptions comported well with previous human studies of intramuscular DMT[43,44] and with "field" reports of smoked free base.[18] The two "hallucinogenic" doses, 0.2 and 0.4 mg/kg, elicited an intensely colored, rapidly moving display of visual images, formed, abstract, or both. Auditory hallucinations were less common and well constituted than the visual ones. A physical rush, commonly progressing to a sense of bodily dissociation, also was noted with the higher doses. Alternating and sometimes simultaneous experiences of fear, anxiety, euphoria, and calm characterized the affective properties of DMT in our subjects. Reality testing was powerfully affected at higher doses, subjects usually ascribing a more compelling nature or greater "validity" to the drug experience than either dreams or everyday waking phenomena. These hallucinogenic doses were where statistically significant differences in biological responses between placebo and active drug, previously described, were seen most consistently.

Lower doses of dimethyltryptamine fumarate, 0.1 and 0.05 mg/kg, were not hallucinogenic, and they produced primarily somaesthetic and emotional responses. The former dose elicited a tensely dysphoric state partaking of the physical stimulation of DMT without providing the desired "breakthrough" into the novel perceptual effects. These results validated "field" data on the unpleasant nature of "too little" DMT.[18] The lowest, 0.05 mg/kg, dose had mildly mood elevating and calming properties, likened by one subject to IV heroin.

Results of the HRS, which must be considered preliminary, provided a quantitative approach to these phenomena. The analysis of these pilot data generated better separation of DMT doses using either clinical clusters or principal components factors of items than did the biological variables (neuroendocrine, cardiovascular, and autonomic) described in the preceding article.

We chose to study DMT in this initial attempt to begin a careful characterization of hallucinogen effects in humans. It has a short duration of action, established clinical safety, and lack of widespread abuse. It also meets electrophysiologic,[45] pharmacologic,[46] and human[47] and animal[48] behavioral criteria for hallucinogenicity. However, there are few data directly comparing human responses to DMT with other hallucinogens, particularly in the same individual(s). Rosenberg et al[41] described "similar subjective and autonomic effects" of DMT and LSD in six prisoner-subjects. The self-experiments of Szara[49] using mescaline, DMT, and LSD revealed the primary differences to be in onset and duration, but not in the quality, of the subjective experiences. However, the situation is not straightforward, as subjects tolerant to LSD showed limited cross-tolerance to DMT.[41]

Of note was the rapid onset and peak effects of IV DMT and its extremely short duration of action. This was in contrast to LSD administered by a 60- to 90-second "slow" infusion, where initial peak effects were not seen until 20 to 30 minutes after injection,[50] when a sudden shift in visual apperception and autonomic response took place.[15] Freedman[15] also described the onset of LSD effects as even quicker (within 2 to 3 minutes) when given by "rapid IV push," and effects were nearly instantaneous after Hoch[51] gave it intraspinally. The "lag" and sudden onset of LSD effects have been evident in rat behavioral studies[52] in which onset can be inferred to correlate with peak brain levels of drug.[53] Thus, the time necessary to reach peak brain LSD levels, that are then promptly followed by a slower clearance of drug, may explain the lag between administration and onset of LSD's "march of effects." In humans after a rapid IV "push," a "rehearsal" of subsequent effects took place during the first 2 to 3 minutes, perhaps related to "equilibration" of LSD with relevant receptors,[15] followed by the march of effects over the subsequent hours as LSD leaves the brain.

The active transport of DMT into rat cortex[54,55] may explain its nearly instantaneous sudden onset. Its rapid metabolism by monoamine oxidase in rat brain[56] is consistent with the brief duration of subsequent effects noted in our and previous studies.

High levels of hallucinogen binding at, and localization of, 5-HT receptor sites exist in human central tissue in areas known to subserve emotional, perceptual, and somatosensory functions.[57] Human in vitro autoradiographic studies on autopsied brain using LSD, with almost equal affinity for the 5-HT_2 and 5-HT_{1A} subtypes,[46] showed high density binding to raphe,[58] presumably a 5-HT_{1A} effect. The 5-HT_2 receptors were found in human cortical areas, mammillary bodies, claustrum, amygdala, caudate, putamen, nucleus accumbens, and hippocampus with in vitro autoradiography,[59-61] while positron-emission tomographic studies with ^{18}F-setoperone suggested 5-HT_2 receptors in cortex and striatum.[62] The 5-HT_{1C} receptors have been found in human choroid plexus, cortex, striatum, hypothalamus, and hippocampus.[60,63,64]

The nonhallucinogenic, but clearly psychoactive, properties of the lower doses of DMT may reflect the relative contributions of several 5-HT receptor subtypes. For example, different levels of 5-HT_{1A} compared with 5-HT_2 agonism on the same cortical cell's electrical activity may selectively enhance responses to stimuli of varying strength.[65]

Although 5-HT mechanisms are currently deemed primary in mediating hallucinogens' effects, older human data were limited by lack of specificity of modifying agents used and lack of careful characterization of "psychological effects" being modulated. Examples include pretreatment protocols using 5-hydroxytryptophan,[66] cyproheptadine,[67] reserpine,[68] monoamine oxidase inhibitors,[69] and 2-bromo-LSD (BOL)[70] (a nonhallucinogenic LSD analogue with poorly characterized subjective effects).

More selective and better characterized serotonergic agonists, with binding profiles overlapping those of the classic hallucinogens, have been administered to humans, but they have not produced classic "hallucinogenic" or "psychedelic" symptoms. For example, *m*-chlorophenylpiperazine (*m*-CPP), with high affinity for the 5-HT_2 and 5-HT_{1C} subtypes,[71] caused anxiety, nausea, activation, "functional deficit," "altered self-reality," depression, and fear in normal subjects.[72,73] Exacerbation of schizophrenic patients' psychotic symptoms by *m*-CPP[74] has not been seen consistently.[75] 6-Chloro-2-(l-piperazinyl) pyrazine (MK-212), another substituted phenlypiperazine with greatest affinity for the 5-HT_3 subtype,[76] but significant affinity for the 5-HT_{1A}, 5-HT_{1C}, and 5-HT_2 subtypes,[77] caused anxiety and dysphoria in normal subjects,[78] but "LSD-like" effects only in alcoholics.[79] This group of observations will require more work before the clinical response picture is understood clearly.

EMPIRICAL TESTING of several hypotheses generated by animal or previous human studies can be performed in humans, using our "normative" dose-response data for DMT, and preliminary results with the HRS. Other psychoactive drugs might be amenable to characterization with the HRS, particularly those with stimulant, dissociative, or less classical hallucinogenic effects; eg, ketamine and PCP, marijuana, sigma opiate agonists, amphetamines and cocaine, methoxylated amphetamines, and anticholinergic deliriants. In addition, "nonhallucinogenic" serotonergic probes' properties could be characterized using this scale.

The phenethylamine hallucinogens, DOM, 2,5-dimethoxy-4-iodo-phenylisopropylamine (DOI), and 2,5-dimethyoxy-4-bromo-phenylisopropylamine (DOB), are often placed together with the tryptamine and lysergamide classic compounds. Psilocybine, DMT, mescaline, and LSD also are believed to be more or less phenomenologically indistinguishable, based on the small number of human studies or extant animal literature. Carefully characterizing effects using well-prepared and experienced hallucinogen users may help determine degree of similarity and areas of differences. Selective blockade of relevant receptors, and noting effects on functions quantified by the HRS, might help tease apart the relative contributions of these receptors in mediating hallucinogens' effects. Patients with psychiatric conditions with presumed abnormalities of serotonergic function could be administered DMT, and differences in sensitivity to its psychological effects could be assessed. These data could help relate hypothetical neurotransmission disorders with subjective symptoms in psychiatric conditions.

Finally, in our study, there was no modulating effect of the extent of prior MDMA exposure on HRS responses to DMT and placebo, and there were minimal modulatory effects on our measured biological variables.[14] 3,4-methylenedioxymethamphetamine is a mammalian serotonergic neurotoxin.[16] Since the 5-HT_2 receptors implicated for hallucinogen effects are postsynaptic,[59] a "functional denervation hypersensitivity"[80] might have been exposed with DMT in MDMA users. Appel and associates[81-83] have shown that the threshold dose for behavioral effects of LSD in rat can be lowered fourfold by pretreatments that reduce presynaptic 5-HT levels; ie, reserpine, *p*-chlorophenylalanine, or raphe lesions. Our data, however, do not suggest functional consequences of prior *moderate* MDMA use. Additional studies using control subjects with no history of drug abuse are necessary for a more rigorous assessment of MDMA effects on human serotonergic function.

Accepted for publication January 25, 1993.

This investigation was supported by grant RO3-DA06524 from the National Institute on Drug Abuse, Rockville, Md; the Scottish Rite Foundation for Schizophrenia Research, NMJ, Lexington, Mass; grant RR00997-13 from the National Institutes of Health General Clinical Research Center, Rockville; the Scott Rogers Fund of the University of New Mexico, Albuquerque; and University of New Mexico Department of Psychiatry research funds.

We thank Cynthia Geist, RN, and the nursing staff of the General Clinical Research Center, 5E, University of New Mexico Hospital, for nursing support; and Paul Salkovskis, PhD, assisted with helpful discussions regarding questionnaire development.

Reprint requests to Department of Psychiatry, University of New Mexico, 2400 Tucker Ave NE, Albuquerque, NM 87131-5326 (Dr Strassman).

REFERENCES

1. Hoffer A, Osmond H. *The Hallucinogens.* Orlando, Fla: Academic Press Inc; 1967.
2. Freedman DX. Effects of LSD-25 on brain serotonin. *J Pharmacol Exp Ther.* 1961;134:160-166.
3. Ahn H, Makman M. Interaction of LSD and other hallucinogens with dopamine-sensitive adenylate cyclase in primate brain: regional differences. *Brain Res.* 1979;162:77-88.
4. Horita A, Hamilton A. Lysergic acid diethylamide: dissociation of its behavioral and hyperthermic effects by DL-alpha-methyl-*p*-tyrosine. *Science.* 1969;164:78-79.
5. Glennon RA, Titeler M, McKenney J. Evidence for 5-HT_2 involvement in the mechanism of action of hallucinogenic agents. *Life Sci.* 1985;35:2505-2511.
6. Buckholtz NS, Zhou D, Freedman DX, Potter WZ. Lysergic acid diethylamide (LSD) administration selectively downregulates $serotonin_2$ receptors in rat brain. *Neuropsychopharmacology.* 1990;3:137-148.
7. Spencer D Jr, Glaser T, Traber J. Serotonin receptor subtype mediation of the interoceptive discriminative stimuli induced by 5-methoxy-N,N-dimethyltryptamine. *Psychopharmacology.* 1987;93:158-166.
8. Yagaloff K, Hartig P. ^{125}I-lysergic acid diethylamide binds to a novel serotonergic site on rat choroid plexus epithelial cells. *J Neurosci.* 1985;5:3178-3183.
9. Fish M, Johnson N, Horning E. Piptadenia alkaloids: indole bases of *P peregrina* (L.) Benth. and related species. *J Am Chem Soc.* 1955;77:5892-5895.
10. Christian ST, Harrison R, Quayle E, Pagel J, Monti J. The in vitro identification of dimethyltryptamine (DMT) in mammalian brain and its characterization as a possible endogenous neuroregulatory agent. *Biochem Med.* 1977;18:164-183.
11. Smythies J, Morin R, Brown G. Identification of dimethyltryptamine and O-methylbufotenin in human cerebrospinal fluid by combined gas chromatography/mass spectrometry. *Biol Psychiatry.* 1979;14:549-556.
12. Deliganis A, Pierce P, Peroutka S. Differential interactions of dimethyltryptamine (DMT) with 5-HT_{1A} and 5-HT_2 receptors. *Biochem Pharmacol.* 1991;41:1739-1744.
13. Jenner P, Marsden C, Thanki C. Behavioral changes induced by N,N-dimethyltryptamine in rodents. *Br J Pharmacol.* 1980;69:69-80.
14. Strassman RJ, Qualls CR. Dose response study of N,N-dimethyltryptamine in humans, I: neuroendocrine, autonomic and cardiovascular effects. *Arch Gen Psychiatry.* 1994;51:85-97.
15. Freedman DX. LSD: The bridge from animal to human. In: Jacobs B, ed. *Hallucinogens: Neurochemical, Behavioral and Clinical Perspectives.* New York, NY: Raven Press; 1984:203-226.
16. Commins DL, Vosmer G, Virus RM, Woolverton WL, Schuster CR, Seiden LS. Biochemical and histological evidence that methylenedioxymethamphetamine (MDMA) is toxic to neurons of the rat brain. *J Pharmacol Exp Ther.* 1987;241:338-345.
17. Price LH, Ricaurte G, Krystal JK, Heninger GR. Neuroendocrine and mood responses to intravenous L-tryptophan in 3,4-methylenedioxymethamphetamine (MDMA) users. *Arch Gen Psychiatry.* 1989;46:20-22.
18. Stafford P. *Psychedelics Encyclopedia: Third Revised Edition.* Berkeley, Calif: Ronin Press; 1992:308-331.
19. Cole JO, Katz MM. The psychotomimetic drugs. *JAMA.* 1964;187:758-761.
20. Sjoberg BM Jr, Hollister LE. The effects of psychotomimetic drugs on primary suggestibility. *Psychopharmacology.* 1965;8:251-262.
21. Mogar RE. Current status and future trends in psychedelic research. *J Humanistic Psychol.* 1965;4:147-166.
22. Strassman RJ. Adverse reactions to psychedelic drugs: a review of the literature. *J Nerv Ment Dis.* 1984;172:577-595.
23. Rinkel M, Atwell CR, DiMascio A, Brown J. Experimental psychiatry, V: psilocybine, a new psychotogenic drug. *N Engl J Med.* 1960;262:295-297.
24. Stockings GT. A clinical study of the mescaline psychosis, with special reference to the mechanism of the genesis of schizophrenic and other psychotic states. *J Ment Sci.* 1940;86:29-47.
25. Savage C. Variations in ego feeling induced by d-lysergic acid diethylamide (LSD-25). *Psychoanal Rev.* 1955;42:1-16.
26. Klee G. Lysergic acid diethylamide (LSD-25) and ego functions. *Arch Gen Psychiatry.* 1963;8:461-474.
27. Greiner T, Burch NR, Edelberg R. Psychopathology and psychophysiology of minimal LSD-25 dosage. *Arch Neurol Psychiatry.* 1958;79:208-210.
28. Belleville R. MMPI score changes induced by lysergic acid diethylamide. *J Clin Psychol.* 1956;12:279-282.
29. Bercel NA, Travis LE, Olinger LB, Dreikurs E. Model psychoses induced by LSD-25 in normals. *Arch Neurol Psychiatry.* 1956;75:612-618.
30. Silverstein AB, Klee GD. Effects of lysergic acid diethylamide (LSD-25) on intellectual functions. *Arch Neurol Psychiatry.* 1958;80:477-480.
31. Hollister LE, Sjoberg BM. Clinical syndromes and biochemical alterations following mescaline, lysergic acid diethylamide, psilocybin and a combination of the three psychotomimetic drugs. *Compr Psychiatry.* 1964;5:170-178.
32. Linton HB, Langs RJ. Subjective reactions to lysergic acid diethylamide (LSD-25) measured by a questionnaire. *Arch Gen Psychiatry.* 1962;6:352-368.
33. Barr HL, Langs RJ, Holt RR, Goldberger L, Klein GS. *LSD: Personality and Experience.* New York, NY: Wiley-Interscience; 1972.
34. Faillace LA, Vourlekis A, Szara S. Clinical evaluation of some hallucinogenic tryptamine derivatives. *J Nerv Ment Dis.* 1967;145:306-313.
35. Abramson HA, Jarvik ME, Kaufman MR, Kornetsky C, Levine A, Wagner M. Lysergic acid diethylamide (LSD-25), I: physiological and perceptual responses. *J Psychol.* 1955;39:3-60.
36. Slater PE, Morimoto K, Hyde RW. The effect of group administration upon

symptom formation under LSD. *J Nerv Ment Dis.* 1957;125:312-315.
37. Isbell H, Belleville RE, Fraser HF, Wikler A, Logan CR. Studies on lysergic acid diethylamide, I: effects in former morphine addicts and development of tolerance during chronic intoxication. *Arch Neurol Psychiatry.* 1956;76:468-478.
38. Haertzen CA, Hickey JE. Addiction Research Center Inventory (ARCI): measurement of euphoria and other drug effects. In: Bozarth MA, ed. *Methods of Assessing the Reinforcing Properties of Abused Drugs.* New York, NY: Springer-Verlag NY Inc; 1987:489-524.
39. Haertzen CA, Hill HE, Belleville RE. Development of the Addiction Research Center Inventory (ARCI): selection of items that are sensitive to the effects of various drugs. *Psychopharmacologia.* 1963;4:155-166.
40. Hill HE, Haertzen CA, Wolbach AB Jr, Miner EJ. The Addiction Research Center Inventory: standardization of scales which evaluate subjective effects of morphine, amphetamine, pentobarbital, alcohol, LSD-25, pyrahexyl and chlorpromazine. *Psychopharmacologia.* 1963;4:167-183.
41. Rosenberg DE, Isbell H, Miner EJ, Logan CR. The effect of N,N-dimethyltryptamine in human subjects tolerant to lysergic acid diethylamide. *Psychopharmacology.* 1964;5:217-227.
42. Angrist B, Rosen J, Gershon S. Assessment of tolerance to the hallucinogenic effects of DOM. *Psychopharmacology.* 1974;36:203-207.
43. Sai-Halasz A, Brunecker G, Szara S. Dimethyltryptamine: ein neues Psychoticum. *Psychiatr Neurol.* 1958;135:285-301.
44. Kaplan J, Mandel L, Stillman R, Walker R, VandenHeuvel W, Gillin J, Wyatt R. Blood and urine levels of N,N-dimethyltryptamine following administration of psychoactive doses to human subjects. *Psychopharmacologia.* 1974;38:239-245.
45. Aghajanian G, Foote W, Sheard M. Action of psychotogenic drugs on single midbrain raphe neurons. *J Pharmacol Exp Ther.* 1970;171:178-187.
46. Pierce P, Peroutka S. Hallucinogenic drug interactions with neurotransmitter receptor binding sites in human cortex. *Psychopharmacology.* 1989;97:118-122.
47. Szara S. DMT (N,N-dimethyltryptamine) and homologues: clinical and pharmacological considerations. In Efron DH, ed. *Psychotomimetic Drugs.* New York, NY: Raven Press; 1970:275-286.
48. Geyer M, Light R, Rose G, Petersen L, Horwitt D, Adams L, Hawkins R. A characteristic effect of hallucinogens on investigatory responding in rats. *Psychopharmacology.* 1979;65:35-40.
49. Szara S. The comparison of the psychotic effect of tryptamine derivatives with the effects of mescaline and LSD-25 in self-experiments. In: Garattini S, Ghetti V, eds. *Psychotropic Drugs.* New York, NY: Elsevier Science Publishing Co Inc; 1957:460-466.
50. Aghajanian GK, Bing OHL. Persistence of lysergic acid diethylamide in the plasma of human subjects. *Clin Pharmacol Ther.* 1964;5:611-614.
51. Hoch P. Studies in routes of administration and counteracting drugs. In: Cholden L, ed. *Lysergic Acid Diethylamide and Mescaline in Experimental Psychiatry.* New York, NY: Grune & Stratton; 1956:8-12.
52. Freedman DX, Appel JB, Hartman FR, Molliver ME. Tolerance to behavioral effects of LSD-25 in rat. *J Pharmacol Exp Ther.* 1964;143:309-313.
53. Rosecrans JA, Lovell RA, Freedman DX. Effects of lysergic acid diethylamide on the metabolism of brain 5-hydroxytryptamine. *Biochem Pharmacol.* 1967;16:2011-2021.
54. Yanai K, Ido T, Ishiwata K, Hatazawa J, Takahashi T, Iwata R, Matsuzawa T. In vivo kinetics and displacement study of a carbon-11-labeled hallucinogen, N,N-[^{11}C]dimethyltryptamine. *Eur J Nucl Med.* 1986;12:141-146.
55. Sangiah S. Gomez MV, Domino EF. Accumulation of N,N-dimethyltryptamine in rat brain cortical slices. *Biol Psychiatry.* 1979;14:925-936.
56. Sitaram BR, Lockett L, Talomsin R, Blackman GL, McLeod WR. In vivo metabolism of 5-methoxy-N,N-dimethyltryptamine and N,N-dimethyltryptamine in the rat. *Biochem Pharmacol.* 1987;36:2235-2237.
57. Azmitia EC. The CNS serotonergic system: progression toward a collaborative organization. In: Meltzer HY, ed. *Psychopharmacology: The Third Generation of Progress.* New York, NY: Raven Press; 1987:61-74.
58. Palacios JM, Probst A, Cortes R. The distribution of serotonin receptors in the human brain: high density of [^{3}H]LSD binding sites in the raphe nuclei of the brainstem. *Brain Res.* 1983;274:150-155.
59. Schotte A, Maloteaux JM, Laduron PM. Characterization and regional distribution of serotonin S_2-receptors in human brain. *Brain Res.* 1983;276:231-235.
60. Hoyer D, Pazos A, Probst A, Palacios JM. Serotonin receptors in the human brain, II: characterization and autoradiographic localization of 5-HT_{1C} and 5-HT_2 recognition sites. *Brain Res.* 1987;376:97-107.
61. Pazos A, Probst A, Palacios JM. Serotonin receptors in the human brain, IV: autoradiographic mapping of serotonin-2 receptors. *Neuroscience.* 1987;21:123-139.
62. Blin J, Sette G, Fiorelli M, Bletry O, Elghozi J, Crouzel C, Braon J. A method for the in vivo investigation of the serotonergic 5-HT_2 receptors in human cerebral cortex using positron emission tomography and ^{18}F-labeled setoperone. *J Neurochem.* 1990;54:1744-1754.
63. Pazos A, Probst A, Palacios JM. Serotonin receptors in the human brain, III: autoradiographic mapping of serotonin-1 receptors. *Neuroscience.* 1987;21:97-122.
64. Waeber C, Dietl MM, Hoyer D, Palacios JM. 5-HT_1 receptors in the vertebrate brain: regional distribution examined by autoradiography. *Naunyn-Schmiedeberg's Arch Pharmacol.* 1989;340:486-494.
65. Araneda R, Andrade R. 5-Hydroxytryptamine$_2$ and 5-hydroxytryptamine$_{1A}$ receptors mediate opposing responses on membrane excitability in rat association cortex. *Neuroscience.* 1991;40:399-412.
66. Brengelmann JC, Pare CMB, Sandler M. Alleviation of the psychological effects of LSD in man by 5-hydroxytryptophan. *J Ment Sci.* 1958;104:1237-1244.
67. Meltzer H, Wiita B, Tricou B, Simonovic M, Fang V. Effects of serotonin precursors and serotonin agonists on plasma hormone levels. In: Ho B, Schoolar J, Usdin E, eds. *Serotonin in Biological Psychiatry.* New York, NY: Raven Press; 1980:117-139.
68. Isbell H, Logan CR. Studies on the diethylamide of lysergic acid (LSD-25), II: effects of chlorpromazine, azacyclonol, and reserpine on the intensity of the LSD-reaction. *Arch Neurol Psychiatry.* 1957;77:350-358.
69. Resnick O, Krus DM, Raskin M. LSD-25 action in normal subjects treated with a monoamine oxidase inhibitor. *Life Sci.* 1964;3:1207-1214.
70. Ginzel KH, Mayer-Gross W. Prevention of the psychological effects of *d*-lysergic acid diethylamide (LSD-25) by its 2-brom derivative, BOL-148. *Nature.* 1956;178:210.
71. Hoyer D. Functional correlates of serotonin 5-HT_1 recognition sites. *J Recept Res.* 1988;8:59-81.
72. Seibyl JP, Krystal JK, Price LH, Woods SW, D'Amico C, Heninger GR, Charney DS. Effects of ritanserin on the behavioral, neuroendocrine, and cardiovascular responses to meta-chlorophenylpiperazine in healthy human subjects. *Psychiatry Res.* 1991;38:227-236.
73. Murphy DL, Mueller EA, Hill JL, Tolliver TJ, Jacobsen FM. Comparative anxiogenic, neuroendocrine, and other physiologic effects of *m*-chlorophenylpiperazine given intravenously or orally to healthy volunteers. *Psychopharmacology.* 1989;98:275-282.
74. Iqbal N, Asnis G, Wetzler S, Kahn RS, Kay SR, van Praag MH. The MCPP challenge test in schizophrenia: hormonal and behavioral responses. *Biol Psychiatry.* 1991;30:770-778.
75. Szymanski S, Mayerhoff D, Lieberman J, Alvir J, Safferman A. The behavioral effect of intravenous *m*CPP in schizophrenia. *Soc Biol Psychiatry Abstr.* 1992;31:78A. Abstract.
76. Glennon RA, Ismaiel A, McCarthy GB, Peroutka SJ. Binding of arylpiperazines to 5-HT_3 serotonin receptors: results of a structure-affinity study. *Eur J Pharmacol.* 1989;168:387-392.
77. Murphy DL, Lesch KP, Aulakh CS, Pigott TA. Serotonin-selective arylpiperazines with neuroendocrine, behavioral, temperature, and cardiovascular effects in humans. *Pharmacol Rev.* 1991;43:527-552.
78. Lowy MT, Meltzer HY. Stimulation of serum cortisol and prolactin secretion in humans by MK-212, a centrally active serotonin agonist. *Biol Psychiatry.* 1988;23:818-828.
79. Lee MA, Meltzer HY. Neuroendocrine responses to serotonergic agents in alcoholics. *Biol Psychiatry.* 1991;30:1017-1030.
80. Heal DJ, Philplot J, Molyneux SG, Metz A. Intracerebral administration of 5,7-dihydroxytryptamine to mice increases both head-twitch response and the number of cortical 5-HT_2 receptors. *Neuropharmacology.* 1985;24:1201-1205.
81. Appel JB, Freedman DX. Chemically-induced alterations in the behavioral effects of LSD-25. *Biochem Pharmacol.* 1964;13:861-869.
82. Appel JB, Lovell RA, Freedman DX. Alterations in the behavioral effects of LSD by pretreatment with *p*-chlorophenylalanine and α-methyl-*p*-tyrosine. *Psychopharmacology.* 1970;18:387-406.
83. Appel JB, Sheard MH, Freedman DX. Alterations in the behavioral effects of LSD by midbrain raphe lesions. *Commun Behav Biol Part A.* 1970;5:237-241.

ORIGINAL ARTICLE

Maintenance Imipramine Therapy for Secondary Depression in Schizophrenia

A Controlled Trial

Samuel G. Siris, MD; Paul C. Bermanzohn, MD; Susan E. Mason, PhD; Mitchell A. Shuwall, PhD

Background: Although recent studies have documented the benefit of adjunctive antidepressant medication for the short-term treatment of certain patients with operationally defined syndromes of postpsychotic depression, the value of maintenance adjunctive antidepressant treatment in this circumstance has not been properly established.

Methods: This study examined 24 schizophrenic or schizoaffective patients with postpsychotic depression or negative symptoms. These patients had all been benefited over the short term by the addition of adjunctive imipramine hydrochloride to their ongoing fluphenazine decanoate/benztropine mesylate regimens, and this adjunctive treatment had been successfully continued for 6 months. In a randomized double-blind protocol, treatment with adjunctive imipramine hydrochloride (mean, 233±72 mg/d) was then either maintained or tapered to placebo for an ensuing 1-year trial, while treatment with fluphenazine and benztropine continued.

Results: Significantly more patients who received placebo substitution relapsed into depression ($P<.001$). Patients who received placebo substitution were also more likely to experience relapses into psychosis ($P<.02$).

Conclusions: These results support the clinical value of maintenance adjunctive imipramine therapy among initially responsive patients with postpsychotic depressions.

(Arch Gen Psychiatry. 1994;51:109-115)

RECENT STUDIES have documented the potential benefit of adding an adjunctive antidepressant medication to the neuroleptic regimen of schizophrenic patients with operationally defined syndromes of secondary depression.[1-3] This seems to be the case particularly for outpatients with symptomatically stable conditions in whom an attempt has been made to rule out the neuroleptic-induced akinesia syndrome, which can present a close clinical phenocopy of depression.[4-7] An anecdotal report suggested that continuation and maintenance treatment with an adjunctive antidepressant may then be valuable for schizophrenic patients who have had an initial favorable response.[8] This impression was also supported by preliminary examination of a subset (N=14) of our own double-blind study data.[9,10] We now present our final and detailed report of that study. To our knowledge, such a definitive test of the utility of maintenance antidepressant treatment among schizophrenic patients with secondary depressions who have responded to short-term trials of adjunctive antidepressant medication has not been published previously.

From the Hillside Hospital Division of the Long Island Jewish Medical Center, Long Island Campus for the Albert Einstein College of Medicine, Glen Oaks, NY.

RESULTS

Twenty-four outpatients personally known by the principal investigator (S.G.S.), with clinically stable conditions, met criteria and entered this study. All were compliant with medications, as documented by pill counts, and were cooperative and familiar with rating procedures. Thirteen patients were randomized to the group continuing to receive maintenance adjunctive imipramine and 11 were randomized to the group whose imipramine was tapered to adjunc-

See Patients and Methods on next page

PATIENTS AND METHODS

Patients who satisfied the following four criteria were included in this study. (1) They met Research Diagnostic Criteria (RDC)[11] for schizophrenia or schizoaffective disorder for their most recent episode of psychotic exacerbation. (2) They had the history, subsequent to that episode, of remission to either a nonpsychotic or residually psychotic state (RDC definition), and of meeting operationalized criteria for either the syndrome of postpsychotic depression (PPD)[1] or negative symptoms.[12] (Stable PPD or negative symptom syndromes were required, meeting the respective criteria for three consecutive weekly ratings, and not remitting under treatment for at least 1 week with adjunctive benztropine mesylate, 2 mg orally three times a day.) (3) That syndrome of PPD or negative symptoms had then responded favorably (physicians's global impression) to a carefully observed treatment trial of adjunctive imipramine hydrochloride added to their clinically best adjusted weekly dose of fluphenazine decanoate and benztropine mesylate, 2 mg orally three times a day, and it had been the treating physician's impression that these patients should be continued on a regimen of adjunctive imipramine on a clinical basis. (4) These patients had then continued to do well clinically during at least 6 months of continuation treatment with the combined regimen of fluphenazine, benztropine, and imipramine, with allowances being made during that interval for "doctor's choice" dosage adjustments leading up to the starting doses for the subsequent double-blind maintenance trial which is the subject of this report. Thus, all patients, clinically, were judged to be candidates for prolonged maintenance treatment with adjunctive imipramine. This study was designed to determine, under these conditions, if such extended treatment would be beneficial and safe.

After having given informed consent, the above patients were randomized under double-blind conditions to one of two treatment groups. One group continued to receive maintenance imipramine with no change of dose. The other group received a tapered dose at a rate of 50 mg/d of imipramine hydrochloride each week to a regimen of matching adjunctive placebo. Both groups were maintained on their regimens of fluphenazine and benztropine as before, and seen by a research psychiatrist at weekly or biweekly intervals as clinically determined. Clinical ratings were done at 4-week intervals with the Clinical Global Impression (CGI)[13] and the Schedule for Affective Disorders and Schizophrenia (SADS)[14] instruments. Side effects were monitored with the Dosage Record and Treatment Emergent Symptoms Scale (DOTES) instrument.[13] These stated treatment strategies were continued for 1 year or until either a depressive or psychotic relapse occurred. A depressive relapse was defined as having a CGI rating of worsening (ie, a rating of 5 or more) and satisfying criteria for PPD.[1] A psychotic relapse was defined as having a CGI rating of worsening, and having a worsening of ratings to "moderate" or more on the SADS hallucinations or delusions item, or any of the SADS thought disorder items.

tive placebo. These patients' clinical and demographic characteristics are shown in **Table 1**. By chance, those patients randomized to the group receiving adjunctive imipramine maintenance were older and were being treated with lower doses of fluphenazine and benztropine. Otherwise, no statistically significant differences were noted between the randomization groups for the Table 1 variables. Also, no significant differences were noted between the randomization groups for the variables shown in **Table 2** (see below) or the responsiveness of the Table 2 variables (analysis of covariance analysis) during the patients' initial short-term 9-week trials of adjunctive imipramine. Specifically, patients subsequently randomized to maintenance adjunctive imipramine or maintenance adjunctive placebo groups, and who completed the reported trial (N=19), had had SADS-Extracted Hamilton Depression Rating Scale scores[16] of 19.4±6.7 vs 19.1±5.6 (mean±SD), respectively, at the start of their short-term treatment trials with adjunctive imipramine, and 12.3±5.3 vs 12.8±7.2, respectively, at the end of these short-term trials. By comparison, these same two groups had SADS-Extracted Hamilton Depression Rating Scale scores of 9.7±3.0 vs 12.6±8.0 at the baseline for their double-blind maintenance trials of adjunctive imipramine or placebo, and 13.1±9.4 vs 23.9±8.0 at the end of this trial. The ANCOVA analysis for this latter comparison is presented in Table 2, which shows the appropriately adjusted means.

The overall results of the double-blind maintenance study are depicted in the **Figure**. Nineteen patients completed their maintenance adjunctive treatment trials with either a relapse or a full year in an unrelapsed state. Two patients, initially assigned to receive adjunctive placebo, were removed in nonrelapsed states, after 8 weeks and 42 weeks, respectively, when they began to receive active imipramine at those points due to pharmacy errors. One patient, assigned to receive active imipramine, was removed after 40 weeks when she began flagrant abuse of cocaine. Another patient, assigned to receive adjunctive active imipramine, was removed in a nonrelapsed state after 2 weeks when he failed to follow instructions properly concerning his taper to a regimen of double-blind medication. The final patient, assigned to receive placebo, was removed from the study in a nonrelapsed state after 4 weeks when she became pregnant.

Table 1. Twenty-Four Patients, Initially Responsive to Adjunctive Imipramine, Entering a Double-blind Maintenance Trial of Adjunctive Imipramine vs Placebo Therapy*

	Imipramine Group (n=13)	Placebo Group (n=11)	t = (χ^2=)	P
Age, y	42.3±12.8	32.3±8.4	2.23	.037
Gender, M/F	6/7	6/5	(.17)	.682
No. of previous hospitalizations	3.5±2.4	4.1±2.6	−0.56	.578
Age first hospitalized, y	29.0±11.5	23.7±7.1	1.31	.206
Fluphenazine decanoate dose, mg/wk	8.5±6.4	18.5±13.5	−2.27	.040
Betztropine mesylate dose, mg/d	4.2±2.2	6.0±0.0	−2.74	.012
Impramine hydrochloride dose, mg/d	242±76	222±68	0.66	.517
SADS-Extracted Hamilton Depression Scale Score[15,16]	10.2±3.0	13.0±8.3	−1.05	.314
SADS-Psychosis Measure†	6.00±2.31	6.64±1.91	−0.73	.475
SADS-Anxiety Measure‡	4.69±1.44	5.91±2.12	−1.67	.109
No. with postpsychotic depression/negative symptoms at time of initial short-term treatment trial with adjunctive imipramine	11/2	10/1	(0.00)§	1.00

*Means are expressed ±SDs. SADS indicates Schedule for Affective Disorders and Schizophrenia.
†Sum of Severity of Hallucinations, Severity of Delusions, and the average of the three Thought Disorder Items (Impaired Understandability, Illogical Thinking, and Loosening of Associations).
‡Sum of SADS items for Somatic Anxiety, Psychic Anxiety, and Phobia.
§Fisher's Exact Test.

Table 2. ANCOVA, Covarying for the Baseline of the Maintenance Trial, of End-Point Ratings for Patients Completing the Double-blind Maintenance Study of Adjunctive Imipramine vs Placebo Therapy*

	Imipramine Group (N=11)	Placebo Group (N=8)	F	P (df=1,17)
CGI Severity Score	3.86±.21	4.70±.25	7.79	.013
SADS-Extracted Hamilton Depression Rating Scale Score[16]	13.7±2.8	23.1±3.4	5.03	.039
SADS Depressive Mood and Ideation Scale Score	11.9±1.1	17.8±1.4	16.15	.001
SADS Endogenous Features Scale Score	21.6±2.0	29.9±2.5	8.48	.010
SADS Depressive-Associated Features Scale Score	27.5±2.3	37.9±2.4	11.03	.004
SADS-Extracted Negative Symptom Score[18]†	11.1±1.6	16.7±1.9	5.64	.030
SADS Severity of Hallucinations	2.00±.38	2.62±.44	1.18	.306
SADS Severity of Delusions	1.97±.34	1.93±.40	.006	.940
SADS Thought Disorder Items‡	3.00±.00	3.12±.35	1.41	.252
SADS Psycho sis Items (sum of above 3 items)	6.82±.59	7.66±.70	0.59	.456
SADS-Derived Anxiety Scale§	5.68±.69	8.44±.85	7.62	.014
DOTES Side Effects Measure‖	5.60±.38	6.16±.44	0.94	.348

*ANCOVA indicates analysis of covariance; CGI, Clinical Global Impression; SADS, Schedule for Affective Disorders and Schizophrenia; and DOTES, Dosage Record and Treatment Emergent Symptoms Scale.
†Sum of ratings for blunted affect, lack of energy, loss of interest, social withdrawal, and diminished concentration.
‡Average of Impaired Understandability, Illogical Thinking, and Loosening of Associations (no variance at baseline, analysis of variance therefore done instead of ANCOVA).
§Sum of SADS items for Somatic Anxiety, Psychic Anxiety, and Phobia.
‖Sum of ratings for dry mouth, blurry vision, constipation, and urinary retention.

A survival analysis of the data for all 24 patients presented in the Figure favored the imipramine-maintained group (Lee-Desu statistic=11.94; *df*=1; *P*=.0005).[17] Further data analysis was carried out, focusing on the 19 study completers. Eleven of these patients had been randomized to receive adjunctive imipramine and eight had been randomized to receive adjunctive placebo. Two of the 11 randomized to receive adjunctive imipramine (18%; 95% confidence interval, 5% to 48%) relapsed into a depression (satisfying RDC criteria). All of the eight randomized to receive adjunctive placebo (100%; 95% confidence interval, 69% to 100%) relapsed into a depression. This difference is highly statistically significant (Fisher's Exact Test, *P*=.0007), with a clinically significant effect size of .82. Furthermore, no imipramine-maintained patients manifested psychotic episodes during the course of the trial, whereas four of the eight patients who received placebo substitution had development of psychotic symptoms meeting RDC criteria for new episodes of psychosis. In all cases, these psychotic relapses occurred at the time of the depressive relapses. This difference in the frequency of psychotic relapses between the two study groups was also statistically significant (Fisher's Exact Test, *P*=.018). The end-point CGI global change measure favored the imipramine-treated group by 1.89 points, which is clinically significant (3.73±1.49 vs 5.62±1.19; *t*=3.09; *P*=.007).

The ANCOVA end-point ratings, covarying for baseline of the double-blind maintenance trial, for the 19 patients who completed the trial or relapsed are shown in Table 2. As shown, those patients maintained on regimens of adjunctive imipramine were found to be less depressed at their study end points. No statistically apparent difference was noted, however, in the psychosis end-point analysis between the two groups, perhaps, in part, because of the small number of relapsers. The ANCOVA

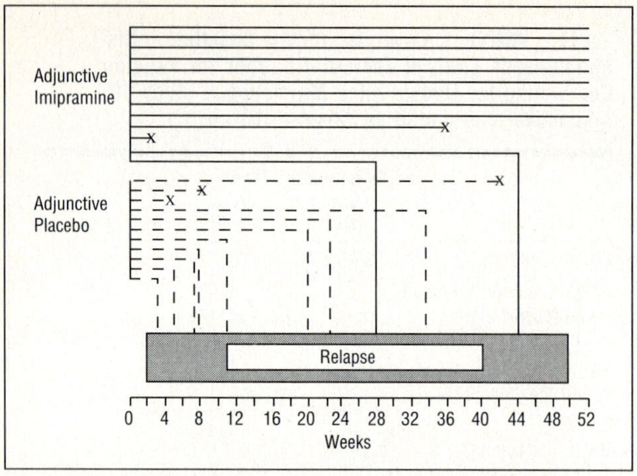

Results of double-blind maintenance trial of adjunctive imipramine hydrochloride vs placebo therapy. X indicates administrative withdrawal.

analysis did find, with statistical significance, that the group that had received placebo substitution exhibited greater symptoms of anxiety at their end points. No differences were found in side effect measures between the two treatment groups.

Since three patients among the initial 24 met criteria for negative symptoms only, and not the specified criteria for PPD, the above-stated analyses were repeated, excluding those three patients. Two of these patients had been randomized to receive adjunctive imipramine and completed the trial without relapse. One had been randomized to receive adjunctive placebo and was among the administrative drops. In this more limited sample, the CGI improvement ratings again favored the imipramine-treated group (3.78 ± 1.64 vs 5.62 ± 1.89; $t=-2.68$, $df=15$; $P=.018$). When a post hoc analysis was then performed of those items in Table 2 for the smaller patient group, few changes were noted. Specifically, the only differences in levels of statistical significance involved the SADS-Extracted Hamilton Depression Scale score, the SADS-Extracted Negative Symptoms Scale score, and the SADS-Derived Anxiety Scale score. Each of these still favored adjunctive imipramine maintenance, but their statistical significances were reduced to trend level. All other depression scales remained statistically significant favoring imipramine maintenance, as did the global CGI severity of illness rating. Psychosis and side effect measures retained their nonsignificant status. The patients with negative symptoms were retained in the rest of the overall data analysis because the primary question in the study design involved the utility of maintenance imipramine therapy among schizophrenic or schizoaffective patients who had initially responded favorably to the short-term administration of this adjunctive medication.

COMMENT

This study demonstrates the benefit and safety of maintenance adjunctive imipramine treatment among neuroleptic-treated schizophrenic or schizoaffective outpatients with stable operationally defined syndromes of secondary depression or negative symptoms, who had been responsive to an initial adjunctive imipramine trial.[1,18,19] Specifically, the benefit applies to the prevention of the return of a syndrome phenotypically similar to depression. Indeed, the magnitude of the differential benefit for maintenance antidepressant treatment over maintenance placebo treatment in this patient cohort is even more dramatic than has been demonstrated to be the case for patients who have recovered from primary depressive disorders.[20-23]

The strength of this finding, however, must be considered in light of the initial care with which these patients were selected as being responders to the adjunctive imipramine therapy.[1] The criteria for ruling out the clinical confound of akinesia[4-7] and for documenting the consistency of the depression before the trial (ie, to rule out potential placebo responders), as well as for assessing the durability of the clinical response throughout the continuation phase before the maintenance trial, were stringent in this study.[24] While some previous studies have shown benefits from the addition of antidepressant medications to the neuroleptic regimen of stably depressed schizophrenic patients,[1-3,25-27] a number of other studies, utilizing alternative definitions and methodologies, have failed to find an advantage in using adjunctive antidepressants for secondary depressive syndromes in schizophrenia[2,28-33] and certainly not all patients with operationally diagnosed syndromes of PPD or negative symptoms by the presently employed criteria respond to adjunctive imipramine therapy.[1-3,18,19] Specifically with the syndrome definition of PPD employed in this study, we have found the response rate with adjunctive imipramine therapy (CGI rating of "2" indicates "much improved" or better) to be in the range of 42%.[1] Therefore, the inclusion of any placebo responders or otherwise spurious cases would have quickly dampened the results. Additionally, schizophrenic patients who were still floridly psychotic at the time of their depressive symptomatology,[34-36] those who were otherwise not in stable conditions,[37] those who were not receiving adequate neuroleptic treatment,[34] or those who were not receiving adequate antiparkinsonian medications[38] would have been poor candidates for the initial adjunctive antidepressant trial.

Nevertheless, a finding suggesting a potentially improved way for treating the secondary depressions that can occur in the course of schizophrenia or schizoaffective disorder is noteworthy. "Postpsychotic depression" is a condition that affects approximately one quarter of schizophrenic individuals at some time during the course of their disorder.[2,39-41] Although estimates have varied with the specific population studied and the specific criteria for the diagnosis of depression employed, this figure represents a modal finding that has withstood the test of time.[2,39-41] Furthermore, the occurrence of such depressive syndromes is important in the life course of these patients, not only because of the suffering and functional impairment it may engender, but also because approximately 10% of schizophrenic lives end in suicide,[42-44] and depressive symptomatology has been noted to be associated with suicidal ideation and acts in schizophrenia.[40,43-47]

The so-called negative symptoms of schizophrenia, which are even more common,[12,48-50] overlap phenomenologically with PPD in ways that can create diagnostic conundrums.[19,51] Although the issue is controversial,[3] some reports indicate they may, at least occasionally, also respond to the addition of adjunctive antidepressant medication[18,19,52,53] in ways that may have unknown implications for commonalities at underlying biological levels. We included such patients in our trial as an empirical test of maintenance treatment among the larger set of schizophrenic or schizoaffective patients initially responsive to adjunctive imipramine therapy. A subsequent post hoc analysis, dropping the few purely negative-symptom patients, led to a loss of significance (to trend level) on several scale items, presumably on the basis of loss of sample size, but did not contradict the overall thrust of the results.

The responsiveness of PPD to a tricyclic antidepressant in no way establishes the case that this condition is identical to primary depression in these patients. To conclude that would represent the use of predicate logic. In fact, studies of the biology of PPD[2,54] have often suggested at least some differences between this state and the condition represented by primary depression. All the same, similarities in pharmacoresponsivity have been found in these patients that parallel their phenomenologic similarities. These various similarities pose intriguing questions with regard to potential commonalities at a syndromal level that may be represented by these conditions.[7]

The continuing of treatment with benztropine mesylate in substantial doses (average 5 mg/d) throughout this maintenance trial is an issue worthy of comment. Long-term continuing treatment with antiparkinsonian medications for neuroleptic-maintained schizophrenic patients has been a controversial topic,[55-60] and the risks of a high anticholinergic burden involved in combining imipramine with benztropine warrant consideration. Nevertheless, our observation during short-term treatment, when we had gradually added imipramine hydrochloride (50 mg/d per week) to a standing fluphenazine decanoate–benztropine regimen, had been that the typical anticholinergic side effects of constipation, dry mouth, blurry vision, and difficulty urinating, did not become problematic.[1] Similarly, in the present maintenance study, we could not detect a difference in these anticholinergic side effects between the fluphenazine-benztropine-imipramine group and the double-blind comparison fluphenazine-benztropine-placebo group. Presumably this lack of difference in side effects was a reflection of a low anticholinergic potency of imipramine compared with benztropine (150 mg of imipramine hydrochloride being equivalent to approximately 2 mg of benztropine mesylate, in vitro[61]), plus the slowness of our increment in dosage. The chance randomization to imipramine, in this study, of a patient group with a slightly lower baseline benztropine dose may have played a role as well—although no side effect differences were found either at baseline or end point between the two treatment groups. (This last finding, no doubt, also helped to preserve the double-blind.)

Slowness of taper from imipramine to placebo in this study may additionally have served to protect patients against any anticholinergic withdrawal reactions. However, we have found that even gradual withdrawal of benztropine therapy during adjunctive imipramine maintenance therapy can be associated with disabling akinesia of the sort easily mistaken for PPD (P. C. Bermanzohn, MD, et al, unpublished data, 1992). Indeed, we had found in earlier work that administering adjunctive imipramine to postpsychotic depressed patients in the absence of benztropine seemed to be associated with an unacceptably high risk of extrapyramidal side effects in general.[38] For these reasons, we advise the continued use of adequate doses of benztropine along with adjunctive imipramine therapy during the maintenance treatment phase of PPD, although a high level of alertness for adverse anticholinergic effects such as memory impairment or anticholinergic psychosis should simultaneously be maintained.

The slowness of taper from imipramine to placebo also lessens the likelihood that the results observed reflected a drug-withdrawal effect rather than an issue of mere nontreatment of a PPD or negative symptom state. That possibility, however, cannot be entirely discounted, since seven of the eight depressive relapses that occurred while receiving adjunctive placebo occurred during the first 6 months while neither of the two relapses that occurred while receiving adjunctive imipramine did.

Counter to suspicions posed in the early literature,[34-41] our observation is of interest that those postpsychotic patients treated with the adjunctive tricyclic antidepressant actually suffered from fewer episodes of psychotic relapse than did their peers treated with neuroleptic and antiparkinsonian drugs alone. Although this finding achieved statistical significance, it must be interpreted with caution because the numbers of patients are small and the corresponding dimensional SADS-derived measure of psychosis, by ANCOVA, did not achieve statistical significance. Additionally, the mechanism for such an outcome is unclear. One possibility is that when treatment with the tricyclic antidepressant was discontinued, the plasma concentrations of neuroleptic were reduced, since these drugs can interfere with each other's metabolism.[62] Arguing against this possibility, however, is the fact that the fluphenazine decanoate doses with which the patients were being treated remained substantial by contemporary standards.[63,64] Indeed, these doses were higher in the group that underwent the imipramine taper. Another possible explanation for the result observed could be a protective effect exerted if the tricyclic drugs interfered with neurons' taking up toxic dopamine metabolites at times of dopamine overproduction.[65] A third set of possibilities involves the ability of long-term tricyclic antidepressant administration to down-regulate β-noradrenergic receptor density and sensitivity.[66,67] Such an action could conceivably be protective, even in the context of the dopamine hypothesis of schizophrenia,[68] because of the role played by β-receptors in epinephrine-mediated dopamine release.[69-71] Yet a fourth speculation would be that by protecting patients from depression, the adjunctive antidepressant was thereby protecting them from a powerful nonspecific stressor that could precipitate psychosis in these vulnerable individuals in accordance with a stress-diathesis model.[72,73] Such a stress-diathesis model could operate at a biological, psychological, and/or a social level, and would be consistent with our finding of increased anxiety in the group that had placebo substituted for imipramine in their regimen. This fourth hypothesis, if substantiated in further studies, could have important implications for the utility of treating any of a variety of secondary syndromes, such as panic,[74-76] obsessive-compulsive,[77,78] or posttraumatic stress,[79,80] any of which may occur in the course of schizophrenia,[81] and which could be an important source of clinical heterogeneity in this condition.[82]

Accepted for publication March 15, 1993.

This study was supported in part by grant MH-34309 from the National Institute of Mental Health, Rockville, Md, and by grant DA05039 from the National Institute on Drug Abuse, Rockville, Md.

Presented in part as a poster at the 30th Annual Meeting of the American College of Neuropsychopharmacology, San Juan, Puerto Rico, December 10, 1991.

Reprint requests to Hillside Hospital, 75-59 263rd St, Glen Oaks, NY 11004 (Dr Siris).

REFERENCES

1. Siris SG, Morgan V, Fagerstrom R, Rifkin A, Cooper TB. Adjunctive imipramine in the treatment of post-psychotic depression: a controlled trial. *Arch Gen Psychiatry.* 1987;44:533-539.
2. Siris SG. Diagnosis of secondary depression in schizophrenia: implications for *DSM-IV. Schizophr Bull.* 1991;17:75-98.
3. Plasky P. Antidepressant usage in schizophrenia. *Schizophr Bull.* 1991;17:649-656.
4. Rifkin A, Quitkin F, Klein DF. Akinesia: a poorly recognized drug-induced extrapyramidal behavioral disorder. *Arch Gen Psychiatry.* 1975;32:672-674.
5. Van Putten T, May PRA. 'Akinetic depression' in schizophrenia. *Arch Gen Psychiatry.* 1978;35:1101-1107.
6. Siris SG. Akinesia and post-psychotic depression: a difficult differential diagnosis. *J Clin Psychiatry.* 1987;48:240-243.
7. Bermanzohn PC, Siris SG. Akinesia: a syndrome common to parkinsonism, retarded depression, and negative symptoms. *Compr Psychiatry.* 1992;33:221-232.
8. Siris SG, Strahan A. Continuation and maintenance treatment trials of adjunctive imipramine in post-psychotic depression. *J Clin Psychiatry.* 1988;49:439-440.
9. Siris SG, Cutler J, Owen K, Mason S, Gingerich S, Lang MP. Adjunctive imipramine maintenance in schizophrenic patients with remitted post-psychotic depressions. *Am J Psychiatry.* 1989;146:1495-1497.
10. Siris SG, Cutler J, Owen K, Lang MP. Maintenance imipramine treatment following post-psychotic depression. *Psychopharmacol Bull.* 1989;25:85-88.
11. Spitzer RL, Endicott J, Robins E. Research Diagnostic Criteria: rationale and reliability. *Arch Gen Psychiatry.* 1978;35:773-782.
12. Andreasen NC, Olsen S. Negative vs positive schizophrenia: definition and validation. *Arch Gen Psychiatry.* 1982;39:789-794.
13. Guy W. *ECDEU Assessment Manual.* Rockville, Md: US Dept of Health, Education, and Welfare; 1976. Alcohol, Drug Abuse, and Mental Health Administration publication 76-338.
14. Endicott J, Spitzer RL. A diagnostic interview: the Schedule for Affective Disorders and Schizophrenia. *Arch Gen Psychiatry.* 1978;35:837-844.
15. Hamilton M. A rating scale for depression. *J Neurol Neruosurg Psychiatry.* 1960;23:56-62.
16. Endicott J, Cohen J, Nee J, Fleiss J, Sarantakos S. Hamilton Depression Rating Scale: extracted from regular and change versions of the Schedule for Affective Disorders and Schizophrenia. *Arch Gen Psychiatry.* 1981;38:98-103.
17. Lee E, Desu M. A computer program for comparing k samples with right-censored data. *Comput Programs Biomed.* 1972;2:315-321.
18. Siris SG, Bermanzohn PC, Gonzalez A, Mason SE, White CV, Shuwall MA. The use of antidepressants for negative symptoms in a subset of schizophrenic patients. *Psychopharmacol Bull.* 1991;27:331-335.
19. Siris SG, Adan F, Cohen M, Mandeli J, Aronson A, Casey E. Post-psychotic depression and negative symptoms: an investigation of syndromal overlap. *Am J Psychiatry.* 1988;145:1532-1537.
20. Prien RF, Kupfer DJ, Mansky PA, Small JG, Tuason VB, Voss CB, Johnson WE. Drug therapy in the prevention of recurrences in unipolar and bipolar affective disorders: report of the NIMH collaborative study group comparing lithium carbonate, imipramine, and a lithium carbonate–imipramine combination. *Arch Gen Psychiatry.* 1984;41:1096-1104.
21. Frank E, Kupfer DJ, Perel JM, Cornes C, Jarrett DB, Mallinger AG, Thase ME, McEachren AB, Grochocinski VJ. Three-year outcomes for maintenance therapies in recurrent depression. *Arch Gen Psychiatry.* 1990;47:1093-1099.
22. Kocsis JH, Sutton BM, Frances AJ. Long-term follow-up of chronic depression treated with imipramine. *J Clin Psychiatry.* 1991;52:56-59.
23. Kupfer DJ, Frank E, Perel JM, Cornes C, Mallinger AG, Thase MA, McEachran AB, Grochocinski VJ. Five-year outcome for maintenance therapies in recurrent depression. *Arch Gen Psychiatry.* 1992;49:769-773.
24. Siris SG, Bermanzohn PC, Mason SE, Shuwall MA, Aseniero MAR. Continuation treatment with adjunctive imipramine in schizophrenia. *Psychopharmacol Bull.* 1992;28:303-307.
25. Singh AN, Saxena B, Nelson HL. A controlled clinical study of trazodone in chronic schizophrenic patients with pronounced depressive symptomatology. *Curr Ther Res.* 1978;23:485-501.
26. Prusoff BA, Williams DH, Weissman MM, Astrachan BM. Treatment of secondary depression in schizophrenia. *Arch Gen Psychiatry.* 1979;36:569-575.
27. Bartels SJ, Drake RE. Depressive symptoms in schizophrenia: comprehensive differential diagnosis. *Compr Psychiatry.* 1988;29:467-483.
28. Waehrens J, Gerlach J. Antidepressant drugs in anergic schizophrenia: a double-blind cross-over study with maprotilitne and placebo. *Acta Psychiatr Scand.* 1980;61:438-444.
29. Johnson DAW. Studies of depressive symptoms in schizophrenia. *Br J Psychiatry.* 1981;139:89-101.
30. Kurland AA, Nagaraju A. Viloxazine and the depressed schizophrenic: methodological issues. *J Clin Pharmacol.* 1981;21:37-41.
31. Becker RE. Implications of the efficacy of thiothixene and a chlorpromazine-imipramine combination for depression in schizophrenia. *Am J Psychiatry.* 1983;140:208-211.
32. Dufresne RL, Kass DJ, Becker RE. Buproprion and thiothixene versus placebo and thiothixene in the treatment of depression in schizophrenia. *Drug Dev Res.* 1988;12:259-266.
33. Becker RE. Depression in schizophrenia. *Hosp Community Psychiatry.* 1988;39:1269-1275.
34. Siris SG, van Kammen DP, Docherty JP. Use of antidepressant drugs in schizophrenia. *Arch Gen Psychiatry.* 1978;35:1368-1377.
35. Kramer MS, Vogel WH, DiJohnson C, Dewey DA, Sheves P, Cavicchia S, Litle P, Schmidt R, Kimes I. Antidepressants in 'depressed' schizophrenic inpatients: a controlled trial. *Arch Gen Psychiatry.* 1989;46:922-928.

36. Docherty JP, vanKammen DP, Siris SG, Marder SR. Stages of onset of acute schizophrenic psychosis. *Am J Psychiatry.* 1978;135:720-726.
37. Siris SG, Rifkin A, Reardon GT, Doddi SR, Strahan A, Hall KS. Stability of the post-psychotic depression syndrome. *J Clin Psychiatry.* 1986;47:86-88.
38. Siris SG, Rifkin A, Reardon GT, November M. Comparative side effects to imipramine, benztropine, or their combination, in patients receiving fluphenazine decanoate. *Am J Psychiatry.* 1983;140:1069-1071.
39. McGlashan TH, Carpenter WT Jr. Postpsychotic depression in schizophrenia. *Arch Gen Psychiatry.* 1976;33:231-239.
40. Breier A, Schreiber JL, Dyer J, Pickar D. National Institute of Mental Health longitudinal study of chronic schizophrenia: prognosis and predictors of outcome. *Arch Gen Psychiatry.* 1991;48:239-246.
41. Bowers MB, Astrachan BM. Depression in acute schizophrenia. *Am J Psychiatry.* 1967;123:976-979.
42. Miles C. Conditions predisposing to suicide: A review. *J Nerv Ment Dis.* 1977; 164:221-246.
43. Roy A. Depression, attempted suicide and suicide in patients with chronic schizophrenia. *Psychiatr Clin North Am.* 1986;9:193-206.
44. Caldwell CB, Gottesman II. Schizophrenics kill themselves too: a review of risk factors for suicide. *Schizophr Bull.* 1990;16:571-589.
45. Drake RE, Gates C, Whitaker A, Cotton PG. Suicide among schizophrenics: a review. *Compr Psychiatry.* 1985;26:90-100.
46. Bartels SJ, Drake RE. Depressive symptoms in schizophrenia: comprehensive differential diagnosis. *Compr Psychiatry.* 1988;29:467-483.
47. Siris SG, Shuwall MA, Mason SE, Roy A. Suicidal ideation in post-psychotic depression. Presented at the 30th Annual Meeting of the American College of Neuropsychopharmacology; December 10, 1991; San Juan, Puerto Rico.
48. Carpenter WT Jr, Heinrichs DW, Alphs LD. Treatment of negative symptoms. *Schizophr Bull.* 1995;11:440-452.
49. Walker E, Lewine RJ. The positive/negative symptom distinction in schizophrenia: validity and etiological relevance. *Schizophr Res.* 1988;1:315-328.
50. Kay SR. Significance of the positive-negative distinction in schizophrenia. *Schizophr Bull.* 1990;16:635-652.
51. Prosser ES, Csernansky JG, Kaplan J, Theiman S, Becker TJ, Hollister LE. Depression, parkinsonian symptoms, and negative symptoms in schizophrenics treated with neuroleptics. *J Nerv Ment Dis.* 1987;175:100-105.
52. Bucci L. The negative symptoms of schizophrenia and the monoamine oxidase inhibitors. *Psychopharmacology.* 1987;91:104-108.
53. Silver H, Nassar A. Fluvoxamine improves negative symptoms in treated chronic schizophrenia: an add-on double-blind, placebo-controlled study. *Biol Psychiatry.* 1992;31:698-704.
54. Siris SG, Frechen K, Strahan A, Cutler J, Owen K, Alvir J, McCorry T. Thyroid-releasing hormone test in schizophrenic patients with post-psychotic depression. *Prog Neuropsychopharmacol Biol Psychiatry.* 1991;15:369-378.
55. Lake CR, Casey DE, McEvoy JP, Siris SG, Boyer WF, Simpson G. Anticholinergic prophylaxis in young adults treated with neuroleptic drugs. *Psychopharmacol Bull.* 1986;22:981-984.
56. Rifkin A, Quitkin F, Kane JM, Klein DF. Are prophylactic antiparkinson drugs necessary? *Arch Gen Psychiatry.* 1978;35:483-489.
57. Manos N, Gkiouzepas J, Logothetis J. The need for continuous use of antiparkinsonian medication with chronic schizophrenic patients receiving long-term neuroleptic therapy. *Am J Psychiatry.* 1981;138:184-188.
58. World Health Organization. Prophylactic use of anticholinergics in patients on long-term neuroleptic treatment: a consensus statement. *Br J Psychiatry.* 1990;156:412.
59. Barnes TRE. Comment on the WHO consensus statement. *Br J Psychiatry.* 1990;156:413-414.
60. Lavin MR, Rifkin A. Prophylactic antiparkinsonian drug use, II: withdrawal after long-term maintenance therapy. *J Clin Pharmacol.* 1991;31:769-777.
61. Snyder SH, Yamamura HI. Antidepressants and the muscarinic acetylcholine receptor. *Arch Gen Psychiatry.* 1977;34:236-239.
62. Siris SG, Cooper TB, Rifkin AE, Brenner R, Lieberman JA. Plasma imipramine concentrations in patients receiving concomitant fluphenazine decanoate. *Am J Psychiatry.* 1982;139:104-106.
63. Kane JM. Treatment of schizophrenia. *Schizophr Bull.* 1987;13:133-156.
64. Marder SR, Van Putten T, Mintz J, Lebell M, McKenzie J, May PRA. Low- and conventional-dose maintenance therapy with fluphenazine decanoate: two-year outcome. *Arch Gen Psychiatry.* 1987;44:518-521.
65. Stein L, Wise CD. Possible etiology of schizophrenia: progressive damage to the noradrenergic reward system by 6-hydroxydopamine. *Science.* 1971;171: 1032-1036.
66. Vetulani J, Sulser F. Action of various antidepressant treatments reduces reactivity of noradrenergic cyclic AMP-generating system in limbic forebrain. *Nature.* 1975;257:495-496.
67. Banerjee SP, Kung LS, Riggi SJ, Chanda SK. Development of beta-adrenergic receptor subsensitivity by antidepressants. *Nature.* 1977;268:455-456.
68. VanKammen DP, Kelley M. Dopamine and norepinephrine activity in schizophrenia: an integrative perspective. *Schizophr Res.* 1991;4:173-191.
69. Anden NE, Grabowska M. Pharmacological evidence for a stimulation of dopamine neurons by noradrenaline neurons in the brain. *Eur J Pharmacol.* 1976; 39:275-282.
70. Langer AZ. Presynaptic regulation of the release of catecholamines. *Pharmacol Rev.* 1981;32:337-362.
71. El-Awar M, Freedman M, Seeman P, Goldenberg L, Little J, Solomon P. Response of tardive and l-dopa-induced dyskinesias to antidepressants. *Can J Neurol Sci.* 1987;14:629-631.
72. Zubin J, Spring B. Vulnerability: a new view of schizophrenia. *J Abnorm Psychol.* 1977;86:103-126.
73. Nuechterlein KH, Dawson ME. A heuristic vulnerability/stress model of schizophrenic episodes. *Schizophr Bull.* 1984;10:300-312.
74. Sandberg L, Siris SG. 'Panic disorder' in schizophrenia: a case report. *J Nerv Ment Dis.* 1987;175:627-628.
75. Kahn JP, Puertollano MA, Schane MD, Klein DF. Adjunctive alprazolam for schizophrenia with panic anxiety: clinical observation and pathogenetic implications. *Am J Psychiatry.* 1988;145:742-744.
76. Cutler JL, Siris SG. 'Panic-like' symptomatology in schizophrenic and schizoaffective patients with post-psychotic depression: observations and implications. *Compr Psychiatry.* 1991;32:465-473.
77. Fenton WS, McGlashan TH. The prognostic significance of obsessive-compulsive symptoms in schizophrenia. *Am J Psychiatry.* 1986;143:437-441.
78. Karno M, Golding JM, Sorenson SB, Vurnam MA. The epidemiology of obsessive-compulsive disorder in five US communities. *Arch Gen Psychiatry.* 1988;45: 1094-1099.
79. Stampfer HG. 'Negative symptoms': a cumulative trauma stress disorder? *Aust N Z J Psychiatry.* 1990;24:516-528.
80. McGorry PD, Chanen A, McCarthy E, Van Riel R, McKenzie D, Singh BS. Post-traumatic stress disorder following recent-onset psychosis: an unrecognized postpsychotic syndrome. *J Nerv Ment Dis.* 1991;179:253-258.
81. Siris SG. Implications of normal brain development for the pathogenesis of schizophrenia. *Arch Gen Psychiatry.* 1988;45:1055.
82. Siris SG. Adjunctive medications in the maintenance treatment of schizophrenia. *Br J Psychiatry.* In press.

ORIGINAL ARTICLE

Striatal D_2 Dopamine Receptor Characteristics in Neuroleptic-Naive Schizophrenic Patients Studied With Positron Emission Tomography

Jarmo Hietala, MD; Erkka Syvälahti, MD; Klaus Vuorio, MD; Kjell Någren, PhD; Pertti Lehikoinen, PhD; Ulla Ruotsalainen, MSc; Viljo Räkköläinen, MD; Ville Lehtinen, MD; Uno Wegelius, MD

Background: According to the D_2 dopamine receptor hypothesis of schizophrenia, there is an increased number of D_2 receptors in the brains of schizophrenic patients than in those of healthy controls. We tested this hypothesis in 13 newly admitted neuroleptic-naive schizophrenic patients and 10 healthy volunteers using positron emission tomography.

Method: The quantification of striatal D_2 dopamine receptor density (B_{max}) and affinity (K_d) was done using an equilibrium model described for raclopride labeled with carbon 11.

Results: No statistically significant alterations were found in D_2 receptor densities or affinities between the patient and control groups. However, a subgroup of four patients with a relatively high striatal D_2 dopamine density was identified. Two patients, especially, had D_2 dopamine densities almost twice as high as the mean control B_{max} value. The K_d values also tended to be higher in this subset of patients than in the controls. No consistent striatal D_2 dopamine receptor laterality was observed in schizophrenic patients or controls. However, an association of high D_2 dopamine density in the left striatum and the mass of raclopride injected in the scan with low-specific radioactivity was observed in patients but not in controls.

Conclusion: There are no general changes in D_2 dopamine receptor B_{max} or K_d values in neuroleptic-naive schizophrenics, but there may be a subgroup of patients with aberrant striatal D_2 dopamine receptor characteristics in vivo.

(Arch Gen Psychiatry. 1994;51:116-123)

THE DOPAMINE hypothesis of schizophrenia postulates that an increase in brain dopaminergic activity, especially in the mesolimbic dopamine pathway, is an etiologic factor in schizophrenia. This hypothesis is mainly supported by several lines of pharmacologic evidence showing that antipsychotic drugs antagonize the dopamine system by blocking D_2 dopamine receptors[1-5] and that dopaminomimetic drugs are able to induce psychotic symptoms resembling paranoid schizophrenia.[6] A more recent suggestion in the hyperdopaminergia hypothesis of schizophrenia is that there is an abnormally high density of D_2 dopamine receptors in the brains of schizophrenic patients compared with those of healthy controls.[7-11] This is also known as the D_2 dopamine receptor hypothesis of schizophrenia. An increased number of D_2 dopamine receptors could contribute to an enhanced dopaminergic neurotransmission in the schizophrenic brain. However, most data supporting an excess of central D_2 dopamine receptors in schizophrenia derive from postmortem studies that are susceptible to a variety of confounding factors. One of the most important factors is previous neuroleptic treatment, which is known to increase the number of brain D_2 dopamine receptors in experimental studies.[12,13] This factor can readily be controlled in studies with positron emission tomography (PET), enabling the quantification of D_2 dopamine receptor characteristics in vivo. In addition, the relationship between clinical condition and D_2 dopamine receptor parameters can be assessed.

From the Department of Pharmacology, University of Turku, Finland (Drs Hietala and Syvälahti); Turku Medical Cyclotron/Positron Emission Tomography Project (Drs Hietala, Syvälahti, Någren, Lehikoinen, and Wegelius and Ms Ruotsalainen); Psychiatric Clinic, Turku City Hospital (Dr Vuorio and Räkköläinen); and Psychiatric Clinic, Turku University Hospital (Dr Lehtinen).

See Subjects and Methods on next page

SUBJECTS AND METHODS

SUBJECTS

The study protocol was approved by the ethics committee of the Turku (Finland) University/University Hospital, Turku. Thirteen newly admitted schizophrenic patients (nine male and four female) from the Psychiatric Clinics of Turku City Hospital and Turku University Hospital were studied. The patients were included in a project on the development of extensive psychotherapeutic care of acute psychosis.[19] In addition, 10 healthy volunteers (six male and four female) with no history of psychiatric disorders or somatic illnesses were recruited. Mean (±SD) ages, heights, and weights were 25.2±6.8 years, 172.8±10.4 cm, and 66.4±9.3 kg, respectively, for patients, and 26.8±7.3 years, 176.1±9.2 cm, and 67.4±8.7 kg, respectively, for controls. All except two patients and two controls were right-handed. Informed consent was obtained in all cases.

The patients met *DSM-III-R* criteria for schizophrenia, schizophreniform disorder, or schizoaffective disorder. The diagnoses were confirmed on follow-up examination. More detailed patient characteristics are shown in the **Table**. Exclusion criteria were previous neuroleptic treatment, previous long-term intensive psychotherapy, serious somatic illness, pregnancy, and lack of adequate cooperation. All patients but one were completely neuroleptic-naive. This was verified by checking the patients' medical records and by careful interviewing of the family members. Patient 2 had received a single 50-mg oral dose of chlorpromazine 1 month before the PET scan. Occasional doses of benzodiazepines (oxazepam, lorazepam, or temazepam) were allowed, except on the day of the PET scan. Eight of the 13 patients received benzodiazepines once or more during the 2 weeks preceeding the PET scan (patients 1 to 4, 8, and 10 to 12). Studies in rodents indicate that occasional doses of benzodiazepines do not alter the characteristics of striatal D_2 dopamine receptors.[20]

The patients stayed at the wards at least 2 weeks before undergoing the PET scan. Patients 9 and 13 were also treated as outpatients before PET study. The clinical condition at the time of the PET scan was assessed using the Brief Psychiatric Rating Scale (BPRS). In addition, a subscale of positive symptoms (disorganization, tension, mannerism and posturing, grandiosity, hostility, suspiciousness, hallucinatory behavior, uncooperativeness, unusual thought content, excitement) was derived from the BPRS.[21]

PET METHOD

The quantification of striatal D_2 dopamine receptor density and affinity was done with [^{11}C]raclopride as a radioligand. The preparation of [^{11}C]raclopride used has been described previously,[22] with some recent modifications.[23] A one-pot procedure[24,25] from [^{11}C]carbon dioxide was used in the preparation of [^{11}C]methyl iodide, which was used in an alkylation reaction of the O-desmethyl precursor (NCQ 259 [hydrobromide], Astra Pharmaceuticals, Södertälje, Sweden). An Efremov 103-cm isochronous cyclotron was used to produce [^{11}C]carbon dioxide. The volume of the formulated (saline) [^{11}C]raclopride solution was determined by weight before and after sterile filtration and by division with the density (1.0046 g/mL) of saline. The concentration of [^{11}C]raclopride was determined with reversed-phase high-pressure liquid chromatography (30% acetonitrile, 70% 0.01 mol/L of phosphoric acid, 2 mL per minute) with ultraviolet detection at 210 nm. Samples of [^{11}C]raclopride and reference solutions (prepared from raclopride tartrate, Astra) were analyzed in triplicate with an SD of less than 2%. For the studies with low-specific-radioactivity [^{11}C]raclopride, a freshly prepared solution of raclopride tartrate in saline was added before sterile filtration of the formulated solution.

The PET experiments were performed using a whole-body PET scanner (ECAT 931/08-12, Computer Technol-

Continued on next page

Two PET studies were published on striatal D_2 dopamine receptor characteristics in neuroleptic-naive schizophrenia. These two studies, using different methods of D_2 dopamine receptor parameter measurement, are highly discrepant, showing either clearly increased[14] or equal[15] D_2 dopamine receptor densities in the striata of neuroleptic-naive schizophrenics compared with those of healthy volunteers. In addition, two PET studies using bromospiperone labeled with bromine 76 and ^{76}Br-bromolisuride have reported unchanged striatal D_2 dopamine binding[16,17] (expressed as striatum-cerebellum [S/C] ratios) in schizophrenics, or marginally but significantly elevated D_2 dopamine values in a small subgroup of patients with acute schizophrenia.[16] These inconsistencies have been discussed with multiple possible explanations ranging from patient selection to the radioligand used.[18] The objective of this study was to compare striatal D_2 dopamine receptor densities and affinities of 13 neuroleptic-naive schizophrenic patients and 10 controls. D_2 dopamine receptor characteristics were measured in vivo using PET and raclopride labeled with carbon 11.

RESULTS

COMPARISON OF STRIATAL D_2 DOPAMINE RECEPTOR CHARACTERISTICS IN SCHIZOPHRENIC PATIENTS AND CONTROLS

There were no statistically significant differences in the striatal density (B_{max}) or apparent affinity (K_d) of D_2 dopamine receptors between the patient population and normal controls (**Figure 2**). Mean (±SD) B_{max} values were 38.7±14.9

ogy & Imaging, Knoxville, Tenn) with 15 slices and a spatial resolution of 6.1 mm on the plane and an axial resolution of 6.7 mm (measured values).[26] Each patient/healthy volunteer underwent two scans in the same day between 10 AM and 4 PM, at least 2 hours apart. The mean injected dose was 104×10^6 Bq. The first scan was done with a high-specific radioactivity of raclopride (mean±SD, $6.14 \times 10^{12} \pm 2.18 \times 10^{12}$ Bq/mmol in patients and $5.10 \times 10^{12} \pm 3.5 \times 10^{12}$ Bq/mmol in controls) and the second with a low-specific radioactivity ($185 \times 10^9 \pm 63 \times 10^9$ Bq/mmol in patients and $190 \times 10^9 \pm 74 \times 10^9$ Bq/mmol in controls). The weight of injected raclopride dose ranged from 2.5 to 443 μg (high- and low-specific activities, respectively).

Head fixation was done by using rapidly hardening polyurethane mass (Insta-foam Productions, Joliet, Ill), which formed an individual headholder, supporting the head from the top, back, and sides. While the mass was hardening, two laser beams parallel to canthomeatal and sagittal lines were used in head positioning. Several points were marked with ink on the skin of the subject to ensure an identical positioning of the head during the first and second PET scans. Before each experiment, a transmission scan was performed with a germanium 68–filled removable ring system. The right and left antecubital veins were cannulated for injection of [^{11}C]raclopride and blood sampling, respectively. A rapid intravenous bolus injection of [^{11}C]raclopride was given (about 5 seconds) and flushed with saline.

The uptake of [^{11}C]raclopride in the brain was measured for 49 minutes using 21 to 24 time frames. As a rule, the striatum was transversed by four slices. Striatal regions of interest were drawn on sum images from 10 to 49 minutes using the two middlemost planes transversing the striatum. The results are expressed as whole striatum because reliable distinction between nucleus caudatus and putamen was not possible in all cases. The volumes of right and left striatal samples were 5.02 ± 0.52 cm^3 and 5.26 ± 0.69 cm^3, respectively, for schizophrenics and 5.14 ± 0.65 cm^3 and 5.16 ± 0.71 cm^3, respectively, for controls (means±SDs), showing no significant differences in striatal sample volumes between schizophrenic patients and controls or between left and right striata within the two groups.

These sizes of striata are well in agreement with an anatomical reference.[27] No attempts were made for partial volume correction. The average decay-corrected levels of radioactivity contained in the left and right striata and the cerebellum were plotted against time and the data analyzed in terms of an equilibrium model using the cerebellum as a receptor-free reference region.[28] An example of radioactivity-time curves is shown in **Figure 1**. D_2 dopamine receptor density and affinity were calculated based on the principles presented by Scatchard.[29]

Routine computed tomographic scans were also obtained parallel to the canthomeatal line. No structural brain defects were observed in these scans. The sizes of lateral (frontal horns) ventricles (linear ventricle index) and the third ventricle–brain ratio were measured. Neither of these parameters differed significantly between control and patient populations, although the third ventricle–brain ratio was almost statistically significantly higher in patients (P=.051 using the Wilcoxon Rank-Sum Test).

STATISTICAL ANALYSIS

The Wilcoxon Rank-Sum Test was used to assess differences in D_2 dopamine receptor characteristics between schizophrenic patients and healthy volunteers. The Wilcoxon Signed-Rank Test was used to test for right-left differences of D_2 receptor parameters within the patient and control populations. Relationships between D_2 receptor characteristics and age, as well as other clinical variables (duration of illness, BPRS), were expressed using Pearson's Product-Moment Correlation Coefficient. Homogeneity of group variances was evaluated with Bartlett's test. A statistical software package (Systat Inc, Evanston, Ill) was used for the statistical analysis. $P<.05$ was considered statistically significant.

pmol/mL and 34.6±7.5 pmol/mL (P=.85), and K_d values were 12.4±4.5 nmol/L and 10.4±2.9 nmol/L (P=.25) for schizophrenic patients and controls, respectively. However, the scatter in D_2 dopamine density was significantly larger in the patient group (P=.04 using the Bartlett Test), and four patients appeared to have relatively high striatal B_{max} values (beyond the 2-SD reach of the control population). Two of these four patients, one with undifferentiated and the other with schizoaffective disorder, had high densities of striatal D_2 dopamine receptors (Table). These four patients, especially patients with the three highest B_{max} values, also had high D_2 dopamine receptor K_d values. Due to the small number of patients in different *DSM-III-R* diagnostic groups, no further subgroup analysis was attempted. It was, however, clear that aberrant D_2 dopamine receptor characteristics appeared across *DSM-III-R* schizophrenia subtypes.

No consistent lateralities in D_2 dopamine receptor density were observed in patients or controls. In general, the controls had 9.5% higher (P=.09) and patients 5.5% higher (P=.34) B_{max} values in the right striatum. Likewise, the K_d value of D_2 dopamine receptors was 7.9% (P=.11) and 2.9% (P=.34) higher in the right striatum in controls and patients, respectively (the Wilcoxon Signed-Rank Test). Thus, no significantly enhanced right-left differences in B_{max} (P=.13) or K_d values (P=.15) were observed between schizophrenic patients and controls (Wilcoxon Rank-Sum Test). Exclusion of the two left-handed controls and two left-handed patients from the analysis resulted in similar statistical probabilities. Interestingly, a subsequent analysis revealed that the five patients with more D_2 dopamine receptors in the left striatum had received more raclopride in the low-specific-radioactivity scan than the remaining eight patients with

Patient Characteristics*

Patient No./Age, y/Sex	*DSM-III-R* Definition	DI, mo	BPRS	B_{max}	K_d
1/23.7/F	Undifferentiated	13	86	68.7	18.3
2/19.7/M	Undifferentiated	11	56	28.8	11.3
3/23.7/F	Undifferentiated	9	68	24.0	7.2
4/25.4/M	Undifferentiated	30	56	26.1	10.1
5/22.8/M	Undifferentiated	6	48	49.8	11.8
6/26.3/M	Undifferentiated	8	57	30.8	14.1
7/30.8/M	Disorganized	54	59	32.8	10.3
8/27.8/M	Disorganized	54	75	33.3	10.0
9/42.6/M	Paranoid	36	42	53.5	20.4
10/19.2/M	Catatonic	7	25	23.5	6.4
11/20.3/F	Schizophreniform	2	21	33.7	9.4
12/20.2/F	Schizophreniform	6	40	35.7	11.8
13/20.9/M	Schizoaffective disorder	7	35	62.1	19.7

**DI* indicates duration of illness and includes prodromal symptoms; BPRS, Brief Psychiatric Rating Scale at the time of positron emission tomography; and B_{max} and K_d, mean right- and left-side values for striatal density and apparent affinity, respectively.*

more D_2 dopamine receptors in the right striatum (332±85 μg vs 173±59 μg, *P*=.002). The K_d value followed a similar pattern. A corresponding phenomenon was not noted in controls despite the fact that some controls also received high doses of raclopride in the low-specific-radioactivity scan. Only one female control had higher D_2 dopamine density in the left striatum. There were no overall differences in the injected mass of raclopride (low-specific-radioactivity scan) in the patients and controls; 234±104 μg and 215±71 μg, respectively.

RELATIONSHIP OF AGE AND DOPAMINE D_2 RECEPTOR CHARACTERISTICS IN SCHIZOPHRENIC PATIENTS AND CONTROLS

No significant correlations between age and B_{max} or K_d values were seen in controls or patients (age ranges were 20 to 44 years and 19 to 43 years for controls and patients, respectively). Correlation coefficients in the control population were .05 and −.11 for right and left B_{max} values, respectively. Corresponding correlations for right and left K_d values were −.15 and −.058. Correlation coefficients for the patient population were .240 and .169 for right and left B_{max} values, respectively. Corresponding correlations were .54 (*P*=.05) and .32 for right and left K_d values, respectively.

RELATIONSHIP OF CLINICAL VARIABLES AND D_2 DOPAMINE RECEPTOR CHARACTERISTICS IN SCHIZOPHRENIC PATIENTS

No correlation was observed between clinical morbidity (indexed by the total BPRS score) and right (*r*=.15; *P*=.62) or left B_{max} values (*r*=.14; *P*=.64) and right (*r*=.12; *P*=.68) or left K_d values (*r*=.07; *P*=.81). Also the subscale consisting only of positive symptoms failed to show any association with D_2 dopamine receptor parameters. In addition, no correlation between duration of illness and B_{max} or K_d values was noted (correlation coefficients between −.17 and .20).

COMMENT

The D_2 dopamine receptor hypothesis of schizophrenia has been intensively studied using postmortem methods. A vast majority of these reports suggest that schizophrenic patients have an elevated D_2 dopamine receptor density in the striatum compared with control subjects.[7-11,30] The largest postmortem study on this issue suggests that schizophrenics can be divided into two populations: one with a modest upregulation (up to 50%) and another with an up to 200% upregulation of striatal D_2 dopamine receptors.[9] However, in that study as well as in most other postmortem studies, previous neuroleptic treatment may affect the results, as it is known from experimental studies that neuroleptics usually induce a 30% to 40% striatal D_2 dopamine receptor upregulation.[12] Thus, the bimodal distribution of D_2 dopamine receptors in schizophrenia may merely reflect differential adaptation of the dopaminergic systems to neuroleptic treatment and not necessarily a basic biochemical disturbance in the schizophrenic brain.

It was hoped that dopamine receptor quantification in vivo using PET in neuroleptic-naive and early-stage schizophrenic patients would overcome the problems associated with postmortem techniques. The following two methods have been used to measure D_2 dopamine receptors in vivo in neuroleptic-naive or neuroleptic-free schizophrenic patients using PET: (1) simple S/C ratio or (2) kinetic or equilibrium models to measure receptor density and affinity. The S/C ratios in schizo-

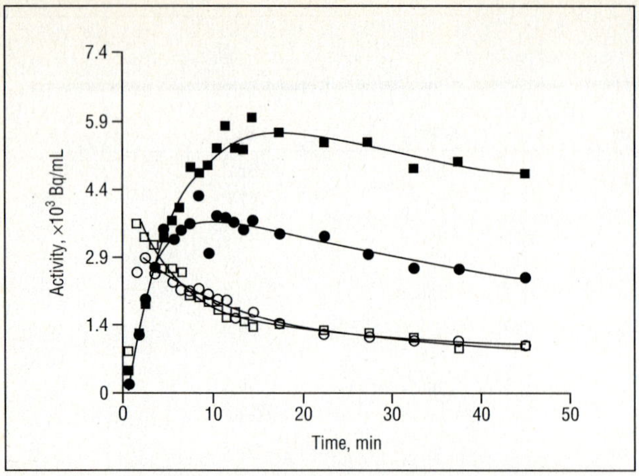

Figure 1. *A representative example of striatal and cerebellar radioactivity time curves after injection of high-specific radioactivity (6.0× 10^{12} Bq/mmol) and low-specific radioactivity (170× 10^9 Bq/mmol) in a 25-year-old female subject. The striatal curve denotes the specific binding curve (cerebellar activity subtracted from total striatal radioactivity). A maximum point (d[Bound]/d[time]=0) was identified on the curves and used as the value for specifically bound ligand. The free (nonspecific) value was taken from the corresponding time point on the cerebellar curve. Open circles and squares represent low- and high-specific radioactivity, respectively, in the cerebellum; closed circles and squares, low- and high-specific radioactivity, respectively, in the striatum.*

phrenics and normal controls have been studied by several groups using PET or single photon emission computed tomography.[16,17,31-33] Typically, a tracer amount of ligand (high-specific radioactivity) is used, and only a small fraction of D_2 dopamine receptors are occupied in the studies measuring the S/C ratio. There are no major discrepancies in these experiments including the high-specific-radioactivity scans between the study by Farde et al[15] and the present study, which suggests unaltered or marginally elevated D_2 dopamine receptor S/C ratios in the striata of drug-naive or drug-free schizophrenic patients. It has, however, been suggested that the measurement of the S/C ratio with only one scan may be confounded by blood flow effects, especially in young patients.[34,35] To measure the actual density of D_2 dopamine receptors, a considerable number of the receptors need to be occupied[14,15] and it appears that differential results begin to arise when subsaturating doses of D_2 dopamine antagonists are used in the quantification procedures.[36]

In this study, the density and affinity of striatal D_2 dopamine receptors in schizophrenics and healthy volunteers were calculated after high- and low-specific-radioactivity scans with [^{11}C]raclopride. The main finding in this study was that neuroleptic-naive schizophrenia is not generally associated with abnormal striatal D_2 dopamine receptor characteristics; however, deviant D_2 dopamine receptor B_{max} and K_d values were observed in four of our patients. This result conforms well with the increasing body of evidence suggesting that not all patients with schizophrenia have an overactive dopamine system.[37] The two previous studies measuring D_2 dopamine receptor characteristics of drug-naive schizophrenic patients yielded contradictory results. The group at The Johns Hopkins University (Baltimore, Md),[14] using a kinetic model for [^{11}C]*N*-methylspiperone, found patients with schizophrenia to have a caudate receptor density that was twofold or threefold higher than that of controls. Although further studies in that laboratory using more patients have not been as convincing as the first one, patients with schizophrenia as a group still have a significantly elevated density of D_2 dopamine receptors despite a considerable overlap with controls (preliminary results by Wong et al[35]). In addition, the increase in the apparent haloperidol inhibition constant seen in these experiments is now taken as evidence of decreased affinity of D_2 dopamine receptors tentatively caused by endogenous dopamine.[38] In contrast, the group at the Karolinska Institute (Stockholm, Sweden), using [^{11}C]raclopride and an equilibrium model for in vivo quantification, showed D_2 dopamine receptor densities and affinities in the nucleus caudatus and putamen to be identical in 18 drug-naive schizophrenic patients and 20 controls.[15] Our results with a corresponding [^{11}C]raclopride method support the findings obtained in the latter study, although four of our patients had relatively high B_{max} values associated with high K_d values in striatal D_2 dopamine receptors.

Several reasons have been suggested to explain the noted discrepancies.[18,36] The two most important factors so far have been the choice of radioligand and model as well as patient-dependent variables. Kinetic and equilibrium models have been used to measure D_2 dopamine receptor characteristics. At least with [^{11}C]raclopride, kinetic and equilibrium models give identical results.[28] It has also been suggested, based on results of animal and in vitro studies, that raclopride may be more easily affected by endogenous dopamine competition[39-41] than [^{11}C]*N*-methylspiperone. In our study, the K_d values tended to be higher in the patients having relatively high D_2 dopamine receptor densities. This observation would be in agreement with a reversible ligand-receptor interaction with interference by endogenous dopamine re-

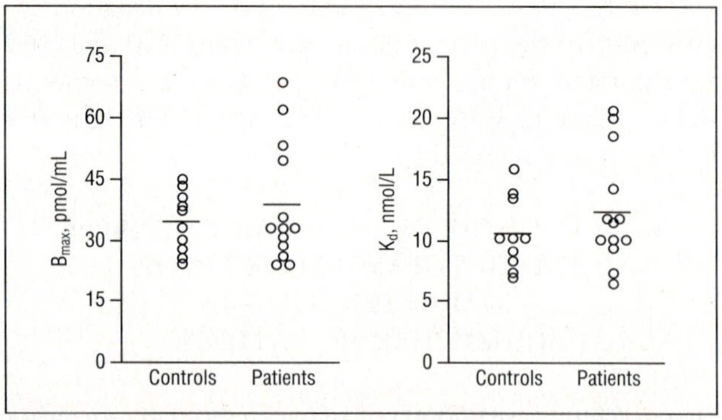

Figure 2. *Striatal D_2 dopamine receptor density (B_{max}) (left) and affinity values (K_d) (right) in schizophrenic patients and normal controls. No significant differences were observed although four patients had high D_2 dopamine densities.*

sulting in an elevated K_d value but an unaltered receptor density. The situation may, however, be more complicated in vivo, as it is clear that the amount of D_2 dopamine antagonist administered in these studies very likely causes an effective D_2 dopamine receptor blockade and increases dopamine release per se in the striatum by interrupting feedback mechanisms. These feedback mechanisms may function differentially in schizophrenic and normal brains. In addition, interaction between the released dopamine and D_2 non–dopamine receptors may further complicate the D_2 dopamine receptor-binding process of radioligands as a reduced D_1-D_2 receptor link has been described in the schizophrenic brain at least in vitro.[42] Although there are undoubtedly definite differences between raclopride and *N*-methylspiperone in vitro[43] and the applied models for quantification, preliminary studies on the use of both ligands in the same schizophrenic patients and controls suggest that no increase in D_2 dopamine density in schizophrenics can be observed with either ligand.[44] This emphasizes the importance of patient-dependent variables.

A POSSIBLE subgroup with aberrant D_2 dopamine receptor characteristics in this study clearly goes across *DSM-III-R* schizophrenia subtypes, as exceptionally high B_{max} values were found in a patient with undifferentiated schizophrenia and another with schizoaffective disorder. Thus, the traditional schizophrenia subtyping appears to be a poor discriminator of a putative dopamine receptor disturbance. The clinical state may contribute to differential results. Preliminary studies suggest that there is a more general association of psychosis (also in bipolar patients) and increased B_{max} values (and decreased D_2 dopamine affinity) in D_2 dopamine receptors.[35] Otherwise, as reported herein and elsewhere,[14,15] no marked correlations were noted between psychiatric rating scales and D_2 dopamine receptor characteristics. This may be due to a lack of sensitivity of BPRS and other clinical rating scales in detecting delicate psychiatric alterations. The BPRS scale consists mainly of positive symptoms that are believed to be associated with hyperdopaminergia in subcortical dopaminergic structures. On the other hand, negative symptoms have been suggested to be linked with hypodopaminergia in cortical (prefrontal) dopaminergic structures.[45,46]

In addition, there are at least four other differences among the patient characteristics in previous studies: age, duration of illness, the clinical setting, and other nonneuroleptic medication. The patients at The Johns Hopkins University are clearly older than the ones investigated at the Karolinska Institute or in the current report. Interestingly, the oldest patient in our study, a 42-year-old patient with paranoid schizophrenia, had a relatively high D_2 dopamine density and the highest K_d value. In this study, with a limited age range, there was no correlation between B_{max} and K_d values and age in controls or patients. In a larger study of normal subjects from our laboratory including a wider age range, a 4.6% decrease per decade in D_2 dopamine density was observed, with no marked change in affinity (Juha Rinne, MD, J.H., unpublished data, 1992).

Duration of illness did not correlate with D_2 dopamine receptor characteristics in this study. A more detailed analysis of duration of illness and D_2 dopamine receptor parameters could not be made as most of our patients had been ill for about a year or less. The duration of illness was in a similar range in the study of Farde et al[15] but considerably longer in the study of Wong et al.[14] Further, the clinical setting was different in all three studies. In our study, patients stayed at the wards at least 2 weeks before undergoing PET scanning, whereas at The Johns Hopkins University, patients underwent scanning immediately after admission; and at the Karolinska Institute, schizophrenic patients were at the wards for several days before PET study was undertaken. During the time before PET scanning, the psychological and physical conditions of patients may change, which may also alter results derived from the PET scanning.[36] In addition, some of our patients, as well as some patients studied by Farde et al,[15] received occasional doses of benzodiazepines. This should not affect D_2 dopamine receptor characteristics in the brain[20]; however, this has not been proven in humans. In our material, the patient with the highest B_{max} value in the D_2 dopamine receptors was given occasional benzodiazepine doses (oxazepam) up to 1 day before PET scanning. On the other hand, patients with the second highest B_{max} value did not receive any benzodiazepines, suggesting that the medication was an unlikely explanation for the deviant D_2 dopamine receptor values.

Several anatomical and functional studies on schizophrenic patients suggest that there may be aberrant anatomical function, especially in the left hemisphere.[47-49] The report by Farde et al[15] suggests that schizophrenic patients have more D_2 dopamine receptors in the left than in the right putamen and that this left-right difference is significantly enhanced compared with controls. The magnitude of this previously detected difference is very small and, as stated previously, may be confounded by partial volume effects. The finding was not supported by this study, showing similar right-left ratios of D_2 dopamine receptors in the striata of patients and controls. In our study, although both patients and controls had more D_2 dopamine receptors in the right side, five patients had clearly more D_2 dopamine receptors in the left striatum. In subsequent analysis of the data, a highly significant association between the weight of injected raclopride in the low-specific-radioactivity scan and left-side lateralization of D_2 dopamine receptor characteristics was found in patients but not in controls. The finding was consistent, regardless of previous benzodiazepine exposure in some patients. It is clear that this discriminatory effect of injected raclopride in the low-specific-radioactivity scan should be regarded with caution because of the fewer patients and the technical limitations of PET, eg, partial volume effects. On the other hand, it may be a true pharmacologic effect of raclopride (with a threshold D_2 dopamine receptor occupancy) and may reflect differential activation of dopaminergic processes in the left and right hemispheres in early-stage neuroleptic-naive schizophrenics compared with healthy controls. This calls for a more detailed analysis on the effects of D_2 dopamine receptor antagonists, such as raclopride and haloperidol, on various aspects of right and left hemisphere function, eg, cortical-striatal interplay, in schizophrenic patients and healthy controls. Interestingly, a recent single photon emission computed tomographic study of blood flow in neuroleptic-naive/neuroleptic-free schizophrenic patients and healthy volunteers suggested that during a cognitive activation task (the Wisconsin Card Sorting Test), there is a failure to increase blood flow in the prefrontal inferior cortex and a corresponding enhanced increase in striatal blood flow in the schizophrenic brain. Both phenomena occurred only in the left hemisphere.[50]

In conclusion, our results suggest that the number of D_2 dopamine receptors is not generally elevated in the striata of newly admitted, neuroleptic-naive schizophrenic patients. However, four of 13 patients in our study had high striatal B_{max} values associated with high K_d values. Thus, there may be a subgroup of schizophrenic patients with abnormalities in striatal D_2 dopamine receptor–binding characteristics in vivo.

Accepted for publication January 25, 1993.

This study was financially supported by the Medical Research Council, Academy of Finland, and the Jalmari and Rauha Ahokas Foundation.

Raclopride and its precursor were donated by Astra Pharmaceuticals, Södertälje, Sweden.

Presented in part as a preannounced discussion at the Fifth World Congress of Biological Psychiatry, Florence, Italy, June 10, 1991.

We thank the staff in the Turku Positron Emission Tomography Laboratory; Curt West, MSc, BM; and Vesa Oikonen, MSc, for data processing.

Reprint requests to Department of Pharmacology, University of Turku, Kiinamyllynkatu 10, 20520-Turku, Finland (Dr Hietala).

REFERENCES

1. Carlsson A, Lindquist M. Effect of chlorpromazine or haloperidol on formation of 3-methoxytyramine and normetanephrine in mouse brain. *Acta Pharmacol Toxicol.* 1963;20:140-144.
2. Seeman P, Lee T, Chau-Wong M, Wong K. Antipsychotic drug doses and neuroleptic/dopamine receptors. *Nature.* 1976;261:717-719.
3. Chiodo LA, Bunney BS. Typical and atypical neuroleptics: differential effects of chronic administration on the activity of A9 and A10 midbrain dopaminergic neurons. *J Neurosci.* 1983;3:1607-1619.
4. White FJ, Wang RY. Differential effects of classical and atypical antipsychotic drugs on A9 and A10 dopamine neurons. *Science.* 1983;221:1054-1057.
5. Farde L, Wiesel F-A, Halldin C, Sedvall G. Central D_2 dopamine receptor occupancy in schizophrenic patients treated with antipsychotic drugs. *Arch Gen Psychiatry.* 1988;45:71-76.
6. Bowers MB. The role of drugs in the production of schizophreniform psychosis and related disorders. In: Meltzer H, ed. *Psychopharmacology: Third Generation of Progress.* New York, NY: Raven Press; 1987;819-823.
7. Lee T, Seeman P, Tourtelotte WW, Farley IJ, Hornykiewicz O. Binding of ^{3}H-neuroleptics and ^{3}H-apomorphine in schizophrenic brains. *Nature.* 1978;274: 897-900.
8. Mackay AVP, Iversen LL, Rossor M, Spokes E, Bird E, Arregui A, Creese I, Snyder SH. Increased brain dopamine and dopamine receptors in schizophrenia. *Arch Gen Psychiatry.* 1982;39:991-997.
9. Seeman P, Bzowej NH, Guan H-C, Bergeron C, Reynolds GP, Bird ED, Riederer P, Jellinger K, Tourtelotte WW. Human brain D_1 and D_2 dopamine receptors in schizophrenia, Alzheimer's, Parkinson's and Huntington's diseases. *Neuropsychopharmacology.* 1987;1:5-15.
10. Joyce JN, Lexow N, Bird E, Winokur A. Organization of dopamine D_1 and D_2 receptors in human striatum: receptor autoradiographic studies in Huntington's disease and schizophrenia. *Synapse.* 1988;2:546-557.
11. Seeman P, Niznik HB. Dopamine receptors and transporters in Parkinson's disease and schizophrenia. *FASEB J.* 1990;4:2737-2744.
12. Burt DR, Creese I, Snyder SH. Antischizophrenic drugs: chronic treatment elevates dopamine receptor binding in brain. *Science.* 1977;196:326-328.
13. Clow A, Jenner P, Theodorou A, Marsden CD. Striatal dopamine receptors become supersensitive while rats are given trifluoroperazine for six months. *Nature.* 1979;278:59-61.
14. Wong DF, Wagner HN, Tune LE, Dannals RF, Pearlson GD, Links JM, Tamminga CA, Broussolle EP, Ravert HT, Wilson AA, Thomas-Toung JK, Malat J, Williams JA, O'Tuama LA, Snyder SH, Kuhar MJ, Gjedde A. Positron emission tomography reveals elevated D_2 dopamine receptors in drug-naive schizophrenics. *Science.* 1986;234:1558-1563.
15. Farde L, Wiesel F-A, Stone-Elander S, Halldin C, Nordström A-L, Hall H, Sedvall G. D_2 dopamine receptors in neuroleptic-naive schizophrenic patients: a positron emission tomography study with [^{11}C]raclopride. *Arch Gen Psychiatry.* 1990;47:213-219.
16. Martinot J-L, Peron-Magnan P, Huret J-D, Mazoyer B, Baron J-C, Boulenger J-P, Loc'h C, Maziere B, Caillard V, Loo H, Syrota A. Striatal D_2 dopaminergic receptors assessed with positron emission tomography and 76-Br-bromospiperone in untreated patients. *Am J Psychiatry.* 1990;147:44-50.
17. Martinot J-L, Paillere-Martinot ML, Loc'h C, Hardy P, Poirier MF, Mazoyer B, Beaufils B, Maziere B, Allilaire JF, Syrota A. The estimated density of striatal D_2 receptors in schizophrenia: a study with positron emission tomography and 76Br-bromolisuride. *Br J Psychiatry.* 1991;158:346-350.
18. Andreasen N, Carson R, Diksic M, Evans A, Farde L, Gjedde A, Hakim A, Lal S, Nair N, Sedvall G, Tune L, Wong D. Workshop on schizophrenia, PET and dopamine D_2 receptors in the human neostriatum. *Schizophr Bull.* 1988;14:471-484.
19. Alanen YO, Lehtinen K, Räkköläinen V, Aaltonen J. Need-adapted treatment of new schizophrenic patients: experiences and results of the Turku project. *Acta Psychiatr Scand.* 1991;83:363-372.
20. Leysen JE, Van Gompel P, de Chaffoy-de Courcelles D, Niemegeers CJ. Opposite regulation of regulation serotonin S_2 and dopamine D_2 receptors in rat brain following chronic receptor blockade. *J Receptor Res.* 1987;7:223-229.
21. Wolkin A, Barouche F, Wolf AP, Rotrosen J, Fowler J, Shiue C-Y, Cooper T, Brodie JD. Dopamine blockade and clinical response: evidence for two biological subgroups of schizophrenia. *Am J Psychiatry.* 1989;146:905-908.
22. Farde L, Pauli S, Hall H, Eriksson L, Halldin C, Högberg T, Nilsson L, Sjögren I, Stone-Elander S. Stereoselective binding of [^{11}C]raclopride in living human brain: a search for extrastriatal central D_2 dopamine receptors by PET. *Psychopharmacology.* 1988;94:471-478.
23. Maziere M, Coenen HH, Halldin C, Någren K, Pike VW. PET radioligands for dopamine receptors and reuptake sites: chemistry and biochemistry. *Nucl Med Biol.* 1992;19:497-512.
24. Långström B, Antoni G, Gullberg P, Halldin C, Någren K, Rimland A, Svärd H.

The synthesis of 1-[^{11}C]labelled ethyl, propyl, butyl and isobutyl iodides and examples of alkylation reactions. *Appl Radiat Isot.* 1986;37:1141-1145.
25. Någren K, Takahashi T, Lehikoinen P, Bergman J. Preparation of the antiestrogenic compound N-[methyl-11-C]toremifene for the study of estrogen-receptor positive tumors in vivo. *J Labeled Comp Radiopharm.* 1991;29:1085-1089.
26. Spinks TJ, Jones T, Gilardi MC, Heather JD. Physical performance of the latest generation of commercial positron scanner. *IEEE Trans Nucl Sci.* 1988;35: 721-725.
27. Aquilonius S-M, Eckernäs SÅ. *A Colour Atlas of the Human Brain Adapted to Computed Tomography.* Uppsala, Sweden: Esselte Studium; 1980.
28. Farde L, Eriksson L, Blomquist G, Halldin C. Kinetic analysis of central [^{11}C]raclopride binding to D_2 dopamine receptors studied by PET: a comparison to the equilibrium analysis. *J Cereb Blood Flow Metab.* 1989;9:696-708.
29. Scatchard G. The attractions of proteins for small molecules and ions. *Ann N Y Acad Sci.* 1949;51:660-672.
30. Kornhuber J, Riederer P, Reynolds GP, Beckmann H, Jellinger K, Gabriel E. 3H-spiperone binding in post-mortem brains of schizophrenic patients: relationship to neuroleptic drug treatment, abnormal movements and positive symptoms. *J Neural Transm.* 1989;75:1-10.
31. Wong DF, Wagner HN Jr, Pearlson G, Dannals RF, Links JM, Ravert HT, Wilson AA, Suneja S, Bjorvvinssen E, Kuhar MJ, Tune L. Dopamine receptor binding of C-11-3-N-methylspiperone in the caudate in schizophrenia and bipolar disorder: a preliminary report. *Psychopharmacol Bull.* 1985;21:595-598.
32. Herold S, Leenders KL, Turton DR, Kensett MJ, Pike VW, Clark JC, Brooks DJ, Crow TJ, Owen F, Cooper S, Johnstone EC. Dopamine receptor binding in schizophrenic patients as measured with ^{11}C-methylspiperone and PET. *J Cereb Blood Flow Metab.* 1985;5:191-192.
33. Crawley JCW, Crow TJ, Johnstone EC, Oldland SRD, Owen F, Owens DGC, Smith T, Veall N, Zanelli GD. Uptake of ^{77}Br-spiperone in the striata of schizophrenic patients and controls. *Nucl Med Commun.* 1986;7:599-607.
34. Wong DF, Gjedde A, Wagner HN. Quantification of neuroreceptors in the living human brain, I: irreversible binding of ligands. *J Cereb Blood Flow Metab.* 1986; 6:137-146.
35. Wong DF, Tune L, Pearlson G, Young T, Shaya E, Ross C, Dannals RF, Wilson AA, Ravert HT, Links J, Wagner HN, Gjedde A. Dopamine receptor elevations in drug-naive schizophrenia and bipolar affective illness measured by [^{11}C]NMSP PET studies: update and methodological considerations. *Clin Neuropharmacol.* 1990;13(suppl):85-86.
36. Sedvall G. PET imaging of dopamine receptors in human basal ganglia: relevance to mental illness. *Trends Neurosci.* 1990;13:302-308.
37. Davis KL, Kahn RS, Ko G, Davidson M. Dopamine in schizophrenia: a review and reconceptualization. *Am J Psychiatry.* 1991;148:1474-1486.
38. Wong DF, Gjedde A, Tune L, Pearlson G, Shaya E, Young T, Young D, Dannals RF, Wilson AA, Ravert HT, Wagner HN. PET results suggest reduced D_2 affinity in psychosis in vivo. *Biol Psychiatry.* 1991:29(suppl);705-706.
39. Seeman P, Guan H-C, Niznik HB. Endogenous dopamine lowers the D_2 dopamine receptor density as measured by 3H-raclopride: implications for positron emission tomography of the human brain. *Synapse.* 1989;3:96-97.
40. Seeman P, Niznik HB, Guan H-C. Elevation of D_2 dopamine receptors in schizophrenia is underestimated by radioactive raclopride. *Arch Gen Psychiatry.* 1990; 47:1170-1172.
41. Young LT, Wong DF, Goldman S, Minkin E, Chen C, Matsumura K, Scheffl U, Wagner HN. Effects of endogenous dopamine on kinetics of 3-H-N-methylspiperone and 3-H-raclopride binding in rat brain. *Synapse.* 1991;9:188-194.
42. Seeman P, Niznik HB, Guan H-C, Booth G, Ulpian C. Link between D_1 and D_2 dopamine receptors is reduced in schizophrenia and Huntington's diseased brain. *Proc Natl Acad Sci U S A.* 1989;86:10156-10160.
43. Hall H, Wedel I, Halldin C, Kopp J, Farde L. Comparison of the in vitro binding properties of N-3H-methylspiperone and 3H-raclopride to rat and human brain membranes. *J Neurochem.* 1990;55:2048-2057.
44. Farde L, Nordström A-L, Eriksson L, Halldin C, Sedvall G. Comparison of methods used with [^{11}C]raclopride and [^{11}C]NMSP for the PET determination of central D_2 dopamine receptors. *Clin Neuropharmacol.* 1990;13(suppl):87-88.
45. Bannon MJ, Roth RH. Pharmacology of mesocortical dopamine neurons. *Pharmacol Rev.* 1983;35:63-68.
46. Pycock CJ, Kerwin RW, Carter CJ. Effect of lesion of cortical dopamine terminals on subcortical dopamine receptors in rats. *Nature.* 1980;286:74-77.
47. Suddath RL, Christison GW, Torrey EF, Casanova MF, Weinberger DR. Anatomical abnormalities in the brains of monozygotic twins discordant for schizophrenia. *N Engl J Med.* 1990;322:789-794.
48. Early TS, Reiman EM, Raichle ME, Spitznagel EL. Left globus pallidus abnormality in never-medicated patients with schizophrenia. *Proc Natl Acad Sci U S A.* 1987;84:561-563.
49. Bracha HS. Asymmetric rotational (circling) behavior, a dopamine-related asymmetry: preliminary findings in unmedicated and never-medicated schizophrenic patients. *Biol Psychiatry.* 1987;22:995-1003.
50. Rubin P, Holm S, Friberg L, Videbech P, Andersen HS, Bendsen BB, Stromso N, Larsen JK, Lassen NA, Hemmingsen R. Altered modulation of prefrontal and subcortical brain activity in newly diagnosed schizophrenia and schizophreniform disorder. *Arch Gen Psychiatry.* 1991;48:987-995.

ORIGINAL ARTICLE

Neuropsychological Deficits in Neuroleptic Naive Patients With First-Episode Schizophrenia

Andrew J. Saykin, PsyD; Derri L. Shtasel, MD; Raquel E. Gur, MD, PhD; D. Brian Kester, MS; Lyn H. Mozley, MS; Paul Stafiniak, MS; Ruben C. Gur, PhD

Background: Medication and chronicity have complicated past attempts to characterize the neuropsychological performance of patients with schizophrenia. There have been inconsistencies regarding the pattern, selectivity, and sources of observed deficits. Our objective was to comprehensively examine neuropsychological function in patients with schizophrenia who had never been exposed to neuroleptic medication, and who were experiencing their first episode (FE) of psychosis.

Methods: Subjects were consecutive recruitments that included 37 patients with FE schizophrenia who were never exposed to neuroleptics. These subjects were compared with 65 unmedicated, previously treated (PT) patients and 131 healthy controls.

Results: The patient groups had nearly identical profiles showing generalized impairment, particularly in verbal memory and learning, attention-vigilance, and speeded visual-motor processing and attention. Verbal memory and learning accounted for most of the variance between patients and controls and removing this effect substantially attenuated all other differences. By contrast, both the FE group and PT group continued to show highly significant deficits in verbal memory and learning after controlling for attention, abstraction, and all other functions. Some functions not typically implicated in schizophrenia (spatial cognition, fine motor speed, and visual memory) were more impaired in the PT group than in the FE group.

Conclusions: Verbal memory, as a primary neuropsychological deficit present early in the course of schizophrenia, implicates the left temporal-hippocampal system. Neuropsychological evaluations before treatment permit differentiation of primary deficits from changes secondary to medication or chronicity. This is essential for developing a neurobehavioral perspective on schizophrenia.

(Arch Gen Psychiatry. 1994;51:124-131)

INVESTIGATIONS OF neuropsychological function in schizophrenia have consistently indicated deficits. However, the characterization and selectivity of impairment have been a source of controversy.[1-9] Major dimensions of impairment include attention-vigilance (ATT),[10,11] abstraction-flexibility (ABS),[7,12,13] verbal intelligence and language function skills (VBL),[14-16] and memory and learning.[9,17-19] Most studies concentrated on one or a few areas of cognition rather than using a comprehensive battery that would permit adequate profiling of test results across neuropsychological dimensions. Medication and chronicity may have influenced past attempts to characterize neuropsychological performance in schizophrenia. Also, effects of demographic variables have often not been appropriately controlled.[20] To address some of these concerns, there has been recent interest in characterization of neuropsychological performance of patients experiencing their first episode (FE) of psychosis.[21-28] Although highly valuable as a way to control for chronicity of illness, prior studies of patients with FE of psychosis all have the limitation of having obtained neuropsychological testing after the introduction of neuroleptic and frequently anticholinergic medications. These agents influence neu-

From the Neuropsychiatry Program, Department of Psychiatry, University of Pennsylvania School of Medicine, Philadelphia. Dr Saykin is now with the Department of Psychiatry, Dartmouth Medical School, Lebanon, NH, and the New Hampshire Hospital, Concord.

See Subjects and Methods on next page

SUBJECTS AND METHODS

We have previously described the methods and procedures used in this study.[9] Herein we summarize them briefly and focus on additional aspects relevant to the study of patients with FE schizophrenia.

All patients were consecutive admissions and recruited by the Mental Health Clinical Research Center on Schizophrenia of the Department of Psychiatry at the University of Pennsylvania, Philadelphia. All patients met *DSM-III-R*[35] criteria for schizophrenia and had no concomitant Axis I or II disorder. Subjects who met *DSM-III-R* criteria for past or present substance abuse and/or substance dependence were excluded from all groups. Patients with FE schizophrenia were followed up for at least 1 year to confirm diagnosis. Recruitment methods and inclusion-exclusion criteria for patients[9,36] and healthy controls are available elsewhere (A.J.S., R.E.G, D.B.K., P.S., and R. C. Gur, PhD, L. H. Mozley, L. J. Robinson, PhD, B. L. Malmut, PhD, B. Watson, PsyD, D. Shtasel, MD, D. Mozley, MD, unpublished data, December 1992).[37] All participants were free of any past or present medical or neurological disorder. Of an initial sample of 108 patients recruited, 37 of 39 patients with FE psychosis and 65 of 69 previously treated (PT) patients were able to complete the core test battery and could be included; 131 of 133 healthy controls had sufficient data for inclusion. Five of the patients with FE psychosis, 25 of the PT patients, and 33 of the controls were also included in our earlier report.[9] All PT subjects were medication free for at least 2 weeks prior to evaluation. Sample characteristics are presented in **Table 1**. The FE and PT groups were comparable in overall severity and positive and negative features. Paranoid and undifferentiated subtypes predominated both groups. Written informed consent was obtained for all subjects.

NEUROPSYCHOLOGICAL BATTERY

The battery, which was described by Saykin et al,[9] was modified as follows (**Table 2**). (1) The continuous performance measures of attention-vigilance[38] are now included in the profile. (2) Because of their high intercorrelation, verbal cognitive measures from the Wechsler Adult Intelligence Scale–Revised[39] Verbal Scale were combined with the language tests as the verbal intelligence and language function skills. (3) Similarly, strongly correlated tests of verbal memory and learning (VBM) were combined. (4) A test of facial recognition memory sensitive to right temporal lobectomy[40] was added to visual memory (VIM). (5) Auditory processing was dropped from the profile. Thus, the areas assessed include attention-vigilance, abstraction-flexibility, verbal intelligence and language function skills, spatial organization (SPT), verbal memory and learning, visual memory, speeded visual-motor processing and attention (VSM), and fine manual motor functions (MOT). Details of test administration, supplementary measures, and scoring procedures were previously reported.[9]

DATA ANALYSIS

Analyses were performed before and after adjustment for age, sex, education, and ethnicity using a multiple linear regression procedure (GLM procedure, SAS Institute)[41] as

robehavioral, cognitive, memory, and psychomotor performance,[29-32] and may cause prolonged alteration in cerebral dopamine-receptor occupancy,[33,34] and thus have likely contributed to some of the previously reported neuropsychological performance data. Herein we report a controlled study using a comprehensive neuropsychological battery to characterize neuroleptic naive patients with FE schizophrenia.

RESULTS

Neuropsychological profiles for both patient groups and controls are shown in **Figure 1**. By definition, the control group mean is represented by the zero line with SD=1 for all functions. Neuropsychological profiles were analyzed by MANOVA for group differences in level, shape, and for interactions. On the overall analysis, both the FE and PT patient groups performed significantly below the healthy controls: $F(2,230)=96.9$, $P<.001$. The profile shape was nonflat for both patient groups indicating a selective pattern of impairment relative to controls. This was reflected by significant group by function interactions (for the contrast between controls and PT patients, $F[7,224]=13.0$, $P<.001$; for controls vs patients with FE schizophrenia, $F[7,224]=10.3$, $P<.001$). The PT group also showed lower mean performance than the patients with FE schizophrenia ($F[1,230]=7.9$, $P=.005$), but there was no difference in profile shape between the FE and PT groups ($F[7,224]=0.9$, not significant). Repeating the above MANOVAs with the addition of maternal and paternal education as covariates did not yield any significant covariate main effects or interactions, nor did it alter the above pattern of significant effects. Results of univariate analyses of variance and pairwise comparisons between groups for the component functions of the overall profile are presented in **Table 3**. After adjustment of α using the Bonferroni method (critical $P=.00625$), both patient groups performed worse than controls ($P<.001$) on all functions, except the FE group for fine manual motor functions. The PT patients performed worse than the FE group ($P<.00625$) on spatial organization and fine manual motor functions, with similar trends noted for all other functions except attention-vigilance and abstraction-flexibility.

Results for the planned mean profile contrasts, used to examine selectivity of differences in profile shape, are presented in **Table 4**. After adjustment of α using the Bonpreviously described.[9] Raw test scores were transformed to standard equivalents (z scores) using the means and SDs (model root mean square error) of the normal control group. The z scores were truncated at −6.0 to prevent rarely occurring, extremely deviant scores on tests with a small raw score SD from distorting profile shape.

Tasks that the patients were unable to perform received a score equal to that of the worst performer among patients who completed the task. Tests that were not administered for technical reasons unrelated to the patient's ability were coded as missing. Most patients had no missing scores and no patient had more than 20% missing values. Since multivariate analysis procedures delete cases with any missing values, possibly affecting the representativeness of an analyzed sample, we used a stepwise regression estimation procedure (BMDP AM)[42] to impute scores for the missing values where they could be reliably estimated from the remaining test scores (one or more variables with F-to-enter >4.0). All analyses were performed with and without the imputed values. Means and SDs were nearly identical after use of this procedure as were all main effects and interactions. As before,[9] multivariate analysis of variance (MANOVA) was used to evaluate profile level and shape with diagnosis (FE, PT, controls) as the between-group factor and neuropsychological function (eg, attention-vigilance, abstraction-flexibility, verbal intelligence and language function) as the within-subject factor. A within-subject contrast was performed to evaluate the selectivity of differences in profile shape between groups. To evaluate selectivity, this procedure (GLM Procedure, Mean Contrast Method)[41] tests the hypothesis that for a patient group a given mean function score (eg, abstraction-flexibility) is higher or lower than the mean of the remaining seven functions relative to the control group. The expected value of the mean contrast for the controls is zero, because of their flat profile. The Bonferroni procedure was used to control experiment-wise type I error for all contrasts by dividing the critical P value by the number of contrasts (eg, α of .05 divided by eight neuropsychological functions=.00625). To further clarify the contribution of each neuropsychological function to between-group differences, in view of their intercorrelation, stepwise multiple discriminant function analysis (BMDP 7M)[42] was also performed. The procedures listed earlier were performed with and without covariance analysis using maternal and paternal education (in years) as covariate markers for parental socioeconomic status.

As a final check on the selectivity of observed deficits, as before,[9] we used the standardized residual score method recommended by Chapman and Chapman.[43] This approach addresses the question: "To what extent is a subject's score on Task B deviant, given that subject's score on Task A?"[43(p363)] Therefore, prior to comparing a subject's scores on two tests, eg, verbal memory and learning and abstraction-flexibility, the score on verbal memory and learning (Test A) was reexpressed to reflect degree of deviation from the score for verbal memory and learning that would be predicted by performance on abstraction-flexibility (Test B). This has the added advantage of taking into account the correlation between the two tests.

ferroni method, the PT group showed selective impairment in verbal memory and learning, speeded visual-motor processing and attention, and attention-vigilance, and relative strengths in verbal intelligence and language function, and in spatial organization and fine manual motor function skills. Like the PT group, the patients with FE schizophrenia also showed selective impairment in verbal memory and learning, attention-vigilance, and speeded visual-motor processing and attention. Spatial organization and fine manual motor function skills, but not verbal intelligence and language function skills, were relative strengths in the FE group's profile.

On the stepwise multiple discriminant function analysis, used to clarify the contribution of each neuropsychological function to overall between-group differences, while controlling for the intercorrelation among these abilities, verbal memory and learning definitively accounted for most of the explained between-group variance (R^2 or accounted for variance=46%). After inclusion of verbal memory and learning in the model, partial correlations for other neuropsychological functions accounted for less than 5% of the between-group variance each. Similarly, in a MANOVA test for group differences in verbal memory and learning after controlling for attention-vigilance, abstraction-flexibility, and all other functions, verbal memory and learning remained a highly significant deficit relative to the control group for both the FE and PT groups ($F[9,223]=15.5$, $P<.0001$, and $F[9,223]=20.6$, $P<.0001$, respectively). Attention-vigilance, after controlling for verbal memory and learning and all other functions, was marginally worse for the FE group only compared with controls ($F[9,223]=3.83$, $P=.052$). No other functions, including abstraction-flexibility, remained significant after controlling for other functions.

We performed a confirmatory check on the selectivity of the deficit in verbal memory and learning using the method of Chapman and Chapman.[43] **Figure 2** illustrates the percent of subjects in each group who show worse verbal memory and learning than abstraction-flexibility, verbal intelligence and language function, or attention-vigilance. The significance of differences in proportion of subjects showing the pattern of worse verbal memory and learning than comparison functions was evaluated by two-tailed, 2×2, Fisher's Exact Tests. Compared with controls, PT patients showed a higher frequency of selective impairment in verbal memory and

Table 1. Demographic and Clinical Characteristics*

Variable	First Episode of Psychosis (n=37)	Previously Treated (n=65)	Controls (n=131)
Age, y	28.64±8.41	31.26±7.00	27.11±7.16
Education, y			
Patient	12.16±1.91	12.91±2.17	14.56±2.04
Mother	12.03±2.78	12.33±2.27	12.84±2.32
Father	12.71±3.17	12.81±3.05	13.04±3.26
Sex, M/F	23/14	48/17	76/55
Ethnicity, W/B	13/24	43/22	87/44
Handedness, R/L/Mixed	29/7/1	60/3/2	123/8/0
Subtype, C/D/P/U	1/1/24/13	4/8/23/34	NA
Age at onset, median y	22	21	N/A
Illness duration, median y	2	9	N/A
No. of hospitalizations, median	0	3	N/A
BPRS, total	50.64±8.71	53.26±10.59	N/A
SANS	2.44±1.08	2.66±1.02	N/A
SAPS	2.49±0.76	2.51±0.83	N/A
MMSE total	26.73±2.66	25.40±5.43	N/A

Values are mean±SD unless noted as median; otherwise, data are frequency counts. FE indicates first episode; PT, previously treated; C, catatonic; D, disorganized; P, paranoid; U, undifferentiated; BPRS, Brief Psychiatric Rating Scale; SANS, Scale for the Assessment of Negative Symptoms; SAPS, Scale for the Assessment of Positive Symptoms; and MMSE, Mini-Mental State Examination. Illness duration is age at evaluation minus age at onset of illness.

learning than abstraction-flexibility (*P*=.0001), VBL (*P*=.006), and attention-vigilance (*P*=.023). Patients with FE schizophrenia, compared with controls, showed more frequent impairment in verbal memory and learning compared with abstraction-flexibility (*P*=.039) and VBL (*P*=.027), but not attention-vigilance. The PT patients and patients with FE schizophrenia did not differ in proportion showing worse verbal memory and learning relative to other functions.

COMMENT

Our findings indicate that there is a characteristic degree and pattern of neuropsychological impairment in patients with schizophrenia, and that this pattern is evident already in patients experiencing FE of psychosis, who have never been exposed to neuroleptics. This supports the hypothesis that there is a characteristic underlying cognitive deficit in schizophrenia. The deficit may reflect genetic vulnerability[10,11,44-46] or may be related to neurodevelopmental complications.[47] Although neuropsychological deficits could be caused by the thought disorder and other primary symptoms of the illness,[35] rather than underlying brain disorder, this is unlikely for two reasons. First, there is temporal stability of these deficits from acute phase to follow-up after clinical stabilization.[21,24,48] Second, the correlations between neuropsychological functions and psychopathology measures such as the Brief Psychiatric Rating Scale, Scale for the Assessment of Negative Symptoms, and Scale for the Assessment of Positive Symptoms are relatively modest.[23,49,50] An alternative interpretation is that neuropsychological deficits may render an individual vulnerable to the development of thought disorder. Future studies could determine whether selective verbal memory and other deficits are present in at-risk relatives. Additional neurocognitive studies of unaffected monozygotic cotwins would be particularly useful.[51]

Even small correlations between neuropsychological and psychopathology measures suggest some relation that is interesting and potentially important. However, in the present sample, psychopathology measures account for a small portion of the explained variance compared with presence of disease itself. We hypothesize that there is an underlying trait deficit in schizophrenia of varying severity, which may be overlaid with state-related cognitive abnormalities. The state-related cognitive abnormalities should covary with measures of psychopathology at a particular time, while the trait-related component should remain relatively stable. In a complete model, trait and state factors and interactions between them should be considered. In a longitudinal framework, the concept of heterogeneity in schizophrenia could be reexamined in terms of trait vs state-related cognitive phenomena.

A recent focus of etiologic hypotheses in schizophrenia research concerns neurodevelopmental vs neurodegenerative models of illness.[48,52,53] Whether early deficits are resolving, static, or progressive remains to be definitively determined. Since cross-sectional studies cannot ascertain whether patients' conditions deteriorate, longitudinal studies will be required to examine temporal stability and disease trajectories. Our data provisionally favor a developmental model in that deficits, observed very early in the disease course, resemble those observed in patients with multiepisode disease. Our preliminary follow-up data indicate that neuropsychological deficits are stable over time, which suggests that these deficits are more a trait than a state-related phenomenon.[48] Prospective genetic and developmental research designs can identify specific risk factors related to disease expression and outcome, as well as precipitating psychosocial stressors.

The overall pattern we observed in patients is one of generalized impairment of approximately 2 SD units magnitude relative to healthy controls of comparable age, gender, ethnicity, and parental education. Additionally, verbal memory and learning is selectively compromised relative to other functions. Attention-vigilance and speeded visual-motor processing and attention were also selectively impaired, but to a lesser extent. After controlling for the substantial intercorrelation among functions, verbal memory and learning was a much better discriminator between controls and patient subgroups than attention-vigilance or speeded visual-motor processing and attention. These data confirm and extend observations of selective cognitive impairment in schizophrenia, particularly for memory processes. We did not find support for the conclusion of some investigators that memory impairment is primarily caused by anticholinergic medications[29,32,54] or that it is attributable to impairment in executive functions such as attention-vigilance or abstraction-flexibility.[19] Controlling for verbal memory greatly attenuated the between-group difference in these functions. By contrast, controlling for attention-vigilance, abstraction-flexibility, and all other neuropsychological functions did not eliminate the group differences in verbal memory. The anatomic implication of the obtained pattern of modality-specific verbal memory impairment is consistent with differential dysfunction of the left temporal-hippocampal system.[41,55,56]

One difference from our prior report[9] is the restriction of selective memory deficits to verbal memory and learning as opposed to the visual modality. Visual memory, although impaired relative to controls, was not a selective deficit. This difference appears to be due to improved procedures for normalizing the data, including use of a larger control group and the inclusion of preadjustment for ethnicity in addition to age, education, and gender. The verbal memory measures we employed may be more sensitive than the visual memory tests, and studies with other visual memory measures may show selective impairment. However, we did not observe such an effect after inclusion of a facial recognition memory test sensitive to acute changes in visual memory after right temporal lobectomy.[40] In view of the present results, additional studies of specific memory processes in schizophrenia appear to be warranted, including remote memory, autobiographical memory, procedural learning, and priming.

Whereas PT patients were slightly, though significantly, more impaired than the FE group overall, the absence of differences in shape of neuropsychological profile suggests consistency of pattern of deficits across stages

Table 2. Neuropsychological Battery With Tests Grouped by Function*

Attention-vigilance (AHTT)
Continuous Performance Test (Gordon Systems Inc) Vigilance and Distractibility Tasks
Abstraction-flexibility (ABS)
Categories and perseveration responses (Wisconsin Card Sorting Test)
Verbal intelligence and language function (VBL)
Information, Vocabulary, Comprehension, Similarities (WAIS-R)
Controlled Oral Word Association (MAE; letters cfl)
Animal Naming and Boston Naming Tests (BDAE)
Comprehension of Complex Ideational Material (BDAE)
Sentence Repetition (MAE)
Reading Recognition (WRAT-R)
Spatial organization (SPT)
Picture Completion, Block Design, Object Assembly (WAIS-R)
Verbal memory and learning (VBM)
Story Recall (Wechsler Memory Scale; immediate and 30-min delay)
Paired Associate Learning (Wechsler Memory Scale)
California Verbal Learning Test (CVLT; sum of trials 1-5)
Visual memory (VIM)
Design Reproduction (Wechsler Memory Scale; immediate and 30-min delay)
Facial Recognition Memory (Saykin et al,[40] 1992; immediate and 30-min delay)
Speeded visual-motor processing and attention (VSM)
Trail Making A and B (HRB)
Digit Symbol (WAIS-R)
Stroop Tests–Word, Color, Color-Word Interference
Fine manual motor functions (MOT)
Thumb-Finger Sequential Touch (Luria; right and left hands)
Finger Tapping (HRB; right and left hands)

**WAIS-R* indicates Wechsler Adult Intelligence Scale–Revised; MAE, Multilingual Aphasia Examination; BDAE, Boston Diagnostic Aphasia Examination; WRAT-R, Wide Range Achievement Test–Revised; and HRB, Halstead-Reitan Battery.*

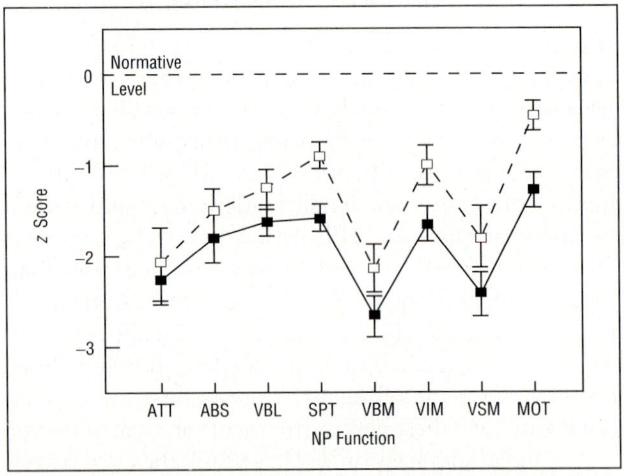

Figure 1. *Neuropsychological profile (NP) (±SEM) for neuroleptic naive patients with first-episode schizophrenia (open squares, n=37) and previously treated patients (solid squares, n=65) relative to healthy controls (dashed line, n=131). ATT indicates attention-vigilance; ABS, abstraction-flexibility; VBL, verbal intelligence and language function; SPT, spatial organization; VBM, verbal memory and learning; VIM, visual memory; VSM, speeded visual-motor processing and attention; and MOT, fine manual motor functions.*

Table 3. Univariate Analyses on Specific Neuropsychological Functions*

Univariate ANOVAs	Overall Model		PT vs Control		FE vs Control		FE vs PT	
	F	*P*	F	*P*	F	*P*	F	*P*
Attention-vigilance	60.3	.0001	96.7	.0001	54.3	.0001	0.3	.5622
Abstraction-flexibility	37.4	.0001	63.5	.0001	29.2	.0001	1.0	.3247
Verbal intelligence and language function	57.7	.0001	105.5	.0001	33.7	.0001	5.4	.0213
Spatial organization	46.9	.0001	91.1	.0001	17.0	.0001	10.9	.0011
Verbal memory and learning	98.8	.0001	170.8	.0001	72.4	.0001	3.8	.0537
Visual memory	40.6	.0001	77.4	.0001	18.2	.0001	6.9	.0092
Speeded visual-motor processing and attention	69.7	.0001	124.9	.0001	44.6	.0001	4.8	.0291
Fine manual motor functions	26.3	.0001	52.5	.0001	3.1	.0793	14.0	.0002

**ANOVA indicates analysis of variance; PT, previously treated; and FE, first episode. For the overall model,* df=*2,230; for all two-group univariate contrasts,* df=*1,230.*

Table 4. Results of Mean Contrast Procedure for Neuropsychological Functions*

	PT vs Control		FE vs Control		FE vs PT	
	F	*P*	F	*P*	F	*P*
Attention-vigilance	7.8	.0055	16.9	.0001	2.7	.1001
Abstraction-flexibility	0.3	.5989	0.6	.4343	1.2	.2742
Verbal intelligence and language function	11.1	.0010	4.6	.0322	0.3	.6163
Spatial organization	11.9	.0006	14.9	.0001	0.9	.3485
Verbal memory and learning	36.1	.0001	24.4	.0001	0.0	.9718
Visual memory	5.3	.0220	6.7	.0102	0.4	.5208
Speeded visual-motor processing and attention	19.1	.0001	8.2	.0045	0.4	.5334
Fine manual motor functions	24.1	.0001	33.8	.0001	2.7	.1013

**PT indicates previously treated; FE, first episode. For the mean contrast procedure, which evaluates selectivity of deficits, statistics (*df=*1,230) are for the contrast between the specific neuropsychological function and the mean of the other remaining functions (see text).*

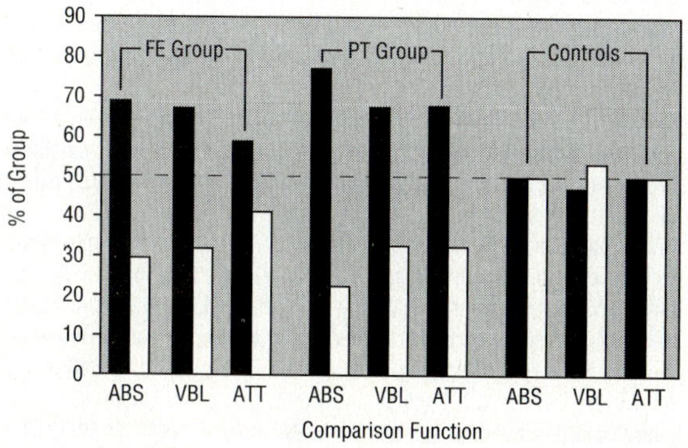

Figure 2. *Percent of subjects in each group who show worse verbal memory and learning (VBM) scores than those on the abstraction-flexibility (ABS), verbal intelligence and language function (VBL), and attention-vigilance (ATT) components of the neuropsychological battery. The verbal memory scores used in this analysis were standardized residual scores that reflect degree of deviation from the predicted VBM score, given the obtained score on the comparison function of interest (ie, ABS, VBL, or ATT), following the procedure recommended by Chapman and Chapman.[43] FE indicates first episode; PT, previously treated; closed bars, verbal memory worse; and open bars, verbal memory better.*

of disease with or without history of neuroleptic administration. Notably, on univariate contrasts, the PT group performed slightly worse than the FE group on speeded visual-motor processing and attention skills, fine manual motor functions, and visual memory. These are infrequently reported deficits in patients with schizophrenia. There were no significant differences in the functions that are most typically associated with schizophrenia (attention-vigilance, abstraction-flexibility, memory, verbal intelligence and language function). The better performance by patients with FE schizophrenia on the nonspecific functions may reflect adverse effects of medication history and chronicity in the PT group. In a study of medicated patients, tested 6 months after treatment onset, Bilder et al[49] found lower performance, but not verbal IQ, in patients with chronic schizophrenia compared with patients who had FE schizophrenia. Hoff and collaborators[23] did not observe significant differences in level of performance between patients with FE and chronic schizophrenia. Differences among the studies in contrasting patients with FE and chronic schizophrenia may be due to influence of medication, and to sample characteristics, selection of measures, and data analysis approaches.

Some characteristics of the present FE patient sample deserve comment, particularly the fact that these patients had been ill for a median of 2 years prior to enrollment. Patients whose onset was acute (35% of the sample) were treated within the first 6 months of illness. The remaining patients in the sample were treated when their symptoms reached the threshold for intervention. For some, the onset of illness was insidious and, with adequate family support, they were able to remain outside of the psychiatric system for a relatively long period. In other cases, the denial of illness by the patients and/or their families contributed to the time gap between the emergence of symptoms and steps to seek help. For these patients, symptoms were often attributed to external factors. A few patients of the paranoid type, mostly female, presented later in life than the majority which accounts for the skew in the distribution of age and age of onset. We do not believe that lack of access to treatment for the FE group was a significant factor in the interval from symptom onset to treatment. Although many patients in the sample were referred from inner-city neighborhoods, these patients were entitled to receive services at their community mental health center and local hospital which are among the most active in the city.

ONE POTENTIAL limitation of the present study is the fact that there were some differences in ethnicity distribution between the FE and other groups, ie, there was a predominance of black subjects in the FE group compared with the PT and control groups which had a majority of white subjects. However, we do not believe that this substantially influenced our findings for three reasons. First, parental education and occupation, the major socioeconomic status markers, did not differ between groups. Second, we performed analyses with and without statistical control for both ethnicity and parental education, which did not change the results. Third, the overall profile shape was similar for the FE and PT groups which differed in the ethnic composition, yet there was a pronounced difference in shape of neuropsychological profile between the PT and control groups which were ethnically comparable.

The presence of a selective deficit in verbal learning and memory in patients with schizophrenia, prominent early in the course of illness, is consistent with other lines of investigation that implicate the temporal-hippocampal system in the pathophysiology of schizophrenia.[57,58] The application of a comprehensive standardized battery has helped focus the search for regional involvement in schizophrenia to the relation between temporal lobe and memory functions. Well-defined experimental neurobehavioral probes combined with physiologic neuroimaging[59] should permit the dissection of components of memory processing that relate to specific regional dysfunction. The relation between such dysfunction and clinical features can guide the development of a neurobehavioral perspective on schizophrenia.

Accepted for publication April 22, 1993.

This research was supported by grants MH-42191, MH-00586, and MH-43880 from the National Institute of Mental Health, and by grants NS-14867 and NS-28813 from the National Institute of Neurological Disorders and Stroke, Bethesda, Md.

Larry Muenz, PhD, and Helena Kraemer, PhD, gave statistical advice.

A table containing means and SDs for individual tests in the neuropsychological battery is available from the authors on request.

Reprint requests to Neuropsychology Program, Department of Psychiatry, Dartmouth Medical School, Lebanon, NH 03756-0001 (Dr Saykin).

REFERENCES

1. Levin S, Yurgelun-Todd D, Craft S. Contributions of clinical neuropsychology to the study of schizophrenia. *J Abnorm Psychol.* 1989;98:341-356.
2. Kolb B, Whishaw IQ. Performance of schizophrenic patients on tests sensitive to left or right frontal, temporal, or parietal function in neurological patients. *J Nerv Ment Dis.* 1983;171:435-443.
3. Goldstein G. Neuropsychological heterogeneity in schizophrenia: a consideration of abstraction and problem-solving abilities. *Arch Clin Neuropsychol.* 1990; 5:251-264.
4. Goldberg E, Seidman L. Higher cortical functions in normals and in schizophrenia: a selective review. In: Steinhauer SR, Gruzelier JH, Zubin J, eds. *Handbook of Schizophrenia: Neuropsychology, Psychophysiology and Information Processing.* New York, NY: Elsevier Science Publishing Co Inc; 1991;5:553-597.
5. Robertson G, Taylor PJ. Laterality and psychosis: neuropsychological evidence. *Br Med Bull.* 1987;43:634-650.
6. Gruzelier J, Seymour K, Wilson L, Jolley A, Hirsch S. Impairments on neuropsychological tests of temporohippocampal and fronto-hippocampal functions and word fluency in remitting schizophrenia and affective disorders. *Arch Gen Psychiatry.* 1988;45:623-629.
7. Flor-Henry P, Fromm-Auch D, Schopflocher D. Neuropsychological dimensions in psychopathology. In: Flor-Henry P, Gruzelier J, eds. *Laterality and Psychopathology.* Amsterdam, the Netherlands: Elsevier Bio-Medical Press; 1983: 59-82.
8. Heaton RK, Baade LE, Johnson KL. Neuropsychological test results associated with psychiatric disorders in adults. *Psychol Bull.* 1978;85:141-162.
9. Saykin AJ, Gur RC, Gur RE, Mozley D, Mozley LH, Resnick SM, Kester DB, Stafiniak P. Neuropsychological function in schizophrenia: selective impairment in memory and learning. *Arch Gen Psychiatry.* 1991;48:618-624.
10. Mirsky AF, Duncan CC. Etiology and expression of schizophrenia: neurobiological and psychosocial factors. *Annu Rev Psychol.* 1986;37:291-319.
11. Asarnow RF, Steffy RA, MacCrimmon DJ, Cleghorn JM. An attentional assessment of foster children at risk for schizophrenia. *J Abnorm Psychol.* 1977;6: 267-275.
12. Weinberger DR, Berman KF, Zec RF. Physiologic dysfunction of dorsolateral prefrontal cortex in schizophrenia, I: regional cerebral blood flow evidence. *Arch Gen Psychiatry.* 1986;43:114-125.
13. Goldberg TE, Weinberger DR, Berman KF, Pliskin NH, Podd MH. Further evidence for dementia of the prefrontal type in schizophrenia? *Arch Gen Psychiatry.* 1987;44:1008-1014.
14. Andreasen NC, Grove W. The relationship between schizophrenic language, manic language and aphasia. In: Gruzelier J, Flor-Henry P, eds. *Hemisphere*

Asymmetries in Function Psychopathology. Amsterdam, the Netherlands: Elsevier/North Holland; 1979.

15. Barr WB, Bilder RM, Goldberg E, Kaplan E, Mukherjee S. The neuropsychology of schizophrenic speech. *J Commun Disord.* 1989;22:327-349.
16. Schwartz S. Is there a schizophrenic language? *Behav Brain Sci.* 1982;5:579-626.
17. Koh SD. Remembering of verbal materials by schizophrenic young adults. In: Schwartz S, ed. *Language and Cognition in Schizophrenia.* Hillsdale, NJ: Lawrence Erlbaum Assoicates Inc; 1978:55-99.
18. Calev A, Venables PH, Monk AF. Evidence for distinct verbal memory pathologies in severely and mildly disturbed schizophrenics. *Schizophr Bull.* 1983;9: 247-264.
19. Goldberg TE, Weinberger DR, Pliskin NH, Berman KF, Podd MH. Recall memory deficit in schizophrenia: a possible manifestation of prefrontal dysfunction. *Schizophr Res.* 1989;2:251-257.
20. Heaton RK, Crowley TJ. Effects of psychiatric disorders and their somatic treatment on neuropsychological test results. In: Filskov SB, Boll TJ, eds. *Handbook of Clinical Neuropsychology.* New York, NY: John Wiley & Sons Inc; 1981: 481-525.
21. Hoff AL, Riordan H, O'Donnell DW, DeLisi LE. Cross-sectional and longitudinal neuropsychological test findings in first episode schizophrenic patients: longitudinal perspectives on the pathophysiology of schizophrenia. *Schizophr Res.* 1991;5:183-210.
22. Hoff AL, Riordan H, O'Donnell DW, Stritzke P, Neale C, Boccio A, Anand A, DeLisi LE. Anomalous lateral sulcus asymmetry and cognitive function in first-episode schizophrenia. *Schizophr Bull.* 1992;18:257-272.
23. Hoff AL, Riordan H, O'Donnell DW, Morris L, DeLisi LE. Neuropsychological functioning in first episode schizophreniform patients. *Am J Psychiatry.* 1992; 149:898-903.
24. Sweeney JA, Haas GL, Keilp JG, Long M. Evaluation of the stability of neuropsychological functioning after acute episodes of schizophrenia: one-year follow-up study. *Psychiatry Res.* 1991;38:63-76.
25. Sweeney JA, Haas GL, Shuhua L. Neuropsychological and eye movement abnormalities in first-episode and chronic schizophrenia. *Schizophr Bull.* 1992; 18:283-293.
26. Bilder RM, Lipschutz-Broch L, Reiter G, Geisler S, Mayerhoff D, Lieberman JA. Neuropsychological deficits in the early course of first episode schizophrenia. *Schizophr Res.* 1991;5:198-199.
27. Bilder RM, Lipschutz-Broch L, Reiter G, Geisler S, Mayerhoff D, Lieberman JA. Intellectual deficits in first episode and chronic schizophrenia: evidence for deterioration? *Schizophr Bull.* 1992;18:437-438.
28. The Scottish Schizophrenia Research Group. The Scottish First Episode Schizophrenia Study, III: cognitive performance. *Br J Psychiatry.* 1987;150:338-340.
29. Spohn HE, Strauss ME. Relation of neuroleptic and anticholinergic medication to cognitive functions in schizophrenia. *J Abnorm Psychol.* 1989;98:367-380.
30. Cassens G, Inglis AK, Appelbaum PS, Gutheil TG. Neuroleptics: effects on neuropsychological function in chronic schizophrenic patients. *Schizophr Bull.* 1990; 16:477-499.
31. Medalia A, Gold J, Merriam A. The effects of neuroleptics on neuropsychological test results of schizophrenics. *Arch Clin Neuropsychol.* 1988;3:249-271.
32. Frith CD. Schizophrenia, memory and anticholinergic drugs. *J Abnorm Psychol.* 1984;98:341-356.
33. Baron JC, Marinot JL, Cambon H, Boulenger JP, Poirier MF, Caillard V, Blin J, Huret J, Loch C, Maziere B. Striatal dopamine receptor occupancy during and following withdrawal from neuroleptic treatment: correlative evaluation by positron emission tomography and plasma prolactin levels. *Psychopharmacology.* 1989;99:463-472.
34. Farde L, Nordstrom A, Wiesel F, Pauli S, Halldin C, Sedvall G. Positron emission tomographic analysis of central D1 and D2 dopamine receptor occupancy in patients treated with classical neuroleptics and clozapine. *Arch Gen Psychiatry.* 1992;49:538-544.
35. American Psychiatric Association, Committee on Nomenclature and Statistics. *Diagnostic and Statistical Manual of Mental Disorders, Revised Third Edition.* Washington, DC: American Psychiatric Association; 1987.
36. Shtasel DL, Gur RE, Gallacher F, Heimberg C, Cannon T, Gur RC. Phenomenology and functioning in first episode schizophrenia. *Schizophr Bull.* 1992; 18:449-462.
37. Shtasel DL, Gur RE, Mozley PD, Richards J, Taleff MM, Heimberg C, Gallacher F, Gur RC. Volunteers for biomedical research: recruitment and screening of normal controls. *Arch Gen Psychiatry.* 1991;48:1022-1025.
38. Gordon M. *Manual, Gordon Diagnostic System.* New York, NY: Gordon Diagnostic Systems Inc; 1986.
39. Wechsler D. *Wechsler Adult Intelligence Scale–Revised, Manual.* Cleveland, Ohio: The Psychological Corporation; 1981.
40. Saykin AJ, Robinson LJ, Stafiniak P, Kester DB, Gur RC, O'Connor MJ, Sperling MR. Neuropsychological effects of temporal lobectomy: acute changes in memory, language, and music. In: Bennett T, ed. *Neuropsychology of Epilepsy.* New York, NY: Plenum Press; 1992:263-290.
41. SAS Institute Inc. *SAS/STAT Software, Version 6.03.* Cary, NC: SAS Institute Inc; 1987.
42. Davidson M, Toporek J. *BMDP P4V (1988 Release).* Los Angeles, Calif: BMDP Statistical Software Inc; 1988.
43. Chapman LJ, Chapman JP. Strategies for resolving the heterogeneity of schizophrenics and their relatives using cognitive measures. *J Abnorm Psychol.* 1989; 98:357-366.
44. Nuechterlein KH. Signal detection in vigilance tasks and behavioral attributes among offspring of schizophrenic mothers and among hyperactive children. *J Abnorm Psychol.* 1983;92:4-28.
45. Nuechterlein KH. Childhood precursors of adult schizophrenia. *J Child Psychol Psychiatry.* 1986;27:133-144.
46. Erlenmeyer-Kimling L, Cornblatt B. Attentional measures in a study of children at high risk for schizophrenia. *J Psychiatr Res.* 1978;14:93-98.
47. Weinberger DR. Implications of normal development for the pathogenesis of schizophrenia. *Arch Gen Psychiatry.* 1987;44:660-669.
48. Saykin AJ, Shtasel D, Gur RE, Kester DB, Mozley LH, Gur RC. Neuropsychology in schizophrenia: state or trait? Presented at the American Psychiatric Association; May 6, 1992; Washington, DC.
49. Bilder RM, Mukherjee S, Rieder RO, Pandurangi AK. Symptomatic and neuropsychological components of defect states. *Schizophr Bull.* 1985;11:409-419.
50. Saykin AJ, Gur RC, Gur RE, Mozley D, Mozley LH, Resnick SE, Kester DB, Stafiniak P. Characterization of neuropsychological dysfunction in schizophrenia: relation to clinical subtypes and positive and negative features. *Arch Clin Neuropsychol.* 1990;5:211.
51. Goldberg TE, Ragland JD, Torrey EF, Gold JM, Bigelow LB, Weinberger DR. Neuropsychological assessment of monozygotic twins discordant for schizophrenia. *Arch Gen Psychiatry.* 1990;47:1066-1072.
52. DeLisi LE, Lieberman J, eds. Longitudinal perspectives on the pathophysiology of schizophrenia. *Schizophr Res.* 1991;5:183-210.
53. Bilder RM. Structure-function relations in schizophrenia: brain morphology and neuropsychology. In: Walker EF, Dworkin RH, Cornblatt BA, eds. *Progress in Experimental Personality and Psychopathology Research.* 1992;15:183-251.
54. Perlick D, Stastny P, Katz I, Mayer M, Mattis S. Memory deficits and anticholinergic levels in chronic schizophrenia. *Am J Psychiatry.* 1986;143:230-232.
55. Milner B. Psychological aspects of epilepsy and its neurosurgical management. *Adv Neurol.* 1975;8:299-321.
56. Squire LR, Butters N. *Neuropsychology of Memory.* New York, NY: Guilford Press; 1984.
57. Crow TJ. Temporal lobe asymmetries as the key to the etiology of schizophrenia. *Schizophr Bull.* 1990;16:433-443.
58. Gray JA, Feldon J, Rawlins JNP, Hemsley DR, Smith AD. The neuropsychology of schizophrenia. *Behav Brain Sci.* 1991;14:1-84.
59. Gur RC, Erwin RJ, Gur RE. Neurobehavioral probes for physiologic neuroimaging studies. *Arch Gen Psychiatry.* 1992;49:409-414.

ORIGINAL ARTICLE

Plasma Homovanillic Acid Levels in First-Episode Schizophrenia

Psychopathology and Treatment Response

Amy R. Koreen, MD; Jeffrey Lieberman, MD; Jose Alvir, DrPH; David Mayerhoff, MD; Antony Loebel, MD; Miranda Chakos, MD; Farooq Amin, MD; Thomas Cooper, MA

Objectives: To examine plasma homovanillic acid (pHVA) levels in first-episode schizophrenia, to compare pHVA levels in patients and controls, and to assess the association of pHVA levels with psychopathology and treatment response.

Methods: Forty-one patients entered the study, and pHVA levels were measured at baseline and on a weekly basis for up to 6 weeks of open standardized neuroleptic treatment. Psychopathology was evaluated with the Schedule for Affective Disorders and Schizophrenia, the Scale for Assessment of Negative Symptoms, and the Clinical Global Impressions scale. Ten healthy controls were used for comparison of baseline pHVA levels.

Results: No differences were observed between patients and controls. Baseline pHVA level was not associated with psychopathology but was associated with time to reach remission. Baseline pHVA levels and week-1 pHVA levels were higher in responders than nonresponders. Regardless of responsiveness, female participants had higher pHVA levels than male participants throughout the study. The pattern of pHVA levels with treatment was similar in all patients with a short-term rise initially and then a decrease toward baseline values.

Conclusions: These findings suggest that pHVA levels have prognostic significance for response and time to reach remission. Qualitative and quantitative differences between first-episode patients' pHVA levels and studies using a long-term, neuroleptic-exposed population suggest that changes occur with neuroleptic treatment or the progression of the illness.

(Arch Gen Psychiatry. 1994;51:132-138)

From Departments of Psychiatry, Hillside Hospital Division of Long Island Jewish Medical Center, Glen Oaks, NY (Drs Koreen, Lieberman, Alvir, Mayerhoff, Loebel, and Chakos), and Bronx (NY) Veterans Administration (Dr Amin); and the Analytical Psychopharmacology Division, Nathan Kline Research Center (Mr Cooper), and the New York Psychiatric Institute (Mr Cooper), New York, NY.

ABNORMALITIES OF dopamine (DA) neurotransmission within the central nervous system have been implicated as important factors in the pathogenesis of schizophrenia.[1] Preclinical[2-5] and subsequent clinical studies[6-21] have suggested that the measurement of plasma homovanillic acid (pHVA) concentrations may reflect brain DA activity, making it a potentially useful tool for studying the pathophysiology of schizophrenia and the pharmacological action of antipsychotic drugs.

Studies examining pHVA levels in patients with schizophrenia have shown that pHVA levels increase with short-term neuroleptic treatment,[9,11,12,16,22-24] decrease with long-term treatment,[6,7,9,18,19,24] and are correlated with psychopathology.[10,13,18-20,25-27] Basal- and neuroleptic-induced changes in pHVA levels have been shown, in some studies, to have prognostic significance, with responders having higher pretreatment levels of pHVA[6-8,10,21,28] and a greater decrease in pHVA levels with continuous neuroleptic treatment[8-10,17,18,29] compared with nonresponders. Of potential concern in interpreting the findings of these studies, which used heterogeneous but predominantly long-term schizophrenic subjects, are the effects of long-term neuroleptic treatment. To our knowledge, only two studies[6,26] included neuroleptic-naive

See Subjects and Methods on next page

SUBJECTS AND METHODS

SUBJECTS

Subjects were drawn from a larger, ongoing prospective study of psychobiology in first-episode schizophrenia, the design and procedures of which have been previously described.[33,34] In summary, the sample was drawn from patients admitted to the inpatient service of Hillside Hospital, Glen Oaks, NY. Eligible patients met research diagnostic criteria[35] for schizophrenia or schizoaffective disorder (mainly schizophrenia), were in the acute phase of their first episode of psychosis, and had no prior or not more than 12 weeks (lifetime) of neuroleptic treatment. Subjects were between 14 and 40 years of age and had no neuromedical contraindications to neuroleptic treatment and no known history of neurological or endocrine disorders. All patients and their families were advised of the study and signed informed consent forms. Healthy volunteers were recruited from the community as controls. Volunteers with significant neuromedical or psychiatric illness were excluded. After a standardized interview was conducted and laboratory and physical examinations were completed, only volunteers who were medically and psychiatrically healthy and who did not have a family history of psychiatric illness were included.

METHODS

Baseline psychopathology was evaluated using the following instruments: the Schedule for Affective Disorders and Schizophrenia (SADS),[36] the Scale for Assessment of Negative Symptoms (SANS),[37] and the Clinical Global Impression scale (CGI).[38] Baseline pHVA levels were obtained through serial sampling with an indwelling catheter between 8 and 9 AM at two different times under standardized conditions.[39] These included a low monoamine diet for 16 hours prior to testing, an overnight fast, and a restriction of activity and smoking prior to sampling.

After completion of baseline procedures, patients received open standardized treatment with fluphenazine hydrochloride (20 mg/d by mouth) for 6 weeks. If patients were nonresponsive, they received further treatment per the study treatment algorithm.[34] Patients underwent assessment by the SADS-Change+Psychotic Disorganization (C+PD), SANS, and CGI biweekly during short-term treatment and then monthly during stabilization and maintenance phases. Remission was defined as when patients received a CGI global improvement rating of 2 or less (much improved) and had a score of 3 or less on any of the critical psychotic items on the SADS-C+PD (severity of delusions, hallucinations, thought disorder, bizarre behavior). Plasma HVA samples were obtained weekly by venipuncture during short-term treatment under standardized conditions.[39] Plasma HVA samples were also obtained from the controls by indwelling catheters between 8 and 9 AM at two different times under standardized conditions,[40] which also included a low monoamine diet for 16 hours prior to testing, an overnight fast, and restriction of smoking and activity prior to sampling.

Plasma samples were assayed by gas chromatography mass spectroscopy using an adaptation of the method of Fri et al[40] for the quantification of spinal fluid HVA levels to the quantification of plasma HVA levels by one of us (T.C.). Using pentadeuterated HVA as an internal standard, 0.5 mL of plasma is diluted with aqueous buffer (pH 4.0) and extracted with ethyl acetate. The ethyl acetate is then placed in a tapered-tip glass tube containing 50-μL pentafluoropropionic anhydride and is taken to dryness via a cavum centrifuge at 40°C. Pentafluoropropionic anhydride and trifluoroethanol (4:1) are then added and incubated at 75°C for 15 minutes and are again taken to dryness. The residue is redissolved in 30-μL cyclohexane, and 1 μL is then injected into a capillary by gas chromatography mass spectroscopy using the cold trapping procedure with the mass spectroscopy operated in the electron impact mode using simultaneous ion monitoring of the molecular ion 410 mol wt+electron (m+e) and the internal standard molecular ion 415 m+e. Secondary ions at 283 m+e and 288 m+e are also monitored for additional specificity. In our study, the method has an intra-assay and interassay coefficient of variation of 4.2% and 6.1%, respectively. Standard curves are linear through 50 ng/mL, with negligible intercept and a lower limit of sensitivity of 0.5 ng/mL.[40] Storage time for the samples ranged from 45 to 160 weeks, with a mean±SD of 70.2±47.9 weeks.

STATISTICAL ANALYSES

Statistical analyses were performed using *t* tests and analysis of variance to compare pHVA levels. Pearson's Product-Moment Correlation coefficients were used to measure associations between baseline pHVA levels and clinical variables as determined by ratings on the SADS-C+PD, SANS, and CGI. Survival analysis using the Cox proportional hazards regression model was used to measure the association between pHVA levels and time to treatment response. A mean baseline pHVA value, which was derived from the pretreatment serial sample values, was used to compare the patients with the controls as well as baseline pHVA levels with pHVA levels in the subsequent short-term treatment weeks.

patients in their sample. Given the importance of the DA hypothesis, surprisingly few studies have compared pHVA levels in schizophrenics and controls. Those studies that have made this comparison show inconsistent results.[18,24,28] Most, but not all, of the studies that examined cerebrospinal fluid HVA levels found lower levels in schizophrenic patients compared with controls.[29-32]

This study compared pHVA concentrations in neuroleptic-naive patients with those in normal healthy volunteers and examined the relationship between pHVA levels and psychopathology, the pharmacological effects of DA antagonists on pHVA levels, and the prognostic significance of absolute and neuroleptic-induced changes in pHVA levels in a neuroleptic-naive schizophrenic population.

RESULTS

STUDY SAMPLE

Forty-one patients who met inclusion criteria and who entered the prospective study of psychobiology had baseline pHVA levels measured. The sample was 59% (24 patients) male, 46% (19) white, and had a mean±SD age at study entry of 24.3±4.9 years. Eighty-five percent (35 patients) met research diagnostic criteria for schizophrenia and 15% (six patients) for schizoaffective disorder, predominantly schizophrenia. Nineteen percent (eight patients) were high school graduates, and 63% (26 patients) had at least some college education. Social class level (determined by the Two-Factor Index of Social Position[41]) included 12% (five patients) from class 1 (upper), 20% (eight patients) from class 2 (upper-middle), 32% (13 patients) from class 3 (middle), 7% (three patients) from class 4 (lower-middle), and 29% (12 patients) from class 5 (lower). Eighty-eight percent of the sample had never been married.

The mean±SD age at onset of psychotic symptoms for the sample was 23.2±4.6 years. The mean±SD number of psychotic symptoms at baseline (defined by the mean of the SADS ratings on severity of delusions, hallucinations, thought disorder, and bizarre behavior) was 3.4±1.1. The mean±SD number of negative symptoms at baseline (defined by the SANS global items) was 2.8±0.9.

Twenty-eight patients (68%) had not received neuroleptic treatment and 13 (32%) had a mean of 13 days of prior lifetime neuroleptic exposure. Patients who had received prior treatment had a minimum of a 2-week washout period prior to baseline evaluation. Patients with prior exposure to neuroleptics did not differ from treatment-naive patients on baseline pHVA levels, age, gender, diagnosis, age of onset, negative symptoms, or Global Assessment Scale. These groups did differ on baseline positive symptoms, with a mean±SD of 3.6±0.9 among the treatment-naive group and of 2.8±1.2 among the treatment-exposed group (*t*=2.43; *df*=37; *P*=.02).

CONTROL SAMPLE

The control patients consisted of 19 healthy volunteers, of whom 13 were male and six were female. Their mean±SD age at study entry was 23.5±4.0 years. Forty-two percent of the control patients had some college education, and 58% were college graduates. Social class level included 30% from class 1 (upper), 20% from class 2 (upper-middle), 30% from class 3 (middle), and 20% from class 5 (lower). Sixty-eight percent of the control sample was white.

PLASMA HVA LEVEL AT BASELINE AND RELATIONSHIP TO CONTROLS

Analysis of variance was performed on baseline pHVA levels with diagnostic group (patients vs controls) and gender as the grouping factors. No differences were noted in baseline mean±SD group pHVA concentrations between patients (6.6±2.8 ng/mL) and controls (6.5±2.0 ng/mL) (F=.046; *df*=1, 56; *P*=.83). However, significant gender differences were noted for patients and controls (F=8.575; *df*=1, 56; *P*=.005). Male patients had baseline mean±SD pHVA concentrations of 5.7±1.1 ng/mL compared with 8.0±3.8 ng/mL in female patients. Male controls had baseline mean±SD pHVA concentrations of 6.3±1.9 ng/mL compared with 7.0±2.3 ng/mL in female controls. Baseline pHVA levels did not correlate with severity of psychopathology as measured by positive symptom items on the SADS-C+PD, the SANS, and the CGI for the group overall or when the patients were subgrouped into drug-naive and drug-exposed samples (**Table**).

RESPONSE

Of the 41 patients with baseline pHVA values, 30 had pHVA levels for at least the first 4 weeks of treatment. Fifty-seven percent (23 patients) met criteria for remission at week 4, while 43% (18 patients) did not meet cri-

Correlations (95% Confidence Intervals) Between Plasma Homovanillic Acid Levels and Psychopathology*

	Overall	Treatment-Naive	Treatment-Exposed
Symptoms			
Positive†	−0.13 (−0.42-0.19)	−0.27 (−0.59-0.13)	0.01 (−0.53-0.54)
Negative‡	−0.11 (−0.42-0.22)	−0.02 (−0.41-0.38)	−0.17 (−0.66-0.43)
CGI severity of illness	−0.07 (−0.39-0.27)	−0.11 (−0.49-0.31)	0.02 (−0.56-0.59)

**None of the correlations were significant at P≤.1. CGI indicates Clinical Global Impression scale.*

†Mean of critical psychotic items of the Schedule for Affective Disorders and Schizophrenia-Change+Psychotic Disorganization (severity of delusions, thought disorder, hallucinations, and bizarre behavior).

‡Mean of Scale for Assessment of Negative Symptoms global items.

teria. During follow-up (up to 3 years), 100% (17) of the females and 68% (16) of the males remitted.

The pattern of pHVA levels during the initial 4 weeks of neuroleptic treatment did not differ between drug-naive and drug-treated patients. Plasma HVA levels rose significantly by week 1 (t=4.46; df=34; P<.001) and decreased toward, but remained above, pretreatment values. By the fourth week, 21 (70%) of the patients still had levels above baseline. When patients were stratified by gender, significant differences were noted (**Figure 1**). Female participants had significantly higher pHVA measurements than male patients at baseline and at week 1 (F=10.01; df=1, 31; P=.002) and tended to have a greater short-term rise in pHVA levels (F=3.36; df=1, 31; P=.08).

Baseline and week-1 pHVA levels were associated with time to reach remission (risk ratio=1.14; 95% confidence interval [CI], 0.98 to 1.32; χ^2=3.01; df=1; P=.08, and risk ratio=1.07; 95% CI, 0.99 to 1.16; χ^2=2.73; df=1; P=.1, respectively) in survival analysis using the Cox proportional hazards model where gender was used as a stratifying variable. The greater the absolute pHVA value at baseline and at week 1, the shorter the time to remission. However, neither the change from baseline to week 1 nor the change from baseline to week 4 was predictive of time to remission. Plasma HVA concentrations at weeks 2 to 4 were not associated with time to reach treatment response. No correlations were found between absolute values or the change in pHVA levels and severity of or the change in psychopathology during treatment.

Mean±SD baseline pHVA levels tended to be higher in responders than nonresponders (7.0±3.9 ng/mL vs 5.7±0.9 ng/mL; $t_{\text{unequal variance}}$=1.24; df=15.9; P=.23), regardless of when they met remission criteria. Male responders at week 4 tended to have higher levels of pHVA throughout their neuroleptic treatment than the male nonresponders, but this was not true for females. The change in pHVA levels from baseline to week 1 was greater in responders (7.0 ng/mL to 10.4 ng/mL) than nonresponders (5.7 ng/mL to 7.0 ng/mL) (F=2.58; df=1, 25; P=.12; test for interaction between response group and time). Responders had slightly higher week 4 pHVA values than nonresponders. When response was stratified by gender, a similar pHVA pattern remained, with responders of the same sex having higher baseline values and a greater increase at week 1 (**Figure 2**). Male responders' pHVA levels remained higher than that of male nonresponders throughout treatment, whereas female responders had lower levels of pHVA during part of their treatment than female nonresponders.

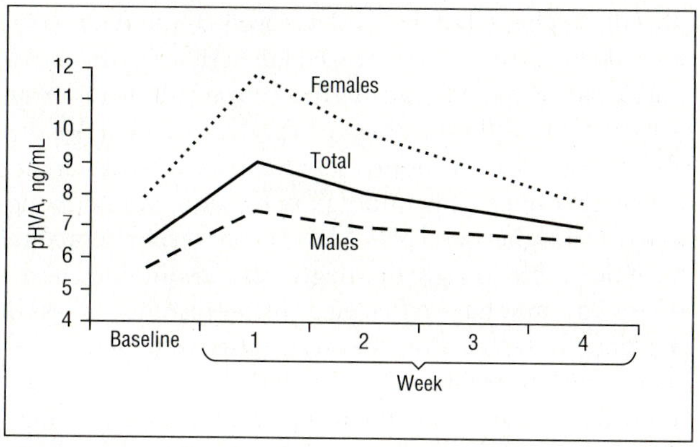

Figure 1. *The pattern of plasma homovanillic acid (pHVA) level during the initial 4 weeks of treatment. For males, n=19; females, n=11; and total, n=30.*

COMMENT

Although previous studies have examined the relationships between pHVA levels, psychopathology, prognosis, treatment response, and normal and schizophrenic subjects, this is, to our knowledge, the first systematic investigation of pHVA levels in treatment-naive schizophrenics studied in their first episode of psychosis. While some of our results are consistent with studies of pHVA levels in more long-term populations, some of our findings that differ suggest that a drug-naive first-episode population may be distinct.

Several studies have found a positive correlation between pHVA levels and psychopathology,[10,13,18-20,27-29] but we did not find such a correlation. Davis et al[1] have suggested that the reason some studies have not found this relationship may be because of methodological differences. Specifically, the negative studies did not have multiple pHVA samples for each time point, whereas the positive ones did. However, we used serial sampling for the baseline pHVA determinations and we did not find an association between pHVA level and severity of psychopathology. This could be due to differences in our patient sample from that of prior studies. It may be that long-term neuroleptic treatment, or a history of neuroleptic treatment, changes DA neuronal activity such that the correlation between psychopathology and pHVA level is enhanced. Clearly, pHVA level is influenced by multiple variables that may decrease the strength of the relationship between pHVA level and psychopathology. The peripheral nervous system is the primary contributor of pHVA, with only 17% of pHVA originating from the brain.[42] Furthermore, pHVA levels can fluctuate in the same individual in short intervals, which may be due to changes in HVA elimination (ie, renal clearance) as opposed to changes in HVA production.[43] Despite these limitations, the measurement of pHVA levels remains the most direct and accurate and least invasive method available to evaluate central DA activity. In fact, considering the many factors that affect pHVA measurements, which are unrelated to the central nervous system it is surprising that any results are replicated.

The pattern of pHVA levels in response to the patient's first treatment with antipsychotics was similar but not identical to the pattern of pHVA levels in patients who have previously received antipsychotic drugs. The short-

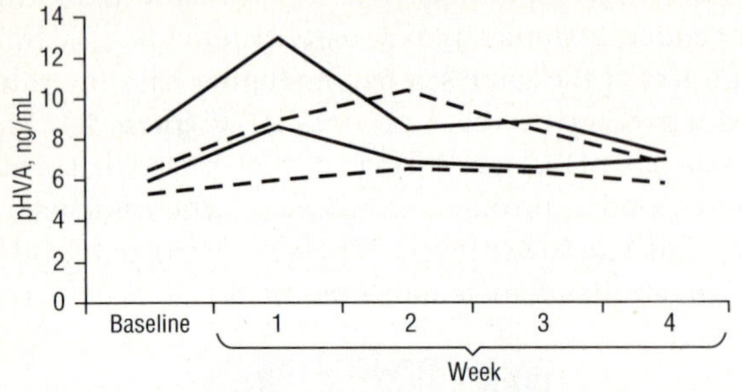

Figure 2. *Plasma homovanillic acid (pHVA) level and response during a 4-week period. The top two lines indicate female patients; bottom two, male patients; solid lines, patients who met remission criteria (Clinical Global Impression scale score ≤2, and Schedule for Affective Disorders and Schizophrenia score ≤3 on critical psychotic items) by week 4; and dashed lines, patients who did not remit by week 4. For male nonresponders, n=8; male responders, n=9; female nonresponders, n=4; and female responders, n=6.*

term increase in pHVA level is consistent with acute blockade of postsynaptic DA receptors and consequent presynaptic synthesis and release of DA. The decrease with long-term treatment is consistent with the development of tolerance to the short-term rise in DA release and turnover and possibly the development of depolarization blockade, as has been described previously.[44] However, the magnitude of these changes is not the same in first-episode patients as in long-term patients. The magnitude of the initial increase in the patients at week 1 is 50% overall (40% in males, 60% in females), 50% in responders (both sexes), and 30% in nonresponders (20% in males, 41% in females), whereas other studies[11,19] have noted less of a short-term increase or even have noted a decrease from baseline in responders.[7-9,26,27] With continued treatment, pHVA levels decreased toward, but never went below, baseline values in our sample, whereas most other studies have found that pHVA levels decreased significantly with treatment to below pretreatment levels. Drug-naive neurons may, in fact, be more responsive to the initial blockade by antipsychotics, causing a greater increase in pHVA levels. In this regard, the pattern of pHVA level response to neuroleptic treatment in our sample is consistent with preclinical studies,[2-4] more so than the pHVA level pattern seen in long-term patients. In addition, drug-naive DA neurons in first-episode patients may have been so pathophysiologically disturbed that it may have taken them longer to develop depolarization blockade and to stabilize. In the latter case, we would expect pHVA levels to fall below pretreatment values with continued treatment beyond our 4-week follow-up.

As other studies have shown,[6-8,10,21,25] we found that pHVA levels tended to differentiate responders from nonresponders and tended to have prognostic significance. Baseline and week-1 pHVA levels tended to be higher in patients who reached remission faster and in patients who responded, although these findings did not reach a level of significance. However, we did not find a greater decrease in pHVA levels with continuous treatment in responders, whereas other studies[8-10,17,18,26] have found a greater decrease. Although baseline pHVA levels and the pattern of response were different between responders and nonresponders, there were no differences between pHVA levels at specific times during treatment (apart from week 1). Thus, neither the magnitude of change (apart from baseline to week 1) nor the absolute pHVA level during subsequent weeks of treatment differentiated responders from nonresponders.

An important and significant finding that was observed in the patients was gender differences. Females had significantly higher baseline and week-1 values and had a greater short-term rise in values than did males. Many studies did not find a gender difference or did not analyze males and females separately, whereas others used only male subjects so that sex would not be a confounding variable.[10,13,17,21,27] Given that female schizophrenics tended to have a more benign course overall, any observed biochemical gender difference is of great importance.

In comparing baseline pHVA levels in patients and controls, no differences were found. Other studies found higher pHVA levels,[18] lower levels,[28] or no overall difference between schizophrenic patients and controls.[24] To our knowledge, only the study by Davidson and Davis[26] accounted for gender. All patients in previous studies had prior neuroleptic treatment. It remains unclear how long it takes neurons to normalize following neuroleptic withdrawal. Thus, the length of the drug-free period and the amount of previous neuroleptic exposure may be important factors accounting for some of the differences in the studies.

Finally, our criteria for response differed from prior studies because the criteria were more stringent in requiring a greater level of response and the sustained remission of psychopathology. These stringent criteria were largely due to our expectation that first-episode patients would be more responsive to antipsychotic treatment than a long-term population.

Current forms of the DA hypothesis suggest that schizophrenia is characterized by decreased DA activity in the mesocortical area and increased DA activity in the mesolimbic pathways.[1] We can interpret our results in two ways to explain the difference between pretreatment pHVA levels in responders and nonresponders based on a difference in degree of hyperdopaminergic or hypodopaminergic activity. The higher basal pHVA level in our responders could have been due to a greater degree of mesolimbic DA activity. This may have reflected a greater responsiveness or plasticity of DA neurons in these patients, which is consistent with the higher short-term rise in DA with neuroleptic treatment seen in the responders relative to nonresponders. Alternatively, nonresponders may have had a greater degree of hypodopaminergic activity than nonresponders, resulting in lower basal pHVA levels.

A number of limitations in this study need to be addressed and at the same time suggest areas for future research. First, our analysis of the difference between patients and controls was limited by the small number of female controls. Given the observed gender difference in pHVA levels and the observed clinical difference between male and female participants, future studies need to control for and stratify by gender. Second, although repeated sampling of pHVA levels was done at baseline, pHVA levels during treatment represented single samples. Considering intraindividual variability of pHVA levels, repeated sampling throughout the study may be necessary when evaluating pHVA levels in this population. Finally, even though most studies only followed up patients for a 6-week period, it may be especially important to evaluate pHVA levels in first-episode patients over a longer period. Six weeks may not have been long enough to detect a continued decrease in pHVA levels to below baseline levels. We should also comment that although our pHVA levels are lower than those in many other published studies,[8,9,11,17,23,28,29] they are certainly comparable with others.[45-48] The low values do not appear to be due to any methodological factors. The assay and blood-collecting procedures are valid, and after reassaying 13 samples, the results were comparable. Storage time was relatively long, but there was no correlation between storage time and mean pHVA level (r=.09).

In summary, our results in a first-episode schizophrenic population are partially consistent with other studies that have examined pHVA levels in long-term schizophrenic patients who have received prior neuroleptic treatment. Pretreatment pHVA levels were not different between controls and patients but tended to differentiate responders from nonresponders and were significantly different between male and female patients. Responders had higher basal pHVA levels and a greater short-term rise with treatment and pHVA levels at baseline and at week 1 predicted time to reach remission. Female patients had significantly higher pHVA levels than male patients and had a greater short-term rise with treatment. No correlations were found between psychopathology and pHVA level, and the pattern of pHVA level response differed from prior reports in that pHVA levels rose more quickly with short-term treatment and never went below pretreatment values in our patients.

Further studies using a drug-naive population are needed to broaden our understanding of DA activity prior to treatment, as well as to help elucidate the changes that occur with long-term treatment and with repeated trials of neuroleptics.

Accepted for publication November 17, 1992.

This study was supported by grant MH 41646 from the National Institute of Mental Health, Rockville, Md, by Research Scientist Development Award MH00537 (Dr Lieberman), and by the Mental Health Clinical Research Center for the Study of Schizophrenia award MH41960.

We are grateful to Sabina Meyer, Judy Dunlop, RN, Rosalind Felber, and Greta Schimmel who assisted in data collection; the Lowenstein III staff who provided inpatient care to study subjects; and Maureen Ward for manuscript preparation.

Reprint requests to Director of Research Psychiatry, Hillside Hospital Division of Long Island Jewish Medical Center, PO Box 38, Glen Oaks, NY 11004 (Dr Lieberman).

REFERENCES

1. Davis KL, Kann RS, Ko G, Davidson M. Dopamine in schizophrenia: a review and reconceptualization. *Am J Psychiatry.* 1991;148:1474-1486.
2. Bacopoulus NG, Hattox SE, Roth RH. 3,4-Dihydroxyphenylactic acid and homovanillic acid in rat plasma: possible indicators of central dopaminergic activity. *Eur J Pharmacol.* 1979;56:225-236.
3. Kendler KS, Heninger GR, Roth RH. Influence of dopamine agonists on plasma and brain levels of homovanillic acid. *Life Sci.* 1982;30:2063-2069.
4. Kendler KS, Davis KL. Acute and chronic effects of neuroleptic drugs on plasma and brain homovanillic acid in the rat. *Psychiatry Res.* 1984;13:51-58.
5. Kopin IJ, Bankiewicz KS, Harvey-White J. Assessment of brain dopamine metabolism from plasma HVA and MHPG during debrisoquin treatment: validation in monkeys treated with MPTP. *Neuropsychopharmacology.* 1988;2:119-125.
6. Bowers MB, Swigar ME, Jatlow PI, Hoffman FJ. Plasma catecholamine metabolites and treatment response at neuroleptic steady state. *Biol Psychiatry.* 1984;25:734-738.
7. Bowers MB, Swigar ME, Jatlow PI, Goicoechen N. Plasma catecholamine metabolites and early response to haloperidol. *J Clin Psychiatry.* 1984;45:248-251.
8. Chang W, Chen T, Lin S, Lung F, Lin W, Hu W, Yeh E. Plasma catecholamine metabolites in schizophrenics: evidence for the two-subtype concept. *Biol Psychiatry.* 1990;27:510-518.
9. Chang W, Chen T, Lee C, Hung J, Hu W, Yeh E. Plasma homovanillic acid levels and subtyping of schizophrenia. *Psychiatry Res.* 1988;23:239-244.
10. Davidson M, Kahn R, Knott P, Kaminsky R, Cooper M, DuMont K, Aptu S, Davis K. Effects of neuroleptic treatment on symptoms of schizophrenia and plasma homovanillic acid concentrations. *Arch Gen Psychiatry.* 1991;48:910-913.
11. Davidson M, Losonczy M, Mohs R, Lester J, Powchik P, Fried L, Davis B, Mykytyn M, Davis K. Effects of debrisoquin and haloperidol on plasma homovanillic acid concentrations in schizophrenic patients. *Neuropsychopharmacology.* 1987;1:17-23.
12. Davila R, Manero E, Zumarraga M, Anclia I, Schweitzer J, Friedhoff A. Plasma homovanillic acid as a predictor of response to neuroleptics. *Arch Gen Psychiatry.* 1988;45:564-567.
13. Davis KL, Davidson M, Mohs RC, Kendler KS, Davis BM, Johns CA, DeNigris Y, Horveth TB. Plasma homovanillic acid concentration and the severity of schizophrenic illness. *Science.* 1985;29:1601-1602.
14. Kaminski R, Powchik P, Warne P, Goldstein M, McQueeney R, Davidson M. Measurement of homovanillic acid concentrations in schizophrenic patients. *Prog Neuropsychopharmacol Biol Psychiatry.* 1990;14:271-287.
15. Kirsch DG, Jaskiw G, Linnoila M, Weinberger DR, Wyatt RJ. Plasma amino metabolites before and after withdrawal from neuroleptic treatment in chronic schizophrenic inpatients. *Psychiatry Res.* 1988;25:233-242.
16. Konicki PE, Owen RR, Litman RE, Pickar D. The acute effects of central and peripheral acting dopamine antagonists on plasma HVA in schizophrenic patients. *Life Sci.* 1991;48:1411-1416.
17. Petrie EC, Faustman WO, Moses JA, Lombrozo L, Csernansky JG. Correlates of rapid neuroleptic response in male patients with schizophrenia. *Psychiatry Res.* 1990;33:171-177.
18. Pickar D, Labarca R, Linnoila M, Roy A, Hommer D, Everett D, Paul S. Neuroleptic-induced decrease in plasma homovanillic acid and antipsychotic activity in schizophrenic patients. *Science.* 1984;25:954-957.
19. Pickar D, Labarca R, Doran AR, Wolkowitz OM, Roy A, Breier A, Linnoila M, Paul S. Longitudinal measurement of plasma homovanillic acid levels in schizophrenic patients. *Arch Gen Psychiatry.* 1986;43:669-676.
20. Sharma R, Javaid JI, Janicak P, Faull K, Comaty J, Davis JM. Plasma and CSF

HVA before and after pharmacological treatment. *Psychiatry Res.* 1989;28:97-104.

21. Van Putten T, Marder SR, Aravagiri M, Chabert N, Mintz J. Plasma homovanillic acid as a predictor of response to fluphenazine treatment. *Psychopharmacol Bull.* 1989;1:89-91.
22. Bjerkenstedt L, Gullberg B, Harnryd C, Sedvall G. Monoamine metabolite levels in cerebrospinal fluid of psychotic women treated with melpesone or thiothixene. *Arch Psychiatr Nervenkr.* 1977;224:107-118.
23. Davila R, Zumarraga M, Perca K, Andia I, Friedhoff AJ. Elevation of plasma homovanillic acid level can be detected within four hours after initiation of haloperidol treatment. *Arch Gen Psychiatry.* 1987;44:837-838.
24. Pickar D, Doran AR, Wolkowitz OM, Labarca R, Breier A, Paul SM. Studies of plasma homovanillic acid in schizophrenia: effects of neuroleptic treatment and evidence for a diurnal rhythm. *New Trends Exp Clin Psychiatry.* 1985;1:187-200.
25. Davidson M, Kahn RS, Powchik P, Warne P, Losonczy MF, Kaminsky R, Aptu S, Jaff S, Davis KL. Changes in plasma homovanillic acid concentrations in schizophrenic patients following neuroleptic discontinuation. *Arch Gen Psychiatry.* 1991;48:73-76.
26. Davidson M, Davis KL. A comparison of plasma homovanillic acid concentrations in schizophrenic patients and normal controls. *Arch Gen Psychiatry.* 1988; 45:561-563.
27. Pickar D, Breier A, Hsiao JK, Doran AR, Wolkowitz OM, Pato CN, Konicki PE, Potter WZ. Cerebrospinal fluid and plasma monoamine metabolites and their relation to psychosis. *Arch Gen Psychiatry.* 1990;47:641-648.
28. Glazer WM, Bowers MB, Charney DS, Heninger GR. The effects of neuroleptic discontinuation on psychopathology, involuntary movements, and biochemical measures in patients with persistant tardive dyskinesia. *Biol Psychiatry.* 1989; 26:224-233.
29. Alfredsson G, Wiesel F. Relationships between clinical effects and monoamine metabolites and amino acids in sulpiride-treated schizophrenic patients. *Psychopharmacology.* 1990;101:324-331.
30. Lindstrom LH. Low HVA and normal 5-HIAA CSF levels in drug-free schizophrenic patients compared to healthy volunteers: correlations to symptomatology and family history. *Psychiatry Res.* 1985;14:265-273.
31. Bowers MB Jr. Central dopamine turnover in schizophrenic syndromes. *Arch Gen Psychiatry.* 1974;31:52-54.
32. Karoum F, Karson CN, Bigelow LB, Lawson WB, Wyatt RJ. Preliminary evidence of reduced combined output of dopamine and its metabolites in chronic schizophrenia. *Arch Gen Psychiatry.* 1987;44:604-607.
33. Lieberman J, Jody D, Ashtari M, Levy D, Bogarts B, Cooper T, Novacenko H, Borenstein M. Brain morphology, dopamine, and eye tracking in first-episode schizophrenia. *Arch Gen Psychiatry.* In press.
34. Lieberman J, Jody D, Geisler S, Syzmanski S, Alvir J, Woerner M. Time course and biological predictors of treatment response in first-episode schizophrenia. *Arch Gen Psychiatry.* In press.
35. Spitzer RL, Endicott J, Robbins E. *Research Diagnostic Criteria (RDC) for a Selected Group of Functional Disorders.* New York, NY: Biometrics Research; 1977.
36. Endicott J, Spitzer RL. A diagnostic interview: the Schedule for Affective Disorders and Schizophrenia. *Arch Gen Psychiatry.* 1978;35:837-844.
37. Andreasen NC. *The Scale for the Assessment of Negative Symptoms in Schizophrenia.* Iowa City: University of Iowa Press; 1983.
38. Guy Wed. *ECDEU Assessment Manual for Psychopharmacology, Revised.* Washington, DC: Dept of Health, Education, and Welfare; 1976:217-222. Publication ADM 76-338.
39. Jody D, Lieberman JA, Geisler S, Vital-Herne J, Alvir JMJ, Walsleben J, Woerner M. Behavioral response to methylphenidate and treatment outcome in first-episode schizophrenia. *Psychopharmacol Bull.* 1990;26:224-230.
40. Fri C-G, Frits-Axel W, Sedvall G. Simultaneous quantification of homovanillic acid and 5-hydroxyindoleacetic acid in cerebrospinal fluid by mass fragmentography. *Life Sci.* 1974;14:2469-2480.
41. Hollingshead AB, Redlich FC. *Social Class and Mental Illness.* New York, NY: John Wiley & Sons Inc; 1958.
42. Lambert GW, Eisenhofer G, Cox HS, Horne M, Kaliff V, Kelly M, Jennings GL, Esker MD. Direct determination of homovanillic acid release from the human brain: an indicator of central dopaminergic activity. *Life Sci.* 1991;49:1061-1072.
43. Amin F, Davidson M, Davis KL. Homovanillic acid measurement in clinical research: a review of methodology. *Schizophr Bull.* 1991;18:123-148.
44. Bunney BS, Grace AA. Acute and chronic haloperidol treatment: comparison of effects on nigral dopaminergic cell activity. *Life Sci.* 1978;23:1715-1728.
45. Contretas SA, Maas JW, Seleshi E, Bowden CL. Urine and plasma levels of dopamine metabolites in response to apomorphine and neuroleptics in schizophrenia. *Biochem Psychol.* 1988;24:815-818.
46. Sharma RP, Javaid J, Pandey G, Easton M, Davis J. Pharmacological effects of methylphenidate on plasma homovanillic acid and growth hormone. *Psychol Res.* 1990;32:9-17.
47. Davis BA, Dawson B, Boulton AA, Yu PH, Durden DA. Investigation of some biological trait markers in migraine: deutrated tyramine challenge test, monoamine oxidase, phenolsulfotransferase and plasma and urinary biogenic amine and acid metabolite levels. *Headache.* 1987;27:384-389.
48. Naber D, Pickar D, Davis GC, Cohen RM, Jinerson DC, Elchisak MA, Defraites EG, Kalin NH, Risch SC, Buchsbaum MS. Naloxone effects on β-endorphin, cortisol, prolactin, growth hormone, HVA and MHPG in plasma of normal volunteers. *Psychopharmacology.* 1981;74:125-128.

NEWS AND VIEWS

Assessing the Validity of an Animal Model of Deficient Sensorimotor Gating in Schizophrenic Patients

Neal R. Swerdlow, MD, PhD; David L. Braff, MD; Navid Taaid; Mark A. Geyer, PhD

Psychiatric researchers need specific animal models to better understand the neurobiology of schizophrenia. Prepulse inhibition (PPI), the reduction in startle produced by a prepulse stimulus, is diminished in schizophrenic patients. Theoretically, deficient PPI in schizophrenic patients reflects a loss of sensorimotor gating that may lead to sensory flooding and cognitive fragmentation. In rats, PPI is disrupted by systemic administration of dopamine agonists or by manipulations of neural circuitry linking the limbic cortex, striatum, pallidum, and pontine reticular formation. This loss of PPI in rats may be a useful model for studying the neurobiology of impaired sensorimotor gating in schizophrenic patients. We assessed the face, predictive, and construct validity of this animal model. *Face validity* was supported: stimulus manipulations produced parallel changes in PPI in humans and rats, and the dopamine agonist apomorphine disrupted PPI in rats, mimicking PPI deficits in schizophrenics. *Predictive validity* was supported: the ability of antipsychotics to restore PPI in apomorphine-treated rats correlated with clinical antipsychotic potency (r_s=.991) and D_2-receptor affinity (r_s=.893). Antipsychotics that restore PPI in apomorphine-treated rats include "typical" antipsychotics and the "atypical" antipsychotic clozapine. *Construct validity* was supported: PPI was disrupted in rats when dopamine was infused into the nucleus accumbens; this effect was blocked by haloperidol. The loss of PPI in dopamine-activated rats may be a valid animal model of sensorimotor gating deficits in schizophrenic patients. This model may help us understand the neurobiology of cognitive deficits in schizophrenic patients.

(Arch Gen Psychiatry. 1994;51:139-154)

Psychiatric researchers have searched for animal models of schizophrenia to better understand the neurobiology of this group of disorders. Since it is unlikely that a "model" of the entire schizophrenic syndrome can be created, much energy has been devoted to identifying models of specific dysfunctions that characterize schizophrenic patients. Schizophrenic patients have a dramatic deficit in the normal inhibition of the startle reflex that occurs when the startling stimulus is preceded by a weak prestimulus.[1-3] This loss of normal "prepulse inhibition" (PPI) may reflect deficient sensorimotor gating[2] that underlies sensory flooding and cognitive fragmentation in these patients.[4] The neural basis of deficient sensorimotor gating[5] is strikingly consistent with findings from neuroimaging[6-8] and neuropathological studies[9-14] in schizophrenic patients that have identified abnormalities within limbic cortico-striato-pallido-thalamic circuitry. By elucidating the neural substrates of impaired PPI, it might be possible to obtain critical information about the contribution of specific brain abnormalities to sensorimotor gating deficits in schizophrenic patients.

Thus, a valid animal model of deficient PPI in schizophrenic patients might be criti-

From the Department of Psychiatry, University of California, San Diego School of Medicine, La Jolla.

cally important for understanding the probable neural substrates of impaired sensorimotor gating in schizophrenia. Prepulse inhibition deficits are produced in rats treated with dopamine agonists such as apomorphine hydrochloride,[15,16] amphetamine,[17,18] or the D_2 agonist quinpirole but not in rats treated with D_1 agonists.[19] This loss of PPI in dopamine-stimulated rats may satisfy three levels of validity as an animal model of sensorimotor gating deficits in schizophrenic patients. First, this loss of PPI in dopamine-stimulated rats may be an animal model with *face validity* for the sensorimotor gating deficits exhibited by schizophrenic patients, since PPI is measured in rats and humans using near-identical stimulus parameters to yield similar response characteristics. Second, the loss of PPI in dopamine-stimulated rats may be an animal model with *predictive validity*, since the apomorphine-induced disruption of PPI in rats is reversed by antipsychotic agents, including drugs that block D_2 receptors, but not by the D_1 antagonist SCH 23390[16]; this apomorphine-induced disruption is not reversed by drugs with clinical antidepressant or anxiolytic properties.[20] Third, the loss of PPI in rats models a psychophysiological construct for the pathophysiology of schizophrenia, ie, impaired sensorimotor gating.[4] In addition, PPI appears to be modulated by neural activity in limbic and mesolimbic cortico-striato-pallido-thalamic circuitry implicated in the pathophysiology of schizophrenia and in the therapeutic mechanisms of antipsychotic agents. Prepulse inhibition can be predictably disrupted or restored in rats with pharmacologic and surgical manipulations of the hippocampus (HPC),[21] the nucleus accumbens (NAC),[22] and the subpallidum.[23] These findings suggest that deficient PPI in these rats may be an animal model with *construct validity* in both psychophysiological and neurochemical domains for sensorimotor gating deficits in schizophrenic patients. Importantly, dopamine-stimulated PPI deficits in rats are clearly not an animal model of schizophrenia per se but may provide a model of *sensorimotor gating deficits* in schizophrenic patients that has face, predictive, and construct validity.

The present studies examine the validity of this animal model. First, to assess the face validity of this model, PPI was measured in humans and rats using near-identical stimulus parameters. These parameters produced strikingly parallel patterns of startle and prepulse latency-modulation and amplitude-modulation across species. Using this paradigm, PPI was disrupted in an orderly and dose-dependent fashion by apomorphine. Second, the predictive value of this model was tested by examining the ability of a wide range of antipsychotic agents to restore PPI in apomorphine-treated rats. The potency of antipsychotic agents, including clozapine, to prevent the PPI-disruptive effects of apomorphine correlate significantly with their clinical potency and D_2 dopamine receptor affinity. Finally, the construct validity of this animal model was studied by measuring PPI in rats after intra-NAC dopamine infusion. Prepulse inhibition was disrupted by intra-NAC dopamine infusion. This effect was prevented by pretreatment with haloperidol. These findings suggest that dopamine-mediated PPI deficits in rats is an animal model with face, predictive, and construct validity for sensorimotor gating deficits in schizophrenic patients. The validity of this model is important since it allows us to use animals to study parametric manipulations to increase the sensitivity of our measures (face validity), to test putative novel antipsychotic compounds (predictive validity), and to identify regions of interest for neuroimaging and postmortem assessment in the brains of schizophrenic patients (construct validity).

SUBJECTS, MATERIALS, AND METHODS

Humans

The 13 subjects (seven women and six men with a mean age of 33.6 years; age range, 25 to 47 years) were staff members at the University of California, San Diego Medical Center, La Jolla. These subjects had no known neurologic or psychiatric illness. Testing occurred in the active (light) circadian phase. Hearing was screened using a screening audiometer (Audiometrics, Interacoustics, Assens, Denmark); no subjects met exclusion criteria of impairment at 40 dB(A) (1000 Hz). The eyeblink component of startle was assessed using electromyographic measurements of orbicularis oculi, as described elsewhere.[3] Stimuli, delivered through headphones (Telephonics, TDH-39-P, Maico, Minneapolis, Minn) with 70-dB(A) background white noise, included a startle pulse (118-dB[A], 40-millisecond white noise burst) presented either alone (P-Alone) or 100 milliseconds after a prepulse (20-millisecond white noise burst) that was either 2, 4, 8, or 16 dB(A) above the background noise level (PP2, PP4, PP8, or PP16, respectively).

Rats

The 238 male Sprague-Dawley rats (weighing between 300 and 400 g; Harlan, Indianapolis, Ind) were housed in pairs, handled daily, and maintained on a reversed 12 hours light/12 hours dark schedule (lights off at 7 AM) with food and water provided ad libitum.

Testing occurred between 9 AM and 3 PM. Some rats had received one subcutaneous injection of placebo or a behaviorally inert dose of an active compound during tests in activity monitors but had been free of drugs for at least 2 weeks before use in the present study.

Apparatus

Each startle chamber (SR-LAB, San Diego Instruments, San Diego, Calif) consisted of an acrylic plastic (Plexiglas) cylinder 8.2 cm in diameter resting on a 12.5×25.5-cm acrylic plastic frame in a ventilated enclosure. Acoustic noise bursts were presented via a speaker mounted 24 cm above the rat.

Statistical Analysis

Several startle variables were analyzed by mixed-design analyses of variance (ANOVAs); specific variables and analyses are described for each experiment. In all cases, $\alpha=.05$.

EXPERIMENT 1

Face Validity: Are the Eliciting Stimuli and Response Patterns of PPI Similar Across Species?

Previous studies have demonstrated that the reduction in startle amplitude caused by an acoustic prepulse increases with prepulse intensity.[24-26] In the present study, PPI was measured in rats and humans using identical startle stimuli and prepulse intensities over a similar range of 2 to 17 dB above background noise. The ability of apomorphine to disrupt PPI in rats using this range of startle and prepulse stimuli was also examined.

Methods

Humans. Test sessions included six trial types (P-Alone, PP2, PP4, PP8, PP16, and no stimulus [NOSTIM]) repeated 12 times in pseudorandom order (72 total trials). Intertrial intervals varied from 15 to 45 seconds (average, 30 seconds). Prepulse inhibition was defined as the percentage of reduction in startle amplitude in the presence of the prepulse compared with the amplitude in the absence of the prepulse (100 − [100 × amplitude on prepulse trial/amplitude on P-Alone trial]). Thus, a high percentage score indicated a high degree of PPI, while a low percentage score indicated less PPI. Prepulse inhibition and startle latency (time from pulse to peak response) were analyzed with a two-way ANOVA with repeated measures on trial type. One subject was excluded from analysis of startle latency because her level of PPI (100% for all prepulse types) precluded an accurate assessment of reflex latency.

Rats. Thirty-four rats were divided into four groups that received subcutaneous injections of 0, 0.1, 0.2, or 0.4 mg/kg of apomorphine hydrochloride (in saline with 0.1 mg/mL of ascorbic acid; n=9, 9, 8, and 8, respectively) immediately before the startle session. After apomorphine treatment, rats were placed in a startle chamber for a 5-minute acclimation period with a 65-dB(A) background noise. Rats were then exposed to a startle pulse (118 dB[A], 40-millisecond white noise burst) either P-Alone or 100 milliseconds after a prepulse (20-millisecond white noise burst) that was 2, 3.5, 5, 6.5, 8, 12, or 17 dB(A) above the background noise level (PP2, PP3.5, PP5, PP6.5, PP8, PP12, or PP17, respectively). Each startle session included eight trial types (P-Alone, PP2, PP3.5, PP5, PP6.5, PP8, PP12, and PP17) repeated eight times in pseudorandom order (64 total trials). Intertrial intervals for all rat studies varied from 11 to 19 seconds (average, 15 seconds). P-Alone amplitude, startle latency (time from pulse to peak response), and PPI were analyzed using a two-way ANOVA with repeated measures on trial type (within-subject variable) and apomorphine dose (between-subject variable).

Results of Experiment 1

Results of experiment 1 are seen in **Figure 1**. Analysis revealed a significant effect of prepulse intensity on PPI in humans ($F=14.76$; *df*, 3,36) and in rats ($F=17.74$; *df*, 6,180; Figure 1, top left). Inspection of the results revealed that the "threshold" sensitivity for reduction of startle amplitude occurred with prepulse intensities approximately 4 dB above background noise in both species, with a less precipitous change occurring at higher prepulse intensities. In humans, startle latency was significantly decreased ("latency facilitation") on PP2 and PP4 trials compared with P-Alone trials. The ANOVA revealed a significant effect of trial type ($F=3.78$; *df*, 2,24); post hoc analysis revealed significant latency facilitation for both PP2 (Student's $t=3.34$; *df*, 11) and PP4 (Student's $t=3.48$; *df*, 11) trials compared with P-Alone trials (Figure 1, bottom left). In rats, startle latency was decreased on PP2 trials compared with P-Alone trials. This latency facilitation was not disrupted by apomorphine. There was a significant effect of trial type ($F=5.79$; *df*, 1,30), no effect of apomorphine ($F<1$), and no trial type × apomorphine interaction ($F<1$). In rats, apomorphine did not change P-Alone amplitude significantly ($F<1$) (Figure 1, top center), but significantly disrupted PPI (Figure 1, bottom center). The ANOVA revealed a significant effect of apomorphine on PPI ($F=20.87$; *df*, 3,30) and a near-significant trial type × apomorphine interaction ($F=1.55$; *df*, 18,180; $P<.08$). Apomorphine reduced PPI to near-zero levels at the two higher doses. Post hoc analyses revealed that the lowest dose of apomorphine hydrochloride (0.1 mg/kg) significantly decreased PPI on PP6.5 and PP8 trials (Student's $t=2.35$ and 2.61, respectively; *df*, 16) but not on trials with weaker or stronger prepulse intensities. This effect approached significance for PP5 trials (Student's $t=2.02$; *df*, 16; $P<.06$).

Comment

These findings have several implications. First, there are clear parallels between the human startle response and the rat startle response to similar eliciting stimuli. Both species (1) exhibited a graded increase in PPI with increasing prepulse intensities; (2) appear to have exhibited a "threshold" range for startle gating at prepulse intensities approximately 4 dB above background noise; and (3) exhibited latency facilitation at the weakest prepulse intensities, even though

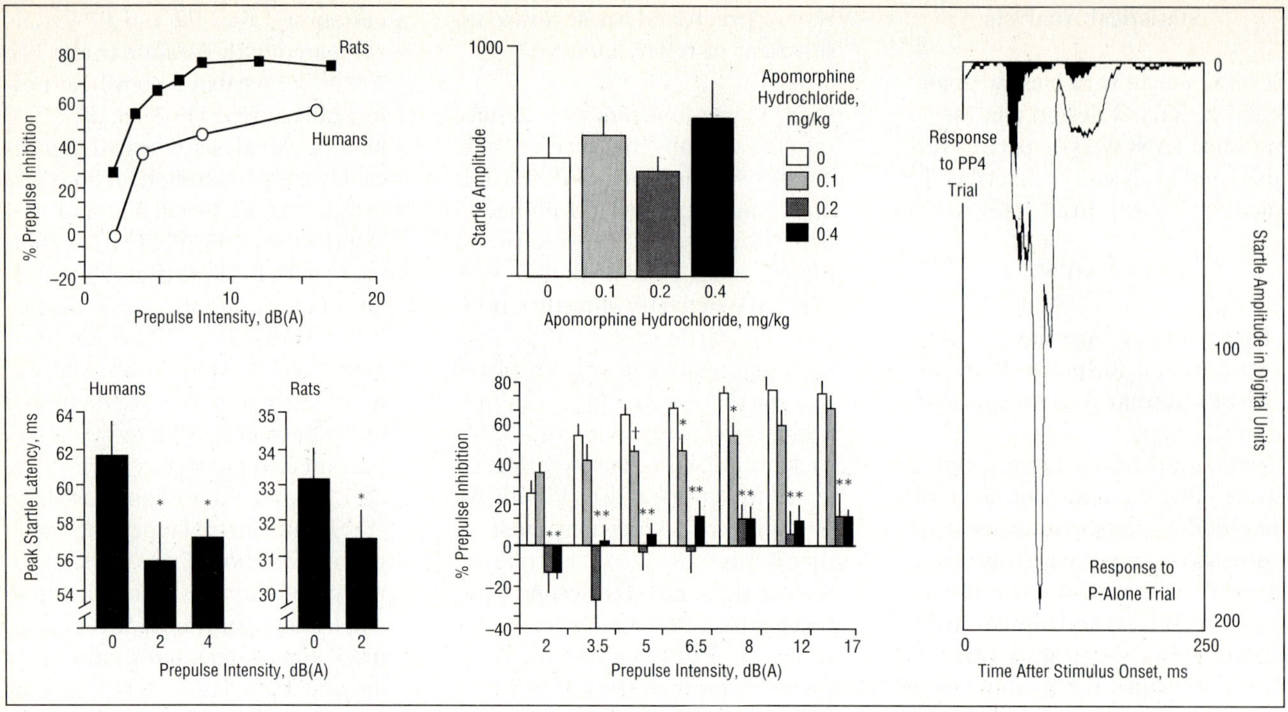

Figure 1. *Top left, Prepulse inhibition in rats and humans, using prepulse stimuli between 2 and 17 dB(A) above background noise. For humans, electromyographic activity was high-pass filtered to minimize electro-oculographic artifact, amplified and digitized via a computerized startle response monitoring system (SR-LAB, San Diego Instruments Inc), and recorded as previously described.[3] Subjects were part of a "control" group in an ongoing study of human sensorimotor gating.[26] For rats, startle was recorded as previously described.[16] The relationship of prepulse intensity to prepulse inhibition (PPI) appears strikingly similar across species, with humans exhibiting approximately 25% less PPI across all prepulse intensities. The difference in the absolute amount of PPI across species might reflect differences in methods of recording startle (see final "Comment" section) or interspecies differences in acoustic spectral sensitivities. Bottom left, Latency from stimulus onset to peak startle amplitude is reduced by prepulse presentation in both humans and rats. The extreme degree of startle inhibition at higher prepulse intensities prevented an accurate measurement of reflex latency; for this reason, latency was analyzed for all pulse-alone (P-Alone) trials and for prepulse trials for which mean PPI did not exceed 50% of maximal PPI values (PP2 and PP4 for humans, and PP2 for rats). Asterisks indicate significant reduction in latency compared with P-Alone trials (*$P<.05$*) by* t *test after significant effect of trial type by analysis of variance. Right, Electromyographic tracings for one human on P-Alone (open tracing: amplitude 193, peak latency 75 milliseconds) and PP4 (solid tracing: amplitude 40, peak latency 53 milliseconds) trials; this demonstrates amplitude reduction and peak latency facilitation on PP4 trial compared with P-Alone trial. Window duration is 250 milliseconds, with stimulus onset at left margin; startle amplitude is in digital units (7.7 μV/U). Center, Effects of apomorphine on startle amplitude (top center) and PPI (bottom center) in rats. Apomorphine hydrochoride (0 to 0.4 mg/kg subcutaneously) had no significant effect on startle amplitude but caused a significant decrease in PPI that was dose-dependent and varied with prepulse intensity. Higher doses of apomorphine hydrochloride (0.2 and 0.4 mg/kg) decreased or eliminated PPI at all prepulse intensities, while the lowest dose of apomorphine hydrochloride (0.1 mg/kg) significantly decreased PPI only when prepulse intensity was 5 to 8 dB(A) over background. Asterisks indicate significantly less than 0 mg/kg dose (*$P<.05$*) by* t *test after significant effect of dose by analysis of variance and near-significant dose $\times$ intensity interaction (*$P<.08$*); dagger,* $P<.06$*, same comparison.*

these weak prepulses do not significantly reduce startle amplitude. Second, PPI in rats is decreased in an orderly and dose-dependent manner by very low doses of apomorphine, while latency facilitation is not decreased by apomorphine. Startle gating in rats appears to be quite sensitive to dopaminergic tone, since a decrease in PPI was evident even at doses of apomorphine that are considered "threshold" doses for postsynaptic dopamine receptor activation (eg, 0.1 mg/kg) and that do not stimulate other obvious forms of behavioral activation.[15] The pharmacologic dissociation between the substrates of PPI and those of latency facilitation suggests that the apomorphine-induced loss of PPI does not appear to reflect a disruption of the rats' ability to "detect" the prepulse, since under conditions where the prepulse does not inhibit startle amplitude (eg, 0.4 mg/kg apomorphine hydrochloride), the prepulse remains behaviorally effective (ie, facilitates latency). A dissociation between these two forms of reflex modulation has been noted in rats treated with intra-NAC dopamine,[27] in patients with Huntington's disease,[28] in schizophrenic patients,[3] and in patients with obsessive-compulsive disorder,[26] all of whom exhibit significantly decreased PPI but exhibit normal latency facilitation. Finally, these findings suggest that PPI in rats is most sensitive to the disruptive effects of increased dopamine tone when prepulse intensity is between 5 and 8 dB above background intensity.

EXPERIMENT 2

Predictive Validity: Can This Model Be Used as a Sensitive and Specific Screen of Antipsychotic Potency?

We have previously reported that the apomorphine-induced loss of PPI in rats is antagonized by antipsychotic agents, including clozapine.[16,29,30] It is thus possible that the ability to restore startle gating in apomorphine-treated rats might serve as a useful screening measure for antipsychotic agents. Several other reports suggest that the apomorphine-induced disruption of PPI might have predictive validity, ie, be a sensitive and specific measure of antipsychotic action. The clinically potent antipsychotics haloperidol,[17] chlorpromazine, and risperidone antagonize the effects of apomorphine on PPI, while buspirone, diazepam, and imipramine—psychoactive agents without antipsychotic properties—do not restore PPI in apomorphine-treated rats,[20] and neither does the opiate antagonist naloxone.[31] While these observations suggest that the ability of a drug to reverse the apomorphine-induced disruption of PPI might predict antipsychotic properties, not enough information is available to assess the ability of this model to accurately predict antipsychotic potency, which is a prerequisite of predictive validity.[32] In experiment 2, a more comprehensive dose-response investigation of several drugs was completed to determine the sensitivity and specificity of this PPI model for predicting antipsychotic potency to assess the predictive validity of this model.

Methods

One hundred eighty-four rats were used in this experiment. Testing occurred during two sessions, with 5 days between sessions. Each rat was pretreated with one dose of haloperidol (0, 0.01, 0.05, or 0.1 mg/kg subcutaneously in distilled water vehicle; n=32), chlorpromazine hydrochloride (0, 1, 5, or 10 mg/kg subcutaneously in saline vehicle; n=24), perphenazine (0, 0.05, 0.1, or 0.05 mg/kg subcutaneously in saline vehicle; n=24), prochlorperazine edisylate (0, 0.05, 0.1, 0.5, or 1.0 mg/kg subcutaneously in saline vehicle; n=32), spiperone (0.001, 0.01, or 0.1 mg/kg subcutaneously in saline vehicle; n=24), or propranolol hydrochloride (0, 1, 5, or 10 mg/kg subcutaneously in saline vehicle; n=24). Injection volume was 1 mL/kg given into the loose tissue on the dorsum over the neck. In a previous experiment, rats treated with these doses of propranolol developed sores, suggesting a regional vasculitis or inflammatory response. To avoid potential problems with drug absorption, propranolol and apomorphine were administered into alternate sides of the neck.

Either 30 minutes (spiperone) or 10 minutes (all other agents) following these pretreatments, animals were treated with apomorphine hydrochloride (0 or 0.5 mg/kg subcutaneously) and then immediately placed in the startle chambers. Five days later, each rat received the identical pretreatment, but apomorphine treatments were reversed, with the number of rats receiving each dose of apomorphine balanced over both sessions. Thus, pretreatment (haloperidol, chlorpromazine, perphenazine, prochlorperazine, spiperone, or propranolol) served as the between-subject variable, while treatment (dose of apomorphine) served as the within-subject variable. The dose ranges were chosen either to incorporate a single dose previously demonstrated to restore PPI in apomorphine-treated rats or because the doses have been reported previously to disrupt other measures of dopamine agonist–induced behavioral changes in the rat.[16,17,20,33] While we have reported a dose-range of spiperone that reverses the apomorphine-induced disruption of PPI, our previous study[16] did not use doses low enough to identify a "threshold" dose of spiperone. The dose range of propranolol was chosen to span a range that should yield blockade of both β-adrenergic receptors (1 mg/kg) and 5-hydroxytryptamine-1A serotonin receptors (10 mg/kg).[34] The dose of apomorphine chosen has been shown to attenuate PPI in rats[16,17]; this dose was also chosen to provide "maximal" disruption of PPI (based on findings in experiment 1) to allow optimal sensitivity of detecting antipsychotic effects.

In contrast to experiment 1, test sessions in experiment 2 were designed to permit analysis of the effects of varying prepulse *intervals* on dopamine-induced changes in startle gating. Previous studies[15] demonstrated that maximal disruption of PPI by dopamine agonists occurred when the intervals between the prepulse and the pulse were 60 to 120 milliseconds, with less robust PPI noted with longer prepulse intervals. Immediately following apomorphine treatment, rats were placed in a startle chamber for a 5-minute acclimation period with a 65-dB(A) background noise. After the acclimation period, rats were exposed to two types of stimuli: P-Alone or a prepulse (80-dB[A], 20-millisecond broad band burst). Each session included five trial types: P-Alone; prepulse followed 60 milliseconds later by P-Alone (60 milliseconds); prepulse followed 120 milliseconds later by P-Alone (120 milliseconds); prepulse followed 500 milliseconds later by P-Alone (500 milliseconds); or NOSTIM. The session consisted of three blocks of five sequences of the five trial types, varied in order; each block thus contained 25 trials. This method is identical to that described in our previous work.[16]

Behavioral data were analyzed in two ways. P-Alone amplitude was analyzed using a three-way ANOVA with repeated measures on dose and block, and PPI, defined as in experiment 1, was analyzed using a four-way ANOVA with repeated measures on dose, prepulse interval, and block. To calculate the median effective dose (ED_{50}) for a test drug, the amount of PPI after apomorphine treatment was compared with the amount of PPI after vehicle treatment. For the purposes of this study, the ED_{50} was defined as the lowest dose of the test drug that restored PPI in apomorphine-treated rats to 50% of what it is in vehicle-treated rats at all prepulse intervals in block 1. This definition was chosen for several reasons. First, since several test drugs appeared to slightly enhance PPI independent of apomorphine treatment, it was important to compare the amount of PPI in apomorphine-treated rats with the amount of PPI in vehicle-treated rats *that had*

Table 1. Drug Effects on Pulse-Alone Startle Amplitude*

Pretreatment	Effect, F Score: Pretreatment	Treatment	T×P	B×P	B×P×T	Other
Haloperidol	NS	4.30†	NS	4.27‡	NS	...
Chlorpromazine hydrochloride	3.15†	NS	4.98†	2.80†	3.12†	T block 1:8.18†
Perphenazine	NS	8.18†	7.57‡	3.57†	2.65†	...
Prochlorperazine edisylate	NS	9.77‡	NS	NS	NS	...
Spiperone	NS	NS	3.77†	NS	NS	T×B:6.3‡, Tblock 1:4.4†§
Propranolol hydrochloride	NS	6.62†	NS	NS	NS	...

**T* indicates treatment; P, pretreatment; B, block; and NS, not significant.*
†*P*<.05.
‡*P*<.005.
§*Main apomorphine-induced* increase *in startle amplitude.*

been given the same dose of the test drug. Second, since we had no a priori reason to identify any one prepulse interval as being most sensitive to the effects of apomorphine or the test drug, we established a uniform criterion that PPI must be restored by 50% in all three intervals. Finally, the first block was chosen because it is most robustly affected by apomorphine. Thus, the reversal of this effect is least likely to be confounded by interactions of test drug effect and duration of apomorphine action or reflex habituation. For all antipsychotics, these ED_{50}s were compared with previously published values of ED_{50}s of clinical potency[33,35-38] and D_2 binding affinity,[33,36,39-41] using a Spearman correlation. Using this definition of ED_{50}, our previous findings using an identical paradigm as described above yielded values of 2.0 mg/kg for clozapine and 0.025 mg/kg for raclopride.[16] We have recently replicated this observation with clozapine using a simplified startle session.[29,30]

Results of Experiment 2

Startle Amplitude. **Figure 2** and **Table 1** summarize analyses of startle amplitudes for all pretreatment (test drug) and treatment (apomorphine) conditions. These analyses revealed three neuroleptic effects on startle amplitude and on apomorphine-induced changes in startle amplitude. First, only chlorpromazine significantly depressed startle amplitude, although several drugs exhibited a nonsignificant trend toward depressing startle. Second, in all studies, apomorphine produced a decrease in startle amplitude that was antagonized by chlorpromazine, perphenazine, and spiperone but not by haloperidol or prochlorperazine. Apomorphine has been reported to increase startle amplitude,[42] decrease startle amplitude,[15] or have no significant effect on startle amplitude[31] (divergent findings that may reflect differences in experi-

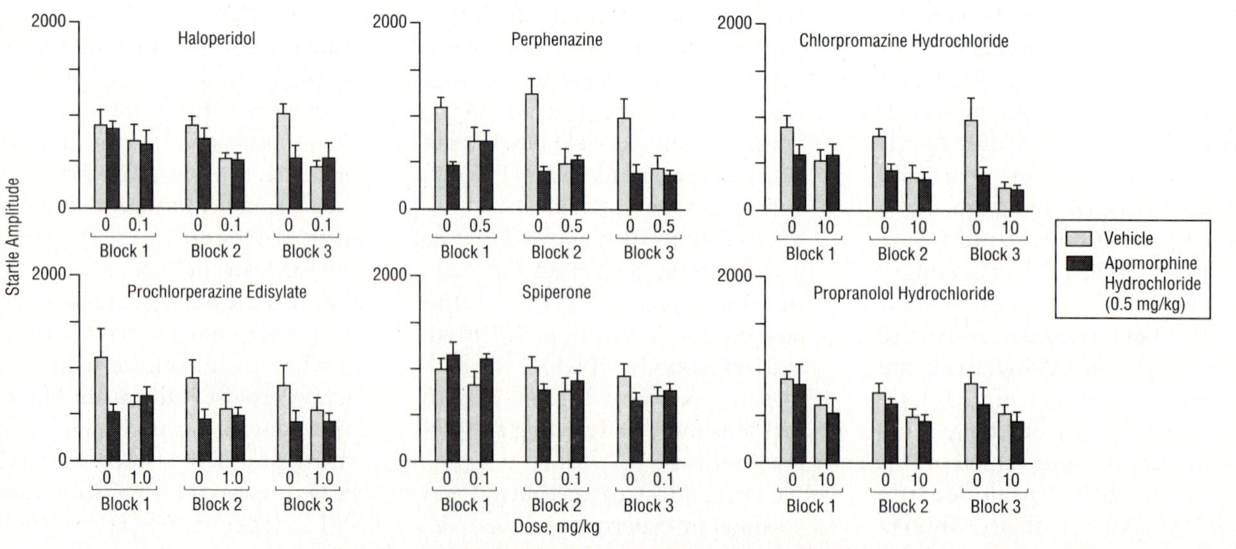

Figure 2. *Effects of apomorphine on startle amplitude in rats pretreated with haloperidol, perphenazine, chlorpromazine, prochlorperazine, spiperone, and propranolol. Statistically significant effects are reported in Table 1. In general, apomorphine treatment tended to decrease startle amplitude. All pretreatments also tended to decrease startle amplitude in vehicle-treated rats, but the antipsychotic pretreatment (all but propranolol) tended to reverse the apomorphine-induced decrease in startle in apomorphine-treated rats. All drugs were administered subcutaneously.*

Table 2. Drug Effects on Prepulse Inhibition (PPI)*

	Effect, F Score					
Pretreatment	**Pretreatment**	**Treatment**	**T×P**	**B×P**	**B×P×T**	**Other**
Haloperidol	9.78†‡	89.97†	19.93†	3.92§	2.19**	Interval, T×I, T×P×I
Chlorpromazine hydrochloride	9.18†‡	16.59§	16.95†	4.91§	2.43‖	I, T×I, P×I, T×P×I
Perphenazine	5.71§‡	43.66†	14.41†	2.69‖	2.92‖	I, T×I, T×P×I
Prochlorperazine edisylate	3.53‖‡	46.64†	5.12§	2.17‖	3.00‖	I, T×I, P×I,T×P×I
Spiperone	8.87†‡	16.90†	NS¶	NS	NS	I, T×I, P×I,T×P×I
Propranolol hydrochloride	NS	135.24†	4.79‖#	2.57‖	NS	I, T×I, P×I,

**T indicates treatment; P, pretreatment; B, block; and NS, not significant.*
†*P<.0005.*
‡*No significant effect of neuroleptic on PPI in rats treated with 0 mg/kg of apomorphine hydrochloride (F<1).*
§*P<.005.*
‖*P<.05.*
¶*T×P at 60-ms interval: 7.91.*
#*Significantly potentiated apomorphine-induced disruption of PPI.*
***P<.06.*

mental design, eg, single vs repeated test sessions, or equipment design, eg, single vs multianimal startle chambers). Spiperone pretreatment actually reversed the effects of apomorphine on startle amplitude. Apomorphine potentiated startle amplitude in spiperone-pretreated rats, an effect that we previously noted with both spiperone and raclopride.[16] Third, chlorpromazine, perphenazine, and haloperidol enhanced startle habituation, an effect manifested by a significant drug-induced decrease in startle amplitude in blocks 2 and 3 but not in block 1. This effect was evident despite the fact that the present paradigm is not designed to be maximally sensitive to changes in response habituation.[43] This delayed reduction of startle amplitude does not simply reflect delayed drug absorption or behavioral activity, since perphenazine blocked the apomorphine-induced reduction of startle amplitude in block 1, and all three drugs antagonized the apomorphine-induced reduction of PPI in block 1 (see below). Specific analyses are reported in Table 1.

Prepulse Inhibition. Drug effects on PPI are seen in **Figure 3** and **Table 2**. Two major drug effects on PPI are notable. First, apomorphine significantly disrupted PPI in all groups. Vehicle-treated rats in all groups exhibited approximately 80% PPI at the 60-millisecond prepulse interval in block 1; this amount of inhibition approximates values for

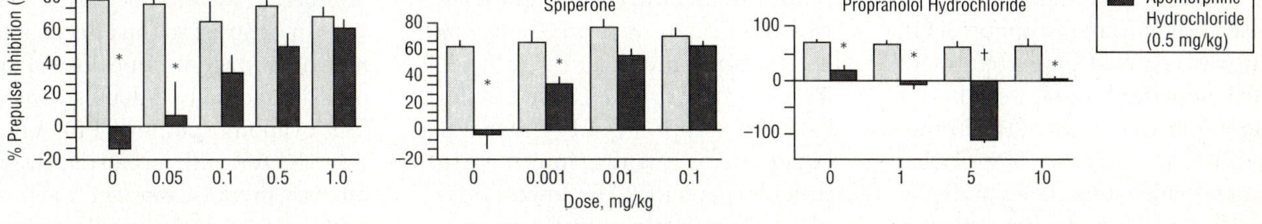

Figure 3. *Effects of apomorphine on prepulse inhibition (PPI) in rats pretreated with haloperidol, perphenazine, chlorpromazine, prochlorperazine, spiperone, and propranolol. Data shown are from 60-millisecond interval in block 1 but are representative of the entire startle session. Statistically significant effects are reported in Table 1. Apomorphine significantly decreased PPI in all groups. This effect was totally reversed by all antipsychotics (all but propranolol), while propranolol actually potentiated this effect of apomorphine. Asterisks indicate significant effect of apomorphine by* t *test after significant main effect of apomorphine by analysis of variance; daggers, significant enhancement of apomorphine-disruption of PPI compared with 0 mg/kg dose of propranolol hydrochloride, by* t *test after significant apomorphine × propranolol interaction by analysis of variance. All drugs were administered subcutaneously.*

"baseline" PPI that we have previously reported using these startle parameters.[5] Apomorphine reduced PPI to approximately 0% in most groups. In some cases, apomorphine-treated rats exhibited startle amplitudes on prepulse trials that greatly exceeded the amplitude on pulse trials. Second, all neuroleptics significantly antagonized the apomorphine-induced disruption of PPI. In contrast, propranolol did not antagonize the apomorphine-induced disruption of PPI, with one dose of propranolol hydrochloride (5.0 mg/kg) actually enhancing the apomorphine-induced disruption of PPI. The magnitude of the neuroleptic restoration of PPI in apomorphine-treated rats resulted in a statistically significant main effect of each neuroleptic agent on PPI (Table 2). Importantly, these results did not reflect independent PPI-enhancing effects of the neuroleptics. Post hoc analyses revealed that neuroleptics did not significantly change PPI in rats treated with 0 mg/kg of apomorphine hydrochloride(Table 2).

HALOPERIDOL completely reversed the effects of apomorphine on PPI. A four-way ANOVA with repeated measures on dose, prepulse interval, and block revealed significant effects of haloperidol and of apomorphine and a significant haloperidol × apomorphine interaction. Other significant two-way, three-way, and four-way interactions are seen in Table 2. Thus, apomorphine caused a significant disruption of PPI that was reversed by pretreatment with haloperidol. The lowest dose of haloperidol that restored PPI in apomorphine-treated rats to 50% of what it was in vehicle-treated rats at all prepulse intervals in block 1 was 0.05 mg/kg.

Chlorpromazine completely reversed the effects of apomorphine on PPI. A four-way ANOVA with repeated measures on dose, prepulse interval, and block revealed significant effects of chlorpromazine and of apomorphine and a significant chlorpromazine × apomorphine interaction. Other significant two-way, three-way, and four-way interactions are seen in Table 2. Thus, apomorphine caused a significant disruption of PPI that was reversed by pretreatment with chlorpromazine. The lowest dose of chlorpromazine hydrochloride that restored PPI in apomorphine-treated rats to 50% of what it was in vehicle-treated rats at all prepulse intervals in block 1 was 1.0 mg/kg.

Perphenazine completely reversed the effects of apomorphine on PPI. A four-way ANOVA with repeated measures on dose, prepulse interval, and block revealed significant effects of perphenazine and of apomorphine and a significant perphenazine × apomorphine interaction. Other significant two-way, three-way, and four-way interactions are seen in Table 2. Thus, apomorphine caused a significant disruption of PPI that was reversed by pretreatment with perphenazine. The lowest dose of perphenazine that restored PPI in apomorphine-treated rats to 50% of what it was in vehicle-treated rats at all prepulse intervals in block 1 was 0.1 mg/kg.

Prochlorperazine completely reversed the effects of apomorphine on PPI. A four-way ANOVA with repeated measures on dose, prepulse interval, and block revealed significant effects of prochlorperazine and of apomorphine and a significant prochlorperazine × apomorphine interaction. Other significant two-way, three-way, and four-way interactions are seen in Table 2. Thus, apomorphine caused a significant disruption of PPI that was reversed by pretreatment with prochlorperazine. The lowest dose of prochlorperazine edisylate that restored PPI in apomorphine-treated rats to 50% of what it was in vehicle-treated rats at all prepulse intervals in block 1 was 0.5 mg/kg.

Spiperone completely reversed the effects of apomorphine on PPI. A four-way ANOVA with repeated measures on dose, prepulse interval, and block revealed significant effects of spiperone and of apomorphine, no significant spiperone × apomorphine interaction, but a significant spiperone × apomorphine × interval interaction. This interaction reflected the fact that spiperone significantly increased PPI in vehicle-treated rats at the 120- and 500-millisecond prepulse intervals. Inspection of the data revealed that in apomorphine-treated rats in block 1, spiperone increased PPI from −3.6%, −27.8%, and 6.4% (0 mg/kg of spiperone at 60-, 120-, and 500-millisecond intervals, respectively) to 60.3%, 59.7%, and 51.5% (0.1 mg/kg spiperone at 60-, 120-, and 500-millisecond intervals, respectively). In the same rats treated with vehicle, spiperone increased PPI from 62.3%, 49.9%, and 41.8% (0 mg/kg of spiperone at 60-, 120-, and 500-millisecond intervals, respectively) to 71.4%, 72.8%, and 65.9% (0.1 mg/kg of spiperone at 60-, 120-, and 500-millisecond intervals, respectively). Thus, while spiperone entirely reversed the effects of apomorphine on PPI at all prepulse intervals, only the effect of spiperone at the 60-millisecond interval distinguished the apomorphine-treated rats from the vehicle-treated rats. Other significant interactions are seen in Table 2. The lowest dose of spiperone that restored PPI in apomorphine-treated rats to 50% of what it was in vehicle-treated rats at all prepulse intervals in block 1 was 0.01 mg/kg.

In contrast to the effects of the neuroleptic agents, one dose of propranolol actually enhanced the effects of apomorphine on PPI. A four-way ANOVA with repeated measures on dose, prepulse interval, and block revealed no significant effect of propranolol, a significant effect of apomorphine, and a significant propranolol × apomorphine interaction. Other significant interactions are seen in Table 1. No three-way or four-way interactions were significant. Post hoc analysis revealed that the apomorphine-induced disruption of PPI was significantly enhanced by 5 mg/kg of propranolol hydrochloride during block 1 only ($F=13.64$; *df*, 1,35; $P<.001$). Thus, apomorphine caused a significant disruption of PPI that was enhanced by pretreatment with 5 mg/kg of propranolol hydrochloride during the initial trial block.

The ability of these drugs to reverse the apomorphine-induced disruption of PPI was compared with their clinical potency (relative antipsychotic potency and average clinical daily dose, from sources listed above) and their D_2 receptor affinity. Values for clozapine and raclopride from our previous study using identical methods were included in this analysis.[16] Spearman rank correlation revealed that the ED_{50}s of these drugs in the present paradigm, as well as ED_{50}s of clozapine and raclopride calculated using an identical paradigm,[16] correlated significantly with their relative antipsychotic potency ($r_s=.991$; $P<.0005$), their average clinical daily dose ($r_s=.964$; $P<.0005$), and their D_2 receptor affinity ($r_s=-0.893$; $P<.01$). Correlations are represented graphically in **Figure 4**.

Comment

These findings suggest that the apomorphine-induced disruption of PPI may be a sensitive and specific tool for screening drugs for antipsychotic potency. This model appears to be "sensitive," since the ability of a wide range of antipsychotics to restore PPI in apomorphine-treated rats is highly predictive of their clinical potency. This correlation was noted with antipsychotics from several different chemical classes, including the dibenzodiazepine clozapine.[16] The fact that propranolol, which lacks antipsychotic potency, did *not* restore PPI in apomorphine-treated rats supports the "specificity" of this model, and extends similar "negative" findings with diazepam, buspirone, imipramine,[20] and naloxone.[31] These findings support the notion that the loss of PPI in apomorphine-treated rats may have predictive validity as an animal model of deficient startle gating in schizophrenic patients.

EXPERIMENT 3

Construct Validity: Repeating and Extending Findings That Specific Mesolimbic Hyperdopaminergia Disrupts PPI in Rats

A model has construct validity if it demonstrates both empirical and theoretical consistency with a proposed physiological construct, related either to the cause of a disorder or to the therapeutic mechanism of drug action.[32] Since impaired sensorimotor gating is proposed to be a critical psychopathological construct in schizophrenic patients,[4] and since impaired sensorimotor gating is exhibited by schizophrenic patients[1-3] and by rats after manipulations of limbic cortico-striato-pallido-pontine circuitry,[5] this animal model of impaired sensorimotor gating has construct validity.[32] In the present experiment, we investigated whether this model has more generalized construct validity by studying the loss of sensorimotor gating after neurochemical manipulations that are consistent with neurochemical constructs for the pathophysiology of schizophrenia and for the mechanism of action of antipsychotic agents. Thus, we examined whether this model with construct validity in a *psychophysiological domain* also satisfies criteria for construct validity in a *neurochemical domain.*

Mesolimbic hyperdopaminergia has long been implicated in the pathophysiology of psychosis and schizophrenia, either as a primary causative insult[6,44] or as a secondary consequence of prefrontal or limbic-cortical dysfunction.[45-47] Other evidence suggests that the blockade of mesolimbic dopamine receptors may be responsible for at least some of the beneficial properties of antipsychotic agents.[48-50] Mesolimbic hyperdopaminergia disrupts PPI in rats. We have reported,[22] and twice replicated,[23,27] the finding that PPI in rats is decreased significantly by direct infusion of dopamine into the NAC, which is the terminal region of mesolimbic dopamine fibers. In the present study, we used mesolimbic hyperdopaminergia as a neurochemical manipulation that disrupts sensorimotor gating in rats and that is consistent with a major construct for the pathophysiology of schizophrenia—the "dopamine hypothesis" of schizophrenia. We further explored whether the reduction in PPI after intra-NAC dopamine infusion is reversed by antipsychotics, since such an effect would be consistent with a major construct for the therapeutic mechanism of antipsychotic action.[48-50] The aim of this study was *not* to demonstrate that mesolimbic hyperdopaminergia is a singular cause of deficient sensorimotor gating in schizophrenia or to imply that blockade of mesolimbic dopamine is the major therapeutic mechanism of antipsychotic action. In fact, we have reported that sensorimotor gating is modulated by neural circuitry linking the HPC, ventral striatum, subpallidum, and pontine tegmentum,[5] and dysfunction at various levels of this circuitry likely accounts for the loss of sensorimotor gating in schizophrenic patients.[6-14,51] Rather, this experiment was designed to assess whether a model with construct validity in a psychophysiological domain also satisfied criteria for construct validity in a neurochemical domain.

Methods

Nineteen rats were anesthetized with pentobarbital sodium (50 mg/kg), placed in a small-animal stereotaxis (model 900, Kopf Instruments, Tujunga, Calif), and prepared with bilateral 23-gauge stainless steel cannulas aimed 3 mm above the NAC as previously described.[22] Testing took place during two sessions, with 1 week between sessions. Before each session, nine rats received a dose of haloperidol found in experiment 2 to re-

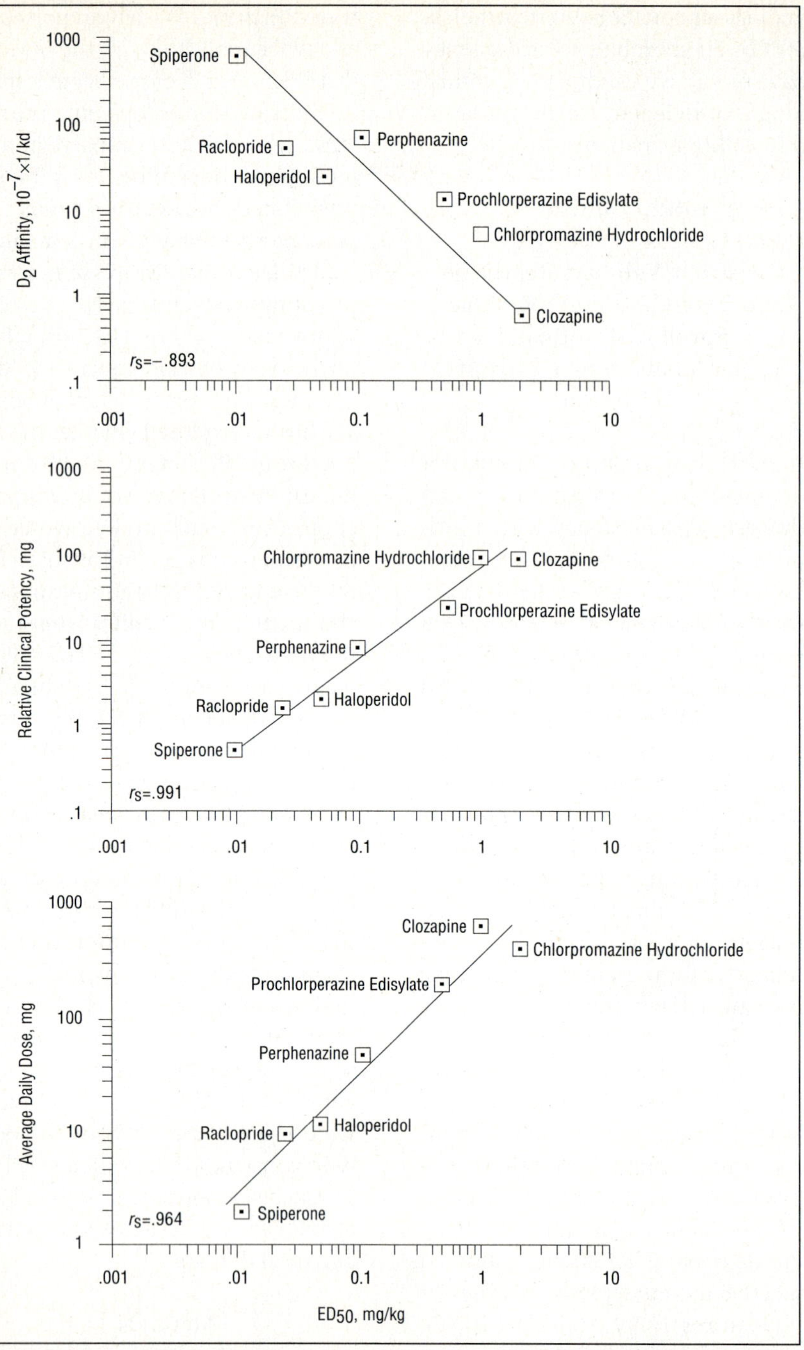

Figure 4. *Relationship between median effective dose (ED_{50}) (to reverse the apomorphine disruption of the prepulse interval) and three other measures: D_2 receptor affinity, relative clinical potency, and average daily antipsychotic dose. Prepulse inhibition data presented are for five antipsychotic compounds from the present study and from clozapine and raclopride[5]; data for clinical antipsychotic potency were extracted from several sources (see text). All drugs were administered subcutaneously.*

store PPI in apomorphine-treated rats (0.05 mg/kg), while the remaining 10 rats received a vehicle injection (all injection parameters as in experiment 2). Ten minutes later, rats received bilateral intra-NAC infusions of dopamine hydrochloride (0 or 40 μg) in a saline vehicle containing 0.1% ascorbic acid. Every rat received each dose once, with the order of dose counterbalanced across the two sessions using methods identical to those previously demonstrated to result in a dopamine-induced disruption of PPI.[22,23]

Test sessions were designed to permit analysis of the effects of different prepulse *intervals and intensities* on dopamine-induced changes in PPI. Immediately after dopamine infusion, rats were placed in a startle chamber for a 5-minute acclimation period with a 65-dB(A) background noise and were then exposed to seven types of stimuli: P-Alone and six types of prepulses (PP5, PP10, PP15, 60 milliseconds, 120 milliseconds, or 500 milliseconds). Sessions included eight trial types: P-Alone, each of the six prepulse trials, followed by the startle pulse or NOSTIM. For each session, 50 trials (10 pulse alone, 10 NOSTIM, and five of each prepulse trial types) were presented in pseudorandom order, with varying prepulse intervals presented in the first half of the session and varying prepulse intensities presented in the second half of the session.

After completion of behavioral testing, all rats were killed with a lethal overdose of pentobarbital and perfused with 10% formalin/saline. Brains were removed and kept in 10% formalin/saline until histologic assessment was performed to verify cannula placement. Intra-NAC needle placements were verified for all cannulas (**Figure 5**). Startle data were analyzed in two ways. To assess P-Alone amplitude, the session was divided into two blocks, with five pulse-alone trials in each block. P-Alone amplitude was analyzed using a two-way ANOVA with repeated measures on dose of dopamine and session block. Level of significance was $P<.05$. Prepulse inhibition, defined as above, was analyzed using a three-way ANOVA with repeated measures on dopamine dose and prepulse interval.

Results of Experiment 3

The results of experiment 3 are seen in Figure 5 and **Figure 6**. Histologic examination revealed that injection sites most often fell within the ventromedial aspect of the NAC, within or bordering on the "shell" region of the NAC[52,53] (Figure 5). Statistical analysis revealed no significant effect on P-Alone amplitude by dopamine

(F=2.92; *df*, 1,17) or haloperidol (F<1); there was a significant effect of block (F=20.36; *df*, 1,17) and no significant two-way or three-way interactions. As previously reported, PPI was reduced significantly by intra-NAC dopamine infusion. There was a significant effect of dopamine dose on PPI (F=4.40; *df*, 1,17; *P*=.05), no significant effect of haloperidol (F<1), and a significant dopamine × haloperidol interaction (F=7.17; *df*, 1,17). Individual ANOVAs revealed that dopamine significantly decreased PPI in vehicle-pretreated rats (F=7.24; *df*, 1,9) (Figure 6, top) but not in haloperidol-pretreated rats (F<1) (Figure 6, bottom). Thus, intra-NAC dopamine infusion significantly decreased PPI; this effect was prevented by pretreatment with a low dose of the D_2 antagonist haloperidol. Consistent with this, we recently reported that intra-NAC infusion of the D_2 agonist quinpirole decreased or eliminated PPI in rats, and this effect was prevented by pretreatment with haloperidol.[54]

Comment

This finding confirms our previous reports[11,12,15] that PPI is disrupted by specific NAC hyperdopaminergia. More importantly, the present findings suggest that the decrease in PPI after intra-NAC infusion reflects dopaminergic activation of D_2 receptors, since this effect is prevented by pretreatment with haloperidol. Thus, while we cannot be certain of the cause(s) of deficient sensorimotor gating in schizophrenic patients, the present findings suggest that the substrates of the dopamine-induced disruption of PPI in rats are consistent with one major—if not predominant—hypothesis for the pathophysiology of schizophrenia: overactivation of mesolimbic D_2 receptors.[6,44] Furthermore, haloperidol appears to "normalize" startle gating in dopamine-activated rats via blockade of mesolimbic D_2 receptors, a mechanism that is consistent with a major hypothesis for the therapeutic activity of these agents.[48-50] This observation *does not* identify mesolimbic hyperdopaminergia as the *single* neural substrate that modulates sensorimotor gating. Instead, these data add to a series of findings suggesting that PPI is modulated by activity in interconnected limbic cortico-striato-pallido-pontine circuitry.[5] Impaired PPI in rats appears to be a valid model for a psychophysiological construct—impaired sensorimotor gating in schizophrenia—and for neurochemical constructs for the pathophysiology of schizophrenia and for the mechanism of antipsychotic action.[6-14,48-50]

COMMENT

The present findings suggest that the loss of PPI of acoustic startle in rats is a model with face, predictive, and construct validity for the loss of sensorimotor gating in schizophrenic patients. This model may be critically important for understanding the neurobiological substrates of schizophrenia, and it may assist in designing novel antipsychotic agents and pharmacological treatment strategies. The PPI model differs from existing animal models since it uses identical methods across species to measure a deficit that is integral to the schizophrenic syndrome (impaired sensorimotor gating), it predicts anti-psychotic potency for both typical and atypical antipsychotics, and it is controlled by a defined neural circuit that has been repeatedly implicated in the pathophysiology of schizophrenia and that can be manipulated and studied in animals.

The search for robust and valid animal models of psychopathological states and abnormal cognitive function is a critically important area of research. Among the features that make the startle reflex a valuable behavioral measure of central nervous system function, two features are most critical to the present discussion. First, this reflex can be modulated by forebrain circuitry and, hence, can be used to study the organization and pathophysiology of brain structures that may be relevant to human psychopathology. In a series of investigations, we have studied the modulation of startle by weak prepulses in rats as a means of understanding the neural substrates of sensorimotor gating.[2,5,21] By delineating the central nervous system control of sensorimotor gating, it might be possible to identify a neural basis for deficient sensorimotor gating in certain disorders, including schizophrenia. Second, startle can be elicited across species using similar or identical stimulus parameters to elicit similar responses. The cross-species comparability of startle is striking, eg, despite the great disparity in body size, the onset latency of acoustic startle in rats (time from auditory nerve stimulation to first electromyographic response) is 8 milliseconds,[55] while in humans, it is approximately 14 milliseconds.[56] This cross-species comparability largely reflects the fact that the "primary" startle response is controlled by simple neural circuitry—at or below the pontine reticular formation—that is similar in

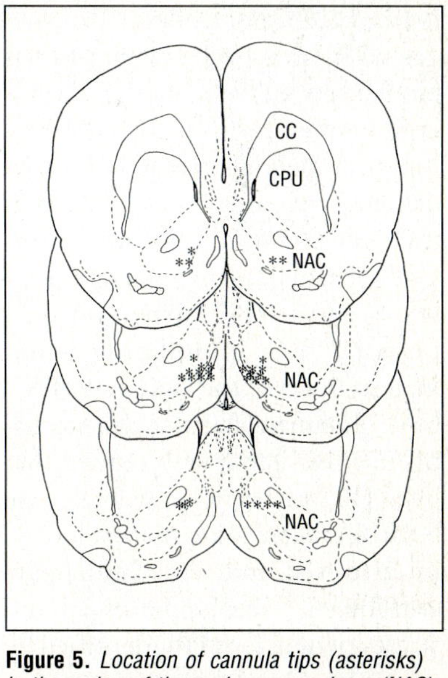

Figure 5. *Location of cannula tips (asterisks) in the region of the nucleus accumbens (NAC), plotted on modified sections from Pellegrino et al.[53] Cannula tracts were visible through the neocortex and striatum, and smaller needle marks penetrated ventral to the striatum, into the NAC. Limited tissue damage was noted to the striatum dorsal to the NAC. Most tips are located in the ventromedial NAC, within or bordering on the "shell" region of the NAC.[52] CPU indicates caudate-putamen; CC, corpus callosum.*

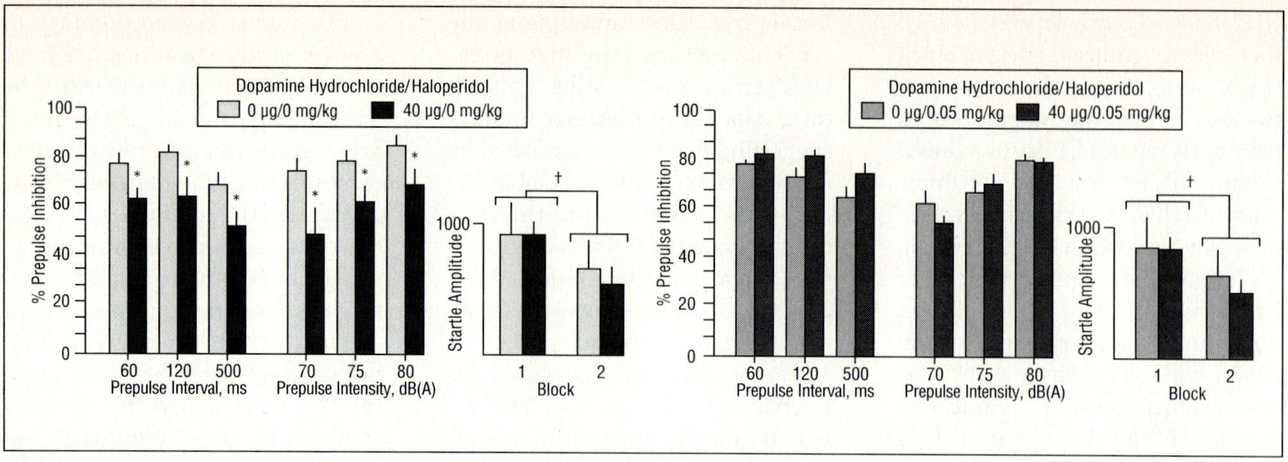

Figure 6. *Left, Effects of intra-nucleus accumbens (NAC) dopamine hydrochloride infusion (0 or 40 µg) on startle amplitude (right) and prepulse inhibition in rats pretreated with vehicle (0 mg/kg of haloperidol). Asterisks indicate significant effect of dopamine on prepulse inhibition by independent analysis of variance after significant main effect of dopamine and dopamine × pretreatment interaction; dagger, significant effect of block. Right, Effects of intra-NAC dopamine hydrochloride infusion (0 or 40 µg) on startle amplitude (right) and prepulse inhibition in rats pretreated with 0.05 mg/kg of haloperidol. In contrast to vehicle-pretreated rats, there was no significant effect of dopamine on prepulse inhibition in haloperidol-pretreated rats. Dagger indicates significant effect of block.*

rats and humans. But it is the startle inhibitory functions rather than the reflex itself that offer special promise in understanding the neurobiology of schizophrenia.

We have reported that the neural modulation of PPI in rats is effected by circuitry linking the HPC, the NAC, the subpallidum, and the pontine reticular formation. A role for the HPC in controlling PPI is suggested by our findings that PPI is blocked by infusion of the cholinergic agonist carbachol into several hippocampal regions (including the dentate gyrus, area CA1, and the ventral subiculum)[21,57] but not by carbachol infusion into parietal cortex.[21] Intra-HPC carbachol may impair PPI by stimulating glutamate release in the NAC via HPC-NAC glutamate fibers; such a mechanism is consistent with reports that intra-HPC carbachol infusions cause behavioral activation that is blocked by intra-NAC infusion of glutamate antagonists.[58] The hippocampal substrates of deficient PPI identified by this animal model may add a functional context for interpreting reports of hippocampal dysfunction in schizophrenia based on neuropsychologic,[59] neuropathologic,[9,13] and neuroimaging studies.[60] Furthermore, the hippocampal substrate links PPI with electrophysiological measures such as P50 gating, which is believed to reflect hippocampal function, is deficient in schizophrenic patients and asymptomatic first-degree relatives,[61] and is significantly correlated with PPI within individual subjects.[62]

Evidence reviewed above suggests that PPI is modulated in part (but not exclusively) by brain dopamine activity. In rats, PPI was reduced by drugs that directly or indirectly activated D_2 receptors but not D_1 receptors.[19,54] Conversely, these effects were reversed by blockade of D_2 receptors but not D_1 receptors.[16] There is evidence that the effects of dopamine agonists on PPI are mediated in part by increased dopamine activity in the NAC. First, low doses of apomorphine that did not decrease PPI in control rats potently disrupted PPI in rats that were regionally altered to have "supersensitive" dopamine receptors in the NAC.[15] Second, the loss of PPI induced by the indirect dopamine agonist amphetamine was reversed by depletion of dopamine in the NAC.[18] Third, PPI was disrupted in rats by dopamine infusion into the NAC or anteromedial striatum (but not the orbital cortex, amygdala, or posterior striatum).[22,23,27] Fourth, in experiment 3, the effects of intra-NAC dopamine infusion on PPI were reversed by systemic treatment with the D_2 antagonist haloperidol and thus likely reflect the action of exogenous dopamine on D_2 receptors.

We have proposed that decreased PPI after NAC dopamine activation reflects decreased activity in γ-aminobutyric acid (GABA) fibers projecting from the NAC to the subpallidal regions that include the ventral pallidum and the substantia innominata.[23] The PPI-disruptive effects of NAC dopamine infusion in rats are reversed by infusion of the GABA agonist muscimol into the subpallidum and are reproduced by subpallidal infusion of the GABA antagonist picrotoxin.[23] This NAC-subpallidal GABAergic projection is a substrate for other behavioral effects of NAC dopamine activation[63-65] and may translate the effects of activity in the amygdala and HPC to lower motor circuitry.[66] While it is not clear how decreased subpallidal GABA activity is translated to the "primary startle circuit" to modulate PPI, one possible route is via subpallidal efferents to the pedunculopontine tegmental nucleus.[67] Others[68] have suggested that the pontine tegmentum is a critical substrate of startle gating. Similarly, we have reported that electrolytic lesions of the pedunculopontine tegmental nucleus significantly reduce PPI in rats.[69]

These findings give initial support for the role of HPC-NAC-subpallidal-pedunculopontine tegmental nucleus circuitry in modulating startle gating in rats. The utility of PPI in elaborating the functional interconnections of limbic-cortical and mesolimbic-subpallidal circuitry, and the potential relevance of this circuitry to the pathophysiology of psychiatric disorders,[58,70] underscores the importance of assessing the validity of this animal model of sensorimotor gating deficits in schizophrenia. Specifically, if the disruption of PPI in rats by manipulations of this circuitry is a valid model of deficient sensorimotor gating in schizophrenics, then gating deficits in schizophrenic patients might reflect pathology in this same neural circuitry. The PPI model would thus be a critical tool for understanding the development and pathophysiology of deficient sensorimotor gating in humans, for identifying general strategies for normalizing gating, and for screening specific compounds for gating-restorative properties.

The present experiments support the validity of this model in three domains: face, predictive, and construct validity. Nonetheless, there are clear limitations to our ability to validate each level of this model. First, startle in humans was measured using electromyographic recordings from orbicularis oculi, while rat startle was measured using whole-body displacement. Whie substantial data support the comparability of startle measures from a wide range of muscle groups,[71] the face validity of this model might be better assessed using identical startle measures in rats and humans. Second, the studies reported herein compared the ability of drugs to restore PPI in rats with their ability *to decrease schizophrenic symptoms in humans*. While one "core" element of schizophrenic pathology is an inability to "inhibit" or "gate" sensory stimuli[4,72] and schizophrenic patients exhibit deficient PPI,[1] the predictive validity of the PPI model would be better assessed by comparing the ability of drugs to restore PPI in dopamine-stimulated rats with their ability to *restore PPI* in schizophrenic patients. Importantly, recent studies have reported that clozapine and haloperidol significantly increase PPI in schizophrenic patients.[73]

FINALLY, THERE are several limitations to assessing the construct validity of this model. These limitations stem from (1) our ignorance regarding the pathophysiology of PPI deficits in schizophrenia or the therapeutic mechanisms of antipsychotic agents, (2) the likelihood that several variations of this disorder reflect different forms of neuropathology that may differ in the extent and substrates of deficient gating, and (3) the construct limitations inherent to modeling cognitive symptoms in infrahumans. For example, the inability of schizophrenic patients to "gate" stimuli may contribute to cognitive flooding and fragmentation,[4] the consequences of which are probably fundamental to psychotic thought processes.[1-3] Obviously, parallel flooding and fragmentation in rats must have a very different impact on a rat's "consciousness" and its integrative social functioning. Furthermore, PPI is deficient in patients with schizotypal personality disorder[74] and in "psychosis-prone" individuals.[75] Thus, deficient PPI may reflect pathology that exists beyond the "nuclear" schizophrenias, and that is expressed in dimensions of personality, temperament, and "ego" function.[76] Particularly in these domains, it will be difficult to demonstrate construct validity of an animal model.

Sensorimotor gating deficits in schizophrenic patients—unlike PPI deficits in apomorphine-treated rats—are not an acute drug response, but instead reflect longitudinal and complex interactions of genetic, developmental, social, and environmental forces. For this reason, it is important that startle gating in rats appears to be sensitive to these same forces. Genetic factors may be critical determinants of sensorimotor gating in rats, since strain-related differences in the dopaminergic modulation of PPI have been reported.[77] If susceptibility to the gating-disruptive effects of dopamine agonists is genetically controlled in rats, this model might offer critical insight into genetic factors mediating the susceptibility to and development of schizophrenia in humans.[78] Studies also indicate that development and stress may significantly alter startle gating in rats. For example, recent studies[79] indicate that isolation-reared rats that exhibit elevated NAC dopamine activity also demonstrate a neuroleptic-reversible deficiency in PPI compared with group-reared controls. Developmental issues may be particularly relevant to understanding PPI deficits in humans. Since PPI appears to develop in children between ages 5 and 8 years,[80] it is conceivable that abnormal developmental processes may contribute to PPI deficits in adult schizophrenics. In a preliminary finding of direct relevance to neurodevelopmental theories of schizophrenia,[78] we have noted impaired PPI and enhanced sensitivity to the PPI-disruptive effects of apomorphine in postpubescent rats that had received neurotoxin lesions of the hippocampus as neonates (M.A.G.; B. K. Lipska, PhD; D. R. Weinberger, MD; D.L.B.; G. E. Jaskiw, MD; and N.R.S.; unpublished data, September 1992). Other findings suggest that social influences may also critically influence the dopaminergic modulation of PPI. The apomorphine-induced disruption of PPI is dramatically reduced in rats that are tested in the presence of other rats compared with rats that are tested alone (M. Davis, PhD, personal communication, August 1991), an effect that may be attributable to changes in sensorimotor gating caused by high-frequency vocal communications between rats.[81] Thus, this model can potentially be used to study the contribution of genetic, developmental, and social forces to the pathophysiology of sensorimotor gating deficits in schizophrenia.

Despite the above caveats, this model has clear strengths, particularly in the domain of predictive validity. Several assets of the PPI model simply reflect the utility of using the startle reflex as a dependent measure: it is an easily and objectively quantified graded response that is under tight stimulus control, is comparable across species, has a nonzero baseline, and is controlled by a simple defined neural circuit.[71] All of these characteristics distinguish the PPI model from other preclinical models of antipsychotic potency, such as the ability of drugs to prevent apomorphine-induced canine emesis[33,82] and rodent stereotypy.[33] Furthermore, the PPI model demonstrates sensitivity to both typical antipsychotics and the atypical antipsychotic clozapine, with the dose of clozapine that reverses the apomorphine-induced disruption of PPI being consistent with its relative potency as an antipsychotic.[16] In contrast, clozapine fails to reverse amphetamine-induced and apomorphine-induced stereotypy in rats, or apomorphine-induced emesis in dogs.[33]

IN ADDITION to its sensitivity, the specificity of the PPI model is supported by previous reports that it predicts no antipsychotic potency for buspirone, diazepam, imipramine, and naloxone, and experiment 2 extends these findings to include the β-adrenergic and serotonergic antagonist propranolol. The properties of propranolol in this model were not entirely expected, since the middle dose of propranolol hydrochloride (5 mg/kg) actually *enhanced* the apomorphine-induced disruption of PPI. This effect clearly resulted from an interaction with apomorphine, since propranolol alone did not significantly change PPI at any dose. This dose of propranolol hydrochloride (5 mg/kg) should antagonize both β_2-adrenergic and serotonergic receptors.[34] Thus, the pharmacologic substrates of this apomorphine-propranolol interaction will likely be complex. We are presently studying the role of noradrenergic and serotonergic systems in the modulation of startle gating and, based on the present findings, will extend these studies to examine interactions of these systems with the dopaminergic control of PPI. Indeed, while our data suggest that D_1 dopamine receptors do not modulate PPI in intact rats, preliminary findings from others suggest that these receptors may be important in the control of PPI in dopamine-denervated rats.[83] This level of pharmacological complexity may be important in a model of schizophrenic pathology since we have moved, in general, from "one transmitter—one locus" theories of the pathophysiology of schizophrenia toward understanding the complex interactions of multiple neurotransmitters in complex neural circuit distributions.[51]

Finally, the strength of this model and its exciting long-term benefits in the predictive domain are enhanced by our ability to define the neural control of PPI "upstream" and "downstream" from the dopamine receptor. The risks of tardive dyskinesia and the prominence of neuroleptic-resistant symptoms in schizophrenics have stimulated efforts to develop antipsychotic compounds that do not act primarily through dopamine receptor blockade. Since the antipsychotic potency of these drugs will not be detected by traditional screening models of dopamine receptor activation,[33] it will be important to develop screening models that measure processes that are central to the pathophysiology of the schizophrenias, but that are not linked exclusively to dopamine receptor activation. The PPI model offers the potential for such utility, since PPI is not controlled exclusively by dopamine receptor activation, but instead is mediated via integrated corticolimbic and basal ganglia circuitry, of which the dopamine receptor is only one—albeit central—element. It is conceivable that variations of the PPI model might be used to predict antipsychotic potency of compounds that act at nondopaminergic receptors at several levels of limbic, mesolimbic, and subpallidal circuitry.

In summary, the present studies assessed the face, predictive, and construct validity of an animal model of deficient sensorimotor gating in schizophrenic patients. This model is based on our consistent observation that PPI of the acoustic startle reflex is impaired in schizophrenic patients[1,3] and in rats after pharmacological or surgical manipulations of neural elements linking the limbic system and basal ganglia.[5] An assessment of the face validity of this model revealed that PPI of acoustic startle can be elicited in humans and rats using near-identical stimuli to produce strikingly similar response patterns. With this measure, weak prepulses produce a comparable reduction of startle amplitude and latency across species. Prepulse inhibition is disrupted in rats in an orderly, dose-dependent fashion by the dopamine agonist apomorphine; a similar disruption of PPI is reported in schizophrenic patients. An assessment of the predictive validity of this model revealed that the apomorphine-induced disruption of PPI was prevented by several antipsychotic compounds but not by propranolol; the ability of typical and atypical antipsychotic agents to prevent this apomorphine effect correlated significantly with their clinical antipsychotic potency and D_2 affinity. An assessment of the construct validity of this model revealed that PPI was significantly decreased by specific mesolimbic hyperdopaminergia produced by direct infusion of dopamine into the NAC, and that this effect was prevented by haloperidol. These findings suggest that the dopamine-stimulated disruption of PPI in rats may be a useful model for understanding the pathophysiology and development of deficient sensorimotor gating in humans and for screening drugs for sensorimotor gating-restorative and putative antipsychotic properties. While the present studies assessed the dopaminergic modulation of PPI, we have reported critical modulatory influences of other transmitter systems within cortico-striato-pallido-pontine circuitry[5] that will continue to be a focus of investigation. In the long run, and in a broader context, it will be important to continue to study how PPI deficits in schizophrenia relate to symptoms, ego function,[76] neuropsychological status,[84] and outcome. In this manner, we will be able to assess how the neurobiology of schizophrenia relates to these critical clinical features of this disorder.

Accepted for publication October 19, 1992.

Dr Swerdlow was supported by a Young Investigator Award from the National Alliance for Research on Schizophrenia and Depression (Chicago, Ill), a Kempf Foundation Award for Research in Psychobiological Psychiatry, American Psychiatric Association (Washington, DC), and FIRST Award MH48381; Drs Braff, Geyer, and Swerdlow were supported by grant MH-42228 from the National Institute of Mental Health, Bethesda, Md.

Some methods in this study were identical to those previously reported by the authors,[16] and the descriptions of these methods may duplicate these previous reports.

The authors gratefully acknowledge the outstanding technical assistance provided by Joyce Sprock and Heidi Hartston.

Reprint requests to 9500 Gilman Dr, La Jolla, CA 92093-0804 (Dr Swerdlow).

REFERENCES

1. Braff D, Stone C, Callaway E, Geyer M, Glick I, Bali L. Prestimulus effects on human startle reflex in normals and schizophrenics. *Psychophysiology.* 1978;15:339-343.
2. Braff DL, Geyer MA. Sensorimotor gating and schizophrenia: human and animal model studies. *Arch Gen Psychiatry.* 1990;47:181-188.
3. Braff DL, Grillon C, Geyer MA. Gating and habituation of the startle reflex in schizophrenic patients. *Arch Gen Psychiatry.* 1992;49:206-215.
4. McGhie A, Chapman J. Disorders of attention and perception in early schizophrenia. *Br J Med Psychol.* 1961;34:102-116.
5. Swerdlow NR, Caine SB, Braff DL, Geyer MA. Neural substrates of sensorimotor gating of the startle reflex: a review of recent findings and their implications. *J Psychopharmacol.* 1991;6:176-190.
6. Wong D, Wagner H, Tune L, Dannals R, Pearlson G, Links J, Tamminga C, Broussolle E, Ravert H, Wilson A, Toung J, Malat J, Williams J, O'Tuama L, Snyder S, Kuhar M, Gjedde A. Positron emission tomography reveals elevated D_2 dopamine receptors in drug-naive schizophrenics. *Science.* 1986;234:1558-1563.
7. Early TS, Relman EM, Raichle ME, Spitzmagel EL. Left globus pallidus abnormality in newly medicated patients with schizophrenia. *Proc Natl Acad Sci U S A.* 1987;84:561-563.
8. Wu JC, Siegel BV, Haier RJ, Buchsbaum MS. Testing the Swerdlow/Koob model of schizophrenia pathophysiology using positron emission tomography. *Behav Brain Sci.* 1990;13:169-170.
9. Altshuler LL, Casanova MF, Goldberg TE, Kleinman JE. The hippocampus and parahippocampus in schizophrenic, suicide, and control brains. *Arch Gen Psychiatry.* 1990;47:1029-1034.
10. Pakkenberg B. Pronounced reduction of total neuron number in mediodorsal thalamic nucleus and nucleus accumbens in schizophrenics. *Arch Gen Psychiatry.* 1990;47:1023-1028.
11. Conrad AJ, Abebe T, Austin R, Forsythe S, Scheibel AB. Hippocampal pyramidal cell disarray in schizophrenia as a bilateral phenomenon. *Arch Gen Psychiatry.* 1991;48:413-417.
12. Seeman P, Ulpian C, Bergeron C, Riederer P, Jellinger K, Babriel E, Reynolds G, Tourtellotte W. Bimodal distribution of dopamine receptor densities in brain of schizophrenics. *Science.* 1984; 225:728-731.
13. Altshuler LL, Conrad A, Kovelman JA, Scheibel A. Hippocampal pyramidal cell orientation in schizophrenia. *Arch Gen Psychiatry.* 1987;44:1094-1098.
14. Bogerts B, Meertz E, Schonfeldt-Bausch R. Basal ganglia and limbic system pathology in schizophrenia: a morphometric study of brain volume and shrinkage. *Arch Gen Psychiatry.* 1985;42: 784-791.
15. Swerdlow NR, Geyer M, Braff D, Koob GF. Central dopamine hyperactivity in rats mimics abnormal acoustic startle in schizophrenics. *Biol Psychiatry.* 1986;21:23-33.
16. Swerdlow NR, Keith VA, Braff DL, Geyer MA. The effects of spiperone, raclopride, SCH 23390 and clozapine on apomorphine-inhibition of sensorimotor gating of the startle response in the rat. *J Pharmacol Exp Ther.* 1991;256:530-536.
17. Mansbach RS, Geyer MA, Braff DL. Dopaminergic stimulation disrupts sensorimotor gating in the rat. *Psychopharmacology.* 1988;94:507-514.
18. Swerdlow NR, Mansbach RS, Geyer MA, Pulvirenti L, Koob GF, Braff DL. Amphetamine disruption of prepulse inhibition of acoustic startle is reversed by depletion of mesolimbic dopamine. *Psychopharmacology.* 1990;100:413-416.
19. Peng RY, Mansbach RS, Braff DL, Geyer MA. A D_2 dopamine receptor agonist disrupts sensorimotor gating in rats: implications for dopaminergic abnormalities in schizophrenia. *Neuropsychopharmacology.* 1990;3:211-218.
20. Rigdon GC, Viik K. Prepulse inhibition as a screening test for potential antipsychotics. *Drug Dev Res.* 1991;23:91-99.
21. Caine SB, Geyer MA, Swerdlow NR. Carbachol infusion into the dentate gyrus disrupts sensorimotor gating of startle in rats. *Psychopharmacology.* 1991;105:347-354.
22. Swerdlow NR, Braff DL, Masten VL, Geyer MA. Schizophrenic-like sensorimotor gating abnormalities in rats following dopamine infusion into the nucleus accumbens. *Psychopharmacology.* 1990;101:414-420.
23. Swerdlow NR, Braff DL, Geyer MA. GABAergic projection from nucleus accumbens to ventral pallidum mediates dopamine-induced sensorimotor gating deficits of acoustic startle in rats. *Brain Res.* 1990;532:146-150.
24. Ison JR, McAdam DW, Hammond GR. Latency and amplitude changes in the acoustic startle reflex produced by variations in auditory prestimulation. *Physiol Behav.* 1973;10:1035-1039.
25. Graham F. The more or less startling effects of weak prestimulation. *Psychophysiology.* 1975; 12:238-248.
26. Swerdlow NR, Benbow CH, Zisook S, Geyer MA, Braff DL. A preliminary assessment of sensorimotor gating in patients with obsessive compulsive disorder. *Biol Psychiatry.* 1993;33:298-301.
27. Swerdlow NR, Caine BC, Geyer MA. Regionally selective effects of intracerebral dopamine infusion on sensorimotor gating of the startle reflex in rats. *Psychopharmacology.* 1992;108:189-195.
28. Swerdlow NR, Caine SB, Geyer MA, Swenson MR, Downs NS, Braff DL. Sensorimotor gating deficits in schizophrenia and Huntington's disease and in rats after manipulation of hippocampus-accumbens circuitry. Presented at the International Congress on Schizophrenia Research; April 21, 1991; Tucson, Ariz.
29. Swerdlow NR, Geyer MA. Clozapine and haloperidol in a novel model for assessing antipsychotic potency. Presented at the meeting of the Society for Neuroscience; October 26, 1992; Anaheim, Calif.
30. Swerdlow NR, Geyer MA. Clozapine and haloperidol in an animal model of sensorimotor gating deficits in schizophrenia. *Pharmacol Biochem Behav.* 1993;44:741-744.
31. Swerdlow NR, Caine B, Geyer MA. Opiate-dopamine interactions in the neural substrates of acoustic startle gating in the rat. *Prog Neuropsychopharmacol Biol Psychiatry.* 1991;15:415-426.
32. Ellenbroek BA, Cools AR. Animal models with construct validity for schizophrenia. *Behav Pharmacol.* 1990;1:469-490.
33. Creese I, Burt DR, Snyder SH. Dopamine receptor binding predicts clinical and pharmacological potencies of antischizophrenic drugs. *Science.* 1976;192:481-483.
34. Sprouse JS, Aghajanian GK. (−)-Propranolol

blocks the inhibition of serotonergic dorsal raphe cell firing by 5HT1A agonists. *Eur J Pharmacol.* 1986;128:295-298.
35. Black JL, Richelson E, Richardson JW. Antipsychotic agents: a clinical update. *Mayo Clin Proc.* 1985;60:777-789.
36. Seeman P, Lee T, Chau-wong M, Wong K. Antipsychotic drug doses and neuroleptic/dopamine receptors. *Nature.* 1976;261:717-719.
37. Richelson E. Pharmacology of neuroleptics in use in the United States. *J Clin Psychiatry.* 1985;46:9-14.
38. Casey DE. Raclopride versus haloperidol: comparative efficacy in a double-blind multicenter investigation. *Biol Psychiatry.* 1991;29:110. Abstract.
39. Hall H, Farde L, Sedvall G. Human dopamine receptor subtypes—in vitro binding analysis using ^{3}H-SCH 23390 and ^{3}H-raclopride. *J Neural Transm.* 1988;73:7-21.
40. Hall H, Kohler C, Gawell L, Farde L, Sedvall G. Raclopride, a new selective ligand for the dopamine D_2 receptors. *Prog Neuropsychopharmacol Biol Psychiatry.* 1988;12:559-568.
41. Madreas BK, Fahey MA, Canfield DR, Spealman RD. D_1 and D_2 dopamine receptors in caudate-putamen of nonhuman primates (*Macaca fascicularis*). *J Neurochem.* 1988;51:934-943.
42. Davis M, Aghajanian GK. Effects of apomorphine and haloperidol on the acoustic startle response in rats. *Psychopharmacology.* 1976;47:217-223.
43. Geyer MA, Tapson GS. Habituation of tactile startle is altered by drugs acting on serotonin-2 receptors. *Neuropsychopharmacology.* 1988;1:135-147.
44. Stevens JR. An anatomy of schizophrenia? *Arch Gen Psychiatry.* 1973;29:177-189.
45. Pycock PJ, Kerwin RW, Carter CJ. Effect of lesions of cortical dopamine terminals on subcortical dopamine receptors in rats. *Nature.* 1990;286:74-77.
46. Weinberger DR, Berman KF, Zec RF. Physiologic dysfunction of dorsolateral prefrontal cortex in schizophrenia, I: regional cerebral blood flow evidence. *Arch Gen Psychiatry.* 1987;44:660-669.
47. Davis KL, Kahn RS, Ko G, Davidson M. Dopamine in schizophrenia: a review and reconceptualization. *Am J Psychiatry.* 1991;148:1474-1486.
48. White FJ, Wang RY. A10 dopamine neurons: role of autoreceptors in determining firing rate and sensitivity to dopamine agonists. *Life Sci.* 1984;34:1161-1170.
49. Rupniak NMJ, Hall MD, Kelly E, Fleminger S, Kilpatrick G, Jenner P, Marsden CD. Mesolimbic dopamine function is not altered during continuous chronic treatment with typical or atypical neuroleptic drugs. *J Neural Transm.* 1985;62:249-266.
50. Tamminga CA, Burrows GH, Chase TN, Alphs LD, Thaker GK. Dopamine neuronal tracts in schizophrenia: their pharmacology and in vivo glucose metabolism. In: Kalivas PW, Nemeroff CB, eds. *The Mesocorticolimbic Dopamine System.* New York, NY: New York Academy of Science; 1988:443-450.
51. Swerdlow NR. Neuropsychology of schizophrenia: the 'hole' thing is wrong. *Behav Brain Sci.* 1991;14:51-53.
52. Heimer L, Zahm DS, Churchill L, Kalivas PW, Wohltmann C. Specificity in the projection patterns of accumbal core and shell in the rat. *Neuroscience.* 1991;41:89-125.
53. Pellegrino LJ, Pellegrino AS, Cushman AJ. *A Stereotaxic Atlas of the Rat Brain.* 2nd ed. New York, NY: Plenum Press; 1979:plates 15-17.
54. Wan FJ, Swerdlow NR. Intra-accumbens infusion of quinpirole impairs sensorimotor gating of acoustic startle in rats. *Psychopharmacology.* In press.
55. Davis M, Gendelman D, Tischler M, Gendelman P. A primary acoustic startle circuit: lesion and stimulation studies. *J Neurosci.* 1982;2:791-805.
56. Meier-Ewert K, Gleitsmann K, Reiter F. Acoustic jaw reflex in man: its relationship to other brain stem and microreflexes. *Electroenceph Clin Neurophysiol.* 1974;36:629-638.
57. Caine SB, Geyer MA, Swerdlow NR. Hippocampal modulation of acoustic startle and prepulse inhibition in rats. *Pharmacol Biochem Behav.* 1992;43:1201-1208.
58. Mogenson GJ, Nielsen M. A study of the contribution of hippocampal-accumbens-subpallidal projections to locomotor activity. *Behav Neural Biol.* 1984;42:52-60.
59. Gray JA, Feldon J, Rawlins JNP, Hemsley DR, Smith AD. The neuropsychology of schizophrenia. *Behav Brain Sci.* 1991;14:1-84.
60. Suddath RL, Christison MD, Torrey EF, Cassanova M, Weinberger DR. Anatomic abnormalities in the brains of monozygotic twins discordant for schizophrenia. *N Engl J Med.* 1990;322:789-794.
61. Siegel C, Waldo M, Mizner G, Adler LE, Freedman R. Deficits in sensory gating in schizophrenic patients and their relatives: evidence obtained with auditory evoked responses. *Arch Gen Psychiatry.* 1984;41:607-612.
62. Schwartzkopf SB, Lamberti JS, Crilly SF, Martin R, Hirt J, Holley L. Combined startle and P50 measures of sensory gating: support for a shared neurophysiology. *Biol Psychiatry.* 1992;31:147. Abstract.
63. Jones DL, Mogenson GJ. Nucleus accumbens to globus pallidus GABA projection subserving ambulatory activity. *Am J Physiol.* 1980;238:R63-69.
64. Swerdlow NR, Koob GF. Separate neural substrates of amphetamine-, caffeine-, and CRF-stimulated locomotor activation. *Pharmacol Biochem Behav.* 1985;23:303-307.
65. Swerdlow NR, Vaccarino FJ, Amalric M, Koob GF. Neural substrates for the motor-activating properties of psychostimulants: a review of recent findings. *Pharmacol Biochem Behav.* 1986;25:233-248.
66. Mogenson GJ. Limbic-motor integration. In: *Progress in Psychobiology and Physiological Psychology.* Orlando, Fla: Academic Press Inc; 1987;12:117-170.
67. Swanson LW, Mogenson GJ, Gerfen CR, Robinson P. Evidence for a projection from the lateral preoptic area and substantia innominata to the 'mesencephalic locomotor region' in the rat. *Brain Res.* 1984;295:161-178.
68. Leitner DS, Powers AS, Stitt CL, Hoffman HS. Midbrain reticular formation involvement in the inhibition of acoustic startle. *Physiol Behav.* 1981;26:259-268.
69. Swerdlow NR, Geyer MA. Prepulse inhibition of acoustic startle in rats after lesions of the pedunculopontine nucleus. *Behav Neurosci.* 1993;107:104-117.
70. Swerdlow NR, Koob GF. Dopamine, schizophrenia, mania and depression: toward a unified hypothesis of cortico-striato-pallido-thalamic function. *Behav Brain Sci.* 1987;10:197-245.
71. Davis M. The mammalian startle response. In: Eaton RC, ed. *Neural Mechanisms of Startle Behavior.* New York, NY: Plenum Press; 1984:287-342.
72. Shagass C. An electrophysiological view of schizophrenia. *Biol Psychiatry.* 1976;11:3-29.
73. Wu JC, Potkin SG, Ploszaj DI, Lau V, Telford J, Richmond G. Clozapine improves sensory gating more than haldol. Presented at the meeting of the American Psychiatric Association; May 6, 1992; Washington, DC.
74. Cadenhead K, Braff DL. Which criteria select 'psychosis-prone' individuals? Presented at the meeting of the Society of Biological Psychiatry; May 1, 1992; Washington, DC.
75. Simmons RF. Schizotypy and startle prepulse inhibition. *Psychophysiology.* 1990;27(suppl):S6.
76. Perry W, Cadenhead K, Braff DL. Thought disorder in the group of schizophrenias. *Biol Psychiatry.* 1992;31:117. Abstract.
77. Rigdon G. Differential effects of apomorphine on prepulse inhibition of acoustic startle reflex in two rat strains. *Psychopharmacology.* 1990;102:419-421.
78. Weinberger DR. Implications of normal brain development for the pathogenesis of schizophrenia. *Arch Gen Psychiatry.* 1987;44:660-669.
79. Geyer MA, Wilkinson LS, Humby TT, Robbins TW. Isolation rearing of rats produces a deficit in sensorimotor gating similar to that in schizophrenia. *Biol Psychiatry.* 1992;31:197. Abstract.
80. Ornitz EM, Guthrie D, Sadeghpour M, Sugiyama T. Maturation of prestimulation-induced startle modulation in girls. *Psychophysiology.* 1991;28:11-20.
81. Miczek KA, Vivian JA, Tornatzky W, Farrell WJ, Sapperstein SB. Withdrawal from diazepam in rats: ultrasonic vocalizations and acoustic startle reflex. Presented at the meeting of the British Association of Psychopharmacology and the European Behavioural Pharmacology Society; August 6, 1992; Cambridge, United Kingdom.
82. Freedman DX, Giarman NJ. Apomorphine test for tranquilizing drugs: effect of dibenamine. *Science.* 1956;124:264.
83. Schwartzkopf SB, Bruno JP, Mitra T. Dopamine D_1/D_2 receptor effects on sensory gating in controls and neonatally dopamine depleted animals. Presented at the meeting of the American College of Neuropsychopharmacology; December 11, 1991; San Juan, Puerto Rico.
84. Braff DL, Heaton R, Kuck J, Cullum M, Moranville J, Grant I, Zisook S. The generalized pattern of neuropsychological deficits in outpatients with chronic schizophrenia with heterogeneous Wisconsin Card Sorting Test results. *Arch Gen Psychiatry.* 1991;48:891-898.

Clinical Response to Clozapine in Patients With Schizophrenia

One of the take-home messages from our recent report regarding the clinical and biological effects of the atypical neuroleptic, clozapine, was that the admixture of clozapine's effects on dopaminergic, serotonergic, and noradrenergic systems may underlie its unique efficacy in otherwise poorly responsive patients with schizophrenia.[1] We agree with a suggestion by R. W. Pies, MD, (unpublished communication to the ARCHIVES, May 1992) that clozapine's diverse pharmacologic properties indicate strategies for augmentation of neuroleptic drugs in treatment-resistant patients and that thioridazine or mesoridazine besylate may be particularly useful, given their relatively low incidence of extrapyramidal side effects.

Whereas much attention has been given to the 5-hydroxytryptamine$_2$ (5-HT$_2$) antagonism of clozapine, including the ratio of 5-HT$_2$ to D$_2$ affinities as a predictor of neuroleptic atypicality,[2] we have noted that clozapine's relatively potent α_2-antagonism (putatively contributing to observed increases in norepinephrine turnover) is distinct among neuroleptics[3] and have used this property as a basis for enhancing neuroleptic treatment. We have observed in pilot investigations that the α_2-antagonist, idazoxan, shows considerable promise as an augmenting agent for the typical neuroleptic, fluphenazine hydrochloride.[4] The **Figure** shows longitudinal behavioral data from one inpatient during a double-blind crossover comparison of fluphenazine and idazoxan augmentation of fluphenazine. Consistent with our experience in other patients, the addition of idazoxan to long-term fluphenazine treatment resulted in clinically significant decrements in symptoms with return to (or above) baseline on discontinuation of idazoxan therapy. Although the crossover design has limitations in establishing efficacy, it is well suited for exploratory studies, and our results suggest that α_2-antagonists be pursued in other investigations in patients with schizophrenia.

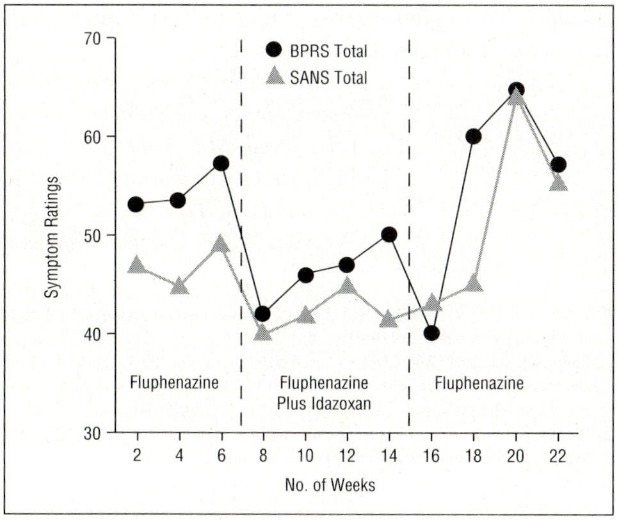

Symptom ratings in an inpatient with schizophrenia who underwent idazoxan augmentation of fluphenazine hydrochloride treatment. BPRS indicates Brief Psychiatric Rating Scale; SANS, Scale for Assessment of Negative Symptoms.

The augmentation of neuroleptic treatment has been tried with at least some success using benzodiazepines and triazolobenzodiazepines,[5] 5-HT$_2$,[6] and opiate antagonists,[7] as well as lithium and anticonvulsants.[8] The inherent difficulty in neuroleptic augmentation studies, including relatively low baseline symptom levels and resultant small drug-induced change, should not preclude attempts to identify potentially useful agents for treating the seriously ill patient. Further, subgroup responsiveness may hold promise for identifying pathophysiologic variants of schizophrenia, which, in turn, may lead to new treatments.[9]

David Pickar, MD
Robert E. Litman, MD
Walter W. Hong, MD
Tom P. Su, MD
Ellen M. Weissman, MD
John K. Hsiao, MD
William Z. Potter, MD, PhD
Experimental Therapeutics Branch, DIRP, NIMH
National Institutes of Health
NIH 10/4N214
9000 Rockville Pike
Bethesda, MD 20892

1. Pickar D, Owen RR, Litman RE, Konicki PE, Gutierrez R, Rapaport MH. Clinical and biological response to clozapine in patients with schizophrenia: crossover comparison with fluphenazine. *Arch Gen Psychiatry.* 1992;49:345-353.
2. Meltzer HY. Clozapine: clinical advantages and biological mechanisms. In: Schulz SC, Tamminga CA, eds. *Schizophrenia: Scientific Progress.* New York, NY: Oxford University Press; 1989:302-309.
3. Richelson E, Nelson A. Antagonism by neuroleptics of neurotransmitter receptors of normal human brain in vitro. *Eur J Pharmacol.* 1984;103:197-204.
4. Litman RE, Hong WW, Weissman EM, Su TP, Potter WZ, Pickar D. Idazoxan, an α_2 antagonist, augments fluphenazine in schizophrenic patients: a pilot study. *J Clin Psychopharmacol.* 1993;13:264-267.
5. Wolkowitz OM, Pickar D. Benzodiazepines in the treatment of schizophrenia: a review and reappraisal. *Am J Psychiatry.* 1991;148:714-726.
6. Bersani G, Grispini A, Marini S, Pasini A, Valducci M, Ciani N. 5-HT$_2$ antagonist ritanserin in neuroleptic-induced parkinsonism: a double-blind comparison with orphenadrine and placebo. *Clin Neuropharmacol.* 1990;13:500-506.
7. Pickar D, Cohen MR, Naber D, Cohen RM. Clinical studies of the endogenous opioid system. *Biol Psychiatry.* 1982;17:1243-1276.

8. Pickar D, Owen RR, Litman RE. New developments in the pharmacotherapy of schizophrenia. In: Tasman A, Goldfinger SM, eds. *American Psychiatric Press Review of Psychiatry*. Washington, DC: American Psychiatric Association; 1991; 10:98-115.
9. Wolkowitz OM, Bartko JJ, Pickar D. Heterogeneity in drug trials in schizophrenia: the mean is not the end. *Biol Psychiatry*. 1990;28:1021-1025.

The Relation of Parenthood to Suicide

Høyer and Lund[1] reported finding only one study "focusing on the importance of parenthood related to suicide," proposing theirs as the "first prospective one [of a large size] focusing on the association between family size and suicide among women." In our review of risk factors for death by suicide,[2] we noted several investigators since Veevers[3] have reported evidence suggesting that parental status is a better demographic marker for decreased suicide risk than marital status (ie, those with responsibility for young children are at lower risk)[4,5] or have offered the same hypothesis as an explanation for their findings.[6]

Nonetheless, the Høyer and Lund study constitutes a remarkable contribution to the epidemiology of suicide. By tracking an entire population of women (almost 1 million) of known marital, childbearing, and parental status for 15 years, they show that married women without children were more likely to die by suicide than married women with children; married women without children were less likely to die by suicide than unmarried women without children; and among married women, suicide risk declined significantly in proportion to the number of children for women who were premenopausal as well as for women who were postmenopausal. They cautioned that childbearing by single women, widows, or divorcées (less than 5% of total births) was not recorded and that their analyses could not take into account parental status changes during the follow-up period.

Although we have cited several overlooked contributions, we too believe that the thought-provoking Høyer and Lund study is the first large-scale population study of the relative contributions of marital status and parental status to female suicide risk and the first to focus on the association between family size and suicide. Like the authors, we are curious to know whether unmarried women with children are at a lower risk for suicide than other unmarried women, whether loss of child custody is associated with an observable increase in risk for suicide, and whether there is any effect of family size on male suicide risk.

David C. Clark, PhD
Jan Fawcett, MD
Rush-Presbyterian-St Luke's Medical Center
1725 W Harrison St, Suite 955
Chicago, IL 60612

1. Høyer G, Lund E. Suicide among women related to number of children in marriage. *Arch Gen Psychiatry*. 1993;50:134-137.
2. Clark DC, Fawcett J. Review of empirical risk factors for evaluation of the suicidal patient. In: Bongar B, ed. *Suicide: Guidelines for Assessment, Management, and Treatment*. New York, NY: Oxford University Press; 1992:16-48.
3. Veevers JE. Parenthood and suicide: an examination of a neglected variable. *Soc Sci Med*. 1973;7:135-144.
4. Kozak CM, Gibbs JO. Dependent children and suicide of married parents. *Suicide Life Threat Behav*. 1979;9:67-75.
5. Fawcett J, Scheftner WA, Clark DC, Hedeker D, Gibbons RD, Coryell W. Clinical predictors of suicide in patients with major affective disorders: a controlled prospective study. *Am J Psychiatry*. 1987;144:35-40.
6. Lindesay J. Age, sex and suicide rates within birth cohorts in England and Wales. *Soc Psychiatry Psychiatr Epidemiol*. 1989;24:249-252.

In reply

We are grateful for the interest in our study. Unfortunately the MEDLINE search we performed did not provide us with references to the articles by Kozak and Gibbs,[1] Fawcett and coworkers,[2] and Lindesay.[3] We have ordered copies of these reports and are looking forward to reading them. We apologize if we have overlooked these prospective studies focusing on the parental status and risk factors for suicide.

We are sorry our data cannot provide any information on the influence of childbearing among unmarried women on suicide rates. As to whether loss of child custody increases the risk for suicide, we think there are (at least) two different situations involved, the first being loss of custody while the children are still cared for by their parents; we are not able to study the impact of such events on suicide rates from our data. Second, when loss of custody occurs as a result of the natural process of children growing up, our study did not support that this kind of loss increased the suicide risk.

The last question—whether there is any effect of family size on male suicide risk—is very interesting. For the time being we have no access to the data that might explore this phenomenon. However, such data could be provided for Norwegian married males, and we hope we will be able to do this analysis in the future.

Georg Høyer, MD, PhD
Eiliv Lund, MD, PhD
Institute of Community Medicine
University of Tromsø
Breivika, 9037 Tromsø, Norway

1. Kozak CM, Gibbs JO. Dependent children and suicide of married parents. *Suicide Life Threat Behav*. 1979;9:67-75.
2. Fawcett J, Scheftner WE, Clark DC, Hedeker D, Gibbons RD, Coryell W. Clinical predictors of suicide in patients with major affective disorders: a controlled prospective study. *Am J Psychiatry*. 1987;144:35-40.
3. Lindesay J. Age, sex and suicide rates within birth cohorts in England and Wales. *Soc Psychiatry Psychiatr Epidemiol*. 1989;24:249-252.

The Third Editor of the ARCHIVES—Jack D. Barchas, MD

THE JULY 1993 issue of the *Archives of General Psychiatry* contained a sad irony for friends of the journal. That issue carried a memorial to the founding editor of the ARCHIVES, Roy R. Grinker, Sr, MD, written by his successor, Daniel X. Freedman, MD.[1] In that same issue was the news that Dr Freedman had died suddenly.

We are pleased to announce the appointment of the third editor of the *Archives of General Psychiatry*: Jack D. Barchas, MD.

Jack David Barchas is an outstanding choice to succeed the two eminent psychiatrists who have edited the journal. A graduate of Yale University School of Medicine, Dr Barchas completed his medical internship at the University of Chicago Pritzker School of Medicine and his psychiatric residency at Stanford University. From 1966 to 1990 he was based at Stanford where he rose to professor of psychiatry and behavioral sciences, director of the Nancy Pritzker Laboratory of Behavioral Neurochemistry, and associate chair of the Department of Psychiatry and Behavioral Sciences. He moved to UCLA in 1990 as associate dean for neuroscience and in 1991 was appointed dean for research development and for neuroscience.

In 1993, Dr Barchas accepted a new challenge as Barklie McKee Henry Professor and chairman of the Department of Psychiatry, Cornell University Medical College, and psychiatrist-in-chief at the New York Hospital, where the ARCHIVES editorial office will now be based.

Dr Barchas's breadth of knowledge in psychiatry is well established. His primary research activities at Stanford centered on the relationship between the brain and behavior, but his interests are wide ranging and embrace the many perspectives within the specialty. He has published more than 400 articles, monographs, and book chapters and is completing a textbook on psychopharmacology. As chairman of the Institute of Medicine's Board of Biobehavioral Science and Mental Disorders, Dr Barchas is well versed in policy issues related to the health sciences.

There is an added poignancy to Jack Barchas's appointment, resulting from his long professional and personal association with Danny Freedman. Jack was a student of Dan's at Yale and did his first research under Dan's preceptorship. He published his first paper with Dan Freedman as coauthor. Years later, Dan took great delight in telling friends that his former student was now his "boss" at UCLA. It was Jack Barchas who, with Myrna Weissman of the editorial board, wrote the farewell tribute to Dan in the August 1993 issue of the ARCHIVES.[2] There is a fitting sense of continuity in entrusting the ARCHIVES to Jack Barchas. We know that while he is mindful of the tradition of excellence that Dan Freedman established, he will bring his own ideas and direction to the journal.

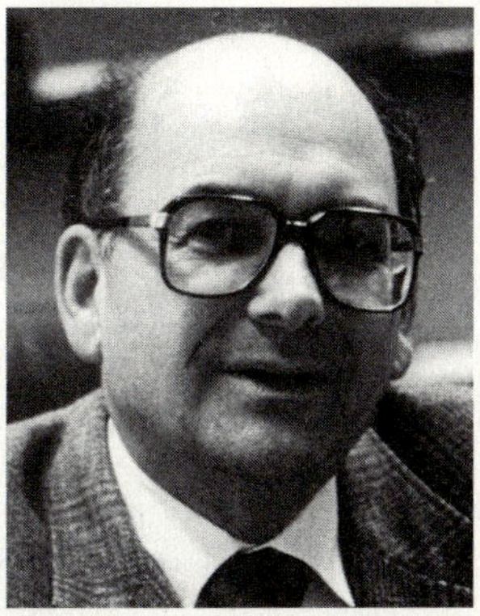

Jack D. Barchas, MD

We could not offer a more eloquent recommendation than this one written by the chair of one of the leading departments of psychiatry:

> I have given careful consideration to the question of the editorship of the ARCHIVES. I personally believe that there are relatively few individuals in the field who could successfully follow in Dan Freedman's footsteps. Dan's encyclopedic knowledge, not only of biological but also psychosocial psychiatry, set a standard that will be hard to match. In addition, his gentle but firm support of junior scientists, as well as his insistence on the highest levels of skills among the senior scientists, suggest the level of diplomacy (perhaps a bit frayed around the edges) that is essential as the overall publication mission of the journal.
>
> In my view, there is only one individual who captures all of the qualities of Dan Freedman. That individual is Jack Barchas, recently of UCLA, and now on his way to being chairman of the Department of Psychiatry of Cornell. Jack could serve in this role admirably and successfully, and he would enjoy the respect and confidence of the field. Having worked with and around Dan, I think that Jack would fully understand the importance and significance of his role as editor of the ARCHIVES.

We trust readers of the ARCHIVES will agree and we wish Dr Barchas the greatest success as editor of this important journal.

Michael D. Springer
Associate Publisher
ARCHIVES *Specialty Journals*
George D. Lundberg, MD
Editor-in-Chief
Scientific Publications

REFERENCES

1. Freedman DX. The founding editor of the *Archives*, Roy R. Grinker, Sr, MD, August 2, 1900, to May 9, 1993. *Arch Gen Psychiatry.* 1993;50:511-513.
2. Weissman MM, Barchas JD. Daniel X. Freedman, MD, August 17, 1921, to June 3, 1993. *Arch Gen Psychiatry.* 1993;50:665-668.

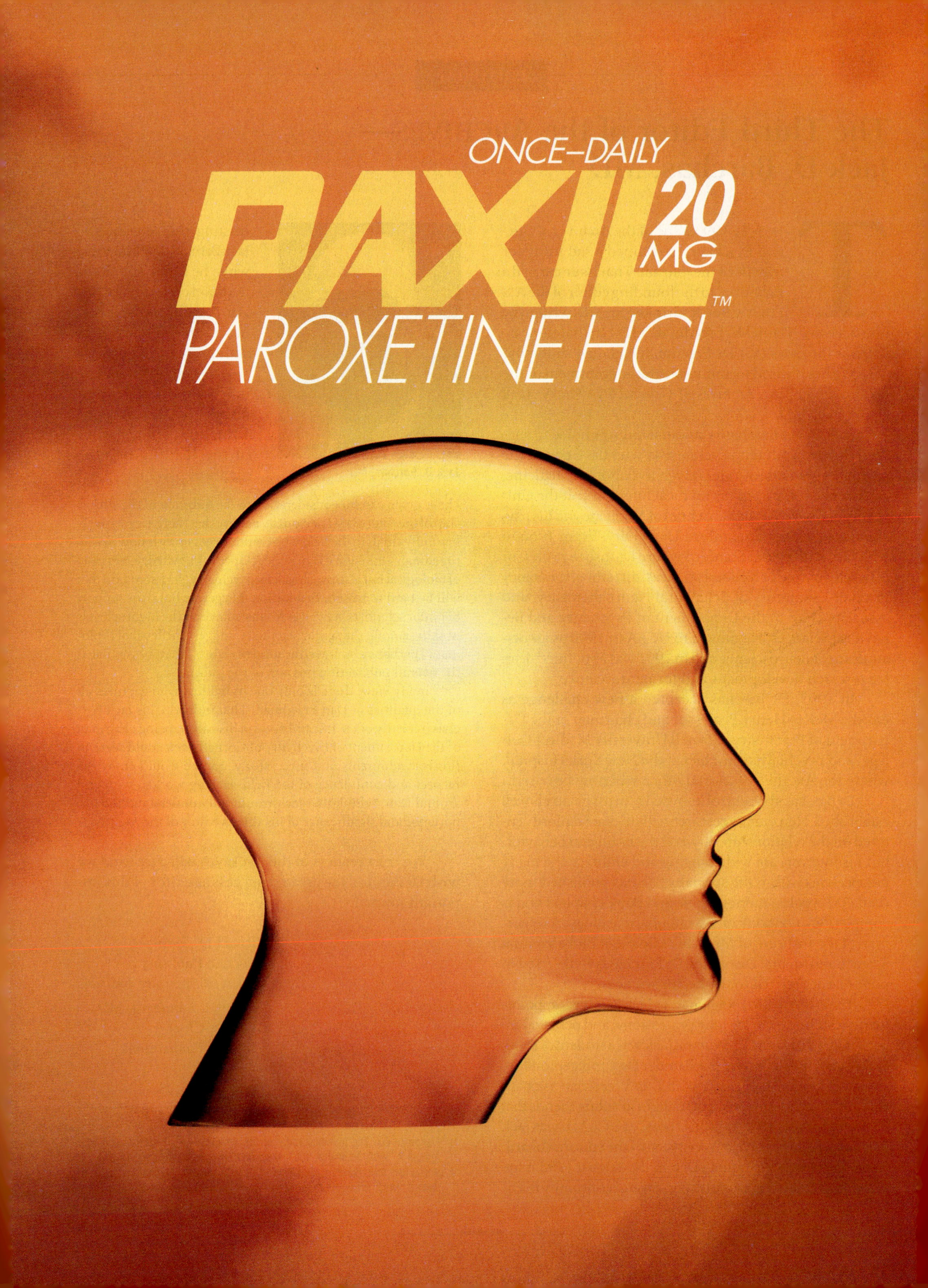
ONCE-DAILY
PAXIL 20 MG™
PAROXETINE HCI

ORIGINAL ARTICLE

Psychotherapy and Pharmacotherapy for Ambulatory Cocaine Abusers

Kathleen M. Carroll, PhD; Bruce J. Rounsaville, MD; Lynn T. Gordon, RN, MPA; Charla Nich, MS; Peter Jatlow, MD; Roseann M. Bisighini; Frank H. Gawin, MD

Background: At present, there is no consensus regarding effective treatment for cocaine abuse or the most productive roles for the two major forms of treatment, pharmacotherapy and psychotherapy. We conducted the first randomized clinical trial evaluating psychotherapy and pharmacotherapy, alone and in combination, as treatment for ambulatory cocaine abusers.

Methods: One hundred thirty-nine subjects were assigned to one of four conditions offered over a 12-week abstinence initiation trial: relapse prevention plus desipramine hydrochloride, clinical management plus desipramine, relapse prevention plus placebo, and clinical management plus placebo. All treatments were manual-guided, delivered by experienced therapists, and monitored to promote the integrity of both forms of treatment.

Results: First, although all groups showed significant improvement, significant main effects for medication or psychotherapy, or their combination, were not found for treatment retention, reduction in cocaine use, or other outcomes at 12 weeks. Second, baseline severity of cocaine use interacted differently with psychotherapy and pharmacotherapy: higher-severity patients had significantly better outcome when treated with relapse prevention than with clinical management, while desipramine was associated with improved abstinence initiation among lower-severity subjects. Third, desipramine was significantly more effective than placebo in reducing cocaine use over 6, but not 12, weeks of treatment. Fourth, depressed subjects had greater reduction in cocaine use than nondepressed subjects and had better response to relapse prevention than to clinical management.

Conclusion: These findings underscore the significance of heterogeneity among cocaine abusers and the need to develop specialized treatments for clinically distinct subgroups of cocaine abusers.

(Arch Gen Psychiatry. 1994;51:177-187)

AT PRESENT, there is no consensus regarding effective treatment for cocaine abuse or the most productive roles for the two major forms of treatment, pharmacotherapy and psychotherapy. The initial promise of heterocyclic antidepressant facilitation of abstinence initiation[1] has not yet been widely replicated in well-controlled clinical trials[2,3]; moreover, the effectiveness of such agents may vary with the subject sample and the ancillary treatment modality in which they are delivered.[4] In addition, as most pharmacologic trials have included psychotherapeutic components (group or individual psychotherapy) intended to encourage treatment retention and enhance compliance with medication, the effectiveness of pharmacotherapies alone, without substantial nonpharmacologic support, is underinvestigated. Moreover, because the role of psychotherapy in pharmacologic trials has been conceived primarily as support to pharmacotherapy, nonpharmacologic aspects of treatment have rarely been specified in terms of content (interventions used), dose (frequency and duration of sessions), agent (experience and training of therapists), or compliance. The potentially unique and specific effects of psychotherapy as treat-

From the Division of Substance Abuse, Departments of Psychiatry (Drs Carroll and Rounsaville and Ms Bisighini) and Laboratory Medicine (Dr Jatlow), Yale University School of Medicine, and the APT Foundation (Mss Gordon and Nich), New Haven, Conn; and Veterans Affairs Medical Center, Brentwood, Calif (Dr Gawin).

See Subjects and Methods on next page

SUBJECTS AND METHODS

SUBJECTS

Subjects were recruited from individuals seeking treatment at the outpatient clinic of the Substance Abuse Treatment Unit of the Connecticut Mental Health Center in New Haven or from respondents to newspaper advertisements or public service announcements. Subjects were initially screened by telephone to establish cocaine as the principal drug of abuse. Subjects were included who met current *DSM-III-R*[8] criteria for cocaine dependence and who reported using at least 12 g of cocaine during the past 3 months. Individuals were excluded who (1) were currently physically dependent on opiates, barbiturates, or alcohol, or whose principal drug of dependence was not cocaine; (2) met current *DSM-III-R*[8] criteria for an Axis I disorder other than depressive or anxiety disorders, met lifetime criteria for schizophrenia or mania, or expressed significant suicidal or homicidal ideation; (3) had a current medical condition that would contraindicate ambulatory tricyclic antidepressant therapy; (4) had been treated for substance abuse during the previous 2 months or were currently involved in psychotherapy or pharmacotherapy for any other psychiatric disorder; or (5) had conditions of probation or parole requiring reports of drug use to officers of the court. In such cases, we believed that these conditions could undercut the validity of subjects' self-reports of substance use.[9,10]

Subjects who passed initial screening were administered sections of the Structured Clinical Interview for *DSM-III-R* (SCID)[11] to rule out major psychiatric disorder. Urinalyses, blood laboratory workups, and electrocardiograms were conducted for medical clearance. One hundred thirty-nine of the 191 individuals who passed telephone screening were eligible for the study and provided informed consent. Primary reasons for ineligibility were (1) failure to complete medical or psychiatric evaluation (n=28), (2) psychiatric or medical illness (n=8), (3) use of less than 1 g of cocaine per week (n=5), (4) decision to seek inpatient treatment (n=5), and (5) inability or unwillingness to take medication (n=2).

THERAPISTS

Eleven experienced therapists (four psychologists and seven psychiatrists) each saw an average of 11 patients (range, 1 to 23). Therapists selected were experienced in and committed to the type of treatment they would be conducting in the trial (four psychologists and one psychiatrist conducted relapse prevention, and six psychiatrists conducted clinical management) and in treating substance users. Therapists averaged 4.4 years of postdoctoral experience. All therapists received training that included (1) a 2-day didactic seminar in which the treatment manual, study aims and procedures, and videotaped case examples were reviewed in detail and (2) successful completion of at least one closely supervised training case. To ensure adherence to manual guidelines and to prevent drift during the main phase of the study, therapists in each condition met weekly with study investigators (K.M.C. for relapse prevention and F.H.G. for clinical management) to discuss case material and review session videotapes.

To evaluate the potential influence of therapist effects on findings, we conducted a one-way analysis of variance (ANOVA) on measures of treatment retention, cocaine use, and patient compliance. The single therapist who saw only one patient was not included in these analyses. No significant effects for therapist were found for any variable, even using liberal ($P<.20$) significance levels as recommended by Crits-Christoph and Mintz.[12] We concluded that the results presented below were not strongly influenced by the unique characteristics of the therapists participating in this trial and would generalize to other groups of therapists with similar backgrounds and training using the treatment manuals and methods presented herein.

TREATMENTS

Each of the study treatments was manual-guided and was delivered to subjects in weekly individual sessions that were offered over 12 weeks. Before meeting with the therapist each week, subjects met with the project coordinator/nurse who dispensed study medication, obtained serum samples for medication blood level assessment, and monitored blood pressure. Subjects also met weekly with an independent clinical evaluator who assessed cocaine use and other clinical symptoms. To maintain a single blind for psychotherapy, the clinical evaluator saw subjects in an office physically separated from the offices in which therapy was conducted and instructed subjects not to disclose details of their therapist or treatment.

DESIPRAMINE

Subjects initiated medication with 50 mg of desipramine hydrochloride at night (or one placebo pill), increasing to an average of 200 mg/d by the end of the first week to a maximum dose of 300 mg/d. Initial target plasma level ranges were 300 to 750 nmol/L. All subjects had plasma drawn weekly for medication level assessments. Dosage adjustments were made by a nonblind study psychiatrist (B.J.R. or F.H.G.) in response to serum blood levels and reported side effects and were yoked to dose changes for subjects receiving placebo to maintain a medication double blind. Standard procedures for time since last medication dose, sample collection, and sample analysis were employed.[13]

COGNITIVE-BEHAVIORAL COPING SKILLS TRAINING

The cognitive-behavioral treatment was based on relapse prevention principles described by Marlatt and Gordon[14] and was adapted for use with cocaine users.[15] The goal of this treatment was abstinence from cocaine and other substances through identification of high-risk situations for relapse and the implementation of more effective coping strategies. As described in the *Manual for Relapse Prevention in the Treatment of Cocaine Abuse* (K.M.C. unpublished data, 1987), primary interventions of this approach include (1) reducing exposure to cocaine and cocaine cues, (2) fostering resolution to stop cocaine use through exploring positive and negative consequences of continued use, (3) self-monitoring to identify high-risk situations for relapse, (4) recognition of conditioned cocaine craving and development of strategies for coping with cocaine craving, (5) identification of seemingly irrelevant decisions that could culminate in high-risk situations, (6) preparation for emergencies and coping with a relapse to cocaine use, and (7) developing alternate activities to cocaine use. Material discussed during sessions was supplemented with extrasession tasks intended to foster implementation and mastery of coping skills.

CLINICAL MANAGEMENT

Clinical management was adapted from the guidelines developed for the National Institute of Mental Health Collaborative Study on the Treatment of Depression by Fawcett et al.[16] The provision of clinical management was intended to provide (1) nonspecific elements of a psychotherapeutic relationship, including a supportive doctor-patient relationship, education, empathy, and the instillation of hope, without providing active ingredients specific to relapse prevention; (2) medication management, as well as an opportunity to monitor subjects' clinical status and treatment response; and (3) a convincing therapeutic rationale to foster greater retention in the protocol and compliance with medication. These features, although desirable in a psychotherapy control condition because they address many ethical and methodologic concerns, may be powerfully therapeutic on their own and, thus, act as much more stringent tests of active psychotherapies than would alternatives such as no-treatment or waiting list–control conditions that would provide neither nonspecific elements nor a persuasive therapeutic rationale.[17]

TREATMENT IMPLEMENTATION

All training and main-phase sessions were videotaped for supervision and process assessment. To evaluate discriminability of the two forms of psychotherapy, session videotapes were rated by independent evaluators using a modification of the Collaborative Study Psychotherapy Rating Scale,[18,19] which assesses therapists' degree of adherence to manual-specified techniques. Ratings of 103 randomly selected sessions, with each session evaluated by two raters who were "blind" to treatment condition, indicated that (1) relapse prevention therapists were significantly more likely to engage in relapse prevention interventions (mean total relapse prevention score for relapse prevention therapists 16.7 vs 4.4 was for clinical management therapists, t=8.2, df=122, P<.001); (2) clinical management therapists were significantly more likely to engage in clinical management interventions (8.4 vs 5.0, t=4.0, df=120, P<.001); and (3) relapse prevention and clinical management therapists engaged in comparable levels of general facilitative interventions such as assessing recent substance use and general functioning, encouraging abstinence, and maintaining session focus (mean score for relapse prevention therapists 8.0 vs 9.2 was for clinical management therapists, not significant).

OUTCOME ASSESSMENT

Subjects were assessed before treatment, weekly during treatment, and at termination. Primary outcome measures were reduction in frequency of cocaine use (percentage of days the subject reported using cocaine while in treatment) and initiation of abstinence (duration of longest period of consecutive abstinence reported in treatment). Subjects' self-reports were verified through urine toxicology screens obtained at every visit. Of 622 urinalyses conducted, 71% (n=442) were consistent with subjects' self-report, 15% (n=93) were negative for cocaine, although the subject reported recent cocaine use, and 14% (n=87) were positive for cocaine in instances where the subject had denied use. In cases of discrepancy between self-report and toxicology reports, the source of data that indicated cocaine use was used in outcome analyses.

SECONDARY OUTCOMES

The Addiction Severity Index (ASI)[20] was administered monthly during treatment to assess multidimensional aspects of outcome and general functioning. We supplemented the drug abuse section of the ASI to calculate separate composite scores for cocaine vs other drug use, resulting in eight rather than seven domains. The Beck Depression Inventory[21] and Hamilton Depression Rating Scale[22] were completed monthly to monitor depressive symptoms.

DATA ANALYSES

The primary analysis of outcome was a factorial ANOVA on continuous measures, with medication and psychotherapy type as the two factors. We used ANOVA rather than analysis of covariance (ANCOVA) because there was significant heterogeneity of regression for baseline severity of cocaine use on primary outcome measures, suggesting that the treatments were differentially effective at different severity levels and the use of pooled regression for the ANCOVA (which assumes a linear relationship between the covariate and outcome) was therefore not justified.

Paired t tests were used to assess change from pretreatment to posttreatment within each of the treatment groups. For analyses of ASI composite scores, end-point analyses, where the subject's status at termination or the

Continued on next page

last rating before leaving the study, were used. To measure change in quantity and frequency of cocaine use over time and to explore possible differences in time to effect for psychotherapy and pharmacotherapy, repeated-measures multivariate analysis of variance (MANOVA) were conducted on continuous variables. To evaluate the effect on outcome of subject's baseline severity of cocaine use and of comorbid psychopathology, exploratory 2×2×3 (medication×psychotherapy×severity/psychopathology) ANOVAs were conducted.

Outcome analyses were conducted on the following samples of subjects:

1. All subjects randomized to treatment (n=139). Analyses for the intention-to-treat sample reflect acceptability and effectiveness of study procedures and treatments for all subjects who met eligibility criteria and provided informed consent.

2. All subjects who completed two or more treatment sessions and who received study medication for at least 1 week (n=110). Analyses for this sample reflect outcome for all subjects with at least minimal exposure to treatment, reflect ability of each treatment to hold subjects, and allow opportunity for medication and psychotherapy effects to emerge.

3. All subjects who completed treatment (n=49), defined as fully complying with psychotherapy (remaining in treatment 12 weeks or completing 12 sessions) and pharmacotherapy (medication blood levels consistently within target range for subjects receiving active medication). Analyses for this sample reflect outcomes for subjects exposed to a full course of treatment.

Findings were highly consistent across the three analysis samples. To simplify presentation of results, analyses are presented herein for the sample on which data are most complete, ie, the 110 subjects who received some exposure to treatment.

ment for cocaine abusers have often gone unsystematized, unmonitored, and perhaps underrecognized in pharmacologic trials.

Similarly, few well-designed clinical trials evaluating the efficacy of psychotherapies as treatment for cocaine abuse have been conducted. Kang et al[5] evaluated the efficacy of weekly psychotherapy, family therapy, or group therapy led by paraprofessionals and reported no differences by treatment type and no association between number of treatment sessions and outcome. However, this study did not make use of many methodologic features that are now standard in psychotherapy efficacy research, such as specification of treatment in manuals, training of experienced and qualified therapists, or monitoring of treatment implementation.[6] Moreover, of 122 subjects observed, 50 (41%) dropped out before beginning treatment and few subjects received even a minimal dose of treatment. In contrast, a study that included methodologic features associated with a technology model of psychotherapy research (which describes psychotherapies to approximate specification of pharmacotherapies in Food and Drug Administration medication trials) found evidence to support the specific effectiveness of psychotherapy among more severely impaired cocaine abusers.[7]

Despite preliminary evaluations of psychotherapy and pharmacotherapy, no study has yet compared these two forms of treatment or systematically evaluated their efficacy when combined. In this article, we report results from a randomized clinical trial evaluating four treatments for ambulatory cocaine abusers: (1) desipramine hydrochloride in combination with relapse prevention, a cognitive-behavioral approach, (2) desipramine in combination with clinical management, a psychotherapy-control condition, (3) relapse prevention plus placebo, and (4) clinical management plus placebo. We hypothesized that both desipramine and relapse prevention would be more effective than placebo and clinical management, respectively. Moreover, the design allowed detection of combined effects of psychotherapy and pharmacotherapy if these were sufficiently robust.

RESULTS

SAMPLE DESCRIPTION

One hundred thirty-nine subjects met study criteria and were randomized to treatment; of these, 121 (87%) began treatment and 110 (79%) completed two sessions or more. As shown in **Table 1**, of the 110 who were exposed to two or more sessions and received medication at least 1 week, 30 were women (27%), 59 were minority (54%), 78 were single or divorced (71%), and 58 were working full or part time (53%). Thirty-seven had some college education (34%), 46 were high school graduates (42%), and 26 did not complete high school (24%). The mean (±SD) age of the sample was 28.8±5.8 years. Subjects reported using a mean of 4.4±3.3 g of cocaine per week for a mean of 4.2 years. Sixty-eight reported predominantly freebase use of cocaine (62%), 32 were intranasal users (29%), and 10 were intravenous users (9%). Thirty-three had some previous exposure to treatment (30%). Forty-eight percent met *DSM-III-R*[8] criteria for a lifetime diagnosis of alcohol dependence, 20% for a lifetime diagnosis of affective disorder, 13% for a lifetime diagnosis of anxiety disorder, 49% for diagnosis of antisocial personality disorder, and 65% for any other personality disorder. Analyses of variance and χ^2 tests revealed that there were no statistically significant differences by treatment group for any of these baseline variables.

Table 1. Pretreatment Characteristics of All Subjects Completing Two or More Sessions (N=110)*

Characteristic	Treatment Group† CM/DMI (n=25)	RP/DMI (n=29)	CM/PLA (n=27)	RP/PLA (n=29)
Demographic				
Age, y	29.2±4.9	28.8±5.7	28.8±5.9	28.6±6.8
Female	8 (32)	6 (21)	10 (37)	6 (21)
Minority	12 (48)	14 (48)	15 (55)	18 (62)
Single/divorced	16 (64)	19 (66)	21 (78)	22 (76)
Unemployed	10 (40)	12 (41)	17 (63)	13 (45)
Education				
Some college	9 (36)	10 (36)	6 (22)	12 (42)
High school graduate	7 (28)	15 (52)	13 (48)	11 (38)
Less than high school	9 (36)	4 (14)	7 (26)	6 (20)
Cocaine use				
Grams per week	4.3±4.3	4.6±3.8	5.1±3.3	3.7±2.7
Years of regular use	3.6±2.5	4.1±4.2	4.6±3.9	4.5±4.6
Previous treatment	9 (36)	7 (24)	8 (29)	9 (31)
Primary route of administration				
Freebase	17 (68)	13 (45)	20 (74)	18 (62)
Intranasal	6 (24)	12 (41)	5 (19)	9 (31)
Intravenous	2 (8)	4 (14)	2 (7)	2 (7)
Severity of cocaine use				
Low (1.00-2.50 g/wk)	9 (36)	8 (28)	5 (19)	13 (45)
Moderate (2.51-4.49 g/wk)	9 (36)	10 (35)	10 (37)	8 (28)
High (≥4.50 g/wk)	7 (28)	11 (38)	12 (44)	4 (28)
Lifetime *DSM-III-R* psychiatric disorders‡				
Any affective disorder	4 (18)	4 (19)	4 (21)	5 (23)
Any anxiety disorder	5 (22)	1 (4)	4 (21)	1 (4)
Alcohol dependence	10 (45)	11 (52)	8 (40)	12 (57)
Antisocial personality disorder	11 (52)	11 (55)	5 (25)	9 (64)
Any non-ASP personality disorder	10 (66)	9 (60)	10 (71)	5 (62)

**Values are reported as mean±SD or number (percent).*

†CM/DMI indicates clinical management plus desipramine hydrochloride; RP/DMI, relapse prevention plus desipramine; CM/PLA, clinical management plus placebo; RP/PLA, relapse prevention plus placebo; and ASP, antisocial personality disorder. There was no statistical significance between treatment groups.

‡From the Structured Clinical Interview for DSM-III-R *(SCID) and the SCID-II interview. N=84 because of missing data due to failure of subjects to complete interviews.*

ATTRITION

For subjects who initiated treatment (n=121), the mean number of sessions completed was 7.2±3.6; 49 subjects (40%) completed treatment (remained in treatment 12 weeks or completed 12 sessions). Four subjects were removed from the protocol because of clinical deterioration, three because of failure to comply with medication, and three because of medication side effects. Of these 10, three were in clinical management plus desipramine, four were in relapse prevention plus desipramine, two were in clinical management plus placebo, and one was in relapse prevention plus placebo. One subject became pregnant during treatment, one initiated azidothymidine treatment, and four moved from the area. The remainder of early terminators were dropouts (n=56).

The relapse prevention plus desipramine group had the highest rate of subjects completing treatment (49%), followed by comparable and lower rates in the clinical management plus placebo, clinical management plus desipramine, and relapse prevention plus placebo groups (39%, 37%, and 36%, respectively). By psychotherapy and medication type, subjects receiving relapse prevention were more likely to complete treatment than subjects receiving clinical management (57% vs 43%), as were subjects who received desipramine as opposed to those receiving placebo (53% vs 47%), although these differences were not statistically significant.

To evaluate whether there were systematic differences between subjects who completed treatment and early terminators, we compared treatment completers (n=49) with early terminators (n=61) on demographic and clinical characteristics at baseline. With respect to dropouts, completers were significantly more likely to be married (41% of the completers were married or cohabitating vs 20% of the dropouts, χ^2=6.1, P<.05) and white (66% vs 34%, χ^2=10.8, P<.001).

OUTCOME ANALYSES

Paired t tests indicated that significant improvement occurred from pretreatment to posttreatment for all treatment groups. Significant effects for time were found across all treatment groups in quantity of cocaine use per week (P<.001) and for four of eight ASI domains (cocaine, alcohol, family/social, and psychological). As shown in **Table 2**, no pretreatment to posttreatment changes were seen for medical, legal, and noncocaine drug use ASI composite scores, as pretreatment scores in each of these areas indicated low baseline severity and were, therefore, unlikely to improve during treatment. Although employment composite scores were elevated at baseline, these showed no significant improvement over time. However, scores improved for subjects treated with relapse prevention and showed some worsening among groups receiving clinical management.

ANALYSIS OF VARIANCE

Table 2 presents means, SDs, and results of ANOVAs for primary (cocaine use) and secondary (ASI composite

Table 2. Treatment Outcome by Treatment Group (N=110)*

	Treatment Group				
	CM/DMI (n=25)	RP/DMI (n=29)	CM/PLA (n=27)	RP/PLA (n=29)	Significance Level†
Cocaine use during treatment					
Longest consecutive days of abstinence‡	24.4±24.1	20.5±17.2	20.6±18.8	18.0±16.0	.67
Percentage abstinent days§	0.79±0.17	0.75±0.20	0.73±0.22	0.71±0.19	.57
Percentage urine toxicology screens positive for cocaine	.33	.33	.27	.39	.18
ASI composite scores‖					
Medical					
Pretreatment	0.17±0.28	0.19±0.25	0.11±0.19	0.16±0.27	
End point	0.17±0.23	0.17±0.29	0.11±0.16	0.11±0.23	.62
Employment					
Pretreatment	0.45±0.36	0.45±0.31	0.53±0.29	0.43±0.33	
End point	0.51±0.37	0.41±0.30	0.59±0.26	0.38±0.30	.06
Alcohol					
Pretreatment	0.11±0.14	0.14±0.19	0.08±0.09	0.12±0.15	
End point	0.06±0.09	0.08±0.17	0.06±0.06	0.10±0.11	.56¶
Cocaine#					
Pretreatment	0.70±0.18	0.69±0.17	0.71±0.18	0.61±0.16	
End point	0.36±0.25	0.43±0.23	0.41±0.24	0.44±0.21	.56¶
Other drug					
Pretreatment	0.02±0.03	0.04±0.04	0.02±0.03	0.02±0.02	
End point	0.01±0.02	0.03±0.04	0.02±0.03	0.02±0.02	.07
Legal					
Pretreatment	0.04±0.08	0.09±0.16	0.08±0.14	0.09±0.14	
End point	0.09±0.17	0.06±0.12	0.05±0.13	0.06±0.11	.68
Family/social					
Pretreatment	0.28±0.18	0.29±0.20	0.29±0.23	0.24±0.19	
End point	0.16±0.17	0.27±0.23	0.20±0.21	0.15±0.15	.12¶
Psychological					
Pretreatment	0.19±0.16	0.27±0.23	0.20±0.22	0.16±0.16	
End point	0.06±0.12	0.15±0.20	0.13±0.21	0.10±0.15	.26¶

*Values are reported as mean±SD except where noted. See Table 1 for explanation of abbreviations.

†Results of 2×2 analysis of variance, significance of F value. For primary outcome variables (consecutive days of abstinence during treatment, percentage of days abstinent, percentage of urine screens positive for cocaine) unadjusted group mean scores are presented. For Addiction Severity Index (ASI) subscale composite scores, pretreatment scores reflect unadjusted means. Posttreatment scores reflect end-point ratings for patients who were early terminators.

‡Duration of longest period of consecutive abstinence during treatment. Range is 0 to 90 days.

§Days of cocaine use as a percentage of total days in treatment.

‖Range is 0 to 1, higher scores indicate higher problem severity.

¶Significant (P<.01) effect for time by paired t test.

#Calculation of separate composite scores for cocaine vs other drug use.

scores) outcome measures for the 110 subjects who completed at least two treatment sessions. There were no significant main effects for psychotherapy or medication type, and there were no significant interactions between psychotherapy and medication.

To facilitate comparison with previous studies[1] that reported significant decreases in cocaine use over 6 rather than 12 weeks of treatment as in the current study, we conducted a repeated-measures MANOVA to evaluate frequency and quantity of cocaine use per week during the first 6 weeks of treatment. There were statistically significant desipramine effects ($F=3.77$, $P<.05$) for grams of cocaine used per week, indicating significant reduction in cocaine use for subjects treated with desipramine over placebo between treatment weeks 2 and 6. This effect, however, was not significant beyond 6 weeks, which may be consistent with recent findings that indicate desipramine treatment beyond 6 weeks countertherapeutically cues relapse due to late onset of cocainelike stimulatory effects.[23]

MEDICATION PLASMA LEVEL AND TREATMENT RESPONSE

The mean desipramine plasma level for the 54 subjects who initiated desipramine treatment was 510 nmol/L. Although medication compliance was monitored weekly by the therapists and by the project nurse, 21 patients did not maintain a blood level within therapeutic range through 80% of medication plasma audits. Analyses that included only the 33 patients whose desipramine levels were consistently within therapeutic range throughout the trial (mean desipramine plasma level, 680 nmol/L) did not reveal a main effect for desipramine on any outcome measure. Compliant subjects whose 1-week plasma levels were above 750 nmol/L were retained significantly longer in treatment than compliant subjects with lower plasma levels (9.2 vs 6.9 weeks, $F=2.4$, $P<.05$), but did not differ on abstinence.

SEVERITY BY TREATMENT INTERACTIONS

As noted above, initial ANCOVAs indicated significant heterogeneity of regression for baseline severity of cocaine use on several primary outcome variables, suggesting the treatments worked differently at different levels of severity. Furthermore, two previous studies by our group[7,24] suggested that severity was potentially an important predictor of treatment response in cocaine abusers. Therefore, to evaluate the relationship between baseline severity of cocaine use and treatment outcome, we stratified the sample into three levels: low (1.00 to 2.50 g of cocaine per week at baseline), moderate (2.51 to 4.49 g), and high severity (≥4.50 g/wk). We chose three levels of severity to sharpen contrasts between high and low severity of cocaine use. Univariate ANOVAs indicated that this classification of severity was associated with chronicity of use ($P=.08$), route of administration (with more

Table 3. Interactions of Treatment Type With Baseline Level of Severity of Cocaine Use, Results of Three-Way Analysis of Variance (ANOVA) (N=110)*

	Treatment Group				
	CM/DMI (n=25)	RP/DMI (n=29)	CM/PLA (n=27)	RP/PLA (n=29)	Significance Level†
Percentage of days abstinent during treatment					
Low‡	0.86±0.19	0.71±0.20	0.74±0.18	0.83±0.12	...
Moderate	0.78±0.13	0.86±0.09	0.76±0.31	0.81±0.07	...
High	0.84±0.10	0.81±0.20	0.80±0.14	0.74±0.32	NS
Consecutive days abstinent during treatment‡					
Low	41.6±26.3	12.4±16.9	17.8±12.0	19.2±13.3	...
Moderate	18.4±22.4	26.1±20.1	31.2±24.9	17.0±7.9	RP/SEV
High	16.3±11.9	23.2±11.9	15.2±10.8	30.2±27.8	.05
Percentage of urine toxicology screens positive for cocaine					
Low	0.09±0.28	0.61±0.05	0.26±0.44	0.46±0.50	...
Moderate	0.30±0.46	0.28±0.45	0.25±0.43	0.42±0.05	RP/SEV
High	0.70±0.46	0.28±0.45	0.32±0.47	0.38±0.45	.01
No. of treatment sessions completed§					
Low	7.6±3.2	5.1±4.3	8.8±2.9	6.6±3.3	...
Moderate	6.7±3.4	9.4±2.2	7.0±3.5	6.8±4.0	RP/SEV
High	6.3±3.5	9.1±3.5	6.1±3.6	7.9±4.5	.05

*Values are reported as mean±SD. See Table 1 for explanation of abbreviations. In addition, NS indicates not significant; SEV, baseline level of severity of cocaine use; low, SEV of 1.00 to 2.50 g/wk; moderate, SEV of 2.51 to 4.49 g/wk; and high, SEV of 4.50 g/wk or greater.

†Results of 2×2×3 ANOVA, significance of F value.

‡Duration of longest period of consecutive abstinence during treatment. Range 0 to 90 days.

§Range is one to 12 sessions.

intravenous users in the high-severity group, $P=.07$), total cocaine use in the past 3 months ($P<.01$), and a lifetime history of opiate dependence ($P<.03$). Nineteen subjects with antisocial personality disorder fell into the high-severity group vs nine and eight in the moderate- and low-severity groups, respectively.

Exploratory 2×2×3 (medication × psychotherapy × severity) ANOVAs are presented in **Table 3**, and the pattern of results is illustrated in **Figure 1**. There were consistent severity of cocaine use by psychotherapy (relapse prevention vs clinical management) interactions, with higher-severity group subjects who received relapse prevention reporting longer consecutive periods of abstinence and lower-severity group subjects reporting briefer periods of abstinence. The inverse was seen for clinical management; clinical management was associated with longer periods of abstinence for low-severity group subjects and shorter periods of abstinence for high-severity group subjects.

Similarly, analyses for treatment retention indicated significant severity by psychotherapy interactions. For relapse prevention, retention was better for higher-severity group subjects, as low-severity group subjects had fewer total sessions (mean, 6.0) and higher-severity group subjects had more sessions (mean, 8.6) ($F=3.6$, $P<.03$). For clinical management, there was better retention for low-severity group subjects (mean, 8.0 sessions) than high-severity group subjects (mean, 6.1 sessions).

There were no significant pharmacotherapy (desipramine plus placebo) by severity interactions for treatment retention or reduction in cocaine use. However, for the subsample who completed at least five sessions and, therefore, had greater opportunity for emergence of medication effects, there was a significant interaction between medication and baseline severity ($F=3.5$, $P=.03$) (**Figure 2**). Low-severity group subjects treated with desipramine had significantly longer periods of consecutive abstinence than low-severity group subjects taking placebo; for moderate- and high-severity group subjects, desipramine and placebo were comparable in effectiveness.

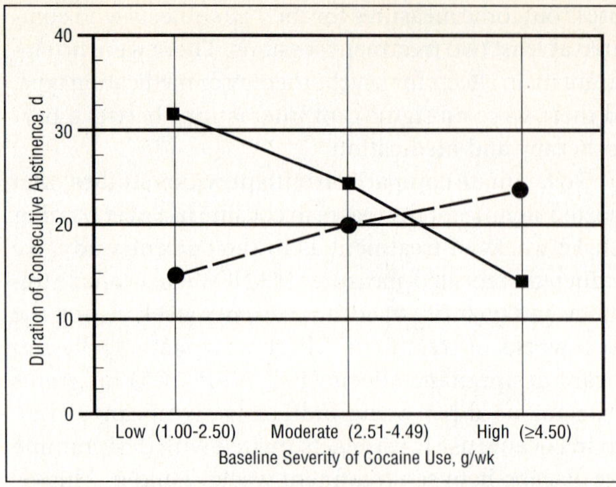

Figure 1. *Severity of cocaine use and response to psychotherapy by subjects completing two or more psychotherapy sessions (n=110). Solid line indicates clinical management; dashed line, relapse prevention.*

COMORBID PSYCHOPATHOLOGY AND TREATMENT OUTCOME

As a number of reports have related the presence of comorbid psychopathology to cocaine-treatment outcome,[24,25] we also explored the relationship between Axis I and II disorders and our primary outcome measures. These are exploratory findings; our exclusion criteria affected the rates and severity of several disorders, and the low rates of current disorders make detection of significant differences in several categories unlikely.

We conducted separate 2×2×2 ANOVAs relating presence of any *DSM-III-R*[8] lifetime nonsubstance use Axis I disorder, any Axis II disorder, lifetime affective disorder (major depression or dysthymia), any lifetime anxiety disorder (generalized anxiety disorder, obsessive-compulsive disorder, panic disorder, or phobia), current or lifetime alcohol abuse or dependence, and antisocial personality disorder to our major outcomes: retention in treatment, longest period of abstinence during treatment, and percentage of abstinent days.

Overall, for most categories, there were few strong or consistent findings, and we report below only those findings that were significant or trends. Subjects with any lifetime affective disorder had significantly longer periods of consecutive abstinence during treatment than subjects without affective disorder (33.5 vs 22.0 days, $P<.05$). The 11 subjects with any lifetime anxiety disorder were more likely to remain in treatment (10.1 vs 8.2 weeks, $t=3.2$, $P<.01$) and had longer periods of consecutive abstinence (39.8 vs 21.3 days, $t=2.1$, $P=.06$). The eight subjects with current alcohol abuse or dependence tended to have a lower percentage of abstinent days (0.69 vs 0.82, $t=2.0$, $P=.07$). There were no main effects for antisocial personality disorder on treatment retention or outcome.

However, level of current depressive symptoms at baseline was more consistently related to outcome. Subjects who reported significant depressive symptoms at baseline, defined as a score of 8 or more on the screening version of the Beck Depression Inventory[21] and 6 or more on the 17-item Hamilton Depression Rating Scale,[22] tended to have higher severity of cocaine use at baseline than nondepressed subjects ($\chi^2=4.9$, $P=.08$), their depression improved significantly over time regardless of treatment received ($F=18.6$, $P<.001$), and their weekly cocaine use decreased significantly between treatment weeks 2 and 12 with respect to nondepressed subjects ($F=4.0$, $P<.01$). Finally, there were consistent significant interactions for depression and psychotherapy, in that

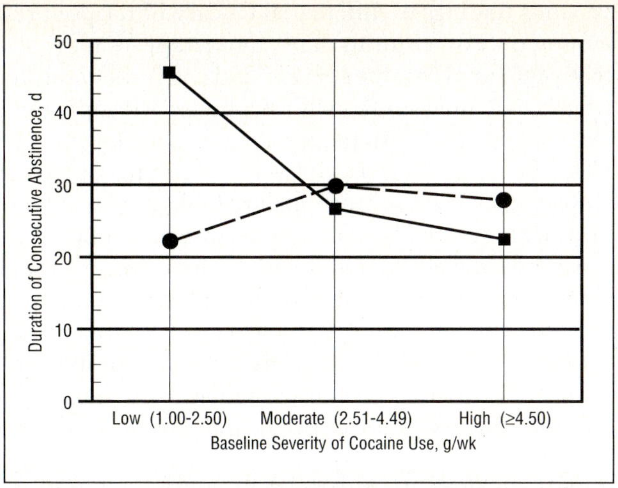

Figure 2. *Severity of cocaine use and response to medication by subjects receiving five or more pharmacotherapy sessions (n=77). Solid line indicates despiramine hydrochloride; dashed line, placebo.*

depressed subjects treated with relapse prevention remained in treatment significantly longer than depressed subjects treated with clinical management (9.7 vs 6.0 weeks, F=10.3, $P<.01$) and maintained longer periods of consecutive abstinence during treatment (28.8 vs 20.2 days, F=28.8, $P=.01$). Significant interactions for depression by pharmacotherapy were not found for cocaine use outcomes.

COMMENT

This study evaluated four treatments for ambulatory cocaine abusers: relapse prevention plus desipramine, clinical management plus desipramine, relapse prevention plus placebo, and clinical management plus placebo. Results indicated first, that all groups showed significant reductions in cocaine use as well as improvement in several other problem areas from pretreatment levels. Second, significant main effects for medication or psychotherapy type were not found, and there were no significant interactions between psychotherapy and pharmacotherapy. Third, baseline severity of cocaine use was found to interact differently with both psychotherapy and pharmacotherapy. Higher-severity subjects were retained longer in treatment, attained longer periods of abstinence, and had fewer urine samples positive for cocaine when treated with relapse prevention vs clinical management. Lower-severity group subjects attained longer periods of abstinence when treated with desipramine rather than placebo.

This study is unique in treatment efficacy research among cocaine abusers in including methodologic features intended to systematize and protect the integrity of both pharmacologic and psychotherapeutic components of treatment. These features included specification of both forms of treatment in manuals, monitoring the delivery of pharmacotherapy through medication plasma levels, and the delivery of psychotherapy through process assessment of session videotapes, delivery of treatment by experienced therapists committed to the type of treatment they conducted, training and ongoing supervision of therapists by investigators who were proponents of the approach they supervised, use of appropriate control groups for each form of treatment, and adequate duration of treatment to allow emergence of specific effects of both forms of treatment.[17,26]

While these features enhanced the likelihood that both psychotherapy and pharmacotherapy received a "fair trial," several design features also precluded unambiguous interpretation of the efficacy of psychotherapy vs pharmacotherapy. For example, all subjects receiving medication also received some form of psychotherapy; hence, the efficacy of pharmacotherapy alone, without nonspecific effects of supportive clinical management or additional active ingredients of relapse prevention, could not be determined. However, without a supportive doctor-patient relationship, it is likely that few subjects would have persisted with a purely pharmacologic approach long enough to evaluate its effectiveness.[27] Similarly, all subjects who received psychotherapy also received active or inert medication that may have influenced their expectations for treatment effects.[28] Nevertheless, empirical evaluations[29,30] have found little evidence of meaningful differences between the efficacy of psychotherapy combined with placebo to that of psychotherapy alone.

Another limitation of the present study is that although baseline severity of cocaine use was strongly associated with outcome and appeared to mediate response to both psychotherapy and pharmacotherapy, these findings emerged from exploratory analyses. While these data are consistent with recent studies that have pointed to the importance of severity of cocaine dependence in influencing extended outcome[24] and response to psychotherapy[7] among cocaine abusers, in this study, severity was not defined a priori as a factor. Although we sought to recruit subjects with a wide range of severity, the sample was not stratified for baseline severity, and findings presented herein may not generalize to other samples with different distributions of severity of cocaine dependence.

The rate of attrition in this study may limit the generalizability of these findings. While we attempted to hold to a minimum the length of time between subjects' application for treatment and first meeting with a therapist, 18 subjects (13%) dropped out before initiating treatment and only 40% of those who began treatment fully complied with and completed a 12-week course of treatment. Although the findings reported herein were consistent across intention to treat, treatment exposed, and completer samples, the poorer retention seen among many high-severity group subjects may suggest the need for more intensive forms of treatment to provide adequate support for initial stabilization of some cocaine abusers.

EFFICACY OF PHARMACOTHERAPY

There was little evidence in this study supporting the efficacy of desipramine over placebo at the end of a 12-week course of treatment. On the other hand, this study was several weeks longer than most pharmacologic trials for cocaine abusers, and time-sensitive analyses demonstrated improved abstinence initiation for desipramine over placebo during the early weeks of treatment (weeks 2 through 6), this effect diminishing in subsequent weeks. These data are consistent with conceptions of the role of desipramine with cocaine abusers as a short-term treatment adjunct intended to foster initial abstinence, to, in effect, "open a window" of abstinence through which other forms of treatment, such as psychotherapy, may have opportunity to take hold.[1]

Exploratory analyses also provide evidence for superior efficacy of desipramine only among low-severity group cocaine abusers. This finding runs counter to simple expectations of greater effectiveness of pharmacotherapy with more severe cocaine abusers. While few studies have reported on severity as a mediator of desipramine effectiveness, such findings might be inferred by the variable findings reported for desipramine efficacy across studies and samples (and presumably varying levels of severity). Similarly, our group has reported on improved outcome with desipramine for depressed methadone-maintained cocaine abusers (whose primary drug of abuse was opiates)[25]; in this sample of primary cocaine abusers, we did not find an interaction between desipramine and depression for reduction of cocaine use. This is, however, consistent with our findings of no difference in efficacy of desipramine in depressed and euthymic primary cocaine abusers.[1]

EFFICACY OF PSYCHOTHERAPY

Results of this study found no evidence of main effects of cognitive-behavioral treatment over clinical management on cocaine use. However, our choice of a psychotherapy-control condition provided a stringent test of relapse prevention; ie, we evaluated the specific effectiveness of relapse prevention over clinical management rather than over a no-psychotherapy–control group. Given the overall rate of improvement of subjects in this study, it appears that clinical management is a fairly effective treatment, associated with improvement in about 70% of subjects. As in the National Institute of Mental Health Treatment of Depression Collaborative Research Program,[31] clinical management in this study involved weekly contacts of 20 to 35 minutes with experienced psychiatrists who offered support, encouragement, and other nonspecific effects of psychotherapy that may powerfully affect outcome.

Results of the present study were consistent with our previous findings of differential efficacy of relapse prevention over other forms of psychotherapy for more severely impaired cocaine abusers[7] and with findings from a priori matching studies with alcoholics.[32] Relapse prevention appeared both to retain higher severity and depressed cocaine users as well as to foster longer periods of abstinence in these more impaired subsamples. Of the treatments studied herein, only relapse prevention displayed specific effectiveness with higher-severity group cocaine abusers. This effect suggests that cocaine abusers with more intense involvement with cocaine may benefit from the additional structure, intensity, or didactic content of relapse prevention, which focused specifically on reducing access to cocaine and avoidance of high-risk situations for relapse, while low-intensity approaches may be effective for the less-severe abusers.

CONCLUSIONS

Overall, these findings do not support the efficacy of a single treatment for all cocaine abusers. Instead, they underscore (1) the significance of heterogeneity among cocaine abusers, as patient characteristics such as severity and psychopathology may influence treatment seeking, treatment retention, and treatment effects[33]; (2) the need to explore patient-treatment matching and the development of specialized treatments for clinically distinct subgroups of cocaine abusers[34]; and (3) the complexity of the relationship between treatment retention and outcome, as more impaired abusers may be differentially retained in some forms of treatment.[24]

Accepted for publication January 25, 1993.

This study was supported by grants RO1-DA04299, RO1-DA04029, R18-DA06963, and K05-DA00089 from the National Institute on Drug Abuse, Bethesda, Md.

We gratefully acknowledge Michael Barrios, PhD; Lisa Fenton, PsyD; Andrew Grunebaum, PhD; Daniel Keller, PhD; Robert Malison, MD; Ismene Petrakis, MD; Glen Pickett, MD; Merrill Rotter, MD; Marlene Steinberg, MD; and Robert Sbriglio, MD, who made many contributions to the success of this project through their work as therapists. Hope Anderson and Glenna King assisted in data collection.

Reprint requests to Yale University, Substance Abuse Treatment Unit, 27 Sylvan Ave, New Haven, CT 06519 (Dr Carroll).

REFERENCES

1. Gawin FH, Kleber HD, Byck R, Rounsaville BJ, Kosten TR, Jatlow PI, Morgan C. Desipramine facilitation of initial cocaine abstinence. *Arch Gen Psychiatry.* 1989;46:117-121.
2. Kosten TR, Morgan CM, Falcione J, Schottenfeld RS. Pharmacotherapy for cocaine-abusing methadone-maintained patients using amantadine or desipramine. *Arch Gen Psychiatry.* 1992;49:894-898.
3. Weddington WW, Brown BS, Haertzen CA, Hess JM, Mahaffey JR, Kolar AF, Jaffe JH. Comparison of amantadine and desipramine combined with psycho-

therapy for treatment of cocaine dependence. *Am J Drug Alcohol Abuse.* 1991; 17:137-152.
4. Levin FR, Lehman AF. Meta-analysis of desipramine as an adjunct in the treatment of cocaine addiction. *J Clin Psychopharmacol.* 1991;11:374-378.
5. Kang SY, Kleinman PH, Woody GE, Millman RB, Todd TC, Kemp J, Lipton DS. Outcomes for cocaine abusers after once-a-week psychosocial therapy. *Am J Psychiatry.* 1991;148:630-635.
6. Elkin I, Parloff MB, Hadley SW, Autry JH. NIMH treatment of depression collaborative research program: background and research plan. *Arch Gen Psychiatry.* 1985;42:305-316.
7. Carroll KM, Rounsaville BJ, Gawin FH. A comparative trial of psychotherapies for ambulatory cocaine abusers: relapse prevention and interpersonal psychotherapy. *Am J Drug Alcohol Abuse.* 1991;17:229-247.
8. American Psychiatric Association, Committee on Nomenclature and Statistics. *Diagnostic and Statistical Manual of Mental Disorders, Revised Third Edition.* Washington, DC: American Psychiatric Association; 1987.
9. Hser Y, Anglin MD, Chou C. Reliability of retrospective self-report by narcotics addicts. *Psychol Assessment.* 1992;4:207-213.
10. O'Malley PM, Bachman JG, Johnston LD. Reliability and consistency in self-reports of drug use. *Int J Addict.* 1983;18:805-824.
11. Spitzer RL, Williams JBW. *Structured Clinical Interview for DSM-III-R.* New York: New York State Psychiatric Institute; 1985.
12. Crits-Christoph P, Mintz J. Implications of therapist effects for the design and analysis of comparative studies of psychotherapies. *J Consult Clin Psychol.* 1991;59:20-26.
13. Nelson JC, Jatlow PI, Mazure C. Rapid desipramine dose adjustment using 24-hour levels. *J Clin Psychopharmacol.* 1987;7:72-77.
14. Marlatt GA, Gordon JR, eds. *Relapse Prevention: Maintenance Strategies in the Treatment of Addictive Behaviors.* New York, NY: Guilford Press; 1985.
15. Carroll KM, Rounsaville BJ, Keller DS. Relapse prevention strategies in the treatment of cocaine abuse. *Am J Drug Alcohol Abuse.* 1991;17:249-265.
16. Fawcett J, Epstein P, Fiester SJ, Elkin I, Autry JH. Clinical management-imipramine/placebo administration manual: NIMH Treatment of Depression Collaborative Research Program. *Psychopharmacol Bull.* 1987;23:309-324.
17. Elkin I, Pilkonis PA, Docherty JP, Sotsky SM. Conceptual and methodological issues in comparative studies of psychotherapy and pharmacotherapy, I: active ingredients and mechanisms of change. *Am J Psychiatry.* 1988;145: 909-917.
18. Hill CE, O'Grady KE, Elkin I. Applying the Collaborative Study Psychotherapy Rating Scale to rate therapist adherence in cognitive-behavior therapy, interpersonal therapy, and clinical management. *J Consult Clin Psychol.* 1992;60: 73-79.
19. Hollon SD, Waskow IE, Evans M, Lowery HA. Systems for rating therapies for depression. Presented at the annual convention of the American Psychiatry Association; May 4, 1984; Los Angeles, Calif.
20. McLellan AT, Luborsky L, Woody GE, O'Brien CP. An improved diagnostic evaluation instrument for substance abuse patients: The Addiction Severity Index. *J Nerv Ment Dis.* 1980;168:26-33.
21. Beck AT, Beck RW. Screening depressed patients in family practice: a rapid technique. *Postgrad Med.* 1972;52:81-85.
22. Hamilton M. A rating scale for depression. *J Neurol Neurosurg Psychiatry.* 1960;23:56-62.
23. Weiss RD. Relapse to cocaine abuse after initiating desipramine treatment. *JAMA.* 1988;260:2545-2546.
24. Carroll KM, Power ME, Bryant KJ, Rounsaville BJ. One-year follow-up status of treatment-seeking cocaine abusers: psychopathology and dependence severity as predictors of outcome. *J Nerv Ment Dis.* 1993;181:71-79.
25. Ziedonis DM, Kosten TR. Depression as a prognostic factor for pharmacological treatment of cocaine dependence. *Psychopharmacol Bull.* 1991;27:337-343.
26. Elkin I, Pilkonis PA, Docherty JP, Sotsky SM. Conceptual and methodological issues in comparative studies of psychotherapy and pharmacotherapy, II: nature and timing of treatment effects. *Am J Psychiatry.* 1988;145:1070-1076.
27. Klerman GL. Assessing the influence of the hospital milieu upon the effectiveness of psychiatric drug therapy: problems of conceptualization and of research methodology. *J Nerv Ment Dis.* 1963;137:143-154.
28. Hollon SD, Beck AT. Psychotherapy and drug therapy: comparision and combinations. In: Garfield SL, Bergin AE, eds. *Handbook of Psychotherapy and Behavior Change.* 2nd ed. New York, NY: John Wiley & Sons Inc; 1978.
29. Klerman GL, DiMascio A, Weissman M, Prusoff B, Paykel ES. Treatment of depression by drugs and psychotherapy. *Am J Psychiatry.* 1974;131:186-190.
30. Frank E, Kupfer DJ. Does a placebo tablet affect psychotherapeutic treatment outcome? Results from the Pittsburgh study of maintenance therapies in recurrent depression. *Psychother Res.* 1992;2:102-111.
31. Elkin I, Shea MT, Watkins JT, Imber SD, Sotsky SM, Collins JF, Glass DR, Pilkonis PA, Leber WR, Docherty JP, Fiester SJ, Parloff MB. National Institute of Mental Health Treatment of Depression Collaborative Research Program: general effectiveness of treatments. *Arch Gen Psychiatry.* 1989;46:971-982.
32. Kadden RM, Cooney NL, Getter H, Litt MD. Matching alcoholics to coping skills or interactional therapies: posttreatment results. *J Consult Clin Psychol.* 1989; 57:698-704.
33. Carroll KM, Rounsaville BJ. Contrast of treatment-seeking and untreated cocaine abusers. *Arch Gen Psychiatry.* 1992;49:464-471.
34. Carroll KM, Ziedonis DM, O'Malley SS, McCance-Katz E, Gordon LT, Rounsaville BJ. Pharmacologic interventions for abusers of alcohol and cocaine: a pilot study of disulfiram versus naltrexone. *Am J Addictions.* 1993;2:77-79.

ORIGINAL ARTICLE

Increased Pressure for Rapid Eye Movement Sleep at Time of Hospital Admission Predicts Relapse in Nondepressed Patients With Primary Alcoholism at 3-Month Follow-up

J. Christian Gillin, MD; Tom L. Smith, PhD; Michael Irwin, MD; Nelson Butters, PhD; Anna Demodena; Marc Schuckit, MD

Objective: To determine whether polygraphic sleep recordings, obtained at the time of admission to an inpatient alcohol treatment program, predict abstinence and relapse 3 months following hospital discharge in nondepressed patients with primary alcoholism.

Design: Two independent, consecutive cohorts of patients (group 1, n=28; group 2, n=17) underwent all-night polygraphic sleep recordings and other clinical evaluations during the first and fourth weeks of a 1-month inpatient treatment program within a Veteran Affairs Medical Center. They were reevaluated 3 months following discharge to the community. None were treated with disulfiram or other medications during or after hospitalization.

Patients: All subjects were male veterans with primary alcoholism and without significant preexisting, secondary, or comorbid diagnoses such as major medical problems, depression, antisocial personality, or drug addiction.

Outcome Measures: Relapse was defined as any alcohol consumption between discharge from the hospital and 3-month follow-up.

Results: Ten (36%) of 28 patients in group 1 were Relapsers at 3-month follow-up. Relapsers in group 1 showed significantly shorter Rapid Eye Movement (REM) latency, increased Rapid Eye Movement percent (REM%), and increased REM Density during their admission sleep studies compared with Abstainers. To replicate these observations, group 2 was then studied as a validation sample. Six (35%) of 17 patients relapsed. As in group 1, Relapsers had significantly shorter REM latency and increased REM% compared with Abstainers; REM Density was not significantly different in the Relapsers as compared with Abstainers in group 2. Using a principal components analysis based on these three REM sleep measures to determine "REM pressure," three separate discriminant function analyses (DFAs) were calculated: one for each group and one for all patients (n=45) together. The DFA from group 1 correctly classified 22 (78.6%) of the 28 patients in group 1 and 13 (76.5%) of the 17 patients in group 2 as Relapsers or Abstainers. The DFA from group 2 correctly classified 13 (76.5%) of the 17 patients in group 2 and 23 (82.1%) of the 28 patients in group 1. The DFA formed from both groups together correctly classified 36 (80%) of the 45 patients. When the REM sleep measures at hospital admission and discharge were compared, no statistically significant effect of time was observed. Abstinence and relapse were not consistently related to other clinical measures at the time of hospital admission such as age, duration and severity of alcoholism, marital status, employment, hepatic enzyme levels, cognitive performance, or depression ratings.

Conclusion: Short REM latency, increased REM%, and, possibly, increased REM Density at the time of admission to a 1-month inpatient alcohol treatment program predict relapse in nondepressed patients with primary alcoholism by 3 months following hospital discharge.

(Arch Gen Psychiatry. 1994;51:189-197)

ALCOHOLIC PATIENTS frequently experience sleep disturbances during periods of heavy drinking as well as during subacute and chronic abstinence.[1-4] Objective sleep abnormalities may continue for 6 months to at least 2 years of abstinence in some recovering alcoholic patients.[5,6] Poor sleep may be associated with relapse, especially since small amounts of alcohol may

From the Psychiatry Service, San Diego Veterans Affairs Medical Center and Department of Psychiatry, University of California, San Diego.

See Patients and Methods on next page

PATIENTS AND METHODS

The alcoholic patients were male veterans who were admitted for 4 weeks to the inpatient Alcohol and Drug Treatment Program at the San Diego (Calif) Veterans Affairs Medical Center and agreed to participate in a multidisciplinary longitudinal study of primary alcoholics that was conducted at the time by a Veterans Affairs–funded Alcohol Research Center. As part of this ongoing study, subjects were invited to participate for three consecutive nights of polygraphically recorded sleep during the first (admission) and fourth (discharge) week of hospitalization, and at 3-, 12-, and 24-month follow-up after discharge. Written informed consent was obtained following a verbal and written explanation of the study.

Patients underwent a full medical and psychiatric history, review of systems, physical examination, routine clinical and hematologic laboratory examinations, and urinalysis. All patients met criteria for primary alcoholism, using a structured diagnostic interview based on *DSM-III* Research Diagnostic Criteria as modified by Schuckit.[17] As part of the diagnostic procedure and 3-month follow-up, a resource person (a close friend or relative of the patient) was also interviewed independently from the patient to corroborate the research and clinical evaluation. Briefly, primary alcoholism refers to patients without a diagnosable psychiatric illness or significant medical problem prior to the onset of major life problems associated with alcoholism. We also excluded primary alcoholics with secondary disorders, such as depression, sedative, or other substance abuse. Hence, in this study, we excluded alcoholic patients with another formal psychiatric diagnosis, such as antisocial personality, borderline personality, major depression, bipolar disorder, substance abuse, and anxiety disorder. Patients were also excluded on the basis of major medical problems or complications related to alcoholism, including delirium tremens or convulsions in the period immediately preceding hospital admission, significant liver dysfunction, peripheral neuropathy, head trauma, or clinically significant cognitive impairment.

This report is based on two consecutive cohorts of patients with primary alcoholism whose clinical outcome (abstinence or relapse) was determined at 3-month follow-up after discharge from the hospital. Further longitudinal studies will be published as the study progresses. Relapse was defined as any reported consumption of alcohol between hospital discharge and 3-month follow-up, based on separate, standardized interviews with the patient and the resource person and corroborated by determination of blood alcohol levels or elevated hepatic enzyme levels.[18] The first cohort, group 1, consisted of 28 patients, 18 Abstainers and 10 Relapsers. As will be explained later, specific sleep measures at baseline were found to distinguish Abstainers from Relapsers. To validate these sleep predictors, we ran a second cohort, group 2, which consisted of 17 patients, 11 Abstainers and six Relapsers.

Subjects were also screened for sleep apnea by finger pulse oximetry and for periodic movements of sleep by tibial electromyogram on the adaptation night in the sleep laboratory; exclusion criteria were 15 or greater desaturation index (number of oxygen saturations greater than 4% for at least 10 s/h of sleep) and 15 or greater for the tibial index (tibial electromyographic events per hour). Data from 18 (64%) of the 28 patients in group 1 have been included in previous reports.[9-11] All subjects were free of psychotropic medications (including major and minor tranquilizers, sleeping pills, disulfiram, etc) for at least 10 days prior to sleep studies and throughout the inpatient treatment program. None of the patients received disulfiram during the 3 months following hospital discharge. None of the 45 patients reported a first-degree relative with depression.

About 1 week following hospital admission, patients slept in individual bedrooms while all-night polygraphically recorded electroencephalograms, electro-oculograms, electromyograms, and electrocardiograms were obtained. Sleep recordings were visually scored according to the criteria of Rechtschaffen and Kales,[19] as previously modified,[10] without knowledge of clinical outcome or the hypotheses of this study. To briefly summarize the scoring method, we defined sleep onset as the first 30-second epoch of stage 2 sleep or REM sleep which is followed by no more than 1 minute of wakefulness in the first 10 minutes of sleep. Rapid Eye Movement latency was the elapsed time from the onset of sleep until the onset of the first REM period. To be counted, the first REM period was required to have a minimum of 3 minutes of REM sleep. *Rapid Eye Movement latency corrected* was calculated by subtracting wake time between sleep onset and the first REM period from REM latency. *Rapid Eye Movement Density* was a measure of ocular activity during REM sleep, scored visually on a scale of 0 to 4 per 30-second epoch

have transient sedative benefits at night in some alcoholics and normal controls.[7,8]

This report is one of a series of studies characterizing the polygraphically recorded sleep disturbances of patients with primary alcoholism.[9-11] Compared with normal controls, patients with relatively "pure" primary alcoholism (no other primary or secondary psychiatric diagnosis, such as major depression) had statistically significantly prolonged sleep latency, diminished total sleep time, non–Rapid Eye Movement (REM) and delta (stages 3 and 4) sleep, and increased REM Density (a measure of ocular activity) during the first REM period.[10] Although patients with uncomplicated primary alcoholism had normal REM sleep time, Rapid Eye Movement percent (REM%), and REM latency (elapsed time from the onset of sleep until the first REM period) compared with normal controls, they differed significantly from patients with either primary depression or patients with primary alcoholism with secondary depression,[9,11] both of whom had short REM latency and increased REM% compared with normal controls.

of REM sleep, but reported on a scale of 0 to 8 per minute of REM sleep. *Rapid Eye Movement percentage* was the percentage of total sleep time spent in REM sleep. Total sleep time was the sum of non-REM and REM sleep. Sleep efficiency was defined as percentage of time in bed spent in sleep. The first night was considered to be adaptation; these data were not included in this study. Data from the second and third night for each subject were averaged for the hospital admission and discharge sleep studies. (Data from the 3-month follow-up will be presented elsewhere for two reasons. First, the focus of this study is the prediction of relapse and abstinence at 3-month follow-up, not the natural course of sleep in alcoholism. Second, the effects of renewed drinking on sleep in the relapsing group is essentially a different scientific question.)

The data on demographic and clinical characteristics, laboratory examinations, cognitive testing, clinical ratings, and sleep were collected during the first week after hospital admission. Cross-sectional data between abstaining and relapsing patients were statistically compared with analysis of variance, with post hoc comparisons by the Newman-Keuls test.

We used two sleep variables from the hospital admission studies to classify Relapsers and Abstainers: (1) Total Sleep Time, which was chosen a priori because poor sleep has traditionally been considered to be predictor of relapse, and (2) increased REM sleep "pressure," a composite statistical variable derived from REM Latency Corrected, REM%, and REM Density. We created a Principal Component Analysis (PCA) for classification of patients as Relapsers and Abstainers for two reasons: (1) short REM latency, increased REM%, and increased REM Density appear to reflect elevated physiologic propensity for REM sleep ("increased REM pressure") and could, therefore, be combined into a single variable, and (2) the three REM sleep measures were used to form a single composite variable, PCA, for statistical reasons to limit the number of predictive measures entered into the discriminant function analysis (DFA). The study of the second group of patients (n=17) was then conducted to (1) confirm the pairwise comparisons indicating short REM latency, increased REM%, and increased REM Density in Relapsers compared with Abstainers, and (2) validate the predictive DFA that was generated from the first group and to cross-validate the hypothesis that increased "REM pressure" predicts relapse.

The PCA, REM pressure, was calculated from a pool of up to 104 subjects: normal controls (n=29), other alcoholics not in this study (n=30), and the alcoholics in the current study (n=45). These 104 subjects had a mean (±SD) age of 48±11 years, mean education of 14±3 years, and were 85% white. The PCA yielded single components under three different conditions: (1) when all 45 patients in the current study were included, (2) when group 1 subjects were included and group 2 subjects were excluded, and (3) when group 2 subjects were included and group 1 subjects were excluded. The three conditions were calculated so that the REM pressure component was not derived from the subjects on whom the DFA would be run using that component. The PCA for all subjects had an eigenvalue of 1.46 accounting for 48.5% of the variance, while the group 2 exclusion for PCA eigenvalue accounted for 48% of the variance and the group 1 exclusion PCA eigenvalue accounted for 50.6% of the variance. The factor loadings for all subjects, group 2 exclusion, and group 1 exclusion runs were as follows, respectively: REM%=0.75, 0.74, and 0.80; REM latency corrected=−0.73, −0.68, and −0.74; and REM Density=0.60, 0.65, and 0.57.

To evaluate whether additional secondary clinical measures might predict relapse or abstinence, we examined neuropsychological deficits, hepatic impairment, smoking, and demographic variables (which have previously been related to relapse). We performed pairwise comparisons on these measures in both group 1 and group 2. In addition, to further determine whether hepatic enzyme level or cognitive impairment correctly classified Abstainers and Relapsers, we calculated two separate PCAs, a neuropsychological component and a liver enzyme component. As with the earlier sleep measures, PCAs were used to limit the number of predictor variables and increase reliability of measurement. The three liver enzymes (γ-glutamyltransferase, aspartate aminotransferase, and alanine aminotransferase) were assessed at the time of hospital admission and produced a single liver enzyme component. Four measurements of neuropsychological functioning (Trails A, Trails B, Digit Symbol Substitution Scaled Scores, and Visual Search Time) were assessed at hospital admission and produced a single neuropsychological component. Other predictor measures, such as marital status, employment, prior hospitalization for alcoholism, and so forth were evaluated by χ^2 or Fisher's Exact Test, as indicated below.

The ability to predict abstinence or relapse in individual patients with alcoholism has been quite poor.[12-16] This study explores the possibility that polygraphic sleep measures, obtained at admission to an inpatient alcohol treatment program, predict abstinence or relapse 3 months following hospital discharge in patients with uncomplicated primary alcoholism. This hypothesis was suggested not only by previous reports linking sleep disturbance to relapse[7,8] but in our own observations on the natural history of sleep disturbances in recovering and relapsing patients with primary alcoholism.

RESULTS

GROUP 1

As shown in **Table 1** and **Table 2**, at the time of admission to the inpatient program, the abstaining patients (n=18) and relapsing (n=10) patients in group 1 did not differ from each other in age, demographic variables, family history of alcoholism, history of alcoholism, recent severity of drinking, or dependency measured by withdrawal symptoms. The relapsing pa-

Table 1. Comparison of Abstainers and Relapsers in Group 1 (n=28): Demographic and Clinical Variables*

	Abstainers (n=18)	Relapsers (n=10)
Age, y	48±8	50±15
Hamilton Depression Rating Scale	8.6±3.2	7.8±4.2
No. days drank per month per past 3 mo	23±9	24±8
No. drinks per drinking day	13±8	13±5
No. days since last drink	16±7	18±11
Maximum No. withdrawal symptoms	5.3±4.2	6.6±3.5
Age at onset of alcoholism, y	36±11	36±13
Duration of alcoholism, y	12±11	14±14
Positive family history for alcoholism (%)	9/17 (52.9)	3/10 (30)
No. of different drugs	1.1±1.4	0.8±1.6
Stable relationship (%)	3/18 (16.7)	4/10 (40)
Employed (%)	7/18 (38.9)	2/10 (20)
Previous alcohol hospitalization (%)	4/18 (22.2)	6/10 (60)
Discharge to alcohol recovery home (%)	11/18 (61.1)	4/10 (40)
Neuropsychiatric component	−0.29±7	0.73±1.3†
Trails A time, s	28.3±7.6	44.4±15.5†
Trails B time, s	89.3±28.9	129.1±73.5
Digit Symbol Substitution Test	9.5±1.8	8.8±3.5
Visual search time, s	157±86	210±76
Liver enzyme component	−0.28±0.7	0.53±1.3
τ-Glutamyltransferase, IU	38±31	132±125†
Aspartate aminotransferase, IU	31±23	43±31
Alanine aminotransaminase, IU	38±39	69±88

*Values are means±SDs.
†$P<.05$.

Table 2. Comparison of Abstainers and Relapsers in Group 1 (n=28): Sleep Variables at Time of Hospital Admission*

Variable	Abstainers (n=18)	Relapsers (n=10)
Total Sleep Time	318±26	307±59
Sleep latency	27±18	21±18
Total WASO	36±21	44±37
Sleep efficiency, %	83.2±5.4	83.0±12.1
Stage 1%	9.8±5.8	8.7±8.1
Stage 2%	59.6±6.2	57.9±12.0
Stage 3%	1.8±3.1	2.2±3.9
Stage 4%	1.6±0.6	0.2±0.5
REM%	27.2±4.3	30.8±6.1†
REM latency	67±29	48±12‡
REM latency corrected	60±24	45±12‡
REM cycle 1 duration	92±17	118±35‡
REM period 1 duration	24±14	24±15
REM density	2.0±0.6	2.5±1.0†
REM period 1 density	2.0±0.9	2.7±1.0†
REM "pressure" component	−0.21±0.8	0.75±0.8§

*All values (means±SD) are in minutes, percentages of Total Sleep Time, or, in the case of Rapid Eye Movement (REM) Density, units (0 to 8 per minute of REM sleep). WASO indicates wake time after sleep onset; REM%, Rapid Eye Movement percent.
†$P<.05$.
‡$P<.02$.
§$P<.003$.

tients, however, had shorter mean REM latency, shorter REM latency corrected, greater REM Density and REM Density first REM period, and greater REM%. The Abstainers and the Relapsers did not differ significantly on other sleep measures, including total sleep time, which was one of our a priori predictor variables.

Both Total Sleep Time and the REM Pressure Component, which were entered as predictors in the DFA, were normally distributed (skewness=0.17 with Shapiro-Wilks P=.36, and skewness=0.41 with Shapiro-Wilks P=.86, respectively). In the DFA, Total Sleep Time did not enter, although the REM Pressure Component did (F=9.09, df=1,26, P=.006) and correctly classified 22 (78.6%) of the 28 patients as to 3-month outcome: 14 (77.8%) of 18 of the abstaining patients and eight (80%) 10 of the relapsing patients.

GROUP 2

To validate the DFA generated on group 1, data were collected from the next 17 consecutively admitted patients who met inclusion criteria for the longitudinal research program, who entered the sleep studies, and whose 3-month outcome had been determined. All were evaluated exactly as the 28 patients in group 1. Clinical, demographic, and laboratory data from group 2 are shown in **Table 3** and **Table 4**. In both group 1 and group 2, Relapsers had significantly higher REM% and shorter REM latency compared with Abstainers (**Figure 1**). While REM Density was statistically higher in Relapsers compared with Abstainers in group 1, the difference was not statistically significant in a pairwise comparison in group 2. No other sleep measures differentiated Abstainers and Relapsers in both groups 1 and 2. In addition, several clinical and demographic measures differentiated Relapsers and Abstainers in one group but not the other (see below).

When the 17 patients in group 2 were classified using the classification function coefficients from the DFA performed on the 28 patients in group 1, 13 (76.5%) of the 17 patients were correctly classified: eight (72.7%) of 11 Abstainers and five (83.3%) of the six Relapsers.

To complete a classic cross-validation procedure, the two a priori chosen predictor variables, Total Sleep Time and the REM Pressure Component, were used to form a new DFA derived from the 17 patients in group 2 to predict classification of patients in both group 2 and group 1. First, as with the DFA derived from group 1, the distributional properties of Total Sleep

Table 3. Comparison of Group 2: Demographic and Clinical Variables*

	Abstainers (n=11)	Relapsers (n=6)
Age, y	52±13	47±12
Hamilton Depression Rating Scale	7.0±3.1	9.8±6.8
No. days drank per month per past 3 mo	23±7	18±11
No. drinks per drinking day	13±7	15±7
No. days since last drink	16±8	11±8
Maximum No. withdrawal symptoms	2.3±1.6	3.3±2.6
Age at onset of alcoholism, y	42±16	30±6†
Duration of alcoholism, y	10±8	18±14
Family history for alcoholism (%)	5/11 (45.5)	1/6 (16.7)
No. of different drugs	0.6±0.8	1.7±1.6
Stable relationship (%)	6/11 (54.5)	2/6 (33.3)
Employed (%)	3/11 (27.3)	3/6 (50)
Previous alcohol hospitalization (%)	2/11 (18.2)	0/6 (0)
Discharge to alcohol recovery home (%)	4/11 (36.4)	1/6 (16.7)
Neuropsychiatric component	0.32±0.8	0.12±0.9
Trails A time, s	35±10	34±16
Trails B time, s	107±35	106±50
Digit Symbol Substitution Test	7.9±2.0	8.5±2.2
Visual search time, s	165±75	141±54
Liver enzyme component	0.34±1.3	0.28±1.6
τ-Glutamyltransferase, IU	161±298	145±176
Aspartate aminotransferase, IU	43±27	41±29
Alanine aminotransaminase, IU	51±43	73±105

*Values are means±SDs.
†P<.05.

Time and the REM Pressure Component were evaluated for group 2 and found to meet criteria for normal distribution (skewness=−0.08 with Shapiro-Wilks *P*=.43, and skewness=0.54 with Shapiro-Wilks *P*=.76, respectively). Second, using the DFA derived from group 2 to classify patients in group 2, Total Sleep Time, as in the first case, did not enter; the REM Pressure Component did enter significantly (F=9.54, *df*=1,15, *P*=.008) and correctly classified 13 (76.5%) of 17 patients in group 2: nine (81.8%) of the 11 Abstainers and four (66.7%) of the six Relapsers. Third, the REM Pressure Component derived from group 2 correctly classified 23 (82.1%) of 28 patients in group 1: 15 (83.3%) of the 18 Abstainers and eight (80%) of the 10 Relapsers. Thus, the results with the various permutations of DFAs from each of the groups fulfilled the classic cross-validation procedures to validate REM pressure as a predictor of outcome.

GROUPS 1 AND 2

Since both groups produced similar DFAs and each group's DFA classification function coefficients cross-

Table 4. Comparison of Abstainers and Relapsers in Group 2 (n=17)*

Variable	Abstainers (n=11)	Relapsers (n=6)
Total Sleep Time	332±51	330±57
Sleep latency	19±10	29±26
Total WASO	42±29	33±10
Sleep efficiency, %	83.9±7.3	83.6±5.8
Stage 1%	10.2±5.3	7.3±3.2
Stage 2%	58.4±6.8	56.8±4.4
Stage 3%	2.7±4.9	1.6±3.6
Stage 4%	0.8±1.5	0.1±0.2
REM%	28.0±4.4	34.2±6.4‡
REM latency	60±17	43±18†
REM latency corrected	57±14	37±15§
REM cycle 1 duration	119±33	104±25
REM period 1 duration	29±13	34±15
REM density	2.1±0.8	2.6±1.0
REM period 1 density	2.0±0.7	2.3±1.3
REM "pressure component"	0.09±0.7	1.27±0.9§

*All values (means±SDs) are in minutes, percentages of Total Sleep Time, or, in the case of Rapid Eye Movement (REM) Density, units (0 to 8 per minute of REM sleep). WASO indicates wake time after sleep onset; REM%, Rapid Eye Movement percent.
†P<.05.
‡P<.02.
§P<.01.

classified the other group's patients well (76.5% and 80%), a final DFA was run with all 45 patients. Once again, Total Sleep Time did not enter while the REM Pressure Component from all patients did (F=18.1, *df*=1,43 *P*=.0001) and correctly classified 36 (80%) of 45 patients: 24 (82.8%) of 29 Abstainers and 12 (75%) of 16 Relapsers. **Figure 2** shows the REM pressure factor for each patient; the mean values were significantly greater in the Relapsers than in the Abstainers (*P*<.0001, Student's *t* test).

POSSIBLE CONFOUNDS

To evaluate the specificity of the apparent predictive power of REM sleep measures, we evaluated potentially confounding variables. None of the following correlated with REM pressure or differentiated Abstainers from Relapsers within group 1 or within group 2 or for all patients: age; education; family history of alcoholism and affective disorder; personal alcohol history, including quantity-frequency of drinking and days since last drink; depressive symptoms; other drug use; neuropsychological performance; and liver enzyme levels. Three measures were different between Relapsers and Abstainers within group 1 but not within group 2 (Neuropsychology Component, Trails A Time, and γ-glutamyltransferase) and one measure (age of onset of alcoholism) was different within group 2 but not within group 1. Furthermore,

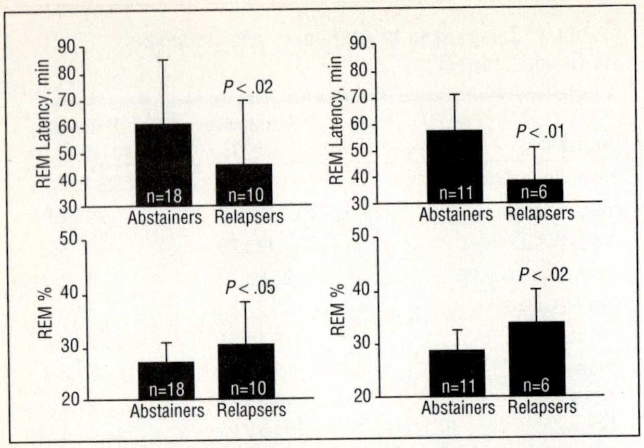

Figure 1. *Elevated Rapid Eye Movement percent (REM%) and shorter Rapid Eye Movement (REM) latency differentiate Relapsers and Abstainers in both group 1 (left) and group 2 (right).*

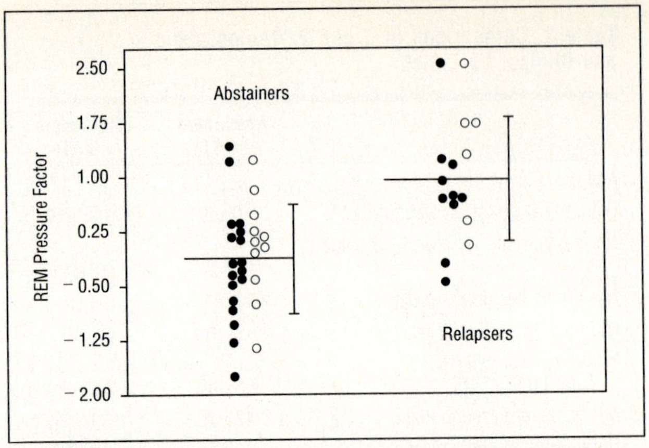

Figure 2. *Rapid Eye Movement (REM) sleep "pressure" at the time of admission to a 1-month inpatient alcoholic treatment program predicts relapse 3 months following discharge in patients with primary alcoholism. The REM sleep pressure is based on a principal component analysis, using REM latency corrected, REM percent, and REM Density, measured during the first week of hospital admission. Two consecutive samples of patients were studied (groups 1 and 2). Mean and SD are shown by horizontal and vertical bars, respectively. Closed circles indicate group 1; open circles, group 2.* P=*.0001.*

of the 32 patients for whom smoking history was known, no relationship was found between smoking and outcome at 3 months: 17 (74%) of 23 Abstainers and six (67%) of nine Relapsers were smokers (*P*=not significant, Fisher's Exact Test); likewise, packs per day did not correlate significantly with any of the REM sleep variables.

Nevertheless, to test whether other variables might do as well in predicting 3-month relapse as the three REM sleep measures, a DFA using the Liver Enzyme Component, the Neuropsychology Component, and the Hamilton Depression Rating Scale (as discussed herein) as potential predictors was run on group 1. The Hamilton Depression Rating Scale did not enter while the Neuropsychology Component (F=5.12, *P*=.034) and the Liver Enzyme Component (F=3.07, *P*=.07) did correctly classify 21 (75%) of the 28 patients in group 1. Using the classification function coefficients, however, from group 1's DFA on the patients of group 2 yielded a correct classification rate of only 40%. Not surprisingly, running the DFA on group 2 first led to none of the potential predictors significantly entering the equation. Thus, the other potential predictors failed in cross-validation.

STABILITY OF SLEEP MEASURES FROM HOSPITAL ADMISSION TO HOSPITAL DISCHARGE

To determine the stability over time of the sleep characteristics of Abstainers and Relapsers, we compared the sleep recordings of 26 Abstainers and 14 Relapsers at the time of hospital admission and discharge (**Table 5**). Data were not available at the time of hospital discharge from five patients for technical reasons.

The analysis revealed no significant changes from the time of hospital admission to discharge in REM latency, REM%, or REM Density (Table 5). The analysis of variance with repeated measures revealed statistically significant greater REM% and shorter REM latency cor-

Table 5. Rapid Eye Movement (REM) Sleep Measures at Time of Hospital Admission and Discharge in Abstainers (n=26) and Relapsers (n=14)

Sleep	Time	Abstainer	Relapser	Statistics*
REM%	Admission	27.8±4.4	32.4±6.4§	Group F=10.4
	Discharge	26.9±5.0	30.7±4.0‡	*P*<.003
REM latency corrected, min	Admission	59±20	43±12‖	Group F=4.2
	Discharge	55±31	44±19	*P*<.05
REM density	Admission	2.0±0.6	2.4±0.9†	GxT, F=3.4
	Discharge	2.0±0.7	2.1±0.7	*P*<.075

*df=*1,38 (two-way analysis of variance with repeated measures); G indicates between group; T, time (admission to discharge); REM%, Rapid Eye Movement percent. Pairwise, between-group comparisons (two-tailed* t *test).*
†P<*.05.*
‡P<*.02.*
§P<*.01.*
‖P<*.005.*

rected in Relapsers than in Abstainers. Rapid Eye Movement Density did not differ between the two groups. No significant interaction (group vs time) effects were observed for any sleep measure. Of the three REM sleep measures, only one between-group comparison was significantly different at session 2: REM% was greater in Relapsers than in Abstainers (30.7%±4.0% vs 26.9%±5.0%, $P<.02$, $t=2.47$, $df=38$).

COMMENT

These results suggest that REM sleep measures from patients with uncomplicated primary alcoholism obtained about 1 week after admission to a 1-month inpatient treatment program predict abstinence or relapse 3 months after discharge. Relapsing patients showed significantly shortened REM latency and elevated REM% compared with Abstainers in two consecutive cohorts of nondepressed primary alcoholics. Relapse was also associated with a composite PCA termed increased REM pressure (short REM latency corrected and elevated REM% and REM Density) at admission in the two separate groups of successively admitted patients. It was verified by successful cross-classification of patients in the two groups based on a DFA derived from each group independently. Interestingly, prognosis was not consistently associated with other clinical or demographic variables, such as age, family history of alcoholism or depression, education, duration and intensity of drinking, number of withdrawal symptoms, severity of depressive symptoms at the time of hospital admission, cognitive or liver enzyme level abnormalities, smoking, employment, marital status, or other polygraphic sleep measures, including Total Sleep Time. Although variables previously related to outcome were not consistently confirmed in this study, this was not unexpected since the percentage of variance they accounted for in previous studies and the number of subjects in the present study were both small. Indeed, one reason for examining sleep variables as outcome predictors was to evaluate whether they would account for a greater percentage of variance. To our knowledge, this is the first study suggesting that short REM latency and increased REM% at the time of hospital admission predict prognosis in patients with primary alcoholism.

Notwithstanding the support provided by the cross-validation procedures in two separate groups, the conclusions must be regarded with caution until larger numbers of alcoholic patients are studied. Moreover, it is important that these data were obtained from patients who completed the follow-up assessments at hospital discharge and 3-month follow-up, who maintained sobriety during the inpatient treatment program, and who did not take other medications, such as disulfiram. It is possible that patients with a more severe clinical course or a more complicated clinical picture (ie, patients who prematurely drop out of the inpatient treatment program, are unavailable for follow-up after hospital discharge, are treated with disulfiram, or have major medical complications, antisocial personality, or secondary depression) might differ from the present patients with relatively pure primary alcoholism.

FURTHERMORE, LARGER sample sizes would be useful to evaluate the predictive value of specific measures that did not cross-validate in our two groups. For example, compared with Abstainers, Relapsers showed an elevated neuropsychological component, Trails A, and γ-glutamyltransferase in group 1 but not group 2, and an earlier age of onset of alcoholism in group 2 but not in group 1. At the present time we have no explanation for these discrepancies between groups 1 and 2.

If we assume that relapse by 3-month follow-up is associated with increased REM pressure at the time of hospital admission, what mechanisms might be involved? One possibility is that both the risk of relapse and increased REM pressure are directly related to individual physical dependence on alcohol. According to this conjecture, the greater the "REM sleep pressure" at the time of hospital admission, the greater the withdrawal ("REM rebound") following the REM sleep-suppressing effects of alcohol. Thus, our REM Pressure Component may reflect individual differences in physical dependence to alcohol. It is thought, for example, that individual genetic or biochemical variability determines susceptibility to some complications of alcoholism, such as Wernicke-Korsakoff syndrome.[20] Previous studies have suggested that relapse is directly related to dependence as assessed by questionnaires and clinical interviews.[15] In this study, however, the relapsing and abstaining patients did not differ from each other on the number of most withdrawal symptoms ever experienced at one time, suggesting that the two groups had similar dependence, at least as measured by this question. Our measure of physical dependence, the most number of withdrawal symptoms at one time, correlates well with the Alcohol Dependence Scale ($r=.68$, $P<.001$, n=453 well-characterized patients with primary alcoholism studied on the Alcohol Research Center). The Alcohol Dependence Scale is an accepted measure of alcohol dependency.

Since alcohol has hypnotic properties, increases REM latency, and reduces total REM sleep, at least over the first part of the night,[7,21] it is logically possible that the patients with elevated REM pressure drink to ameliorate a physiologic sleep disturbance or even the negative subjective experiences associated with increased dreaming sleep. Again, we have no direct data to address these hypotheses, but other investigators have reported that poor subjective sleep may predispose to increased rates of relapse.[1,5,7,8]

In terms of possible neurochemical mechanisms underlying both poor prognosis in alcoholism and increased REM pressure, one possibility involves insufficient serotonergic neurotransmission. Current hypotheses about the regulation of normal REM sleep implicate cholinergic promoting and aminergic inhibitory control over REM sleep.[22,23] A relative deficiency of serotonergic neurotransmission may be involved in the symptoms of alcoholism, including craving, depression, and sleep disturbance.[3] Some previous studies have provided modest evidence that administration of zimeldine hydrochloride or citalopram, both serotonin reuptake blockers, may prolong abstinence and reduce drinking in nondepressed alcoholic patients.[24] Most of these medications prolong REM latency and reduce REM% in patients with depression or normal volunteers.[25]

THESE PATIENTS showed little change in their REM sleep measures from the time of hospital admission to discharge (Table 5). Whether the present REM sleep abnormalities predate the onset of alcoholism, have traitlike qualities, or have a genetic component are not known. Some limited evidence from sleep studies of depressed patients suggests that short REM latency, for example, is found in first-degree relatives of depressed patients[26] and persists in remission.[27] Alternatively, these abnormalities could reflect a persistent withdrawal syndrome in recovering alcoholic patients, which would eventually wane. Longer periods of follow-up study are needed but will be difficult if patients resume drinking, since renewed alcoholism will presumably affect sleep measures.

Short REM latency characterizes patients with major depressive disorder and primary alcoholism with secondary depression. It has also been reported in some patients with schizophrenia, mania, eating disorders, borderline personality, obsessive-compulsive disorder, and substance abusers during acute withdrawal.[28] The presence of short REM latency in these later diagnostic groups has often been attributed to the presence of secondary or comorbid depression or dysthymia. In contrast, the Relapsers in the present study are a group of well-documented patients without depression who have short REM latency.

Short REM latency may have prognostic value, not only in primary alcoholism, as in this study, but in depression. Giles et al[29] have previously reported that depressed patients with short REM latency (defined as ≤65 minutes) prior to treatment were statistically more likely to relapse following maintenance therapy than patients with a longer REM latency prior to treatment. Rush et al[30] also reported that short REM latency predicts successful treatment with tricyclic antidepressants. Perhaps in contrast, Cartwright et al[31] recently reported that short REM latency (<60.5 minutes) at baseline was associated with good adjustment 1 year later in depressed divorcees.

These current results require us to reevaluate our interpretation of the earlier findings we reported in relative pure primary alcoholics, specifically, that as a group they did not show abnormal values for REM latency or REM%.[10] On the basis of the current data, we now suggest that a clinically meaningful subgroup of nondepressed patients with primary alcoholism, the Relapsers, have short REM latency and elevated REM% compared with both Abstainers and normal controls. The overall mean for the entire group in this report, both Relapsers and Abstainers, is within normal limits, however, consistent with the earlier publication.

In summary, these results suggest that relapse within 3 months after discharge from a 1-month inpatient alcohol treatment program may be predicted during the first week of hospitalization on the basis of short REM latency and increased REM%, and, possibly, increased REM Density in patients with uncomplicated primary alcoholism. Taken together as a statistical measure, these three REM sleep variables correctly predicted relapse or abstinence in 36 (80%) of the 45 patients in this study. While additional data will be necessary to confirm these observations, the present findings may help clinicians predict prognosis in nondepressed patients with primary alcoholism early during hospitalization and tailor treatment programs accordingly. These observations may also help researchers to understand physiologic mechanisms associated with prognosis in alcoholism.

Accepted for publication April 8, 1993.

This investigation was supported in part by the Department of Veterans Affairs, the Alcohol Research Center, and grants MH 30914 and MH 38738 (J.C.G.) from the University of California, San Diego Mental Health Clinical Research Center.

Regina Ciambrone, Kathy Resovsky, RN, Jeannie Moore, RN, David Namie, Laura Sutton, RN, Caroline Ruiz, Frederick Storch, and Arlene Naldowski provided technical assistance.

Reprint requests to Department of Psychiatry (0603), University of California, San Diego, 9500 Gilman Dr, La Jolla, CA 92093-0603 (Dr Gillin).

REFERENCES

1. Gross MM, Hastey JM. Sleep disturbances in alcoholism. In: Tarter RE, Sugarman A, eds. *Alcoholism: Interdisciplinary Approaches to an Enduring Problem.* Reading, Mass: Addison-Wesley Publishing Co; 1976:257-309.
2. Lester B, Rundell OH, Cowden LC, Williams HL. Alcohol and sleep in the chronic alcoholic. In: Burch N, Altshuler HL, eds. *Behavior and Brain Electrical Activity.* New York, NY: Plenum Press; 1975:55-80.
3. Zarcone V. Alcoholism and sleep. In: Passonant P, Oswald I, eds. *Pharmacology of the State of Alertness.* Oxford, England: Pergamon Press; 1979:9-38.
4. Snyder S, Karacan I. Sleep patterns of sober chronic alcoholics. *Neuropsychobiology.* 1985;13:97-100.

5. Allen RP, Faillace LA, Wagman A. Recovery time for alcoholics after prolonged alcohol intoxication. *Johns Hopkins Med J.* 1971;128:158-164.
6. Rundell OH, Williams HL, Lester BK. Sleep in alcoholic patients: longitundinal findings. *Adv Exp Med Biol.* 1977;85B:389-340.
7. Skoloda TE, Alterman AI, Gottheil E. Sleep quality reported by drinking and non-drinking alcoholics. In: Gottheil EL, ed. *Addiction Research and Treatment: Converging Trends.* Elmsford, NY: Pergamon Press Inc; 1979:102-112.
8. Gross MM, Hastey JM. The relation between baseline slow wave sleep and the slow wave sleep response to alcohol in alcoholics. *Adv Exp Med Biol.* 1975; 59:467-475.
9. Gillin JC, Smith TL, Irwin M, Kripke DF, Brown S, Schuckit M. Short REM latency in primary alcoholics with secondary depression. *Am J Psychiatry.* 1990; 147:106-109.
10. Gillin JC, Smith TL, Irwin M, Kripke DF, Schuckit M. EEG sleep studies in 'pure' primary alcoholism during subacute withdrawal: relationships to normal controls, age, and other clinical variables. *Biol Psychiatry.* 1990;27:447-488.
11. Moeller FG, Gillin JC, Irwin M, Golshan S, Kripke DF, Schuckit M. A comparison of sleep EEGs in patients with primary major depression and major depression secondary to alcoholism. *J Affect Disord.* 1993;27:39-42.
12. Vaillant GE, Milofsky ES. Natural history of male alcoholism, IV: paths to recovery. *Arch Gen Psychiatry.* 1982;39:127-133.
13. Ornstein P, Cherepon JA. Demographic variables as predictors of alcoholism treatment outcome. *J Stud Alcohol.* 1985;46:425-432.
14. Schuckit MA, Schwei MG, Gold E. Prediction of outcome in inpatient alcoholics. *J Stud Alcohol.* 1986;47:151-155.
15. Rounsaville BJ, Dolinsky ZS, Babor TF, Meyer RE. Psychopathology as a predictor of treatment outcome in alcoholics. *Arch Gen Psychiatry.* 1987;44:505-513.
16. Schuckit MA, Morrison CR, Gold EO. A pragmatic alcoholism treatment outcome scale. *Am J Drug Alcohol Abuse.* 1984;10:125-131.
17. Schuckit MA. The clinical implications of primary diagnostic groups among alcoholics. *Arch Gen Psychiatry.* 1985;42:1043-1049.
18. Irwin M, Baird SM, Smith TL, Schuckit M. Use of laboratory tests to monitor heavy drinking by men discharged from a treatment program. *Am J Psychiatry.* 1988;145:595-599.
19. Rechtschaffen A, Kales AA. *A Manual of Standardized Terminology, Techniques, and Scoring System for Sleep Stages of Human Subjects.* Washington, DC: Public Health Service; 1968.
20. Charness ME, Simon RP, Greenber DA. Ethanol and the nervous system. *N Engl J Med.* 1989;321:442-454.
21. Yules RB, Lippman ME, Freedman DX. Alcohol administration prior to sleep: the effect of EEG sleep stages. *Arch Gen Psychiatry.* 1967;16:94-97.
22. Luebke JI, Greene RW, Semba K, Kamondi A, McCarley RW, Reiner PB. Serotonin hyperpolarizes cholinergic low-threshold burst neurons in the rat laterodorsal tegmental nucleus in vitro. *Proc Natl Acad Sci U S A.* 1992;89: 743-747.
23. Jones BE. Paradoxical sleep and its chemical/structural substrates in the brain. *Neuroscience.* 1991;40:637-656.
24. Naranjo CA, Sellers EM, Lawrin MO. Modulation of ethanol intake by serotonin uptake inhibitors. *J Clin Psychiatry.* 1986;47(suppl):16-22.
25. Vogel GW, Buffenstein A, Minter K, Hennessey A. Drug effects on REM sleep and on endogenous depression. *Neurosci Biobehav Rev.* 1990;14:49-63.
26. Giles DE, Kupfer DJ, Roffwarg HP, Rush AJ, Biggs MM, Etzel BA. Polysomnographic parameters in first-degree relatives of unipolar probands. *Psychiatry Res.* 1989;27:127-136.
27. Rush AJ, Erman MK, Giles DE. Polysomnographic findings in recently drug free and clinically remitted depressed patients. *Arch Gen Psychiatry.* 1986;43: 878-884.
28. Benca RM, Obermeyer WH, Thisted RA, Gillin JC. Sleep and psychiatric disorders: a meta-analysis. *Arch Gen Psychiatry.* 1992;49:651-668.
29. Giles DE, Jarrett RB, Roffwarg HP, Rush AJ. Reduced REM latency: a predictor of recurrence in depression. *Neuropsychopharmacology.* 1988;1:33-39.
30. Rush AJ, Giles DE, Jarrett RB, Feldman-Koffler F, Debus JR, Weissenburger J, Orsulak PJ, Roffwarg HP. Reduced REM latency predicts response to tricyclic medication in depressed outpatients. *Biol Psychiatry.* 1989;26: 61-72.
31. Cartwright RD, Kravitz HM, Eastman CI, Wood E. REM latency and the recovery from depression: getting over divorce. *Am J Psychiatry.* 1991;148: 1530-1535.

ORIGINAL ARTICLE

Subanesthetic Effects of the Noncompetitive NMDA Antagonist, Ketamine, in Humans

Psychotomimetic, Perceptual, Cognitive, and Neuroendocrine Responses

John H. Krystal, MD; Laurence P. Karper, MD; John P. Seibyl, MD; Glenna K. Freeman; Richard Delaney, PhD; J. Douglas Bremner, MD; George R. Heninger, MD; Malcolm B. Bowers, Jr, MD; Dennis S. Charney, MD

Background: To characterize further behavioral, cognitive, neuroendocrine, and physiological effects of subanesthetic doses of ketamine hydrochloride in healthy human subjects. Ketamine, a phencyclidine hydrochloride derivative, is a dissociative anesthetic and a noncompetitive antagonist of the *N*-methyl-D-aspartate subtype of excitatory amino acid receptor.

Methods: Nineteen healthy subjects recruited by advertisements from the community participated in this randomized, double-blind, placebo-controlled study. Subjects completed three test days involving the 40-minute intravenous administration of placebo, ketamine hydrochloride (0.1 mg/kg), or ketamine hydrochloride (0.5 mg/kg). Behaviors associated with the positive and negative symptoms of schizophrenia were assessed by using the Brief Psychiatric Rating Scale. Changes in perception and behaviors associated with dissociative states were assessed by the Perceptual Aberration Subscale of the Wisconsin Psychosis Proneness Scale and the Clinician-Administered Dissociative States Scale. Cognitive function was assessed by using the (1) Mini-Mental State Examination; (2) tests sensitive to frontal cortical dysfunction, including a continuous performance vigilance task, a verbal fluency task, and the Wisconsin Card Sorting Test; and (3) tests of immediate and delayed recall. Plasma levels of cortisol, prolactin, homovanillic acid, and 3-methoxy-4-hydroxyphenethyleneglycol were measured.

Results: Ketamine (1) produced behaviors similar to the positive and negative symptoms of schizophrenia; (2) elicited alterations in perception; (3) impaired performance on tests of vigilance, verbal fluency, and the Wisconsin Card Sorting Test; (4) evoked symptoms similar to dissociative states; and (5) preferentially disrupted delayed word recall, sparing immediate recall and postdistraction recall. Ketamine had no significant effect on the Mini-Mental State Examination at the doses studied. Ketamine also had no effect on plasma 3-methoxy-4-hydroxyphenethyleneglycol levels, although it blunted a test day decline in plasma homovanillic acid levels at the higher dose. It also dose dependently increased plasma cortisol and prolactin levels. Ketamine produced small dose-dependent increases in blood pressure.

Conclusions: These data indicate that *N*-methyl-D-aspartate antagonists produce a broad range of symptoms, behaviors, and cognitive deficits that resemble aspects of endogenous psychoses, particularly schizophrenia and dissociative states.

(Arch Gen Psychiatry. 1994;51:199-214)

From the Department of Psychiatry, Yale University School of Medicine, New Haven, Conn (Drs Krystal, Karper, Seibyl, Delaney, Bremner, Heninger, Bowers, and Charney and Ms Freeman), the Psychiatry Service, West Haven (Conn) Department of Veterans Affairs Medical Center (Drs Krystal, Karper, Seibyl, Delaney, Bremner, and Charney and Ms Freeman), the Connecticut Mental Health Center, New Haven (Dr Heninger), and the Grace Education Building, Yale University (Dr Bowers).

EARLY REPORTS suggested that the cyclohexylamine anesthetics, phencyclidine hydrochloride (PCP) and ketamine hydrochloride, produced behavioral effects resembling schizophrenia and dissociative states.[1-7] Both agents altered sensory perception and produced bizarre and impoverished thought and speech, impaired attention, disrupted memory, and interfered with thought processes in healthy individuals. Phencyclidine abuse was associated with agitation, catatonia, and protracted psychosis.[8] Phencyclidine also exacerbated symptoms in schizophrenic patients.[1,9,10] Because phencyclidine produced a spectrum of symptoms and deficits associated with schizophrenia, a prominent theory, the "phencyclidine model of schizophrenia," suggested that the mechanism of ac-

See Subjects and Methods on next page

SUBJECTS AND METHODS

SUBJECTS

Subjects were recruited for participation in this study through public advertisement and they were paid for their participation. Healthy subjects were selected for participation after obtaining written informed consent and following a two-step process to exclude individuals with a history of psychiatric illness, substance abuse disorders, or significant current life stress. The first step involved a structured psychiatric interview that excluded subjects who gave evidence of a psychiatric or substance abuse disorder, history of consultation for an emotional difficulty, psychiatric illness in a first-degree relative, or clinically significant current life stress defined operationally as 3 or greater on the Severity of Psychosocial Stressors Scale for Adults employed in Axis IV of *DSM-III-R*.[52] The second step was a telephone interview conducted with an individual identified by the subject to confirm the information collected in the first stage of screening. No subject was excluded due to the history obtained during the informant interview. Subjects were instructed to abstain from consuming psychoactive medications for the 4 weeks before testing. Compliance with this request was supported with urine toxicology screens at initial screening and on test days. None of the subjects reported a history of serious medical illness. All of the subjects had normal results on physical examination and laboratory testing, including liver and thyroid function tests. Subjects were all within normal limits on two measures of vulnerability to psychosis, the Bell Reality Testing Inventory,[53,54] and the Wisconsin Scales of Psychosis Proneness.[55-57]

Twelve male (mean age±SEM, 23.7±0.9 years; mean±SEM weight, 79.4±3.2 kg) and seven female (mean±SEM age, 25.9±0.9 years; mean±SEM weight, 65.9±4.7 kg) subjects completed ketamine hydrochloride (0.1 and 0.5 mg/kg, respectively, intravenously during 40 minutes) and placebo testing. One subject dropped out after completing his first test day in which he received ketamine hydrochloride, 0.5 mg/kg. Gender did not appear to influence responses to ketamine; thus, data were collapsed across gender. On their first day, six subjects received placebo, five subjects received ketamine hydrochloride, 0.1 mg/kg, and eight subjects received ketamine hydrochloride, 0.5 mg/kg.

KETAMINE TEST PROCEDURES

Ketamine Administration

Subjects completed 3 test days in a randomized order during which they received saline solution (0.9% sodium chloride, USP), ketamine hydrochloride (0.1 mg/kg, Parke-Davis, Kalamazoo, Mich), or ketamine hydrochloride (0.5 mg/kg) intravenously during 40 minutes. These doses were selected on the basis of pilot data and published reports[6,7] suggesting that they affected behavior but were subanesthetic. Before each test day, potential responses to ketamine were reviewed with subjects to decrease discomfort during the test day. Assessments began 10 minutes following the initiation of drug infusion and continued for the remaining 30 minutes of infusion. Ketamine blood levels were not measured in this study. Published pharmacokinetic parameters[45] were fitted into established equations for describing blood levels during constant drug infusion[58] to estimate ketamine plasma levels during this study. Plasma ketamine levels during the 0.1-mg/kg dose (0.0025 mg/kg per minute) were predicted to range between 0.025 and 0.05 mg/L and during the 0.5-mg/kg dose (0.0125 mg/kg per minute) were estimated to be between 0.1 and 0.25 mg/L.

Behavioral Ratings

Symptoms and behaviors that are characteristic of schizophrenia were assessed by using the Brief Psychiatric Rating Scale (BPRS).[59] Four key BPRS items were selected as an index of the positive symptoms of schizophrenia based on previous reports that indicated their utility and validity[60-62] and inclusion within the empirically derived thought disorder factor of the BPRS.[63] These four key positive symptoms were conceptual disorganization, hallucinatory behavior, suspiciousness, and unusual thought content. Three key BPRS items, blunted affect, emotional withdrawal, and motor retardation were selected as a measure of the negative symptoms of schizophrenia based on a report of their reliability and validity[64] and their inclusion within the empirically derived withdrawal-retardation factor of the BPRS.[63] Activation and hostility were also assessed by using factors derived from the BPRS.[63] The items associated with each factor are listed as follows: (1) activation—tension, mannerisms and posturing, and excitement; and (2) hostility-suspiciousness—hostility, suspiciousness, uncooperativeness, and grandiosity.

Anger, anxiety, drowsiness, high, and sadness were assessed by using clinician-rated visual analog scales. These scales were scored in millimeters from the left-hand side of a 100-mm line to a perpendicular mark made by the clinician at a point corresponding to the apparent magnitude of the feeling state reported and exhibited by the subject (range: 0, "not at all," to 100, "most ever").[65] The BPRS and analog scales were administered at 30 and 15 minutes before ketamine administration, 10 minutes into the ketamine administration, and 40, 70, and 190 minutes following the termination of ketamine infusion (80-, 110-, and 230-minute time points). Ratings assessed the period following the previous assessment. Thus, the 80-minute time point reflected the last 30 minutes of ketamine infusion.

Perceptual alterations that are characteristic of schizophrenia and dissociative disorders were also assessed. The Perceptual Aberration Subscale of the Wisconsin Psychosis Proneness Scale was a self-rated measure utilized to evaluate the presence of perceptual changes reported by schizophrenic patients.[55,56] The Perceptual Aberration Subscale was administered at 30 minutes before ketamine infusion and at the 10-, 80-, and 110-minute time points. The Clinician-Administered Dissociative States Scale (CADSS)[66] was a clinician-administered measure of perceptual, behavioral, and attentional alterations occurring during dissociative experiences that had been validated in healthy subjects and patients with posttraumatic stress disorder. This scale involved 19 self-report questions and eight observer ratings scored from 0 (not at all) to 4 (extremely). To characterize dissociative responses to ketamine better, CADSS items were sorted into five subscales with apparent face validity and based on published scales that assessed dissociative states[67,68]: body perception, environmental perception, feelings of unreality, memory impairment, and time perception (items in each subscale available on request). The CADSS was administered at the −30-, 10-, 80-, and 110-minute time points. General aspects of cognitive function were assessed by using the Mini-Mental State Examination (MMSE).[69] This study slightly modified this examination to add an assessment of word recall following a 10-minute delay. For the memory assessment, separate sets of words, selected on the basis of their comparable frequency of use in the English language and comparable difficulty,[70] were presented at each time point. Thus, each set of words was presented once, but recall was assessed three times: (1) immediately following presentation, (2) following a distracting task, and (3) following a 10-minute delay. The MMSE, including memory testing, was presented 85 minutes before ketamine infusion and at the 10-, 80-, 110-, and 230-minute time points.

Frontal lobe function was assessed by using the Wisconsin Card Sorting Test, a verbal fluency test, and a continuous performance test of vigilance. The Wisconsin Card Sorting Test is a task in which cards are sorted by the number, color, and shape of objects depicted on the card. This task requires the subject to determine the rule governing the matching of cards and to adapt when these rules shift during the task. Patients with frontal lobe lesions[71] and schizophrenia[72,73] exhibit increased perseverative error and fewer categories successfully completed on this task. Computerized versions of the Wisconsin Card Sorting Test have been used as a test of frontal lobe function in schizophrenic patients undergoing studies of cerebral blood flow.[74] The current study utilized a computerized version of the Wisconsin Card Sorting Test (developed and validated by Donald Quinlan, PhD, unpublished data, September 1990). The verbal fluency task requires subjects to generate as many words as possible, beginning with a specified letter during a 1-minute interval.[75] Equivalent versions of this task were administered on the 3 test days by using letters equated for frequency in English.[75] Verbal fluency tasks are sensitive to frontal lobe damage, particularly of the left frontal lobe.[71]

Vigilance to visual stimuli, an attentional task that also involves the frontal lobes,[76-78] was measured by using a continuous performance task[79] in which subjects attended to numbers that were presented sequentially on a screen. The subject pushed a button to signal when a "9" was preceded by a "1." This test was introduced after four subjects had entered the study (n=14).

The frontal lobe tasks were presented in a fixed order to increase comparability between test days. The tests began 20 minutes after starting the ketamine infusion and were completed before the termination of the ketamine infusion. The order of presentation was continuous performance task, Wisconsin Card Sorting Test, and verbal fluency test. Ketamine effects rapidly declined following the termination of drug infusion. As a result, verbal fluency data on three subjects were not analyzed because their tests were not completed before the termination of ketamine infusion.

Subjects were contacted on the day following the infusion of ketamine hydrochloride (0.5 mg/kg). They were also interviewed on subsequent weeks when ketamine hydrochloride, 0.5 mg/kg, was administered as the first or second test day.

BIOCHEMICAL METHODS

Radioimmunoassay kits were utilized for determining plasma levels of prolactin (Serono Diagnostics Inc, Norwell, Mass, intra-assay and interassay coefficients of variance [CVs] were 3%, and 7%, respectively) and cortisol (Baxter Travenol Diagnostics Inc, Incstar Corp, Stillwater, Minn, intra-assay and interassay CVs were 3% and 5%, respectively). Plasma samples for hormonal analysis were run in duplicate pairs. Plasma free levels of homovanillic acid (HVA)[80] and 3-methoxy-4-hydroxyphen ethyleneglycol (MHPG)[81] were measured by gas chromatography and mass spectrometry with the use of deuterated internal standards. The intra-assay and interassay CVs were 4% and 8%, respectively, for HVA and 6% and 11%, respectively, for MHPG.

DATA ANALYSIS

Data were analyzed by using repeated-measures analyses of variance (ANOVAs) with time and ketamine dose as within-subjects variables (SPSS V4.0, SPSS Inc, Chicago, Ill). When the ANOVA dose×time interactions were significant, post hoc multiple comparisons of postinfusion time points to baseline were conducted by using Dunnett's multiple *t* test.[82] Dunnett's tests were also performed on the change from baseline at each time point to compare each ketamine dose with placebo. In data analyses, baseline values were defined as the meaned preinfusion values. Comparison of baseline values were conducted by using Dunnett's *t* tests, comparing the baseline values on the placebo day with baseline values on the other 2 test days. To adjust for placebo day responses, the change from baseline at each time point on the placebo day was subtracted from the change from baseline at each time point on the ketamine day. Placebo-corrected increases from baseline were also analyzed by using Dunnett's test. When significant differences in baseline values emerged, data were reanalyzed by covarying for the baseline values. The Wisconsin Card Sorting Test cannot be repeated in individuals who learn the rules of the test.[71] As a result, Wisconsin Card Sorting Test data in this report are solely from the first test day for each subject. These data were compared by using an ANOVA in a between-subjects design. Post hoc testing of Wisconsin Card Sorting Test results were conducted by using the Student-Newman-Keuls multiple comparison test. The relationship between baseline demographical and descriptive data and peak change after infusion at the highest dose of ketamine was explored by using Pearson correlation coefficients.

tion of phencyclidine was fundamentally related to the neurobiology of schizophrenia.[1,11] Despite this theory, there has been limited direct study of the behavioral and neuropsychological effects of drugs related to phencyclidine in humans since the 1960s. Three possible reasons for the reluctance of investigators to study this class of agent include (1) greater interest in other pharmacological models for schizophrenia; (2) little understanding, until recently, of their mechanism of action; and (3) concern that phencyclidine or ketamine administration was associated with an unacceptable risk of adverse psychological reactions.

Alternatives to the phencyclidine model of schizophrenia, based on the behavioral effects of amphetamine, lysergic acid diethylamide (LSD), and dimethyltryptamine (DMT), have contributed greatly to the study of schizophrenia.[12-18] While these agents produce symptoms resembling acute psychosis,[19] they do not produce the full range of symptoms associated with schizophrenia, particularly cognitive deficits and negative symptoms such as blunted affect and concrete thinking.[4,5,9,16,20] There is increasing awareness that negative symptoms and neuropsychological deficits are relatively resistant to available pharmacotherapies,[21] are the source of significant distress, and are associated with social-vocational impairment.[22] Thus, there is heightened interest in pharmacological strategies, such as the study of ketamine effects, that might provide insight into these cognitive deficits and symptoms.

Molecular mechanisms underlying phencyclidine and ketamine effects have now been identified. These agents interfere with the action of the excitatory amino acid (EAA) neurotransmitters, including glutamate and aspartate. The EAAs are the most prevalent excitatory neurotransmitters in the brain and are particularly important in corticocortical and cortical-subcortical interactions.[23] The EAAs act via four main types of receptors. Three EAA receptor subtypes contain ion channels: the N-methyl-D-aspartate (NMDA), kainate, and 3-hydroxy-5-methyl-4-isoxazole–propionic acid (AMPA) receptors.[23-25] The fourth principal EAA subtype is a metabotropic glutamate receptor coupled by G proteins to the inositol signal transduction pathway.[26,27] In the human brain, the NMDA receptor is most densely localized in the cerebral and hippocampal cortices,[28] where EAA binding activates neurons by opening a voltage-dependent cation channel that is permeable to calcium.[11,23] Phencyclidine and ketamine are noncompetitive NMDA antagonists. They bind to a site that is distinct from NMDA within the ion channel and block calcium influx.[11,23,29] At subanesthetic doses, phencyclidine is a selective noncompetitive antagonist of the NMDA receptor with a median effective dose (ED_{50}) of approximately 0.07 to 0.08 μmol/L.[11] Ketamine binds to the NMDA receptor complex at the same site as phencyclidine, with an affinity of approximately 35 μmol/L.[30] It is 10 to 50 times less potent than phencyclidine in blocking NMDA-mediated neurotoxicity,[31] seizures,[32] and physiological effects,[33] and in substituting for phencyclidine in drug discrimination paradigms.[11] Ketamine is clinically available as a racemic mixture of two enantiomers. The S-isomer has two to four times greater affinity for the NMDA receptor[34,35] and clinical potency[36] than the R-isomer. Both ketamine isomers are more than 10 times more potent at the NMDA receptor than the σ receptor,[34] a receptor that is neither an opiate receptor nor the principal mediator of the psychotomimetic effects of phencyclidine.[37] Consistent with the limited contributions of the σ receptor to the dissociative anesthetic properties of ketamine, the R-isomer of ketamine has an approximately sevenfold greater affinity for the σ receptor than the S-isomer.[34] Ketamine binds to the μ opiate receptor with less than one fifth the potency with which it binds to the NMDA receptor.[34,38] The small contribution of the μ receptor to the behavioral effects of ketamine is consistent with the limited capacity of naloxone hydrochloride to reverse the analgesic and behavioral effects of ketamine.[38-41] Ketamine has less potent, but significant affinity at monoamine transporter sites.[42] Ketamine also weakly inhibits acetylcholinesterase.[43]

KETAMINE HAS advantages over phencyclidine as an agent to study NMDA receptor function in humans. The intensity and disturbing nature of the behavioral effects of phencyclidine, the reports of protracted phencyclidine-induced psychosis or exacerbations in psychotic symptoms in patients, and its abuse liability contributed to its removal from the clinical armamentarium. Ketamine has a shorter half-life than phencyclidine,[44,45] thus reducing the likelihood of lingering behavioral effects. Also, the detrimental impact of perceptual alterations associated with the emergence from ketamine anesthesia may be minimized by psychological preparation[46] and premedication with benzodiazepines[47] or neuroleptics.[48] High doses of phencyclidine in rats produce pathological neuronal changes in brain regions, such as the cingulate cortex.[49] However, ketamine is less potent than phencyclidine in producing these changes, and subanesthetic doses of ketamine are far lower than those studied in the toxicity studies. Overall, there is little evidence of long-term adverse effects of ketamine anesthesia in humans despite extensive clinical experience with this drug.[50,51]

The current study characterized the dose dependency of the perceptual, cognitive, behavioral, neuroendocrine, and physiological effects of subanesthetic doses of ketamine in healthy human subjects. In doing so, this study further defined the contributions of NMDA receptor function to behavior in humans.

RESULTS

BPRS SCORES

Positive Symptoms of Schizophrenia

As indicated in **Figure 1**, ketamine produced a dose-related increase in the four key positive symptoms of schizophrenia in healthy subjects (n=18). In the repeated-measures ANOVA, the effects of ketamine dose ($F_{2,34}$=72.0, *P*=.0001), time ($F_{4,68}$=19.3, *P*=.0001), and the interaction of dose and time ($F_{8,136}$=22.9, *P*=.0001) were significant. There were no significant differences in baseline scores between test days. Placebo and low-dose ketamine did not produce significant changes from baseline in the four key positive symptoms score. Post hoc testing of the high-dose ketamine day, by using Dunnett's test, revealed significant increases from baseline ($P<.01$) at 10 ($t_{5,\ 136}$=9.4) and 80 ($t_{5,\ 136}$=12.8) minutes following the initiation of ketamine infusion. These increases remained significant ($P<.01$) when adjusting for changes on the placebo day at these time points. Positive symptom scores returned to baseline generally within 15 minutes following the termination of ketamine infusion.

When analyzed separately, each of the four key symptom items were increased by ketamine (all dose×time interaction effects were significant, $P<.0001$). At the ketamine doses reported in this study, hallucinatory behavior was limited to illusory experiences in all sensory domains. Subjects experienced alterations in perception of both self and environment. For example, one person perceived that his legs were floating in the air when they were resting on his bed. Another subject felt that music quietly playing in another room sounded inordinately loud—"like a transistor radio implanted in (his) ear." Several subjects developed ideas of reference, and these individuals often had related paranoid thought content about staff in neighboring rooms talking about them in ominous ways. Formal thought disorder was also noticeable on the high-dose ketamine day with loosening of association, derailment, stilted speech, and other alterations contributing to the conceptual disorganization item of the four key positive symptoms.

None of the pretest predictors of vulnerability to psychosis, the Bell Reality Testing Inventory, any of its subscales, or the Wisconsin Psychosis Proneness Scale correlated significantly ($r<.25$) with the placebo-controlled peak increase in the BPRS four key positive symptoms score.

Negative Symptoms of Schizophrenia

Ketamine also dose dependently increased the three key negative symptom scores in healthy subjects (n=18, Figure 1). The ANOVA revealed significant effects of dose ($F_{2,34}$=34.6, *P*=.0001), time ($F_{4,68}$=28.0, *P*=.0001), and the dose×time interaction ($F_{8,136}$=18.0, *P*=.0001). There were no significant differences in baseline scores between test days. Placebo did not elicit increases from baseline at any

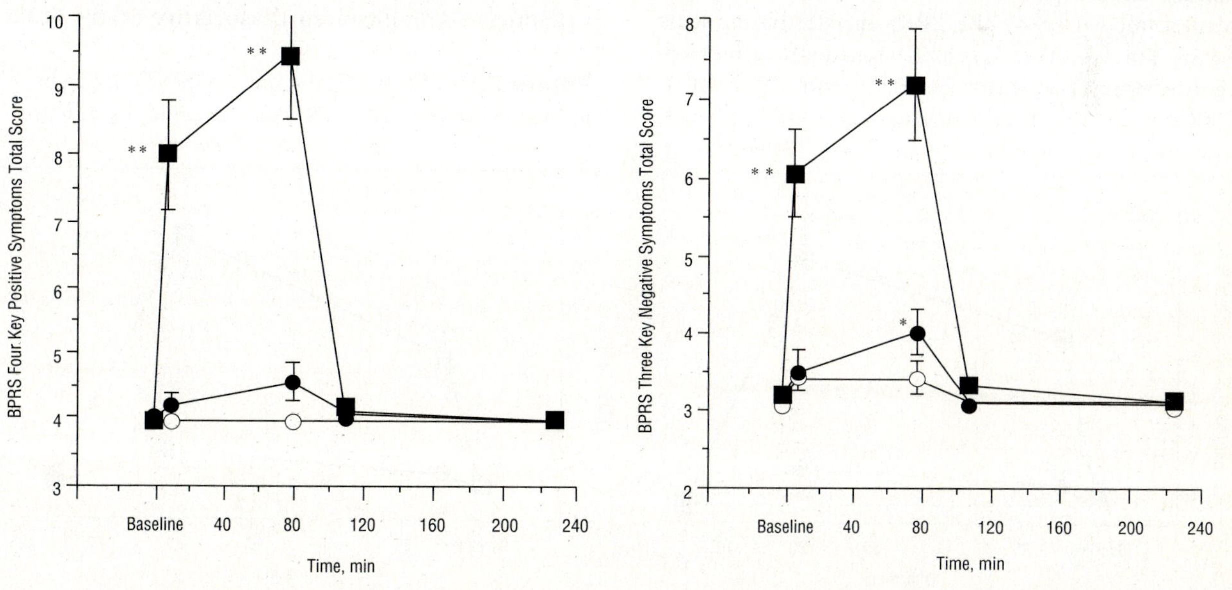

Figure 1. *Left, Ketamine hydrochloride effects on the Brief Psychiatric Rating Scale (BPRS) four key positive symptoms in healthy subjects (n=18). Cluster scores (mean±SEM) are presented for placebo (open circles), ketamine hydrochloride (0.1 mg/kg) (closed circles), and ketamine hydrochloride (0.5 mg/kg) (closed squares) test days. Individual time point increases from baseline, by Dunnett's* t *test: two asterisks,* P<.01. *All other statistics are presented in the text. Right, Ketamine effects on the BPRS three key negative symptoms in healthy subjects (n=18). Cluster scores (mean±SEM) are presented for placebo (open circles), ketamine hydrochloride (0.1 mg/kg) (closed circles), and ketamine hydrochloride (0.5 mg/kg) (closed squares) test days. Individual time point increases from baseline, by Dunnett's* t *test: one asterisk,* P<.05; *two asterisks,* P<.01. *All other statistics are presented in the text.*

time point. The low-dose ketamine day significantly increased negative symptom scores only at 80 minutes following the initiation of the infusion ($t_{5,136}$=2.56, *P*<.05). Ketamine hydrochloride (0.5 mg/kg), significantly increased negative symptoms from baseline at 10 ($t_{5,136}$=9.1, *P*<.01) and 80 ($t_{5,136}$=12.6, *P*<.01) minutes after initiating the ketamine infusion. These increases from baseline remained significant (*P*<.01) after adjusting for the placebo response.

When analyzed separately, the ANOVA dose×time interaction effects were significant (*P*<.0001) for each of the three key negative symptoms. On the high-dose day, subjects felt detached from their surroundings. Subjects described an amotivational state in which they had difficulty with initiating or sustaining concentration on tasks or interpersonal interactions. When effortful maintenance of attention lapsed, task performance suffered and subjects withdrew emotionally. Emotional responses were blunted on the high-dose ketamine day, and subjects frequently appeared emotionally dulled. Despite this blunting, ketamine evoked intense emotional responses in several subjects (see below). Psychomotor retardation was evident during the high-dose ketamine infusion. The degree of psychomotor retardation evoked by ketamine was disproportionate to the feeling of drowsiness, which was only modestly increased by ketamine (see below). Subjects felt awake but detached from the external environment rather than sleepy.

BPRS ACTIVATION FACTOR SCORE

Ketamine dose dependently increased behavioral activation as measured by the BPRS in healthy subjects (n=18). The ANOVA revealed significant effects of ketamine dose ($F_{2,34}$=11.8, *P*=.0001), time ($F_{4,68}$=10.1, *P*=.0001), and the dose×time interaction ($F_{8,136}$=6.1, *P*=.0001). There were no significant differences in baseline values between test days. Neither placebo nor ketamine hydrochloride (0.1 mg/kg) produced significant increases in activation from baseline. However, high-dose ketamine increased activation scores from baseline (mean±SEM, 3.2±0.1) at 10 (mean±SEM, 3.9±0.2; $t_{5,136}$=3.4; *P*<.01) and 80 (mean±SEM, 4.7±0.5; $t_{5,136}$=7.3; *P*<.01) minutes after beginning the ketamine infusion. The high-dose effects of ketamine were still significant (*P*<.01) after adjusting for placebo day effects.

BPRS HOSTILITY-SUSPICIOUSNESS FACTOR SCORE

Ketamine dose dependently increased hostility and suspiciousness as measured by the BPRS in healthy subjects (n=18). The ANOVA revealed significant effects of ketamine dose ($F_{2,34}$=6.7, *P*=.004), time ($F_{4,68}$=5.1, *P*=.001), and the dose×time interaction ($F_{8,136}$=6.1, *P*=.0001). There were no significant differences in baseline scores between test days. Neither placebo nor ketamine hydrochloride, 0.1 mg/kg, produced significant increases in activation from baseline. However, high-dose ketamine increased activation scores from baseline (mean±SEM, 3.2±0.1) at the 80-minute time point (mean±SEM, 4.7±0.5; $t_{5,136}$=6.9; *P*<.01). This effect was still significant (*P*<.01) after adjusting for placebo day effects.

PERCEPTUAL ALTERATIONS

Clinician-Administered Dissociative States Scale

Figure 2 presents the total scores on the CADSS in healthy subjects (n=17). The ANOVA revealed significant ef-

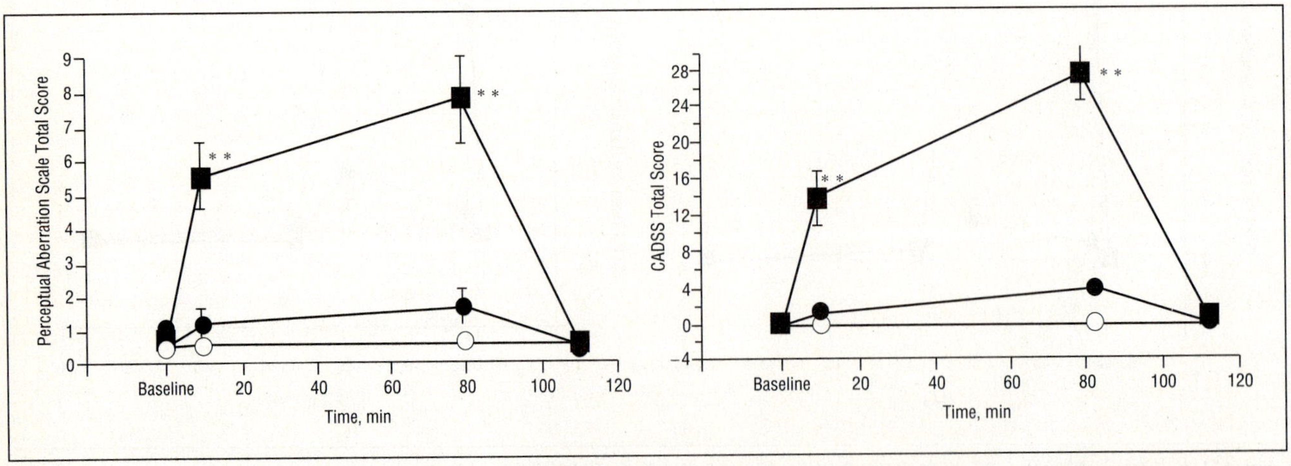

Figure 2. *Left, Ketamine hydrochloride effects on the Wisconsin Psychosis Proneness Perceptual Aberration Subscale scores in healthy subjects (n=18). Subscale scores (mean± SEM) are presented for placebo (open circles), ketamine hydrochloride (0.1 mg/kg) (closed circles), and ketamine hydrochloride (0.5 mg/kg) (closed squares) test days. Individual time point increases from baseline, by Dunnett's* t *test: two asterisks,* P<.01. *All other statistics are presented in the text. Right, Ketamine effects on the Clinician-Administered Dissociative States Scale (CADSS) in healthy subjects (n=18). The CADSS scores (mean± SEM) are presented for placebo (open circles), ketamine hydrochloride (0.1 mg/kg) (closed circles), and ketamine hydrochloride (0.5 mg/kg) (closed squares) test days. Individual time point increases from baseline, by Dunnett's* t *test: two asterisks,* P<.01. *All other statistics are presented in the text.*

fects of dose ($F_{2,32}$=65.0, P=.0001), time ($F_{3,48}$=46.8, P=.0001), and the dose×time interaction ($F_{6,96}$=46.0, P=.0001). There were no significant differences in baseline scores between test days. Placebo did not elicit increases from baseline at any time point. The low-dose ketamine day produced a nonsignificant increase in perceptual alterations from baseline at 80 minutes following the initiation of the infusion ($t_{4,96}$=2.56, P<.1). Ketamine hydrochloride, 0.5 mg/kg, significantly affected perception at 10 ($t_{4,96}$=9.4, P<.01) and 80 ($t_{4,96}$=18.8, P<.01) minutes after initiating the ketamine infusion. These increases from baseline remained significant (P<.01), adjusting for changes on the placebo day.

DOSE-RELATED effects of ketamine were also observed within all five CADSS subscales. The body perception subscale showed significant effects of ketamine dose ($F_{2,32}$=26.0, P=.0001), time ($F_{3,48}$=24.5, P=.0001), and the dose×time interaction ($F_{6,96}$=17.6, P=.0001). Subjects reported alterations in the shape or position of body parts. The ANOVA for the environmental perception subscale also showed significant effects of dose ($F_{2,32}$=55.2, P=.0001), time ($F_{3,48}$=33.2, P=.0001), and the dose×time interaction ($F_{6,96}$=30.0, P=.0001). In this category, subjects reported alterations in sensory intensity and disruption of the integrity of sensory experience. Individuals experienced themselves as having a constricted field of attention that ranged from inches to feet, outside of which, environmental stimuli seemed distant or difficult to attend to. Yet, spatially distant, weak, or insignificant stimuli were often perceived as disproportionately loud or close. Similarly, colors within a field of focused attention seemed more vivid than usual, and colors beyond the range of focused attention seemed dulled in intensity. Feelings of unreality were also significantly increased by ketamine: dose ($F_{2,32}$=29.7, P=.0001), time ($F_{3,48}$=20.2, P=.0001), and the dose×time interaction ($F_{6,96}$=21.0, P=.0001) effects were significant. Subjects reported altered self-observation, feeling that things were unreal. Depersonalization was evident, with some subjects reporting a feeling of emptiness or "feeling dead inside." A few subjects transiently lost the perspective that they were participating in a study in which they received a drug. Most subjects described a loss of control over thought processes. The ANOVA for memory impairment indicated significant effects of dose ($F_{2,32}$=41.8, P=.0001), time ($F_{3,48}$=31.1, P=.0001), and the dose×time interaction ($F_{6,96}$=29.0, P=.0001). Time perception was significantly slowed by ketamine. The ANOVA revealed significant dose ($F_{2,32}$=36.2, P=.0001), time ($F_{3,48}$=30.3, P=.0001), and the dose×time interaction ($F_{6,96}$=26.5, P=.0001) effects.

Perceptual Aberration Subscale of the Wisconsin Psychosis Proneness Questionnaire

As indicated in Figure 2, ketamine produced a dose-related increase in self-rated perceptual alterations (n=18). In the repeated-measures ANOVA, the effects of the ketamine dose ($F_{2,34}$=35.4, P=.0001), time ($F_{3,51}$=26.7, P=.0001), and the interaction of dose and time ($F_{6,102}$=20.0, P=.0001) were significant. There were no significant differences in baseline scores between test days. Placebo and low-dose ketamine did not produce significant changes from baseline scores. Post hoc testing, by using Dunnett's test, revealed significant increases from baseline (P<.01) at 10 ($t_{4,102}$=12.9) and 80 ($t_{4,102}$=18.7) minutes following the initiation of the high-dose ketamine infusion. These increases remained significant when adjusting for changes on the placebo day at these time points (P<.01). As with positive symptoms, perceptual alteration scores returned to baseline generally within 15 minutes following the termination of ketamine infusion.

The CADSS is clinician-rated, and the Perceptual Aberration Subscale is self-rated. Although both scales measured perceptual alterations, peak increases in both scales on the ketamine hydrochloride (0.5-mg/kg) test day were not significantly correlated.

MINI-MENTAL STATE EXAMINATION

Ketamine did not produce statistically significant effects on the MMSE, which is a brief bedside evaluation of global cognitive function in healthy subjects (n=18). Neither the dose×time interaction effect for MMSE data ($F_{8,136}$=1.4, P=.2) nor comparisons of the peak decrease from baseline for each test day (placebo, 0.7±0.4 [mean±SEM]; low, 0.2±0.1; high, 0.3±0.2; dose effect: $F_{2,34}$=1.6, P=.2), reached statistical significance.

MEASURES OF FRONTAL LOBE FUNCTION

Vigilance, Verbal Fluency, and the Wisconsin Card Sorting Test

Vigilance. Ketamine had small dose-related effects on vigilance in healthy subjects (n=14). The number of items correctly identified on the continuous performance test was decreased only on the high-dose day (placebo, 29.7±0.1 [mean±SEM]; low, 29.6±0.2; high, 28.5±0.4; dose effect: $F_{2,26}$=8.6, P=.001). The number of errors of omission was increased only on the ketamine hydrochloride (0.5-mg/kg) day (placebo, 0.3±0.1 [mean±SEM]; low, 0.4±0.2; high, 1.5±0.4; dose effect: $F_{2,26}$=8.6, P=.001). Commission errors were also significantly increased only on the high-dose ketamine day (placebo, 0.1±0.1 [mean±SEM]; low, 0.2±0.2; high, 0.6±0.3; dose effect: $F_{2,26}$=4.3, P=.03). Reaction time during the vigilance test was not significantly affected by either ketamine dose (pla-

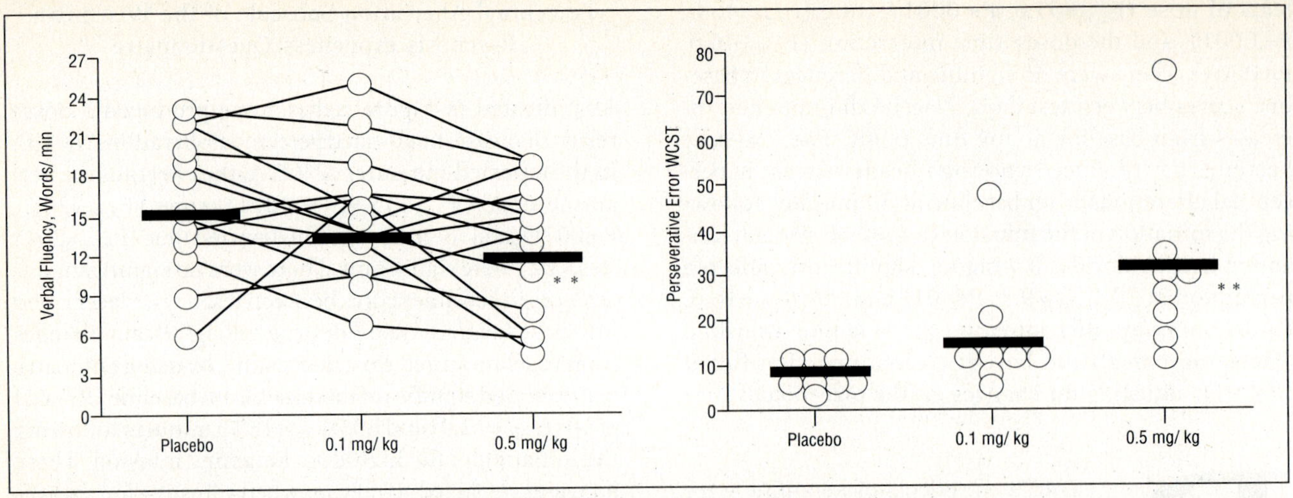

Figure 3. *Left, Ketamine hydrochloride effects on verbal fluency in healthy subjects (n=15). Open circles represent individual subjects. Comparisons of ketamine test days with placebo test day, by a within-subjects post hoc contrast: two asterisks,* P<.01. *All other statistics are presented in the text. Right, Ketamine effects on the Wisconsin Card Sorting Test (WCST) perseverative error in healthy subjects (n=19) on their first test day. Open circles represent individual subjects. Comparisons of ketamine test days with placebo test day, by Student-Newman-Keuls test: two asterisks,* P<.01. *All other statistics are presented in the text.*

cebo, 0.48±0.03 [mean±SEM] seconds; low, 0.46±0.02 seconds; high, 0.51±0.03 seconds; dose effect: $F_{2,24}$=1.8, P=.2).

Verbal Fluency. Ketamine produced dose-dependent decreases in verbal fluency (n=15; placebo, 16.1±1.3 [mean±SEM]; low, 15.1±1.2; high, 12.9±1.3; dose effect: $F_{2,28}$=4.4, P=.02). Within-subjects post hoc contrasts revealed that word productivity was significantly lower on the high-dose day compared with that on the placebo day (F_1=8.4, P=.007), but there was only a trend toward a difference on the low- and high-dose days (F_1=3.8, P=.06).

Wisconsin Card Sorting Test. As presented in **Figure 3**, ketamine dose dependently increased perseverative errors on the Wisconsin Card Sorting Test in healthy subjects on their first test day (placebo [n=6], 0.1 mg/kg [n=5], 0.5 mg/kg [n=8]). The ANOVA revealed a significant dose effect (placebo, 6.5±0.8 [mean±SEM]; low, 16.8±7.9; high, 31.9±7.0; dose effect: $F_{2,16}$=4.6, P=.03). Post hoc testing using the Student-Newman-Keuls test revealed that a ketamine hydrochloride dose of 0.5 mg/kg produced significantly more perseverative errors than placebo. There was a dose-related ketamine effect on the number of trials to the first category completion (placebo, 13.5±1.9 [mean±SEM]; low, 14.6±2.5; high, 35.1±7.8; dose effect: $F_{2,16}$=4.6, P=.03) and the total number of errors (placebo, 12.8±2.2 [mean±SEM]; low, 25.6±10.0; high, 53.4±8.4; dose effect: $F_{2,16}$=8.0, P=.004). Perhaps because of the increased total errors, the ketamine effect on percent perseverative error did not reach statistical significance (placebo, 54%±5% [mean±SEM]; low dose, 62%±5%; high dose, 58%±4%; dose effect: $F_{2,16}$=0.7, P=not significant [NS]). However, all subjects completed all six categories correctly, and the number of correct items (placebo, 70.8±3.9 [mean±SEM]; low, 68.8±1.8; high, 65.6±5.0; dose effect: $F_{2,16}$=0.4, P=.7) and the number of losses of set ($F_{2,16}$=2.0, P=.2) did not differ between dose groups.

Since the Wisconsin Card Sorting Test cannot be repeated, correlations between performance on this test and other measures were determined for the first test day only. Wisconsin Card Sorting Test perseverative error scores significantly correlated with the peak increases from baseline in three key negative symptom scores (r=.5, P=.05) and CADSS scores (r=.6, P=.008). Nonsignificant trends toward correlation also emerged between the Wisconsin Card Sorting Test perseverative error scores and peak increases in the four key positive symptoms (r=.5, P<.06) and the perceptual aberration subscale (r=.4, P=.06).

Memory

Analysis of memory data, presented in **Figure 4**, indicated an interaction between the time within the session that memory was tested (before, during, or after ketamine administration), the dose of ketamine administered, and the delay following stimulus exposure (immediate recall, postdistraction recall, and following a 10-minute delay). The overall repeated-measures ANOVA revealed significant main effects of ketamine dose (n=16; $F_{2,30}$=60.6, P=.0001), delay ($F_{2,30}$=4.9, P=.02), time ($F_{4,60}$=3.0, P=.02), and the interaction of ketamine dose, time, and delay ($F_{16,240}$=2.7, P=.0006). Post hoc analyses of the different periods of delay revealed a particular vulnerability of the 10-minute delay to disruption by high-dose ketamine. There was no significant dose×time interaction for immediate recall

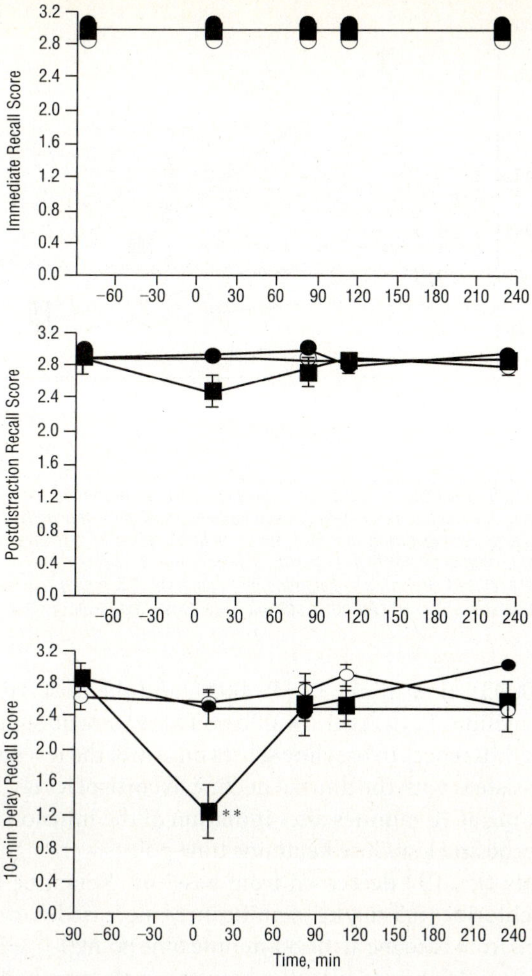

Figure 4. *Ketamine hydrochloride effects on recall in healthy subjects (n=16). Cluster scores (mean±SEM) are presented for placebo (open circles), ketamine hydrochloride (0.1 mg/kg) (closed circles), and ketamine hydrochloride (0.5 mg/kg) (closed squares) test days. Top, Immediate recall data. Center, Postdistraction recall data. Bottom, Effect of a 10-minute delay on word recall. Different three-word sets were presented at each time point for immediate recall. However, the same set of words was assessed at comparable time points for immediate, postdistraction, and delayed recall data. Individual time point decreases from baseline, by Dunnett's* t *test: two asterisks,* $P<.01$. *All other statistics are presented in the text.*

($F_{8,120}$=0.0, P=NS), a nonsignificant trend for the postdistraction recall to be disrupted by high-dose ketamine ($F_{8,120}$=1.7, P=.1), and a clear dose×time interaction for the 10-minute delayed recall ($F_{8,120}$=3.4, P=.002). On the ketamine hydrochloride (0.5 mg/kg) test day, impairments in delayed recall did not significantly correlate with increases in positive symptoms (r=.2), negative symptoms (r=.07), or CADSS scores (r=.2).

VISUAL ANALOG SCALES OF MOOD STATES

As illustrated in **Figure 5**, there were dose-related increases in anxiety and high.

Anxiety

There was evidence of a biphasic ketamine dose effect on anxiety, with the low dose decreasing anxiety and the higher dose increasing it. In the repeated-measures ANOVA, the effects of time ($F_{3,51}$=16.3, P=.0001) and the interaction of dose and time ($F_{6,102}$=2.5, P=.03) were significant. There were no significant differences in baseline scores on any of the test days. Post hoc testing suggested that low-dose ketamine produced a significant decline in anxiety from baseline at the 10-minute time point ($t_{4,102}$=2.4, $P<.05$), while the decline did not reach significance at any time point on the placebo day. Controlling for the placebo day decline in anxiety eliminated the significance of the anxiolytic effect of low-dose ketamine. On the high-dose ketamine day, subjects reported a reduction in anxiety from baseline levels at 80 ($t_{4,102}$=5.5, $P<.01$) minutes following the initiation of ketamine infusion. However, relative to the placebo day decline in anxiety, high-dose ketamine significantly increased anxiety levels 10 minutes following the initiation of ketamine administration ($t_{3,102}$=4.7, $P<.01$).

High

The ANOVA revealed significant effects of dose ($F_{2,34}$=6.8, P=.003), time ($F_{3,51}$=13.6, P=.0001), and the dose×time interaction ($F_{6,102}$=5.1, P=.0001). There were no significant differences in baseline scores on any of the test days. Neither placebo nor ketamine hydrochloride, 0.1 mg/kg, produced significant changes in high from baseline. Ketamine hydrochloride, 0.5 mg/kg, significantly increased the feeling of high from baseline at 10 ($t_{4,102}$=6.8, $P<.01$) and 80 ($t_{4,102}$=5.1, $P<.01$) minutes after initiating the ketamine infusion. Adjusting for the placebo response, only the 10-minute time point remained significant ($P<.01$). Although not systematically assessed, before the emergence of perceptual and cognitive changes on the high-dose ketamine day, several subjects anecdotally reported similarities between the ketamine high and alcohol intoxication.

The drug×time effects in the ANOVAs did not reach significance for anger ($F_{6,102}$=0.7, P=.7), drowsiness ($F_{6,102}$=1.8, P=.1), or sadness ($F_{6,102}$=1.1, P=.4). Although the drug×time effect in the overall ANOVA was not significant for drowsiness, an ANOVA performed on peak increases from baseline (peak−meaned baseline values) showed a significant dose-related sedative effect for ketamine (0- to 100-mm scale: placebo, 6.2±4.3 mm [mean±SEM]; low, 15.5±4.4 mm; high, 22.9±6.9 mm; dose: $F_{2,34}$=4.3, P=.02).

NEUROENDOCRINE INDEXES

Homovanillic Acid

The initial ANOVA revealed significant main effects of ketamine dose ($F_{2,26}$=6.1, P=.007), time ($F_{4,52}$=30.3,

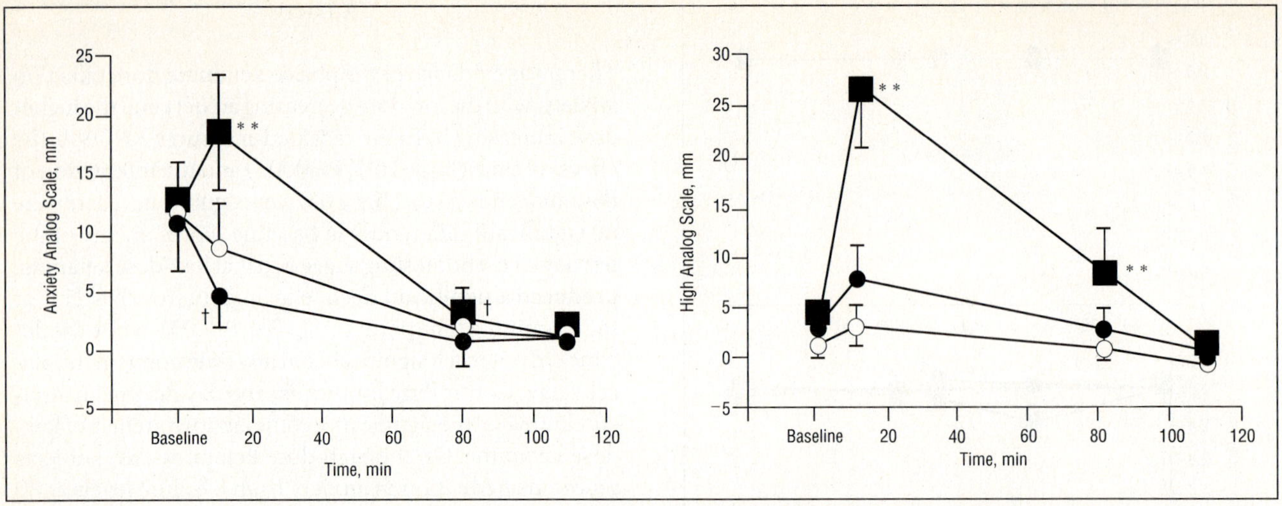

Figure 5. *Left, Ketamine hydrochloride effects on the visual analog scale for anxiety in healthy subjects (n=18). Scores (mean±SEM) are presented for placebo (open circles); ketamine hydrochloride, 0.1 mg/kg (closed circles); and ketamine hydrochloride, 0.5 mg/kg (closed squares) test days. Individual time point changes from baseline, by Dunnett's* t *test: dagger. Comparison of ketamine and placebo changes from baseline, by Dunnett's* t *test: two asterisks,* $P<.01$. *All other statistics are presented in the text. Right, Ketamine effects on the visual analog scale for high in healthy subjects (n=18). Scores (mean±SEM) are presented for placebo (open circles); ketamine hydrochloride, 0.1 mg/kg (closed circles); and ketamine hydrochloride, 0.5 mg/kg (closed squares) test days. Individual time point changes from baseline, by Dunnett's* t *test: two asterisks,* $P<.01$. *All other statistics are presented in the text.*

P=.0001), and the dose×time interaction ($F_{8,104}$=3.8, P=.0007) in healthy subjects (n=14). Comparison of baseline values for each test day (placebo, 14.7±1.6 [mean±SEM] ng/mL; low, 13.4±1.2 ng/mL; high, 10.3±1.0 ng/mL) revealed that the baseline plasma HVA level on the ketamine hydrochloride (0.5-mg/kg) test day was significantly lower than the baseline values on the placebo (t_{13}=4.1, P=.001) and low-dose ketamine (t_{13}=3.1, P=.009) test days. As a result, an analysis of covariance (ANCOVA) was performed utilizing baseline values for each test day as covariates. Although the main effect of the ketamine dose was no longer significant ($F_{2,25}$=0.9, P=.4), the time effect ($F_{3,39}$=19.1, P=.0001) and the dose×time interaction ($F_{6,78}$=3.1, P=.008) remained significant. Consistent with the ANCOVA, peak decreases from baseline (placebo, −0.9±0.4 [mean±SEM] ng/mL; low, −1.2±0.6 ng/mL; high, 0.3±0.6 ng/mL) suggested that ketamine blunted the test day decline in HVA (placebo vs high: t_{13}=2.4, P=.03).

3-Methoxy-4-Hydroxyphenethyleneglycol

Neither the dose×time interaction of the initial ANOVA ($F_{8,112}$=1.1, P=.4) nor the dose effect in the ANOVA for peak increases from baseline (n=15; placebo, 0.4±0.09 [mean±SEM]; low, 0.6±0.3; high, 0.3±0.1; dose effect: $F_{2,28}$=0.5, P=.6) were significant.

Cortisol

As presented in **Figure 6**, ketamine produced a dose-related increase in cortisol levels in healthy subjects (n=16). The ANOVA revealed significant effects of dose ($F_{2,30}$=10.6, P=.0003), time ($F_{4,60}$=4.1, P=.005), and the dose×time interaction ($F_{8,120}$=10.1, P=.0001). There were no significant differences in baseline scores on any of the test days. Consistent with the diurnal decline in cortisol levels, beginning at 40 minutes after initiation of the infusion, all placebo and low-dose ketamine time points were significantly (P<.01) decreased from baseline. Ketamine hydrochloride, 0.5 mg/kg, significantly increased cortisol levels from baseline at the 80-minute time point ($t_{5,120}$=3.8, P<.01). Relative to placebo, however, ketamine hydrochloride, 0.5 mg/kg, produced significant (P<.01) increases at the 40-, 80-, and 100-minute time points.

Prolactin

The initial analysis of prolactin levels revealed significant or near-significant effects of dose ($F_{2,34}$=4.9, P=.01), time ($F_{4,68}$=2.1, P=.09), and the dose×time interaction ($F_{8,136}$=3.7, P=.0007). There were no significant baseline differences between test days. There were no significant increases from baseline on either the placebo or low-dose ketamine days. On the high-dose ketamine day, prolactin levels increased from baseline at 40 minutes following the initiation of ketamine infusion ($t_{5,136}$=2.49, P<.05). This increase remained significant when adjusting for responses on the placebo day (P<.05).

The relationship of peak increases in neurotransmitter metabolite levels (MHPG, HVA) and hormones (prolactin, cortisol) to the peak increase in four key positive symptoms, three key negative symptoms, and CADSS scores was examined on the high-dose ketamine day. No significant correlations emerged in this analysis.

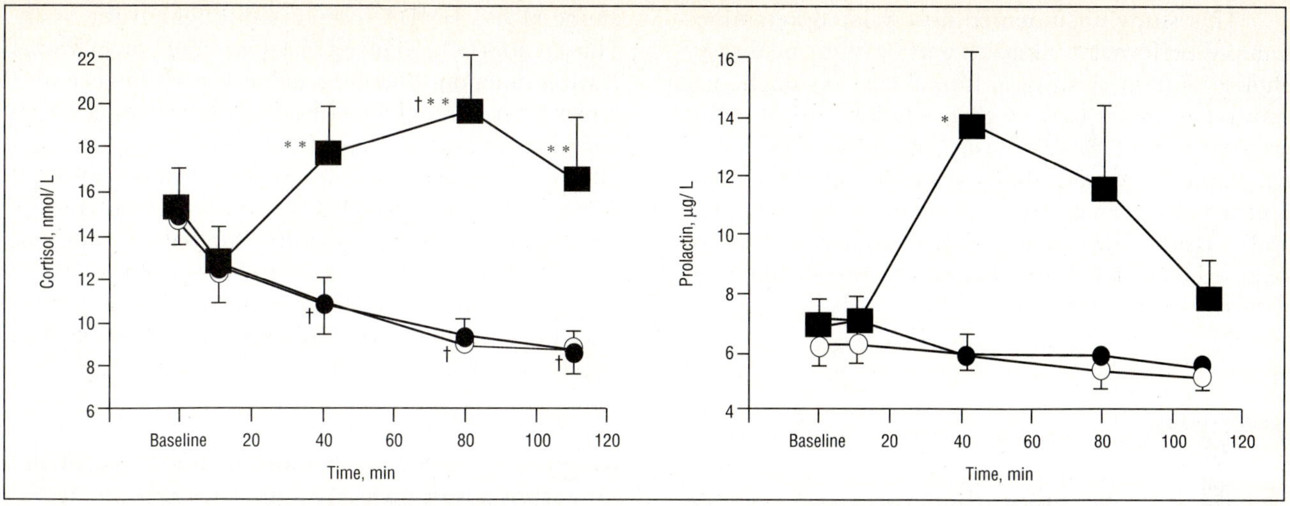

Figure 6. *Left, Ketamine effects on plasma cortisol levels in healthy subjects (n=18). Scores (mean±SEM) are presented for placebo (open circles); ketamine hydrochloride, 0.1 mg/kg (closed circles); and ketamine hydrochloride, 0.5 mg/kg (closed squares) test days. Individual time point changes from baseline, by Dunnett's* t *test: dagger,* P<.05. *Comparison of ketamine and placebo changes from baseline, by Dunnett's* t *test:* P<.01. *All other statistics are presented in the text. Right, Ketamine effects on plasma prolactin levels in healthy subjects (n=18). Scores (mean±SEM) are presented for placebo (open circles); ketamine hydrochloride, 0.1 mg/kg (closed circles); and ketamine hydrochloride, 0.5 mg/kg (closed squares) test days. Individual time point changes from baseline, by Dunnett's* t *test: one asterisk,* P<.05; *two asterisks,* P<.01. *All other statistics are presented in the text.*

BLOOD PRESSURE AND PULSE

Ketamine produced a dose-related increase in systolic blood pressure. The ANOVA revealed a significant drug×time interaction ($F_{12,204}$=2.2, *P*=.01), a finding loosely supported by analysis of peak increases from baseline (placebo, 11.3±1.9 [mean±SEM] mm Hg; low, 13.2±1.9 mm Hg; high, 18.6±2.6 mm Hg; dose effect: $F_{2,34}$=2.9, *P*=.07). Ketamine also produced a dose-related increase in diastolic blood pressure (dose×time interaction: $F_{12,204}$=3.6, *P*=.0001) and a dose-dependent peak increase in diastolic blood pressure from baseline (placebo, 5.9±1.3 mm Hg; low, 6.9±0.9 mm Hg; high, 12.5±2.2 mm Hg; dose effect: $F_{2,34}$=4.7, *P*=.02). Analysis of resting pulse did not reveal a significant interaction of drug and time effects ($F_{12,204}$=1.1, *P*=.3).

OTHER RESPONSES

Eight (44%, four males and four females) of the 18 subjects complained of blurred vision on the high-dose ketamine test day. In approximately half of these cases, blurred vision was associated with horizontal nystagmus. Subjects felt that they could complete the tasks requiring visual perception despite the blurred vision. Two women vomited during a high-dose ketamine test day, and both women had blurred vision and nystagmus at the time of vomiting. On follow-up interview, no subject had lingering or recurrent physiological or psychological effects, such as nightmares, flashbacks, or perceptual alterations following a test day.

COMMENT

This study further characterized effects of subanesthetic doses of the NMDA antagonist, ketamine, in healthy human subjects. Consistent with previous reports suggesting that NMDA antagonists produced psychosis in healthy individuals,[1-7] ketamine dose dependently altered the form and content of thought in healthy subjects. Ketamine elicited paranoia, loose associations, tangentiality, concreteness, ideas of reference, and unusual thought content. The higher dose of ketamine had significant perceptual effects, including alterations of body perception, perception of the environment, and time perception. It also produced derealization, depersonalization, and a subjective sense that memory was impaired. Supporting some,[7,36] but not all,[83] previous studies, ketamine influenced all domains of sensory function. Previous reports suggested that ketamine, usually at higher doses than those in the current study, produced hallucinations in individuals who did not have preexisting psychoses.[7,83,84] However, consistent with a previous report,[85] at the doses studied, ketamine distorted the perception of identifiable sensory stimuli, producing illusions rather than hallucinations.

Ketamine also produced emotional withdrawal, blunting of affective responses, and psychomotor retardation. As previously reported,[7] subjects reported feeling emotionally detached rather than sedated following the administration of the higher dose of ketamine. Subjects were not somnolent during the study. Following the higher ketamine dose, they noted that greater effort was required to initiate and sustain attention and emotional investment in tasks. Subjects also reported that initiating or sustaining interpersonal interactions demanded increased effort. A mild to moderate degree of psychomotor retardation was observed, consistent with the dissociative anesthetic properties of ketamine.[7] However, this motor retardation was not evident in the reaction time of subjects recorded during the vigilance task.

This study documented dose-related ketamine-induced performance impairments on three neuropsychological tests sensitive to frontal lobe dysfunction: a continuous performance vigilance task,[77,78] a verbal fluency test,[75,76] and the Wisconsin Card Sorting Test.[71] Ketamine produced small, but statistically significant decrements in vigilance, resulting in errors of commission and omission. This subtle decrement in attention was not reflected in MMSE scores, but may have contributed to reductions in performance on both the verbal fluency task and the Wisconsin Card Sorting Test.

THE HIGHER dose of ketamine impaired inductive or trial-and-error learning on the Wisconsin Card Sorting Test. Subjects failed to modify their behavior in response to feedback. They took longer to learn the initial sorting rule and showed increased perseveration of previously correct sorting principles. In addition, they were more likely to sort cards seemingly randomly, without an identifiable strategy. Ketamine did not, however, decrease the number of categories obtained or increase the failure to persist in employing correct strategies. Decrements in executive functions on the Wisconsin Card Sorting Test were paralleled by clinical evaluations that indicated impaired insight and disruption of thought processes as assessed by the BPRS. One link between the clinical and neuropsychological assessments comes from the work of Goldman-Rakic,[86] who suggested that the frontal lobes contribute to the generation of mental representations. Applying this metaphor to the current data, blockade of NMDA receptor function appeared to disrupt thought structure and impair one's capacity to utilize abstract representations to generate or improve problem-solving strategies.

Previous clinical studies have implicated the cerebral cortex in the behavioral effects of NMDA antagonists. Frontal lobotomy, for example, reduced the psychotomimetic responses to phencyclidine in schizophrenic patients.[10] One early theory suggested that perceptual alterations associated with phencyclidine result from a drug-induced sensory deprivation state arising through blockade of thalamocortical projections.[87] The initial sensory evoked potentials study of ketamine in humans[7] suggested that ketamine had specific disruptive effects on sensory integration rather than on sensory perception. The notion that subanesthetic ketamine primarily disturbs sensory integration rather than sensory perception is consistent with findings that sensory deprivation reduces the psychotomimetic and perceptual effects of phencyclidine.[88]

Preclinical data support a modulatory role for NMDA receptors in cortical function. Ketamine could act at several sites to produce a chemically induced performance impairment on tests sensitive to frontal lobe damage. Ketamine blocks NMDA receptors throughout the brain. Thus, it does not produce a selective reduction in frontal NMDA function. Ketamine-induced performance decrements on frontal lobe tasks could reflect an effect on cortical networks involving frontal, parietal, and temporal lobe structures.[86] Also, ketamine could modulate frontal cortical function via effects on a circuit involving the cortex, striatum, globus pallidus, subthalamic nucleus, and thalamus, in which EAAs play prominent roles.[86,89] Ketamine actions at multiple brain regions could produce impairments on the Wisconsin Card Sorting Test, consistent with reports that diffuse brain dysfunction may increase perseverative errors.[90]

Ketamine produced a preferential dose-related impairment in delayed word recall with little effect on immediate or postdistraction recall. Preclinical studies indicated that NMDA antagonists impair spatial memory[91-93] and molecular processes that are implicated in learning.[94-96] Previous clinical studies reported ketamine-induced disruption of learning and memory in humans.[36,83,97,98] In contrast, ketamine doses that did not affect memory in the current study were reported to enhance memory in patients with Alzheimer's disease.[99] The current study did not find ketamine effects on a simple test of immediate recall, ie, learning three words. However, a study by Ghoneim et al[83] found that ketamine impaired immediate recall on the more difficult memory task of learning 24 words. It is possible that the task employed by Ghoneim et al[83] was sufficiently challenging to demonstrate ketamine effects on immediate recall, perhaps consistent with disruption of "scratch pad" or working memory.[86] Alternatively, the immediate recall impairment found by Ghoneim and colleagues[83] using the more difficult task could have reflected ketamine interference with attention rather than with memory.

The clinical literature does not clearly indicate whether ketamine preferentially impairs retrieval, the capacity to recall learned information, or the consolidation of learned information from transient to long-term memory. If retrieval is selectively impaired, information that cannot be recalled may be recognized. Ghoneim et al[83] found dose-related ketamine-induced impairments in immediate and delayed recall with a relative sparing of recognition memory. They also referred to data, not presented, suggesting that retrieval of information learned before ketamine administration was impaired following ketamine administration. However, another study failed to replicate the ketamine-induced retrieval deficit for stimuli presented before ketamine infusion by using a task that was less dependent on sustained attention.[36] Interpretation of the data from the study by Ghoneim et al[83] is also limited by the utilization of multiple memory assessments during periods when ketamine blood levels were decreasing. Further complicating interpretations of ketamine effects on learning, a recent preclinical study[100] suggested that NMDA antagonists make learning state-dependent. Thus, it is not currently possible to characterize the relative contributions of impaired attention, consolidation, or retrieval to ketamine-induced memory impairments.

Ketamine dose dependently altered mood states. Subjects generally felt high following ketamine administration. On low-dose days, the high was perceived as a mildly euphoric "buzzing" feeling and tingling in their face and extremities, while the ketamine hydrochloride dose, 0.5 mg/kg, produced much stronger responses. Consistent with previous reports with phencyclidine,[1] there may be similarities between the ketamine "high" and alcohol intoxication. These reports are in agreement with laboratory data indicating that alcohol has NMDA antagonist properties[101] and that NMDA antagonists have alcohol-like discriminative properties in rodents.[102] Most subjects found the ketamine hydrochloride (0.1 mg/kg) test day fairly pleasant, and consistent with the preclinical literature,[103] anxiolytic effects were noted at this dose. However, subjects had diverse reactions to the ketamine hydrochloride dose of 0.5 mg/kg, ranging from enjoyment to fear. As suggested by the literature on psychedelic drugs,[15] subjects who disliked loss of control of cognitive functions seemed to be most disturbed by ketamine administration. Some subjects enjoyed the altered state of consciousness produced by ketamine and felt that it produced novel experiences or perspectives. These descriptions complemented reports from individuals who self-administered ketamine on a recreational basis.[104] Overall, the higher dose of ketamine was anxiogenic in the subjects studied.

This study also documented neuroendocrine and physiological responses to ketamine. At the higher dose, ketamine blunted a test day decline in plasma HVA levels. The slight enhancement of dopamine turnover in this study could be related to blockade of dopamine reuptake.[42] In light of studies questioning a direct relationship between plasma HVA levels and central dopaminergic function,[105] future studies will be needed to determine the locus of ketamine effects on plasma HVA levels. Ketamine did not significantly alter plasma MHPG levels. In humans, a transient rise in plasma norepinephrine associated with ketamine-induced hypertension has been attributed to peripheral mechanisms.[106] However, ketamine effects on norepinephrine turnover were not observed at the doses evaluated in this study. Ketamine produced dose-related increases in both prolactin and cortisol. Studies in the rodents and primates have generally,[107-110] but not uniformly,[111] found small NMDA antagonist-induced enhancements in prolactin and cortisol release. These findings are consistent with the presence of NMDA receptors in hypothalamic regions that modulate hormone release,[112] although non-NMDA receptors appear to play a predominant role in neuroendocrine regulation.[113] Direct and indirect mechanisms underlying the increases in prolactin and cortisol levels observed in this study need further characterization. Ketamine also had clear, but modest, physiological effects throughout the dose range studied. Consistent with findings of previous reports,[6,7,114] ketamine dose dependently increased systolic and diastolic blood pressures, with less clear effects on pulse.

This study also provided further evidence that subanesthetic doses of ketamine may be administered to healthy subjects in controlled laboratory settings without significant risk of untoward psychological consequences. None of the subjects in this study experienced any problematic sequelae reported to be associated with phencyclidine abuse, including protracted psychosis, flashbacks, or agitation.[8] Several steps were taken to minimize the risk of an adverse response to ketamine in this study. Given reports that mood disturbance before the administration of ketamine might increase the risk of an unpleasant reaction to ketamine,[115] individuals with personal or family psychiatric histories were excluded from this study. Perhaps because this group was so carefully screened, neither of the pretest assessments predicted the positive symptom response to ketamine. In addition, subjects were carefully prepared for the full range of ketamine effects before testing and debriefed following each session. This approach has previously been shown to reduce the risk of psychiatric morbidity associated with ketamine administration.[46]

ONE QUESTION raised by these data is whether ketamine effects mimic the signs and symptoms of psychiatric illnesses, particularly schizophrenia and dissociative states. The pathophysiologies of these conditions are little understood but, particularly for schizophrenia, under intensive study. A conservative initial evaluation of the data would suggest that ketamine does not produce a behavioral state that is identical to either schizophrenia or dissociative states. Unlike many patients with schizophrenia, the behavioral state produced by ketamine was associated with a sense of intoxication, dissociative symptoms, and the absence of hallucinations. Unlike most dissociative states, ketamine was associated with paranoia, thought disorder, and a sense of intoxication.

If ketamine effects are to guide studies of clinical pathophysiology, then one might begin by drawing parallels between aspects of the behavioral effects of ketamine and components of clinical disorders. There are similarities between ketamine effects and some aspects of psychosis. Despite the failure to generate hallucinations, ketamine produces many symptoms associated with endogenous psychosis. Ketamine also produces symptoms in healthy subjects that resemble the negative symptoms of schizophrenia. However, this study could not determine the degree to which the negative symptoms elicited by ketamine in healthy subjects share biological mechanisms with the negative symptoms in schizophrenic patients. Some schizophrenic patients perform poorly on tests of abilities impaired by frontal lobe dysfunction, exhibiting decreased vigilance,[74,116] reduced verbal fluency,[73,117] and increased perseverative errors on the Wisconsin Card Sorting Test.[71-74] They also exhibit impairments in temporohippocampal function, particularly memory.[73,118] The higher dose of ketamine impaired healthy subject performance on neuropsychological tests sensitive to frontotemporal dysfunction. The elicitation of negative symptoms and cognitive deficits by ketamine contrast with the psychedelic experiences associated with acute psychosis[19] and more closely resemble deficit syndromes associated with schizophrenia. Ketamine also produced symptoms associated with dissociative states, including slowed time perception; tunnel vision; changes in the intensity, shape, or color of environmental stimuli; alterations in body perception; derealization, depersonalization; and memory deficits.[67,68]

THE PHENCYCLIDINE model of schizophrenia suggested that this drug mimicked endogenous deficits in NMDA function associated with schizophrenia.[11] While the current study could not evaluate NMDA deficit models of mental illness, it heightens interest in excitatory amino acid neurotransmitter systems and their contributions to psychotic and dissociative states.

Accepted for publication April 22, 1993.

This study was supported by funding from the Department of Veterans Affairs through the Schizophrenia Biological Research Center, Department of Veterans Affairs–Yale Alcoholism Research Center, West Haven, Conn, and by a Merit Review Grant from the Department of Veterans Affairs (Dr Krystal). Additional funding came from research grant MH-30929 from the National Institute of Mental Health, Bethesda, Md.

The authors wish to acknowledge the critical contributions to this research program made by the staff of the Biological Studies Unit and the Schizophrenia Biological Research Center, West Haven (Conn) Veterans Affairs Medical Center. Kristen Morrissey is particularly acknowledged for her contributions in data collection and data analysis. Alexandre Bennett, PhD, is also thanked for consultations during the preparation of the manuscript. Pedro Mendia, MS, provided helpful assistance with statistical analyses. The authors also acknowledge the assistance of Morris Bell, PhD, and Paul Lysaker, PhD, in utilizing the Bell Reality Testing Inventory. Consultations with Elliot Luby, MD, Hsing-Cheng Loh, MD, and Edward Domino, MD, are gratefully acknowledged. Pharmacokinetic consultations provided by Anissa Abi-Dargham, MD, are also greatly appreciated.

Reprint requests to Psychiatry Service, West Haven Veterans Affairs Medical Center, 950 Campbell Ave, West Haven, CT 06516 (Dr Krystal).

REFERENCES

1. Luby ED, Cohen BD, Rosenbaum G, Gottlieb JS, Kelley R. Study of a new schizophrenomimetic drug—sernyl. *Arch Neurol Psychiatry.* 1959;81:363-369.
2. Bakker CB, Amini FB. Observations on the psychotomimetic effects of sernyl. *Compr Psychiatry.* 1961;2:269-280.
3. Davies BM, Beech HR. The effect of 1-arylcyclohexylamine (sernyl) on twelve normal volunteers. *J Ment Sci.* 1960;106:912-924.
4. Cohen BD, Rosenbaum G, Luby ED, Gottlieb JS. Comparison of phencyclidine hydrochloride (sernyl) with other drugs: simulation of schizophrenic performance with phencyclidine hydrochloride (sernyl), lysergic acid diethylamide (LSD-25), and amobarbital (Amytal) sodium, II: symbolic and sequential thinking. *Arch Gen Psychiatry.* 1962;6:79-85.
5. Rosenbaum G, Cohen BD, Luby ED, Gottlieb JS, Yelen D. Comparison of sernyl with other drugs: simulation of schizophrenic performance with sernyl, LSD-25, and amobarbital (Amytal) sodium, I: attention, motor function, and proprioception. *Arch Gen Psychiatry.* 1959;1:651-656.
6. Domino EF, Chodoff P, Corssen G. Pharmacologic effects of CI-581, a new dissociative anesthetic, in man. *Clin Pharmacol Ther.* 1965;6:279-291.
7. Corssen G, Domino EF. Dissociative anesthesia: further pharmacologic studies and first clinical experience with phencyclidine derivative CI-581. *Anesth Analg.* 1966;45:29-40.
8. Fauman B, Aldinger G, Fauman M, Rosen P. Psychiatric sequelae of phencyclidine abuse. *Clin Toxicol.* 1976;9:529-538.
9. Ban TA, Lohrenz JJ, Lehmann HE. Observations on the action of sernyl—a new psychotropic agent. *Can J Psychiatry.* 1961;6:150-157.
10. Itil T, Keskiner A, Kiremitci N, Holden JMC. Effect of phencyclidine in chronic schizophrenia. *Can J Psychiatry.* 1967;12:209-212.
11. Javitt DC, Zukin SR. Recent advances in the phencyclidine model of schizophrenia. *Am J Psychiatry.* 1991;148:1301-1308.
12. Angrist B, Gershon S. The phenomenology of experimentally induced amphetamine psychosis—preliminary observations. *Biol Psychiatry.* 1970;2:95-107.
13. Janowsky DS, Risch SC. Amphetamine psychosis and psychotic symptoms. *Psychopharmacology (Berl).* 1979;65:73-77.
14. Lieberman JA, Kane JM, Alvir J. Provocative tests with psychostimulant drugs in schizophrenia. *Psychopharmacology (Berl).* 1987;91:415-433.
15. Freedman DX. On the use and abuse of LSD. *Arch Gen Psychiatry.* 1968;18:330-347.
16. Freedman DX. LSD: the bridge from human to animal. In: Jacobs BL, ed. *Hallucinogens: Neurochemical, Behavioral, and Clinical Perspectives.* New York, NY: Raven Press; 1984:203-226.
17. Gillin JC, Kaplan J, Stillman R, Wyatt RJ. The psychedelic model of schizophrenia: the case of N,N-dimethyltryptamine. *Am J Psychiatry.* 1976;133:203-208.
18. Bowers MB Jr. The role of drugs in the production of schizophreniform psychoses and related disorders. In: Meltzer HY, ed. *Psychopharmacology: The Third Generation of Progress.* New York, NY: Raven Press; 1987:819-823.
19. Bowers MB, Freedman DX. 'Psychedelic' experiences in acute psychoses. *Arch Gen Psychiatry.* 1966;15:240-248.
20. Angrist B, Sathananthan G, Wilk S, Gershon S. Amphetamine psychosis: behavioral and biochemical aspects. *J Psychiatr Res.* 1974;11:13-23.
21. Andreasen ND, Olsen SA. Negative vs positive schizophrenia: definition and validation. *Arch Gen Psychiatry.* 1982;39:789-794.
22. Mueser KT, Douglas MS, Bellack AS, Morrison RL. Assessment of enduring deficit and negative symptom subtypes in schizophrenia. *Schizophr Bull.* 1991;17:565-582.
23. Cotman CW, Monaghan DT. Chemistry and anatomy of excitatory amino acid systems. In: Meltzer HY, ed. *Psychopharmacology: The Third Generation of Progress.* New York, NY: Raven Press; 1987:197-210.
24. Moriyoshi K, Masu M, Ishii T, Shigemoto R, Mizuno N, Nakanishi S. Molecular cloning and characterization of the rat NMDA receptor. *Nature.* 1991;354:31-37.
25. Dingledine R. New wave of non-NMDA excitatory amino acid receptors. *Trends Pharmacol Sci.* 1991;12:360-362.

26. Schoepp D, Bockaert J, Sladeczek F. Pharmacological and functional characteristics of metabotropic excitatory amino acid receptors. *Trends Pharmacol Sci.* 1990;11:508-514.
27. Masu M, Tanabe Y, Tsuchida K, Shigemoto R, Nakanishi S. Sequence and expression of a metabotropic glutamate receptor. *Nature.* 1991;349:760-765.
28. Kornhuber J, Mack-Burkhardt F, Riederer P. Regional distribution of [^{3}H]MK-801 binding sites in the human brain. *Brain Res.* 1989;489:397-399.
29. Thomson AM, West DC, Lodge D. An N-methylaspartate receptor–mediated synapse in rat cerebral cortex: a site of action of ketamine? *Nature.* 1985; 313:479-481.
30. Hampton RY, Medzihradsky F, Woods JH, Dahlstrom PJ. Stereospecific binding of ^{3}H phencyclidine in brain membranes. *Life Sci.* 1982;30:2147-2154.
31. Rothman SM, Olney JW. Excitotoxicity and the NMDA receptor. *Trends Neurosci.* 1987;10:299-302.
32. Willetts J, Balster RL, Leander JD. The behavioral pharmacology of NMDA receptor antagonists. *Trends Pharmacol Sci.* 1990;11:423-428.
33. Byrd LD. Effects of phencyclidine and ketamine on cardiovascular activity and temperature in the squirrel monkey. *Life Sci.* 1987;41:7-13.
34. Øye N, Hustveit O, Moberg ER, Pausen O, Skoglund LA. The chiral forms of ketamine as probes for NMDA receptor function in humans. In: Kameyama T, Nabeshima T, Domino EF, eds. *NMDA Receptor Related Agents: Biochemistry, Pharmacology, and Behavior.* Ann Arbor, Mich: NPP Books; 1991:381-389.
35. Zeilhofer HU, Swandulla D, Geisslinger G, Brune K. Differential effects of ketamine enantiomers on NMDA receptor currents in cultured neurons. *Eur J Pharmacol.* 1992;213:155-158.
36. Øye N, Paulsen O, Maurset A. Effects of ketamine on sensory perception: evidence for a role of *N*-methyl-D-aspartate receptors. *J Pharmacol Exp Ther.* 1992;260:1209-1213.
37. Quirion R, Chicheportiche R, Contreras PC, Johnson KM, Lodge D, Tam SW, Woods JH, Zukin SR. Classification and nomenclature of phencyclidine and sigma receptor sites. *Trends Neurosci.* 1987;10:444-446.
38. Smith DJ, Westfall DP, Adams JD. Ketamine interacts with opiate receptors as an agonist. *Anesthesiology.* 1980;53:anesthetic action I. Abstract.
39. Fratta W, Casu M, Balestrieri A, Loviselli A, Biggio G, Gessa GL. Failure of ketamine to interact with opiate receptors. *Eur J Pharmacol.* 1980;61:389-391.
40. Byrd LD, Standish LJ, Howell LL. Behavioral effects of phencyclidine and ketamine alone and in combination with other drugs. *Eur J Pharmacol.* 1987; 144:331-341.
41. Chan MY. Naloxone interaction with some CNS depressants. *Pharmacology.* 1985;31:294-297.
42. Smith DJ, Azzaro AJ, Zaldivar SB, Palmer S, Lee HS. Properties of the optical isomers and metabolites of ketamine on the high affinity transport and catabolism of monoamines. *Neuropharmacology.* 1981;20:391-396.
43. Cohen ML, Chan SL, Bhargava HN, Trevor AJ. Inhibition of mammalian brain acetylcholinesterase by ketamine. *Biochem Pharmacol.* 1974;23:1647-1652.
44. Kammerer RC, Cho AK. The biotransformation of phencyclidine. In: Domino EF, ed. *PCP (Phencyclidine): Historical and Current Perspectives.* Ann Arbor, Mich: NPP Books; 1981:177-189.
45. Wieber J, Gugler R, Hengstmann JH, Dengler HJ. Pharmacokinetics of ketamine in man. *Anesthetist.* 1975;24:260-263.
46. Sklar GS, Zukin SR, Reilly TA. Adverse reactions to ketamine anesthesia: abolition by a psychological technique. *Anesthesia.* 1981;36:183-187.
47. Freuchen I, Ostergaard J, Kuhl JG, Mikkels BO. Reduction of psychotomimetic side effects of ketalar (ketamine) by Rohypnol (flunitrazepam). *Acta Anaesthesiol Scand.* 1976;20:97-103.
48. Geist ET, Gross BD. Reduction of ketamine-induced emergence phenomena by preoperative promethazine. *J Oral Maxillofac Surg.* 1982;40:549-550.
49. Olney JW, Labruyere J, Price MT. Pathological changes induced in cerebrocortical neurons by phencyclidine and related drugs. *Science.* 1989;244:1360-1362.
50. Schorn TOF, Whitman JG. Are there long-term effects of ketamine on the central nervous system? *Br J Anaesth.* 1980;52:967-968.
51. Moretti RJ, Hassan SZ, Goodman LI, Meltzer HY. Comparison of ketamine and thiopental in healthy volunteers: effects on mental status, mood, and personality. *Anesth Analg.* 1984;63:1087-1096.
52. American Psychiatric Association. *Diagnostic and Statistical Manual of Mental Disorders, Third Edition, Revised.* Washington, DC: American Psychiatric Association; 1987.
53. Bell M. *An Introduction to the Bell Object Relations Reality Testing Inventory.* Los Angeles, Calif: Western Psychological Services; 1991.
54. Bell M, Billington R, Becker B. A scale for the assessment of reality testing: reliability, validity, and factorial invariance. *J Consult Clin Psychol.* 1985;53: 506-511.
55. Chapman LJ, Chapman JP, Raulin ML. Body image aberration in schizophrenia. *J Abnorm Psychol.* 1978;87:399-407.
56. Chapman LJ, Edell WS, Chapman JP. Physical anhedonia, perceptual aberration, and psychosis proneness. *Schizophr Bull.* 1980;6:639-653.
57. Chapman LJ, Chapman JP, Miller EN. Reliabilities and intercorrelations of eight measures of proneness to psychosis. *J Consult Clin Psychol.* 1982;50: 187-195.
58. Rowland M, Tozer TN. *Clinical Pharmacokinetics: Concepts and Applications.* 2nd ed. Philadelphia, Pa: Lea & Febiger; 1989.
59. Overall JE, Gorham DR. The Brief Psychiatric Rating Scale. *Psychol Rep.* 1962; 10:799-812.
60. Bowers MB, Heninger GR, Sternberg D, Meltzer HY. Clinical processes and central dopaminergic activity in psychotic disorders. *Comm Psychopharmacol.* 1980;4:177-188.
61. Kane J, Honigfeld G, Singer J, Meltzer H, and the Clozaril Collaborative Study Group. Clozapine for the treatment-resistant schizophrenic: a double-blind comparison with chlorpromazine. *Arch Gen Psychiatry.* 1988;45:789-796.
62. Krystal JH, Seibyl JP, Price LH, Woods SW, Heninger GR, Aghajanian GK, Charney DS. *m*-Chlorophenylpiperazine (MCPP) effects in neuroleptic-free schizophrenic patients: evidence implicating serotonergic systems in the positive symptoms of schizophrenia. *Arch Gen Psychiatry.* In press.
63. Hedlund JL, Vieweg BW. The Brief Psychiatric Rating Scale (BPRS): a comprehensive review. *J Operational Psychiatry.* 1980;11:48-64.
64. Thiemann S, Csernansky JG, Berger PA. Rating scales in research: the case of negative symptoms. *Psychiatry Res.* 1987;20:47-55.
65. Charney DS, Woods SW, Goodman WK, Heninger GR. Serotonin function in anxiety, II: effects of the serotonin agonist MCPP in panic disorder patients and healthy subjects. *Psychopharmacology (Berl).* 1987;92:14-24.
66. Bremner JD, Putnam F, Southwick SM, Krystal JH, Hansen C, Roach L, Johnson DR, Charney DS. The Clinician-Administered Dissociative States Scale: studies on the reliability and validity in use in the assessment of patients with psychiatric disorders. In: *1992 New Research Program and Abstracts.* Washington, DC: American Psychiatric Association; 1992. Abstract NR157.
67. Sanders S. The perceptual alteration scale: a scale measuring dissociation. *Am J Clin Hypn.* 1986;29:95-102.
68. Steinberg M, Rounsaville B, Cicchetti DV. The structure clinical interview for *DSM-III-R* dissociative disorder: preliminary report on a new diagnostic instrument. *Am J Psychiatry.* 1990;147:76-82.
69. Folstein MF, Folstein SE, McHugh PR. 'Mini-mental state': a practical method of grading the cognitive state of patients for the clinician. *J Psychiatr Res.* 1975;12:189.
70. Kucera H, Francis WN. *Computational Analysis of Present Day American English.* Providence, RI: Brown University Press; 1967.
71. Milner B. Some effects of frontal lobectomy in man. In: Warren JM, Akert K, eds. *The Frontal Granular Cortex and Behavior.* New York, NY: McGraw-Hill International Book Co; 1964:313-334.
72. Malmo HP. On frontal lobe functions: psychiatric patient controls. *Cortex.* 1974;10:231-237.
73. Kolb B, Whishaw IQ. Performance of schizophrenic patients on tests sensitive to left or right frontal, temporal, or parietal function in neurological patients. *J Nerv Ment Dis.* 1983;171:435-443.
74. Weinberger DR, Berman, KF, Zec RF. Physiological dysfunction of dorsolateral prefrontal cortex in schizophrenia. *Arch Gen Psychiatry.* 1986;43:114-124.
75. Borkowski JG, Benton AL, Spreen O. Word fluency and brain damage. *Neuropsychologia.* 1967;5:135-140.
76. Frith CD, Friston KJ, Liddle PF, Frackowiak SJ. A PET study of word finding. *Neuropsychologia.* 1991;29:1137-1148.
77. Wilkins AJ, Shallice T, McCarthy R. Frontal lesions and sustained attention. *Neuropsychologia.* 1987;25:359-365.
78. Salmaso D, Denes G. Role of the frontal lobes on an attention task: a signal detection analysis. *Percept Mot Skills.* 1982;54:1147-1150.
79. Gordon M. *The Gordon Diagnostic System.* DeWitt, NY: Gordon Systems; 1983.
80. Bacopoulos NG, Redmond DE, Roth RH. Serotonin and dopamine metabolites in brain regions and cerebrospinal fluid of a primate species: effects of ketamine and fluphenazine. *J Neurochem.* 1979;32:1215-1218.
81. Maas JW, Hattox SE, Landis DH, Roth RH. The determination of a brain ar-

teriovenous difference for 3-methoxy-4-hydroxyphenylethylene glycol (MHPG). *Brain Res.* 1976;118:167-173.
82. Winer BJ. *Statistical Principles in Experimental Design.* 2nd ed. New York, NY: McGraw-Hill International Book Co; 1971.
83. Ghoneim MM, Hinrichs JV, Mewaldt SP, Petersen RC. Ketamine: behavioral effects of subanesthetic doses. *J Clin Psychopharmacol.* 1985;5:70-77.
84. Collier BB. Ketamine and the conscious mind. *Anaesthesia.* 1972;27:120-134.
85. Garfield JM, Garfield FB, Stone JG, Hopkins D, Johns LA. A comparison of psychologic responses to ketamine and thiopental-nitrous oxide-halothane anesthesia. *Anesthesiology.* 1972;36:329-338.
86. Goldman-Rakic PS. Circuitry of primate prefrontal cortex and regulation of behavior by representational memory. In: Plum F, ed. *Handbook of Physiology. Section I: Higher Functions of the Brain.* New York, NY: Oxford University Press Inc; 1987:373-417.
87. Meyer JS, Griefenstein F, Devault M. A new drug causing symptoms of sensory deprivation. *J Nerv Ment Dis.* 1959;129:54-61.
88. Cohen BD, Luby ED, Rosenbaum G, Gottlieb JS. Combined sernyl and sensory deprivation. *Compr Psychiatry.* 1960;1:345-348.
89. Carlsson M, Carlsson A. Schizophrenia: a subcortical neurotransmitter imbalance syndrome? *Schizophr Bull.* 1990;16:425-432.
90. Robinson AL, Heaton RK, Lehman RAW, Stilson DW. The utility of the Wisconsin Card Sorting Test in detecting and localizing frontal lobe lesions. *J Consult Clin Psychol.* 1980;48:605-614.
91. Shapiro ML, Caramano Z. NMDA antagonist MK-801 impairs acquisition but not performance of spatial working and reference memory. *Psychobiology.* 1990;18:231-243.
92. Parada-Turska J, Turski WA. Excitatory amino acid antagonists and memory: effect of drugs acting at *N*-methyl-D-aspartate receptors in learning and memory tasks. *Neuropharmacology.* 1990;29:1111-1116.
93. Danysz W, Wroblewski JT, Costa E. Learning impairment in rats by *N*-methyl-D aspartate receptor antagonists. *Neuropharmacology.* 1988;27:653-656.
94. Morris RGM, Enderson E, Lynch GS, Baudry M. Selective impairment of learning and blockade of long-term potentiation by *N*-methyl-D-aspartate receptor antagonist AP5. *Nature.* 1986;319:774-776.
95. Harris EW, Ganong AH, Cotman CW. Long-term potentiation in the hippocampus involves activation of *N*-methyl-D-aspartate receptors. *Brain Res.* 1984; 323:132-137.
96. Muller D, Joly M, Lynch G. Contributions of quisqualate and NMDA receptors to the induction and expression of LTP. *Science.* 1988;242:1694-1697.
97. McCarthy DA, Chen G, Kaump DH, Ensor CJ. General anesthetic and other pharmacological properties of 2-(O-chlorophenyl)-2-methylamino cyclohexanone HCl (CI-581). *J New Drugs.* 1965;5:21-33.
98. Harris AJ, Biersner RJ, Edwards D, Bailey LW. Attention, learning, and personality during ketamine emergence: a pilot study. *Anesth Analg.* 1975;54: 169-172.
99. Foster NL, Giordani B, Mellow A, Aronson S, Berent S. Memory effects of low-dose ketamine in Alzheimer's disease. *Neurology.* 1991;41(suppl 1):214. Abstract 349P.
100. Jackson A, Koek W, Colpaert FC. NMDA antagonists make learning and recall state dependent. *Behav Pharmacol.* 1992;3:415-421.
101. Lovinger DM, White G, Weight FF. Ethanol inhibits NMDA-activated ion currents in hippocampal neurons. *Science.* 1989;243:1721-1724.
102. Colombo G, Grant KA. NMDA receptor complex antagonists have ethanol-like discriminative stimulus effects. *Ann N Y Acad Sci.* 1992;654:421-423.
103. Willetts J, Balster RL, Leander JD. The behavioral pharmacology of NMDA receptor antagonists. *Trends Pharmacol Sci.* 1990;11:423-428.
104. Siegel RK. Phencyclidine and ketamine intoxication: a study of four populations of recreational users. In: Petersen RC, Stillman RC, eds. *Phencyclidine (PCP) Abuse: An Appraisal.* NIDA Research Monograph 21. Rockville, Md: National Institute on Drug Abuse; 1978:119-147.
105. Elsworth JD, Leahy DJ, Roth RH, Redmond DE Jr. Homovanillic acid concentrations in brain, CSF, and plasma as indicators of central dopamine function in primates. *J Neural Trans.* 1987;68:51-62.
106. Zsigmond EK, Kelsch RC, Kothary SP. Rise in plasma free-norepinephrine during anesthetic induction with ketamine. *Behav Neuropsychiatry.* 1975;6: 81-84.
107. Arslan M, Pohl CR, Smith MS, Plant TM. Studies of the role of the *N*-methyl-D-aspartate (NMDA) receptor in the hypothalamic control of prolactin secretion. *Life Sci.* 1991;50:295-300.
108. Elvidge H, Challis JRG, Robinson JS, Roper C, Thorburn GD. Influence of handling and sedation on plasma cortisol in rhesus monkeys (*Macaca mulatta*). *J Endocrinol.* 1976;70:325-326.
109. Aidara D, Tahiri-Zagret C, Robyn C. Serum prolactin concentrations in magabey (*Cercocebus atys lunulatus*) and patas (*Erythrocebus patas*) monkeys in response to stress, ketamine, TRH, sulpiride, and levodopa. *J Reprod Fertil.* 1981;62:165-172.
110. Ferin M, Carmel PW, Warren MP, Himsworth R, Frantz AG. Phencyclidine sedation as a technique for handling rhesus monkeys: effects on LH, GH, and prolactin secretion. *Proc Soc Exp Biol Med.* 1976;151:428-433.
111. Castro MI, Rose J, Green W, Lehner N, Peterson D, Taub D. Ketamine-HCl as a suitable anesthetic for endocrine, metabolic, and cardiovascular studies in *Macaca fascicularis* monkeys. *Proc Soc Exp Biol Med.* 1981;168:389-394.
112. Gribkoff VK. Electrophysiological evidence for *N*-methyl-D-aspartate excitatory amino acid receptors in the rat supraoptic nucleus in vitro. *Neurosci Lett.* 1991;131:260-262.
113. van den Pol AN, Wuarin J-P, Dudek FE. Glutamate, the dominant excitatory transmitter in neuroendocrine regulation. *Science.* 1990;250:1276-1278.
114. Tweed WA, Minuck M, Mymin D. Circulatory responses to ketamine anesthesia. *Anesthesiology.* 1972;37:613-619.
115. Biersner RJ, Harris JA, Ryman DH. Emotional predisposition to psychotropic drug effects. *J Consult Clin Psychol.* 1977;45:943-945.
116. Strauss ME, Novakovic T, Tien AY, Bylsma F, Pearlson GD. Disengagement of attention in schizophrenia. *Psychiatry Res.* 1991;37:139-146.
117. Gruzelier J, Seymour K, Wilson L, Jolley A, Hirsch S. Impairments on neuropsychologic tests of temporohippocampal and frontohippocampal functions and word fluency in remitting schizophrenia and affective disorders. *Arch Gen Psychiatry.* 1988;45:623-629.

ORIGINAL ARTICLE

The International Personality Disorder Examination

The World Health Organization/Alcohol, Drug Abuse, and Mental Health Administration International Pilot Study of Personality Disorders

Armand W. Loranger, PhD; Norman Sartorius, MD, PhD; Antonio Andreoli, MD; Peter Berger, MD; Peter Buchheim, MD; S. M. Channabasavanna, MD; Bina Coid, PhD; Alv Dahl, MD; Rene F. W. Diekstra, PhD; Brian Ferguson, MD; Lawrence B. Jacobsberg, MD, PhD; W. Mombour, MD; Charles Pull, MD; Yutaka Ono, MD; Darrel A. Regier, MD

Background: One of the aims of the World Health Organization/Alcohol, Drug Abuse, and Mental Health Administration joint program on psychiatric diagnosis and classification is the development and standardization of diagnostic assessment instruments for use in clinical research worldwide. The International Personality Disorder Examination (IPDE) is a semistructured clinical interview compatible with the *International Classification of Diseases, Tenth Revision,* and the *DMS-III-R* classification systems. This is the first report of the results of a field trial to investigate the feasibility of using the IPDE to assess personality disorders worldwide.

Methods: The IPDE was administered by 58 psychiatrists and clinical psychologists to 716 patients enrolled in clinical facilities at 14 participating centers in 11 countries in North America, Europe, Africa, and Asia. To determine interrater reliability, 141 of the IPDEs (20%) were independently rated by a silent observer. To determine temporal stability, 243 patients (34%) were reexamined after an average interval of 6 months.

Results: The IPDE proved acceptable to clinicians and demonstrated an interrater reliability and temporal stability roughly similar to instruments used to diagnose the psychoses, mood, anxiety, and substance use disorders.

Conclusion: It is possible to assess personality disorders with reasonably good reliability in different nations, languages, and cultures using a semistructured clinical interview that experienced clinicians find relevant, meaningful, and user-friendly.

(Arch Gen Psychiatry. 1994;51:215-224)

From the Department of Psychiatry, Cornell University Medical College, New York, NY (Drs Loranger and Jacobsberg); World Health Organization (Dr Sartorius), and Institutions Universitaires de Psychiatrie-Genève (Dr Andreoli), Geneva, Switzerland; Psychiatrische Universitätsklinik, Vienna, Austria (Dr Berger); Nervenklinik der Universität Munchen, Munich, Germany (Dr Buchheim); National Institute of Mental Health and Neurosciences, Bangalore, India (Dr Channabasavanna); Institute of Psychiatry, London, England (Dr Coid); Universitetet I Oslo Psychiatrisk Institutt, Oslo, Norway (Dr Dahl); Rijksuniversiteit Te Leiden, Leiden, the Netherlands (Dr Diekstra); Stonebridge Research Centre, Nottingham, England (Dr Ferguson); Max-Planck-Institut für Psychiatrie, Munich (Dr Mombour); Centre Hospitalier de Luxembourg, Luxembourg (Dr Pull); Keio University School of Medicine, Tokyo, Japan (Dr Ono); and National Institute of Mental Health, Rockville, Md (Dr Regier).

In 1979, the World Health Organization (WHO) and US Alcohol, Drug Abuse, and Mental Health Administration (ADAMHA) joined forces in mounting a large-scale review and assessment of the knowledge base of psychiatric diagnosis and classification. One consequence of this review was the establishment of a long-term program of activities aimed at developing a battery of standardized diagnostic assessment instruments for use in clinical and epidemiologic research worldwide.[1] This was intended to facilitate comparisons of clinical and research findings from different nations and cultures.

One instrument developed in this program, the Composite International Diagnostic Interview (CIDI),[2] a modification of the Diagnostic Interview Schedule (DIS),[3] is highly structured, computer scored, and designed for use by lay interviewers in epidemiologic studies. Another, the Schedules for Clinical Assessment in Neuropsychiatry (SCAN),[4] a descendant of the ninth edition of the Present State Examination (PSE),[5] is intended for use by clinicians, ie, those capable of making independent psychiatric diagnoses. Except for the inclusion of antisocial disorder in the CIDI, neither interview provides coverage of the personality disorders.

This is the first report of the results of a field trial to investigate the feasibility of using a semistructured clinical interview developed within the WHO/ADAMHA program to diagnose personality disorders in different languages and cultures. The principal objectives of the trial were to determine the cultural acceptability, user friendliness, inter-

See Subjects and Methods on next page

SUBJECTS AND METHODS

STUDY SITES

The sites for the field trial were selected to provide a broad representation of different nations, languages, and cultures. An additional consideration was the availability of interested and experienced investigators who were able to devote their time and clinical resources to the venture. There were 14 participating centers located in 11 countries in North America, Europe, Africa, and Asia.

TRAINING

During the development of the IPDE from 1985 to 1987, the principal investigators at each center had participated in several meetings and workshops concerning the instrument. After they had acquired proficiency in its administration and scoring, they assumed responsibility for the training and supervision of the psychiatrists and clinical psychologists who served as examiners at their centers. In early 1988, the coordinator of the project (A.W.L.) visited each site and conducted workshops that used videotaped demonstrations and lengthy discussions of principles of administration and problems in scoring. The examiners were required to administer a minimum of 10 interviews before they were considered sufficiently experienced to evaluate study subjects. To monitor scoring practices during the study, videotaped interviews conducted in English were circulated for rating by the participating clinicians.

PATIENT SELECTION

The investigators were asked to select approximately 50 patients, ranging between ages 21 and 55 years, from admissions to their facilities. In the judgment of a senior screening clinician, the patients should have had either a personality disorder according to *ICD-10* and/or *DSM-III-R* criteria or another common mental disorder important in the differential diagnosis of a personality disorder. To ensure an adequate test of the discriminating properties of the IPDE, the screening clinicians were asked to provide a sample that approximated a 3:2 ratio of those with and without a personality disorder. Exclusion criteria included below-normal intelligence, organic brain disease, language or communication difficulties, alcohol or other drug intoxication that might interfere with the examination, and delusional or psychotic disorders likely to have altered personality functioning. Sampling of consecutive admissions was not feasible, and patients were selected within the guidelines specified above according to their availability and at the convenience of the examiners. At each site, the goal was to have 10 of the interviews observed and independently rated by another clinician and to have 25 of the patients reexamined several months later.

CLINICAL AND IPDE EVALUATIONS

Without knowledge of the diagnostic conclusions of the screening clinicians, the psychiatrists and clinical psychologists who administered the IPDE also conducted a general clinical evaluation of the patients and provided the *ICD-10* diagnoses of any disorders other than personality disorders. At several centers, this evaluation included a semistructured interview: DIS[3] at Rijksuniversiteit Te Leiden, Leiden, the Netherlands; Schedule for Affective Disorders and Schizophrenia—Lifetime version[10] at Institute of Psychiatry, London, England; and Structured Interview for *DSM-III-R* (SCID)[11] at Cornell Medical Center, New York, NY; Stonebridge Research Centre, Nottingham, England; Universitetet I Oslo Psychiatrisk Institutt, Oslo, Norway; and Keio University School of Medicine, Tokyo, Japan.

COURSE OF THE TRIAL

The first patients entered the study in April 1988 and the last patient was examined in December 1990. After the project coordinator verified all of the forms returned by the centers, the information was entered in a computer at the ADAMHA data processing facility in Rockville, Md. In August 1991, the investigators met at WHO headquarters in Geneva, Switzerland, to analyze and discuss the results. They also reviewed the replies to a questionnaire completed by all the participants about the strengths and limitations of the IPDE, including its user friendliness, cultural relevance, and apparent clinical validity.

rater reliability, and temporal stability of the instrument. When the study was planned, it was considered inappropriate to undertake the development of a highly structured lay-administered interview such as the CIDI. The state of the art of standardized interviews for personality disorders was in its infancy and considerably behind that of the clinical assessment of other mental disorders. The complexity of the diagnostic criteria and the level of inference and clinical sophistication that is required to make personality disorder diagnoses, especially in those with other mental disorders, were additional reasons for favoring an instrument for use by clinicians rather than trained lay interviewers.

THE INTERNATIONAL PERSONALITY DISORDER EXAMINATION

The International Personality Disorder Examination (IPDE) is an outgrowth of the Personality Disorder Examination (PDE)[6] that was modified for international use and compatibility with the *International Classification of Diseases, Tenth Revision (ICD-10)*[7] and the *DSM-III-R*[8] classification systems. A detailed history of its development, rationale, structure, and translations is available elsewhere.[9] In brief, the IPDE surveys the behavior and life experiences relevant to the more than 150 criteria used in making personality

Table 1. Sample Sizes and IPDE Field Trial Centers*

Location	Center	No. of IPDE Examiners	No. of Patients			
			Men	Women	Inpatient	Outpatient
Bangalore, India	National Institute of Mental Health and Neurosciences	3	31	16	7	40
Geneva, Switzerland	Institutions Universitaire de Psychiatrie-Genève	3	11	21	2	30
Leiden, the Netherlands	Rijksuniversiteit Te Leiden	6	34	31	55	10
London, England	Institute of Psychiatry	3	23	29	26	26
Luxembourg, Luxembourg	Centre Hospitalier de Luxembourg	5	28	24	46	6
Munich, Germany	Max-Planck-Institut für Psychiatrie Nervenklinik der Universität Munchen Bezirkskrankenhaus Kaufbeuren	11	58	55	54	59
Nairobi, Kenya	Kenyatta National Hospital	1	30	20	10	40
New York, NY	Cornell Medical Center	10	48	52	56	44
Nottingham, England	Stonebridge Research Centre	4	26	24	0	50
Oslo, Norway	Universitetet I Oslo Psychiatrisk Institutt	4	20	28	20	28
Tokyo, Japan	Keio University School of Medicine	3	28	29	5	52
Vienna, Austria	Psychiatrische Universitätsklinik	5	27	23	14	36
Total		**58**	**364**	**352**	**295**	**421**

**IPDE indicates International Personality Disorder Examination.*

disorder diagnoses according to *DSM-III-R* and *ICD-10*. Although it contains a prescribed set of carefully selected and researched questions, the examiner is expected to conduct an adequate clinical examination of the subject to provide clarification and confirmatory examples, anecdotes, and details. A manual defines the scope and meaning of each criterion and provides guidelines and anchor points for scoring.

The IPDE requires that a behavior or trait be present at least 5 years before it should be considered a manifestation of personality. This conservative and somewhat arbitrary convention is intended to reflect the relatively enduring nature of personality traits and to avoid confusing them with transient or situational phenomena and episodic abnormalities of mental state and behavior. The IPDE also requires that at least one criterion of a disorder be fulfilled before age 25 years, before that particular disorder can be diagnosed. This is in keeping with clinical tradition and *DSM-III-R* and *ICD-10*, which date the first indications of a personality disorder to childhood, adolescence, or the early adult years. Age 25 years rather than an earlier age was selected to allow more informed and accurate judgments about many of the adult-oriented personality disorder criteria in the *DSM* and *ICD* systems.

Scoring of the 157 items was as follows: absent or within normal range, 0; present to an accentuated degree, 1; pathological/meets criterion, 2. The final algorithmic integration of the individually scored items was done clerically or by computer. It included the following information for each disorder: the presence or absence of each criterion, whether the scoring of a criterion was based solely on the interview or included information from informants, the number of criteria met for each disorder, and the diagnostic decision about each disorder (definite, probable, or negative). It also provided a dimensional score for all subjects on each disorder, regardless of whether they receive the diagnosis or meet any of the criteria for the disorder. It is calculated by summing the individual scores for all of the criteria on the disorder.

RESULTS

FINAL PATIENT SAMPLE

At the conclusion of the study, 716 patients had been examined, 243 reexamined, and 141 of the interviews rated by an observer. The average interval between the initial and second IPDE was 6 months, with approximately 85% of the repetitions occurring between 2 months and 1 year. **Table 1** provides details of the sample sizes at each center. Tables containing the demographic characteristics of the sample and the clinical *ICD-10* diagnoses, exclusive of personality disorders, are available on request. **Table 2** provides the IPDE personality disorder diagnoses in the *DSM-III-R* and *ICD-10* systems. They are based on the examiner's scoring of the initial interview.

IPDE INTERRATER RELIABILITY AND TEMPORAL STABILITY

Intraclass correlation coefficients[12] were used to determine the examiner-observer agreement in scoring each of the 157 items on the IPDE and their stability from the initial to the second examinations. To provide a more accurate estimate of stability per se, with adjustment for the less-than-perfect interrater reliability of the instrument, correlations with a correction for attenuation[13] are also included with the sta-

Table 2. IPDE *DSM-III-R* and *ICD-10* Diagnoses (N=716)*

Personality Disorder Diagnosis	No. (%) of Patients
DSM-III-R	
Paranoid	42 (5.9)
Schizoid	20 (2.8)
Schizotypal	25 (3.5)
Obsessive compulsive	22 (3.1)
Histrionic	51 (7.1)
Dependent	32 (4.5)
Antisocial	46 (6.4)
Narcissistic	9 (1.3)
Avoidant	79 (11.0)
Borderline	104 (14.5)
Passive aggressive	36 (5.0)
Sadistic	2 (0.3)
Self-defeating	9 (1.3)
Other†	92 (12.8)
Any personality disorder	366 (51.1)
ICD-10	
Paranoid	17 (2.4)
Schizoid	13 (1.8)
Dissocial	23 (3.2)
Emotionally unstable	
Impulsive	32 (4.5)
Borderline	107 (14.9)
Histrionic	31 (4.3)
Anankastic	26 (3.6)
Anxious	109 (15.2)
Dependent	33 (4.6)
Other‡	49 (6.8)
Any personality disorder	283 (39.5)

**IPDE indicates International Personality Disorder Examination;* ICD-10, International Classification of Diseases, Tenth Revision. *Personality disorder diagnoses include patients with more than one type of personality disorder. Of the 366 patients with a* DSM-III-R *personality disorder, 111 (30.3%) had more than one type of disorder, including 55 (15.0%) with two disorders, 32 (8.7%) with three disorders, and 24 (6.6%) with more than three disorders. Of the 283 patients with an* ICD-10 *personality disorder, 96 (33.9%) had more than one type of disorder, including 57 (20.1%) with two disorders, 27 (9.5%) with three disorders, and 12 (4.2%) with more than three disorders.*

†*Did not fulfill diagnostic criteria for any specific personality disorder but met 10 or more of the 110* DSM-III-R *personality disorder criteria.*

‡*Did not fulfill diagnostic criteria for any specific personality disorder but met 10 or more of the 56* ICD-10 *personality disorder criteria.*

bility coefficients. The same statistics were also used to measure the examiner-observer agreement regarding the dimensional scores and the number of criteria met on each disorder and their stability from the initial to the second examinations. These correlations are presented in **Table 3**.

We used κ[14] to measure the interrater agreement and temporal stability of the personality disorder diagnoses. Because of its known instability when based on samples with an infrequent number of cases of a disorder, the recommendation was followed that it be calculated only when the prevalence of a disorder is at least 5%.[15] To provide more opportunities for the calculation of κ, it was also determined by combining definite and probable diagnoses. A probable diagnosis was assigned when the subject met one criterion less than the number required for the diagnosis. An overall weighted κ is also reported for all personality disorders, including those with a base rate of less than 5%. It was calculated by weighing each category of personality disorder by the total number of cases assigned a diagnosis in that category by either rater, regardless of whether the raters agreed on the diagnosis. The numerator is the sum of the product of the diagnostic weight and κ for each disorder; the denominator is the sum of the weights. The κ values are presented in **Table 4**.

COMMENT

This investigation is the first attempt to assess personality disorders on a worldwide basis with contemporary methods of diagnosis. To some extent, it is reminiscent of *The International Pilot Study of Schizophrenia*,[16] a project undertaken by WHO more than two decades ago. The present study, however, was more challenging in some respects. Unlike schizophrenia, the personality disorders have rarely occupied center stage in psychiatry and have long been a source of frustration to diagnosticians and nosologists. The assessments in the present study were also undertaken within the framework and guidelines of two distinct but overlapping classification systems: *DSM-III-R*, which was designed for use in the United States, is primarily the product of American psychiatric opinion, and *ICD-10*, which is intended for use worldwide, reflects the views and needs of the international psychiatric community.

INTERRATER AGREEMENT

The validity of any diagnostic instrument presupposes a reasonable degree of interrater reliability in its application. The IPDE was administered in different languages, in a wide variety of national and cultural settings, and by a large number of clinicians. This was an unusually exacting test of reliability to which no other interview for personality disorders has been subjected. The results, nevertheless, compare quite favorably with published reports on semistructured interviews that are used to diagnose the psychoses, mood, anxiety, and substance use disorders. Such comparisons, however, should be viewed as rough approximations. There are differences in the heterogeneity of the patient samples and the base rates of the individual disorders and variations in the methods used to determine reliability.

With these caveats in mind, we compared the results of the present study with those of the SCID Axis I field trial.[17] That study involved 390 patients at four locations in the United States and one in Germany. The median κ values for those individual disorders with a base rate of at least 5% were 0.64 for current diagnoses and 0.68 for lifetime diagnoses. In the present study, the median κ values for the individual personality disorders (diagnosis definite) with base rates

Table 3. Interrater Reliability and Temporal Stability of 157 IPDE Items, Number of Criteria Met, and Dimensional Scores*

	Interrater Reliability (N=141)		Temporal Stability (N=243)†		
Intraclass *R*	No. (%) of Items	Cumulative, %	No. of Items	%	Cumulative, %
.90-1.00	13 (8.3)	...	0 (2)	0 (1.3)	...
.80-.89	72 (45.9)	54.2	2 (13)	1.3 (8.3)	1.3 (9.6)
.70-.79	52 (33.1)	87.3	14 (42)	8.9 (26.8)	10.2 (36.3)
.60-.69	12 (7.6)	94.9	62 (62)	39.5 (39.5)	49.7 (75.8)
.50-.59	4 (2.5)	97.4	53 (27)	33.8 (17.2)	83.4 (93.0)
.40-.49	1 (0.6)	98.0	19 (5)	12.1 (3.2)	95.5 (96.2)
<.40	3 (1.9)	...	7 (6)	4.5 (3.8)	...

	Intraclass *R*			
	No. of Criteria Met		Dimensional Score	
Disorder	Interrater Reliability (N=141)	Temporal Stability (N=243)†	Interrater Reliability (N=141)	Temporal Stability (N=243)†
		DSM-III-R		
Paranoid	.75	.58 (.67)	.85	.68 (.74)
Schizoid	.83	.72 (.79)	.86	.76 (.82)
Schizotypal	.82	.69 (.76)	.87	.81 (.87)
Obsessive compulsive	.82	.75 (.83)	.89	.80 (.85)
Histrionic	.81	.75 (.83)	.87	.78 (.84)
Dependent	.89	.67 (.71)	.92	.72 (.75)
Antisocial	.88	.74 (.79)	.94	.92 (.95)
Narcissistic	.83	.71 (.78)	.90	.75 (.79)
Avoidant	.82	.71 (.78)	.89	.77 (.82)
Borderline	.89	.84 (.89)	.93	.87 (.91)
Passive aggressive	.92	.72 (.75)	.89	.78 (.83)
Sadistic	.80	.61 (.69)	.88	.76 (.81)
Self-defeating	.71	.74 (.88)	.79	.75 (.84)
		ICD-10		
Paranoid	.78	.56 (.72)	.87	.66 (.71)
Schizoid	.79	.62 (.78)	.87	.74 (.80)
Dissocial	.88	.55 (.62)	.92	.69 (.72)
Emotionally unstable				
Impulsive	.87	.74 (.85)	.89	.78 (.83)
Borderline	.91	.82 (.90)	.93	.86 (.90)
Histrionic	.84	.69 (.82)	.88	.80 (.85)
Anankastic	.73	.74 (1.00)	.86	.77 (.83)
Anxious	.83	.74 (.89)	.88	.77 (.82)
Dependent	.88	.58 (.66)	.91	.65 (.71)

**IPDE indicates International Personality Disorder Examination;* ICD-10, International Classification of Diseases, Tenth Revision. *For temporal stability, the average interval between test and retest was 6 months.*

†For temporal stability, data in parentheses are corrected for attenuation.

of at least 5% were 0.70 in *DSM-III-R* and 0.72 in *ICD-10*. The overall weighted κ values in the SCID study were 0.61 for current diagnoses and 0.68 for lifetime diagnoses. In the present study, the overall weighted κ values for the definite diagnoses of the specific personality disorders were 0.57 in *DSM-III-R* and 0.65 in *ICD-10*. The median κ values for an IPDE diagnosis that was definite or probable were 0.73 for *DSM-III-R* and 0.77 for *ICD-10*. The corresponding IPDE weighted κ values for a diagnosis that was definite or probable were 0.65 for *DSM-III-R* and 0.72 for *ICD-10*. The SCID study did not identify probable cases.

The SCID study involved a test-retest design in which the interview was given by different examiners at least 1 day but no more than 2 weeks apart. This is likely to result in somewhat lower reliabilities than when an examiner and observer rate the same interview, as in the present study. The pursuit of an additional objective in the IPDE study (the determination of temporal stability over an extended period) weighed against the use of a similar test-retest method because of the practical and methodological problems associated with too frequent repetitions of a lengthy interview.

The IPDE also fared well compared with other criteria-

Table 4. Interrater Agreement (κ), Temporal Stability (κ), and Base Rate (%) of IPDE *DSM-III-R* and *ICD-10* Diagnoses*

Disorder	Interrater Agreement † (N=141) Definite	Interrater Agreement † (N=141) Definite/Probable	Temporal Stability † (N=243) Definite	Temporal Stability † (N=243) Definite/Probable
DSM-III-R				
Paranoid	... (5)	.51 (12)	.24 (5)	.28 (10)
Schizoid	... (3)	.87 (6)	... (2)	.68 (5)
Schizotypal	... (1)	... (3)	... (3)	.68 (5)
Obsessive compulsive	... (2)	.60 (6)	... (2)	... (4)
Histrionic	.34 (6)	.66 (13)	.45 (5)	.46 (12)
Dependent	.70 (5)	.82 (9)	... (4)	.43 (9)
Antisocial	... (5)	.73 (9)	.59 (5)	.62 (9)
Narcissistic	... (1)	... (3)	... (1)	... (4)
Avoidant	.71 (10)	.78 (17)	.48 (10)	.56 (19)
Borderline	.80 (10)	.76 (16)	.70 (13)	.72 (19)
Passive aggressive	... (2)	... (4)	... (3)	.41 (6)
Sadistic	... (1)	... (1)	... (0)	... (2)
Self-defeating	... (0)	... (3)	... (2)	.71 (7)
Any specific personality disorder	.59 (27)	.70 (46)	.62 (34)	.63 (51)
ICD-10				
Paranoid	... (2)	.43 (7)	... (2)	.30 (8)
Schizoid	... (1)	... (5)	... (1)	... (3)
Dissocial	... (4)	1.00 (6)	... (2)	... (4)
Emotionally unstable				
Impulsive	... (4)	.79 (7)	... (4)	.60 (7)
Borderline	.76 (12)	.78 (16)	.65 (14)	.62 (15)
Histrionic	... (3)	.64 (7)	... (2)	.53 (7)
Anankastic	... (2%)	.53 (6)	... (2)	.60 (7)
Anxious	.72 (11)	.77 (22)	.64 (15)	.65 (24)
Dependent	... (4)	.81 (13)	... (3)	.36 (11)
Any specific personality disorder	.64 (25)	.71 (43)	.59 (29)	.60 (44)

**IPDE indicates International Personality Disorder Examination;* ICD-10, *International Classification of Diseases, Tenth Revision. The κ statistic was calculated only when the base rate was 5% or greater according to both raters; base rates in table are means of both raters. Average interval between test and retest (temporal stability) was 6 months. Probable diagnosis assigned when patient met one criterion less than required number. For interrater agreement, the overall weighted κ values for the definite and definite/probable diagnoses were 0.57 and 0.69 in* DSM-III-R *and 0.65 and 0.72 in* ICD-10, *respectively. For temporal stability, the overall weighted κ values for the definite and definite/probable diagnoses were 0.50 and 0.53 in* DSM-III-R *and 0.54 and 0.53 in* ICD-10, *respectively.*

†*Values in parentheses are percents.*

based interviews for personality disorders that have been developed in recent years.[18,19] However, reports of large-scale reliability studies conducted outside of the facilities where these other interviews were developed are rare or nonexistent. The other interviews differ from the IPDE in several ways: they do not provide coverage of *ICD-10*; are not available in so many languages; and do not have a detailed, item-by-item scoring manual.

TEMPORAL STABILITY

Not only should a personality disorder instrument demonstrate adequate interrater reliability but it should also have temporal stability. This is because "personality" refers to a person's long-term functioning. Before imputing a particular criterion to a patient, the IPDE requires a minimum duration of 5 years, including some manifestation of the behavior during the current year (past 12 months). Since the study patients were reexamined after an average interval of 6 months, temporal stability required that they provide essentially similar information on both occasions. The only exceptions were patients who might have failed to manifest the behavior in both segments of the nonoverlapping portions of the previous 12 months or the rare patient who might have fallen a few months short of meeting the 5-year requirement at the time of the initial interview. Naturally, these patients would adversely affect the measurement of stability. The determination of temporal stability is also influenced by the less-than-perfect reliability associated with the single administration of an instrument. Adjustments for the effect on the stability of the individual items, the number of criteria met, and the dimensional scores were made by calculating additional correlations with a correction for attenuation.

There are comparatively few reports on the temporal stability of the semistructured interviews that are used to make lifetime diagnoses of the psychoses, mood, anxiety, and substance use disorders.[20-24] **Table 5** summarizes them for one popular instrument, the Schedule for Affective Disorders and Schizophrenia–Lifetime version. The findings reflect moderate, but at times disappointing, stabilities that are not consistently superior to many of those obtained in this study with the personality disorders. Given the beleaguered history of the diagnosis and classification of personality disorders, this may come as a surprise to some. It should be acknowledged, however, that four[21-24] of the five studies involved longer time intervals than 6 months. The one study[20] within that timeframe reported a κ of 0.63 for the presence or absence of any Schedule for Affective Disorders and Schizophrenia–Lifetime diagnosis. This compares with 0.62 in *DSM-III-R* and 0.59 in *ICD-10* for the presence or absence of any specific personality disorder on the IPDE. The studies in Table 5 did not report an overall weighted κ, thus precluding comparisons based on that statistic. Another potentially relevant difference is that in most of these studies, the initial and second interviews were conducted by different interviewers. One study, however, did not find significant differences in stability when the same and different interviewers were used[21]; another study[22] reported an inconsistent effect.

There is very little literature on the temporal stability of criteria-based personality disorders diagnosed with semistructured interviews. There appear to be only three studies that involved more than a brief test-retest interval. One was based on an early trial version of the PDE,[25]

Table 5. Temporal Stability of SADS-L Diagnoses*

Disorder	Andreasen et al[20] (N=50)	Bromet et al[21] (N=391)	Fendrich et al[22] (N=69)	Rice et al[23] (N=50)	Rice et al[24] (N=1669)
Major depression	0.75	0.41	0.54	0.56	0.61
Mania	0.88	...	...	0.48	0.60
Hypomania	0.06	...	...	0.09	0.33
Generalized anxiety	0.15	...	...	...	0.30
Phobic	...	...	0.33	...	0.34
Separation anxiety	...	...	0.26	...	...
Panic	...	...	0.66	...	0.37
Obsessive compulsive	...	...	0.66	...	0.27
Alcoholism	0.72	...	...	0.73	0.70
Drug use	...	...	...	...	0.56
Substance abuse	...	...	0.66	...	...
Any diagnosis	0.63	...	0.62	...	...

*SADS-L indicates Schedule for Affective Disorders and Schizophrenia—Lifetime version. All coefficients are κ values except the study by Andreasen et al,[20] which reported intraclass correlation. Four[21-24] of the five studies involved longer time intervals than did one[20] study. The time frame for those four studies were 18 months and 2, 5, and 6 years, respectively.

which is no longer extant. Pfohl et al[26] reported on the stability of the Structured Interview for *DSM-III* Personality Disorders in 36 depressed inpatients after 6 to 12 months. The κ values, which ranged from 0.16 to 0.84, are problematic because of the small sample sizes of the individual disorders. Similar findings with the Structured Interview for *DSM-III* Personality Disorders were obtained in a study in the Netherlands.[27]

The belief that interviewers are perfectly interchangeable would seem naive in view of the potential influence that the age, sex, and personality of an interviewer might have on the information volunteered by a patient. The assumption made by those who use semistructured interviews is that such factors ordinarily are not a major source of error. In planning the present study, consideration was given to a design in which half of the interviews would be repeated by the same examiner and half by a different examiner. This would have helped to determine how much the interviewers themselves, in addition to their ratings, contributed to the instability of the measures. However, concerns about scheduling influenced the decision to use the same interviewer whenever possible. As a result, 93% of the interviews were given by the same examiner on both occasions.

A second interview, whether conducted by the same or a different person, may be contaminated by the experience of the first interview. Repetitions can lead to boredom and decreased motivation. Patients may believe that the interviews are no longer for their benefit but for that of the examiner. Repetitions can also produce fantasies that the interviewer is dissatisfied with the previous interview or is checking on the consistency of the responses. Patients may also refrain from providing as many positive replies as previously owing to a heightened awareness that these invite further probing and prolong the interview. Elsewhere,[25] one of us (A.W.L.) has argued that the problem of attempting to measure the precise degree to which interviewers are interchangeable is reminiscent of the Heisenberg principle in physics: one cannot study the phenomenon without somehow tampering with it in the process.

Another source of instability is the possibility that patients in a dysphoric state may have a selective recall or distorted perception of certain personality traits. They may also confuse them with the symptoms of another (Axis I) mental disorder. An earlier version of the PDE proved resistant to changes in symptoms of anxiety and depression during the course of treatment.[25] In that study, the majority of patients had mood or anxiety disorders of mild to moderate severity. The finding has since been replicated with the present version of the PDE (A.W.L. and Mark F. Lenzenweger, PhD, unpublished data, February 1992). There is, however, a contradictory report based on a group of depressed patients treated with cognitive therapy.[28] That study used an earlier version of the PDE and the authors failed to specify the professional status of the interviewers, a potentially relevant variable. It may require an experienced psychiatrist or clinical psychologist to distinguish personality traits from transient pathological mental states and the symptoms of other disorders. The reliability and validity of the IPDE, like that of any semistructured interview, cannot be judged apart from the qualifications of the interviewers. At times, semistructured interviews have assumed a mystique of their own, and that caveat is all too often ignored. The IPDE is intended for use by those who have the clinical sophistication and training required to make psychiatric diagnoses independently, ie, without a semistructured interview. This is not to imply that the IPDE or any other personality disorder interview is necessarily impervious to the influence of abnormal mental states, particularly those characterized by severe symptoms. We are encouraged, however, by the evidence that some clinical states do not appear to invalidate the assessment of personality. In any event, no attempt was made to determine the extent to which trait-state artifacts may have affected the stability of the IPDE in the present study.

CATEGORIES AND DIMENSIONS

The prevailing systems of disease classification are categoric. They define the features of disorders, and ideally the categories have points of rarity with normality and other disorders. Although such nosologies sometimes fall short of the ideal, their value as a shorthand form of communication accounts for their widespread acceptance. However, proponents of what has come to be known as the "dimensional" approach question the applicability of the categorical method to personality disorders.[29-31] One argument is that if personality disorders are not truly dichotomous in nature, reliability should improve with the use of dimensions because their measurement would incorporate more information than that provided by categories alone.

Critics sometimes overlook the fact that categories and dimensions need not be mutually exclusive, witness their harmonious coexistence in the classification of mental retardation and hypertension. Following that tradition, the IPDE was designed to provide categorical diagnoses and dimensional scores based on the categories. The results of the present study demonstrate the favorable effect of these scores on the reliability of the IPDE. This is illustrated, eg, by paranoid personality, the disorder with the least stability. Although the *DSM-III-R* κ was only 0.24, the stability of the paranoid dimensional scores was 0.68 (0.74 with correction for attenuation). The stability of all of the *DSM-III-R* dimensional scores ranged from 0.68 to 0.92 (0.74 to 0.95 corrected), with a median of 0.77 (0.83 corrected). The corresponding correlations for the *ICD-10* dimensions ranged from 0.65 to 0.86 (0.71 to 0.90 corrected), with a median of 0.77 (0.82 corrected).

These findings provide a striking example of the advantage of supplementing a categorical conclusion about the presence or absence of a specific personality disorder with dimensional information about the traits that underlie the decision-making process. The IPDE dimensional scores include information about accentuated normal traits below the threshold required for a personality disorder. A measure based on pathological traits alone consists of the actual number of criteria that a patient meets on a particular disorder. Table 3 reveals that this coarser measure is almost invariably associated with lower reliabilities than the dimensional scores, although the differences are not usually great.

CLINICAL ACCEPTABILITY OF THE IPDE

At the conclusion of the study, a questionnaire concerning the IPDE was completed by all of the interviewers and discussed at length at the meeting of principal investigators in Geneva. The only significant reservation about the instrument concerned its length, a necessary consequence of the decision to systematically inquire about all of the personality disorder criteria in the *ICD-10* and *DSM-III-R* classification systems. The mean length of the interview was 2 hours 20 minutes, and there was considerable variation around that figure. If a patient acknowledged many criteria, the subsequent inquiry for confirmatory examples and anecdotes prolonged the interview. If few of the behaviors were endorsed, then the IPDE went comparatively rapidly. If it became evident that the interview was likely to exceed 1½ to 2 hours, an effort was made to administer it in more than one sitting to prevent erosion of the quality of the interview from fatigue or boredom.

To offset the concern about the length of the interview and to make it more acceptable to a wider range of clinicians and investigators, it was decided to issue it in modules. The complete IPDE would continue to assess all of the disorders in *ICD-10* and *DSM-III-R*. Separate modules would also be available for those who wished to limit the examination to only one of the two classification systems. There would also be modules for the individual types of personality disorders for those whose interests were confined to only certain disorders. A *DSM-IV* is also now available.

Consideration was also given to the use of a self-administered screening version of the IPDE, which would eliminate the need to interview patients who are unlikely to receive a diagnosis of personality disorder. This assumes, of course, that false-negative cases could be kept to a minimum, something that would have to be demonstrated by additional field trials. The literature indicates that clinical interviews and inventories do not provide equivalent information.[32] The latter are especially prone to false-positive findings. For that reason, we are currently examining the data based on the 716 patients in the present study to determine whether a few interview items might also be used as a screen. A limitation of both screening methods is that they do not provide dimensional scores, at least ones that are comparable with those based on an interview. The low literacy rate in some cultures also limits the use of inventories.

The problems associated with establishing the validity of semistructured interviews remain intractable because of the absence of an acceptable gold standard.[33] The ultimate validation may prove to be a pragmatic one. Does the interview provide more replicable and useful answers to questions about etiology, course, and treatment than the assessments provided by clinicians without one? It was the impression of the examiners who used the IPDE in this study that it was clinically valid. There was also evidence that it tended to make fewer personality disorder diagnoses than some of the clinicians who screened the patients. After discussion of whether this should lead to the adoption of less stringent scoring standards, there was general agreement among the examiners that clinicians were often inclined to diagnose personality disorders without strict adherence to the criteria and the requirement that the maladaptive behavior be relatively enduring (with onset by early adulthood). The participants unanimously decided not to relax or alter the present method of conducting and scoring the interview. There were, however, some suggestions for minor alterations in the wording of some items.

There are cultural variations in what is considered maladaptive behavior. No attempt was made to modify any of the criteria in *DSM-III-R* or *ICD-10* to accommodate a particular culture. However, the clinicians at each site were instructed to judge the meaning of the behavior in the context of their particular culture. This proved to be a significant issue in surprisingly few instances. Examples include the *DSM-III-R* criteria pertaining to monogamous relationships (antisocial) and harsh treatment of spouses and children (sadistic). Otherwise, the clinicians viewed the two classification systems as applicable to their particular cultures.

FREQUENCY OF PERSONALITY DISORDER SUBTYPES

The study was not intended to be an epidemiological survey of residents in the community or those under treatment. The principal objective was to determine the acceptability and reliability of the personality disorder component of the WHO instrumentation package. The sampling did not involve consecutive admissions, and there are obviously different thresholds associated with the request for mental health care in different cultures. We have reported the overall rates of the individual disorders for all of the centers combined and believe that it would be potentially misleading to report the rates for each center. It is noteworthy, however, that the overwhelming majority of personality disorder subtypes were diagnosed in most of the 11 nations represented in the study.

It is also of interest that the two most frequently diagnosed types in the sample as a whole are disorders that were not included in the *ICD-9*, or the *DSM-II*. They are borderline (*DSM-III-R*) or emotionally unstable, borderline type (*ICD-10*), and avoidant (*DSM-III-R*) or anxious (*ICD-10*). At least one case of these two disorders occurred at every center with the exception of Bangalore, India (no avoidant diagnosis) and Nairobi, Kenya (no borderline diagnosis).

Two controversial disorders, sadistic and self-defeating, are not included in *ICD-10* and have been relegated to the appendix of *DSM-III-R*. Both were among the three least frequent diagnoses in the entire sample. Interestingly, the third one, narcissistic, was not included in *DSM-II* and is still not recognized in *ICD-10*. It occurred in only 1.3% of study patients. This contrasts with the findings regarding passive aggressive, which is also not included in *ICD-10* but was diagnosed in 5% of study patients and appeared in all centers but one.

ICD-10 AND *DSM-III-R*

As previously noted, *ICD-10* and *DSM-III-R* are different but overlapping classification systems. There are slight differences in nomenclatures: anankastic/obsessive compulsive, anxious/avoidant, and dissocial/antisocial. In *ICD-10*, borderline and impulsive are viewed as subtypes of emotionally unstable; schizotypal is located with schizophrenia and delusional disorders; and narcissistic, passive aggressive, and the two disorders in the appendix of *DSM-III-R*, sadistic and self-defeating, do not appear. There are also several significant differences in the criteria in the two systems and some minor variations in their wording. Except for emotionally unstable, *ICD-10* requires four of seven criteria for a diagnosis; and except for antisocial, *DSM-III-R* requires four or five from a list that varies from seven to nine criteria.

This report will not attempt a more detailed comparison of the two classification systems for personality disorders. However, mention should be made of the extent to which *ICD-10* and *DSM-III-R* tend to produce similar results. First, within the limitations imposed by the sample sizes of the individual disorders, no statistically significant ($P<.05$) differences were observed in the base rates with which the corresponding specific personality disorders were diagnosed in the overall sample of 716 patients. There was a trend, albeit statistically not significant, for *DSM-III-R* to identify more cases of antisocial, paranoid, and histrionic behavior and for *ICD-10* to diagnose more cases of anxious/avoidant behavior. Both systems provide a residual category for cases judged to have a personality disorder that does not meet the requirements for any of the specific types. There is no method of identifying these patients without invoking some arbitrary standard. The IPDE assigns a residual diagnosis to anyone who does not meet the requirements for a specific disorder, but nevertheless accumulates 10 or more criteria from the various disorders. There are more opportunities to obtain the diagnosis in *DSM-III-R* than in *ICD-10* because the former has 110 criteria and the latter only 56. It is not surprising, then, that approximately twice as many patients received a nonspecific diagnosis of personality disorder in *DSM-III-R* as in *ICD-10* (12.8% vs 6.8%).

This, of course, does not address the question of whether the two classification systems actually identified the same patients as having a particular disorder. That can be determined by the κ statistic, particularly for those disorders with a prevalence of at least 5%. There are only two of them; the κs are 0.66 (borderline) and 0.52 (anxious/avoidant), evidence of moderate but far from perfect agreement. With the distribution of cases in the sample of 716 patients, these κs were associated with 92% agreement regarding the diagnosis of borderline and 89% for anxious/avoidant. The κ values for the remaining disorders should be viewed as relatively unstable because of the base rate problem. They range from 0.32 (dissocial/

antisocial) to 0.61 (anankastic/obsessive-compulsive disorder), with a median of 0.52. The *DSM-III-R* and *ICD-10* comparisons should not be affected by the less-than-perfect interrater reliability of the IPDE since the same examiner conducted the interview and rated the information on which the *ICD-10* and *DSM-III-R* diagnoses for a particular patient were based.

The substantial disagreement regarding the dissocial and antisocial diagnoses is not entirely unexpected considering the different approaches the two classification systems have taken regarding the disorder. The *DSM-III-R* emphasizes lawbreaking and criminal acts, while *ICD-10* is more concerned with generic concepts such as lack of empathy, inability to profit from experience, and inability to maintain enduring relationships.

It is also possible to judge the overall agreement between *DSM-III-R* and *ICD-10* for the eight disorders they share in common. This can be done by calculating an overall weighted κ based on all of these disorders, regardless of whether they meet the criterion of a 5% base rate. That κ is .54, an indication of only moderate agreement. In conclusion, there appears to be sufficient disagreement regarding the cases of personality disorders identified by *ICD-10* and *DSM-III-R* to justify the prior decision of the WHO/ADAMHA steering committee to develop an instrument that would accommodate both classification systems. The two, however, provide roughly similar interrater agreement and temporal stability when assessed by the IPDE.

Accepted for publication September 28, 1993.

Reprint requests to The New York Hospital–Cornell Medical Center, Westchester Division, 21 Bloomingdale Rd, White Plains, NY 10605 (Dr Loranger).

REFERENCES

1. Jablensky A, Sartorius N, Hirschfeld R, Pardes H. Diagnosis and classification of mental disorders and alcohol- and drug-related problems: a research agenda for the 1980s. *Psychol Med.* 1983;13:907-921.
2. Robins LN, Wing J, Wittchen HU, Helzer JE, Babor TF, Burke J, Farmer A, Jablenski A, Pickens R, Regier DA, Sartorius N, Towle LH. The Composite International Diagnostic Interview: an epidemiologic instrument suitable for use in conjunction with different diagnostic systems and in different cultures. *Arch Gen Psychiatry.* 1988;45:1069-1077.
3. Robins LN, Helzer JE, Croughan J, Ratcliff KS. National Institute of Mental Health Diagnostic Interview Schedule: its history, characteristics, and validity. *Arch Gen Psychiatry.* 1981;38:381-389.
4. Wing JK, Babor T, Brugha T, Burke J, Cooper JE, Giel R, Jablenski A, Regier D, Sartorius N. SCAN: Schedules for Clinical Assessment in Neuropsychiatry. *Arch Gen Psychiatry.* 1990;47:589-593.
5. Wing JK, Cooper JE, Sartorius N. *The Measurement and Classification of Psychiatric Symptoms.* England: Cambridge University Press; 1974.
6. Loranger AW. *Personality Disorder Examination (PDE) Manual.* Yonkers, NY: DV Communications; 1988.
7. World Health Organization. *I.C.D.-10 Chapter V: Mental and Behavioural Disorders (Including Disorders of Psychological Development), Diagnostic Criteria for Research, Draft for Field Trials.* Geneva, Switzerland: World Health Organization; 1990.
8. American Psychiatric Association, Committee on Nomenclature and Statistics. *Diagnostic and Statistical Manual of Mental Disorders, Revised Third Edition.* Washington, DC: American Psychiatric Association; 1987.
9. Loranger AW, Hirschfeld RMA, Sartorius N, Regier DA. The WHO/ADAMHA International Pilot Study of Personality Disorders: background and purpose. *J Pers Disord.* 1991;5:296-306.
10. Spitzer RL, Endicott J. *Schedule for Affective Disorders and Schizophrenia (SADS).* 3rd ed. New York: New York State Psychiatric Institute; 1978-1979.
11. Spitzer RL, Williams JBW, Gibbon M, First M. *User's Guide for the Structured Clinical Interview for DSM-III-R.* Washington, DC: American Psychiatric Association Press; 1990.
12. Ebel RL. Estimation of the reliability of ratings. *Psychometrika.* 1951;16:407-423.
13. Nunnally JC. *Psychometric Theory.* New York, NY: McGraw-Hill International Book Co; 1978:219-220, 237-239.
14. Fleiss JL. *Statistical Methods for Rates and Proportions.* 2nd ed. New York, NY: John Wiley & Sons Inc; 1981:217-220.
15. Grove WM, Andreasen NC, McDonald-Scott P, Keller MB, Shapiro RW. Reliability studies of psychiatric diagnosis: theory and practice. *Arch Gen Psychiatry.* 1981;38:408-413.
16. World Health Organization. *Report on the International Pilot Study of Schizophrenia.* Geneva, Switzerland: World Health Organization; 1973.
17. Williams JBW, Gibbon M, First MB, Spitzer RL, Davies M, Borus J, Howes MJ, Kane J, Pope HG Jr, Rounsaville B, Wittchen H-U. The Structured Clinical Interview for *DSM-III-R* (SCID), II: multisite test-retest reliability. *Arch Gen Psychiatry.* 1992;49:630-636.
18. Stangl D, Pfohl B, Zimmerman M, Bowers W, Cornethal C. A structured interview for *DSM-III* personality disorders: a preliminary report. *Arch Gen Psychiatry.* 1985;42:591-596.
19. Zanarini MC, Frankenburg FR, Chauncey DL, Gunderson JG. The Diagnostic Interview for Personality Disorders: interrater and test-retest reliability. *Compr Psychiatry.* 1987;28:467-480.
20. Andreasen NC, Grove WM, Shapiro RW, Keller MB, Hirschfeld RMA, McDonald-Scott P. Reliability of lifetime diagnosis: a multicenter collaborative perspective. *Arch Gen Psychiatry.* 1981;38:400-405.
21. Bromet EJ, Dunn LO, Connell MM, Dew MA, Schulberg HC. Long-term reliability of diagnosing lifetime major depression in a community sample. *Arch Gen Psychiatry.* 1986;43:435-440.
22. Fendrich M, Weissman MM, Warner V, Mufson L. Two-year recall of lifetime diagnoses in offspring at high and low risk for major depression: the stability of offspring reports. *Arch Gen Psychiatry.* 1990;47:1121-1127.
23. Rice JP, McDonald-Scott P, Endicott J, Coryell W, Grove WM, Keller MB, Altis D. The stability of diagnosis with an application to bipolar II disorder. *Psychiatry Res.* 1986;19:285-296.
24. Rice JP, Rochberg N, Endicott J, Lavori PW, Miller C. Stability of psychiatric diagnoses: an application to the affective disorders. *Arch Gen Psychiatry.* 1992;49:824-830.
25. Loranger AW, Lenzenweger MF, Gartner AF, Lehmann Susman V, Herzig J, Zammit GK, Gartner JD, Abrams RC, Young RC. Trait-state artifacts and the diagnosis of personality disorders. *Arch Gen Psychiatry.* 1991;48:720-728.
26. Pfohl B, Black DW, Noyes R, Coryell WH, Barrash J. Axis I and Axis II comorbidity findings: implications for validity. In: Oldham JM, ed. *Personality Disorders: New Perspectives on Diagnostic Validity.* Washington, DC: American Psychiatric Press; 1991:147-161.
27. van den Brink W. *Meting van* DSM-III *persoonlijkheidspathologie: Betrouwbaarheid en validiteit van de SIDP-R as II van de* DSM-III. Groningen, the Netherlands: Drukkerij Van Denderen BV; 1989.
28. Stuart S, Simons AD, Thase ME, Pilkonis P. Are personality disorders valid in acute major depression? *J Affect Disord.* 1992;24:281-290.
29. Widiger TA. Categorical versus dimensional classification: implications from and for research. *J Pers Disord.* 1992;6:287-300.
30. Cloninger CR. A systematic method for clinical description and classification of personality variants: a proposal. *Arch Gen Psychiatry.* 1987;44:573-588.
31. Frances A. Categorical and dimensional systems of personality diagnosis: a comparison. *Compr Psychiatry.* 1982;23:516-527.
32. Loranger AW. Are current self-report and interview measures adequate for epidemiological studies of personality disorders? *J Pers Disord.* 1992;6:313-325.
33. Loranger AW. Diagnosis of personality disorders: general considerations. In; Michels R, ed. *Psychiatry.* Philadelphia, Pa: JB Lippincott; 1991;1(chap 15):1-14.

Diagnosing Personality Disorders

A Review of Issues and Research Methods

Mark Zimmerman, MD

Many questions face researchers conducting personality disorder research. Which measure should be used? When should patients be evaluated—at initial presentation when they are still symptomatic, or after symptom resolution? Can a patient accurately describe his or her personality, or must an informant be contacted? What do you do when personality traits change during an individual's lifetime? I discuss these and other issues of personality disorder assessment in the *DSM-III/DSM-III-R* era, and examine the empiric literature bearing on these questions. First, I review studies of diagnostic reliability and stability, because studies of the above questions can only be interpreted in the context of the limitations imposed by modest reliability. *(Arch Gen Psychiatry. 1994;51:225-245)*

Since the publication of the *DSM-III* personality disorder (PD) criteria, research in this area has grown markedly.[1] This system of diagnosing PDs essentially is being retained in *DSM-IV* (albeit with some modification); therefore, it will continue to influence American psychiatric thinking for at least the next 15 to 20 years.

Subsequent to the development of the taxonomy came the development of measures to assess the PD criteria. I have been involved in the development and validation of one of these instruments,[2] and in the course of designing our studies, my colleagues and I were faced with several decisions regarding assessment methods. Should we evaluate patients at the time of initial presentation or wait until symptom abatement? Should we interview the patient or speak to someone who knows the patient well? How should we evaluate aspects of personality that reportedly changed during the patient's lifetime? Although we were not faced with a choice regarding the instrument to be used, present-day researchers need to choose among the five interviews[2-6] and eight self-administered questionnaires[7-14] that diagnose these disorders. Are these measures more or less equivalent and therefore interchangeable?

The purpose of this article is to review the issues and research bearing on the assessment of PDs. After reviewing the literature on the reliability of Axis II diagnoses, I turn to the empiric literature on the who, what, and when of *DSM-III/DSM-III-R* PD measurement. Issues such as diagnostic stability, state-trait artifacts, the use of informants, interviews vs questionnaires, what to do when personality changes, the retest artifact, and interviewer training, are examined. Some issues, though, are not addressed. Specifically, I omitted discussion of the categoric/dimensional debate, and whether other conceptualizations of abnormal personality are superior to those of *DSM-III/DSM-III-R* because these are more theoretic, than practical, assessment issues. The interested reader is referred to the excellent reviews of these topics by Frances and Widiger.[15-17]

To interpret studies of the agreement between different measures, or between different sources of information, it is necessary to consider first the reliability of the measurement procedure. Only if the diagnostic

From the Medical College of Pennsylvania at Eastern Pennsylvania Psychiatric Institute, Philadelphia.

Table 1. Joint-Interview Reliability of *DSM-III/DSM-III-R* Personality Disorders*

Investigator(s)	Sample	Measure	PD κ Coefficient											
			Any PD	PAR	ZOID	TYPAL	COMP	HIST	DEP	ANTI	NARC	AVOID	BORD	PASS
Arntz et al[22]	70 outpatients	SCID-II†	...	.77	...	.65	.72	.85	1.00	...	...	.82	.79	.66
Brent et al[23]‡	17 inpatients or outpatients	SIDP	...	.58	...	1.00	.69	.62	.43	...	.32	.34	.40	.53
Brooks et al[24]	30 outpatients with panic disorder and agoraphobia	SCID-II†	...	.77	...	.89	.66	.43	.84	...	.78	.56	.64	.50
Jackson et al[25]	39 inpatients	SIDP	...	.54	...	.72	...	.80	.48	1.00	...	...	.66	.72
Loranger et al[26]	60 inpatients	PDE	.80	...	...	.80	.88	.77	...	.70	...	...	.96	...
Loranger[27]	141 inpatients or outpatients	IPDE	...	...	...	...	...	...	...	...	...	.71	.80	...
Renneberg et al[28]	32 anxious outpatients	SCID-II†	.75	.61	...	...	.71	...	...	...	...	.81	.63	...
Standage and Ladha[29]	20 inpatients	PDE	.41	.41	...	.62	.62	.77	.70	.38	.63	.69	.78	...
Stangl et al[30]	43 inpatients	SIDP	.71	...	...	.55	.36	.84	.88	...	.85	.45	.95	...
Stanley et al[31]‡	13 obsessive-compulsive outpatients	SCID-II†	...	...	.75	.79	.63	.85	.71	...	.63	.61	.63	...
Widiger et al[5]	67 inpatients with PDs	PIQ	...	.71	.71	.64	.67	.71	.52	.83	.77	.69	.75	.52
Widiger et al[32]	47 inpatients	PIQ-II†	...	.69	.76	.45	...	.59	.82	.83	.70	.91	.58	.92
Wonderlich et al[33]	14 patients with eating disorder	SCID-II†	...	...	...	...	.77	.75	.66	...	...	.56	.74	...
Zanarini et al[6]	43 inpatients with PDs	DIPD	.89	.52	...	.86	.92	.87	.92	1.00	.87	1.00	.94	.95
Zimmerman and Coryell[34]	104 nonpatients	SIDP	.93	...	...	1.0	.66	1.00	1.00	.66	...	...	...	.80

**PD indicates personality disorder; PAR, paranoid; ZOID, schizoid; TYPAL, schizotypal; COMP, compulsive; HIST, histrionic; DEP, dependent; ANTI, antisocial; NARC, narcissistic; AVOID, avoidant; BORD, borderline; PASS, passive-aggressive; SCID-II, Structured Clinical Interview for* DSM-III *Axis II; SIDP, Structured Interview for* DSM-III *Personality Disorders; PDE, Personality Disorders Examination; IPDE, International Personality Disorders Examination; PIQ, Personality Interview Questions; and DIPD, Diagnostic Interview for Personality Disorders.*

†*Diagnoses based on* DSM-III-R.

‡*Patients categorized as having the trait or the disorder vs not having the disorder.*

methods are reliable can we infer that diagnostic discordance is a function of the parameter that is being varied.

For example, if two independent raters demonstrate only modest agreement by using the same measure, then no more than modest agreement can be expected between the index instrument and another measure, or between independent interviews of the patient and a close informant. Thus, I will begin with a review of the reliability literature.

RELIABILITY OF PD DIAGNOSES

Issues in Reviewing the Literature

Numerous studies report interrater reliability coefficients for isolated PDs, or for the presence of any PD; however, I focused my review on the studies that assessed the full range of the *DSM* disorders.

Some of the samples are small—four studies had fewer than 20 patients, and half had 40 or fewer. When the sample size is small, κ coefficients have a large SE of measurement and thus are less stable.[18] Although there was no evidence that small sample size was associated with poorer reliability, the results based on small samples should be interpreted more cautiously.

Authors varied in their sample size and base rate requirements of positive cases for calculating κ. Kappa is influenced by the illness base rate, such that a few diagnostic disagreements have a more pronounced effect on reliability when the base rate is either very low or high. Some authors labeled this the "base rate problem" of κ,[19,20] though Shrout and colleagues[21] convincingly argued that this phenomenon should not be interpreted as a problem with κ but as a problem with establishing diagnostic reliability in homogeneous samples. Nevertheless, because of these concerns, some investigators calculated κ only if the base rate was greater than 5%. Other researchers required a minimum number of cases to be diagnosed (usually at least five individuals by at least one rater). And some had no sample size or base rate requirement, or made no reference to such a requirement.

In tabulating the results of the reliability studies (**Table 1** through **Table 3**), I included all κ values that were reported by the authors of the studies, except in those instances where no patient had a positive diagnosis. For several studies, I computed the κ coefficients from the raw data that were given in the article (or provided to me

Table 2. Short-Interval Test-Retest Reliability Studies of *DSM-III/DSM-III-R* Personality Disorders*

			PD κ Coefficient											
Investigator(s)	Sample	Measure	Any PD	PAR	ZOID	TYPAL	COMP	HIST	DEP	ANTI	NARC	AVOID	BORD	PASS
Hurt et al[35]	40 outpatients with PDs	PDQ	...	.59		.56	.75	.30	.04	.74	.11	.70	.63	−.25
Stangl et al[30]	20 inpatients	SIDP	.66	...		.77	...	.43	...	.77	...	.77	.58	...
Zanarini et al[6]	54 inpatients with PDs	DIPD	.58	.54		.61	.56	.68	.77	.84	.78	.67	.85	.46
First et al[36]	103 inpatients or outpatients	SCID-II	.51	.68		...	.24	.74	.42	.71	.43	.71	.40	.59
	181 symptomatic nonpatients	...	.48	.47		...	.24	.51	.59	...	.42	.35	.57	.31

**PDQ indicates Personality Diagnostic Questionnaire. For explanation of rest of abbreviations, see first footnote to Table 1.*

Table 3. Long-Interval Test-Retest Reliability Studies of *DSM-III/DSM-III-R* Personality Disorders*

				PD κ Coefficient											
Investigator(s)	Sample	Measure	Interval	Any PD	PAR	ZOID	TYPAL	COMP	HIST	DEP	ANTI	NARC	AVOID	BORD	PASS
Ames-Frankel et al[37]	30 bulimic outpatients	PDE	6 wk	.48	...	...	.00	...	.26	−.04	...	.27	.25	.67	...
O'Boyle and Self[38]	17 depressed inpatients	PDE	63 d (mean)	.35	...	...	...	...	...	.00	...	...	.46	.11	...
		SCID-II		.65	.49	...	...	.77	...	−.08	...	...	.34	.30	...
Loranger et al[39]	84 inpatients	PDE	1 wk-6 mo	.55	...	...	...	.26	.47	.57	...	.36	.57	.57	...
Loranger[27]	243 inpatients or outpatients	IPDE	6 mo (mean)	...	...	...	...	...	...	...	...	...	.48	.70	...
Pfohl et al[40]	36 depressed inpatients	SIDP	6-12 mo	...	.64	...	.22	...	.46	...	.84	...	...	.58	.16
Piersma[41]	109 inpatients	MCMI	30.4±10.5 d	...	...	...	.27	.09	...	.44	...	.35	.27	.11	.01
Reich[42]	70 outpatients	PDQ	8 wk	...	.55	...	.55	.39	.17	.75	...	...	.50	.50	...
Barasch et al[43]	30 PD outpatients	Unspecified†	3 y	...	−.04	...	−.09	...	.24	.30	...	−.06	.39	.46	.00

**MCMI indicates Millon Clinical Multiaxial Inventory. For explanation of rest of abbreviations, see first footnote to Table 1.*
†Unspecified standardized interview used at intake and retest.

by the authors). Because some of these studies already had small samples, I used a conservative standard and required a base rate of approximately 10%. Studies that only reported reliability coefficients for dimensional scores, and not for categoric diagnoses, were excluded.[44]

Reliability of Diagnoses Based on Unstructured Interviews

In the *DSM-III* field trials,[45] the κ coefficient for the presence or absence of any PD was .61 based on a joint-interview design, and it was .54 in a test-retest situation. Reliability coefficients for the individual disorders were not reported. Mellsop and colleagues[46] reported even poorer agreement for the presence of any PD (κ=.41); the κ coefficients for the individual disorders ranged from .01 to .49, with a median of .23. In the National Institute of Mental Health Collaborative Study for the Treatment of Depression,[47] the Personality Assessment Form was used to determine PD diagnoses.[48] On the Personality Assessment Form, the interviewer rates how characteristic of the patient's long-term personality are the features of each PD. The ratings are on a scale of 1 through 6, and they are not based on a standard set of questions asked of the patient. A threshold of 4 on any dimension was used to identify patients with a probable or definite PD.

In the Collaborative Study, the chance-corrected reliability coefficient for the presence of any PD was .48.[48] In another study of the Personality Assessment Form in depressed patients, the κ coefficient was .36 for any PD diagnosis made at intake, and it was .44 for diagnoses made at a 6-month follow-up evaluation.[49]

Joint-Interview Interrater Reliability of Diagnoses Based on Semistructured Interviews

Compared with the four studies that did not use semistructured interviews, the reliability coefficients in the 15 joint-interview studies are considerably higher (Table 1). Nearly 80% (92/

116) of the κ values are above .60, and nearly 60% (68/116) are .70 and above. Summarizing across studies, the mean κ for each disorder, except paranoid PD, was between .69 and .77. For paranoid PD, the mean κ was .62, and for any PD, the mean κ was .75.

Six of the 15 studies were conducted by the personnel that developed the instrument. Of the nine remaining studies, five used the Structured Clinical Interview for *DSM-III* Axis II (SCID-II) for which there are currently no published reliability data from its developers (though unpublished test-retest data are summarized below). Only four replication studies have been published. The raters in the studies by Brent et al[23] and Jackson et al[25] less reliably diagnosed PD based on the Structured Interview for the *DSM-III* Personality Disorders (SIDP) than the raters in the study by Stangl et al.[30] Standage and Ladha,[29] using the initial version of Loranger's Personality Disorders Examination (PDE), were unable to achieve the same level of reliability as in the original report (any PD, .41 vs .80; mean κ for the five specific diagnoses reported in both studies, .63 vs .82). However, the revised 1988 version of the PDE significantly differs from the original, and for the two disorders diagnosed in at least 5% of the sample, the reliability of the international PDE used in the World Health Organization's multinational study of PDs was high.[27]

Short-Interval Test-Retest Reliability

A more rigorous examination of reliability is the test-retest approach in which the two raters separately interview the patient. Whereas there is only one source of unreliability in a joint-interview study (ie, rater variance in criteria interpretation), there are three sources of error in a test-retest study (ie, rater variance in criteria interpretation, rater variance in the elicitation of information, and patient variance across interviews). It is therefore not surprising that both Stangl et al[30] and Zanarini et al[6] found lower test-retest than joint-interview reliabilities (Table 2). Stangl et al[30] evaluated 43 inpatients conjointly and 20 inpatients in a test-retest design, and they reported that the κ for the presence of any PD decreased from .71 to .66. Although they did not calculate test-retest reliability coefficients for specific disorders, they provided the raw data in their article to do so. For the five disorders diagnosed in at least three of the 20 patients by one or both raters, the mean κ decreased from .73 to .66. The findings by Zanarini et al[6] were analogous though the drop-off in reliability from the joint-interview to the test-retest situation was greater (any PD, .89 vs .56; mean κ for 10 specific PDs, .89 vs .68).

First et al,[36] Spitzer et al,[50] and Williams et al[51] recently completed a large multicenter test-retest reliability study of the SCID. Approximately half of the patients in the SCID Axis I reliability study also participated in the SCID-II substudy.[36] No joint-interview reliability data were collected. There were two major methodologic limitations of the study. First, the interviewers received very little training. The authors noted that the focus of their training sessions was the Axis I SCID to the relative neglect of the SCID-II. A lack of adequate training should reduce diagnostic reliability. Second, the SCID-II interview may have been limited to those criteria that were checked positive by the patient on a preinterview questionnaire. To reduce SCID-II administration time, the patient first completed a screening self-administered inventory. The interviewer inquired only about those criteria that were positive on the questionnaire, unless data from the SCID Axis I Interview were inconsistent with the questionnaire responses, or the patient was within one criterion of the threshold for a positive diagnosis. In these cases, the interviewer was encouraged to ask all of the SCID-II questions for the section. The questionnaire was only given once, and the same information was used by both interviewers to guide their SCID-II interviews. This might have artificially increased test-retest reliability because the raters would have agreed on all criteria that were answered in the nonpathologic direction on the self-report scale. Despite this bias, the test-retest reliability of the SCID-II was generally not as good as that found by Stangl et al[30] and Zanarini et al.[6] Whether this was due to inadequate training, better reliability when instruments were used by their developers, or inherently better reliability of the SIDP and Diagnostic Interview for Personality Disorders (DIPD) is impossible to determine. The joint-interview reliability of the SCID-II is as good as that of other instruments (Table 1), so the third hypothesized explanation is unlikely.

There is also one study of the test-retest reliability of a self-administered questionnaire designed to diagnose the *DSM* PDs. (Because my emphasis is on the reliability of categoric diagnoses, studies of the Millon Clinical Multiaxial Inventory [MCMI] that report only Pearson correlation coefficients of dimensional scores are not summarized here.) Hurt et al[35] administered the Personality Diagnostic Questionnaire (PDQ) to 40 outpatients with clinically diagnosed PDs two times at 1 month apart. The reliability of the PDQ was comparable with that found in the test-retest interview studies, conducted by Stangl et al[30] and Zanarini et al,[6] for six PDs (paranoid, schizotypal, compulsive, antisocial, avoidant, and borderline), and much lower for four disorders (histrionic, dependent, narcissistic, and passive-aggressive) (Table 2).

Longer-Interval Test-Retest Reliability Coinciding With Changes in Psychiatric State

The biasing effect of the depressed state on self-report personality inventories has been repeatedly demonstrated,[52-57] and this effect is present even when patients are instructed to describe what they are like when they are their usual, normal selves. In the four test-retest reliability studies described above, psychiatric state was purportedly relatively stable. Stangl et al,[30] Zanarini et al,[6] and First et al[36] retested patients within a week of the first assessment, and Hurt et al[35] studied outpatients with PDs who did not have a concurrent Axis I disorder. All but one of the studies summarized in Table 3, in contrast, tested patients when they presented for treatment and after symptom reduction. In this section, I only discuss diagnostic reliability and κ coefficients. Below, in the section entitled "When Should the Assessment Be Done?" I discuss the influence of psychiatric state on PD prevalence rates.

O'Boyle and Self[38] interviewed 17 depressed inpatients with both the PDE and the SCID-II at admission and again just before or after discharge. All patients were clinically judged to be recovered, and the mean (±SD) Hamilton Rating Scale for Depression scores (HRSD) had decreased from 23.5±5.8 to 7.9±5.3. The authors did not calculate test-retest reliability coefficients; however, they presented the raw data to do so. I calculated κ coefficients only for those PDs diagnosed in three or more patients by at least one of the raters. On the PDE, diagnostic consistency was poor (any PD, κ=.35). The test-retest reliability of any SCID-II diagnosis was good (κ=.65); however, agreement for the individual PDs was low (Table 3).

Loranger and colleagues[39] interviewed 84 patients with the PDE within 2 weeks of hospital admission and again at 1 week to 6 months later. At each interview, a silent observer independently rated the PDE, and concordance between the initial and repeated interview required all raters to agree on the diagnosis. Initially, patients were minimally-moderately depressed (mean [±SD] HRSD scores, 11.1±7.9; mean [±SD] Beck Depression Inventory [BDI] scores, 19.5±11.3) or anxious (mean [±SD] Clinical Anxiety Scale scores, 6.7±4.8), and symptom levels decreased significantly at follow-up (HRSD scores, 7.0±7.4; BDI scores, 11.8±11.0; Clinical Anxiety Scale scores, 4.4±4.3). The test-retest reliability for the presence or absence of any PD and most of the individual disorders was fair-moderate. Their sample was heterogeneous with regard to the Axis I diagnosis, baseline levels of anxiety and depressive symptoms, and the amount of change from initial to repeated testing in these symptom levels. Of importance, they found no evidence that a change in the level of anxiety or depression affected diagnostic stability.

Pilkonis et al[49] also used the PDE to interview 31 depressed patients on presentation to treatment (HRSD scores, 15.6±7.3; BDI scores, 23.2±10.7) and at a 6-month follow-up evaluation (HRSD scores, 8.8±8.1; BDI scores, 12.5±11.8). The κ coefficient for the presence of any PD was nearly identical to the value found by Loranger et al[39] (.52 vs .55). They did not report reliability coefficients for the individual PDs.

Ames-Frankel and colleagues[37] administered the PDE to 30 bulimic outpatients before and after 6 weeks of treatment with desipramine hydrochloride or placebo. They noted that for "many" patients the same interviewer conducted both evaluations, and this might have increased test-retest agreement. From the data provided in their article, I calculated the κ for the presence or absence of any PD (κ=.48); this is comparable with the values reported by Loranger et al[39] and Pilkonis et al.[49] From the raw data provided to me by the authors (M. Devlin, MD, written communication, July 1992), I calculated κ coefficients for disorders diagnosed at least three times by one or more raters, and only borderline PD achieved good reliability (Table 3).

In the International Pilot Study of PDs, 241 inpatients and outpatients with a mixture of Axis I disorders were interviewed with the International PDE two times—an average of 6 months apart.[27] As with the study by Ames-Frankel et al,[37] a major methodologic weakness was that the same interviewer administered the International PDE on the two occasions. This lack of blindness would increase diagnostic reliability. Loranger et al[39] presented reliability coefficients for those disorders present in at least 5% of the sample and found that borderline PD was diagnosed with good reliability, but avoidant PD achieved only fair reliability. They also broadened the definition of a case to include individuals who had one fewer than the threshold level of criteria. The test-retest reliability of probable and definite PDs could be calculated for more PDs, and it was somewhat higher than for definite PD only (histrionic, κ=.46; antisocial, κ=.62; avoidant, κ=.66; and borderline, κ=.72).

Pfohl et al[40] interviewed 36 depressed inpatients with the SIDP during the first week of hospitalization and at 6 to 12 months later. In contrast to the above studies, information from informants supplemented patient interviews. They did not describe the severity level of depressive symptoms, though other reports from this group indicated that patients were significantly less depressed at follow-up.[58-60] The authors found that the test-retest reliability coefficients for the disorders diagnosed at least four times by either rater ranged from .16 to .84. They did not report the κ coefficient for the presence of any PD.

Piersma[41] gave 151 consecutively admitted inpatients (major depression [n=83], bipolar disorder [n=12], dysthymia [n=19], adjustment reaction [n=21], anxiety disorder [n=15], and schizophrenia [n=1]) the MCMI at admission and at 1 to 2 days before hospital discharge (mean interval, 30.4 days). Agreement for the presence of any PD was little better than chance, and reliability coefficients for the specific diagnoses were all below .45. In his updated review of PD instruments, Reich[42] briefly described a study in which he administered the PDQ to 70 patients when they were clinically ill and at 8 weeks after recovery, and he found good reliability for some, but only poor-fair agreement for most of the PDs. (Reich[42] also reported reliability data for the MCMI, but it was not stated whether the coefficients represented correlations of dimensional scores or κ values.)

Long-term Test-Retest Reliability/Diagnostic Stability

Although the distinction between "longer-interval test-retest reliability" and "diagnostic stability" is somewhat arbitrary, the studies summarized in the section above and in this section differ in three ways. First, in the above studies, there was usually a documented change in symptoms from the time of the first to the second evaluation, and the effect of psychiatric state on personality assessments was a focus of the research. Second, the interval between assessments was generally longer in the diagnostic stability studies reviewed below. And finally, some of the diagnostic stability studies, particularly those of borderline PD, are follow-up studies of patient cohorts that examined the frequency of patients who continued to meet the diagnostic criteria. This is not a test-retest reliability design, and κ coefficients cannot be computed.

A longitudinal perspective is essential in diagnosing PDs, and in validating them. Personality (and PDs) refer to individuals' long-standing characteristic style of thinking, acting, interacting, and reacting. Longitudinal studies of personality in normal adults have demonstrated that personality traits are fairly stable during 2 to 30 years. The mean of the stability coefficients of personality dimensional scores on self-administered questionnaires across the eight longitudinal studies reviewed by Costa and McCrae[61] was .57. As high a level of stability may not be found for PDs because of individuals' desire to change their maladaptive and distressing traits. However, if PD diagnoses are not stable throughout relatively short intervals, such as 6 months or a year, then something is wrong with the diagnostic method, the diagnostician, or perhaps the diagnostic criteria.

European developers of standardized personality schedules, despite not using a criteria-based system to make a PD diagnosis, have reported fair-good temporal reliability. Mann et al[62] interviewed the informants of 62 patients on two occasions at 1 year apart, and the mean correlation for five personality types according to the *International Classification of Diseases* was .43. Tyrer and colleagues[63] interviewed 28 patients at an average of 2.9 years apart and found excellent agreement for diagnosing the presence or absence of any PD (κ=.72), though the individual types were less stable.

Overholser[64] administered the MCMI to 25 psychiatric inpatients during separate hospitalizations that occurred at least 3 months apart (mean, 379 days), and the average correlation across the personality scales was .69. Murphy et al[65] also tested psychiatric inpatients with the MCMI across hospitalizations (mean, 176 days), and the mean correlation for the 11 personality scales was .66. Neither of these studies reported categoric diagnostic stability coefficients. The problem in interpreting studies of the MCMI is that psychiatric state has a strong influence on MCMI personality scores (see below). Thus, stability reported in these studies might just as well reflect consistency of mood across hospitalizations rather than personality.

Barasch and colleagues[43] interviewed 30 patients 3 years after they received a standardized PD interview. They did not describe their assessment procedure in detail, and it is not clear from their report if the same or different methods were used at the baseline and repeated evaluations. The focus of their report was on borderline PD; however, they presented the Axis II diagnoses for all 30 patients, and stability coefficients for all diagnoses could be calculated. Seven disorders were diagnosed in four or more patients, and the highest diagnostic stability coefficient was found for borderline PD (κ=.46). All other κ coefficients were below .40 (Table 3).

Estimates of the diagnostic stability of borderline PD have ranged widely. Paris and coworkers[66] interviewed 100 borderline patients from a general hospital inpatient unit with the Diagnostic Interview for Borderlines (DIB) at 15 years after index hospitalization, and they found that 25% still met DIB criteria for a borderline diagnosis. Diagnostic stability in the Chestnut Lodge study of McGlashan[67] was somewhat higher—44% of *DSM-III* and 50% of patients who met the criterion proposed by Gunderson were similarly diagnosed after an average interval of 15 years. Pope and colleagues[68] reported that two thirds of borderline patients (most of whom had other PDs as well) retained the diagnosis (and retained the other PD diagnoses as well) after a 4- to 7-year interval. In all three of these studies, initial diagnoses were based on chart review, and only Paris and colleagues[66] used a widely used structured PD interview at follow-up. Barasch et al[43] reported that six of 10 borderline patients met *DSM-III* criteria (ie, had five or more borderline features) 3 years later (and three others met four of the eight *DSM-III* criteria).

Antisocial PD has been the most frequently studied PD from a diagnostic stability perspective. Two follow-up studies of heterogeneous patient samples included antisocial PD as one of the index disorders. Robins et al[69] reevaluated 57 patients diagnosed as having antisocial PD in a psychiatry emergency department at an average of 18 months after the baseline interview. Fifty-four were similarly diagnosed (κ=.93). In the follow-up study of female criminals by Martin and associates,[70] 19 of the 26 women who initially met antisocial PD criteria continued to do so 6 years later (κ=.65). In both studies, a small number of individuals met antisocial PD only at follow-up (Robins et al,[69] three of 242; Martin et al,[70] one of 16).

Four long-interval test-retest reliability studies of the Diagnostic Interview Schedule (DIS)[71] and Sched-

Table 4. Summary of Reliability Studies of *DSM-III/DSM-III-R* Personality Disorders Diagnosed by Standardized Interviews—Frequency Distribution of κ Coefficients Across Studies*

			% (n) of κ Coefficients				
Study Design	**No. of Studies**	**No. of κ**	**<.40**	**.40-.49**	**.50-.59**	**.60-.69**	**≥.70**
Joint interview	15†	116	3.4 (4)	6.9 (8)	10.3 (12)	20.7 (24)	58.6 (68)
Short-interval test-retest	4‡	36	11.1 (4)	22.2 (8)	25.0 (9)	13.9 (5)	27.8 (10)
Long-interval test-retest	5§	27	44.4 (12)	18.6 (5)	18.6 (5)	11.1 (3)	11.1 (3)

**For explanation of abbreviations, see first footnote to Table 1.*

†Includes the 15 studies listed in Table 1. The table should be read as follows: 3.4% of the 116 κ coefficients reported in the 15 studies of joint-interview reliability were below .40, 6.9% were between .40 and .49, 10.3% were between .50 and .59, and so on.

‡Includes the four interview studies listed in Table 2. The two samples from First et al[36] are counted as separate studies.

§Includes the five interview studies using standardized interviews listed in Table 3. For the study of O'Boyle and Self,[38] the SCID-II rather than the PDE data were used because κ coefficients were available for more disorders.

Table 5. Summary of Reliability Studies of *DSM-III/DSM-III-R* Personality Disorders Diagnosed by Standardized Interviews—Unweighted Mean κ Coefficients of Specific PDs Across Studies*

		Mean PD κ Coefficient											
Study Design	**No. of Studies†**	**Any PD**	**PAR**	**ZOID**	**TYPAL**	**COMP**	**HIST**	**DEP**	**ANTI**	**NARC**	**AVOID**	**BORD**	**PASS**
Joint interview	15	.75	.62	.74	.75	.69	.76	.75	.77	.69	.68	.73	.70
Short-interval test-retest	4	.56	.56	...	.69	.35	.59	.59	.77	.54	.63	.60	.45
Long-interval test-retest	5	.56	.57	...	.11	.52	.40	.15	.84	.32	.41	.56	.16

**For explanation of abbreviations, see first footnote to Table 1.*

†See Table 4 footnotes for clarification of studies included.

ule for Affective Disorders and Schizophrenia (SADS)[72] included data on antisocial PD. Prusoff et al[73] interviewed 143 probands and their relatives with the SADS two times at an average of 4 years apart. One person met Research Diagnostic Criteria[74] for antisocial PD at both interviews, and one only received the diagnosis at the second assessment (κ=.66). Rounsaville et al[75] also used the SADS to interview 117 opiate addicts. They diagnosed antisocial PD, according to Research Diagnostic Criteria, in 20 patients at baseline and again at 6 months later. Six patients were positive only at the first evaluation, and 16 only at the second (κ=.52). Two studies of the DIS examined the *DSM-III* antisocial PD criteria. In the 1-year follow-up of 370 community subjects by Helzer et al,[76] 17 were positive on both interviews, eight only on the first, and three only on the second (κ=.74). Vandiver and Sher[77] administered the DIS to 486 college students at 9 months apart, and the reliability of a lifetime antisocial PD diagnosis was .65. Twelve students met criteria both times, seven only on the first interview, and five only on the second.

SUMMARY AND DISCUSSION OF RELIABILITY STUDIES

The development of standardized assessment schedules has clearly improved diagnostic reliability. Joint-interview interrater reliability is very good, at least when the instruments are used by their developers. When used by independent researchers reliability may be lower,[78] though the results of the World Health Organization cross-cultural study indicated that good reliability could be achieved by interviewers of diverse cultures and languages who were not involved in the development of the instrument. The average κ coefficient of interrater agreement across the 15 studies in Table 1 was above .60 for all PDs. As expected, test-retest reliability coefficients were lower than joint-interview coefficients. In **Table 4** and **Table 5**, I summarize the results across studies, and in these tables, the effects of study design are readily apparent. The κ coefficients above .60 were nearly twice as common in joint-interview as in short-interval test-retest reliability studies (79.3% vs 41.7%) (Table 4). Likewise, poor-fair reliability (κ<.50) was only one third as frequent (10.3% vs 33.3%). I computed the unweighted mean κ coefficient for the specific disorders, and for every PD, except antisocial PD, the joint-interview reliability was higher (Table 5).

The length of the follow-up interval also seems to affect test-retest reliability. The mean κ coefficients of five disorders decreased by more than .20 from the short- to the long-interval test-retest design, and poor agreement (κ<.40) was four times more frequent in the long-interval studies (Tables 4 and 5).

It is not clear if reliability is poorer still when the retest interval coincides with a change in psychiatric state. Reliability in the study by

O'Boyle and Self,[38] in which they administered the SCID-II to 17 depressed patients during the acute phase and an average of 2 months later after they all were judged to be recovered, was comparable with the 1-week test-retest reliability of the SCID-II reported by First et al.[36] (It is possible, though, that the reliability of the SCID-II was underestimated by First et al[36] because their raters were inadequately trained.) Similarly, histrionic, antisocial, and borderline PD were as reliably diagnosed by the SIDP in the study of depressed patients by Pfohl et al,[40] in which these patients were reinterviewed 6 to 12 months after the initial evaluation, as in the report by Stangl et al[30] of 20 inpatients who were reassessed within a week of the initial interview. Schizotypal PD, however, was more reliably diagnosed when the retest interval was brief. In the only direct study of diagnostic reliability as a function of changing state, Loranger and colleagues[39] found no evidence of a state effect. In contrast to these studies are those that found that the prevalence of PDs sharply declines when patients are reevaluated after symptom improvement. This is discussed in greater detail below.

To understand fully the effect of changing state on diagnostic reliability, it is first necessary to obtain estimates of joint-interview reliability and test-retest reliability in situations where there is no change in the patient's current mental state. Reliability estimates under these conditions will provide upper bounds to the reliability coefficients that are obtained under more rigorous testing situations, such as when psychiatric state also changes. In the study by O'Boyle and Self,[38] the joint-interview reliability coefficients for the presence or absence of any PD were .74 and .63 for the SCID-II and PDE, respectively. It is therefore somewhat encouraging that the test-retest reliability for the SCID-II in depressed patients whose depression significantly improved was as high as .65. In the study by Loranger et al,[39] the joint-interview reliability coefficients were .80 at the initial interview and .83 for the repeated interview. The κ coefficients in the study by Pilkonis et al[49] were nearly identical (.79 and .84, respectively). Since short-interval (eg, <1 week) test-retest reliability coefficients would be lower than joint-interview coefficients, perhaps long-interval test-retest κ values that coincide with a change in psychiatric state should not be expected to be much higher than .5 to .6. Whether the test-retest reliability of PD is a function of the length of the retest interval has not been studied directly.

The falloff in reliability from a joint-interview to a brief-interval test-retest to a long-interval test-retest design may vary by PD. The reliability of antisocial PD seems to be relatively independent of study design (Table 5). The unweighted mean κ across the seven studies of joint-interview reliability was .77. In the three brief-interval test-retest reliability studies of interviews, it was also .77. In the only test-retest study that coincided with a change in state, κ was equal to .84,[40] and across the six diagnostic stability studies, the mean κ was .69.[69,70,73,75-77] The reliability of paranoid PD also is stable across study design (Table 5). In contrast, the reliability of all of the remaining disorders, except compulsive PD, drops from the joint-interval to the short-interval test-retest to the long-interval test-retest studies.

The follow-up studies of borderline PD suggest that diagnostic stability is related to the length of the follow-up interval. However, some caution is warranted in interpreting the findings from these studies. Patients whose conditions are diagnosed according to retrospective chart review are likely to be prototypic examples of the PD. Conditions of patients with a clinically diagnosed PD usually are similarly diagnosed on research assessments, but the reverse is frequently not true. Thus, patients whose conditions are diagnosed according to chart review may be at the most pathologic end of the spectrum. A similar bias may operate in studies of severely character-disordered samples. The patients in the sample of Barasch et al[43] were chosen because of their high degree of personality pathology.

Before concluding this section on the reliability of Axis II, I wish to highlight the potential importance of sample selection. Diagnostic reliability is related to prototypicality, ie, the more criteria met on the initial interview, the more likely the patient will again score above the diagnostic threshold on retesting. Both Helzer et al[76] and Martin et al[70] commented that individuals whose conditions are unreliably diagnosed tended to have threshold levels of symptoms. Vandiver and Sher[77] empirically demonstrated this phenomenon. They found that the antisocial individuals whose conditions were reliably diagnosed averaged one to two more antisocial criteria than the inconsistently diagnosed cases. Analogously, in their study of the concordance between the PDE and SCID-II, Skodol and colleagues[79] found that the paranoid PD dimensional score was highest for patients who were diagnosed as having paranoid PD on both measures, lowest for patients who were diagnosed as not having paranoid PD on both measures, and in the middle of these extremes for patients diagnosed as having paranoid PD on only one of the two interviews. Robins et al[80] looked at this phenomenon from a different perspective. They subdivided patients who did not meet criteria for antisocial PD according to a psychiatrist's interview into those with no or only one antisocial feature vs those with more than one feature. They found that reliability was higher in the clear-cut noncases (none or one feature) than the threshold noncases (two or more features) (.51 vs .78). (A similar analysis based on a subdivision of the positive cases into clear-cut and threshold cases was not done because there were too few cases.) In light of these data, studies of reliability using severely character-disordered samples, or patients with significant personality pathology presenting for long-term psychodynamic therapy, may achieve higher reliability than studies of patients who are consecutively admitted to a tertiary care center or general hospital unit or who are consecutively presenting to an outpatient clinic, because the character-disordered patients are more likely to be prototypic cases.

THE WHO, WHAT, AND WHEN OF PD ASSESSMENT

Who Should Be Questioned?

Who should be questioned in assessing PDs—the patient or someone who knows the patient well?

Clinical evaluations of psychiatric patients are frequently based on multiple sources of information. The clinician generally judges the reliability of the patient as a historian and, depending on the patient's mental status and apparent forthrightness, uses collaterals as either the primary or secondary source. The evaluation of PDs, however, presents special problems that may require the routine use of informants. In contrast to the symptoms of major Axis I disorders, the defining features of PDs are based on an extended longitudinal perspective of how individuals act in different situations, how they perceive and interact with a constantly changing environment, and the perceived reasonableness of their behaviors and cognitions. Only a minority of the PD criteria are discrete, easily enumerated behaviors. For *any* individual to describe validly his or her normal personality, he or she must be somewhat introspective and aware of the effect his or her attitudes and behaviors have on himself or herself and others. This task is more formidable for acutely ill psychiatric patients because state effects color their perceptions of their usual personality.

Tyrer and colleagues[81] interviewed 15 outpatients (11 with depressed neurosis and four with anxiety neurosis) and their corresponding informants and found very poor agreement in their ratings of 24 personality factors. Of interest, informant-based ratings were significantly higher on three of the 24 scales. In a study of 11 patients with obsessive-compulsive disorder, patients and informants completed the PDQ, and the diagnostic frequencies were higher according to the informant ratings.[82] In the study by Dowson[83,84] of 60 psychiatric patients who were considered by their primary clinicians to have significant PD pathology, there was poor correspondence between the patients' and their informants' responses on the PDQ (all κ values, $\leq .40$). In the largest study to date, Zimmerman et al[85] made *DSM-III* PD diagnoses in 66 depressed inpatients based on independent SIDP interviews of the patient and a close informant. The level of agreement between the two sources of information was poor (any PD, $\kappa = .13$; for all individual PDs, $\kappa < .35$), and informants reported more pathology—PDs were diagnosed in 57.6% of the patients based on the informant interview and in 36.4% based on the patient interview. Importantly, the two raters in this study had previously demonstrated high test-retest interrater reliability with each other ($\kappa = .80$); therefore, the poor agreement between patient and informant interviews could not be attributed to rater variance.

In three of the four studies, more personality pathology was elicited from the informant. This should be considered in the context of the self-administered personality questionnaire literature, in which studies consistently find evidence that patients overreport pathology when they are acutely ill. In fact, some researchers have recommended that only informants be used because the bias due to psychiatric state invalidates patient reports.[62,81]

There are several possible reasons why informants may describe more pathology than patients. Perhaps patients are better able to distinguish their normal personality from their episodic Axis I disorder. In our study of acutely ill depressed inpatients,[85] we found that many of the features reported significantly more often by informants reflected aspects of depressive disorder (eg, low self-esteem, lack of self-confidence, overreaction to minor events, hypersensitivity to criticism, social anxiety, seeking of reassurance, and lacking a sense of humor). Thus, the patient's depressed state may have had a greater bias on the informant's perception. Alternatively, the patient may be describing an idealized usual self-personality, and the informant's report is a more accurate description of the patient's normal personality. Even patients with chronic depressions have brief periods when they are feeling and functioning better, and these atypical intervals may be viewed by the patient as their "normal" baseline. A third possibility is that patients may lack insight into the effect their behavior has on others, or even that certain behaviors are characteristic of them. Individuals may not realize that they do not accept blame, that they look for hidden meanings, or that they are stubborn and insistent that things be done their way. Finally, one cannot rule out the possibility that patients lie and deny negative attributes (although we found that antisocial behaviors, perhaps the most socially undesirable features, were reported equally frequently by patients and informants).

So, who should be interviewed? That is, which source of information is the more valid one? Or, should the patient and an informant both be questioned? As noted above, agreement between the two information sources is generally poor. If two descriptions of a patient's personality are to be obtained, a method of combining information from discrepant reports is needed. We have always relied on our "best clinical judgment." Admittedly, this is a vague and unsatisfying description of our research methods. However, despite our failure to develop operational guidelines for resolving contradictory information, we found that the reliability of PD assessment was as high based on two sources of information as compared with that based on the patient interview alone.[86]

Regarding validity, we compared the validities of the patient and informant interviews in our 66 depressed patients, and the results were inconclusive.[87] The predicted demographic, psychosocial, family history, and outcome differences between depressed patients with and without a PD were greater when the diagnoses were based on the patient interview alone. However, subtyping based on the informant interview was also valid.

There are insufficient data to recommend one source of information over the other, or whether it is cost-effective to interview both patients and informants. It is likely that for some characteristics (eg, affective, cognitive), patients must be interviewed, whereas for others (eg, interpersonal, behavioral), informants may be more appropriate. In the psychology literature, studies of normal personality and emotional traits have demonstrated that the magnitude of self-other correlations is affected by the reliability of observer ratings, the visibility of the behavior or trait, and how well the informant knows the individual.[88-91] Traits that are more overt and visible are more reliably rated, and the self-other correlation is higher. Greater acquaintanceship between the informant and individual is also associated with higher self-other correlations.[88] This type of research has not yet been conducted in the PD field.

What Instrument Should Be Used?

What type of measure should be used—an interview or a questionnaire? And after this is decided, which of the five interviews and eight questionnaires should be chosen? For that matter, does it make a difference? Do the different measures tend to diagnose patients similarly, or are there major discrepancies between them? There are several recent reviews that describe in detail the development and characteristics of the instruments used to make PD diagnoses, and the reader is referred to these reviews for a more complete discussion of the individual measures.[42,92-96] From these reviews, and my overall literature review, I have identified nine features that distinguish the measures:

Coverage. Some measures assess only one or two PDs,[97-102] whereas others cover all of the *DSM-III-R* disorders.[2-14] The International PDE,[27] used in the World Health Organization–sponsored international cross-cultural study of PDs, covers *DSM-III-R* and the *International Classification of Diseases, 10th Revision.*

Correspondence to *DSM-III-R*. Many instruments measure PD constructs that are related, but not identical, to those of the *DSM-III-R* criteria. For example, the DIB of Gunderson et al[97] was developed before the publication of the *DSM-III/DSM-III-R* criteria, and its content overlaps with, but does not fully correspond to, these criteria. Consequently, some DIB-positive cases do not meet the *DSM* criteria, and some DIB-negative cases do.[103-107] The correspondence of the MCMI to *DSM-III/DSM-III-R* has been the subject of debate.[108-111] In contrast, other measures, such as the PDE, SCID-II, DIPD, PDQ, and SIDP, were explicitly developed to assess the *DSM* criteria.

Method of Administration. Both self-administered questionnaires and semistructured interviews have been developed and are in common use. Unique to the SCID-II is the concurrent use of a screening questionnaire that is completed by the respondent and reviewed by the interviewer before the interview. The interviewer only inquires about criteria that are endorsed on the questionnaire; thus, the length of the interview is shortened. To date, there is one published study of the screening ability of this questionnaire, and the results are encouraging.[112]

Interviewer Requirements. The recommended clinical experience required for interviewer competence greatly varies. The Personality Interview Questionnaire was designed for use by lay interviewers, thereby minimizing the effect of preconceived clinical prejudices at the price of losing the benefits of clinical experience and judgment.[5] At the other end of the experience spectrum, the PDE was designed for use by experienced psychiatrists, clinical psychologists, or other professionals with comparable training. The PDE manual[3] explicitly states that it should not be used by research assistants, nurses, students, or clinicians early in their training. The authors of the SIDP recommend an intermediate level of experience, ie, an undergraduate degree in the social sciences, at least 6 months' experience in interviewing psychiatric patients, and about 1 month of specific training in using the SIDP.

Organization. The questions in the SIDP and PDE are grouped into thematically organized sections, such as interpersonal relationships, emotions, etc. In contrast, the SCID-II, DIPD, and PDQ are organized by diagnosis. Each approach has its respective advantages. A topically oriented interview is smoother and less redundant, and should facilitate rapport between the subject and interviewer. In addition, it is less prone to halo effects in which ratings of individual criteria are influenced by how close the individual is to meeting the criteria for the disorder, or ratings of certain disorders are influenced by whether criteria for other disorders are already met. Because the bias of halo effects is minimized, thematically organized instruments are more appropriate for studies of comorbidity. The developers of the SCID-II suggested that a diagnosis-organized interview corresponds more closely to the clinical interview format. It can be argued that it is appropriate for the interviewer to be aware of how close an individual is to meeting the diagnostic criteria because the depth of probing *should* increase for threshold cases. This is not possible with thematically organized measures. Diagnosis-oriented interviews can be shortened by omitting questions of all of the criteria after it is determined that the diagnosis cannot be present, though studies of the convergent and discriminant validity of individual criteria would be compromised. In addition, abbreviated interviews cannot be used to determine dimensional scores.

Time Frame. On the PDQ, the respondent is instructed to consider the "past several years." The DIPD evaluates attitudes and behaviors for the 2 years before the interview, the SCID-II and the PDE for the past 5 years, whereas the SIDP focuses on the individual's "usual self," and if there is a dramatic recent change in the individual's personality, then the functioning that predominated for the greatest amount of time during the past 5 years is considered typical. On the PDE, the interviewer also inquires about the age of onset of pathologic attitudes and behavior, and at least one criterion must be present before the age of 25 years to make a PD diagnosis. Thus, the PDE emphasizes persistence and early onset more than the other measures, and it is most concordant with the *DSM-III/DSM-III-R* definition of a PD.

Rating Guidelines. The PDE is the only interview that is accompanied by a detailed item-by-item scoring manual. The items are scored from 0 through 2 with descriptors provided for each severity level. The SIDP items are also scored from 0 through 2 with accompanying anchor point descriptions. In contrast, the SCID-II interviewer rates whether the item is absent, subthreshold, or present at the threshold level, and there are general guidelines for distinguishing subthreshold and threshold severity levels. The DIPD ratings follow the same format as that of the SCID-II.

Scoring. On the SIDP, several criteria are listed at the end of each section, and their ratings are based on the responses to all of the questions in the section, though specific questions are identified as corresponding most closely to specific criteria. On the other interviews, the questions used to rate each criterion are listed immediately below or to the side of the item.

Content. The above eight characteristics of PD measures primarily refer to the structural and procedural aspects of the instruments. A ninth difference between the measures is in their content. That is, different questions are used to assess the same criteria. This is illustrated in **Table 6** with a listing of the questions from the SIDP, PDE, and the items from the PDQ to evaluate selected *DSM-III-R* PD criteria. The questions are sufficiently different so that it cannot be assumed that individuals who are rated positive on one measure will be positive on the others.

A study of the comparability of two different interviews is technically difficult. It requires independent administration of the measures so that the results of one do not influence the other. Thus, at least two raters who are trained to conduct both interviews are needed. These raters must demonstrate high levels of test-retest reliability with each measure; otherwise, interinstrument diagnostic discordance might be due to rater variance. As summarized above, these measures have only modest short-interval test-retest reliability. It is therefore not surprising that the only studies comparing two different interviews found generally poor-fair agreement.[38,79,113,114] In the largest study, Skodol and colleagues[79] interviewed 100 applicants for long-term inpatient treatment of personality pathology with the SCID-II and PDE. The mean κ for the 11 *DSM-III-R* PDs was .45, and only dependent PD achieved a κ above .60. (Although it is beyond the scope of this review to discuss in detail the literature on Axis I assessment, it should be noted that the agreement between different diagnostic interviews for major Axis I disorders is no better than the agreement for Axis II.[115-117])

Comparisons of interviews and self-report questionnaires are more frequent. Hyler et al[113] included the PDQ-Revised (PDQ-R) in their study of the PDE and SCID-II, and they found poor agreement between the questionnaire and both of the interviews (PDQ-R–SCID-II, mean κ=.41; PDQ-R–PDE, mean κ=.36). In a replication study with 59 outpatients with less severe personality pathology, the agreement was even poorer (PDQ-R–SCID-II, mean κ=.34; PDQ-R–PDE, mean κ=.27). In a study of 40 outpatients with panic disorder, social phobia, or obsessive-compulsive disorder, Hunt and Andrews[118] found that 7.5% had a PD according to the PDE and 67.5% had a PDQ-R diagnosis. Because of the wide disparity in prevalences, and the low rate of PD on the PDE, they did not compute agreement coefficients. Hogg et al[119] interviewed 40 recent-onset schizophrenics with the SIDP and found poor agreement with MCMI diagnoses (all κ values, <.35), and Reich et al[120] found poor agreement among the SIDP, PDQ, and MCMI in a sample of psychiatric outpatients. Jackson et al[121] Torgersen and Alnaes,[122] and Nazikian et al[123] found poor agreement between the SIDP and MCMI, and Renneberg et al[28] found low concordance between the SCID-II and MCMI.

The poor agreement between self-report and interview measures extends to nonpatient samples. Zimmerman and Coryell[124] reported poor diagnostic concordance between the SIDP and PDQ in 696 relatives of psychiatric patients and healthy controls. We also conducted detailed item analyses and concluded that the lack of agreement between the measures was largely due to differences in content. The PDQ includes items that are reverse-scored (ie, a response of "no" indicates pathology) to reduce the effect of a yea-saying/nay-saying response set. However, comments in the side margins of the PDQ form suggested that respondents were confused by these questions. For example, several subjects wrote that they never threatened suicide, and simultaneously they answered no to the question: "I have never threatened to kill myself." In addition to the problems due to negatively worded items, some reverse-scored PDQ items did not ac-

Table 6. Assessment of Selected *DSM-III-R* PD Criteria by the SIDP, PDE, and PDQ*

Criterion	SIDP	PDE	PDQ
Schizoid, item 2: almost always chooses solitary activities	1. What kinds of activities do you usually enjoy? (If solitary): Are there any activities you enjoy doing with others?	1. Do you almost always choose the kind of activities that you can do all by yourself rather than with other people? (If yes): Give me some examples.	1. I enjoy myself most when I'm with other people.
Passive-aggressive, item 1: procrastinates, ie, puts off things that need to be done so that deadlines are not met	1. There is a saying, "Never put off 'til tomorrow what you can do today." Are you the kind of person who puts things off? (If yes): Do you put things off because you are irritated with being asked to do them? What problems does this cause? Do you miss deadlines because of procrastinating?	1. When there is something that you're expected to do but you would rather not do, do you usually put it off until the last minute, so that it doesn't get done on time? (If yes): Tell me about it.	1. I procrastinate so much that I have trouble meeting deadlines.
Narcissistic, item 2: is interpersonally exploitative, takes advantage of others to achieve his or her own ends	1. Some successful people have commented privately that the world is a jungle, and that to survive, you must be tough, even if it means occasionally stepping on some other people. Are there any examples in your own life that show this to be true? 2. Have you ever wanted something so badly that you misled someone about what they could expect from you? (If yes): How often have experiences like that happened? How do you feel afterwards?	1. Some people are skillful at using others or taking advantage of them to get what they want. Are you able to do that? (If yes): Give me some examples. (If no): Have you been told that you are? (If yes): Why do you think people have said that? 2. Do you ever find yourself losing interest in people after they've served their purpose? (If yes): Tell me about it.	1. When I'm involved with people I use them. 2. Some people think I take advantage of others.
Narcissistic, item 5: is preoccupied with fantasies of unlimited success, power, brilliance, beauty, or ideal love	1. When people imagine what their life would be like if they could have anything they want, they may think of such things as power, success, brilliance, or beauty. What do you daydream about? If you were to add it all up, how much time would you spend thinking about these things in a typical day? # Hours _________. Has this ever caused problems at home or work?	1. Do you daydream a lot about being successful, powerful, brilliant, or famous? (If yes): Do those daydreams prevent you from concentrating or accomplishing things, or make you feel like a failure? (If yes): Tell me about it. 2. Do you daydream a lot about having an ideal love affair or a storybook romance? (If yes): Do those daydreams prevent you from concentrating or accomplishing things, or make you feel like a failure? (If yes): Tell me about it. 3. Do you daydream a lot about being very beautiful (handsome)? (If yes): Do those daydreams prevent you from concentrating or accomplishing things, or make you feel like a failure? (If yes): Tell me about it.	3. I often find myself thinking about how great a person I am, or will be.
Histrionic, item 4: expresses emotion with inappropriate exaggeration	1. Some people are very expressive. They cry at weddings, embrace people, show their fear and their joy. Would you say you are more or less likely than most people to show your emotions? (If more): Has this ever caused you problems or embarrassment? 2. Has anyone ever said anything about how you show your emotions? (If yes): What did they say? Do you agree?	1. Do you almost always show your feelings in a very obvious way for others to see? (If yes): Do you ever get carried away and exaggerate the way you feel? (If yes): Give me some examples. 2. Have people told you that you're dramatic or theatrical? (If yes): Why do you think they've said that?	1. I often act very emotionally when little things go wrong. 2. If I don't get my way I get angry and behave childishly.

(continued)

curately reflect the *DSM-III* criteria. For example, responding no to "I find it easy to relax" or "I am usually self-confident" is not the same as responding yes to "I find it difficult to relax" or "I usually lack self-confidence."

In both patient and nonpatient samples, the questionnaires tend to overdiagnose PDs. In the initial study of Hyler et al,[113] for each of the PDs, the PDQ-R prevalence rate was higher than the PDE or SCID-II rates (and many of these differences were quite large, eg, avoidant [24% vs 1%] and passive-aggressive [31% vs 7%]). In their replication study[125] of less severely personality-disordered outpatients, the results were the same (and again the prevalence of PDs was sometimes markedly higher on the PDQ-R, eg, paranoid [39% vs 3%], histrionic

Table 6. Assessment of Selected *DSM-III-R* PD Criteria by the SIDP, PDE, and PDQ* (cont)

Criterion	SIDP	PDE	PDQ
Histrionic, item 7: is self-centered, actions being directed toward obtaining immediate satisfaction; has no tolerance for the frustration of delayed gratification	1. Has anyone ever accused you of only thinking of yourself? (If yes): What caused them to say that? 2. Do you see yourself as self-centered? (If yes): What kinds of problems has this caused? 3. Do you frequently insist on having what you want right now, even when waiting a little longer would get you something much better? Do you find it hard to keep working for long-term goals? 4. Do you get irritable if you have to stand in line to get into a movie or event that you are anxious to see? Do you ever try to get in without waiting? (If yes): What do you do? 5. How do you react when someone refuses to do a favor for you? (If reacts negatively): Does this happen often? (If has not happened): How do you think you would react?	1. When there's something you really want, do you try to get it right away? (If yes): Do you ever feel very frustrated or angry when you don't get what you want right away? (If yes): When that happens does it ever cause problems for you or for others? (If yes): Give me some examples.	1. People say that I'm self-centered. 2. I have great difficulty delaying gratification.
Dependent, item 1: is unable to make everyday decisions without an excessive amount of advice or reassurance from others	1. Some people enjoy making decisions and other people prefer to have someone they trust tell them what to do. Which do you prefer? (If someone else): Do you often check with someone else about everyday decisions like what to have for lunch or what clothes to buy?	1. Are you usually able to make ordinary, everyday decisions without turning to others for advice or reassurance? (If no): Give me some examples.	1. I would rather make my own decisions than rely on the advice of others.
Borderline, item 8: frantic efforts to avoid real or imagined abandonment (do not include suicidal or self-mutilating behavior)	1. Are you concerned that people you depend on might leave you? (If yes): Are there times when you can't stop thinking about this? (If yes): How often does this happen? What do you do to keep them from leaving?	1. Do you ever find yourself frantically trying to do something to stop someone close to you from abandoning you? (If yes): Give me some examples.	1. If I know a relationship is going to end I'll let it end peacefully.

**For explanation of abbreviations, see first footnote to Table 1.*

[37% vs 7%], and narcissistic [32% vs 5%]). In a series of studies of patients with panic disorder and major depression, Reich and Noyes[126] reported much higher PD rates on the MCMI and PDQ than on the SIDP. Some of the MCMI prevalence rates seem particularly excessive. In a sample of putative healthy controls, 42.5% were judged to have a PD.[127] In a separate study of relatives of psychiatric outpatients, Reich[128] found that 54.9% had an MCMI PD diagnosis in comparison with 18.2% based on the SIDP and 20.4% based on the PDQ. And, as noted above, Hunt and Andrews[118] found that anxious outpatients were nine times more frequently diagnosed as having a PD on the PDQ than on the PDE.

The overdiagnoses of PD by questionnaire is not necessarily a condemning feature because the instrument may be useful in screening for pathology (rather than diagnosing it). In both studies by Hyler et al,[113,125] the PDQ could not substitute for structured interviews because of its tendency to overdiagnose PDs; however, its high sensitivity and moderate specificity for most of the disorders made it potentially useful as a screening instrument. Compared with the findings of Hyler et al,[113,125] Dubro et al[129] found the PDQ had lower sensitivity and higher specificity (using SIDP diagnoses as the standard). Dubro et al[129] also examined the diagnostic efficiency of the MCMI and Minnesota Multiphasic Personality Inventory PD scales, and they found that no measure distinguished itself as superior to the others across all of the PDs. Other studies of the MCMI have noted its limited utility as a screening measure because of its high false-positive rate.[130-132]

So, WHICH measure should be used? Intuitively, one would expect interviews to be more valid than self-administered questionnaires. On interviews, questions can be clarified, examples of pathology can be elicited, positive responses can be followed up to verify that the pathology was not situation or state specific but instead characteristic of long-term functioning, and the rater has the respondent's demeanor and presentation during the interview as available data. However, there is a long tradition in personality research of using paper-and-pencil questionnaires to evaluate normal and abnormal personality characteristics, and it is reasonable to assume that this method can be applied to the *DSM* PD constructs. Aside from tradition, and their low cost, an advantage of self-report scales is that they are free from systematic biases and tendencies of interviewers. A vexing problem in the *DSM-III/DSM-III-R* era of specified inclusion and exclusion diagnostic criteria is the differential application of these criteria.[133-136] In a review of the literature on the frequency of PDs in patients with major depressive disorder (MDD), the variation in rates was nearly as wide as is possible, ranging from a low of 9.3% to a high of 100%.[137] Part of the variability could be ascribed to overt methodologic factors (eg, chart review vs clinical evaluations vs questionnaire vs standardized interview). However, even in studies that used essentially the same method, the rates varied greatly. For example, using the SIDP, we found that 40% to 50% of individuals with MDD had a PD,[137] whereas Alnaes and Torgersen[138] reported a rate of 85%. Why is there a twofold difference? True sample differences may exist, or there may have been systematic differences in the use of the instrument or interpretation of the criteria. As described elsewhere, self-report scales could be useful in detecting systematic differences in diagnostic practices between centers.[136]

Studies of the MCMI suggest that it overdiagnoses PD to too great an extent to be useful as either a diagnostic or screening measure. The developers of the PDQ have concluded that it has more utility as a screening than as a diagnostic instrument. In our studies of the PDQ, we have noted some problems with the wording of some items, and in my opinion, some of the diagnostic criteria are not adequately assessed by the PDQ items (see Table 6). The other self-report scales[10-14] have not yet received much study.

Of the five interviews, only three (SIDP, SCID-II, PDE) have been used in published studies by researchers outside of the center in which they were developed. These three measures have generally similar reliabilities (Tables 1 through 3). Comparative studies of their validities are almost nonexistent and, as suggested above, are likely to remain few in number because of the practical difficulties in conducting such studies.

In fact, the conceptual basis for studying the validity of PD measures is itself an unsettled topic. Spitzer[139] suggested that newly developed diagnostic measures be validated against expert clinical diagnoses that are based on a longitudinal evaluation encompassing multiple sources of data (ie, a LEAD standard). Two research groups used this strategy to validate PD instruments.[49,79] A major problem with the LEAD standard in PD research, though, is that the reliability of clinically based PD diagnoses is poor.[46,48,49,140] The reason for developing standardized PD interviews was to improve on the poor interrater diagnostic reliability of unstructured clinical evaluations. If clinicians cannot reliably diagnose PD, their diagnoses cannot serve as a standard of comparison. The poor concordance between LEAD and semistructured diagnostic interview–based diagnoses may be due to the poor reliability of the LEAD diagnoses, or it may be due to validity problems with the instrument. Skodol et al[79] acknowledged this interpretative problem and indicated that a reliability study of their LEAD standard was ongoing.

The validity of instruments diagnosing PDs needs to be examined in terms of the predicted correlates of the PD construct. However, the associated features described in the *DSM-III* and *DSM-III-R* text are not based on studies of the specified operational criteria; rather, they are derived from rich clinical descriptions of the phenomena, studies of non–criteria-based clinical diagnoses, and studies of self-report scales of the personality dimensions. Thus, it remains to be demonstrated that the operational criteria proposed in the *DSM-III* and *DSM-III-R* are themselves valid, and researchers of PDs are therefore faced with the dual task of validating instruments as well as validating the diagnostic criteria. Because of this, negative studies are difficult to interpret—do they indicate that the criteria are invalid or that the instrument fails to measure validly the criteria?

This dilemma was not faced by the developers of instruments evaluating Axis I disorders. Axis I diagnoses are primarily based on the signs and symptoms presented in the evaluation or occurring in the recent past. Measures such as the SADS and SCID essentially standardize the unstructured clinical interview, and thus improve the reliability and comprehensiveness of the diagnostic process.

In contrast to Axis I disorders, PDs represent stable, long-term, maladaptive characteristics based on how individuals act in different situations, on how they perceive and interact with the environment, and on the reasonableness of their behaviors and attitudes. It is unknown whether relatively brief 1½- to 2-hour interviews, or self-report scales, are capable of validly evaluating long-standing personality traits and associated problems. Thus, the issue of face validity, which is more or less taken for granted in designing instruments to evaluate Axis I disorders, cannot be likewise assumed to exist for Axis II measures because the criteria for Axis II disorders are more inferential than those for Axis I syndromes. This difficulty is reflected in the different questions on independently developed instruments to assess the same criteria (Table 6).

Despite these caveats, returning to the question of which measure to use, at present, the only reasonable recommendation is to use any of the interviews already in common use, and to also use a self-administered questionnaire to serve as a *paper standard* with which interviewer-derived diagnoses can be compared.[136]

When Should the Assessment Be Done?

When should personality evaluations be done? Assessing PDs soon after presentation for treatment may result in inflated estimates of morbidity. However, this is the time when treatment decisions are usually made, and if PD assessments are to have treatment implications, they should be made at this early date. For many Axis I disorders, the presence of a comorbid PD has unfavorable prognostic significance.[141] Thus, if symptom abatement was a prerequisite for PD assessment, then the sample would be biased toward including individuals without personality pathology. Several studies have administered PD measures before and after treatment to determine the effect of state on PD evaluation. Before considering these studies, it is first necessary to discuss briefly a possible confound of studies using multiple evaluations—*the retest artifact.* A basic assumption of studies measuring a variable on more than one occasion is that all measurements are of comparable validity. However, in studies using repeated evaluations, there is evidence that less pathology is reported on retest.[142,143] Proposed explanations for this phenomenon include (1) respondents realize that symptom denial shortens the interview, and therefore, they attempt to abbreviate the second interview by denying symptoms; (2) respondents have a greater need to present themselves more favorably on retest; (3) respondents are bored, disinterested, and less motivated the second time around; and (4) respondents do not fully understand the purpose of the retest and assume that the second interview is meant to supplement the first, and therefore, they do not report pathology previously described.[39,143-146]

The empiric literature demonstrating a retest artifact for Axis I disorders is mixed. Bromet et al[146] interviewed 391 women with the SADS two times, at 18 months apart, and the lifetime prevalence of MDD dropped from 29.4% for the first interview to 21.5% for the second. Of the 89 individuals whose conditions were diagnosed inconsistently on the two interviews, two thirds met criteria for MDD at the first interview only, and one third met criteria only at the second interview. In the Epidemiologic Catchment Area Study, lay interviewers administered the DIS at 1 year after their initial interview. Helzer and colleagues[147] noted that the lifetime prevalence rates were lower at the retest; however, they did not test statistically the difference in prevalence rates. In their comparison of lay interviewers' and psychiatrists' administrations of the DIS, no disorder was diagnosed significantly less frequently on retest. Interpretation of this nonsignificant finding was compromised by the study's methods—the psychiatrist always did the second interview, and the greater prestige of this second rater may have offset the retest artifact. However, in the test-retest study of the Spanish DIS by Burnam et al,[148] in which lay interviewers administered the DIS on both occasions, there was no significant retest bias. Other studies have found evidence of the retest artifact for one or two of the many disorders examined, or that the mean number of symptoms reported was lower on the second than on the initial interview.[77,149,150] However, many test-retest studies of Axis I disorders have failed to find evidence of a significant retest artifact.[148,151-155]

Turning to studies of Axis II, Loranger et al[39] suggested that the retest bias may have been responsible for the small, albeit significant reduction in the mean dimensional score for 10 of the 12 PDs. To explore this issue further, I used the raw data presented in the test-retest reliability studies by Stangl et al[30] and Zanarini et al[6] to compute McNemar's χ^2, which tests for bias. No disorder in either study was diagnosed significantly less frequently at the second interview. In the study by Stangl et al,[30] somewhat more patients had a PD at the retest (65% vs 70%), and across all 20 patients, more diagnoses were given (20 vs 26). These trends were reversed in the study by Zanarini et al[6] (83.3% vs 77.8%; 128 vs 113).

To summarize, if a retest artifact biases diagnostic reevaluations, it is neither a large nor a consistent effect. Consequently, in studies that demonstrate a significant decrement in personality pathology in patients who were retested after Axis I symptom resolution, this is likely to represent a state effect rather than retest artifact. However, this conclusion is limited to studies using diagnostic interviews, and may not be generalizable to self-report questionnaires. Self-report scales have generally not been used to make lifetime diagnoses, their susceptibility to a retest artifact is unknown, and the findings from studies administering the MCMI or PDQ to patients before and after symptom resolution should be interpreted more cautiously.

Compared with pretreatment evaluations, less personality pathology is reported on self-report scales after treatment. Two studies of the MCMI in depressed patients found that the frequency of PD diagnoses was dramatically higher when the scale was completed while the patients were acutely depressed.[156,157] Kennedy et al[158] found similar results in patients with eating disorders, and they also noted that changes in the MCMI scores between admission and discharge were significantly correlated with changes on the BDI. In the only study of the revised MCMI, ie, the MCMI-II, Stankovic et al[159] found that the depressed state had only a modest biasing effect. In their study of 43 depressed outpatients, there were no significant changes in the prevalences of any of the PDs from pretreatment to posttreatment, and only four-dimensional scale scores were significantly lower after treatment. Mavissakalian and colleagues[160,161] reported similar results with the PDQ in patients with agoraphobia and obsessive-compulsive disorder, though the magnitude of the pretreatment-posttreatment changes were not as great as in the studies of the MCMI.

There are seven studies assessing PDs with interviews before and after treatment. Gartner et al[162] interviewed 27 patients who had eating disorders with the PDE within 1 week of hospital admission and shortly before discharge. A similar number of patients had at least one PD at both times (57.1% vs 55.5%), though there was a significant decrease in the total number of criteria met. Ames-Frankel et al[37] administered the PDE to 30 bulimic outpatients who were treated with desipramine or placebo for 6 weeks. Similar to the results found by Gartner et al,[162] the total number of patients with at least one PD did not change (30% vs 27%), though the overall number of PD diagnoses in the sample decreased from 27 at the first interview to 16 at the second. For those patients with a PD, the mean number of PDs dropped from 3.0 to 2.0, and eight of the 12 PD dimensional scores were significantly lower on retest. Of note, there were significant correlations between improvement in the eating disorder and reduction in cluster A and cluster B dimensional scores. O'Boyle and Self[38] administered both the PDE and SCID-II to 17 depressed patients during the acute and recovery phases, and they found no change in the prevalence of PDs on either measure, though two of the 12 PDE dimensional scores significantly decreased. Loranger et al[39] found a significant decrease on all but the schizoid and antisocial dimensional scores at retest; however, the reductions were not a function of changes in depression or anxiety symptom levels, and there was no change in diagnostic frequencies. Ricciardi et al[163] readministered the SIDP to 17 patients with obsessive-compulsive disorder and a comorbid PD after 4 months of treatment and found that one of the 10 treatment responders, in contrast to five of the seven nonresponders, continued to meet criteria for a PD. Stuart et al[164] reported similar findings in their study of unipolar depressives treated with cognitive therapy. Considering their entire sample, the prevalence of PD decreased from 26.4% (pretreatment) to 9.4% after treatment. Subdividing the sample by treatment response, they found that all three treatment nonresponders with a pretreatment PDE diagnosis were again diagnosed as having a PD after treatment. In contrast, only one of the 11 treatment responders with a pretreatment PD were similarly diagnosed after successful treatment. Finally, Pilkonis et al[49] also found that the overall prevalence of PDE PDs dropped from intake to 6-month follow-up (63% vs 39%) in a sample of patients with MDD. For the entire sample, symptom levels were significantly lower at follow-up; however, they did not examine whether the reduction in personality pathology only occurred in patients with symptom improvement.

Thus, the available data suggest that *both* PD interviews and self-report inventories are susceptible to the overreporting bias due to the acute psychiatric state. All 12 studies found some evidence of a decrement of personality pathology on retest. Moreover, there is evidence that this is not a general phenomenon due to a retest artifact, but instead it reflects a state-biasing effect. In three studies using interviews, "normalization" of personality was associated with Axis I symptom reduction. This was found in patients with obsessive-compulsive disorder,[163] MDD[164] and bulimia.[37] Only Loranger et al[39] failed to find evidence of a state effect, and this may be due to the methodologic differences between this study and the others. The three studies that found a state effect included homogeneous samples with the same Axis I disorder, and symptom improvement reflected a change in the target symptoms (ie, obsessions, compulsions, eating binges, depression). In contrast, the sample described by Loranger et al[39] was heterogeneous with respect to Axis I diagnoses (MDD [n=40], depressive disorder not otherwise specified [n=5], anxiety disorder [n=20], eating disorder [n=17], substance use disorder [n=15], adjustment disorder [n=1], and no Axis I disorder [n=16]). Perhaps a state effect on personality measurement is evident only when there is a change in the primary Axis I pathology. Thus, a reduction in depression or anxiety in patients with eating or substance use disorders may be irrelevant. Consistent with this, Ames-Frankel et al[37] found a significant association between changes in personality scores and eating-related variables, but there was no association with a change in depression scores. Another possible difference between studies may be the level of expertise of the interviewers. Loranger[3] recommended that the PDE be used by "experienced psychiatrists, clinical psychologists, and those with comparable training," and the raters in his study were so experienced. Although all of the raters in the other studies were said to have received extensive training, some were BA degree–level research assistants, one was a masters' degree–level social worker, and the education credentials of the others were not specified. It is possible that the raters in the study by Loranger et al[39] were more skilled, and thus better able to tease apart state and trait when they administered the initial PDE.

WHAT DO YOU DO WHEN PERSONALITY CHANGES?

The *DSM-III* and *DSM-III-R* identify three aspects of the life course of PDs: (1) their first manifestations occur by adolescence, (2) the traits are enduring and characteristic of long-term functioning, and (3) the features (ie, the diagnostic criteria) are characteristic of present functioning. How then do you diagnose PDs when attitudes, behaviors, and cognitive styles change? This occurs frequently in individuals with Axis I disorders whose recent functioning is not characteristic of their "usual personality." The *DSM*s note that a PD diagnosis should not be made when the personality pathology is limited to discrete episodes of illness, and on the SIDP (as well as other interviews), we attempt to disentangle state and trait by frequently reminding the ill patients that the questions refer to their normal selves, not what they are like just when they are ill.

But what if the patient has been chronically or subchronically ill from an Axis I disorder? On the SIDP, we focus on the personality features characteristic of the 5 years before the interview. Thus, we do not assess *premorbid* personality in the strict sense, and this is at variance with how *DSM-III/DSM-III-R* defines a PD. In a 40-year-old woman who has had a major depression for nearly all of the past 10 years, we would focus on functioning during these 10 years. We might, therefore, diagnose a PD in this woman even though the initial manifestations of abnormal personality did not occur during adolescence. In fact, we do not inquire about the onset of personality disturbance. Only the PDE includes specific questions to determine the onset of character pathology.

The reverse may also occur. Individuals, as they age, might modify their maladaptive behaviors and no longer "meet criteria." I can recall several interviews with elderly individuals who reported they "used to act that way." Because I followed our 5-year rule, I did not diagnose a PD in these individuals. Follow-up studies indicate that many individuals may outgrow their personality pathology. The studies summarized above indicated that many patients with borderline PD no longer met diagnostic criteria several years after the initial evaluation.[66-68] Unless the questions on a semistructured interview were reworded to elicit a lifetime history of pathology, these individuals would not be diagnosed as being borderline. The PDE allows for a lifetime diagnosis in individuals who have outgrown their pathology; however, the reliability and validity of these diagnoses have not been studied.

The rules used to diagnose PDs when personality changes have implications for epidemiologic and family studies. The usual approaches to diagnosing PD yield point-prevalence estimates because individuals who were cases only in the past are considered noncases. This is consistent with the *DSM-III-R* suggestion that the PD diagnostic criteria "refer to behaviors or traits that are characteristic of the person's recent (past year) and long-term functioning." However, of the 24 disorders with specified criteria in *DSM-III* and *DSM-III-R*, only the *DSM-III* definition of antisocial PD includes a criterion regarding the continued expression of pathologic behavior. Criterion D was as follows:

> A pattern of continuous antisocial behavior in which the rights of others are violated, with no intervening period of at least five years without antisocial behavior between age 15 and the present time (except when the individual was bedridden or confined in a hospital or penal institution).

This criterion was dropped in *DSM-III-R* for unspecified reasons. In our study of *DSM-III* PDs among 808 relatives of controls and psychiatric patients, we found that when this criterion was suspended, the number of individuals with antisocial PD increased from 26 to 30—a 15% increase.[165] Moreover, the mean age of the four added antisocial individuals was nearly 10 years greater than the mean age of the other 26 (41.0 vs 32.5 years).

So what should be done when personality changes? The answer may depend on the purpose of the assessment. In family and genetic studies, it is important to determine lifetime rates of disorder. Consequently, individuals who no longer meet criteria for a PD diagnosis, whether it is because they develop more adaptive cognitive styles, behaviors, and attitudes as they age, or the physical changes of growing old limit their behavior repertoire of dysfunction, should nonetheless be counted as cases. On the other hand, for clinical purposes, current PD diagnoses are more important, even though there is probably a tendency to confound Axis I and Axis II pathology, with some presumed manifestations of a PD in fact being the result of a (chronic) Axis I disorder. Despite this confound, the diagnosis of a comorbid PD consistently has been found to have prognostic implications, and this has been true across Axis I disorders.[141] The degree to which the chronicity of Axis I pathology confounds the assessment of PDs, and thus is responsible for the prognostic validity of Axis II, has not been adequately addressed.

This issue of changing personality also raises interesting theoretic questions that are not easily answered. Can an Axis I disorder *cause* a PD? That is, can chronic anxiety, depression, or substance use that begins by early adulthood and persists produce a PD? Or should the chronic mood disturbance and substance use be interpreted as manifestations of PD? For that matter, what is "personality" and what is "illness"?

INTERVIEWER TRAINING

After deciding who will serve as the source of information, when to conduct the evaluation, and which instrument to use, if an interview is chosen, it is probably prudent for the raters to be trained in the interview's administration. The interviews provide a standard set of questions and guidelines to interpret the responses; however, additional probes frequently are needed to clarify answers, and the threshold for scoring responses as pathologic often is not clear-cut. Training helps to standardize the diagnostic process further. There is disagreement among scale developers regarding the qualifications necessary to be a skilled interviewer. Widiger et al[5] used trained and supervised college seniors to administer the Personality Interview Questionnaire. In contrast, Loranger[3] emphasized that the PDE should be used by experienced clinicians, and he explicitly cautioned against its use by research assistants, nurses, and medical or graduate students. Our recommended minimum level of experience for SIDP interviewers falls between these extremes—an undergraduate degree in the social sciences and 6 months' experience with interviewing psychiatric patients. The effect of different levels of expertise and experience on Axis II assessment has not been studied.

Unfortunately, even extensive training does not guarantee consistency in interview administration and scoring. Two family studies of healthy controls were conducted at the University of Iowa, using similar recruitment and assessment procedures. Yet, in one study, the rate of PDs was a little less than 15%, and in the other, it was nearly 34%.[166,167] There was a concern that the personality of one of the raters might influence his or her evaluations. We believe that it did because the groups were similar in the rates of Axis I diagnoses based on the fully structured DIS and of Axis II diagnoses based on the self-administered PDQ.[168] It is disconcerting to consider that interviewers' personalities may affect their evaluations. Other interviewer characteristics, such as age, sex, and race, and the interaction between these and patient demographic characteristics might also affect rapport and, thus, data collection. Potentially, this is a major limitation of interviews, and it is likely to account for some failures to replicate original research. Hopefully, as we gain more experience in assessing PDs, we will develop criteria, instruments, and training programs to reduce interviewer variance.

CONCLUSIONS

The evaluation of the Axis II PDs has posed challenges generally not faced in the assessment of major Axis I disorders. In studies of psychosis, mania, depression, anxiety disorders, etc, there is relatively little disagreement about who to interview, when to interview, or even what measure to use. In contrast, there is no consensus as to how to assess the PDs. In the present article, I have reviewed these issues and the data bearing on them. The following conclusions are suggested:

1. The reliability of unstandardized clinical evaluations is poor-fair. Whether clinicians more reliably diagnose particular PDs has only been addressed in one study of *DSM-III*, which found poor reliability in diagnosing all of them.

2. Using standardized interviews, joint-interview interrater reliability is generally good-excellent, at least when the measures are used by their developers. It is unclear if reliability is as good when these instruments are used by independent researchers.

3. Test-retest reliability coefficients are lower than joint-interview values, especially when the interval between the interviews is greater than a couple of weeks or coincides with an improvement in psychiatric state.

4. The effect of study design on reliability (ie, joint-interview vs short-interval test-retest vs long-interval test-retest) probably varies by PD (eg, antisocial PD is less affected than other PDs).

5. Patients and informants differ in their descriptions of patients' usual personality. There are insufficient data examining which source of information is more valid, or whether it is cost-effective to interview both patients and informants.

6. There is variability among PD instruments in terms of the extent of coverage of the *DSM* disorders, correspondence to *DSM-III-R* criteria (ie, face validity), method of administration (self-report vs interview), the recommended level of clinical experience required for interviewer competence, organization of the measure (topically vs diagnostically), the time frame covered, scoring, and guidelines for rating the criteria.

7. A content analysis of three widely used instruments identified sufficient differences between measures so that it cannot be assumed that individuals who are rated positive on one measure will be positive on the others. Consistent with this, studies comparing instruments have found poor diagnostic concordance.

8. Both self-report personality inventories and semistructured interviews are biased by the patient's acute state.

9. The directions for interview administration focus the interviewer on the personality features characteristic of the past few years before the evaluation, thus yielding current, not lifetime, PD diagnoses. When personality changes, this time frame focus can result in overdiagnosing or underdiagnosing PD. That is, PD may be overdiagnosed when the personality pathology, though present for several years, coincides with a chronic or subchronic Axis I disorder. Likewise, PD may be "underdiagnosed" in individuals who, over the years, modified their maladaptive attitudes and behaviors, and no longer meet criteria for the disorder. The problem of overdiagnosis is more relevant to clinical studies, whereas that of underdiagnosis is more relevant to epidemiologic and family studies where the emphasis is on lifetime prevalence rates.

It has been only 8 years since the publication of the first article describing an instrument evaluating the full range of the *DSM-III* PDs[30]; thus, there has been relatively little time to research many questions. During the next decade, we should acquire a greater understanding of the most reliable and valid method to diagnose PDs.

Accepted for publication March 24, 1993.

The author thanks Armand Loranger, PhD, for his comments on an earlier version of the manuscript.

Reprint requests to Medical College of Pennsylvania/Eastern Pennsylvania Psychiatric Institute, 3200 Henry Ave, Philadelphia, PA 19129 (Dr Zimmerman).

REFERENCES

1. Blashfield RK, McElroy RA. The 1985 journal literature on the personality disorders. *Compr Psychiatry.* 1987;28:536-546.
2. Pfohl B, Blum N, Zimmerman M, Stangl D. *Structured Interview for* DSM-III-R *Personality SIDP-R.* Iowa City, Iowa: Department of Psychiatry, University of Iowa; 1989.
3. Loranger AW. *Personality Disorder Examination (PDE) Manual.* Yonkers, NY: DV Communications; 1988.
4. Spitzer RL, Williams JBW, Gibbon M, First M. *User's Guide for the Structured Clinical Interview for* DSM-III-R. Washington, DC: American Psychiatric Association Press; 1990.
5. Widiger TA, Trull TJ, Hurt SW, Clarkin J, Frances A. A multidimensional scaling of the *DSM-III* personality disorders. *Arch Gen Psychiatry.* 1987; 44:557-563.
6. Zanarini MC, Frankenburg FR, Chauncey DL, Gunderson JG. The Diagnostic Interview for Personality Disorders: interrater and test-retest reliability. *Compr Psychiatry.* 1987;28:467-480.
7. Hyler SE, Rieder RD, Williams JBW, Spitzer RL, Hendler J, Lyons M. The Personality Diagnostic Questionnaire: development and preliminary results. *J Pers Disord.* 1988;2:229-237.
8. Millon T. The MCMI provides a good assessment of *DSM-III* disorders: the MCMI-II will prove even better. *J Pers Assess.* 1985;49:379-391.
9. Morey LC, Blashfield RK, Webb WW, Jewell J. MMPI scales for *DSM-III* personality disorders: a preliminary validation study. *J Clin Psychol.* 1988;44:47-50.
10. Clark LA. Toward a consensual set of symptom clusters for assessment of personality disorder. In: Butcher JN, Spielberger CD, eds. *Advances in Personality Assessment.* Hillsdale, NJ: Erlbaum; 1990;8:243-266.
11. Burgess JW. The Personality Inventory Scales: a self-rating clinical instrument for diagnosis of personality disorder. *Psychol Rep.* 1991;69:1235-1246.
12. Coolidge FL, Merwin MM. Reliability and validity of the Coolidge Axis II Inventory: a new inventory for the assessment of personality disorders. *J Pers Assess.* 1992;59:223-238.
13. Morey LC. *Personality Assessment Inventory.* Lutz, Fla: Psychological Assessment Resources; 1991.
14. Klein MH, Benjamin LS, Rosenfeld R, Treece C, Husted J, Greist JH. The Wisconsin Personality Disorders Inventory, I: development, reliability, and validity. *J Pers Disord.* In press.
15. Frances A. Categorical and dimensional systems of personality diagnosis: a comparison. *Compr Psychiatry.* 1982;23:516-527.
16. Widiger TA, Frances A. Axis II personality disorders: diagnostic and treatment issues. *Hosp Community Psychiatry.* 1985;36:619-627.
17. Widiger T, Frances A. The *DSM-III* personality disorders: perspectives from psychology. *Arch Gen Psychiatry.* 1985;42:615-623.
18. Fleiss JL. *Statistical Methods for Rates and Proportions.* 2nd ed. New York, NY: John Wiley & Sons Inc; 1981.
19. Grove WM, Andreasen NC, McDonald-Scott P, Keller MB, Shapiro RW. Reliability studies of psychiatric diagnosis: theory and practice. *Arch Gen Psychiatry.* 1981;38:408-413.
20. Spitznagel EL, Helzer JE. A proposed solution to the base rate problem in the kappa statistic. *Arch Gen Psychiatry.* 1985;42:725-728.
21. Shrout PE, Spitzer RL, Fleiss JL. Quantification of agreement in psychiatric diagnosis revisited. *Arch Gen Psychiatry.* 1987;44:172-177.
22. Arntz A, van Beijsterveldt B, Hoekstra R, Hofman A, Eussen M, Sallaerts S. The interrater reliability of a Dutch version of the Structured Clinical Interview for *DSM-III-R* personality disorders. *Acta Psychiatr Scand.* 1992;85:394-400.
23. Brent DA, Zelenak JP, Bukstein O, Brown RV. Reliability and validity of the Structured Interview for Personality Disorders in adolescents. *J Am Acad Child Adolesc Psychiatry.* 1990;29:349-354.
24. Brooks RB, Baltazar PL, McDowell DE, Munjack DJ, Bruns JR. Personality disorders cooccurring with panic disorder with agoraphobia. *J Pers Disord.* 1991;5:328-336.
25. Jackson HJ, Whiteside HL, Bates GW, Bell R, Rudd RP, Edwards J. Diagnosing personality disorders in psychiatric inpatients. *Acta Psychiatr Scand.* 1991;83:206-213.
26. Loranger AW, Susman VL, Oldham JM, Russakoff LM. The Personality Disorder Examination: a preliminary report. *J Pers Disord.* 1987;1:1-13.
27. Loranger AW. The World Health Organization/Alcohol, Drug Abuse and Mental Health Administration International Pilot Study of Personality Disorders. Presented at the 145th Annual Meeting of the American Psychiatric Association; May 1992; Washington, DC.
28. Renneberg B, Chambless DL, Dowdall DJ, Fauerbach JA, Gracely EJ. The Structured Clinical Interview for *DSM-III-R,* Axis II and the Millon Clinical Multiaxial Inventory: a concurrent validity study of personality disorders among anxious outpatients. *J Pers Disord.* 1992;6:117-124.
29. Standage K, Ladha N. An examination of the reliability of the Personality Disorder Examination and a comparison with other methods of identifying personality disorders in a clinical sample. *J Pers Disord.* 1988;2:267-271.
30. Stangl D, Pfohl B, Zimmerman M, Bowers W, Corenthal C. A structured interview for the *DSM-III* personality disorders: a preliminary report. *Arch Gen Psychiatry.* 1985;42:591-596.
31. Stanley MA, Turner SM, Borden JW. Schizotypal features in obsessive-compulsive disorder. *Compr Psychiatry.* 1990;31:511-518.
32. Widiger TA, Freiman K, Bailey B. Convergent and discriminant validity of personality disorder prototypic acts. *Psychol Assess J Consult Clin Psychol.* 1990;2:107-113.
33. Wonderlich SA, Swift WJ, Slotnick HB, Goodman S. *DSM-III-R* personality disorders in eating-disorder subtypes. *Int J Eating Disord.* 1990;9:607-616.
34. Zimmerman M, Coryell W. The reliability of personality disorder diagnoses in a nonpatient sample. *J Pers Disord.* 1989;3:53-57.
35. Hurt SW, Hyler SE, Frances A. Assessing borderline personality disorder with self-report, clinical interview, or semi-structured interview. *Am J Psychiatry.* 1984;141:1228-1231.
36. First MB, Spitzer RL, Gibbon M, Williams JBW, Davies M, Borus J, Howes MJ, Kane J, Pope HG, Rounsaville B. The Structured Clinical Interview for *DSM-III-R* personality disorders (SCID-II), II: multisite test-retest reliability study. *J Pers Disord.* In press.
37. Ames-Frankel J, Devlin MJ, Walsh BT, Strasser TJ, Sadik C, Oldham JM, Roose SP. Personality disorder diagnoses in patients with bulimia nervosa: clinical correlates and changes with treatment. *J Clin Psychiatry.* 1992;53:90-96.
38. O'Boyle M, Self D. A comparison of two interviews for *DSM-III-R* personality disorders. *Psychiatry Res.* 1990;32:85-92.
39. Loranger AW, Lenzenweger MF, Gartner AF, Susman VL, Herzig J, Zammit GK, Gartner JD, Abrams RC, Young RC. Trait-state artifacts and the diagnosis of personality disorders. *Arch Gen Psychiatry.* 1991;48:720-728.
40. Pfohl B, Black DW, Noyes R, Coryell WH, Barrash J. Axis I/Axis II comorbidity findings: implications for validity. In: Oldham J, ed. *Axis II: New Perspectives on Validity.* Washington, DC: American Psychiatric Association Press; 1990:147-161.
41. Piersma HL. The MCMI as a measure of *DSM-III* Axis II diagnoses: an empirical comparison. *J Clin Psychol.* 1987;43:478-483.
42. Reich JH. Update on instruments to measure *DSM-III* and *DSM-III-R* personality disorders. *J Nerv Ment Dis.* 1989;177:366-370.
43. Barasch A, Frances A, Hurt S, Clarkin J, Cohen S. Stability and distinctiveness of borderline personality disorder. *Am J Psychiatry.* 1985;142:1484-1486.
44. Trull TJ. *DSM-III-R* personality disorders and the five-factor model of personality: an empirical comparison. *J Abnorm Psychol.* 1992;101: 553-560.
45. Spitzer RL, Forman JBW, Nee J. *DSM-III* field trials, I: initial interrater diagnostic reliability. *Am J Psychiatry.* 1979;136:815-817.
46. Mellsop G, Varghese F, Joshua S, Hicks A. The reliability of Axis II of *DSM-III. Am J Psychiatry.* 1982;139:1360-1361.
47. Elkin I, Parloff MB, Hadley SW, Autry JH. NIMH treatment of depression Collaborative Research Program: background and research plan. *Arch Gen Psychiatry.* 1985;42:305-316.
48. Shea MT, Pilkonis PA, Beckham E, Collins JF, Elkin I, Sotsky SM, Docherty JP. Personality disorders and treatment outcome in the NIMH treatment of depression: Collaborative Research Program. *Am J Psychiatry.* 1990;147: 711-718.
49. Pilkonis PA, Heape CL, Ruddy J, Serrao P. Validity in the diagnosis of personality disorder: the use of the LEAD standard. *Psychol Assess J Consult Clin Psychol.* 1991;3:46-54.
50. Spitzer RL, Williams JBW, Gibbon M, First MB. The Structured Clinical Interview for *DSM-III-R* (SCID), I: history, rationale, and description. *Arch Gen Psychiatry.* 1992;49:624-629.
51. Williams JBW, Gibbon M, First MB, Spitzer RL, Davies M, Borus J, Howes MJ, Kane J, Pope HG, Rounsaville B, Wittchen HU. The Structured Clinical Interview for *DSM-III-R* (SCID), II: multisite test-retest reliability. *Arch Gen Psychiatry.* 1992;49:630-636.
52. Coppen A, Metcalf M. Effect of a depressive illness on MPI scores. *Br J Psychiatry.* 1965;17: 236-239.
53. Hirschfeld RMA, Klerman GL, Clayton PJ, Keller MB, McDonald-Scott P, Larkin BH. Assessing personality: effects of the depressive state on trait measurement. *Am J Psychiatry.* 1983;140:695-699.
54. Kerr TA, Schapira K, Roth M, Garside RF. The relationship between the Maudsley Personality Inventory and the course of affective disorders. *Br J Psychiatry.* 1970;116:11-18.
55. Lumry AE, Gottesman II, Tuason VB. MMPI state dependency during the course of bipolar psychosis. *Psychiatry Res.* 1982;7:59-67.
56. Liebowitz MR, Stallone F, Dunner DL, Fieve RR. Personality features of patients with primary affective disorder. *Acta Psychiatr Scand.* 1979; 60:214-224.
57. Reich J, Noyes R, Hirschfeld R, Coryell W, O'Gorman

T. State and personality in depressed and panic patients. *Am J Psychiatry.* 1987;144:181-187.
58. Pfohl B, Stangl D, Zimmerman M. The implications of *DSM-III* personality disorders for patients with major depression. *J Affect Disord.* 1984;7:309-318.
59. Pfohl B, Coryell W, Zimmerman M, Stangl D. Prognostic validity of self-report and interview measures of personality disorder in depressed inpatients. *J Clin Psychiatry.* 1988;45:468-472.
60. Zimmerman M, Coryell W, Pfohl B, Corenthal C, Stangl D. ECT response in depressed patients with and without a *DSM-III* personality disorder. *Am J Psychiatry.* 1986;143:1030-1032.
61. Costa PT, McCrae RR. Personality stability and its implications for clinical psychology. *Clin Psychol Rev.* 1986;6:407-423.
62. Mann AH, Jenkins R, Cutting JC, Cowen PJ. The development and use of a standardized assessment of abnormal personality. *Psychol Med.* 1981;11:839-847.
63. Tyrer P, Strauss J, Cicchetti D. Temporal reliability of personality in psychiatric patients. *Psychol Med.* 1983;13:393-398.
64. Overholser JC. Retest reliability of the Millon Clinical Multiaxial Inventory. *J Pers Assess.* 1990;55:202-208.
65. Murphy TJ, Greenblatt RL, Mozdzierz GJ, Trimakas KA. Stability of the Millon Clinical Multiaxial Inventory among psychiatric inpatients. *J Psychopathol Behav Assess.* 1990;12:143-150.
66. Paris J, Brown R, Nowlis D. Long-term follow-up of borderline patients in a general hospital. *Compr Psychiatry.* 1987;28:530-535.
67. McGlashan TH. The Chestnut Lodge Follow-up Study, II: long-term outcome of borderline personalities. *Arch Gen Psychiatry.* 1986;43:20-30.
68. Pope HG, Jonas JM, Hudson JI, Cohen BM, Gunderson JG. The validity of *DSM-III* borderline personality disorder: a phenomenologic, family history, treatment response, and long-term follow-up study. *Arch Gen Psychiatry.* 1983;40:23-30.
69. Robins E, Gentry KA, Munoz RA, Marten S. A contrast of the three more common illnesses with the ten less common in a study and 18-month follow-up of 314 psychiatric emergency room patients, III: findings at follow-up. *Arch Gen Psychiatry.* 1977;34:285-291.
70. Martin RL, Cloninger CR, Guze SB. The evaluation of diagnostic concordance in follow-up studies, II: a blind prospective follow-up of female criminals. *J Psychiatr Res.* 1979;15:107-125.
71. Robins LN, Helzer JE, Croughan J, Ratcliff KS. National Institute of Mental Health Diagnostic Interview Schedule: its history, characteristics, and validity. *Arch Gen Psychiatry.* 1981;38:381-389.
72. Endicott J, Spitzer RL. A diagnostic interview: the Schedule for Affective Disorders and Schizophrenia. *Arch Gen Psychiatry.* 1978;35:837-844.
73. Prusoff BA, Merikangas KR, Weissman MM. Lifetime prevalence and age of onset of psychiatric disorders: recall 4 years later. *J Psychiatr Res.* 1988;22:107-117.
74. Spitzer RL, Endicott J, Robins E. Research Diagnostic Criteria: rationale and reliability. *Arch Gen Psychiatry.* 1978;35:773-782.
75. Rounsaville BJ, Cacciola J, Weissman MM, Kleber HD. Diagnostic concordance in a follow-up study of opiate addicts. *J Psychiatr Res.* 1981;16:191-201.
76. Helzer JE, Spitznagel EL, McEvoy L. The predictive validity of lay Diagnostic Interview Schedule diagnoses in the general population: a comparison with physician examiners. *Arch Gen Psychiatry.* 1987;44:1069-1077.
77. Vandiver T, Sher KJ. Temporal stability of the Diagnostic Interview Schedule. *Psychol Assess: J Consult Clin Psych.* 1991;3:277-281.
78. Marin DB, Widiger TA, Frances AJ, Goldsmith S, Kocsis J. Personality disorders: issues in assessment. *Psychopharmacol Bull.* 1989;25:508-514.
79. Skodol AE, Oldham JM, Rosnick L, Kellman HD, Hyler SE. Diagnosis of *DSM-III-R* personality disorders: a comparison of two structured interviews. *Int J Methods Psychiatr Res.* 1991;1:13-26.
80. Robins LN, Helzer JE, Ratcliff KS, Seyfried W. Validity of the Diagnostic Interview Schedule, version II: *DSM-III* diagnoses. *Psychol Med.* 1982;12:855-870.
81. Tyrer P, Alexander MS, Cicchetti D, Cohen MS, Remington M. Reliability of a schedule for rating personality disorders. *Br J Psychiatry.* 1979;135:168-174.
82. Steketee G. Personality traits and disorders in obsessive-compulsives. *J Anxiety Disord.* 1990;4:351-364.
83. Dowson JH. *DSM-III-R* narcissistic personality disorder evaluated by patients' and informants' self-report questionnaires: relationships with other personality disorders and a sense of entitlement as an indicator of narcissism. *Compr Psychiatry.* 1992;33:397-406.
84. Dowson JH. Assessment of *DSM-III-R* personality disorders by self-report questionnaire: the role of informants and a screening test for comorbid personality disorders (STCPD). *Br J Psychiatry.* 1992;161:344-352.
85. Zimmerman M, Pfohl B, Coryell W, Stangl D, Corenthal C. Diagnosing personality disorder in depressed patients: a comparison of patient and informant interviews. *Arch Gen Psychiatry.* 1988;45:733-737.
86. Zimmerman M, Pfohl B, Stangl D, Corenthal C. Assessment of *DSM-III* personality disorders: the importance of interviewing an informant. *J Clin Psychiatry.* 1986;47:261-263.
87. Zimmerman M, Pfohl BM, Coryell WH, Stangl D, Corenthal C. Personality disorder diagnoses: who should be interviewed? Presented at the 143rd Annual Meeting of the American Psychiatric Association; May 1990; New York, NY.
88. Clark LA, Watson D. Tripartite model of anxiety and depression: psychometric evidence and taxonomic implications. *J Abnorm Psychol.* 1991;100:316-336.
89. Watson D, Clark LA. Self- versus peer ratings of specific emotional traits: evidence of convergent and discriminant validity. *J Pers Soc Psychol.* 1991;60:927-940.
90. Funder DC, Dobroth KM. Differences between traits: properties associated with interjudge agreement. *J Pers Soc Psychol.* 1987;52:409-418.
91. Watson D. Strangers' ratings of five robust personality factors: evidence of a surprising convergence with self-report. *J Pers Soc Psychol.* 1989;57:120-128.
92. Reich JH. Instruments measuring *DSM-III* and *DSM-III-R* personality disorders. *J Pers Disord.* 1987;1:220-240.
93. Standage K. Structured interviews and the diagnosis of personality disorders. *Can J Psychiatry.* 1989;34:906-912.
94. Tyrer P, Casey P, Ferguson B. Personality disorder in perspective. *Br J Psychiatry.* 1991;159:463-471.
95. Widiger TA, Frances A. Interviews and inventories for the measurement of personality disorders. *Clin Psychol Rev.* 1987;7:49-75.
96. Loranger AW. Diagnosis of personality disorders: general considerations. In: Michels R, ed. *Psychiatry.* Philadelphia, Pa: JB Lippincott; 1991: chap 15.
97. Gunderson JG, Kolb JE, Austin V. The diagnostic interview for borderlines. *Am J Psychiatry.* 1981;138:896-903.
98. Gunderson JG, Ronningstam E, Bodkin A. The diagnostic interview for narcissistic patients. *Arch Gen Psychiatry.* 1990;47:676-680.
99. Hare R. Comparison of procedures for the assessment of psychopathy. *J Consult Clin Psychol.* 1985;53:7-16.
100. Conte H, Plutchik R, Karasu T, Jerrett I. A self-report borderline scale. *J Nerv Ment Dis.* 1980;168:428-435.
101. Kendler KS, Lieberman JA, Walsh D. The structured interview for schizotypy (SIS): a preliminary report. *Schizophr Bull.* 1989;15:559-571.
102. Claridge G, Hewitt JK. A biometrical study of schizotypy in a normal population. *Pers Indiv Diff.* 1987;8:303-312.
103. Frances A, Clarkin JF, Gilmore M, Hurt SW, Brown R. Reliability of criteria for borderline personality disorder: a comparison of *DSM-III* and the diagnostic interview for borderline patients. *Am J Psychiatry.* 1984;141:1080-1084.
104. Ono Y, Okonogi K. Borderline personality disorder in Japan: a comparative study of three diagnostic criteria. *J Pers Disord.* 1988;2:212-220.
105. Kavoussi RJ, Coccaro EF, Klar HM, Bernstein D, Siever LJ. Structured interviews for borderline personality disorder. *Am J Psychiatry.* 1990;147:1522-1525.
106. Loranger AW, Oldham JM, Russakoff LM, Susman V. Structured interviews and borderline personality disorder. *Arch Gen Psychiatry.* 1984;41:565-568.
107. Angus LE, Marziali E. A comparison of three measures for the diagnosis of borderline personality disorder. *Am J Psychiatry.* 1988;145:1453-1454.
108. Widiger TA, Williams JBW, Spitzer RL, Frances A. The MCMI as a measure of *DSM-III*. *J Pers Assess.* 1985;49:366-378.
109. Millon T. The MCMI provides a good assessment of *DSM-III* disorders: the MCMI-II will prove even better. *J Pers Assess.* 1985;49:379-391.
110. Widiger TA, Williams JBW, Spitzer RL, Frances A. The MCMI and *DSM-III:* a brief rejoinder to Millon (1985). *J Pers Assess.* 1986;50:198-204.
111. Millon T. The MCMI and *DSM-III:* further commentaries. *J Pers Assess.* 1986;50:205-207.
112. Nussbaum D, Rogers R. Screening psychiatric patients for Axis II disorders. *Can J Psychiatry.* 1992;37:658-660.
113. Hyler SE, Skodol AE, Kellman D, Oldham JM, Rosnick L. Validity of the Personality Diagnostic Questionnaire–Revised: comparison with two structured interviews. *Am J Psychiatry.* 1990;147:1043-1048.
114. Oldham JM, Skodol AE, Kellman D, Hyler SE, Rosnick L, Davies M. Diagnosis of *DSM-III-R*

personality disorders by two structured interviews: patterns of comorbidity. *Am J Psychiatry.* 1992;149:213-220.
115. Hesselbrock V, Stabenau J, Hesselbrock M, Mirkin P, Meyer R. A comparison of two interview schedules: the Schedule for Affective Disorders and Schizophrenia–Lifetime and the National Institute for Mental Health Diagnostic Interview Schedule. *Arch Gen Psychiatry.* 1982; 39:674-677.
116. Hasin DS, Grant BF. Psychiatric diagnosis of patients with substance abuse problems: a comparison of two procedures, the DIS and the SADS-L. *J Psychiatr Res.* 1987;21:7-22.
117. Hasin DS, Grant BF. Diagnosing depressive disorders in patients with alcohol and drug problems: a comparison of the SADS-L and the DIS. *J Psychiatr Res.* 1987;21:301-311.
118. Hunt C, Andrews G. Measuring personality disorder: the use of self-report questionnaires. *J Pers Disord.* 1992;6:125-133.
119. Hogg B, Jackson HJ, Rudd R, Edwards J. Diagnosing personality disorders in recent-onset schizophrenia. *J Nerv Ment Dis.* 1990;178:194-199.
120. Reich J, Noyes R, Troughton E. Lack of agreement between instruments measuring *DSM-III* personality disorders. In: Millon T, ed. *Proceedings from the First Millon Clinical Multiaxial Inventory Conference.* Minnetonka, Minn: National Computer Systems; 1987: 223-234.
121. Jackson HJ, Gazis J, Rudd RP, Edwards J. Concordance between two personality disorder instruments with psychiatric inpatients. *Compr Psychiatry.* 1991;32:252-260.
122. Torgersen S, Alnaes R. The relationship between the MCMI personality scales and *DSM-III,* Axis II. *J Pers Assess.* 1990;55:698-707.
123. Nazikian H, Rudd RP, Edwards J, Jackson HJ. Personality disorder assessment for psychiatric inpatients. *Aust N Z J Psychiatry.* 1990;24:37-46.
124. Zimmerman M, Coryell WH. Diagnosing personality disorders in the community: a comparison of self-report and interview measures. *Arch Gen Psychiatry.* 1990;47:527-531.
125. Hyler SE, Skodol AE, Oldham JM, Kellman D, Doidge N. Validity of the Personality Diagnostic Questionnaire–Revised: a replication in an outpatient sample. *Compr Psychiatry.* 1992;33:73-77.
126. Reich JH, Noyes R. A comparison of *DSM-III* personality disorders in acutely ill panic and depressed patients. *J Anxiety Disord.* 1987;1:123-131.
127. Reich J, Troughton E. Frequency of *DSM-III* personality disorders in patients with panic disorder: comparison with psychiatric and normal control subjects. *Psychiatry Res.* 1988;26:89-100.
128. Reich JH. A family history method for *DSM-III* anxiety and personality disorders. *Psychiatry Res.* 1988;26:131-139.
129. Dubro AF, Wetzler S, Kahn MV. A comparison of three self-report questionnaires for the diagnosis of *DSM-III* personality disorders. *J Pers Disord.* 1988;2:256-266.
130. Cantrell JD, Dana RD. Use of the Millon Clinical Multiaxial Inventory (MCMI) as a screening instrument at a community mental health center. *J Clin Psychol.* 1987;43:366-375.
131. Repko GR, Cooper R. The diagnosis of personality disorder: a comparison of MMPI profile, Millon Inventory, and clinical judgment in a workers' compensation population. *J Clin Psychol.* 1985;41:867-881.
132. Wetzler S, Dubro A. Diagnosis of personality disorders by the Millon Clinical Multiaxial Inventory. *J Nerv Ment Dis.* 1990;178:261-263.
133. Helzer JE, Coryell W. More on *DSM-III:* how consistent are precise criteria? *Biol Psychiatry.* 1983;18:1201-1203.
134. Winokur G, Zimmerman M, Cadoret R. Cause the Bible tells me so. *Arch Gen Psychiatry.* 1988; 45:683-684.
135. Zimmerman M, Coryell W, Black DW. Variability in the application of contemporary diagnostic criteria: endogenous depression as an example. *Am J Psychiatry.* 1990;147:1173-1179.
136. Zimmerman M, Coryell W, Black DW. A method to detect intercenter differences in the application of contemporary diagnostic criteria. *J Nerv Ment Dis.* 1993;181:130-134.
137. Zimmerman M, Pfohl B, Coryell WH, Corenthal C, Stangl D. Major depression and personality disorder. *J Affect Disord.* 1991;22:199-210.
138. Alnaes R, Torgersen S. Personality and personality disorders among patients with major depression in combination with dysthymic or cyclothymic disorders. *Acta Psychiatr Scand.* 1989;79:363-369.
139. Spitzer RL. Psychiatric diagnosis: are clinicians still necessary? *Compr Psychiatry.* 1983;24:399-411.
140. Sartorius N, Kaelber CT, Cooper JE, Roper MT, Rae DS, Gulbinat W, Üstrün TB, Regier DA. Progress toward achieving a common language in psychiatry: results from the field trial of the clinical guidelines accompanying the WHO classification of mental and behavioral disorders in *ICD-10. Arch Gen Psychiatry.* 1993;50: 115-124.
141. Reich JH, Green AI. Effect of personality disorders on outcome of treatment. *J Nerv Ment Dis.* 1991;179:74-82.
142. Wilson VL, Putnam RR. A meta-analysis of pretest sensitization effects in experimental design. *Am Educ Res J.* 1982;19:249-258.
143. Jorm AF, Duncan-Jones P, Scott R. An analysis of the re-test artefact in longitudinal studies of psychiatric symptoms and personality. *Psychol Med.* 1989;19:487-493.
144. Robins LN. Epidemiology: reflections on testing the validity of psychiatric interviews. *Arch Gen Psychiatry.* 1985;42:918-924.
145. Henderson AS, Byrne DG, Duncan-Jones P. *Neurosis and the Social Environment.* Orlando, Fla: Academic Press Inc; 1981.
146. Bromet EJ, Dunn LO, Connell MM, Dew MA, Schulberg HC. Long-term reliability of diagnosing lifetime major depression in a community sample. *Arch Gen Psychiatry.* 1986;43:435-440.
147. Helzer JE, Spitznagel EL, McEvoy L. The predictive validity of lay Diagnostic Interview Schedule diagnoses in the general population. *Arch Gen Psychiatry.* 1987;44:1069-1077.
148. Burnam, MA, Karno M, Hough RL, Escobar JI, Forsythe AB. The Spanish Diagnostic Interview Schedule: reliability and comparison with clinical diagnoses. *Arch Gen Psychiatry.* 1983;40:1189-1196.
149. Semler G, Wittchen HU, Joschke K, Zaudig M, von Geiso T, Kaiser S, von Cranach M, Pfister H. Test-retest reliability of a standardized psychiatric interview (DIS/CID). *Eur Arch Psychiatry Clin Neurosci.* 1987;236:214-222.
150. Blouin AG, Perez EL, Blouin JH. Computerized administration of the Diagnostic Interview Schedule. *Psychiatry Res.* 1987;23:335-344.
151. Kisely SR, Faragher B, Gask L, Goldberg DP. Measuring psychiatric disorder in the recent past: the use of the Psychiatric Assessment Schedule retrospectively. *Psychol Med.* 1992;22:457-463.
152. Paulsen AS, Crowe RR, Noyes R, Pfohl B. Reliability of the telephone interview in diagnosing anxiety disorders. *Arch Gen Psychiatry.* 1988;45:62-63.
153. Prusoff BA, Merikangas KR, Weissman MM. Lifetime prevalence and age of onset of psychiatric disorders: recall 4 years later. *J Psychiatr Res.* 1988;22:107-117.
154. Wells KB, Burnam MA, Leake B, Robins LN. Agreement between face-to-face and telephone-administered versions of the depression section of the NIMH Diagnostic Interview Schedule. *J Psychiatr Res.* 1988;22:207-220.
155. Harrington R, Hill J, Rutter M, John K, Fudge H, Zoccolillo M, Weissman M. The assessment of lifetime psychopathology: a comparison of two interviewing styles. *Psychol Med.* 1988;18:487-493.
156. Joffe RT, Regan JJ. Personality and depression. *J Psychiatr Res.* 1988;22:279-288.
157. Libb JW, Stankovic S, Freeman A, Sokol R, Switzer P, Houck C. Personality disorders among depressed outpatients as identified by the MCMI. *J Clin Psychol.* 1990;46:277-284.
158. Kennedy SH, McVey G, Katz R. Personality disorders in anorexia nervosa and bulimia nervosa. *J Psychiatr Res.* 1990;24:259-269.
159. Stankovic SR, Libb JW, Freeman AM, Roseman JM. Posttreatment stability of the MCMI-II personality scales in depressed outpatients. *J Pers Disord.* 1992;6:82-89.
160. Mavissakalian M, Hamann MS, Jones B. *DSM-III* personality disorders in obsessive-compulsive disorder: changes with treatment. *Compr Psychiatry.* 1990;31:432-437.
161. Mavissakalian M, Hamann MS. *DSM-III* personality disorder in agoraphobia, II: changes with treatment. *Compr Psychiatry.* 1987;28: 356-361.
162. Gartner AF, Marcus RN, Halmi K, Loranger AW. *DSM-III-R* personality disorders in patients with eating disorders. *Am J Psychiatry.* 1989;146:1585-1591.
163. Ricciardi JN, Baer L, Jenike MA, Fischer SC, Sholtz D, Buttolph ML. Changes in *DSM-III-R* Axis II diagnoses following treatment of obsessive-compulsive disorder. *Am J Psychiatry.* 1992;149: 829-831.
164. Stuart S, Simons AD, Thase ME, Pilkonis P. Are personality assessments valid in acute major depression? *J Affect Disord.* 1992;24:281-290.
165. Zimmerman M, Coryell W. *DSM-III* personality disorder diagnoses in a nonpatient sample: demographic correlates and comorbidity. *Arch Gen Psychiatry.* 1989;46:682-689.
166. Coryell W, Zimmerman M. Personality disorder in the families of depressed, schizophrenic and never-ill probands. *Am J Psychiatry.* 1989;146: 496-502.
167. Black DW, Noyes R, Pfohl B, Goldstein R, Blum N. Personality disorder in obsessive-compulsive volunteers, well comparison subjects, and their first-degree relatives. *Am J Psychiatry.* 1993;150:1226-1232.
168. Zimmerman M, Coryell W, Black D. A major problem in diagnosing personality disorder. Presented at the 146th Annual Meeting of the American Psychiatric Association; May 1993; San Francisco, Calif.

Psychoneuroimmunology and Human Immunodeficiency Virus Type 1 Infection Revisited

In the May 1992 issue of the ARCHIVES, Perry et al[1] reported on the relationship between psychosocial and immune variables in human immunodeficiency virus type 1 (HIV-1) seropositive individuals. This is the second ARCHIVES article devoted to this area that did not find significant associations on the whole.[1,2] We are impressed by the efforts involved in the generation of these two studies. However, we are concerned that the conclusion of Perry et al[1] suggesting no relationship between psychosocial and immune variables is premature. Thus, we raise the following four points.

First, there was no discernible theoretical rationale interrelating the broad set of psychosocial and psychiatric measures assessed and driving the statistical hypotheses tested. In other reports, a theoretically driven psychosocial model interrelating stressful life events, social support, and coping style has demonstrated associations with psychological distress,[3] immune measures,[4-11] and clinical health status.[11,12] In addition, both prior studies in the ARCHIVES[1,2] focused more on measures aimed at individuals with psychopathological behavior than on those in the normal range, despite the fact that most HIV-1 seropositive individuals followed in longitudinal studies do not manifest a current psychiatric disorder.

Second, in both studies[1,2] there was a need for additional controls for other behavioral influences on immune measures. These influences included alcohol use and nonparenteral substance use (outside a diagnosis of dependence), nutritional status, cigarette smoking, caffeine intake, physical exercise, sexual activity, and sleep deprivation. All of these have been previously described for psychoneuroimmunological research[13] but were not employed by Perry et al.[1]

Third, the selection of immunological measures was largely limited to the CD4 cell count, which has already been criticized by Stein et al[14] regarding the study by Rabkin et al.[2] Although other immune measures were assessed here (percentage of CD4, CD4/CD8 ratio, and CD8 cell count), the percentage of CD4 cells and the CD4/CD8 ratio are dependent on the CD4 cell count, and the CD8 cell count has only infrequently been examined as an outcome in psychoneuroimmunological studies. Psychosocial factors have been related to the CD4 cell count in other studies of HIV-1–infected individuals[5,6] as well as to functional immunological measures, which are directly affected by HIV-1 disease progression such as mitogen response to phytohemagglutinin [PHA],[6,7,11] a functional measure of T cells, and natural killer cell cytotoxicity.[4,6,7] Regarding bereavement, associations with decrements in mitogen response to PHA and natural killer cell cytotoxicity have been shown. The decrement in natural killer cell cytotoxicity occurred at the first assessment following the loss, whereas mitogen response to PHA showed decrements only after a lag of 6 months.[7] This may be due to differential neuroendocrine mediation by the sympathetic adrenomedullary system and the limbic-hypothalamic-pituitary-adrenal axis, respectively. We are currently studying the impact of a bereavement support group intervention in HIV-1 seropositive homosexual men to replicate these immunological changes, support their neuroendocrine mediation, and determine their potential response to therapy. Further, immunological effects of the following therapeutic interventions have already been reported in asymptomatic HIV-1 seropositive homosexual men: cognitive behavioral stress management training,[8,11] experiential group therapy,[9] and aerobic exercise training.[10]

Fourth, stage of disease may have been relevant to control in this study. In contrast to the suggestion made in the report by Perry et al,[1] the subjects did appear to have symptoms that qualified for Centers for Disease Control and Prevention (CDC) stage IVA (constitutional disease) as well as IVC-2. Such symptoms do not require a diagnosis of acquired immunodeficiency syndrome (AIDS) but are consistent with symptomatic stages prior to AIDS that are currently defined by CDC stage B in the recent revision of CDC staging.[15] This difference between symptomatic and asymptomatic subjects could account for differences in effects observed across other studies as well.

Undoubtedly, as the data of Perry et al[1] support, a bidirectional theoretical model must be posited in which symptoms are also related to subsequent psychological distress. However, our conclusion differs with that of Perry et al, who caution clinicians against recommending that HIV-1 seropositive patients focus on stressor management because of a putative direct effect between "stress" and "T cells." In fact, evidence to date points to a greater contribution to variance accounted for by this pathway rather than by the converse. That is, the evidence supports psychoneuroimmunological mediation of relationships between distress and subsequent level of physical symptoms. Moreover, these relationships highlight the potential importance of mental health and behavioral interventions not only for improved self-care, compliance with medical regimens, and quality of life but also possibly for effects on the disease process itself. We note with interest the finding of Perry et al[1] of the association of hopelessness with CD4 cell count (maintained after post hoc confirmatory analyses) and that of Rabkin et al[2] of an association between stressful life events, distress, depressive disorders, and number of HIV-1–related symptoms. Interestingly, regarding both of these findings, it has now been reported that depressed mood was associated with a more rapid rate of decline in CD4 cell count[16,17] and with more rapid progression to AIDS and death over 4 years.[16] We agree that future research is required to extend the data gathered to date and suggest that these studies should account for the four points described herein.

Karl Goodkin, MD, PhD
Department of Psychiatry (D-22)
University of Miami School of Medicine
1425 NW 10th Ave, 3rd Floor
Miami, FL 33136
C. L. Mulder, MD
Rotterdam, the Netherlands
Nancy T. Blaney, PhD
Gail Ironson, MD, PhD
Mahendra Kumar, PhD
Mary Ann Fletcher, PhD
Miami, Fla

1. Perry S, Fishman B, Jacobsberg L, Frances A. Relationships over 1 year between lymphocyte subsets and psychosocial variables among adults with infection by human immunodeficiency virus. *Arch Gen Psychiatry.* 1992;49:396-401.
2. Rabkin JG, Williams JBW, Remien RH, Goetz RR, Kertzner R, Gorman JM. Depression, lymphocyte subsets, and human immunodeficiency virus symptoms on two occasions in HIV-positive homosexual men. *Arch Gen Psychiatry.* 1991;48:111-119.
3. Blaney NT, Goodkin K, Morgan RO, Feaster D, Millon C, Szapocznik J, Eisdorfer C. A stress-moderator model of distress in early HIV infection: concurrent analysis of life events, hardiness, and social support. *J Psychosom Res.* 1991;35:297-305.
4. Goodkin K, Blaney NT, Feaster D, Fletcher MA, Baum MK, Mantero-Atienza E, Klimas N, Millon C, Szapocznik J, Eisdorfer C. Active coping style is associated with natural killer cell cytotoxicity in asymptomatic HIV-1 seropositive homosexual men. *J Psychosom Res.* 1992;36:635-650.
5. Goodkin K, Fuchs I, Feaster D, Leeka J, Dickson-Rishel D. Life stressors and coping style are associated with immune measures in HIV-1 infection: a preliminary report. *Int J Psychiatry Med.* 1992;22:155-172.
6. Goodkin K, Blaney NT, Feaster D, Baum M, Fletcher MA, Antoni MH, Ironson G, Goldstein D, Szapocznik J, Eisdorfer CE. The association of a stress moderator model and immunological measures in asymptomatic HIV-1 infected homosexual men. In: Abstracts of Research Perspectives in Psychoneuroimmunology III; September 12-13, 1991; Columbus, Ohio.
7. Goodkin K, Blaney NT, Feaster D, Fletcher MA, Baum M, Szapocznik J, Eisdorfer CE. Bereavement is associated with changes in cellular immune function in asymptomatic HIV-1 seropositive gay men. In: Abstracts of the 7th International Conference on AIDS; June 16-21, 1991; Florence,Italy. Abstract MC3179.
8. Antoni MH, Baggett L, Ironson G, LaPerriere A, August S, Klimas NG, Schneiderman N, Fletcher MA. Cognitive-behavioral stress management intervention buffers distress responses and immunologic changes following notification of HIV-1 antibody seropositivity. *J Consult Clin Psychol.* 1991;59:906-915.
9. Mulder CL, Emmelkamp PMG, Mulder JW, Antoni MH, Sandfort T, Heijnen C, de Vries MJ. Immunological and psychosocial effects of a cognitive behavioral vs. an experiential group therapy program for asymptomatic HIV seropositive homosexual men. In: Abstracts of the 8th International Conference on AIDS; July 19-24, 1992; Amsterdam, the Netherlands. Abstract PoB3809.
10. LaPerriere AR, Antoni MH, Schneiderman N, Ironson G, Klimas NG, Caralis P, Fletcher MA. Exercise intervention attenuates emotional distress and natural killer cell decrements following notification of positive serologic status for HIV-1. *Biofeedback Self Regul.* 1990;15:229-242.
11. Ironson G, Friedman A, Klimas N, Antoni M, Fletcher MA, LaPerriere A, Simoneau J, Schneiderman N. Distress, denial, and low adherence to behavioral interventions predict faster disease progression in HIV infected gay men. *Int J Behav Med.* In press.
12. Blaney NT, Goodkin K, Feaster D, Morgan R, Baum M, Wilkie F, Szapocznik J, Eisdorfer C. Life events and active coping style predict health status in early HIV-1 infection. In: Abstracts of the 8th International Conference on AIDS; July 19-24, 1992; Amsterdam, the Netherlands. Abstract PuB7213.
13. Kiecolt-Glaser JK, Glaser R. Methodological issues in behavioral immunology research with humans. *Brain Behav Immun.* 1988;2:67-78.
14. Stein M, Miller AH, Trestman RL. Depression, the immune system, and health and illness: findings in search of meaning. *Arch Gen Psychiatry.* 1991;48:171-177.
15. Centers for Disease Control and Prevention. 1993 revised classification system for HIV infection and expanded surveillance case definition for AIDS among adolescents and adults. *MMWR Morb Mortal Wkly Rep.* 1992;41(RR-17):1-19.
16. Burack JH, Stall RD, Barrett DC, Coates TJ. Depression predicts accelerated CD4 decline among gay men in San Francisco. In: Abstracts of the 8th International Conference on AIDS; July 19-24, 1992; Amsterdam, the Netherlands. Abstract WeC1031.
17. Solomon GF, Kemeny ME, Temoshok L. Psychoneuroimmunological aspects of human immunodeficiency virus infection. In: Ader R, Felten DL, Cohen N, eds. *Psychoneuroimmunology.* 2nd ed. San Diego, Calif: Academic Press Inc; 1991:1081-1113.

In reply

There is currently a debate regarding how liberally or conservatively researchers in psychoimmunology should interpret occasional and inconsistent correlations between psychosocial and immune variables.[1] We thank Goodkin et al because their impassioned letter and our more cautious tone[2,3] capture the nature of this debate.

In their first criticism, our Miami colleagues are concerned that we did not use the right hypotheses or measures. Another reading of our articles should help assure them that we tested hypotheses based on the cited psychoimmune literature and that we used a broad set of standardized psychiatric and psychosocial measures used in psychoimmune research. Many of our instruments did not assess psychopathology, but rather assessed the same constructs used by the Miami group (eg, social support, hardiness, and life stressors).

In response to their second criticism, we believe it was not necessary to control for all the many factors that may affect immune measures, such as coffee, exercise, or sleep. Any clinically relevant relationship between numerous psychosocial and immune measures should be detectable as a signal above the noise created by these various behavioral influences.

The third point raised by our colleagues appears to be a combination of criticizing our immune measures and summarizing their past, present, and future psychoimmune research. In regard to our immune measures, we can only repeat that although we extensively analyzed possible psychoimmune relationships involving total lymphocytes, total CD8, and the CD4/CD8 ratio, we primarily reported correlations involving the total CD4 count because it remains the most commonly used marker of disease progression among HIV-infected adults. For now, we contend that among this population, total CD4 cell count is a more meaningful immune measure than, for example, in vitro responses of peripheral blood cells to PHA,[4] a measure that has no established pathophysiological meaning or health consequences.

In regard to the Miami group's published and unpublished findings, we agree that their preliminary results are interesting. Even though our results were based on over 200 HIV-infected subjects prospectively followed for as long as 1 year, we were cautious about generalizing from our results. We recommend that the Miami investigators exercise similar caution, especially because their peer-reviewed reports are based on only 11 HIV-infected men assessed cross-sectionally[5] and on only six HIV-infected men briefly followed after assignment to a stress-reduction intervention.[4]

We agree that clinically significant psychoimmune effects among HIV-infected adults, if they exist and if they can be detected, may vary according to the degree of immune impairment. We do not agree that past or current CDC staging is the best way to examine for this possibility. An HIV-infected adult can have chronic debilitating physical symptoms and still not meet the old or revised CDC criteria for AIDS or, conversely, may have fully recovered from an AIDS-defining diagnosis and currently be without physical symptoms. In our prospective analyses, we chose to sidestep such nosological problems by measuring concurrent severity of physical symptoms and by controlling for a reliable marker of disease progression—baseline CD4 cell count at entry.

We looked long and hard for psychoimmune effects in our HIV-infected populations. If we had any bias, it was toward hoping to find such relationships, but after extensive analyses, we simply did not find any compelling correlations, certainly none that would withstand correction for chance significant findings. We therefore do not share the view of our Miami colleagues that "the evidence supports psychoneuroimmunological mediation of relationships between distress and subsequent level of physical symptoms."

As a final note, we did not recommend that clinicians avoid referrals to programs that might be helpful in reducing distress. We did, however, recommend that clinicians be cautious in telling their HIV-infected patients that distress will adversely affect their immune system and thereby accelerate disease progression. We still contend that current knowledge does not support such statements and may prompt self-accusation when physical symptoms inevitably occur.

Samuel Perry, MD
The New York Hospital
Cornell University Medical Center
525 E 68th St
New York, NY 10021
Judith Rabkin, PhD
New York, NY

1. Stein M, Miller AH, Trestman RL. Depression, the immune system, and health and illness: findings in search of meaning. *Arch Gen Psychiatry*. 1991;48:171-177.
2. Rabkin JG, Williams JBW, Remien RH, Goetz RR, Kertzner R, Gorman JM. Depression, lymphocyte subsets, and human immunodeficiency virus symptoms on two occasions in HIV-positive homosexual men. *Arch Gen Psychiatry*. 1991;48:111-119.
3. Perry S, Fishman B, Jacobsberg L, Frances A. Relationships over 1 year between lymphocyte subsets and psychosocial variables among adults with infection by human immunodeficiency virus. *Arch Gen Psychiatry*. 1992;49:396-401.
4. Antoni MH, Baggett L, Ironson G, LaPerriere A, August S, Klimas N, Schneiderman N, Fletcher MA. Cognitive-behavioral stress management intervention buffers distress responses and immunologic changes following notification of HIV-antibody seropositivity. *J Consult Clin Psychol*. 1991;59:906-915.
5. Goodkin K, Fuchs I, Feaster D, Leeka J, Dickson-Rishel D. Life stressors and coping style are associated with immune measures in HIV-l infection: a preliminary report. *Int J Psychiatry Med*. 1992;22:155-172.

Pindolol Induces a Rapid Improvement of Depressed Patients Treated With Serotonin Reuptake Inhibitors

Preclinical evidence indicates that repeated treatment with antidepressant drugs (serotonin [5-HT] reuptake or monoamine oxidase [MAO] inhibitors) potentiates the ascending brain serotonergic pathways.[1,2] Also, clinical data show that the inhibition of 5-HT synthesis results in a marked worsening of patients recovering from depression who are treated with these drugs.[3-5] These findings suggest that the antidepressant effects of uptake and MAO inhibitors emerge when serotonergic activity increases.

Using intracerebral microdialysis in the awake, freely moving rat, a single treatment with 5-HT uptake blockers, such as clomipramine[6] or fluvoxamine,[7] was reported to cause little or no increase of 5-HT concentration in frontal cortex at doses comparable with or higher than those used clinically. In contrast, extracellular 5-HT concentration is dramatically augmented by the same doses in the vicinity of cell bodies of serotonergic neurons, in the midbrain raphe nuclei, a preferential increase also observed after a single treatment with MAO inhibitors.[8] This increase may be common to different types of antidepressants acting on the serotonergic system. These results have been replicated using other selective 5-HT reuptake inhibitors (SSRI).[9,10] In contrast, repeated treatment for 2 weeks with a low dose of fluvoxamine maleate (1 mg/kg) results in a sixfold increase in extracellular 5-HT concentration in frontal cortex,[11] indicating a potentiation of the serotonergic system by repeated (but not a single) treatment with uptake inhibitors, perhaps due to autoreceptor subsensitivity and changes in reuptake efficacy.

It is very likely that the limited action of uptake inhibitors in serotonergic projection areas after a single treatment is caused by the activation at the raphe nuclei of the somatodendritic receptors (5-HT_{1A}) by the excess of 5-HT that follows reuptake blockade. The function of somatodendritic autoreceptors is to slow down the activity of serotonergic neurons. Their activation reduces neuronal firing, 5-HT synthesis, and terminal release. Long-term treatment with uptake blockers dramatically decreases 5-HT cell firing in rats,[1] which suggests an impairment of the firing-dependent release of 5-HT at projection areas. Thus, low, clinically relevant doses of 5-HT uptake inhibitors may not increase the synaptic availability of the amine after a single treatment, due to this negative feedback mechanism operating at the cell body level. This view appears to be confirmed by two types of evidence: (1) the local application of clomipramine into the midbrain raphe nuclei reduces 5-HT release in frontal cortex,[6] mimicking the transynaptic effects of its systemic administration, and (2) the blockade of 5-HT_1 raphe receptors enables low doses of uptake inhibitors to increase extracellular 5-HT concentration in cortex or hippocampus.[9,12]

From all the above, it appears that blocking 5-HT_{1A} somatodendritic receptors could augment the antidepressant efficacy of 5-HT uptake blockers by enabling serotoninergic terminals to release more 5-HT. Hence, in an extrapolation of these animal data, we attempted to increase the serotonin function in patients with depression by antagonizing the somatodendritic 5-HT_{1A} receptors. Although no selective antagonists of 5-HT_{1A} receptors are available for human use, some β-blockers (ie, pindolol) have a high affinity for this subtype of 5-HT receptors[13] and antagonize 5-HT_{1A}–mediated responses in rats and humans.[13-15] Therefore, we used this compound in a pilot, open study to examine its effects in patients with depression who were being treated with SSRIs or MAO inhibitors.

Methods. Two groups of patients were selected to examine the effects of pindolol on reduction of the latency period (group 1) and potentiation of the antidepressant response in resistant patients (group 2). Inclusion criteria were as follows: (1) occurrence of a major depressive disorder (single or recurrent based on *DSM-III-R* diagnosis) with a minimum score on the Hamilton Depression Rating Scale (HDRS) of 20 (group 1) or insufficient response after treatment with SSRI or MAO inhibitors (minimum HDRS score in this group was 14), and (2) absence of any physical illness or pregnancy. Patients in group 2 had been treated for at least 6 weeks with SSRIs or MAO inhibitors without full antidepressant response. They were chosen from among those attending the Department of Psychiatry of the Hospital de Sant Pau (Barcelona, Spain) between October 1992 and February 1993 (all except two were outpatients). Patients were informed of the purpose of the study and gave their consent to participate. The characteristics of the patients are shown in the **Table**. Patients in group 1 were prescribed 20 mg of paroxetine and 2.5 mg of pindolol three times a day. Patients in group 2 were given stabilized antidepressant medication (Table) at the time of admission. Pindolol was added at the same doses as for group 1. Outpatients were advised to call one of us (V.P.) as soon as they started to feel better and were examined on the following days.

Results. The Table shows the characteristics of the patients who experienced a rapid improvement. Four of the seven patients in group 1 experienced a complete remission of symptoms in less than 1 week. Another patient had a partial recovery (decrease in HDRS score from 30 to 13) in 5 days. The other two patients did not show any marked improvement in 2 weeks. Also, five patients of group 2 recovered completely in 1 week while another patient experienced a partial recovery (reduction of HDRS score from 27 to 13). Two other patients did not improve in 2 weeks. The following two cases illustrate a good response to the addition of pindolol.

Report of Cases. *Case 2 (Group 1).* This was a female patient aged 38 years, who was married and had a son, with no family history of psychiatric disorders. She had a depressive episode in 1988, with a complete remission after treatment for 2 months with amitryptiline. She was euthymic since December 1992. Her mood worsened rapidly, with a clear pattern of melancholia, feelings of worthlessness, guilt, personal ruin and loss of hope, psychic anxiety, and late insomnia. Her mood improved in the evenings. She also lost weight and had a reduction of the libido. The HDRS score at admission was 26 and she was prescribed 20 mg/d of paroxetine and 7.5 mg/d (2.5 mg three times a day) of pindolol. She experienced a complete remission in 1 week (HDRS score, 9).

Case 1 (Group 2). This was a married, childless female patient, with a family history of affective disorders. She experienced her first depressive episode at age 35 years, after a hysterectomy, and had a complete remission of symptoms with tricyclic treatment. Ten years later, she had another episode that required hospitalization, resulting in partial recovery with treatment with 60 mg/d of phenelzine. One year later, while still taking phenelzine, her depression worsened. Her therapy was then sequentially changed to clomipramine (up to 200 mg/d) which resulted in no response and iproniazid (100 mg/d) which resulted in full response. Since her episodes in 1987 and 1992, she had four episodes with only minor improvements with different SSRI or MAO inhibitors. The latter were withdrawn because of side effects. Lithium could not be added due to intolerance. In 1992, owing to her lack of response to pharmacotherapies, she was treated with electroconvulsive therapy. Her depressive symptoms went into remission after 18 treatments but relapsed after 3 months, and she was given a second series of electroconvulsive therapy. In September 1992, she was hospitalized owing to a high risk of suicide while treatment with paroxetine was being tested. She was then selected for the present study and pindolol was added to paroxetine. A very important remission (decrease in HDRS score from 36 to 11) was achieved in 4 days. She was discharged. Two weeks later, pindolol was discontinued, and she experienced a relapse 10 weeks later (HDRS score, 30). Pindolol was added again to paroxetine and she recovered in 6 days (HDRS score, 9). Since then (January 1993) she has been euthymic while receiving pindolol.

Comment. These data indicate that pindolol, a β-blocker with a strong antagonistic activity at $5\text{-}HT_{1A}$ receptors,[13-15] induces a dramatic and rapid improvement of the antidepressant efficacy of SSRIs and MAO inhibitors. The onset of action was reduced and, more importantly, a rapid and full antidepressant response was observed in patients resistant to treatment with SSRIs or MAO inhibitors. On average, the effectiveness of pindolol was similar in both groups (five of seven patients improved in group 1; six of eight in group 2) although the most impressive effects were observed in resistant patients. Pindolol appears to make the serotonergic neuron respond to the combination of pindolol with an uptake inhibitor in the same manner that it does after long-term treatment with an uptake inhibitor alone and to obtain a response in the unresponsive neurons of the treatment-refractory patient that cannot be obtained with the uptake inhibitor alone. The negative isomers of some β antagonists (pindolol, propanolol, penbutolol) but not others (betaxolol, ICI 118.551, metoprolol) exhibit an antago-

Patient Characteristics*

Case No./Sex/Age, y	Diagnosis	Previous Resistant Treatments/Dose, mg/d	Current Treatment/Dose, mg/d	HDRS/NCI Score Before Pindolol	Latency Period, d	HDRS Score After Pindolol
			Group 1 (Reduction of Latency Period)†			
1/F/42	MDE-nm	...	Paroxetine/20	27/5	4	4
2/F/38	MDR-m	...	Paroxetine/20	26/8	6	9
3/F/32	MDE-nm	...	Paroxetine/20	27/4	5	4
4/M/55	MDR-m	...	Paroxetine/20	30/9	5	13
5/F/16	MDE-nm	...	Paroxetine/20	21/4	3	4
			Group 2 (Resistant Patients)†			
6/F/48	MDR-m	Clomipramine/200 Phenelzine/45 Phenelzine and imipramine Iproniazid Imipramine, carbamazepine, tyronine; methylphenidate Fluoxetine, carbamazepine ECT (12 sessions)	Paroxetine/40 (6 wk)	36/9	4	11
6/F/48‡	...	...	Paroxetine/40 (4 mo)	30/9	6	7
7/F/31	BDD	Clomipramine/200 Fluoxetine/60, carbamazepine; lithium; valproic acid	Paroxetine/20 (6 wk)	32/4	3	3
8/M/45	MDR-m	Fluvoxamine maleate/300, lithium	Phenelzine/60 (6 wk)	27/8	6	13
9/M/57	MDR-nm	Clomipramine/200, lithium Phenelzine/60, lithium Fluoxetine/40, lithium	Paroxetine/20 (6 wk)	14/4	6	4
10/F/80	MDE-nm	Fluvoxamine maleate/200, lithium; maprotiline	Fluvoxamine maleate/200 (8 wk)	18/1	7	6
11/F/51	MDR-m	Imipramine/250 Imipramine, lithium ECT (6 sessions) Imipramine, fluvoxamine	Imipramine/200 (8 wk)	17/7	7	5

**HDRS indicates Hamilton Rating Scale for Depression; NCI, Newcastle Index; MDE, major depressive episode; m, melancholic type; nm, nonmelancholic type; MDR, major depression (recurrent); BDD, bipolar disorder (depressed); and ECT, electroconvulsive therapy.*

†Includes only patients who responded to the addition of pindolol.

‡Patient 6 2.5 months later.

nistic action at postsynaptic and presynaptic 5-HT_{1A} receptors.[13-16] Therefore, antagonism of the 5-HT_{1A}–mediated function may be accountable. However, a concurrent blockade of β-adrenergic receptors is also possible, particularly since it has been known for years that uptake inhibitors and MAO inhibitors induce a down-regulation of the density of β-adrenoceptors,[17] an effect requiring the functional integrity of the serotoninergic system.[18,19] More experimental work is certainly needed to examine the influence of pindolol in serotoninergic brain systems. The present clinical results should, of course, be replicated in a larger, double-blind study before a final conclusion on the potentiation caused by pindolol can be reached.

Francesc Artigas, PhD
Victor Perez, MD
Enric Alvarez, MD
Department of Neurochemistry, CID, CSIC
Department of Psychiatry
Hospital de Sant Pau
Centre d'Investigació i Desenvolupament, CSIC
Jordi Girona 18-26
08034 Barcelona, Spain

This work was supported by grant 92/0268 from the Fondo de Investigación Sanitaria (Dr Artigas). Dr Perez is the recipient of a training fellowship from the Fondo de Investigación Sanitaria.

Reprint requests to F. Artigas, PhD, Department of Neurochemistry, CID, CSIC, Jordi Girona 18-26, 08034 Barcelona, Spain.

1. Blier P, De Montigny C, Chaput Y. Modifications of the serotonin system by antidepressant treatments: implications for the therapeutic response in major depression. *J Clin Psychopharmacol.* 1987;7(suppl):24-35.
2. Chaput Y, De Montigny C, Blier P. Presynaptic and postsynaptic modifications of the serotonin system by long-term administration of antidepressant treatments. *Neuropsychopharmacology.* 1991;5:219-229.
3. Shopsin B, Gershon S, Goldstein M, Friedman E, Wilk S. Use of synthesis inhibitors in defining a role for biogenic amines during imipramine treatment in depressed patients. *Psychopharmacol Commun.* 1975;1:239-249.
4. Shopsin B, Friedman E, Gershon S. Parachlorophenylalanine reversal of tranylcypromine effects in depressed patients. *Arch Gen Psychiatry.* 1976;33:811-819.
5. Delgado PL, Charney DS, Price LH, Aghajanian GK, Landis H, Heninger GR. Serotonin function and the mechanism of antidepressant action. *Arch Gen Psychiatry.* 1990;47:411-418.
6. Adell A, Artigas F. Differential effects of clomipramine given locally or systemically on extracellular 5-hydroxytryptamine in raphe nuclei and frontal cortex: an in vivo microdialysis study. *Naunyn-Schmiedeberg's Arch Pharmacol.* 1991;343:237-244.
7. Bel N, Artigas F. Fluvoxamine preferentially increases extracellular 5-hydroxytryptamine in the raphe nuclei: an in vivo microdialysis study. *Eur J Pharmacol.* 1992;229:101-103.
8. Celada P, Artigas F. Effects of local and systemic MAO inhibitors on extracellular brain 5-hydroxytryptamine and 5-hydroxyindoleacetic acid in the frontal cortex and raphe nuclei of freely moving rats: an in vivo microdialysis study. *Naunyn-Schmiedeberg's Arch Pharmacol.* 1993;347:583-590.
9. Invernizzi R, Belli S, Samanin R. Citalopram's ability to increase the extracellular concentration of serotonin in the dorsal raphe prevents the drug's effect in frontal cortex. *Brain Res.* 1992;584:321-326.
10. Wozniak K, Pert A, Linnoila M. Alterations in raphe and frontal cortex serotonin overflow following focal and systemic administration of fluoxetine. *Soc Neurosci Abs.* 1992;18;1525.
11. Bel N, Artigas F. Chronic treatment with fluvoxamine increases extracellular serotonin in frontal cortex but not in raphe nuclei. *Synapse.* 1993;15:243-245.
12. Hjorth S. Serotonin 5-HT_{1A} autoreceptor blockade potentiates the ability of the 5-HT reuptake inhibitor citalopram to increase nerve terminal output of 5-HT in vivo: a microdialysis study. *J Neurochem.* 1992;60:776-779.
13. Hoyer D. 5-HT receptors: subtypes and second messengers. *J Recept Res.* 1991;11:197-214.
14. Middlemiss DN, Neill J, Tricklebank MD. Subtypes of the 5-HT receptor involved in hypothermia and forepaw treading induced by 8-OH-DPAT. *Br J Pharmacol.* 1985;85:251P.
15. Lesch KP, Poten B, Söhnle K, Schulte HM. Pharmacology of the hypothermic response to 5-HT_{1A} receptor activation in humans. *Eur J Clin Pharmacol.* 1990;39:17-19.
16. Hjorth S, Sharp T. In vivo microdialysis evidence for central serotonin$_{1A}$ and serotonin$_{1B}$ autoreceptor blocking properties of the beta adrenoceptor antagonist (-) penbutolol. *J Pharmacol Exp Ther.* 1993;265:707-712.
17. Baker GB, Greenshaw AJ. Effects of long-term administration of antidepressants and neuroleptics on receptors in the central nervous system. *Cell Mol Neurobiol.* 1989;9:1-44.
18. Barbaccia ML, Brunello N, Chuang DM, Costa E. On the mode of action of imipramine: relationship between serotonergic axon terminal function and down-regulation of beta-adrenergic receptors. *Neuropharmacology.* 1983;22:373-383.
19. Manier DH, Gillespie DD, Sanders-Bush E, Sulser F. The serotonin/noradrenaline link in brain, I: role of noradrenaline and serotonin in the regulation of density and function of beta adrenoceptors and its alteration by desipramine. *Naunyn-Schmiedeberg's Arch Pharmacol.* 1987;335:109-114.

The Diagnostic Interview Schedule and Anorexia Nervosa in Hong Kong

The February 1993 ARCHIVES article by Chen et al[1] is an important step toward a methodologically sound approach to the epidemiological study of psychiatric disorders in the Chinese community of Hong Kong. Only one female with *DSM-III* diagnosis for anorexia nervosa among 7229 subjects (3786 females and 3443 males; age range, 18 to 64 years) was identified, giving a low lifetime prevalence of 0.03% in females. It confirms the customary belief that anorexia nervosa is a condition "bound" to western cultures and is extremely rare in Chinese people.

However, such a presumptive belief should be tempered until factors relating to patients' presenting mode of distress, help-seeking behavior, investigators' alertness to abnormal eating behavior as psychiatric morbidity, and the diagnostic criteria used are elucidated. Regarding the Chinese, besides recent reports from Taiwan and Hong Kong[2] on anorexia nervosa and bulimia nervosa, Song and Fang[3] described nine females with anorexia nervosa who were admitted to the Institute of Mental Health of Beijing (China) Medical University between 1982 and 1988. Furthermore, Chen[4] reported that seven children with anorexia nervosa were treated with behavioral therapy in Anding Hospital, another mental institution in Beijing, between 1979 and 1986. Although detailed case histories are often not available, these reports signify that some type of eating disorder exists in contemporary Chinese societies.

Recent reports from Asian countries such as India, Malaysia, Singapore, and Hong Kong concurrently suggest that while young females with food refusal, self-imposed emaciation, and amenorrhea undoubtedly exist, a significant proportion of them do not exhibit the fear of obesity, which is the sine qua non of contemporary western anorexia nervosa.[5] Of seven Chinese patients systematically studied in Singapore, Ong and Tsoi[6] reported that the fear of fatness was obvious in three, slight in two, and completely absent in two others. In India, according to Khandelwal and Saxena,[7] anorectic patients "are also young females showing decreased appetite, excessive weight loss and amenorrhea. But a clear body image disturbance or fear of becoming fat is hardly ever seen." From 1970 through 1988 at a university hospital in West Malaysia, Goh et al[8] identified 15 females with anorexia nervosa, six of whom did not demonstrate the fear of fatness. A recent study of 70 Chinese anorectic patients in Hong Kong reaffirms that although they were similar to western anorexics in most other ways, 41 (58.6%) of them did not exhibit any fear of fatness throughout their course of illness. Instead, these nonfat phobic patients used epigastric bloating (31.4%), loss of appetite/hunger (15.7%), or simply eating less (12.9%) as legitimating rationales for food refusal and emaciation. The possible explanations for this intriguing absence of the fear of fatness and the interpretive dilemma it provokes have been discussed from historical, pathoplastic, and cultural anthropological perspectives.[2] Historically, it was only until about 1960 that the now characteristic fear of fatness appeared regularly as a predominant motive for self-imposed starvation in scientific writings on anorexia nervosa.[9]

As the Diagnostic Interview Schedule (eg, Have you ever thought that you were too fat or in danger of becoming too fat?) is fully structured and based on *DSM-III* diagnoses, which require an intense fear of obesity as an obligatory criterion for the diagnosis of anorexia nervosa, Chinese anorexics without the fear of fatness could have been missed by lay interviewers. This suspicion may be strengthened by clinical experience also in Shatin, Hong Kong, that less restrictively defined anorexia nervosa does not appear to be as rare as suggested by the survey.[2] It is possible that an inquiry mode that connected more directly with indigenous Chinese concepts of alimentation, body weight, and shape might have uncovered more anorectic patients. Using the more flexible criteria of "complete unconcern regarding extreme thinness" and "a distorted attitude and behaviour toward eating" for case identification at the screening and interview stages respectively, Mizushima and Ishii[10] identified 16 females with anorexia nervosa out of a high school population of 36 403 in Ishikawa, Japan. At clinical assessment, only four of these 16 females exhibited a "thin ideal" and one of them continued to do so at 9-month follow-up.

Nonwestern cultures make up about 80% of the world. If half of their anorectic patients should present without the fear of fatness, the Diagnostic Interview Schedule clearly needs contextually appropriate modifications to be validly used in the cross-cultural study of anorexia nervosa. The imposition of the criterion of the fear of fatness on all fasting patients from nonwestern cultures that are not preoccupied with slimness, without regard for its contextual validity, constitutes a "category fallacy." When less ethnocentrically defined, anorexia nervosa may not be as rare as suggested by the Shatin community mental health survey.[1] The formulation of a culture-flexible set of diagnostic criteria for anorexia nervosa will enhance patient-practitioner negotiation and the use of individually tailored therapeutics, as well as epidemiological research. It will also encourage the reporting of a greater variety of "typical" and "atypical" subjects with morbid starvation from different countries in the world.

Sing Lee, MRCPsych
Department of Psychiatry
The Chinese University of Hong Kong
Shatin, NT, Hong Kong

1. Chen C-N, Wong J, Lee N, Chang-Ho M-W, Lau J, Fung M. The Shatin community mental health survey in Hong Kong, II: major findings. *Arch Gen Psychiatry*. 1993;50:125-133.
2. Lee S, Ho TP, Hsu LKG. Fat phobic and non-fat phobic anorexia nervosa: a comparative study of 70 Chinese patients in Hong Kong. *Psychol Med*. In press.
3. Song YP, Fang YK. A clinical report of nine cases of anorexia nervosa. *Chin Ment Health J*. 1990;4:24-25.
4. Chen J. Behavioural therapy of seven cases of childhood anorexia nervosa. *Chin Ment Health J*. 1990;4:26.
5. American Psychiatric Association, Committee on Nomenclature and Statistics. *Diagnostic and Statistical Manual of Mental Disorders, Third Edition*. Washington, DC: American Psychiatric Association; 1980.
6. Ong YL, Tsoi WF. A clinical and psychosocial study of seven cases of anorexia nervosa in Singapore. *Singapore Med J*. 1982;23:255-261.
7. Khandelwal SK, Saxena S. Anorexia nervosa in people of Asian extraction. *Br J Psychiatry*. 1990;157:784.
8. Goh SE, Ong SBY, Subramaniam M. Eating disorders in Hong Kong. *Br J Psychiatry*. 1993;162:276-277.
9. Casper RC. On the emergence of bulimia nervosa as a syndrome: a historical view. *Int J Eating Dis*. 1983;2:3-16.
10. Mizushima N, Ishii Y. The epidemiology of anorexia nervosa in junior and senior high school students in Ishikawa Prefecture. *Jpn J Psychosom Med*. 1983;23:311-319.

Schizophrenia and Temporal Lobe Epilepsy

A Neuropsychological Analysis

James M. Gold, PhD; Bruce P. Hermann, PhD; Christopher Randolph, PhD; Alan R. Wyler, MD; Terry E. Goldberg, PhD; Daniel R. Weinberger, MD

Background: Recent neuroimaging studies have reported structural abnormalities of mesial temporal lobe structures in schizophrenia. This study compared the neuropsychological performance of patients with schizophrenia with patients with either left or right temporal lobe epilepsy to determine if lateralized, developmental temporal lobe dysfunction provides a model of the cognitive impairments observed in schizophrenia.

Methods: A total 66 patients with schizophrenia and 101 patients with medically intractable focal temporal lobe epilepsy (48 left temporal, 53 right temporal) received a comprehensive neuropsychological battery.

Results: The three groups did not differ on age, years of education, or Full-Scale IQ. However, clear differences were noted in performance profiles. Patients with schizophrenia scored significantly higher than either epilepsy group on a measure of word reading thought to reflect premorbid competence. Patients with schizophrenia demonstrated greater attentional impairment and motor slowing than either epilepsy group. The patients with schizophrenia had superior semantic knowledge and verbal memory compared with the left temporal lobe group. On the Wisconsin Card Sorting Test the patients with schizophrenia obtained significantly fewer categories than either temporal lobe group, but were not significantly more perseverative.

Conclusions: Data suggest lateralized temporal lobe dysfunction does not provide an adequate model of the cognitive impairments seen in schizophrenia. The disorders seem to follow different developmental paths: In early-onset epilepsy, the acquisition of cognitive skills and academic knowledge is compromised, while in schizophrenia congnitive functions are lost. Extratemporal pathologic features, most likely of the frontal lobe, are implicated in the cognitive dysfunction of schizophrenia.

(Arch Gen Psychiatry. 1994;51:265-272)

From the Clinical and Research Services Branch (Dr Gold) and the Clinical Brain Disorders Branch (Drs Goldberg and Weinberger), Division of Intramural Research Programs, National Institute of Mental Health, Washington, DC; the EpiCare Center, Baptist Memorial Hospital, Departments of Psychiatry and Neurosurgery, University of Tennessee, and Semmes-Murphey Clinic, Memphis (Drs Hermann and Wyler); and the Experimental Therapeutics Branch, National Institute of Neurological Diseases and Stroke, National Institutes of Health, Bethesda, Md (Dr Randolph).

THERE HAVE been numerous demonstrations of neuropsychological deficits among patients with schizophrenia.[1-6] Interpretation, however, remains controversial, with varied proposals that temporal, frontal, frontal-striatal, or a combination of prefrontal-temporal lobe dysfunction accounts for the range and nature of the deficits.[6-10] The lateralization of dysfunction is also actively debated.[11-14]

In part, the controversy is attributable to the basic methodologic approach used. The typical design contrasts the performance of patients to normal controls on a collection of tasks validated on subjects with neurological disorders.[4,5,8] Tasks sensitive to focal lesions in patients with neurological disorders purportedly support inferences about areas of maximal dysfunction in patients with schizophrenia. There are two basic problems with this approach in the study of schizophrenia.

First, the neuropsychological deficits noted with focal lesions are acquired impairments, the result of stroke, tumor, or trauma in an adult brain, which, until that point, had undergone normal development. It is uncertain that the neurophysiological dysfunction in schizophrenia is acquired in adulthood; in fact, evidence suggests

See Subjects and Methods on next page

early developmental compromise in the pathogenesis of the disorder.[15-18] The behavioral expression of a focal lesion that occurs in a developing brain is likely to be different from that of an anatomically identical lesion acquired as an adult.[19] This limits the validity of inferences derived from adult patients with neurological disorders. The second problem stems from the fact that schizophrenic patients tend to perform below the level of normal subjects on a variety of tests.[20] This precludes the derivation of differential deficit profiles due to the variation in reliability, difficulty, sensitivity, and specificity among neuropsychological tests.[21] Tasks equally sensitive to effects of different types of focal damage, but that differ in their sensitivity to the more general effects of brain damage, may falsely implicate localized dysfunction. Further, the distribution of scores on different tests in brain-damaged populations varies widely, and the use of standard scores from normal controls does not account for this fact, particularly if "floor" effects are present on some measures.[22] Until a reference scaling method is developed to permit such comparisons among tests, it is unlikely that the comparison of normal controls and schizophrenic patients will yield much new information.

A potentially more fruitful approach is to directly compare the cognitive performance of schizophrenic patients with that of patients with well-defined lesions. Older studies with this approach tended to use diagnostically hetereogeneous brain-damaged samples and did not focus on patient populations with developmental lesions that might be most relevant to schizophrenia.[23] Direct comparisons allow for an evaluation of the cognitive consequences of brain damage per se, and may also yield evidence of distinctive performance patterns across cognitive domains. Thus, the primary question of interest is how overall cognitive profiles compare, not if a particular test result is "most" abnormal. Finding superior performance by schizophrenic patients in one domain relative to a contrast population coupled with significantly impaired performance in another domain would be the most direct evidence that the generalized deficit observed in patients with schizophrenia does not fully account for their profile of cognitive strengths and weaknesses.

In this study, we directly compared the neuropsychological performance of schizophrenic patients and patients with focal right or left temporal lobe epilepsy (TLE) to determine if lateralized temporal lobe dysfunction provides an adequate model of the cognitive

SUBJECTS AND METHODS

We studied 66 patients with a *DSM-III-R*[41] diagnosis of schizophrenia and 101 patients with TLE. Schizophrenic patients were research volunteers assessed at the National Institute of Mental Health Neuropsychiatric Research Hospital, Washington, DC. Consensus research diagnosis was made by ward physicians in consultation with senior clinical-research staff following review of past records and extended clinical observation (generally greater than 6 months, and often including an extended drug-free period) and repeated interviews. Approximately 40% (27) of the patients also received a Structured Clinical Interview for *DSM-III* as this became standard hospital procedure. The patients received the following subtype diagnosis: paranoid, 17; undifferentiated, 38; disorganized, eight; and residual, three. All were tested as part of their initial clinical-research assessment while receiving stable medication regimens. In all but one patient this included neuroleptics alone (n=8), in conjunction with anticholinergic medication (n=35), or in combination with other medications such as lithium carbonate or carbamazapine (n=22). Patients also received complete medical, laboratory, neurological, and neuroimaging studies to rule out other possible sources of neuropsychological compromise.

The epilepsy sample was composed of 101 consecutive referred nonretarded patients (Full-Scale IQ >70) older than 16 years with medication-resistant epilepsy of unilateral temporal lobe origin. Patients were tested as part of an evaluation to determine their suitability for anterior temporal lobectomy. The evaluation included 24-hour video-electroencephalographic monitoring with scalp electrodes to record spontaneous seizures. To provide precise localization of ictal onset, almost every patient also underwent invasive monitoring with subdural strip electrodes; those patients with only scalp electrode monitoring had unequivocal localization of seizure onset. Only patients with left hemisphere speech dominance determined by intracarotid amobarbital sodium testing were included in the study. Patients with structural lesions (tumors, infarcts) as determined by magnetic resonance imaging or computed tomographic scan were eliminated. Determination of ictal onset localization was made without knowledge of the neuropsychological results. The presurgery cognitive testing, which provides the data of this study, was done with patients not receiving anticonvulsant medications for 24 to 72 hours except in patients with a history of status epilepticus who were tested while receiving half doses of their medications.

The epilepsy sample was composed of 48 patients with a left (dominant) temporal lobe ictal focus (left TLE [LTLE]) and 53 patients with a right (nondominant) ictal focus (right TLE [RTLE]). Demographics of the three patient groups are shown in **Table 1**. The groups did not differ in age or years of education completed. The two epilepsy groups did not differ in their early age of onset of chronic seizures. Age of onset is dated from first hospitalization for the schizophrenic group, which had a 2:1 male-to-female ratio; the epilepsy samples were composed of nearly equal gender numbers. Each of the three groups included 10% to 11% of subjects who used their left hands for writing.

Patients were administered a neuropsychological test battery composed of the following: Wide Range Achievement Test–Revised (WRAT-R) reading subtest,[42] Wechsler Adult Intelligence Scale–Revised (WAIS-R),[43] Wisconsin Card Sorting Test (WCS),[44] Trail Making Test A and B,[45] Finger Tapping,[45] Controlled Oral Word Association Test (verbal fluency),[46] Token Test,[46] Facial Recognition Test,[47] Judgment of Line Orientation,[47] and California Verbal Learning Test (CVLT).[48] Tests were administered and scored as described in the manuals (**Table 2**). For the WCS at the National Institute of Mental Health (NIMH), 26 subjects received a standard administration and 23 were tested with a computer version. No significant differences were noted in WCS performance indexes between these groups and they are combined for all the analyses reported below. Different, but equivalent, letter cues were used for verbal fluency across sites.[49] Complete data sets were available for almost every patient with TLE, with a maximum of two missing subjects on several tests. The variability in subject number in the NIMH sample is due to changing the composition of the test battery over the several years that these data were collected. The 32 schizophrenic patients who received the CVLT did not differ from the rest of the sample on demographic variables or IQ.

To protect against type I error, we first performed multivariate analyses of variance (MANOVAs) with an α level of .01 on tests grouped by the cognitive domain they are traditionally believed to measure (ie, language, motor speed). If the MANOVA was significant, univariate analyses of variance (ANOVAs) and post hoc *t* tests with an α level of .05 were then performed. To further reduce the total number of comparisons, we used factor scores from the WAIS-R, used only two measures from the WCS (categories achieved and percent perseverative error), and performed a factor analysis of the 19 scores from the CVLT. We obtained a six-factor solution for the CVLT that closely resembled the factor analysis of the original normative sample.[48] The first factor, accounting for 31% of the variance, was a general verbal learning factor with loading on total recall over the five learning trials and the short- and long-delay recall trials. The next five factors (and proportion of variance) reflect the following: intrusion of nonlist words (11%), the consistency of recall and learning slope (10%), primacy-recency effects (9%), interference list recall (8%), and tendency to recall items in serial order (8%). We performed a MANOVA on the six factor scores. Univariate ANOVAs were performed on measures that did not fit into any of the test clusters. To ensure that differences in sample gender composition were not responsible for the between-group findings, the between-group analyses were repeated after randomly deleting female subjects from both epilepsy groups (12 from the group with LTLE, 13 from the group with RTLE) to create equal gender ratios across the three groups. All of the epilepsy-schizophrenia contrasts that were significant in the entire sample remained significant in the sex-balanced samples. In light of this fact, we are reporting the findings from the total sample.

impairments observed in patients with schizophrenia. This comparison is of interest given recent evidence of structural changes in medial temporal lobe regions in patients with schizophrenia,[16,24-26] regions consistently implicated in TLE.[27] Further, in both schizophrenic patients and patients with TLE, it is likely that the anatomic abnormalities occurred early in development and both groups demonstrate impairments in memory and problem solving.[28-34] Indeed, TLE has long been seen as a potential biological model for schizophrenia given that there may be an increased frequency of interictal psychosis among patients with TLE, and some of the perceptual abnormalities that occur as "auras" or that may be elicited by direct electrical stimulation of medial temporal structures resemble schizophrenic symptoms.[35-40] Thus, these study populations appear to share important anatomic, phenomenologic, and cognitive features.

RESULTS

IQ AND ACADEMIC ACHIEVEMENT

The three groups did not differ on Full-Scale IQ. An overall group effect was noted on the WRAT-R reading subtest ($F=8.3, P<.001$). Post hoc *t* tests revealed that the schizophrenic patients performed better than both epilepsy groups (both $P<.005$), which did not differ from each other.

To evaluate the WAIS-R data, factor scores were calculated as suggested by Kaufman.[50] The verbal comprehension factor was composed of the Information, Vocabulary, Comprehension, and Similarities subtests; the perceptual organization factor was composed of the Picture Completion, Block Design, and Object Assembly subtests; and the freedom from distractibility factor (or attentional factor) was composed of the Digit Span and Arithmetic subtests. As seen in **Figure 1**, there was a

Table 1. Demographic Features*

	Patients With Right TLE	Patients With Left TLE	Patients With Schizophrenia
Age, y	29.9±9.7	29.8±9.8	32.3±7.6
Education, y	12.4±2.9	12.5±2.2	12.3±2.0
Age of onset, y	13.8±10.1	11.1±10.9	20.2±4.0
Sex, No.			
M	26	23	44
F	27	25	22

**TLE indicates temporal lobe epilepsy. Unless otherwise indicated, values are mean±SD.*

Table 2. Neuropsychological Test Performance*

	Patients With Right TLE, Mean±SD	Patients With Left TLE, Mean±SD	Patients With Schizophrenia	
			N	Mean±SD
WRAT-R Reading	88.2±16.8	84.1±18.7	63	96.4±13.9
Full-Scale IQ	90.7±11.6	87.9±13.5	66	87.7±11.5
Trails, s				
A	37.7±13.7	37.6±17.1	66	47.0±24.5
B	84.7±32.3	84.6±35.7	65	119.3±67.8
Tapping				
Dominant	49.0±6.6	48.0±7.5	65	44.5±7.3
Nondominant	44.7±7.1	44.6±7.0	65	40.9±7.2
Token Test	41.8±3.0	40.7±3.6	51	40.6±2.6
Fluency	35.2±10.4	33.0±11.6	66	36.6±9.4
Line Orientation	23.8±5.3	22.8±5.1	65	23.9±5.1
Facial Recognition	46.5±3.9	43.9±6.1	65	44.4±4.6
WCST				
Categories	4.3±2.0	4.3±2.1	49	3.3±2.2
% PE	19.6±13.6	19.3±11.7	49	24.2±16.3

WCST indicates Wisconsin Card Sorting Test; % PE, percent perseverative errors; TLE, temporal lobe epilepsy; and WRAT-R, Wide Range Achievement Test–Revised.

clear difference in performance pattern across groups, the overall MANOVA being significant (Wilks' λ F=8.01, *P*<.0001). On the verbal factor there was a significant overall difference (F=5.46, *P*<.005), with the schizophrenic patients and the RTLE group, who did not differ from each other, both significantly outperforming the LTLE group as determined by post hoc tests (both *P*<.04). On the attentional factor, there was a significant overall group effect (F=5.00, *P*<.01), and the schizophrenic patients performed significantly worse than either TLE group on post hoc *t* tests (both *P*<.01). The epilepsy groups did not differ from one another. The three groups did not differ on the perceptual organization factor.

ATTENTIONAL AND MOTOR PERFORMANCE

A MANOVA was performed on Trails A, Trails B, and the Digit Symbol subtest of the WAIS-R, considering them measures of attention, and obtained a Wilks' λ of 4.09 (*P*<.001). Univariate ANOVAs on all three measures were significant (all *P*<.02), and in post hoc *t* tests both TLE groups, who did not differ from each other, performed significantly better than the schizophrenic patients (all *P*<.02). A MANOVA combining the two-finger tapping conditions was significant (Wilks' λ F=3.41, *P*<.01). Both univariate ANOVAs were significant (both *P*<.005), and in post hoc *t* tests both TLE groups, who did not differ from each other, significantly outperformed the schizophrenic group in both conditions (all *P*<.02).

LANGUAGE

The overall MANOVA combining the Token and Verbal Fluency tests approached significance (Wilks' λ F=2.42, *P*<.048).

VISUAL SPATIAL

The MANOVA combining the Judgment of Line Orientation Test and the Facial Recognition Test approached significance (Wilks' λ F=2.22, *P*<.067).

ABSTRACTION

The MANOVA combining the categories achieved and percent perseverative error scores from the WCS was not significant (*P*<.11). In light of the importance of this measure in the literature, we performed univariate ANOVAs on both measures. An overall group effect was noted on the categories measures (F=3.8, *P*<.03) and post hoc tests revealed that both epilepsy groups performed significantly better than the schizophrenic patients (*P*<.03). The groups did not differ on the perseveration measure (*P*<.15).

MEMORY

Performance of the three groups on the CVLT is shown in **Figure 2**. The MANOVA on the six-factor scores was significant (Wilks' λ F=2.43, *P*<.005). Univariate ANOVAs were significant only for factor 1, general verbal memory (F=4.78, *P*<.01), and factor 4, primacy-recency (F=4.99, *P*<.01). Post hoc *t* tests for factor 1 revealed that both the patients with RTLE and the schizophrenic patients, who did not differ from each other, performed better than the patients with LTLE (both *P*<.02). This first factor includes the total recall score over the five learning trials as well as the short- and long-delay, free and cued, recall scores shown in Figure 2. Post hoc tests for factor 4 revealed that both TLE groups, which did not differ from each other, scored higher than the schizophrenic groups (both *P*<.03). This factor reflects primacy and recency effects in recall. Examination of raw data reveals that the schizophrenic patients tended to recall more material from the recency portion (last four of the 16 words) and less material from the primacy portion (first four of the 16 words) of the list than either TLE group. Thus, both the patients with RTLE and schizophrenia evidenced better verbal memory than the patients with LTLE, but the schizophrenic patients differed from both TLE groups on this qualitative indicator of learning style.

To further evaluate the pattern of results, we performed a stepwise discriminant analysis between the schizophrenic patients and the combined TLE sample. We entered all the variables discussed above that significantly separated the schizophrenic patients from the two TLE groups except for the CVLT factor 4 score, which

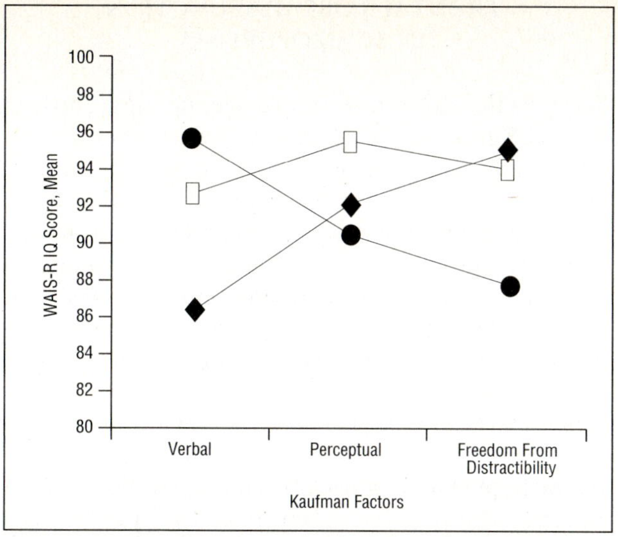

Figure 1. *Wechsler Adult Intelligence Scale–Revised (WAIS-R) Verbal Comprehension, Perceptual Organization, and Freedom From Distractibility factor scores for schizophrenic patients (circles), patients with right temporal lobe epilepsy (rectangles), and patients with left temporal lobe epilepsy (diamonds). See text for subtest composition of factor scores.*

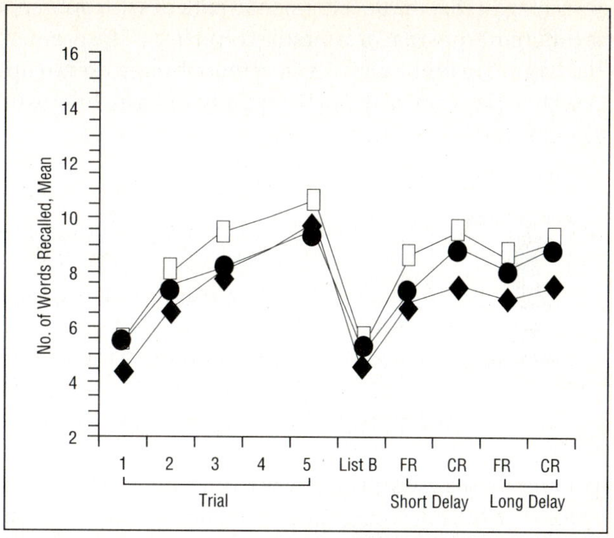

Figure 2. *California Verbal Learning Test performance of schizophrenic patients (circles), patients with right temporal lobe epilepsy (rectangles), and patients with left temproal lobe epilepsy (diamonds). Trials 1 through 5 indicate free recall trials for initial list; list B, free recall of interference list; FR, free recall; and CR, cued recall.*

would have reduced the sample size significantly. In addition, we examined the 11 WAIS-R subtests. The overall MANOVA on these 11 subtests was significant ($P<.0001$) and the subsequent ANOVAs (all $P<.01$) and *t* tests (all $P<.03$) revealed that four subtests were significantly different between the groups: the schizophrenic group performed significantly better than either TLE group on Information, and significantly worse than both TLE groups on three subtests (Arithmetic, Picture Arrangement, and Digit Symbol). These tests were used in the discriminant analysis. The sample size for this analysis was 47 schizophrenic patients and 92 patients with TLE. A seven-variable solution emerged that included, in order of entry, Trails B, WAIS-R Information, Arithmetic, Picture Arrangement, Digit Symbol, WRAT-R Reading, and preferred-hand Finger Tapping. This combination of variables correctly classified 83% (39/47) of the schizophrenic subjects and 89% (81/92) of the TLE group. Thus, it seems to be the pattern of impaired attention and motor speed coupled with relatively elevated reading and semantic memory in the schizophrenic group that best distinguishes them from the TLE group.

COMMENT

These data suggest that there are limits to a lateralized, developmental temporal lobe lesion model of schizophrenic cognitive impairment. Patients with schizophrenia demonstrate a degree of attentional impairment in both auditory (WAIS-R attentional factor) and visual tasks (Digit Symbol, Trails) that was not observed in either TLE group. These tasks do not appear to be highly dependent on medial temporal lobe structures given the near-normal performance of the TLE groups on the WAIS-R attentional factor and are consistent with extratemporal involvement in schizophrenia.

The limits of the temporal lobe model are also evident when considering the WRAT-R reading and WAIS-R verbal factor scores. Intractable TLE, particularly LTLE, seems to interfere with the acquisition or availability of basic linguistic and semantic knowledge. In contrast, these functions seem to be an area of relative cognitive strength in patients with schizophrenia. Given the clear effects of laterality of seizure focus on these verbal functions, it appears that the left temporal lobe "model" of schizophrenia has definite limitations.

This finding also has important developmental implications. The performance pattern in both TLE groups is suggestive of developmentally based neuropsychological compromise consistent with their relatively early age of onset. We base this conclusion on the fact that basic linguistic skills such as single-word reading and knowledge of word meanings are at subnormal levels, and are at or below the level seen in other areas of intellectual function. A different pattern is often observed in adult-acquired brain damage where measures of word reading and "crystallized intelligence" such as the WAIS-R verbal factor often are maintained at, or near, premorbid levels.[51-53] Using this model, the schizophrenic performance profile is suggestive of a deterioration of function from premorbid levels as word reading and knowledge are superior to other intellectual abilities.

This does not imply that schizophrenia develops de novo in adulthood. Evidence of premorbid cognitive abnormalites is abundant in many schizophrenic patients.[54] However, the contrasts in neuropsychological pattern suggest that the developmental path of schizophrenia is different from that of lateralized epilepsy. The premorbid cognitive abnormalities in schizophrenia do not appear to compromise the development of basic linguistic skills and semantic knowledge.

THE WCS and CVLT findings are more ambiguous than the WAIS-R and WRAT-R data. Both epilepsy groups obtained significantly more categories on the WCS than did the schizophrenic patients, but the schizophrenic patients did not perseverate significantly more. Insofar as the WCS categories achieved score is a measure of frontal function, then the schizophrenic patients seem to have a degree of frontal compromise that cannot be fully accounted for by a temporal lobe lesion. However, it is clear that the WCS performance of the TLE groups is below that reported for normal control populations,[33,44] suggesting either that frontal function is impaired based on connectivity of frontal and medial temporal regions or that the task is also sensitive to nonfrontal lesions. These data are consistent with other recent studies demonstrating WCS impairment in nonfrontal lesion groups.[55,56]

All three groups demonstrate memory impairments when contrasted with the CVLT normative sample. However, there is a clear laterality effect on the first, and by far the most powerful factor of this test, with the LTLE group performing more poorly than the RTLE group. On this measure, the schizophrenic group also performed better than the LTLE group, additional evidence that a left lateralized model of schizophrenia is limited. The schizophrenic-TLE difference on the primacy-recency factor raises the possibility that the path to poor memory in schizohrenia patients may be somewhat different than in patients with TLE and suggests a more passive learning style in the schizophrenic group. The fact that the three groups did not differ on four of the six factor scores suggests that there are important similarities as well. However, in the absence of an additional nontemporal lesion sample, these data remain ambiguous as the overall profile level and qualitative features may simply reflect "bad memory" of any origin.

Thus, our overall conclusion is that the present data do not fit a model of selective lateralized temporal-limbic dysfunction in schizophrenia. This conclusion, however, is qualified in light of several important facts. While the epilepsy sample had lateralized ictal foci, both groups demonstrate generalized dysfunction, perhaps reflective of the early age of onset of chronic seizures. For example, the Verbal IQ of the RTLE group is clearly below average, as is the Performance IQ of the LTLE group. Thus, treatment-refractory epilepsy appears to involve a degree of generalized impairment despite the fact that a clearly lateralized seizure focus can be ascertained.

FRONTAL LOBE DYSFUNCTION IN SCHIZOPHRENIA

The tests that differentiate the schizophrenic group from both TLE groups generally involve some type of manipulation and sequencing of information, as in performing arithmetic computations or in Trail Making and the WCS. While the construct of working memory eludes precise definition, it appears to be relevant to this pattern where impairments are observed on tasks that require the active maintenance of information over time so that additional cognitive operations can be performed.[57] In essence, there is a loss of attentional control in schizophrenia that is manifest in a variety of tasks involving multiple component cognitive operations. This attentional impairment, which has been one of the primary concerns of cognitive research in schizophrenia,[54,58] cannot be explained exclusively on the basis of temporal lobe abnormalities given the current data, except perhaps by implicating disease-specific indirect effects on prefrontal function.[59]

The frontal lobe has been suggested as a critical part of a widely distributed system that subserves working memory.[60] The basic attentional impairments in schizophrenia may have an important relationship to the compromise of complex executive controls demanded by the WCS and typically associated with frontal lobe function.[61] The WCS did not contribute to the discriminant function after attentional measures had been entered. Thus, impairments at simpler levels of information maintenance and manipulation as required by Trail Making and Arithmetic may underlie the compromise of more complex cognitive operations. Thus, we would suggest that the overall pattern of findings does imply a distinctive frontal contribution to the impairment observed in schizophrenia in the form of attentional dyscontrol.

LIMITATIONS

Our patient groups came from tertiary care or research facilities. Specifically, the patients with epilepsy had medication-resistant disorders and all subsequently underwent surgical procedures. Thus, they are not representative of the broader population of patients with TLE, most of whom can be treated satisfactorily with antiseizure medications. However, the relatively "extreme" nature of these patients underscores the implications of finding neuropsychological functions that were more impaired in the patients with schizophrenia.

The NIMH schizophrenic group also has sampling biases; the "good outcome" end of the spectrum is underrepresented. The NIMH sample has a 2:1 male-to-female ratio, while broader epidemiologic studies suggest a nearly equal sex ratio.[62] About 25% of our sample requires nearly continuous inpatient care. However, many of the cognitive findings in this sample are similar to those seen in patients with first-episode schizophrenia.[63,64] Thus, the sample may be more representative than would otherwise be inferred.

An additional interpretive issue is the role of medication effects. Most patients with TLE were unmedicated for at least 24 hours at the time of assessment and it is probable that the cognitively "toxic" effects of antiseizure medications were modest by that point.[65] More critically, the impairments sometimes attributed to these medications such as in attention, motor speed, and memory include the areas where the TLE patient groups performed better than the schizophrenic patients.

The schizophrenic patients were receiving stable medication regimens at the time of testing. There is little evidence that the schizophrenic-TLE differences on attention, graphomotor speed, and abstracting can be attributed to neuroleptics.[66-69] Neuroleptics, in fact, may improve some attentional functions.[68] Anticholinergic activity may have played a role in the memory data[68] but was not examined in this sample as the assignment of medications was not under experimental control. Yet, memory impairments were reported in schizophrenia during the preneuroleptic era[70] and have also been observed in high-risk populations.[71] We lacked standard ratings of tardive dyskinesia on our sample, a variable that may influence cognitive performance.[72,73]

In summary, the neuropsychological comparison of patients with schizophrenia and TLE suggests that lateralized, developmental temporal lobe dysfunction does not provide by itself an adequate account of the cognitive abnormality of schizophrenia. Schizophrenic patients demonstrated a degree of attentional dyscontrol that was not observed in the TLE samples and may be evidence of frontal lobe dysfunction. The schizophrenic patients have superior verbal memory and verbal knowledge when compared with the patients with LTLE, evidence against the hypothesis that schizophrenia is a selective left medial temporal lobe disorder. Based on measures of reading and acquired knowledge, it appears that schizophrenia and epilepsy follow different developmental paths. Epilepsy interferes with either the aquisition or access to basic verbal skills and knowledge whereas schizophrenia appears to spare these functions.

Accepted for publication October 13, 1992.

Rex Cowdry provided encouragement for this project, Constance Carpenter assisted with the manuscript, and Teresa Blaxton helped on a related project that led to the current study.

Reprint requests to NIMH Neuroscience Center at St Elizabeths, 2700 Martin Luther King Ave SE, Washington, DC 20032 (Dr Gold).

REFERENCES

1. Goldberg TE, Gold JM, Braff DL. Neuropsychological functioning and time-linked information processing in schizophrenia. In: Tasman A, Goldfinger SM, eds. *Review of Psychiatry.* Washington DC: American Psychiatric Press; 1991:10:60-78.
2. Goldberg E, Seidman LJ. Higher cortical functions in normals and schizophrenics: a selective review. In: Steinhaurer SR, Gruzelier JH, Zubin J, eds. *Handbook of Schizophrenia.* Amsterdam, the Netherlands: Elsevier Science Publishers; 1991:5:553-598.
3. Levin S, Yurgelun-Todd D, Craft S. Contributions of clinical neuropsychology to the study of schizophrenia. *J Abnorm Psychol.* 1989;98:341-356.
4. Braff DL, Heaton R, Kuck J, Cullum M, Moranville J, Grant I, Zisook S. The generalized pattern of neuropsychological deficits in outpatients with chronic schizophrenia with heterogeneous Wisconsin Card Sorting Test results. *Arch Gen Psychiatry.* 1991;48:891-898.
5. Saykin AJ, Gur RC, Gur RE, Mozley PD, Mozley LH, Resnick SM, Kester DB, Stafniak P. Neuropsychological impairment in schizophrenia: selective impairment in memory and learning. *Arch Gen Psychiatry.* 1991;48:618-624.
6. Goldberg TE, Ragland JD, Torrey EF, Gold JM, Bigelow LB, Weinberger DR. Neuropsychological assessment of monozygotic twins discordant for schizophrenia. *Arch Gen Psychiatry.* 1990;47:1066-1072.
7. Goldberg TE, Weinberger DR, Berman KF, Pliskin NH, Podd M. Further evidence for dementia of the prefrontal type in schizophrenia? *Arch Gen Psychiatry.* 1987;44:1008-1014.
8. Kolb B, Whishaw IQ. Performance of schizophrenic patients on tests sensitive to left or right, frontal, temporal or parietal function in neurological patients. *J Nerv Ment Dis.* 1983;171:435-443.
9. Gruzelier J, Seymour K, Wilson L, Jolley A, Hirsch S. Impairments on neuropsychological tests of temporohippocampal and fronto-hippocampal functions and word fluency in remitting schizophrenia and affective disorders. *Arch Gen Psychiatry.* 1988;45:623-629.
10. Robbins TW. The case for frontostriatal dysfunction in schizophrenia. *Schizophr Bull.* 1990;16:391-402.
11. Posner MI, Early TS, Reiman E, Pardo PJ, Dhawan M. Asymmetries in hemispheric control of attention in schizophrenia. *Arch Gen Psychiatry.* 1988;45:814-821.
12. Cutting J. *The Right Cerebral Hemisphere and Psychiatric Disorders.* New York, NY: Oxford University Press Inc; 1990.
13. Gur RE. Left hemisphere dysfunction and left hemisphere overactivation in schizophrenia. *J Abnorm Psychol.* 1978;87:226-238.
14. Flor-Henry P, Fromm-Auch D, Schopflocher D. Neuropsychological dimensions in psychopathology. In: Flor-Henry P, Gruzelier J, eds. *Laterality and Psychopathology.* Amsterdam, the Netherlands: Elsevier Science Publishers; 1983:59-82.
15. Weinberger DR. Implications of normal brain development for the pathogenesis of schizophrenia. *Arch Gen Psychiatry.* 1987;44:660-669.
16. Jakob H, Beckman H. Prenatal developmental disturbances in the limbic allocortex in schizophrenics. *J Neural Transm.* 1986;65:303-326.
17. Crow TJ, Ball J, Bloom SR, Brown R, Bruton CD, Colter N, Frith CD, Johnstone EC, Owens DGC, Roberts GW. Schizophrenia as an anomaly of development of cerebral asymmetry: a post-mortem study and a proposal concerning the genetic basis of the disease. *Arch Gen Psychiatry.* 1989;46:1145-1150.
18. Murray RM, Lewis SW. Is schizophrenia a neurodevelopmental disorder? *BMJ.* 1988;285:681-682.
19. Chadwick O, Rutter M, Thompson J, Shaffer D. Intellectual performance and reading skills after localized head injury in childhood. *J Child Psychol Psychiatry.* 1981;22:117-139.
20. Chapman LJ, Chapman JP. *Disordered Thought in Schizophrenia.* East Norwalk, Conn: Appleton & Lange; 1973.
21. Chapman LJ, Chapman JP. Problems in the measurement of cognitive deficit. *Psychol Bull.* 1973;79:380-385.
22. Randolph C, Goldberg TE, Weinberger DR. The neuropsychology of schizophrenia. In: Heilman KM, Valenstein E, eds. *Clinical Neuropsychology.* 3rd ed. New York: Oxford University Press Inc. In press.
23. Heaton RK, Baade LE, Johnson KL. Neuropsychological test results associated with psychiatric disorders in adults. *Psychol Bull.* 1979;85:141-162.
24. Brown R, Colter N, Corsellis JAN, Crow TJ, Frith CD, Jagoe R, Johnstone EC, Marsh L. Post-mortem evidence of structural brain changes in schizophrenia: differences in brain weight, temporal horn area, and parahippocampal gyrus compared with affective disorder. *Arch Gen Psychiatry.* 1986;43:36-42.
25. Suddath RL, Christison GW, Torrey EF, Weinberger DR. Cerebral anatomical abnormalites in monozygotic twins discordant for schizophrenia. *N Engl J Med.* 1990;322:789-794.
26. Bogerts B, Ashtari M, Degreef G, Alvir JMJ, Bilder RM, Lieberman JA. Reduced temporal limbic structure volumes on magnetic resonance images in first episode schizophrenia. *Psychiatry Res.* 1990;35:1-13.

27. Babb TL, Brown WJ. Pathological findings in epilepsy. In: Engel J, ed. *Surgical Treatment of the Epilepsies.* New York, NY: Raven Press; 1987:511-540.
28. McKenna PJ, Tamlyn D, Lund CE, Mortimer AM, Hammond S, Baddely AD. Amnesic syndrome in schizophrenia. *Psychol Med.* 1990;20:967-972.
29. Gold JM, Randolph C, Carpenter CJ, Goldberg TE, Weinberger DR. Forms of memory failure in schizophrenia. *J Abnorm Psychol.* 1992;101:487-494.
30. Rausch R, Babb TL. Evidence for memory specialization within the medial temporal lobe in man. In: Engel J, Ojemannn GA, Luders HO, Williamson PD, eds. *Fundamental Mechanisms of Human Brain Function.* New York, NY: Raven Press; 1987:103-109.
31. Novelly RA, Augustine EA, Mattson RH, Glaser G, Williamson PD, Spencer DD, Spencer SS. Selective memory improvement and impairment in temporal lobectomy for epilepsy. *Ann Neurol.* 1984;15:64-67.
32. Jones-Gotman M. Psychological evaluation: testing hippocampal function. In: Engel J, ed. *Surgical Treatment of the Epilepsies.* New York, NY: Raven Press; 1987:203-211.
33. Hermann BP, Wyler AR, Richey ET. Wisconsin Card Sorting Test performance in patients with complex partial seizures of temporal-lobe origin. *J Clin Exp Neuropsychol.* 1988;10:467-476.
34. Rausch R. Cognitive strategies in patients with unilateral temporal lobe excisions. *Neuropsychologia.* 1977;15:385-395.
35. Gloor P, Olivier A, Quesney LF, Andermann F, Horowitz S. The role of the limbic system in experiential phenomena of temporal lobe epilepsy. *Ann Neurol.* 1982; 12:129-144.
36. Halgren E, Walter RD, Cherlow DG, Crandall PH. Mental phenomena evoked by electrical stimulation of the human hippocampal formation and amygdala. *Brain.* 1978;101:83-117.
37. Slater E, Beard AW. The schizophrenia-like psychosis of epilepsy. *Br J Psychiatry.* 1963;109:95-150.
38. Perez MM, Trimble MR, Murray NMF, Reider I. Epileptic psychosis: an evaluation of PSE profiles. *Br J Psychiatry.* 1985;146:155-163.
39. Roberts GW, Done DJ, Bruton C, Crow TJ. A 'mock up' of schizophrenia: temporal lobe epilepsy and schizophrenia-like psychosis. *Biol Psychiatry.* 1990;28:127-143.
40. Stevens JR. Psychosis and the temporal lobe. In: Smith D, Treiman M, Trimble M, eds. *Advances in Neurology.* New York, NY: Raven Press; 1991:79-96.
41. American Psychiatric Association, Committee on Nomenclature and Statistics. *Diagnostic and Statistical Manual of Mental Disorders, Revised Third Edition.* Washington, DC: American Psychiatric Association; 1987.
42. Jastak S, Wilkinson GS. *The Wide Range Achievement Test–Revised.* Wilmington, Del: Jastak Associates; 1984.
43. Wechsler D. *Wechsler Adult Intelligence Scale–Revised.* New York, NY: Psychological Corp; 1981.
44. Heaton RK. *Wisconsin Card Sorting Test, Manual.* Odessa, Fla: Psychological Assessment Resources; 1981.
45. Reitan RM, Wolfson D. *The Halstead-Reitan Neuropsychological Test Battery.* Tucson, Ariz: Neuropsychology Press; 1985.
46. Benton AL, Hamsher K. *Multilingual Aphasia Examination.* Iowa City, Iowa: University of Iowa; 1976.
47. Benton AL, Hamsher K, Varney N, Spreen O. *Contributions to Neuropsychological Assessment: A Clinical Manual.* New York, NY: Oxford University Press Inc; 1983.
48. Delis DC, Kramer JH, Kaplan E, Ober BA. *California Verbal Learning Test, Research Edition.* San Antonio, Tex: Psychological Corp; 1983.
49. Borkowski JG, Benton AL, Spreen O. Word fluency and brain damage. *Neuropsychologia.* 1967;5:135-140.
50. Kaufman AS. *Assessing Adolescent and Adult Intelligence.* Boston, Mass: Allyn & Bacon Inc; 1990.
51. Russell EW. Three patterns of brain damage on the WAIS. *J Clin Psychol.* 1979; 35:611-620.
52. Dalby JT, Williams R. Preserved reading and spelling ability in psychotic disorders. *Psychol Med.* 1986:16:171-175.
53. Nelson HE, McKenna P. The use of current reading ability in the assessment of dementia. *Br J Soc Clin Psychol.* 1975;14:259-267.
54. Nuechterlein KH, Dawson ME. Information processing and attentional functioning in the developmental course of schizophrenic disorders. *Schizophr Bull.* 1984;10:160-203.
55. Anderson SW, Damasio H, Jones RD, Tranel D. Wisconsin Card Sorting Test performance as a measure of frontal lobe damage. *J Clin Exp Neuropsychol.* 1991;13:909-922.
56. Grafman J, Jonas B, Salazar A. Wisconsin Card Sorting Test performance based on location and size of neuroanatomic lesion in Vietnam veterans with penetrating head injury. *Percept Mot Skills.* 1990;71:1120-1122.
57. Baddely AD. *Working Memory.* New York, NY: Oxford University Press Inc; 1986.
58. Mirsky AF. Research on schizophrenia in the NIMH Laboratory of Psychology and Psychopathology, 1954-1987. *Schizophr Bull.* 1988;14:151-156.
59. Weinberger DR, Berman KF, Suddath R, Torrey EF. Evidence of dysfunction of a prefrontal-limbic network in schizophrenia: a magnetic resonance imaging and regional cerebral blood flow study of discordant monozygotic twins. *Am J Psychiatry.* 1992;149:890-897.
60. Goldman-Rakic PS. Circuitry of primate prefrontal cortex and regulation of behavior by representational knowledge. In: Plum F, Mountcastle V, eds. *Handbook of Physiology: The Nervous System V.* Washington, DC: American Physiological Society; 1987:373-417.
61. Stuss DT, Benson DF. *The Frontal Lobes.* New York, NY: Raven Press; 1985.
62. Jablensky A, Sartorious N, Ernberg G, Anker M, Korten A, Cooper JE, Day R, Bertelson A. Schizophrenia: manifestations, incidence and course in different cultures: a World Health Organization 10-country study. *Psychol Med Monogr Suppl.* 1991;20:1-97.
63. Bilder RM, Lipschutz-Broch L, Reiter G, Geisler S, Meyerhoff D, Lieberman JA. Neuropsychological deficits in the early course of first episode schizophrenia. *Schizophr Res.* 1991;5:198-199.
64. Bilder RM, Lipschutz-Broch L, Reiter G, Geisler S, Mayerhoff D, Lieberman JA. Intellectual deficits in first episode and chronic schizophrenia: evidence for progressive deterioration? *Schizophr Bull.* 1992;18:437-448.
65. Trimble MR, Thompson PJ. Neuropsychological aspects of epilepsy. In: Grant I, Adams KM, eds. *Neuropsychological Assessment of Neuropsychiatric Disorders.* New York, NY: Oxford University Press Inc; 1986:321-346.
66. Medalia A, Gold J, Merriam A. The effects of neuroleptics on neuropsychological test results of schizophrenics. *Arch Clin Neuropsychol.* 1988;3:249-271.
67. Heaton RK, Crowley TJ. Effects of psychiatric disorders and their somatic treatment on neuropsychological test results. In: Filskov SB, Boll TJ, eds. *Handbook of Clinical Neuropsychology.* New York, NY: John Wiley & Sons Inc; 1981: 481-525.
68. Spohn HE, Strauss ME. Relation of neuroleptic and anticholinergic medication to cognitive functions in schizophrenia. *J Abnorm Psychol.* 1989;98:367-380.
69. Gold JM, Hurt SW. The effects of haloperidol on thought disorder and IQ in schizophrenia. *J Pers Assess.* 1990;54:390-400.
70. Rapaport D, Gill M, Schafer R. *Diagnostic Psychological Testing.* Chicago, Ill: Year Book Medical Publishers Inc; 1945;1.
71. Rutschmann J, Cornblatt B, Erlenmeyer-Kimling L. Auditory recognition memory in adolescents at risk for schizophrenia: report on a verbal continuous recognition task. *Psychiatry Res.* 1980;3:151-161.
72. Spohn HE, Coyne L, Lacoursiere R, Mazur D, Hayes K. Relation of neuroleptic dose and tardive dyskinesia to attention, information-processing, and psychophysiology in medicated schizophrenics. *Arch Gen Psychiatry.* 1985;42:849-859.
73. Waddington JL, Youssef HA, Dolphin C, Kinsella A. Cognitive dysfunction, negative symptoms, and tardive dyskinesia in schizophrenia. *Arch Gen Psychiatry.* 1987;44:907-912.

ORIGINAL ARTICLE

Cannabis Abuse and the Course of Recent-Onset Schizophrenic Disorders

Don H. Linszen, MD, PhD; Peter M. Dingemans, PhD; Marie E. Lenior, MA

Objective: We sought to examine the relation between cannabis abuse and the symptomatic course of recent-onset schizophrenia and related disorders.

Design: A prospective cohort study over a year using monthly Brief Psychiatric Rating Scale assessments.

Participants: Cannabis-abusing patients (n=24) were compared with nonabusers (n=69). Eleven patients were mild and 13 were heavy cannabis-abusing patients.

Results: Significantly more and earlier psychotic relapses occurred in the cannabis-abusing group (P=.03). This association became stronger when mild and heavy cannabis abuse were distinguished (P=.002). No confounding effect of other variables, eg, other street drugs, was found. In all but one patient, cannabis abuse preceded the onset of the first psychotic symptoms for at least 1 year.

Conclusions: Cannabis abuse and particularly heavy abuse can be considered a stressor eliciting relapse in patients with schizophrenia and related disorders and possibly a premorbid precipitant.

(Arch Gen Psychiatry. 1994;51:273-279)

STUDIES EXAMINING the relationship between cannabis use and schizophrenic symptoms among patients with schizophrenic disorders have found the following: (1) an increase in psychotic (positive) symptoms[1-6]; (2) no difference in psychotic symptoms in comparison to non–cannabis-abusing schizophrenic populations[7,8]; and (3) a decrease in negative symptoms.[7,8] Studies are needed to continue systematic study of this relationship to understand these discrepant findings. Clarification of the relationship would have both theoretical benefits of elucidating the mechanisms of psychotic relapse and practical applications for treatment of mentally ill substance abusers. Questions such as, "Do variable amounts of cannabis consumption render different symptomatic impact on schizophrenic patients?" or "Do positive consequences such as relief of psychotic or negative symptoms occur with some level of cannabis use?" might be answered.

However, the available studies consisted of case series, in which possible relationships between cannabis abuse and psychotic symptoms were difficult to test. In a few case-control studies, psychotic symptoms were evaluated retrospectively, using hospital files.[4] Also, the observation period was only 1 week[7] and schizophrenic symptoms were evaluated once.[8]

This study seeks to make improvements over past efforts. Therefore, data were analyzed from the present prospective 1-year outpatient follow-up study to examine the relationship between reported cannabis abuse and the symptomatic course of psychotic, negative, and affective symptoms in young patients consecutively admitted to the hospital with recent-onset schizophrenia and related disorders.

See Subjects and Methods on next page

From the Psychiatric Center of the Academic Medical Center and the Department of Psychiatry, University of Amsterdam, the Netherlands.

SUBJECTS AND METHODS

Patients were eligible for the study if they were diagnosed as having schizophrenia or a related disorder using *DSM-III-R* criteria,[9] were in need of continuous antipsychotic medication, were between 15 and 26 years of age, and were living with or in close contact with parents or other relatives. Patients with primary alcohol or drug dependence or brief drug-related psychoses who needed detoxification were excluded. All included patients participated in a 15-month treatment program. This program was composed of an inpatient phase (3 months), in which baseline data were collected. An important issue during the inpatient treatment was trying to maximize antipsychotic medication compliance. After hospital discharge, treatment was continued in a 12-month outpatient phase, composed of day hospital treatment (3 months) and community care (9 months).

The present study took place during the outpatient phase, in which patients were maintained on a regimen of optimal antipsychotic medication and received individual supportive treatment. During day treatment, patients received medication management training. Patients were seen biweekly during day hospital treatment and during the first 2 months of outpatient care. The last 7 months, individual treatment contacts took place monthly. In addition, half of the patients received an additional psychoeducative family treatment by family therapists designed to reduce family stress. Patients and their families in the latter condition were seen with the same frequency as with the individual treatment contacts.

INSTRUMENTS

Parents or relatives of the patients were interviewed with the Psychiatric and Social History Schedule.[10] In this interview, data were elicited about present and past illness as well as prognostic factors and premorbid social attainment,[11] substance abuse, medication, family history of mental disorder, and other prognostic factors.

Cannabis abuse was described according to the cannabis dependence criterion of the *DSM-III-R*, defined as daily or almost daily use of cannabis.[9] Abuse was rated as present if it was reported by (1) the patient and parents or former treatment summaries as having existed prior to hospital admission *and* (2) during the 12-month outpatient treatment phase, as reported both by the patient and the treatment staff. If in any one case these criteria were not met, cannabis abuse was rated as absent. During the study, no systematic laboratory confirmation of cannabinoid derivatives in urine was made that could have verified abuse. The combined self-reports as well as reports of relatives and therapists over an extended period (with a minimum of more than 1 year) were likely to be valid, since the use of cannabis, though officially illegal, is practically not restricted in Holland. The use was and is discussed freely and it seems unlikely that nonabusers were, in fact, abusers. Within the abusing group, two subgroups were defined: mild or heavy cannabis abuse. Patients with heavy abuse smoked more than one cigarette a day before hospital admission and during the 12-month outpatient treatment period. Patients with mild abuse smoked between once a week and once a day.

Psychopathologic symptoms were assessed by an independent clinical evaluator who saw patients on a monthly basis using the Brief Psychiatric Rating Scale (BPRS).[12] The BPRS interviewer (P.M.D.) had been trained at the University of California, Los Angeles (UCLA, Department of Psychology), before and the test was recalibrated for reliability again halfway into the study. The interrater agreement between the interviewer and standardized UCLA BPRS ratings was satisfactory (κ=0.79). He was blind to cannabis abuse.

The monthly collected BPRS data were used to evaluate relapses in the present study. The monthly BPRS ratings allowed us to formulate objective quantitative criteria for relapse or exacerbations of psychotic episodes. Nuechterlein et al[10] introduced a precise system for evaluating psychotic relapse. Relapse or significant exacerbation of psychotic symptoms was defined according to the following criteria.

Remission Followed by Relapse

The patient maintained a 3 or below on all BPRS relapse scales (hallucinations, conceptual thought disorder, formal thought disorder) during the first month of the outpatient treatment phase and a score of 6 or 7 was noted on

RESULTS

Of the 97 patients consecutively admitted to the hospital, four patients dropped out before psychopathologic conditions on the BPRS could be assessed; hence, evaluations for 93 patients were available. The experimental family treatment condition did not affect the relapse rate (*P*=.87) nor did any treatment condition influence cannabis abuse (*P*=.25). The patients had a clinical hospital discharge diagnosis of schizophrenia (52 patients), schizoaffective (19 patients), schizophreniform (11 patients), and other (delusional disorder, nine patients; atypical psychosis, two patients) psychotic disorders (11 patients). Compliance with antipsychotic medication was deemed high throughout the study, as the mean (±SD) rating during day treatment was 3.8±0.58 and during community care it was 3.8±0.58.

According to our definition, 24 (26%) of the patients were cannabis abusers. The frequency of abuse varied from once a week to four to five cigarettes a day. The mean (±SD) age when they started cannabis abuse was 16±2.2 years and the mean duration of abuse before hospital admission was 3.9±2.3 years. All but one of the cannabis-abusing patients started their habit at one of these scales during the other 11 months of the outpatient treatment.

Remission Followed by Significant Exacerbation

The patient maintained at least a 3 or below on relapse scales for at least 1 month and the patient also (1) scored 5 on a relapse scale at some point following this period, plus an increase of two points on another conceptually related scale; or she or he (2) scored 5 on a relapse scale for more than 1 month.

Persisting Symptoms Followed by Significant Exacerbation

The patient scored 4 or 5 on a relapse scale during the first month and (1) she or he maintained this state throughout the following period and subsequently showed an increase of two points on this scale; or (2) showed one-point increase on this scale (to a 6 or 7), accompanied by two-point increase on another conceptually related scale. In other reports on this sample,[13] data collected regularly by treating clinicians were also used to form a composite relapse criterion. However, since these clinicians contributed data to the estimate of cannabis abuse, these data could have influenced their relapse judgments. Thus, only the BPRS data were truly independent of the cannabis status of patients in the study.

Negative symptoms were operationalized with the anergy factor of the BPRS items (factor 2).[12] This factor has been found to be a parsimonious description of the negative symptom complex.[14,15] Again, a mean was calculated monthly for the anergy items for a period of 12 months; the mean was used as the negative symptom score. Affective symptoms were operationalized with the anxiety-depression factor of the BPRS items (factor 1).[12] A mean was also calculated monthly for a year for the affective items; the mean was used as the affective symptom score.

Antipsychotic medication compliance was indexed by the treating psychiatrist and the social psychiatric nurse in their regular contacts with the patient during the 12-month study period. Both interviewed the patient about compliance and compliance estimates were recorded. The social psychiatric nurse did occasional pill counts. A research assistant reviewed the compliance data for each month of the study and made ratings on a four-point scale: 1, 0% to 24% compliance: no or irregular; 2, 25% to 49%: rather irregular; 3, 50% to 74%: rather regular; and 4, 75% to 100%: regular, including depot. The recorded antipsychotic medication was rated from 1 (not prescribed) to six (more than 15 equivalents) in daily haloperidol equivalents.

PROCEDURE

During the intake before hospital admission, the Psychiatric and Social History Schedule was assessed by a research psychologist (P.M.D.). During the inpatient phase, a research assistant and a psychiatrist (D.H.L.) verified parental Psychiatric and Social History Schedule data with psychiatric case notes, the patient's own reports, and former treatment hospital discharge summaries. Conflicting data were presented to the informants. Cannabis abuse and the use of alcohol and other psychoactive drugs during outpatient treatment were independently assessed by the treating psychiatrist and nursing personnel. From hospital admission until the end of the 12-month study period (15 months), the patients were assessed monthly with the BPRS.[12]

DATA ANALYSIS

Analyses of psychotic, negative, and affective symptoms were based on the scores of 12 monthly BPRS-E interviews during the outpatient treatment period. The data were analyzed with Statistical Package for the Social Sciences (SPSS Inc, Chicago, Ill)[16] and Biomedical Computer Programs (BMDP)[17] programs. Relapses or significant exacerbations of psychotic symptoms were analyzed by product-limit survival analyses. Survival time until the first incidence of relapse or exacerbation was analyzed with treatment condition, cannabis abuse, intensity of cannabis abuse, and duration of cannabis abuse before hospital admission as grouping variables. The effect of covariates was analyzed using proportional hazards analysis: "Cox regression" (likelihood ratio tests). Analysis of variance for repeated measures and incomplete data was carried out on the means of negative and affective symptom item scores of the BPRS.

least 1 year prior to their first psychotic symptoms (mean, 3 years; range, 0 to 7 years). Within the group of cannabis abusers, 13 (54%) heavy cannabis-abusing patients could be distinguished. The mild cannabis-abusing group consumed between one cigarette a week and one a day. Hard drug abuse was rare (two patients used cocaine and 3,4-methylenedioxymetamphetamine ["ecstasy"]; one of these patients used hard drugs sporadically in combination with heavy cannabis abuse). The characteristics of the patient group and comparisons of the nonabusing and abusing group are summarized in the **Table**.

The two groups showed no statistically significant differences in variables of clinical importance: *DSM-III-R* diagnoses, history of illness course, sum score of positive and negative symptoms on the BPRS at the start of the study,[18] and compliance with and dosage of antipsychotic medication during treatment. Moreover, there were no differences in familial social class,[19] education, and race (data not shown). Statistically significant differences between abusers of cannabis and nonabusers were found for age at the time of hospital admission, sex, and alcohol use. No differences were found between the heavy and mild cannabis-abusing group, in particular not for

Demographic, Psychiatric, and Drug Characteristics of All Patients and of the Cannabis-Abusing and Nonabusing Groups

Variable	All Patients (N=93)	Nonabusers (N=69)	Abusers (N=24)	P Value*
		Demographic		
Mean (±SD) age, y at admission	20.6±2.44	20.8±2.5	19.8±1.98	.04
Sex, No. (%)				
F	26 (28)	23 (33)	3 (13)	.05
M	67 (72)	46 (67)	21 (88)	
Mean (±SD) prognostic scale score (Strauss and Carpenter)[20]	61.7±11.08	62.2±11.55	60.4±9.70	.52
		Psychiatric		
Mean (±SD) age, y at onset of schizophrenia	19.1±2.56	19.3±2.70	18.8±2.11	.38
Psychotic episodes, No. (%)				
1	52 (56)	37 (54)	15 (63)	.45
>1	41 (44)	32 (46)	9 (38)	
Schizophrenia (*DSM-III-R*), No. (%)				
No	41 (44)	30 (44)	11 (46)	.84
Yes	52 (56)	39 (57)	13 (54)	
Mean (±SD) sum score of positive and negative symptoms (BPRS)†	15.1±4.77	14.6±4.70	16.3±4.85	.13
		Drugs		
Abuse of alcohol, No. (%)				
No	84 (91)	67 (97)	17 (74)	.00
Yes	8 (9)	2 (3)	6 (26)	
Mean compliance to antipsychotic medication, No. (%)				
0-24	3 (3)	2 (3)	1 (4)	.23
25-49	2 (2)	1 (1)	1 (4)	
50-74	13 (14)	7 (10)	6 (25)	
75-100	75 (81)	59 (86)	16 (67)	
Mean (±SD) dosage of antipsychotic medication‡	3.6±1.2	3.5±1.2	3.8±1.0	.27

**P value for difference between nonabusers of cannabis.*

†These Brief Psychiatric Rating Scale (BPRS) items[12] were scored from 1 (not present) to 7 (very severely); the mean item scores of the last 2 months of inpatient treatment were taken.

‡The mean dosage (in haloperidol [Haldol] equivalents) during inpatient and outpatient treatment was taken. Dosage was scored from 1 (no prescription) to 6 (>15 haloperidol equivalents) (3, four to six equivalents; 4, seven to nine equivalents).

compliance with medication (*P*=.55) or dosage of antipsychotic medication (*P*=.47).

In the cannabis-abusing group, 10 (42%) of 24 patients suffered relapses, whereas of the 69 patients who did not abuse cannabis, 12 patients (17%) suffered relapses or exacerbations during the 12-month study period. As compared with patients without abuse, a significant difference in time until relapse was observed (*P*=.03), indicating that cannabis abusers suffered relapses more frequently and earlier than nonabusers (**Figure**).

Eight patients (61%) in the heavy cannabis-abusing group of 13 patients suffered relapses, whereas of the 11 mild cannabis-abusing patients only two (18%) suffered relapses. With the cannabis-abusing group divided in mild and heavy abusers, an ordered effect was revealed (*P*=.002).

To test the effect of the duration of cannabis abuse prior to hospital admission, a survival analysis was conducted for three groups: no cannabis abuse, 3 years or less of cannabis abuse before hospital admission, and more than 3 years of cannabis abuse. Again an ordered effect was found (*P*=.02), revealing that with a longer period of abuse the risk of relapse increased.

The cannabis effects were tested again with age at time of hospital admission, sex, and use of alcohol as covariates. A strong trend of cannabis abuse remained, if corrected for the differences between the two groups (*P*=.06). Also, the intensity of cannabis abuse was analyzed, revealing that the effect of the intensity of cannabis abuse (no, mild, and heavy abuse) remained highly significant (*P*=.01). Finally, the effect of the duration of cannabis abuse before hospital admission was reduced when corrected for differences between abusers and nonabusers (*P*=.08). This was caused by the fact that duration of cannabis abuse was shorter for younger patients (20 years or younger) than for older patients

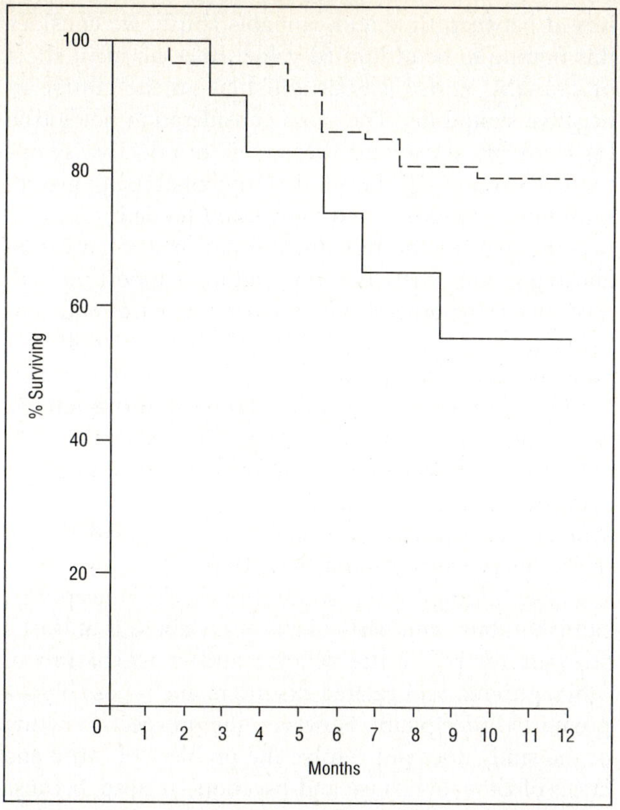

Survival curves of time until psychotic relapse (Brief Psychiatric Rating Scale) by no abuse (dashed line) and abuse (solid line) of cannabis.

(*P*=.01). With regard to sex and alcohol, no significant differences were found between the two groups according to duration of cannabis abuse. Likelihood tests demonstrated no significant effects of sex, age at the time of hospital admission, and alcohol use on the survival function or any interaction effect.

One may find the diagnosis of the sample too heterogeneous. Therefore, we carried out analyses in a subsample of patients with schizophrenia only (*DSM-III-R* criteria: N=52 [56%]). Post hoc analyses revealed that the relation between the intensity of cannabis abuse (no abuse, 10 of 39 patients suffering a relapse; mild abuse, one of six patients suffering a relapse; heavy abuse, five of seven patients suffering a relapse) and the time until psychotic relapse remained highly significant (*P*=.01). This effect remained when corrected for age, sex, and alcohol (*P*=.01).

NO MAIN EFFECT of cannabis abuse for the course of negative symptom scores was found (*P*=.286). However, negative symptoms generally decreased over 12 months, with a significant increase at month 2 and a decrease at month 10. There was an interaction effect between cannabis and time (*P*=.03). The interaction effect became stronger when the cannabis-abusing group was divided into mild and heavy abusers (*P*=.002). A significant interaction effect was found at month 10 for mild abusers and nonabusers of cannabis. At this point, the mean negative symptom score was increasing for nonabusers while decreasing for mild abusers.

Also, no effect of cannabis abuse for the course of affective symptom scores was found (*P*=.53). However, a trend was found with the intensity of cannabis abuse (*P*=.09). In the mild cannabis-abusing group, there was a trend for less anxiety and depression than in the nonabusing and heavy cannabis-abusing group.

COMMENT

The most relevant finding of this prospective study in patients with recent-onset schizophrenia and schizophrenia-related disorders was the occurrence of significantly more and earlier psychotic relapses or exacerbations in the group of cannabis-abusing patients. When a distinction with respect to the intensity of abuse was made, it appeared that particularly heavy cannabis-abusing patients had more and earlier relapses. This finding was not confounded by exposure to alcohol and/or any other (psychoactive) drugs, nor by differences in antipsychotic medication compliance and dosage. Baseline symptom status, prognostic scale score,[20] or history of prior relapse rates were similar for cannabis abusers and nonabusers. No other demographic or clinical factors could be identified that affected this relationship. Another finding was that all cannabis-abusing patients but one started their habit at least 1 year prior to the first psychotic symptoms, suggesting that cannabis abuse can possibly be a premorbid precipitant.

These findings could have been more convincing when this study had included systematic laboratory confirmation of cannabinoid derivatives in urine. Martin et al,[21] however, found that the information on use of soft drugs given by patients is reliable. Moreover, evaluation of cannabis abuse in the present study was based on information given by various sources: the reports of the patients, parents, psychiatrist, and nursing staff. Also, the reader may not be familiar with cannabis use patterns in Amsterdam. Though not officially sanctioned, the use of cannabis products is not restricted by legislation; however, hard drugs are much more difficult to get. Levels of antipsychotic medication in the blood of the patients under study should have been measured to provide the compliance data with a solid base.

Two additional findings indicate a possible causal relation between cannabis and psychotic relapse. First, 14 of 24 cannabis-abusing patients reported an immediate increase of psychotic symptoms after cannabis abuse. Thirteen of these 14 patients were clinically in remission when they reported the increase of psychotic symptoms. Six patients noted no such increase and only one patient reported a decrease of psychotic symptoms when abusing cannabis, which is in agreement with earlier case reports.[2,3,6] Second, in all but one patient, cannabis abuse preceded the initial onset of psychotic episodes for at least 1 year. This finding is congruent with the observations of a Swedish epidemiologic study[22] that revealed that cannabis abuse prior to illness was an independent risk factor for schizophrenia.

A BIOLOGIC EXPLANATION of the demonstrated relation between psychotic symptoms of schizophrenic patients and cannabis abuse may be found in recent pharmacologic studies.[23] Delta (9)-tetrahydrocannabinol (δ-9-THC), the principal psychoactive constituent of cannabis, was found to act as a dopamine agonist in dopaminergic projections of the medial forebrain bundles.

Dopaminergic hyperactivity is generally thought to be related to the presence of psychotic symptoms of schizophrenia,[24] although other neurotransmitters may be affected as well. An increase of dopamine could undo the dopamine receptor blockade of antipsychotic medication. In our study, the intensity of abuse was correlated with an increase of psychotic relapses, suggesting that δ-9-THC acts as a dopamine agonist in the projections of the medial forebrains of the patients as well. Future studies with brain imaging techniques applied to heavy abusing and nonabusing schizophrenic patients with standard antipsychotic medication may be indicated to reveal these differences in dopamine receptor blockade or in other neurotransmission systems. Cannabis abuse may also have influenced the antipsychotic drug metabolism, lowering plasma levels of active metabolites. Thus, cannabis abusers could have been relatively undertreated, despite the finding of a lack of differences in antipsychotic dosage between heavy and mild abusers. Of course, it may not be the biologic action alone that increases the risk for relapse in these young patients. Those patients who used cannabis heavily both before and after the onset of their psychosis may represent a different population of cases from those who were nonabusers. While it is true that most of our background measures do not discriminate cannabis abusers from nonabusers, it is possible that those persons who use cannabis regularly are more vulnerable to or have less effective coping mechanisms for dealing with intercurrent life events. This same vulnerability to stress may produce a lower threshold for recurrence of the psychiatric disorder, even if these patients discontinued cannabis use.

As for cannabis abuse and negative symptoms, even though a significant interaction effect was observed between time and cannabis abuse, we consider this finding to be of limited value, since no main effect of cannabis abuse was established on the course of negative symptoms. The same consideration holds true for cannabis abuse and the course of affective symptoms. However, in the mild cannabis-abusing group, symptoms of anxiety and depression tended to be less present than in the nonabusing and heavy cannabis-abusing group. Therefore, our findings support the self-medication hypothesis only for patients with mild cannabis abuse.[25] According to this theory, schizophrenic patients succesfully try to reduce their negative and affective symptoms[8,26] or side effects of antipsychotic medication[6] by using street drugs. The existence of an amotivational syndrome with an increase of negative symptoms in the cannabis-abusing group of young schizophrenic patients was not tenable, particularly not in the heavy cannabis-abusing group.

The findings of this study support the concept that cannabis abuse and particularly heavy abuse is at least a stressor for psychotic relapse and exacerbation in schizophrenia and related disorders and—possibly—a premorbid precipitant. However, the prospective nature of the study does not resolve the problem of cause and effect of cannabis abuse and psychotic relapse, because the needed nonschizophrenic cannabis-abusing controls were lacking. Nevertheless, treatment strategies have to be developed to discourage cannabis abuse by schizophrenic patients. Further studies should include cannabis abuse intervention programs, a quantitative estimation of cannabis abuse repeated in time, laboratory confirmation of cannabis abuse, and repeated assessments of dose-response effects as soon after abuse as possible in cannabis-abusing patients.[27]

Accepted for publication July 30, 1993.

This study was funded in part by grant 28-1241 from the "Praeventiefonds," the Hague, the Netherlands.

Jitse Verhoeff, MD, provided continuous support of the study and Harry Büller, MD, PhD, gave a critical review of the article.

Reprint requests to Psychiatric Center AMC, Tafelbergweg 25, 1105 BC Amsterdam, the Netherlands (Dr Linszen).

REFERENCES

1. Weil AT. Adverse reactions to marijuana, classification and suggested treatment. *N Engl J Med.* 1970;282:997-1000.
2. Chopra GS, Smith JW. Psychotic reactions following cannabis use in East Indians. *Arch Gen Psychiatry.* 1974;30:24-27.
3. Treffert DA. Marijuana use in schizophrenia: a clear hazard. *Am J Psychiatry.* 1978;135:1213-1215.
4. Negrete JC, Knapp WP, Douglas DE, Smith B. Cannabis affects the severity of schizophrenic symptoms: results of a clinical survey. *Psychol Med.* 1986;16:515-520.
5. Cleghorn JM, Kaplan RD, Szechtman B, Szechtman H, Brown GM, Franco S.

Substance abuse and schizophrenia: effect on symptoms but not on neurocognitive function. *J Clin Psychiatry.* 1991;52:26-30.
6. Knudsen P, Vilmar T. Cannabis and neuroleptic agents in schizophrenia. *Acta Psychiatr Scand.* 1984;69:162-174.
7. Rottanburgh D, Robins AH, Ben-Arie O, Teggin A, Elk R. Cannabis-associated psychosis with hypomanic features. *Lancet.* 1982;2:1364-1366.
8. Peralta V, Cuesta MJ. Influence of cannabis abuse on schizophrenic psychopathology. *Acta Psychiatr Scand.* 1992;85:127-130.
9. American Psychiatric Association, Committee on Nomenclature and Statistics. *Diagnostic and Statistical Manual of Mental Disorders, Revised Third Edition.* Washington, DC: American Psychiatric Association; 1987.
10. Nuechterlein KH, Snyder KS, Dawson ME, Rappe S, Gitlin M, Fogelson D. Expressed emotion, fixed dose fluphenazine decanoate maintenance and relapse in recent-onset schizophrenia. *Psychopharmacol Bull.* 1986;22:663-639.
11. Kokes R, Strauss J, Klorman R. Measuring premorbid adjustment: the instruments and their development. *Schizophr Bull.* 1977;3:186-213.
12. Overall JE, Gorham DR. The Brief Psychiatric Rating Scale. *Psychol Rep.* 1962;10:799-812.
13. Linszen DH, Dingemans PMAJ, Scholte WF, et al. Behandeling, 'expressed emotion' en recent ontstane schizofrenie en verwante stoornissen. *Tijdschr Psychiatr.* 1993;9:625-640.
14. Thiemann S, Csernansky JG, Berger PA. Rating scales in research: the case of negative symptoms. *Psychiatry Res.* 1987;20:47-55.
15. Czobor P, Bitter I, Volavka J. Relationship between Brief Psychiatric Rating Scale for the assessment of negative symptoms: a study of their correlation and redundancy. *Psychiatry Res.* 1991;36:129-139.
16. Norusis MJ. *SPSSPC+ 4.0 Base Manual for the IBM PC/XT/AT and PS/2.* Chicago, Ill: SPSS Inc; 1990.
17. Dixon MJ, Brown MB, Engelman L, et al, eds. *BMDP Statistical Software Manual.* Berkeley: University of California Press; 1990;1-2.
18. Breier A, Schreiber JL, Dyer J, Pickar D. National Institute of Mental Health Longitudinal Study of Chronic Schizophrenia: prognosis and predictors of outcome. *Arch Gen Psychiatry.* 1991;48:239-246.
19. Hollingshead AB, Redlich FC. *Social Class and Mental Illness.* New York, NY: John Wiley & Sons Inc; 1968:387-397.
20. Strauss JS, Carpenter WT. Prediction of outcome in schizophrenia, III: Five-year outcome and its predictors. *Arch Gen Psychiatr.* 1977;34:159-163.
21. Martin GW, Wilkinson A, Kapur BM. Validation of self-reported cannabis use by urine analysis. *Addict Behav.* 1988;13:147-150.
22. Andreasson S, Allebeck P, Engström A, Rydberg U. Cannabis and schizophrenia: a longitudinal study of Swedish conscripts. *Lancet.* 1987;2:1483-1486.
23. Gardner EL, Lowinson JH. Marijuana's interaction with brain reward systems: update 1991. *Pharmacol Biochem Behav.* 1991;40:571-580.
24. McKena PJ. Pathology, phenomenology and the dopamine hypothesis of schizophrenia. *Br J Psychiatry.* 1987;151:288-301.
25. Schneier FR, Siris SG. A review of psychoactive substance use and abuse in schizophrenia: patterns of drug choice. *J Nerv Ment Dis.*1987;175:641-652.
26. Dixon L, Haas G, Weiden PJ, Sweeney J, Frances AJ. Drug abuse in schizophrenic patients: clinical correlates and reasons for use. *Am J Psychiatry.* 1991;148:224-230.
27. Thornicroft G. Cannabis and psychosis: is there epidemiological evidence for an association? *Br J Psychiatry.* 1990;157:25-33.

Fluphenazine vs Placebo Supplementation for Prodromal Signs of Relapse in Schizophrenia

Stephen R. Marder, MD; William C. Wirshing, MD; Theodore Van Putten, MD†; Jim Mintz, PhD; Joanne McKenzie, RN; Kathleen Johnston-Cronk, MS; Malca Lebell, PhD; Robert P. Liberman, MD

Background: We studied the effectiveness of treating patients with low doses of fluphenazine decanoate and supplementing them with oral fluphenazine when there was evidence of prodromal symptoms of psychotic exacerbations.

Methods: Eighty schizophrenic patients who were receiving 5 to 10 mg of fluphenazine decanoate every 2 weeks were monitored for prodromal symptoms using an idiosyncratic prodromal rating scale. When patients met our criteria for a prodromal episode, they were randomly assigned to a double-blind comparison of oral fluphenazine hydrochloride (5 mg twice daily) or a placebo for the current and future prodromal episodes. We compared rates of psychotic exacerbations in the two treatment groups.

Results: Thirty-six patients (45%) met the criteria for a prodrome at some point during the trial and were randomized to drug or placebo. Using survival analysis during the entire 2 years, we did not find a significant difference between fluphenazine and placebo in the likelihood that a prodrome would continue to an exacerbation. Survival analysis beginning at the start of the second year of treatment did indicate a significant reduction in exacerbation risk for patients receiving drug supplementation ($P=.032$). Similarly, there was no difference between the two groups in the proportion of time at risk spent in exacerbation during the first year, but patients receiving active drug supplementation spent less time in an exacerbated state in the second year ($P=.05$).

Conclusions: Our treatment strategy appeared to be effective for some patients, particularly those who were able to remain in the study beyond the first year. Although the occurrence of a prodrome was a fairly good marker that a patient was at high risk of ultimate exacerbation with our low-dose maintenance protocol, prodromes were not highly sensitive indicators of imminent exacerbation.

(Arch Gen Psychiatry. 1994;51:280-287)

From the West Los Angeles (Calif) Veterans Affairs Medical Center, Brentwood Division (Drs Marder, Wirshing, Van Putten, Mintz, Lebell, and Liberman, and Ms McKenzie), and the Department of Psychiatry and Biobehavioral Sciences, UCLA, Los Angeles, Calif (Drs Marder, Wirshing, Van Putten, Mintz, and Liberman and Ms Johnston-Cronk).
†Deceased.

RECENT STUDIES have encouraged clinicians to treat schizophrenic patients with the lowest effective dose of antipsychotic medications. Finding an effective low dose may be of considerable importance for long-term maintenance therapy since even mild extrapyramidal side effects may interfere with a patient's compliance with maintenance pharmacotherapy and response to rehabilitation. A number of recent studies[1-3] have evaluated both the benefits and disadvantages of dosage reduction. Kane et al[1] found that patients receiving a very low dose of fluphenazine decanoate (1.25 to 5 mg every 2 weeks) had less blunting of affect and emotional withdrawal, but higher relapse rates when compared with patients who received 12.5 to 50 mg every 2 weeks. Hogarty and coworkers[3] found that patients who received substantial dosage reductions were more improved in their instrumental and interpersonal role performance than were patients who received standard doses. They also noted that patients who received low doses were more vulnerable to mild psychotic episodes during the second year following randomization. In our study,[1] patients who received 5 mg of fluphenazine decanoate every 2 weeks experienced less anxiety and depression, as well as less akathisia and retardation, than those who re-

See Methods on next page

METHODS

The subjects were 80 male outpatients at the Brentwood Division of the West Los Angeles (Calif) Veterans Affairs Medical Center with a schizophrenic disorder diagnosed by *DSM-III-R*. The symptom profiles of all patients were documented using the Present State Examination. Patients were candidates for maintenance neuroleptic therapy. Each individual had at least two documented episodes of acute schizophrenic illness or at least 2 years of continuing psychotic symptoms. Before study entry, each patient was stabilized with a low dose of fluphenazine decanoate (5 to 10 mg every 14 days). The dose was set at 5 mg unless there was a history that a higher dose was needed to prevent psychotic exacerbations. Patients who could not be stabilized for 2 or more months with 10 mg or less of fluphenazine decanoate every 2 weeks for a 2-month period were dropped from the study during the stabilization period.

It is difficult to assess how representative our patients were of schizophrenic patients living in the community. We evaluated 42 patients who fulfilled our diagnostic criteria, but did not enter the study. These patients were not entered because they could not be stabilized with low doses or because they were viewed as poor candidates for dosage reduction study. Also, our referral sources tended to select patients who were already well stabilized with moderate or low doses of an antipsychotic.

MONITORING FOR PRODROMAL SYMPTOMS

During the stabilization phase, study staff met separately with the patient and an informant—usually a family member—who had observed the patient at the time of previous relapses. A detailed history of events that preceded relapses was taken. From this history, research staff attempted to define early indicators of relapse. Both the patient and an informant were given a list of items (derived from the work of Herz et al[6]) that included both the hypothesized prodromal symptoms and a number of other symptoms, and they were asked to check which items were the earliest indicators of relapse. From the items checked, an individualized scale was organized—the Idiosyncratic Prodromal Scale—that contained the three symptoms that were reported to occur most reliably before relapses. The most common prodromal symptoms that we monitored were as follows: (1) trouble with sleeping; (2) trouble with concentrating; (3) withdrawn, isolated, or avoiding people; (4) impatient, irritable, easily angered, or argumentative; (5) feeling depressed or worthless; (6) thoughts you cannot get rid of; and (7) drinking more or using more drugs. Each symptom was assigned a number from 1 to 100 that indicated the present severity of the symptom and the preset criteria for when a "prodromal" period was defined. The scale items for each individual were revised following exacerbations if new symptoms were identified.

Following 2 months of stabilization, patients were followed up with weekly ratings of prodromal symptoms using the Idiosyncratic Prodromal Scale. When a patient was considered to have fulfilled previously established Idiosyncratic Prodromal Scale criteria for a prodrome, the individual was randomly assigned to receive 5 mg twice daily of fluphenazine hydrochloride or a matching placebo until the patient was stable or fulfilled criteria for a "psychotic exacerbation." The study criteria for a psychotic exacerbation was a worsening of four points or more on the sum of the BPRS cluster scores for thought disturbance and paranoia or an increase of three or more points on either cluster. This is the same definition of a "psychotic

Continued on next page

ceived 25 mg. However, the patients who received the lower dose were more likely to experience exacerbations of their illness duringthe second year following randomization.

We[2] also reported that when patients were treated with 5 mg of fluphenazine decanoate administered every 2 weeks, an increase in dose at the first signs of psychotic worsening substantially improved survival rates. In that study, we prescribed additional long-acting fluphenazine decanoate when patients worsened. However, since long-acting depot neuroleptics require a much longer time to reach steady state when compared with that of oral drugs,[4] intervention with oral fluphenazine would, in theory, be more effective. As a result, we tested the efficacy of treating patients with low doses of supplemental oral fluphenazine at the first signs of psychotic exacerbations.

Others have tested the usefulness of "intermittent" treatment. In this approach, patients are gradually withdrawn from their antipsychotic medications. Drug treatment is resumed when patients show signs of incipient relapse or a symptomatic exacerbation. The four studies[5-8] that have compared intermittent treatment with continuous therapy have found that this is a feasible management strategy that does reduce the amount of antipsychotic medications. On the other hand, all of the studies have found that this strategy is also associated with an increased risk of symptomatic relapse. The treatment strategy that we studied differs in that we maintained patients with a stable, but low dose of medication (5 to 10 mg of fluphenazine decanoate every 14 days) and intervened at the earliest sign that patients were relapsing with either supplemental oral fluphenazine or a placebo.

In implementing an early intervention strategy, it is important to identify accurately patients who are in the early stages of relapse. Retrospective and prospective studies[9-15] have reported that both patients and their relatives could detect prodromal signs that occurred well in advance of a relapse. In the study of Herz and Melville,[10] 52% of the patients and 68% of their relatives reported retexacerbation" that we have used in prior studies. Many of these events were relatively mild compared with what is commonly considered a psychotic relapse and were seldom a cause for hospitalization or other interventions. In contrast with a previous study,[2] we did not define relapse as an outcome.

If patients demonstrated multiple prodromes during the course of the study, they were treated under the same condition (that is, fluphenazine or placebo) as they were for the first prodrome. Patients who initially experienced exacerbations without prodromes and later experienced a prodrome were then randomized to one of the two double-blind conditions and continued in that condition for the remainder of the 2 years. Patients in both the active oral fluphenazine- and placebo-treated groups, as well as those who never had a prodrome and were never assigned, were treated with 5 mg twice daily of open-labeled oral fluphenazine hydrochloride during exacerbations.

PSYCHOSOCIAL TREATMENT

At the beginning of the study, all 80 patients were randomly assigned to receive either behavioral skills training or twice-weekly supportive group therapy. A description of the psychosocial conditions and the effects of these interventions on patient outcomes will be the subject of a separate report.

THE OVERALL DATA ANALYTIC STRATEGY

The data analyses addressed two specific research questions: first, the usefulness of monitoring prodromal symptoms as a method for determining when schizophrenic patients were vulnerable to psychotic exacerbations; and second, the effectiveness of supplemental oral fluphenazine in preventing psychotic exacerbations during these periods of presumed increased vulnerability.

The drug trial occurred in the context of a larger study that included a psychosocial treatment component, but this report focuses only on the drug treatment findings. Our decision to delimit this report was based on the following considerations. The randomized trial of the drug supplementation strategy is a distinct component of the overall treatment study, both in terms of the sample available and the methods. Clinical outcome data relevant to the evaluation of the drug supplementation were obtained only from the subsample of patients who experienced a prodrome and were randomly assigned to drug or placebo supplementation. Since these patients represent just under half of the total sample who participated in the trial of psychosocial treatments, their outcomes clearly do not fairly test the efficacy of the psychosocial treatments.

Furthermore, tracking of clinical outcomes for this component began only at the point of the first prodromal episode, ie, the point at which the patients entered this phase of the experiment. Only exacerbations that occurred after the point of drug randomization bear on the issue of efficacy of the drug intervention. However, exacerbations did occur in a number of individuals before drug randomization, and those events are relevant to an overall assessment of the psychosocial modules.

We performed preliminary survival analyses, using both the total sample of 80 patients who entered the overall study, and the subsample of 36 patients who entered the randomized drug trial, to rule out confounding effects of psychosocial treatment assignment on the major outcome variable, ie, psychotic exacerbation. Neither main nor interaction effects were found to approach statistical significance. We concluded that the outcome analyses reported here were not influenced to any substantial degree by the psychosocial treatments, and defer fuller consideration of their efficacy to another report.

rospectively that prodromes could be detected more than a week before the patient relapsed. Birchwood et al[9] found that 75% of patients and families observed a prodrome 2 weeks or more before a relapse. Subotnick and Nuechterlein[14] found that relatively small increases in odd thought content, unusual perceptual experiences, depression, somatic concern, and guilt commonly preceded a psychotic relapse. Hirsch and Jolley[12] reported that dysphoric and neurotic symptoms occur frequently in the weeks before relapse. Using receiver operating characteristic methods, we[16] recently reported that two scales, ie, the Anxiety-Depression Cluster of the Brief Psychiatric Rating Scale (BPRS) and the Idiosyncratic Prodromal Scale, were significantly better than chance at identifying patients who were on the verge of psychotic exacerbations. The latter of these two scales was utilized in the current study.

In our study, patients were randomized to either active oral fluphenazine or a placebo supplementation during periods when they fulfilled our prodromal criteria. This permitted us to study the validity of our prodromal criteria on the one hand, and to study the usefulness of oral supplementation during these periods of presumed increased vulnerability on the other.

RESULTS

STUDY SUBJECTS

Of the 80 patients entered, 36 (45%) met the criteria for a prodrome at some point during the trial and were randomized to drug or placebo. **Figure 1** displays the number of patients in the different treatment conditions: (1) never randomized (n=44) (that is, patients who either remained stable or experienced exacerbations without prodromes); (2) patients who fulfilled our criteria for a prodromal episode and were randomly assigned to active fluphenazine (n=17); and (3) patients who fulfilled prodromal criteria and were assigned to placebo (n=19). **Table 1** provides the demographics of the three groups. None of the demographic differences among the groups were statistically significant.

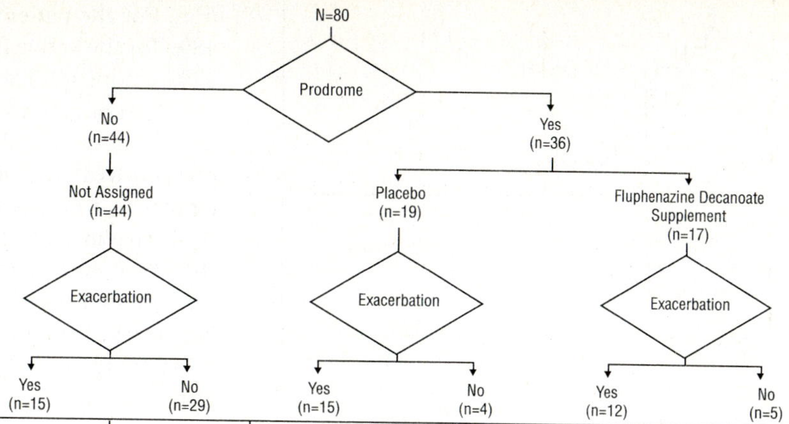

	Not Assigned: Yes (n=15)	Not Assigned: No (n=29)	Placebo: Yes (n=15)	Placebo: No (n=4)	Fluphenazine: Yes (n=12)	Fluphenazine: No (n=5)
Prodromes (N=60)	0	0	29	4	18	9
Exacerbations (N=88)	22	0	32	0	34	0
"Sensitivity": Proportion of exacerbations preceded by a prodrome	0/22=0%		16/32=50%		10/34=29%	
PPV: Proportion of prodromes followed by an exacerbation	N/A		16/33=48%		10/27=37%	

Figure 1. *Overview of clinical course during the trial. The 36 patients who fulfilled criteria for a prodrome were randomly assigned to either supplemental oral fluphenazine hydrochloride (5 mg twice daily) or placebo. PPV indicates positive predictive value.*

We did, however, find a statistically significant difference in the dose of antipsychotic that patients received before entering the study stabilization period. For this analysis, drug doses were converted to haloperidol equivalents using previously published guidelines.[17] Patients ultimately randomized to placebo supplementation had somewhat higher prestudy doses (mean=16.8 mg, SD=11.0 mg) than either those randomized to drug supplementation (mean=12.2 mg, SD=5.5 mg) or those never randomized (mean=11.9 mg, SD=6.2; the Savage nonparametric test, used because of unequal variances, yielded χ^2=9.8, *df*=2, $P<.01$).

Survival models were computed, stratifying by drug condition, to evaluate the importance of prestudy dosage as a covariate. The association of prestudy dosage and exacerbation did not approach statistical significance in either the first (χ^2=0.60, *P*=.44) or second (χ^2=0.06, *P*=.80) year of the study. Separate analyses of the association of prestudy dose and outcome within each drug condition yielded similar results (year 1: χ^2=0.28, *P*=.60 within the drug supplementation group, χ^2=1.29, *P*=.26 in the placebo supplementation group; year 2: χ^2=0.01, *P*=.93 for drug-treated patients and χ^2=0.06, *P*=.81 for placebo-treated patients). On the basis of these preliminary analyses, we concluded that the differences in prestudy dose did not affect conclusions about treatment effects on exacerbation rates, ie, the study's major dependent variable.

Table 1. Demographic Characteristics*

	Never Randomized (n=44)	Drug (n=17)	Placebo (n=19)
Age, y	37.9 (8.3)	40.4 (9.4)	39.1 (8.6)
Education, y	12.7 (1.7)	12.8 (1.2)	13.5 (1.7)
Duration of illness, mo	144.6 (105.8)	187.0 (114.2)	152.6 (99.0)
No. of hospitalizations	3.8 (1.9)	3.9 (2.0)	3.6 (1.9)
Age at onset, y	24.9 (5.0)	24.0 (6.0)	25.9 (5.3)
Single, %	77	71	79
Nonwhite, %	70	71	79
Total BPRS, baseline	31.5 (9.1)	31.7 (7.9)	32.1 (7.3)
Prestudy dose, haloperidol equivalent	11.9 (6.2)	12.2 (5.5)	16.8† (11.0)

**Data are given as mean (SD) throughout, except for single and nonwhite characteristics. BPRS indicates Brief Psychiatric Rating Scale.*
†χ^2=9.79, df=2, $P<.01$.

PRODROMAL EPISODES AS PREDICTORS OF PSYCHOTIC EXACERBATIONS

During the 2-year trial, there were a total of 88 exacerbations that occurred in 42 individuals (20 patients had one exacerbation, seven had two, 10 had three, and five had more than three). As displayed in Figure 1, 15 of the patients who had exacerbations never had prodromes and were in the not assigned group. These patients actually had 22 of the 88 exacerbations. Using survival analysis, we found that the risk of having an exacerbation was significantly lower in this unassigned group compared with that in the patients who were randomized after they experienced prodromes (19.9% of the patients assigned to either drug or placebo survived without exacerbations during the 2 years, whereas 54.8% survived in the unassigned group [χ^2=4.94, *P*=.026]).

Among the 36 patients who had prodromes and were randomized, the 17 who were assigned to active drug supplementation had 34 exacerbations, 10 of which (29%)

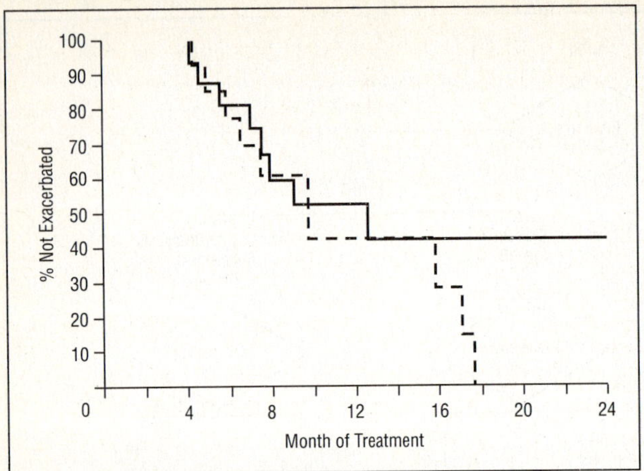

Figure 2. *Survival without psychotic exacerbations in patients who were randomized to receive either oral fluphenazine hydrochloride supplementation (n=17) (solid line) or placebo supplementation (n=19) (dashed line). The time to the first exacerbation was measured from the week that the patient first met prodromal criteria, at which time the patient was randomized to a drug treatment group. The χ^2 value (exponential model)=1.89, not significant.*

were preceded by a prodrome. The 19 patients who were assigned to placebo had 32 exacerbations, of which 16 (50%) were preceded by a prodrome.

We evaluated the sensitivity of prodromes as a means of predicting psychotic exacerbations. The "sensitivity" of a screening test (eg, prodrome evaluation) refers to the probability that a targeted condition (or event, eg, exacerbation) will be identified by the test. For this report, we computed the probability that a psychotic exacerbation was immediately preceded by a prodrome. Computing the overall sensitivity of prodromes was complicated by the study design. The fact that the proportion of exacerbations preceded by prodromes was somewhat lower in the active fluphenazine–treated group is as would be expected if active treatment reduced the likelihood of subsequent exacerbations. Inclusion of this group would thus result in an artificially low estimate of sensitivity. We accordingly estimated overall sensitivity using only the patients who had never been assigned, and those who had been assigned to placebo. Appropriate weighting of these two strata yielded an overall sensitivity of 37%.

POSITIVE PREDICTIVE VALUE OF PRODROMES

The 36 patients who were randomized to either active fluphenazine supplementation or placebo supplementation experienced 60 prodromes. (One patient who dropped out during a prodromal episode and another who reached the 2-year end point during a prodrome were not included in the analysis.) We computed the likelihood that when a prodrome occurred, it would be followed by an exacerbation—that is, the positive predictive value (PPV) of prodromes. Across both treatment groups, 34 (57%) of these prodromes resolved without an exacerbation (ie, were followed by a return to clinical stability), whereas 26 (43%) were immediately followed by an exacerbation. For the patients assigned to placebo, the PPV was 48%; for the active fluphenazine–treated patients, it was 37%, a nonsignificant (NS) difference (χ^2=0.79, *P*=.32).

Post hoc, however, we noted that there appeared to be a change in the PPV over time in the two groups. The placebo-treated group had a PPV of 29% during the first 6 months, followed by 63% during the final 18 months; the active drug–treated group had a PPV of 50% during the first 6 months and 29% during the final 18 months. The interaction of treatment by time (ie, the difference between year 1 and year 2 outcomes) was statistically significant (Breslow-Day test: χ^2=4.47, *df*=1, *P*=.034). We also studied this interaction using logistic regression. In these data, each patient typically contributed more than one data point (in fact, there were 60 prodromes from 36 subjects). Because this is a violation of the assumption of independence of observations, we analyzed the significance of the data displayed using two variants of robust analysis based on bootstrap resampling.[18] In the first analysis, we analyzed 100 replications, each of which was created by sampling only one prodrome randomly from each subject. Each replication thus had a total N of 36. In each replication, we computed a logistic regression analysis, including drug group, week of prodrome onset, and their interaction as independent variables, and we also computed successful resolution of the prodromal episode (ie, return to stability) as the outcome. The interaction parameter was distributed normally in the 100 replications, and it was less than zero in all of them (ie, *P*<.01). In the second method, we used conventional bootstrap resampling of the original data set of N=60 prodromes, yielding 100 random replications with N=60 in each. In all but one of these analyses, the interaction parameter was negative (ie, *P*=.01). Thus, both methods of analysis yielded essentially the same results. The negative interaction parameter indicated the likelihood of a successful resolution of a prodrome (ie, a return to stability rather than an exacerbation) increased over time in the drug-treated group. In the early stages of the trial, there was a nonsignificant advantage associated with being assigned to a placebo, whereas during the later part of the study, there was a statistically significant advantage to being assigned to the active fluphenazine.

EFFECT OF FLUPHENAZINE AND PLACEBO TREATMENT ON THE OUTCOME OF PRODROMES

We used survival analysis as a method for determining any differences between fluphenazine and placebo supplementation in preventing exacerbations. For this method, the time to the first exacerbation was calculated, beginning with the occasion when the patient first met prodromal criteria and was randomized. For this analysis, only the first exacerbation was counted, and subsequent events were ignored. Across the whole study period, there was a nonsignificant advantage associated with being assigned to fluphenazine supplementation using time to first exacerbation as the outcome variable (log-rank χ^2=1.32, NS). As displayed in **Figure 2**, there was no apparent difference in the two groups during the first year, but there was a suggestion of a higher risk of exacerbations in the placebo-treated group during the second year. We therefore analyzed group differences separately for the first and second years of the study. This data analytic strategy is conceptually similar to stratification based on time (described by Kalbfleisch and Prentice[19] in 1980), but it differs in that all patients who were treated during the second year were entered into the analysis of second-year survival, including those who had exacerbations in the first year. In the first year, the difference between groups was not significant. Among patients who entered the second year of the study, however, we found that 58% of fluphenazine-treated patients (n=14) and 16% of placebo-treated patients (n=14) survived without exacerbations (likelihood ratio: χ^2=4.61, *P*=.032).

Finally, we compared the effects of supplemental fluphenazine and placebo on the amount of time that patients were in an exacerbated state or a prodrome. In contrast to survival analysis that only included outcome up until the first exacerbation, this method provides information regarding the patient's illness course for the entire period that the patient remained in the trials. For this analysis, we computed the percent of the time at risk spent in either state. For example, if a patient was randomized at week 26 (and therefore at risk for the next 26 weeks of the first year) and spent weeks 30 to 35 in an exacerbation, the percent of time in exacerbation for the first year was (5/26)×100 or 19.2%. For the purpose of statistical analysis, these proportions were arcsine transformed to stabilize variance. As noted in **Table 2**, there were no statistically significant differences during the first year between patients assigned to active fluphenazine and those assigned to placebo although there was a tendency for active drug–treated patients to spend less time in prodrome and more time in exacerbation. During the second year (**Table 3**), patients who received active fluphenazine supplementation spent significantly less time in an exacerbated state (F=4.34; *df*=1, 27; *P*=.05).

AMOUNT OF SUPPLEMENTAL ORAL FLUPHENAZINE

We computed the amount of supplemental fluphenazine prescribed in the two treatment groups by adding the amount of active fluphenazine prescribed during prodromes and exacerbations. Patients assigned to placebo only received supplemental fluphenazine during exacerbations. In Tables 2 and 3, data are expressed as the mean amount of daily fluphenazine prescribed following randomization (for statistical analysis, data were the square roots transformed to stabilize variance). In year 1

Table 2. Outcome in Randomized Patients During Year 1

	Fluphenazine Decanoate (n=17)		Placebo (n=19)		
	Mean	SD	Mean	SD	*P**
Prodrome (as % of time at risk)	10.5	15.9	19.4	22.3	NS
Exacerbation (as % of time at risk)	11.8	15.0	7.2	10.7	NS
Mean daily fluphenazine total oral supplement	2.26	2.60	0.87	1.38	.014†

*NS indicates not significant.
†Data square root transformed to stabilize variance (t=2.59, df=34).

(Table 2), significantly more fluphenazine was prescribed in the active drug–treated group (*t*=2.59, *df*=34, *P*=.014), primarily because of the additional fluphenazine prescribed during prodromal periods in the active group. There was not a significant difference in the amount prescribed to the two groups during year 2.

EFFECT OF FLUPHENAZINE OR PLACEBO SUPPLEMENTATION ON PSYCHOPATHOLOGY AND SIDE EFFECTS

We also evaluated whether assignment to fluphenazine or placebo during prodromes had an effect on rates of change in psychopathology or side effects. We computed mean slopes for patients in the two treatment groups for the total BPRS and BPRS cluster scores for thought disturbance, paranoid suspiciousness, anxiety-depression, and withdrawal-retardation. We found in most cases that slopes were relatively flat, indicating no change, or were in the direction of slight improvement. There were no significant differences between the drug groups in slopes. We were also unable to find significant differences in side effects or in social adjustment. For the latter, we monitored mean slopes on the global items of the Social Adjustment Scale II.

COMMENT

This study was designed to evaluate the effectiveness of a maintenance strategy aimed at increasing the safety of dosage reduction. If such an early intervention strategy is to be effective, two things are necessary. First, the clinician must be able to identify patients at the time that they are at an increased risk for relapse. Second, an effective treatment must be available that can forestall progression to a full exacerbation of symptoms. Our results indicate that we were limited in our ability to predict when patients were at greatest risk. For example, a considerable number of patients in our study never experienced prodromes. For these patients, an early intervention strategy would obviously not be effective. Even among those

Table 3. Outcome in Randomized Patients During Year 2

	Fluphenazine Decanoate (n=14)		Placebo (n=15)		
	Mean	SD	Mean	SD	P*
Prodrome (as % of time at risk)	2.8	3.8	4.9	5.7	NS
Exacerbation (as % of time at risk)	5.5	10.4	12.9	13.6	.05†
Mean daily fluphenazine total oral supplement	0.80	1.02	1.07	1.17	NS

*NS indicates not significant.
†Data were arcsine transformed to stabilize variance ([θ=2 arc sin $\sqrt{p}$], F=4.34, df=1, 27).

patients who did experience prodromes, our data from the placebo-treated group indicated that 50% of exacerbations were not preceded by a prodrome (and thus could not be treated with supplementation). The data from the placebo-treated group also indicated that only 47% of the prodromes would end in an exacerbation if these events were untreated.

These findings are consistent with those of an earlier prospective study[13] in which we found that changes in psychopathology ratings and scores from self-rating scales could be used to predict which patients were on the verge of psychotic exacerbations. Although these symptoms could predict most psychotic exacerbations, the method had a substantial number of false positives. In a more recent study[16] (using the same population as in this report), we used receiver operating characteristic methods[20] for evaluating our prodromal scale and the BPRS cluster score for anxiety-depression as methods for predicting whether patients would or would not demonstrate a psychotic exacerbation in the 4 weeks following the assessment. We found that both scales were only modestly better than chance at correctly identifying periods of vulnerability to psychotic exacerbation. The sensitivity of both methods was improved when unstable patients were dropped. This latter finding is also consistent with this report in which we found that the PPV of prodromes increased during the second year, a time when more unstable individuals had left the study.

Others have encountered similar problems in the early detection of psychotic relapses. Subotnick and Nuechterlein[14] found that they could correctly classify 59% of relapses, but with a false-positive rate of 26%. However, Birchwood et al,[9] using instruments for detecting prodromes that were completed by both patients and an observer, found that their scale predicted relapse with an overall accuracy of 79%.

A number of research groups have used similar methods for studies of intermittent treatment. Herz et al[6] also reviewed each patient's idiosyncratic early signs with the patient and significant others. Heinrichs and Carpenter[11] asked clinicians to report when they believed that patients were beginning to have exacerbations, and this event was considered a prodrome. Patients and relatives in the study of Jolley et al[7] participated in training sessions that included instructions about prodromal symptoms. All of the above studies included intervention with antipsychotics when prodromal symptoms were detected and, as a result, the sensitivity of their methods for detecting untreated episodes could not be evaluated.

An interesting finding in this study was that the relative risk for exacerbations in the two experimental groups of patients appeared to change over time. For the patients who were randomized to active fluphenazine, the risk decreased during the second year. The patients assigned to placebo demonstrated a relatively constant risk during the 2 years. Since this finding emerged in post hoc analyses, we understand that it can only be proposed tentatively at this point. Nevertheless, this finding is very reminiscent of a similar observation from our prior study,[2] as well as from a study by Hogarty et al,[3] in which there were differences in exacerbation rates between two doses in the second year, but not in the first.

Our interpretation from that study was that some individuals had exacerbations within a few weeks following dosage assignment because they either experienced side effects on too high a dose or their psychosis was not adequately suppressed on too low a dose. This may have been a factor in this study in that some patients may have exacerbations early because they were not adequately stabilized with our low dose of fluphenazine decanoate (5 to 10 mg every 14 days). These patients, as a result of their dosage requirements, or because of the nature of their illness that included considerable personal discomfort, may not have reached a stable state that could readily be distinguished from a prodromal episode. These patients—at least at the time that we evaluated them—were poor candidates for this strategy. Conceivably, the predictive value of a prodrome improved because these patients left the study.

Another possible explanation of the changes between years 1 and 2 is based on the pharmacokinetics of long-acting depot drugs. Patients who have received these drugs for many months may maintain therapeutic plasma concentrations for more than 6 months after the drug is discontinued.[4] It is possible that prodromes and exacerbations during the first year were being suppressed by circulating drug levels. However, this explanation could only be valid for a subgroup of our patients since the rates of prodromes and exacerbations were higher in year 1 than in year 2.

We believe that there were other factors that contributed to the decreasing risk of exacerbations in the fluphenazine supplementation group. That is, for an early intervention strategy to be effective, patients and clinicians should accurately identify prodromal episodes. We observed that both patients and their clinicians improved over time in their ability to detect true prodromes. The evidence for this is the increase in the PPV of a prodrome from 29% in the first 6 months to 63% in the last 18 months. This appeared to be a result of the regular prodromal rating occasions during which the patient and a nurse would review and revise the prodromal symptom rating list. We believe that these interactions led both parties to become better at predicting when a patient was on the verge of an exacerbation. This may have occurred because their combined efforts at discriminating nuances in prodromal symptoms were positively reinforced by the successful preventive intervention with supplemental fluphenazine. The decrease in the PPV of the active fluphenazine–treated patients was probably related to the effectiveness of the supplementation—during the second year—in preventing exacerbations. This may have resulted from earlier recognition of prodromes and, hence, more timely drug intervention.

This change in effectiveness of the strategy over time suggests an interesting limitation of an early intervention strategy in patients receiving low doses, and possibly in those receiving intermittent or targeted treatment. These treatments may have a period of early risk that is followed by a period of increasing effectiveness. If a clinician views a patient as a candidate for a strategy that involves low-dose medication and supplementation when patients show early signs, the first few months may constitute a "trial" period. At this time, the clinician should evaluate whether the patient can be stabilized with a low dose, and if so, the patient and the treatment team should begin the initial stages of improving their abilities to detect prodromes.

Our study has important differences from the four studies of intermittent treatment.[5-8] All of our patients received continuous low doses of fluphenazine decanoate, whereas patients in the other studies were withdrawn from their medications. Low-dose treatment may have influenced the course of exacerbations and the sensitivity of the monitoring system.

In summary, we found both advantages and limitations for our form of early intervention for patients receiving low doses of fluphenazine decanoate. For patients who met our criteria for being well stabilized or for those who were able to remain in the study for more than 6 months, there appeared to be a significant advantage of fluphenazine over placebo in forestalling psychotic exacerbations. For those who could not be stabilized or those who tended to have exacerbations without warning, our strategy was ineffective. In any case, further attention should be given to improving the ability to detect early signs and symptoms of relapse.

Accepted for publication July 6, 1993.

This investigation was supported by the Medical Research Service of the Department of Veterans Affairs, Washington, DC, by grant MH-41573 from the National Institute of Mental Health, Bethesda, Md, and by the UCLA Mental Health Clinical Research Center for Schizophrenia, grant MH-30911 from the National Institute of Mental Health.

Reprint requests to Psychiatry Service (116A), West Los Angeles Veterans Affairs Medical Center, Brentwood Division, 11301 Wilshire Blvd, Los Angeles, CA 90073 (Dr Marder).

REFERENCES

1. Kane JM, Rifkin A, Woerner M, Reardon G, Sarantakos S, Schiabel D, Ramos-Lorenzi J. Low dose neuroleptic treatment of outpatient schizophrenics, I: preliminary results for relapse rates. *Arch Gen Psychiatry.* 1983;40:893-896.
2. Marder SR, Van Putten T, Mintz J, Lebell M, McKenzie J, May PRA. Low and conventional dose maintenance therapy with fluphenazine decanoate: two year outcome. *Arch Gen Psychiatry.* 1987;44:518-521.
3. Hogarty GE, McEvoy JP, Munetz M, DiBarry AL, Bartone P, Cather R, Cooley SJ, Ulrich RF, Carter M, Madonia MJ. Environmental/personal indicators in the course of schizophrenia research group: dose of fluphenazine, familial expressed emotion, and outcome in schizophrenia: results of a two-year controlled study. *Arch Gen Psychiatry.* 1988;45:797-805.
4. Marder SR, Hubbard JW, Van Putten T, Midha KK. The pharmacokinetics of long-acting injectable neuroleptic drugs: clinical implications. *Psychopharmacology (Berl).* 1989;98:433-439.
5. Carpenter WT, Heinrichs DW, Hanlon TE. A comparative trial of pharmacologic strategies in schizophrenia. *Am J Psychiatry.* 1987;144:1466-1470.
6. Herz MI, Glazer WM, Mostert MA, Sheard MA, Szymanski HV, Hafez H, Mirza M, Vana J. Intermittent vs maintenance medication in schizophrenia: two-year results. *Arch Gen Psychiatry.* 1991;48:333-339.
7. Jolley AG, Hirsch SR, McRink A, Manchanda R. Trial of brief intermittent neuroleptic prophylaxis for selected schizophrenic outpatients: clinical outcome at one year. *BMJ.* 1989;298:985-990.
8. Muller P, Bandelow B, Gaebel W, Kopcke W, Linden M, Muller-Spahn F, Pietzcker A, Schafer E, Tegeler J. Intermittent medication, coping and psychotherapy: interactions in relapse prevention and course modification. *Br J Psychiatry.* 1992; (suppl 18):140-144.
9. Birchwood M, Smith J, Macmillan F, Hogg B, Prasad R, Harvey C, Bering S. Predicting relapse in schizophrenia: the development and implementation of an early signs monitoring system using patients and families as observers. *Psychol Med.* 1989;19:649-656.
10. Herz MI, Melville C. Relapse in schizophrenia. *Am J Psychiatry.* 1980;137:801-812.
11. Heinrichs DW, Carpenter WT. Prospective study of prodromal symptoms in schizophrenic relapse. *Am J Psychiatry.* 1985;142:371-373.
12. Hirsch SR, Jolley AG. The dysphoric syndrome in schizophrenia and its implications for relapse. *Br J Psychiatry.* 1989;155:46-50.
13. Marder SR, Mintz J, Van Putten T, Lebell M, McKenzie J. Prodromal symptoms as predictors of relapse. In: Lieberman JA, Kane JM, eds. *Predictors of Relapse in Schizophrenia.* Washington, DC: American Psychiatric Press Inc; 1986:chap 4.
14. Subotnick KL, Nuechterlein KH. Prodromal signs and symptoms of schizophrenic relapse. *J Abnorm Psychol.* 1988;97:405-412.
15. Docherty JP, van Kammen DP, Siris SG, Marder SR. Stages of onset of schizophrenic psychosis. *Am J Psychiatry.* 1978;135:420-426.
16. Marder SR, Mintz J, Van Putten T, Lebell M, Wirshing WC, Johnson-Cronk K. Early prediction of relapse in schizophrenia: an application of receiver operating characteristic (ROC) methods. *Psychopharmacol Bull.* 1991;27:79-82.
17. Kane JM. Schizophrenia: somatic treatment. In: Kaplan HI, Sadock BJ, eds. *Comprehensive Textbook of Psychiatry/V.* Baltimore, Md: Williams & Wilkins; 1989:777-792.
18. Efron B. Bootstrap methods: another look at the jackknife. *Ann Stat.* 1979;7:1-26.
19. Kalbfleisch JD, Prentice RL. *The Statistical Analysis of Failure Time Data.* New York, NY: John Wiley & Sons Inc; 1980.
20. Hsiao JK, Bartko JJ, Potter WZ. Diagnosing diagnoses: receiver operating characteristic methods and psychiatry. *Arch Gen Psychiatry.* 1989;46:664-667.

ORIGINAL ARTICLE

Analysis of the D_4 Dopamine Receptor Gene Variant in an Italian Schizophrenia Kindred

Fabio Macciardi, MD, PhD; Arturas Petronis, MD, PhD; Hubert H. M. Van Tol, PhD; Cecilia Marino, MD; M. Cristina Cavallini, MD; Enrico Smeraldi, MD; James L. Kennedy, MD

Background: Among the different dopamine receptors, the D_4 dopamine receptor is of particular interest in schizophrenia because of its high affinity for the atypical neuroleptic clozapine. Recently, the gene for the D_4 dopamine receptor has been cloned and a new and intriguing polymorphism has been described. Different versions of the receptor have varying affinity for clozapine, and thus variant forms of D_4 with differing pharmacologic activity exist in the human population. Our hypothesis was that these variants play a role in susceptibility to psychotic illness. Thus, our objective was to test the D_4 dopamine receptor genes for linkage to schizophrenia.

Methods: Our genetic linkage study was carried out in a large Italian kindred segregating schizophrenia. Diagnoses were made by using a structured clinical interview and a consensus diagnosis was established. For the computer analysis, 80 members of the family were constructed into a linked set of relatives with 15 of these individuals affected by schizophrenia. The functional variants of the D_4 dopamine receptor gene were identified by a combination of Southern blot techniques and the polymerase chain reation. The gene for tyrosine hydroxylase (TH) was also tested for linkage to schizophrenia in this family. Linkage analyses were done with both a single-locus and a two-locus model.

Results: Our results revealed significantly negative lod scores in the region of the D_4 dopamine receptor gene and the TH gene. The application of different models of transmission for schizophrenia had an effect on the magnitude of the lod scores, but did not modify the direction of the results.

Conclusions: Our results provide significant evidence for exclusion for linkage between schizophrenia and the dopamine D_4 receptor gene and the TH gene under the models specified. Furthermore, we tabulated the distribution of D_4 dopamine gene variants in the diseased vs healthy individuals in the family and the results showed that no specific form of the receptor gene is significantly asociated with the presence of schizophrenia in the family. Our study does not exclude the possibility that regulatory elements of the D_4 dopamine gene located elsewhere in the genome may be involved in the etiology of schizophrenia.

(Arch Gen Psychiatry. 1994;51:288-293)

From the Istituto Scientifico H San Raffaele, Department of Neuroscience, University of Milano (Italy) School of Medicine (Drs Macciardi, Marino, Cavallini, and Smeraldi); and the Sections of Neurogenetics (Drs Petronis and Kennedy) and Molecular Psychobiology (Dr Van Tol), the Clarke Institute of Psychiatry, University of Toronto, Ontario.

ALTHOUGH THE genetics of schizophrenia has had a long history, some six decades at least, few conclusions have been established. However, these 60 years have been productive because adoption, twin, and family studies have all pointed to strong genetic factors in schizophrenia.[1-3] Additional epidemiologic studies have been performed to illuminate the genetic determinants of the disease and have produced interesting but conflicting results.[4,5] New technology now provides progressively more informative markers for DNA investigators to test genetic hypotheses of schizophrenia at the molecular level.

In 1988, Sherrington et al[6] reported evidence for linkage of two markers to schizophrenia in Icelandic and British families. At the same time, Kennedy et al[7] found no evidence for linkage of schizophrenia to seven chromosome 5 markers in a Swedish kindred. A reevaluation of the posi-

See Patients, Materials, and Methods on next page

PATIENTS, MATERIALS, AND METHODS

CLINICAL AND DNA MARKER DATA

The family used in these analyses is a kindred from northern Italy, previously described by Macciardi et al.[10] The affected members of this family exhibit the full range of symptoms of schizophrenia, including the subtypes of paranoid, undifferentiated, and mixed. The family has a low level of schizophrenia spectrum disorders such as schizotypal personality and a low level of affective disorders. Diagnoses were made using the structured clinical interview Schedule for Affective Disorders and Schizophrenia, Lifetime version (SADS-L).[30] The interview was administered by psychiatrists on our team who were experienced with the Italian version of this instrument. The results of the SADS-L interview plus medical charts were reviewed separately by two additional research psychiatrists, and a consensus diagnosis was established.

For the computer analyses, 80 members of the family were constructed into a linked set of relatives, with 15 of these individuals affected by schizophrenia. Forty individuals had provided DNA samples. The functional variants of *DRD4* were identified by a combination of Southern blot techniques and polymerase chain reaction (PCR). The clone used to detect the polymorphism for the original *DRD4* RFLP[24] was pB28, which recognizes a four-allele system with *Hinc*II (A1=0.04, A2=0.15, A3=0.20, A4=0.61). The RFLP for TH was detected using the probe TY7. This probe detects a three-allele RFLP with allele frequencies A1=0.56, A2=0.03, and A3=0.41. Standard procedures for Southern blotting and RFLP analysis were used throughout.[31] Southern blot procedures for the new *DRD4* polymorphism using the probe pD2S10 are described by Van Tol et al.[27]

The PCR methods for *DRD4* are described by Lichter et al.[32] Eight alleles (classified herein as number of repeats) have been revealed, with the following frequencies: 2=0.11, 3=0.04, 4=0.68, 5=0.01, 6=0.02, 7=0.13, 8=0.01, and one individual has been found with 10 repeats. Tyrosine hydroxylase has a tetrameric nucleotide repeat (adenosine, adenosine, thymidine, guanosine [AATG]) that can be faithfully amplified with PCR, using the appropriate primers. The product size ranges between 183 and 207 bp, according to the number of tandem repeats present in the amplification product.[33] Seven alleles are detected: their frequencies are variable across four populations studied by Edwards et al.[34] Two alleles, A1 and A7, with respectively, the higher and lower number of repeats of the tetranucleotide, are very rare in white persons; frequencies of the other alleles are as follows: A2=0.23; A3=0.16; A4=0.11; A5=0.14; and A6=0.35. The estimated heterozygote frequency in whites is 0.87. Mutation rates were estimated and were not significant.[34]

Tyrosine hydroxylase was typed using conditions described by Edwards et al[33] with some modifications for the PCR machine (Perkin-Elmer model 9600). Amplification was performed with one cycle at 95°C for 3 minutes, followed by denaturing at 94°C for 45 seconds, annealing at 55°C for 45 seconds, and extension at 72°C for 45 seconds. The concentration of primers was 0.1 μmol/L; DNA template, 50 ng/μL; deoxyadenosine triphosphate, deoxyguanosine triphosphate, deoxythymidine triphosphate, at 200 μmol/L each, deoxycytidine triphosphate at 50 μmol/L, and deoxycytidine triphosphate labeled with radioactive phosphorus at 50 μmol/L; 50-mmol/L potassium chloride; 1% gelatin; 15-mmol/L magnesium chloride, at a pH of 8.0, in a 10-μL reaction volume. Two microliters of the amplification product was electrophoresed through a denaturing 6% polyacrylamide sequencing gel at 1800 V for approximately 2 hours; roentgenograms were exposed overnight. We tested the TH microsatellite polymorphism in 42 healthy unrelated northern Italians and detected five alleles with frequencies comparable to those found in the literature. All five of these alleles were observed among the 38 DNAs typed from our family with schizophrenia.

LINKAGE ANALYSIS

Segregation analyses were performed on the family in an attempt to determine the best mode of inheritance in this kindred and these analyses pointed to an unrestricted model. However, the unrestricted model could not be distinguished from a single-locus model, which, for all practical purposes, fits the data equally as well (data not shown). For the computer analysis of the genotyping data, we selected genetic parameters as follows: autosomal dominant with penetrance=0.70; phenocopies=0.001; and frequency of the disease allele (q)=0.0085. For the recessive single major locus (SML) model, q=0.05. Both recessive and dominant models were employed in light of work by Clerget-Darpoux et al[35,36] suggesting that errors in the model parameters may lead to erroneous estimates in the recombination fraction, but that linkage to a disease gene is still detectable, provided that both dominant and recessive models are tested. Parameters of the models were derived either by estimates in the Italian population or from the recent literature on segregation for schizophrenia.[37,38] Pairwise analyses were done with the computer program MLINK. The program LINKMAP was used for the multipoint analyses.[39]

Continued on next page

tive linkage result in the Icelandic and British families led to lod scores falling to very negative values in some families and to indeterminate positive values in others.[8,9] Other investigators have explored the chromosome 5 hypothesis in schizophrenia and have found consistently negative results,[10] indicating that linkage of schizophrenia to chromosome 5 is unlikely. However, it remains a possibility that chromosome 5 is playing a role

TWO-LOCUS ANALYSIS

The data were subjected to a model that incorporates two loci acting epistatically. This oligogenic model of disease was suggested recently by Risch[40] as a reasonable model to explain the observed pattern of schizophenia occurrence in affected families. Thus, a computer program (TLINK)[41] was used to hypothesize that a second locus was linked to the disease and interacting with the first locus in an epistatic manner. The estimation of the TLINK parameter values most appropriate for schizophrenia can be described as follows. The epistatic model suggests that the two potential loci conferring risk for schizophrenia act in a multiplicative manner. Assuming both locus A and B as autosomal dominant with two alleles (A2 and B2 are disease alleles) and disease genotypes as A1A2, A2A2, B1B2, B2B2, then the disease is manifested only where locus A=A1A2 or A2A2 *and* locus B=B1B2 or B2B2, otherwise a given subject is healthy.[42] In other words, this model requires that the disease allele at locus A and the disease allele at locus B must both be present for the disease to be manifested. Penetrance values were formatted in a 3×3 matrix, using the three possible genotypes at each locus.[42,43] We estimated values for model parameters in our family incorporating the recent suggestions from Vieland et al[44]: gene frequencies were 0.20 and 0.01 for the two loci, while the penetrance used for the two-locus model was assigned values of 1.00 for the cells of the matrix corresponding to presence of the risk alleles at both of the loci.

in a small fraction of families with schizophrenia. In Alzheimer's disease, for example, the codon 717 mutation of the amyloid precursor protein gene has been found in only eight of more than 250 families examined.[11]

Following these initial linkage studies of schizophrenia, it became clear that additional strategies were needed to study the role of genes involved in the origin of the disorder. The candidate gene approach provided a hypothesis-driven alternative to a search across the entire human genome for a potential etiologic gene. The hypothesis for a candidate gene usually stems from a priori knowledge about a given biologic measure that is viewed as correlated with pathologic factors in the disease. If a gene expressing the putative etiologic genetic factor has been identified, cloned, and mapped, then this gene is a potentially powerful candidate to explore the genetic basis of a disease. The candidate gene strategy has valuable attributes and the most important is that the hypothesis to be tested is specific and thus falsifiable. Biologically based genetic models that are known to be of interest for schizophrenia can be effectively tested. However, in the absence of a meaningful a priori hypothesis, the process of selecting a candidate gene might be endless, given the estimate of 30 000 to 50 000 genes expressed in brain.[12]

For schizophrenia, the dopamine hypothesis has had substantial support and is of sufficient interest to require investigation of genes involved in the major components of the dopamine system. Based primarily on the fact that the neuroleptic drugs used to treat schizophrenia bind to dopamine receptors, the dopamine hypothesis has emerged from more than 25 years of pharmacologic research in schizophrenia.[13,14] The efficacy of neuroleptic drugs is tightly correlated with their affinity for the D_2 dopamine receptor.[15] Using positron emission tomography, some groups have found an increase in D_2 dopamine receptors in unmedicated schizophrenic patients.[16-18] Other investigators have not been able to replicate this result.[19] Moises et al[20] evaluated the D_2 dopamine receptor gene for linkage in the Swedish schizophrenia kindred, but no evidence was found for linkage of the D_2 gene, or its surrounding region on 11q, to schizophrenia.

The D_4 dopamine receptor is of particular interest in schizophrenia because of its high affinity for the atypical neuroleptic clozapine. The dramatic clinical success of clozapine in a subset of patients with schizophrenia has led to a great deal of interest in the medication in recent years.[21,22] This also leads to direct interest in the use of the D_4 dopamine gene (*DRD4*) as a candidate in linkage studies for schizophrenia. Other evidence for the role of *DRD4* in schizophrenia comes from the fact that the anatomic distribution of the receptor is primarily in the limbic system,[23] a localization consistent with neuroanatomic theories of schizophrenia.

A restriction fragment length polymorphism (RFLP) for *DRD4* was discovered[24] and used to map the gene to the tip of the short arm of chromosome 11 in proximity to the gene for tyrosine hydroxylase (TH).[25] The TH gene is an interesting locus both due to the previous finding by Leboyer et al[26] of a positive association with bipolar disorder in a French population, and for its rate-limiting role in the pathway of catecholamine biosynthesis. Because TH is the rate-limiting step in the synthesis of dopamine, and because the genes for TH and D_4 are located close together, we were prompted to perform genetic studies of this region to evaluate the dopamine hypothesis of schizophrenia.

The new and intriguing polymorphism for *DRD4* that is the focus of this study has been recently noted by Van Tol et al[27] and further evaluated by Petronis et al[28] and Kennedy et al.[29] This polymorphism consists of a set of variants in the portion of the gene coding for the third cytoplasmic loop of the receptor. The variation occurs as a result of a variable number of copies of a 48–base pair (bp) sequence inserted into the third exon. Petronis et al[28] have genotyped more than 250 individuals and now document seven different forms of the *DRD4* gene con-

Table 1. Pairwise Linkage Analysis Results for *DRD4* and TH vs Schizophrenia Under the SML Dominant and Recessive Models With RFLP and PCR-Based Polymorphisms*

	Locus				
	θ=0.0	θ=0.1	θ=0.2	θ=0.3	θ=0.4
SML Dominant					
RFLPs					
DRD4	−0.4266	−0.1721	−0.0638	−0.0225	−0.0077
TH	−1.1133	−0.5327	−0.2575	−0.1048	−0.0251
PCR-based polymorphisms					
DRD4	−0.2449	−0.1755	−0.1632	−0.1356	−0.0766
TH	−2.6156	−0.8415	−0.3472	−0.1274	−0.0324
SML Recessive					
RFLPs					
DRD4	−0.7153	−0.4932	−0.2868	−0.1255	−0.0274
TH	−1.7169	−0.4273	−0.1594	−0.0594	−0.0147
PCR-based polymorphism					
DRD4	−2.4894	−0.7388	−0.2496	−0.0724	−0.0141
TH	−2.9182	−1.0526	−0.4461	−0.1718	−0.0416

*DRD4 *indicates D_4 dopamine receptor; TH, tyrosine hydroxylase; SML, single major locus; RFLP, restriction fragment length polymorphism; and PCR, polymerase chain reaction. Gene frequency for the dominant model is 0.01; homozygote and heterozygote penetrance is 72%. Gene frequency for the recessive model is 0.05; homozygote penetrance is 90%.*

sisting of two to eight repeats of the 48-bp sequence. Most important is the fact that different variants of the gene code for D_4 dopamine receptor proteins that exhibit significant differences in pharmacologic affinity for clozapine and spiperone. Immediately the hypothesis arises that these variable functional forms of *DRD4* in the human population may play a role in susceptibility to psychotic illness. For this reason we investigated the *DRD4* polymorphism in our Italian family, segregating for schizophrenia.

RESULTS

Table 1 shows the results of the pairwise linkage analyses for *DRD4* and TH vs schizophrenia under the SML dominant model with the RFLP and PCR-based marker typing for each locus. In both cases lod score results are negative and point to an exclusion of *DRD4* and TH as candidate genes for schizophrenia in our family. The application of different hypotheses of transmission for schizophrenia, for example, varying penetrance parameters in an SML autosomal dominant model or testing an SML recessive model with higher q values, had an effect on the absolute magnitude of the lod scores, but did not modify the direction of the results (Table 1). Assuming a 6-centiMorgan (cM) distance between *DRD4* and TH,[25,28] we performed a multipoint analysis where the locus for susceptibility to schizophrenia was moved across a fixed map of *DRD4* and TH. The results remained negative with a minimum lod score of −2.9 at the TH location. The area for exclusion of linkage also includes *DRD4* (lod score of -2.1) and extends for approximately 10 cM across the 11p15 region (**Figure**). The presence of one crossover between *DRD4* and TH in our family is consistent with the genetic map. The two-locus models show a major reduction of goodness of fit in the lod score estimates for *DRD4*. The values are in the negative range, but no single lod score for different θ values achieved a significant exclusion level (**Table 2**).

In view of the fact that the *DRD4* polymorphism represents a variation in the coding region of the gene, and that different variants appear to have different pharmacologic activity,[27] we tabulated the distribution of *DRD4* variants in diseased vs healthy individuals (**Table 3**). The

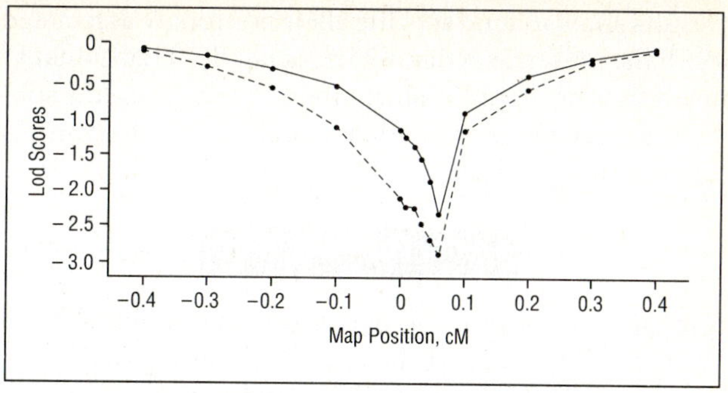

Multipoint linkage for schizophrenia across a fixed map of D_4 dopamine receptor gene and tyrosine hydroxylase. Solid line indicates restriction fragment length polymorphism; dotted line, microsatellites. D_4 dopamine receptor gene is arbitrarily fixed at 0.0 centiMorgan (cM); tyrosine hydroxylase is located 6 cM centromeric to the D_4 dopamine receptor gene.

Table 2. Two-Locus Linkage Analysis Results for *DRD4* and TH Schizophrenia: Two-Locus Model Double Dominant*

	Locus				
	θ=0.0	θ=0.1	θ=0.2	θ=0.3	θ=0.4
DRD4	−0.478	−0.299	−0.189	−0.133	−0.073
TH	−0.922	−0.475	−0.244	−0.102	−0.025

**Results are shown for restriction fragment length polymorphism (RFLP) only.* DRD4 *indicates D_4 dopamine receptor; TH, tyrosine hydroxylase. Gene frequencies are 0.2 for Q1, 0.01 for Q2.*

Table 3. *DRD4* Variants in Schizophrenic Individuals (n=28 Chromosomes) and Controls (n=44 Chromosomes)*

No. of 48 bp Repeats	Schizophrenic Individuals	Controls
2	3 (10.7)	0 (0.0)
4	13 (46.4)	24 (54.5)
7	10 (35.7)	12 (27.3)
8	2 (7.1)	8 (18.2)

**Results are from PCR genotypes, and percentages are given in parentheses.* DRD4 *indicates D_4 dopamine receptor; PCR, polymerase chain reaction; and bp, base pair.*

results show that no specific allele is strongly associated with the presence of disease in the family. Traditional χ^2 analysis is not appropriate for these data because the subjects are related to each other, and thus the observations are not independent.

COMMENT

Linkage analysis for the hypothesis of a schizophrenia susceptibility locus in the 11p15 region showed negative results in both pairwise and multipoint analyses. It is helpful to employ both pairwise and multipoint strategies because each strategy has advantages and disadvantages. Pairwise analyses are not able to use all of the polymorphic information across several loci, but they are more robust to errors in the parameter estimates of the model. Multipoint analyses are able to benefit from the polymorphic information from several loci in a given region, but the results are more sensitive to errors in parameter estimates, and quite sensitive to errors in order of loci in the chromosomal map.[45] The results of the more robust pairwise analyses in our data are consistent with the multipoint results, and therefore, it is less likely that the exclusion of linkage to schizophrenia is due to artifact from misspecification of model parameters.

The multipoint results in the Figure are influenced by the accuracy of the map location of *DRD4* and TH relative to each other. The precise map location for *DRD4* has not been established. In our Italian kindred, there was one crossover noted between *DRD4* and TH, although the number of informative meioses was relatively small. Petronis et al[28] have noted a definitive crossover in reference family 1341 (taken from the Centre d'Etude Polymorphism Humain [CEPH] collection) between *DRD4* and HRAS, and no crossovers between the *DRD4* PCR marker and the TH microsatellite marker, thus placing *DRD4* between TH and Harvey-RAS (HRAS). The *DRD4 Hinc*II RFLP is not in tight disequilibrium with the new *DRD4* PCR marker (data not shown), which could be a result of errors in reading the Southern blot due to the difficulty in distinguishing the bands for the lower three alleles of the *Hinc*II RFLP. The fine mapping of *DRD4* would be assisted by the use of fluorescent in situ hybridization to further define the location of *DRD4* relative to TH and HRAS.[46] The results for the two-locus model of schizophrenia are indeterminate (Table 2), but it must be remembered that this model is very complex and still represents a relatively unexplored approach to linkage analysis. Even though we have reasonable basis to hypothesize that schizophrenia is resulting from an oligogenic model of transmission,[40] the extension of the mathematical model from segregation analyses to an experimental test for linkage must be performed cautiously. The larger number of parameters needed to describe the two-locus model, compared with SML, is assumed in order to allow for a better fit of the model to illness transmission, and errors in parameter estimates have a deleterious effect only on the recombination values. Other unknown factors could be responsible for the results produced using the two-locus model. We do not know, for example, whether a two- or a three-locus hypothesis best describes the trait of schizophrenia and, moreover, we do not know whether the effects of multiple loci plus additional reduced penetrance may limit the power of the analysis to such a degree that linkage is undetectable. Applying more complex models emphasizes the point that simple genetic models, even allowing for incomplete penetrance and sporadic cases, generally do not fit satisfactorily the family data for psychiatric disorders.[47]

In conclusion, *DRD4* does not appear to be linked to schizophrenia in this large multigenerational, partially isolated Italian family, at least under the model conditions specified. The new PCR-based repeated polymorphism for *DRD4* used in this linkage analysis is unique in that it detects a repeat of 48 bp in the coding sequence. Association studies of the functionally important variant may be an interesting alternative to linkage analyses. If the variant determines a portion of the variance for susceptibility to schizophrenia, then an association study with a large sample size may be able to detect the increased risk conferred by one or more of the *DRD4* alleles.

Since the *DRD4* variants exhibit a different affinity for dopamine antagonists (ie, antipsychotic drugs), it will be especially interesting to look at covariation between *DRD4* variants and antipsychotic medication response. The patients in the family that we have analyzed respond relatively well to haloperidol, as measured by their low level of rehospitalization after treatment, if they remain compliant with the medication. Other families with different pharmacologic response profiles may have a corresponding difference in the distribution of *DRD4* alleles. At the present state of our knowledge, it is premature to draw conclusions about the precise involvement of *DRD4* in schizophrenic disorders, and further investigations into the molecular structure of this gene and its significance are required.

Accepted for publication July 16, 1993.

Jaques Mallet, PhD, provided the TY7 probe to detect the RFLP for TH.

Reprint requests to the Clarke Institute of Psychiatry, Section of Neurogenetics, 250 College St, Toronto, Ontario, Canada M5T 1R8 (Dr Kennedy).

REFERENCES

1. Gottesman II, Shields J. *Schizophrenia: The Epigenetic Puzzle.* New York, NY: Cambridge University Press; 1982.
2. Kendler K. The genetics of schizophrenia and related disorders: a review. In: Dunner D, Gershon E, Barret J, eds. *Relative at Risk for Mental Disorders.* New

York, NY: Raven Press; 1988:247-266.
3. Kennedy JL, Giuffra L. Recent developments in genetic linkage studies of schizophrenia. In: Tamminga CA, Schultz SC, eds. *Advances in Neuropsychiatry and Psychopharmacology.* New York, NY: Raven Press; 1991:21-31.
4. Smeraldi E, Macciardi F, Gasperini M, Orsini A, Bellodi L, Fabio G, Morabito A. Genetic modelling in schizophrenia according to HLA typing. *Clin Genet.* 1986; 30:157-166.
5. Tsuang MT, Lyons MJ, Faraone SV. Clinical phenotypes: problem in diagnosis. In: Mendlewicz J, Hippius H, eds. *Genetic Research in Psychiatry.* Berlin, Germany: Springer-Verlag; 1992:173-192.
6. Sherrington R, Brynjolfsson J, Peturson H, Potter M, Dudleston K, Barraclough B, Wasmuth J, Dobbs M, Gurling H. Localization of a susceptibility locus for schizophrenia on chromosome 5. *Nature.* 1988;336:164-167.
7. Kennedy JL, Giuffra L, Moises H, Cavalli-Sforza L, Pakstis A, Kidd J, Castiglione C, Sjogren B, Wetterberg L, Kidd KK. Evidence against linkage of schizophrenia to markers on chromosome 5 in a northern Swedish pedigree. *Nature.* 1988;336:167-170.
8. Risch N. Genetic linkage and complex disease with special reference to psychiatric disorders. *Genet Epidemiol.* 1990;7:3-16.
9. Mankoo B, Sherrington R, Brynjolfsson J, Kalsi G, Petursson H, Sigmundsson T, Read T, Murphy P, Curtis D, Melmer G, Gurling H. New microsatellite polymorphisms provide a highly polymorphic map of chromosome 5 bands q11.2-q13.3 for linkage analysis of Icelandic and English families affected by schizophrenia. *Psychiatr Genet.* 1991;2:17.
10. Macciardi F, Kennedy JL, Ruocco L, Giuffra L, Carrera P, Marino C, Rinaldi V, Smeraldi E, Ferrari M. A genetic linkage study of schizophrenia to chromosome 5 markers in a northern Italian population. *Biol Psychiatry.* 1992;31:720-728.
11. Schellenberg GD, Anderson L, O'Dahl S, Wijsman EM, Sadovnick AD, Ball MJ, Larson EB, Kukull WA, Martin GM, Roses AD, Bird TA. APP717, APP693, and PRIP gene mutations are rare in Alzheimer disease. *Am J Hum Genet.* 1991; 49:511-517.
12. Milner RJ, Sutcliff JG. Gene expression in rat brain. *Nucleic Acid Res.* 1983; 11:5497-5520.
13. Seeman P. Dopamine receptors and the dopamine hypothesis of schizophrenia. *Synapse.* 1987;1:133-152.
14. Losonczy MF, Davidson M, Davis KL. The dopamine hypothesis of schizophrenia. In: Meltzer HY, ed. *Psychopharmacology: The Third Generation of Progress.* New York, NY: Raven Press;1987:715-726.
15. Seeman P, Lee T. Antipsychotic drugs: direct correlation between clinical potency and presynaptic action on dopamine neurons. *Science.* 1975;188:1217-1219.
16. Lee T, Seeman P, Tourtellotte WW, Farley IJ, Hornikiewicz O. Binding of 3H-neuroleptics and 3H-apomorphine in schizophrenic brain. *Nature.* 1978;274: 897-900.
17. Seeman P, Ulpian C, Bergeron C, Riederer P, Jellinger K, Gabriel E, Reynolds GP, Tourtellotte WW. Bimodal distribution of dopamine receptor densities in brains of schizophrenics. *Science.* 1984;225:728-730.
18. Kornhuber J, Riederer P, Reynolds GP, Beckmann H, Jellinger K, Gabriel E. 3H-Spiperone binding sites in post-mortem brains from schizophrenic patients: relationship to neuroleptic drug treatment, abnormal movements, and positive symptoms. *J Neural Transm.* 1989;75:1-10.
19. Farde L, Wiesel FA, Stone-Elander S, Sedvall G. No D2 receptor increase in PET study of schizophrenia. *Arch Gen Psychiatry.* 1987;44:671-672.
20. Moises HW, Gelernter J, Giuffra LA, Zarcone V, Wetterberg L, Civelli O, Kidd KK, Cavalli-Sforza LL, Grandy DK, Kennedy JL, Vinogradov S, Mauer J, Litt M, Sjogren B. No linkage between D2 dopamine receptor gene region and schizophrenia. *Arch Gen Psychiatry.* 1991;48:643-647.
21. Kane J, Honigfeld G, Singer J, Meltzer HY. Clozapine for the treatment-resistant schizophrenic. *Arch Gen Psychiatry.* 1988;45:789-796.
22. Meltzer HY. Clozapine: clinical advantages and biologic mechanisms. In: Schultz SC, Tamminga CA, eds. *Schizophrenia: Scientific Progress.* New York, NY: Oxford University Press; 1989:302-309.
23. Van Tol HHM, Bunzow JR, Guan HC, Sunahara RK, Seeman P, Niznik HB, Civelli O. Cloning of the gene for a human dopamine D4 receptor with high affinity for the antipsychotic clozapine. *Nature.* 1991;350:610-614.
24. Kennedy JL, Sidenberg DG, Van Tol HHM, Kidd KK. A *Hinc*II RFLP in the human D4 dopamine receptor locus (DRD4). *Nucleic Acids Res.* 1991;19:5805.
25. Gelernter J, Kennedy JL, Van Tol HHM, Civelli O, Kidd KK. The D4 dopamine receptor (DRD4) maps to distal 11p close to HRAS. *Genomics.* 1992;13:208-210.
26. Leboyer M, Malafosse A, Boularand S, Campion D, Gheysen F, Samolyk D, Henriksson B, Denise E, Des Lauriers A, Lepine JP, Zarifian E, Clerget-Darpoux F, Mallet J. Tyrosine hydroxylase polymorphisms associated with manic-depressive illness. *Lancet.* 1990;335:1219.
27. Van Tol HHM, Wu CM, Guan HC, Ohara K, Bunzow JR, Civelli O, Kennedy JL, Seeman P, Niznik HB, Jovanovic V. Multiple dopamine D4 receptor variants in the human population. *Nature.* 1992;358:149-152.
28. Petronis A, Van Tol HHM, Livak KJ, Lichter J, Macciardi FM, Sidenberg DG, Kennedy JL. Genetic analysis of variable repeat sequence in DRD4 gene exon. *Am J Hum Genet.* 1992;51:A198. Abstract.
29. Kennedy JL, Van Tol HHM, Petronis A, Sidenberg DG, Honer WG, Macciardi FM, Bassett AS. Genetic linkage studies of DRD4 variants in schizophrenia. *Am J Hum Genet.* 1992;51(suppl):A365. Abstract.
30. Spitzer RL, Endicott J. *Schedule for Affective Disorders and Schizophrenia (SADS).* New York, NY: New York State Psychiatric Institute; 1978.
31. Southern EM. Detection of specific sequences among DNA fragments separated by gel electrophoresis. *J Mol Biol.* 1975;98:503-517.
32. Lichter JB, Barr CL, Kennedy JL, Van Tol HHM, Kidd KK, Livak KJ. A hypervariable segment in the human dopamine receptor (DRD4) gene. *Hum Mol Genet.* 1993;2:767-773.
33. Edwards A, Civitello A, Hammond HA, Caskey CT. DNA typing and genetic mapping with trimeric and tetrameric tandem repeats. *Am J Hum Genet.* 1991;49: 746-756.
34. Edwards A, Hammond HA, Jin L, Caskey CT, Chakraborty R. Genetic variation at five trimeric and tetrameric tandem repeat loci in four human population groups. *Genomics.* 1992;12:241-253.
35. Clerget-Darpoux F, Bana:ti-Pellie' C, Hochez J. Effects of misspecifying genetic parameters in lod score analysis. *Biometrics.* 1986;42:393-399.
36. Clerget-Darpoux F, Babron MC, Bana:ti-Pellie' C. Assessing the effect of multiple linkage tests in complex diseases. *Genet Epidemiol.* 1990;7:245-253.
37. Vogler GP, Gottesman II, McGue MK, Rao DC. Mixed model segregation analysis of schizophrenia in the Lindelius Swedish pedigrees. *Behav Genet.* 1990; 20:461-472.
38. Asherson P, Parfitt E, Sargeant M, Tidmarsh S, Buckland P, Taylor C, Clements A, Gill M, McGuffin P, Owen M. No evidence for a pseudoautosomal locus for schizophrenia: linkage analysis of multiple affected families. *Br J Psychiatry.* 1991;161:63-68.
39. Lathrop M, Lalouel JM, Julier C, Ott J. Multilocus linkage analysis in humans: detection of linkage and estimation of recombination. *Am J Hum Genet.* 1985; 37:482-498.
40. Risch N. Linkage strategies for genetically complex traits, I: multilocus model. *Am J Hum Genet.* 1991;46:219-221.
41. Lathrop GM, Ott J. Analysis of complex diseases under oligogenic models and intrafamilial heterogeneity by the LINKAGE programs. *Am J Hum Genet.* 1990; 47:A188. Abstract.
42. Macciardi F, Cavallini MC. A 2-locus model for Alzheimer's disease? Read before the Eighth Genetic Analysis Workshop; November 9, 1992; San Francisco, Calif.
43. Merette C, Lehner T, Leal S, Ott J. Two approaches toward linkage heterogeneity of FAD: age of onset and the two locus model of epistasis. Read before the Eighth Genetic Analysis Workshop; November 9, 1992; San Francisco, Calif.
44. Vieland VJ, Hodge SE, Greenberg DA. Adequacy of single-locus approximations for linkage analyses of oligogenic traits. *Genet Epidemiol.* 1992;9:45-60.
45. Risch N, Giuffra L. Model misspecifications and multipoint linkage analysis. *Hum Hered.* 1992;42:77-92.
46. Lawrence JB. A fluorescence in situ hybridization approach for gene mapping and the study of nuclear organization. In: Davies KE, Tilghman SM, eds. *Genetic and Physical Mapping.* Cold Spring Harbor, NY: Cold Spring Harbor Laboratory Press; 1990:1-38.
47. Smeraldi E, Macciardi F. The 'candidate gene' approach to the genetics of schizophrenia and other psychoses. In: Racagni G, Brunell N, Fukuda T, eds. *Biological Psychiatry: Proceedings of the Fifth World Congress of Biological Psychiatry.* Amsterdam, the Netherlands: Elsevier Science Publishers; 1991;2:465-468.

ORIGINAL ARTICLE

Epidemiology of Nonaffective Acute Remitting Psychosis vs Schizophrenia

Sex and Sociocultural Setting

Ezra Susser, MD, DrPH; Joseph Wanderling, MA

Background: This article first examines the epidemiology of nonaffective acute remitting psychosis with respect to variation in incidence by sex and sociocultural setting. Second, it examines whether nonaffective acute remitting psychosis can be epidemiologically differentiated from schizophrenia.

Methods: The data were drawn from the World Health Organization Determinants of Outcome Study. Sex-specific incidence rates were obtained for two sites in the developing-country setting and for six sites in the industrialized-country setting.

Results: For nonaffective acute remitting psychosis, the incidence in men was about one-half the incidence in women, and the incidence in the developing-country setting was about 10-fold the incidence in the industrialized-country setting. These associations with sex and with setting were sharply distinct from those of schizophrenia.

Conclusions: The epidemiologic patterns of this form of psychosis may be distinct from those of schizophrenia and could yield clues to its causes.

(Arch Gen Psychiatry. 1994;51:294-301)

From the New York State Psychiatric Institute, Department of Psychiatry, Columbia University, New York (Dr Susser), and the Department of Statistical Sciences and Epidemiology, Nathan Kline Institute for Psychiatric Research, Orangeburg, NY (Mr Wanderling).

THIS ARTICLE reports epidemiologic findings on *nonaffective acute remitting psychosis* (NARP). We introduce this term to describe precisely the subject of our attention, namely, nonaffective psychoses that are characterized by very acute onset and full remission but that resemble schizophrenia sufficiently to be given at least an *International Classification of Diseases, Ninth Revision* (*ICD-9*) diagnosis of schizophrenia.[1] We first examine the epidemiologic characteristics of NARP with respect to variation in incidence by sex and by sociocultural setting. Second, we examine whether NARP can be epidemiologically differentiated from other cases diagnosed as schizophrenia by *ICD-9* in terms of variation in incidence, sex ratios, and sex differences in age of onset.

The data were drawn from the World Health Organization Determinants of Outcome Study, which included 13 sites in two contrasting sociocultural settings, namely, the developing-country setting and the industrialized-country setting.[2,3] Incidence rates were obtained from two sites in the developing-country setting and from six sites in the industrialized-country setting. Sex ratios and sex differences in age of onset were obtained from all 13 sites.

For at least three quarters of a century, investigators have tried to differentiate forms of acute remitting psychosis under a variety of names, for instance, reactive psychosis, schizophreniform psychosis, and cycloid psychosis.[4-13] Nonetheless, the demarcation of these conditions from schizophrenia and from one another remains a critical area of uncertainty in psychiatric diagnosis.[14] For instance, the *DSM-III-R*[15] excludes from schizophrenia all remitting psychoses with less than 6 months of continuous illness, whereas the *ICD-10*[16] excludes only those with acute onset

See Methods on next page

METHODS

The methods of the Determinants of Outcome Study are described in detail elsewhere.[2,3] Briefly, in defined catchment areas in 13 sites, investigators were to include over a 2-year period all patients aged 15 to 54 years with a psychotic disorder at their first contact with a helping agency. To focus on schizophrenia, patients with *ICD-9* affective diagnoses were later excluded unless they had prominent psychotic symptoms on the Present State Examination (ie, CATEGO classification of S, P, or O).[2,3,24] The five developing-country sites were Agra, India; Cali, Colombia; urban Chandigarh, India; rural Chandigarh; and Ibadan, Nigeria. The eight industrialized-country sites were Århus, Denmark; Dublin, Ireland; Honolulu, Hawaii; Moscow, Russia; Nagasaki, Japan; Nottingham, England; Prague, the Czech Republic; and Rochester, NY.

In practice, ascertainment was sufficiently complete to calculate incidence rates in only eight of the 13 sites: two developing-country sites (rural Chandigarh and urban Chandigarh) and six industrialized-country sites (Århus, Dublin, Honolulu, Moscow, Nagasaki, and Nottingham). In the other five sites, a significant number of cases may have been missed. In all 13 sites, however, the study cohort included only patients making a first-treatment contact for a psychotic disorder.

Patients were followed up for 2 years. In the eight sites with incidence data, 840 patients were included in the study and 646 (77%) had a full 2-year follow-up assessment. In all 13 sites, 1379 patients were included in the study and 1078 (78%) had a full 2-year follow-up assessment.

RESEARCH INSTRUMENTS

At the initial evaluation and the 2-year follow-up, patients had a full clinical assessment that included the ninth edition of the Present State Examination,[24] the Psychiatric and Personal History Schedule (usually completed with a key informant), and the Diagnostic and Prognostic Schedule. A psychiatrist administered the Present State Examination and made an *ICD-9* diagnosis.

Research teams were trained to rate mode of onset (five categories[3(pp24-25)]) and pattern of course over the 2-year follow-up period (eight categories[3(pp57-58)]) in a standardized fashion. Interrater reliability has been previously reported[3]; for mode of onset, pairwise percentage agreement was 0.90 in 63 patients, and for pattern of course, it was similarly high in 23 patients. (More subjects were included in reliability studies at initial assessment when mode of onset was rated than at follow-up when pattern of course was rated.)

For inclusion as NARP, we required both an acute onset and a remitting course. The mode of onset we defined as acute in this analysis was that in which a psychotic state developed within 1 week without any prodrome. The courses we defined as remitting were those in which there was a single psychotic episode followed by complete remission or two or more psychotic episodes with complete remissions between all or most of the episodes. Complete remission meant "the patient is virtually symptom-free and shows his or her usual premorbid personality."[3]

STUDY SUBJECTS

In the eight sites with incidence data, 444 patients met all criteria for inclusion in the present study, namely, a full initial evaluation and a 2-year follow-up assessment, an *ICD-9* schizophrenia diagnosis at study entry, and no clear-cut affective (or other nonpsychotic) syndrome during the follow-up period. Of these 444 patients, 57 (13%) had NARP and 387 (87%) had other *ICD-9* schizophrenia. Thirty-five (35%) of the 101 patients in the developing-country setting had NARP com-

Continued on next page

and less than 1 or 3 months of psychotic symptoms, depending on subtype. Again, some of the diagnoses for remitting psychoses in the *DSM-III-R* are not given the full status of a diagnosis in the *ICD-10* (eg, brief reactive psychosis), and some of the diagnoses for remitting psychoses in the *ICD-10* do not appear at all in the *DSM-III-R* (eg, cycloid psychosis).

From previous reports, it appears that some acute remitting psychoses may have distinctive associations with sex[11] and with sociocultural setting[14,17-21] and may differ from schizophrenia in this regard. Epidemiologic data on these conditions, however, are sparse. Studies generally did not use clearly specified and replicable criteria to define the form of acute remitting psychosis under investigation, lacked incident samples, or were based on small numbers.

With the data from the Determinants of Outcome Study, we were able to apply explicit and reliable criteria for NARP, derive sex-specific incidence rates for NARP in both the developing- and the industrialized-country settings, and study a larger number of cases of NARP than has been possible in most prior research on acute remitting psychoses. Furthermore, these data enabled us to compare demographic patterns for NARP and other cases diagnosed as schizophrenia by *ICD-9*. We reasoned that if NARP and other cases of *ICD-9* schizophrenia show different patterns of association with sex and with setting, they are more likely to constitute a distinct entity. This type of comparison of demographic patterns is a time-honored epidemiologic method for clarifying the relation between two potentially distinct forms of a disorder.[22,23]

It should be emphasized at the outset that unlike the *DSM-III-R* but in accord with the *ICD-10*, for the purposes of this analysis, we do not exclude nonacute remitting psychoses from the schizophrenia category. The literature suggests that the acute-onset form of remitting psychosis is more likely than the nonacute pared with 22 (6%) of the 343 patients in the industrialized-country setting (χ^2=55.61, *df*=1, *P*<.001).

In all 13 sites taken together, 794 patients met all criteria for inclusion in the present study. One hundred forty (18%) had NARP, and 654 (82%) had other *ICD-9* schizophrenia. One hundred four (28%) of the 376 patients in the developing-country setting had NARP compared with 36 (9%) of the 418 patients in the industrialized-country setting (χ^2=48.14, *df*=1, *P*<.001).

The 140 cases of NARP had been assigned to the following *ICD-9* schizophrenia subtypes: acute schizophrenia, 58 (41%); catatonic schizophrenia, 24 (17%) (all but one were in developing countries); paranoid schizophrenia, 21 (15%); schizoaffective schizophrenia, nine (6%); other schizophrenia (eg, atypical), 13 (9%); hebephrenic schizophrenia, nine (6%); unspecified schizophrenia (eg, schizophreniform not otherwise specified), four (3%); and latent schizophrenia, two (1%). At the 2-year follow-up, only 12 of these 140 patients with NARP were given an *ICD-9* diagnosis different from schizophrenia (three were given diagnoses of affective psychoses; four, other nonorganic psychoses; three, transient organic psychoses; one, paranoid psychoses; and one, neurosis). Ninety-eight (70%) of the 140 had a single episode of psychosis during the 2-year period of the study, and 42 (30%) had more than one episode. Eighty-six (61%) of the 140 had a combined total duration of psychosis and incomplete remission of less than 6 months. Eighty (57%) of the 140 were treated with antipsychotic medication for less than half of the follow-up period: 69 (66%) of the 104 in the developing-country setting and 11 (31%) of the 36 in the industrialized-country setting.

DATA ANALYSIS

Data from the developing- and the industrialized-country settings were analyzed separately. Because numbers tended to be small in individual sites, results are presented for the developing-country sites combined and for the industrialized-country sites combined for most analyses.

Incidence Rates

Incidence rates could be derived in two sites in the developing-country setting and in six sites in the industrialized-country setting. For both NARP and other cases of *ICD-9* schizophrenia, we compared available incidence rates in men and women and in the developing- and the industrialized-country settings. The 95% confidence limits for incidence rate differences and incidence rate ratios were calculated using a standard approach.[25(pp170-171)] In addition, a χ^2 statistic was used to test the statistical significance of differences in incidence.

Sex Ratios

Sex ratios (male to female) for the number of new cases of treated psychosis that entered this study could be derived in all 13 sites. A χ^2 statistic was used to test the statistical significance of the association between gender and NARP.

Sex ratios may reflect sex differences in population denominators and in ascertainment of cases for this study as well as sex differences in incidence rates. Although more open to bias than incidence rates, they are based on larger numbers of patients and are useful for examining the consistency of findings across a variety of developing- and industrialized-country sites.

Age of Onset

The mean age of onset could be derived at all 13 sites. The mean age of onset of NARP in men vs women and the mean age of onset of other cases of *ICD-9* schizophrenia in men vs women were compared using *t* tests. (Seven respondents whose ages of onset were unknown were excluded from this analysis; none had NARP.)

form to be clearly differentiated from schizophrenia.[6,7,17,18] It should also be noted that the *ICD-9*, which was used to classify all cases in this study, defines schizophrenic symptoms in much the same way as does the *ICD-10*. The main difference is that the *ICD-10* excludes cases with very acute onset and brief duration of schizophrenic symptoms from schizophrenia. The *ICD-9* assigns these cases to schizophrenia and therefore proved convenient for this analysis of NARP.

RESULTS

Results are given first for incidence rates by sex and by setting (eight sites), second for sex ratios (all 13 sites), and third for sex differences in age of onset (all 13 sites). The results of statistical tests are fully reported in the tables; for clarity of exposition, only the *P* values from these tests are reported in the text.

INCIDENCE RATES FOR NARP

The annual incidence per 10 000 people of NARP in men was about half that in women (in the developing-country setting, 0.486 vs 0.878, respectively, *P*=.07; in the industrialized-country setting, 0.040 vs 0.104, respectively, *P*=.04). In the developing-country setting, the incidence was about 10-fold that in the industrialized-country setting for both sexes (men, 0.486 vs 0.040, respectively, *P*<.001; women, 0.878 vs 0.104, respectively, *P*<.001). Incidence rate differences and ratios and χ^2 tests are shown in **Table 1**.

INCIDENCE RATES FOR OTHER CASES OF *ICD-9* SCHIZOPHRENIA

The incidence rates for other cases of *ICD-9* schizophrenia are shown in **Table 2**. The incidence rate of other *ICD-9* schizophrenia was higher in men than in women

Table 1. Nonaffective Acute Remitting Psychosis: Differences in Incidence (Annual Rate per 10 000) Between Men and Women and Between Developing (DEV)- and Industrialized (IND)-Country Settings*

	DEV-Country Settings†	IND-Country Settings‡
Incidence rates (n)		
Male	0.486 (15)	0.040 (6)
Female	0.878 (20)	0.104 (16)
Sex		
Incidence rate difference, M−F (95% CL)	−0.393 (−0.849, +0.064)	−0.064 (−0.126, −0.003)
Incidence rate ratio, M/F (95% CL)	0.55 (0.28, 1.08)	0.38 (0.15, 0.98)
χ^2, *P*(*df*=1)	3.1, .07	4.2, .04
	Male	**Female**
DEV- vs IND-country settings		
Incidence rate difference, DEV−IND (95% CL)	+0.446 (+0.198, +0.694)	+0.774T(+0.386, +1.163)
Incidence rate ratio, DEV/IND (95% CL)	12.24 (4.75, 31.54)	8.45 (4.38, 16.30)
χ^2, *P*(*df*=1)	42.2, <.001	56.2, <.001

*CL indicates confidence limits.
†Developing-country settings include urban and rural Chandigarh, India.
‡Industrialized-country settings include Århus, Denmark; Moscow, Russia; Dublin, Ireland; Nagasaki, Japan; Honolulu, Hawaii; and Nottingham, England.

(in the developing-country setting, 1.328 vs 1.098, respectively, *P*=.45; in the industrialized-country setting, 1.190 vs 0.880, respectively, *P*=.03). Incidence rates were similar in the developing- and industrialized-country settings for both sexes.

SEX RATIOS

Sex ratios are shown in **Table 3**. In the developing-country setting, the male-female ratio was 0.96 for NARP and 1.96 for other cases of *ICD-9* schizophrenia (*P*=.002). In the industrialized-country setting, the male-female ratio was 0.44 for NARP and 1.12 for other cases of *ICD-9* schizophrenia (*P*=.010). In 12 of the 13 sites, the male-female ratio for NARP was lower than the male-female ratio for other cases of *ICD-9* schizophrenia. The other site, Honolulu, had only one (male) case of NARP.

For both NARP and other cases of *ICD-9* schizophrenia, the male-female ratio was higher in the developing- than in the industrialized-country setting.

AGE OF ONSET

The mean age of onset of NARP did not differ significantly between men and women in either setting (**Table 4**). The mean age of onset of other cases of *ICD-9* schizophrenia was significantly younger in men than in women in both the developing-country setting (23.0 years vs 25.7 years, *P*=.003) and the industrialized-country setting (26.0 years vs 30.7 years, *P*<.001).

The mean age of onset of NARP was similar to the mean age of onset of other cases of *ICD-9* schizophrenia in men and somewhat younger in women in both the developing- and the industrialized-country settings. For both NARP and other cases of *ICD-9* schizophrenia, the mean age of onset was somewhat younger in the developing- than in the industrialized-country setting.

COMMENT

In these data, incidence rates of NARP vary significantly by sex and by setting. Thus, the incidence in men was about one half that in women; and the incidence in the developing-country setting was about 10-fold that in the industrialized-country setting. There was no difference between men and women in age of onset of NARP in either setting.

The demographic patterns of other cases of *ICD-9* schizophrenia are clearly different from those of NARP. For other cases of *ICD-9* schizophrenia, the incidence rate was higher in men than in women in both settings. Incidence did not differ significantly by setting. The average age of onset was significantly younger in men than in women in both settings. Further evidence for a different demographic pattern is found in the sex ratios, which were available for all five developing-country sites and for eight industrialized-country sites and which confirm that NARP and other cases of *ICD-9* schizophrenia differed consistently across a wide variety of individual sites in each setting.

These results are consistent with the results of previous studies. Reports on acute remitting psychoses generally suggest a female predominance[11,26-28] and a higher frequency in developing than in industrialized countries.[17-21,29] The majority of epidemiologic studies of schizophrenia have found the incidence to be somewhat higher in men than in women,[30,31] have not found wide variation in incidence across sociocultural

Table 2. *ICD-9* Schizophrenia After Exclusion of Cases of NARP: Differences in Incidence (Annual Rate per 10 000) Between Men and Women and Between Developing (DEV)- and Industrialized (IND)-Country Settings*

	DEV-Country Settings†	IND-Country Settings†
Incidence rates (n)		
Male	1.328 (41)	1.190 (177)
Female	1.098 (25)	0.880 (144)
Sex		
Incidence rate difference, M−F (95% CL)	+0.230 (−0.362, +0.822)	+0.310 (+0.072, +0.548)
Incidence rate ratio, M/F (95% CL)	1.21 (0.74, 1.99)	1.35 (1.09, 1.69)
χ^2, *P* (*df*=1)	0.56, .45	4.6, .03
	Male	**Female**
DEV- vs IND-country settings		
Incidence rate difference, DEV−IND (95% CL)	+0.138 (−0.306, +0.582)	+0.218 (−0.240, +0.676)
Incidence rate ratio, DEV/IND (95% CL)	1.12 (0.79, 1.57)	1.25 (0.82, 1.91)
χ^2, *P*(*df*=1)	0.25, .62	0.40, .53

*ICD-9 *indicates* International Classification of Diseases, Ninth Revision; *NARP, nonaffective acute remitting psychosis; and CL, confidence limits.*
†*See footnotes to Table 1 for explanation of developing- and industrialized-country settings.*

settings,[32] and have found a younger average age of onset in men than in women.[33-35]

IMPLICATIONS

This analysis suggests that NARP may represent either a distinct disorder or a valid subgroup of schizophrenia. Therefore, the results tend to support the separation in diagnosis of some remitting psychoses with schizophrenic symptoms from schizophrenia, as in *DSM-III-R*, *DSM-IV*, and *ICD-10*. The results of most,[10,29,36-40] although not all,[41] earlier studies of conditions that can present as acute remitting psychoses, including family/genetic studies, also are compatible with a distinction from schizophrenia. However, the results for NARP do not necessarily support the specific *DSM-III-R*, *DSM-IV*, or *ICD-10* criteria for the demarcation of acute remitting psychoses from schizophrenia. The criteria of these systems differ from one another, and none of them corresponds precisely to the criteria used to demarcate NARP from schizophrenia in this study.

This analysis also suggests that there may be a psychotic condition or group of conditions that can be differentiated from schizophrenia and that have a 10-fold higher incidence in the developing- than in the industrialized-country setting. Surely, in the search for the causes of NARP or other forms of acute remitting psychosis, it would be useful to focus attention on the developing-country setting and on those potential risk factors for psychotic disorders that are more prevalent in that setting (eg, certain prenatal exposures[42]).

LIMITATIONS

First, the incidence rates reported in this study were based on patients making a first-treatment contact. Differences in selection into treatment by sex and by setting are a potential source of bias. It is highly unlikely that this type of selection bias accounts for the main findings reported herein. Bias in treatment selection would have to be extremely different for these two psychotic conditions to produce for NARP but not for other cases of *ICD-9* schizophrenia a twofold higher incidence in women than in men and a 10-fold higher incidence in the developing- than in the industrialized-country setting. Treatment selection also cannot readily explain the absence of a gender difference in age of onset for NARP or the consistency of the main findings across diverse sites with different types of selection bias.

Second, incidence rates were available for only two of the five developing-country sites and for six of the eight industrialized-country sites. In particular, it still needs to be established that the finding of a high incidence rate of NARP in urban and rural Chandigarh is generalizable to the diverse array of countries and cultures that compose the developing-country setting. Indeed, some differences were evident between the urban and rural sites in Chandigarh, although both the urban and rural sites provided a contrast with the industrialized-country sites. For instance, the ratio of NARP to other cases of *ICD-9* schizophrenia was 14:16 in rural Chandigarh and 21:50 in urban Chandigarh (Table 3). A generally high incidence of NARP in the developing-country setting is compatible, however, with the consistent finding that acute remitting psychoses are a large proportion of treated psychoses in developing countries. This finding has been reported by several prior studies[17-21,29] as well as by this study and has been reported for a wide variety of countries and cultures.

In the five sites that lacked incidence data, we relied perforce on indirect indicators of differences in frequency by sex and by setting. Therefore, results from these

Table 3. Numbers and Male-Female Ratio of NARP and Other Cases of *ICD-9* Schizophrenia: Developing- and Industrialized-Country Settings*

	Male/Female, No.	Male-Female Ratio	No. in Individual Centers, Male/Female							
			AGR	CAL	CHR	CHU	IBA			
Developing-Country Settings										
NARP	51†/53†	0.96	19/13	6/6	8/6	7/14	11/14			
Other *ICD-9* schizophrenia	180†/92†	1.96	24/12	78/35	11/5	30/20	37/20			
Industrialized-Country Settings										
			AAR	DUB	HON	MOS	NAG	NOT	PRA	ROC
NARP	11‡/25‡	0.44	0/1	1/2	1/0	2/5	1/2	1/6	4/8	1/1
Other *ICD-9* schizophrenia	202‡/180‡	1.12	20/10	21/16	12/5	51/68	33/29	40/16	13/25	12/11

**NARP indicates nonaffective acute remitting psychosis;* ICD-9, International Classification of Diseases, Ninth Revision*; AGR, Agra, India; CAL, Cali, Colombia; CHR, rural Chandigarh, India; CHU, urban Chandigarh; IBA, Ibadan, Nigeria; AAR, Århus, Denmark; DUB, Dublin, Ireland; HON, Honolulu, Hawaii; MOS, Moscow, Russia; NAG, Nagasaki, Japan; NOT, Nottingham, England; PRA, Prague, the Czech Republic; ROC, Rochester, NY.*

†χ^2=9.33, df=1, P=.002.

‡χ^2=6.56, df=1, P=.010.

sites were more open to bias. For instance, in the three developing-country sites that lack incidence data, there may have been more complete ascertainment of men than women,[43] and young men seeking work may have been a relatively large proportion of the mainly urban catchment populations. These sources of bias could explain why, for both NARP and other cases of *ICD-9* schizophrenia, male-female ratios were higher in the developing- than in the industrialized-country setting. Nonetheless, the results from these sites provided confirmation that the demographic patterns of NARP and other cases of *ICD-9* schizophrenia differ consistently across a wide variety of sites within each of the two settings.

Third, we relied on an *ICD-9* diagnosis of schizophrenia to select remitting psychoses with schizophrenic symptoms. Neither *ICD-10* nor *DSM-III-R* diagnoses were available for these data. Schizophrenic symptoms are defined similarly in *ICD-9* and *ICD-10*. With respect to the *DSM-III-R*, symptom criteria for schizophrenia differ from both *ICD-9* and *ICD-10*. There is no firm evidence that remitting psychoses that meet *DSM-III-R* criteria (schizophreniform by *DSM-III-R*) differ epidemiogically from those that meet *ICD-9* or *ICD-10* criteria.

Fourth, this study did not address the relationship of NARP to the affective disorders.[38,44] All patients with a clear-cut affective syndrome at onset or during the follow-up period were excluded. We found no indication that affective symptoms were especially prominent in cases of NARP. For instance, in the initial evaluation, only nine (6%) of the 140 subjects with NARP were diagnosed as having schizo-affective schizophrenia by *ICD-9*. Only a small minority of patients with NARP were rated as being significantly depressed, elated, or irritable on the Present State Examination (results not shown).

Fifth, we were not able to compare NARP and other cases of *ICD-9* schizophrenia in terms of other factors, for instance, familial aggregation and biological correlates.[45] Therefore, we cannot entirely rule out the possibility that NARP represents only a mild course of schizophrenia. Conceivably, NARP is more common in women because schizophrenia is more likely to have a remitting course in women.[46-48] This explanation is not consistent, however, with the findings of this study. Sex differences in the course of psychosis were neither prominent nor consistently present across the two settings.[3] Moreover, if NARP were a mild course of schizophrenia, one would expect the sex difference in age of onset that is typical for schizophrenia to also be apparent for NARP.

Sixth, under the best of circumstances, it can be difficult to detect prodromal and residual symptoms of schizophrenia. We cannot rule out the possibility that in some cases an apparently acute onset was preceded by subtle prodromal symptoms or that an apparently complete remission was associated with subtle residual symptoms. Misclassification of mode of onset and of pattern of course would tend to diminish the striking associations of NARP with sex and sociocultural setting. Intersite variation in misclassification, which is also a possibility in a multicenter study, could lead to artifactual associations, but it is highly unlikely that such bias accounts for the consistent and large effects reported herein.

Finally, in some cases, the remission of cases classified as NARP may have been related to effective treatment, for instance, with medication. Effective treatment, like misclassification, would tend to suppress the associations reported here. In the developing-country setting, only one third of the patients with NARP were prescribed antipsychotic medication for more than half of the follow-up period compared with two thirds of the patients with NARP in the industrialized-country setting.

Table 4. Gender Differences in Age of Onset of NARP and Other Cases of Schizophrenia: Developing- and Industrialized-Country Settings*

	Mean Age of Onset, y (n)	Percentage in Age of Onset Group			
		<24 y	25–34 y	35–44 y	45–54 y
		Developing-Country Setting			
NARP					
Male	22.4 (51)†	73	24	4	0
Female	22.4 (53)†	70	25	4	2
Other *ICD-9* schizophrenia					
Male	23.0 (178)‡	68	24	7	1
Female	25.7 (92)‡	51	33	14	2
		Industrialized-Country Setting			
NARP					
Male	25.5 (11)§	64	18	18	0
Female	24.9 (25)§	56	40	0	4
Other *ICD-9* schizophrenia					
Male	26.0 (198)‖	55	29	13	4
Female	30.7 (179)‖	38	28	20	15

*NARP indicates nonaffective acute remitting psychosis; ICD-9, International Classification of Diseases, Ninth Revision.
†$t=-0.05$, $df=102$, $P=.96$.
‡$t=-3.0$, $df=268$, $P=.003$.
§$t=0.24$, $df=34$, $P=.81$.
‖$t=-4.7$, $df=375$, $P<.001$.

Therefore, remissions due to effective treatment would tend to reduce the difference in incidence between the developing- and the industrialized-country settings.

RELATION TO PREVIOUS REPORT

In the primary report on the Determinants of Outcome Study,[3] the authors compared cases initially diagnosed as the acute schizophrenic episode subtype of *ICD-9* schizophrenia with cases initially diagnosed as other subtypes of *ICD-9* schizophrenia.[3(p86)] A limited analysis of presenting symptoms did not find significant differences between these two groups. In this study, we demarcated NARP from other cases of *ICD-9* schizophrenia according to reliable standardized ratings of mode of onset and course of disorder rather than according to an initial clinical impression as to *ICD-9* subtype. Cases of NARP were then compared with other cases of *ICD-9* schizophrenia in terms of incidence rates and sex differences in age of onset rather than in terms of presenting symptoms. This approach has provided new evidence in support of a nosologic distinction.

CONCLUSIONS

In these data, NARP shows striking associations with sex and with setting that are sharply distinct from those of schizophrenia. The number of cases of NARP in the sites with incidence data was not large enough and the follow-up period was not long enough for these results to be definitive. Nonetheless, they provide important support for the view that cases of NARP constitute an entity distinct from schizophrenia or at least a valid subgroup of schizophrenia. The findings also underscore the potential usefulness of cross-cultural studies in yielding clues to the causes of psychotic disorders. It is our hope that future family/genetic, biological, and epidemiological studies will further elucidate the characteristics of acute remitting psychoses and their relation to schizophrenia and investigate whether there may be distinct causes of acute remitting psychoses that are related to sex and to setting.

Accepted for publication October 11, 1993.

This work was supported by grant MH47154-02 from the National Institute of Mental Health, Rockville, Md, a grant from the Laureat Mental Health Association, Tulsa, Okla, and by the World Health Organization, Geneva, Switzerland.

The views expressed herein are the authors' own and do not necessarily present the opinions of the other investigators participating in the Determinants of Outcome Study project or the views or policy of the sponsoring agencies.

We would like to acknowledge the contribution of the 12 World Health Organization Field Research Centers that carried out the Determinants of Outcome Study. The chief collaborating investigators were E. Stromgren, Århus; K. C. Dube, Agra; C. Leon, Cali; N. N. Wig and V. Varma, Chandigarh; D. Walsh, Dublin; A. Marsella and M. Katz, Honolulu; M. Olatawura, Ibadan; R. A. Nadzharov and N. N. Zharikov, Moscow; R. Takahashi and Y. Nakane, Nagasaki; J. Cooper, Nottingham; L. Hanzlicek and J. Gebhart, Prague; and L. C. Wynne and T. Gift, Rochester. At the World Health Organization Headquarters, the study was coordinated by N. Sartorius, principal investigator, and A. Jablensky, co–principal investigator. We thank Jack Gorman, MD, for helpful comments on the manuscript.

Reprint requests to the New York State Psychiatric Institute, Department of Psychiatry, Columbia University, Unit 24, 722 W 168th St, New York, NY 10032 (Dr Susser).

REFERENCES

1. World Health Organization. *Mental Disorders: Glossary and Guide to Their Classification in Accordance With the Ninth Revision of the International Classification of Diseases.* Geneva, Switzerland: World Health Organization; 1978.
2. Sartorius N, Jablensky A, Korten A, Ernberg G, Anker M, Cooper JE, Day R. Early manifestations and first-contact incidence of schizophrenia in different cultures. *Psychol Med.* 1986;16:909-928.
3. Jablensky A, Sartorius N, Ernberg G, Anker M, Korten A, Cooper JE, Day R, Bertelsen A. Schizophrenia: manifestations, incidence and course in different cultures: a World Health Organization Ten Country Study. *Psychol Med Monogr Suppl.* 1992;20:97.
4. Procci WR. Schizo-affective psychosis: fact or fiction? *Arch Gen Psychiatry.* 1976;33:1167-1178.
5. Kasanin J. The acute schizoaffective psychoses. *Am J Psychiatry.* 1933;13: 97-126.
6. Manschreck TC, Petri M. The atypical psychoses. *Cult Med Psychiatry.* 1978; 2:233-268.
7. Menuck M, Legault S, Schmidt P, Remington G. The nosologic status of the remitting atypical psychoses. *Compr Psychiatry.* 1989;30:53-73.
8. Langfeldt G. The prognosis in schizophrenia and the factors influencing the course of the disease. *Acta Psychiatr Neurol Scand.* 1937;13(suppl):1-228.
9. Leonhard K. Cycloid psychoses—endogenous psychoses which are neither schizophrenic nor manic-depressive. *J Ment Sci.* 1961;197:633-648.
10. McCabe MS, Stromgren E. Reactive psychoses: a family study. *Arch Gen Psychiatry.* 1975;32:447-454.
11. Stephens JH, Shaffer JW, Carpenter WT Jr. Reactive psychoses. *J Nerv Ment Dis.* 1982;170:657-663.
12. Pichot P. The concept of 'bouffee delirante' with special reference to the Scandinavian concept of reactive psychosis. *Psychopathology.* 1986;19:35-43.
13. Leonhard classification of psychoses. *Psychopathology.* 1990;23(special issue):331-338.
14. Cooper JE, Jablensky A, Sartorius N. W.H.O. collaborative studies on acute psychoses using the SCAAPS schedule. In: Stefanis CN, Rabavilas AD, Soldatos CR, eds. *Psychiatry: A World Perspective.* Amsterdam, the Netherlands: Elsevier Science Publishers; 1990;1:185-192.
15. American Psychiatric Association, Committee on Nomenclature and Statistics. *Diagnostic and Statistical Manual of Mental Disorders, Revised Third Edition.* Washington, DC: American Psychiatric Association; 1987.
16. World Health Organization. *The ICD-10 Classification of Mental and Behavioral Disorders.* Geneva, Switzerland: World Health Organization; 1992.
17. Lambo TA. Further neuropsychiatric observations in Nigeria with comments on the need for epidemiological study in Africa. *BMJ.* December 10, 1960:1696-1704.
18. Wig NN, Singh G. A proposed classification of psychiatric disorders for use in India. *Indian J Psychiatry.* 1967;9:158-171.
19. German GA. Aspects of clinical psychiatry in Sub-Saharan Africa. *Br J Psychiatry.* 1972;121:461-479.
20. World Health Organization. *Schizophrenia: An International Follow-up Study.* New York, NY: John Wiley & Sons Inc; 1979.
21. Malhotra S, Varma VK, Malhotra A. Classification of acute nonorganic psychotic states in India. *Int J Ment Health.* 1992;21:16-32.
22. Morris JN. *Uses of Epidemiology.* Edinburgh, Scotland: E & S Livingstone; 1957.
23. Susser M. *Epidemiology, Health, and Society.* New York, NY: Oxford University Press; 1987.
24. Wing JK, Cooper JE, Sartorius N. *The Measurement and Classification of Psychiatric Symptoms.* London, England: Cambridge University Press; 1974.
25. Rothman KL. *Modern Epidemiology.* Boston, Mass: Little Brown & Co Inc; 1986.
26. Perris C. A study of cycloid psychoses. *Acta Psychiatr Scand Suppl.* 1974; 253:7-77.
27. Cutting J. Relationship between cycloid psychosis and typical affective psychosis. *Psychopathology.* 1990;23:212-219.
28. Lindvall M, Hagnell O, Ohman R. Epidemiology of cycloid psychosis. *Psychopathology.* 1990;23:228-232.
29. Sartorius N, Jablensky A, Shapiro R. Cross-cultural differences in the short-term prognosis of schizophrenic psychoses. *Schizophr Bull.* 1978;4:102-103.
30. Castle D, Murray R. The neurodevelopmental basis of sex differences in schizophrenia. *Psychol Med.* 1991;21:565-575.
31. Iacono WG, Beiser M. Are males more likely than females to develop schizophrenia? *Am J Psychiatry.* 1992;149:1070-1074.
32. Eaton WW. Epidemiology of schizophrenia. In: Szklo M, Gordis L, Gregg MB, Levine MM, eds. *Epidemiology Reviews.* Baltimore, Md: The Johns Hopkins University School of Hygiene and Public Health; 1985:105-126.
33. Lewine RRJ, Strauss JS, Gift TE. Sex differences in age at first hospital admission for schizophrenia: fact or artifact? *Am J Psychiatry.* 1981;138:440-444.
34. Angermeyer MC, Kuhn L. Gender differences in age at onset of schizophrenia: an overview. *Eur Arch Psychiatry Neurol Sci.* 1988;237:351-364.
35. Hafner H, Riecher A, Maurer K, Loeffler W, Munk-Jorgenesen P, Stromgren E. Does gender influence age at first hospitalization for schizophrenia? *Psychol Med.* 1989;19:903-918.
36. Mitsuda H. The concept of 'atypical psychoses' from the aspect of clinical genetics. *Acta Psychiatr Scand.* 1965;41:372-377.
37. Tsuang MT, Dempsey M, Rauscher F. A study of 'atypical schizophrenia.' *Arch Gen Psychiatry.* 1976;33:1157-1160.
38. Fogelson DL, Cohen BM, Pope HG. A study of DSM-III schizophreniform disorder. *Am J Psychiatry.* 1981;139:1281-1285.
39. Beiser M, Fleming JAE, Iacono WG, Lin TY. Refining the diagnosis of schizophreniform disorder. *Am J Psychiatry.* 1988;145:695-700.
40. Gottesman II, Bertelsen A. Dual mating studies in psychiatry: offspring of inpatients with examples from reactive (psychogenic) psychoses. *Int Rev Psychiatry.* 1989;1:287-296.
41. Kendler KS, Gruenberg AM, Tsuang MT. A DSM-III family study of the non-schizophrenic psychotic disorders. *Am J Psychiatry.* 1986;143:1098-1105.
42. Susser ES, Shang PL. Schizophrenia after prenatal exposure to the Dutch Hunger Winter of 1944-1945. *Arch Gen Psychiatry.* 1992;49:983-988.
43. Hoenig J, Sreenivasan U. Mental hospital admissions in Mysore State, India. *J Ment Sci.* 1959;105:124-141.
44. Guldberg CA, Dahl AA, Hansen H, Mina Bergem AL. Were Langfeldt's schizophreniform psychoses really affective? *Psychopathology.* 1991;24:270-276.
45. Robins E, Guze S. Establishment of diagnostic validity in psychiatric illness: its application to schizophrenia. *Am J Psychiatry.* 1970;126:983-989.
46. Riecher A, Maurer K, Loeffler W, Fatkenheuer B, an-der Heiden W, Munk-Jorgensen P, Stromgren E, Hafner H. Gender differences in age at onset and course of schizophrenic disorders. In: Hafner H, Gattaz WF, eds. *Search for the Causes of Schizophrenia.* Heidelberg, Germany: Springer-Verlag; 1990;2:14-33.
47. Bardenstein K, McGlashan TH. Gender differences in affective, schizoaffective, and schizophrenic disorders: a review. *Schizophr Res.* 1990;3:159-172.
48. Gender and Schizophrenia. *Schizophr Bull.* 1990;16(special issue):171-354.

Haloperidol Addition in Fluvoxamine-Refractory Obsessive-Compulsive Disorder

A Double-blind, Placebo-Controlled Study in Patients With and Without Tics

Christopher J. McDougle, MD; Wayne K. Goodman, MD; James F. Leckman, MD; Nicole C. Lee, MSNC; George R. Heninger, MD; Lawrence H. Price, MD

Background: To determine the efficacy of adding haloperidol to the treatment of patients with obsessive-compulsive disorder (OCD), with or without a comorbid chronic tic disorder, who were refractory to adequate treatment with the serotonin-uptake inhibitor fluvoxamine alone. It was hypothesized that OCD patients with a concurrent chronic tic disorder would preferentially respond to this treatment.

Methods: Sixty-two patients with a primary *DSM-III-R* diagnosis of OCD received placebo fluvoxamine for 1 week, followed by 8 weeks of active fluvoxamine. Thirty-four of these patients were refractory to fluvoxamine and were randomized in a double-blind fashion to 4 weeks of treatment with either haloperidol (n=17) or placebo (n=17) added to ongoing fluvoxamine treatment. The placebo-treated group included five women and 12 men, six inpatients and 11 outpatients, and eight patients with a comorbid chronic tic disorder. The haloperidol-treated group consisted of two women and 15 men, three inpatients and 14 outpatients, and seven patients with a comorbid chronic tic disorder. All 34 patients completed the entire study. The Yale-Brown Obsessive Compulsive Scale (Y-BOCS) and the Clinical Global Impression scale were the principal measures of treatment outcome.

Results: Haloperidol addition was significantly better than placebo in reducing the severity of obsessive-complusive symptoms as measured by the Y-BOCS. Eleven of 17 patients responded to the haloperidol, compared with none of 17 patients given placebo. Eight of eight patients with comorbid chronic tic disorders, such as Tourette's disorder, responded to double-blind haloperidol addition to ongoing fluvoxamine treatment. Haloperidol addition was of little benefit in treating OCD patients without tics. Fluvoxamine blood levels were not related to treatment response.

Conclusions: The results of this study suggest that OCD patients with a comorbid chronic tic disorder constitute a clinically meaningful subtype of OCD that might require conjoint serotonin-uptake inhibitor/neuroleptic therapy for effective symptom reduction.

(Arch Gen Psychiatry. 1994;51:302-308)

SEROTONIN-UPTAKE inhibitors (SUIs) are the most effective primary drug treatment for patients with obsessive-compulsive disorder (OCD).[1] However, obsessive-compulsive symptoms in up to 40% to 60% of patients are unimproved after treatment with these drugs.[1] Adding lithium carbonate[2] or buspirone hydrochloride[3] to ongoing SUI therapy is not usually an effective approach in such cases. This has suggested that pharmacotherapy targeted at more than one neurochemical system may be necessary to treat some forms of OCD.[4]

Preliminary reports have described the use of combined SUI/neuroleptic treatment in OCD patients with comorbid chronic tic disorders, such as Tourette's disorder (Tourette's syndrome [TS]).[5-7] This placebo-controlled study was designed to determine the efficacy of fluvoxamine, a potent and selective SUI, in combination with haloperidol in treating OCD patients who were refractory to fluvoxamine alone. It was hypothesized that OCD patients with a concurrent chronic tic disorder would preferentially respond to this treatment.

From the Department of Psychiatry, Yale University School of Medicine (Drs McDougle, Goodman, Leckman, Heninger, and Price and Ms Lee), the Clinical Neuroscience Research Unit, Abraham Ribicoff Research Facilities, Connecticut Mental Health Center (Drs McDougle, Goodman, Heninger, and Price and Ms Lee), and The Yale Child Study Center (Drs McDougle and Leckman), New Haven, Conn.

See Patients and Methods on next page

PATIENTS AND METHODS

PATIENTS

All patients gave voluntary written informed consent and were free of medical illness based on results of a physical examination, electrocardiogram, and screening tests of blood and urine. Patients were free of psychotropic medications for at least 3 weeks (5 weeks for fluoxetine) before starting the study. A semistructured interview modeled after the Schedule for Affective Disorders and Schizophrenia was administered to ascertain that all patients met *DSM-III-R*[8] criteria for a principal diagnosis of OCD. Only patients with obsessive-compulsive symptoms of at least 1 year's duration and of at least moderate severity on the Clinical Global Impression scale[9] were included.

Patients were categorized as "depressed" (secondary to OCD) if they met *DSM-III-R* criteria for major depression or received a baseline score on the modified Hamilton Rating Scale for Depression (HAM-D)[10] of greater than 20. Relevant portions of the Schedule for Tourette and Other Behavioral Syndromes[11] were used to diagnose tic disorders. Patients with chronic tics (motor or phonic) were included, provided that obsessive-compulsive symptoms, rather than tics, constituted the predominant presenting complaint. Obsessive-compulsive disorder patients with comorbid tic disorders were specifically sought from the community. None of the patients participated in our prior open-label trial.[7]

STUDY DESIGN

Sixty-two patients received placebo for 1 week, followed by 8 weeks of fluvoxamine in identical-appearing capsules. There were no 1-week placebo responders. Patients and raters were blind to drug assignment during this fluvoxamine treatment phase, although the prescribing physician was open to assignment. Fluvoxamine treatment was started at 50 mg/d, and the dosage was increased by 50 mg every day, to a maximum of 300 mg/d. Thus, patients were receiving the maximum dose of fluvoxamine for more than 7 weeks before entering the haloperidol-addition phase.

Thirty-four patients were refractory to fluvoxamine and were entered into the 4-week double-blind, placebo-controlled haloperidol-addition phase. Criteria for refractoriness to fluvoxamine included (1) less than 35% improvement on the Yale-Brown Obsessive Compulsive Scale (Y-BOCS)[12,13] or a Y-BOCS score of 16 or greater, (2) no better than "minimal" improvement on the Clinical Global Impression scale, and (3) consensus of the treating clinician and two of the authors (C.J.M. and W.K.G.) that the patient's condition was unimproved.

The 34 fluvoxamine-refractory patients continued with the same dose of fluvoxamine during the haloperidol-addition phase. Assignment to haloperidol (2 mg per capsule) or placebo was random, with patients, treating staff (including prescribing physicians), and raters blind to assignment. Patients were given haloperidol 2 mg/d for 3 days, with the dosage then increased by 2 mg every 3 days, to a maximum of 10 mg/d. Patients were given benztropine mesylate, 0.5 mg twice daily, as prophylaxis against extrapyramidal symptoms and in an attempt to preserve blind treatment conditions. When patients reported significant "restlessness," propranolol hydrochloride (10 mg three times daily to 20 mg four times daily) was given by a nonrating physician blind to drug allocation. With the exception of low-dose benzodiazepines for sleep, no other drugs were administered. Patients were not instructed in formal behavior therapy techniques. The clinical characteristics of each treatment group are summarized in the **Table**.

RATINGS

Patients were assessed once (outpatients) or twice (inpatients) weekly by raters blind to drug assignment. Obsessive-compulsive symptoms were measured with the Y-BOCS. Depression was rated with a 24-item version of the HAM-D, which excludes an item for rating obsessive-compulsive symptoms. Anxiety was measured by using the Hamilton Rating Scale for Anxiety.[14] The frequency dimension of the Yale Global Tic Severity Scale[15] (rated from 0="none" to 5="always") was used to measure change in tic frequency. Tics were distinguished from "ticlike" compulsions (such as compulsive touching or blinking) based on whether the patient attached a meaning or purpose to the behavior. This definition allowed raters to distinguish true tics from "ticlike" compulsions so that Y-BOCS scores reflected changes in severity of obsessions and compulsions rather than tics. A clinician-rated global treatment response of OCD was obtained by using the Clinical Global Impression scale. The Patient-Rated Anxiety Scale[16] (rated from 0="not at all anxious" to 4="extremely anxious") was also administered.

TREATMENT RESPONSE CRITERIA

Criteria for response to the fluvoxamine-haloperidol combination included (1) 35% or greater improvement on the Y-BOCS from the beginning of the haloperidol-addition trial *and* a final Y-BOCS score of less than 16, (2) a final Clinical Global Impression scale rating of "much" or "very much improved," *and* (3) consensus of the treating clinician and two of the primary investigators (C.J.M. and W.K.G.) that the patient's condition was improved. Patients who met all three criteria were classified as "marked" responders, those who met two thirds of the criteria were "partial" responders, and those who met less than two thirds of the criteria were nonresponders.

DETERMINATION OF FLUVOXAMINE BLOOD LEVELS

Blood samples were collected before and after the 4-week double-blind trial to determine if coadministration of halo-

Continued on next page

peridol increased fluvoxamine blood levels. Fluvoxamine levels were determined by high-performance liquid chromatography with fluorescence detection (method available on request).

STATISTICAL ANALYSIS

All 34 refractory patients received 4 weeks of haloperidol or placebo and were included in the analyses. Baseline ratings were obtained after 8 weeks of single-blind fluvoxamine treatment. Testing with the Shapiro-Wilks statistic showed that Y-BOCS scores could be approximated by the normal distribution at all assessment time points in both the haloperidol- and placebo-treated groups. The haloperidol- and placebo-treated groups were compared by using analysis of variance (ANOVA) with repeated measures to determine significant drug×time interactions. Student's *t* tests of the difference scores from baseline were computed to determine when significant drug-placebo differences occurred. The ANOVA with repeated measures was also calculated within each condition for the 4 weeks of haloperidol and placebo treatment to determine if significant effects occurred over time. Following significant main effects of time in these ANOVAs, paired *t* tests were calculated to determine at which weeks significant changes from baseline occurred.

The χ^2 test was used to compare the two treatment groups for rate of responders (marked or partial) vs nonresponders. The relationship between response vs nonresponse to active haloperidol and the presence or absence of a comorbid chronic tic disorder was analyzed by using Fisher's Exact Test or the χ^2 test, depending on sample size. Fisher's Exact Test was used to compare the response to haloperidol vs placebo among OCD patients without tics. Shapiro-Wilks testing showed that fluvoxamine blood levels were not normally distributed. Therefore, Wilcoxon Signed-Rank and Mann-Whitney tests were used to compare fluvoxamine blood levels within and between treatment groups. Spearman's correlation was used to assess the relationship between fluvoxamine blood levels and treatment response. Data are presented as mean±SD, and are reported as significant when $P<.05$ (two tailed).

RESULTS

CLINICAL CHARACTERISTICS OF TREATMENT GROUPS

Of the 28 patients who did not enter the haloperidol-addition phase, 16 responded to fluvoxamine alone, seven had side effects to fluvoxamine (anxiety, n=2; rash, n=1; sedation, n=2; psychosis, n=1; general malaise, n=1), four were noncompliant with treatment, and one had exacerbation of motor tics while receiving fluvoxamine. Only one patient with a comorbid chronic tic disorder showed significant improvement in obsessive-compulsive symptoms during fluvoxamine monotherapy. No significant reduction in frequency of motor or phonic tics occurred in patients with comorbid chronic tic disorders during fluvoxamine treatment.

Seventeen patients were randomized to haloperidol and 17 to placebo. The two groups did not differ significantly in age, gender, treatment setting, prevalence of secondary major depression, age at onset of OCD, or duration of OCD (Table). There was no significant difference between groups in the dose of fluvoxamine (300.0±0.0 mg/d vs 282.4±49.8 mg/d, respectively) before the double-blind addition trial. No significant differences between groups were found in the Y-BOCS, HAM-D, Hamilton Rating Scale for Anxiety, or Patient-Rated Anxiety Scale scores at baseline. There was no significant difference in the dose of haloperidol between patients randomized to haloperidol (6.2±3.0 mg/d) and placebo (7.4±2.8 mg/d).

RESPONSE OF OBSESSIVE-COMPULSIVE, DEPRESSIVE, AND ANXIETY SYMPTOMS

As measured by a reduction in total Y-BOCS scores, haloperidol addition was superior to placebo in OCD patients who were refractory to fluvoxamine (**Figure 1**). The baseline Y-BOCS scores in the haloperidol- and placebo-treated groups were 25.4±5.0 and 24.9±4.0, respectively. The ANOVA revealed significant interaction effects of drug and time (F=3.89, *df*=4, 128, $P<.005$) for the 4-week haloperidol- vs placebo-addition phase. In comparing the effects of haloperidol and placebo on obsessive-compulsive symptoms, Student's *t* test showed that haloperidol was significantly better than placebo beginning at week 4 of treatment ($t=-2.9$, *df*=24, $P<.008$) (Figure 1). The ANOVA showed that there was a highly significant decrease in total Y-BOCS scores from baseline in the haloperidol-treated group (F=9.24, *df*=4, 64, $P<.0001$). A trend ($P<.10$) toward a significant decrease in Y-BOCS ratings appeared as early as week 2 of haloperidol treatment. By week 3, the reduction in total Y-BOCS scores was highly significant ($t=3.2$, *df*=16, $P<.006$), and by week 4, the decrease was even greater ($t=4.3$, *df*=16, $P<.001$) (Figure 1), representing a 26% reduction from baseline. In contrast, paired *t* tests showed no significant changes in Y-BOCS scores for any week following baseline in the placebo-treated group (Figure 1).

Haloperidol addition was not associated with a significant change in scores on the HAM-D (−0.9±5.5), Hamilton Rating Scale for Anxiety (−1.1±4.2), or Patient-Rated Anxiety Scale (1.9±13.8). Placebo addition also had no effect on these measures.

Clinical Characteristics of Patients With OCD Treated With Haloperidol or Placebo Addition to Fluvoxamine*

Patient/Type/Sex/Age, y	Age at Onset of OCD, y	Duration of OCD, y	Comorbid Tic Disorders	Baseline Tic Frequency†	DEP	No. of Past Medication Trials	Previous SUIs	Previous Behavior Therapy
			Active Haloperidol					
1/OUT/M/30	14	16	TS	3	Y	5	CMI, FLUOX	N
2/IN/M/31	16	15	TS	4	N	3	FLUOX	N
3/IN/M/32	25	7	CMT	1	Y	3	FLUOX	Y
4/IN/M/38	33	5	TS	2	Y	2	None	Y
5/OUT/M/52	16	36	N	...	N	8	FLUOX	N
6/OUT/M/40	12	28	N	...	Y	1	FLUOX	N
7/OUT/M/49	7	42	CMT	2	N	3	FLUOX	Y
8/OUT/F/36	23	13	N	...	N	4	CMI, FLUOX	Y
9/OUT/M/37	15	22	N	...	Y	4	FLUOX	Y
10/OUT/M/24	8	16	N	...	N	5	CMI, FLUOX	N
11/OUT/F/43	19	24	N	...	Y	3	FLUOX	N
12/IN/M/20	14	6	TS	4	N	2	None	N
13/IN/M/20	11	9	CMT	3	N	4	FLUOX	N
14/OUT/F/30	29	1	N	...	Y	2	None	Y
15/IN/M/18	16	2	CMT	4	N	3	CMI, FLUOX	N
16/OUT/F/39	7	32	N	...	Y	2	FLUOX	Y
17/OUT/F/65	23	42	N	...	Y	4	FLUOX	Y
Mean±SD/.../.../.../35.0±12.0	17.0±7.5	18.6±13.5	...	...	...	3.4±1.6	...	...
			Placebo Haloperidol					
18/OUT/F/58	11	47	N	...	Y	4	FLUOX	Y
19/IN/M/26	12	14	CMT	3	N	5	CMI, FLUOX	Y
20/OUT/M/24	13	11	TS	2	N	2	None	Y
21/OUT/M/25	14	11	N	...	N	2	FLUOX	Y
22/IN/M/24	13	11	N	...	Y	3	None	N
23/OUT/F/25	19	6	N	...	Y	4	CMI, FLUOX	N
24/OUT/M/18	14	4	CMT	2	N	2	FLUOX	Y
25/OUT/M/48	18	30	CMT	3	Y	6	CMI, FLUOX	Y
26/OUT/M/68	16	52	N	...	N	1	FLUOX	N
27/OUT/M/41	10	31	TS	4	Y	3	FLUOX	N
28/OUT/M/34	22	12	N	...	N	2	FLUOX	Y
29/OUT/M/25	7	18	N	...	N	3	CMI, FLUOX	N
30/OUT/M/32	10	22	TS	4	N	2	FLUOX	N
31/OUT/M/38	15	23	N	...	N	2	FLUOX	Y
32/IN/M/35	12	23	TS	3	Y	4	CMI, FLUOX	N
33/OUT/F/47	24	23	N	...	Y	1	None	N
34/OUT/M/22	18	4	N	...	N	2	FLUOX	N
Mean±SD/.../.../.../34.7±14.0	14.5±4.4	20.1±13.8	...	...	...	2.8±1.3	...	...

**OCD indicates obsessive-compulsive disorder; DEP, major depression; SUIs, serotonin-uptake inhibitors; CMI, clomipramine, FLUOX, fluoxetine; OUT, outpatient; TS, Tourette's syndrome; Y, yes; N, no; IN, inpatient; CMT, chronic motor tic disorder; and ellipses, data not supplied.*

†Yale Global Tic Severity Scale: frequency dimension—0=none to 5=always.

GLOBAL TREATMENT RESPONSE

Eleven (65%) of 17 haloperidol-treated patients had a response (seven marked, four partial). In responders, Y-BOCS scores decreased by 39%, from a baseline of 25.3±6.0 to a final score of 15.5±9.1 (t=6.1, df=10, P<.0001), following 4 weeks of haloperidol treatment. None of 17 placebo-treated patients responded (χ^2=13.4, P<.0002).

After completing the 4-week double-blind phase of the study, 14 of 17 placebo-treated patients received open haloperidol addition to fluvoxamine for 4 weeks. In this group, haloperidol addition caused a significant improvement in scores on the Y-BOCS (−5.1±5.8, t=3.3, df=13, P<.006) but not on the HAM-D (−1.3±8.0), Hamilton Rating Scale for Anxiety (−1.2±6.1), or Patient-Rated Anxiety Scale (−1.4±7.6). Eight (57%) of 14 patients who were given 4 weeks of open haloperidol addition showed a response (five marked, three partial).

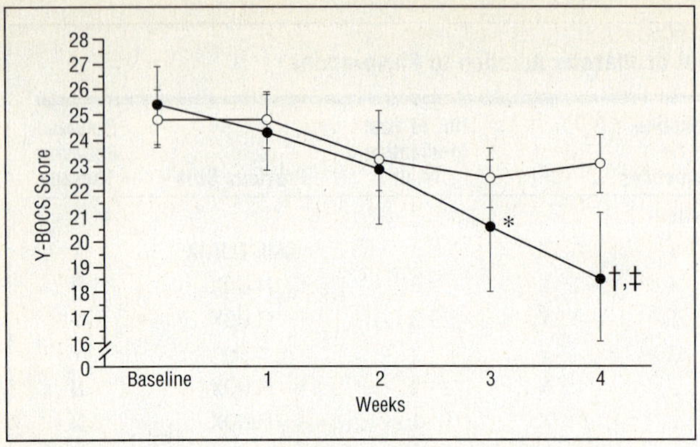

Figure 1. *Change in severity of obsessive-compulsive symptoms in patients given haloperidol (closed circles) or placebo (open circles) for 4 weeks, as measured on the Yale-Brown Obsessive Compulsive Scale (Y-BOCS; range: 0=no symptoms, 40=most severe). Asterisk indicates* P<*.006, change from baseline (haloperidol), paired* t *test; dagger,* P<*.001, change from baseline (haloperidol), paired* t *test; and double dagger,* P<*.008, change from baseline, haloperidol vs placebo, Student's* t *test. All tests are two tailed.*

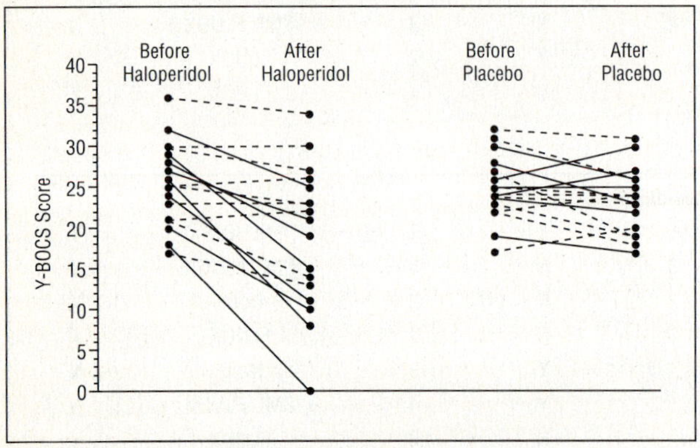

Figure 2. *Change in Yale-Brown Obsessive Compulsive Scale (Y-BOCS) scores for obsessive-compulsive disorder patients with (solid lines) and without (dotted lines) comorbid chronic tic disorder given haloperidol or placebo for 4 weeks in addition to ongoing fluvoxamine treatment.*

TREATMENT RESPONSE AND COMORBID CHRONIC TIC DISORDER

Eight (100%) of eight patients with a current comorbid tic disorder (TS, n=4; chronic motor tic disorder, n=4) were responders (five marked, three partial) to the double-blind addition of haloperidol, whereas three (33%) of nine without tics (two females, one male; no known family history of tics) responded (none marked, three partial) (*P*=.007, Fisher's Exact Test) (**Figure 2**). In comparing the effects of haloperidol on obsessive-compulsive symptoms between patients with and without tics, haloperidol proved to be significantly better in patients with tics beginning at week 2 of treatment (Student's *t*=2.3, *df*=15, *P*<.04) (**Figure 3**). This effect was even more pronounced after 3 (*t*=4.0, *df*=15, *P*<.001) and 4 (*t*=5.6, *df*=15, *P*<.0001) weeks. Within the group of patients with tics, Y-BOCS scores decreased significantly beginning at week 2 of haloperidol (*t*=−2.4, *df*=7, *P*<.05), an effect that continued to increase at weeks 3 (*t*=−4.9, *df*=7, *P*<.003) and 4 (*t*=−7.2, *df*=7, *P*<.0002) (Figure 3). This represented a 47% decrease in Y-BOCS scores, from 25.5±4.7 to 13.6±8.0, following 4 weeks of haloperidol addition (Figure 3). During the 4-week open haloperidol phase for patients crossed over from placebo, four (80%) of five patients with tics (TS, n=2; chronic motor tic disorder, n=2) were responders, whereas four (44%) of nine without tics responded (*P*=.21, Fisher's Exact Test). Of the 31 patients who were given 4 weeks of haloperidol (double-blind phase, n=17; open haloperidol phase, n=14), 12 (92%) of 13 with tics responded (eight marked, four partial), whereas seven (39%) of 18 without tics were responders (two marked, five partial) (χ^2=7.0, *P*<.008). In patients without tics, there was a trend toward a significant response to haloperidol compared with placebo (*P*=.09, Fisher's Exact Test).

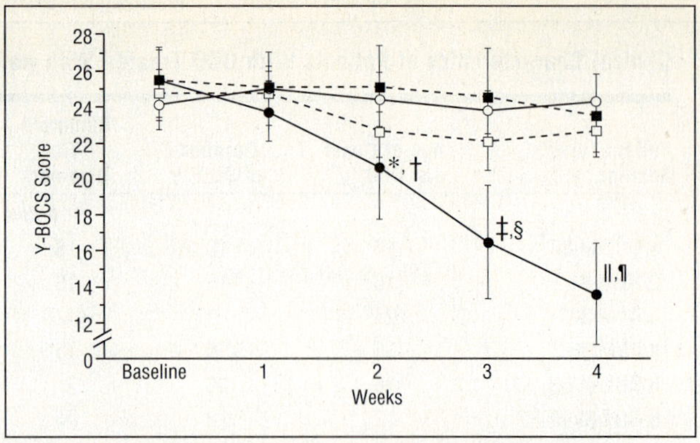

Figure 3. *Change in severity of obsessive-compulsive symptoms on the Yale-Brown Obsessive Compulsive Scale (Y-BOCS) in patients with tics given haloperidol (closed circles with solid line) or placebo (open circles with solid line) and in patients without tics given haloperidol (closed squares with dotted line) or placebo (open squares with dotted line) for 4 weeks. Asterisk indicates* P<*.05, change from baseline in patients with tics (haloperidol), paired* t *test; dagger,* P<*.04, change from baseline, patients with vs without tics (haloperidol), Student's* t *test; double dagger,* P<*.003, change from baseline in patients with tics (haloperidol), paired* t *test; section mark,* P<*.001, change from baseline, patients with vs without tics (haloperidol), Student's* t *test; parallels,* P<*.0002, change from baseline in patients with tics (haloperidol), paired* t *test; and paragraph mark,* P<*.0001, change from baseline, patients with vs without tics (haloperidol), Student's* t *test. All tests are two tailed.*

During the double-blind phase, the eight patients with tics who were randomized to haloperidol showed a significant reduction in tic frequency as measured by the Yale Global Tic Severity Scale (2.9±1.1 to 1.4±0.5, *t*=5.6, *df*=7, *P*<.001).

TOLERABILITY OF FLUVOXAMINE/ HALOPERIDOL TREATMENT

The fluvoxamine/haloperidol treatment was well tolerated. No acute dystonic reactions or other serious medical complications occurred. Nine of 31 patients who received haloperidol experienced akathisia that responded to propranolol hydrochloride (74.4±16.7 mg/d). Other than mild anticholinergic side effects, no additional adverse reactions occurred.

RESULTS OF FLUVOXAMINE BLOOD LEVEL DETERMINATION

There were no significant differences in fluvoxamine blood levels between groups before randomization to haloperidol (408.5±243.8 ng/mL) or placebo (282.4±236.1 ng/mL). Although fluvoxamine levels increased after 4 weeks of haloperidol (436.9±272.1 ng/mL) and placebo (331.2±273.1 ng/mL), these increases were not significant, nor did changes in levels between the two groups differ. In the nine patients who were given concomitant propranolol, fluvoxamine levels before (204.7±155.2 ng/mL) and after (240.9±162.6 ng/mL) haloperidol addition did not significantly differ. Fluvoxamine blood levels did not correlate with treatment response.

COMMENT

The response of OCD patients to fluvoxamine/haloperidol treatment in this investigation supports findings of our previous open-label study.[7] As hypothesized, OCD patients with a concurrent chronic tic disorder showed preferential response to combination treatment, with eight of eight such patients responding to double-blind haloperidol addition and none of seven responding to placebo. In contrast, combination treatment was of benefit in significantly fewer OCD patients without comorbid tics, usually effecting only partial improvement when any response occurred, so that the data provide little support for the use of neuroleptic addition in treating these individuals.

POTENTIAL STUDY LIMITATIONS

The design of this study does not exclude the possibility that treatment response was due to haloperidol alone. Based on a review[4] of the sparse literature on this topic, and on extensive clinical experience, this seems unlikely. We are not aware of any placebo-controlled studies of neuroleptic monotherapy in *DSM-III-R* OCD.

The possibility that response was simply due to a longer duration of fluvoxamine is unlikely, since none of the 17 patients who were randomized to placebo responded. The possibility that fluvoxamine blood levels played some role in treatment response cannot be entirely excluded: the six lowest prerandomization and the seven lowest postrandomization fluvoxamine blood levels fell within the placebo-treated group, and the mean fluvoxamine blood levels were lower in the placebo-treated group before and after randomization. However, these differences between the active and placebo-treated groups were not statistically significant, and fluvoxamine blood levels did not correlate with treatment response. Because significant pharmacokinetic interactions between propranolol and fluvoxamine have been reported,[17] this possibility was also assessed. However, there was no significant difference in fluvoxamine levels before or after 4 weeks of haloperidol in the nine patients who received concomitant propranolol. Fluvoxamine levels were not correlated with treatment response, making it unlikely that haloperidol with or without propranolol exerted a therapeutic effect through a pharmacokinetic interaction.

Finally, due to haloperidol's side-effect profile, it is difficult to be certain that assessments were truly double blind. In attempts to preserve blind conditions, we prophylactically treated all patients with benztropine and had side effects assessed and treated by a nonrating physician blind to treatment assignment.

RELATIONSHIP BETWEEN OCD AND TS

Pitman et al[18] reported that 38% of OCD patients studied met criteria for a tic disorder. Obsessive-compulsive symptoms occur in 52% to 74% of TS patients.[19] Family genetic studies indicate that some forms of OCD and TS are etiologically related.[20] Although perturbations in other neurochemical systems have been demonstrated in TS,[21] most evidence supports a dysregulation of dopamine neurotransmission.[22] Indirect evidence suggests that dopamine may contribute to the pathophysiology of some forms of obsessive-compulsive behavior.[4] Interestingly, the basal ganglia and frontal cortex, ie, the same brain regions that have been implicated in the pathophysiology of OCD,[23] appear to be the prime anatomic loci of the neuropathology of TS.[24]

IMPLICATIONS

Obsessive-compulsive disorder patients with a comorbid chronic tic disorder may require conjoint SUI/neuroleptic therapy for effective symptom reduction. Combined with differences in the clinical phenomenology between OCD patients with and without tics,[25] these treatment response data support the hypothesis that OCD patients with a comorbid chronic tic disorder may be a clinically meaningful subtype.

Neuroleptic treatment should not be used indiscriminately in the treatment of OCD. Because of the risks of tardive dyskinesia, adequate trials of available SUIs should be completed before neuroleptic addition is considered. Should neuroleptic addition be initiated, only a time-limited trial should be attempted, with reassessment of the risk-benefit ratio at regular intervals. Additional research is necessary to investigate further the role of dopamine and its interactions with 5-hydroxytryptamine in obsessive-compulsive phenomena, and to identify homogeneous clinical and biologic subgroups of patients with OCD.

Accepted for publication April 28, 1993.

This study was supported in part by grants MH30929 and MH45802 from the National Institute of Mental Health, Bethesda, Md, by the State of Connecticut, Hartford, by the 1990-1991 Lilly Psychiatric Research Fellowship (Dr McDougle), and by a 1990-1992 National Alliance for Research on Schizophrenia and Affective Disorders Young Investigators Award (Dr McDougle).

Fluvoxamine was generously provided by Solvay Pharmaceuticals, Marietta, Ga. Pete Pullen, MS, and Menno Barrs, MS, of the Solvay Analytical R&D Group, determined the fluvoxamine blood levels. We thank the research, clinical, pharmacy, and clerical staff of the Clinical Neuroscience Research Unit, Connecticut Mental Health Center, New Haven, for their expert assistance: Deborah Herbst, Sally Trufan, Beth Ruff, and Betsy Kyle.

Reprint requests to Clinical Neuroscience Research Unit, Abraham Ribicoff Research Facilities, Connecticut Mental Health Center, 34 Park St, New Haven, CT 06519 (Dr McDougle).

REFERENCES

1. Goodman WK, Price LH, Rasmussen SA, Delgado PL, Heninger GR, Charney DS. Efficacy of fluvoxamine in obsessive-compulsive disorder: a double-blind comparison with placebo. *Arch Gen Psychiatry.* 1989;46:36-43.
2. McDougle CJ, Price LH, Goodman WK, Charney DS, Heninger GR. A controlled trial of lithium augmentation in fluvoxamine-refractory obsessive compulsive disorder: lack of efficacy. *J Clin Psychopharmacol.* 1991;11:175-184.
3. McDougle CJ, Goodman WK, Leckman JF, Holzer JC, Barr LC, McCance-Katz E, Heninger GR, Price LH. Limited therapeutic effect of addition of buspirone in fluvoxamine-refractory obsessive compulsive disorder. *Am J Psychiatry.* 1993; 150:647-649.
4. Goodman WK, McDougle CJ, Price LH, Riddle MA, Pauls DL, Leckman JF. Beyond the serotonin hypothesis: a role for dopamine in some forms of obsessive compulsive disorder? *J Clin Psychiatry.* 1990;51(suppl):36-43.
5. Riddle MA, Leckman JF, Hardin MT, Anderson GM, Cohen DJ. Fluoxetine treatment of obsessions and compulsions in patients with Tourette's syndrome. *Am J Psychiatry.* 1988;145:1173-1174.
6. Delgado PL, Goodman WK, Price LH, Heninger GR, Charney DS. Fluvoxamine/pimozide treatment of concurrent Tourette's and obsessive-compulsive disorder. *Br J Psychiatry.* 1990;157:762-765.
7. McDougle CJ, Goodman WK, Price LH, Delgado PL, Krystal JH, Charney DS, Heninger GR. Neuroleptic addition in fluvoxamine-refractory obsessive-compulsive disorder. *Am J Psychiatry.* 1990;147:652-654.
8. American Psychiatric Association, Committee on Nomenclature and Statistics. *Diagnostic and Statistical Manual of Mental Disorders, Revised Third Edition.* Washington, DC: American Psychiatric Association; 1987.
9. Guy W. *ECDEU Assessment Manual for Psychopharmacology.* Washington, DC: US Dept of Health, Education, and Welfare; 1976. Publication 76-338.
10. Mazure C, Nelson JC, Price LH. Reliability and validity of the symptoms of major depressive illness. *Arch Gen Psychiatry.* 1986;43:451-456.
11. Pauls D, Hurst C. *Schedule for Tourette and Other Behavioral Syndromes.* New Haven, Conn: Yale University, Child Study Center; 1991. Version AI, March.
12. Goodman WK, Price LH, Rasmussen SA, Mazure C, Fleischmann R, Hill C, Heninger GR, Charney DS. The Yale-Brown Obsessive Compulsive Scale (Y-BOCS), I: development, use, and reliability. *Arch Gen Psychiatry.* 1989;46: 1006-1011.
13. Goodman WK, Price LH, Rasmussen SA, Mazure C, Delgado P, Heninger GR, Charney DS. The Yale-Brown Obsessive Compulsive Scale (Y-BOCS), II: validity. *Arch Gen Psychiatry.* 1989;46:1012-1016.
14. Hamilton M. The assessment of anxiety states by rating. *Br J Med Psychol.* 1959;32:50-55.
15. Leckman JF, Riddle MA, Hardin MT, Ort SI, Swartz KL, Stevenson J, Cohen DJ. The Yale Global Tic Severity Scale: initial testing of a clinician-rated scale of tic severity. *J Am Acad Child Adolesc Psychiatry.* 1989;4:566-573.
16. Woods SW, Charney DS, Loke J, Goodman WK, Redmond DE, Heninger GR. Carbon dioxide sensitivity in panic anxiety: ventilatory and anxiogenic response to CO_2 in healthy subjects and panic disorder patients before and after alprazolam treatment. *Arch Gen Psychiatry.* 1986;43:900-909.
17. Benfield P, Ward A. Fluvoxamine: a review of its pharmacodynamic and pharmacokinetic properties, and therapeutic efficacy in depressive illness. *Drugs.* 1986;32:313-334.
18. Pitman RK, Green RC, Jenike MA, Mesulam MM. Clinical comparison of Tourette's disorder and obsessive-compulsive disorder. *Am J Psychiatry.* 1987;144:1166-1171.
19. Frankel M, Cummings JL, Robertson MM, Trimble MR, Hill MA, Benson DF. Obsessions and compulsions in Gilles de la Tourette's syndrome. *Neurology.* 1986;36:378-382.
20. Pauls DL, Leckman JF. The inheritance of Gilles de la Tourette's syndrome and associated behaviors: evidence for autosomal dominant transmission. *N Engl J Med.* 1986;315:993-997.
21. Leckman JF, Riddle MA, Berrettini WH, Anderson GM, Hardin M, Chappell P, Bissette G, Nemeroff CB, Goodman WK, Cohen DJ. Elevated CSF dynorphin A [1-8] in Tourette's syndrome. *Life Sci.* 1988;43:2015-2023.
22. Shapiro E, Shapiro AK, Fulop G, Hubbard M, Mandeli J, Nordlie J, Phillips RA. Controlled study of haloperidol, pimozide, and placebo for the treatment of Gilles de la Tourette's syndrome. *Arch Gen Psychiatry.* 1989;46:722-730.
23. Rapoport JL, Wise SP. Obsessive-compulsive disorder: evidence for basal ganglia dysfunction. *Psychopharmacol Bull.* 1988;24:380-384.
24. Singer HS, Hahn I-H, Moran TH. Abnormal dopamine uptake sites in postmortem striatum from patients with Tourette's syndrome. *Ann Neurol.* 1991; 30:558-562.
25. Holzer JC, Goodman WK, McDougle CJ, et al. Obsessive complusive disorder with and without a chronic tic disorder: a comparison of symptoms in 70 patients. *Br J Psychiatr y.* In press.

ORIGINAL ARTICLE

Tryptophan Depletion in Patients With Obsessive-Compulsive Disorder Who Respond to Serotonin Reuptake Inhibitors

Linda C. Barr, MD; Wayne K. Goodman, MD; Christopher J. McDougle, MD; Pedro L. Delgado, MD; George R. Heninger, MD; Dennis S. Charney, MD; Lawrence H. Price, MD

Methods: The effects of short-term tryptophan depletion were examined in 15 patients with *DSM-III-R* obsessive-compulsive disorder who had demonstrated symptom reduction following treatment with serotonin reuptake inhibitors. Patients received a 24-hour, low-tryptophan (160-mg/d) diet followed the next morning by a drink of 15 amino acids. A double-blind, placebo-controlled crossover design was used.

Results: The diet and the amino acid drink reduced free plasma tryptophan levels by a mean of 84% 5 hours later. Short-term tryptophan depletion did not significantly change mean ratings of obsessions and compulsions. In contrast, mean depression ratings were significantly increased with tryptophan depletion compared with the control (tryptophan-supplemented) testing.

Conclusion: Maintenance of serotonin reuptake inhibitor–induced improvement of obsessive and compulsive symptoms, unlike remission of depressive symptoms, may not depend on ongoing short-term availability of serotonin.

(Arch Gen Psychiatry. 1994;51:309-317)

From the Clinical Neuroscience Research Unit, the Abraham Ribicoff Research Facilities, the Connecticut Mental Health Center (Drs Barr, Goodman, McDougle, Heninger, and Price) and the West Haven (Conn) Veterans Affairs Medical Center, (Drs Delgado and Charney), Department of Psychiatry, Yale University School of Medicine, New Haven. Dr Goodman is currently with the University of Florida School of Medicine, Gainesville. Dr Delgado is currently with the Veterans Affairs Medical Center, University of Arizona School of Medicine, Tucson.

THE FACT that serotonin reuptake inhibitors (SRIs) reduce obsessive and compulsive (OC) symptoms in patients with obsessive-compulsive disorder (OCD) indicates the important role of the serotonin (5-hydroxytryptamine [5-HT]) system in the mechanism of action of these agents. The potent, clinically available SRIs clomipramine,[1] fluoxetine,[2] fluvoxamine,[3] and sertraline[4] all produce clinically significant reductions in OC symptoms. The 5-HT reuptake inhibition appears to be central to the mechanism of action of these drugs because agents without significant SRI properties (eg, desipramine) are ineffective.[5-7]

Studies that link changes in the indexes of 5-HT function with treatment response provide additional support for the role of the 5-HT system in the anti–obsessive-compulsive mechanism of these agents. Clomipramine-induced reductions in both platelet 5-HT content[8] and cerebrospinal fluid 5-hydroxyindoleacetic acid levels[9] have been correlated with reductions in OC symptoms. However, other demonstrated changes in 5-HT function that are produced by SRI treatment have not been linked with treatment response. Long-term fluoxetine treatment in patients with OCD attenuates their hypothermic and neuroendocrine responses to the 5-HT_{1a} partial agonist ipsapirone, but this attenuation does not correlate with symptom reduction.[10] Administration of the mixed agonist-antagonist *m*-chlorophenyl piperazine does not worsen OC symptoms in patients with OCD who were treated with clomipramine[11] or fluoxetine,[12] whereas administration of the 5-HT antagonist metergoline may worsen OC symptoms relative to a placebo in clomipramine-treated patients.[13] Thus, although action on the 5-HT system appears important, the exact mechanisms responsible for the improvement of symptoms remain unclear.

See Patients and Methods on next page

PATIENTS AND METHODS

PATIENTS

Fifteen patients meeting *DSM-III-R* criteria[35] for OCD for at least 2 years participated (eight men and seven women; mean±SEM age, 36±2.2 years [range, 26 to 54 years]; 13 outpatients and two inpatients). Diagnosis was established by the best estimate method,[36] which included a semistructured interview based on *DSM-III-R* criteria and sections of the Yale-Brown Obsessive Compulsive Disorders Scale (Y-BOCS).[37,38] Those with serious medical or neurological conditions as determined by a history, physical examination, and screening laboratory tests were excluded, as were patients with a history of substance abuse in the past 6 months. Patients whose OC symptoms occurred exclusively in their home were excluded. A lifetime history of depression and other psychiatric diagnoses were determined using a semistructured interview based on *DSM-III-R*. Ten patients had a lifetime history of major depression, two had a history of chronic motor tic disorder, two had a history of alcohol abuse (but had not abused alcohol during the 6 months prior to the study), and one patient each had a diagnosis of Gilles de la Tourette's syndrome, body dysmorphic disorder, and avoidant personality disorder. Four patients were receiving adjunctive medications in addition to an SRI (two were receiving buspirone hydrochloride; one, lithium carbonate; and one, clonazepam). Patients were recruited both from the community (n=2) and following successful treatment in the Yale OCD Clinic, New Haven, Conn, (n=13). Treatment response was defined as a 35% decrease in pretreatment score when this was available, a Y-BOCS score of less than 16 on entry into the study, and a Clinician Global Impression Scale rating of much or very much improved. The mean±SEM Y-BOCS score at the time of challenge was 8.2±1.1 (range, 0 to 14). Patients had been treated with fluvoxamine maleate (n=8; dosage range, 150 to 300 mg/d), clomipramine hydrochloride (n=5; dosage range, 100 to 200 mg/d) and fluoxetine hydrochloride (n=2; dosage range, 40 to 60 mg/d); the mean±SEM duration of treatment was 50±15.8 weeks (range, 5 to 104 weeks). The **Table** summarizes the clinical characteristics of the patients and the SRI treatments. All patients gave written informed consent after the procedures were fully described.

PROCEDURE

Control and short-term TRP depletion were preceded by a 24-hour low-TRP diet (10 500 kJ, 7% protein, 27% fat, 64% carbohydrate) supplemented with either placebo (depletion diet) or 1.5 g of TRP (control diet). After the patients consumed the 24-hour diet, on the morning of the challenge, patients received a 15-AA drink that was supplemented with either placebo (depletion drink) or 2.3 g of TRP (control drink). A detailed description of the diet and AA drink appears elsewhere.[33] The sequence of control and depletion testing was randomly assigned in a double-blind fashion with tests separated by 7 to 10 days. Ten patients received the TRP depletion first and the control diet and drink second. Normal TRP intake resumed 8 hours after the AA drink was given. Behavioral ratings were obtained by trained research nurses or a research psychiatrist immediately before starting the diet (day 1, 9 AM), and 15 minutes prior to and 5 and 7 hours following administration of the AA drink (day 2, 8:45 AM, 2 PM, and 4 PM).

Preclinical studies demonstrate diverse effects of long-term SRI administration on the 5-HT system. Observed effects vary according to brain region, response measure (electrophysiologic response, radioligand binding, and measures of putative 5-HT–mediated behaviors), and the specific SRI investigated. Long-term administration of SRIs increases net 5-HT transmission as assessed by CA3 hippocampal neuron firing,[14] possibly by producing desensitization of somatodendritic[15] and terminal autoreceptors.[16] Long-term administration of clomipramine,[17] fluoxetine,[17] and fluvoxamine[18] reduces radioligand binding to postsynaptic 5-HT_2 receptors, though this has not been demonstrated consistently.[19-21] The role these effects may play in the anti–obsessive-compulsive action of the SRIs is unknown.

A short-term tryptophan (TRP) depletion paradigm was developed to evaluate the effects produced by a temporary reduction of brain 5-HT in humans.[22] Under physiologic conditions, availability of the 5-HT–precursor TRP limits synthesis of 5-HT.[23] Orally administered amino acid (AA) mixtures induce protein synthesis. If the AA mixture is deficient in TRP, it reduces plasma TRP by stimulating protein synthesis and incorporation of plasma and other body stores of TRP into new proteins. Preclinical studies demonstrate that changes in plasma TRP levels produce parallel alterations in brain 5-HT levels[24-26] without a change in tyrosine, homovanillic acid, or 3-methoxy-4-hydroxyphenylglycol levels.[27] Increased competition by other large neutral AAs for active transport across the blood-brain barrier may produce additional reductions in brain 5-HT.[28] Preclinical evidence suggests that TRP depletion that is accomplished by administration of a TRP-free diet or an AA mixture devoid of TRP produces functionally significant decreases in brain 5-HT.[29]

Functional changes associated with short-term TRP depletion have also been demonstrated in humans. In healthy men, short-term TRP depletion causes reduced concentration and negative mood[30,22] and blocks morphine-induced analgesia.[31] Untreated depressed patients show a variable response to TRP depletion,[32] with some demonstrating a worsening of mood and some improving following depletion. Short-term TRP depletion exacerbates depressive symptoms in up to 60% of drug-remitted depressed patients; remitted patients treated with SRIs appear especially vulnerable.[33,34]

The OC symptoms were reviewed on the morning of the challenge, and principal obsessions and compulsions were identified via the Y-BOCS symptoms checklist. Because the Y-BOCS has not been demonstrated to be sensitive to short-term changes in the severity of OC symptoms, a 15-point clinician-rated global OC severity scale (GOCS) (range, 0 [no symptoms] to 14 [extreme]) was devised. Global ratings of obsessions and compulsions were obtained on day 2 after the patient had acclimated to the testing environment by the same interviewer during both TRP depletion and control testing. Clinician global ratings incorporated aspects of frequency, distress, interference, resistance, and control in obtaining the global rating. Patients also completed a self-reported version of the GOCS. Other behavioral ratings consisted of the 24-item modified Hamilton Depression Rating Scale (HDRS),[39] the Beck Depression Inventory,[40] and sixteen 100-mm visual analog scale items (talkative, happy, drowsy, nervous, sad, calm, depressed, anxious, energetic, fearful, mellow, high, angry, irritable, tired, hungry). Patients also completed a physical symptom checklist consisting of 23 self-rated items, each scored from 0 (not at all) to 3 (severe).[41] Free and total plasma TRP levels were obtained prior to starting the 24-hour diet, 15 minutes prior to the administration of the AA drink, and 5 hours following it.

BIOCHEMICAL METHODS

Total plasma TRP was assayed by high-performance liquid chromatography with fluorometric detection. Free plasma TRP was assayed by obtaining the ultrafiltrate of plasma from cellulose-based filters (30 000–molecular weight cutoff) (1000g) at room temperature and subjecting the ultrafiltrate to the high-performance liquid chromatography with fluorometric detection method.[42]

DATA ANALYSIS

Change in TRP levels and behavioral ratings were analyzed by means of an analysis of variance (ANOVA) with repeated measures. Main effects of challenge type (control vs TRP depletion) and time (changes over the time points sampled) were determined, as was the interaction of challenge type×time (indicating the overall effect of the TRP depletion during the study). The reported *P* values for all ANOVAs employed the Huynh-Feldt correction factor. This correction factor decreases the *df* used in the ANOVA to reflect lack of independence in the variance of measures across time points; for clarity, uncorrected *df* are presented. Post hoc *t* tests were employed to examine significant interactions revealed by ANOVA. Additionally, the difference between the change in HDRS scores over time during control testing (the rating at 4 PM minus the rating at 9 AM) and TRP depletion (the rating at 4 PM minus the rating at 9 AM) (double difference) was examined. If significant effects of ANOVA were identified for a total scale score, ANOVA of the individual items of the scale was employed to identify which items were changing. Obsessive and compulsive symptom exacerbation was categorically defined as a 2-point or greater increase in GOCS ratings; depressive symptom exacerbation was defined as a 50% increase from the day 2, 9 AM HDRS total score and an HDRS score that was greater than or equal to 17. Results were considered significant when $P<.05$ (two-tailed *t* test). Data analysis used SAS OS/2 (SAS Institute Inc, Cary, NC)[43] and BMDP statistical software (BMDP Statistical Software, Berkeley, Calif).[44]

The purpose of this study was to further investigate the mechanism of action of the potent SRIs in the treatment of OC symptoms. The effects of short-term TRP depletion were studied in patients with OCD who were identified as SRI treatment responders to determine whether a short-term reduction in plasma TRP (and presumably brain 5-HT) would result in a return of OC symptoms.

RESULTS

CHANGES IN FREE AND TOTAL PLASMA TRP

Administration of the low-TRP diet and TRP-free AA drink reduced mean total and free plasma TRP levels when compared with the control diet and drink (total TRP: $F=105$; $df=2,24$; $P<.002$; and free TRP: $F=41$; $df=2,24$; $P<.0002$) (**Figure 1**). As shown in Figure 1, top, depletion decreased the mean±SEM total TRP level from 50.0±13.2 μmol/L before the diet was begun to 5.9±4.9 μmol/L 5 hours after the TRP-free AA drink was administered (89% decrease) ($t=11.8$; $df=1,12$; $P<.0001$). With control testing, the mean±SEM total TRP level increased from 55.8±12.2 μmol/L before the diet was begun to 104.8±33.3 μmol/L 5 hours after the TRP-supplemented drink was administered ($t=6.0$; $df=1,13$; $P<.0001$). As shown in Figure 1, bottom, depletion decreased the mean±SEM free TRP level from 9.3±3.9 μmol/L before the diet was begun to 1.5±1.5 μmol/L 5 hours after the TRP-free AA drink was administered (84% decrease) ($t=6.8$; $df=1,12$; $P<.0001$). In contrast, the mean±SEM free TRP level increased from 11.3±5.4 μmol/L before the diet was begun to 21.9±7.8 μmol/L after the TRP-supplemented drink was administered ($t=6.0$; $df=1,12$; $P=.001$). Total and free plasma TRP decreased in every patient during TRP depletion and increased in every patient during control testing.

BEHAVIORAL EFFECTS

OC Symptoms

The OC ratings for one patient did not employ the GOCS; the ratings for this patient are not included in the subsequent analysis. Short-term TRP depletion had no significant effect on OC symptoms in these SRI-treatment

Patient Characteristics*

Patient No./Sex	Age at Challenge, y	Age of Onset, y	Medication, mg/d†	Treatment, wk	Y-BOCS Before Treatment	Y-BOCS Before Challenge	HDRS Before Challenge	Lifetime History of MDD	Additional Diagnosis (Current)
1/F	42	38	Fluvoxamine, 300	13	20	13.5	8.5	No	Bulimia
2/M	30	29	Fluvoxamine, 300	8	21	5.5	10	Yes	Avoidant PD
3/F	31	15	Fluvoxamine, 300	12	23	7	2	No	None
4/F	36	15	Fluvoxamine, 300	24	30	10.5	8.5	Yes	None
5/M	25	24	Fluoxetine, 40	5	26	9	1.5	No	None
6/F	42	37	Clomipramine, 200; buspirone, 60	240	22	10.5	14	Yes	BDD
7/F	47	37	Fluoxetine, 60; lithium, 900	91	24	14	6	No	Past ETOH
8/M	46	38	Clomipramine, 175	24	NA	10.5	7.5	Yes	Past ETOH
9/M	30	23	Fluvoxamine, 200; clonazepam, 3	104	NA	0	0	No	Tourette's syndrome
10/M	28	22	Fluvoxamine, 300	13	17	14.5	1.5	Yes	Motor tics
11/M	37	35	Clomipramine, 175; buspirone, 60	76	NA	8	8.5	Yes	None
12/M	53	52	Clomipramine, 150	26	25	5.5	2	Yes	None
13/M	26	13	Fluvoxamine, 250	56	22	7	2	Yes	Motor tics
14/F	33	24	Clomipramine, 100	46	20	8	11	Yes	None
15/F	27	21	Fluvoxamine, 150	12	14	0	1	Yes	None
Mean or Total/ 8 M, 7 F	36	28	...	50	22.0	8.23	5.6	10 Yes 5 No	...
SEM	2.2	2.8	...	15.8	1.21	1.13	1.14	...	...

*Y-BOCS indicates Yale-Brown Obsessive Compulsive Scale; HDRS, Hamilton Rating Scale for Depression; MDD, major depressive disorder; PD, personality disorder; BDD, body dysmorphic disorder; ETOH, alcohol abuse; NA, data not available; and ellipses, not applicable.

†The salt for fluvoxamine was maleate; for fluoxetine, hydrochloride; for clomipramine, hydrochloride; for buspirone, hydrochloride; and for lithium, carbonate.

responders (**Figure 2**). An ANOVA of OC symptoms as reflected in the clinician-rated GOCS showed decreases over time (main effect of time) in obsessions (F=4.8; *df*=2,26; *P*<.02), compulsions (F=3.4; *df*=2,26; *P*<.05), and the sum of these (F=4.12; *df*=1,13; *P*<.03). However, there were no main effects of challenge type or challenge type×time interactions for these ratings. There were no significant changes in patient-rated OC symptoms. A categorically defined worsening of OC symptoms (>2-point increase in clinician-rated GOCS) was observed in only one of 15 patients during TRP depletion. The GOCS ratings of obsessions and compulsions before the AA drink (day 2, 9 AM) and the net change in ratings 7 hours after the drink (day 2, 4 PM) are shown in Figure 2.

Mood

Short-term TRP depletion was associated with increased depressive symptoms in contrast to OC symptoms. Patients reported depressed mood, impaired concentration, and decreased energy and interest. Two patients became tearful during TRP depletion; others became noticeably more quiet and withdrawn. An ANOVA revealed a significant challenge type×time interaction for HDRS ratings (F=4.6; *df*=3,42; *P*<.007) (**Figure 3**). Paired *t* tests revealed significantly increased HDRS ratings 7 hours following the administration of the AA drink on the depletion day when compared with both day 1 (*t*=3.4; *df*=1,14; *P*<.005) and day 2, 9 AM (*t*=2.22; *df*=1,14; *P*<.04). Control testing produced no significant change from day 1 for any subsequent time point. The difference between the change in HDRS scores over time when control testing and TRP depletion were compared (day 1, 9 AM compared with day 2, 4 PM; double difference) was significant (*t*=2.6; *df*=1,14; *P*<.03). An ANOVA of individual items of the HDRS score revealed that changes in mood (F=3.56; *df*=3,33; *P*<.03) and concentration (F=3.19; *df*=3,33; *P*<.05) primarily accounted for the overall change in HDRS scores. There was a trend for increased ratings of loss of pleasure associated with TRP depletion (F=2.49; *df*=3,33; *P*<.08). An ANOVA of total HDRS scores revealed no main effects of challenge type or time. The HDRS scores before the AA drink (day 2, 9 AM) and the change in HDRS scores 7 hours after the drink are shown in Figure 3. There were no significant effects of challenge, time, or the interaction on self-rated depressive symptoms as reflected in the Beck Depression Inventory scores. Five patients met categorical criteria for depressive symptom exacerbation (50% increase from the day 2, 9 AM HDRS rating and an HDRS score greater than 17) during TRP depletion. One patient fulfilled these criteria during control testing.

Analog Scale Ratings

As reflected by significant challenge type×time interactions, clinician ratings were increased for the visual analog scale items nervous (F=6.5; *df*=2,28; *P*<.005), sad (F=5.7; *df*=2,28; *P*<.01), and depressed (F=5.2; *df*=2,28; *P*<.002) and were decreased for mellow (F=4.5; *df*=2,28; *P*<.02) during TRP depletion compared with control testing. Subsequent *t* tests of the double difference (day 2, 9 AM compared with day 2, 4 PM) of these measures showed that ratings of sad (*t*=2.72; *df*=1,14; *P*<.02), nervous (*t*=−3.5; *df*=1,14; *P*<.004) and depressed (*t*=−2.8; *df*=1,14; *P*<.02) were increased and ratings of mellow (*t*=2.5; *df*=1,14; *P*<.03) decreased with TRP depletion as compared with control testing. Clinician analog ratings of drowsiness increased over time with both TRP depletion and control testing (F=3.6; *df*=2,28; *P*<.04).

An ANOVA of the patient-rated analog scales revealed a significant main effect of time on patient ratings of hungry (F=6.6; *df*=2,20; *P*<.006), which increased during both control and depletion tests. A significant challenge type×time interaction for this rating (F=7.5; *df*=2,20; *P*<.004) was largely accounted for by differing baseline ratings of hungry at the day 2, 9 AM time point during control and TRP depletion testing.

FACTORS ASSOCIATED WITH THE RETURN OF DEPRESSION

The HDRS ratings for patients with and without a lifetime history of major depression were also examined separately, although interpretation of these analyses was limited by the small sample sizes. An ANOVA of total HDRS scores for those patients with a lifetime history of depression (n=10) revealed a significant challenge type×time interaction (F=5.1; *df*=3,27; *P*<.007). An ANOVA of total HDRS scores for those patients without a history of major depression (n=5) showed no significant interaction effect. No relationship between the duration of SRI treatment and peak change in HDRS ratings was identified (*r*=−.11, not significant). There also was no correlation between free plasma TRP 5 hours after the TRP-free AA drink was administered and HDRS scores 7 hours after the drink was administered (*r*=.1, not significant). There was no significant interaction between challenge type×time×sequence of testing with HDRS score as the dependent variable (F=.19; *df*=3,39; *P*<.90), which suggests that the sequence of testing was not an important effect.

PHYSICAL SYMPTOMS

An ANOVA of the 23-item self-reported physical symptom checklist demonstrated main effects of challenge type on symptoms of headache (F=7.37; *df*=1,11; *P*<.02), drowsiness (F=11.3; *df*=1,11; *P*<.006), and faintness (F=8.7; *df*=1,11; *P*<.01), which were greater during TRP depletion than during control testing. Nonspecific ef-

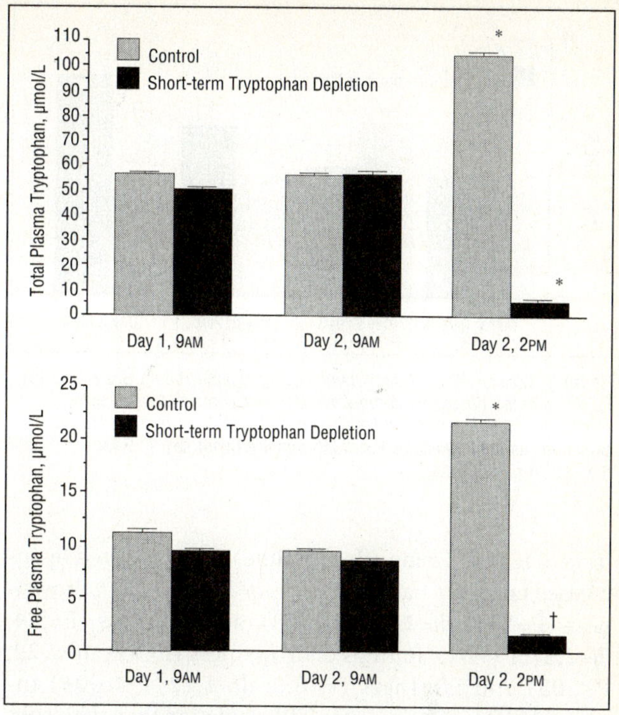

Figure 1. *Mean±SEM total (top) and free (bottom) plasma tryptophan levels during control and tryptophan depletion. Asterisk indicates* P*<.0001 compared with day 1, 9 AM (two-tailed paired* t *test). Dagger indicates* P*<.0009 compared with day 1, 9 AM (two-tailed paired* t *test).*

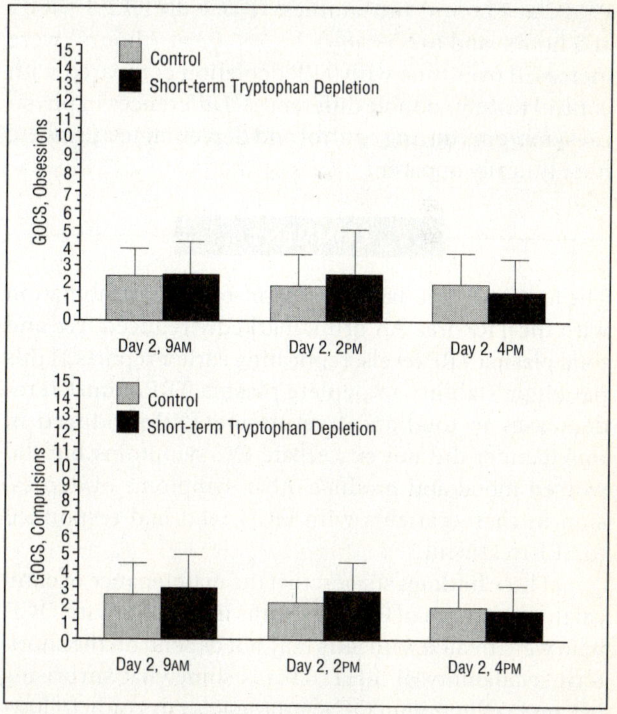

Figure 2. *Mean±SEM global obsessions and compulsions scale (GOCS) obsessions (top) and compulsions (bottom) subscale scores for day 2, 9 AM, 2 PM, and 4 PM.*

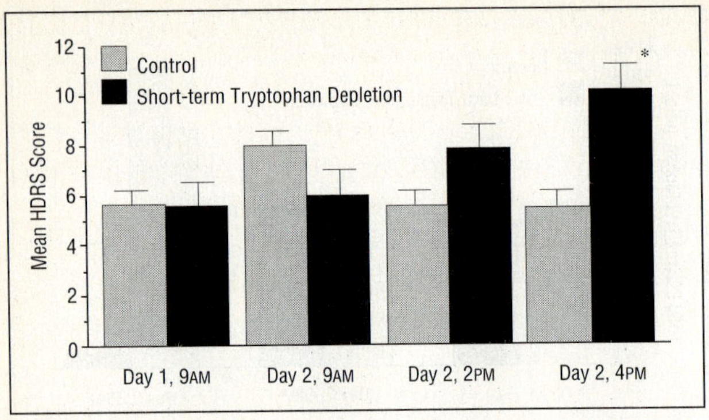

Figure 3. *Mean±SEM 24-item Hamilton Depression Rating Scale (HDRS) for 15 remitted obsessive-compulsive disorder patients treated with serotonin uptake inhibitors following control and short-term tryptophan depletion. Asterisk indicates* $P<.005$ *compared with day 1, 9 AM (two-tailed paired* t *test).*

fects of testing (main effect of time) were reflected by increased ratings of nausea ($F=3.9$; $df=2,22$; $P<.03$), drowsiness ($F=10.0$; $df=2,22$; $P<.002$), and faintness ($F=5.4$; $df=2,22$; $P<.01$). Ratings of drowsiness ($F=5.8$; $df=2,22$; $P<.02$) and faintness ($F=8.0$; $df=2,22$; $P<.004$) increased more over time with TRP depletion than with control testing (challenge type×time interaction). Subsequent t tests demonstrated that ratings of drowsiness ($t=2.2$; $df=1,12$; $P<.05$ at 5 hours; and $t=2.7$; $df=1,12$; $P<.02$ at 7 hours) and faintness ($t=3.4$; $df=1,12$; $P<.005$ at 5 hours; and $t=2.54$; $df=1,12$; $P<.03$ at 7 hours) were increased over time with TRP depletion compared with control testing (double difference). Differences in physical symptoms during control and depletion testing were not clinically apparent.

COMMENT

The low-TRP diet that was administered in combination with the TRP-free AA drink markedly reduced free and total plasma TRP levels, replicating earlier reports of this paradigm's ability to deplete plasma TRP. Short-term decreases in total and free plasma TRP produced in this manner did not exacerbate OC symptoms but did worsen mood and produce other symptoms of depression in these patients with OCD who had responded to SRI treatment.

These findings suggest that the maintenance of clinical improvement of OC symptoms in patients with OCD who were treated with SRIs may not depend on the short-term availability of 5-HT. This is somewhat surprising because reduction in OC symptoms occurs only following SRI treatment and not with other antidepressant treatments. However, the conclusion that maintenance of improvement of OC symptoms may be independent of short-term changes in 5-HT function is not inconsistent with the findings of other studies examining putative 5-HT alterations in drug-treated patients with OCD. These results suggest that treatment with SRIs may produce downstream effects not immediately reversed by a temporary reduction in 5-HT transmission. Possibly, the anti-OC effect of the SRIs results from changes in a non–5-HT system that is functionally coupled to 5-HT. Indeed, preclinical evidence suggests that the SRIs may affect the dopamine system with long-term administration.[45] Clomipramine, which five of the participants received, inhibits reuptake of dopamine[46,47] and binds at the D_2 dopamine receptor.[48] Clomipramine's major metabolite, desmethylclomipramine, is also a potent inhibitor of norepinephrine reuptake. It is possible that these properties contributed to the observed lack of exacerbation of OC symptoms.

ALTERNATIVE EXPLANATIONS for the study's failure to find a worsening of OC symptoms following TRP depletion warrant consideration. Possibly, OC symptoms and depressive symptoms differ in the rate at which they recur following TRP depletion; more extended periods of TRP depletion might be necessary to produce a worsening of OC symptoms. Patients became drowsy following administration of both the control and the TRP-free AA drinks; it is possible that this may have contributed to the time-dependent decrease in OC symptoms observed. The degree of drowsiness reported by patients was greater during TRP depletion than during control testing; however, there was no clinically apparent difference in the degree of drowsiness produced. Thus, it seems unlikely that this effect could have masked a worsening of OC symptoms produced by depletion. Patients were studied within the confines of the research unit; the OC symptoms may have been more likely to worsen in other environments, such as in the patients' homes. It is unlikely that this could completely account for the observed lack of exacerbation because patients with highly context-dependent symptoms were excluded from the study. Transient changes in symptom severity may not have been detected because symptoms were assessed over fairly long intervals (5 and 7 hours). No validated instrument exists for the assessment of short-term changes in OC symptoms; possibly, the global ratings scales employed lacked sufficient sensitivity to detect a worsening. The instrument employed did detect an improvement of OC symptoms over the course of both test days, demonstrating sensitivity in detecting improvement of symptoms. Sample size may have limited detection of small changes in OC symptoms associated with TRP depletion. Power analysis indicates that a 25% worsening of the obsessions and compulsions associated with TRP depletion would have been detected with the sample size employed ($\alpha=.05$, $\beta=.20$); smaller changes in the severity of symptoms would not have been detected.

Clinical characteristics and heterogeneity of participating patients also limit conclusions based on the current finding. Participating patients demonstrated a range of responses to SRI treatment (from complete absence of symptoms to a level of symptoms just meeting the study criteria for treatment response), and this may have contributed to the observed lack of exacerbation of OC symptoms. It is possible that a worsening with short-term TRP depletion might be more easily detected in those patients with very robust responses to SRI treatment. However, such a group of patients would not reflect the usual range of responses that are experienced by patients with OCD who are receiving SRI treatment. The possibility that the adjunctive medications taken by four patients contributed to the lack of exacerbation also cannot be excluded. Study participants had been receiving SRIs for a mean of 50 weeks; early treatment response of symptoms may be more dependent on availability of 5-HT than is the long-standing improvement that was experienced by the majority of patients in this sample.

LIMITATIONS OF the paradigm to produce changes in brain 5-HT must be considered. Decreases in plasma TRP of the degree produced in this study have been demonstrated to produce parallel decreases in brain 5-HT levels in preclinical studies,[24] making it unlikely that brain 5-HT levels were unaffected. Moreover, the development of depressive symptoms in these patients also suggests that brain 5-HT levels were reduced. In rats, administration of a TRP-free AA mixture reduces by 30% cortical extracellular 5-HT as measured by in vivo microdialysis.[49] A greater reduction in 5-HT than can be achieved by administration of TRP-free AA mixtures may be required to alter OC symptoms. Reductions in brain 5-HT may also not affect net 5-HT transmission uniformly. Brain regions that are particularly implicated in the mediation of OC symptoms (eg, orbitofrontal cortex[50] and caudate nuclei[51]) may be resistant to the effects of TRP depletion. Molliver and Molliver[52] have documented differential sensitivity to *p*-chloroamphetamine treatment in neurons in the dorsal as compared with the median raphe. Tryptophan depletion could also differentially affect some 5-HT neurons and spare others.

Despite these caveats, the stability of improvement of OC symptoms in the face of short-term TRP depletion is notable. This stability suggests that although OC symptoms may specifically require SRI treatment for improvement, these symptoms are not as sensitive to perturbations in 5-HT transmission as are depressive symptoms. This finding is especially interesting in light of the capacity of the short-term TRP depletion paradigm to induce symptoms of depression in these patients with OCD who have improved. This parallels the production of depressive symptoms by TRP depletion in remitted depressed patients treated with SRIs,[33] suggesting a similar vulnerability to short-term TRP depletion in both disorders.

On the other hand, the differences in the quality of mood exacerbation seen in depressed patients and in these patients with OCD were apparent. Most patients with OCD, although noting a worsening of their mood and reductions of energy and interest, did not report the development of cognitive changes other than impaired concentration. A typical comment was "I don't know why I feel sad, I have nothing to feel sad about." In contrast, Delgado et al[33] reported the return of content-specific ruminations and negative thoughts with the return of depressed mood. Perhaps the lack of cognitive disturbances such as guilt, hopelessness, and worthlessness reflects a difference between patients with the primary diagnosis of OCD and those with primary depression. Lack of accompanying cognitive changes with the development of depressed mood may explain the lack of significant change in the Beck Depression Inventory total scores. Free plasma TRP levels did not correlate with HDRS scores during TRP depletion in these patients with OCD, which is another difference between these patients and remitted depressed patients.[33] The long duration of SRI treatment prior to TRP depletion may have produced a more variable depressive response to TRP depletion in this study; the depressed patients reported by Delgado et al[33] were tested after they remained clinically stable for a mean of 4 weeks. Additional studies in patients with OCD with and without a lifetime history of depression may help to clarify whether the induction of depressive symptoms by short-term TRP depletion is restricted to patients with a depressive diathesis.

Although the possibility that physical symptoms contributed to the ratings of depressive symptoms cannot be excluded (patient ratings of physical symptoms of drowsiness and faintness were increased with both TRP depletion and control testing, but were more so with TRP depletion), the time course for the development of depressive symptoms appears consistent with the hypothesis that the increase in depressive symptoms is related to reductions in brain 5-HT in these patients. Furthermore, TRP depletion does not increase symptoms of depression or OC symptoms in unmedicated patients with OCD (L.C.B., W.K.G., C.J.M., P.L.D., G.R.H., D.S.C., and L.H.P., unpublished data, January 1993). Analysis of individual items of the HDRS demonstrated that changes in mood and interest primarily accounted for the overall change in HDRS scores with TRP depletion, rather than changes in items that might be more directly influenced by physical symptoms (eg, hypersomnia and energy).

It is conceivable that SRI treatment per se might induce a vulnerability to depressive symptoms following short-term TRP depletion. That is, could long-term administration of an SRI produce a 5-HT–dependent mood state? If so, mood worsening with TRP depletion will be observed in patients with a variety of diagnoses who receive treatment with these agents. Investigations of the effects of short-term TRP depletion in normal subjects before and after long-term administration of an SRI may clarify whether this phenomenon is produced solely by exposure to these drugs or, alternatively, is produced by an interaction between drug treatment and underlying pathophysiologic processes.

Short-term TRP depletion highlights both differences and similarities in the mechanism of action of the SRIs in the treatment of OCD and major depression. Depressive symptoms of major depression do not require SRI treatment for improvement, yet they are sensitive to short-term TRP depletion in SRI-treated patients. Obsessive and compulsive symptoms are unaffected by short-term TRP depletion, but the depressive symptoms that are associated with OCD are sensitive to TRP depletion. These findings further differentiate the mechanism of action of the SRIs in the treatment of OCD and major depression while simultaneously underscoring a similar depressive response to short-term TRP depletion in these illnesses.

Accepted for publication September 28, 1993.

This study was supported in part by grants MH 36229, MH 14276, MH 30929, and MH 45802 from the National Institute of Mental Health, Bethesda, Md, and by the State of Connecticut.

This work was previously presented, in part, at the American Psychiatric Association 145th Annual Meeting, Washington, DC, May 4, 1992.

We thank the staff of the Clinical Neuroscience Research Unit for their expert assistance.

Reprint requests to the Connecticut Mental Health Center, Third Floor, 34 Park St, New Haven, CT 06519 (Dr Barr).

REFERENCES

1. DeVeaugh-Geiss J, Katz R, Landau P, Akiskal H, Ananth J, Ballenger J, Betts WC, Diamond B, Feiger A, Foa E, Fogelson D, Goodman W, Greist J, Himmelhoch J, Hoehn-Saric R, Jenike M, Kim SW, Liebowitz M, Mavissakalian M, Noyes R, Rasmussen S, Ringold A, Shear K. Clomipramine in the treatment of patients with obsessive-compulsive disorder. *Arch Gen Psychiatry.* 1991;48:730-738.
2. Pigott TA, Pato MT, Bernstein SE, Grover GN, Hill JL, Tollier TJ, Murphy DL. Controlled comparison of clomipramine and fluoxetine in the treatment of obsessive-compulsive disorder: behavioral and biological results. *Arch Gen Psychiatry.* 1990;47:926-993.
3. Goodman WK, Price LH, Rasmussen SA, Delgado PL, Heninger GR, Charney DS. Efficacy of fluvoxamine in obsessive-compulsive disorder: a double-blind comparison with placebo. *Arch Gen Psychiatry.* 1989;46:36-44.
4. Chouinard G, Goodman W, Griest J, Jenike M, Rasmussen S, White K, Hackett E, Gaffney M, Bick P. Obsessive-compulsive disorder-treatment with sertraline: a multicenter study. *Psychopharmacol Bull.* 1990;26:278-284.
5. Zohar J, Insel TR. Obsessive-compulsive disorder: psychobiological approaches to diagnosis, treatment, and pathophysiology. *Biol Psychiatry.* 1987;22:667-687.
6. Leonard HL, Swedo SE, Rapoport JL, Coffey M, Cheslow D. Treatment of obsessive-compulsive disorder with clomipramine and desipramine in children and adolescents: a double-blind crossover comparison. *Arch Gen Psychiatry.* 1989;46:1088-1092.
7. Goodman WK, Price LH, Delgado PL, Palumbo J, Krystal JH, Nagy LM, Rasmussen SA, Heninger GR, Charney DS. Specificity of serotonin reuptake inhibitors in the treatment of obsessive compulsive disorder: comparison of fluvoxamine and desipramine. *Arch Gen Psychiatry.* 1990;47:577-585.
8. Flament MF, Rapoport JL, Murphy DL, Berg CJ, Lake CR. Biochemical changes during clomipramine treatment of childhood obsessive-compulsive disorder. *Arch Gen Psychiatry.* 1987;44:219-225.
9. Thoren P, Asberg M, Bertelsson L. Clomipramine treatment of obsessive-compulsive disorder, II: biochemical aspects. *Arch Gen Psychiatry.* 1980;37:1289-1294.
10. Lesch KP, Hoh A, Schulte HM, Osterheider M, Müller T. Long-term fluoxetine treatment decreases 5-HT1a receptor responsivity in obsessive compulsive disorder. *Psychopharmacology (Berl).* 1991;105:415-420.
11. Zohar J, Insel TR, Zohar-Kadouch RC, Hill JL, Murphy DL. Serotonergic responsivity in obsessive-compulsive disorder: effects of chronic clomipramine treatment. *Arch Gen Psychiatry.* 1988;45:167-172.
12. Hollander E, DeCaria CM, Nitescu A, Gully R, Suckow RF, Cooper TB, Gorman JM, Klein DF, Liebowitz MR. Serotonergic function in obsessive-compulsive disorder: behavioral and neuroendocrine responses to oral *m*-chlorophenylpiperazine and fenfluramine in patients and healthy volunteers. *Arch Gen Psychiatry.* 1992;49:21-28.
13. Benkelfat C, Murphy DL, Zohar J, Hill JL, Grover G, Insel TR. Clomipramine in obsessive-compulsive disorder: further evidence for a serotonergic mechanism of action. *Arch Gen Psychiatry.* 1989;46:22-28.
14. Chaput Y, Blier P, de Montigny C. Acute and long-term effects of antidepressant serotonin (5-HT) reuptake blockers on the efficacy of 5-HT neurotransmission: electrophysiological studies in the rat central nervous system. *Adv Biol Psychiatry.* 1988;17:1-17.
15. Blier P, Chaput Y, de Montigny C. Long-term 5-HT reuptake blockade, but not monoamine oxidase inhibition, decreases the function of terminal 5-HT autoreceptors: an electrophysiological study in the rat brain. *Naunyn Schmiedebergs Arch Pharmacol.* 1988;337:246-254.
16. Blier P, de Montigny C, Chaput Y. A role for the serotonin system in the mechanism of action of antidepressant treatments: preclinical evidence. *J Clin Psychiatry.* 1990;51(suppl 4):14-20.
17. Stolz JF, Marsen CA, Middlemiss DN. Effect of chronic antidepressant treatment and subsequent withdrawal on 3H-spiperone binding in rat frontal cortex and serotonin receptor mediated behavior. *Psychopharmacology.* 1983;80:150-155.
18. Bradford LD, Tulp MTM, Schipper J. Biochemical effects in rats after long term treatment with fluvoxamine and clovoxamine: post synaptic changes. In: Society for Neuroscience abstracts; October 20-25, 1985; Dallas, Tex. Abstract 223.12.
19. Peroutka SJ, Snyder SH. Chronic antidepressant treatment decreases spiroperidol-labeled serotonin receptor binding. *Science.* 1980;210:88-90.
20. Claassen V. Review of the animal pharmacology and pharmacokinetics of fluvoxamine. *Br J Clin Pharmacol.* 1983;15(suppl):349S-355S.
21. Armstrong NA, Stockmeier CA, Kellar KJ. Neurochemical effects of repeated administration of sertraline. *Fed Proc.* 1985;44:887.
22. Young SN, Smith SE, Pihl R, Ervin FR. Tryptophan depletion causes a rapid lowering of mood in normal males. *Psychopharmacology.* 1985;87:173-177.
23. Cooper JR, Bloom FE, Roth RH. *The Biochemical Basis of Neuropharmacology.* New York, NY: Oxford University Press; 1991:338-380.
24. Moja EA, Cipollo P, Castoldi D, Tofanetti O. Dose-response decrease in plasma tryptophan and in brain tryptophan and serotonin after tryptophan-free amino acid mixtures in rats. *Life Sci.* 1989;44:971-976.
25. Curzon G. Relationships between plasma, CSF and brain tryptophan. *J Neural Transm.* 1979;15(suppl):81-92.
26. Fernstrom JD. Effects of the diet on brain neurotransmitters. *Metabolism.* 1977;26:207-223.
27. Young SN, Ervin FR, Pihl RO, Finn P. Biochemical aspects of tryptophan depletion in primates. *Psychopharmacology.* 1989;98:508-511.
28. Gessa GL, Biggio G, Fadda F, Corsini GV, Tagliamonte A. Effect of the oral administration of tryptophan-free amino acid mixtures on serum tryptophan, brain tryptophan and serotonin metabolism. *J Neurochem.* 1974;22:869-870.
29. Walters JK, Davis M, Sheard MH. Tryptophan-free diet: effects on the acoustic startle reflex in rats. *Psychopharmacology.* 1979;62:103-109.
30. Smith SE, Pihl RO, Young SW, Ervin FR. A test of possible cognitive and en-

vironmental influences on the mood lowering effect of tryptophan depletion in normal males. *Psychopharmacology.* 1987;91:451-457.

31. Abbott FV, Etienne P, Franklin KBJ, Morgan MJ, Sewitch MJ, Young SN. Acute tryptophan depletion eliminates morphine analgesia in the cold-pressor test in humans. *Psychopharmacology.* 1992;108:60-66.
32. Delgado PL, Charney DS, Price LH, Aghajanian GK, Heninger GR. Tryptophan depletion alters mood in depression. In: The American Psychiatric Association's new research abstracts; May 12-17, 1990; New York, NY. Abstract NR412.
33. Delgado PL, Charney DS, Price LH, Aghajanian GK, Landis H, Heninger GR. Serotonin function and the mechanism of antidepressant action. *Arch Gen Psychiatry.* 1990;47:411-418.
34. Delgado PL, Charney DS, Miller H, Licinio J, Salomon R, Heninger GR. Serotonin function and antidepressant action. In: The American Psychiatric Association's new research abstracts; May 11-16,1991; New Orleans, La. Abstract NR631.
35. American Psychiatric Association, Committee on Nomenclature and Statistics. *Diagnostic and Statistical Manual of Mental Disorders, Revised Third Edition.* Washington, DC: American Psychiatric Association; 1987.
36. Leckman JF, Sholomskas D, Thompson WD, Belanger A, Weissman MM. Best estimate of lifetime psychiatric diagnoses: a methodological study. *Arch Gen Psychiatry.* 1982;39:879-883.
37. Goodman WK, Price LH, Rassmussen SA, Mazure C, Fleischman RL, Hill CL, Heninger GR, Charney DS. The Yale-Brown Obsessive-Compulsive Scale, I: development, use, and reliability. *Arch Gen Psychiatry.* 1989;46:1006-1011.
38. Goodman WK, Price LH, Rassmussen SA, Mazure C, Delgado P, Heninger GR, Charney DS. The Yale-Brown Obsessive-Compulsive Scale, II: validity. *Arch Gen Psychiatry.* 1989;46:1012-1016.
39. Mazure CM, Nelson JC, Price LH. Reliability and validity of the symptoms of major depressive illness. *Arch Gen Psychiatry.* 1986;43:451-456.
40. Beck AT, Ward CH, Mendelson M, Mock J, Erbaugh J. An inventory for measuring depression. *Arch Gen Psychiatry.* 1961;4:561-571.
41. Woods SW, Charney DS, Goodman WK, Heninger GR. Carbon dioxide-induced anxiety. *Arch Gen Psychiatry.* 1988;45:43-52.
42. Anderson GM, Young JG, Cohen DJ, Schlicht KR, Patel N. Liquid-chromatographic determination of serotonin and tryptophan in whole blood and plasma. *Clin Chem.* 1981;27:775-776.
43. *SAS/STAT Users Guide.* Cary, NC: SAS Institute Inc; 1990.
44. Dixon WJ, Brown MB, Engelman L, Jennrich RI. *BMDP Statistical Software.* Berkeley, Calif: University of California Press; 1990.
45. Baldessarini RJ, Marsh E. Fluoxetine and side effects. *Arch Gen Psychiatry.* 1990;47:191-192.
46. Halaris AE, Belendiuk KT, Freedman DX. Antidepressant drugs affect dopamine uptake. *Biochem Pharmacol.* 1975;24:1896-1898.
47. Halaris AE, Freedman DX. Psychotropic drugs and dopamine uptake inhibition. In: Freedman DX, ed. *Biology of the Major Psychoses.* New York, NY: Raven Press; 1975:247-258.
48. Austin LS, Lydiard RB, Ballenger JC, Cohen BM, Laraia MT, Zealberg JJ, Fossey MD, Ellinwood EH. Dopamine blocking activity of clomipramine in patients with obsessive-compulsive disorder. *Biol Psychiatry.* 1991;30:225-232.
49. Heslop K, Portas CM, Curzon G. Effect of alternate tryptophan availability on tissues and extra-cellular serotonin in the rat cortex. In: Rollema J, Westerink B, Drijshout WJ, eds. *Molecules in Neuroscience.* Neppel, the Netherlands: Kriptsreproduction; 1991:259-261.
50. Swedo SE, Pietrini P, Leonard HL, Schapiro MB, Rettew DC, Goldberger EL, Rapoport SI, Rapoport JL, Grady CL. Cerebral glucose metabolism in childhood-onset obsessive-compulsive disorder: revisualization during pharmacotherapy. *Arch Gen Psychiatry.* 1992;49:690-694.
51. Baxter LR Jr, Schwartz JM, Bergman KS, Szuba MP, Guze BH, Mazziotta JC, Alazraki A, Selin CE, Ferng H-K, Munford P, Phelps ME. Caudate glucose metabolic rate changes with both drug and behavior therapy for obsessive-compulsive disorder. *Arch Gen Psychiatry.* 1992;49:681-689.
52. Molliver LA, Molliver ME. Evidence for dual serotonergic projections to neocortex: axons from the dorsal raphe nuclei are differentially vulnerable to the neurotoxin p-chloroamphetamine PCA. *Exp Neurol.* 1988;102:23-36.

Familial Correlates of Reduced Central Serotonergic System Function in Patients With Personality Disorders

Emil F. Coccaro, MD; Jeremy M. Silverman, PhD; Howard M. Klar, MD; Thomas B. Horvath, MD; Larry J. Siever, MD

Background: To test the hypothesis that evidence of reduced central serotonergic (5-HT) system function in probands with personality disorders is associated with an elevated morbid risk of psychopathological conditions putatively associated with 5-HT dysfunction in first-degree relatives of these probands.

Methods: Data were collected during a study of the 5-HT correlates of behavior in male patients with *DSM-III* personality disorders conducted at a Veterans Affairs medical center. Probands in this study were selected from those patients who had undergone both a fenfluramine hydrochloride challenge and a family history assessment. Axis II diagnoses were made acording to *DSM-III* criteria after a structured interview of the proband, using the Structured Interview for Diagnosing Personality Disorders, given by two raters and a similar interview with a knowledgeable informant by another rater.

Results: Reduced prolactin responses to the 5-HT releasing/uptake inhibiting agent fenfluramine was associated with an elevated morbid risk of impulsive personality disorder traits in the first-degree relatives of patients with a primary *DSM-III* diagnosis of a personality disorder. Quantitative scores on assessments of impulsive aggression in the probands were not correlated with an increased morbid risk for impulsive personality disorder traits. A trend in the same direction was noted for affective personality disorder traits and alcoholism.

Conclusions: These results suggest that a central 5-HT system abnormality in probands is associated with an increased risk of impulsive aggression in their first-degree relatives, and that assessment of central 5-HT system function in probands may be a more sensitive parameter for identification of this familial trait than the presence of impulsive aggressive behaviors in the proband.

(*Arch Gen Psychiatry. 1994;51:318-324*)

From the Clinical Neuroscience Research Unit, Department of Psychiatry, Medical College of Pennsylvania, Philadelphia (Dr Coccaro); the Department of Psychiatry, Mt Sinai School of Medicine, New York, NY (Drs Silverman and Siever); the Department of Psychiatry, St Lukes-Roosevelt Medical Center, New York, NY (Dr Klar); and the Northport Veterans Affairs Medical Center, Northport, NY (Dr Horvath).

REDUCED CENTRAL serotonin (5-HT) system function, as reflected by reduced concentrations of lumbar cerebrospinal fluid 5-hydroxyindolacetic acid (CSF 5-HIAA) or reduced prolactin (PRL) responses to short-term challenge with various central 5-HT agents, has frequently been associated with aggressive, suicidal, and impulsive aggressive behaviors in patients with personality disorders.[1-7] This, along with experimental data from animal studies, suggests an inverse relationship between indices of central 5-HT system function and of impulsive aggressive behaviors.[8] Evidence for similar relationships between central 5-HT system function and other behaviors or affects, such as the magnitude of a depressive state, has also been reported[9-11] but with less consistency compared with that of suicidal and/or impulsive aggressive behavior.

Indices of reduced central 5-HT system function thus appear to reflect a trait vulnerability toward suicidal and/or impulsive aggressive behavior given a sufficient adverse stimulus.[8] Reductions in CSF 5-HIAA concentrations[1-3,12] or in neuroendocrine responses to central 5-HT agents correlate with lifetime history, or by self-assessment, of these behaviors.[4-7] Since indices of central 5-HT system function[13-17] and of impulsive aggressive behavior[18] ap-

See Subjects and Methods on next page

SUBJECTS AND METHODS

PROBAND SAMPLE

This study is based on data collected during a study of the serotonergic correlates of behavior in male patients with *DSM-III* personality disorder (10 white, seven Hispanic, one black) conducted at the Bronx (NY) Veterans Affairs Medical Center of the Mt Sinai School of Medicine. Probands in this study were selected from those patients who had undergone a fenfluramine challenge[4] and a family history assessment,[22,23] as previously reported. Informed consent, as approved by the institutional review board, was granted by all subjects for all procedures reported. Axis I diagnoses were made according to *DSM-III* criteria[24] after a structured interview,using the Schedule for Schizophrenia and Affective Disorders–Lifetime Version[25] given by a reliable rater (κ coefficient for two reliable raters for major depression was 0.87). Axis II diagnoses were made according to *DSM-III* criteria after a structured interview of the proband, using the Structured Interview for Diagnosing Personality Disorders,[26] given by two reliable raters (κ coefficients for two reliable raters was 0.81 for borderline personality disorder) and a similar interview with a knowledgeable informant by another rater. A final diagnosis was made by consensus of all available ratings in a meeting chaired by a senior clinician who was blind to the biologic and familial data (H.M.K. or T.B.H.). All probands had a primary *DSM-III* diagnosis of an Axis II personality disorder. Fifteen met *DSM-III* criteria for one or more specific personality disorders (eight each for borderline, histrionic, schizotypal, and paranoid personality disorder and five or less for compulsive, narcissistic, and avoidant personality disorder); three met criteria for a mixed personality disorder. While many probands had current (n=6) or past (n=8) Axis I diagnoses of major depression, the presence of a personality disorder always preceded the onset of the first (or only) episode of major depression and was always the primary cause of functional morbidity.

FENFLURAMINE CHALLENGE STUDY

The methods for this procedure have been described in detail elsewhere.[4] Each subject underwent a fenfluramine challenge procedure after being free of all psychotropic medication for at least 2 weeks and after being on a low-monoamine diet for at least 3 days. All subjects were medically healthy as determined by a comprehensive medical evaluation. Each procedure began at 8 AM after an overnight fast since midnight. At 8 AM an intravenous catheter was placed in a forearm vein and was kept open with normal saline solution. Baseline samples for plasma PRL were obtained at 9:45 and 9:55 AM. Fenfluramine hydrochloride, 60 mg, was given orally at 10 AM. Postfenfluramine samples for plasma PRL were then obtained hourly until 3 PM. Peak delta PRL (ie, peak PRL after fenfluramine minus the averaged baseline PRL; hereafter referred to as PRL-fenfluramine) was used as the main outcome measurement of PRL response to the fenfluramine challenge. This measurement has been found to correlate extremely highly with the PRL response over time (ie, PRL response as expressed as the delta area under the curve) to fenfluramine challenge.[4] Prolactin was assayed by radioimmunoassay[27]; intra-assay and interassay coefficients of variation were 4% and 8%, respectively.

FAMILY HISTORY DIAGNOSES IN THE FIRST-DEGREE RELATIVES OF PROBANDS WITH PERSONALITY DISORDERS

Family history data were collected during the same period that fenfluramine challenge studies were being performed. The family history rater (J.M.S.), proband, and/or family history informant(s) were not aware of the PRL-fenfluramine values of the probands during the family history assessment phase of the study. The specifics of the family history interview methods have been described in detail elsewhere.[22,23] Diagnostic information, blind to proband diagnosis, was collected on all first-degree relatives of all probands primarily through telephone interviews with knowledgeable informants. The families of 18 of the total 20 probands were assessed with at least one or two family informants. In addition to the Family History Research Diagnostic Criteria, supplementary family history criteria for impulsive, affective,[23] and schizophrenia-related[22,28] personality disorder traits were assessed (these criteria are available from the authors on request).

Family history criteria for impulsive personality disorder (IPD) traits were designed to characterize individuals with chronic impulsive and aggressive behaviors and are similar to the impulsivity, intense anger, and aggressive-related items found in the diagnostic criteria for *DSM-III* borderline and antisocial personality disorder. Family history criteria for affective personality disorder (APD) traits were designed to characterize individuals with chronic affective instability not due to a concurrent major mood disorder. These items are similar to the Research Diagnostic Criteria diagnosis of labile personality. Finally, family history criteria for schizophrenia-related personality disorder traits were designed to characterize individuals with chronic cognitive/perceptual distortions and/or social deficits not attributable to schizophrenia or any other chronic psychotic disorder. These items represent a condensation of the *DSM-III* criteria for schizotypal and paranoid personality disorder.

A diagnosis was considered present in relatives who met criteria for at least a "probable" diagnosis. This diagnosis was assigned if there was any uncertainty about the presence of one, and only one, criterion in a diagnostic category. As described elsewhere,[22,23] good interrater reliability was found for all family history diagnoses assessed together, and for each of the supplementary personality disorder diagnostic categories taken individually (κ range, 0.67 to 1.00).

Continued on next page

ASSESSMENT OF IMPULSIVE AGGRESSIVE BEHAVIOR AND DEPRESSION IN PROBANDS

As in previous studies,[4-6] historical (Brown-Goodwin Assessment for Life History of Aggression[1] [BGA] and Hamilton Depression Rating Scale[29]) and self-report (Buss-Durkee Hostility Inventory[30] [BDHI]) data regarding impulsive aggression (BGA, n=17; BDHI, n=18) and state severity of depression (Hamilton Depression Rating Scale, n=18) were available from the probands.

MORBID RISK ANALYSES

The morbid risk for a disorder in first-degree relatives of a proband group was assessed using the Weinberg Abridged Method.[31] Morbid risk is the proportion of the "number of cases with the disorder" to the "number of individuals at risk for developing the disorder." The figure for the "individuals at risk" is corrected by the "age of risk." Individuals with the disorder in question or individuals beyond the age of risk were counted as a single "lifetime of risk"; individuals within the age of risk and without the disorder in question were counted as half a lifetime of risk. The age of risks employed were 15 to 59 years for major affective disorder and 15 to 39 years for schizophrenia, alcoholism, drug-use disorder, and IPD, APD, and schizophrenia-related personality disorder traits. Individuals older than 15 years were considered to have lived through their age of risk for antisocial personality disorder. Differences in the relative morbid risks were assessed using the "Test of the Difference Between Two Proportions" as described by Fleiss[32]:

$$z=\frac{MR_1-MR_2}{\sqrt{pq\left(\frac{1}{n_1}+\frac{1}{n_2}\right)}}$$

where p equals the number of "cases" in the total sample divided by the number of lifetimes of risk in the total sample; q equals $1-p$; and n_1 and n_2 equal the number of relatives in the two samples, respectively.

For the main analyses, probands were divided into two groups by median split as a function of PRL-fenfluramine values. The median PRL-fenfluramine value divided this sample at 6.5 ng/mL. Hence, patients with values below this cutoff fell into a "reduced" PRL-fenfluramine group (mean [±SD], 3.6±2.2 ng/mL) while those above this cutoff fell into the "nonreduced" PRL-fenfluramine group (mean, 10.7±4.1 ng/mL). For purposes of comparison, the mean PRL-fenfluramine value in a comparable group of healthy male volunteers (n=14; mean age, 35.9±7.9 years), as previously reported with this sample,[4] was 12.5±6.9 ng/mL.

A secondary analysis, comparing the morbid risk of IPD traits as a function of BDHI (ie, "assault+irritability" and BDHI "A+I") and BGA scores in probands was similarly performed to compare the aggregation of biologic and phenomenologic variables with these traits in first-degree biologic relatives of patients with personality disorders.

pear to be relatively stable over time, it is possible that the relationship between these two variables represents an enduring, and possibly heritable, psychobiologic trait.

An association between reductions in indices of central 5-HT system function and familial psychopathologic conditions has been reported for healthy volunteers,[19] depressed patients,[20] and alcoholic violent offenders.[21] In one study,[19] reduced lumbar CSF 5-HIAA concentrations in healthy nonpsychiatric probands was associated with a family history of depression. In another study, depressed patients with family history of alcoholism had reduced lumbar CSF 5-HIAA concentration compared with similar patients without this family history.[20] Finally, a trivariate relationship between reduced lumbar CSF 5-HIAA concentration, family history of alcoholism, and life history of impulsive aggression is suggested by data in a study of alcoholic violent offenders and impulsive arsonists.[21] Hence, there is preliminary evidence indicating that reductions of central 5-HT system function in humans are associated with familial psychopathologic conditions that have been associated with an abnormality in central 5-HT system function (eg, depression or alcoholism).

To explore the familial correlates of reduced central 5-HT function, we examined the morbid risk of a variety of major psychiatric (ie, Axis I) disorders and of personality traits (ie, Axis II) reflective of chronic impulsive aggression, chronic affective instability, chronic cognitive/perceptual distortions, and/or social deficits, in the first-degree biologic relatives of 18 male patients with a primary *DSM-III* diagnosis of personality disorder who had undergone a fenfluramine hydrochloride challenge procedure. Fenfluramine, a central 5-HT–releasing/uptake-inhibiting agent, produces a robust PRL response, on short-term single-dose challenge, which can be used as an index of overall function of limbic and hypothalamic 5-HT synapses.[4] Based on previous data, we hypothesized that reduced PRL responses to fenfluramine challenge would be associated with an increased morbid risk of impulsive aggressive behavior, affective lability, and alcohol abuse in the first-degree relatives of personality-disordered probands.

RESULTS

CHARACTERISTICS OF THE PROBAND SAMPLE

Selected demographic, biologic, and phenomenologic data for the proband sample are displayed in **Table 1**. There were no significant differences between the reduced and nonreduced PRL-fenfluramine groups on any variable except for higher BDHI A+I scores in the reduced PRL-fenfluramine group. As previously reported,[4] PRL-fenfluramine values

Table 1. Characteristics of Personality Disordered Probands as a Function of 'Reduced' and 'Nonreduced' Prolactin (PRL)-Fenfluramine Values*

	Personality Disorder Reduced PRL-Fenfluramine (N=9)	Personality Disorder Nonreduced PRL-Fenfluramine (N=9)	*P*
PRL-fenfluramine, ng/mL	3.6±2.2	10.7±4.1	...
Basal PRL, ng/mL	5.1±3.0	5.5±2.5	NS
Fenfluramine level, ng/mL	87.6±8.9 (n=5)	87.0±15.0 (n=7)	NS
Age, y	34.6±8.1	38.9±8.0	NS
BDHI ("A+I") score	16.8±2.6	13.0±4.6	.05†
BGA score	19.7±7.3 (n=9)	14.1±8.8 (n=8)	NS
History of major affective disorder (current/past/none)	4/4/1	2/4/3	NS
Hamilton Depression Rating Scale score	17.3±5.6	12.3±8.1	NS

**BDHI indicates Buss-Durkee Hostility Inventory; BGA, Brown-Goodwin Assessment for Life History of Aggression; A+I, Assault plus Irritability; and NS, not significant.*
†By t *test.*

Table 2. Relative Morbid Risks for Research Diagnostic Criteria Family History Axis I and II Disorders and Traits in First-Degree Relatives* as a Function of 'Reduced' and 'Nonreduced' Prolactin (PRL) Responses to Fenfluramine Challenge

	Reduced PRL-Fenfluramine Group		Nonreduced PRL-Fenfluramine Group	
	No. of Cases Among Relatives	Morbid Risk†	No. of Cases Among Relatives	Morbid Risk†
All disorders				
Axis I and/or II	25	0.725§	13	0.481
Axis I only	12	0.393	11	0.415
Axis II only	19	0.551‖	6	0.207
Axis I				
Major affective disorder	6	0.214	9	0.353
Schizophrenia‡	0	0.000	0	0.000
Drug use disorder	1	0.032	1	0.034
Alcoholism	7	0.215§	2	0.070
Axis II				
Antisocial personality disorder	2	0.046	0	0.000
Impulsive personality disorder traits	8	0.254¶	2	0.068
Affective personality disorder traits	10	0.299§	4	0.138
Schizophrenia-related personality disorder traits	6	0.185¶	1	0.035

**Relatives of probands in the "reduced" PRL-fenfluramine group: n=43 ("age-corrected lifetimes of risk" for antisocial personality disorder [AsPD], 43.0; major affective disorder [MAD], 28.0; and for all other categories, 30.5 to 34.5). Relatives of probands in the "nonreduced" PRL-fenfluramine group: n=33 ("age-corrected lifetimes of risk" for AsPD, 33.0; for MAD, 25.5; and for all other categories, 26.5 to 29.0).*
†Morbid risk indicates cases divided by the "age-corrected lifetimes of risk."
‡Includes chronic schizoaffective and chronic undifferentiated functional psychosis.
§P<.1 (two tailed).
‖P<.01 (two tailed).
¶P<.05 (two tailed).

were inversely correlated with BDHI A+I and BGA scores (BDHI A+I, *r*=−.79, n=18, *P*<.001; BGA, *r*=−.56, n=17, *P*<.05), which were also correlated (*r*=.81, n=17, *P*<.001); there was no correlation with Hamilton Depression Rating Scale scores (*r*=−.25, n=18, *P*=not significant).

MORBID RISK ANALYSES OF THE PROBAND SAMPLE: OVERALL FINDINGS

Table 2 shows the family history diagnoses of the proband sample and the morbid risks for the Axis I and Axis II (disorders and traits), as global categories and as specific disorders and/or traits, examined as a function of reduced and nonreduced PRL-fenfluramine values. Overall, the morbid risk of any familial Axis I or II condition was increased in probands with reduced PRL-fenfluramine values (*z*=2.18, *P*<.03). This was due to the increased morbid risk of familial personality disorder traits (*z*=3.04, *P*<.002); morbid risk of familial Axis I disorders was not elevated as a function of PRL-fenfluramine values (*z*=.19, *P*=not significant).

MORBID RISK ANALYSES OF THE PROBAND SAMPLE: PRL-FENFLURAMINE CORRELATES WITH SPECIFIC DISORDERS AND/OR PERSONALITY DISORDER TRAITS

Among the personality disorder traits studied, there was a significantly increased morbid risk of IPD traits among

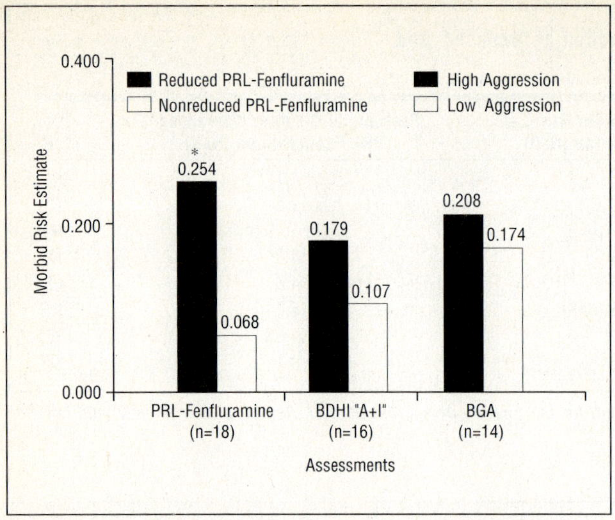

Comparison of morbid risk estimates for impulsive personality disorder traits in first-degree relatives as a function of pathologic prolactin (PRL)–fenfluramine hydrochloride values (ie, low vs high by median split), Buss-Durkee Hostility Inventory "Assault+Irritability" (BDHI A+I) scores (ie, high vs low by median split), and Brown-Goodwin Assessment for Life History of Aggression (BGA) (ie, high vs low by median split) in the personality-disordered proband subjects. Asterisk indicates P<.029.

the relatives of probands with reduced PRL-fenfluramine values (z=2.19, P<.029). A marginally increased morbid risk for APD traits in the biologic relatives of probands with reduced PRL-fenfluramine values was also noted (z=1.68, P<.093), as was a significantly increased morbid risk for schizophrenia-related personality disorder traits (z=2.06, P<.039). The latter observation, however, may be explained by the fact that four (67%) of the six relatives who were positive for schizophrenia-related personality disorder traits in the reduced PRL-fenfluramine group came from only one proband, without whom the difference in morbid risk for familial schizophrenia-related personality disorder traits was not statistically significant (0.073 vs 0.035, z=0.71, P=not significant).

Among the Axis I disorders studied, a marginally increased morbid risk of familial alcoholism was noted among probands with reduced PRL-fenfluramine values (z=1.77, P=.077). Reduced PRL-fenfluramine values in probands were not associated with an increased morbid risk of major affective disorder, schizophrenia, antisocial personality disorder, or drug use disorder among their relatives.

RELATIONSHIP BETWEEN FAMILIAL IPD/APD TRAITS AND FAMILIAL ALCOHOLISM

The comorbid frequency of IPD traits, APD traits, and/or alcoholism was low (eight of 18; 44% of cases with any familial diagnoses) and evenly distributed: IPD with APD, three cases (17%); IPD with alcoholism, two cases (11%); and APD with alcoholism, three cases (17%) (no case had all three). Hence, alcoholism, IPD, and APD traits appeared to aggregate independently within families of these probands.

MORBID RISK ANALYSES FOR IPD TRAITS: COMPARISON WITH DIMENSIONAL MEASURES OF IMPULSIVE AGGRESSION

To determine how the morbid risk of familial IPD traits associated with reduced PRL-fenfluramine values compared with dimensional indices of the impulsive aggressive behaviors that correlated so highly in probands, we also calculated the morbid risks associated with BDHI A+I and BGA scores split by the median for the proband sample (**Figure**). Unlike reduced PRL-fenfluramine values, neither "high" BDHI A+I nor high BGA scores demonstrated a significantly increased morbid risk for familial IPD traits.

COMMENT

In this study, evidence of reduced central 5-HT system function in probands, reflected by reduced PRL-fenfluramine values, was associated with an aggregation of personality disorder traits in first-degree biologic relatives. Among these, traits reflective of impulsive aggression were most clearly associated with reduced PRL-fenfluramine values in the probands. Since reduced PRL-fenfluramine values correlated highly with indices of impulsive aggression in the probands, these data raise the possibility that the IPD traits rated in the relatives of probands (parents as well as siblings) with reduced PRL-fenfluramine values are also correlated with indices of central 5-HT system function and that the abnormalities in central 5-HT system function demonstrated in the probands are heritable. This hypothesis can be tested at a later time by examination of indices of central 5-HT system function in relatives of patients with personality disorders.

The observation that familial IPD "traits" did not aggregate in probands with elevated scores on the assessments of impulsive aggressive behavior suggests that an index of central 5-HT system function in probands may be more sensitive as a predictor of IPD traits in relatives than assessments of the behavior in the proband. This may reflect a greater error variance in our assessments of impulsive aggression. Alternately, this observation may reflect the fact that impulsive aggressive behavior is biologically overdetermined and is not invariably associated with reduced central 5-HT system function in all probands.[33] Under this model, individuals with reduced central 5-HT system function may manifest impulsive aggressive behavior while the converse in impulsive aggressive individuals might not be true in as many cases.

The observation that reduced PRL responses to fenfluramine challenge were not associated with an increased morbid risk of familial Axis I disorders, in general, or of familial major affective disorder, schizophrenia, drug use disorder, or antisocial personality disorder, specifically, suggests that reduced PRL responses to fenfluramine challenge in probands are not associated with an increased risk of familial psychopathologic conditions in a nonspecific manner. However, reduced PRL responses to fenfluramine challenge in these probands were associated with a trend toward an increased morbid risk of familial APD traits and familial alcoholism. Since familial IPD traits and these two variables appeared to sort independently of each other, it is unlikely that the increased morbid risk of familial IPD traits in reduced PRL-fenfluramine probands accounts for these findings. Moreover, the family history method used herein may not have had sufficient sensitivity to identify all true cases of familial APD or alcoholism.[34] It is possible that direct interview of all relatives (ie, family study) would have identified additional cases of familial APD traits and familial alcoholism in the probands with reduced PRL-fenfluramine values and that a significantly increased morbid risk for these familial diagnoses would have been found.

THE DATA suggesting an association of increased morbid risk of familial alcoholism and/or APD traits are consistent with those of other studies. Reduced concentrations of CSF 5-HIAA in probands of healthy volunteers and of psychiatric patients have previously been shown to correlate with an increased incidence of familial affective disorder[19] and alcoholism.[20,21] Experimental evidence suggesting an important role for central 5-HT in the maintenance of mood[10,11] and in the regulation of alcohol intake[35] makes this possibility highly likely, particularly if aspects of central 5-HT function are under genetic control.[36] Accordingly, it is possible that reduced central 5-HT function in probands represents a risk factor for IPD traits, APD traits, and alcoholism in family members. Under this model, the phenotypic expression of any (ie, one or more) of these conditions within individual family members would be determined by other factors (eg, related to other neuronal systems, gender) as yet unknown. Further research will be required to more fully test these hypotheses.

The implication of these data is that reduced central 5-HT system function in probands, associated with an increased incidence of familial IPD traits (and perhaps affective instability and alcoholism), is also present in the biologic relatives of these probands. Hence, these results raise the possibility that central 5-HT system function is under partial genetic control, although environmental factors modifying central 5-HT system function cannot be ruled out in a family history study. Since receptors and other cellular components involved in central 5-HT neurotransmission represent products of the genetic code, central serotonergic system function must be influenced by genetic factors. Indeed, central 5-HT receptor number in rodents is under genetic control.[35] Moreover, CSF 5-HIAA concentrations correlate well over time in rodents[36] and across developmental periods in nonhuman primates,[37] suggesting stability that is consistent with genetic influence on these factors. In humans, CSF 5-HIAA concentrations have been shown to be relatively stable over time in some studies,[13-16] but to vary with the season of study in others.[38,39] On the other hand, CSF 5-HIAA concentrations have been shown to correlate highly on repeated measurement within subjects[16] and to be heritable in a study of monozygotic and dizygotic twins.[40]

Evidence for similar characteristics regarding PRL responses to central 5-HT probes is limited. Prolactin responses to amphetamine challenge have been reported to demonstrate statistically significant ($P<.05$) concordance in monozygotic twins.[41] While PRL responses to amphetamine do not reflect 5-HT stimulation specifically, this finding was interpreted as reflecting a heritable component of 5-HT function.[41] More specifically, PRL responses to fenfluramine were highly correlated within a small group of patients with major affective disorder studied many months apart in the euthymic and depressed state[42] and across a period of at least 1 week in adolescents.[43] This raises the possibility that PRL responses to fenfluramine challenge may be stable enough over time to reflect a trait characteristic of central 5-HT function in humans. Prospective studies examining PRL response to fenfluramine challenge over weeks to years within the same individuals and others employing monozygotic and dizygotic twins will be necessary to assess the stability and heritability of this index of central 5-HT function.

A number of limitations merit further comment. First, the use of the family history method to assess personality traits in first-degree relatives, and our relatively small sample, requires that our conclusions remain tentative at this time. The validity of the family history method to identify impulsive aggressive behavior in family members has not yet been firmly established. As with other behavioral variables (eg, depression), it is possible that this method may underestimate the true frequency of relevant behaviors in family members.[34] Second, family history data cannot establish the presence of a common genetic influence underlying the phenotypic relationship between reduced central 5-HT system function and impulsive aggressive (or other) behaviors in probands. Hence, the nature of familial transmission of impulsive aggressive behavior, and/or 5-HT system function, cannot be determined from this type of analysis regardless of specific methodologic considerations or sample size. However, with these caveats in mind, these data suggest the presence of a common familial, possibly genetic, influence to impulsive aggressive behaviors and reduced central 5-HT system function in patients with personality disorders. Further work will be necessary to confirm this hypothesis and to eluicdate the nature of this influence if present.

Accepted for publication January 11, 1993.

Reprint requests to Department of Psychiatry, MCP/EPPI, Clinical Neuroscience Unit, 3200 Henry Ave, Philadelphia, PA 19129 (Dr Coccaro).

REFERENCES

1. Brown GL, Goodwin FK, Ballenger JC, Goyer PF, Major LF. Aggression in humans correlates with cerebrospinal fluid amine metabolites. *Psychiatry Res.* 1979;1:131-139.
2. Brown GL, Ebert MH, Goyer PF, Jimerson DC, Klein WJ, Bunney WE, Goodwin FK. Aggression, suicide and serotonin: relationships to CSF amine metabolites. *Am J Psychiatry.* 1982;139:741-746.
3. Linnoila M, Virkkunen M, Scheinin M, Nuutila A, Rimon R, Goodwin FK. Low cerebrospinal fluid 5-hydroxyindolacetic acid concentration differentiates impulsive from nonimpulsive violent behavior. *Life Sci.* 1983;33:2609-2614.
4. Coccaro EF, Siever LJ, Klar HM, Maurer G, Cochrane K, Cooper TB, Mohs RC, Davis KL. Serotonergic studies in affective and personality disorder patients: correlates with behavioral aggression and impulsivity. *Arch Gen Psychiatry.* 1989;46:587-599.
5. Coccaro EF, Siever LJ, Kavoussi R, Davis KL. Impulsive aggression in personality disorder: evidence for involvement of 5-HT-1 receptors. *Biol Psychiatry.* 1989;25:86A. Abstract.
6. Coccaro EF, Gabriel S, Siever LJ. Buspirone challenge: preliminary evidence for a role for central 5-HT-1a receptor function in impulsive aggressive behavior in humans. *Psychopharmacol Bull.* 1990;26:393-405.
7. Moss HB, Yao JK, Panzak G. Serotonergic responsivity and behavioral dimensions in antisocial personality disorder with substance abuse. *Biol Psychiatry.* 1990;28:325-338.
8. Coccaro EF. Central serotonin and impulsive aggression. *Br J Psychiatry.* 1989;155:52-62.
9. Asberg M, Thoren P, Traksman L, Bertilsson L, Ringberger V. 'Serotonin depression'—a biochemical subgroup within the affective disorders? *Science.* 1976;191:478-480.
10. Young SN, Smith SE, Pihl RO, Ervin FR. Tryptophan depletion causes a rapid lowering of mood in normal males. *Psychopharmacology.* 1985;87:173-177.
11. Delgado PL, Charney DS, Price LH, Aghajanian GK, Landis H, Heninger GR. Serotonin function and the mechanism of antidepressant action: reversal of antidepressant-induced remission by rapid depletion of plasma tryptophan. *Arch Gen Psychiatry.* 1990;47:411-418.
12. Asberg M, Schalling D, Traksman-Bendz L, Wagner A. Psychobiology of suicide, impulsivity, and related phenomena. In: Meltzer HY, ed. *Psychopharmacology: Third Generation of Progress.* New York, NY: Raven Press; 1987:655-688.
13. Coppen AJ, Prange AJ, Whybrow PC, Noguera R. Abnormalities of indoleamines in affective disorders. *Arch Gen Psychiatry.* 1972;26:474-478.
14. Van Pragg HM. Significance of biochemical parameters in the diagnosis, treatment, and prevention of depressive disorders. *Biol Psychiatry.* 1977;12:101-131.
15. Post RM, Ballenger JC, Goodwin FK. Cerebrospinal fluid studies of neurotransmitter function in manic and depressive illness. In: Wood JH, ed. *Neurobiology of Cerebrospinal Fluid.* New York, NY: Plenum Press; 1980:685-717.
16. Traksman-Benz I, Asberg M, Bertilsson L, Thoren P. CSF monoamine metabolites of depressed patients during illness and after recovery. *Acta Psychiatr Scand.* 1984;69:333-342.
17. Coccaro EF, Siever LJ, Owen KR, Davis KL. Serotonin function in mood and personality disorder. In: Coccaro EF, Murphy DL, eds. *Serotonin in Major Psychiatric Disorders.* Washington, DC: American Psychiatric Press; 1990:71-97.
18. Olweus D. Stability of aggressive reaction patterns in males: a review. *Psychol Bull.* 1979;86:852-875.
19. Sedvall G, Fyro B, Gullberg B, Nyback H, Wiesel FA, Wode-Helgodt B. Relationships in healthy volunteers between concentrations of monoamine metabolites in cerebrospinal fluid and family history of psychiatric morbidity. *Br J Psychiatry.* 1980;136:366-374.
20. Rosenthal NE, Davenport Y, Cowdry RW, Webster MH, Goodwin FK. Monoamine metabolites in cerebrospinal fluid of depressive subtypes. *Psychiatry Res.* 1980;2:113-119.
21. Linnoila M, De Jong J, Virkkunen M. Family history of alcoholism in violent offenders and impulsive fire setters. *Arch Gen Psychiatry.* 1989;46:613-616.
22. Siever LJ, Silverman JM, Horvath T, Klar H, Coccaro E, Keefe RS, Pinkham L, Rinaldi P, Mohs RC, Davis KL. Increased morbid risk of schizophrenia-related disorders in relatives of schizotypal personality disordered patients. *Arch Gen Psychiatry.* 1990;47:634-640.
23. Silverman JM, Pinkham L, Horvath TB, Coccaro EF, Klar H, Schear S, Apter S, Davidson M, Mohs RC, Siever LJ. Affective and impulsive personality disorder traits in the relatives of borderline personality disorder patients. *Am J Psychiatry.* 1991;148:1378-1385.
24. American Psychiatric Association, Committee on Nomenclature and Statistics. *Diagnostic and Statistical Manual of Mental Disorders, Third Edition.* Washington, DC: American Psychiatric Association; 1980.
25. Spitzer RL, Endicott J. *Schedule for Affective Disorders and Schizophrenia.* New York, NY: New York State Psychiatric Institute; 1978.
26. Stangl D, Pfohl B, Zimmerman M. Structured interview for *DSM-III* personality disorder. *Arch Gen Psychiatry.* 1985;42:591-598.
27. Davis BM, Mathe AA, Mohs RC, Levy MI. Effects of probantheline bromide on basal growth hormone, cortisol, and prolactin levels. *Psychoneuroendocrinology.* 1983;8:103-107.
28. Kendler KS, Masterson CC, Ungaro R, Davis KL. A family history study of schizophrenia-related personality disorders. *Am J Psychiatry.* 1984;141:424-427.
29. Guy W. *ECDEU Manual for Psychopharmacology.* Washington, DC: Superintendent of Documents; 1976. US Dept of Health, Education, and Welfare publication ADM 766-338.
30. Buss AJ, Durkee A. An inventory for assessing different kinds of hostility. *J Consult Psychol.* 1957;21:343-348.
31. Slater E, Cowie V. *The Genetics of Mental Disorders.* London, England: Oxford University Press; 1971.
32. Fleiss JL. *Statistical Methods for Rates and Proportions.* New York, NY: John Wiley & Sons Inc; 1981.
33. Eichelman B. Neurochemical and psychopharmacologic aspects of aggressive behavior. In: Meltzer HY, ed. *Psychopharmacology: Third Generation of Progress.* New York, NY: Raven Press; 1987:697-704.
34. Andreasen NC, Rice J, Endicott J, Reich T, Coryell W. The family history approach to diagnosis: how useful is it? *Arch Gen Psychiatry.* 1986;43:421-429.
35. Roy A, Virkkunen M, Linnoila M. Serotonin in suicide, violence and alcoholism. In: Coccaro EF, Murphy DL, eds. *Serotonin in Major Psychiatric Disorders.* Washington, DC: American Psychiatric Press; 1990:187-208.
36. Boehme RE, Ciaranello RD. Genetic control of dopamine and serotonin receptors in brain regions of inbred mice. *Brain Res.* 1983;266:51-65.
37. Degrell I, Zenner K, Kummer P, Stock G. Monamine metabolites in CSF of conscious and unrestrained cats. *Brain Res.* 1983;277:283-287.
38. Higley JD, Suomi SJ, Linnoila M. Developmental influences on the serotonergic system and timidity in the nonhuman primate. In: Coccaro EF, Murphy DL, eds. *Serotonin in Major Psychiatric Disorders.* Washington, DC: American Psychiatric Press; 1990:29-46.
39. Loscenczy MF, Mohs RC, Davis KL. Seasonal variation of human lumbar CSF neurotransmitter metabolite concentration. *Psychiatry Res.* 1984;12:79-87.
40. Brewerton TD, Berrittini WH, Nurnberger JI, Linnoila M. Analysis of seasonal fluctuations of CSF monoamine metabolites and neuropeptides in normal controls: findings with 5-HIAA and HVA. *Psychiatry Res.* 1988;23:257-265.
41. Oxenstierna G, Edman G, Iselius L, Oreland L. Concentrations of monoamine metabolites in the cerebrospinal fluid of twins and unrelated individuals—a genetic study. *J Psychiatr Res.* 1986;20:19-29.
42. Nurnberger JI, Gershon ES, Simmons S, Ebert M, Kessler LR, Dibble ED, Jimerson DC, Guroff JJ, Storch FL. Behavioral, biochemical and neuroendocrine responses to amphetamine in normal twins and 'well-state' bipolar patients. *Psychoneuroendocrinology.* 1982;7:163-176.
43. Stoff DM, Pasatiempo A, Yeung J, Bridger WH, Rabinovich H. Test-retest reliability of the prolactin and cortisol responses to fenfluramine challenge in disruptive behavior disorders. *Psychiatry Res.* 1992;42:62-72.

ORIGINAL ARTICLE

Incidence of Dementia in a Population Older Than 75 Years in the United Kingdom

Eugene S. Paykel, MD, FRCP, FRCPsych; Carol Brayne, MSc, MD, MRCP, MFPHM; Felicia A. Huppert, PhD; Caroline Gill, MSc; Claire Barkley, MB, ChB, MRCPsych; Eric Gehlhaar, MB, MRCPsych, DGM; Lynn Beardsall, PhD; Deborah M. Girling, MA, MB, BChir, MRCPsych; Penelope Pollitt, PhD; Daniel O'Connor, MD, FRANZCPsych

Background: Incidence studies have been relatively neglected in psychiatric epidemiology. They are particularly important for dementia, since prevalence rates are affected by length of survial, which itself falls with increasing age and presence of dementia.

Methods: Two-wave community study of 1195 elderly subjects aged older than 75 years, restudied 2.4 years after a community prevalence study. A two-stage method was used, comprising the Mini-Mental State Examination followed in a stratified sample by the Cambridge Examination for Mental Disorders of the Elderly (CAMDEX) interview. Incidence rates were based on person-years at risk.

Results: Annual incidence rates for dementia were 2.3% for subjects initially aged 75 to 79 years, 4.6% for ages 80 to 84 years, and 8.5% for ages 85 to 89 years, approximately doubling every 5 years. Rates did not differ significantly by sex, educational level, or social class. Twice as many additional individuals received a diagnosis of minimal dementia not reaching case threshold.

Conclusions: The findings show high rates of new onset dementia, increasing markedly with age, and suggest rapid acceleration of one or more processes that is common in advanced age.

(Arch Gen Psychiatry. 1994;51:325-332)

From the Departments of Psychiatry (Drs Paykel, Huppert, Barkley, Beardsall, Gehlhaar, and Girling) and Community Medicine (Dr Brayne), University of Cambridge (England); MRC Biostatistics Unit, Cambridge (Ms Gill); Department of Old Age Psychiatry, Monash University, Melbourne, Australia (Dr O'Connor); and the Australian National University, Canberra (Dr Pollitt).

THERE HAVE been many studies of the prevalence of dementia.[1,2] Rates double with age approximately every 5 years. In the Epidemiologic Catchment Area Study, severe cognitive impairment was based solely on the Mini-Mental State Examination (MMSE),[3] which can include transient causes of cognitive impairment, such as toxic confusion or depression. Prevalences were 1.29% (aged 65 to 74 years), 3.83% (aged 75 to 84 years), and 10.14% (85 years and older).[4]

Prevalence studies, although valuable in estimating service needs, have limitations. Prevalence is affected not only by onset of the disorder but also by its persistence and by survival of cases. In dementia, survival is reduced both by increasing age and by dementia itself. Unbiased comparison can be achieved only with incidence studies. Also, because dementia implies cognitive decline, it is best demonstrated by measurement of change between two or more points rather than from a single low level of performance. The effects of such potential confounding factors on cognitive test scores as education and culture can also best be controlled for in this way.

Incidence studies of dementia are difficult. Large samples must be followed up and examined at two or more time points to eliminate prevalent cases and then establish new cases. High death rates lead to much sample attrition and there are liable to be few subjects aged older than 75 years, because they have very high death rates and the base sample distribution is skewed to the younger elderly. Reliable rates require a diagnostic interview rather than solely a cognitive test, but since there are not precise cutoff points between

See Methods on next page

METHODS

THE PREVALENCE WAVE

The prevalence wave for this study was the Hughes Hall Project for Later Life, carried out and fully reported by O'Connor et al.[9] The sampling frame, often used in epidemiologic studies,[10,11] was based on the fact that each United Kingdom resident is registered with a specific general practitioner to obtain health care. All those aged 75 years and older on the lists of six group practices in the City of Cambridge and one in three of a seventh practice were approached. Cambridge is a small, stable city and in the elderly, with high medical needs, nonregistration was very unlikely except in long-term residents of institutions, which were therefore checked separately for residents' last general practitioners. Subjects (response rate 93%) received a structured interview from trained lay interviewers, which included the MMSE[3] and some other information.

All those who scored below 24 on the MMSE (scored using the best of serial sevens or WORLD spelled backward) and a 23% sample of those who scored 24 or 25 received further interview from a psychiatrist using the Cambridge Examination for Mental Disorders of the Elderly (CAMDEX).[12,13] Those who scored 26 or above were assumed to be nondemented.

INCIDENCE WAVE: THE SAMPLE

Sampling for the incidence wave is shown in the **Figure**. The basic sample constituted 1778 initially nondemented subjects. They were derived from an initial cohort of 1968 subjects, of whom 190 had satisfied criteria for mild or greater prevalent dementia and were therefore excluded. Thirty-seven subjects with minimal dementia were included. The initial sample differed from that in the main prevalence report[9] by the following: including one additional practice, excluding one practice in which a different approach (only those who replied to an initial letter were interviewed) had resulted in a high refusal rate that might have produced bias, and also excluding subjects resident in rural areas outside the city (N=92) so as to provide a homogeneous urban sample, spouses of prevalent dements (N=22) because they were involved in an intervention study, and the accidental exclusion of some subjects later found to have been wrongly coded as demented (N=82). Subjects were interviewed in the prevalence wave between August 1985 and July 1987, and they were restudied in March 1988 to March 1990, a mean of 2.4 years later. Deaths were ascertained. Subjects who had moved were traced and interviewed. At the time of original study most (87.8%) had been resident in the community, with a further 8.3% in warden-assisted accommodation, 3.1% in residential homes, and 0.8% in long-stay hospitals.

The Figure shows the results of the follow-up. A total of 305 (17.2%) of the original sample had died, leaving 1473 survivors of whom 1195 (81.1% of survivors, 67.2% of total prevalence nondemented sample) were successfully restudied. The main unavailability of follow-up in survivors was due to refusal (190, 12.9% of survivors). Sixty-one individuals were away from home and could not be contacted, and 27 were too ill to be interviewed.

THE SCREENING INTERVIEW

The incidence wave used the same two-stage method, but with more extensive sampling. The screening interview was administered by six trained lay interviewers. Quality control was monitored by regular meetings with review of audiotapes of field interviews. The interview was similar to the prevalence screening interview, comprising questions on perceived physical health and well-being, activities of daily living, medication, questions on any change in circumstances, together with the MMSE. There were 19 additional questions complying with Medical Research Council guidelines on Alzheimer's disease,[14] but they were not involved in this report. In the first two general practices the cognitive section of the CAMDEX, CAMCOG, was administered but only the MMSE score, within it, was used. The MMSE was administered without the item spelling WORLD backward because of complexity of scoring (M. Folstein, MD, oral communication). As the alternative serial sevens item is more difficult, scores are shifted downward[15] and the cut point was adjusted to 21. For subsequent sampling, prevalence wave MMSEs were also recalculated.

SELECTION FOR DIAGNOSTIC ASSESSMENT

Following screening, subjects were selected for diagnostic assessment. At this point 114 subjects (9.5% of the restudied sample) refused any further participation. Among 548 selected for interview, 74 refused the interviewer; 13 died before interview or were too ill to test. A total of 483 subjects (40.4% of those screened) were interviewed in the diagnostic stage, an average of 1.8±1.5 months (mean±SD) after screening.

The sampling strategy for diagnostic interview was designed to provide reliable incidence estimates and to enable further neuropsychological study of certain groups (2, 3, 4, and 6 below). The samples (numbers interviewed/numbers screened in parentheses) were as follows: (1) those scoring 21 or less on MMSE (131 of 204); (2) those declining four or more on MMSE (with increased risk of dementia), but still above 21 (62 of 84); (3) those scoring 29 or 30 on both occasions (to study good preservation) (45 of 68); (4) those with incomplete MMSE (five of 35); (5) those aged 87 years and older at the incidence wave (to provide sufficient very old) (69 of 91); (6) subjects who had previously received special neuropsychological study in the prevalence wave[16] (41 of 49); (7) subjects minimally demented in the prevalence wave (all received CAMDEX approximately annually from the original investigators; the 2-year interview was used for this study [22 of 22]); and (8) a random selection (108 of 642) taken from those who remained, sampled by age and general practice. In the first two practices, a high sampling fraction of one in two was used to identify sampling for the remaining practices that would produce sufficient but not too large interview numbers (1:15 for ages 77 to 82 years, 1:6 for ages 83 to 86 years).

THE DIAGNOSTIC ASSESSMENT

This comprised CAMDEX administered by psychiatrists and one research nurse supervised by a psychiatrist. CAMDEX[12,13] is a structured interview, including a mental state examination, medical and psychiatric history, detailed cognitive testing, brief physical examination, and interview with an informant. In this study, additional items included the Hamilton Depression Scale,[17] the Clinical Interview for Depression,[18] the Nottingham Life Satisfaction Index,[19] more detailed family history, and possible risk factors. Venipuncture was undertaken where possible to assist exclusion of thyroid disorder and diabetes. Some subjects subsequently received detailed neuropsychological testing and magnetic resonance imaging, to be reported separately.

At the end of CAMDEX, a clinical diagnosis is made by the interviewing psychiatrist using all the information collected. Criteria for dementia of minimal, mild, moderate, and severe degree are specified. Alternative excluding causes of cognitive impairment can be diagnosed such as depression or toxic confusion. The method has established validity in the community.[9,20,21] Our main findings use the criteria for mild dementia that are similar to criteria for dementia and somewhat similar to those for mild severity in *DSM-III-R*.[22] In the prevalence study[9] these gave rates close to the review by Jorm et al.[1] The CAMDEX criteria for minimal dementia were also applied separately. Since these are nonstandard they are reproduced as follows:

Limited and variable impairment in acquisition of new information and in recalling recent events. An increased tendency to misplace and lose possessions. Minor and variable errors in orientation. Some blunting in the capacity to follow or pursue a reasoned argument and to solve problems. Occasional errors (but of slowly advancing frequency) in occupational tasks and/or housework. Errors in judgement on occasion in professional or highly skilled tasks or socially responsible roles requiring difficult decisions or choices. Self care unimpaired. Emotional life and responses well preserved. Clinical examination usually yields negative results except for manifest anxiety when asked to carry out demanding tasks.

Training for CAMDEX was by viewing videotapes and by observing interviews in the field, together with some joint interviewing at various points in the study. In a small interrater reliability study on 15 interviews between two psychiatrists, 10 subjects were diagnosed as normal by both and three were diagnosed as demented (with agreement on severity in these), while two were diagnosed as demented by one and normal or depressed by the other. While this study was small, in the prevalence wave and in another small study by one of the present investigators, good reliability was found.[20,23] One US study[24] has reported good reliability of CAMDEX items.

ESTIMATION OF INCIDENCE

Incidence rates were estimated as the number of new cases divided by the person-years at risk. Age bands were based on age at entry to the study. Person-years for nondements were calculated as the time between prevalence screen and incidence screen. For dements, the time of incidence was assumed to be the midpoint between screening interviews and person-years were calculated accordingly. Subjects unavailable for study before the incidence wave were excluded, because neither MMSE nor CAMDEX information was available.

By means of weighting, incidence rates representative of the entire rescreened population were derived. First, 165 subjects scoring 25 or less at prevalence wave had not received a diagnostic interview then, and because in this range risk of being an undetected prevalent case was considerable, their follow-up data were not used but the diagnostic data for subjects scoring in this range who did have a prevalence diagnostic interview were weighted upward. Subjects with prevalence MMSE score of 26 or more were assumed not to have been demented then.

The subsequent main procedure was to weight up rates for those subjects not receiving a diagnostic interview at follow-up. This was done separately for the 14 different CAMDEX sampling groups (the eight original sampling groups, but with six groups rather than one from those in the remainder group because of sampling rates by practice). Sometimes, in subgroup analyses, no diagnostic information was available within a sampling group and these groups were excluded from the particular analysis. Full details of the procedure are available on request.

For comparison of rates and testing of differences for significance, rate ratios (ratios of the two rates) and their confidence intervals were calculated.[25] Since age was a key variable, rates were adjusted for age by standardization to the England and Wales age distribution, when used for this purpose.

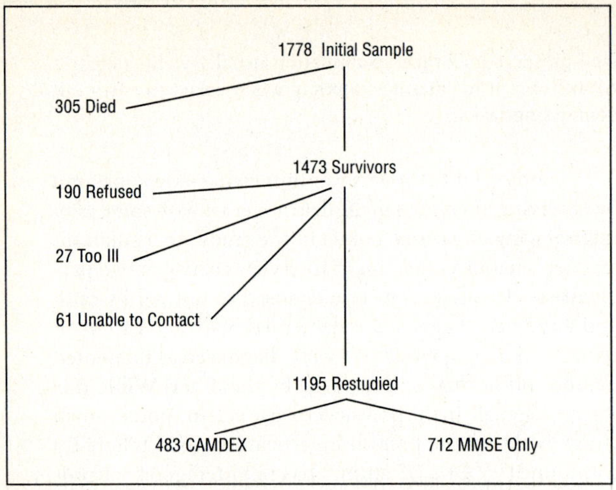

Results of the follow-up. CAMDEX indicates Cambridge Examination for Mental Disorders of the Elderly; and MMSE, Mini-Mental State Examination.

dementia and normality,[5] it is preferable to incorporate alternative definitions and severity thresholds.

Some studies have simply enumerated new cases reaching services, but these give spuriously low rates[6] because of low service take-up.[7,8] The few field studies have found considerably higher rates,[6] which rise with age, but with small older samples.

This article is the first in a series from the Cambridge Project for Later Life, a two-wave community incidence study employing a diagnostic interview after screening and focusing on subjects older than 75 years. This article reports the main incidence rates using both a standard and a wider criterion.

RESULTS

SAMPLE CHARACTERISTICS

The age and sex distributions of the subjects studied are given in **Table 1**. Two thirds were women. The social class distribution (Registrar General's method[26]) reflected that of Cambridge, in which a greater proportion of people are in social class II than in the United Kingdom nationally: 3.5% were in social class I, 21.3% were in class II, 13.5% were in class IIIa (nonmanual), 31.5% were in class IIIb (manual), 21.6% were in class IV, 5.8% were in class V, and 2.8% were unclassified.

The mean ages and MMSE scores of those unavailable for follow-up between prevalence and incidence waves (screening stage) are given in **Table 2**. Differences of groups unavailable for follow-up vs completers were tested by the Mann-Whitney *U* Test. Those who died, were too ill, or refused had significantly lower initial MMSE scores and, except for refusers, they were older than those who were successfully restudied.

Table 1. Age at Prevalence Wave and Sex of the Sample Followed Up

Age,* y	Women, No. (%)	Men, No. (%)	All, No. (%)
75-79	405 (51.6)	224 (54.6)	629 (52.6)
80-84	253 (32.2)	134 (32.7)	387 (32.4)
85-89	96 (12.2)	45 (11.0)	141 (11.8)
90+	31 (4.0)	7 (1.7)	38 (3.2)
Total	**785 (100)**	**410 (100)**	**1195 (100)**

**In all tables, age refers to age at time of prevalence wave.*

Table 2. Age and MMSE Scores at Prevalence Wave of Subjects Studied and Unavailable for Incidence Wave*

Sample	No.	Age, y, Mean±SD	MMSE, Mean±SD
Completed	1195	80.8±4.2	25.8±3.0
Died	305	82.1†±4.6	24.8†±3.6
Refused	190	80.4±4.1	24.4‡±3.9
Away or untraced	61	80.8±3.5	25.2±3.4
Too ill to study	27	84.4†±5.3	23.0§±5.6

**MMSE indicates Mini-Mental State Examination.*
†P<.001 vs completed.
‡P<.05 vs completed.
§P<.01 vs completed.

Table 3. Average Annual Incidence of Dementia of Mild or Greater Severity

	No. of Dements From Diagnostic Assessment	No. of Weighted Person-Years at Risk	Annual Incidence Rates, %	95% Confidence Intervals
Overall	49	2579	4.3	3.0-6.1
By age, y				
75-79	16	1346	2.3	1.5-3.6
80-84	20	855	4.6*	2.9-7.3
85-89	9	267	8.5†	5.3-13.5
90+	4	73	8.2*	3.3-20.6
By gender				
Men	16	915	3.2‡	2.0-5.1
Women	33	1663	4.8	3.1-7.3
By age and gender				
Men, y				
75-79	5	800	1.5	0.7-3.5
80-84	9	280	7.1†	3.8-13.2
85-89	2	89	2.9	0.8-11.0
90+	0	7	...	...
Women, y				
75-79	11	846	2.7	1.7-4.5
80-84	11	543	3.6	1.9-7.2
85-89	7	178	11.2†	6.8-18.5
90+	4	66	8.9*	3.5-22.2

**Differs significantly from age 75 to 79 years, P<.05.*
†Differs significantly from age 75 to 79 years, P<.01.
‡After standardization for age: men = 3.5%; women = 4.6%, not significant.

Table 4. Average Annual Incidence of Dementia of Mild or Greater Severity by Age at Leaving School and by Social Class

	No. of Dements From Diagnostic Assessment	No. of Weighted Person-Years at Risk	Annual Incidence Rates, %	95% Confidence Intervals
Overall	49	2579	4.3	3.0-6.1
By age at leaving school, y				
>14	13	834	2.7‡	1.7-4.3
≤14	36	1738	4.9	3.4-7.2
By social class				
Class I-IIIa*	20	1013	3.6§	2.5-5.2
Class IIIb-V†	28	1488	4.4	2.9-6.8

*Nonmanual.

†Manual.

‡After age standardization: older than 14 years = 3.5%; 14 years and younger = 4.7%, not significant.

§After age standardization: class I-IIIa = 4.3%; class IIIb-V = 4.5%, not significant.

INCIDENCE OF DEMENTIA

Table 3 shows the average annual incidence rates for dementia of mild or greater severity by age and sex. Among the 49 cases of dementia in the subjects receiving CAMDEX, 41 were mild, seven were moderate, and one was severe. As can be seen in the table, numbers in older age groups were low, and confidence limits were very wide for the older than 90 years age group and in men older than 85 years, so that no conclusions could be drawn for these. For the remainder, the rates showed a consistent rise with age, doubling approximately in each 5-year age band. Rates did not differ significantly between men and women, and the suggestive difference decreased after standardization for age, reflecting the tendency for women in the sample to be older.

EDUCATION AND SOCIAL CLASS

Table 4 shows the rates of mild or greater dementia broken down by age at school leaving and social class (I-IIIa, IIIb-V). When this cohort was educated, the usual age of school leaving was 14 years. None of the differences were significant and the effects of age adjustment were to reduce the trends. The education effect was almost significant before adjustment.

To check these findings a logistic regression was carried out for dements vs normal subjects, based only on subjects who received CAMDEX (since weighting of rates to the full sample was not possible). Independent variables were age (as a continuous variable), sex, social class, and years of schooling (as a continuous variable). After fitting age and sex, neither social class nor education showed significant effects.

Table 5. Average Annual Incidence of Dementia of Minimal and Greater Severity

	No. of Dements From Diagnostic Assessment	No. of Weighted Person-Years at Risk	Annual Incidence Rates, %	Minimal Dementia Alone,* % (Imputed Rate)	95% Confidence Intervals (Minimal and Greater Rates)
Overall	91	2363	9.7	5.4	7.7-12.1
By age, y					
75-79	27	1285	5.1	2.8	3.6-7.2
80-84	37	762	12.5†	7.9†	9.0-17.4
85-89	20	238	16.4†	7.9†	11.4-23.7
90+	7	42	36.9†	28.7†	20.7-65.9
By gender					
Men	31	855	7.7	4.5	5.4-11.0
Women	60	1509	10.5	5.7	8.0-13.7
By age and gender					
Men, y					
75-79	8	493	2.4	0.9	1.2-4.7
80-84	17	241	18.7†	11.6†	11.6-30.0
85-89	6	75	13.8†	10.9†	6.0-31.7
90+	0	7	...	...	...
Women, y					
75-79	19	791	6.8	4.1	4.6-10.1
80-84	20	495	9.3	5.7	6.2-13.8
85-89	14	161	19.5†	8.3†	12.8-29.7
90+	7	34	44.9†	36.0†	25.2-80.1

*By subtraction of rates in this table from Table 3.

†Differs significantly from age 75 to 79 years, $P<.01$.

MINIMAL DEMENTIA

Table 5 shows rates for dementia of minimal and greater severity. For this analysis subjects with minimal dementia at the prevalence wave were excluded, as they were not at risk. In this sample, there were 52 subjects with new minimal dementia, 34 subjects with mild dementia, and five subjects with moderate dementia. Rates for minimal dementia alone were not estimated directly, but they were imputed by subtraction from rates for mild and greater dementia, and these are also shown in the table. The rates of minimal dementia rose markedly with age. In almost every group at least as many subjects were diagnosed as having minimal dementia as were diagnosed as having mild or more severe dementia (Table 3). Average annual incidence rates for dementia of any severity were very high in those aged 85 to 89 years (16.4%) and 90+ years (36.9%).

COMMENT

The special features of this study were the use of incidence rather than prevalence, and a rare opportunity for concentration on a very elderly population that tends to be poorly represented in studies. We found high-onset rates for dementia, rising steeply with age.

METHODS

We used a two-wave design so that incidence could be based on those known not to be demented earlier. Response rates for the original prevalence study were very high. Some unavailablity for follow-up was inevitable, particularly because of high mortality in the elderly. The loss of approximately 600 subjects from the original 1778 was half due to death and about one third due to refusal, probably due to dislike of repeated cognitive assessment. The follow-up period was aimed to produce sufficient incident cases, without too much loss through death.

BECAUSE LOSS was associated with older age and lower prevalence wave MMSE scores, the incidence rates may have been underestimates, although the degree of bias implied by the small differences in Table 2 would have been small. Also, those who had development of dementia in the intervening period are more likely to have died. It was not possible to correct for loss prior to incidence screening, even by interviewing relatives, since cognitive impairment reported could have other causes such as terminal illness. However, measurement error in a follow-up study can bias rates upward.[27] The two opposite effects may balance and we believe that our estimates are reasonably accurate.

Almost all incident cases were mild, as expected over 2.5 years. The diagnosis of mild dementia in the community is not easy,[28] and eliminating other transient causes of cognitive impairment is harder. CAMDEX incorporates extensive cognitive testing, questions and an informant interview to exclude other causes, and explicit diagnostic criteria. Reliability and validity in other studies employing CAMDEX after MMSE screening have been good.[9,20,23,24,29] In this article we have confined results to the diagnosis of dementia, rather than attempting differentiation between Alzheimer's and vascular types, which also adds unreliability, but results to be reported separately suggest that about two thirds of cases were of Alzheimer's disease.

The two-stage method of screening, full assessment in a subsample and standard weighting methods[30] for rates, is efficient for field data collection. The lack of diagnostic interview for high prevalence MMSE scores meant that some apparent new dements might have been demented previously. O'Connor and colleagues[29] estimated in the prevalence wave that 5% of those scoring 26 and 1% to 2% of those scoring 27 or more might have been demented. These would not greatly distort the incidence figures.

FINDINGS

We found high incidence rates of dementia that rose markedly with age. Differences by sex, education, or social class were not significant after age correction. Rates at higher age were limited by sample size but a rise with age in the larger number of women was clearly demonstrated up to age 89 years at prevalence wave. Onset of minimal dementia was particularly common and rates rose rapidly with age. Overall the rates doubled approximately in each 5-year age band. This increase roughly parallels that in prevalence studies.[1,2] If prevalence increases rapidly with age, when both increasing age and the disorder shorten life expectation, many new cases must develop.

There have only been a few previous studies, using methods varying from cognitive scale performance[31] to full diagnostic interview with collateral sources and in one study,[32] information on those who died. In studies using two-wave designs with adequate field methods,[6,10,11,32-36] rates have been comparable but samples older than 80 years have been limited. In two studies employing comparable 5-year age bands,[11,36] rates for 75 to 79 years were 2.8% and 5.2%, respectively; for 80 to 84 years, rates were 4.8% and 9.0%, respectively; and for 85 to 89 years, rates were 9.2% and 8.7%, respectively, of the same order as ours.

Only two incidence studies have come from the United States.[35,36] Can the rates be generalized to a US population? Further studies are needed to answer this question. One prevalence study[37] has suggested higher rates in New York, NY, than London, England, but differences were probably not outside possible effects of methods or sampling.

It has been argued that the very old show a falloff in rates of dementia. Prevalence fell in those older than 85 years in two studies.[38,39] However, most studies and pooled reports[1,2] show marked acceleration with age, as did the prevalence wave of this study.[9] Our incidence findings confirm this trend. Overall the findings suggest rapid acceleration of one or more processes that are widespread in advanced age.

THE ASSOCIATIONS of social class and education with cognitive function are problematic. Many studies, including the Epidemiologic Catchment Area Study[40,41] and this study's prevalence wave[42] have found associations with cross-sectional MMSE scores. However, cognitive test scores have an element that is dependent on general and verbal knowledge and hence related to education and social group. A diagnostic interview assists in excluding such effects. Education and social class were not related to rates for diagnosed dementia in this or another CAMDEX prevalence study.[43,44] An incidence study assessing change should be even better for excluding baseline effects. We did not find either variable significantly related to incidence.

MINIMAL DEMENTIA

Our main incidence rates are for mild dementia, but we have also reported rates for CAMDEX minimal dementia. This threshold is less precise or reliable and is vulnerable to transient cognitive impairment. Some confirmation that it does represent early progressive dementia comes from the fate in this study of subjects who were diagnosed as having minimal dementia in the prevalence wave. Among 22 such individuals studied in the incidence wave, seven were diagnosed as normal, five still had a diagnosis of minimal dementia, seven had a diagnosis of mild dementia, two had a diagnosis of moderate dementia, and one had a diagnosis of severe dementia, giving a high rate of more definite dementia.

The incidence rates of minimal dementia were at least as high as those for mild and above. There are two possible interpretations. One is that thresholds for dementia are artificial, and there is a continuous distribution of cognitive decline from minor to major. Brayne and Calloway[5] have argued for this and presented supporting data from test scores. The distribution of MMSE change in our study, to be reported elsewhere, approximated to normality. The frequency of new minimal dementia in this population, although not conclusive in itself, is in keeping with a continuous distribution in which onset of more clear-cut dementia lies in the distribution tail.

The rates of minimal dementia increased rapidly with age. A second possibility is that minimal dementia is a different phenomenon from more frank dementia, particularly in the very elderly. It has been argued that the old show a mild nonprogressive "benign senescent forgetfulness."[45,46] Japanese centenarians who showed some cognitive dysfunction did not show the full clinical picture of dementia.[47] A related concept, but not limited to the very elderly, is that of age-associated memory impairment.[48] The criteria of minimal dementia in CAMDEX are intended to select a greater degree of impairment than this very common phenomenon and the high rates of progression support this difference. One postmortem study[49] found that 10 subjects in their 70s and 80s with very mild dementia showed typical Alzheimer's abnormalities. Further follow-up of our subjects is being undertaken and postmortem examinations are being carried out.

Accepted for publication April 22, 1993.

This study was supported by Special Project Grant 8712116 from the Medical Research Council, London, England.

Thanks are due to the general practitioners and practice staff; the study administrator, Eileen Richardson; the team of interviewers; Beryl Jones, Lynn Daly, MB, ChB, Istra Toner, BSc, Bernard Reiss, MB, BS, FRCGP, and Peter Brook, MD, FRCPsych; and particularly to our respondents. Statistical advice and consultation was provided by David Clayton, MRC Biostatistics Unit, and help with the data files was provided by Diane Mathewson.

Reprint requests to Department of Community Medicine, Institute of Public Health, University Forvie Site, Robinson Way, Cambridge CB2 2SR, England (Dr Brayne).

REFERENCES

1. Jorm AF, Korten AE, Henderson AS. The prevalence of dementia: a quantitative integration of the literature. *Acta Psychiatr Scand.* 1987;76:465-479.
2. Hofman A, Rocca WA, Brayne C, Breteler MMB, Clarke M, Cooper B, Copeland JRM, Dartigues JF, Da Silva Droux A, Hagnell O, Heeren TJ, Engedal K, Jonker C, Lindesay J, Lobo A, Mann AH, Molsa PK, Morgan K, O'Connor DW, Sulkava R, Kay DWK, Amaducci L. The prevalence of dementia in Europe: a collaborative study of 1980-1990 findings. *Int J Epidemiol.* 1991;20:736-748.
3. Folstein MF, Folstein SE, McHugh PR. Mini-Mental State: a practical method for grading the cognitive stage of patients for the clinician. *J Psychiatr Res.* 1975;12:189-198.
4. George LK, Landoman R, Blazer DG, Anthony JC. Cognitive impairment. In: Robins LN, Regier DA, eds. *Psychiatric Disorders in America.* New York, NY: Free Press; 1991:291-327.
5. Brayne C, Calloway P. Normal ageing, impaired cognitive function, and senile dementia of the Alzheimer's type: a continuum? *Lancet* 1988;1:1265-1267.
6. Bickel H, Cooper B. Incidence of dementing illness among persons aged over 65 in an urban population. In: Cooper B, Helgason T, eds. *Epidemiology and the Prevention of Mental Disorders.* London, England: Routledge; 1989:59-76.
7. Williamson J, Stokoe IH, Gray S, Fisher M, Smith A, McGhee A, Stephenson E. Old people at home: their unreported needs. *Lancet.* 1964;1:1117-1120.
8. O'Connor DW, Pollitt PA, Hyde JB, Brook CPB, Reiss BB, Roth M. Do general practitioners miss dementia in elderly patients? *BMJ.* 1988;297:1107-1110.
9. O'Connor DW, Pollitt PA, Hyde JB, Fellows JL, Miller ND, Brook CPB, Reiss BB, Roth M. The prevalence of dementia as measured by the Cambridge Mental Disorders of the Elderly Examination. *Acta Psychiatr Scand.* 1989;79:190-198.
10. Copeland JRM, Davidson IA, Dewey ME, Gilmore C, Larkin BA, McWilliam C, Saunders PA, Scott A, Sharma V, Sullivan C. Alzheimer's disease, other dementias, depression and pseudo-dementia: prevalence, incidence and 3-year outcome in Liverpool. *Br J Psychiatry.* 1992;161:230-239.

11. Morgan K, Lilley J, Arie T, Byrne J, Jones R, Waite J. Incidence of dementia: preliminary findings from the Nottingham Longitudinal Study of Activity and Ageing. *Neuroepidemiology.* 1992;11:80-83.
12. Roth M, Tym E, Mountjoy CQ, Huppert FA, Hendrie H, Verma S, Goddard R. CAMDEX: a standardised instrument for the diagnosis of mental disorder in the elderly, with special reference to the early detection of dementia. *Br J Psychiatry.* 1986;149:698-709.
13. Roth M, Huppert FA, Tym E, Mountjoy CQ. *CAMDEX.* Cambridge, England: Cambridge University Press; 1988.
14. Medical Research Council. *Report From the MRC Alzheimer's Disease Workshop.* London, England: Medical Research Council; 1987.
15. Brayne C, Calloway P. The case identification of dementia in the community: a comparison of methods. *Int J Geriatric Psychiatry.* 1990;5:309-316.
16. Beardsall L, Huppert FA. A comparison of clinical psychometric and behavioural memory tests: findings from a community study of the early detection of dementia. *Int J Geriatric Psychiatry.* 1991;6:295-306.
17. Hamilton M. Development of a rating scale for primary depressive illness. *Br J Soc Clin Psychol.* 1967;6:278-296.
18. Paykel ES. The Clinical Interview for Depression: development, reliability and validity. *J Affect Disord.* 1985;9:85-96.
19. Neugarten BL, Hayhurst RJ. The measurement of life satisfaction. *J Gerontol.* 1961;16:134-143.
20. O'Connor DW, Pollitt PA, Jones BJ, Hyde JB, Fellowes JL, Miller ND. Continued clinical validation of dementia diagnosed in the community using the Cambridge Mental Disorders of the Elderly Examination. *Acta Psychiatr Scand.* 1991;83:41-45.
21. Brayne C, Calloway P. The case identification of dementia in the community: a comparison of methods. *Int J Geriatric Psychiatry.* 1990;5:309-316.
22. American Psychiatric Association, Committee on Nomenclature and Statistics. *Diagnostic and Statistical Manual of Mental Disorders, Third Revised Edition.* Washington, DC: American Psychiatric Association; 1987.
23. Brayne C. *A Study of Dementia in a Rural Population.* London, England: London University; 1990. Thesis.
24. Hendrie HC, Hall KS, Brittain HM, Austrom MG, Farlow M, Parker J, Kane M. The CAMDEX: a standardized instrument for the diagnosis of mental disorder in the elderly: a replication with a US sample. *J Am Geriatr Soc.* 1988;36:402-408.
25. Clayton D, Hills M. *Statistical Models in Epidemiology.* Oxford, England: Oxford University Press; 1993.
26. Office of Population and Censuses. *Classification of Occupations.* London, England: Her Majesty's Stationery Office; 1980.
27. Eaton WW, Kramer M, Anthony JC, Chee EML, Shapiro S. Conceptual and methodological problems in estimation of the incidence of mental disorders from field survey data. In: Cooper B, Helgason T, eds. *Epidemiology and Prevention of Mental Disorders.* London, England: Routledge; 1989:108-131.
28. Henderson AS, Huppert FA. The problem of mild dementia. *Psychol Med.* 1984; 13:5-11.
29. O'Connor DW, Pollitt PA, Hyde JB, Fellows JL, Miller ND, Brook CPB, Reiss BB. The reliability and validity of the Mini-Mental State in a British community survey. *J Psychiatr Res.* 1989;23:87-96.
30. Armitage P, Berry G. *Statistical Methods in Medical Research.* Boston, Mass: Blackwell Scientific Publications Inc; 1987.
31. Jagger C, Clarke M, Cook AJ. Mental and physical health of elderly people: five year follow-up of total population. *Age Ageing.* 1989;18:77-82.
32. Hagnell O, Ojesjo L, Rorsman B. Incidence of dementia in the Lundby Study. *Neuroepidemiology.* 1977;11(suppl 1):61-66.
33. Nielsen JA, Biorn-Henriksen T, Bork BR. Incidence and disease expectancy for senile and arteriosclerotic dementia in a geographically delimited Danish rural population. In: Magnussen J, Nielsen J, Buch J, eds. *Epidemiology and Prevention of Mental Illness in Old Age.* Hellerup, Denmark: EGV; 1982:52-53.
34. Nilsson LV. Incidence of severe dementia in an urban sample followed up from 70 to 79 years of age. *Acta Psychiatr Scand.* 1984;70:478-486.
35. Katzman R, Aronson M, Fuld P, Kawas C, Brown T, Morgenstern H, Frishman W, Gidez L, Eder H, Ooi WL. Development of dementing illness in an 80-year-old volunteer cohort. *Ann Neurol.* 1989;25:317-324.
36. Hebert LE, Scherr PA, Smith LA, Evans DA. Age-specific incidence of Alzheimer's disease. *Am J Epidemiol.* 1991;139:786-787.
37. Copeland JRM, Gurland BJ, Dewey ME, Kelleher MJ, Smith AMR, Davidson IA. Is there more dementia, depression and neurosis in New York? a comparative study of the elderly in New York and London using the computer diagnosis AGECAT. *Br J Psychiatry.* 1987;151:466-473.
38. Essen-Moller E. Individual traits and morbidity in a Swedish rural population. *Acta Psychiatr Neurol Scand.* 1956;100(suppl).
39. Nielsen J. Geronto-psychiatric period-prevalence investigation in a geographically delimited population. *Acta Psychiatr Scand.* 1962;38:307-330.
40. Holzer CE, Tischler GL, Leaf PJ, Myers JK. An epidemiologic assessment of cognitive function in a community population. *Res Commun Ment Health.* 1984;4:3-32.
41. Folstein MF, Anthony JC, Parhad I, Duffy B, Gruenberg EM. The meaning of cognitive impairment in the elderly. *J Am Geriatr Soc.* 1985;33:228-235.
42. O'Connor DW, Pollitt PA, Treasure FP, Brook CPB, Reiss BB. The influence of education, social class and sex on Mini-Mental State scores. *Psychol Med.* 1989;19:771-776.
43. O'Connor DW, Pollitt PA, Treasure FP. The influence of education and social class on the diagnosis of dementia in a community population. *Psychol Med.* 1991;21:219-224.
44. Brayne C, Calloway P. The association of education and socioeconomic status with the Mini Mental State Examination and the clinical diagnosis of dementia in elderly people. *Age Ageing.* 1990;19:91-96.
45. Kral VA. Senescent forgetfulness, benign and milignant. *Can Med Assoc J.* 1962;86:257-260.
46. Kral VA. Benign senescent forgetfulness. In: Katzman R, Terry RD, Bick KL, eds. *Alzheimer's Disease: Senile Dementia and Related Disorders.* New York, NY: Raven Press; 1978:47-51.
47. Karasawa A, Kawashima K, Kasahara H. Mental aging and its medico-psychosocial background in the very old Japanese. *J Gerontol.* 1979;14:680-686.
48. Crook T, Bartus RT, Ferris SH, Whitehouse P, Cohen GD, Gershon S. Age-associated memory impairment: proposed diagnostic criteria and measures of clinical change—report of a National Institute of Mental Health Work Group. *Dev Neuropsychol.* 1986;2:261-276.
49. Morris JC, McKeel DW, Storandt M, Rubin EH, Price JL, Grant EA, Ball MJ, Berg L. Very mild Alzheimer's disease: informant-based clinical, psychometric and pathologic distinction from normal aging. *Neurology.* 1991;41:469-478.

Schizophrenia After Prenatal Exposure to the Dutch Hunger Winter of 1944-1945

Susser and Lin[1] report the remarkable finding of an increased risk for hospitalized schizophrenia in women whose mothers were among the population exposed to severe famine during the Dutch Hunger Winter of 1944 through 1945 and who were members of a risk set alive at 19 years of age. The authors' broad consideration of the limitations of their analysis is to be commended, and the result is discussed in the context of other lines of evidence in favor of antenatal risk factors for schizophrenia, albeit at various and contradictory periods of gestation. However, I am curious as to one point of detail and take issue with their conclusion regarding gender differences in the increased relative risk.

It is unclear whether the numerator for exposed and unexposed groups consists of true incident cases of schizophrenia, ie, first hospital admissions, or the total number of admissions for schizophrenia, including readmissions, appearing in the Dutch psychiatric registry. If it is the latter, the only conclusion that can be drawn from the data is that putative exposure to famine during the first trimester is associated not with increased incidence of schizophrenia but with increased rates of hospitalization for women in their middle-to-late 30s, perhaps indicating more severe illness in the exposed group.

If the data do refer to true incidence rates, the conclusion regarding a gender difference in the effect is, surely, unsafe, owing to the age of the cohort during the period of assessment (1978 to 1989) and the differential ages at onset for men and women. Members of the risk set would have been between 32 and 45 years of age during this period. The men would have lived through a greater proportion of their period of risk for schizophrenia than would the women, who would have only just passed their mean age at onset and entered the tail of age at onset stretching into middle age and beyond.[2] Thus, the majority of men, exposed or not, had already developed their schizophrenia by the time Susser and Lin[1] made their assessments. The data are therefore entirely compatible with an effect in men at least as large as that demonstrated in women, but one would predict that the excess illness in men would have occurred in the previous decade. Even without the appropriate age correction, the confidence limits betray the same possibility and raise the specter of a type II statistical error rather than a gender effect.

Gender differences are popular in schizophrenia research.[3] Given that men are different from women in many ways, schizophrenic or not, researchers must be alert to the possibility of confounding, particularly from the well-established gender difference in mean age at onset; once this is adequately controlled for, many apparent gender differences may melt away.[4,5] Small sample sizes leading to type II errors are usually a problem for analysis of data from women. It is possible that the balance between the sexes has been inadvertently restored in this study and that the true effect was not, in fact, discriminatory.

Peter Jones, MD
London, England

1. Susser ES, Lin SP. Schizophrenia after exposure to the Dutch Hunger Winter of 1944-1945. *Arch Gen Psychiatry.* 1992;49:983-988.
2. Loranger AW. Sex differences in age at onset of schizophrenia. *Arch Gen Psychiatry.* 1984;41:157-161.
3. Goldstein JM, Tsuang MT. Gender and schizophrenia: an introduction and synthesis of findings. *Schizophr Bull.* 1990;16:179-184.
4. DeLisi LE. The significance of age at onset for schizophrenia. *Schizophr Bull.* 1992;18:209-215.
5. Eaton WW, Mortensen PB, Herrman H, Freeman H, Bilker W, Burgess P, Wooff K. Long-term course of hospitalisation for schizophrenia, I: risk for rehospitalisation. *Schizophr Bull.* 1992;18:217-228.

In reply

Dr Jones asks for clarification of case ascertainment, suggesting that there may have been an undetected effect in men as well as in women because of low statistical power, ie, a type II error.

Our numerators are the number of individuals who were hospitalized for schizophrenia during the period 1978 through 1989 in the birth cohorts exposed and unexposed to famine in the first trimester. No individual is counted twice (ie, an individual with five admissions during 1978 through 1989 is still counted as one case). This is not a true incident sample of cases of new onset because some individuals may also have had hospitalizations prior to the study period (these birth cohorts were from 32 to 45 years of age). As noted by Dr Jones, an effect of prenatal exposure to famine on the course of illness as well as on incidence could conceivably produce an increase in the number of patients hospitalized for schizophrenia after 32 years of age.

A large effect on the incidence of schizophrenia prior to 32 years of age could translate into only a small effect on hospitalized schizophrenia after 32 years of age. This effect would occur, for instance, if patients with onset prior to 32 years of age do not require hospitalization after 32 years of age. Effects could be diminished more in men than in women because schizophrenia on average has an earlier onset in men than in women. It is possible, then, that a large effect on incidence in men produced only a small effect on hospitalized schizophrenia in men after 32 years of age and that the effect was not found to be significant in our data due to low statistical power.

We did not suggest this interpretation in our report. We were cautious because, while there was a trend toward increased risk for "restricted" schizophrenia in men, there was no trend for "broad" schizophrenia in men. In addition, there were no prior studies of this prenatal exposure to famine in schizophrenia.

We have now extended our findings to include the following: (1) the association with exposure in the first trimester to famine was specific to schizophrenia among psychiatric disorders; (2) focusing on the years 1978 through 1983, the relative risks (RRs) for restricted schizophrenia are larger in both men (RR, 1.8) and women (RR, 3.3); (3) separate studies suggest that a focus on restricted schizophrenia is justified; and (4) among men aged 18 years in these birth cohorts, the prevalence of abnormalities that could represent early signs of schizophrenia was higher in birth cohorts exposed to famine in the first trimester than in unexposed birth cohorts.

In light of these new data, a type II error in men seems more plausible. Statistically, it is not unlikely: the probability of a type II error in men for restricted schizophrenia—given a rate in the unexposed population (1.4 per 1000), an RR (1.4) as in our data, and an α of .05—was about 50%. We are currently testing this possibility in a further study, for which we have obtained data from an earlier Dutch psychiatric registry.

Ezra Susser, MD, DrPH
New York, NY
Shang P. Lin, PhD
Orangeburg, NY

Age of Onset in Familial Schizophrenia

The age of onset of schizophrenia characteristically peaks in early adulthood, although spanning at least four decades of life among unrelated individuals, and on average, it peaks a few years earlier in males than females.[1,2] It also has been previously shown that the age of onset, rather than the time of onset, is highly correlated among affected sibling pairs,[3] thus suggesting a genetic determination of the age of onset. There recently have been reports of a curious lack of gender differences in the age of onset when only schizophrenic individuals with a positive family history of schizophrenia (ie, multiplex families) are examined.[4-6] However, L. S. Penrose, in a large cohort of familial mental illness, previously observed that the age of onset for males was lower than for females (mean difference, 3.7 years), with a wider scatter in male ages at first admission than in female and a lower correlation of the age of onset among brother-sister pairs than among same-sex siblings.[7] While some of these findings lack consistency, they are worth further focus as clues to the genetic basis for schizophrenia.[8,9]

If there is a genetic mechanism for determining the age of onset and, within nuclear families, the same genetic mechanism is likely to be present despite the overall sex differences noted above, there may not be a difference in the age of onset between males and females within the same family. If so, this would imply that genetic control of the age of onset somehow contributes to gender differences. The gender effect may only be observed in populations of unrelated individuals, ie, an "early-onset" gene, more likely expressed in males, and a "late-onset" gene, more likely expressed in females.

We have been ascertaining multiplex families with schizophrenia by recruiting families with at least two siblings with chronic *DSM-III-R* schizophrenia or schizoaffective disorder. The age of onset among ill sibling sets of mixed sex were examined. The age of onset was based on the age of first hospitalization, since this is the most reliable retrospective indicator of the approximate age of onset and is correlated with the age at first psychotic symptoms. Fifty-eight mixed-sex sets of siblings were obtained from 162 consecutively recruited multiplex families from the United States, England, and Italy. There were 52 male-female pairs, two male-male-female sets, three male-female-female sets, and one set of four ill siblings (three males and one female). In the six families with more than two ill siblings, the average age of onset for same-sex individuals was used in analyses. The mean ($\pm$SD) age of onset for males was 21.1$\pm$4.9 years and for females, 22.3$\pm$6.1 years (paired t test, 1.37; $P<.18$). Twenty-nine sets of siblings had an earlier age of onset in the males than the females (by a mean difference of 6.2 years); 25 sets had an earlier age of onset in the females than the males (by a mean difference of 4.5 years); and four sets of siblings had the same age of onset. The age of onset was modestly correlated in sibships (r=.254; P=.05).

The above results suggest that no significant gender differences in the age of onset are present within families with "familial" schizophrenia. The age of onset among ill sibling pairs appears to be correlated but differs by a few years regardless of sex. These data confirm that the genetic determination of the age of onset may be stronger than any sex-related hormonal and/or environmental or nongenetic effects and that the gender differences

in the age of onset could be determined by the nature of the genetic locus for schizophrenia.

Lynn E. DeLisi, MD
New York, NY
Nick Bass, MD
Harrow, England
Angela Boccio, MS
Gail Shields, MD
New York, NY
Carla Morganti, MD
Antonio Vita, MD
Milan, Italy

This project is partially funded by grant ROlMH44245 from the National Institute of Mental Health, Rockville, Md; by the Medical Research Centre, Harrow, England; and by the Department of Psychiatry, University of Milan, Italy.

1. Lewine RRJ, Strauss JS, Gift TE. Sex differences in age at first admission for schizophrenia: a fact or artifact? *Am J Psychiatry*. 1981;138:440-444.
2. Loranger AW. Sex differences in age of onset of schizophrenia. *Arch Gen Psychiatry*. 1984;41:157-161.
3. Crow TJ, Done J. Age of onset of schizophrenia: a test of the contagion hypothesis. *Psychiatry Res*. 1986;18:107-117.
4. DeLisi LE, Goldin LR, Maxwell E, Kazuba DM, Gershon ES. Clinical features of illness in siblings with schizophrenia or schizoaffective disorder. *Arch Gen Psychiatry*. 1987;44:891-896.
5. Walsh CM, Asherson P, Castle D, Sham P, Williams J, Taylor C, Clements A, Owen M, Gill M, McGuffin P, Murray RM. Age of onset of schizophrenia in multiply affected families. Poster presentation at the European Science Foundation Collaborative Network on Schizophrenia and Affective Disorder Annual Workshop; January 8, 1993; Aussois, France.
6. Leboyer M, Filteau M-J, Jay M, Campion D, Rochet T, D'Amato T, Feingold J, Des Lauriers A, Widlocher D. No gender effect on age of onset in familial schizophrenia? *Am J Psychiatry*. 1992;149:1409.
7. Crow TJ. A note on 'Survey of Cases of Familial Mental Illness' by L. S. Penrose. *Eur Arch Psychiatry Clin Neurosci*. 1991;240:314-324.
8. Crow TJ. The age of onset of psychosis as a clue to a defect in the cerebral dominance gene. *Schizophr Res*. 1991;5:194-195.
9. DeLisi LE. The significance of age of onset for schizophrenia. *Schizophr Bull*. 1992;18:209-215.

Naltrexone and Alcohol Dependence: Some Methodological Issues

Volpicelli et al[1] presented an interesting study on the use of naltrexone in the treatment of alcohol dependence. We make two observations that although seemingly minor nevertheless have an impact on design and reporting in research.

First, we fail to understand why the Brief Psychiatric Rating Scale (BPRS),[2] which is customarily used to rate psychosis, was applied to assess psychiatric status; did the authors expect their alcoholic subjects to become psychotic during naltrexone therapy? The futility of having used this scale is apparent from the mean scores in the two groups: 24.3 and 23.3 at baseline and 21.6 and 19.9 at end point. Considering that the BPRS version that was used scores the subject at 17 in the total absence of psychopathology, this scale probably measured emotionality with little sensitivity. More appropriate would have been specific anxiety, depression, and other scales. Also curious is that interrater reliability for the BPRS was not reported despite the use of a nonweighted (and hence subjectively rated) version of the instrument.

Second, none of the χ^2 values reported on page 879 of the article are correct. With Yates' correction for continuity, as is considered necessary in all 2×2 contingency tables, the correct χ^2 values for alcohol sampling, relapse (overall), and relapse (in alcohol samplers) in the two groups are 0.51, 6.03, and 7.35, respectively, and not 1.15, 8.51, and 10.5, respectively, as reported. Of note, the low expected frequencies in the last contingency table would have prompted most statisticians to use a two-tailed Fisher Exact Test and not the χ^2 statistic as was actually applied. When authors err with basic statistics, how much reliance can readers place on their remaining inferences, which cannot be cross-checked?

Chittaranjan Andrade, MD
N. Sanjay Kumar Rao, MBBS
Bangalore, India

1. Volpicelli JR, Alterman AI, Hayashida M, O'Brien CP. Naltrexone in the treatment of alcohol dependence. *Arch Gen Psychiatry*. 1992;49:876-880.
2. Overall JE, Gorman DE. The Brief Psychiatric Rating Scale in psychopharmacologic research. *Psychol Res*. 1961;10:799-812.

In reply

The letter by Andrade and Rao provides two criticisms of our article.[1] The first concerns use of the BPRS with alcohol-dependent subjects. The BPRS measures a broad range of psychopathologic symptoms, including paranoid ideation, psychosis, depression, and anxiety. Because this was the first systematic study in which naltrexone was given to alcoholics, we were interested in general psychopathology rather than in specific symptoms. Also, we had used the BPRS and the Symptom Checklist-90 routinely for several years in our clinic and therefore had extensive experience with obtaining baseline norms in this population.

We were not surprised that neither instrument showed group differences. There may be subtle psychological symptoms caused by naltrexone, and symptom-specific instruments such as the Hamilton Depression or Anxiety Scales would be appropriate instruments. We did not intend to test that specific hypothesis in this study.

Second, Andrade and Rao state that the Yates correction is required for all 2×2 contingency tables and Fisher's Exact Test is preferred when there are low expected frequencies. We agree that standard texts often suggest these procedures. Empirically, however, these assumptions may not be correct. For example, Camilli and Hopkins[2] determined the proportion of Type I errors for the χ^2 test of independence with and without Yates' correction for 10 000

Results of Volpicelli et al[1] Using χ^2, χ^2 With Yates' Correction, and Fisher's Exact Test*

	χ^2 (*P*)	χ^2 With Yates' Correction (*P*)	*P* Value for Fisher's Exact Test
Alcohol sampling	0.915 (NS)	0.51 (NS)	.473
Relapse rates (overall)	7.30 (<.01)	6.03 (<.025)	.013
Relapse rates (alcohol samplers)	9.60 (<.01)	7.35 (<.01)	.004

**NS indicates not significant.*

computer-generated replications. They conclude:

Both the chi-square test of homogeneity and the chi-square test of independence for 2×2 contingency tables give accurate Type I error probability statements even when the expected frequencies in one or two cells are as low as 1 or 2 when N is 20 or more. The conclusion applies when the marginal frequencies are equal or unequal. In all instances, the Yates correction decreases the accuracy of the probability statements; its use causes the proportion of Type I errors to be far less than the nominal value of alpha.

In further response, we recalculated our χ^2 values and present our corrected values and, for comparison, the χ^2 values using the Yates correction and P values for Fisher's Exact Test. As the **Table** *shows, the conclusions of the article remain the same regardless of the statistic used.*

Joseph R. Volpicelli, MD, PhD
Arthur I. Alterman, PhD
Charles P. O'Brien, MD, PhD
Philadelphia, Pa

1. Volpicelli JR, Alterman AI, Hayashida M, O'Brien CP. Naltrexone in the treatment of alcohol dependence. *Arch Gen Psychiatry*. 1992;49:876-880.
2. Camilli G, Hopkins KD. Applicability of chi-square to 2×2 contingency tables with small expected cell frequencies. *Psychol Bull*. 1978;85:163-167.

The Time Course of Nonchronic Major Depressive Disorder: Uniformity Across Episodes and Samples 405
William Coryell, MD; Hagop S. Akiskal, MD; Andrew C. Leon, PhD; George Winokur, MD; John D. Maser, MD; Timothy I. Mueller, MD; Martin B. Keller, MD; for the National Institute of Mental Health Collaborative Program on the Psychobiology of Depression—Clinical Studies

Sympathetic Nervous System Activity in Major Depression: Basal and Desipramine-Induced Alterations in Plasma Norepinephrine Kinetics 411
Richard C. Veith, MD; Nancy Lewis, RN; Oscar A. Linares, MD; Robert F. Barnes, MD; Murray A. Raskind, MD; Enrique C. Villacres, MD; M. Michele Murburg, MD; E. Alexandra Ashleigh, MD; Sonia Castillo, PhD; Elaine R. Peskind, MD; Marcella Pascualy, MD; Jeffrey B. Halter, MD

Letters to the Editor

No Evidence of a Schizophrenia Locus in a Second Pseudoautosomal Region 427
Zhe Wu Wang, MD; Donald W. Black, MD; Nancy Andreasen, MD, PhD; Raymond R. Crowe, MD

Lower-Dose Therapy With Traditional Neuroleptics in Chronically Hospitalized Schizophrenic Patients 427
Robert C. Smith, MD, PhD

Correction and Amplification 429
Hector R. Bird, MD

Alcohol Dependence May Be the Missing Link Between Posttraumatic Stress Disorder and Panic 429
Eve J. Wiseman, MD

In Reply 430
John H. Krystal, MD; Steven M. Southwick, MD; Dennis S. Charney, MD

Familial Obsessive-Compulsive Disorder Presenting as Pathological Jealousy Successfully Treated With Fluoxetine 430
Simon Wright, MB, ChB, MRCPsych

Biologic Theories of Sexual Orientation 431
Nathaniel McConaghy, DSc, MD

Theories of Sexual Orientation: A Reappraisal 432
Douglas Berger, MD; Hiroyuki Suematsu, MD; Yutaka Ono, MD

In Reply 432
William Byne, MD, PhD, Bruce Parsons, MD, PhD

Departments

Correction 422

Classified Advertising 430

**Instructions for Authors—
See January 1994 issue, page 6.**

ARCHIVES OF GENERAL PSYCHIATRY

Standardized Assessment for Panic Disorder Research

A Conference Report

M. Katherine Shear, MD, Jack D. Maser, PhD

Lively controversies related to panic disorder are under active investigation by research groups around the world. However, publications from different laboratories are difficult to compare since there has been little consistency in measures or even in types of assessment used to characterize and follow up patients. Participants in the recently convened National Institutes of Health Consensus Development Conference on the Treatment of Panic Disorder noted this problem and recommended establishment of procedures to ensure comparability of studies. We organized a conference of clinical investigators whose objective was to develop a standard assessment package. Participants represented biological and psychosocial panic disorder treatment research sites in the United States and Canada. The 2-day conference resulted in agreement on a battery of assessments considered essential for panic disorder studies. The purposes of our report are to disseminate the conference conclusions and to encourage adoption of the proposed standards by clinical researchers, journal editors, Public Health Service peer review committees, and the Food and Drug Administration. We also identify some problematic issues that require further work.
(Arch Gen Psychiatry. 1994;51:346-354)

Recent progress in pharmacologic and psychosocial treatment of panic disorder indicates efficacy of both modalities, within limits.[1] However, meaningful comparison of these approaches is difficult because of the bewildering array of assessment procedures and instruments, inconsistent and incomplete descriptions of study samples (unreported, even when these data have been collected), and inconsistent definitions for terms such as "responder" and "recurrence."

Comparable assessment procedures across different settings are necessary to conduct meta-analyses and to interpret individual study results within the context of the field. Standard procedures would ensure consistency in measurement and reporting of results among investigators studying treatment outcome as well as the origins and pathophysiologic and psychopathologic features. Assessment needs to be standardized for the array of panic symptoms and other clinical and subclinical phenomena with which patients with panic disorder present.

Diagnostic criteria for panic disorder are among the most simple and clear in the *DSM-III-R*.[2] Nevertheless, patients vary in the severity and frequency of panic episodes, anticipatory anxiety, and phobic avoidance. Functional impairment varies, as does overall severity. Clinical and epidemiologic studies indicate a very high prevalence of comorbidity among patients with panic disorder.[3] Populations seen in different settings may vary in the severity, characteristics and type, and prevalence of coexisting disorders. Consistent and complete characterization of samples is necessary for ensuring accuracy in the design of replication studies, generalizability of results, and confidence in the soundness of the database.

The field suffers from a lack of operational criteria for different types of success-

From the Department of Psychiatry, University of Pittsburgh, Pa (Dr Shear) and the National Institute of Mental Health, Bethesda, Md (Dr Maser).

ful outcome in treatment studies. The term responder is used inconsistently to indicate either some response to treatment or achievement of remission; recovery and remission often are not distinguished; and relapse criteria vary. While some investigators use a criterion of full reemergence of the *DSM-III-R* syndrome to identify relapse and to trigger a referral for further treatment, others place the threshold for intervention lower and consider recurrence of limited-symptom episodes an indication for further treatment. Since different investigators tend to use different criteria, referral for intervening treatment varies and published relapse rates are not comparable.

The objectives of the 2-day conference that we organized were to obtain agreement on a minimum set of assessments considered essential to the conduct of any study of panic disorder and to ensure agreement on the definitions of key symptoms. Such agreement would define for investigators, journal editors, and reviewers a set of standards whose implementation would ensure consistency and comparability of studies.

PROCEDURES

Participants representing major panic disorder research sites in the United States and Canada were invited to a 2-day conference. Those invitees who were unable to attend were sent drafts of our report and asked for comments and concurrence. Forty-three individuals representing 26 different research sites participated at some level in the preparation of our report. Eight topics were chosen for discussion. Attendees were divided into four subcommittees, each of which was asked to make specific recommendations in two topic areas to the conference as a whole.

The topics included (1) structured diagnostic assessment, (2) panic attacks and limited-symptom episodes, (3) anticipatory anxiety, (4) phobic symptoms, (5) overall functional impairment, global severity, and improvement, (6) comorbidity and coexisting symptoms, (7) definitions of responder, remission, and relapse, and (8) follow-up. Each subcommittee included approximately equal representation of biologically and psychosocially oriented investigators and approximately equal representation of psychiatric and psychological researchers.

We developed a questionnaire consisting of forced-answer questions in each of the eight topic areas. The questionnaire was circulated to conference participants prior to the meeting. The subcommittees were asked to answer these questions and then to discuss additional issues relevant to the assigned topic that they considered important. A reporter was designated from each subcommittee to present to the conference as a whole a summary of the subcommittee's deliberations. The large group then discussed each topic and decided which assessments should be designated as essential. The recommendations reported herein are those of the overall group of conference participants.

Audiotape records of large group meetings were transcribed and used in preparing our report. We also invited meeting participants as well as individuals who were unable to attend to provide written answers to the questionnaire and to comment on a draft of our report. The group achieved almost unanimous agreement on almost all issues. There was discussion of appropriate instruments that could be used for each assessment, but the group did not identify as essential any specific one. The purposes of our report are to describe the outcome of the conference and to encourage adoption of the proposed standards by clinical researchers, journal editors, Public Health Service peer review committees, and the Food and Drug Administration.

RESULTS

STRUCTURED DIAGNOSTIC ASSESSMENT

There was clear consensus that a structured diagnostic interview is essential to ensure uniformity of the

Conference Participants

W. Stewart Agras, MD, Palo Alto, Calif; James Ballenger, MD, Charleston, SC; David H. Barlow, PhD, Albany, NY; Timothy Brown, PsyD, Albany; Alexander Bystritsky, MD, Los Angeles, Calif; Oliver G. Cameron, MD, PhD, Ann Arbor, Mich; Diane Chambless, PhD, Washington, DC; Duncan B. Clark, MD, PhD, Pittsburgh, Pa; Bernard S. Coleman, MD, Kalamazoo, Mich; George Curtis, MD, Ann Arbor; Stephen Dager, MD, Seattle, Wash; Jean Endicott, PhD, New York, NY; Abby Fyer, MD, New York; George Heninger, MD, New Haven, Conn; Craig S. Holt, PhD, Iowa City, Iowa; Jeffrey Jonas, MD, Kalamazoo; Samuel J. Keith, MD, Rockville, Md; Donald Klein, MD, New York; Hillary Lee, PhD, Rockville; R. Bruce Lydiard, MD, Charleston, SC; Jack D. Maser, PhD, Rockville; Matig Mavissikalian, MD, Columbus, Ohio; Richard J. McNally, PhD, Cambridge, Mass; Cory Newman, PhD, Philadelphia, Pa; G. Ronald Norton, PhD, Winnipeg, Manitoba; Emmeline Otey, PhD, Rockville; Ashok Raj, MD, Tampa, Fla; Karl Rickels, MD, Philadelphia, Pa; Jerrold Rosenbaum, MD, Boston, Mass; M. Katherine Shear, MD, Pittsburgh; Edward Schweizer, MD, Philadelphia; Michael Telch, PhD, Austin, Tex; Myrna Weissman, PhD, New York; Barry Wolfe, PhD, Rockville.

Further comments provided by: Martin Keller, MD, Providence, RI; Andrew C. Leon, PhD, New York, NY; Larry Michelson, PhD, State College, Pa; S. Rachman, PhD, Vancouver, British Columbia; Diane Sholomskas, PhD, New Haven; David Sheehan, MD, Tampa, Fla; Richard Swinson, MD, Toronto, Ontario; Thomas Uhde, MD, Bethesda, Md.

samples studied at different times and places. There was a strong recommendation that current and lifetime comorbidity also be assessed by this type of instrument. Patients who meet criteria for panic disorder frequently have comorbid illness,[3] and different studies may include patients with different patterns of comorbidity. Current and/or lifetime comorbid conditions may account for differences in the origins, pathophysiologic and psychopathologic features, and/or treatment outcome.

There was some discussion of potential pitfalls in the use of structured interviews. The group noted that the structured format and the time-consuming nature of these interviews have led to the practice of hiring junior individuals, with little or no clinical experience, to conduct these interviews. There was concern that such a practice, while understandable, could lead to significant error. One participant cited an example of watching a videotape of a structured interview being administered by a doctoral student. The student followed the interview guide admirably but failed to explore sufficiently a comment by the patient that would have been considered significant by an experienced clinician.

Conferees made a recommendation that an experienced clinician have input into the final diagnostic decision. This input might be accomplished by use of a trained junior rater to conduct the interview and provide a completed rating form. An accompanying written narrative description of the patient would document the rater's understanding of the clinical presentation and highlight possible problem areas in the diagnosis. A senior clinician would then review this information to ensure accuracy of the diagnosis. Alternatively, two experienced clinicians might assess the patient independently, with at least one using a structured interview. In this case, the final diagnosis would be made by consensus of the two interviewers.

The group found acceptable the Anxiety Disorders Interview Schedule–Revised,[4] the Composite International Diagnostic Interview,[5] the Diagnostic Interview Schedule,[6] the Schedule for Affective Disorders–Lifetime, Anxiety(SADS–LA),[7] and the Structured Clinical Interview for *DSM-III-R*.[8] In the absence of evidence to the contrary, conferees assumed that these instruments are comparable in obtaining a valid diagnosis but noted that the scales differ in the level and type of elaboration on the basic diagnostic criteria. Some expressed preference for one instrument, but most participants held the view that different instruments would be preferred for different purposes and that each would be acceptable. There was a general sentiment that structured interviews should be made more user-friendly and streamlined.[9]

PANIC ATTACKS

A daily, self-reported measure of panic attacks (sometimes referred to as a panic diary) is essential to all studies of panic disorder. Limited-symptom episodes, including autonomic surges, are monitored along with full panic episodes. The self-report should include such information as the time of day, the duration and severity of panic episodes, the severity of each of the individual symptoms, and an indication of whether the episode was unexpected situation bound or situation predisposed. There should also be a way to register the degree of the increment over the baseline anxiety. Several participants noted that compliance with daily self-reported measures can be difficult to obtain. There was agreement that this problem needs to be addressed, but the group still decided that collecting a daily panic report is essential.

Accurate assessment of panic attacks requires a discussion with the patients to establish that they understand how to identify and monitor panic. Different patients and clinicians use terms like "panic" and "anxiety" without necessarily meaning the same thing. A script, perhaps with a graphic illustration of the type of onset and escalation of panic sensations, is helpful. Although the question of putting words in the patient's mouth was raised, it was concluded that the potential problem of noncommunication is more serious. A discussion between patient and clinician that serves to establish accurate communication is essential.

Panic frequency is highly variable and, in general, when an unstable signal is being measured, longer time frames are preferable. The group considered a 1-month monitoring period optimal to obtain a stable baseline. However, 1 month may not be practical, especially for pretreatment monitoring. The group recommended that the minimum length of monitoring time for panic frequency should be 2 weeks, although 4 weeks is preferable. Of course, if there is a specific interest in a phenomenon such as benzodiazepine withdrawal, the time frame for reporting panic might be as short as a day.

Conference participants concluded that an entry criterion for panic frequency is important in studies where panic is the main target symptom. Concern was raised that such a requirement could lead to a high placebo response rate, due to the statistical tendency of regression toward the mean. However, one participant reported that when an entry criterion for panic frequency was used, there was a lower placebo response rate for a requirement of two than for one panic episodes per week (J. Ballenger, MD, oral communication, February 10, 1993). This finding suggests that a requirement for panic attacks may select for more severe illness, counteracting, to some degree, the problem of regression to the mean. The outcome of this discussion was to recommend a criterion of panic frequency of at least one panic attack per week for at least 2 weeks for treatment studies using panic as the main outcome. It is con-

ceivable that someone may wish to study treatment of panic disorder in patients with clinically significant anticipatory anxiety and/or phobic avoidance, even if current panics are infrequent. In this case, an entry criterion for panic frequency would not be used.

THERE WAS a strong recommendation that some effort be made to address the identification and definition of subthreshold panic symptoms. Individuals with subthreshold panic may be distressed and impaired and may respond to treatment known to be effective for panic disorder. Conferees thought that the threshold for panic disorder is probably above the level associated with clinically important symptoms; however, too little is known about subthreshold phenomena to determine what the definition of a subthreshold panic disorder should be. Nevertheless, in certain studies such as family, epidemiologic, and treatment follow-up it is particularly important to register subthreshold panic (eg, limited-symptom panic attacks, as well as full panic attack(s) that fail to meet diagnostic criteria for the disorder).

ANTICIPATORY ANXIETY

Anticipatory anxiety is a central symptom of panic disorder, and the group consensus was that its measurement is essential. Careful thought was given to defining what is meant by anticipatory anxiety. There are at least three separate constructs embedded in the idea of fear of panic: (1) the worried or apprehensive preoccupation with having a panic attack; (2) the specific expectation or prediction that a panic attack will occur and will be dangerous; and (3) the ongoing tendency to fear and/or fear-related bodily sensations.

Most current treatment studies include a daily rating of the degree of preoccupation, worry, or anxious anticipation about having a panic episode, and conference participants considered this type of measure essential. Anticipatory anxiety was considered variable enough to lead to a strong endorsement of the use of a daily self-report. Both the frequency (ie, percent of the day spent worrying about having a panic attack) and the intensity of the anxiety should be recorded. A standard time frame for assessing anticipatory anxiety, matched to the panic time frame (ie, 2 weeks), is highly recommended.

A single measure of anxiety related to the prediction of panic may produce a conflation of two different phenomena: the expectation or prediction of having a panic attack and how bad it would be to have one. Treatments may affect these two dimensions differentially. For example, if panic attacks are suppressed with imipramine hydrochloride, the patient may predict or expect panic less but still dread it. Cognitive behavior therapies may have the opposite effect: panic may still occur and still be predicted, while the dread of panic is markedly diminished. A measure of prediction or expectation of having a panic episode in the near future (eg, in the next week) is recommended, as is a measure of prediction of panic severity. The expectation of panic could be measured with Likert scales incorporated into the daily diary. The subject would be asked to rate the likelihood of experiencing a panic episode in the next week (subjective probability of panic, panic expectancy) and to rate its expected aversiveness.

The group considered essential a measure of the tendency to fear the bodily sensations related to anxiety. Cognitive behavioral treatments target this fear, and some researchers believe that such fearfulness may be a traitlike characteristic different from statelike preoccupation (worry, anxious apprehension) or expectancy. Data suggest that the presence of anxiety focused on bodily sensations may be predictive of posttreatment outcome in both medication and psychosocial treatments.[10] There are several measures available to rate this dimension of anticipatory anxiety, including the Anxiety Sensitivity Inventory,[11,12] the Agoraphobic Cognitions and the Body Sensations questionnaires,[13] the Panic Appraisal Inventory,[14] and the Panic Belief Questionnaire.[14] The latter two measures are still under development. As in other areas, the group believed that it is the fear of anxiety construct, rather than the specific instrument, that should be viewed as essential.

Participants noted other dimensions of anticipatory anxiety that might be measured by Likert scales. Examples include the likelihood of a panic episode if the person engages in no avoidance (conditional subjective probability), how bad it would be if the person experienced panic (negative valence), and the degree of confidence that the person could cope if a panic episode occurred.

PHOBIC SYMPTOMS

The group agreed that a measure of phobic symptoms is essential. Phobic fear and avoidance should be measured separately, since they occur with different frequency and respond differently to treatment. Assessment of phobic severity must always refer to fear avoidance when the patient is unaccompanied, ie, alone. The most important consideration in rating phobic symptoms in a population with panic disorder is whether or not the phobia is panic related. However, extant phobia scales rate phobias according to diagnostic groups, ie, agoraphobia, simple phobia, and social phobia. Panic-related phobias often include social or specific phobic as well as agoraphobic situations and occur in response to internal as well as to external cues. In general, patients with panic disorder tend to avoid situations or activities because they fear that the situation or activity will provoke a panic

attack or because they are afraid of the consequences (physical and/or social) if an unexpected panic attack occurs.

Rating fear of internal sensations and the set of situations and activities that provoke these sensations was viewed as essential. Fear of bodily sensations and avoidance of situations that provoke these sensations occur with regularity in patients with panic disorder and are not usually included in the agoraphobic cluster. The importance of systematic assessment of fear of sensations was expressed by one participant, who said: "If we don't ask, we do not hear about it. I don't think I have ever asked a patient, 'Are you afraid of exercising?' But I can think of people who are afraid of exercising." Inquiry should be made about situations in which uncomfortable bodily sensations (cardiac, vestibular, or respiratory) are evoked. Examples are various forms of exercise, using saunas, or drinking coffee.

Since there is no existing, broadly focused, panic-related phobic rating scale, the subcommittee suggested the following five core characteristics of an "ideal" scale: (1) it separates fear and avoidance; (2) it adequately samples both interoceptive and external fear cues; (3) it meets acceptable psychometric standards; (4) it has an adequate database for making cross-study comparisons; and (5) it includes data from populations.

Even though there is not yet an ideal instrument, the group still believed phobia ratings to be necessary. Based on the fact that there is a large database for the brief Marks and Mathews Fear Questionnaire,[15,16] this questionnaire should be used for now. There was strong support for the development of a new scale to accomplish more effectively the rating of panic-related phobia that is essential to studies of panic disorder.

Phobic assessments can be based on self-report, clinician ratings, reporting by significant others, self-monitoring, psychophysiologic measures, or behavioral approach testing. The group endorsed the usefulness of all these methods but considered it essential that all studies of panic disorder should include a self-report scale and a clinician rating, encompassing both fear and avoidance. There was a recommendation that studies have a direct behavioral assessment of the patient's fear response to internal cues. Examples might include running in place, spinning in a desk chair, hyperventilation, or a sudden change in posture. A direct behavioral assessment of fear response to external cues is recommended only if agoraphobia is a major component of the study.

There are subtleties in the assessment of phobias that might be addressed, but they are considered optional for studies at this point in time. For example, whether the patient avoids a feared situation even when accompanied and whether recovery from avoidance occurs only when the patient is using medication could be important to consider.

OVERALL IMPAIRMENT, GLOBAL SEVERITY, AND IMPROVEMENT

There was consensus that a diagnosis-based, composite, global rating of severity is essential. A composite scale should include episodes of panic and limited symptoms, anticipatory anxiety phobic symptoms, and illness-related impairment, rated separately. The recently developed Multicenter Panic Anxiety Scale is an example of such a scale (available from M.K.S.). A measure of overall global severity and improvement was also considered essential, with separate panic and phobic rating scales.

A rating of functional impairment is essential and should include social, work, and family impairment, utilization of medical care (including psychiatric and nonpsychiatric care), and use of alcohol and other drugs.[17] There are several measures available to accomplish these goals, such as the Social Adjustment Scale,[18] but the group did not endorse any one of them as best. There was agreement that ratings of severity and impairment should be completed by the patient and the treating clinician. An additional rating by an independent evaluator (clinician) was recommended.

COMORBIDITY

Pretreatment assessment of current and lifetime comorbid Axis I disorders, especially including other anxiety disorders, mood disorders, substance abuse and dependence, and somatoform disorders is considered essential. Documentation of a history of childhood anxiety disorder may be of interest because of pathophysiologic and/or treatment implications of this history. The group recommended that childhood anxiety be assessed despite the limitations of retrospective data collection. Suggestions about how to conduct this assessment included using a modified version of the Schedule for Affective Disorders and Schizophrenia for School-Age Children,[19] using the parent version of a childhood structured assessment interview to rate the person as a child or using the section on childhood anxiety in the SADS-LA.

There was discussion of the need to define the criteria used to decide on panic disorder as the primary diagnosis in patients with comorbid disorders. This determination may be based on the clinical predominance, focus of help seeking, degree of impairment, or temporal sequence. There are multiple definitions of the distinction between primary and secondary disorders,[20] so it is important that investigators make explicit which one they are using. Since it is unknown whether treatment of panic disorder also results in improvement of concurrent comorbid disorders, conferees recommended reassessment of concurrent diagnoses posttreatment.

Attention to Axis III diagnoses

was considered essential. The group concluded that medical assessment should be documented and the presence of any Axis III disorder be recorded. There was a recommendation that women be assessed for the presence of late luteal-phase dysphoric disorder (*DSM-III-R*) and/or for the possibility of exacerbation of menstrual-related symptoms.

An assessment of personality disorder was recommended. Several considerations explained the conclusion that personality assessment is not essential. One problem is that the presence of an Axis I disorder may influence the assessment of the personality disorder, raising a question about the usefulness of conducting such assessments before treatment. A second problem is that the quality of existing assessment instruments is only fair. Self-reported measures of personality are sensitive but not specific, and interview methods are cumbersome and not well validated.[21] The group concluded that, in spite of the difficulties, it is meaningful to obtain information on personality disorders. Pretreatment personality assessment was recommended and posttreatment assessment was optional.

The discussion of comorbidity included agreement that it is essential to include dimensional measures of general anxiety and depression. General anxiety is defined as a state of activation or arousal, both cognitive and physiologic, not necessarily linked to the anticipation of panic. This dimension is not fully captured by any of the categorical diagnoses of anxiety disorder, nor is it covered by the concept of anticipatory anxiety. However, general anxiety was seen as a core feature of panic disorder that is essential to measure. Instruments such as the Hamilton Anxiety Rating Scale,[22] the Zung Anxiety Scales,[23] the Beck Anxiety Scale,[24] the Sheehan Patient Rated Anxiety Scale,[25] or Bystritsky's Four Dimensional Anxiety Scale[26] might be used.

Depression, in particular its atypical form, may be present to a substantial degree in patients who do not meet diagnostic criteria for a mood disorder. Thus, a dimensional rating of depression was considered essential. It was advised that a depression measure be used that is not heavily contaminated with anxiety items and that rates the atypical depressive items.

RESPONSE, REMISSION, RECOVERY, RELAPSE, AND RECURRENCE

Definitions of the terms response, remission, recovery, relapse, and recurrence are central to dialogue about treatment efficacy. However, there are no standard definitions, and investigators have used these terms idiosyncratically, virtually ensuring that different studies will use different definitions of these important concepts.

A MacArthur Foundation work group recently identified and addressed this problem for affective disorders.[27] Conference participants might have chosen to adopt criteria for remission, recovery, relapse, and recurrence in parallel with the affective disorder recommendations. However, recovery from an affective disorder is predicated on the known episodic nature of the disorder. Panic disorder is different because an episodic course is not established. For this reason, participants were unwilling to use the proposed criteria for affective disorders. It was believed that more discussion (and/or data) is needed to provide alternative definitions.

Whether recovery from panic disorder occurs is unclear. While data documenting symptom remission has been published[28] and some researchers interpret this as full recovery, others suggest that panic disorder resembles diabetes: current treatments allow for the disease to be controlled, but there is never recovery. One participant commented that remission implies a total absence of symptoms, and that state is seldom true for patients with panic disorder. Some studies of nonclinical populations document occasional panic in a low-to-moderate percentage of individuals.[29-31] However, it is not known if even occasional panic is worthy of clinical consideration.

Once the idea of defining recovery was abandoned, the group struggled with a definition of remission or response. However, agreement on a definition of these terms was not possible either since it was acknowledged that remission or response would depend on which symptom was being considered. For example, an individual might respond on a measure of panic but not respond on a measure of anticipatory anxiety or phobic avoidance. Data are not yet available to determine criteria for panic remission, eg, the time required to be free from panic, whether a patient with occasional panic could be "remitted" and whether the absence of limited-symptom episodes is required for remission.

Although the group agreed that it is important to acknowledge the possibility of remission and to determine an appropriate definition of remission, it was not possible to do so at this time. When the proposal to define remission as "asymptomatic" was put forward, there was controversy whether this term would mean asymptomatic without medication or whether it is possible to achieve remitted status while receiving medication. The conference concluded with this area unresolved. Further work is clearly needed to better define and operationalize these concepts. For the present, it is essential that investigators clearly define how these terms are used in their settings.

FOLLOW-UP

The kind and frequency of assessments following a treatment intervention was the last subject considered. Conferees noted that there is too little information about the long-term course of panic disorder and long-term effects of treatment inter-

ventions. There was agreement that it is essential to conduct a 12-month follow-up assessment after almost any treatment study. A follow-up assessment soon after the end of a treatment comparison was also recommended.

Consideration of practical issues related to conducting follow-up assessments resulted in the following essential areas to be measured: (1) a structured interview diagnosis, including panic disorder and other comorbid Axis I conditions, (2) severity of panic attacks, anticipatory anxiety, and phobic symptoms, (3) degree of impairment, global severity, and improvement, (4) type and frequency of interval treatments, and (5) interval medical conditions.

Additional measures recommended for follow-up assessment were a panic diary, other symptom ratings, life events, and quality of life information. Participants made note of the need for follow-up information about patients in clinical treatment settings who meet diagnostic criteria for panic disorder, but who are either not eligible for or are unwilling to enter research protocols. Recommendations are summarized as follows:

Summary of Recommendations: Essential Measures

- Structured interview diagnosis of panic disorder
- Daily self-monitoring of panic and limited-symptom episodes
  - Baseline period of at least 2 weeks
  - Establishing that the patient understands the definition of panic
- Anticipatory anxiety assessment
  - Daily self-monitoring of worry about panic and/or fear intensity
  - Measuring tendency to fear bodily sensations
- Panic-related phobias
  - Fear and avoidance rated separately
  - Social, specific, and agoraphobic situations included
  - Situations and/or activities in which uncomfortable bodily sensations are evoked included
- Overall illness severity
  - Composite rating of panic, limited-symptom episodes, anticipatory anxiety, phobic symptoms, and impairment
  - Rating by both patient and clinician
  - Global severity and improvement
- Social, work, and family impairment, medical care utilization, and use of alcohol and other drugs
- Comorbidity
  - Lifetime and current comorbid Axis I disorders
  - Axis III diagnoses
    - Record of type of medical assessment performed
    - Record of all Axis III disorders
  - Dimensional measures of anxiety and depressive symptoms
- Remission, relapse, response, and recovery
  - Define terms
- Follow-up
  - Structured interview diagnosis, including both panic disorder and other diagnoses
  - Measurement of frequency and severity of panic attacks, degree of anticipatory anxiety, and panic-related phobia
  - Measurement of impairment, global severity, and improvement
  - Measurement of type and frequency of interval treatment
  - Measurement of interval medical outcomes

Summary of Recommendations: Recommended and Optional Measures

- Structured diagnostic assessment, recommended
  - Structured interview diagnosis of current and lifetime comorbidity
  - Inclusion of an experienced clinician in the diagnostic decision making
- Panic attack assessment, recommended
  - Four weeks of monitoring of panic attacks
  - Criterion of one or more panic attack per week for 2 weeks for studies targeting panic as the main outcome
  - Registration of subthreshold panic in studies for which this is appropriate
- Anticipatory anxiety assessment, recommended
  - Daily self-monitoring of anticipatory anxiety for at least 2 weeks
  - Measurement of prediction or expectation of having a panic episode in the near future (eg, in the next week)
- Phobic symptom assessment, recommended
  - Measurement of social phobia
  - Direct behavioral measurement of fear of internal cues
  - Direct behavioral measurement of panic-related, external fear cues, for agoraphobia studies
- Phobic symptom assessment, optional
  - Measurement of simple phobia
  - Measurement of influence on phobic symptoms by factors such as being with someone or receiving medication
- Overall impairment, global severity, and improvement, recommended
  - Ratings by an independent evaluator
- Comorbidity, recommended
  - Posttreatment assessment of comorbid diagnoses identified at pretreatment
  - Definition of explicit criteria for determining primary or predominant diagnoses
  - Assessment of women for late luteal-phase dysphoric disorder and/or exacerbation of menstrual-related symptoms

Assessment of personality disorders
Assessment of childhood anxiety disorders

- Follow-up assessment, recommended
  Panic diary
  Information about major life events and quality of life
  Follow-up soon after the end of a treatment study

COMMENT

To our knowledge, this conference was one of the first attempts to bring together a group of active investigators from diverse backgrounds to decide on a standardized battery of assessments for a *DSM-III-R* disorder. The group of anxiety researchers assembled for this conference represented both psychosocial and biological perspectives. While there were some differences among attendees regarding which assessments were essential, conference participants were united in their strong agreement with the need for developing standardized procedures. This sentiment led to a willingness to compromise and made it possible to achieve unanimity on an assessment package considered essential. The group did not endorse any instrument as the best one for rating any of the dimensions considered essential. In some cases, there was a conclusion that no instrument exists that serves the purpose. This was true, in particular, for the assessment of panic-related phobic symptoms.

How should the terms essential, recommended, and optional be used in peer review of grant applications and journal articles? The sense of the group was that for research to be considered of highest quality and rigorous, and for publication in the best journals, assessments deemed essential are essential. Recommended and optional assessments are intended more for the investigator than for the peer reviewer.

On one prominent issue the group could reach no agreement. This issue was the question of definitions of remission, recovery, recurrence, relapse, and response. Although there was agreement on the need for defining these concepts, it was not possible to resolve the central problem of uncertainty about the course of illness that is the basis for the definition of recovery or about the level of symptom relief that should be considered "remission."

Discussion and endorsement of standard assessment brought to the fore several problematic issues in the field. Three deserve to be highlighted. First, there has been a strong movement toward the use of scheduled, structured interviews as the "gold standard" for assessment of diagnosis. The group endorsed this procedure but emphasized the need for input by a senior, experienced clinician, in addition to appropriate training and certification of the interviewers.

A second issue relates to the concept of anticipatory anxiety. The *DSM-III-R* criteria for panic disorder include the presence of panic attacks and/or of persistent fear of having a panic episode. The *DSM-IV* criteria will continue to include anticipatory anxiety in the diagnostic criteria. However, the meaning of anticipatory anxiety and the ways of assessing fear of panic are ambiguous. The conference subcommittee pointed out that anxiety related to fear of panic is different from the general level of arousal and from generalized anxiety. Fear of panic is a specific, focused anxiety that may be manifest in a variety of ways, such as preoccupation or worry about having a panic attack, the degree of expectation or prediction that a panic attack may occur, and a tendency to fear panic, the consequences of panic, or the bodily sensations associated with panic. It has now been established that fear of the bodily sensations is a consistent characteristic of patients with panic disorder, but there is controversy over whether this is a cause or a consequence of panic, or both. To ensure further investigation of this important question, conference participants endorsed as essential a measure of the tendency to fear anxiety and anxiety-related bodily sensations.

The relationship between panic and phobic avoidance was the third issue addressed. While panic disorder is linked to agoraphobia in *DSM-III*, *DSM-III-R*, and *DSM-IV*, conferees considered assessment of any area of panic-related phobic symptoms to be essential. This requirement refers to the fact that patients with panic disorder fear and avoid situations that do not meet diagnostic criteria for agoraphobia. Agoraphobia is defined in *DSM-III-R* as "fear of being in places or situations from which escape might be difficult (or embarrassing) or in which help might not be available"[2(p241)] and is associated with a typical constellation of situations such as public transportation, crowds, tunnels, bridges, open spaces, travel far from home, and being home alone. Most agoraphobics fear these situations because of fear of having a panic or a limited-symptom episode. However, patients with panic disorder commonly fear other situations as well. Many have phobias about situations such as physical exercise or emotionally arousing events that provoke physiologic arousal of feared bodily sensations. Others may be fearful predominantly in social situations in which they feel embarrassed or otherwise in danger if a panic episode occurs; a patient with panic disorder may also experience a specific fear and avoidance reaction, such as a driving phobia, as the phobic complication. Thus, the group concluded that it is essential for assessment procedures for panic disorder to include measures of any panic-related phobia, not simply agoraphobia. It was acknowledged that a new instrument is needed to measure such phobias.

Another issue of importance was communicated after the conference by Robert Prien, PhD, and by Hillary Lee, PhD, and Gregory Dubitsky, MD. These experts pointed out that there are serious, but seldom attended to, issues related to the

control and design of follow-up studies. They questioned whether it would be possible to evaluate rigorously the 12-month outcomes since there would be no control over what the patients did during the interval. They suggested that questions be included to assess what treatments may have been obtained by the subject between the end of the research protocol and follow-up and whether the patient had continued "homework" instructions given during and/or at the end of the formal protocol. When the patient comes in for assessment at the time of follow-up, the rater should be blind to the earlier condition of treatment. The science of follow-up studies is not well thought through and deserves a separate program of discussion. This conference did not address follow-up methods in depth.

It seems logical that the requirements developed by this conference should not persist indefinitely. An end date was not discussed, but a reasonable time limit of 5 to 8 years after the date of this publication would be appropriate. At that time the impact of the decisions made in 1993 can be judged for their effectiveness, and investigators can reconsider what is essential for the assessment of panic.

In conclusion, this group of researchers was united in a belief that standardized assessment procedures are needed for advancing our understanding of panic disorder, especially its treatment. At the same time, there was a healthy respect for the need to preserve a substantial degree of freedom for investigators to decide which assessments are most appropriate for the study that they plan to conduct. No rule or standard can substitute for good judgment in research. Clearly, establishment of standards for assessment in no way prevents the creative application of additional assessment procedures, and, with reasonable justification, any of the essential measures can be omitted.

Accepted for publication July 30, 1993.

Supported in part by an unrestricted grant from the Upjohn Company, Kalamazoo, Mich, to the University of Pittsburgh, Pa.

This article reports the results of a conference held from October 29, 1992, to October 30, 1992, in Pentagon City, Va, sponsored by the National Institute of Mental Health (NIMH), Bethesda, Md.

The opinions expressed are those of the participants as understood by the authors and do not necessarily represent the views of the NIMH.

Reprint requests to Western Psychiatric Institute and Clinic, 3811 O'Hara St, Pittsburgh, PA 15213 (Dr Shear).

REFERENCES

1. Wolfe B, Maser JD, eds. *The Treatment of Panic Disorder: A Consensus Development Conference.* Washington, DC: American Psychiatric Press. In press.
2. American Psychiatric Association. *Diagnostic and Statistical Manual of Mental Disorders, Third Edition Revised.* Washington, DC: American Psychiatric Association; 1987.
3. Maser JD, Cloninger CR, eds. *Comorbidity of Mood and Anxiety Disorders.* Washington, DC: American Psychiatric Press; 1990.
4. DiNardo PA, Barlow DH. *Anxiety Disorders Interview Schedule, Revised (ADIS-R).* New York, NY: Graywinds Publications; 1988.
5. Robins LN, Wing J, Wittchen H-U, Helzer JE, Babor TF, Burke J, Farmer A, Jablensky A, Pickens R, Regier DA, Sartorius N, Towle LH. The composite international diagnostic interview: an epidemiologic instrument suitable for use in conjunction with different diagnostic systems and in different cultures. *Arch Gen Psychiatry.* 1989; 45:1069-1077.
6. Robins LN, Helzer JE, Croughan J, Ratliffe KS. National Institute of Mental Health Diagnostic Interview Schedule: its history, characteristics, and validity. *Arch Gen Psychiatry.* 1981;38:381-389.
7. Manuzza S, Fyer A, Klein D, Endicott J. Schedule for Affective Disorders–Lifetime, Anxiety (SADS-LA): rationale and conceptual development. *J Psychiatr Res.* 1986;20:317-325.
8. Spitzer RL, Williams JBW, Gibbon M, First MB. *Structured Clinical Interview for DSM-III-R: Patient Version (SCID-P 6/1/88).* New York, NY: Biometrics Research Department, New York State Psychiatric Institute; 1988.
9. Page AC. An assessment of structured diagnostic interviews for adult anxiety disorders. *Int Rev Psychiatry.* 1991;3:265-278.
10. Clark DM. Cognitive therapy for panic disorder. In: Wolfe B, Maser JD, eds. *The Treatment of Panic Disorder: A Consensus Development Conference.* Washington, DC: American Psychiatric Press. In press.
11. Reiss S, Peterson RA, Gursky DM, McNally RJ. Anxiety sensitivity, anxiety frequency, and the prediction of fearfulness. *Behav Res Ther.* 1986;24: 1-8.
12. Peterson RA, Reiss S. *Manual for the Anxiety Sensitivity Index.* 2nd ed. Worthington, Ohio: International Diagnostic Services, Inc; 1992.
13. Chambless DL, Caputo GC, Bright P, Gallagher R. The assessment of fear of fear in agoraphobics: the Body Sensations Questionnaire and the Agoraphobic Cognitions Questionnaire. *J Consult Clin Psychol.* 1984;52:1090-1097.
14. Greenberg RL. Panic disorder and agoraphobia. In: Scott J, Williams JMG, Beck AT, eds. *Cognitive Therapy in Clinical Practice: An Illustrative Casebook.* London, England: Routledge and Kegan Paul; 1989:25-49.
15. Marks IM, Mathews AM. Brief standard self-rating for phobic patients. *Behav Res Ther.* 1979; 17:263-267.
16. Mizes JS, Crawford J. Normative values on the Marks and Mathews Fear Questionnaire: a comparison as a function of age and sex. *J Psychopathol Behav Assessment.* 1986;8:253-262.
17. Markowitz JS, Weissman MM, Ouellette R, Lish JD, Klerman JL. Quality of life in panic disorder. *Arch Gen Psychiatry.* 1989;46:984-992.
18. Weissman MM, Bothwell S. The assessment of social adjustment patient self-report. *Arch Gen Psychiatry.* 1976;33:1111-1115.
19. Puig-Antich J, Chambers W. *The Schedule for Affective Disorders and Schizophrenia for School-Age Children (Kiddie-SADS).* New York, NY: New York State Psychiatric Institute; 1978.
20. Maser JD, Weise R, Gwirtsman H. Depression and its boundaries with selected axis I disorders. In: Beckham EE, Leber WR, eds. *Handbook of Depression.* 2nd ed. Homewood, Ill: The Dorsey Press. In press.
21. Perry JC. Problems and considerations in the valid assessment of personality disorders. *Am J Psychiatry.* 1992;149:1645-1653.
22. Hamilton M. The assessment of anxiety states by rating. *Br J Med Psychol.* 1959;32:50-55.
23. Zung WWK. A rating instrument for anxiety disorders. *Psychosomatics.* 1971;12:371-379.
24. Riskind JH, Beck AT, Brown GB, Steer RA. Taking the measure of anxiety and depression: validity of reconstructed Hamilton Scales. *J Nerv Ment Dis.* 1987;175:474-479.
25. Sheehan DV. *The Anxiety Disease.* New York, NY: Charles Scribner's Sons; 1983:126-128.
26. Bystritsky A, Linn LS, Ware JE. Development of a multidimensional scale of anxiety. *J Anxiety Disorders.* 1990;4:99-115.
27. Frank E, Prien RF, Jarrett R, Keller MB, Kupfer DJ, Lavori PW, Rush AJ, Weissman MM. Conceptualization and rationale for consensus definitions of terms in major depressive disorder. *Arch Gen Psychiatry.* 1991;48:851-855.
28. Margraf J, Barlow D, Clark D, Telch M. Psychological treatment of panic: work in progress on outcome, active ingredients, and follow-up. *Behav Res Ther.* 1993;31:1-9.
29. Norton GR, Dorward J, Cox BJ. Factors associated with panic attacks in nonclinical subjects. *Behav Ther.* 1986;17:239-252.
30. Norton GR, Harrison B, Hauch J, Rhodes L. Characteristics of people with infrequent panic attacks. *J Abnorm Psychol.* 1985;94:216-222.
31. Wilson KG, Sandler LS, Asmundson GJG, Ediger JM, Larson DK, Walker JR. Panic attacks in the nonclinical population: an empirical approach to case identification. *J Abnorm Psychol.* 1992;101:460-468.

DSM-III-R Generalized Anxiety Disorder in the National Comorbidity Survey

Hans-Ulrich Wittchen, PhD; Shanyang Zhao, PhD; Ronald C. Kessler, PhD; William W. Eaton, PhD

Background: Nationally representative general population data are presented on the current, 12-month, and lifetime prevalence of *DSM-III-R* generalized anxiety disorder (GAD) as well as on risk factors, comorbidity, and related impairments.

Methods: The data are from the National Comorbidity Survey, a large general population survey of persons aged 15 to 54 years in the noninstitutionalized civilian population of the United States. *DSM-III-R* GAD was assessed by lay interviewers using a revised version of the Composite International Diagnostic Interview.

Results: Generalized anxiety disorder was found to be a relatively rare current disorder with a current prevalence of 1.6% but was found to be a more frequent lifetime disorder affecting 5.1% of the US population aged 15 to 45 years. Generalized anxiety disorder was twice as common among women as among men. Multivariate logistic regression analysis showed that being older than 24 years, separated, widowed, divorced, unemployed, and a homemaker are significant correlates of GAD. Consistent with studies in treatment samples, we found that GAD was frequently associated with a wide spectrum of other mental disorders, with a lifetime comorbidity among 90.4% of the people who had a history of GAD.

Conclusion: Contrary to the traditional view that GAD is a mild disorder, we found that the majority of people with GAD, whether they were comorbid or not, reported substantial interference with their life, a high degree of professional help seeking, and a high use of medication because of their GAD symptoms. Although lifetime GAD is highly comorbid, the proportion of current GAD that is not accompanied by any other current diagnosis is high enough to indicate that GAD should be considered an independent disorder rather than exclusively a residual or prodrome of other disorders.

(Arch Gen Psychiatry. 1994;51:355-364)

From the Max-Planck-Institut fur Psychiatrie Clinical Institute, Munich, Germany (Dr Wittchen); the Institute for Social Research (Drs Zhao and Kessler) and the Department of Sociology (Dr Kessler), the University of Michigan, Ann Arbor; and the Department of Mental Hygiene, The Johns Hopkins University School of Hygiene and Public Health, Baltimore, Md (Dr Eaton).

GENERALIZED Anxiety disorder (GAD) is usually regarded as prevalent in both the primary care and mental health specialty care sectors. However, the high comorbidity of GAD with other disorders has led to considerable disagreement concerning whether GAD should be conceptualized as an independent disorder or as a residual or prodrome of other disorders.[1] There are only few, rather contradictory epidemiologic data available to address this question and to provide basic data about the prevalence, associated risk factors, and comorbidity of GAD in the general population.

As shown in **Table 1**,[2-9] community prevalence studies based on *DSM-III* diagnoses reported current prevalences of GAD that ranged from 1.2%[6] to 6.4%[3] and lifetime prevalences between 4.0%[7] and 6.6%.[6] The Epidemiologic Catchment Area (ECA) Study was the only one of these studies to report detailed findings on the associated features of GAD.[5] However, an assessment of GAD was included in only three of the five ECA sites, and no nationwide projection of the prevalence of GAD was reported. The three ECA sites that assessed GAD varied somewhat in their questions and criteria, which led to a lack of precision in the findings regarding GAD

See Methods on next page

METHODS

SAMPLE

The data presented herein come from the NCS, a congressionally mandated survey of the United States designed to produce data on the prevalence, risk factors, and consequences of psychiatric morbidity and comorbidity. The 8098 respondents, aged 15 to 54 years, were selected from a stratified sample of small areas in 172 counties in 34 states throughout the United States by use of probability methods. The survey was administered by the staff of the Survey Research Center at the University of Michigan, Ann Arbor. The field period was between September 14, 1990, and February 6, 1992. The response rate was 82.4%. The data reported herein have been weighted to adjust for variation in within-household probabilities of selection and systematic nonresponse and have been poststratified by means of an iterative procedure to approximate the national population distributions of the cross-classification of age, sex, race/ethnicity, marital status, education, living arrangements, region, and urbanicity as defined by the 1989 US National Health Interview Survey.[20] A more detailed description of the NCS sampling design is reported elsewhere.[21]

DIAGNOSTIC ASSESSMENT

The *DSM-III-R* diagnoses were based on a modified version of the Composite International Diagnostic Interview (CIDI),[22] a fully structured diagnostic interview developed in a collaborative project of the World Health Organization, Geneva, Switzerland, and the Alcohol, Drug Abuse, and Mental Health Administration, Washington, DC,[23] to foster epidemiologic and cross-cultural comparative research by producing diagnoses according to the definitions and criteria of both *DSM-III-R*[24] and the Diagnostic Criteria for Research of the *ICD-10*.[25] The CIDI uses the same basic architecture as the Diagnostic Interview Schedule.[26] Diagnoses were generated by the use of the CIDI diagnostic program.[22,27-29]

There are five diagnostic criteria for GAD in the *DSM-III-R*. Criterion A requires unrealistic or excessive anxiety and worry about two or more life circumstances more days than not over a period of at least 6 months.[24] This criterion was translated in a series of CIDI questions that began by asking about the lifetime occurrence of a period lasting 6 months or more when "most of the time you felt worried or anxious." This was followed by a question about whether the worries were ever about "things that were not likely to happen" or "things that were not really serious." A third question then asked whether the respondent ever had "different worries" on his or her mind "at the same time." Among respondents who answered all three of these criterion A questions positively, information was collected about the content of the worries ("What sorts of things did you worry about?"). This information was used to classify respondents according to the requirement of criterion B that "if another Axis I disorder is present, the focus of the anxiety and worry in A is unrelated to it." Based on this requirement, respondents who reported that their worries were exclusively about having a recurrence or a worsening of some other psychiatric disorder were excluded from further questioning. The remaining respondents were then asked whether they experienced any of 18 psychophysiological symptoms. Exclusion probes were used to determine whether any of these symptoms could be due entirely to physical illness, injury, medications, or alcohol or other drugs. These exclusion probes were meant to assess criterion E, which stipulates that "it cannot be established that an organic factor initiated and maintained the disturbance." A count of the symptoms endorsed as occurring typically during the periods of anxiety and worry and not due to organic causes was then used to match criterion D, which requires that at least six of the remaining 18 symptoms are present during periods of worry and anxiety. Symptoms that were also present during panic attacks were excluded from this count to meet the stipulation in criterion D that symptoms present only during panic attacks should not be counted among the six required for a diagnosis of GAD. Finally, respondents in whom a mood disorder and/or psychotic disorder was diagnosed were asked additional questions to assess the diagnostic hierarchy rule in criterion C that the anxiety cannot occur "only during the course of a mood disorder or a psychotic disorder."

The reliability and validity of the GAD section in the

in comparison with other ECA findings. Furthermore, the major study on the ECA findings[5] reported most of the findings only for the subset of respondents with GAD who did not have a history of either major depression or panic disorder.

Since the introduction of the *DSM-III-R* in 1987, only two small regional epidemiologic studies have reported *DSM-III-R* prevalences for GAD. Faravelli et al[8] reported a current prevalence of 2.8% and a lifetime prevalence of 5.4% in a population survey of Florence, Italy. Wacker et al[9] reported a lifetime prevalence of 1.9% without using diagnostic hierarchy rules in a survey of Basel, Switzerland. The latter study, which, to our knowledge, is the only epidemiologic survey to compare prevalence according to the definitions and criteria of both the *DSM-III-R* and the *International Classification of Diseases, Tenth Revision* (*ICD-10*), found the lifetime prevalence to be over four times higher (9.2%) using *ICD-10* criteria.

This considerable heterogeneity of prevalence findings can be explained partly by the fact that there have been many changes and revisions in the diagnostic criteria for GAD between the *DSM-III* and the *DSM-III-R*. Whereas the *DSM-III* required a 1-month duration of symptoms, the *DSM-III-R* requires a 6-month duration. The *DSM-III-R* also requires more specific cognitive elements (unrealistic and excessive anxiety and worry) than

CIDI has been examined in a series of international studies that were, in large part, conducted as part of the World Health Organization field trials of the CIDI.[26] These results are relevant to the present investigation because the modifications of the CIDI in the NCS did not involve any changes in the GAD section. The CIDI field trials documented good acceptance and the cultural appropriateness of the CIDI,[30,31] excellent interrater reliability,[32,33] and good test-retest reliability in two independent investigations with a time interval of 1 to 3 days.[12,31] Good validity of the CIDI was also documented with regard to concordance with clinical diagnoses,[34-37] procedural validity compared with the Present State Examination,[34,38,39] as well as specific issues such as the validity of time-related information compared with well-documented clinical records,[40] the validity of the probe questions,[37] and assessments of comorbidity (H-U.W. and A. Gnutzman, Dipl Psych, unpublished data, September 1992). The interrater reliability for GAD was found to be excellent with a κ value of 0.96 (n=575).[31] The test-retest reliability for the diagnosis of GAD was found to be good with a κ value of 0.69 (n=158),[41] whereas κ values for symptom reliability ranged from 0.5 to 0.96 (n=60).[34]

INTERVIEWERS AND INTERVIEWER TRAINING

The Survey Research Center interviewing staff was highly experienced. The 158 interviewers working on the NCS had an average of 5 years prior interviewing experience with the Survey Research Center. In addition, the NCS interviewers completed a 7-day study-specific training program for the NCS consisting of 2 days of self-study followed by a 5-day group training session in Ann Arbor. Interviewer performance was closely monitored throughout the NCS field period. Three aspects of monitoring are particularly noteworthy. First, all interviews were edited by field supervisors as soon as they were completed to allow rapid detection of missing data and unclear responses. The interviews were returned to the field for recontact with the respondent whenever problems of this sort were detected. Second, the field edits were reviewed at the national field office as soon as the interviews were received to provide a second check on the interviewer's performance as well as a check on the accuracy of the supervisor's editing. Supervisors were contacted whenever errors were found, and the interview was sent back to the field for resolution. Third, a random subsample of respondents were recontacted by the field supervisors to verify the accuracy of the interviewer reports and to check on the care and accuracy with which the interviews were carried out. The interviewers were aware of the fact that this random checking was being done and that their continued participation in the study required high ratings when the checks were made, thus leading to the expectation that this quality-control mechanism led to improved data in all interviews rather than only in the subsample of interviews that were checked.

ANALYSIS PROCEDURES

The analyses included the estimation of prevalences of GAD, of prevalences of other disorders in the subsample of respondents with GAD for the purpose of studying comorbidity, and of the prevalence of various types of impairment. In addition, odds ratios (ORs) were calculated to describe comorbidity between GAD and other disorders and to describe the strength of demographic correlates of GAD.

Because the data analyzed were obtained from a stratified multistage sample with weights, estimates of the SEs based on the usual assumptions of equal-probability simple random sampling are biased. More complex analysis methods are needed to obtain appropriate SEs. Estimates of the SEs of the prevalences and proportions reported herein were obtained using the Taylor series linearization method.[42] The PSRATIO program in OSIRIS[43] was used to make these calculations. Estimates of confidence intervals of ORs were obtained using the method of Balanced Repeated Replications.[44] The LOGISTIC program in SAS[45] was used to estimate the ORs. An SAS macro was used to replicate these estimates in subsamples, to compute estimates of the SEs of the logits from the distribution of the coefficients across these replications, and to use this design-based estimate of the SEs to compute confidence intervals of the ORs. The Balanced Repeated Replications estimates take into account the clustering and weighting in the design without the linearization constraint required in the Taylor series method, yielding somewhat less biased estimates of the SEs in nonlinear models such as logistic regression.[46,47]

did the *DSM-III* and requires six specific symptoms from a slightly different symptom criteria group than the three required in the *DSM-III*. Furthermore, a narrower diagnostic hierarchy rule (GAD should not be diagnosed when it only occurs during the course of a mood or psychotic disorder) was introduced in the *DSM-III-R*. Based on these changes, we would expect to find a lower prevalence of GAD using *DSM-III-R* criteria.[10]

Comparisons are also made below between the *DSM-III-R* and the new *ICD-10* criteria[11] for GAD. Although the two systems agree on requiring a 6-month duration, the *ICD-10* criteria are broader in that worrying, which must be unrealistic or excessive in the *DSM-III-R* system, can include prominent tension, worry, and feelings of apprehension about everyday events and problems whether or not they are justified. Furthermore, a lower symptom threshold is used in the *ICD-10* (four symptoms, of which at least one must be an autonomous arousal symptom) compared with the six-symptom threshold in the *DSM-III-R*. In light of these diagnostic differences, we would expect to find a higher prevalence of *ICD-10* GAD compared with *DSM-III-R* GAD, which is consistent with the results of Wacker et al.[12]

In addition to general population surveys, there have been several studies that documented considerably higher prevalences of *DSM-III-R* GAD relative to the general popu-

lation in samples of psychiatric outpatients,[13] patients infected with the human immunodeficiency virus,[14] and patients in a specialty clinic.[15] These service-oriented studies also found a high current comorbidity of GAD with major depression and dysthymia.[12,16,17] These results are consistent with clinical reports that describe GAD as a generally mild but chronic disorder that primarily comes to clinical attention if a comorbid condition, such as depression, develops.[17] Some authors also consider GAD conceptually as a possible characterological disorder.[16,18] It is also noteworthy that there are several authors who suggest that GAD is especially prevalent in primary care settings.[19] However, there are no empirical studies that investigate this assumption.

With regard to risk factors, the only stable finding across all studies is a 2:1 female-male preponderance of GAD. The ECA Study was the only study that investigated other risk factors and associated impairments.[5] The ECA investigators found that GAD (defined without using the *DSM-III* hierarchy rules) is more prevalent in women, in blacks, and in persons under the age of 30. However, no multivariate risk factor analysis was carried out in the ECA. Nor was a systematic attempt made to study the comorbidity of GAD with other disorders.

The current report attempts to advance our understanding of GAD beyond these earlier investigations by reporting results from the National Comorbidity Survey (NCS), the first survey to administer a structured psychiatric interview to a representative national sample of the US population. We report estimates of the prevalence of GAD in the United States based on *DSM-III-R* criteria. We also evaluate differences in these results using *ICD-10* criteria and assess risk factors for GAD, comorbidity between GAD and other disorders, and the severity and impairments associated with GAD.

Table 1. Prevalence of GAD in Previous General Population Survey*

Source, y	Period	Prevalence: Total	Females	Males
RDC/*DSM-III* studies				
Weissman et al,[2] 1978	Current	2.5	NA	NA
Uhlenhuth et al,[3] 1983	Current	6.4	NA	NA
Angst et al,[4] 1982	12 mo	3.8	NA	NA
Blazer et al,[5] 1991				
ECA, Durham, NC[6]	Current/ lifetime	1.2/6.6	7.3	5.7
ECA, St Louis, Mo[6]	Current/ lifetime	1.3/6.6	7.8	5.2
ECA, Los Angeles, Calif[6]	Current/ lifetime	1.4/4.1	5.5	2.6
Wittchen et al,[7] 1992	Current/ lifetime	2.4/4.0	NA	NA
DSM-III-R studies				
Faravelli et al,[8] 1989	Current/ lifetime	2.8/5.4	NA	NA
Wacker et al,[9] 1992	Lifetime *DSM-III-R*	1.9	NA	NA
	Lifetime *ICD-10*	9.2	NA	NA

**GAD indicates generalized anxiety disorder; RDC, Research Diagnostic Criteria; NA, not available; ECA, Epidemiologic Catchment Area; and* ICD-10, International Classisication of Diseases, Tenth Revision.

RESULTS

THE PREVALENCE OF GAD

The NCS prevalence estimates for *DSM-III-R* GAD are reported in **Table 2**. These estimates were made without using diagnostic hierarchy rules. Prevalence in the total sample was 1.6% for current GAD (defined as the most recent 6-month period of anxiety still going on in the 30 days prior to the interview), 3.1% for 12-month GAD, and 5.1% for lifetime GAD. In all three time frames there was a clear predominance of women, with a female-to-male ratio of approximately 2:1. The lowest prevalence in all three time frames was found for the age group of 15 to 24 years (current, 0.8%; lifetime, 2.0%). Considerably higher prevalences were found for women aged 45 or older (current, 3.5%; lifetime, 10.3%). This suggests that GAD is rare in adolescence and early adulthood (although the lifetime prevalence of 2.0% among respondents in the age range from 15 to 24 years shows that GAD can occur early in life) and is more common among adults, especially women.

Prevalence estimates did not change much when diagnostic hierarchy rules were imposed to exclude respondents whose GAD occurs exclusively during episodes of a mood disorder or a psychotic disorder. This is striking, in light of the fact that 72.2% of NCS respondents with a lifetime history of GAD also had a history of a mood or psychotic disorder. Only 8% of these respondents, however, reported that their GAD occurs exclusively during episodes of these other disorders. As a result, our estimate of the lifetime prevalence of GAD was reduced by only about 5% of the base (from 5.1% to 4.8%) when *DSM-III-R* diagnostic hierarchy rules were imposed ($5.1-5.1\times0.722\times0.08=4.8$). In comparison, prevalence estimates were considerably lower when we followed the ECA investigators in reporting the prevalence of GAD, excluding respondents with comorbid major depression and/or panic disorder. The estimated prevalences of GAD without major depression or panic disorder were 1.6% (lifetime), 1.1% (12 month), and 0.8% (current). These prevalences are only between one third (lifetime, 1.6/5.1=0.31; 12 month, 1.1/3.1=.35) and one half (current, 0.8/1.6=0.50) as large as the unrestricted prevalences in Table 2. The higher ratio for the most recent period suggests that the comorbidity of GAD with major depression or panic disorder is associated with a more chronic course of GAD.

Table 2. Current (30 Days), 12-Month, and Lifetime Values for Generalized Anxiety Disorder (GAD) by Age and Sex (Weighted)

	Men			Women			Total		
Age, y	**Percentage***	**SE**	**No.**	**Percentage***	**SE**	**No.**	**Percentage***	**SE**	**No.**
Current (30 days)									
15-24	0.8	0.4	8	0.8	0.4	10	0.8	0.3	18
25-34	1.6	0.5	18	2.5	0.8	25	2.1	0.5	43
35-44	1.0	0.4	16	1.9	0.6	18	1.4	0.3	34
≥45	0.4	0.2	9	3.5	1.0	19	1.9	0.5	28
Total	1.0	0.2	**51**	2.1	0.4	**72**	1.6	0.2	**123**
12 month									
15-24	1.3	0.5	11	1.5	0.6	13	1.4	0.4	24
25-34	3.2	0.7	32	5.0	0.9	53	4.1	0.6	85
35-44	2.3	0.6	27	4.5	1.0	43	3.4	0.6	70
≥45	0.9	0.3	14	6.3	1.3	35	3.5	0.7	49
Total	2.0	0.3	**84**	4.3	0.4	**144**	3.1	0.3	**228**
Lifetime									
15-24	1.5	0.6	14	2.5	0.7	24	2.0	0.5	38
25-34	4.7	0.8	54	7.1	1.0	90	6.0	0.6	144
35-44	4.6	0.8	58	7.2	1.2	81	5.9	0.8	139
≥45	3.6	1.1	28	10.3	1.5	66	6.9	0.8	94
Total	3.6	0.5	**154**	6.6	0.5	**261**	5.1	0.3	**415**

**The proportion of respondents with GAD.*

DIFFERENCES BETWEEN *DSM-III-R* AND *ICD-10* CRITERIA

The NCS did not collect data on symptoms of GAD for respondents whose anxiety never lasted as long as 6 months, so we have no way of computing *DSM-III* prevalence estimates. We can, however, investigate the difference between *DSM-III-R* and *ICD-10* prevalence estimates. As noted above, the most important difference between these two systems is whether extreme worry or anxiety in the face of real situations is considered normal (*DSM-III-R*) or part of the GAD psychopathological spectrum (*ICD-10*). This distinction can be expected to have a substantial effect on prevalence estimates because there are presumably a great many people who have objectively severe problems that lead to justifiable worries. In an effort to shed some light on this issue, we looked separately at the people who met the criteria for *DSM-III-R* GAD and those who met only the *ICD-10* criteria for GAD. The lifetime prevalence of GAD was considerably higher when defined according to the definitions and criteria of the *ICD-10* (8.9%) than those of the *DSM-III-R* (5.1%), although the ratio of these two prevalence estimates (8.9/5.1=1.74) was considerably lower than the ratio reported by Wacker and colleagues[9] (4.84). It is also noteworthy that 12-month *ICD-10* GAD had roughly the same relative prevalence as 12-month *DSM-III-R* GAD (5.0% compared with 3.1%, which produces a prevalence ratio of 1.61).

COMORBIDITY

Ignoring the *DSM-III-R* diagnostic hierarchy rules, 90.4% of the respondents with lifetime GAD reported having at least one of the other lifetime disorders listed in **Table 3**, whereas 66.3% of those with current GAD reported at least one other disorder during the past 30 days. These results changed only modestly when the analysis was replicated with the imposition of diagnostic hierarchy rules for GAD (lifetime comorbidity, 89.8%; current comorbidity, 65.0%). The strongest comorbidities, with ORs between 9.91 and 13.52 for lifetime disorders and between 13.86 and 26.98 for current disorders, were with affective disorders, panic disorder, and (for current comorbidity only) agoraphobia. Analyses not reported here showed that these ORs were not strongly affected by diagnostic hierarchy rules. Detailed results of all comorbidity analyses with hierarchy rules are available from one of us (H-U.W.). For example, the OR between lifetime GAD and dysthymia was 13.52 when GAD was defined without hierarchy rules and 12.81 when it was defined with hierarchy rules.

The extremely high comorbidity of GAD with other disorders raises questions concerning whether GAD should be considered an independent disorder. It is informative in this regard to note that in addition to the 9.6% of people with GAD who reported that this was their only lifetime disorder, another 12.2% reported that the age of onset of GAD was earlier than that of any other disorder. To-

Table 3. Comorbidity of 30-Day and Lifetime *DSM-III-R* GAD Without Hierarchy*

Comorbid Disorder	30-Day GAD†				Lifetime GAD‡			
	Percentage§	SE	OR	95% CI	Percentage§	SE	OR	95% CI
Mania	12.1	4.1	19.64	7.24-53.27	10.5	2.0	9.91	5.34-18.38
Major depression	38.6	6.0	13.86	7.93-24.25	62.4	4.2	9.72	6.68-14.12
Dysthymia	22.1	5.3	24.78	12.40-49.53	39.5	3.6	13.52	10.01-14.12
Panic disorder	22.6	5.7	26.08	9.83-68.22	23.5	2.2	12.32	9.20-16.50
Agoraphobia	26.7	6.8	19.21	9.05-40.77	25.7	2.8	5.80	4.39-7.66
Simple phobia	24.5	6.2	5.91	2.77-12.59	35.1	3.5	4.88	3.43-6.89
Social phobia	23.2	4.6	6.87	4.33-10.90	34.4	3.4	3.77	2.83-5.03
ALC	11.2	3.1	1.68	1.19-6.27	37.6	3.7	2.04	1.46-2.87
Drug	5.1	2.1	1.99	0.68-11.41	27.6	2.6	3.08	2.28-4.15
Any of the above	66.3	6.9	10.18	5.42-19.05	90.4	1.6	11.56	7.87-16.98

**GAD indicates generalized anxiety disorder; OR, odds ratio; CI, confidence interval of the OR; ALC, alcohol abuse and dependence; and Drug, drug abuse and dependence.*
†Thirty-day results refer to the 30-day prevalence of other disorders among respondents with 30-day GAD.
‡Lifetime results refer to the lifetime prevalence of other disorders among respondents with lifetime GAD.
§The proportion of respondents with GAD who reported the other disorder indicated in the row heading.

gether, these people with primary GAD made up approximately one fifth (21.8%) of all GAD cases.

CORRELATES OF GAD

Table 4 summarizes the results of the logistic regression analyses for a number of sociodemographic correlates of lifetime GAD. The results in the first column show the crude effects of each predictor taken one at a time, whereas the results in the second column are based on a multivariate analysis that adjusts for overlap among the predictors. Results are reported as ORs. As noted above, the 95% confidence intervals are based on complex variance estimation techniques that adjust for the weighting and clustering of the sample data.

Consistent with the pattern in Table 2, the results show that women are significantly more likely than men (OR=1.89 in the crude model and OR=1.63 in the adjusted model) to have lifetime GAD and that the lowest prevalence of GAD is in the 15- to 24-year age group (OR=0.28 in the crude model and OR=0.36 in the adjusted model). We also found that GAD is inversely related to income in the crude model, although this effect disappears when we adjust for covariates. In the crude model, previously married people had a significantly higher lifetime prevalence of GAD than either married or never married people. This effect held up in the adjusted model (OR=1.95). A higher prevalence among married than among never married people in the crude model (OR=2.71), in comparison, disappeared when we adjusted for covariates. More detailed analysis (the results are available from one of us [H-U.W.]) shows that this disappearance of the married vs never married effect is due to a strong association between being young (aged 15 to 24 years) and never married. Homemakers and other unemployed respondents, who consisted primarily of the permanently disabled and early retirees, had significantly higher prevalences of GAD than other respondents in both the crude model (OR=2.24 for homemakers and OR=2.11 for the unemployed) and the adjusted model (OR=2.25 for homemakers and OR=2.45 for the unemployed). A significantly lower prevalence among students than among employed respondents in the crude model (OR=0.45), in comparison, disappeared in the adjusted model, again because of a powerful association between young age (15 to 24 years) and being a student. Finally, there was a significant regional difference in GAD, with a higher lifetime prevalence in the Northeast than in other parts of the country in both the crude (OR=1.45) and adjusted (OR=1.39) models. We also examined the effects of other predictors, including education, religion, and urbanicity, and found them not to be statistically significant in either the crude or the adjusted model.

Parallel logistic regression analyses were also carried out to study the differences between pure (no other lifetime disorder) and comorbid GAD and between primary (GAD had an earlier age of onset than any other disorder) and secondary GAD. None of the predictors described above was significant in discriminating these subtypes of GAD. This means that pure GAD, primary GAD, and secondary GAD do not differ in their associations with age, sex, race, social class, or the other biosocial variables considered here.

PROFESSIONAL HELP SEEKING, MEDICATION, AND INTERFERENCE WITH LIFE

Although the *DSM-III-R* does not specifically require the impairment of role functioning in GAD, there is considerable interest in the extent to which GAD causes role

impairment. To address this question, we asked all respondents who met the criteria for lifetime *DSM-III-R* GAD whether the disorder ever interfered a lot with their life and activities, whether they ever sought professional help for the disorder, and whether they ever took medication for the disorder. As shown in **Table 5**, 82.0% of the respondents with lifetime GAD met at least one of these severity criteria, suggesting that GAD has a high probability of creating significant role impairment. Because some authors suggest that any impairment associated with GAD is largely associated with comorbidity, results are also presented separately for respondents with pure GAD and those with comorbid GAD. The results show that comorbidity is associated with a significantly greater probability of professional help seeking for GAD (67.9% of the comorbid cases compared with 48.2% of the pure cases), receiving medications (46.2% of the comorbid cases compared with 24.1% of the pure cases), and interference with daily activities (51.2% of the comorbid cases compared with 28.1% of the pure cases). It is important to note, however, that 59.2% of the respondents with pure GAD reported at least one of these impairments.

As described earlier, several authors have suggested that GAD is especially prevalent in primary care settings.[19] However, to our knowledge, there have been no empirical studies until now that investigated this assumption. The results in Table 5 focus on help seeking in general, either in the general medical sector or in the specialty mental health sector of the health care system. A breakdown of these results shows that 43.3% of the respondents with pure GAD and 50.8% of those with comorbid GAD have sought help for their anxiety in the general medical sector at some time in their life, whereas 29.2% of those with pure GAD and 49.6% of those with comorbid GAD have sought help for their anxiety in the specialty mental health sector. It is noteworthy that the ratio of primary care to specialty care help seeking is much greater among respondents with pure (43.3/29.2=1.48) rather than comorbid (50.8/49.6=1.02) GAD.

Table 4. Sociodemographic Correlates of Lifetime *DSM-III-R* GAD*

	Crude†		Adjusted‡	
	OR	95% CI	OR	95% CI
Sex				
M	1.00	. . .	1.00	. . .
F	1.89	1.34-2.67	1.63	1.13-2.37
Age, y				
15-24	0.28	0.17-0.45	0.36	0.21-0.56
25-35	0.87	0.59-1.26	1.00	. . .
35-44	0.84	0.58-1.22	1.00	. . .
45-55	1.00	. . .	1.00	. . .
Race				
W	1.43	0.82-2.49		
B	0.74	0.25-2.17		
Hispanic	1.00	. . .		
Other	1.30	0.51-3.37		
Income§				
0-19	2.10	1.32-3.33		
20-34	1.35	0.86-2.13		
35-69	1.25	0.78-2.01		
≥70	1.00	. . .		
Marital status				
Married	2.71	1.96-3.73	1.00	. . .
Separated/ widowed/ divorced	5.25	3.37-8.18	1.95	1.43-2.66
Never married	1.00	. . .	1.00	. . .
Employment				
Working	1.00	. . .	1.00	. . .
Student	0.45	0.26-0.80	1.00	. . .
Homemaker	2.47	1.50-4.08	2.25	1.35-3.73
Other	2.11	1.18-3.79	2.45	1.41-4.27
Region				
Midwest	1.09	0.77-1.55	1.00	. . .
Northeast	1.45	1.10-1.92	1.39	1.07-1.80
West	1.11	0.74-1.55	1.00	. . .
South	1.00	. . .	1.00	. . .

**GAD indicates generalized anxiety disorder; OR, odds ratio; CI, confidence interval of the OR.*

†Zero-order odds ratios with only one predictor in the model.

‡Odds ratios of a given predictor after adjusting the effect of other predictors in the model (predictors were put into the adjusted model only when they had been significant at the zero-order level).

§In thousands of dollars.

COMMENT

The results presented herein suggest that GAD is a relatively rare current disorder (current prevalence, 1.6%) but one that affects over 5% of the population at some time in their life. Our 12-month prevalence estimate for *DSM-III-R* GAD (3.1%; SE, 0.3%) is only slightly lower than the prevalence estimates for *DSM-III* GAD that were reported in three sites of the ECA Study,[6] which ranged from 3.4% to 4.9%. Our lifetime prevalence estimate, in comparison, appears to be much lower than that in the ECA Study. This comparison is complicated by the fact that the lifetime prevalence of GAD in the ECA Study was reported only after excluding cases with comorbid major depression or panic disorder. The range of estimates with these restrictions applied was between 4.1% and 6.6%. When we imposed the same restrictions to the NCS data, we arrived at an estimated lifetime prevalence of 1.6% for GAD without major depression or panic disorder. Our much lower lifetime prevalence estimate presumably reflects the fact that the *DSM-III-R* criteria are more strict than the *DSM-III* criteria and reflects differences in the sampling designs, administrative procedures, and years of administration of the ECA Study and the NCS. It is less clear why the 12-month prevalence estimates in the ECA Study and the NCS should be so similar. One possibility is that the more serious anxiety captured in the

Table 5. Lifetime Generalized Anxiety Disorder (GAD): Interference, Help Seeking, and Use of Medication

	Interference		Help Seeking		Medication		Any of the Three	
	Percentage*	SE	Percentage*	SE	Percentage*	SE	Percentage*	SE
Pure GAD	28.1	0.08	48.2	0.10	24.1	0.08	59.2	0.10
Comorbid GAD	51.2	0.04	67.9	0.04	46.2	0.04	84.4	0.03
Total	49.0	0.04	66.0	0.03	44.0	0.04	82.0	0.02

**The proportion of respondents with lifetime GAD who reported particular types of impairment.*

DSM-III-R criteria is, as the designers of the *DSM-III-R* intended, more chronic than the anxiety captured in the *DSM-III* criteria. We were unable to investigate this possibility directly because we did not collect information about periods of anxiety that lasted less than 6 months. However, the one comparison that we could make between the NCS and the ECA Study suggests that *DSM-III-R* GAD is more chronic than is *DSM-III* GAD; namely, that whereas 69% (1.1/1.6) of NCS respondents with a lifetime history of *DSM-III-R* GAD but not major depression or panic disorder reported a 12-month prevalence of GAD, only between 44% (2.9/6.6 in St Louis) and 55% (3.6/6.6 in Durham) of comparable ECA cases did so.

Consistent with the findings of Wacker et al,[12] we found that the lifetime prevalence of GAD was considerably higher when defined according to the definitions and criteria of the *ICD-10* (8.9%) than according to those of the *DSM-III-R* (5.1%), although the ratio of these two prevalence estimates (8.9/5.1=1.74) was considerably lower than the ratio reported by Wacker and colleagues[12] (4.84). The fact that 12-month *ICD-10* GAD had roughly the same relative prevalence as 12-month *DSM-III-R* GAD suggests that the course of the two disorders is comparable. This last result is unexpected, as the *ICD-10* definition of GAD would be expected to include less severe disorders with presumably a more benign course.

Our analysis of comorbidity documented that the vast majority of people with GAD also have at least one other disorder (current comorbidity, 66.3%; lifetime comorbidity, 90.4%). Generalized anxiety disorder is commonly associated with a wide spectrum of other mental disorders. The strongest comorbidities were found for affective disorders, panic disorder, and (for current comorbidity only) agoraphobia. Because we know from previous research that comorbidity is, in general, more common in treatment samples than in community samples,[48,49] it is somewhat surprising that the extent of comorbidity found among persons with GAD in the NCS is similar to that reported in treatment samples.[50] For example, 62.4% of the NCS respondents with lifetime GAD also had lifetime major depression, and 39.5% had lifetime dysthymia. These percentages are similar to those reported by Lépine et al[13] and Brown and Barlow[16] for a wide variety of treatment samples. The substantial comorbidity of GAD means that pure lifetime GAD is extremely rare (lifetime prevalence, 0.5%). This raises the question of how frequently GAD is merely a residual or a prodrome of some other disorder rather than an independent disorder, a question that has been the subject of considerable debate in the recent literature.[1,51] Our finding that a full third of the people with current GAD did not carry any other recent diagnosis argues that GAD is independent in at least some cases, but a more definitive analysis of how often this is the case would require a study in which cases of pure current GAD are followed up over time to see if an episode of some other disorder occurs shortly thereafter. Although this type of investigation cannot be carried out with the NCS data, future comorbidity analyses with these data will attempt to shed some light on this important nosological issue by investigating the chronicity of current pure vs comorbid cases and comparing levels of impairment and patterns of help seeking.

Our results concerning risk factors confirm the findings of other studies[5,52] that women have a higher prevalence of GAD than do men. Multivariate logistic regression analysis also identified being older than 24, being previously married, being unemployed, being a homemaker, and living in the Northeast as significant correlates of current GAD. The fact that the effect of being a homemaker was stronger than the effect of being female in the adjusted model suggests that characteristics associated with sex roles might be important determinants of GAD. It is also possible that selection factors are at work. In particular, women with GAD might be too tense and worried to handle a job and, as a result, structure their lives in a way that allows them to stay at home. This could also help explain the effect of being unemployed. We hope to shed some light on this issue in more detailed age-of-onset analyses that determine whether the onset of GAD occurs prior to the age of making decisions about entering the labor force and, if so, whether GAD influences this decision. In light of the fact that employment status is such a powerful correlate of GAD, this might be a fruitful area of further analysis.

The finding that lifetime GAD was lowest among the youngest NCS respondents is not surprising. However, the results in Table 2 show that young people also have the lowest current prevalence of GAD, and this was unexpected in light of the fact that the ECA Study found that the youngest age group had the highest prevalence

of current GAD. It is important to remember in this regard that the ECA analysis was based on *DSM-III* criteria, which require only a 1-month duration, whereas the NCS required the minimum 6-month duration specified in the *DSM-III-R*. The difference in the two studies regarding the effects of age might reflect the fact that young people are more likely to have short episodes that do not meet the 6-month duration requirement of the *DSM-III-R*. We were unable to investigate this possibility directly because the NCS did not collect data on episodes of GAD with durations of less than 6 months. It is relevant in this regard to note that recent twin research suggests that the etiologic role of genetic factors is similar in GAD with 1-month and 6-month duration requirements, suggesting that there may be a single underlying disorder with different determinants of onset and duration.[53] This being the case, the juxtaposition of the ECA Study results and the NCS results concerning age might be taken to suggest that young people are more likely to have short periods of anxiety but older people are more likely to have persistent GAD. Future research should investigate this by examining the precipitating factors for GAD in adolescents and young adults compared with those of older respondents and determining whether age is differentially associated with GAD with onset of 1-month (*DSM-III*) and subsequent duration.

Generalized anxiety disorder is traditionally seen as a frequently occurring disorder that is typically chronic and associated with only minor impairment.[50] It is also thought that GAD usually comes to the attention of the treatment system only when it occurs in conjunction with some other, more debilitating, disorder.[54] Although we found that impairment is positively associated with the comorbidity of GAD, our results also show that the majority of people with GAD, whether comorbid or not, report substantial interference with their lives and have a high probability of seeking professional help. The high proportion of people with GAD who seek professional help might partly explain why many primary care physicians emphasize that GAD is one of the most prevalent psychiatric disorders seen in their patient population,[55] although misdiagnosis may also be involved in this claim. Our finding that a full half of the people with GAD seek help for their anxiety in the primary care sector of the medical care system also means that there is a need for programs for primary care physicians to help detect and treat GAD.

Accepted for publication January 6, 1994.

The NCS is a collaborative epidemiologic investigation of the prevalence, causes, and consequences of psychiatric morbidity and comorbidity in the United States. The NCS is supported by grant 5 R01 MH46376 from the US Alcohol, Drug Abuse, and Mental Health Administration with supplemental support from grant 90135190 from the W. T. Grant Foundation, New York, NY.

Ronald C. Kessler, PhD, is the principal investigator of the NCS. Collaborating NCS sites and investigators are Robin Room, PhD, The Addiction Research Foundation, Toronto, Ontario; Dan Blazer, MD, and Marvin Swartz, MD, Duke University Medical Center, Durham, NC; James Anthony, PhD, William Eaton, PhD, and Philip Leaf, PhD, The Johns Hopkins University, Baltimore, Md; Hans-Ulrich Wittchen, PhD, the Max-Planck-Institute of Psychiatry Clinical Institute, Munich, Germany; Kenneth S. Kendler, MD, the Medical College of Virginia/Virginia Commonwealth University, Richmond; Lloyd Jonston, PhD, and Ronald Kessler, PhD, the University of Michigan; Darrell Kirsch, MD, and Darrel Regier, MD, the National Institute of Mental Health, Bethesda, Md; Patrick Shrout, PhD, New York (NY) University; Evelyn Bromet, PhD, State University of New York–Stony Brook; R. Jay Turner, PhD, the University of Toronto (Ontario); and Linda Cottler, PhD, Washington University School of Medicine, St Louis, Mo. A complete list of NCS publications can be obtained from the NCS Study Coordinator, Room 1006, Institute for Social Research, the University of Michigan, Box 1248, Ann Arbor, MI 48106-1248.

Reprint requests to Max-Planck-Institut fur Psychiatrie, Klinisches Institut, Kraepelinstr 2 D-8000, Munchen 40, Germany (Dr Wittchen).

REFERENCES

1. Cooper JE. The classification of anxiety states in the *International Classification of Diseases*. In: Sartorius N, Andreoli V, Cassano G, Eisenberg L, Kielholz P, Pancheri P, Racagni G, eds. *Anxiety: Psychobiological and Clinical Perspectives*. Washington, DC: Hemisphere Publishing Co; 1990:147-152.
2. Weissman MM, Myers JK, Harding PS. Psychiatric disorders in a US urban community: 1975-1976. *Am J Psychiatry*. 1978;135:459-462.
3. Uhlenhuth EH, Balter MB, Mellinger GG, Cisin IH, Clinthorpe J. Symptom checklist syndromes in the general population: correlations with psychotherapeutic drug use. *Arch Gen Psychiatry*. 1983;40:1167-1173.
4. Angst J, Dobler-Mikola A, Scheidegger P. A panel study of anxiety states, panic attacks, and phobia among young adults. Presented at the Research Conference on Anxiety Disorders, Panic Attacks and Phobia; December 9, 1982; Key Biscayne, Fla.
5. Blazer DG, Hughes D, George LK, Swartz M, Boyer R. Generalized anxiety disorder. In: Robins LN, Regier DA, eds. *Psychiatric Disorders in America: The Epidemiologic Catchment Area Study*. New York, NY: The Free Press; 1991; 180-203.
6. Robins LN, Regier DA, eds. *Psychiatric Disorders in America: The Epidemiologic Catchment Area Study*. New York, NY: The Free Press; 1991.
7. Wittchen H-U, Essau CA, von Zerssen D, Krieg CJ, Hecht H. Lifetime and six-month prevalence of mental disorders in the Munich Follow-up Study. *Eur Arch Psychiatry Clin Neurosci*. 1992;241:247-258.
8. Faravelli C, Guerinni Degl'Innocenti BG, Giardinelli L. Epidemiology of anxiety disorders in Florence. *Acta Psychiatr Scand*. 1989;79:308-312.
9. Wacker HR, Mullejans R, Klein KH, Battegay R. Identification of cases of anxiety disorders and affective disorders in the community according to *ICD-10* and *DSM-III-R* by using the Composite International Diagnostic Interview (CIDI). *Int J Methods Psychiatr Res*. 1992;2:91-100.
10. Breslau N, Davis GC. Generalized anxiety disorder: an empirical investigation of more stringent criteria. *Psychiatry Res*. 1985;14:231-238.
11. Lépine JP, Wittchen H-U, Essau CA. Lifetime and current comorbidity of anxiety and depressive disorders: results from the International WHO/ADAMHA CIDI Field Trials. *Int J Methods Psychiatr Res*. 1993;3:67-77.
12. Wacker HR, Battegay R, Mullejans R, Schlosser C. Using the CIDI-C in the

general population. In: Stefanis CN, Rabavilas AD, Soldatos CR, eds. *Psychiatry: A World Perspective.* Amsterdam, the Netherlands: Elsevier Science Publishers BV; 1990:138-143.

13. Lépine JP, Pariente P, Boulenger J-P, Hardy P, Zarifian E, Lemperiere T, Lellouch J. Anxiety disorders in a French general psychiatric outpatient sample: comparison between *DSM-III* and *DSM-III-R* criteria. *Soc Psychiatry Psychiatr Epidemiol.* 1989;24:301-308.
14. Atkinson JH, Grant I, Kennedy CJ, Richman DD, Spector SA, McCutchan JA. Prevalence of psychiatric disorders among men infected with human immunodeficiency virus: a controlled study. *Arch Gen Psychiatry.* 1988;45:859-864.
15. Barlow DH, Blanchard EB, Vermilyea JA, Vermilyea BB, DiNardo PA. Generalized anxiety and generalized anxiety disorder: description and reconceptualization. *Am J Psychiatry.* 1986;143:40-44.
16. Brown TA, Barlow DH. Comorbidity among anxiety disorders: implications for treatment and *DSM-IV. J Consult Clin Psychol.* 1992;60:835-844.
17. Wittchen H-U, von Zerssen D, eds. *Verlaufe Behandelter und Unbehandelter Depressionen und Angstsorungen: Eine Klinisch-Psychiatrische und Epidemiologische Verlaufsuntersuchung.* Berlin, Germany: Springer-Verlag; 1988.
18. Sanderson WC, Wetzler S. Chronic anxiety and generalized anxiety disorder: issues in comorbidity. In: Rapee RM, Barlow DH, eds. *Chronic Anxiety, Generalized Anxiety Disorder, and Mixed Anxiety Depression.* New York, NY: Guilford Press; 1992:119-135.
19. Sartorius N, Goldberg D, de Girolamo G, Costa e Silva JA, Lecrubier Y, Wittchen H-U, eds. *Psychological Disorders in General Medical Settings.* Bern, Switzerland: Hogrefe and Huber Publishers; 1990.
20. Dept of Health and Human Services. *National Health Interview Survey: 1989 (Computer File).* Hyattsville, Md: National Center for Health Statistics; 1992.
21. Kessler RC, McGonagle KA, Zhao S, Nelson CB, Hughes M, Eshleman S, Wittchen H-U, Kendler KS. Lifetime and 12-month prevalence of *DSM-III-R* psychiatric disorders in the United States: results from the National Comorbidity Survey. *Arch Gen Psychiatry.* 1994;51:8-19.
22. World Health Organization. *Composite International Diagnostic Interview.* Geneva, Switzerland: World Health Organization; 1990.
23. Robins LN, Wing J, Wittchen H-U, Helzer JE. The Composite International Diagnostic Interview: an epidemiological instrument suitable for use in conjunction with different diagnostic systems and in different cultures. *Arch Gen Psychiatry.* 1988;45:1069-1077.
24. American Psychiatric Association, Committee on Nomenclature and Statistics. *Diagnostic and Statistical Manual of Mental Disorders, Revised Third Edition.* Washington, DC: American Psychiatric Association; 1987.
25. World Health Organization. *The* ICD-10 *Classification of Mental and Behavioral Disorders: Diganostic Criteria for Research.* Geneva, Switzerland: World Health Organization; 1993.
26. Wittchen H-U. Reliability and validity studies of the WHO Composite International Diagnostic Interview (CIDI): a critical review. *J Psychiatr Res.* In press.
27. World Health Organization. *Composite International Diagnostic Interview: User Manual.* Geneva, Switzerland: World Health Organization; 1990.
28. World Health Organization. *Composite International Diagnostic Interview: Training Manual.* Geneva, Switzerland: World Health Organization; 1990.
29. World Health Organization. *Composite International Diagnostic Interview: Computer Programs.* Geneva, Switzerland: World Health Organization; 1990.
30. Cottler LB, Robins LN, Helzer JE. The reliability of the CIDI-SAM: a comprehensive substance abuse interview. *Br J Addict.* 1989;84:802-814.
31. Wittchen H-U, Robins LN, Cottler L, Sartorius N, Altamura AC, Andrews G, Dingemanns R, Droux A, Essau CA. *Interrater Reliability of the Composite International Diagnostic Interview (CIDI): Results of the Multicenter WHO/ADAMHA Field Trials (Wave I).* Amsterdam, the Netherlands: Excerpta Medica; 1990.
32. Wittchen H-U, Robins LN, Cottler LB, Sartorius N, Burke JD, Regier DA, Participants in the Multicenter WHO/ADAMHA Field Trials. Cross-cultural feasibility, reliability and sources of variance in the Composite International Diagnostic Interview (CIDI). *Br J Psychiatry.* 1991;159:645-653.
33. Cottler LB, Robins LN, Grant B, Blaine J, Towle I, Wittchen H-U, Sartorius N, Burke J, Regier D, Helzer J, Janca A. The CIDI-CORE substance abuse and dependence questions: cross-cultural and nosological issues. *Br J Psychiatry.* 1991;159:653-658.
34. Semler G. *Reliabilitat und Validitat des Composite International Diagnostic Interview (CIDI).* Regensburg, Germany: S Roderer Verlag; 1990.
35. Spengler P, Wittchen H-U. Procedural validity of standardized symptom questions for the assessment of psychotic symptoms: a comparison of the DIS with two clinical methods. *Compr Psychiatry.* 1988;29:309-322.
36. Janca A, Robins LN, Cottler LB, Early TS. Clinical observation of CIDI assessments: an analysis of the CIDI field trials: wave II at the St Louis site. *Br J Psychiatry.* 1992;160:815-818.
37. Leitmeyer P. *Zur Symptomerfassung mit dem standardisierten Interview CIDI-C in der Allgemeinpraxis.* Mannheim, Germany: Universität Mannheim; 1990.
38. Farmer AE, Katz R, McGriffin P, Bebbington P. A comparison between the Present State Examination and the Composite International Diagnostic Interview. *Arch Gen Psychiatry.* 1987;44:1064-1068.
39. Farmer AE, Jenkins PL, Katz R, Ryder L. Comparison of CATEGO-derived *ICD-8* and *DSM-III* classifications using the composite international diagnostic interview in severely ill subjects. *Br J Psychiatry.* 1991;158:177-182.
40. Wittchen H-U, Burke JD, Semler G, Pfister H, von Cranach M, Zaudig M. Recall and dating of psychiatric symptoms: test-retest reliability of time-related symptom questions in a standardized psychiatric interview (CIDI/DIS). *Arch Gen Psychiatry.* 1989;46:437-443.
41. Semler G, Wittchen H-U, Joschke K, Zaudig M, Geiso T, Kaiser S, von Cranach M, Pfister H. Test-retest reliability of a standardized psychiatric interview (DIS/CIDI). *Eur Arch Psychiatry Clin Neurosci.* 1987;236:214-222.
42. Woodruff RS, Causey BD. Computerized method for approximating the variance of a complicated estimate. *J Am Stat Assoc.* 1976;71:315-321.
43. University of Michigan. *OSIRIS VII.* Ann Arbor: Institute of Social Research, the University of Michigan; 1981.
44. Kish L, Frankel MR. Balanced repeated replications for standard errors. *J Am Stat Assoc.* 1970;65:1071-1094.
45. SAS Institute Inc. *SAS Users' Guide 6.03.* Cary, NC: SAS Institute Inc; 1988.
46. Kalton G. Practical methods for estimating survey sampling errors. *Bull Int Stat Inst.* 1977;47:495-514.
47. Eaton WW, Kessler RC, Wittchen H-U, Magee WJ. Panic and panic disorder in the United States. *Am J Psychiatry.* In press.
48. Glass SB, Jackson P. Maudsley-hospital survey: prevalence of alcohol-problems and other psychiatric-disorders in a hospital population. *Br J Addict.* 1988;83:1105-1111.
49. Wolf AW, Schubert DSP, Patterson MB, Marion B, Grande TP. Associations among major psychiatric diagnoses. *J Consult Clin Psychol.* 1988;56:292-294.
50. Wittchen H-U, Essau CA, Krieg JC. Anxiety disorders: similarities and differences of comorbidity in treated and untreated groups. *Br J Psychiatry.* 1991;159(suppl 12):23-33.
51. Frances A, Pincus H, Manning D, Widiger T. Classification of anxiety states in *DSM-III* and perspectives for its classification in *DSM-IV.* In: Sartorius N, Andreoli V, Cassano G, Eisenberg L, Kielholz P, Pancheri P, Racagni G, eds. *Anxiety: Psychobiological and Clinical Perspectives.* Washington, DC: Hemisphere Publishing Co; 1990:139-146.
52. Essen-Möller E, Larsson H, Uddenberg CE, White G. Individual traits and morbidity in a Swedish rural population. *Acta Psychiatr Neurol Scand.* 1965;702(suppl 100):1-160.
53. Kendler KS, Neale MC, Kessler RC, Heath AC, Eaves LJ. Generalized anxiety disorder in women: a population-based twin study. *Arch Gen Psychiatry.* 1992;49:267-272.
54. Goldberg D. Reasons for misdiagnosis. In: Sartorius N, Goldberg D, de Girolamo G, Costa e Silva JA, Lecrubier Y, Wittchen H-U, eds. *Psychological Disorders in General Medical Settings.* Bern, Switzerland: Hogrefe and Huber; 1990:139-145.
55. Sartorius N, Andreoli V, Cassano G, Eisenberg L, Kielholz P, Pancheri P, Racagni G, eds. *Anxiety: Psychological and Clinical Perspectives.* Washington, DC: Hemisphere Publishing Co; 1990.

Childhood-Onset Dysthymic Disorder

Clinical Features and Prospective Naturalistic Outcome

Maria Kovacs, PhD; Hagop S. Akiskal, MD; Constantine Gatsonis, PhD; Phoebe L. Parrone, MS

Objectives: To characterize the clinical presentation, course, and outcome of childhood-onset dysthymic disorder and assess the predictive validity of this diagnosis.

Design: As part of a longitudinal prospective study, school-age, clinically referred youngsters (n=55) whose first depression was dysthymic disorder and a comparison group of youngsters (n=60) whose first affective episode was major depressive disorder (MDD) were repeatedly examined during a 3- to 12-year interval. The diagnoses were based on *DSM-III* criteria.

Results: Dysthymic disorder was associated with earlier age at onset than MDD, similarly frequent symptoms of affective dysregulation, but low rates of anhedonia and neurovegetative symptoms and greater overall risk of any subsequent affective disorder. The affective disorders that dysthymic children developed, including first-episode MDD (76%) and bipolar disorder (13%), far outnumbered nonaffective conditions. After the first episode of MDD, the clinical course of the initially dysthymic youths was similar to the course of the comparison patients with regard to rates of recurrent major depression, bipolar disorder, and certain nonaffective disorders.

Conclusions: Childhood-onset dysthymic disorder is an early marker of recurrent affective illness. Although on long-term follow-up, dysthymic disorder and MDD are associated with similar rates of certain outcomes, there exist sufficient differences to warrant diagnosis of each disorder. Dysthymic children who have subsequent mood disorders are most likely first to have an episode of MDD, and that episode appears to be the "gateway" to recurrent affective illness. The interval between the onset of dysthymia and the first major depression provides a window of opportunity for intervention and possible prevention of later episodes.

(Arch Gen Psychiatry. 1994;51:365-374)

THE NEW diagnostic category of dysthymic disorder (DD), introduced in *DSM-III*,[1] is believed to subsume several chronic depressive conditions that are heterogeneous with respect to cause, age at onset, clinical presentation, psychobiologic correlates, and treatment response.[2-5] As posited by Akiskal,[2,3] one type of dysthymia is a variant or precursor of bona fide affective disorder and is characterized by comparatively early onset, protracted course, eventual episodes of major depression, and bipolar tendencies. Indeed, the existence of such a subtype is supported by accumulating evidence from studies of adults.[6-14] For example, the pattern of comorbidity involving major depression superimposed on dysthymic disorder, also called "double depression,"[8] is now increasingly recognized.[9,10,15-19] There also is a growing body of literature supporting the link between dysthymia or chronic depression and bipolarity among some individuals, as evidenced in clinical course, development of hypomania during antidepressant pharmacotherapy, and family history.[10-14]

However, the nosologic significance of some of the aforementioned findings has been debated. For example, on the one hand, the co-occurrence of DD and major

From the Department of Psychiatry, University of Pittsburgh (Pa) School of Medicine, and Western Psychiatric Institute and Clinic (Dr Kovacs and Ms Parrone); University of California at San Diego, La Jolla (Dr Akiskal); and Department of Health Care Policy, Harvard Medical School, Boston, Mass (Dr Gatsonis).

See Patients and Methods on next page

PATIENTS AND METHODS

DESIGN

We review aspects of our research methods that are relevant to the present article. For more detailed descriptions, see previous publications.[24-26,31,32] Subjects for the main longitudinal investigation were recruited primarily from among sequentially referred patients to the child psychiatry outpatient service of the University of Pittsburgh and the general medical clinics of the Children's Hospital of Pittsburgh. These two sites contributed 83% and 15%, respectively, of all depressed subjects described in the present article; a few cases were obtained through other avenues. Subjects were screened and assessed by our own research staff, irrespective of referral reason or the service provider's diagnosis. To be considered for the study, each child had to meet the following criteria: 8 to 13 years old; not mentally retarded; no major systemic medical illness; ambulatory status; and living with parent or legal guardian within commuting distance of greater Pittsburgh. Signed consents were obtained from parents and children for the intake interview, an initial 5-year follow-up period, and then further follow-up periods. Families received monetary reimbursement at each assessment. The protocol stipulated three postintake assessments in the first year of study participation, and no more than two interviews per year thereafter. Because of logistic problems (eg, canceled appointments, staff shortage, families moving away), the intervals between interviews varied across cases.

PSYCHIATRIC EVALUATION AND DIAGNOSIS

At each clinical assessment, first the parent was interviewed alone about the child, then the child was interviewed separately by the same research clinician. The interviewers were mental health professionals (MSW and PhD level) who received individually supervised training in psychiatric assessment and differential diagnosis. The clinical evaluations were conducted with the semistructured, symptom-oriented Interview Schedule for Children and Adolescents and its diagnostic addenda. The interrater reliability of the symptom ratings has been reported as satisfactory.[33] Demographic and other information were gathered from parents via structured data sheets. Interviewers were aware of the outcome of previous assessments.

Subsequent to each interview, a subject's psychiatric diagnosis was based on pertinent historical information and the clinician's final symptom ratings, according to the data supplied by both parent and child. Only symptoms at operationally predefined levels of severity were counted.[24] The data were reviewed by the research clinicians and *DSM-III* diagnoses were consensually assigned or updated at each interview. These decisions were further reviewed by one of us (M.K.), who also resolved any disagreements. To supplement the *DSM-III*,[1] we also had additional operational rules: (1) a protracted, partially remitted MDD was never diagnosed as DD, (2) to diagnose "bipolar II" disorder, we used the *DSM-III* symptom criteria for hypomania,[1(p220)] with at least a 1-week duration, and (3) hierarchical diagnostic rules were not routinely followed. For example, anxiety disorders secondary to depressive disorders were diagnosed as separate conditions.

We have illustrated elsewhere our approach to diagnosing concurrent disorders that had overlapping symptoms.[24,25] However, we briefly review the diagnosis of MDD superimposed on DD. To meet *DSM-III* criteria for DD, the required dysthymic syndrome had to be evident for at least 1 year. The diagnosis of a superimposed MDD was assigned if the *subsequent* clinical course involved one of the following: (1) the child with DD evidenced new symptoms by virtue of which he or she also met criteria for MDD (eg, in addition to the preexisting dysthymic symptoms, the child developed appetite disturbance, fatigue, and guilt), or (2) a dysthymic symptom changed sufficiently (eg, inability to respond with pleasure to praise merged into anhedonia) and/or previous subclinical symptoms exacerbated to criterion levels such that the child qualified for the additional diagnosis of MDD. Thus, patients with "double depression"[8] usually had a 1-year history of DD *before* their first MDD, although after the MDD was superimposed on it, some symptoms were necessarily counted toward both diagnoses.

DEFINITION OF ONSET AND RECOVERY FROM A DISORDER

Onset and recovery have been defined operationally.[24,25] For onset and offset dates of disorders, parents were the primary informants. The onset of a disorder was dated to the time when the child had the full *DSM-III*-specified syndrome. Offset, or recovery, was defined as (1) the absence of the symptoms of a syndrome or, at most, one clinically significant symptom and few, if any, subclinical symptoms remaining, and (2) maintenance of the foregoing state for at least 2 months. If the subject recovered from a disorder, but became symptomatic again in 2 months or less, he or she was viewed as still in the previous episode of illness. If an MDD was superimposed on a DD, the "offset" date of the MDD corresponded to the time when the child no longer had those additional depressive symptoms by vir-

depressive disorder (MDD) has been viewed as supporting the thesis that dysthymia is an attenuated form of affective illness.[6] On the other hand, given the symptomatic overlap of these two disorders, it has been questioned whether they can be distinguished from one another and whether both should be diagnosed.[15,20,21] Additionally, the retrospective accounts of adult patients supporting histories of early-onset, protracted depressive symptoms, and subsequent florid affective episodes, could be erroneous (see reviews[22,23]). Finally, although the type of dysthy-

tue of which he or she had met criteria for major depression. The baseline DD still could be present.

The 2-month asymptomatic period required to assign an offset date for an episode was waived if the disorder switched to a different diagnostic entity. For example, if a child switched from the index DD directly into an episode of mania, the date of the switch was defined as the offset of the index dysthymia and the onset of the bipolar disorder. If a date could not be readily determined, a calendar interval was delimited during which the problems emerged or remitted, respectively (eg, "between Christmas and Easter"). The date in question was then set at the midpoint of that interval. Onset and offset dates also were consensually assigned, using all available information.

COHORT

The subjects of the present article were 55 children who had an index diagnosis of DD (with or without superimposed MDD), as determined within the first 6 months of study entry. Another sample of 60 children with the index diagnosis of MDD, but no history of DD at study entry, served as a comparison group. The index diagnoses of all patients were verified within the first 6 months of study entry. Portions of these samples and their early course have been characterized in previous publications.[24-26,31,32] The most up-to-date information on the rates and correlates of recovery for the full DD group is summarized elsewhere.[34]

The dysthymic sample included 28 girls and 27 boys, of whom 69% were white, 27% were black, and 4% were biracial. At study entry, their ages ranged from 8.0 to 13.9 years (mean, 11.15 years). The head of household's socioeconomic status was estimated by means of Hollinghead's (unpublished copyrighted manuscript, 1957) two-factor index. Of the sample, 7% were in categories I and II (highest), 22% were in category III, and 71% were in categories IV and V (lowest). The DD and MDD groups were similar in gender distribution (χ^2=0.38, *df*=1, *P*=.54), mean age at study entry (*t*=1.04, *df*=113, *P*<.30), and socioeconomic status distribution, dichotomized as high (I, II, and III) vs low (IV and V) (χ^2=0.01, *df*=1, *P*=.92).

At study entry, 30 dysthymic children (55%) were living in two-parent households, but only 14 (26%) were in intact families of origin. Four (7%) had a history of psychiatric hospitalization, 20 (36%) had past outpatient psychologic treatment, and five (9%) had received psychotropic medications. A substantial number already had been suspended from school (24%) or had failed a school grade (36%). There were no significant differences between the DD and MDD groups on the foregoing variables (*P*=.25 to .96).

FOLLOW-UP INTERVAL

Patients were recruited as they became available, during the period from April 1978 through March 1987. Before completing the first 5 years of the project, five dysthymic subjects dropped out and four became unavailable for the study because of multiple geographic moves. Subject attrition did not significantly differ across the DD and MDD groups (χ^2=0.04, *df*=1, *P*=.84), and the follow-up periods were comparable for the nine patients with DD who dropped out or became unavailable (mean, 0.7 year; range, 0.1 to 1.7 years) and the nine patients with MDD who dropped out or became unavailable (mean, 1.4 years; range, 0.0 to 2.6 years). For the remaining youths, the data in the present article cover interviews up to September 1, 1990 (called the *cutoff interview*). Because recruitment spanned 9 years, the follow-up intervals ranged from 3 to 12 years for patients with DD, with a mean of 6.4 years, and from 1 to 12 years (mean, 6.3 years) for the patients with MDD. At the cutoff interview, mean age was 17.7 years (range, 12.5 to 23.7 years).

STATISTICAL PROCEDURES

Between-group differences on continuous variables (eg, age at onset) were examined by means of the Mann-Whitney *U* test, and categorical variables (eg, presence or absence of certain symptoms) were subjected to χ^2 tests. Rates of development of MDD, bipolar disorder, and selected nonaffective disorders are summarized up to the cutoff interview. These outcomes also are estimated longitudinally, by means of survival analytic methods, to accommodate censored observations.[35] Censored observations refer to the fact that some subjects may not have experienced the outcome of interest during the follow-up interval, while other subjects may have completed or dropped out of the study before having developed the outcome. Taking censorship into account, these longitudinal statistics provide an estimate of the survival (time to disorder onset) distribution for the entire cohort. In separate analyses, the start point was the onset date of the index DD, and the end point was the onset date of another specific disorder (eg, anxiety disorder), or the date of censorship if the criterion disorder had not occurred. Nonparametric tests also were used to compare the DD and MDD samples on illness-related dimensions. Proportions of time free of certain disorders during the follow-up were compared across the two samples via the Mann-Whitney *U* test. Odds ratios for selected psychiatric outcomes were derived from logistic regression analyses,[36] controlling for the length of time from the onset of the index disorder (DD or MDD) to the date of the cutoff interview.

mia that is linked to bona fide affective illness presumably originates during childhood or adolescence,[6] typologies of chronic depression and data supporting the association of DD, MDD, and bipolar disorder were derived from studies of adults. The validity of the relevant nosologic formulations and clinical accounts therefore should be tested through the prospective study of patients with childhood-onset chronic depressions.

One of the first reports on dysthymia diagnosed according to *DSM-III*[1] in clinically referred, school-age

Table 1. Preexisting *DSM-III* Psychiatric Disorders in the Dysthymic Sample (n=55)*

Variable	No. (%)
Had preexisting disorder	26 (47.3)
1 disorder	18 (32.7)
≥2 disorders	8 (14.6)
Type of disorder†	
Attention deficit disorder	13 (23.6)
Enuresis or encopresis	8 (14.6)
Overanxious disorder	6 (10.9)
Separation anxiety disorder	4 (7.3)
Other anxiety disorders	2 (3.6)
Developmental and personality disorders	3 (5.5)

*Adjustment disorders and V codes were excluded.
†Some children had multiple disorders; therefore, the total rate by types of disorder exceeds 47.3%.

youngsters[24] derived from the present Pittsburgh (Pa) longitudinal investigation of childhood-onset depressive disorders. Preliminary findings indicated that early-onset DD has a protracted course, with a superimposed episode of major depression as a frequent complication, and a notable risk of bipolar outcome.[24-26] The existence of DD in childhood and adolescence and its co-occurrence with major depression have now been reconfirmed in other clinical as well as nonclinical and epidemiologic samples.[16,27-30] However, questions still remain about the presenting characteristics of childhood-onset DD and the extent to which it is symptomatically distinct from major depression. Additionally, the clinical outcomes of dysthymic children in late adolescence and young adulthood have not yet been examined. If childhood-onset dysthymia is a bona fide affective disorder, then it should run true to form; that is, as years pass, new-onset affective disorders among previously dysthymic children should clearly outnumber other psychiatric conditions.

In the present article, several clinical and nosologic issues are addressed concerning the characteristics and diagnostic validity of DD in childhood, diagnosed according to *DSM-III*.[1] More specifically, DD is characterized in terms of age at onset, rate of preexisting disorders, and symptomatic picture, extending earlier findings from the Pittsburgh longitudinal investigation of early-onset depressions.[24-26] Clinical course and outcome during a 3- to 12-year follow-up are then examined from multiple related perspectives. The predictive validity of the initial diagnosis is evaluated in terms of the actual rates, as well as the estimated longitudinal cumulative probabilities of the development of MDD, bipolar disorder, and nonaffective disorders. In the latter category, we included anxiety and conduct disorders because of their prevalence among depressed youths,[31,32] and substance use/abuse disorder because it has been noted to be a complication of DD.[13] Long-term outcomes of our childhood-onset dysthymic patients also are characterized as proportions of "well time," or disorder-free days during the observation period. The clinical features of dysthymia and specificity of outcomes were evaluated by comparison with a sample of children whose first affective episode was a major depression.

RESULTS

CHARACTERISTICS OF INDEX DD

All 55 children with a DD at study entry were in their first episodes. Age at onset of the DD ranged from 5.1 to 12.8 years (mean, 8.7 years). Children with dysthymia were significantly younger when they became depressed than were the comparison patients whose first episode of depression was MDD (mean, 8.7 vs 10.9 years, respectively; Mann-Whitney *U* test, $P<.0001$). At study entry, 32 of the dysthymic children (58.2%) already had a superimposed MDD. However, age at onset of DD was essentially the same for the children with and those without superimposed major depression (mean±SD, 8.7±1.68 and 8.7±1.99 years, respectively).

Preexisting Disorders

As indicated in **Table 1**, 29 children (53%) had primary dysthymia. For the rest of the children whose dysthymia was secondary to some other psychiatric disorder (47%), all the preexisting conditions predated the DD by 2 months or more. Attention deficit disorder was the most prevalent preexisting condition (24%). In the MDD comparison group, a similarly high proportion of patients had preexisting disorders in general (62%) and attention deficit disorder in particular (17%).

Symptomatic Profile

To determine whether DD can symptomatically be distinguished from MDD, the longitudinal data of each patient with DD was searched for the first interview at which the child met *full DSM-III*[1] criteria for DD but was *free* of current or recent MDD. (Thus, an interview would not qualify if a subject had DD and partially remitted MDD.) Rates of selected symptoms, meeting operational definition of clinical severity at the pertinent assessment, are presented in **Table 2** for the resultant 36 subjects. Rates of the same symptoms also are presented for 45 children in a full-blown episode of MDD (but no concurrent dysthymia) selected from among the comparison cases.

Dysthymia is predominantly characterized by gloomy and depressed mood, brooding about feeling unloved, and additional manifestations of affective dysregulation, including irritability and anger (Table 2). The other prominent feature is the "cognitive" symptom of self-deprecation or negative self-esteem. As compared with MDD, dysthymia is distinguished by the virtual *absence*

Table 2. Prevalence of Depressive and Other Symptoms in a Subsample of Children With Index Dysthymic Disorder and With Index Major Depressive Disorder*

Variable	Dysthymic Disorder, % (n=36)	Major Depressive Disorder, % (n=45)
Depressed or sad mood	91.7	80.0
Feeling unloved	55.6	48.9
Feeling friendless	41.7	40.0
Irritability	55.6	71.1
Anger	63.9	62.2
Self-deprecation	55.6	64.4
Anhedonia	5.6	71.1†
Guilt	13.9	31.1‡
Social withdrawal	8.3	53.3†
Impaired concentration	41.7	67.4†§
Thoughts of wanting to die	16.7	42.2†
Reduced sleep	22.2	62.2†
Reduced appetite	5.6	46.7†
Fatigue	22.2	64.4†
Temper tantrums	44.4	28.9
Pessimism/hopelessness	36.1	42.2
Suicidal ideation	16.7	22.2
Increased sleep	11.1	22.2
Increased appetite	16.7	13.3
Excess energy	8.3	8.9
Somatic complaints	36.1	66.7†
Generalized anxiety	28.6§	43.2§
Separation anxiety	36.1	40.0
Disobedience	58.3	43.2§
Physical fighting	19.4	20.0
Lying	13.9	22.2

**Meeting full* DSM-III *criteria.*
†*P between .00001 and .01 for* χ^2 *statistics, with* df=*1 for each contrast.*
‡*P=.07.*
§*Percentage adjusted for missing data.*

and significantly lower prevalence of anhedonia and social withdrawal, and comparatively lower rates of guilt, morbid preoccupation, and impaired concentration. Practically none of the dysthymic children had reduced appetite, and few had hyposomnia and fatigue (Table 2). Disobedient behavior was the most prevalent associated feature of DD. A Bonferroni correction[37] for the 19 depressive symptom contrasts (included in Table 2), at an overall $P=.05$, requires $P<.003$ for definite significance. Five depressive symptom contrasts met this criterion: anhedonia, social withdrawal, reduced sleep, reduced appetite, and fatigue.

CLINICAL COURSE AND OUTCOME OF INDEX DD

Secondary Disorders

The rates of major depression, bipolar disorder, and the targeted nonaffective disorders that developed after the onset of DD (up to the cutoff interview) are presented in **Table 3**; bipolar I and II disorders are combined, and substance use/abuse includes both alcohol and other drug-related diagnoses. Major depression was the most frequent "new-onset" disorder in the dysthymic sample (it developed in 42 patients). The MDD was *superimposed* on the DD in 38 of the 42 cases, and in four others, the major depression developed *after* the index DD remitted.

Table 3. Selected Further Psychiatric Disorders in the Sample With Index Dysthymic Disorder and the Sample With Index Major Depressive Disorder

Variable*	Dysthymic Disorder, % (n=55)	Major Depressive Disorder, % (n=60)
Any further affective disorder	80	48
Major depressive disorder (1st episode)	76	...
Bipolar disorder	13	15
Substance use/abuse disorder	7	22
Anxiety disorder	40	43
Conduct disorder	31	35

**Summary of longitudinal outcomes secondary to the onset of the specified depressive disorder, not taking into account variable observation lengths; outcomes are not mutually exclusive.*

The outcome data for the DD and MDD groups in Table 3 are not directly comparable because dysthymic children had an earlier onset of their disorder than did those with index MDD. Accordingly, children with DD were at risk for secondary outcomes for longer periods. **Table 4** therefore presents the relative odds of the various outcomes derived from logistic regression analyses, controlling for the length of time elapsed from the onset of the respective index depressive disorder to the cutoff interview. As indicated in Table 4, children whose first affective disorder was DD significantly differed in two regards from children whose first affective episode was MDD. When dysthymia was the first depressive episode, there was about fourfold greater odds of any subsequent affective disorder, but significantly lower odds of eventual substance use/abuse disorders. However, the subsequent risk for *recurrent* MDD, bipolar, anxiety, and conduct disorders was comparable whether or not the affective disorder history commenced with DD or MDD.

The cumulative, time-dependent risk of each new-onset disorder *separately* also was estimated for the dysthymic sample by means of survival analytic techniques. Once again, MDD emerged as the outcome of highest likelihood (**Figure 1**). In other words, if all dysthymic children in the present sample were to be followed up for at least 9 years since DD onset, an estimated 81% of them would be expected to have a first episode of MDD (in contrast to the cross-sectional summary rate of 76%). The second and third years of dysthymia represented a high-risk

Table 4. Odds of Further Psychiatric Disorders in the Sample With Index Dysthymic Disorder (n=55) Compared With the Sample With Index Major Depressive Disorder (n=60)

Variable	Ajusted Odds Ratio*	*P*	95% Confidence Interval
Any further affective disorder	3.70	.0027	1.58-8.71
Recurrent major depressive disorder	0.87	NS†	0.38-2.00
Bipolar disorder	0.59	NS	0.19-1.88
Substance use/abuse disorder	0.18	.0110	0.05-0.68
Anxiety disorder	0.71	NS	0.32-1.56
Conduct disorder	0.62	NS	0.27-1.45

Using logistic regression, and controlling for time elapsed from onset of specified depressive disorder to the last (cutoff) interview by September 1, 1990.

†*NS indicates not significant.*

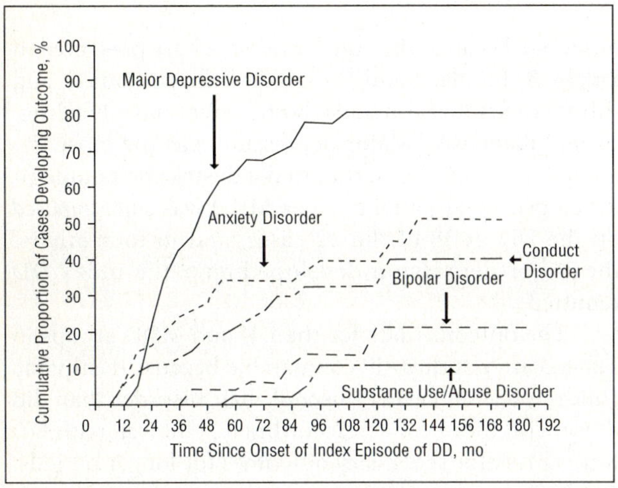

Figure 1. *Cumulative probability of first-episode major depressive, bipolar, and selected nonaffective disorders developing among children with index dysthymic disorder (DD) (n=55).*

period for major depression (shown in the steep rise of the corresponding function in Figure 1), with a median time to first MDD episode of 38 months. The cumulative probability of bipolar illness over time was estimated at 0.21. Consistent with the cross-sectional summaries, secondary substance use disorder was associated with the lowest cumulative risk over time (0.11), and secondary conduct disorder (0.40) and anxiety disorder (0.51) remained less likely than affective disorders.

Chronology of Affective Disorders

The chronology or *sequential unfolding* of affective disorders among the dysthymic and comparison cases is schematically shown in **Figure 2** (up to the cutoff interview). The depicted rates are not corrected for variable follow-up periods across the cases. The most notable finding is that for dysthymic children who proceeded to develop subsequent affective episodes (n=44), the first major depression appeared to be a "gateway." That is, all but two of the children with DD whose dysthymia culminated in new bouts of affective illness *first had an episode of major depression.*

The other notable finding is that *after* the first episode of major depression, the rates of affective disorders for the two groups of depressed patients were similar (see Figure 2). For example, among the children whose affective disorder history started with MDD, approximately one third developed a second episode of MDD and about 15% developed bipolar illness. As already noted (Table 4), the odds of recurrent MDD and bipolar disorder were similar for the index DD and comparison groups, when the at-risk periods were controlled. Dysthymia did not affect the age at onset of first MDD (Mann-Whitney *U* test, *P*=.31); for dysthymic children with this outcome (n=42), the average age (±SD) at first MDD was 11.4±1.9 years and was similar to the mean age of 10.9±1.7 years at the onset of first MDD in the comparison sample (n=60).

Well Time

As an alternative way to characterize long-term outcome and to correct for the variable follow-up intervals across subjects, we derived five indexes of "well time." For each subject, the number of days free of a particular disorder during the follow-up (counting from the date of intake to the cutoff interview) was divided by the number of days of observation, yielding proportions. According to the results (**Table 5**), the initially dysthymic youths were free of *affective* disorder close to 50% of the time during the follow-up. Thus, an episode of childhood-onset DD does not persist into late adolescence and young adulthood. However, these youths were well, or free of *any* disorder, only about one third of the time, on average, suggesting that comorbid and secondary conditions complicate the prospective course of childhood-onset DD. Regarding the five definitions of well time in Table 5, children with DD were significantly different from the patients with index MDD in two regards: dysthymic youths evidenced fewer days free of any affective disorder on average (Mann-Whitney *U* test, *P*=.0015) but more days free of substance use/abuse disorder (Mann-Whitney *U* test, *P*=.0341).

COMMENT

By means of a combination of retrospective data and prospectively observed course, *DSM-III* DD could be distinguished from MDD in the present study of clinically referred school-age children, in terms of age at onset and symptoms. However, both disorders were characterized by high rates of preexisting, comorbid psychiatric diagnoses and similar long-term clinical outcomes on selected dimensions. Confirming Akiskal's thesis[2-4] of the

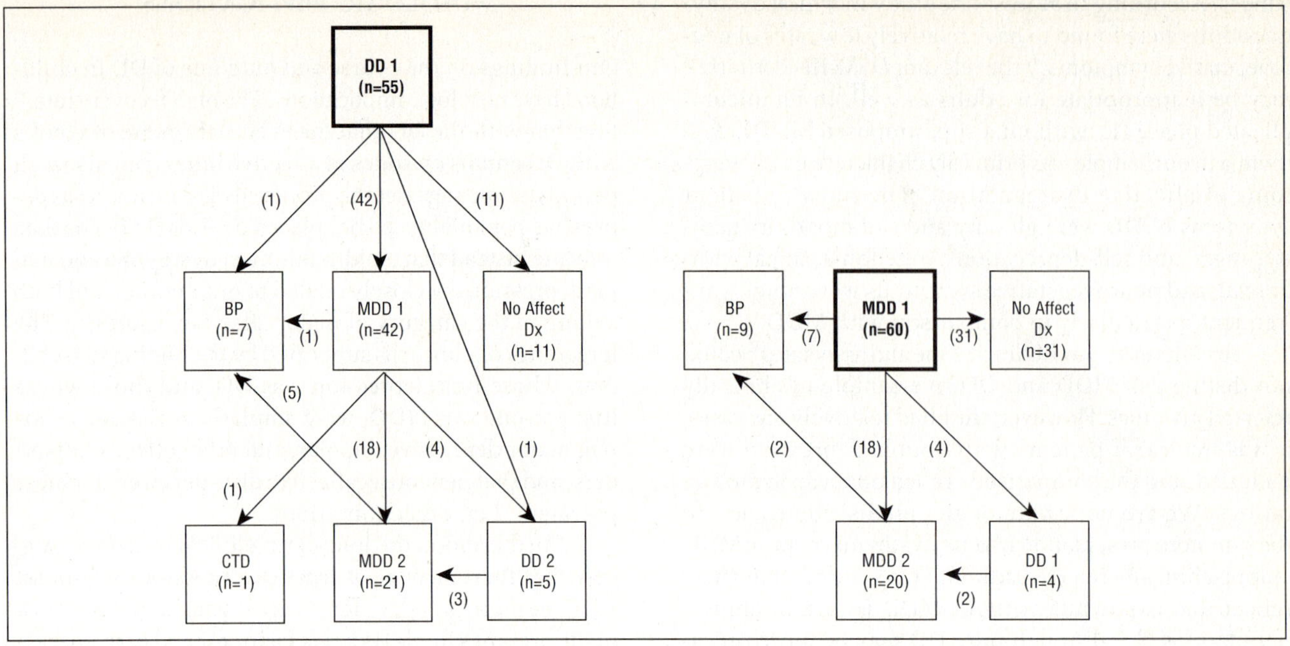

Figure 2. *Sequence of affective disorders in the sample with index dysthymic disorder (DD) and the comparison sample with index major depressive disorder (MDD) (from onset of specified depressive disorder to cutoff interview by September 1, 1990). BP indicates bipolar disorder; CTD, cyclothymic disorder; and Affect Dx, affective disorder diagnosis. From both the index DD and index MDD groups, one patient each who developed BP after the third episode of major depression was included in the "MDD 2" box for the purpose of simplification.*

nosologic standing of early-onset "subsyndromal" depression, DD in childhood was associated with a high risk of subsequent affective illness. The first episode of major depression appeared to be a gateway to further affective disorders. However, the interval between the onset of the dysthymia and the first MDD provides a window of opportunity for early identification and intervention. Furthermore, although childhood dysthymics developed multiple affective episodes, they were free of mood disorders almost 50% of the time while under observation. We comment below on the clinical, nosologic, and public health implications of these findings.

AGE AT ONSET AND PREEXISTING DISORDERS

The age at onset of first depression may help to differentiate types of affective disorder. Our patients, whose first affective episode was dysthymia, were younger at its onset than were the patients whose first episode was MDD (means, 8.7 vs 10.9 years, respectively). Lewinsohn and associates[16] similarly found in their community-based investigation of adolescents (aged 14 to 18 years) that dysthymia started about 3 years earlier than MDD. It is notable, however, that in the present study, dysthymia did not affect the age at which the first episode of major depression developed. Conversely, age at the onset of dysthymia was essentially the same for patients who developed an MDD and those who did not.

Among our school-age patients, DD was often secondary to other psychiatric conditions, underscoring the high rate of comorbidity associated with childhood-onset affective illness in clinically referred populations.[27,31,32] The finding that attention deficit disorder was the most frequent preexisting condition may reflect its high base rate in clinical populations and does not provide information about whether it is a risk factor for dysthymia. Furthermore, the likelihood of preexisting disorders in general, and of attention deficit disorder in particular, did not appear to differentiate children whose first depression was DD as compared with MDD.

Table 5. 'Well Time' for Dysthymic Youths During Study Observation*

Definition of Well Time by Absence of *DSM-III* Disorders	Proportion of Days Meeting Definition: Mean	Range
Free of Axis I/II disorder†	0.31	0.00-0.99
Free of affective disorder	0.48	0.00-0.99
Free of substance use/abuse disorder	0.97	0.57-1.00
Free of anxiety disorder	0.81	0.00-1.00
Free of conduct disorder	0.83	0.00-1.00

*Computed for the interval from study entry to last (cutoff) interview by September 1, 1990.
†Not counting adjustment disorders, V codes, developmental disorders, and enuresis-encopresis.

SYMPTOMATIC PROFILE OF DD

Our findings suggest that the *DSM-III-R*[38] symptom set for dysthymia is probably invalid for younger age groups because of the weight given to neurovegetative distur-

bances. According to at least one study in which dysthymic adults were found to have relatively low rates of neurovegetative symptoms,[39] the relevant *DSM-III-R* criteria[38] may be inappropriate for adults as well. In its uncomplicated phase (ie, without a superimposed MDD), dysthymia in our sample was primarily characterized by symptoms of affective dysregulation. The most prevalent symptoms of DD were gloomy and sad mood, irritability, anger, and self-deprecation. Anhedonia, social withdrawal, and neurovegetative symptoms were notably infrequent, particularly in comparison with MDD.

In contrast to our findings, Fine and associates[40] could not distinguish MDD and DD in a sample of clinically referred juveniles. However, they had relatively few cases, it was unclear if patients with double depression were included, and the comparisons relied on mean symptom ratings. We are not aware of any published articles on the symptom presentation of pure dysthymia vs pure MDD among clinically referred adults. This state of affairs may reflect that dysthymia without MDD is rare in clinical populations,[20,23] although pure DD may be more prevalent in community samples.[15,17,41]

LONG-TERM CLINICAL COURSE

Reconfirming and extending our preliminary findings,[24] we recently reported that, although dysthymia is protracted, with a mean episode length of about 4 years, almost all of these children recover from it.[34] Other investigators likewise have found that juvenile-onset DD has a lengthy course.[16,28] Nonetheless, over the years, our young patients generally were free of affective disorders close to 50% of the time, underscoring that childhood-onset, first-episode DD does *not* persist into adulthood.

Yet, dysthymia is not as benign a diagnosis as it has been hitherto thought. The vast majority of children with DD develop major depression, and from among those youths, a substantial portion then is at risk for recurrent MDD, bipolar disorder, and other forms of affective illness. Along with episodes of mood disorder, many of these young patients have secondary nonaffective conditions, including anxiety disorders (40%) and conduct disorders (31%). The prevalence of dysthymia with superimposed major depression (69%), or double depression, in the present sample is similar to the rates among depressed, psychiatrically referred adults[8-10] and also is consistent with figures for nonreferred, depressed adolescents and adults in community and other settings.[16,28,30]

The rate of switch to bipolarity among our dysthymic patients was 13%, and the estimated cumulative risk of bipolar disorder was 0.21. The foregoing figures are notably high for a pediatric sample. However, the results are entirely consistent with reports of bipolar outcomes among adults who had had chronic low-grade depressions.[11-14]

NOSOLOGIC IMPLICATIONS

Our findings on the course and outcome of DD in childhood have nosologic implications. The high recovery rate,[34] together with the fact that the eventual course of youths with DD entails episodes of affective illness but also well periods, argues against the proposed classification "as depressive personality [to be] placed on Axis II."[42] The data indicate instead that childhood-onset dysthymia and major depression are closely related to one another and both belong in the category of major affective disorders. The foregoing conclusion is supported by the finding that children whose first depression was DD, and those whose first episode was MDD, were similarly at risk for *recurrent* major depressive, bipolar, and other affective disorders, and that new-onset affective disorders were far more prevalent than other conditions.

Furthermore, the long-term clinical outcomes suggest that there may be at least two types of early-onset DD. The more prevalent form (as evidenced by about 80% of the present sample) is a risk factor for and early marker of recurrent affective illness. This type of low-grade, chronic, early-onset depression is probably the same clinical entity that received various names over the years: Kraepelin[43] called it one of the "fundamental states" that underlies bona fide affective illness, Kretschmer[44] labeled it as "affective temperament," and Akiskal[4] designated it "subsyndromal" affective illness or "subaffective" disorder. The results of the present study are therefore consistent with Akiskal's theory and systematic clinical observations,[2-7,11,12,45] and more recent conceptual arguments and empiric work by Akiskal and associates and others[46-49] that one form of early-onset mild depression or dysthymia aggregates with the major affective disorders.

The results of the present study also bear on the much debated issue of whether MDD, DD, and their co-occurring forms warrant separate diagnoses. This debate has been fueled by the fact that cases of pure dysthymia are rare among clinically referred adults,[2,20,21] and that patients with double depression vs those with pure recurrent MDD or other affective disorder do not consistently differ on historical or cross-sectional variables.[9,10,18,19,50] However, early-onset dysthymia should be separately diagnosed from MDD for several reasons: DD appears to have a characteristic earlier age at onset and symptom constellation; about 20% of dysthymic youths did *not* develop further affective disorders; compared with MDD, first-episode DD was associated with different odds of later affective and substance use/abuse disorders; and, concomitantly, DD (with or without subsequent major depression) was associated with shorter affective disorder–free periods than was major depression without dysthymia. Although it is not clear from the present study whether MDD superimposed on dysthymia is etiologically distinct from MDD without dysthymia, the fact remains that the diagnoses of DD and MDD have somewhat different information values.

POTENTIAL PUBLIC HEALTH IMPLICATIONS

The finding that childhood-onset DD is a risk factor for major depressive and other affective disorders could have implications for secondary and tertiary prevention. That is, one possible interpretation of our results is that if children with DD are identified promptly and treated successfully, the first episode of major depression, as well as bouts of affective illness after that first episode, may be delayed or prevented. Recall that for those dysthymic children who had subsequent mood disorders, the latter outcomes were almost always mediated by their first MDD (the gateway episode). The gateway episode usually occurred after the second year of dysthymia. Therefore, identification of dysthymic youngsters *before* their first episode of MDD could provide a unique temporal window for therapeutic intervention. According to a recent report from the Epidemiologic Catchment Area study,[51] adults with dysthymia also are at high risk for developing new-onset, first-episode major depression. Thus, one hypothesis to be tested is that early recognition and successful treatment of DD may help to reduce the rates of first-episode MDD across the age span. In the treatment of dysthymic adult patients, both pharmacologic agents (see review[52]) and psychotherapy[53,54] have been explored, although their efficacy still must be demonstrated. However, there is a complete lack of empiric data regarding the applicability and effectiveness of any intervention for dysthymia in childhood. Consequently, the development and systematic testing of treatments for young dysthymic patients remains a priority.

METHODOLOGIC ISSUES

Several methodologic features of the present study should be highlighted. Because, in our sample, dysthymia was *not* a residual condition of earlier affective disorders, the findings are probably not generalizable to prolonged, partially remitted depressive states that characterize approximately 15% to 20% of adult patients[23,42,48] and close to 10% of juveniles[34] with MDD. Furthermore, it is not known whether our findings are applicable to nonreferred and/or untreated populations. Additionally, because the follow-up assessments were not blind to the results of previous research interviews, some degree of unintentional diagnostic bias cannot entirely be ruled out. Importantly, our conclusions are constrained by the comparatively small sample size and the overrepresentation of patients with lower socioeconomic status, and thus the findings require replication by other investigators. Finally, it would be important to study diagnostic validators of childhood-onset DD other than clinical course, including the usefulness of biologic variables.[55,56]

Accepted for publication September 27, 1993.

This study was supported by grant MH33990 from the National Institute of Mental Health, Health and Human Services Administration, Bethesda, Md, and by a grant from the W. T. Grant Foundation, New York, NY.

We thank David S. Obrosky, MS, for computational assistance.

Reprint requests to Western Psychiatric Institute and Clinic, 3811 O'Hara St, Pittsburgh, PA 15213 (Dr Kovacs).

REFERENCES

1. American Psychiatric Association, Committee on Nomenclature and Statistics. *Diagnostic and Statistical Manual of Mental Disorders, Third Edition.* Washington, DC: American Psychiatric Association; 1980.
2. Akiskal HS. Dysthymic disorder: psychopathology of proposed chronic depressive subtypes. *Am J Psychiatry.* 1983;140:11-20.
3. Akiskal HS. Chronic depression. *Bull Menninger Clin.* 1991;55:156-171.
4. Akiskal HS. An integrative perspective on recurrent mood disorders: the mediating role of personality. In: Becker J, Kleinman A, eds. *Psychosocial Aspects of Depression.* Hillsdale, NJ: Lawrence Erlbaum Assoc Inc; 1991:215-235.
5. Akiskal HS. Clinical subtypes of chronic-resistant depression. In: Feighner JP, Boyer WF, eds. *Diagnosis of Depression.* New York, NY: John Wiley & Sons Inc; 1991:149-162.
6. Akiskal HS, Rosenthal TL, Haykal RF, Lemmi H, Rosenthal RH, Scott-Strauss A. Characterological depressions: clinical and sleep EEG findings separating 'subaffective dysthymias' from 'character spectrum disorders.' *Arch Gen Psychiatry.* 1980;37:777-783.
7. Akiskal HS, King D, Rosenthal TL, Robinson D, Scott-Strauss A. Chronic depressions, 1: clinical and familial characteristics in 137 probands. *J Affective Disord.* 1981;3:297-315.
8. Keller MB, Lavori PW, Endicott J, Coryell W, Klerman GL. 'Double depression': two-year follow-up. *Am J Psychiatry.* 1983;140:689-694.
9. Kocsis JH, Voss C, Mann JJ, Frances A. Chronic depression: demographic and clinical characteristics. *Psychopharmacol Bull.* 1986;22:192-195.
10. Klein DN, Taylor EB, Harding K, Dickstein S. Double depression and episodic major depression: demographic, clinical, familial, personality, and socioenvironmental characteristics and short-term outcome. *Am J Psychiatry.* 1988; 145:1226-1231.
11. Rosenthal TL, Akiskal HS, Scott-Strauss A, Rosenthal RH, David M. Familial and developmental factors in characterological depressions. *J Affective Disord.* 1981;3:183-192.
12. Akiskal HS, Walker P, Puzantian VR, King D, Rosenthal TL, Dranon M. Bipolar outcome in the course of depressive illness: phenomenologic, familial, and pharmacologic predictors. *J Affective Disord.* 1983;5:115-128.
13. Rihmer Z. Dysthymia: a clinician's perspective. In: Burton SW, Akiskal HS, eds. *Dysthymic Disorder.* London, England: Royal College of Psychiatrists; 1990: 112-125.
14. Wicki W, Angst J. The Zurich Study, X: hypomania in a 28- to 30-year old cohort. *Eur Arch Psychiatry Clin Neurosci.* 1991;240:339-348.
15. Angst J, Wicki W. The Zurich Study, XI: is dysthymia a separate form of depression? Results of the Zurich cohort study. *Eur Arch Psychiatry Clin Neurosci.* 1991;240:349-354.
16. Lewinsohn PM, Rohde P, Seeley JR, Hops H. Comorbidity of unipolar depression, I: major depression with dysthymia. *J Abnorm Psychol.* 1991;100:205-213.
17. Weissman MM, Bruce ML, Leaf PJ, Florio LP, Holzer C. Affective disorders. In: Robins LN, Regier DA, eds. *Psychiatric Disorders in America: The Epidemiologic Catchment Area Study.* New York, NY: Free Press; 1991:53-80.
18. Alnaes R, Torgersen S. Characteristics of patients with major depression in combination with dysthymic or cyclothymic disorders. *Acta Psychiatr Scand.* 1989;79:11-18.
19. Miller IW, Norman WH, Dow MG. Psychosocial characteristics of 'double depression.' *Am J Psychiatry.* 1986;143:1042-1044.
20. Keller MB, Lavori PW. Double depression, major depression, and dysthymia:

distinct entities or different phases of a single disorder? *Psychopharmacol Bull.* 1984;20:399-402.
21. Kocsis JH, Frances AJ. A critical discussion of *DSM-III* dysthymic disorder. *Am J Psychiatry.* 1987;144:1534-1542.
22. Akiskal HS, Weise RE. The clinical spectrum of so-called 'minor' depressions. *Am J Psychother.* 1992;46:9-22.
23. Keller MB, Sessa FM. Dysthymia: development and clinical course. In: Burton SW, Akiskal HS, eds. *Dysthymic Disorder.* London, England: Royal College of Psychiatrists; 1990:13-23.
24. Kovacs M, Feinberg TL, Crouse-Novak MA, Paulauskas SL, Finkelstein R. Depressive disorders in childhood, I: a longitudinal prospective study of characteristics and recovery. *Arch Gen Psychiatry.* 1984a;41:229-237.
25. Kovacs M, Feinberg TL, Crouse-Novak M, Paulauskas SL, Pollock M, Finkelstein R. Depressive disorders in childhood, II: a longitudinal study of the risk for a subsequent major depression. *Arch Gen Psychiatry.* 1984b;41:643-649.
26. Kovacs M, Gatsonis C. Stability and change in childhood-onset depressive disorders: longitudinal course as a diagnostic validator. In: Robins L, Barrett J, eds. *The Validity of Psychiatric Diagnosis.* New York, NY: Raven Press; 1989:57-75.
27. Mitchell J, McCauley E, Burke PM, Moss SJ. Phenomenology of depression in children and adolescents. *J Am Acad Child Adolesc Psychiatry.* 1988;27:12-20.
28. Keller MB, Beardslee W, Lavori PW, Wunder J, Drs DL, Samuelson H. Course of major depression in non-referred adolescents: a retrospective study. *J Affective Disord.* 1988;15:235-243.
29. Anderson JC, Williams S, McGee R, Silva PA. *DSM-III* disorders in preadolescent children: prevalence in a large sample from the general population. *Arch Gen Psychiatry.* 1987;44:69-76.
30. Kashani JH, Carlson GA, Beck NC, Hoeper EW, Corcoran CM, McAllister JA, Fallahi C, Rosenberg TK, Reid JC. Depression, depressive symptoms, and depressed mood among a community sample of adolescents. *Am J Psychiatry.* 1987;144:931-934.
31. Kovacs M, Paulauskas S, Gatsonis C, Richards C. Depressive disorders in childhood, III: a longitudinal study of comorbidity with and risk for conduct disorders. *J Affective Disord.* 1988;15:205-217.
32. Kovacs M, Gatsonis C, Paulauskas SL, Richards C. Depressive disorders in childhood, IV: a longitudinal study of comorbidity with and risk for anxiety disorders. *Arch Gen Psychiatry.* 1989;46:776-782.
33. Kovacs M. The Interview Schedule for Children (ISC). *Psychopharmacol Bull.* 1985;21:991-994.
34. Kovacs M. Chronic depression or dysthymic disorder in childhood. In: Akiskal HS, Cassano GB, eds. *Chronic Depression and Their Treatment.* New York, NY: Guilford Press. In press.
35. Kalbfleisch JD, Prentice RL. *The Statistical Analysis of Failure Time Data.* New York, NY: John Wiley & Sons Inc; 1980.
36. Hosmer DW, Lemeshow S. *Applied Logistic Regression.* New York, NY: John Wiley & Sons Inc; 1989.
37. Snedecor GW, Cochran WG. *Statistical Methods.* 7th ed. Ames, Iowa: Iowa State University Press; 1980.
38. American Psychiatric Association, Committee on Nomenclature and Statistics. *Diagnostic and Statistical Manual of Mental Disorders, Revised Third Edition.* Washington, DC: American Psychiatric Association; 1987.
39. McCullough JP, Kasnetz MD, Braith JA, Carr KF, Cones JH, Fielo J, Martelli MF. A longitudinal study of an untreated sample of predominantly late onset characterological dysthymia. *J Nerv Ment Dis.* 1988;176:658-667.
40. Fine S, Moretti M, Haley G, Marriage K. Affective disorders in children and adolescents: the dysthymic disorder dilemma. *Can J Psychiatry.* 1985;30:173-177.
41. McCullough JP, Braith JA, Chapman RC, Kasnetz MD, Carr KF, Cones JH, Fielo J, Shoemaker OS, Roberts WC. Comparison of early and late onset dysthymia. *J Nerv Ment Dis.* 1990a;178:577-581.
42. Frances A, Kocsis J, Marin D, Manning D, Markowitz J, Mason B, Widiger T. Implications of recent research on dysthymic disorder: diagnostic criteria for dysthymic disorder. *Psychopharmacol Bull.* 1989;25:325-329.
43. Kraepelin E; Barclay RM, trans. *Manic-Depressive Insanity and Paranoia.* Edinburgh, Scotland: ES Livingstone; 1921.
44. Kretschmer E; Sprott WJH, trans. *Physique and Character.* New York, NY: Harcourt Brace & Co; 1936.
45. Akiskal HS, Khani MK, Scott-Strauss A. Cyclothymic temperamental disorders. *Psychiatr Clin North Am.* 1979;2:527-554.
46. Akiskal HS, Downs J, Jordan P, Watson S, Daugherty D, Pruitt DB. Affective disorders in referred children and younger siblings of manic-depressives: mode of onset and prospective course. *Arch Gen Psychiatry.* 1985;42:996-1003.
47. Akiskal HS, Cassano GB, Musetti L, Perugi G, Tundo A, Mignani V. Psychopathology, temperament, and past course in primary major depressions, 1: review of evidence for a bipolar spectrum. *Psychopathology.* 1989;22:268-277.
48. Cassano GB, Musetti L, Perugi G, Soriani A, Mignani V, McNair DM, Akiskal HS. A proposed new approach to the clinical subclassification of depressive illness. *Pharmacopsychiatry.* 1988;21:19-23.
49. Depue RA, Slater JF, Wolfstetter-Kausch H, Klein D, Goplerud E, Farr D. A behavioral paradigm for identifying persons at risk for bipolar depressive disorder: a conceptual framework and five validation studies. *J Abnorm Psychol.* 1981;90:381-437.
50. McCullough JP, Braith JA, Chapman RC, Kasnetz MD, Carr KF, Cones JH, Fielo J, Roberts WC. Brief reports: comparison of dysthymic major and non-major depressives. *J Nerv Ment Dis.* 1990b;178:596-597.
51. Horwath E, Johnson J, Klerman GL, Weissman MM. Depressed symptoms as relative and attributable risk factors for first-onset major depression. *Arch Gen Psychiatry.* 1992;49:817-823.
52. Howland RH. Pharmacotherapy of dysthymia: a review. *J Clin Psychopharmacol.* 1991;11:83-92.
53. Weissman MM, Akiskal HS. The role of psychotherapy in chronic depressions: a proposal. *Compr Psychiatry.* 1984;25:23-31.
54. McCullough JP. Psychotherapy for dysthymia: a naturalistic study of ten patients. *J Nerv Ment Dis.* 1991;179:734-740.
55. Howland RH, Thase ME. Biological studies of dysthymia. *Biol Psychiatry.* 1991;30:283-304.
56. Brambilla F, Musetti C, Tacchini C, Fontanillas J, Guareschi-Cazzullo A. Neuroendocrine investigation in children and adolescents with dysthymic disorders: the DST, TRH and clonidine tests. *J Affective Disord.* 1989;17:279-284.

ORIGINAL ARTICLE

Psychiatric and Medical Effects of Anabolic-Androgenic Steroid Use

A Controlled Study of 160 Athletes

Harrison G. Pope, Jr, MD, David L. Katz, MD, JD

Background: We sought to expand on preliminary findings suggesting that anabolic-androgenic steroids produce psychiatric effects in some athletes who use them.

Methods: We compared 88 athletes who were using steroids with 68 nonusers, using the Structured Clinical Interview for *DSM-III-R* to diagnose psychiatric syndromes occurring in association with steroid use (if applicable) and in the absence of steroid use. Demographic, medical, and laboratory measures were also performed.

Results: Steroid users displayed more frequent gynecomastia, decreased mean testicular length, and higher cholesterol–high-density lipoprotein ratios than nonusers. Most strikingly, 23% of steroid users reported major mood syndromes—mania, hypomania, or major depression—in association with steroid use. Steroid users displayed mood disorders during steroid exposure significantly more frequently than in the absence of steroid exposure ($P<.001$) and significantly more frequently than nonusers ($P<.01$). Users rarely abused other drugs simultaneously with steroids.

Conclusion: Major mood disturbances associated with anabolic-androgenic steroids may represent an important public health problem for athletes using steroids and sometimes for the victims of their irritability and aggression.

(Arch Gen Psychiatry. 1994;51:375-382)

RECENT YEARS have seen mounting scientific and public interest in the effects of anabolic-androgenic steroid use (hereafter abbreviated as "steroids"). These drugs, which include testosterone and its many synthetic analogues, produce not only well-documented medical effects[1] but also psychiatric effects.[2] Given recent evidence suggesting that hundreds of thousands of Americans—many of them teenagers—have illicitly used anabolic steroids,[3-5] it is important to assess whether these psychiatric effects represent a public health problem.

Evidence for the psychiatric effects of steroid use derives from three sources: clinical studies of steroids in the treatment of psychiatric and medical disorders, laboratory studies of steroids in normal volunteers, and naturalistic studies of athletes. The clinical studies include many early psychiatric reports of the antidepressant properties of testosterone[6,7]; one study found that four of five depressed men developed paranoid delusions when methyltestosterone was added to their imipramine hydrochloride treatment.[8] By contrast, studies of steroids in the treatment of anemias,[9] muscular dystrophy,[10] and hypogonadism[11,12] have rarely noted prominent psychiatric effects. However, these studies have used only physiologic or modestly supraphysiologic doses of steroids—doses far lower than the massive doses often used illicitly by athletes.[2]

More than 25 laboratory studies have evaluated the effects of various steroids on athletic performance.[1,13-15] Many of these studies also used modest steroid dosages, and most did not sys-

From the Biological Psychiatry Laboratory, McLean Hospital, Belmont, Mass, and the Department of Psychiatry, Harvard Medical School, Boston, Mass.

See Subjects and Methods on next page

SUBJECTS AND METHODS

We advertised in four gymnasiums in the Boston, Mass, area and in three gymnasiums in the Santa Monica, Calif, area to recruit subjects. We offered $60 for a confidential interview to any male aged 16 years or older who had lifted weights for at least 2 years. The advertisement mentioned that steroid use, if any, would be discussed during the interview, but neither the specific hypotheses to be tested nor the study's emphasis on psychological effects was revealed. Gymnasiums with a large percentage of steroid users were selected in both sites to ensure that respondents would be approximately evenly distributed between the two groups.

All participating subjects were required to sign informed consent for the study as approved by the McLean Hospital (Belmont, Mass) Institutional Review Board. The interview began with demographic questions, followed by steroid history, if applicable. The latter covered drugs used, dates, doses, and durations, together with observed changes in body weight and strength, assessed in the same manner as in our earlier uncontrolled study.[21] Most steroid users provided remarkably detailed accounts of the steroid "cycles" (courses) that they had taken. Next, subjects were administered the Structured Clinical Interview for *DSM-III-R* (SCID),[34] including the questions on antisocial personality disorder. For reasons of time, the sections on other personality disorders were not included. For the steroid users, as in our previous study,[21] the SCID was administered twice: first, for the "on-steroid" period, defined as the time during which the subject was actually using steroids or withdrawing from their use (considered as the 3-month period after a cycle had ended), and second, for the "off-steroid" period, defined as all other times in the subject's life. If a given psychiatric syndrome occurred exclusively during the on-steroid period or exclusively during the off-steroid period, it was recorded under that heading; syndromes occurring during both periods were classified under the "off-steroid" heading. Finally, subjects were interviewed regarding their medical history, including any problems possibly attributable to steroid use (if applicable), and current tobacco, alcohol, and other drug use; family history of psychiatric disorders, using the methods described in our previous epidemiologic studies[35,36]; and history of violent or criminal behavior during steroid use and during periods of no steroid exposure.

Following the interview, subjects received a physical examination, with particular attention paid to abnormalities possibly associated with steroid use, such as hypertension, edema, acne, gynecomastia, and testicular atrophy.[1] The latter was assessed by measuring the length of the long axis of the right testicle with calipers. Subjects' height and weight were measured, and body fat as a percentage of total body weight was approximated from caliper measurements of skinfolds by the method of Jackson and Pollock[37]:

$$\% \text{ Body Fat} = 0.217X_1 - 0.00029X_1^2 + 0.133X_2 - 5.73,$$

where X_1 is the sum of six skinfold measurements (chest, thigh, ilium, abdomen, triceps, and scapula) in millimeters and X_2 is age in years.

All subjects provided urine samples (50 mL), which were stored at 4°C until analyzed for conjugated and unconjugated anabolic-androgenic steroids and for testosterone and epitestosterone by gas chromatography and mass spectrometry.[38] Testosterone use was assessed by the ratio of testosterone to epitestosterone.[39] The urine samples were analyzed by the UCLA Olympic Analytical Laboratory, Los Angeles, Calif, or by American Biotest Laboratories, Santa Clara, Calif. Subjects were also sent to a neighboring commercial laboratory (SmithKline Laboratories in Waltham, Mass, and Van Nuys, Calif) to provide blood samples for standard chemistry screens, including high-density lipoprotein and low-density lipoprotein cholesterol, complete blood cell count and differential cell count, standard urinalysis, and urine screens for drugs of abuse other than steroids. It should be noted that muscle trauma from weight lifting can elevate levels of so-called liver enzymes, such as lactic dehydrogenase and the transaminases (aspartate aminotransferase and alanine aminotransferase), since these enzymes are present in skeletal muscle and in the liver.[40] Therefore, to assess hepatic function, the chemistry screen also measured γ-glutamyl transferase, an enzyme present exclusively in the liver.[40]

Most of the above psychiatric and medical assessments are familiar or self-explanatory. However, the choice of the SCID,[34] the principal psychiatric measure in the study, deserves comment. The SCID offered several advantages. First, it generates diagnoses according to the widely used criteria of *DSM-III-R*.[41] Second, the SCID has been assessed for test-retest reliability in a large multicenter study[42] in which one of us (H.G.P.), who interviewed the 160 athletes in the present study, established interrater reliability against other interviewers from McLean Hospital and other centers. The κ values for interrater reliability at McLean Hospital for all major *DSM-III-R* Axis I disorders in this study have been published.[42] Third, unlike most rating scales, the SCID is designed to assess lifetime history of psychiatric syndromes rather than merely current levels of psychiatric symptoms. Thus, the SCID seemed better suited than a rating scale for subjects who were generally describing past rather than current psychiatric symptoms.

Differences between steroid users and controls were assessed by Fisher's Exact Test for 2×2 comparisons and by Wilcoxon's Rank Sum Test for comparisons of continuous variables. All findings significant at $P<.05$ (two-tailed significance) are noted. However, these values are not corrected for the effect of multiple comparisons because of the lack of a uniformly accepted method for calculating a correction factor for many different types of comparisons spread over different tables. Thus, some findings, particularly those with modest levels of significance, may represent chance associations.

Within the steroid-user group, the hypothesis that specific psychiatric syndromes were associated with steroid use was assessed by the McNemar or marginal χ^2 test,[43] which generates a χ^2 value from a 2×2 table of the number of users reporting the syndrome (1) during steroid exposure; (2) during periods of no steroid use; (3) under both conditions; or (4) under neither condition. This procedure would be expected to produce conservative significance estimates since the total duration of a user's on-steroid period(s) was usually much less than half of his total lifetime duration of risk for the psychiatric syndrome in question.

tematically assess psychiatric effects. One recent laboratory study,[16] however, specifically assessed the psychiatric effects of markedly supraphysiologic doses of steroids. Su et al[16] administered placebo, methyltestosterone (40 mg/d), and methyltestosterone (240 mg/d), for 3 days each, to 20 normal men. For the sample as a whole, the high-dose methyltestosterone treatment produced modest but significant psychiatric effects. Interestingly, however, one subject developed an acute manic episode to the point where he requested to be placed in seclusion.

In contrast to the often subtle psychiatric effects noted in clinical and laboratory studies, naturalistic studies of athletes have often reported marked psychiatric symptoms with steroids. These studies began with anecdotal reports of psychotic or manic symptoms[17-19] associated with steroid exposure and depressive symptoms[20] on steroid withdrawal. Subsequently, six groups of investigators[21-26] have assessed samples of steroid users, using diagnostic interviews and/or rating scales for mood, hostility, and other measures. These studies have generally documented significant increases in irritability, aggressiveness, euphoria, and other maniclike symptoms during steroid exposure and depressive symptoms during steroid withdrawal. These differences have been demonstrated by using steroid users as their own controls (comparing periods of steroid exposure with nonexposure)[21-24,26] and by using nonsteroid–using athletes as controls.[23-26] Further details of these studies are provided later in this article.

Several investigators have suggested that steroids may induce dependence or "addiction" in susceptible individuals.[27,28] Also, several groups[22,29-31] have described individuals who committed violent or criminal acts, including attempted murder or actual murder, while using steroids. None of these latter individuals reported comparable behavior before steroid use.

Not all investigators, however, have found psychiatric changes in athletes using steroids. Bahrke and colleagues[32,33] compared 53 current or past steroid users with 40 nonusers. Although users reported subjective increases in enthusiasm, aggression, and irritability while taking steroids, these changes could not be documented on two rating scales for mood and hostility.

In summary, the weight of evidence from medical, laboratory, and particularly naturalistic studies suggests that steroid use and steroid withdrawal may produce psychiatric effects. These effects appear subtle when steroids are administered in physiologic or modestly supraphysiologic doses, as in most medical and laboratory studies, but become more prominent with markedly supraphysiologic doses, as often reported by athletes in naturalistic study designs.

However, previous naturalistic studies are subject to several methodologic limitations. First, they necessarily rely on subjects' retrospective reports of the effects of illicitly obtained drugs of uncertain authenticity. Most studies have not used urine testing to confirm which steroids or other drugs were used by subjects. Second, self-selection may produce subjects who are not representative of the overall population of steroid users. Third, it is unclear whether reported psychiatric symptoms are attributable to the steroids themselves or to other concomitantly used psychoactive drugs, premorbid psychiatric disorder in the subjects, expectancy effects, or social influences from the gymnasium subculture. These limitations could be fully resolved only by a double-blind, placebo-controlled laboratory study, but ethics preclude mimicking illicit use by administering massive doses of several steroids simultaneously over prolonged periods to volunteers. Thus, only naturalistic study designs can be used to assess the full psychiatric effects of steroid use among athletes. We conducted a controlled study of 88 steroid users and 68 control athletes to provide further data in this area, with attention to the methodologic limitations described above.

RESULTS

One hundred sixty males, 97 in the Boston area and 63 in the Los Angeles area, were studied. Composition of the sample of evaluable subjects follows.

	No. (%) of Subjects		
	Boston (n=96)	Los Angeles (n=60)	Total (N=156)
Steroid nonusers	39 (41)	29 (48)	**68** (44)
Steroid users	57 (59)	31 (52)	**88** (56)
Current users	28 (29)	9 (15)	**37** (24)
Past users	29 (30)	22 (37)	**51** (33)

Four subjects were excluded from analysis: one subject had been prescribed steroids for the treatment of hypogonadism and three had used small amounts of steroids or probable counterfeit steroids and thus could not easily be classified as "users" or "nonusers." Several other subjects also appeared to have used counterfeit steroids at some time, but each of these latter subjects had taken several cycles (courses) of steroids or had "stacked" (combined) several steroids during a cycle. Therefore, these subjects had almost certainly used genuine steroids in addition to any possibly counterfeit ones, and thus, were classified as "users."

Thirty-seven (42%) of the 88 evaluable users were classified as "current" users. To be classified as current, it was required that a user (1) report use of either an orally active steroid within the past week or an injectable depot steroid preparation within the past month, and (2) display a urine sample positive for steroids or have a testosterone to epitestosterone ratio of greater than 6:1. Forty-two (48%) of the 88 users met the first criterion, and of these, 37 (88%) displayed positive urine samples. Of the five discrepant subjects,

three had just begun a cycle of low-dose testosterone (two patients) or boldenone (one patient) and thus might not have ingested a cumulative steroid dose adequate to test positive. The other two subjects were likely using counterfeit steroids at the time of testing. All five of these subjects, however, had used previous cycles of steroids during which they made large muscle gains. Thus, they were retained in the study as users, but classified as "past" rather than current. Among the 68 self-described nonusers, none produced a urine sample positive for steroids.

The steroids taken by the 37 current users were ascertained by self-report and by urine testing.

	Frequency of Use, No. (%)	
Drug	**Self-report**	**Urine Testing**
Testosterone	25 (68)	15 (41)
Nandrolone	20 (54)	21 (57)
Oxymetholone	12 (32)	4 (11)
Stanozolol	11 (30)	5 (14)
Methenolone	9 (24)	6 (16)
Boldenone	7 (19)	4 (11)
Oxandrolone	2 (5)	1 (3)
Methandrostenolone	2 (5)	1 (3)
Mesterolone	2 (5)	2 (5)
Methyltestosterone	1 (3)	6 (16)
Other	12 (32)	0

Differences in the frequencies of different drugs between the "self-report" and "urine testing" columns were not unexpected. Subjects often reported using illicit steroids of uncertain identity or steroids that they suspected to be deliberately mislabeled. Boston and Los Angeles users did not differ significantly on drugs reportedly used or found in urine samples.

The 88 steroid users ranged from high school students who had briefly experimented with steroids to elite athletes with extensive steroid histories. The latter group included several men who had competed nationally or internationally in bodybuilding contests. Among all users, the duration of lifetime steroid use ranged from a single cycle lasting 2 weeks to 28 cycles totaling 336 weeks. The mean (±SD) duration of lifetime steroid use was 43±42 weeks for Boston users and 99±88 weeks for Los Angeles users (P=.004). Most users had stacked two or more steroids during their cycles, and some had taken as many as eight steroids simultaneously. It was usually impossible to calculate precisely the maximum steroid dose that subjects had used, especially since many subjects had included veterinary steroids and illicit "basement laboratory" steroids in their regimens. Also, different steroids may not be equipotent on a milligram basis, although this assumption is often used owing to the lack of a more precise method.[23,33] Recognizing these limitations, we approximated subjects' maximum steroid dosage as "low" (estimated as <300 mg/wk), "medium" (300 to 1000 mg/wk), or "high" (>1000 mg/wk). This classification, performed while "blind" to all other data on each user, is as follows:

	No. (%) of Users		
Dose	**Boston (n=57)**	**Los Angeles (n=31)**	**Total (N=88)**
Low	9 (16)	3 (10)	**12** (14)
Medium	32 (56)	19 (61)	**51** (58)
High	16 (28)	9 (29)	**25** (28)

As indicated in this tabulation, the Boston and Los Angeles subsamples of steroid users did not differ significantly on maximum dose of steroids used. In subsequent analyses, these subsamples are combined, but on variables where they differed significantly; the difference is presented in the text.

Several demographic characteristics distinguished users from nonusers.

Characteristic	**Users (N=88)**	**Nonusers (N=68)**	***P***
Age, y	25.5±7.0	28.3±10.0	. . .
Duration of weight lifting, y	9.0±7.2	6.7±5.9	<.01
Height, cm	179.3±7.1	180.6±7.4	. . .
Weight, kg	92.3±12.3	84.1±13.6	<.001
Body fat, %	13.1±4.7	13.7±6.2	. . .
White	81 (92)	65 (96)	. . .
Married	11 (13)	13 (19)	. . .
Currently using tobacco	13 (15)	18 (26)	. . .
Currently drinking >6 alcoholic drinks per week	12 (14)	18 (26)	. . .

(The first five variables are given as mean±SD and the last four as number [percentage]).

Users weighed significantly more and had lifted weights for a significantly longer time than nonusers. Current users compared with past users weighed significantly less (88.6 vs 94.5 kg; P=.02) and leaner (11.4% vs 14.4% body fat; P=.002) and had lifted weights for a shorter period (7.7 vs 10.0 years; P=.02). Boston subjects were significantly younger than Los Angeles subjects (23.8 vs 32.7 years; P<.001) and had lifted weights for a shorter period (6.1 vs 11.1 years; P<.001). Differences between the subsamples on all other variables in the above tabulation were not significant.

Medical history, findings on physical examination, and laboratory test results were generally unremarkable in all types of subjects; only three findings differed significantly between users and nonusers (**Table 1**). Gynecomastia was equally common among current and past users, whereas testicular atrophy and elevated ratios of total cholesterol to high-density lipoprotein cholesterol were significantly more prominent among current users than among past users. This finding is consistent with previous observations that steroid-induced gynecomastia is often irreversible,[44] whereas testicular size and ratios of total cholesterol to high-density lipoprotein cholesterol tend to normalize after steroid use.[45]

Other physical and laboratory findings, including some abnormalities previously reported in certain indi-

Table 1. Medical and Laboratory Findings That Differed Significantly Between Groups

	Users			
	Current (n=37)	Past (n=51)	Total (N=88)	Nonusers
Mean (±SD) testicular length, mm	42.1 (6.5)*†	46.1 (5.5)*	44.4 (6.2)*	49.5 (6.3)
Gynecomastia, No. (%)	9 (24)‡	16 (31)*	25 (28)*	2 (3)
Total cholesterol–high-density lipoprotein ratio, mean (±SD)	5.4 (1.8)‡§	4.3 (1.1)	4.7 (1.5)‖	4.1 (1.4)

*P<.001 vs nonusers.
†P<.01 vs past users.
‡P<.01 vs nonusers.
§P<.05 vs past users.
‖P<.05 vs nonusers.

Table 2. *DSM-III-R* Diagnoses in Steroid Users vs Nonusers

	No. (%) of Subjects		
	Users (N=88)		
	When Taking Steroids*	When Not Taking Steroids*	Nonusers (N=68)
Mood disorders			
Manic episode	4 (5)	0	0
Major depression	11 (13)†	4 (5)	3 (4)
Hypomanic episode	9 (10)‡§	1 (1)	0
Depressive disorder not otherwise specified	0	1 (1)	1 (1)
Dysthymia	0	2 (2)	0
Any mood disorder	20 (23)§‖¶	7 (10)¶	4 (6)
Psychotic symptoms	3 (3)	0	0
Anxiety disorders			
Panic disorder	2 (2)	3 (3)	1 (1)
Obsessive-compulsive disorder	1 (1)	2 (2)	1 (1)
Generalized anxiety disorder	1 (1)	0	0
Eating disorders			
Anorexia nervosa	0	3 (3)	1 (1)
Bulimia nervosa	0	1 (1)	0
Eating disorder not otherwise specified	1 (1)	1 (1)	0
Reverse anorexia nervosa*	6 (7)	10 (11)	0#
Substance abuse or dependence, if any	1 (1)	28 (32)¶	15 (22)¶
Antisocial personality disorder	NA	9 (10)	2 (3)

*See text for definitions of these terms. NA indicates not applicable.
†P=.06 vs users not taking steroids.
‡P<.01 vs users not taking steroids.
§P<.01 vs nonusers.
‖P<.001 vs users not taking steroids.
¶Total is less than the sum of the individual diagnoses because some subjects had more than one diagnosis within the same category.
#For all users (taking or not taking steroids) vs all nonusers, P<.001.

viduals using steroids,[1] such as hypertension, edema, acne, hair loss, and abnormalities on liver function tests, were not significantly more frequent among current users, past users, or all users than among nonusers. Indeed, among the 19 current users and 34 past users who underwent laboratory testing, only one displayed an abnormal elevation of the liver-specific enzyme γ-glutamyl transferase (84 U/L; normal, 0 to 65 U/L). However, 18 (49%) of the 37 current users and 17 (33%) of the 51 past users, as well as 15 (22%) of the 68 nonusers failed to report for their laboratory tests, so that other individuals with abnormal laboratory findings might have been missed. On physical examination, no steroid user displayed evidence of liver disease or other major abnormalities possibly attributable to steroids. On medical history, however, one 22-year-old current user reported a past hospital admission for renal dysfunction that developed while he was stacking five steroids totaling about 2000 mg/wk. His hospital records revealed a peak serum creatinine level of 5.1 mg/dL (450 μmol/L) on hospital day 3; his creatinine level normalized within several days after discontinuing steroids.

Among psychiatric diagnoses noted in the 156 subjects (**Table 2**), major mood disorders were significantly associated with steroid use—both in the comparison of users with nonusers and in the comparison of users while receiving steroids with these same users when not taking steroids. Three users reported mood disorders with psychotic features; of these, two developed paranoid and grandiose delusions during manic episodes associated with steroid use. One of these two required treatment with perphenazine. A third subject, during a depression associated with steroid withdrawal, developed delusions that his thoughts were being controlled by outside forces. No psychotic symptoms were found in nonusers or in the users when not taking steroids.

Aggressive or violent behavior often accompanied steroid-associated manic or hypomanic episodes. For example, one user, using his fists and a metal bar, seriously damaged three cars, all with their drivers cowering inside, because he had become annoyed by a traffic delay. Another was arrested for causing $1000 of property damage during a fit of anger at a sports event; another was arrested for assaulting a motorist; another rammed his head through a wooden door; another became involved in a nearly successful murder plot; and another beat and almost killed his dog. Several users reported that they were expelled from their homes by parents, wives, or girlfriends because they became intolerably aggressive. Nearly all of these individuals denied comparable behavior before steroid use.

Major mood disorder among relatives did not predict major mood syndromes among steroid users them-

Table 3. Relationship of Weekly Steroid Dose to Prevalence of Mood Disorders

	No. (%) of Subjects Displaying Mood Disorders*			
	Manic Episode	Hypomanic Episode	Major Depression	Total†
Weekly steroid dose‡ (No. of users)				
Low (n=12)	0	1 (8)	0	1 (8)
Medium (n=51)	0	5 (10)	3 (6)	7 (14)
High (n=25)	4 (16)	3 (12)	7 (28)	11 (44)

**Significance of relationship between increasing doses of steroids and prevalence of mood disorders by two-sided trend test: manic episode, P=.0104; major depression, P=.0033; total, P=.0037.*

†Total is less than sum of individual categories because some individuals displayed both a manic or hypomanic episode and a major depressive episode in association with steroids.

‡Low represents less than 300 mg/wk; medium, 300 to 1000 mg/wk; and high, more than 1000 mg/wk.

selves. Of the 20 users reporting a steroid–associated major mood syndrome, five (25%) described at least one first-degree relative with a major mood disorder. This frequency compares with 12 (18%) of the remaining 68 steroid users and 12 (18%) of the 68 nonusers (differences not statistically significant).

Other psychiatric disorders generally did not differ significantly between users and nonusers. One unusual disorder, which we have termed "reverse anorexia nervosa," was found exclusively among steroid users. Individuals with this disorder believed that they looked small and weak, even though they were large and muscular. They declined to be seen in public, refused invitations to the beach, or wore baggy sweatclothes even in summer to avoid being seen as "small." Remarkably, two of the individuals with reverse anorexia nervosa had experienced actual anorexia nervosa when younger. These opposite body-image disorders and their possible role in inducing or perpetuating steroid use are discussed in detail elsewhere.[46]

Antisocial personality disorder and substance dependence or abuse (other than steroids) were slightly but not significantly more common among steroid users than nonusers ($P>.1$ in both comparisons). Of note, however, only two (2%) of the users reported dependence on another substance while taking steroids; one displayed alcohol dependence only during his steroid cycles and the other displayed cannabis dependence both when using and when not using steroids (which was hence classified as off-steroids by our convention). All other users displayed substance abuse or dependence only while not using steroids. The results of urine drug screens supported these reports: cannabinoids were found in the urine sample of only one current user (the individual with cannabis dependence described above), three past users, and one nonuser. No urine samples contained amphetamines, barbiturates, benzodiazepines, methaqualone, opiates, phencyclidine, or cocaine metabolites.

Approximately 25% of the users appeared to show a syndrome of dependence on steroids. However, we did not make a formal diagnosis of steroid dependence based on the responses to the SCID substance abuse questions, although other groups have elected to use this method.[26,28]

Finally, a highly significant relationship was found between the total weekly dose of steroids used (estimated as low, medium, or high, as described earlier) and the prevalence of mood disorders, as shown in **Table 3**. All four individuals with manic episodes and all three individuals with psychotic symptoms fell into the high-dose group.

COMMENT

We obtained demographic, medical, and psychiatric data from 88 athletes who had used anabolic-androgenic steroids and 68 control athletes who had not used steroids, all recruited from gymnasiums in the Boston and Los Angeles areas. Steroid users had lifted weights for a longer period than nonusers, and they were 8 kg heavier than nonusers. Steroid users generally exhibited few medical abnormalities but displayed more frequent gynecomastia, decreased testicular size, and elevated ratios of total cholesterol to high-density lipoprotein cholesterol compared with nonusers. The most striking difference between users and nonusers, and the principal focus of this study, was in psychiatric morbidity: 23% of users displayed major mood syndromes, including mania, hypomania, and major depression, in association with steroid use. These mood syndromes often created significant problems for the users themselves and sometimes for the victims of their irritability or aggression.

In assessing these findings, however, several methodologic limitations should be considered. First, the study relied on retrospective self-reports of athletes using steroids under nonblind conditions. Although retrospective assessment of psychiatric syndromes, using structured diagnostic interviews such as the SCID, has been shown to be reliable,[42] it cannot control for the fact that the subjects were knowingly taking steroids within a gymnasium subculture. Thus, expectational effects or subcultural influences may have contributed to the psychiatric syndromes reported. Nevertheless, it would seem difficult to explain the protracted and often striking syndromes described by many subjects, the similar frequency of the syndromes in subjects from different gymnasiums in different metropolitan areas, or the significant association of the syndromes with steroid dose if these syndromes were attributable purely to psychosocial influences. Moreover, the one small study that administered high-dose steroids on a blind basis found diagnosable mood disturbances in three of 20 subjects.[16]

Second, it was often impossible to establish the ex-

act dose or even identity of steroids that subjects had used. However, urine test results indicated that the great majority of subjects who claimed to be taking steroids were in fact doing so, although sometimes the specific steroids that they believed that they were taking were not those found in their urine samples.

Third, it is difficult to assess possible effects of subject self-selection. For example, it might be speculated that users with prominent psychiatric symptoms or users who had taken high doses of steroids might be more likely or less likely to respond to the study advertisement than users as a whole. Similarly, subjects who had experienced prominent medical side effects from steroids and who had perhaps abandoned steroid use as a result might have been less likely to participate—possibly causing us to underestimate the adverse medical effects of steroids. Several observations, however, argue against a serious psychiatric selection bias. First, a similar range of steroid dosage and similar rates of psychiatric symptoms were found in both metropolitan areas. Also, the lifetime rates of mood disorders and other psychiatric disorders in users when they were not taking steroids and the corresponding rates in the nonusers resemble the rates found in young men in community studies using structured interviews, such as the Epidemiologic Catchment Area Study.[47] This observation weighs against the possibility that the sample of subjects who presented for interview was seriously biased for or against psychiatric symptoms.

Fourth, several possible confounding variables should be considered. Do bodybuilders in general or steroid users in particular possess characteristic personality traits, such as insecurity or narcissism, that might predispose them to mood disorders? In agreement with the recent findings of Moss et al,[25] we did not note any characteristic personality traits among the males in the sample, although it should be acknowledged that personality traits, other than antisocial traits, were not assessed in a formal manner. However, even if such traits did exist, they would not explain the relative absence of mood disorders in the nonusers or in the users at times when they were not taking steroids. Antisocial personality disorder, as noted earlier, was slightly more common among users than nonusers, but antisocial users did not display any greater prevalence of mood disorders than other users. Similarly, use of other illicit drugs might cause mood syndromes, and many subjects reported substantial use of other drugs, including cannabis, cocaine, amphetamines, opiates, and hallucinogens. But as noted earlier, steroid users largely abstained from other drugs while using steroids, and almost all cases of diagnosable mood disorders occurred in conjunction with steroids and not with other substances.

In short, despite the methodologic limitations inherent in retrospective naturalistic studies, it would be difficult to explain as an artifact the association of psychiatric syndromes with steroid use observed in this investigation. Further support for this association is found

Table 4. Relationship of Steroid Dose to Steroid-Induced Psychiatric Symptoms*

Source, y	No./Sex of Steroid Users	Mean Weekly Steroid Dose, mg (No. of Cases/Grade)*	Psychiatric Effects†
Pope and Katz,[21] 1988	39/M, 2/F	750 (12/L, 15/M, 14/H)	+ to +++‡
Choi et al,[22] 1990	3/M	300 (1/L, 2/M)	+ to +++§
Lefavi et al,[23] 1990	31/M	550 (5/L, 23/M, 2/H, 1/U)	++
Perry et al,[24] 1990	20/M	480 (5/L, 14/M, 1/H)	++/0‖
Moss et al,[25] 1992	25/M	436 (9/L, 15/M, 1/H)	+
Malone et al,[26] 1991	71/M, 6/F	513 (18/L, 9/M, 4/H)¶	++
Bahrke et al,[33] 1992	53/M	318 (low to medium)#	0
Present study	88/M	700 (12/L, 51/M, 25/H)	+ to +++**

*L indicates low dose (<300 mg/wk); M, medium (300-1000 mg/wk); H, high (>1000 mg/wk); U, unknown. All dose estimates based on text of studies and on personal communications with each author.

†One plus sign indicates slight psychiatric effect; two plus signs indicate moderate psychiatric effects; three plus signs, marked psychiatric effects; and 0, no significant psychiatric effects.

‡All cases of psychosis, mania, and major depression occurred in subjects in the medium- and high-dose groups; subjects in the low-dose group exhibited only one case of hypomania.

§Slight effects in one subject taking a low dose and one subject taking a medium dose; marked effects in the other subject.

‖Moderate steroid effects found on rating scales, but no steroid-associated psychiatric disorders diagnosed on diagnostic interviews.

¶These data are for the 31 current users only. Note that these estimates are more conservative than those in the other studies, in that steroids reported, but not found in subjects' urine samples, were not counted.

#Number of subjects taking a low or medium dose cannot be calculated from the data given. No subject reported using more than 620 mg/wk.

**One plus sign indicates the psychiatric effect found in the low-dose group; two plus signs, psychiatric effects found in the medium-dose group; and three plus signs, psychiatric effects found in the high-dose group. See text and Table 3 for details.

when comparing the present study with the six series previously reported,[21-26] taking the issue of steroid dose into account. As **Table 4** illustrates, apparent discrepancies between different studies may be related to differences in the steroid dosages used by the subjects. For example, the study by Pope and Katz,[21] which included the largest percentage of high-dose users, also found the highest levels of steroid-associated psychiatric symptoms: a 12% prevalence of both manic episodes and psychotic symptoms. The eight subjects exhibiting mania and/or psychosis in this study reported an average weekly dose of about 900 mg. At the other extreme are the 53 users studied by Bahrke et al[33] who reported a mean weekly dose of only 318 mg and in whose study even the heaviest user reached only 620 mg/wk. These users displayed minimal psychiatric effects. A similar relationship of dose to psychiatric effects appears within the present study, as previously shown in Table 3. It is not possible, however, to judge which of the various study populations is most representative of steroid users as a whole.

In conclusion, this investigation augments a growing literature suggesting that steroids, particularly when used in very large doses by athletes, may cause serious mood disorders, with substantial morbidity for the user and possibly for the victims of his irritability or aggression. Indeed, these psychiatric effects, at least in the cohort studied here, may account for greater overall morbidity than the adverse medical effects of steroids. Further studies of these effects under rigorous and carefully supervised conditions, together with more sophisticated field studies of the doses of steroids actually used by athletes, are needed to assess the extent of this public health problem.

Accepted for publication October 6, 1993.

This study was supported by grant DA-06543 from the National Institute of Drug Abuse, Rockville, Md.

Presented in part at the 145th Annual Meeting of the American Psychiatric Association, Washington, DC, May 5, 1992.

The authors thank Michael Bahrke, Don Catlin, Precilla Choi, Karl Friedl, Caroline Hatton, Robert Lefavi, Donald Malone, George Panzak, Paul Perry, William Yates, and Charles Yesalis for their assistance.

Reprint requests to Biological Psychiatry Laboratory, McLean Hospital, 115 Mill St, Belmont, MA 02178-9106 (Dr Pope).

REFERENCES

1. Haupt HA, Rovere GD. Anabolic steroids: a review of the literature. *Am J Sports Med.* 1984;12:469-484.
2. Pope HG Jr, Katz DL. Psychiatric effects of anabolic steroids. *Psychiatr Ann.* 1992;22:24-29.
3. Pope HG Jr, Katz DL, Champoux R. Anabolic-androgenic steroid use among 1010 college men. *Physician Sportsmed.* 1988;16:75-81.
4. Buckley WA, Yesalis CE, Friedl KE, Anderson W, Streit A, Wright J. Estimated prevalence of anabolic steroid use among male high school seniors. *JAMA.* 1988;260:3441-3445.
5. DuRant RH, Rickert VI, Ashworth CS, Newman C, Slavens G. Use of multiple drugs among adolescents who use anabolic steroids. *N Engl J Med.* 1993;328:922-926.
6. Altschule MD, Tillotson KJ. The use of testosterone in the treatment of depressions. *N Engl J Med.* 1948;239:1036-1038.
7. Vogel W, Klaiber EL, Braverman DM. A comparison of the anti-antidepressant effect of a synthetic androgen (mesterolone) and amitriptyline in depressed men. *J Clin Psychiatry.* 1985;46:6-8.
8. Wilson IC, Prange AJ Jr, Lara PP. Methyltestosterone with imipramine in men: conversion of depression to paranoid reaction. *Am J Psychiatry.* 1974;131:21-24.
9. Shahidi NT, Diamond LK. Testosterone-induced remission in aplastic anemia of both acquired and congenital types: further observations in 24 cases. *N Engl J Med.* 1961;264:953-967.
10. Griggs RC, Pandya S, Florence JM, Brooke MH, Kingston W, Miller JP, Chutkow J, Herr BE, Moxley RT. Randomized controlled trial of testosterone in myotonic dystrophy. *Neurology.* 1989;39:219-222.
11. O'Carroll R, Shapiro C, Bancroft J. Androgens, behavior, and nocturnal erection in hypogonadal men: the effects of varying the replacement dose. *Clin Endocrinol.* 1985;23:527-538.
12. Davidson JM, Cavhargo CA, Smith ER. Effects of androgen on sexual behavior in hypogonadal men. *J Clin Endocrinol Metab.* 1979;48:955-958.
13. Alén M, Häkkinen K, Komi PV. Changes in neuromuscular performance and muscle fiber characteristics of elite power athletes self-administering androgenic and anabolic steroids. *Acta Physiol Scand.* 1984;122:535-544.
14. Crist DM, Peake GT, Egan PA, Waters DL. Body composition response to exogenous GH during training in highly conditioned adults. *J Appl Physiol.* 1988;65:579-584.
15. Friedl KE, Dettori JR, Hannan CJ, Patience THE, Plymate SR. Comparison of the effect of high-dose testosterone and 19-nortestosterone to a replacement dose of testosterone on strength and body composition in normal men. *J Steroid Biochem Mol Biol.* 1991;40:607-612.
16. Su TP, Pagliaro M, Ollo C, Pickar D, Wolkowitz O, Rubinow DR. Neuropsychiatric effects of anabolic steroids. *JAMA.* 1993;269:2760-2764.
17. Annitto WR, Layman WA. Anabolic steroids and acute schizophrenic episode. *J Clin Psychiatry.* 1980;41:143-144.
18. Freinhar JP, Alvarez W. Androgen-induced hypomania. *J Clin Psychiatry.* 1985;46:354-355.
19. Pope HG Jr, Katz DL. Bodybuilders' psychosis. *Lancet.* 1987;i:863.
20. Tennant F, Black DL, Voy RO. Anabolic steroid dependence with opioid-type features. *N Engl J Med.* 1988;319:578.
21. Pope HG Jr, Katz DL. Affective and psychotic symptoms associated with anabolic steroid use. *Am J Psychiatry.* 1988;145:487-490.
22. Choi PYL, Parrott AC, Cowan D. High-dose anabolic steroids in strength athletes: effects upon hostility and aggression. *Hum Psychopharmacol.* 1990;5:349-356.
23. Lefavi RG, Reeve TG, Newland MC. Relationship between anabolic steroid use and selected psychological parameters in male bodybuilders. *J Sport Behav.* 1990;13:157-166.
24. Perry PJ, Yates WR, Andersen KH. Psychiatric symptoms associated with anabolic steroids: a controlled, retrospective study. *Ann Clin Psychiatry.* 1990;2:11-17.
25. Moss HB, Panzak GL, Tarter RE. Personality, mood, and psychiatric symptoms among anabolic steroid users. *Am J Addictions.* 1992;1:315-324.
26. Malone DA Jr, Dimeff R, Lombardo JA. The psychiatric effects of anabolic steroids. Presented at the 144th Annual Meeting of the American Psychiatric Association; May 13, 1991; New Orleans, La.
27. Kashkin KB, Kleber HD. Hooked on hormones?: an anabolic steroid addiction hypothesis. *JAMA.* 1989;262:3166-3170.
28. Brower KJ. Addictive potential of anabolic steroids. *Psychiatr Ann.* 1992;22:30-34.
29. Conacher GN, Workman DG. Violent crime possibly associated with anabolic steroid use. *Am J Psychiatry.* 1989;146:679.
30. Pope HG Jr, Katz DL. Homicide and near-homicide by anabolic steroid users. *J Clin Psychiatry.* 1990;51:28-31.
31. Dalby JT. Brief anabolic steroid use and sustained behavioral reaction. *Am J Psychiatry.* 1992;149:271-272.
32. Bahrke MS, Wright JE, O'Connor JS, Strauss RH, Catlin DH. Selected psychological characteristics of anabolic-androgenic steroid users. *N Engl J Med.* 1990;323:834-835.
33. Bahrke MS, Wright JE, Strauss RH, Catlin DH. Psychological moods and subjectively perceived behavioral and somatic changes accompanying anabolic-androgenic steroid use. *Am J Sports Med.* 1992;20:717-724.
34. Spitzer RL, Williams JBW, Gibbon M. *Structured Clinical Interview for DSM-III-R (SCID).* New York: New York State Psychiatric Institute; 1989.
35. Linden R, Jonas JM, Pope HG Jr. Pathological gambling and major affective disorder: preliminary findings. *J Clin Psychiatry.* 1986;47:201-203.
36. Hudson JI, Pope HG Jr, Jonas JM, Yurgelun-Todd D, Frankenburg FR. A controlled family history study of bulimia. *Psychol Med.* 1987;17:883-890.
37. Jackson AS, Pollock ML. Generalized equations for predicting body density of man. *Br J Nutr.* 1978;40:497-504.
38. Catlin DH, Kammerer RC, Hatton CK, Sekera MH, Merdink JM. Analytical chemistry at the games of the XXIIIrd Olympiad in Los Angeles, 1984. *Clin Chem.* 1987;33:319-327.
39. Catlin DH, Cowan DA. Detecting testosterone administration. *Clin Chem.* 1992;38:1685-1686.
40. Tilkian SM, Conover MB, Tilkian AG. *Clinical Implications of Laboratory Tests.* 3rd ed. St Louis, Mo: Mosby–Year Book Inc; 1983.
41. American Psychiatric Association, Committee on Nomenclature and Statistics. *Diagnostic and Statistical Manual of Mental Disorders, Revised Third Edition.* Washington, DC: American Psychiatric Association; 1987.
42. Williams JBW, Gibbon M, First MB, Spitzer RL, Davies M, Borus J, Howes MJ, Kane J, Pope HG Jr, Rounsaville B, Wittchen H-U. The Structured Clinical Interview for *DSM-III-R* (SCID), II: multisite test-retest reliability. *Arch Gen Psychiatry.* 1992;49:630-636.
43. MacMahon B, Pugh TF. *Epidemiology: Principles and Methods.* Boston, Mass: Little Brown & Co Inc; 1970:276.
44. Friedl K, Yesalis CE. Self-treatment of gynecomastia in bodybuilders who use anabolic steroids. *Physician Sportsmed.* 1989;17:67-79.
45. Lenders JWM, Demacher PNM, Vos JA, Jansen PLM, Hoïtsma AJ, van't Laar A, Thien T. Deleterious effects of anabolic steroids on serum lipoproteins, blood pressure and liver function in amateur bodybuilders. *Int J Sports Med.* 1988;9:19-23.
46. Pope HG Jr, Katz DL, Hudson JI. Anorexia nervosa and 'reverse anorexia' among 108 male bodybuilders. *Compr Psychiatry.* 1993;34:406-409.
47. Robins LN, Regier DA, eds. *Psychiatric Disorders in America: The Epidemiologic Catchment Area Study.* New York, NY: Free Press; 1991.

ORIGINAL ARTICLE

Psychiatric Disorders in Relatives of Probands With Panic Disorder and/or Major Depression

Risë B. Goldstein, PhD, MPH; Myrna M. Weissman, PhD; Phillip B. Adams, PhD; Ewald Horwath, MD; Jennifer D. Lish, PhD; Dennis Charney, MD; Scott W. Woods, MD; Christina Sobin, PhD; Priya J. Wickramaratne, PhD

Background: Panic disorder and major depression (MDD) are both highly familial disorders that co-occur in individuals but do not cosegregate in families. Evidence concerning their familial aggregation with other psychiatric disorders, including phobias, substance abuse, and antisocial personality, has been contradictory. In part, the contradictory findings may be due to failure to account for the effects of proband comorbidity on risks in relatives.

Methods: A family study of 1047 adult first-degree relatives of 193 probands in four diagnostic groups (panic disorder without MDD, panic disorder plus MDD, early-onset MDD, and screened normal controls) was used to determine the range of psychiatric disorders associated with panic disorder and MDD and the effects of proband comorbidity on the rates of disorders in relatives.

Results: Compared to relatives of normal controls, relatives of probands with panic disorder or panic disorder and MDD showed significantly increased risks of panic disorder, but relatives of probands with early-onset MDD did not. After proband comorbidity was controlled for, relatives of probands with panic disorder were also at a significantly increased risk for social phobia but not for any other psychiatric disorders. Relatives of probands with early-onset MDD were at significantly increased risks for MDD, dysthymia, abuse of or dependence on alcohol and other drugs, and antisocial personality disorders but not for any other psychiatric disorders.

Conclusions: We conclude that panic disorder is a specific familial entity that is not associated with a broad range of other anxiety or other psychiatric disorders, with the possible exception of social phobia. Dysthymia, substance abuse, and antisocial personality appear to be on the spectrum of early-onset MDD.

(Arch Gen Psychiatry. 1994;51:383-394)

From the Division of Clinical and Genetic Epidemiology, the New York State Psychiatric Institute, New York (Drs Goldstein, Weissman, Adams, Sobin, and Wickramaratne), and the Departments of Psychiatry, College of Physicians and Surgeons, Columbia University, New York (Drs Weissman, Adams, Horwath, Sobin, and Wickramaratne), the University of Pennsylvania School of Medicine, Philadelphia (Dr Lish), Yale University School of Medicine (Drs Charney and Woods), and the Connecticut Mental Health Center (Dr Woods), New Haven. Dr Lish is currently with the Medical College of Pennsylvania, Philadelphia.

IN THIS article, we examine the range of psychiatric disorders associated with panic disorder and major depression (MDD) using data from a family study originally designed to determine the relationship between panic disorder and MDD. Included were the first-degree relatives (FDRs) of probands in four diagnostic groups: panic disorder and no MDD (n=30); panic disorder and MDD (n=77); MDD with onset before age 30 years (early-onset MDD) and no panic disorder (n=41); and screened normal controls (n=45). Both panic disorder and MDD are highly familial.[1-10] Furthermore, the high level of comorbidity between panic disorder and MDD has been well documented in epidemiologic,[11,12] clinical,[13,14] longitudinal, and cross-sectional studies of adults and children.[15-17] In the first publication from this study, we showed that panic disorder and MDD are two separate disorders which are independently and specifically transmitted and that the comorbid presentation of panic disorder and MDD does not seem to be a single, distinct disorder.[18]

There is also evidence suggesting the familial occurrence of social and simple phobias.[19,20] However, findings regarding the aggregation of phobias in relatives of probands with other disorders are contradictory. In our earlier studies at Yale,[1,21] we found increased risks for phobias in relatives of probands with MDD and either generalized anxiety disorder (GAD)

See Methods on next page

METHODS

PROBAND ASCERTAINMENT

The study methodology has been described in detail by Weissman et al.[18] In brief, potential probands were ascertained consecutively from specialty treatment clinics for depression or anxiety disorders affiliated with Yale University and from the New Haven site of the Epidemiologic Catchment Area study (ECA). By design, about two thirds of the ill probands were recruited from the clinics and one third were recruited from the ECA sample; this strategy was deliberate in order to determine whether probands recruited from treatment clinics had an overrepresentation of ill relatives. The probands selected had to be white and aged 18 to 70 years, in addition to meeting the diagnostic criteria for one of the four cells of interest. After giving informed consent, potential probands who initially met inclusion criteria were reinterviewed blindly by a member of the research team using the Schedule for Affective Disorders and Schizophrenia–Lifetime Version for Anxiety Disorders (SADS-LA).[34] Probands were accepted if they met the diagnostic and demographic criteria on reinterview and agreed to participate; a total of 229 probands were admitted to the study. Acceptance was blind to the willingness of the proband to have family members interviewed, as well as to family size and the diagnoses of relatives.

DIAGNOSTIC CRITERIA FOR PROBANDS

Probands were excluded from all diagnostic groups if they met the criteria for schizophrenia, mania, Briquet's disease, antisocial personality disorder, or anorexia nervosa. The initial exclusion criteria of abuse of or dependence on alcohol and other drugs for the ill groups were dropped because of the small number of potential probands without these conditions. As a result, these disorders were not exclusionary if they were chronologically secondary to the primary diagnosis, chronologically primary but mild, or followed by substantial periods of recovery before the onset of the inclusion diagnosis. The specific inclusion criteria for each proband group will now be described.

Panic Disorder With or Without MDD

Probands were required to meet the *DSM-III* panic disorder criteria based on the SADS-LA. For MDD, the RDC, which were modified to require a duration of illness of at least 4 weeks and impairment of functioning in the major social role, were used. In addition to meeting the exclusion criteria for all groups, probands in the panic disorder without MDD group could have no evidence of MDD by any diagnostic criteria at any level of certainty at any time. They could, however, carry a diagnosis of dysthymia.

Early-Onset MDD

Probands were required to have a history of MDD according to the modified RDC as described above, with the first episode occurring before age 30 years. Furthermore, in addition to meeting the exclusion criteria listed above, probands in this group could have no evidence of any panic disorder or panic attacks by any diagnostic criteria at any level of certainty. The cutoff onset age of 30 years was used as the criterion because of our previous work,[35] which indicated that this form of MDD was the most familial.

Never Mentally Ill Controls

These probands had received no lifetime psychiatric diagnosis during any of the three waves of the ECA interviews based on the Diagnostic Interview Schedule[36] or at blind reinterview with the SADS-LA.

ASSESSMENT OF RELATIVES

Following the acceptance of the proband into the study, all FDRs were enumerated systematically from the proband using the Pedigree Collection Form,[37] and permission to contact the relatives was obtained from the proband. All consenting relatives were directly interviewed either in person or by telephone, depending on their proximity to the study site and their preferences for telephone or face-to-face interviews. As shown by Sobin et al,[38] no differences were found in amount or quality of information obtained between face-to-face and telephone interviews. During the interview, information on the FDRs of probands was obtained from all probands and relatives who were interviewed. Relatives about whom family history information was to be obtained were listed individually by name on the Pedigree Collection Form with the relationships reoriented to the particular informant.

All interviews with probands and relatives aged 17.5 years and older were based on the SADS-LA as previously described.

or panic disorder, and Coryell et al[22] found increased risks for phobias among relatives of probands with primary panic disorder and secondary MDD but not among relatives of probands with MDD and panic attacks. However, these three studies reported Research Diagnostic Criteria (RDC) diagnoses, which do not differentiate specific subtypes of phobias (eg, social vs simple), and they did not consider the role of comorbid phobias among probands in this aggregation. By contrast, neither Noyes et al[6] nor Mendlewicz et al[23] found elevated rates of phobia among relatives of probands with panic disorder, GAD, or agoraphobia compared to relatives of controls.

Discrepancies in findings may be accounted for by methodologic differences among the studies, including proband selection criteria and the use of diagnostic hierarchies in reporting the rates of disorders in relatives.[24] The studies[1,6,22,25] also involved comparatively small numbers of probands in each group with anxiety disorders. Moreover, our earlier studies grouped probands according to a hierarchy of anxiety disorders, with agora-

Interviewers had clinical experience with psychiatric patients and had master's degrees in social work or doctorates in clinical psychology or were advanced graduate students in clinical psychology doctoral programs. In addition, they underwent 40 hours of training in the administration of the study interviews.[18] A family history on all FDRs, including the proband, was collected using a modified family history method for RDC, which was initially developed by Andreasen et al,[39] following the interview with the proband or relative about herself or himself. An earlier version of this modification was used in previous family studies by Weissman et al,[2] and a further revision has been made by Mannuzza et al.[40] All assessments were performed by interviewers who were blind to proband diagnoses.

BEST-ESTIMATE DIAGNOSES

Best-estimate diagnoses on probands and relatives were based on all available information, including direct interviews, family history data from multiple informants, and/or medical records.[18] These diagnoses were made separately by a psychiatrist or a clinical psychologist with a PhD degree who was blind to proband status, unaware of whether the subject was a proband or a relative, and not involved in data collection. So that we could compare our findings to those of previous family studies and evaluate the effects of changes in diagnostic systems, diagnoses were made according to RDC, *DSM-III*, and *DSM-III-R* criteria. Diagnoses were assigned one of three levels of certainty: possible, probable, and definite.[41] Diagnostic hierarchies (eg, under RDC and *DSM-III*, exclusion of anxiety disorders manifest in the presence of MDD) were not applied. Age at onset and severity of impairment due to each disorder were also estimated. Probands who did not meet the original cell assignment on best estimates were formally reassigned or excluded without any knowledge of the data concerning relatives. Data concerning the reliability of the best-estimate diagnoses have been reported elsewhere.[18]

This article reports probable and definite *DSM-III-R* diagnoses in relatives. In analyzing the familial aggregation of agoraphobia without a history of panic disorder, we also consider subsyndromic panic symptoms, including isolated spontaneous (not precipitated by exposure to a phobic stimulus), situational (precipitated by exposure to a phobic stimulus), and limited symptom attacks (intense subjective anxiety and one to three panic symptoms, not precipitated by exposure to a phobic stimulus). Also included in this category is *near panic*, which is defined as any of the following: (1) a sudden onset of intense subjective anxiety or fear for no apparent reason without the accompanying physical symptoms that are characteristic of typical panic attacks; (2) one or more discrete periods of sudden onset of at least one physical symptom that is typical of a panic attack (eg, dyspnea, palpitations, paresthesias, or gastrointestinal discomfort) but without intense subjective anxiety or fear; (3) feeling the ground as unsteady; (4) a combination of sudden subjective anxiety or fear and only one somatic symptom, or (5) depersonalization episodes with sudden onset.

FINAL SAMPLE OF PROBANDS AND RELATIVES

The 193 probands, who had a total of 1047 adult (aged 17.5 years and older) FDRs, were included. Fifty-two percent of all living adult FDRs were directly interviewed, and this percentage did not differ significantly by proband group. An average of 2.3 relatives per proband were interviewed for a total of 435 interviewed adult FDRs. In addition, information on each relative was available from multiple informants; for 77% of all adult relatives, information was obtained from two or more informants.[18]

DATA ANALYSIS

Crude lifetime rates (LTRs) of disorders were compared using χ^2 tests. Age-corrected LTRs were estimated using product-limit survival curves,[42] and the survival curves of the four proband groups were compared using log-rank tests. Survival analysis can be used to estimate LTRs by treating age at onset of a disorder as a failure time and by regarding censoring as occurring when the disorder does not appear by the end of the follow-up period.[43] To control for the potentially confounding effects of gender, age, and interview status of relatives as well as proband source, proportional hazards (PH) regressions[44] were fit for each disorder. The PH model is a quasi-parametric multivariable model which applies the multiple regression method to a survival distribution or another one-time event, such as the onset of a disorder. The PH procedure yields a ratio of the hazards, or age-specific incidences, of the outcome variable (eg, a particular disorder in relatives) while simultaneously controlling for potentially confounding variables. All analyses were performed using SAS statistical software, version 6.06 (SAS Institute Inc, Cary, NC).[45]

phobia superseding panic disorder, panic disorder superseding GAD, and GAD superseding other anxiety disorders. Therefore, some probands with other anxiety disorders may also have had comorbid phobias, and the observed aggregation of phobias among their relatives may have been due to proband comorbidity.

Findings that pertain to the aggregation of alcohol disorders among relatives of probands with panic disorder and probands with MDD are also inconsistent. Mendlewicz et al[23] found no aggregation of alcoholism in relatives of probands with either panic disorder or MDD but included probands with both early- and late-onset MDD. Noyes et al[6] found elevated rates among relatives of agoraphobics but, interestingly, not among relatives of probands with panic disorder. However, although 12 of their 40 agoraphobics and three of their 40 probands with panic disorder carried secondary diagnoses of alcohol or sedative abuse, they did not compare rates of alcohol-use disorders in relatives of probands with comorbid substance abuse to rates in relatives of probands without comorbid substance abuse. By

contrast, Maier et al[10] found elevated rates of alcohol disorders in relatives of probands with panic disorder who were screened to rule out alcohol-abuse comorbidity.

With respect to relatives of probands with MDD, Winokur et al[25] found elevated rates of alcoholism, especially in male relatives of probands whose onset of MDD occurred before age 40 years. Other studies, which did not consider the age of probands at mood disorder onset, report a range of results. Winokur and Coryell[26] found increased rates of alcohol disorders in relatives of female but not male probands who participated in the National Institute of Mental Health Collaborative Study and had primary unipolar MDD and no personal history of alcoholism, but they did not present data on the gender of relatives. Similarly, in a study based on psychiatric hospitalization records, Ingraham and Wender[27] and Wender et al[28] found elevated rates of substance abuse disorders, most of which involved alcohol and not other drugs (Paul Wender, MD, oral communication, January 1993), among biologic but not adoptive relatives of adoptees with major affective disorders, even after excluding relatives of adoptees with comorbid substance abuse disorders. Conversely, Weissman et al[2] and Gershon et al[29] did not find elevated rates of substance abuse disorders in relatives of probands with depression. Cloninger et al,[30] in a review of studies published between 1951 and 1976, concluded that primary depressives, including those with secondary alcoholism, have fewer alcoholic and more depressed relatives than do primary alcoholics, suggesting that secondary alcoholism may be less familial than primary alcoholism. However, the Yale studies[31,32] found significantly higher rates of alcoholism in relatives of probands with both primary MDD (not divided by age at onset) and secondary alcoholism than among relatives of controls or probands with MDD alone, and they concluded that depression does not transmit alcoholism disorders in the absence of comorbid alcoholism in probands. Coryell et al[33] also reported elevated rates of alcohol disorders in male but not female relatives of probands with primary MDD and secondary alcoholism compared to relatives of nonalcoholic depressed probands.

In this article, we examine the rates of a range of psychiatric disorders in relatives to determine the spectrum of disorders associated with panic disorder and/or MDD. This work differs from most previously published family studies in that we have multiple comparison groups and we test the effect of proband comorbidity on the aggregation of disorders in relatives.

RESULTS

DEMOGRAPHIC AND CLINICAL CHARACTERISTICS OF PROBANDS

The demographic and clinical characteristics of the probands and relatives have already been described in detail.[18] To summarize, there were no differences among the proband groups in age, marital status, number of times married, social class, education, or religion. Proband groups were initially matched on gender and age; however, gender differences emerged when best-estimate diagnoses required reclassification or elimination of probands because they did not meet the diagnostic criteria. Specifically, there were significantly more female probands in the panic disorder and MDD and in the early-onset MDD groups. Probands were typically in their mid-40s, married, and in the lower-middle to middle class. Sixty percent had attended or graduated from college or had graduate or professional education. The largest religious group was Roman Catholic, which also represents the largest religious group in the region from which the probands were drawn.

UNADJUSTED LTRs OF PSYCHIATRIC DISORDERS IN RELATIVES

All Adult FDRs

Table 1 shows crude lifetime prevalences of *DSM-III-R* psychiatric disorders by proband diagnostic group among all adult FDRs. We report global tests of statistical significance based on 2×4 contingency tables; however, all possible two-group comparisons were performed, and results are available from one of us (R.B.G.) on request. Some two-group comparisons did show significant differences, especially between the relatives in the ill proband groups and the relatives of the normal controls; however, most of these differences disappeared once potential confounders were controlled for in the PH models. The rates of panic disorder and of MDD will differ slightly from those initially reported by Weissman et al,[18] where rates of RDC MDD and *DSM-III* panic disorder and not *DSM-III-R* diagnoses were presented. However, the patterns of results using *DSM-III-R* diagnoses are similar.

Panic disorder with or without agoraphobia was significantly increased in relatives of probands with panic disorder or panic disorder and MDD; the rate in the former group was about twice that in the latter. Conversely, MDD and dysthymia were most significantly increased in relatives of probands with early-onset MDD, although they were also elevated in the relatives of probands with panic disorder or panic disorder and MDD compared to the relatives of normal controls. Interestingly, the rates of MDD in relatives of probands with panic disorder and relatives of probands with panic disorder and MDD were virtually identical. However, when the panic disorder and MDD group was subdivided by age at onset of MDD (≤30 vs >30 years) in probands, rates of MDD in relatives of probands with panic disorder and early-onset MDD were found to be nonsignificantly greater than those in relatives of probands with panic disorder (28.5% vs 24.8%) and to be significantly greater than those in relatives of

Table 1. Unadjusted Lifetime Rates per Relatives of Selected *DSM-III-R* Disorders in Interviewed and Uninterviewed Relatives (N=1047) by Proband Group

	Proband Group			
	Panic Disorder and No MDD*	Panic Disorder and MDD	Early-Onset MDD	Never Mentally Ill
No. of probands	30	77	41	45
No. of relatives	141	442	209	255
Disorder in relatives				
Bipolar disorders	1.42	2.71	2.39	0.78
Cyclothymia	0	1.13	0.48	0.39
MDD	24.82	23.76	35.41	14.51†
Dysthymia	5.67	5.43	11.96	1.57†
Panic disorder with or without agoraphobia	14.18	7.47	2.39	1.18†
Agoraphobia with subsyndromic panic symptoms‡	2.84	1.13	0.96	0.39
Social phobia	5.67	1.58	1.91	1.57§
Simple phobia	10.64	7.24	6.70	3.92‖
Obsessive-compulsive disorder	0.71	0.45	0	0
Generalized anxiety disorder	2.84	3.85	1.91	0.78‖
Psychotic disorders¶	0	0.23	0.48	0
Drug abuse/dependence	7.09	7.24	10.05	3.92‖
Alcohol abuse/dependence	21.28	20.14	22.49	10.59#
Antisocial personality disorder	2.13	2.94	3.35	0§
No. of diagnoses in relatives†				
0	51.06	52.04	44.02	72.55
1	22.70	23.76	25.36	16.47
≥2	26.24	24.21	30.62	10.98

*MDD indicates major depression.
†$P<.0001$.
‡Includes any evidence of limited symptom, near, spontaneous, and situational panic attacks in agoraphobics who do not meet the full criteria for panic disorder.
§$P<.05$.
‖$.05<P<.10$.
¶Includes schizophrenia, schizoaffective disorder, and brief reactive psychosis.
#$P<.01$.

probands with panic disorder and late-onset MDD (28.5% vs 18.7%, $P<.05$).

In an attempt to explain the comparatively high rate of MDD in relatives of probands with panic disorder, we examined comorbidity between panic disorder and MDD in relatives in each group. Consistent with previous findings of high comorbidity within individuals between panic disorder and MDD, including findings previously reported from this study,[18] we found that approximately one third of the relatives of probands with panic disorder who had MDD also had panic disorder, which suggests that at least some of the MDD in the panic disorder group reflects the high prevalence of comorbidity between panic disorder and MDD within individual relatives. Furthermore, as will be shown below, PH models which control for several potentially confounding variables showed no increase in the risk for MDD in relatives of probands with panic disorder compared to relatives of normal controls.

To determine whether proband comorbidity for dysthymia could account for the elevated rates of either dysthymia or MDD, the lifetime prevalences were compared within ill proband groups between relatives of probands with and relatives of probands without comorbid dysthymia. In the panic disorder and the early-onset MDD groups, dysthymia was significantly more prevalent among the relatives of probands with dysthymia than among relatives of probands without dysthymia, but this result did not hold in the panic disorder and MDD group (not shown). Moreover, there were no differences in any ill proband group in the rates of MDD between relatives of probands with dysthymia and relatives of probands without dysthymia.

Social phobia was significantly increased in relatives of probands with panic disorder. To determine whether proband comorbidity might account for this finding, rates in relatives of probands with vs without comorbid social phobias were compared within proband groups. There were no differences within any of the ill groups in the rates of social phobia in relatives of comorbid vs noncomorbid probands. However, these findings should be regarded cautiously because there were few cases of social phobia among relatives in each proband group. Therefore, the statistical power of this set of comparisons to detect differences related to pro-

Table 2. Age-Corrected Lifetime Rates per Relatives of *DSM-III-R* Disorders in Interviewed and Uninterviewed Relatives (N=1047) by Proband Group*

	Proband Group			
	Panic Disorder and No MDD	Panic Disorder and MDD	Early-Onset MDD	Never Mentally Ill
No. of probands	30	77	41	45
No. of relatives	141	442	209	255
Disorder in relatives				
Bipolar disorders	1.48	2.74	3.30	0.83
Cyclothymia	0	0.92	0.66	0.39
MDD	35.61	33.04	43.88	20.58†
Dysthymia	6.11	5.90	14.84	1.86†
Panic disorder with or without agoraphobia	16.14	9.28	2.61	1.82†
Agoraphobia with subsyndromic panic symptoms‡	4.47	1.24	0.51	0.39§
Social phobia	5.93	1.62	2.00	1.59‖
Simple phobia	10.73	7.15	8.14	4.14
Obsessive-compulsive disorder	0.71	0.47	0	0
Generalized anxiety disorder	3.32	3.96	7.76	0.78
Psychotic disorders¶	0	0.23	0.48	0
Drug abuse/dependence	7.20	7.39	10.09	4.25§
Alcohol abuse/dependence	25.01	21.98	25.16	11.83#
Antisocial personality disorder	2.13	2.50	2.88	0§

**MDD indicates major depression.* P *values obtained by log-rank test for differences across proband diagnostic groups (*df=*3).*
†*P*<*.001.*
‡*Includes any evidence of limited symptom, near, spontaneous, and situational panic attacks in agoraphobics who do not meet the full criteria for panic disorder.*
§*.05<*P*<.10.*
‖*P*<*.05.*
¶*Includes schizophrenia, schizoaffective disorder, and brief reactive psychosis.*
#*P*<*.01.*

band comorbidity may be limited. Furthermore, 40% to 50% of the relatives with social phobia in each ill proband group had comorbid panic disorder, raising the possibility that the association of panic disorder in probands with social phobia in relatives may be accounted for by comorbidity with panic disorder in the relatives. However, exclusion of the relatives with social phobia and comorbid panic disorder left too few cases to allow for reanalyses.

Although uncommon in all groups, antisocial personality disorder was significantly increased in relatives of probands with early-onset MDD. Because antisocial personality disorder was an exclusionary diagnosis for probands, proband comorbidity by definition could not account for this result. Alcohol disorders were significantly more frequent among relatives of all three groups of ill probands compared to the relatives of the normal controls. Comparisons of rates of disorder within proband groups among the relatives of probands with vs relatives of probands without comorbid alcohol diagnoses showed a significant difference only in the panic disorder and MDD group (27.97% in relatives of comorbid vs 17.28% in relatives of noncomorbid probands, $P<.05$). Nevertheless, the number of adult FDRs in the panic disorder and MDD group was substantially larger than in the other three groups. Therefore, the statistical power to detect differences in the other ill proband groups is likely to be considerably lower.

No statistically significant aggregation in any ill group compared to the normal control group was observed for drug, generalized anxiety, bipolar, cyclothymic, obsessive-compulsive, or psychotic disorders. Bipolar, cyclothymic, obsessive-compulsive, and psychotic disorders were uncommon in all groups.

Interviewed Adult FDRs Only

Not shown here, the data were examined separately in the interviewed subgroup of adult FDRs. The patterns of unadjusted rates of disorders in the interviewed subgroup of adult FDRs were generally similar to those observed in all adult FDRs, although the rates themselves were generally 1.5 to 2.5 times higher in the interviewed subsample.

AGE-CORRECTED LTRs

All Adult FDRs

Table 2 presents the age-corrected LTRs derived from Kaplan-Meier survival curves for all adult FDRs. Again,

Table 3. Adjusted Hazard Ratios (95% Confidence Limits) for *DSM-III-R* Diagnoses Among Adult First-degree Relatives (N=1047)*

Diagnosis in Relative	Panic Disorder and No MDD vs NMI	Panic Disorder and MDD vs NMI	Early-Onset MDD vs NMI
Bipolar disorders	1.25 (0.13, 11.97)	2.41 (0.39, 14.97)	1.91 (0.31, 11.72)
Cyclothymia	. . .†	3.31 (0.29, 37.76)	1.61 (0.09, 30.05)
MDD	1.41 (0.80, 2.48)	1.53 (0.94, 2.49)‡	2.46 (1.61, 3.77)§
Dysthymia	3.80 (0.99, 14.57)‡	3.24 (0.99, 10.64)‡	5.54 (1.83, 16.84)‖
Panic disorder with or without agoraphobia	8.77 (2.28, 33.78)‖	5.66 (1.51, 21.16)¶	2.14 (0.49, 9.34)
Agoraphobia with subsyndromic panic symptoms	8.62 (0.96, 77.45)	2.51 (0.28, 22.52)	1.31 (0.08, 21.02)
Social phobia	5.44 (1.38, 21.54)¶	1.52 (0.37, 6.27)	0.98 (0.21, 4.52)
Simple phobia	1.95 (0.70, 5.40)	1.57 (0.62, 3.97)	1.06 (0.42, 2.70)
GAD	5.89 (0.95, 36.60)‡	6.19 (1.19, 32.04)¶	2.28 (0.39, 13.57)
Drug abuse/dependence	1.02 (0.34, 3.10)	1.33 (0.50, 3.55)	3.09 (1.38, 6.90)‖
Alcohol abuse/dependence	1.81 (0.96, 3.40)‡	1.82 (1.04, 3.19)¶	2.28 (1.35, 3.85)‖

**MDD indicates major depression; NMI, no mental illness; and GAD, generalized anxiety disorder. Adjusted from proportional hazard models controlling for proband source and age, gender, and interview status of relative.*

†*This parameter could not be estimated because there were no cases of cyclothymia among relatives of probands with panic disorder and no MDD.*

‡$.05<P<.10$.

§$P<.001$.

‖$P<.01$.

¶$P<.05$.

we report global tests of statistical significance which compare the survival functions in all four proband groups; however, all possible two-group comparisons were performed, and results are available from one of us (R.B.G.) on request. As with the unadjusted rates, some two-group comparisons did show significant differences, especially between relatives in the various ill proband groups and the relatives of normal controls; however, most of these differences disappeared once the potential confounders were controlled for in the PH models. Relatives whose age at onset of a disorder was unknown were not included in the calculation of the survival function; the total number of FDRs excluded from the Kaplan-Meier curves on this basis was small, ranging from none for panic disorder, social phobia, and psychotic disorders to seven for simple phobia. The age-corrected LTRs for MDD are about 1.5 times greater than those indicated by the unadjusted prevalences in all proband groups. For other disorders, however, there appeared to be no consistent pattern of differences between unadjusted and age-adjusted results.

The pattern of the results with the adjusted figures is essentially the same as that with the unadjusted figures, although the absolute magnitude of the LTRs and the levels of statistical significance of differences in some diagnoses across proband groups differ. A notable exception was GAD, of which the age-corrected and unadjusted rates were similar to one another in the panic disorder, the panic disorder and MDD, and the normal groups, but the age-corrected rate was almost four times higher than the unadjusted rate in the early-onset MDD group, possibly because many relatives had not yet passed through the age of risk for this disorder. Significant familial aggregation of panic disorder was observed in relatives of probands with panic disorder or panic disorder and MDD; of social phobia, in relatives of probands with panic disorder; of MDD and dysthymia, in relatives of probands with early-onset MDD; and of alcohol disorders, in all three ill groups compared to relatives of normal controls.

Interviewed Adult FDRs

Not shown here, the patterns of age-corrected LTRs in the interviewed relatives are generally similar to those observed among all adult FDRs, although the magnitudes of the LTRs themselves and, in some instances, their levels of statistical significance, differed, possibly because of the reduced sample size and the consequent loss of statistical power.

RESULTS OF PH REGRESSIONS

Table 3 presents the hazard ratios obtained from the PH regression models with 95% confidence intervals for the disorders in the full sample among relatives in the three ill proband groups compared to the relatives of the normal controls after controlling for the effects of source from which the proband was recruited, age and gender of the relative, and whether the relative was directly interviewed. The referent proband source was the ECA sample, and the referent age category was younger than 30 years old. The hazard ratios indicate the magnitude of the specified main effect adjusted for the effects of the other variables in the model. Because there were no onsets of obsessive-compulsive, psychotic, or antisocial personality disorders among relatives of normal controls, PH mod-

els could not be fit for these disorders and, therefore, they are not considered herein.

Proband-Group Effects

In general, proband-group effects on hazards for specific disorders resembled those from the unadjusted and age-corrected LTRs presented previously. Panic disorder aggregated in relatives of probands with panic disorder or panic disorder and MDD. Although rates of MDD were elevated in relatives of probands with panic disorder compared to relatives of normal controls in the unadjusted and age-corrected analyses, this difference disappeared once age, gender, and interview status of relatives and recruitment source of probands were controlled. Major depression aggregated in relatives of probands with early-onset MDD; in the panic disorder and MDD group, the elevation in the hazard for MDD was only at trend level ($P=.087$). Social phobia aggregated in relatives of probands with panic disorder. Agoraphobia with subsyndromic panic symptoms also showed some evidence of aggregation in relatives of probands with panic disorder, but only at trend level ($P=.055$) and based on only 12 FDRs in the entire sample with that diagnosis.

In contrast to what was observed in the unadjusted and age-corrected analyses, GAD aggregated significantly in relatives of probands with panic disorder and MDD in the multivariable model. Dysthymia and drug abuse and dependence aggregated significantly in relatives of early-onset MDD probands. Alcohol abuse and dependence aggregated significantly both in the panic disorder and MDD and in the early-onset MDD groups, but they aggregated more strongly in the latter. Bipolar disorders, cyclothymia, and simple phobia did not aggregate in relatives of any ill proband group compared to relatives of normal controls.

Effects of Proband Comorbidity on Observed Familial Aggregation

To determine the extent to which proband comorbidity accounted for the familial aggregation of the disorders described in the preceding paragraph, the PH models for disorders of which significant aggregation was observed were refit with relatives of probands comorbid for the respective disorders excluded from the analysis samples. These results are not shown but are available on request from one of us (R.B.G.). When the model for social phobia was refit excluding relatives of probands who were comorbid for social phobia, aggregation in the panic disorder group remained statistically significant. By contrast, when the model for GAD was refit excluding relatives of probands who were comorbid for GAD, there was no aggregation in any ill group.

Because hazard ratios for dysthymia were elevated at trend level ($.05<P<.10$) in the relatives of probands with panic disorder and MDD as well as, unexpectedly, with panic disorder and no MDD, we also refit the PH model for dysthymia with relatives of probands with dysthymia excluded. Aggregation remained only in the relatives of probands with early-onset MDD. Likewise, aggregation of abuse of and dependence on both alcohol and other drugs remained only in the early-onset MDD group after relatives of probands with the respective comorbid disorders were excluded.

Gender, Age, and Interview Status of Relatives

Female gender of relative was associated with increased hazards of MDD, of agoraphobia with subsyndromic panic symptoms, of simple phobia, and of GAD, and with decreased hazards of alcohol and other drug disorders. Significant associations with age were found for MDD, panic disorder, and social phobia, as well as alcohol- and other drug-use disorders, with relatives older than 45 years displaying the lowest hazards of these disorders developing. Source of proband, ie, treatment clinic compared to ECA sample, was not independently associated with the hazards of any disorders. As expected, rates of disorders were higher in interviewed relatives (not shown).

COMMENT

When proband comorbidity, source of proband recruitment, and age, gender, and interview status of the relative were controlled for, the family study results showed the following:

1. Panic disorder and social phobia aggregate in the relatives of probands with panic disorder.

2. Major depression, dysthymia, and alcohol and other drug disorders aggregate in the relatives of probands with early-onset MDD.

3. Panic disorder and MDD both aggregate in the panic disorder and MDD group but to a lesser degree than that seen for panic disorder in the relatives of probands with panic disorder and for MDD in relatives of probands with early-onset MDD. The elevation in the hazard for MDD in the panic disorder and MDD group is only at trend level ($P=.087$), possibly because of differences in the distributions of ages at onset in relatives with MDD across the proband groups.

4. Generalized anxiety, bipolar disorders, cyclothymia, and simple phobia do not aggregate in any of the ill proband groups, whereas obsessive-compulsive and psychotic disorders were too rare to allow detection of aggregation.

5. Consistent with prior epidemiologic studies, risks for MDD, agoraphobia with subsyndromic panic symptoms, simple phobia, and GAD are higher and rates of alcohol and other drug disorders are lower in female relatives.

6. The patterns of findings in relatives were not affected by the source of the proband, ie, whether the pro-

band was recruited from the treatment clinic or an epidemiologic sample, or by interview status of relatives (directly interviewed vs family history information only).

COMPARISONS WITH OTHER FAMILY STUDIES

Familial Transmission in Relatives of Probands With Panic Disorder, Panic Disorder and MDD, and Early-Onset MDD

The separation of panic disorder and MDD in terms of familial transmission is consistent with other family studies,[1-10] including those previously reported from this study by Weissman et al.[18] The present findings, using *DSM-III-R*, further support the hypothesis that panic disorder and MDD represent separate disorders because each aggregated in relatives of probands with that disorder, either with or without the other, but not in relatives of probands with the other disorder alone.

The heterogeneity of panic disorder comorbid with MDD in probands may explain the finding that the rate of panic disorder in the panic disorder group was approximately twice that in the panic disorder and MDD group. In particular, there may be forms of MDD in which syndromic panic disorder exists as a manifestation of MDD, whereas other cases of panic disorder and MDD might represent patients with syndromic MDD occurring as a complication of panic disorder. A third subtype of the comorbid condition might represent a true co-occurrence of panic disorder and MDD. Evidence currently available, including data from the present study, does not allow us to distinguish among these possibilities.

Other Anxiety Disorders in Relatives of Probands With Panic Disorder. The *DSM-III-R* lists agoraphobia without a history of panic disorder as a diagnostic entity that is distinct from panic disorder or attacks. Of the 16 FDRs in our sample who carried this diagnosis, only four had no history of panic attacks, whereas 12 had subsyndromic panic symptoms. These results are consistent with those reported from the New Haven ECA data by Horwath et al,[46] which suggest that although agoraphobia with no history of either panic disorder or attacks does occur, it is uncommon. Furthermore, our findings suggest that agoraphobia with subsyndromic panic symptoms is on the spectrum of panic disorder, based on evidence of increased familial risk in relatives of probands with panic disorder. However, the number of relatives with this disorder was too small to draw firm conclusions. An alternative explanation for our findings involves possible limitations in retrospective recall of symptoms. For example, a person with agoraphobia who actually met the full criteria for panic disorder but only recalled and reported sudden anxiety and three (instead of the four required by *DSM-III-R*) symptoms or three (instead of four) attacks in 4 weeks would be classified as having subsyndromic panic symptoms but not panic disorder because of incomplete recall.

To our knowledge, the aggregation of social phobia in relatives of probands with panic disorder has not been reported previously. These findings are inconsistent with those reported by the Iowa group,[4,6,47] which showed no statistically significant aggregation of this disorder in relatives either of agoraphobics or of probands with panic disorder compared to relatives of controls. Rates of social phobia in relatives could not be determined from the results reported by Mendlewicz et al,[23] our earlier studies,[1,21] and Coryell et al[22] because social phobia was not considered separately from other phobias. Data on social phobia were not presented by Maier et al.[10]

Our finding that social phobia aggregates in relatives of probands with panic disorder is not accounted for by comorbid social phobia in probands. Moreover, aggregation was not found in relatives of probands with panic disorder and MDD. The lack of aggregation of social phobia in relatives of probands with panic disorder and MDD argues against a simple association between panic disorder and social phobia and may also reflect the heterogeneity of the panic disorder and MDD group that was noted previously.[18] The association between panic disorder in the probands with panic disorder and social phobia in their relatives may be accounted for by the high rates of comorbidity between social phobia and panic disorder in relatives and by diagnostic imprecision. As already noted, nearly half of the relatives with social phobia in each ill proband group had comorbid panic disorder; 25% to 50% had comorbid agoraphobia. Moreover, the differential diagnosis of social phobia vs agoraphobia can be difficult, raising the possibility that individuals diagnosed with social phobia may actually have agoraphobia.[48] Alternatively, social phobia may be an epiphenomenon of panic disorder in some cases.

Based on data obtained from the ECA, Horwath et al[49] concluded that boundaries between social phobia and agoraphobia are unclear when the disorders are not complicated by panic disorder but become sharply demarcated by comorbid panic disorder. Furthermore, a recent family study of social phobia[50] has shown that social phobia does not transmit panic disorder. Thus, social phobia may not be a distinct disorder on the spectrum of panic disorder. We are currently examining this issue in greater detail and will report our findings separately.

That no other anxiety disorders aggregated in relatives of probands with panic disorder is consistent with the results of both the Iowa[5] and the Belgium[23] groups. These findings lend further support to the hypothesis that panic disorder is a specific familial entity that is not associated with increased familial risk for a broader spectrum of anxiety disorders.

Other Disorders in Relatives of Probands With Early-Onset MDD. Previous reports[2,51,52] suggest the aggregation of dysthymia in relatives of probands with MDD. The

aggregation of dysthymia in relatives of probands with early-onset MDD remained significant when relatives of probands with comorbid dysthymia were excluded. This finding is consistent with the results reported by Weissman et al,[2] Gershon et al,[52] and Klein et al[51] and lends further support to the notion that dysthymia is on the spectrum of early-onset MDD. If this is the case, some or all of the probands with panic disorder and comorbid dysthymia and their relatives may in the future be expected to manifest MDD as part of that spectrum of illness. Indeed, dysthymia has been identified as a risk factor for the subsequent development of MDD in both clinical and community samples.[53,54]

The apparent aggregation of alcohol disorders in the panic disorder and MDD group seems to be accounted for by proband comorbidity. However, aggregation in the early-onset MDD group remained after the relatives of probands with comorbid alcohol disorders were excluded, in contrast to what was found by Mendlewicz et al[23] and by Merikangas et al[31,32] in our previous Yale family study, both of which involved relatives of probands with both early- and late-onset MDD. Some probands in all groups who have not yet passed through the period of risk for alcohol disorders may develop them in the future. However, the aggregation of alcohol as well as antisocial disorders in relatives of predominantly female probands with early-onset, nonbipolar MDD is also consistent with Winokur's[55,56] concept of depression spectrum disease. This disorder is typically manifest in women as depression, possibly with an increased propensity toward secondary alcoholism, and in men as alcoholism and/or antisocial personality disorder. As noted earlier, Coryell et al[33] found increased risks of alcoholism and antisocial personality in male but not female relatives of probands with primary MDD and secondary alcoholism, although proband gender did not influence the results. Conversely, Winokur and Coryell[26] found elevated rates of alcoholism in relatives of female but not male probands with primary MDD and without personal histories of alcoholism, but they did not examine the effect of the gender of relatives.

When we reanalyzed the data and fit separate PH models for male and female relatives, we found a significant aggregation of alcohol disorders among male but not female relatives of probands with early-onset MDD. In contrast to the findings of Coryell et al[33] but consistent with the findings of Winokur and Coryell,[26] this aggregation remained even after relatives of probands with alcohol comorbidity were excluded. Consistent with the results of Coryell et al[33] and in contrast to those of Winokur and Coryell,[26] however, we found no effect of proband gender.

To our knowledge, aggregation of drug abuse and dependence in relatives of early-onset MDD probands has not previously been reported. However, it appears consistent with the finding by Winokur and Coryell[57] that patients with depression spectrum disease showed an increased risk of both alcohol and other drug disorders over a 5-year follow-up. In particular, as already shown, many of our probands with early-onset MDD have FDRs with alcohol and/or antisocial personality disorders (the definition of depression spectrum disease). Some of these probands have also not passed through the period of risk for drug disorders. Drug disorders have been shown to be familial, at least in relatives of opiate addicts.[58] Aggregation of these disorders in the relatives of our probands with early-onset MDD might thus be expected if drug abuse or dependence were to develop in the probands themselves at a later date.

It would therefore be of interest to assess the extent to which expanding the definition of depression spectrum disease to include primary unipolar depressives with family histories of drug abuse or dependence would yield a similar or a different affected group. That such an expanded definition might capture a similar affected group is suggested by the fact that 20% to 30% of the FDRs in each of our proband groups with alcohol disorders also carried diagnoses of drug abuse or dependence; conversely, 65% to 80% of the FDRs in each group with other drug disorders also carried diagnoses of alcohol abuse or dependence.

Disorders Showing No Familial Aggregation

Our finding that the elevated rates of GAD in relatives of probands with panic disorder and MDD were apparently due to proband comorbidity appears to contradict those reported by Leckman et al[1] in our previous Yale family study and by Coryell et al.[22] As already noted, Leckman et al classified probands with respect to anxiety disorders using a hierarchy in which both agoraphobia and panic disorder superseded GAD. Therefore, probands with MDD and agoraphobia or panic disorder but also with GAD would be classified as having MDD and agoraphobia or as having MDD and panic disorder but not as having MDD and GAD. Similarly, Coryell et al[22] did not assess comorbidity for GAD in their probands.

We reanalyzed the aggregation of GAD in our previous family study, assigning probands to four nonhierarchic diagnostic groups: panic disorder and MDD, early-onset (before age 30 years) MDD, late-onset MDD, and never mentally ill. Generalized anxiety disorder aggregated in relatives of probands with panic disorder and MDD or with late-onset MDD but not in relatives of probands with early-onset MDD when relatives of probands with comorbid GAD were included in the sample. When relatives of comorbid probands were excluded, GAD aggregated only in relatives of probands with early-onset MDD. Although this finding is at variance with those of the present study, the differences between RDC and *DSM-III-R* criteria for GAD limit the interpretability of the differences between the two sets of results. Furthermore,

as already noted, the previous study did not include probands with panic disorder and no MDD. Our findings are, in any event, consistent with the lack of aggregation of GAD reported in relatives of probands with panic disorder by the Iowa[4-6,47] and Belgium[23] groups. They also are consistent with the aggregation of GAD in relatives of probands with GAD reported by Noyes et al.[47] As such, they give further support to the differentiation of panic disorder from GAD.

The lack of aggregation of bipolar disorders, cyclothymia, and simple phobia in any ill proband group is consistent with a number of prior studies of relatives of probands with panic disorder with or without nonbipolar MDD and relatives of probands with nonbipolar MDD.[2,4,6,19,52,59] Bipolar disorders and cyclothymia have been observed to aggregate in relatives of probands with bipolar but not unipolar disorders. The rarity of obsessive-compulsive disorder in the families of our probands with panic disorder is also consistent with the results of both the Iowa[4,6] and the Belgium[23] groups.

Limitations

The limitations of the study include the fact that it was limited to white families. The demographic selection criteria necessarily precluded attempts to examine heterogeneity in patterns of familial aggregation across racial and ethnic groups. However, we made the decision to study white families in an attempt to reduce the heterogeneity of genetic markers that could affect the validity of linkage analyses involving a proportion of these families.

An additional limitation is that many relatives could not be directly interviewed. However, the patterns in our results remained similar when only the interviewed relatives were considered. Moreover, the availability of family history information from more than one source on 77% of all relatives should partially mitigate this limitation.[60] In addition, although the overall sample size and the number of probands and relatives in each group were comparatively large, the number of probands with the comorbid disorders (phobias, GAD, and substance-use disorders) that we assessed in detail and their relatives, especially in the interviewed subsample, were relatively small. As a result, the statistical power of our within-group comparisons of rates of disorders between relatives of probands with and without the relevant comorbidity is limited.

A third potential limitation involves the fact that not all probands had completely passed through the age of risk for disorders that would have been either exclusionary or indicative of comorbidity that is possibly relevant to study findings (eg, MDD in the "pure" panic disorder group, especially among probands with comorbid dysthymia, and alcohol disorders). Although ideally one would do a follow-up on the probands past the age of risk and ascertain the development of these disorders, doing so would require so large a commitment of time and resources that it might not be feasible.

Accepted for publication October 11, 1993.

This research was supported by grants MH-438781, MH-28274, and MH-30906 from the National Institute of Mental Health, Bethesda, Md.

Address reprint requests to Director, Clinical and Genetic Epidemiology, New York State Psychiatric Institute, 722 W 168th St, Unit 14, New York, NY 10032 (Dr Weissman).

REFERENCES

1. Leckman JF, Weissman MM, Merikangas KR, Pauls DL, Prusoff BA. Panic disorder and major depression: increased risk of depression, alcoholism, panic, and phobic disorders in families of depressed probands with panic disorder. *Arch Gen Psychiatry.* 1983;40:1055-1060.
2. Weissman MM, Gershon ES, Kidd KK, Prusoff BA, Leckman JF, Dibble E, Hamovit J, Thompson WD, Pauls DL, Guroff JJ. Psychiatric disorders in the relatives of probands with affective disorders. *Arch Gen Psychiatry.* 1984;41:13-21.
3. Pauls DL, DiBenedetto AM. The familial relationship between panic disorder and major depressive disorder. In: Racagni G, Smeraldi E, eds. *Anxious Depression: Assessment and Treatment.* New York: Raven Press; 1987:73-79.
4. Harris EL, Noyes R, Crowe RR, Chaudhry DR. Family study of agoraphobia: report of a pilot study. *Arch Gen Psychiatry.* 1983;40:1061-1064.
5. Crowe RR, Noyes R, Pauls DL, Slymen D. A family study of panic disorder. *Arch Gen Psychiatry.* 1983;40:1065-1069.
6. Noyes R, Crowe RR, Harris EL, Hamra BJ, McChesney CM, Chaudhry DR. Relationship between panic disorder and agoraphobia: a family study. *Arch Gen Psychiatry.* 1986;43:227-232.
7. Hopper JL, Judd FK, Derrick PL, Burrows GD. A family study of panic disorder. *Genet Epidemiol.* 1987;4:33-41.
8. Moran C, Andrews G. The familial occurrence of agoraphobia. *Br J Psychiatry.* 1985;146:262-267.
9. McGuffin P, Katz R, Aldrich J, Bebbington P. The Camberwell Collaborative Depression Study, II: investigation of family members. *Br J Psychiatry.* 1988;152:766-774.
10. Maier W, Lichtermann D, Meyer A, Oehrlein A, Klingler T. A controlled family study in panic disorder. *J Psychiatr Res.* 1993;27(suppl 1):79-87.
11. Angst J, Vollrath M, Merikangas KR, Ernst C. Comorbidity of anxiety and depression in the Zurich cohort study of young adults. In: Maser JD, Cloninger CR, eds. *Comorbidity of Mood and Anxiety Disorders.* Washington, DC: American Psychiatric Press Inc; 1990:123-137.
12. Boyd JH, Burke JD, Gruenberg E, Holzer CE, Rae DS, George LK, Karno M, Stoltzman R, McEvoy L, Nestadt G. Exclusion criteria of *DSM-III*: a study of co-occurrence of hierarchy-free syndromes. *Arch Gen Psychiatry.* 1984;41:983-989.
13. Barlow DH, DiNardo PA, Vermilyea BB, Vermilyea J, Blanchard EB. Comorbidity and depression among the anxiety disorders: issues in diagnosis and classification. *J Nerv Ment Dis.* 1986;174:63-72.
14. Breier A, Charney DS, Heninger GR. Major depression in patients with agoraphobia and panic disorder. *Arch Gen Psychiatry.* 1984;41:1129-1135.
15. Biederman J, Rosenbaum JF, Bolduc EA, Faraone SV, Hirschfeld DR. A high risk study of young children of parents with panic disorder and agoraphobia with and without comorbid major depression. *Psychiatry Res.* 1991;37:333-348.
16. Strauss CC, Last CG, Hersen M, Kazdin AE. Association between anxiety and depression in children and adolescents with anxiety disorders. *J Abnorm Child Psychol.* 1988;16:57-68.
17. Weissman MM. Evidence for comorbidity for anxiety and depression: family and genetic studies of children. In: Maser JD, Cloninger CR, eds. *Comorbidity of Mood and Anxiety Disorders.* Washington, DC: American Psychiatric Press Inc; 1990:349-365.
18. Weissman MM, Wickramaratne P, Adams P, Lish J, Horwath E, Charney D, Woods SW, Leeman E, Frosch E. The relationship between panic disorder and major depression: a new family study. *Arch Gen Psychiatry.* 1993;50:767-780.
19. Reich J, Yates WR. Family history of psychiatric disorders in social phobia. *Compr Psychiatry.* 1988;29:72-75.
20. Fyer AJ, Mannuzza S, Gallops MS, Martin LY, Aaronson C, Gorman JM, Liebowitz MR, Klein DF. Familial transmission of simple phobias and fears: a preliminary report. *Arch Gen Psychiatry.* 1990;47:252-256.

21. Weissman MM, Leckman JF, Merikangas KR, Gammon GD, Prusoff BA. Depression and anxiety disorders in parents and children: results from the Yale Family Study. *Arch Gen Psychiatry.* 1984;41:845-852.
22. Coryell WH, Endicott J, Andreasen NC, Keller MB, Clayton PJ, Hirschfeld RMA, Scheftner WA, Winokur G. Depression and panic attacks: the significance of overlap as reflected in follow-up and family study data. *Am J Psychiatry.* 1988; 145:293-300.
23. Mendlewicz J, Papadimitriou G, Wilmotte J. Family study of panic disorder: comparison with generalized anxiety disorders, major depression, and normal subjects. *Psychiatr Genet.* 1993;3:73-78.
24. Leckman JF, Weissman MM, Merikangas KR, Pauls DL, Prusoff BA. Methodologic differences in major depression and panic disorder studies. *Arch Gen Psychiatry.* 1984;41:722-723.
25. Winokur G, Cadoret R, Dorzab J, Baker M. Depressive disease: a genetic study. *Arch Gen Psychiatry.* 1971;24:135-144.
26. Winokur G, Coryell W. Familial alcoholism in primary unipolar major depressive disorder. *Am J Psychiatry.* 1991;148:184-188.
27. Ingraham L, Wender PH. Risk for affective disorder and alcohol and other drug abuse in the relatives of affectively ill adoptees. *J Affect Disord.* 1992;26:45-52.
28. Wender PH, Kety SS, Rosenthal D, Schulsinger F, Ortman J, Lunde I. Psychiatric disorder in the biological and adoptive families of adopted individuals with affective disorders. *Arch Gen Psychiatry.* 1986;43:923-929.
29. Gershon ES, Mark A, Cohen N, Belizon M, Baron M, Knobe KE. Transmitted factors in the morbid risk of affective disorders: a controlled study. *J Psychiatr Res.* 1975;12:283-299.
30. Cloninger CR, Reich T, Wetzel R. Alcoholism and affective disorders: familial associations and genetic models. In: Goodwin DW, Erickson CK, eds. *Alcoholism and Affective Disorders: Clinical, Genetic, and Biochemical Studies.* New York, NY: SP Medical and Scientific Books; 1979:57-86.
31. Merikangas KR, Leckman JF, Prusoff BA, Pauls DL, Weissman MM. Familial transmission of depression and alcoholism. *Arch Gen Psychiatry.* 1985;42:367-372.
32. Merikangas KR, Weissman MM, Prusoff BA, Pauls DL, Leckman JF. Depressives with secondary alcoholism: psychiatric disorders in offspring. *J Stud Alcohol.* 1985;46:199-204.
33. Coryell WH, Winokur G, Keller M, Scheftner W, Endicott J. Alcoholism and primary major depression: a family study to co-existing disorders. *J Affect Disord.* 1992;24:93-99.
34. Mannuzza S, Fyer AJ, Klein DF, Endicott J. Schedule for Affective Disorders and Schizophrenia-Lifetime Version (modified for the study of anxiety disorders); rationale and conceptual development. *J Psychiatr Res.* 1986;20:317-325.
35. Weissman MM, Wickramaratne P, Merikangas KR, Leckman JF, Prusoff BA, Caruso KA, Kidd KK, Gammon GD. Onset of major depression in early adulthood: increased familial loading and specificity. *Arch Gen Psychiatry.* 1984;41:1136-1143.
36. Robins LN, Helzer JE, Croughan J, Ratcliff KS. National Institute of Mental Health Diagnostic Interview Schedule: its history, characteristics, and validity. *Arch Gen Psychiatry.* 1981;38:381-389.
37. Thompson WD, Kidd JR, Weissman MM. A procedure for the efficient collection and processing of pedigree data suitable for genetic analysis. *J Psychiatr Res.* 1980;15:291-303.
38. Sobin C, Weissman MM, Goldstein RB, Adams PB, Wickramaratne PJ, Warner V, Lish JD. Diagnostic interviewing for family studies: comparing telephone and face-to face methods for the diagnosis of lifetime psychiatric disorders. *Psychiatr Genet.* 1993;3:227-233.
39. Andreasen NC, Endicott J, Spitzer RL, Winokur G. The family history method using diagnostic criteria: reliability and validity. *Arch Gen Psychiatry.* 1977; 34:1229-1235.
40. Mannuzza S, Fyer AJ, Endicott J, Klein DF. *Family Informant Schedule and Criteria (FISC).* New York, NY: Anxiety Disorders Clinic, New York State Psychiatric Institute; 1985.
41. Leckman JF, Sholomskas D, Thompson WD, Belanger A, Weissman MM. Best estimates of lifetime psychiatric diagnosis: a methodological study. *Arch Gen Psychiatry.* 1982;39:879-883.
42. Kaplan EL, Meier P. Nonparametric estimation from incomplete observations. *J Am Stat Assoc.* 1958;53:457-481.
43. Weissman MM, Merikangas KR, John K, Wickramaratne P, Prusoff BA, Kidd KK. Family-genetic studies of psychiatric disorders: developing technologies. *Arch Gen Psychiatry.* 1986;43:1104-1116.
44. Cox DR. Regression models and life tables (with discussion). *J R Stat Soc.* 1972;34:187-220.
45. SAS Institute Inc. *SAS/STAT User's Guide, Version 6.* 4th ed. Cary, NC: SAS Institute Inc; 1989.
46. Horwath E, Lish JD, Johnson J, Hornig CD, Weissman MM. Agoraphobia without panic: clinical reappraisal of an epidemiologic finding. *Am J Psychiatry.* 1993;150:1496-1501.
47. Noyes R, Clarkson C, Crowe RR, Yates WR, McChesney CM. A family study of generalized anxiety disorder. *Am J Psychiatry.* 1987;144:1019-1024.
48. Liebowitz MR, Gorman JM, Fyer AJ, Klein DF. Social phobia: review of a neglected anxiety disorder. *Arch Gen Psychiatry.* 1985;42:729-736.
49. Horwath E, Johnson J, Hornig CD, Weissman MM. Social phobia diagnostic subtypes and the relationship between social phobia and panic disorder/agoraphobia. In: Frances A, Widiger TA, eds. *DSM-IV Source Book.* Washington, DC: American Psychiatric Association. In press.
50. Fyer AJ, Mannuzza S, Chapman TF, Liebowitz MR, Klein DF. A direct interview family study of social phobia. *Arch Gen Psychiatry.* 1993;50:286-293.
51. Klein DN, Clark DC, Dansky L, Margolis ET. Dysthymia in the offspring of parents with primary unipolar affective disorder. *J Abnorm Psychol.* 1988;97:265-274.
52. Gershon ES, Hamovit J, Guroff JJ, Dibble E, Leckman JF, Sceery W, Targum SD, Nurnberger JI, Golden LR, Bunney WE Jr. A family study of schizoaffective, bipolar I, bipolar II, unipolar, and normal controls. *Arch Gen Psychiatry.* 1982;39:1157-1167.
53. Kovacs M, Feinberg TL, Crouse-Novak M, Paulauskas SL, Pollock M, Finkelstein R. Depressive disorders in childhood, II: a longitudinal study of the risk for a subsequent major depression. *Arch Gen Psychiatry.* 1984;41:643-649.
54. Horwath E, Johnson J, Klerman GL, Weissman MM. Depressive symptoms as relative and attributable risk factors for first onset major depression. *Arch Gen Psychiatry.* 1992;49:817-823.
55. Winokur G. The division of depressive illness into Depression Spectrum Disease and Pure Depressive Disease. *Int Pharmacopsychiatry.* 1974;9:5-13.
56. Winokur G. Unipolar depression: is it divisible into autonomous subtypes? *Arch Gen Psychiatry.* 1979;36:47-52.
57. Winokur G, Coryell W. Familial subtypes of unipolar depression: a prospective study of familial pure depressive disease compared to depression spectrum disease. *Biol Psychiatry.* 1992;32:1012-1018.
58. Rounsaville BJ, Kosten TR, Weissman MM, Prusoff BA, Pauls DL, Anton SF, Merikangas KR. Psychiatric disorders in relatives of probands with opiate addiction. *Arch Gen Psychiatry.* 1991;48:33-42.
59. Andreasen NC, Rice J, Endicott J, Coryell W, Grove WM, Reich T. Familial rates of affective disorder: a report from the National Institute of Mental Health Collaborative Study. *Arch Gen Psychiatry.* 1987;44:461-469.
60. Andreasen NC, Rice J, Endicott J, Reich T, Coryell W. The family history approach to diagnosis: how useful is it? *Arch Gen Psychiatry.* 1986;43:421-429.

ORIGINAL ARTICLE

Cognitive Behavioral Treatment Compared With Nonprescriptive Treatment of Panic Disorder

M. Katherine Shear, MD; Paul A. Pilkonis, PhD; Marylene Cloitre, PhD; Andrew C. Leon, PhD

Background: The efficacy of cognitive behavioral treatment for panic disorder has been established in controlled studies. However, little is known about the efficacy of other psychological treatments. We report the results of a study comparing cognitive behavioral treatment with a focused nonprescriptive treatment for panic.

Methods: Three sessions of panic-related information were provided in each treatment, followed by 12 sessions of either nonprescriptive, reflective listening (nonprescriptive treatment) or a treatment package that included breathing retraining, muscle relaxation, cognitive reframing, and exposure to interoceptive and agoraphobic stimuli (cognitive behavioral treatment).

Results: Posttreatment and 6-month follow-up assessments revealed a good response to both treatments. We observed a high rate of panic remission and significant improvement in associated symptoms in subjects in each treatment group.

Conclusion: These findings raise questions about the specificity of cognitive behavioral treatment.

(Arch Gen Psychiatry. 1994;51:395-401)

THE EFFICACY of cognitive behavioral treatment (CBT) for panic disorder has been reported[1-3] and endorsed as a standard treatment by the National Institutes of Health Consensus Development Conference.[4] Cognitive behavioral treatment for panic disorder is based on a model described by Barlow,[5] Beck,[6] and Clark.[7] The basic premise is that individuals who meet diagnostic criteria for panic disorder have a heightened tendency to react with fear to ordinary bodily sensations. This sensitivity is thought to be a consequence of interoceptive conditioning and/or catastrophic misinterpretation of bodily sensations. Since the usual fear reaction is accompanied by autonomic arousal, an individual who is fearful of bodily sensations will be susceptible to feed-forward escalation of fear.[8] The cognitive behavioral model predicts remission of panic *if* the link is broken between bodily sensations and fear. The CBT intervention, currently thought to be the preferred strategy to accomplish this, includes a focused cognitive therapy and interoceptive exposure.

Several articles attest to the efficacy of such a treatment,[9-13] but it is not yet clear if CBT is the only psychological approach that can reliably achieve panic remission, and the mechanism of antipanic effects has not been elucidated. To test the specificity of CBT in the treatment of panic disorder, we compared a 15-session manualized CBT with a manualized nonprescriptive treatment (NPT) that used techniques of reflective listening. The first three sessions of each treatment included information about panic. This was done because such information is generally provided when a patient seeks treatment in an anxiety disorders specialty clinic. We also believed this information would ensure credibility of the control treatment

See Subjects and Methods on next page

From the Western Psychiatric Institute and Clinic, University of Pittsburgh, Pa (Drs Shear and Pilkonis), and the Department of Psychiatry, Cornell University Medical College, New York, NY (Drs Cloitre and Leon).

SUBJECTS AND METHODS

SUBJECTS

Sixty-five subjects who met *DSM-III-R* criteria for panic disorder with (n=61) or without (n=4) agoraphobia gave informed consent and were randomly assigned to receive a 15-week treatment with CBT or NPT. All subjects participated in structured diagnostic interviews using the Anxiety Disorders Interview Schedule–Revised (ADIS-R)[15] conducted by raters trained by the authors of the instrument.[16] Forty-five subjects (CBT=24, NPT=21) completed the 15-week treatment. Forty-three subjects (CBT=23, NPT=20) completed the follow-up assessments.

All subjects were required to discontinue psychotropic medication for at least 2 weeks before study entry and to refrain from using medication or any other psychotherapeutic treatment during the study.

TREATMENT PROCEDURES

Both treatments began with three sessions in which an ethological model of panic was presented and fully explained. An anxiety reaction, according to this model, consists of separable components of thoughts, physical sensations, and behaviors. Anxiety is considered to be an inborn, potentially adaptive reaction, not inherently dangerous. Physiologic symptoms of anxiety or panic occur as a result of activation of the sympathetic nervous system. Likewise, hyperventilation occurs frequently during anxiety and often plays a role in triggering and/or maintaining panic.

The role of misconceptions about the meaning of having panic symptoms was discussed. This discussion included reassurance that panic is not an indication of character weakness or of serious mental or physical illness. Therapists tried to help the subject identify any obvious triggers for individual episodes and pointed out that the onset of a panic disorder often occurs at the time of a life stress. A handout titled "Causes of Anxiety and Panic" was distributed at the second session. The handout reviewed the basic principles described in these introductory sessions.

The remaining 12 treatment sessions differed, depending on whether the subject was assigned to CBT or NPT. The rationale for CBT was that panic can be blocked by application of specific, prescribed techniques targeting each component of the panic reaction. Breathing retraining and progressive muscle relaxation were used to control physiologic symptoms. Identification and countering of cognitive errors, especially catastrophic misinterpretation and probability overestimation, were used to control escalation of symptoms. Exposure to interoceptive cues was used to practice cognitive and physiologic coping strategies and for habituation of conditioned reactivity to bodily sensations. Exposure to agoraphobic situations was used if subjects had significant levels of agoraphobic avoidance. Homework, which was assigned weekly, was reviewed by the therapist at each session. Homework assignments required 30 to 60 min/d and included practice in breathing and relaxation techniques, monitoring and countering cognitions, and practicing exposure.

The rationale for NPT was different. Subjects were told that panic disorder often begins as a reaction to life stress. However, recurrent panic attacks tend to focus attention on the frightening symptoms, interfering with effective management and sometimes awareness of the importance of the stressor. This means that the stress is likely to continue to exacerbate the panic. If the role of stress can be understood and reactions effectively managed, overall anxiety decreases and vulnerability to panic lessens. The subject was told that the NPT intervention would focus on life problems and stresses. The therapist's role was to listen reflectively to help the subject recognize and cope with hidden feelings. Direct advice and prescriptive interventions were excluded from this treatment. The subject matter discussed in sessions differed among subjects. The only exception to reflective listening was that if the subject asked a direct question about panic or anxiety symptoms, the therapist might answer the question by repeating some of the information provided in the initial three sessions. This could include an explicit reassurance that panic is not dangerous.

Treatment manuals were used for both treatment conditions. The manual for CBT was developed by the Albany Stress and Anxiety Clinic research group, State University of New York, in 1987, and is similar to the current *Panic Control Treatment (PCT) Manual*.[17] The manual for NPT, which was far less detailed, was written for this study by Janet Klosko, PhD, and one of us (M.K.S). (A more detailed manual of this treatment has now been written and is available from one of us [M.K.S.]). Treatment credibility was rated by all subjects after the second session.

Treatments were conducted by therapists with at least 2 years' experience in CBT, who had participated in previous treatment research using these techniques. Each therapist also had at least 2 years' experience in NPT techniques. All treatments were supervised by one of us (M.K.S.)

necessary for a meaningful comparison of the two treatments.

The primary aim of our study was to test the hypothesis that a treatment that includes interoceptive exposure and specific cognitive techniques for correction of misinterpretation of bodily sensations would be significantly more effective in achieving relief of panic than a credible psychotherapy that does not use rigidly prescribed interventions. Although we were aware that comparisons of different psychotherapies often fail to show significant differences,[14] in this case CBT, but not NPT, was targeted specifically at hypothesized panic-maintaining processes. Thus, we predicted a significantly better response to CBT.

in weekly meetings. The CBT sessions were rated for treatment adherence by Michelle Craske, PhD, and Karla Moras, PhD, from the Albany Stress and Anxiety Clinic. The NPT sessions were rated for absence of CBT material.

ASSESSMENT MEASURES AND DATA ANALYSIS

All subjects participated in a structured diagnostic interview (ADIS-R) before and after treatment and 6 months following treatment termination. Most pretreatment and all posttreatment and follow-up interviews were conducted by an independent evaluator who was "blind" to the treatment condition, study aims, and methods. The person rating the ADIS-R was a graduate of the State University of New York, Albany, and had been trained for reliability by the Stress and Anxiety Clinic research team. Reliability checks conducted at our clinic confirmed that this rater matched with another rater, who was also trained at the State University of New York, on the primary diagnosis on each of four corated interviews.

Panic episodes and anticipatory anxiety were monitored daily by diary beginning 2 weeks before the first treatment visit and continuing for 2 weeks after treatment termination. Self-report scales were administered before and after treatment to assess phobic symptoms (Brief Fear Questionnaire[18] and the Mobility Inventory[19]), depression (Beck Depression Inventory[20]), overall symptoms (Hopkin's Symptom Checklist [SCL-90][21]), and overall impairment (Sheehan Disability Scale[22]). In addition, the ADIS-R incorporates scores from the Hamilton Rating Scale for Anxiety[23] and Hamilton Rating Scale for Depression.[24]

To explore possible underlying mechanisms, we measured anxiety proneness (State-Trait Anxiety Inventory[25]), anxiety sensitivity (Reiss Epstein Gursky Anxiety Sensitivity Inventory[26]), and panic-related cognitions and fear of somatic sensations (the Agoraphobic Cognitions Questionnaire and the Body Sensations Questionnaire,[27] respectively). Subjects were asked to report any medication use, and an unexpected urine drug screen was performed within 2 to 3 weeks of the 10th session.

Pretreatment assessment was conducted 2 weeks before the first treatment visit. Posttreatment assessment was conducted 2 weeks following the final treatment visit. A follow-up assessment was conducted at approximately 6 months following treatment termination. For the follow-up assessment, diaries and questionnaires were sent by mail and subjects were asked to monitor panic and anxiety for 2 weeks before the final evaluation interview. The ADIS-R was conducted by the independent evaluator in person or, if necessary, by telephone.

Since we found that our control group showed active treatment effects, we undertook in-depth statistical analyses to confirm equivalence to CBT and to exclude the possibility that subtle differences between the treatments were present. The data analytic strategy involved several steps. First, to explore the characteristics of dropouts, completers were compared with noncompleters for the overall sample and then separately for each treatment group. Next, to test the effectiveness of the randomization, completers from each group were compared at pretreatment. We then conducted a one-way analysis of variance (ANOVA) to compare outcome scores between treatments, and a one-way analysis of covariance (ANCOVA) was used with baseline symptom severity scores as covariates to determine the effect of baseline symptom levels on outcome.

To determine whether the treatments differed in effectiveness for different symptom groups, we conducted multivariate ANCOVA analyses using three symptom groups, panic attacks (full panic and limited symptom episodes), other panic disorder symptoms (anticipatory anxiety, agoraphobic avoidance, anxiety sensitivity and agoraphobic cognitions, illness-related impairment, and Hamilton Rating Scale for Anxiety), and general illness measures (Beck Depression Inventory, Hamilton Rating Scale for Depression, SCL-90, and State-Trait Anxiety Inventory). Before conducting ANCOVA and multivariate ANCOVA, we inspected pretreatment vs posttreatment scatterplots to confirm homogeneity of regression. Some variables (panic, limited symptom episodes, and agoraphobia) were highly positively skewed, so we used a logarithmic $(X + 1)$ transformation in the analysis. Examination of the regression lines revealed a small number of individuals (CBT=2, NPT=1) who appeared to worsen during treatment and whose standardized residual scores were 1.96 or greater ($P \leq .05$). We calculated regression curves with these individuals included in, and removed from, the analysis. When the subjects who worsened (eg, the obvious outliers) were removed from the analysis, there was no evidence of significant heterogeneity of regression on any of the 14 measures we tested, using a liberal standard of $P \leq .10$.

Lastly, to explore the relationship between fear of bodily sensations and panic, we conducted a two-way ANOVA of scores on the Anxiety Sensitivity Inventory (ASI) by group and panic remitter status, in which panic remitter was defined as a subject who had no panic episodes in the 2-week posttreatment monitoring period.

RESULTS

BASELINE CHARACTERISTICS AND BETWEEN-GROUP COMPARISONS

The mean ($\pm$SD) age of completers was 34.7$\pm$9.7 years. Pretreatment data were obtained on 45 subjects (CBT=24, NPT=21). Forty-one subjects completed posttreatment assessments (CBT=20, NPT=21) and 43 subjects completed the follow-up assessments (CBT=23, NPT=20). The mean ($\pm$SD) age of the three men and 21 women in the CBT group was 32.3$\pm$6.5 years. The mean ($\pm$SD) age of the five men and 16 women in the NPT group was 37.4$\pm$12.0 years. Study subjects had a moderate level of

Table 1. Treatment Group Comparisons*

Measure	CBT Pretreatment	CBT Posttreatment	CBT 6-mo Follow-up	NPT Pretreatment	NPT Posttreatment	NPT 6-mo Follow-up
Panic	4.0±4.1	1.2±3.2	0.3±0.7	4.2±4.2	0.4±0.8	0.8±1.8
Limited symptom episodes	5.4±3.8	1.4±3.0	1.1±1.6	5.1±5.1	0.8±1.1	0.2±0.6
Anticipatory anxiety	30.5±20.0	16.3±17.2	10.7±15.5	27.6±21.6	12.6±14.0	9.2±15.2
Phobic avoidance	63.1±17.7	48.0±17.3	45.0±14.8	67.5±16.4	54.1±14.5	48.5±17.2
State-Trait Anxiety Inventory	44.6±12.6	41.2±3.0	41.8±10.5	49.9±13.4	44.3±14.0	36.8±11.9
Hamilton Rating Scale for Anxiety	21.8±7.5	14.1±6.7	11.8±5.7	23.0±5.8	13.5±6.8	11.8±6.9
Anxiety sensitivity	30.8±15.0	20.7±10.5	17.9±9.6	31.6±11.2	21.4±13.8	13.7±11.8
Brief Fear Questionnaire (Total)	42.5±26.1	31.7±29.9	27.3±13.4	33.8±11.3	22.8±13.6	22.3±17.3
Brief Fear Questionnaire (Agoraphobia)	11.5±6.9	7.5±7.3	6.2±5.1	12.1±6.9	6.2±4.6	4.8±6.0
ADIS-R Ag	20.4±17.0	10.2±8.8	3.7±5.1	16.4±15.2	4.9±6.8	5.3±7.5
Beck Depression Inventory	12.1±7.0	7.8±7.2	7.3±6.0	13.9±9.4	8.1±7.1	4.5±4.4
Hamilton Rating Scale for Depression	13.3±5.8	8.9±6.4	6.9±5.6	14.4±5.5	8.0±6.8	6.6±6.0
Hopkins Symptom Checklist	1.1±0.8	0.6±0.5	0.6±0.5	1.2±0.6	0.6±0.5	0.3±0.3
Sheehan Disability Scale	11.5±6.3	6.3±5.2	5.5±4.6	12.8±7.2	5.4±5.2	3.0±4.1

**CBT indicates cognitive behavioral treatment; NPT, nonprescriptive treatment; and ADIS-R Ag, total agoraphobic avoidance from Anxiety Disorders Interview Schedule–Revised. Data are given as mean±SD. For an explanation of measures, see "Assessment Measures and Data Analysis" subsection of "Subject and Methods" section.*

agoraphobia, with a mean score on the ADIS-R Agoraphobic Avoidance Scale of 21.5. A score of 14 or less indicates mild agoraphobia. Subjects in the NPT group had a higher rate of comorbid social phobia (28.6% vs 8.3%) and dysthymia (28.6% vs 4.2%). Otherwise, the two groups were similar with respect to demographics, illness history, and illness severity.

One-way ANOVA comparing treatment groups at baseline showed no significant pretreatment group differences in panic disorder severity, panic frequency, or any other clinical measures (**Table 1**).

POSTTREATMENT RESULTS

Panic, limited symptom episodes, and anticipatory anxiety were measured using a daily self-report diary. The values reported are the mean number of panic and limited symptom episodes per 2 weeks and the mean percentage of the day spent worrying about having a panic episode during the same period. The "phobic avoidance" measure was the Mobility Inventory,[19] a self-report evaluation. Values reported are the mean ratings of avoidance when alone.

At posttreatment, 66% of subjects in the CBT group and 78% of those in the NPT group had been free of panic for 2 weeks, while two (10%) subjects in the CBT group and no subjects in the NPT group had four or more panic episodes in the 2-week monitoring period. At 6 months, 75% of subjects in the CBT group and 68% of those in the NPT group were free of panic. Both groups showed significant pretreatment to posttreatment differences and pretreatment to follow-up differences on each measure of panic disorder symptoms. Results of urine drug screens revealed one subject in the NPT group had evidence of benzodiazepine use (a panic nonremitter) and one had evidence of tricyclic antidepressant use. One subject in the CBT group had evidence of benzodiazepine use.

One-way ANOVA revealed no significant differences between groups before treatment, after treatment, or at 6-month follow-up. Analysis of covariance was conducted for baseline to posttreatment and baseline to follow-up ratings. There were significant effects of baseline symptom levels on all posttreatment measures and no significant differences between groups. Table 1 shows means (±SDs) for all assessment measures at pretreatment, posttreatment, and at 6-month follow-up. The numbers vary somewhat due to missing observations.

Inspection of regression plots for CBT and NPT reveal strong and consistent treatment effects on panic (CBT slope=.25, r=.68; NPT slope=.08, r=.53) and limited symptom episodes (CBT slope=.19, r=.41; NPT slope=.08, r=.40) when clear outliers (CBT=2, NPT=1) are removed. Treatment effects are consistent, but less strong, for other panic disorder measures (eg, anticipatory anxiety, phobic avoidance, and anxiety sensitivity). For ancillary symptoms such as depression, trait anxiety (State-Trait Anxiety Inventory), and SCL-90, treatment effects are least strong. Most striking is the similarity of the treatments in each analysis. These results provide further support for the conclusion that NPT and CBT were equivalent in almost every way. Our results also indicate that both treatments were most powerful in achieving relief of panic symptoms.

SIX-MONTH FOLLOW-UP RESULTS

Treatment gains were maintained at 6-month follow-up for both groups. However, subjects in the CBT group showed further improvement in panic symptoms, while those in the NPT group showed slight worsening (Table

Table 2. Mean Anxiety Sensitivity Ratings*

	CBT		NPT	
	Remitter (n=16)	Nonremitter (n=8)	Remitter (n=16)	Nonremitter (n=5)
Pretreatment	28.8	31.0	31.1	37.2
Posttreatment	19.7	23.0	19.8	28.2
6-mo follow-up	17.5	17.8	12.8	16.5

**CBT indicates cognitive behavioral treatment; NPT, nonprescriptive treatment.*

1). At 6-month follow-up, 75% of subjects in the CBT group were free of panic compared with 68% of those in the NPT group. On the other hand, subjects in the NPT group showed further marked improvement on several ancillary symptoms, while those in the CBT group showed no or minimal further improvement. Analysis of covariance showed no significant covariate findings and no between-group differences at 6-month follow-up.

DROPOUTS

Study subjects included 53 females and 13 males. Thirty-seven females and eight males completed the study. There were 21 dropouts, 13 of whom had been assigned to CBT and eight to NPT. We were not able to obtain posttreatment measures on most dropouts. A two-way ANOVA (treatment group by completers) revealed a significant main effect for pretreatment trait anxiety level (State-Trait Anxiety Inventory, F=4.0, *P*=.02) and a nearly significant main effect for pretreatment depression (Beck Depression Inventory, F=2.7, *P*=.07). On both measures, completers had significantly lower scores than dropouts (F=6.6, *P*=.01 vs F=5.1, *P*=.03). There were no significant group effects or group-by-completer interactions.

We experienced a somewhat higher dropout rate than in most other reported studies. Our clinic was located in a tertiary care hospital in New York City where alternative treatment was easily available to subjects who did not complete our protocol. Seven of the dropouts had the onset of life stresses that precluded continuation in a symptom-focused treatment. Twelve of the 22 dropouts were minorities, and we had no minority therapist on our staff. Seven of the 12 were Hispanic. These factors may have contributed to our high dropout rate. Perhaps of importance, dropouts had significantly higher levels of trait anxiety and depression and were generally more symptomatic than completers.

TREATMENT FIDELITY RESULTS

Treatment fidelity measures were conducted with reference to treatment credibility, adherence to CBT manualized techniques, and absence of CBT techniques in NPT sessions 4 through 16. Treatment credibility ratings were completed by all subjects at week 2. On a scale of 1 through 10,[28] the mean (±SD) ratings for CBT were as follows: how logical the treatment seemed, 8.4±0.9; confident the treatment would be helpful, 6.7±1.9; confidence in recommending the treatment, 7.5±1.9; and predicted success in treating problems unrelated to panic, 6.2±2.2. Comparable ratings for the NPT group were 8.4±1.0, 7.2±1.2, 7.6±2.0, and 7.1±1.6, respectively. There were no significant differences between the two groups.

Treatment adherence ratings were conducted by Craske and Moras. The CBT intervention was rated separately for protocol adherence, general skill, and specific skill on a scale of 0 through 8. The NPT intervention was screened for absence of CBT. Thirty audiotapes were randomly selected from each condition. The mean adherence ratings for CBT sessions was 4.5 on a scale of 0 through 8. The mean general skill was 5.3, and the mean specific skill was 5.5. There was no indication that NPT sessions 3 through 16 included CBT techniques. The NPT intervention was not rated for adherence or skill in this study.

ANALYSES OF MEASURES OF BODILY SENSATION FEARS

We conducted two-way ANOVA to compare treatment group by panic remission status on pretreatment, posttreatment, and follow-up bodily sensation fears, as measured by the ASI. There was no significant difference between panic remitters and those who did not remit in mean ASI score at any measurement period. There were no differences in ASI ratings between CBT and NPT remitters. Both treatments led to a significant decrease in ASI after treatment and a further decrease at 6-month follow-up (**Table 2**).

COMMENT

Our CBT results are consistent with those in previous studies showing the efficacy of this approach in the treatment of panic disorder. There are little data with which to compare our NPT results; however, some evidence is consistent with our findings. Klein et al[29] reported similar results with either systematic hierarchical desensitization or supportive psychotherapy in agoraphobics, and Borkovec and Mathews[30] reported equivalent outcome of CBT and a nondirective reflective listening treatment in a mixed group of subjects with panic or generalized anxiety. Case reports suggest that brief psychodynamic psychotherapy may be effective in panic disorder.[31-34]

On the other hand, a prospective comparative study, similar to ours, compared focused cognitive treatment (CT) in 17 subjects with nondirective treatment in 16 and showed a significant difference between treatments.[35] However, there were important design differences between that study and ours. In the previous study, CT involved 12 weekly sessions with a trained cognitive therapist who followed a de-

tailed treatment manual. Four subjects required up to four sessions beyond the 12-week protocol. The supportive treatment given to the control group was administered in 30-minute sessions by postdoctoral therapists for only 8 weeks. Nondirective therapy included review of the panic diary, using a nondirective, empathic, reflective listening approach. On occasion, nonpanic issues were addressed if they were pressing. The treatments were compared at the 8-week point, when the nondirective group was given a choice to switch to CT and the CT group was given a choice to switch to nondirective treatment. The study was conducted at a world-renowned cognitive therapy clinic, and it is unlikely that the training or expertise of the nondirective therapists was comparable to that of the CT therapists. Our study was different in that CBT and NPT were matched for credibility, session number and duration, and therapist skill. Both treatments were administered for 15 weeks. Furthermore, we included a three-session psychoeducation intervention in the NPT cell. It is likely that these differences account for the difference in our results.

In any case, our results showing equivalent outcome of CBT and NPT were unexpected and need to be explained. One possibility is that the positive outcome achieved by both treatments is related to a nonspecific psychotherapy effect. An increase in self-efficacy has been reported to be an important mediator of good outcome in agoraphobics.[36] A decrease in sense of demoralization may be common to all conditions amenable to psychotherapy[37] and may mediate the improvement in symptoms that we observed.

Another possibility is that panic remission in both treatment groups resulted from decreased fear of bodily sensations. As noted, CBT directly targets this fear. Nonprescriptive treatment may also decrease bodily sensation fears. The informational material included in the focused NPT for panic is aimed at correcting misconceptions about panic, especially regarding fear of bodily sensations. Bodily sensation fears may also have been reduced through the discussions of distressing emotions that occurred during reflective listening sessions.[38] These discussions identified previously unrecognized feelings with associated somatic sensations and provided an explanation for the occurrence of sensations, previously seen as emerging "out of the blue." In-session experiencing of emotions in NPT often included experience of the somatic aspect of the emotion. This would have constituted an exposure to feared interoceptive cues that might have decreased conditioned interoceptive fear responses.

Another possibility is that study subjects used medication covertly. Previous studies suggest occult medication use might be responsible for pill-placebo response.[39] Urine drug screens in our subjects did not support this possibility.

Whatever the mechanism of action of NPT (or CBT), NPT and CBT clearly represent different therapeutic approaches. Our results do not support the specificity of CBT techniques in blocking panic. Instead, the results of our study suggest that CBT techniques are not necessary to achieve relief of panic disorder symptoms.

Our results also do not fully support the hypothesis that breaking the link between bodily sensations and fear is necessary for panic remission, as predicted by the cognitive behavioral model. Fear of bodily sensations was markedly reduced in both treatment groups, but there was no statistically significant difference in anxiety sensitivity between panic remitters and nonremitters. This could mean that a decrease in bodily sensation fear is necessary but not sufficient for panic remission, but other explanations are also possible. Other evidence that targeting fear of bodily sensations may not be crucial for panic remission is that Ost[40] reported good outcome with applied relaxation, a different type of behavioral intervention. Further work is needed in this area.

The main study limitation was that there was no inactive treatment cell. The NPT group was initially planned to be a control psychotherapy, but we found it to be equivalent to CBT. Thus, it is possible that our findings reflect a high placebo response rate in our clinic and/or in the sample we studied. However, this seems unlikely since our remission rate was far higher than in previous placebo studies, and the subjects in this study had been ill for a long time and had undergone previous treatment. Furthermore, our results were stable during a 6-month posttreatment period.

Another study limitation was that CBT treatment adherence ratings were only moderately high, and this may mean that CBT was not delivered optimally. However, even if CBT ratings were higher and the CBT outcome was better, the results we obtained from NPT would still be far better than we expected and need to be explained.

The inclusion in NPT in the initial three sessions of information also limits conclusions we may draw from our study. It is possible that this psychoeducational component is the active ingredient of NPT. However, provision of such information is now standard in most specialized anxiety settings, and if this were the active ingredient, it still would indicate that specific cognitive and/or exposure techniques are not needed for panic remission.

Our findings of NPT efficacy are important in documenting the usefulness of a psychological treatment for panic. Beutler et al[41] have recently shown that an NPT approach is superior to CBT for subjects who score high on "reactance," a measure of the tendency to resist threatened loss of interpersonal control.[42] We have evidence that at least some subjects with panic disorder achieved high scores on a measure of need for interpersonal control,[43] a trait that may be similar to reactance. Nonprescriptive treatment may be the best treatment for this subgroup. It may also be useful in broadening the range of target symptoms in psychological treatment of panic disorder or in combination with medication in subjects whose panic does not remit fully.

Subjects with panic disorder are a heterogeneous group.

It is likely that inborn vulnerability and learned responses play a role in the diathesis of panic and that generating and/or ameliorating panic can occur via neurophysiologic changes or a change in psychological functioning or conditioned reactivity. Patient characteristics and life stress may influence short- and long-term expression of symptoms and play a role in treatment responsiveness. In addition, there are patients for whom standard treatment is not fully effective. Confirmation of NPT effectiveness and study of its usefulness in combination with other approaches would broaden the therapeutic horizon for these patients.

Accepted for publication October 27, 1993.

This study was supported in part by grant MH42430 from the National Institute of Mental Health, Rockville, Md (Drs Shear and Cloitre).

Presented in part at the American Psychiatric Association 144th Annual Meeting Poster Presentation, New Orleans, La, May 14, 1991.

The authors acknowledge the contributions of study therapists Bonnie Gitlin, MSW, and Janet Klosko, PhD; independent evaluator Jane Rygh, PhD; and study coordinator Jane Levitan, RN. We also thank Beth Zboran, MS, Laura Portera, and Lisa Spielman, PhD, for their roles in data management and analysis, and Sandy Barbieri and Juanita Beltran for secretarial assistance in preparing the manuscript.

Reprint requests to the Western Psychiatric Institute and Clinic, University of Pittsburgh, 3800 O'Hara St, Pittsburgh, PA 15213 (Dr Shear).

REFERENCES

1. Barlow DH, Craske MG, Cerny J, Klosko J. Behavioral treatment of panic disorder. *Behav Ther.* 1989;20:261-282.
2. Craske MG. Cognitive behavioral treatment of panic. In: Frances A, Hale R, eds. *Annual Review of Psychiatry.* Washington, DC: American Psychiatric Press; 1988;7:121-137.
3. Clark DM. A cognitive approach to panic. *Behav Res Ther.* 1986;24:461-470.
4. Wolfe B, Maser JD, eds. *The Treatment of Panic Disorder: A Consensus Development Conference.* Washington, DC: American Psychiatric Press; 1994.
5. Barlow D. *Anxiety and Its Disorders.* New York, NY: Guilford Press; 1988:405-474.
6. Beck A. Cognitive approaches to panic disorder. In: Rachman S, Maser J, eds. *Panic: Psychological Perspectives.* Hillsdale, NJ: Lawrence Erlbaum Assocs Pub; 1988:91-111.
7. Clark DM. A cognitive model of panic attacks. In: Rachman S, Maser J, eds. *Panic: Psychological Perspectives.* Hillsdale, NJ: Lawrence Erlbaum Assocs Pub; 1988:71-91.
8. Clark DM, Salkovskis PM, Gelder M, Koehler C, Martin M, Anastasiades P, Hackmann A, Middleton H, Jeavons A. Tests of a cognitive theory of panic. In: Hand I, Wittchen HU, eds. *Panic and Phobias.* New York: Springer-Verlag NY Inc; 1988;2:149-158.
9. Klosko JS, Barlow D, Tassinari R, Cerny JA. A comparison of alprazolam and behavior therapy in treatment of panic disorder. *J Consult Clin Psychol.* 1990; 58:77-84.
10. Michelson L, Marchione K, Greenwald M, Glanz L, Testa S, Marchione N. Panic disorder: cognitive-behavioral treatment. *Behav Res Ther.* 1990;28:141-153.
11. Margraf J, Schneider S. Outcome and active ingredients of cognitive behavioral treatments for panic disorder. Presented at the 25th Annual American Association of Behavioral Therapy Meeting; November 23, 1991; New York, NY.
12. Salkovskis PM, Jones DRO, Clark DM. Respiratory control in the treatment of panic attacks: replication and extension with concurrent measurement of behavior and Pco_2. *Br J Psychiatry.* 1986;148:526-532.
13. Shear MK, Fyer AJ, Ball G, Josephson S, Fitzpatrick M, Gorman J, Liebowitz M, Klein DF, Frances AJ. Vulnerability to sodium lactate in panic disorder patients given cognitive-behavior therapy. *Am J Psychiatry.* 1991;148:795-797.
14. Beutler LE. Have all won and must all have prizes? revisiting Luborsky et al.'s verdict. *J Consult Clin Psychol.* 1991;59:226-232.
15. Di Nardo PA, Barlow DH. *Anxiety Disorders Interview Schedule-Revised (ADIS-R).* Albany, NY: Phobia and Anxiety Disorders Clinic, State University of New York; 1988.
16. Di Nardo PA, O'Brien GT, Barlow DH, Waddell MT, Blanchard EB. Reliability of *DSM-III* anxiety disorders categories using a new structured interview. *Arch Gen Psychiatry.* 1983;40:1070-1074.
17. Barlow DH, Craske M. *Mastery of Your Anxiety and Panic.* Albany, NY: Graywinds Publishing; 1990.
18. Marks IM, Mathews AM. Brief standard self-rating for phobic patients. *Behav Res Ther.* 1979;17:263-267.
19. Chambless DL, Caputo GC, Jasin SE, Gracely EJ, Williams C. The Mobility Inventory for agoraphobia. *Behav Res Ther.* 1985;23:35-44.
20. Beck AT. *Depression Inventory.* Philadelphia, Pa: Center for Cognitive Therapy; 1978.
21. Derogatis LR. *SCL-90: Administration Scoring and Procedures Manual—I for the (Revised) Version.* Baltimore, Md: Clinical Psychometrics Research Unit, Johns Hopkins University School of Medicine; 1977.
22. Leon AC, Shear MK, Portera L, Klerman GL. Assessing impairment in patients with panic disorder: The Sheehan Disability Scale. *Soc Psychiatry Psychiatr Epidemiol.* 1992;27:78-82.
23. Hamilton M. The assessment of anxiety states by rating. *Br J Med Psychol.* 1959;32:50-55.
24. Hamilton M. A rating scale for depression. *J Neurol Neurosurg Psychiatry.* 1960;23:56-62.
25. Spielberger C, Gorsuch A, Lushene R. *The State-Trait Anxiety Inventory.* Palo Alto, Calif: Consulting Psychologist Press; 1970.
26. McNally RJ, Lorenz M. Anxiety sensitivity in agoraphobics. *J Behav Ther Exp Psychiatry.* 1987;18:3-11.
27. Chambless DL, Caputo GC, Bright P, Gallagher R. Assessment of fear in agoraphobics: the Body Sensations Questionnaire and the Agoraphobic Cognitions Questionnaire. *J Consult Clin Psychol.* 1984;52:1090-1097.
28. Borkovec TD, Nau SD. Credibility of analogue therapy rationales. *J Behav Ther Exp Psychiatry.* 1972;3:257-260.
29. Klein DF, Zitrin CM, Woerner MG, Ross DC. Treatment of phobias, II: behavioral therapy and supportive psychotherapy: are there any specific ingredients? *Arch Gen Psychiatry.* 1983;40:139-145.
30. Borkovec TD, Mathews AM. Treatment of nonphobic anxiety disorders: a comparison of nondirective, cognitive, and coping desensitization therapy. *J Consult Clin Psychol.* 1988;56:877-884.
31. McDougall J. *Theaters of the Mind.* New York, NY: Basic Books Inc Publishers; 1985.
32. Malan D. *The Frontier of Brief Psychotherapy.* New York, NY: Plenum Medical Book Co; 1976.
33. Mann J. *Time Limited Psychotherapy.* Cambridge, Mass: Harvard University Press; 1973.
34. Sifneos PE. *Short-Term Psychotherapy and Emotional Crisis.* Cambridge, Mass: Harvard University Press; 1972:147-167.
35. Beck AT, Sokol L, Clark D, Berchick R, Wright F. A crossover study of focused cognitive therapy for panic disorder. *Am J Psychiatry.* 1992;149:778-784.
36. Williams SL, Kinney PJ, Falbo J. Generalization of therapeutic changes in agoraphobia: the role of perceived self-efficacy. *J Consult Clin Psychol.* 1989;57:436-442.
37. Frank JD. *Persuasion and Healing.* Baltimore, Md: The Johns Hopkins University Press; 1973.
38. Mathieu-Coughlin PL, Klein MH. Experiential psychotherapy: key events in client-therapist interaction. In: Rice LN, Greenberg LS, eds. *Patterns of Change: Intensive Analysis of Psychotherapy Process.* New York, NY: Guilford Press; 1984:213-248.
39. Clark DB, Taylor CB, Roth WT, Hayward C, Ehlers A, Margraf J, Agras WS. Surreptitious drug use in panic disorder. *Am J Psychiatry.* 1990;4:507-509.
40. Ost L. Applied relaxation vs. progressive relaxation in the treatment of panic disorder. *Behav Res Ther.* 1988;26:13-22.
41. Beutler LE, Engle D, Mohr D, Daldrup RJ, Bergan J, Meredith K, Merry W. Predictors of differential response to cognitive, experiential and self-directed psychotherapeutic procedures. *J Consult Clin Psychol.* 1991;59:333-340.
42. Asendorpf JB, Scherer KR. The discrepant repressor: differentiation between low anxiety, high anxiety, and repression of anxiety by autonomic-facial-verbal patterns of behavior. *J Pers Soc Psychol.* 1983;45:1334-1346.
43. Heckleman LR, Spielman LA, Shear MK. Focusing on retrospective views of parenting and current interpersonal difficulties in patients with panic disorder. Presented at the 1992 Annual International Meeting Society for Psychotherapy Research; June 24, 1992; San Francisco, Calif.

The First in a New Chemical Class of Non-benzodiazepine Sleep Agents

AMBIEN™

(ZOLPIDEM TARTRATE) CIV

5-MG & 10-MG TABLETS

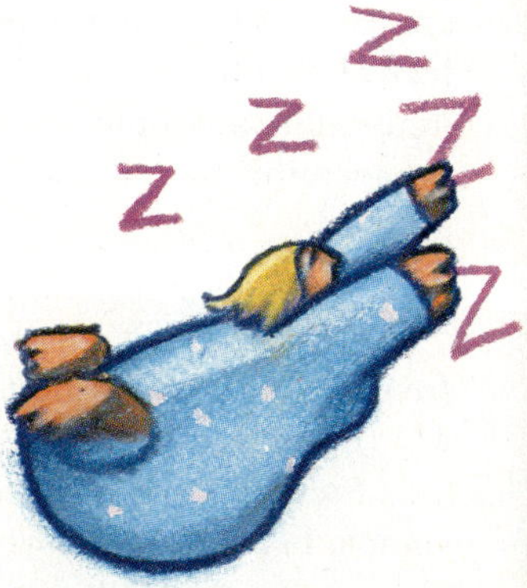

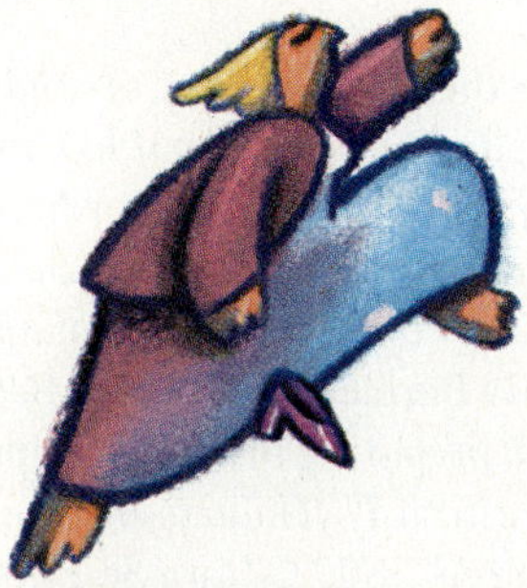

- AMBIEN—an imidazopyridine, chemically unrelated to benzodiazepines or any other sleep agent
- Extensive clinical experience—over 500 million doses prescribed throughout Europe[1]

With AMBIEN, Patients Fall Asleep Fast and Get a Full Night's Sleep

AMBIEN Generally Preserves Normal Sleep Physiology[2-5]

Mean Percentage of Time in Each Sleep Stage[2]

	Stage 1	Stage 2	Stages 3&4	REM
AMBIEN	8.8%	56.5%	16.1%	18.6%
Natural Sleep	8.8%	56.7%	14.3%	20.5%

No statistically significant difference from natural sleep (at baseline) for all sleep stages, in a double-blind, controlled study of 12 healthy volunteers.[2] The clinical significance is unknown.

With AMBIEN, Patients Awaken Refreshed and Alert

- A short half-life — mean 2.5 hours, with no active metabolites
- No evidence of significant daytime sedation or psychomotor impairment[1,2,5,6]

Although AMBIEN is generally not associated with next-day effects, until your patients know how they will react to this sleep agent, they should not engage in activities requiring mental alertness or motor coordination after taking AMBIEN (eg, driving or operating hazardous machinery). Potential impairment of the performance of such activities may occur the day following ingestion of AMBIEN

SEARLE

Please see references and brief summary of prescribing information on last page of this advertisement.

For more information, call **1-800-AMBIEN-1** (1-800-262-4361)

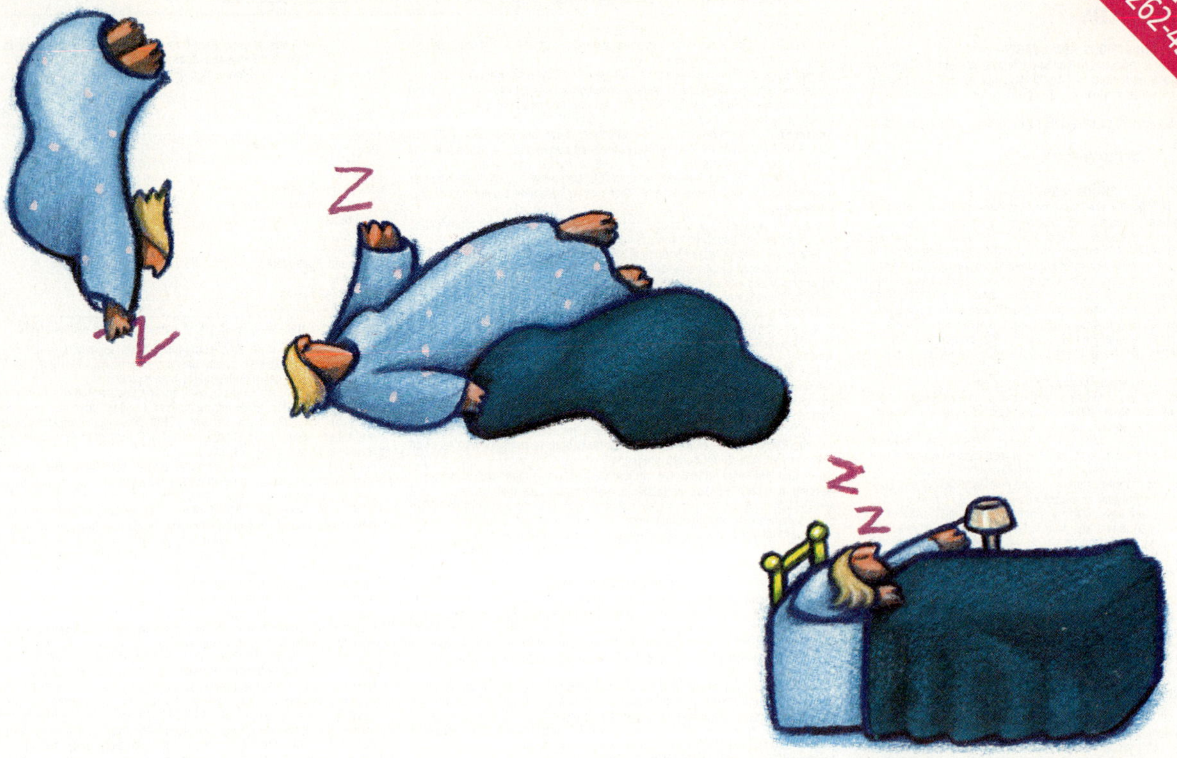

A Favorable Safety Profile

- No rebound insomnia in studies of up to 35 nights at recommended doses[1-4]
- No evidence of tolerance in sleep latency in studies of up to 35 nights[1,3]
- A low incidence of adverse events

  In short-term treatment (up to 10 nights) with AMBIEN at doses ≤ 10 mg, the adverse events seen at statistically significant differences from placebo were: drowsiness (2%), dizziness (1%), and diarrhea (1%); and in longer-term treatment (28 to 35 nights): dizziness (5%) and drugged feelings (3%).
- Because of additive effects, AMBIEN should not be combined with alcohol. Dosage adjustments may be necessary when AMBIEN is coadministered with CNS depressants.

Indicated For Short-Term Management of Insomnia

- Prescriptions for AMBIEN should not exceed a 1-month supply. Hypnotics should generally be limited to 7 to 10 days of use, and reevaluation of the patient is recommended if they are taken for more than 2 to 3 weeks.

Recommended Dosage:

For normal adults:	one **10-mg** tablet
For elderly/debilitated patients:	one **5-mg** tablet

Patients should take AMBIEN right before going to bed and when ready for sleep.

- In patients with hepatic dysfunction, dosage should be reduced and appropriate monitoring instituted.

The First in a New Chemical Class of Sleep Agents

AMBIEN™ (ZOLPIDEM TARTRATE) CIV
5-MG & 10-MG TABLETS

References: **1.** Data on file, Searle. **2.** Merlotti L, Roehrs T, Koshorek G, et al. The dose effects of zolpidem on the sleep of healthy normals. *J Clin Psychopharmacol.* 1989;9:9-14. **3.** Vogel GW, Scharf M, Walsh J, et al. Effects of chronically administered zolpidem on the sleep of health insomniacs. *Sleep Research.* 1989;18:80. Abstract. **4.** Scharf MB, Mayleben DW, Kaffeman M, et al. Dose response effects of zolpidem in normal geriatric subjects. *J Clin Psychiatry.* 1991;52:77-83. **5.** Walsh JK, Schweitzer PK, Sugerman JL, et al. Transient insomnia associated with a 3-hour phase advance of sleep time and treatment with zolpidem. *J Clin Psychopharmacol.* 1990;10:184-189. **6.** Oswald I, Adam K. A new look at short-acting hypnotics. In: Sauvanet JP, Langer SZ, Morselli PL, eds. *Imidazopyridines in Sleep Disorders.* New York, NY: Raven Press; 1988:253-259.

Ambien™ CIV
(zolpidem tartrate)
BRIEF SUMMARY

INDICATIONS AND USAGE

Ambien (zolpidem tartrate) is indicated for the short-term treatment of insomnia. Hypnotics should generally be limited to 7 to 10 days of use, and reevaluation of the patient is recommended if they are to be taken for more than 2 to 3 weeks.

Ambien should not be prescribed in quantities exceeding a 1-month supply (see *Warnings*).

CONTRAINDICATIONS

None known.

WARNINGS

Since sleep disturbances may be the presenting manifestation of a physical and/or psychiatric disorder, symptomatic treatment of insomnia should be initiated only after a careful evaluation of the patient. The failure of insomnia to remit after 7 to 10 days of treatment may indicate the presence of a primary psychiatric and/or medical illness which should be evaluated. Worsening of insomnia or the emergence of new thinking or behavior abnormalities may be the consequence of an unrecognized psychiatric or physical disorder. Such findings have emerged during the course of treatment with sedative/hypnotic drugs, including Ambien. Because some of the important adverse effects of Ambien appear to be dose related (see *Precautions* and *Dosage and Administration*), it is important to use the smallest possible effective dose, especially in the elderly.

A variety of abnormal thinking and behavior changes have been reported to occur in association with the use of sedative/hypnotics. Some of these changes may be characterized by decreased inhibition (eg, aggressiveness and extroversion that seemed out of character), similar to effects produced by alcohol and other CNS depressants. Other reported behavioral changes have included bizarre behavior, agitation, hallucinations, and depersonalization. Amnesia and other neuropsychiatric symptoms may occur unpredictably. In primarily depressed patients, worsening of depression, including suicidal thinking, has been reported in association with the use of sedative/hypnotics.

It can rarely be determined with certainty whether a particular instance of the abnormal behaviors listed above are drug induced, spontaneous in origin, or a result of an underlying psychiatric or physical disorder. Nonetheless, the emergence of any new behavioral sign or symptom of concern requires careful and immediate evaluation.

Following the rapid dose decrease or abrupt discontinuation of sedative/hypnotics, there have been reports of signs and symptoms similar to those associated with withdrawal from other CNS-depressant drugs (see *Drug Abuse and Dependence*).

Ambien, like other sedative/hypnotic drugs, has CNS-depressant effects. Due to the rapid onset of action, Ambien should only be ingested immediately prior to going to bed. Patients should be cautioned against engaging in hazardous occupations requiring complete mental alertness or motor coordination such as operating machinery or driving a motor vehicle after ingesting the drug, including potential impairment of the performance of such activities that may occur the day following ingestion of Ambien. Ambien showed additive effects when combined with alcohol and should not be taken with alcohol. Patients should also be cautioned about possible combined effects with other CNS-depressant drugs. Dosage adjustments may be necessary when Ambien is administered with such agents because of the potentially additive effects.

PRECAUTIONS

General

Use in the elderly and/or debilitated patients: Impaired motor and/or cognitive performance after repeated exposure or unusual sensitivity to sedative/hypnotic drugs is a concern in the treatment of elderly and/or debilitated patients. Therefore, the recommended Ambien dosage is 5 mg in such patients (see *Dosage and Administration*) to decrease the possibility of side effects. These patients should be closely monitored.

Use in patients with concomitant illness: Clinical experience with Ambien in patients with concomitant systemic illness is limited. Caution is advisable in using Ambien in patients with diseases or conditions that could affect metabolism or hemodynamic responses. Although preliminary studies did not reveal respiratory depressant effects at hypnotic doses of Ambien in normals, precautions should be observed if Ambien is prescribed to patients with compromised respiratory function, since sedative/hypnotics have the capacity to depress respiratory drive. Data in end-stage renal failure patients repeatedly treated with Ambien did not demonstrate drug accumulation or alterations in pharmacokinetic parameters. No dosage adjustment in renally impaired patients is required; however, these patients should be closely monitored (see *Pharmacokinetics*). A study in subjects with hepatic impairment did reveal prolonged elimination in this group; therefore, treatment should be initiated with 5 mg in patients with hepatic compromise, and they should be closely monitored.

Use in depression: As with other sedative/hypnotic drugs, Ambien should be administered with caution to patients exhibiting signs or symptoms of depression. Suicidal tendencies may be present in such patients and protective measures may be required. Intentional overdosage is more common in this group of patients; therefore, the least amount of drug that is feasible should be prescribed for the patient at any one time.

Information for patients: Patient information is printed in the complete prescribing information and is available in pads for distribution to patients.

Laboratory tests: There are no specific laboratory tests recommended.

Drug interactions

CNS-active drugs: Ambien was evaluated in healthy volunteers in single-dose interaction studies for several CNS drugs. A study involving haloperidol and zolpidem revealed no effect of haloperidol on the pharmacokinetics or pharmacodynamics of zolpidem. Imipramine in combination with zolpidem produced no pharmacokinetic interaction other than a 20% decrease in peak levels of imipramine, but there was an additive effect of decreased alertness. Similarly, chlorpromazine in combination with zolpidem produced no pharmacokinetic interaction, but there was an additive effect of decreased alertness and psychomotor performance. The lack of a drug interaction following single-dose administration does not predict a lack following chronic administration.

An additive effect on psychomotor performance between alcohol and zolpidem was demonstrated.

Since the systematic evaluations of Ambien in combination with other CNS-active drugs have been limited, careful consideration should be given to the pharmacology of any CNS-active drug to be used with zolpidem. Any drug with CNS-depressant effects could potentially enhance the CNS-depressant effects of zolpidem.

Other drugs: A study involving cimetidine/zolpidem and ranitidine/zolpidem combinations revealed no effect of either drug on the pharmacokinetics or pharmacodynamics of zolpidem. Zolpidem had no effect on digoxin kinetics and did not affect prothrombin time when given with warfarin in normal subjects. Zolpidem's sedative/hypnotic effect was reversed by flumazenil; however, no significant alterations in zolpidem pharmacokinetics were found.

Drug/Laboratory test interactions: Zolpidem is not known to interfere with commonly employed clinical laboratory tests.

Carcinogenesis, mutagenesis, impairment of fertility

Carcinogenesis: Zolpidem was administered to rats and mice for 2 years at dietary dosages of 4, 18, and 80 mg/kg/day. In mice, these doses are 26 to 520 times or 2 to 35 times the maximum 10-mg human dose on a mg/kg or mg/m^2 basis, respectively. In rats these doses are 43 to 876 times or 6 to 115 times the maximum 10-mg human dose on a mg/kg or mg/m^2 basis, respectively. No evidence of carcinogenic potential was observed in mice. Renal liposarcomas were seen in 4/100 rats (3 males, 1 female) receiving 80 mg/kg/day and a renal lipoma was observed in one male rat at the 18 mg/kg/day dose. Incidence rates of lipoma and liposarcoma for zolpidem were comparable to those seen in historical controls and the tumor findings are thought to be a spontaneous occurrence.

Mutagenesis: Zolpidem did not have mutagenic activity in several tests including the Ames test, genotoxicity in mouse lymphoma cells in vitro, chromosomal aberrations in cultured human lymphocytes, unscheduled DNA synthesis in rat hepatocytes in vitro, and the micronucleus test in mice.

Impairment of fertility: In a rat reproduction study, the high dose (100 mg base/kg) of zolpidem resulted in irregular estrus cycles and prolonged precoital intervals, but there was no effect on male or female fertility after daily oral doses of 4 to 100 mg base/kg or 5 to 130 times the recommended human dose in mg/m^2. No effects on any other fertility parameters were noted.

Pregnancy

Category B. Studies to assess the effects of zolpidem on human reproduction and development have not been conducted.

Teratology studies were conducted in rats and rabbits.

In rats, adverse maternal and fetal effects occurred at 20 and 100 mg base/kg and included dose-related maternal lethargy and ataxia and a dose-related trend to incomplete ossification of fetal skull bones.

In rabbits, dose-related maternal sedation and decreased weight gain occurred at all doses tested. At the high dose, 16 mg base/kg, there was an increase in postimplantation fetal loss and underossification of sternebrae in viable fetuses.

This drug should be used during pregnancy only if clearly needed.

Nonteratogenic effects: Studies to assess the effects on children whose mothers took zolpidem during pregnancy have not been conducted. However, children born of mothers taking sedative/hypnotic drugs may be at some risk for withdrawal symptoms from the drug during the postnatal period. In addition, neonatal flaccidity has been reported in infants born of mothers who received sedative/hypnotic drugs during pregnancy.

Labor and delivery: Ambien has no established use in labor and delivery.

Nursing mothers: Studies in lactating mothers indicate that between 0.004 and 0.019% of the total administered dose is excreted into milk, but the effect of zolpidem on the infant is unknown.

The use of Ambien in nursing mothers is not recommended.

Safety and effectiveness in children below the age of 18 have not been established.

ADVERSE REACTIONS

Associated with discontinuation of treatment: Approximately 4% of 1,701 patients who received zolpidem at all doses (1.25 to 90 mg) in U.S. premarketing clinical trials discontinued treatment because of an adverse clinical event. Events most commonly associated with discontinuation from U.S. trials were daytime drowsiness (0.5%), dizziness (0.4%), headache (0.5%), nausea (0.6%), and vomiting (0.5%).

Approximately 6% of 1,320 patients who received zolpidem at all doses (5 to 50 mg) in similar foreign trials discontinued treatment because of an adverse event. Events most commonly associated with discontinuation from these trials were daytime drowsiness (1.6%), amnesia (0.6%), dizziness (0.6%), headache (0.6%), and nausea (0.6%).

Incidence in controlled clinical trials

Most commonly observed adverse events in controlled trials: During short-term treatment (up to 10 nights) with Ambien at doses up to 10 mg, the most commonly observed adverse events associated with the use of zolpidem and seen at statistically significant differences from placebo-treated patients were drowsiness (reported by 2% of zolpidem patients), dizziness (1%), and diarrhea (1%). During longer-term treatment (28 to 35 nights) with zolpidem at doses up to 10 mg, the most commonly observed adverse events associated with the use of zolpidem and seen at statistically significant differences from placebo-treated patients were dizziness (5%) and drugged feelings (3%).

Incidence of Treatment-Emergent Adverse Experiences in Short-term Placebo-Controlled Clinical Trials
(Percentage of patients reporting)

Body System/ Adverse Event*	Zolpidem (≤10 mg) (N=685)	Placebo (N=473)
Central and Peripheral Nervous System		
Headache	7	6
Drowsiness	2	–
Dizziness	1	–
Gastrointestinal System		
Nausea	2	3
Diarrhea	1	–
Musculoskeletal System		
Myalgia	1	2

*Events reported by at least 1% of Ambien patients are included.

Incidence of Treatment-Emergent Adverse Experiences in Long-term Placebo-Controlled Clinical Trials
(Percentage of patients reporting)

Body System/ Adverse Event*	Zolpidem (≤10 mg) (N=152)	Placebo (N=161)
Autonomic Nervous System		
Dry mouth	3	1
Body as a Whole		
Allergy	4	1
Back pain	3	2
Influenza-like symptoms	2	–
Chest pain	1	–
Fatigue	1	2
Cardiovascular System		
Palpitation	2	–
Central and Peripheral Nervous System		
Headache	19	22
Drowsiness	8	5
Dizziness	5	1
Lethargy	3	1
Drugged feeling	3	–
Lightheadedness	2	1
Depression	2	1
Abnormal dreams	1	–
Amnesia	1	–
Anxiety	1	1
Nervousness	1	3
Sleep disorder	1	–
Gastrointestinal System		
Nausea	6	6
Dyspepsia	5	6
Diarrhea	3	2
Abdominal pain	2	2
Constipation	2	1
Anorexia	1	1
Vomiting	1	1
Immunologic System		
Infection	1	1

Incidence of Treatment-Emergent Adverse Experiences in Long-term Placebo-Controlled Clinical Trials (Cont'd)
(Percentage of patients reporting)

Body System/ Adverse Event*	Zolpidem (≤10 mg) (N=152)	Placebo (N=161)
Musculoskeletal System		
Myalgia	7	7
Arthralgia	4	4
Respiratory System		
Upper respiratory infection	5	6
Sinusitis	4	2
Pharyngitis	3	1
Rhinitis	1	3
Skin and Appendages		
Rash	2	1
Urogenital System		
Urinary tract infection	2	2

*Events reported by at least 1% of patients treated with Ambien.

There is evidence from dose comparison trials suggesting a dose relationship for many of the adverse events associated with zolpidem use, particularly for certain CNS and gastrointestinal adverse events.

Adverse events are further classified and enumerated in order of decreasing frequency using the following definitions: frequent adverse events are defined as those occurring in greater than 1/100 subjects; infrequent adverse events are those occurring in 1/100 to 1/1,000 patients; rare events are those occurring in less than 1/1,000 patients.

Frequent: abdominal pain, amnesia, ataxia, confusion, depression, diarrhea, diplopia, dizziness, dreaming abnormal, drowsiness, drugged feeling, dry mouth, dyspepsia, euphoria, fatigue, headache, insomnia, lethargy, lightheadedness, myalgia, nausea, upper respiratory infection, vertigo, vision abnormal, vomiting.

Infrequent: agitation, allergy, anorexia, anxiety, arthralgia, arthritis, asthenia, back pain, bronchitis, cerebrovascular disorder, chest pain, constipation, coughing, cystitis, decreased cognition, detached, difficulty concentrating, dysarthria, dysphagia, dyspnea, edema, emotional lability, eye irritation, falling, fever, flatulence, gastroenteritis, hallucination, hiccup, hyperglycemia, hypertension, hypoaesthesia, infection, influenza-like symptoms, malaise, menstrual disorder, migraine, nervousness, pallor, palpitation, paresthesia, pharyngitis, postural hypotension, pruritus, rash, rhinitis, scleritis, SGPT increased, sinusitis, sleep disorder, sleeping (after daytime dosing), stupor, sweating increased, tachycardia, taste perversion, tinnitus, tooth disorder, trauma, tremor, urinary incontinence, urinary tract infection, vaginitis.

Rare: abdominal body sensation, abscess, acne, acute renal failure, aggressive reaction, allergic reaction, allergy aggravated, anaphylactic shock, anemia, appetite increased, arrhythmia, arteritis, arthrosis, bilirubinemia, breast fibroadenosis, breast neoplasm, breast pain female, bronchospasm, bullous eruption, BUN increased, circulatory failure, corneal ulceration, delusion, dementia, depersonalization, dermatitis, dysphasia, dysuria, edema periorbital, enteritis, epistaxis, eructation, esophagospasm, ESR increased, extrasystoles, eye pain, face edema, feeling strange, flushing, furunculosis, gastritis, glaucoma, gout, hemorrhoids, hepatic function abnormal, herpes simplex, herpes zoster, hot flashes, hypercholesteremia, hyperhemoglobinemia, hyperlipidemia, hypertension aggravated, hypotension, hypotonia, hypoxia, hysteria, illusion, impotence, injection site inflammation, intestinal obstruction, intoxicated feeling, lacrimation abnormal, laryngitis, leg cramps, leukopenia, libido decreased, lymphadenopathy, macrocytic anemia, manic reaction, micturition frequency, muscle weakness, myocardial infarction, neuralgia, neuritis, neuropathy, neurosis, otitis externa, otitis media, pain, panic attack, paresis, personality disorder, phlebitis, photopsia, photosensitivity reaction, pneumonia, polyuria, pulmonary edema, pulmonary embolism, purpura, pyelonephritis, rectal hemorrhage, renal pain, restless legs, rigors, saliva altered, sciatica, SGOT increased, somnambulism, suicide attempt, syncope, tendinitis, tenesmus, tetany, thinking abnormal, thirst, tolerance increased, tooth caries, urinary retention, urticaria, varicose veins, ventricular tachycardia, weight decrease, yawning.

DRUG ABUSE AND DEPENDENCE

Controlled substance: Schedule IV.

Abuse and dependence: Studies of abuse potential in former drug abusers found that the effects of single doses of zolpidem tartrate 40 mg were similar, but not identical, to diazepam 20 mg, while zolpidem tartrate 10 mg was difficult to distinguish from placebo.

Sedative/hypnotics have produced withdrawal signs and symptoms following abrupt discontinuation. These reported symptoms range from mild dysphoria and insomnia to a withdrawal syndrome that may include abdominal and muscle cramps, vomiting, sweating, tremors, and convulsions. The U.S. clinical trial experience from zolpidem does not reveal any clear evidence for withdrawal syndrome. Nevertheless, the following adverse events included in DSM-III-R criteria for uncomplicated sedative/hypnotic withdrawal were reported at an incidence of ≤1% during U.S. clinical trials following placebo substitution occurring within 48 hours following last zolpidem treatment: fatigue, nausea, flushing, lightheadedness, uncontrolled crying, emesis, stomach cramps, panic attack, nervousness, and abdominal discomfort.

Individuals with a history of addiction to, or abuse of, drugs or alcohol are at risk of habituation and dependence; they should be under careful surveillance when receiving any hypnotic.

OVERDOSAGE

Signs and symptoms: In European postmarketing reports of overdose with zolpidem alone, impairment of consciousness has ranged from somnolence to light coma, with one case each of cardiovascular and respiratory compromise. Individuals have fully recovered from zolpidem tartrate overdoses up to 400 mg (40 times the maximum recommended dose). Overdose cases involving multiple CNS-depressant agents, including zolpidem, have resulted in more severe symptomatology, including fatal outcomes.

Recommended treatment: General symptomatic and supportive measures should be used along with immediate gastric lavage where appropriate. Intravenous fluids should be administered as needed. Flumazenil may be useful. Respiration, pulse, blood pressure, and other appropriate signs should be monitored and general supportive measures employed. Sedating drugs should be withheld following zolpidem overdosage. Zolpidem is not dialyzable.

The possibility of multiple drug ingestion should be considered.

Caution: Federal law prohibits dispensing without prescription.

5/27/93

Manufactured and distributed by
G.D. Searle & Co.
Chicago, IL 60680
by agreement with
Lorex Pharmaceuticals
Skokie, IL

Address medical inquiries to:
G.D. Searle & Co.
Medical & Scientific Information Department
4901 Searle Parkway
Skokie, IL 60077

SEARLE *Box 5110*
Chicago, IL 60680-5110

C93AB8570T

The Time Course of Nonchronic Major Depressive Disorder

Uniformity Across Episodes and Samples

William Coryell, MD; Hagop S. Akiskal, MD; Andrew C. Leon, PhD; George Winokur, MD; John D. Maser, MD; Timothy I. Mueller, MD; Martin B. Keller, MD; for the National Institute of Mental Health Collaborative Program on the Psychobiology of Depression—Clinical Studies

Background: Most natural history studies of affective disorders have emphasized the prediction of eventual recovery. Little is known of changes over time in the immediate probability of recovery.

Methods: To identify regularities in the timing of recovery from nonbipolar major depressive disorders, we considered only episodes that began during follow-up to increase the accuracy with which onsets were timed and to limit the study sample to individuals who had a demonstrably episodic course. Five participating centers conducted baseline assessments and followed probands (N=605) and nonclinical subjects (relatives, controls, and spouses, N=826) up for 6 years. During that time, 359 probands had at least one prospectively observed episode, and 181 had two episodes; corresponding numbers for the nonclinical subjects were 216 and 78, respectively. Our analyses considered the distribution of episode lengths across ascertainment source (probands vs nonclinical subjects), center, and episode number (first vs second prospectively observed episode).

Results: Distribution was remarkably uniform. Regardless of ascertainment source, center, or episode number, recovery occurred within 3 months in 40% of episodes, within 6 months in 60%, and within 1 year in 80%; 20% had more protracted courses.

Conclusions: Once triggered, the immediate likelihood of recovery changes over time in a predictable fashion. This has practical implications for the study of antidepressant efficacy and theoretical implications for factors involved in affective dysregulation.

(Arch Gen Psychiatry. 1994;51:405-410)

A THOROUGH knowledge of the natural history of an illness is critical to understanding its origins and to optimizing its management. Many follow-up studies of the affective disorders now exist in the literature, but most of these have based their conclusions on single follow-up assessments. Measures were consequently limited to the likelihood of recovery from the index episode and to the final outcome as reflected in symptoms and social adjustment measured at the end of follow-up. However, a fundamental attribute of affective disorders, episodicity, demands a closer look. How does the immediate likelihood of recovery or of recurrence change with time, and how regular or generalizable are these patterns? Many factors might influence episode and remission lengths. If reproducibility in the timing of remission and recurrence can be appreciated despite these highly variable influences, then these temporal patterns could be viewed as inherent and biologically fundamental aspects of the illness.

In 1978, the National Institute of Mental Health Collaborative Program on the Psychobiology of Depression—Clinical Studies (CDS) undertook to chart the course of the affective disorders with frequent follow-up assessments. The initial reports from this effort emphasized the course of the illness over the first 1 to 2 years, and later publications described the course of the first 5 years. Most of these publications described

From the Department of Psychiatry, University of Iowa College of Medicine, Iowa City (Drs Coryell and Winokur); the National Institute of Mental Health, Rockville, Md (Drs Akiskal and Maser); the Department of Psychiatry, New York (NY) Hospital, Cornell University Medical Center (Dr Leon); and the Department of Psychiatry, Butler Hospital, Providence, RI (Drs Mueller and Keller).

See Methods on next page

METHODS

Probands entered the study shortly after hospital admission or within 2 months of their first outpatient visit at one of the following five participating centers: Massachusetts General Hospital and Harvard University, Boston; Rush Presbyterian–St Luke's Medical Center, Chicago, Ill; University of Iowa College of Medicine, Iowa City; New York State Psychiatric Institute and Columbia University, New York; and Washington University School of Medicine, St Louis, Mo. Baseline assessments, detailed elsewhere,[9] included the full Schedule for Affective Disorders and Schizophrenia (SADS).[10] Baseline diagnoses were based on the Research Diagnostic Criteria[11] and reflected not only the structured patient interview but also the review of all available medical records and interviews with physicians. The following analysis will be limited to those probands who, at the baseline assessment, had a lifetime diagnosis of nonbipolar MDD; those with a history of mania, schizoaffective mania, or hypomania were excluded.

Follow-up evaluations took place at 6-month intervals over the ensuing 5 years and at yearly intervals thereafter. Raters structured their interviews with the Longitudinal Interval Follow-up Evaluation (LIFE)[12] and made ratings based both on the patient interviews and a review of medical records. According to LIFE conventions, the number and the severity of symptoms were rated on a six-point scale for each week of follow-up. To make this rating, the interviewer first identified change points, or times at which significant improvement or worsening took place. "Recovery" required at least 8 contiguous weeks during which symptoms were absent or limited to one or two of a mild degree; the beginning of recovery was the first of these weeks. "Recurrence" presumed recovery and required the reappearance of the full syndrome of MDD. Typically, subsyndromal symptoms appeared before the full syndrome and were initially scored as minor depressive disorder. The onset of the episode then was considered to begin at the first week in which symptoms satisfied criteria for definite minor depressive disorder, if these criteria were contiguous. A New Episode/New Condition Report (available on request) was used to further characterize new episodes.

The study protocol did not determine or influence treatment. Treatment was, however, carefully monitored and characterized on a weekly basis. The resulting data were subsequently converted to drug equivalencies and these, in turn, were condensed to one of three six-point scales meant to reflect the intensity of somatic therapy appropriate for MDD.[13]

Approximately two thirds of the probands participated in a family substudy in which raters, blind to proband diagnosis, used the SADS-Lifetime[10] (SADS-L) to interview all first-degree relatives 17 years of age or older.[14] The spouses of probands were similarly interviewed, as were controls matched to a subset of relatives through an acquaintance method.[14] These individuals were reassessed 6 years later and at that time underwent interviews with a SADS-L and an Interval SADS-L. The latter of these evaluations was an instrument modified to more fully characterize episodes that had occurred since the previous assessment. Previous reports have described the success of this follow-up and the rates of onset and recurrence within this sample.[15-17] As with probands, the following analyses will be limited to subjects who at baseline had a history of MDD but no history of mania, schizoaffective mania, or hypomania. Although some of these subjects sought treatment when they developed depressive episodes during follow-up, treatment seeking was not a requisite for inclusion, as it has been in most follow-up studies. For this reason, we refer to this group of relatives, controls, and spouses as the "nonclinical" sample.

These analyses used life-table methods[18] and a complement of the Kaplan-Meier product-limit estimator to provide a visual depiction of time to recovery.[19] These techniques describe all subjects over time to the event of interest, in this case recovery, or until they are lost to further follow-up (censored). In this way, the techniques minimize the effects of censored data by including all subjects who began the observation period regardless of whether they finished it. Further analyses used hazard functions to determine interval-specific probabilities of recovery, the likelihood that an individual who had not recovered by a given point would recover in the next time interval. All tests of significance were two-tailed.

the likelihood and the timing of recovery from the index episode and of recurrence into the next episode.

Patterns differed by clinical grouping. Nonbipolar[1] and secondary[2] subtypes were associated with lower likelihoods of recovery within limited follow-up periods, as were preexisting chronicity,[2,3] coexisting panic attacks,[4] obsessive-compulsive symptoms,[5] and high neuroticism scores.[6] Patients with bipolar illness,[1] secondary depression,[7] or more than three previous episodes[2] relapsed more quickly after index episodes had resolved. However, certain elements in the timing of recovery and recurrence held across these groups. The likelihood of recovery was greatest in the first 4 to 6 months of follow-up, whether observations began with study intake or with the beginning of a prospectively observed episode.[1] This likelihood decreased in the second 6 months and then fell further, such that recoveries accumulated at a relatively slow pace after 1 year.[1,2,8] Risks for recurrence also declined with time, but these changes were more gradual.[1]

The following analyses were undertaken to further explore these patterns and to determine whether nonbipolar major depressive disorder (MDD) has certain inherent and robust temporal characteristics. Are there aspects in the timing of episodes that are manifest regularly

Table 1. Probands and Nonclinical Subjects: Demographics and Previous Episodes of Major Depressive Disorder (MDD)

	Probands	Nonclinical Subjects
No. of subjects with at least one prospectively observed episode of MDD	359	216
Female, No. (%)	233 (64.9)	154 (71.3)
Mean (SD) age at intake, y	37.4 (14.5)	35.0 (12.1)
Marital status, No. (%)		
Single	123 (34.3)	53 (24.5)
Married	148 (41.2)	129 (59.7)
Divorced, separated, or widowed	88 (24.5)	34 (15.7)
Median No. of episodes of MDD before intake	2	1
Median length of longest episode of MDD before intake, wk	35	34.5

* χ^2=12.8; df=1; P =.0003 by the Kruskal-Wallis test.

across sequential episodes, sites, and both clinically and nonclinically based samples?

A study well suited to describe the robust temporal features of a recurrent illness should be of a length sufficient to allow for the prospective observation of two episodes from start to finish. This requirement is important in several respects. First, the episode present at the time of patient recruitment may be an atypical one because patients may seek treatment for only the more persistent of their episodes. Such episode biases are particularly powerful at the academic referral centers where most follow-up studies originate. Second, many of the index episodes may have begun 1 or more years before intake, and this will compromise recall accuracy. Third, the study of prospectively observed episodes limits a sample to subjects who indeed display a remitting course.

The prospective observation period must also be sufficient to encompass nearly all recoveries. Otherwise, episode lengths will be biased toward those short enough to be observed within a limited time frame. Finally, the sample must contain enough diversity to allow generalizability. Findings can be considered robust if they arise regularly across broad groupings.

The CDS is unique in meeting all of these specifics. Included in it are patients with major affective disorders recruited at tertiary care centers across five diverse sites and followed up at frequent intervals for 10 years. Also included are relatives, controls, and spouses, likewise recruited at five sites but followed up with a single reassessment 6 years after the baseline evaluation. Characteristic times to recovery and recurrence can thus be viewed across sites, episodes, and clinical and nonclinical sources of recruitment.

RESULTS

Of 605 probands and 826 nonclinical subjects who entered the study, 431 (71.2%) and 589 (71.3%), respectively, completed 6 years of follow-up. Thirty of the probands failed to recover from their index episode during that interval, and another 42 had no prospectively observed episodes. Among the nonclinical subjects, 29 were in episodes of MDD when first interviewed, and six of these failed to recover during the follow-up interval. Thus, of those who completed 6 years of follow-up and who recovered from any episode of MDD present at the first evaluation, 89.5% (359/401) of the probands and 37.0% (216/583) of the nonclinical subjects developed new episodes (χ^2=269.0; *df*=1; *P*<.0001).

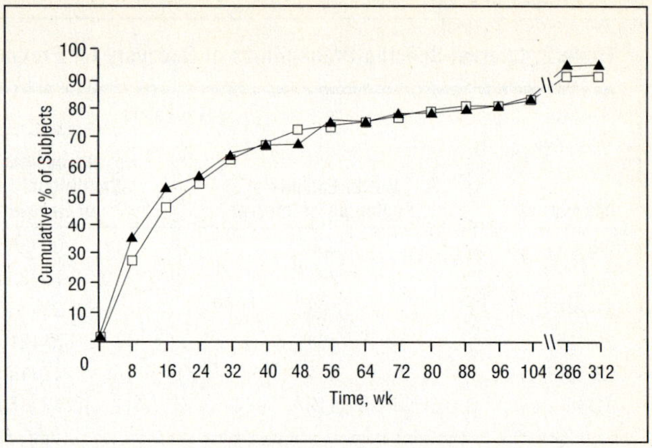

Figure 1. *Comparison of the time to recovery from the first prospectively observed episode of major depressive disorder in probands (squares) (N=359) and nonclinical subjects (triangles) (N=216).*

Proband times to recovery from the first prospectively observed episode of MDD were not significantly different across the five centers. Likewise, times to recovery among nonclinical subjects at the different centers were nearly identical, and differences did not approach statistical significance.

Despite large dissimilarities in the liability to develop new episodes of MDD (**Table 1**) between probands and nonclinical subjects, these groups showed very similar time courses once MDD developed (**Figure 1**). In particular, 55% of the probands and 57% of the nonclinical subjects had recovered by 6 months; 73% and 69%, respectively, by 1 year; 83% and 87%, respectively, by 2 years; and 97% of both groups by the end of follow-up. Within the nonclinical sample, the 164 relatives, 20 spouses, and 32 controls also showed very similar distributions and times to recovery. The likelihood of recovery at 6 months in these three groups was 62%, 55%, and 58%, respectively; at 1 year, 74%, 71%, and 73%, respectively, had recovered.

Interval-specific probabilities offer another clinically relevant view of the likelihood of recovery over time (**Table 2**). The odds that recovery would begin within 2 months of onset appeared to be at least one in four. Those subjects who had not recovered at the end of 8 weeks had a one-in-three chance of recovery during the next 2 months. However, the odds of recovery in any 2 of the next 8 months then dropped to one in five or six. Beyond this point, hazard functions became unstable due

Table 2. Interval-Specific Probabilities of Recovery for Probands and Nonclinical Subjects

	Probands		Nonclinical Subjects	
Interval, wk	No. in Episode at Beginning of Interval	No. Recovered in Interval (Conditional Probability of Recovery, %)	No. in Episode at Beginning of Interval	No. Recovered in Interval (Conditional Probability of Recovery, %)
0-8	359	83 (26.2)	216	57 (30.8)
9-16	274	79 (33.8)	154	47 (36.4)
17-24	193	28 (15.7)	104	13 (13.3)
25-32	163	31 (21.1)	91	13 (15.7)
33-40	131	17 (14.0)	75	8 (11.4)
41-48	112	17 (16.5)	65	4 (6.4)

to low event rates, but the overall resemblance between the probands and the nonclinical subjects persisted. The average likelihood of recovery in any 2-month period in the second year of observation for episodes that had lasted at least a year was 7.2% for the probands and 7.4% for the nonclinical subjects (one in 14).

Survival curves depicting recovery from the second prospectively observed episode were nearly identical to those for the first prospectively observed episode, both for the probands and for the nonclinical subjects. **Figure 2** illustrates this finding for the probands. **Table 3** shows that the distribution of episode durations for the first prospectively observed episodes closely resembled that for the second prospectively observed episodes. High intraindividual regularity across episodes did not account for this finding; the correlation of episode durations within individuals (first vs second prospectively observed episode) did not approach statistical significance (Pearson r=.08; P=.29).

Because probands were recruited at tertiary care centers, all received treatment for MDD at the time of intake. Ascertainment of prospectively observed episodes did not depend on treatment-seeking behavior; in fact, 114 (31.8%) of 359 probands received no somatic antidepressant therapy for the first prospectively observed episode. Those probands who sought and received such therapy had significantly longer times to recovery than did those who sought no therapy. Mean times to recovery were 50.9 weeks and 26.5 weeks for those who did and those who did not receive antidepressant therapy, respectively (Wilcoxon χ^2=18.5; df=1; P=.0001). The same pattern held for nonclinical subjects, of whom more than half (59.3% [128/216]) received no antidepressant therapy. The time until recovery for these individuals was significantly shorter than for nonclinical subjects who received somatic treatment (Wilcoxon χ^2=12.8; df=1; P=.0003).

To recapitulate, the distribution of episode lengths for prospectively observed recurrences did not differ significantly by the number of episodes (first or second) or by center, either among probands or among the nonclinical sample of controls, spouses, and relatives. Moreover, episode lengths did not differ across controls, spouses, and relatives, nor did perceptible differences emerge when probands were compared with members of the nonclinical sample. On the other hand, treatment seeking was associated with significantly longer episodes, both among the probands and in the nonclinical sample.

COMMENT

The immediate likelihood of recovery from episodes of MDD apparently declines in a highly regular fashion. Once triggered, episode duration seems to follow a time course with predictable qualities, at least among individuals whose illness follows a clearly episodic course. When the sampling of episodes is not dependent on treatment-seeking behavior, one fourth of all episodes end within 2 months and over 80% end within 1 year. Only 6% to 8% last 2 years or longer.

Earlier descriptions of this cohort found that certain depressive subtypes and phenomena predicted longer times to recovery. These subtypes and phenomena included the secondary diagnostic subtype,[2] panic attacks,[3] and obsessions or compulsions.[4] Does the similarity between the probands and the nonclinical subjects in episode duration necessarily imply an equal distribution of these characteristics?

In fact, these groups did differ modestly but not significantly by percent with secondary depression; 148 (41.2%) of 359 probands and 74 (34.2%) of 216 nonclinical subjects had a lifetime diagnosis of one or more nonaffective disorders at the beginning of follow-up (χ^2=2.8; df=1; P=.097). Apparently the effects of this disproportion were not sufficient to produce group differences in the time to recovery. The follow-up instruments for the nonclinical subjects did not allow us to determine the proportion of those with panic attacks or obsessions or compulsions in prospectively observed episodes. However, panic attacks have a relatively modest effect on episode length[3]; obsessions and compulsions seem more important prognostically but are relatively uncommon. Thus, any disproportion across samples probably had little impact on comparative lengths of episodes. The apparent importance of these factors may have also been lessened by our selective focus on patients who showed a clearly episodic

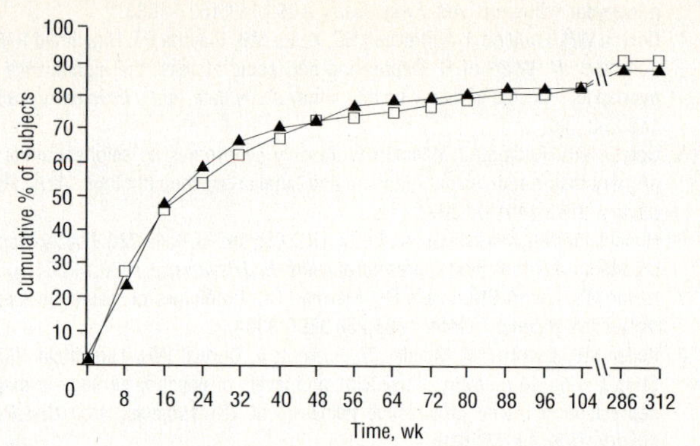

Figure 2. *Time to recovery from the first (squares) and second (triangles) prospectively observed episodes of major depressive disorder in probands.*

Table 3. Duration Distributions Among Probands Who Recovered From First and Second Prospectively Observed Episodes of Major Depressive Disorder

Duration of Episode	First Episode, No. (%) (N=314)	Second Episode, No. (%) (N=181)
<4 wk	25 (8.0)	16 (8.8)
4-7 wk	58 (18.5)	29 (16.0)
8-11 wk	42 (13.4)	30 (16.6)
12-23 wk	65 (20.7)	48 (26.5)
24-51 wk	69 (22.0)	31 (17.1)
52-103 wk	31 (9.9)	16 (8.8)
≥2 y	24 (7.6)	11 (6.1)

course. Patients for whom these prognostic factors were important were probably overrepresented among those eliminated from the analysis, because they were less likely to recover from the index episode.

Probands were more likely to seek treatment than were the nonclinical subjects, yet these two groups had very similar episode durations. Several factors may have acted together to lessen the impact of treatment differences. First, according to predictions based on numerous controlled trials, approximately one third of patients given antidepressants will fail to respond and another one third will show a placebo effect.[20] Thus, drug effects may have been evident in only 23% of probands (one third of the 69% who were treated) and 13% of the nonclinical subjects (one third of the 40.7% who were treated). Second, probands may have sought treatment more readily because of their earlier experiences in treatment and their established contact with mental health care providers. If so, the placebo response may have been more prevalent among probands than among nonclinical subjects, and this difference may have further narrowed any apparent group differences in course produced by the uneven proportions with treatment.

The relationships between the presence or absence of treatment and the episode durations seem counterintuitive at first glance. However, these findings simply highlight the fact that some time passes before individuals seek help for any problem. This time will vary markedly by individual and by problem, but, generally, difficulties that persist are more likely to result in treatment seeking than are those that do not. In the case of MDD, the more persistent episodes are likely to be overrepresented among treatment-seeking populations. Symptoms may then be relieved by treatment, but treatment cannot shorten a preexisting duration. Thus, the relationship between episode duration and treatment seeking may overshadow direct treatment effects on subsequent episode duration.

If, as the patterns described above strongly suggest, the immediate likelihood of recovery from depression falls rapidly, then those who present for treatment after, for instance, 4 months of symptoms may be much less likely to recover spontaneously in the next 4 weeks than would patients who had had symptoms for only 1 month. Thus, the placebo response may be more likely among patients who begin treatment shortly after the onset of symptoms. Indeed, those studies that have described both the duration of preexisting episodes and the likelihood of the placebo response have consistently indicated that this is so.[21-24] Because the placebo response may account for 30% to 50% of responders in antidepressant treatment trials,[22,25,26] this rapidly declining risk for spontaneous remission may account for the reported negative association between episode duration and treatment outcome.[27-29] As a further consequence, true medication effects (outcome differences between patients given active medication and patients given placebo) may be more robust among patients with episode durations exceeding 4 months at treatment onset. The few studies that have considered true medication effects as a function of episode duration have found larger medication effects among those patients whose episodes had been present longer at the outset of treatment.[21,23]

The relationship between the episode duration and the size of medication effect has important implications for the design of antidepressant trials and for clinical decisions. Trials of new antidepressants, whether they involve comparisons to standard medications or placebo, should be designed to reveal the maximum medication effect possible. Inclusion criteria that specify a minimum duration of 2 to 4 months might help to accomplish this. Likewise, clinicians might wish to include episode duration among the factors they consider in their decisions to initiate antidepressant treatment.

These data also have implications for the methods of follow-up studies. Probands were followed up at intervals of 6 months or 1 year, but the nonclinical subjects were assessed only at the 6-year follow-up. Despite this marked difference in ascertainment interval, the shapes of the survival curves for prospectively observed episodes were very similar in the two samples. Rice et al[30] showed that the recall of whether previous episodes occurred or not is quite unstable, particularly for episodes with fewer symptoms,

Study Participants

FROM THE NATIONAL INSTITUTE OF MENTAL HEALTH COLLABORATIVE PROGRAM ON THE PSYCHOBIOLOGY OF DEPRESSION—CLINICAL STUDIES

Investigators

M. B. Keller, MD, Boston / Providence, Mass (*Chairperson*); W. Coryell, MD, Iowa City (*Cochairperson*); J. D. Maser, PhD, H. S. Akiskal, MD, Washington, DC; P. W. Lavori, PhD, M. T. Shea, PhD, Boston / Providence; J. A. Fawcett, MD, W. A. Scheftner, MD, Chicago, Ill; J. Haley, Iowa City; J. Endicott, PhD, J. Loth, MSW, New York, NY; J. Rice, PhD, T. Reich, MD, St Louis, Mo.

Other Contributors

N. C. Andreasen, MD, PhD; P. J. Clayton, MD; J. Croughan, MD; G. L. Klerman, MD; R. M. A. Hirschfeld, MD; M. M. Katz, PhD; E. Robins, MD; R. W. Shapiro, MD; R. L. Spitzer, MD; G. Winokur, MD; M. Young, PhD.

shorter durations, and/or no treatment. The results described here, however, suggest that the duration and perhaps other aspects of those episodes that are recalled may be remembered with relative accuracy.

The apparent uniformity in the distribution of episode durations does not imply a common origin of the illness. Major depressive disorder is widely assumed to have various origins, and these findings do not challenge that assumption. However, once this syndrome is triggered, for whatever reason, certain predictions regarding its likely duration seem feasible. While the high interindividual variability of psychosocial contexts implies that triggering factors are highly variable, the determinants of episode persistence may be more biologically determined. If so, the inherent propensity to recovery (the likelihood of recovery in the immediate future) dissipates rapidly and in a temporally regular fashion. Investigations into the nature of this propensity should emphasize correlations between episode duration and biological measures believed to underlie periodicity and affective dysregulation.

Accepted for publication January 6, 1994.

Reprint requests to Department of Psychiatry, University of Iowa College of Medicine, 1-457 Medical Education Bldg, Iowa City, IA 52242 (Dr Coryell).

REFERENCES

1. Coryell WH, Keller MB, Endicott J, Andreasen NC, Clayton PJ, Hirschfeld RMA. Bipolar II illness: course and outcome over a five-year period. *Psychol Med.* 1989;19:129-141.
2. Keller MB, Klerman GL, Lavori PW, Coryell WH, Endicott J, Taylor J. Long-term outcome of episodes of major depression. *JAMA.* 1984;252:788-792.
3. Coryell WH, Endicott J, Keller MB. Chronic affective disorder: outcome during a five-year follow-up. *Am J Psychiatry.* 1990;147:1627-1633.
4. Coryell WH, Endicott J, Andreasen NC, Keller MB, Clayton PJ, Hirschfeld RMA, Scheftner W, Winokur G. Depression and panic attacks: the significance of overlap as reflected in follow-up and family study data. *Am J Psychiatry.* 1988; 145:293-300.
5. Coryell WH, Endicott J, Winokur G. Anxiety syndromes as epiphenomena of primary major depression: outcome and familial psychopathology. *Am J Psychiatry.* 1992;149:100-107.
6. Hirschfeld RMA, Klerman GL, Andreasen NC, Clayton PJ, Keller MB. Psycho-social predictors of chronicity in depressed patients. *Br J Psychiatry.* 1986;148:648-654.
7. Keller MB, Lavori PW, Lewis CE, Klerman GL. Predictors of relapse in major depressive disoder. *JAMA.* 1983;250:3299-3304.
8. Keller MB, Lavori PW, Mueller TI, Endicott J, Coryell WH, Hirschfeld RMA, Shea T. Time to recovery, chronicity, and levels of psychopathology in major depression: a 5-year prospective follow-up of 431 subjects. *Arch Gen Psychiatry.* 1992;49:809-816.
9. Andreasen NC, Grove WM, Endicott J, Coryell WH, Scheftner WA, Hirschfeld RMA, Keller MB. The phenomenology of depression. *Psychiatry Psychobiol.* 1988;3:1-10.
10. Endicott J, Spitzer RL. A diagnostic interview: the Schedule for Affective Disorders and Schizophrenia. *Arch Gen Psychiatry.* 1978;35:837-844.
11. Spitzer RL, Endicott J, Robins E. *Research Diagnostic Criteria.* 3rd ed. New York, NY: Biometrics Research, New York State Dept of Mental Hygiene; 1978.
12. Keller MB, Lavori PW, Friedman B, Neilsen E, Endicott J, McDonald-Scott P, Andreasen NC. The Longitudinal Interval Follow-up Evaluation. *Arch Gen Psychiatry.* 1987;44:540-548.
13. Keller MB, Lavori PW, Klerman GL, Andreasen NC, Endicott J, Coryell WH, Fawcett J, Hirschfeld RMA. Low levels and lack of predictors of somatotherapy and psychotherapy received by depressed patients. *Arch Gen Psychiatry.* 1986; 43:458-466.
14. Andreasen NC, Rice J, Endicott J, Coryell WH, Grove WM, Reich T. Familial rates of affective disorders. *Arch Gen Psychiatry.* 1987;44:461-469.
15. Coryell WH, Endicott J, Andreasen NC, Keller MB. A comparison of bipolar I, bipolar II and nonbipolar major depression among the relatives of affectively ill probands. *Am J Psychiatry.* 1985;142:817-821.
16. Coryell WH, Endicott J, Keller MB. Major depression in a nonclinical sample: demographic and clinical risk factors for first onset. *Arch Gen Psychiatry.* 1992; 49:117-125.
17. Coryell WH, Endicott J, Keller MB. Predictors of relapse into major depressive disorder in a nonclinical population. *Am J Psychiatry.* 1991;148:1353-1358.
18. Kalbfleisch JD, Prentice RL. *The Statistical Analysis of Failure Time Data.* New York, NY: John Wiley & Sons Inc; 1980:12-15.
19. Kaplan EL, Maier P. Nonparametric estimation from incomplete observations. *J Am Stat Assoc.* 1958;53:457-481.
20. Baldessarini RJ. *Chemotherapy in Psychiatry.* Cambridge, Mass: Harvard University Press; 1985:162.
21. Downing RW, Rickels K. Predictors of response to amitriptyline and placebo in three outpatient treatment settings. *J Nerv Ment Dis.* 1973;156:109-129.
22. Fairchild CJ, Rush AJ, Vasavada N, Giles DE, Khatami M. Which depressions respond to placebo? *Psychiatry Res.* 1986;18:217-226.
23. Kahn A, Dager SR, Cohen S, Avery DM, Scherzo B, Dunner DL. Chronicity of depressive episode in relation to antidepressant-placebo response. *Neuropsychopharmacology.* 1991;4:125-130.
24. Brown WA, Johnson MF, Chen MG. Clinical features of depressed patients who do and do not improve with placebo. *Psychiatry Res.* 1992;41:203-214.
25. Medical Research Council Psychiatry Committee. Clinical trial of the treatment of depressive illness. *BMJ.* 1965;1:881-886.
26. Brown W, Doranseif B, Wernicke J. Placebo response in depression: a search for predictors. *Psychiatry Res.* 1988;26:259-264.
27. Moller H, Fischer G, Von Zerssen D. Prediction of therapeutic response in acute treatment with antidepressants. *Eur Arch Psychiatry Neurol Sci.* 1987;236: 349-357.
28. Black DW, Goldstein RB, Nasrallah A, Winokur G. The prediction of recovery using a multivariate model in 1471 depressed inpatients. *Eur Arch Psychiatry Clin Neurosci.* 1991;241:41-45.
29. Coryell WH, Zimmerman M. Outcome following ECT for primary unipolar depression: a test of newly proposed response predictors. *Am J Psychiatry.* 1984; 141:862-867.
30. Rice JP, Rochberg N, Endicott J, Lavori PW, Miller C. Stability of psychiatric diagnoses: an application to the affective disorders. *Arch Gen Psychiatry.* 1992; 49:824-830.

ORIGINAL ARTICLE

Sympathetic Nervous System Activity in Major Depression

Basal and Desipramine-Induced Alterations in Plasma Norepinephrine Kinetics

Richard C. Veith, MD; Nancy Lewis, RN; Oscar A. Linares, MD; Robert F. Barnes, MD; Murray A. Raskind, MD; Enrique C. Villacres, MD; M. Michele Murburg, MD; E. Alexandra Ashleigh, MD; Sonia Castillo, PhD; Elaine R. Peskind, MD; Marcella Pascualy, MD; Jeffrey B. Halter, MD

Background: To determine whether elevations of plasma norepinephrine (NE) in major depression represent increased sympathetic nervous system (SNS) activity and to assess the effects of desipramine hydrochloride on sympathetic function.

Methods: SNS activity was assessed in depressed patients and controls by an isotope-dilution, plasma NE kinetic technique using mathematical modeling and compartmental analysis. This approach provided estimates of the rate of NE appearance into an extravascular compartment, which is the site of endogenous NE release from SNS nerves, the corresponding rate of NE appearance into plasma, and the rate of NE clearance from plasma.

Results: Norepinephrine appearance into the extravascular and vascular compartments was significantly elevated in 17 depressed patients compared with that in 36 controls. The rate of NE clearance from plasma was similar in both groups. This is compatible with increased SNS activity in major depression. Desipramine, given for 2 days, significantly reduced the concentration of NE in plasma of patients and controls by markedly suppressing the rates of extravascular and vascular NE appearance, compatible with a short-term reduction in SNS activity. Desipramine prolonged the rate of NE clearance from plasma, consistent with a blockade of NE re-uptake into SNS nerve terminals. The initial suppression of SNS activity by desipramine was reversed by long-term (28 days) treatment of patients, with extravascular and vascular NE appearance rates returning to approximately basal levels. An associated rise in plasma NE concentrations compared with the baseline was attributable to a progressive reduction in plasma NE clearance.

Conclusion: Sympathetic nervous system activity is elevated in major depression and is suppressed by short-term desipramine administration. The demonstration of SNS reactivation occurring with prolonged desipramine treatment is compatible with the theory that long-term treatment desensitizes CNS α_2-adrenergic receptors and emphasizes the value of examining the temporal course of responses to pharmacological challenges of neuroendocrine systems. Previously reported elevations of plasma NE during prolonged administration of tricyclic antidepressants are probably the result of a reduction in plasma NE clearance, not an increase in SNS activity.

(Arch Gen Psychiatry. 1994;51:411-422)

From the Geriatric Research, Education, and Clinical Center (GRECC) (Drs Veith, Raskind, and Castillo and Ms Lewis) and Psychiatry Service (Drs Barnes, Villacres, Murburg, Ashleigh, Peskind, and Pascualy), Seattle (Wash) VAMC; the Department of Psychiatry and Behavioral Sciences, University of Washington, Seattle (Drs Veith, Raskind, Barnes, Villacres, Murburg, Ashleigh, Peskind, and Pascualy); GRECC, Ann Arbor (Mich) VAMC (Drs Linares and Halter); and the Division of Geriatric Medicine, Department of Internal Medicine, University of Michigan, Ann Arbor (Drs Linares and Halter).

WE[1,2] AND others[3-11] have previously reported that plasma norepinephrine (NE) concentrations are increased in some patients with major depression and, moreover, that prolonged tricyclic antidepressant (TCA) treatment elevates plasma NE concentrations.[12-15] Most investigators attribute the baseline increase to central nervous system (CNS) mechanisms and ascribe the drug response to a combination of effects on clearance and release of NE peripherally. Direct data in depressed patients are, however, limited.

Because the concentration of plasma NE generally parallels the level of activity of the sympathetic nervous system (SNS),[16,17] the elevation of plasma NE in depressed patients suggests that SNS activity is increased in major depression. However, the interpretation of plasma NE concentrations is complex.[16-22] The total concentration of NE in plasma is deter-

See Methods on next page

METHODS

STUDY SUBJECTS

The following protocols were approved by the Human Subjects Review Committee of the University of Washington, Seattle.

Baseline Plasma NE Kinetic Study

Informed consent was obtained from 36 healthy volunteers (25 men, 11 women; mean [±SEM] age, 40±3 years) and 17 depressed patients (12 men, five women; mean age, 56±4 years) who participated in plasma NE kinetic studies. All of the depressed patients met *DSM-III* criteria for major depression, and eight met criteria for melancholia.[29] One patient was bipolar, and the remainder had unipolar depression; three were inpatients, and 14 were outpatients. The minimum criterion for entry into the study was a score of 18 or greater on the 17-item Hamilton Depression Rating Scale.[30] None had other Axis I *DSM-III* diagnoses or a history of active alcohol or drug abuse. All patients had discontinued psychotropic medications with the occasional exception of as-needed chloral hydrate use for at least 3 weeks before study, and none had received hypnotic medication for 48 hours before study participation. Four of the depressed patients were considered dexamethasone nonsuppressors, as defined by a plasma cortisol value of 138 nmol/L (5.0 μg/dL) or greater at 8 AM or 4 PM on the day following an 11 PM, 1.0-mg oral dexamethasone dose.

The 36 control subjects were free of psychiatric disorders or substance abuse. Patients and controls were normotensive, were within 125% of ideal body weight (1959 Metropolitan Life Tables), and were free of significant medical disease thought to influence SNS function; none were taking medications that might influence the SNS.

Effect of Short- and Long-term Desipramine Administration on Plasma NE Kinetics

Following completion of baseline studies of plasma NE kinetics, 23 of the normal control subjects and 16 of the depressed patients repeated the ^{3}H-NE kinetic study following desipramine or placebo administration (see below). Data from five of the control subjects were excluded from the analysis because technical problems interfered with blood sampling for the kinetic analysis. Of the remaining controls, 13 subjects (seven men, six women; mean age, 31±4 years) received desipramine, and five subjects (two men, three women; mean age, 30±13 years) received placebo.

STUDY PROTOCOLS

Studies were performed in the Special Studies Unit of the Seattle (Wash) Veterans Affairs Medical Center. Study subjects were admitted at 8 AM following a 12-hour fast, and two intravenous lines were placed—one in an antecubital vein for infusion of a tracer and one in a dorsal hand vein for blood sampling. All blood samples during these studies were taken from indwelling lines that were placed at least 30 minutes before blood sampling. Plasma samples were obtained from arterialized blood, which provides a more accurate assessment of systemic NE activity than does antecubital venous blood.[19,31,32] Arterialized samples are obtained by drawing blood from a dorsal hand vein after warming the hand in a warming box. Under these conditions, the NE samples obtained in "arterialized" venous blood closely approximate NE samples obtained from the radial artery,[19] which is a much more invasive method to obtain systemic arterial samples. This approach has been used for studying the kinetics of a variety of substrates and hormones.[19,33,34] Studies were performed with subjects in a supine position. Heart rate and blood pressure measurements were obtained by using automated methods (DinaMap, Critikon Co, Tampa, Fla). Mean arterial pressure (MAP) was calculated with the formula: MAP=Diastolic Blood Pressure+(1/3 [Systolic−Diastolic] Pressure). During the 12-hour period before the studies, subjects were prohibited from using known stimuli of catecholamine release, including nicotine, caffeine, and marijuana.[3]

^{3}H-NE Plasma NE Infusions

The ^{3}H-NE tracer was infused via an indwelling intravenous catheter that was placed in an antecubital vein. Arterialized plasma samples were obtained from a 19-gauge scalp vein needle that was placed retrograde in a dorsal vein of the hand, which was placed in a heated box (60°C). After a 30-minute stabilization period, baseline samples were obtained for plasma NE and epinephrine, and blood pressure and heart rate were measured. Subjects were administered a 15-μCi/m^2 bolus of ^{3}H-NE (specific activity, 40 to 60 Ci/mmol, New England Nuclear, Boston, Mass), followed immediately by a constant intravenous infusion of ^{3}H-NE at the rate of 0.35 μCi/m^2 per minute for 30 minutes by using a syringe pump (Harvard Apparatus, S Natick, Mass) to allow distribution of the tracer. Three sets of arterialized blood samples (10 mL) were then obtained at 5-minute intervals for determination of steady-state ^{3}H-NE and NE concentrations, and the reported values are the mean of these measurements. The ^{3}H-NE infusion was then stopped, and blood samples were collected at 1, 2, 4, 6, 8, 10, 15, and 20 minutes after stopping the ^{3}H-NE infusion.

Desipramine Administration

After completion of the baseline studies, 16 depressed patients repeated the plasma NE kinetic study following the administration of desipramine hydrochloride, 50 mg orally at bedtime for 2 nights (short-term desipramine treatment). Thereafter, desipramine treatment was continued for 28 days (long-term desipramine treatment) with individual dosing increments adjusted according to clinical re-

sponse (day 28 mean daily dose, 120±12 mg). After 28 days of treatment, the NE kinetic study was repeated as described above. Sixteen patients completed both the short- and long-term desipramine studies, but three patients were excluded from the day 28 analysis because technical problems interfered with blood sampling for the kinetic analysis.

Thirteen control subjects participated in baseline and short-term desipramine studies as described above for the depressed patients with the exception that desipramine or placebo was administered single-blind and that the order of the basal and postdesipramine studies was randomized, with at least 7 days separating the two studies. In addition, four of the control subjects were randomly assigned to receive desipramine hydrochloride, 100 mg orally at bedtime instead of 50 mg. Because there was no difference in their responses, these subjects were combined with the controls who received 50 mg for this analysis. Five additional control subjects were randomly assigned, single-blind to receive placebo for 2 days instead of desipramine. Long-term desipramine studies were not performed in the control subjects.

ANALYTICAL METHODS

Blood samples for measurement of plasma catecholamines and plasma ^{3}H-NE were collected in prechilled glass tubes containing ethyleneglycol-bis-β aminoethyl ether N,N′-tetraacetic acid (EGTA) and reduced glutathione and placed on ice. Samples were centrifuged promptly at 4°C and stored at −70°C until assay. In each sample, catecholamines were measured in duplicate by a single isotope enzymatic assay.[35] All plasma samples from an individual subject were run in the same assay. The intra-assay coefficient of variation is 6%. The ^{3}H-NE concentrations were determined by liquid scintillation counting of radiolabeled catecholamines after alumina extraction as previously described.[19,36,37] The tracer doses of ^{3}H-NE that were used did not contribute significantly to the circulating NE levels. The ^{3}H-NE infusion rate (equal to 0.01 nmol/min of NE) was 50 times smaller than an NE infusion rate that was previously shown to have no measurable effects on heart rate, blood pressure, or metabolic parameters.[38] It has previously been shown that the high specific activity triple-labeled ring ^{3}H-NE that was used in this study did not produce a significant in vivo isotope effect on the NE kinetic parameters estimated from compartmental analysis.[21] For both groups, the plasma NE and ^{3}H-NE concentrations during the ^{3}H-NE infusion were constant over the time of the experiments, which is compatible with the assumption that the NE system and ^{3}H-NE infusion were at steady state.

An important requirement for the use of tracer ^{3}H-NE in the measurement of plasma NE kinetics is the assumption that the plasma radioactivity recovered after alumina extraction is in the form of ^{3}H-NE and does not contain any labeled metabolic products of catecholamines that would falsely increase the apparent concentration of labeled NE. We have previously shown that the amount of radioactivity recovered as alumina-extractable NE metabolites during an ^{3}H-NE infusion is negligible.[37]

DATA ANALYSIS

A physiologically based, two-compartment differential equation model was the minimal model necessary to fit all the data for each subject. The development of this model has been described elsewhere.[18] In this minimal model, the vascular compartment (plasma-containing compartment) includes circulating NE and is accessible for sampling (**Figure 1**). The extravascular compartment is a lumped compartment that includes body tissues that locally release, take up, metabolize, and "spill" NE into the circulation (eg, SNS neurons, heart). The NE mass in the extravascular compartment most likely represents NE anywhere in the vicinity of, and/or at a distance from, the neuroeffector junctions of SNS nerve synapses but does not include NE contained within SNS nerve terminals.[18]

The unknown compartmental parameters estimated by this model that are of primary interest in this report include the steady-state rate of NE appearance into the extravascular compartment (nanomoles per square meter per minute), the rate of NE spillover from the extravascular to the vascular compartment (plasma NE appearance rate, nanomoles per square meter per minute), the rate of NE clearance from the vascular compartment (liters per minute per square meter), and the NE mass in the extravascular compartment (nanomoles per square meter).

These parameters were estimated by solving simultaneously a series of differential equations that corresponded to the known physiology of plasma NE kinetics and that fit all of the basal and postdesipramine ^{3}H-NE and NE data. For example, the rate of NE appearance into the extravascular compartment represents the net sum of sources of NE input into that compartment (ie, release of NE from SNS nerves and transfer of NE back into the extravascular compartment from the vascular compartment) *minus* the sources of NE removal from the extravascular compartment (ie, NE neuronal uptake [uptake$_1$], nonneuronal uptake [uptake$_2$], and spillover into the vascular compartment). Because under steady-state conditions the rate of spillover of NE into the vascular compartment (extravascular NE mass × the transfer coefficient) must equal the rate of NE returning to the extravascular compartment from the vascular compartment (vascular NE mass × the transfer coefficient), these values cancel each other out. Thus, the equation defining the rate of NE appearance into the extravascular compartment at steady state is as follows: $NE_2=Q_2L_{02}+Q_2L_{12}-Q_1L_{21}$; since $Q_2L_{12}=Q_1L_{21}$; then, $NE_2=Q_2L_{02}$, where NE_2 is the rate of NE appearance into the extravascular compartment; Q_2 and Q_1 represent the mass of NE in the extravascular (2) and vascular (1) compartments, respectively; and L represents the NE transfer coefficients that regulate transport of NE from the extravascular to the vascular compartment (L_{12}), the vascular

Continued on next page

to the extravascular compartment (L_{21}), or irreversible removal from the extravascular compartment by neuronal and nonneuronal uptake (L_{02}). Compartmental analysis was performed on a computer (VAX 11/730, Digital Equipment Corp, Maynard, Mass) by using the SAAM[39] and CONSAM[40] simulators. All of the model parameter values for each subject were derived by using the method of weighted nonlinear least squares.[39]

STATISTICAL ANALYSIS

Values are presented as mean±SEM. Statistical analyses were performed by using a data analysis system (PC!Info, Retriever Data Systems, Seattle, Wash). Assessment of baseline differences between the depressed patients and controls was performed by using analysis of covariance, with age as the covariate. The assessment of the short-term effects of desipramine on NE kinetic and cardiovascular measures in the patients and controls was performed by using two-way analysis of variance with repeated measures. The analysis of the effect of placebo was performed by using paired *t* tests.

The study components investigating the effects of long-term desipramine treatment on plasma NE kinetics in depressed patients were designed to test the hypothesis that desipramine would acutely suppress SNS activity and that prolonged treatment would be associated with a return of some parameters toward basal levels. Because these interval changes were the subject of specific hypotheses, it was determined a priori that planned comparisons among basal and short- and long-term studies would be performed by using paired *t* tests.[41] To minimize the potential α error due to multiple comparisons, the Bonferroni correction was used, and the minimum criterion for statistical significance was considered $P=.025$ for the comparisons of the day 28 findings with baseline and with short-term desipramine findings. For other analyses, the minimum criterion was $P=.05$. Analyses performed on parameters for which directional hypotheses were assumed a priori, ie, NE, plasma NE appearance rate, extravascular NE appearance rate, NE clearance rate, and heart rate, were performed by using one-tailed tests. Correlations between cardiovascular and NE kinetic measures were performed by linear regression.

mined not only by the rate of NE release from SNS nerves, but also by its synaptic re-uptake, local metabolic degradation, and redistribution into more than one physiological space.[18] It is possible, for instance, that a reduction in the rate of removal of NE from plasma, not an increase in its release, accounts for plasma NE elevations among depressed patients. Our first goal was to determine whether elevations of plasma NE in depressed patients represent increased SNS activity or a reduction in the clearance of NE from plasma.

The observation that prolonged TCA treatment increases plasma NE is also open to several interpretations. This finding could indicate that TCAs act to stimulate SNS activity, possibly through influencing CNS regulatory mechanisms or, alternatively, by acting peripherally at the SNS nerve terminals to enhance NE release. However, TCAs block re-uptake of NE at postganglionic SNS nerve terminals. This effect alone should increase plasma NE because synaptic re-uptake is the major route of removal of NE from plasma. To interpret accurately the physiological effects of TCAs on the peripheral NE system, our second objective was to examine the effects of desipramine hydrochloride on plasma NE by using methods that allow discrimination of the rates of appearance of NE following release from postganglionic SNS nerves from changes in plasma NE clearance.

Extensive preclinical research investigating the effects of antidepressants on neuronal, neurotransmitter, and receptor function indicates that responses to short-term administration often differ from those of long-term exposure.[23-27] The adaptive responses of *prolonged* TCA administration on CNS receptor systems correspond temporally to the onset of the therapeutic effects of these drugs and are, accordingly, those most likely to yield insights into the mechanisms responsible for their clinical efficacy.[23-27] Thus, the third goal of this study was to compare the effects of short-term (2 days) and prolonged (28 days) administration of desipramine on plasma NE kinetics in humans and to determine whether responses to treatment *change* over time.

In this study, we employed a tritiated (^3H)–NE isotope dilution technique for measuring plasma NE kinetics and mathematical modeling of the kinetic data with compartmental analysis.[18] Compartmental analysis is now commonly used in studies of metabolic and endocrine processes to estimate physiological parameters that cannot be assayed directly.[18,20,21,28] Application of this methodology to the NE system has resulted in the demonstration that a two-compartment kinetic model closely approximates the kinetics of NE metabolism in plasma.[18,20,21] This model (Figure 1) includes a vascular compartment (the circulating blood pool where NE is sampled) and an extravascular compartment (into which NE is released from SNS nerves). This methodology provides estimates of such parameters as the rate of appearance of NE into the extravascular compartment following release from postganglionic SNS nerves, the rate of NE appearance or spillover into plasma, and the rate of NE clearance from plasma. Each of these factors is an important determinant of the overall concentration of NE in plasma and a potential source of information regarding SNS activity in depression and the effects of TCAs on peripheral NE metabolism.

RESULTS

BASELINE NE KINETIC INFUSION STUDY

Baseline NE Kinetics—Patients vs Controls

Plasma NE kinetic studies were performed in 17 depressed patients and 36 normal volunteers. The depressed patients were significantly older than the control subjects (56±4 vs 40±3 years, *P*=.003). Because plasma NE and SNS activity are increased in older individuals,[21,36] baseline comparisons between the depressed and control groups were performed by controlling for age effects, by using analysis of covariance. Baseline plasma NE kinetic parameters for the two groups are summarized in **Table 1**.

Plasma Catecholamines, Blood Pressure, and Heart Rate

The mean plasma NE concentration was higher in the depressed patients, but the difference from control values was not statistically significant when controlled for age. Plasma epinephrine levels were similar in the two groups (depressed patients, 0.31±0.04 nmol/L vs controls, 0.30±0.03 nmol/L; *P*=not significant [NS]). There was an NS trend for higher mean arterial blood pressure in the patients (depressed patients, 89±2 mm Hg vs controls, 85±2 mm Hg; *P*=NS). The mean heart rate was greater in the patients (depressed patients, 66±2 beats per minute vs controls, 59±1 beats per minute; *P*=.003).

NE Extravascular Appearance, Plasma Appearance, and Plasma Clearance Rates

The estimated steady-state extravascular NE appearance rate in the depressed patients was 29% higher than that in controls (*P*=.04). There was also a 32% increase in the rate of NE appearance into plasma in the depressed patients (*P*=.03). The plasma NE clearance rate was similar in the two groups. The total NE mass in the extravascular compartment was increased in the depressed patients, but the difference between groups was not statistically significant (600±111 vs 411±59 nmol/m^2, *P*=NS).

NE Kinetics in Melancholic vs Nonmelancholic Patients

Patients who fulfilled *DSM-III* criteria for melancholia (n=8) were significantly older than patients without melancholia (n=9) (65±4 vs 47±5 years, *P*=.01). Patients with melancholia tended to have higher mean plasma NE concentrations (melancholic, 2.04±0.29 nmol/L vs nonmelancholic, 1.39±0.18 nmol/L; *P*=NS), rates of extravascular NE appearance (melancholic, 12.47±1.42 nmol/min per square meter vs nonmelancholic, 10.10±1.85 nmol/min per square meter; *P*=NS), plasma NE appearance rates (melancholic, 2.76±0.40 nmol/min per square meter vs nonmelancholic, 1.97±0.24 nmol/min per square meter; *P*=NS), and MAP (melancholic, 93±3 mm Hg vs nonmelancholic, 85±3 mm Hg; *P*=NS) compared with that in nonmelancholic patients (n=9), but these differences were not statistically significant when controlled for age. The mean plasma NE clearance rate was similar in the melancholic and nonmelancholic patients (melancholic, 1.09±0.02 L/min per square meter vs nonmelancholic, 1.25±0.22 L/min per square meter; *P*=NS). There was no significant difference in heart rate in the two groups (68±2 vs 64±2 beats per minute, *P*=NS).

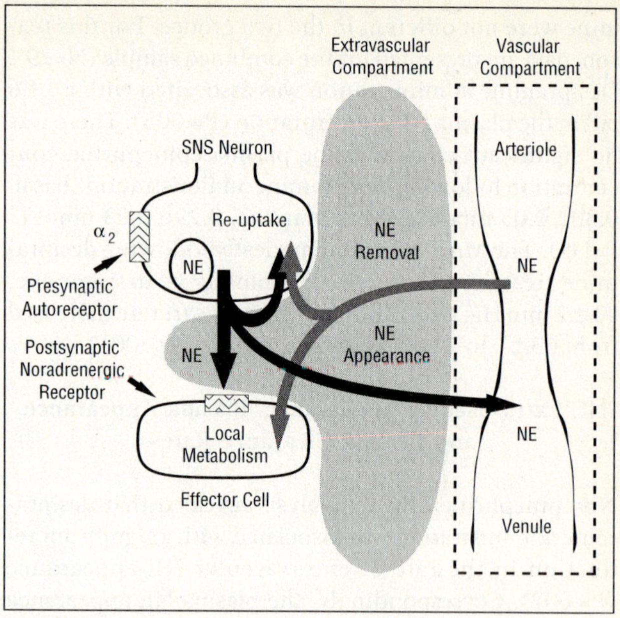

Figure 1. *Schematic presentation of the plasma norepinephrine (NE) kinetic two-compartment model. NE released from postganglionic sympathetic nervous system (SNS) nerves activates presynaptic and postsynaptic receptors, is inactivated by neuronal re-uptake mechanisms and storage or by extraneuronal metabolism, and spills over into the circulation. The concentration of NE in the circulation is determined by the rates of appearance of NE into plasma and clearance from plasma. The "extravascular compartment" is a lumped compartment that includes body tissues that locally release, take up, metabolize, and "spill" NE into the circulation (eg, SNS neurons, heart). Norepinephrine in the extravascular compartment most likely represents NE anywhere in the vicinity of neuroeffector junctions of SNS nerve synapses but does not represent NE within SNS nerve endings themselves. The "vascular compartment" represents plasma and some part of the extracellular space.*

SHORT-TERM DESIPRAMINE STUDY

Plasma Catecholamines, Blood Pressure, and Heart Rate

The effects of 2 days of desipramine or placebo administration on arterialized plasma NE kinetics in patients and normal controls are described in **Table 2**. Two-way analysis of variance with repeated measures revealed no statistically significant group × time effects among the variables tested, indicating that the effects of desipra-

mine were not different in the two groups. For this reason, data are presented for the combined sample (N=29). Desipramine administration was associated with a 14% fall in the plasma NE concentration (*P*=.005). There was no significant change in the plasma epinephrine concentration following desipramine administration (basal, 0.30±0.03 nmol/L vs desipramine, 0.29±0.03 nmol/L; *P*=NS). The MAP increased modestly following desipramine treatment (basal, 86±2 mm Hg vs desipramine, 91±2 mm Hg; *P*<.001). The resting heart rate increased from 63±1 to 71±2 beats per minute (*P*<.001).

NE Extravascular Appearance, Plasma Appearance, and Plasma Clearance Rates

Norepinephrine kinetic analysis revealed that desipramine administration was associated with a significant reduction in the rate of extravascular NE appearance (*P*=.002). Correspondingly, the plasma NE appearance rate was significantly reduced (*P*=.001). Desipramine administration was associated with a fall in plasma NE clearance (*P*=.001). The NE mass in the extravascular compartment was significantly reduced (488±72 vs 251±56 nmol/m², *P*<.006).

Placebo Control Group

Five control subjects were randomly assigned to placebo administration as an additional control for the effects of time on the variables of interest (the sequence of the baseline and postdesipramine study days was also randomized in all control subjects). The absence of an effect of placebo on the parameters of interest is demonstrated in Table 2.

LONG-TERM DESIPRAMINE STUDY

The effects of 2 days' and 28 days' desipramine administration on arterialized plasma NE kinetics among the depressed patients are summarized in **Table 3**. As noted above, analysis of the effects of long-term desipramine administration and comparisons with basal and short-term desipramine findings were performed by using paired *t* tests and the Bonferroni correction (*P*≤.025 was required for statistical significance for these analyses).

Plasma Catecholamines, Blood Pressure, and Heart Rate

Following long-term (28 days) desipramine treatment, the plasma NE value rose above baseline (*P*=.035). Although the difference from baseline was of borderline statistical significance, the change from the short-term desipramine (2 days) value was highly significant (*P*=.003). The mean plasma epinephrine concentration following long-term desipramine treatment was higher than basal, but neither this difference nor the change from the short-term desipramine condition was statistically significant (basal, 0.31±0.04 nmol/L vs short-term desipramine, 0.32±0.04 nmol/L, *P*=NS; vs long-term desipramine, 0.40±0.08 nmol/L, *P*=NS). The increase in MAP noted in the depressed patients and controls following short-term desipramine treatment persisted in the depressed patients following long-term desipramine treatment (basal, 89±3 mm Hg vs long-term desipramine, 95±2 mm Hg; *P*=.04). The mean heart rate increased further to 78±2 beats per minute following long-term desipramine treatment (*P*=.001 vs basal; *P*=.001 vs short-term desipramine treatment).

Table 1. Baseline Plasma NE Kinetics in Depressed Patients and Controls*

	Depressed Patients (n=17)	Controls (n=36)	*P*†
Plasma NE, nmol/L	1.70±0.18	1.22±0.10	>.1
Extravascular NE appearance, nmol/min per square meter	11.22±1.19	7.97±0.70	.04
Plasma NE appearance, nmol/min per square meter	2.35±0.24	1.58±0.12	.03
Plasma NE clearance, L/min per square meter	1.17±0.11	1.09±0.04	>.1

*All values are given as mean±SEM, except for P values. NE indicates norepinephrine.
†Analysis of covariance.

NE Extravascular Appearance, Plasma Appearance, and Plasma Clearance Rates

Following the initial suppression by short-term desipramine treatment, the rate of extravascular NE appearance returned toward baseline following long-term desipramine treatment (*P*=NS vs basal), but this change from the short-term to the long-term desipramine condition fell short of statistical significance (*P*=.044). Similarly, the mean plasma NE appearance rate returned to approximately basal levels (*P*=NS vs basal) following long-term desipramine treatment. The rise in plasma NE appearance from the short-term to the long-term desipramine study was statistically significant (*P*=.018). Despite the return of extravascular and plasma NE appearance to basal levels, the total NE mass remained approximately 20% below baseline following long-term desipramine treatment (basal, 632±112 nmol/m² vs short-term desipramine, 372±87 nmol/m² [*P*<.013]; vs long-term desipramine, 491±89 nmol/m² [*P*=NS]), although this difference from basal was not statistically significant. The plasma NE clearance rate fell to 29% below baseline following long-term desipramine treatment (*P*=.016 vs

Table 2. Effect of 2 Days' Desipramine or Placebo on NE Kinetics*

	Desipramine Hydrochloride Treatment			Placebo Treatment		
	Basal (n=29)	Desipramine (n=29)	P†	Basal (n=5)	Placebo (n=5)	P‡
Plasma NE, nmol/L	1.39±0.13	1.19±0.11	.005	0.85±0.07	0.82±0.19	>.1
Extravascular NE appearance, nmol/min per square meter	9.59±0.90	6.53±0.71	.002	7.62±1.24	7.03±0.59	>.1
Plasma NE appearance, nmol/min per square meter	1.98±0.18	1.37±0.14	.001	1.12±0.12	1.05±0.18	>.1
Plasma NE clearance, L/min per square meter	1.18±0.07	0.90±0.03	.001	1.23±0.08	1.10±0.08	>.1

**All values are given as mean±SEM, except for* P *values. NE indicates norepinephrine.*
†*Two-way analysis of variance with repeated measures.*
‡*Paired* t *test vs basal.*

Table 3. Effect of 2 Days' and 28 Days' Desipramine on NE Kinetics in Depressed Patients*

	Desipramine Hydrochloride				
	Basal (n=16)	Short-term (n=16)	Long-term (n=13)	P,† Long-term vs Basal	P,† Long-term vs Short-term
Plasma NE, nmol/L	1.72±0.19	1.48±0.15	2.25±0.40	.035	.003
Extravascular NE appearance, nmol/min per square meter	11.52±1.24	8.63±0.95	10.93±1.48	>.1	.044
Plasma NE appearance, nmol/min per square meter	2.41±0.24	1.74±0.24	2.21±0.36	>.1	.018
Plasma NE clearance, L/min per square meter	1.20±0.12	1.02±0.11	0.85±0.08	.016	>.1

**All values are given as mean±SEM, except for* P *values. NE indicates norepinephrine.*
†*Paired* t *test (*$P<.025$ *required for statistical significance due to Bonferroni correction for multiple comparisons).*

basal). The reduction in NE clearance from the short-term to the long-term study was not statistically significant.(Figures depicting changes in these kinetic parameters that show data points for individual subjects are available on request.)

Relationship Between the Changes in NE Appearance and Mean Arterial Blood Pressure

We investigated the possibility that the apparent reduction in SNS outflow following short-term desipramine administration in controls and patients was related to the increase in blood pressure. There was no significant correlation between the change in blood pressure and the change in the rate of plasma NE appearance following short-term desipramine administration for the normal controls ($r=-.28$, P=NS) or the depressed patients ($r=.18$, P=NS) nor was there a significant correlation between the changes in these variables from baseline in the depressed patients following long-term desipramine administration ($r=.14$, P=NS). Similarly, there was no significant correlation between the change in blood pressure and the change in the rate of extravascular NE appearance following short-term desipramine administration in the controls ($r=-.15$) or patients ($r=.21$), or following long-term desipramine administration in the patients ($r=.24$).

COMMENT

BASELINE NE KINETICS STUDY—PATIENTS VS CONTROLS

A major objective of these studies was to define the mechanisms underlying elevated plasma NE concentrations in major depressive illness. We[1,2] and others[3-11] have demonstrated previously that venous plasma NE concentrations are increased in some patients. Our NE kinetic analysis revealed an increased rate of NE appearance into the extravascular and vascular compartments in depressed patients but similar rates of NE clearance from plasma in patients and controls. These findings provide direct support for increased SNS activity in major depression.

Earlier studies of depressed patients[1,2,5,42] have shown an association between elevations of plasma NE and the presence of melancholia or increased hypothalamic-pituitary-adrenal activity, suggesting that increased SNS activity is related to severity of illness. Eight of our 17 patients were melancholic, four of whom were dexamethasone nonsuppressors, and 14 were outpatients.

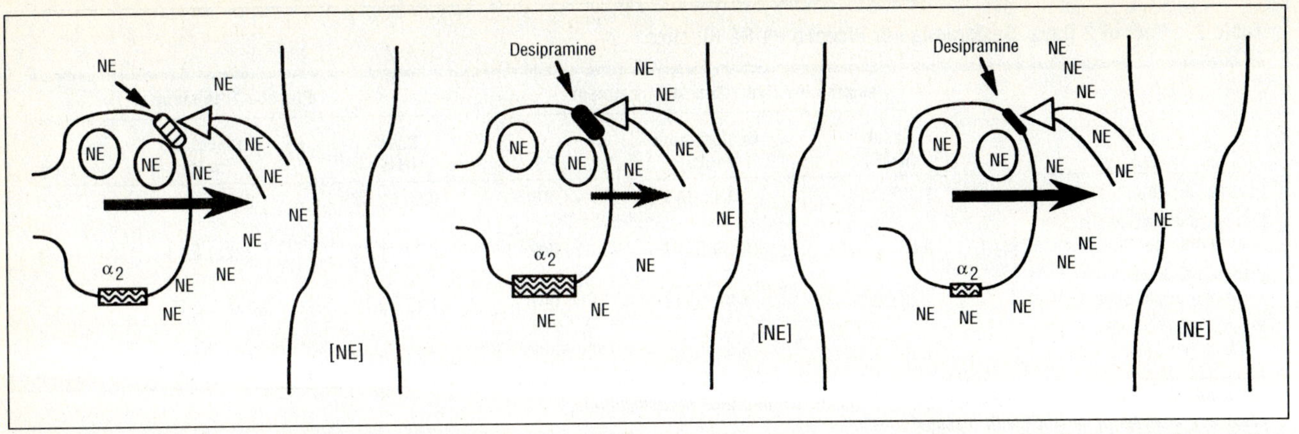

Figure 2. *Schematic representation of short- and long-term effects of desipramine hydrochloride on plasma norepinephrine (NE) kinetics. This Figure depicts a postganglionic sympathetic nerve terminal, neuronal re-uptake transporter, inhibitory α_2-autoreceptor, NE release, and overall plasma NE concentration. Left, Baseline: the plasma NE concentration is determined by the rates of sympathetic nervous system tone, NE release into an extravascular compartment, extravascular NE removal by neuronal re-uptake or local metabolism, and NE appearance into plasma. Center, Short-term desipramine hydrochloride treatment: plasma NE concentration falls despite a reduction in NE clearance; NE release, extravascular NE appearance, and vascular NE appearance are reduced. The reduction in NE clearance is consistent with the known effect of desipramine to block the NE uptake transporter. The fall in extravascular and plasma NE appearance suggests an overall suppression of sympathetic nervous system tone, possibly due to central nervous system mechanisms. Alternatively, re-uptake blockade by desipramine could increase the local NE concentration in the vicinity of the inhibitory α_2-autoreceptor and diminish NE release. Right, Long-term desipramine treatment: plasma NE concentration is elevated compared with baseline, and NE clearance is further reduced. Extravascular NE appearance and plasma NE appearance return to baseline levels, indicating that a reduction in NE clearance is primarily responsible for any increase in plasma NE compared with baseline. The increases in extravascular (trend) and plasma NE appearance compared with those of short-term desipramine treatment are compatible with sympathetic nervous system reactivation via central nervous system mechanisms. Alternatively, desensitization of the terminal α_2-autoreceptor could have occurred, leading to a reduction in the inhibitory restraint on NE release.*

Thus, our patients were highly representative of the majority of depressed individuals, who are generally mildly to moderately depressed outpatients with normal hypothalamic-pituitary-adrenal function. It is, therefore, significant that even in this less severely affected population, we detected the presence of increased SNS activity.

Our findings are consistent with those of the report by Maas et al,[43] who compared the differential urinary excretion of NE and its metabolites in depressed patients and healthy controls and suggested that the release of NE into the circulation is increased in major depression. Our methods, however, allow a much closer approximation of the actual source of NE release into the circulation than can be achieved by using urinary sampling. The observed increase in the plasma NE appearance rate in our patients is also compatible with the finding by Esler et al,[3] who demonstrated an increased plasma NE appearance rate in a small number of depressed patients. We extend their findings by including estimates of NE appearance into the extravascular compartment, ie, the site of endogenous NE release from the SNS neuroeffector junction.

The presence of increased SNS tone in depressed patients might have clinical implications. For example, major depression is associated with an increased risk of death from cardiovascular causes.[44-46] In addition, the presence of depression following myocardial infarction is a powerful predictor of subsequent cardiovascular morbidity, eg, arrhythmias, myocardial infarction, or death.[47] Because it has been shown that cardiac SNS activity is increased in cardiac patients with sustained ventricular arrhythmias[48] who are at high risk for sudden death, the present findings raise the possibility that increased SNS activity might play a role in the increased cardiovascular morbidity and mortality associated with major depression. Finally, it is intriguing to consider that increased SNS activity might contribute to the weight loss associated with depression, since the SNS is an important component of the neuroendocrine systems that regulate caloric metabolism.[49,50]

We cannot make specific inferences regarding the CNS mechanisms that might underlie SNS hyperactivity in depression. However, several possible explanations deserve further exploration. Nemeroff et al[51] have demonstrated elevated concentrations of corticotropin-releasing factor in the cerebrospinal fluid of depressed patients, and it has been proposed that increased corticotropin-releasing factor activity in the CNS could account for hypothalamic-pituitary-adrenal hyperactivity in major depression.[52,53] Corticotropin-releasing factor–containing neurons in the hypothalamus provide stimulatory input to several autonomic centers involved in regulating peripheral sympathetic activity.[54-57] Thus, increased activity of corticotropin-releasing factor pathways in the CNS is also compatible with increased SNS activity in depressed patients. Our findings also agree with long-standing theories that hypothesize a reduction in CNS noradrenergic activity[58,59] and/or an increase in CNS cholinergic activity[60] in depression. Norepinephrine pathways that involve α_2-receptors *inhibit* SNS outflow.[19,61-66] Therefore, if depression were associated with low CNS NE activity, at least at the level of the brain stem, this would be expected to diminish α_2-mediated, inhibitory restraint on SNS outflow. Similarly, CNS choliner-

gic input to brain-stem autonomic nuclei mechanisms are thought to *stimulate* the SNS in animals and humans.[67-70] Of course, SNS hyperactivity in depression could represent a nonspecific, physiological response to the stress of the illness. However, individuals suffering from panic disorder, who are often as distressed and functionally impaired as depressed patients, do not generally exhibit an increased plasma NE concentration[71] or NE appearance rate.[72] This argues against ascribing our findings to nonspecific stress.

It is possible to explain increased peripheral NE appearance in our patients without invoking CNS mechanisms. Presynaptic α_2-autoreceptors on SNS nerve terminals inhibit NE release and regulate the amount of NE that is released with firing of the nerve. Because the NE kinetic methodology does not specifically measure the firing rate of SNS nerves, we cannot exclude the possibility that a defect in the functioning of these receptors, separate from an increase in SNS nerve activity, might account for or contribute to increased NE release.

SHORT-TERM DESIPRAMINE STUDY

Our second major objective was to define the effects of short- and long-term desipramine administration on SNS activity in patients with depression (these findings are represented schematically in **Figure 2**). We found that desipramine administration for 2 days suppressed plasma NE in both controls and depressed patients. A potentially greater fall in plasma NE was offset by a simultaneous reduction in plasma NE clearance, which likely reflects a desipramine-induced blockade of NE neuronal uptake at SNS postganglionic nerves. These findings are in agreement with those of other studies of plasma NE kinetics in controls given single doses of desipramine.[73-75] A significant fall in extravascular and plasma NE appearance indicates that SNS activity was suppressed by desipramine in the patients and controls. This is supported by findings from recent animal studies demonstrating that short-term desipramine administration reduces SNS nerve activity.[76-79]

Both CNS and peripheral mechanisms must be considered to explain the apparent suppression of SNS activity by desipramine. In animal studies, TCAs consistently suppress the firing rate of the locus coeruleus following short-term administration,[80-83] probably due to an increase in the local concentration of NE at inhibitory α_2-autoreceptors on locus coeruleus neurons. A corresponding increase in local NE concentrations at inhibitory α_2-mechanisms that regulate SNS outflow would also be expected to reduce SNS activity. The same effect of re-uptake blockade at α_2-autoreceptors on SNS nerve terminals could possibly reduce release of NE from SNS nerves by a peripheral mechanism. Two factors lead us to believe, however, that CNS rather than peripheral effects of desipramine account for the suppression of plasma NE appearance. First, the function of the α_2-autoreceptor on SNS nerve terminals is probably to inhibit the amount of NE released per unit of firing, not to regulate the firing rate of the nerve. Second, desipramine has acutely suppressed the firing rate of SNS nerves in animal studies.[76-79]

LONG-TERM DESIPRAMINE STUDY

In an earlier study that served as a major impetus for this investigation,[12] we found that long-term (4 weeks) TCA treatment increased plasma NE concentrations. In the present study, analysis of NE kinetics revealed a progressive fall in NE clearance with desipramine treatment, most likely reflecting blockade of NE re-uptake at postganglionic SNS nerves.[84] Although the plasma NE concentration after prolonged desipramine administration was not significantly greater than baseline in the present study, the rise in plasma NE appeared to be due to a reduction in plasma NE clearance because the rate of NE appearance into the extravascular compartment and the rate of plasma NE appearance closely approximated basal values.

Extravascular and plasma NE appearance rates were not significantly different from baseline following 28 days of desipramine treatment, but the apparent recovery of NE appearance following the initial suppression is potentially meaningful. Prolonged TCA administration produces subsensitivity and downregulation of α_2-noradrenergic receptors,[80,82,85,86] presumably by blocking NE re-uptake and increasing the local NE concentration in the vicinity of these receptors. This is the putative mechanism whereby short-term suppression of locus coeruleus activity by desipramine is attenuated by prolonged treatment.[80,82,83,87] If this occurred at brain-stem cardiovascular centers in humans, it would be reflected initially by suppression of SNS outflow due to increased NE availability at inhibitory brain-stem α_2-receptors. If subsensitivity then developed at these receptors, this might result in attenuation of the inhibitory restraint on SNS outflow and reactivation of SNS activity. We cannot exclude alternative CNS mechanisms, but our findings are compatible with this model.

PERIPHERAL MECHANISMS must also be considered, however. Prolonged desipramine administration might downregulate α_2-autoreceptors on SNS nerve terminals and reduce inhibitory influences on NE release, thereby accounting for or contributing to the apparent increase in extravascular and plasma NE appearance. Finally, it is notable that we would have concluded that desipramine had no significant effect on SNS activity had we performed only baseline and day 28 assessments. This illustrates the importance of employing study

designs that will detect temporal changes in neuroendocrine functioning in future investigations of this type.

Prolonged TCA treatment has been associated with an overall reduction in urinary excretion of NE and its major metabolites.[85-90] In our study, short-term desipramine treatment was associated with an apparent suppression of peripheral NE release but, following prolonged treatment, extravascular and plasma NE appearance returned to approximately basal values. Although our findings appear to contradict the results of earlier urinary studies (which suggest that prolonged TCA administration suppresses peripheral SNS activity), the total NE mass in the extravascular compartment estimated by the two-compartment model was 20% lower than baseline after long-term desipramine administration. Since the mass of NE is estimated to be 100 times greater in the extravascular compartment than in the plasma-containing, vascular compartment,[16] it is possible that total urinary excretion of NE and its metabolites would indeed have been reduced by long-term desipramine in our subjects, despite a return of NE appearance rates to basal levels.

Nevertheless, the present study does resolve one dilemma arising from the urinary excretion studies of long-term TCA use, ie, how to account for a simultaneous *increase* in the plasma NE concentration and *reduction* in urinary excretion of NE and its metabolites. It has been proposed that long-term TCA administration reduces sympathetic activity but also delays the plasma clearance of the NE that *is* released from SNS nerves by blocking neuronal uptake, thereby causing a rise in the overall plasma NE concentration.[89] Our findings confirm that a reduction in plasma NE clearance is the likely explanation for increased plasma NE associated with long-term desipramine administration.

We observed a small increase in blood pressure associated with both short-term and prolonged administration, as has been demonstrated previously.[75,91] Although the suppression of NE release following short-term desipramine administration could be a reflex response to baroreceptor activation, the absence of a correlation between the changes in blood pressure and NE appearance into the extravascular or vascular compartments suggests otherwise. Moreover, SNS tone returned to approximately basal values with prolonged desipramine administration whereas the mean blood pressure remained elevated. This also argues against a primary effect of desipramine on blood pressure to explain the suppression of SNS activity by short-term administration. Interestingly, the rise in blood pressure associated with short-term treatment does not appear to have been mediated by a generalized SNS activation. We cannot exclude the possibility that desipramine caused a regional increase in cardiac noradrenergic activity, thereby increasing heart rate, cardiac output, and blood pressure, as has been suggested by Esler et al.[75]

CONCLUSION

In summary, analysis of plasma NE kinetics suggests that increased SNS activity is present in major depression, even in relatively mildly depressed outpatients. Short-term desipramine administration appears to suppress SNS activity in depressed patients and normal controls, most likely via a CNS mechanism. A reduction in peripheral clearance of NE from plasma is the likely explanation for earlier reports of plasma NE elevations following long-term TCA treatment. The apparent recovery of plasma NE release following an initial suppression by desipramine in the present study parallels a similar effect of TCAs on locus coeruleus activity in animals and is compatible with models suggesting that downregulation of α_2-adrenergic receptor function may be important in the mechanism of action of TCAs.

Accepted for publication March 13, 1993.

This work was supported in part by the Medical Research Service of the Department of Veterans Affairs, Washington, DC.

The authors appreciated the skillful technical assistance of David Flatness, David Federighi, and Carl Sikkema. David Foster, PhD, and Carol Harris provided valuable training and computer resources for the mathematical modeling methodology. Peter Roy-Byrne, MD, provided incisive reviews of earlier versions of the manuscript.

Reprint requests to Geriatric Research, Education, and Clinical Center (182B), Department of Veterans Affairs Medical Center, 1660 S Columbian Way, Seattle, WA 98108 (Dr Veith).

REFERENCES

1. Veith RC, Barnes RF, Villacres EC, Murburg MM, Raskind MA, Borson S, Backus F, Halter JB. Plasma catecholamines and norepinephrine kinetics in depression and panic disorder. In: Belmaker R, ed. *Catecholamines: Clinical Aspects.* New York, NY: Alan R Liss Inc; 1988:197-202.
2. Barnes RF, Veith RC, Borson S, Verhey J, Raskind MA, Halter JB. High levels of plasma catecholamines in dexamethasone-resistant depressed patients. *Am J Psychiatry.* 1983;140:1623-1625.
3. Esler M, Turbott J, Schwarz R, Leonard P, Bobik A, Skews H, Jackman G. The peripheral kinetics of norepinephrine in depressive illness. *Arch Gen Psychiatry.* 1982;39:295-300.
4. Lake CR, Pickar D, Ziegler MG, Lipper S, Slater S, Murphy DL. High plasma norepinephrine levels in patients with major affective disorder. *Am J Psychiatry.* 1982;139:1315-1318.
5. Roy A, Pickar D, Linnoila M, Potter WZ. Plasma norepinephrine level in affective disorders: relationship to melancholia. *Arch Gen Psychiatry.* 1985;42:1181-1185.
6. Siever LJ, Pickar D, Lake R, Cohen RM, Uhde TW, Murphy DL. Extreme elevations in plasma norepinephrine associated with decreased alpha-adrenergic responsivity in major depressive disorder: two case reports. *J Clin Psychopharmacol.* 1985;3:39-41.
7. Wyatt RJ, Portnoy B, Kupfer DJ, Snyder F, Engelman K. Resting plasma catecholamine concentrations in patients with depression and anxiety. *Arch Gen Psychiatry.* 1971;24:65-70.
8. Roy A, Pickar D, DeJong J, Karoum F, Linnoila M. Norepinephrine and its metabolites in cerebrospinal fluid, plasma and urine: relationship to hypothalamic-pituitary-adrenal axis function in depression. *Arch Gen Psychiatry.* 1988;45:849-857.

9. de Villiers AS, Russell VA, Carstens ME, Aalbers C, Gagiano CA, Chalton DO, Taljaard JJF. Noradrenergic function and hypothalamic-pituitary-adrenal axis activity in primary unipolar major depressive disorder. *Psychiatry Res.* 1987; 22:127-140.
10. Louis WJ, Doyle AE, Anavekar SN. Plasma noradrenaline concentration and blood pressure in essential hypertension, phaeochromocytoma and depression. *Clin Soc.* 1975;48:239s-242s.
11. Rudorfer MV, Ross RJ, Linnoila M, Sherer MA, Potter WZ. Exaggerated orthostatic responsivity of plasma norepinephrine in depression. *Arch Gen Psychiatry.* 1985;42:1186-1192.
12. Veith RC, Raskind MA, Barnes RF, Gumbrecht G, Ritchie JL, Halter JB. Tricyclic antidepressants and supine, standing and exercise plasma norepinephrine levels. *Clin Pharmacol Ther.* 1983;33:763-769.
13. Ross RJ, Zavadil AP, Calil HM, Linnoila M, Kitanaka I, Blombery P, Kopin IJ, Potter WZ. Effects of desmethylimipramine on plasma norepinephrine, pulse, and blood pressure. *Clin Pharmacol Ther.* 1983;33:429-437.
14. Lake CR, Mikkelsen EJ, Rapoport JL, Zavadil AP, Kopin IJ. Effect of imipramine on norepinephrine and blood pressure in enuretic boys. *Clin Pharmacol Ther.* 1979;26:647-653.
15. Cameron OG, Smith CB, Hollingsworth PJ, Nesse RM, Curtis GC. Platelet alpha-2 adrenergic receptor binding and plasma catecholamines. *Arch Gen Psychiatry.* 1984;41:1144-1148.
16. Lake CR, Chernow B, Feuerstein G, Goldstein DS, Ziegler MG. The sympathetic nervous system in man: its evaluation and measurement of plasma norepinephrine. In: Ziegler MG, Lake CR, eds. *Norepinephrine.* Baltimore, Md: Williams & Wilkins; 1984:70-80.
17. Kopin IJ, Lake RC, Ziegler MG. Plasma levels of norepinephrine. *Ann Intern Med.* 1978;88:671-680.
18. Linares OA, Jacquez JA, Zech LA, Smith MJ, Sanfield JA, Morrow LA, Rosen SG, Halter JB. Norepinephrine metabolism in humans: kinetic analysis and model. *J Clin Invest.* 1987;80:1332-1341.
19. Veith RC, Best JD, Halter JB. Dose-dependent suppression of norepinephrine appearance rate in plasma by clonidine in man. *J Clin Endocrinol Metab.* 1984; 59:151-155.
20. Linares OA, Zech LA, Jacquez JA, Rosen SG, Sanfield JA, Morrow LA, Supiano MA, Halter JB. Effect of sodium-restricted diet and posture on norepinephrine kinetics in humans. *Am J Physiol.* 1988;254:E222-E230.
21. Supiano MA, Linares OA, Smith MJ, Halter JB. Age-related differences in norepinephrine kinetics: effect of posture and sodium-restricted diet. *Am J Physiol.* 1990;259:E422-E431.
22. Esler M, Jennings G, Korner P, Willett I, Dudley F, Hasking G, Anderson W, Lambert G. Assessment of human sympathetic nervous system activity from measurements of norepinephrine turnover. *Hypertension.* 1988;11:3-20.
23. Baker GB, Greenshaw AJ. Effects of long-term administration of antidepressants and neuroleptics on receptors in the central nervous system. *Cell Mol Neurobiol.* 1989;9:1-44.
24. Nestler EJ, McMahon A, Sabban EL, Tallman JF, Duman RS. Chronic antidepressant administration decreases the expresssion of tyrosine hydroxylase in the rat locus coeruleus. *Proc Natl Acad Sci U S A.* 1990;87:7522-7526.
25. Curtis AL, Valentino RJ. Acute and chronic effects of the atypical antidepressant mianserin on brain noradrenergic neurons. *Psychopharmacology.* 1991; 103:330-338.
26. Brady LS, Whitfield HJ, Fox RJ, Gold PW, Herkenham M. Long-term antidepressant administration alters corticotropin-releasing hormone, tyrosine hydroxylase, and mineralocorticoid receptor gene expression in rat brain. *J Clin Invest.* 1991;87:831-837.
27. Lacroix D, Blier P, Curet O, de Montigny C. Effects of long-term desipramine administration on noradrenergic neurotransmission: electrophysiological studies in the rat brain. *J Pharmacol Exp Ther.* 1991;257:1081-1090.
28. Carson ER, Cobelli C, Finkelstein L. *Mathematical Modeling of Metabolic and Endocrine Systems.* New York, NY: John Wiley & Sons Inc; 1983:1-393.
29. American Psychiatric Association. *Diagnostic and Statistical Manual of Mental Disorders, Third Edition.* Washington, DC: American Psychiatric Association Press; 1981.
30. Hamilton M. A rating scale for depression. *J Neurol Neurosurg Psychiatry.* 1960;23:56-63.
31. Best JD, Halter JB. Blood pressure and norepinephrine spillover during propranolol infusion in man. *Am J Physiol.* 1985;248:R400-R406.
32. Hjemdahl P, Freyschuss U, Juhlin-Dannfelt A, Linde B. Differential sympathetic activation during neutral stress evoked by the Stroop test. *Acta Physiol Scand Suppl.* 1984;527:25-29.
33. Abumrad NN, Rabin D, Diamond MP, Lacy WN. Use of a heated superficial hand vein as an alternative site for the measurement of amino acid concentrations and for the study of glucose and alanine kinetics in man. *Metabolism.* 1981;30:936-940.
34. McGuire EAH, Helderman JH, Tobin JD, Andress R, Berman M. Effects of arterial versus venous sampling of glucose kinetics in man. *J Appl Physiol.* 1976; 41:565-573.
35. Evans MI, Halter JB, Porte D. Comparison of double- and single-isotope derivative methods for measuring catecholamines in human plasma. *Clin Chem.* 1978;24:567-570.
36. Veith RC, Featherstone JA, Linares OA, Halter JB. Age differences in plasma norepinephrine kinetics in humans. *J Gerontol.* 1986;41:319-324.
37. Featherstone JA, Veith RC, Flatness D, Murburg M, Villacres EC, Halter JB. Age and alpha-2 adrenergic regulation of plasma norepinephrine kinetics in humans. *J Gerontol.* 1987;42:271-276.
38. Silverberg AB, Shah SD, Hammond MW, Cryer PE. Norepinephrine: hormone and neurotransmitter in man. *Am J Physiol.* 1978;234:E252-E255.
39. Berman M, Weiss MF. *SAAM Manual.* Washington, DC: US Dept of Health, Education, and Welfare; 1978. US Dept of Health, Education, and Welfare publication NIH 78-180.
40. Berman M, Beltz WF, Grief PC, Chabay R, Boston RC. *CONSAM Users Guide.* Washington, DC: US Government Printing Office; 1984. Publication 1983-421-132:3279.
41. Keppel G. *Design and Analysis: A Researchers' Handbook.* Englewood Cliffs, NJ: Prentice-Hall International Inc; 1973:89-94.
42. Rubin AL, Price LH, Charney DS, Heninger GR. Noradrenergic function and the cortisol response to dexamethasone in depression. *Psychiatry Res.* 1985;15: 5-15.
43. Maas JW, Koslow SH, Davis J, Katz M, Frazer A, Bowden CL, Berman N, Gibbons R, Strokes P, Landis H. Catecholamine metabolism and disposition in healthy and depressed subjects. *Arch Gen Psychiatry.* 1987;44:337-344.
44. Malzberg B. Mortality among patients with involution melancholia. *Am J Psychiatry.* 1937;93:1231-1238.
45. Avery D, Winokur G. Mortality in depressed patients treated with electroconvulsive therapy and antidepressants. *Arch Gen Psychiatry.* 1976;33:1029-1037.
46. Rabins PV, Harvis K, Koven S. High fatality rates of late-life depression associated with cardiovascular disease. *J Affect Disord.* 1985;9:165-167.
47. Carney RM, Rich MW, Freedland KE, Saini J, teVelde A. Major depressive disorder predicts cardiac events in patients with coronary artery disease. *Psychosom Med.* 1988;50:627-633.
48. Meredith IT, Broughton A, Jennings GL, Esler MD. Evidence of a selective increase in cardiac sympathetic activity in patients with sustained ventricular arrhythmias. *N Engl J Med.* 1991;325:618-624.
49. Schwartz RS, Jaeger L, Silberstein SS, Veith RC. Sympathetic nervous system activity and the thermic effect of feeding. *Int J Obes.* 1987;11:141-149.
50. Landsberg L, Young JB. Diet-induced changes in sympathoadrenal activity: implications for thermogenesis and obesity. *Life Sci.* 1981;28:1801-1819.
51. Nemeroff CB, Widerlov E, Bissette G, Walleus H, Karlsson I, Eklund K, Kilts CD, Loosen PT, Vale W. Elevated concentrations of CSF corticotropin-releasing factor-like immunoreactivity in depressed patients. *Science.* 1984;266:1342-1343.
52. Gold PW, Goodwin FK, Chrousos GP. Clinical and biochemical manifestations of depression: relation to the neurobiology of stress (second of two parts). *N Engl J Med.* 1988;319:413-420.
53. Gold PW, Chrousos G, Kellner C, Post R, Roy A, Augerinos P, Schulte H, Oldfield E, Loriaux DL. Psychiatric implications of basic and clinical studies with corticotropin-releasing factor. *Am J Psychiatry.* 1984;141:619-627.
54. Swanson LW, Sawchenko PE. Paraventricular nucleus: site for the integration of neuroendocrine and autonomic mechanisms. *Neuroendocrinology.* 1980; 31:410-417.
55. Swanson LW, Sawchenko PE, Rivier J, Vale WW. Organization of ovine corticotropin-releasing factor immunoreactive cells and fibers in the rat brain: an immunohistochemical study. *Neuroendocrinology.* 1983;36:165-186.
56. Merchenthaler I, Vigh S, Petrusz P, Schally AV. Immunocytochemical localization of corticotropin-releasing factor (CRF) in the rat brain. *Am J Anatomy.* 1982;165:385-396.
57. Cummings S, Elde R, Ells J, Lindall A. Corticotropin-releasing factor immunoreactivity is widely distributed within the central nervous system of the rat: an immunohistochemical study. *J Neurosci.* 1983;3:1355-1368.

58. Janowsky DS, El-Yousef MK, Davis JM, Sekerke HJ. A cholinergic-adrenergic hypothesis of mania and depression. *Lancet.* 1972;2:632-635.
59. Bunney WE Jr, Davis JM. Norepinephrine and depressive reactions: a review. *Arch Gen Psychiatry.* 1965;13:483-494.
60. Schildkraut JJ. The catecholamine hypothesis of affective disorders: a review of supporting evidence. *Am J Psychiatry.* 1965;122:509-522.
61. Brezenoff HE. Cardiovascular regulation by brain acetylcholine. *FASEB J.* 1984; 43:17-20.
62. Sawchenko PE, Swanson LW. Central noradrenergic pathways for the integration of hypothalamic neuroendocrine and autonomic responses. *Science.* 1981; 214:685-687.
63. Kennedy B, Janowsky DS, Risch SC, Ziegler MG. Central cholinergic stimulation causes adrenal epinephrine release. *J Clin Invest.* 1984;74:972-975.
64. Sundaram K, Hreday S. Cholinergic nerve terminals in the ventrolateral medullary pressor area: pharmacological evidence. *J Auton Nerv Syst.* 1988;22: 221-228.
65. Reis DJ, Morrison S, Ruggiero DA. The C1 area of the brainstem in tonic and reflex control of blood pressure: state of the art lecture. *Hypertension.* 1988; 11(suppl I):8-13.
66. Kobinger W. Alpha-adrenoceptors in cardiovascular regulation. In: Ziegler MG, Lake CR, eds. *Norepinephrine.* Baltimore, Md: Williams & Wilkins; 1984:307-326.
67. Unnerstall JR, Kopajtic TA, Kuhar MJ. Distribution of alpha2-agonist binding sites in the rat and human central nervous system: analysis of some functional, anatomic correlates of the pharmacologic effects of clonidine and related adrenergic agents. *Brain Res.* 1984;319:69-101.
68. Morrison SF, Milner TA, Reis DJ. Reticulospinal vasomotor neurons of the rat rostral ventrolateral medulla: relationship to sympathetic nerve activity and the C1 adrenergic cell group. *J Neurosci.* 1988;8:1286-1301.
69. Elam M, Yao T, Svensson TH, Thoren P. Regulation of locus coeruleus neurons and splanchnic, sympathetic nerves by cardiovascular afferents. *Brain Res.* 1984; 290:281-287.
70. Brown DL, Guyenet PG. Cardiovascular neurons of brain stem with projections to spinal cord. *Am J Physiol.* 1984;247:R1009-R1016.
71. Veith RC. Sympathetic nervous system disturbances in psychiatric illness. In: Brown MR, Rivier C, Koob G, eds. *The Neuroendocrinology and Neurobiology of Stress.* New York, NY: Marcel Dekker Inc; 1990:395-435.
72. Villacres EC, Hollifield M, Katon WJ, Veith RC. Sympathetic nervous system activity in panic disorder. *Psychiatry Res.* 1987;21:313-321.
73. Esler M, Jackman G, Leonard P, Skews H, Bobik A, Korner P. Effect of norepinephrine uptake blockers on norepinephrine kinetics in depressive illness. *Clin Pharmacol Ther.* 1981;29:12-20.
74. Stromberg JS, Linares OA, Supiano MA, Smith MJ, Foster AN, Halter JB. The effect of desipramine on norepinephrine metabolism in humans: interaction with aging. *Am J Physiol.* 1991;261:R1484-R1490.
75. Esler MD, Wallin G, Dorward PK, Eisenhofer G, Westerman R, Meredith I, Lambert G, Cox HS, Jennings G. Effects of desipramine on sympathetic nerve firing and norepinephrine spillover to plasma in humans. *Am J Physiol.* 1991;260: R817-R823.
76. Cohen MD, Finberg J, Dibner-Dunlap M, Yuih SN, Thames MD. Effects of desipramine hydrochloride on peripheral sympathetic nerve activity. *Am J Physiol.* 1990;258:R876-R882.
77. Szabo B, Schultheiss A. Desipramine inhibits sympathetic nerve activity in the rabbit. *Naunyn Schmiedebergs Arch Pharmacol.* 1990;342:469-476.
78. Lavian G, DiBona G, Finberg JPM. Inhibition of sympathetic nerve activity by acute administration of the tricyclic antidepressant desipramine. *Eur J Pharmacol.* 1991;194:153-159.
79. Eisenhofer G, Saigusa T, Esler MD, Cox HS, Angus JA, Dorward PK. Central sympathoinhibition and peripheral neuronal uptake blockade after desipramine in rabbits. *Am J Physiol.* 1991;260:R824-R832.
80. Svensson TH, Usdin T. Feedback inhibition of brain noradrenaline neurons by tricyclic antidepressants: alpha-receptor mediation. *Science.* 1978;202:1089-1091.
81. Haskins JT, Moyer JA, Muth EA, Sigg EB. DMI, Wy-45,030, WY-45,881 and ciramadol inhibit locus coeruleus neuronal activity. *Eur J Pharmacol.* 1985; 115:139-146.
82. McMillin BA, Warnack W, German D, Shore PA. Effects of chronic desipramine treatment on rat brain noradrenergic responses to alpha-adrenergic drugs. *Eur J Pharmacol.* 1980;61:239-246.
83. Valentino RJ, Curtis AL, Parris DG, Wehby RG. Antidepressant actions on brain noradrenergic neurons. *J Pharmacol Exp Ther.* 1990;253:833-840.
84. Trendelenburg U. A kinetic analysis of the extraneuronal uptake and metabolism of catecholamines. *Rev Physiol Biochem Pharmacol.* 1980;87:33-115.
85. Sulser F, Vetulani J, Mobley PL. Mode of action of antidepressant drugs. *Biochem Pharmacol.* 1978;27:257-261.
86. Charney DS, Menkes DB, Heninger GR. Receptor sensitivity and the mechanism of action of antidepressant treatment. *Arch Gen Psychiatry.* 1981;38: 1160-1180.
87. Scubee-Moreau JJ, Dresse AE. Effect of various antidepressant drugs on the spontaneous firing rate of locus coeruleus and raphe dorsalis neurons of the rat. *Eur J Pharmacol.* 1979;57:219-225.
88. Linnoila M, Guthrie S, Lane EA, Karoum F, Rudorfer M, Potter WZ. Clinical studies on norepinephrine metabolism: how to interpret the numbers. *Psychiatry Res.* 1986;17:229-239.
89. Linnoila M, Karoum F, Calil HM, Kopin IJ, Potter WZ. Alteration of norepinephrine metabolism with desipramine and zimelidine in depressed patients. *Arch Gen Psychiatry.* 1982;39:1025-1028.
90. Golden RN, Markey SP, Risby ED, Rudorfer MV, Cowdry RW, Potter WZ. Antidepressants reduce whole-body norepinephrine turnover while enhancing 6-hydroxymelatonin output. *Arch Gen Psychiatry.* 1988;45:150-154.
91. Ross RJ, Zavadil AP, Calil HM, Linnoila M, Kitanaka I, Blombery P, Kopin IJ, Potter WZ. Effects of desmethylimipramine on plasma norepinephrine, pulse, and blood pressure. *Clin Pharmacol Ther.* 1983;33:429-437.

Correction

Incorrect Wording. In the article "Naturalistic Follow-up of a Behavioral Treatment for Chronically Parasuicidal Borderline Patients" published in the December issue of the ARCHIVES (1993;50:971-974), the second sentence in the "Results" section on page 973 should read as follows: Throughout the follow-up year, both the parasuicide repeat rate (DBT=26%, TAU=60%; z=2.12; P<.01) and the likelihood of any psychiatric hospitalization (DBT=11%, TAU=40%; z=1.43; P<.07) were lower for subjects completing DBT than for subjects remaining in TAU. The ARCHIVES regrets the error.

No Evidence of a Schizophrenia Locus in a Second Pseudoautosomal Region

We have previously reported that we found no evidence of linkage between schizophrenia and the pseudoautosomal region of the X and Y chromosomes in our series of pedigrees.[1] The pseudoautosomal region we tested is located at the telomere of the short arms. Recently, a second pseudoautosomal region has been found at the telomere of the long arms as well.[2] This latter region spans over 400 kilobases in physical distance and approximately 2 centimorgans in map distance. A highly polymorphic marker, sDF-1 (*DXYS154*), has been identified in this region.

To search for a schizophrenia vulnerability locus in the second pseudoautosomal region, we tested for linkage to the above marker in our 12 pedigrees.[1] The polymerase chain reaction conditions are essentially as those described previously.[2] The models used in the linkage analyses were also the same as those previously reported,[1] except that the male-to-female recombination ratio was assumed to be equal, since the true value is unknown and this assumption is conservative. The results of these linkage analyses in our pedigrees provided strong evidence against linkage of schizophrenia to a locus in the second pseudoautosomal region (**Table**).

Zhe Wu Wang, MD
Donald W. Black, MD
Nancy Andreasen, MD, PhD
Raymond R. Crowe, MD
University of Iowa College of Medicine
Department of Psychiatry
Iowa City, IA 52242

1. Wang ZW, Crowe RR, Black D, Andreasen N. Pseudoautosomal locus for schizophrenia excluded in 12 pedigrees. *Arch Gen Psychiatry.* 1993;50:199-204.
2. Freije D, Helms C, Watson MS, Donis-Keller H. Identification of a second pseudoautosomal region near the Xq and Yq telomeres. *Science.* 1992;258:1784-1787.

Results of Linkage Analyses to Locus *DXYS154**

	Recombination Fraction						
	0.00	0.01	0.02	0.03	0.04	0.05	0.10
Model							
DOM	−6.83	−4.64	−3.69	−3.06	−2.60	−2.22	−1.07
REC	−7.67	−5.36	−4.19	−3.40	−2.80	−2.33	−0.91

**DOM indicates autosomal dominant transmission with a disease allele frequency of 0.008 and homozygote and heterozygote penetrance of 0.70; REC, autosomal recessive transmission with disease allele frequency of 0.10 and homozygote penetrance of 0.70. The affected phenotype is assumed to be the schizophrenia spectrum as defined by Wang et al.[1]*

Lower-Dose Therapy With Traditional Neuroleptics in Chronically Hospitalized Schizophrenic Patients

Several recent studies have shown that relatively low doses and low blood levels of neuroleptics are often as effective as high doses of these drugs both in the treatment of an acute exacerbation of schizophrenia[1-3] and in the maintenance treatment of stabilized outpatients with schizophrenia.[4,5] Yet, some patients with chronic schizophrenia or related disorders, hospitalized for extended periods, are treated with relatively high doses of neuroleptics for many years. The efficacy of low doses vs standard or high doses of traditional neuroleptics in this group of patients has not been extensively investigated and thus represents an important gap in the low-dose research and treatment strategy. This letter reports an attempt to address this important clinical question.

Patients and Methods. In the course of clinical management of a service of chronically psychotic female patients, a program of neuroleptic dosage reduction combined with quantitative monitoring of their psychopathologic condition was instituted. This report summarizes the results of 16 patients (mean age, 46.5 years; diagnoses: schizophrenia in 14, schizoaffective disorder in two) who had been hospitalized a mean of 11.5 years during their current hospitalization. Patients were clinically assessed monthly or bimonthly by both

standardized rating scales (Brief Psychiatric Rating Scale [BPRS], Scale for the Assessment of Positive Symptoms, Scale for the Assessment of Negative Symptoms) and a review of clinical notes and medications administered on an as needed (prn) basis in the patients' records. The number of patients taking different types of neuroleptics were as follows: decanoate, four; oral—high potency, four; oral—medium potency, five; oral—low potency (aliphatic), three. Patients were maintained on the same neuroleptic drug regimen, but the patients' doses of that neuroleptic were reduced by approximately one fifth to one third of the current dose every 1 or 2 months if the patient's psychopathological condition did not appreciably worsen. If an exacerbation of psychosis appeared that was persistent or very disorganizing, the neuroleptic dosage was temporarily increased and then lowered again as clinically feasible. If the patient was taking multiple psychotropic medications, the dosage of only one of the medications was altered at a time. Patients were followed up for a mean of 10.3 months (range, 5 to 14 months).

Results and Comment. The mean (±SD) initial neuroleptic dosage (chlorpromazine hydrochloride equivalents in milligrams per day) was 1290±305 and the final dosage was 437±291. The mean percent decrease in neuroleptic dosage at the last evaluation was 62% (range, 37% to 83%), and at the "best dose" (ie, the dose at which the patient achieved the lowest BPRS Psychosis score), it was 60%. In no patient did the BPRS total or psychosis factor (sum of thought disorder and hostility-suspiciousness factors) scores show a consistent increase during dosage reduction, although in some patients the scores fluctuated from month to month and showed transient increases in some months. Three patients showed a greater than 10-point fluctuation in their BPRS total scores in different months while receiving the same neuroleptic dose. Overall, at the best lower dose, there was a statistically significant reduction in BPRS and Scale for the Assessment of Positive Symptoms scores (**Table**). There was no significant increase in the administration of neuroleptics or benzodiazepines on a prn basis during the months of neuroleptic dose reduction. Only one patient had a slightly higher number of doses administered on a prn basis, and two other patients had a similar or decreased pattern of doses administered on a prn basis. Verbal complaints and clinical notes by mental health aides suggested that some patients were less cooperative with ward rules and staff directives, or were seen as more angry or transiently upset or agitated. However, as noted above, use of medication administered on a prn basis was not increased in these patients during low-dose treatment. Furthermore, clinical interview evaluations by two psychiatrists (R.C.S. and a colleague) did not confirm an increase in psychotic symptoms in most cases.

The results of our quantitative clinical monitoring suggest that some chronically hospitalized schizophrenic patients do not show increased psychopathological scores when treated with relatively low doses of neuroleptics, but rather they show small decreases in their psychotic symptoms. These results are consistent with the clinical observations of five patients reported by Cohen et al,[6] and 13 patients in a preliminary report by Kuehnel et al.[7] The latter group reported a similar reduction in dosage (66% decrease) but stated that there was no statistically significant change in either positive or negative symptoms (although no quantitative data were presented). The data presented here should be interpreted with caution because of the small number of patients and the clinical monitoring design. Two sources of potential bias are (1) the nonblind ratings of psychopathological status, and (2) the shorter length of time the patients were followed up compared with some previous studies. Some studies of lower-dose neuroleptics in maintenance therapy for outpatient schizophrenics have shown a substantial increase in exacerbation of symptoms and a slight in-

Changes in Neuroleptic Dose and Psychopathology Scores at Best and Final Doses*

	Absolute Change		% Change	
	Final Dose	Best Dose	Final Dose	Best Dose
Neuroleptic dose, chlorpromazine hydrochloride equivalents in milligrams per day	−778±625†	−668±435†	−62±14†	−60±13†
BPRS Total score	−3.2±6.3	−4.7±6.4‡	−8.0±14.7§	−12.6±15.0‡
BPRS Psychosis score	−2.8±3.8‡	−3.6±5.1‖	−14.0±22.3§	−19.4±23.8‡
SAPS Total score	−12.7±10.0†	−11.9±9.8‡	−32.9±29.5†	−35.6±31.3‡

Values are presented as mean±SD. Because of missing values, the N's of all the means are not 16: N (final dose)= 13-16; N (best dose)= 11-16. BPRS indicates Brief Psychiatric Rating Scale; SAPS, Scale for the Assessment of Positive Symptoms; best dose, dose at which patients achieved the lowest BPRS Psychosis score.

†P<.001, two-tailed paired t test.
‡P<.01, two-tailed paired t test.
§P<.05, two-tailed paired t test.
‖P<.02, two-tailed paired t test.

crease in relapse during the second year of treatment.[8] These preliminary findings suggest the need for more systematic studies that can address these questions.

Robert C. Smith, MD, PhD
Department of Psychiatry
NYU Medical School and
Manhattan Psychiatric Center
PO Box 316
Hewlett, NY 11557

1. Baldessarni RJ, Cohen BM, Teicher MH. Significance of neuroleptic dose and plasma level in the pharmacological treatment of psychoses. *Arch Gen Psychiatry*. 1988;45:79-91.
2. Rifkin A, Doddi S, Karajgi B, Waschspress M. Dose of haloperidol for schizophrenia. *Arch Gen Psychiatry*. 1991;48:166-170.
3. McEnvoy JP, Hogarty GE, Steingrad S. Optimal dose of neuroleptic in acute schizophrenia. *Arch Gen Psychiatry*. 1991;48:739-745.
4. Schooler, NR. Maintenance medication for schizophrenia: strategies for dose reduction. *Schizophr Bull*. 1991;17:311-324.
5. Burnett PL, Galley CA, Moyke RJ, Clark CR. Low-dose depot medication in schizophrenia. *Schizophr Bull*. 1993;19:155-164.
6. Cohen BM, Benes FM, Baldessarini RJ. Atypical neuroleptics, dose-response relationships, and treatment-resistant psychosis. *Arch Gen Psychiatry*. 1989;46:381-383.
7. Kuehnel TG, Liberman RP, Marshall BD, Bowen L. Optimal drug and behavior therapy for treatment-refractory institutionalized schizophrenics. In: Liberman RP, ed. *Effective Psychiatric Rehabilitation, New Directions for Mental Health Services*. San Francisco, Calif: Jossey-Bass; 1992;53:67-77.
8. Marder SR, Van Putten T, Mintz J, Lebell M. Low and conventional-dose maintenance therapy with fluphenazine decanoate: two-year outcome. *Arch Gen Psychiatry*. 1987;44:518-521.

Correction and Amplification

In reexamining the data on comorbidity from the Puerto Rico Child Psychiatry Epidemiologic Study that appeared in the December 1988 issue of the ARCHIVES, we have discovered an error in Table 5 (page 1124) of that article[1] in the number of children reported as having anxiety disorders. Because of a computer programming error, only those with separation anxiety disorder and phobias (n=18) were originally included as having anxiety disorders on this table. Fifteen children with other anxiety disorders had been left out (correct total, n=96). A revised **Table** appears here.

Comorbidity of Four Diagnostic Domains*

	Weighted, % (Unweighted, n)			
	Affective	Conduct/ Oppositional	ADD	Anxiety
Affective	. . . (60)	51.7 (27)	30.7 (18)	35.9 (23)
Conduct/ oppositional	23.9 (27)	. . . (118)	44.7 (55)	36.9 (39)
ADD	17.0 (18)	53.6 (55)	. . . (96)	25.3 (27)
Anxiety	16.5 (23)	36.8 (39)	21.0 (27)	. . . (96)

**ADD indicates attention deficit disorder.*

For the same reason, the overall comorbidity rates appearing in the text on page 1124 of the article were also misstated. Of the 265 children who were classified as having one or more *DSM-III* diagnoses, 221 (rather than 215) fell into one or more of the supraordinate domains of psychopathology. Of those, 48.9% (53.2% weighted) fell into only one domain, whereas the remaining 51.1% (46.8% weighted) fell into two or more domains. Except for the comorbidity rates for anxiety disorders and the numbers of children with the anxiety disorder comorbid combinations appearing on the diagram on page 1125, no other data reported in the article were affected. We regret this error and any inconvenience that it may have caused the reader.

Hector R. Bird, MD
Department of Psychiatry
Columbia University
New York, NY 10032

1. Bird HR, Canino G, Rubio-Stipec M, et al. Estimates of the prevalence of childhood maladjustment in a community survey in Puerto Rico. *Arch Gen Psychiatry*. 1988;45:1120-1126.

Alcohol Dependence May Be the Missing Link Between Posttraumatic Stress Disorder and Panic

In their article, Southwick et al[1] did not discuss the ramifications of the high rate (85%) of lifetime alcohol dependence in their subjects. They concluded that posttraumatic stress disorder (PTSD) and panic disorder may "share a common neurobiological abnormality that is related to altered sensitivity of the noradrenergic system."[1] However, the authors did not mention what impact alcohol dependence might have on panic disorder or on the noradrenergic system.

In a review of the relationship between alcohol problems and anxiety disorders, it was suggested that symptoms of panic disorder often result from, rather than cause, problem drinking.[2] Kushner et al[2] speculated that the cumulative effects of alcohol withdrawal (autonomic nervous system hyperexcitability), toxic effects of long-term alcohol use, and negative alcohol-related consequences (social, legal, and interpersonal) may trigger symptoms of panic disorder. It has also been proposed that the chemical and cognitive changes from repeated alcohol withdrawals may kindle panic attacks.[3] The "chemical changes" referred to included sympathetic (noradrenergic) nervous system activation from alcohol withdrawal and acute effects of alcohol on functioning of norepinephrine.

Therefore, it is reasonable to consider the ramifications of a high rate of alcohol dependence in subjects with-

PTSD, panic disorder, and abnormal noradrenergic function. Perhaps alcohol dependence will prove that "common neurobiological abnormality related to altered sensitivity of the noradrenergic system"[1] of patients with PTSD and panic disorder.

Eve J. Wiseman, MD
Special Treatment Section
John L. McClellan Memorial Veterans Affairs Hospital
4300 W 7th St, Slot 116-E
Little Rock, AR 72205

1. Southwick SM, Krystal JH, Morgan CA, Johnson D, Nagy LM, Nicolaou A, Heninger GR, Charney DS. Abnormal noradrenergic function in posttraumatic stress disorder. *Arch Gen Psychiatry.* 1993;50:266-274.
2. Kushner MG, Sher KJ, Beitman BD. The relation between alcohol problems and anxiety disorders. *Am J Psychiatry.* 1990;147:685-695.
3. George DT, Nutt DJ, Dwyer BA, Linnoila M. Alcoholism and panic disorder: is the comorbidity more than coincidence? *Acta Psychiatr Scand.* 1990;81: 97-107.

In reply

We appreciate Dr Wiseman's effort to highlight the possible neurobiological significance of substance abuse for patients with PTSD and panic disorder. Similar to the clinical reports on patients with panic disorder that she cited, we and others previously described cases in which acute alcohol or opiate withdrawal exacerbated PTSD symptoms in dually diagnosed patients.[1,2]

The hypothesis that activation of noradrenergic systems might increase panic or PTSD symptoms was studied in a series of investigations using the α_2*-adrenergic antagonist, yohimbine. We found that this drug elicited panic attacks in some patients with panic disorder and PTSD, but not in healthy subjects or patients with other major psychiatric disorders including generalized anxiety disorder, major depression, and schizophrenia.*[3,4]

While it is likely that the cycle of alcohol consumption and withdrawal affects the course of panic disorder and PTSD, there is little evidence to support the hypothesis that subacute alcohol withdrawal produces a vulnerability to yohimbine-induced panic attacks. We directly studied this question by evaluating the reactivity to yohimbine (0.4 mg/kg administered intravenously over 10 minutes under double-blind placebo-controlled conditions) in healthy subjects (n=15) and alcoholic patients (n=22, studied 12 to 26 days after their last drink) who did not meet diagnostic criteria for PTSD or panic disorder.[5] *Preliminary data analyses suggested that there was a nonsignificant trend for increased anxiety levels following yohimbine administration relative to placebo but that patients did not show increased anxiogenic responses compared with healthy subjects. Also, yohimbine did not precipitate panic attacks in the patient group.*

Dr Wiseman cites evidence of subacute or long-term effects of alcoholism on noradrenergic regulation. One cannot rule out the possibility that the sensitization of noradrenergic systems by long-term alcoholism might be found only in alcoholic patients with comorbid panic disorders, a group excluded from the study described here. However, the failure of yohimbine to precipitate panic attacks in recently detoxified alcoholics suggests that yohimbine-induced panic attacks in patients with panic disorder or PTSD reflect the pathophysiologic characteristics of these disorders rather than the effects of comorbid alcohol abuse.

John H. Krystal, MD
National Center for Posttraumatic Stress Disorder
West Haven Veterans' Affairs Medical Center
West Haven, CT 06516
Steven M. Southwick, MD
Dennis S. Charney, MD
West Haven

1. Kosten TR, Krystal JH. Biological mechanisms in post traumatic stress disorder: relevance for substance abuse. In: Galanter M, ed. *Recent Developments in Alcoholism.* New York, NY: Plenum Press; 1988;6:49-68.
2. Salloway S, Southwick S, Sadowsky M. Opiate withdrawal presenting as posttraumatic stress disorder: a case of malingering following the L-Ambiance Plaza Building disaster. *Hosp Comm Psychiatry.* 1990;41:666-667.
3. Charney DS, Woods SW, Price LH, Goodman WK, Glazer WM, Heninger GR. Specificity of noradrenergic dysregulation in panic disorder. In: Belmaker RH, Sandler M, Dahlstrom A, eds. *Progress in Catecholamine Research, Part C: Clinical Aspects.* New York, NY: Alan R. Liss Inc; 1988:343-347.
4. Southwick SM, Krystal JH, Morgan CA, Johnson D, Nagy LM, Nicolaou A, Heninger GR, Charney DS. Abnormal noradrenergic function in posttraumatic stress disorder. *Arch Gen Psychiatry.* 1993;50:266-274.
5. Krystal JH, Webb E, Kranzler H, Cooney N, Southwick S, Heninger GR, Charney DS. Yohimbine and MCPP effects in alcoholics and healthy subjects. *Alcoholism: Clin Exp Res.* 1992;16:234.

Familial Obsessive-Compulsive Disorder Presenting as Pathological Jealousy Successfully Treated With Fluoxetine

Pathological jealousy in some patients is hypothesized as a variant of obsessive-compulsive disorder (OCD).[1] A patient is presented herein who belonged to a pedigree of multiply affected members, suffered from pathological jealousy and features of OCD, and responded successfully to treatment with high-dose fluoxetine hydrochloride.

A 36-year-old twice-married woman presented in 1990 suffering from marital problems. Previous assessments noted the presence of pathological jealousy with no additional diagnosis given. She reported anxiety when she was separated from her husband, obsessional fears of his infidelity, and an obsessional thought that he was being unfaithful. These symptoms, evident 15 years ago during her first marriage, were more severe since her second marriage in 1986.

A family history revealed three relatives reported as having excessive jealousy to a degree that affected social relationships. Her maternal grandmother would cut out all the pictures of women from any literature to prevent

her husband from seeing them, moved their household several times to prevent the feared infidelity, and was described as obsessionally tidy. The patient's mother was excessively jealous of her partners. She displayed a need for correctness and symmetry and was preoccupied with her health. Her maternal uncle refused to let his wife out of his sight and was convinced she was attracted to other men.

Other members of the family exhibited more common features of OCD. Her son was obsessionally tidy and suffered from fear of contamination. Her daughter had a compulsive need to tell and ask, was excessively concerned with illness, and engaged in repeated examinations of her body. Her brother was often anxious and preoccupied with his health.

At the initial interview, the patient had a comorbid diagnosis of dysthymic disorder and was started on therapy with fluoxetine hydrochloride (20 mg, every day). She then failed to return to outpatient facilities for 13 months.

On her return to the clinic, her symptoms persisted. She viewed these thoughts as irrational and senseless and resisted them unsuccessfully. These ideas never became delusional in nature and were acted on in an attempt to reduce anxiety. She exhibited a compulsion to ask her husband repeatedly if he had been unfaithful, and her day was dominated by behaviors to investigate this. For example, she would take all the phones out of the house when she was away to prevent her husband from calling another woman. She would mark his penis with a pen and examine it later to see if it had been touched. She would accompany her husband to work and stay in the car for hours at a time to stop any possible illicit liaison. While at home, she forbade him to look out of the curtains, which were perpetually drawn.

Other features of OCD were prominent, including a fear of harming others, intrusive violent images, perverse sexual thoughts and nonsense words, an excessive concern with morality, an excessive concern about illness and disease, counting compulsions, rereading and rewriting, onychophagia, and compulsive picking of her toenails.

She reported a lifting of her mood during her previous 6 weeks of treatment with 20 mg of fluoxetine hydrochloride every day but no change in her other symptoms. She was prescribed fluoxetine hydrochloride at a dose of up to 60 mg every day, but severe anxiety developed above 40 mg/d. She received 20 mg/d for 2 weeks and 40 mg/d for 6 weeks. She then reported a marked decrease in her symptoms. In particular, her obsessional fear and thoughts of her husband's infidelity had almost completely subsided with only an occasional questioning remark made to him. She no longer engaged in compulsive behavior to alleviate her anxiety. Her other features of OCD also remitted with only moderate onychophagia still remaining. She remains well at 9 months' follow-up.

This case illustrates several points of note. The history of pathological jealousy in this pedigree with other features of OCD supports the belief that the syndrome of pathological jealousy is in some people a variant of OCD. This belief is strengthened by this patient's need for a higher dose of fluoxetine to ameliorate her symptoms, which is similar to other reported cases of OCD.[2] Finally, this pedigree shows that pathological jealousy can exist as a familial disorder and that there may well be a genetic component operating as a prominent etiologic factor.

Simon Wright, MB, ChB, MRCPsych
Department of Psychiatry
Northern General Hospital
Sheffield S5 7AU, England

1. Rasmussen SA, Eisen LE. The epidemiology and differential diagnosis of obsessive compulsive disorder. *J Clin Psychiatry.* 1992;53(suppl):4-10.
2. Frenkel A, Rosenthal J, Nezu A, Winston A. Efficacy of long-term fluoxetine treatment of obsessive-compulsive disorder. *Mt Sinai J Med.* 1990;57:349-352.

Biologic Theories of Sexual Orientation

In their review of the literature concerning biologic theories of human sexual orientation, Byne and Parsons[1] overlooked some issues of relevance. Biologic theories can account for the feelings that motivate behaviors; the behaviors themselves will be strongly determined by environmental factors—in the case of sexual orientation such factors as available opportunities and social and legal sanctions. A number of men who identify and express their sexuality mainly or exclusively as heterosexual report strong or predominant homosexual feelings.[2] In a US national probability sample, 14% of men considered homosexual sex offered them some possibility of enjoyment and 12% of men considered that heterosexual sex offered them none.[3] Yet, only 6.7% of the men reported homosexual contacts resulting in orgasm after age 19 years, and in half of these, the contacts were rare.[4] Contrary to the statement by Byne and Parsons[1(p229)] concerning "the pattern of essentially exclusive male homosexuality familiar to us," the majority of self-identified male and female homosexuals give a history of heterosexual romantic attachments and arousal.[2] Investigations of subjects identified as homosexual based on their behavior rather than their ratio of sexual interest in males vs females will minimize the possibility of demonstrating biologic influences.

Byne and Parsons[1] suggested that a biologic model could not account for findings that although

child hood gender nonconformity is shown by a greater proportion of identified homosexual than heterosexual men, it is not shown by all homosexual men and is shown by some heterosexual men. Studies were overlooked that found relationships in men aware of predominant heterosexual feelings between the degrees of their childhood gender nonconformity and ratios of homosexual to heterosexual feelings.[5] This finding would be predicted by the biologic model, postulating that both variables are influenced by the ratio of same- to opposite-sex hormones to which individuals are exposed at critical periods in brain development in utero. Most people would show minimal changes from the hormone ratio producing exclusive heterosexual feelings and gender conformity, with an increasingly small proportion experiencing greater changes. This model, but not the common psychological model that homosexuality is due to a fear of heterosexuality, accounts for the consistent finding that most subjects who are aware of homosexual feelings are also aware of predominant heterosexual feelings.[2]

In considering a biologic influence on sexual orientation incompatible with findings of a large proportion of monozygotic twins discordant for homosexuality, Byne and Parsons incorrectly considered that monozygotic twins share the same prenatal environment. A discussion[6] of monozygotic twins discordant for homosexual feelings pointed out that the increased risk of fetal death and congenital malformations in monozygotic compared with dizygotic twins could be attributed at least in part to the 15% to 30% of monochorial twins with transfusion syndrome. In this syndrome, blood is shunted from one twin to the other so that it differentially stresses the two members of the monozygotic twinship and could produce differences in their prenatal hormonal balance.

Nathaniel McConaghy, DSc, MD
School of Psychiatry
University of New South Wales
Anzac Parade
PO Box 1
Kensington, New South Wales, Australia 2033

1. Byne W, Parsons B. Human sexual orientation: the biologic theories reappraised. *Arch Gen Psychiatry*. 1993;50:228-239.
2. McConaghy N. *Sexual Behavior: Problems and Management*. New York, NY: Plenum Press; 1993:103-129.
3. Klassen AD, Williams CJ, Levitt EE. *Sex and Morality in the U.S.* Middletown, Conn: Wesleyan University Press; 1989:419.
4. Fay RE, Turner CF, Klassen AD, Gagnon JH. Prevalence and patterns of same-gender sexual contact among men. *Science*. 1989;243:338-348.
5. McConaghy N, Silove D. Opposite sex behaviors correlate with degree of homosexual feeling in the predominantly heterosexual. *Aust N Z J Psychiatry*. 1991;25:77-83.
6. McConaghy N, Blaszczynski A. A pair of monozygotic twins discordant for homosexuality: sex-dimorphic behavior and penile volume responses. *Arch Sex Behav*. 1980;9:123-131.

Theories of Sexual Orientation: A Reappraisal

The article by Byne and Parsons[1] in the March 1993 issue of the ARCHIVES proposed an interesting "interactionist model" of sexual orientation after a thorough review of the biologic research in this area. While they criticized the biologists (and to a much lesser degree the psychosocial theories) for not integrating the two theoretical approaches, they too seem to be inflexible for not allowing for the possibility that not all homosexual individuals need to necessarily fit into one model.

Inconsistencies in the data may be reflective of different subpopulations of homosexuals, some whose sexual orientation may be only biologically determined, some only psychosocially determined, and some who are better described by an interactionist model.

We agree with their statement that it is imperative to "resist the urge to search for simplistic explanations,"[1(p236)] and stress the need to be flexible when considering the determinants of sexual orientation for any one individual—a point also relevant to clinical work. Because the topic of homosexuality is emotionally charged, there may be a tendency to try to package all homosexual behavior into one model (even if it permits interactions among other models). Allowance for individual variation would do well for a field where the bias among the workers is also varied and where the data are still inconclusive.

Douglas Berger, MD
Hiroyuki Suematsu, MD
Department of Psychosomatic Medicine
Tokyo University Branch Hospital
3-28-6 Mejirodai, Bunkyo-ku
Tokyo, Japan 112
Yutaka Ono, MD
Department of Psychiatry
Keio University
Tokyo

1. Byne W, Parsons B. Human sexual orientation: the biologic theories reappraised. *Arch Gen Psychiatry*. 1993;50:228-239.

In reply

As biological psychiatrists, we believe that everything we do, think, or feel has an ultimate biological substrate. Although we are interested in delimiting these substrates and their interactions with experiential factors, we realize that if we are to progress in this endeavor, we must rigorously question our methods and our data, as well as our hypotheses and the assumptions on which they rest. Unfortunately, one cannot offer constructive criticism of the bio-

logical theories of sexual orientation without being perceived by some as rejecting the hypothesis that biology plays any role.

We did not, as McConaghy concludes, consider "a biological influence on sexual orientation incompatible with findings of a large proportion of monozygotic twins discordant for homosexuality." Our conclusion was that, while genes are not irrelevant, "the large proportion of discordant pairs undersciores our ignorance of the factors that are involved . . . in the emergence of sexual orientation."[1(p230)] *Logically, the* as yet unknown *factors could turn out to be biological, psychosocial, or both. Similarly, we did not imply that the prenatal uterine environments of identical twins are identical, as McConaghy suggests we did. Moreover, we merely pointed out that "any model" for the development of sexual orientation must be able to account for adult heterosexuals with histories of childhood gender nonconformity as well as for adult homosexuals with gender-typical childhood histories. This applies equally to biological, psychosocial, and interactional models and does not, as McConaghy suggests, challenge the notion of a biological contribution.*

While McConaghy is correct that the majority of self-identified homosexuals give a history of heterosexual attachments and arousal, he fails to mention that such experiences are often limited to their early sexual explorations. We certainly do not endorse, nor did we even mention in our article, the model that homosexuality is due to fear of heterosexuality. It is surprising that McConaghy should introduce that model in the present context.

McConaghy's emphasis on feelings of sexual attraction is well placed; however, biology need not "determine" such feelings to influence sexual orientation. Our interactional model poses a plausible alternative in which the influence of biological factors would be exerted on temperamental variables rather than on sexual orientation per se. Acting through psychodynamic processes in a context-dependent manner, temperament would then influence the objective and subjective aspects of familial and peer relationships that contribute to the development of sexual attractions and orientation. Most important, this interactional model addresses the genesis of feelings of sexual attraction. The environmental impact would not, as McConaghy suggests, merely influence whether one chooses to act on particular biologically determined attractions.

We fully agree with the concerns of Berger et al regarding the heterogeneity of homosexuality. Our interactional model was intended only to illustrate that biological factors could conceivably influence sexual orientation indirectly through an influence on temperament rather than in the direct manner by which hormones act on the developing rodent brain to determine whether the adult will display predominantly male-typical or female-typical motor patterns of copulation. We certainly did not want to suggest a single origin of homosexuality. In fact, we commented on "numerous patterns of homosexuality" and suggested that our model would allow for multiple developmental pathways.

It seems implausible to us that any mental phenomenon as complex and as socially embedded as sexual orientation could be "only biologically determined" as Berger et al suggest may be the case for some individuals. Moreover, we suggest that in speaking of "determinants" rather than of "influences," they may unwittingly be perpetuating the simplistic explanations their letter criticizes.

William Byne, MD, PhD
Albert Einstein College of Medicine
Department of Pathology
Bronx, NY 10461

Bruce Parsons, MD, PhD
Department of Psychiatry
Columbia University
College of Physicians and Surgeons
New York, NY

1. Byne W, Parsons B. Human sexual orientation: the biologic theories reappraised. *Arch Gen Psychiatry.* 1993;50:228-239.

The Panicogenic Effects of Cholecystokinin-Tetrapeptide Are Antagonized by L-365,260, a Central Cholecystokinin Receptor Antagonist, in Patients With Panic Disorder 486
Jacques Bradwejn, MD, FRCPC; Diana Koszycki, MA; Anne Couëtoux du Tertre, MD; Harold van Megen, MD; Johan den Boer, MD; Herman Westenberg, PhD; Lawrence Annable, DipStat

Increased Density of Guanine Nucleotide–Binding Proteins in the Postmortem Brains of Heroin Addicts 494
Pablo V. Escriba, PhD; Magdalena Sastre, PhD; Jesús A. García-Sevilla, MD

Letters to the Editor

Lithium Prophylaxis in American Patients With Unipolar Disorder 502
Mogens Schou, MD

In Reply 502
Mitchell S. Nobler, MD, Harold A. Sackeim, PhD

Maintenance Therapy in Depression 503
Gary J. Barnes, FRANZCP, Quentin Jones

In Reply 504
Ellen Frank, PhD, David J. Kupfer, MD

Klein's Suffocation Theory of Panic 505
Steven Taylor, PhD, S. Rachman, PhD

In Reply 506
Donald F. Klein, MD

Departments

Classified Advertising 508

Instructions for Authors—See January 1994 issue, page 6.

ARCHIVES OF GENERAL PSYCHIATRY

ORIGINAL ARTICLE

Mental Illness in the Biological and Adoptive Relatives of Schizophrenic Adoptees

Replication of the Copenhagen Study in the Rest of Denmark

Seymour S. Kety, MD; Paul H. Wender, MD; Bjørn Jacobsen, MD; Loring J. Ingraham, PhD; Lennart Jansson, MD; Britta Faber, MD; Dennis K. Kinney, PhD

Background: Our previous investigation of the prevalence of mental illness among the biological and adoptive relatives of schizophrenic adoptees in Copenhagen, Denmark, showed a significant concentration of chronic schizophrenia (5.6%) and what Bleuler called "latent schizophrenia" (14.8%) in the biological relatives of chronic schizophrenic adoptees, indicating the operation of heritable factors in the liability for schizophrenic illness.

Methods: We now report the results of a replication of that study in the rest of Denmark (the "Provincial Sample").

Results: In this sample, the corresponding prevalences were 4.7% and 8.2%. In the combined "National Sample" of adoptees with chronic schizophrenia, that disorder was found exclusively in their biological relatives and its prevalence overall was 10 times greater than that in the biological relatives of controls.

Conclusions: This study and its confirmation of previous results in the Copenhagen Study speak for a syndrome that can be reliably recognized in which genetic factors play a significant etiologic role. These findings provide important and necessary support for the assumption often made in family studies: observed familial clustering in schizophrenia is an expression of shared genetic factors.

(Arch Gen Psychiatry. 1994;51:442-455)

From the Laboratory of Psychology and Psychopathology, Intramural Research Program, National Institute of Mental Health, Bethesda, Md (Drs Kety and Ingraham); the Department of Psychiatry, University of Utah, Salt Lake City (Dr Wender); the Institute of Preventative Medicine, Kommunehospitalet, Copenhagen, Denmark (Dr Jacobsen); Hvidovre Hospital, Hvidovre, Denmark (Dr Jansson); Hospitalet Fjorden, Roskilde, Denmark (Dr Faber); and the Mailman Research Center, McLean Hospital, Harvard University, Belmont, Mass (Dr Kinney).

David Rosenthal, PhD, formerly Chief of the Laboratory of Psychology and Psychopathology, Intramural Research Program, National Institute of Mental Health, was a major contributor at the beginning of this study; illness prevented his continued participation.

THE TENDENCY displayed by several of the psychiatric syndromes to occur in other members of the patient's family has been recognized since these syndromes were first described and has been used variously to support genetic or environmental inferences of origin. To what extent the symptoms, syndromes, and diagnoses in the natural relatives of patients reared together are affected by genetic or environmental factors, enhanced in frequency by ascertainment and subjective bias, and molded or confounded by the relatives' close association with the patient, is difficult to specify, leaving conclusions regarding origin indeterminate and controversial. Where adoption has separated the genetic and familial environmental influences, they can more readily be differentiated and evaluated. Mental disorders, when they occur in the adoptee and some of the biological relatives, have developed independently and can be ascertained and diagnosed without interference from relatives' behavior or diagnosis. An increased prevalence of the disorder or one of the characteristics that constitute it in the biological or adoptive relatives when compared with suitable matched control groups would be compatible with the operation in them of genetic or family-associated environmental factors, respectively.

In 1963 a compilation of adoptees was begun in Denmark designed to provide the basis for an examination of the prevalence of schizophrenia in the nuclear biological and adoptive families of individuals adopted at an early age who eventually developed schizophrenia.[1] To our knowledge, adoption strategies had not been applied previously to the problem of schizophrenia and it seemed likely that

See Methods on next page

METHODS

Completion of the adoption register for the remainder of Denmark (the Provincial Sample), selection of probands, gathering of clinical information, and analysis of results proceeded in a manner similar to that involved in the Copenhagen Sample,[1] and it began with a search of the records of the Department of Justice that documents every legal adoption. The compilation of the Provincial Sample, designed to complete the national sample, started with a chronological search of the department's records from 1924 through 1947, and included every adoption granted by the courts outside of the city and county of Copenhagen to others than biological relatives of the adoptee, for a total of 8944 adoptees. (The Copenhagen Sample, selected earlier, had comprised 5483 adoptees, for a combined total for Denmark of 14 427.) The name, sex, and birth date of the adoptee were recorded and a code number was assigned that served to identify the adoptee, rather than the name, through subsequent processing. The same demographic information with the inclusion of occupation was recorded for the biological and adoptive parents, usually the father, and, for adoptive parents, their income and financial status around the time of the adoption.

STUDY OF THE PROVINCIAL SAMPLE BASED ON INSTITUTIONAL RECORDS

To identify the adoptees who had developed schizophrenia (the "index" adoptees), a search was made of the National Psychiatric Register and of individual hospital files for those adoptees who had ever been admitted to a mental hospital or psychiatric service of a general hospital. All of these facilities are part of the National Health Insurance system and report, with rare exceptions, to the Psychiatric Register, maintained by Eric Stromgren and Annalise Dupont at the Institute of Psychiatric Demography in Risskov, Denmark. The experience in Copenhagen indicated that about 95% of admissions to psychiatric facilities would thus be recovered.[1] The dates of hospital admission and discharge and each hospital discharge diagnosis were recorded. Where the information was compatible with the possibility that the subject's disorder was schizophrenia, an abstract of the institutional records was prepared in English by a Danish psychiatrist and edited to remove any family-related information.

Independent diagnoses were made by three raters in America (S.S.K., P.H.W., D. Rosenthal, PhD), who then conferred to formulate a consensus diagnosis of schizophrenic or nonschizophrenic disorder according to an agreed-on set of criteria for chronic, latent, and acute schizophrenia or for other diagnoses, based on the descriptions of Bleuler[9] and the *Diagnostic Manual* then in use in the United States (*DSM-II*[10]). This yielded 41 presumptive index adoptees with preliminary diagnoses of chronic, latent, or acute schizophrenia, based only on the Psychiatric Register and abstracts of hospital records.

To arrive at an estimate of the prevalence of schizophrenia and other diagnoses that would result from the application of our search and diagnostic techniques in the populations of biological and adoptive relatives of adoptees without mental illness in this sample, presumptive controls were chosen who had no record of admission to a psychiatric facility.[1] From a group of four or five such adoptees who approximated each index adoptee in age, sex, and socioeconomic class of the adoptive family, one was selected who most closely matched the index proband in time spent with a biological parent and in placement before transfer to adoptive parents, as well as the time of that transfer. Time spent with biological parents was generally short, with a mean of 5 weeks and a median of 1 week; index and control probands did not differ significantly in time spent with biological parents before placement. Since later interviews indicated that individuals with no history of psychiatric hospitalization were not necessarily free of current or past mental illness, the final controls comprised only those who were interviewed and found to be free of affective or schizophrenic spectrum disorders, current or past. Screening control probands for diagnoses other than those by which index probands are selected introduces a possible bias toward the observation of an excess of screened disorders among the biological relatives of the unscreened index probands, which may be incorrectly interpreted as evidence for coaggregation among disorders.[11] In the present study, eliminating control probands with diagnoses other than chronic schizophrenia introduces a potential bias toward observation of coaggregation of these disorders among the relatives of index probands with chronic schizophrenia who were not screened for the presence of latent schizophrenia or nonbipolar affective disorder. However, screening control probands allows more accurate estimation of the magnitude of risk for chronic schizophrenia in the biological relatives of controls.

Identification of relatives proceeded through the adoption and population registers as was the case with the Copenhagen Study. The adoption records identified the adoptive parents and the biological mother and putative biological father. Confidence in the latter information was enhanced by the requirement that the mother name the father and that he contribute to the costs of maternity care and the adoption process. In one instance the biological mother named two putative fathers and it was decided that the more conservative choice, made blindly, was to include both and their offspring, if any, in the subsequent analyses.

Offspring of the biological and adoptive parents were then identified through the Folkeregister, a remarkably comprehensive population register, which lists for each resident the present and all previous home addresses and members of the household, thus permitting the identification of siblings and half-siblings of the proband, both biological and adoptive, and often, the other biological parent in the case of half-siblings. The dates of death or emigration of any of the relatives were also noted.

Continued on next page

DIAGNOSES IN RELATIVES BASED ON ABSTRACTS OF HOSPITAL RECORDS

The Psychiatric Register was then searched for admission of any relative to a psychiatric facility, and an English abstract was prepared from the institutional record and edited to remove any information regarding relationship to an index or control proband. Military or police records that had been searched in the Copenhagen Study had not yielded sufficient new information to warrant their continued use. The edited abstracts were read by three raters (S.S.K., P.H.W., and D. Rosenthal, PhD) in the United States, who made blind independent diagnoses, followed by consensus diagnoses. Agreement among raters' independent diaqnoses of schizophrenia, latent schizophrenia, acute schizophrenia, or other diagnosis in probands and relatives ranged from κ=0.71 to κ=0.77 by the κ statistic of Cohen.[12] These were the basis of a preliminary report on the Provincial Sample, based only on institutional records, which appeared in 1978.[13]

THE PSYCHIATRIC INTERVIEWS

Experience with the Copenhagen Sample indicated the desirability of augmenting the clinical information available on probands and relatives in the sample through careful follow-up and extensive personal interviews.[2] Nearly 90% of the relatives alive and known to be residing in Denmark or a neighboring Scandinavian country agreed to participate in a personal interview by a physician. Initial contact was through a letter to each living relative residing in Denmark, Norway, or Sweden, which if not answered was followed by a telephone call or visit by one of us (B.J.). The detailed interview was usually conducted in the subject's home and lasted from 1 to sometimes more than 3 hours. In the 6% to 9% of available relatives who refused to be interviewed, the circumstances surrounding the refusal and information from the subject prior to refusal were reported. In one instance the information was sufficient for the raters to make a blind diagnosis that was included in the analyses. All of the control adoptees and those index adoptees who were not in hospital were included, without being identified as such, among those asked to participate in an interview, and a large majority did so. The distribution of subjects who were interviewed, who refused to participate, who died prior to the study, or who were unavailable for follow-up is presented in **Table 1**.

Refusals were distributed nonsystematically among groups, but a greater proportion of adoptive relatives (both index and control) had died, reflecting older adoptive and younger biological parents. The smaller number of adoptive relatives compared with biological relatives also reflects the smaller size of adopting families. These observations duplicate those found in the Copenhagen Study.[2]

The structured interviews and hospital record summaries were more comprehensive than the Schedule for Affective Disorders and Schizophrenia–Lifetime version (SADS-L),[14] which had become available by that time, extending to 40 or more pages with numerous checklists and extensive narrative elaborations, designed to elicit information on a complete range of medical, psychological, and psychiatric symptoms and manifestations, particularly those that had been described in the literature for schizophrenia and schizophrenialike syndromes. The questions covered the major aspects of the life experience: sociological, interpersonal, educational, occupational, and marital; peer relationships; medical background; and a careful mental status examination. The observations were recorded in English soon after the interview and transcribed. The standard Schedule for Affective Disorders and Schizophrenia–Lifetime version questionnaire (in Danish) was also completed as were various notations of cognitive ability, verbal activity, and social functioning.

The interviews were conducted by one of the authors (L.J. or B.F.), psychiatrists trained in Copenhagen by interviewing patients on the ward to achieve reliable ratings, and who periodically met to ensure that reliability was maintained. The interviewers, when the interview began, did not know whether the subject was a proband or relative, index or control, biological or adoptive, or what relationship to a proband, and did not raise the issues of adoption or of mental illness in the subject's family. If the subject gave such unsolicited information, however, the semistructured interview required that it be noted in a particular place on the interview form. This, as well as other potentially biasing information, was deleted from copies of the interviews that were used for diagnosis. For every index proband, in addition to the original abstract of institutional records, more exhaustive summaries of these records were prepared on forms similar to the interview forms and were edited in the same manner. These were recognized as those of presumptive index probands, although which proband and the relationship to other subjects remained unknown. These as well as the edited interview transcripts were then read by

schizophrenic adoptees who shared their genetic endowment with their biological relatives but their family environment with others would make it possible to disentangle the genetic from the family-related environmental influences. The goal was a maximal national sample in which ascertainment of illness was based on exhaustive surveys of total population groups with the expectation that such a sample would provide an adequate number of schizophrenic probands with a minimum of ascertainment bias. If, in addition, diagnoses in probands and relatives were made without knowledge of their relationship, subjective bias would also be minimized.

Demographically matched controls who had no history of psychiatric hospitalization and appeared free of significant mental illness on interview were selected from the adoption register to arrive at an estimate of the prevalence of schizophrenia and other diagnoses that would result from the application of the same search and diagnostic techniques in the relatives of adoptees without mental illness in this sample. The probands were adults who

two of the American authors (S.S.K. and P.H.W.), who made independent global diagnoses. The raters' independent diagnoses of the interviews agreed moderately well (κ=0.68) for the diagnoses of chronic schizophrenia, latent schizophrenia, acute schizophrenia, or other and no diagnosis. Following independent diagnoses, the raters conferred and made a consensus interview diagnosis for each subject.

A final comprehensive diagnosis was arrived at for probands and relatives, based on all of the consensus diagnoses made from abstracts and summaries of institutional records, refusal reports, and psychiatric interviews conducted without knowledge of the identity or relationship of any subject to another. In previous reports we have presented results based on hospital records and psychiatric interviews separately; in the present study we have based our diagnoses on a final comprehensive diagnosis for each individual.

DIAGNOSTIC CRITERIA

Diagnoses, as in the case of the Copenhagen Study, represented global judgments based on symptom clusters described by Kraepelin[15] for dementia praecox and by Bleuler[9] for schizophrenia, less clearly demarcated by him for latent schizophrenia, and on the succinct encapsulations of *DSM-II*[10] for these and cognate disorders. Certain minor modifications evolved in our criteria or in their use after the earlier studies. These included a decreased utilization of the *DSM-II* diagnoses "acute schizophrenia" or "pseudoneurotic schizophrenia," probably because of their infrequency and lack of association with schizophrenia in the Copenhagen Study. There was also the recognition that the distinction between chronic and "latent" schizophrenia was demonstrable and significant for these diagnoses, whereas that between "definite" and "uncertain" or "probable" was not. Since classical schizophrenia and latent schizophrenia were to become the only forms of schizophrenic illness to be identified as such, there was no longer a need to characterize the former as "chronic." The diagnosis "schizoaffective" was rarely used since adherence to the classic descriptions of schizophrenia and manic-depressive disorder diminished its applicability. This was borne out by the independent *DSM-III* ratings on the Copenhagen interviews,[16] where the separate proband grouping of "schizoaffective, mainly schizophrenic" could not be differentiated from "schizophrenia" in the prevalence of schizophrenic illness in the results.

The negative features of schizophrenia and traits similar to them continued to play a major role in the characterization of schizophrenia and latent schizophrenia, and when they were present, affective disturbances were not exclusionary, in conformity with the following argument of Bleuler[9(p304)]: "All the phenomena of manic-depressive psychosis may also appear in our disease; the only decisive factor is the presence or absence of schizophrenic symptoms."

However, a description of the criteria we used in making the global diagnoses remains to be made and incorporated into an operational form. As a first step, the criteria regarded as important in our diagnosis of schizophrenia and their presence or absence in the probands for whom we made that diagnosis are presented in **Table 2**.

The diagnosis of latent schizophrenia, analogous but not identical with the *DSM-III*[17] diagnoses of schizotypal and paranoid personality disorders, was made following the *DSM-II*[10] description of latent schizophrenia, which emphasizes the presence of symptoms of schizophrenia in the absence of a psychotic episode, and following the description by Bleuler[9(pp238-239)] of latent schizophrenia:

> If one observes the relatives of our patients, one often finds in them peculiarities which are qualitatively identical with those of the patients themselves, so that the disease appears to be only a quantitative increase of the anomalies seen in the parents and siblings.
>
> There is also a latent schizophrenia, and I am convinced that this is the most frequent form, although admittedly these people hardly ever come for treatment. It is not necessary to give a detailed description of the various manifestations of latent schizophrenia. In this form, we can see in nuce all the symptoms and all the combination of symptoms that are present in the manifest type of the disease.

A diagnosis of latent schizophrenia was made where social withdrawal, affective flattening, changes in the form of thought and speech, or delusional (including paranoid) tendencies characteristic of chronic schizophrenia were present in the absence of frank delusions or other psychotic symptoms. The presence of characteristics important in making our diagnoses of latent schizophrenia among relatives of index and control probands is presented in **Table 3**. A diagnosis of schizoid personality in the present study most frequently reflected severe introversion, suspicious or referential symptoms in otherwise psychiatrically unremarkable individuals, and was not identical to the *DSM-III* diagnosis of schizoid personality.

Table 1. Interview Participation by Provincial Sample Relatives*

Relatives of Proband Type	No. (%) of Total: Unavailable for Follow-up	Died	Refused	Interviewed	Total No.	Interviewed, % of Available
Biological index	7 (2.9)	44 (18.0)	22 (9.0)	172 (70.2)	**245**	88.6
Adoptive index	2 (2.0)	52 (51.0)	6 (5.9)	42 (41.2)	**102**	87.5
Biological control	7 (3.3)	38 (17.5)	17 (7.8)	155 (71.4)	**217**	90.1
Adoptive control	0 (0.0)	46 (44.2)	7 (6.7)	51 (49.0)	**104**	87.9

**Includes only relatives at least 15 years old.*

Table 2. Course and Symptoms of Chronic Schizophrenia in Adoptee Probands

Good premorbid adjustment	Insidious onset	Schizoid features observed premorbidly	Age at first psychiatric hospitalization, y	Chronic course observed	Withdrawal from social interaction	Autistic behavior	Poverty of thought/speech	Loose associations	Flat affect	Suspicious/ideas of reference	Delusions	Auditory hallucinations	Other hallucinations	Family No.
	x		35	x		x			x	x	x	x		369
		x	34	x	x	x		x	x	x	x	x	x	420
			24			x	x		x			x		794
	x	x	25	x	x				x	x	x	x		241
x			26	x				x		x	x	x	x	368
x	x		25	x	x	x	x		x	x	x	x	x	830
	x		33	x		x		x	x	x	x	x	x	936
	x	x	27	x	x	x		x	x	x				974
x	x	x	19	x	x				x	x	x			078
x	x		36	x	x				x	x	x	x	x	258
x	x		25	x				x	x	x	x	x	x	991
	x		26	x				x	x	x	x	x		055
x	x	x	20	x	x			x		x				828
	x		25	x				x			x			871
x	x	x	27	x	x	x		x	x	x	x	x	x	975
	x	x	21	x	x	x			x	x	x	x	x	042
x	x	x	21	x	x					x	x	x	x	141
	x	x	17	x	x			x	x	x	x	x		831
x	x	x	19	x	x	x	x	x	x	x	x	x		069
	x	x	22	x	x	x	x	x	x	x	x	x	x	462
	x	x	11	x	x	x			x	x	x	x		592
x	x		12	x				x		x	x	x	x	913
	x	x	20	x	x	x			x	x	x	x	x	940
	x	x	14	x	x	x		x	x	x	x	x	x	782
x	x	x	19	x	x	x	x	x	x	x	x	x	x	806
	x	x	17	x	x				x	x	x	x	x	900
x	x		21				x	x	x	x	x			020
	x	x	24	x	x				x					139
x	x		20	x				x		x	x	x		388

had been adopted early in life, separating, to the maximal extent possible, their genetic and environmental endowments and making possible independent evaluations of the significance of genetic and family-associated environmental factors in the development of their disorder. Results of the studies based on the adoptions granted in the city and county of Copenhagen, Denmark (the Copenhagen Sample), have been published previously using psychiatric information from institutional records[1] and from extensive personal interviews.[2]

Another strategy that the register of adoptions would serve was to be an examination of the risk for schizophrenia in the adopted-away offspring of a schizophrenic biological parent, compared with the risk in an adoptee whose biological parents were free of the disease.[3,4] There have been several studies by others of adopted-away offspring of schizophrenic mothers,[5-8] but to our knowledge, the Copenhagen Study of adoptees' families and the present replication in the rest of Denmark represent the only examinations of schizophrenia and other mental illness in the biological and adoptive relatives of schizophrenic adoptees that have been conducted.

RESULTS

The interviews, detailed review of hospital records, and follow-up information on the initial group of potential proband adoptees made possible the selection of a final set of index probands who exemplified schizophrenia or latent schizophrenia, and a comparable set of control adoptees who had been interviewed by a psychiatrist and found to be free from serious or confounding mental illness (major affective disorder, chronic or latent schizophrenia, or schizoid personality). This decreased the number of control probands to 24 since a psychiatric interview was refused or unobtained in five patients and in 13 patients it identified a confounding illness among putative control probands who had never been hospitalized on a psychiatric service. The review identified 29 index probands with chronic schizophrenia and four index probands with latent schizophrenia among the original sample of potential schizophrenic probands on the basis of interviews, updated information, or new information.

At the same time that the interviews, hospital records, and follow-up information on the proband adoptees in the present (Provincial) sample were reviewed, the records of the Copenhagen sample of probands, augmented by the same additional information, were also reviewed in an effort to use all available information in identifying index probands with chronic (or latent) schizophrenia and control probands free from serious or confounding illness. Overall, this resulted in one additional proband with chronic schizophrenia and one fewer proband with latent schizophrenia (two probands diagnosed as having acute schizophrenia some 15 years earlier were now found to be better characterized by chronic schizophrenia, as was one proband with latent schizophrenia; for two probands, review indicated that the previous diagnosis of chronic schizophrenia should be revised to latent schizophrenia, as was the case for one proband previously diagnosed as having acute schizophrenia; four probands previously diagnosed as having latent schizophrenia were, on review, diagnosed as having nonschizophrenia spectrum diagnoses). Updated diagnoses were always made without knowledge that could identify the subjects or their relatives.

Study of the biological relatives of these schizophrenic and control probands permitted an examination of the hypothesis that there are one or more clinical syndromes genetically related to schizophrenia as well as the primary hypothesis that genetic factors operate in the familial transmission of schizophrenia. We removed from our analysis relatives who had died or emigrated before the age of 15 years to exclude relatives who had not entered the age of risk for schizophrenia.

Figure 1 and **Figure 2** present the pedigrees of probands with chronic and latent schizophrenia in the Provincial Sample and the diagnoses of their biological and adoptive relatives. **Figure 3** similarly diagrams pedigrees and diagnoses in the families of control probands.

Table 4 and **Table 5** summarize the results presented in Figures 1 and 3. Table 4 compares the prevalence of schizophrenia and latent schizophrenia (definite or probable) as well as schizoid and paranoid personality disorder in the biological and adoptive relatives of chronic schizophrenic index and control probands.

The figures and tables present the observed prevalence of schizophrenic illness in our sample, rather than a hypothetical lifetime prevalence. An age-corrected morbid risk can be estimated with the abridged Weinberg method (age of risk of 15 to 39 years).[18(pp38-42)] The age-corrected morbid risks for chronic schizophrenia and latent schizophrenia among the biological relatives of chronic schizophrenic index adoptees are 9.9% and 5.7%, respectively; the age-corrected risk for latent schizophrenia among the relatives of control probands is 2.9%.

Schizophrenia and latent schizophrenia are significantly more common in the biological relatives of adoptees with chronic schizophrenia than in the biological relatives of controls, and they are absent in adoptive relatives. The prevalence of schizoid and paranoid personality is not significantly different among groups.

Table 5 compares the prevalence of major affective disorder, other psychotic disorders, minor affective disorder, and all other diagnoses, and indicates that they occur at similar rates in the biological relatives of index and control probands. Among adoptive relatives, there are no significant differences between the adoptive relatives of schizophrenic or control adoptees. **Table 6** presents for comparison the results from the updated Copenhagen Sample, and **Table 7** presents the results of the combined Copenhagen and Provincial Samples as the National Sample.

FAMILIES AFFECTED

It is possible to express the results in terms of biological families affected rather than relatives. Of the 29 biological families of probands with chronic schizophrenia, five had at least one schizophrenic member and 14 had one or more members with schizophrenia or latent schizophrenia. These frequencies are significantly different from

Table 3. Course and Symptoms of Latent Schizophrenia in Relatives of Probands With Chronic Schizophrenia and in Relatives of Control Probands

Referential delusive tendency	Social anxiety	Odd beliefs/magical thinking	Unusual perceptual experiences	Odd/eccentric/unkempt	No close friends/seclusive/withdrawn	Odd or digressive speech	Inappropriate or constricted affect	Suspicious/paranoid ideation	Anhedonic	Impaired reality testing	Age at psychiatric hospitalization, y	Family No.
							x					420
x							x					794
					x		x	x				794
	x				x		x	x				368
							x	x				368
					x		x		x	x		487
		x								x	28	830
						x					66	936
	x	x			x		x	x	x			974
					x	x	x	x				258
		x									46	837
					x			x				871
				x			x					497
		x						x				940
		x			x		x	x	x			940
x		x			x	x		x			44	782
				x	x	x	x					388

those in the control families, which were zero and three of 24 (*P*=.041 and *P*=.006), respectively.

FIRST- AND SECOND-DEGREE RELATIVES

A focus on the first-degree relatives of schizophrenic probands finds an excess of schizophrenia (six of 81) compared with those of controls (none of 60; *P*=.033). In disorders in which genetic influences appear to play a role, the distribution of illness between first- and second-degree biological relatives may be pertinent if the size of the samples involved is large enough to achieve statistical power. Since the abortion and placement policies in Denmark reduced the observed incidence of schizophrenia in parents of adoptees, our examination of the relative incidence of schizophrenia in first- and second-degree relatives focused on adoptees' full and half siblings. The Copenhagen Sample suffered from a paucity of full biological siblings that prevented a meaningful estimate

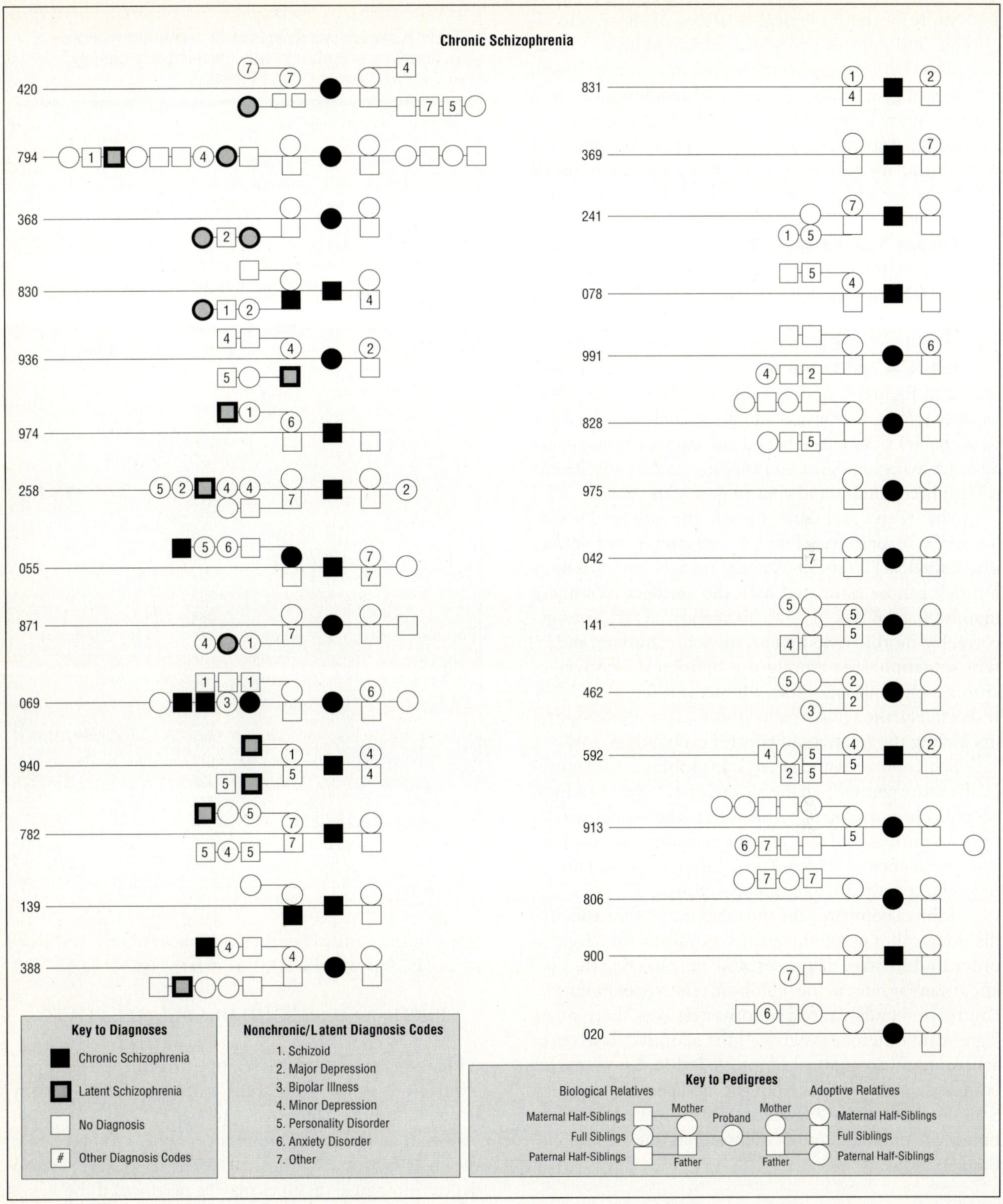

Figure 1. *Pedigrees of adoptees with chronic schizophrenia.*

of disease prevalence in first-degree relatives, but in the Provincial Sample there were a substantial number of full siblings (24 biological index siblings compared with three in the Copenhagen Sample), probably the result of differences in lifestyle from that of the large city. Schizophrenia was found in three (12.5%) of the 24 full siblings, nearly six times the rate in the half-siblings (two [2.2%] of 90) (one-tailed *P*=.062). (The less specific marginal syndrome [latent schizophrenia] was evenly distributed between full siblings and half-siblings [12.5%

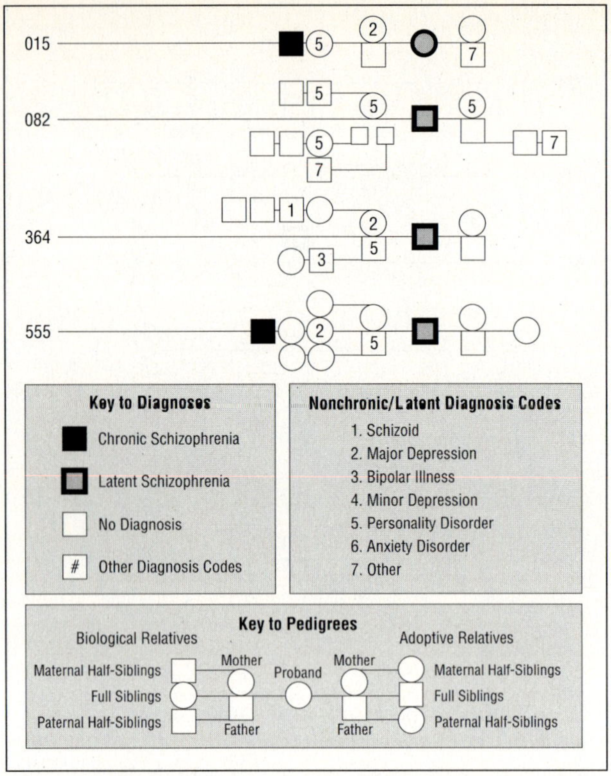

Figure 2. *Pedigrees of adoptees with latent schizophrenia*

vs 11.1%, respectively], suggesting a greater degree of heterogeneity and of nongenetic influence within that syndrome.)

SPECIFICITY OF LATENT SCHIZOPHRENIA

The 8.2% prevalence of latent schizophrenia in the biological relatives of index probands was significantly higher than the 2.5% in the relatives of controls (*P*=.032), while paranoid or schizoid personality did not show significantly different prevalence, confirming similar findings in the Copenhagen Sample. Since a higher than expected prevalence of the features of schizotypal personality disorder (the *DSM-III* diagnosis derived from and comparable to our latent schizophrenia) was reported in the adolescent children of parents with affective disorder,[19] the occurrence of latent schizophrenia in the biological relatives of adoptees with affective disorder in this sample became of interest. Eight such adoptees had been identified through the psychiatric interviews (seven unipolar depressed and one bipolar manic) and among their 37 biological relatives a prevalence of 13.5% of latent schizophrenia was found, significantly higher (*P*=.015) than the prevalence in relatives of normal controls and not significantly different from the prevalence of that syndrome in the relatives of schizophrenics.

Another approach to investigating the relationship between chronic and latent schizophrenia focuses on whether there is an increased risk of chronic schizophrenia among the relatives of individuals with latent schizophrenia, as would be expected if they share common genetic liabilities.[20-22] In our limited sample of four probands with latent schizophrenia, we observed two instances of chronic schizophrenia among their 29 biological relatives (Figure 2), a prevalence of 6.9%; we did not observe latent schizophrenia among these relatives.

In sum, our present results find a substantial risk for latent schizophrenia among the biological relatives of probands with chronic schizophrenia, indicate that latent schizophrenia is not seen exclusively among the biological relatives of individuals with chronic schizophrenia, and suggest that latent schizophrenia may be associated with an increased liability to chronic schizophrenia among biological relatives. While the existence of a link between chronic schizophrenia and latent schizophrenia is supported by our results, further elucidation of the nature of the relationship between schizophrenia and latent schizophrenia is necessary.

COMMENT

EVIDENCE FOR THE OPERATION OF GENETIC FACTORS IN THE ETIOLOGY OF SCHIZOPHRENIA

The most striking finding in both this and the Copenhagen Study is the highly significant concentration of classical schizophrenia in the biological relatives of the adoptees with the same severe disorder: 4.7% and 5.6%, respectively. This is significantly higher than that found in the biological relatives of adoptees free of serious mental illness: 0% and 0.9%, respectively. For all of Denmark, schizophrenia was found in 14 (5.0%) of 279 biological relatives of schizophrenic adoptees compared with one (0.4%) of 234 biological relatives of controls (*P*=.0013). Moreover, schizophrenia was found almost exclusively in the biological relatives of index adoptees with classical schizophrenia in both this and the Copenhagen Study. Schizophrenia was found in 12.5% of the first-degree relatives (full siblings) compared with 2.2% of second-degree relatives in this study, also consistent with genetic transmission. The classical schizophrenia syndrome was found in five of 29 index families in this sample compared with none in 24 control families. All of these differences speak for a syndrome that can be reliably recognized, in which genetic factors play a significant etiological role. It should also be noted that this prevalence in the biological relatives of schizophrenic adoptees who were not reared by or with them, matching that in the relatives of naturally reared schizophrenics, provides important and needed support for the assumption usually made in family studies: that the familial clustering is an expression of genetic factors.

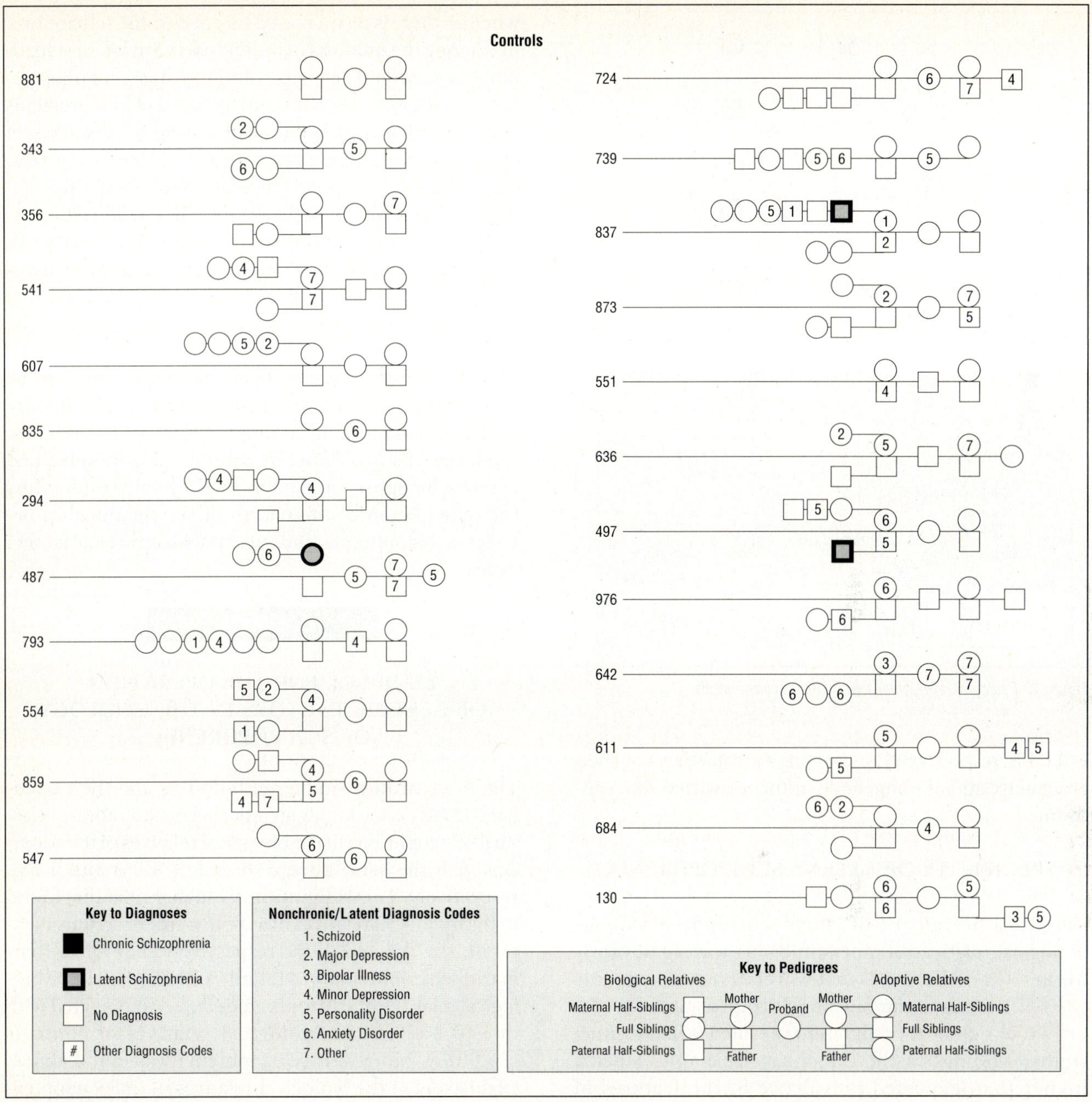

Figure 3. *Pedigrees of control adoptees.*

LIMITS TO THE SCHIZOPHRENIA SPECTRUM

The marginal syndrome (latent schizophrenia) seen by Bleuler[9] in the relatives of schizophrenics is also found in the biological relatives of the schizophrenic adoptees in this and the Copenhagen sample: 8.2% and 14.8% compared with 2.5% and 0.9%, respectively, in the relatives of control adoptees, with a prevalence for the combined national sample of 10.8% vs 1.7% (P=.00002). Furthermore, chronic schizophrenia was found in two biological siblings of probands with latent schizophrenia in the Provincial Sample. While these results support the genetic relationship of this marginal syndrome to schizophrenia, its increased prevalence in the biological relatives of adoptees with affective disorders renders it less than completely specific to schizophrenia. It is possible that more precise diagnostic criteria could characterize a specifically schizophrenia-related syndrome.

Neither schizoid or paranoid personality nor any diagnosis outside of the schizophrenia spectrum appeared in significantly higher frequency in the relatives of index vs control adoptees. This suggests that increased risk for psychiatric illness in the biological relatives of schizophrenic individuals is limited to the diagnoses of schizophrenia and latent schizophrenia, rather than a risk for psychopathologic features in general or for a range of mild

Table 4. Provincial Sample: Chronic Schizophrenia and Potentially Related Diagnoses in Relatives of Adoptees With Chronic Schizophrenia and in Relatives of Control Adoptees With No History of Major Mental Illness

Relative Groups	Paranoid, No. (%)	Schizoid, No. (%)	Latent Schizophrenia, No. (%)*	Chronic Schizophrenia, No. (%)†	Total No. of Relatives
Biological relatives of 29 adoptees with chronic schizophrenia	3 (1.8)	7 (4.1)	14 (8.2)	8 (4.7)	171
Biological relatives of 24 control adoptees	1 (0.8)	4 (3.3)	3 (2.5)	0	121
Adoptive relatives of 29 adoptees with chronic schizophrenia	0	0	0	0	71
Adoptive relatives of 24 control adoptees	1 (1.8)	0	0	0	55

*One-tailed P=.0321 for biological index vs control (Fisher's Exact Test).
†One-tailed P=.0129 for biological index vs control (Fisher's Exact Test).

Table 5. Provincial Sample: Affective, Other Psychotic, and Any Other Diagnoses in Relatives of Adoptees With Chronic Schizophrenia and in Relatives of Control Adoptees With No History of Major Mental Illness

Relative Groups	Major Affective, No. (%)	Other Psychotic, No. (%)	Minor Affective, No. (%)	Any Other, No. (%)	Total No. of Relatives
Biological relatives of 29 adoptees with chronic schizophrenia	19 (11.1)	1 (0.6)	5 (2.9)	32 (18.7)	171
Biological relatives of 24 control adoptees	12 (9.9)	0	4 (3.3)	26 (21.5)	121
Adoptive relatives of 29 adoptees with chronic schizophrenia	7 (9.9)	0	1 (1.4)	9 (12.6)	71
Adoptive relatives of 24 control adoptees	2 (3.6)	0	2 (3.6)	10 (18.2)	55

syndromes with features resembling some aspect of schizophrenia.

If schizophrenia were simply the extreme end of a normal and continuous distribution of a set of behaviors that ranged from normalcy through schizoid personality to latent and chronic schizophrenia, one might expect the diagnosis of schizoid personality to be more common than the diagnosis of latent schizophrenia, as there are more individuals near the center of a normal distribution. Such was not the case in the present report. Schizophrenic illness appears to be characterized by the definable and identifiable syndromes of chronic and latent schizophrenia, rather than being a variation of normalcy as may be the case for schizoid personality.

PREVALENCE OF NONFAMILIAL SCHIZOPHRENIA

In this study, as in the Copenhagen Study, very close to half (14 of 29) of the probands with chronic schizophrenia had one or more instances of schizophrenia or latent schizophrenia among their biological relatives, consistent with the operation of genetic factors in the transmission of schizophrenic illness. The remaining 15 index probands whose biological families appeared to be free of those disorders could exemplify a nongenetic, nonfamilial form of schizophrenia or forms in which nongenetic influences predominate. However, the relatively low risk for schizophrenia in the biological relatives of schizophrenic individuals alternatively suggests that these unaffected families of schizophrenic probands were the consequence of small family size and low familial risk for illness rather than evidence of nonfamilial schizophrenia.

Specifically, in the present study we observed a mean family size of 6.0 biological relatives per index proband, and found the risk of either chronic or latent schizophrenia in a biological relative to be 12.9%, similar to the values found in other studies of familial risk.[23(p96)] Given such an observed family size and risk, one would predict that by chance 44% of the families would be unaffected even if all probands had a familial form of the disorder (calculated via the binomial probability distribution).[24(pp126-129)] We observed that 52% of the families appeared to be unaffected, a difference from expectation that is not significant. Thus, the observed distribution of schizophrenia and latent schizophrenia in the families of the probands is quite compatible with an inference that all cases were familial. The alternative hypothesis, that the risk of chronic or latent schizophrenia among the relatives of probands with familial chronic schizophrenia is on the order of 24%, while absent among the probands with putatively nonfamilial schizophrenia (accounting for the observation of illness in only about one half of our families), would require that consistency in familial risk for schizophrenia observed in different samples be accounted for by stability in the ratio of familial to nonfamilial probands.

THE SEPARATION OF GENETIC AND ENVIRONMENTAL FACTORS

There are possible biases and sources of error to be considered in evaluating the results of this study. These are

Table 6. Copenhagen Sample: Diagnoses in Relatives of Adoptees With Chronic Schizophrenia and in Relatives of Control Adoptees With No History of Major Mental Illness

Relative Groups	Paranoid, No. (%)	Schizoid, No. (%)	Latent Schizophrenia, No. (%)*	Chronic Schizophrenia, No. (%)†	Total No. of Relatives
Biological relatives of 18 adoptees with chronic schizophrenia	1 (0.9)	9 (8.3)	16 (14.8)	6 (5.6)	108
Biological relatives of 23 control adoptees	1 (0.9)	15 (13.3)	1 (0.9)	1 (0.9)	113
Adoptive relatives of 18 adoptees with chronic schizophrenia	0	1 (2.5)	2 (5.0)	0	40
Adoptive relatives of 23 control adoptees	0	4 (6.5)	2 (3.2)	0	62

*One-tailed P=.00006 for biological index vs control (Fisher's Exact Test).
†One-tailed P=.0526 for biological index vs control (Fisher's Exact Test).

Table 7. National Sample: Diagnoses in Relatives of Adoptees With Chronic Schizophrenia and in Relatives of Control Adoptees With No History of Major Mental Illness

Relative Groups	Paranoid, No. (%)	Schizoid, No. (%)	Latent Schizophrenia, No. (%)*	Chronic Schizophrenia, No. (%)†	Total No. of Relatives
Biological relatives of 47 adoptees with chronic schizophrenia	4 (1.4)	16 (5.7)	30 (10.8)	14 (5.0)	279
Biological relatives of 47 control adoptees	2 (0.9)	19 (8.1)	4 (1.7)	1 (0.4)	234
Adoptive relatives of 47 adoptees with chronic schizophrenia	0	1 (0.9)	2 (1.8)	0	111
Adoptive relatives of 47 control adoptees	1 (0.9)	4 (3.4)	2 (1.7)	0	117

*One-tailed P=.00002 for biological index vs control (Fisher's Exact Test).
†One-tailed P=.0013 for biological index vs control (Fisher's Exact Test).

essentially the same as those pertinent to the Copenhagen Study, which were discussed in our original reports of that study[1,2] and in our response[25-27] to questions raised by others. The research design of these studies minimizes subjective and selective bias in ascertainment and diagnosis, and independent diagnosis by another group using widely accepted operational criteria[16] has essentially confirmed the findings. The problem of selective placement that is often cited in connection with adoption studies is not as applicable to these for a number of reasons, many peculiar to the Danish adoption sample.

The adoption strategy depends on the ability of that approach to dissociate and randomize the genetic and family-dependent rearing variables in the transmission of the disorders studied. There are circumstances, however, that could make that dissociation imperfect. One circumstance that could operate to diminish the complete separation or randomization of genetic and environmental variables is the possibility of selective placement. Since the etiological role of environmental variables remains obscure at present, it is not likely that a social agency, even if it set about doing so deliberately, could find sufficient of the unknown variables in the prospective adoptive parents to materially affect the risk of illness in the adoptee. One environmental variable, however, that appears to be correlated with the prevalence of schizophrenia is socioeconomic status (SES), although conclusive evidence that it plays an etiological role is lacking. A study of this question, carried out in the Copenhagen adoption sample, found that adoptees who came from low SES biological parents or were placed in low SES adoptive homes were no more likely to develop schizophrenia than adoptees from high SES biological parents or those placed with high SES adoptive homes. Schizophrenic adoptees, however, tended to move into lower socioeconomic strata.[28] The correlation between SES of biological and adoptive parents provides some measure of the degree of selective placement based on that measure. Where such correlations have been measured in Denmark and elsewhere, they have been low. In one study of 206 adoptions in Colorado,[29] average weighted correlations between biological and adoptive parents for education and occupation were .19 and .13, respectively. Teasdale[30] found a correlation coefficient of .15 between SES of biological and adoptive fathers in 11 094 adoptions in the national sample in Denmark, where both data were available. These correlations, though statistically significant, are both small and indicate that selective placement on the basis of SES would not account for more than 3% of the variance. In neither the Copenhagen nor the Provincial Sample was there a significant correlation between socioeconomic class of biological and adoptive parents. Furthermore, in these samples of adoptees, selective placement on the basis of mental illness in the parents could hardly have occurred, since social and legal processes were operating that would select biological and adoptive parents quite free of mental illness. Prospective adoptive parents were screened for mental health and economic stability by the courts and a history or current indication of mental illness in either biological parent would favor a legal abortion or a decision not to place the child for adoption.

The Mothers' Aid Organization, a state social agency

that counseled the biological mother and arranged for adoption or other outcome was the repository of information its staff had gathered on the mental status and psychiatric history of the biological and adoptive parents. As a result of the restrictive policies regarding adoption, only two of the 84 initial probands had a biological parent with a history of admission to a mental hospital in the records of the Mothers' Aid Organization at the time of adoption. In neither of these instances, one each among the index and control probands, was the selection of the adoptive parents made by that organization nor did the parental history of mental disturbance play a role in the placement.

Thus, mental illness found in the biological and adoptive parents developed, in practically every case, well after the placement of the adoptee took place. Subsequent search of the Psychiatric Register for dates of all mental hospital admissions of relatives indicated that the average interval between the date of birth of the adoptee and the date of first psychiatric admission for the relatively few biological parents ever hospitalized was 15.5 years and 11.3 years for the Provincial and Copenhagen studies, respectively. A major advantage of the means of ascertainment used in these studies, from a total sample of adoptees rather than from the adopted-away offspring of schizophrenic mothers, was to minimize the effect of schizophrenia in a biological parent, on placement, rearing, personality development, and the recognition of mental illness or its diagnosis in the adoptee. It should also be pointed out that these factors as well as the possibility of nonrandom or selective placement, pertinent, if not adequately controlled, to the development and diagnosis of schizophrenia in adoptees, will have little effect on the prevalence of schizophrenia in the relatives of schizophrenics, which it is the aim of family studies such as this one to ascertain.

More important than selective placement is the possibility of knowledge on the part of adoptive parents, adoptees, and mental health personnel regarding the presence of mental illness in the biological parents and the effect such knowledge could have on the occurrence, perception, and diagnosis of mental illness in the adoptee. Although this problem could be of some significance in studies where the adoptee sample represented children born of mentally ill mothers, it would be negligible in the Danish adoptee sample for reasons that have been discussed.

In contrast to the potential problems in separating genetic and environmental influences that have been discussed above, and that, in Denmark, are minimized, there is the period of time before separation in which the child shared the environment of the biological parents. Ideally this should have been as short as possible, but because of the expected small size of the sample we were reluctant to limit the sample to those adoptees separated immediately after birth. There were, however, more than 80% of the index and control adoptees who were separated from their biological mothers during the first month, 60% within the first week. Restricting the analysis to the 22 index and the 20 control adoptees who spent no more than 4 weeks with their biological families, we find eight of the 128 biological index relatives who developed schizophrenia and none of the 105 biological control relatives (Fisher's Exact Test, one-tailed P=.0075). A similar pattern is observed for latent schizophrenia (eight of 128 index relatives vs three of 105 control relatives), which is not statistically significant. These results, similar to those found in the Copenhagen Study, indicate that the striking concentration of schizophrenia found in the biological relatives of schizophrenic adoptees is not accounted for by the period of time spent with the biological mother or parents. All of the adoptees in the present study who were found to have schizophrenia in their biological relatives had stayed with the natural mother for 2 weeks or less.

However, every adopted child has spent 9 months in the uterus of its biological mother, where it shares with her a number of environmental influences, and, in most cases, has had a certain amount of early mothering at her hands. It is possible to disentangle that conjunction of genes and environment by examining the prevalence of the disorder in the biological paternal half-siblings of the adoptees. These shared neither the same uterus nor the same early mothering with the adoptee, but a certain amount of genetic overlap. In both the Copenhagen and the Provincial Samples, the prevalence of chronic or latent schizophrenia in the paternal biological half-siblings was at least as high as in the maternal half-siblings, and significantly higher than in their controls.

DIAGNOSTIC VALUE OF GLOBAL CRITERIA COMPARED WITH THOSE BASED ON *DSM-III*

A serious deficiency in psychiatric diagnosis is its dependence on current usage in the absence of independent criteria for validity. Pathognomonic features and laboratory findings of proved specificity have served as valuable support for the structure of diagnostic systems in medicine and much of the confusion that has accompanied the diagnosis and study of schizophrenia would have been obviated had there been a serological, chemical, psychological, or clinical test with acceptable sensitivity and specificity. The development of *DSM-III* and its successors, operational diagnostic systems endorsed by the American Psychiatric Association, has improved the interrater reliability and communicability of many psychiatric diagnoses, as was to be expected. The question of validity, however, has not often been addressed or adequately answered.

The prevalence of schizophrenia in the biological relatives of schizophrenic adoptees and its relative absence in normal control relatives can be a test not only of hypotheses of genetic transmission, but also of the sensitivity and specificity with which that syndrome is de-

tected by the diagnostic criteria chosen. Diagnoses in the Copenhagen Study were global judgments based on the descriptions in *DSM-II*, the diagnostic manual then in use. For schizophrenia the original and more complete descriptions of Kraepelin[15] and Bleuler[9] were employed. It was important to use the same global diagnostic system in the Provincial Study if it was to be a replication of the Copenhagen Study in a new Danish sample.

Despite the fact that *DSM-III* became available about the time that the diagnoses on the relatives in the present study were to be made, it did not supplant the global diagnoses in this study for several additional reasons. The focus of *DSM-III* on a minimum number of putative characteristics made it useful for quick and economic diagnosis, but its necessary neglect of a large number of potentially important features diminished its sensitivity and usefulness in research. Interrater reliability would be enhanced, as expected, for any system using criteria agreed on in advance by the raters, and our diagnostic system had criteria previously agreed on by the raters and with comparable interrater reliability. Furthermore, the validity of the *DSM-III* diagnosis of schizophrenia and cognate diagnoses, in common with that of other operational diagnoses, had not been tested independently. When Kendler and Gruenberg[16] asked to review the interviews from our Copenhaqen sample to determine whether a genetic relationship between schizophrenia and anxiety neurosis was observable, an opportunity became available for independent diagnoses of schizophrenic illness using *DSM-III* and a comparison with global diagnoses. They were encouraged to extend their diagnostic ratings into the schizophrenia spectrum as well.

The Copenhagen adoption study provided a means of evaluating the validity of the global and *DSM-III* diagnoses of schizophrenia and related syndromes and comparing them for sensitivity and specificity. The *DSM-III* diagnoses made independently by Kendler and Gruenberg[16] from the interviews alone in the Copenhagen Study appeared to confirm but did not improve the results of our global diagnoses on the same interviews,[2] which encouraged us to continue to use global diagnoses in the present study.

CONCLUSION

This communication reports the results of the second phase of a national study, replicating the design of the first phase that was confined to the city and county of Copenhagen and offers the advantage of testing hypotheses examined or derived in the first study in an additional and independent sample. The design of both studies involves matched case-controls, minimizes ascertainment and subjective bias, and is unaffected by selective placement. Results from these two major divisions of the Danish adoption sample at the level of the family and at the level of individual family members, each involving specific diagnoses, support the presence of a strong genetic liability in a major segment of schizophrenia.

Since no excess of such liability has been observed among natural families when compared with the adoption samples we have investigated, the familial tendency in schizophrenia appears to be largely an expression of genetic factors, lending important justification to the use of natural pedigrees for investigating the genetics of schizophrenia. The observation that in both population samples a syndrome based on the classic descriptions of Kraepelin[15] and Bleuler[9] is found in certain adoptees and in their biological relatives consistently and almost exclusively is evidence for the reliability and validity of their concept of schizophrenia as well as its genetic transmission.

Investigation of the sensitivity and specificity of diagnostic criteria to identify illness in the biological families of adoptees has the potential to provide an empirical basis for diagnosis. Furthermore, such studies provide an approach for assessing the validity of psychiatric diagnoses in reflecting the operation of genetically determined underlying biological mechanisms. If comparison between our global diagnoses and *DSM-III* diagnoses in the Provincial Sample mirrors the results of the previous comparison of diagnostic systems in the Copenhagen Study, this will provide further indication that global diagnoses are capable of greater sensitivity and equal specificity when compared with operational diagnoses exemplified by *DSM-III*. In both the Copenhagen and Provincial studies, a milder syndrome, latent schizophrenia, was found significantly concentrated in the biological relatives of schizophrenic adoptees at an even greater prevalence than classical schizophrenia. This speaks for a genetic relationship between the two syndromes. The lack of specificity of latent schizophrenia to the biological relatives of individuals with chronic schizophrenia suggests heterogeneity of latent schizophrenia as presently defined.

The results suggest that inconsistencies in the familial distribution of schizophrenia due to nongenetic, sporadic schizophrenia are probably of minor importance. Nevertheless, clarifying the potential existence (and origin) of a putative nongenetic form of schizophrenia remains a valid goal.

The demonstration of a genetic liability for schizophrenia in no way diminishes the role that the environment plays in the initiation, course, and outcome of schizophrenic illness and is not incompatible with external physical and chemical, or viral, autoimmune, and developmental etiological influences and processes. Continued investigation of the genetic and extragenetic contributions will be necessary to elucidate the modes of genetic transmission and expression, and to identify and define the large number of environmental influences operating in tandem with them in the development of this disorder.

Accepted for publication February 25, 1994.

This research was supported in part by the Intramural and Extramural Research Programs of the National Insti-

tute of Mental Health, Bethesda, Md, the MacArthur Foundation, the Foundations' Fund for Research in Schizophrenia, and the Scottish Rite Schizophrenia Research Program.

The authors wish to acknowledge the invaluable contribution made by Prof Fini Schulsinger, formerly chief of the Psychiatric Service, Kommunehospitalet, Copenhagen, who directed the work in Denmark until 1983 and played an essential role in the early phases of the Copenhagen and Provincial studies. Vera Hildebrande translated the SADS-L into Danish and Dr Jean Endicott demonstrated the administration of that instrument to the interviewing psychiatrists. Sandra Cole was responsible for the maintenance of records, editing, and coding of interviews and abstracts of hospital records; Thalene Mallus and Peter Kim carried out statistical analyses; and Tina Chan assisted in the preparation of figures.

Reprint requests to Room 4C110, Bldg 10, National Institutes of Health, Bethesda, MD 20892 (Dr Kety).

REFERENCES

1. Kety SS, Rosenthal D, Wender PH, Schulsinger F. The types and prevalence of mental illness in the biological and adoptive families of adopted schizophrenics. In: Rosenthal D, Kety SS, eds. *The Transmission of Schizophrenia.* Oxford, England: Pergamon Press; 1968:345-362. Also in: *J Psychiatr Res.* 1968;6 (suppl):345-362.
2. Kety SS, Rosenthal D, Wender PH, Schulsinger F, Jacobsen B. Mental illness in the biological and adoptive families of adopted individuals who have become schizophrenic: a preliminary report based upon psychiatric interviews. In: Fieve R, Rosenthal D, Brill H, eds. *Genetic Research in Psychiatry.* Baltimore, Md: The Johns Hopkins University Press; 1975:147-165.
3. Rosenthal D, Wender PH, Kety SS, Schulsinger F, Welner J, Ostergaard L. Schizophrenics' offspring reared in adoptive homes. In: Rosenthal D, Kety SS, eds. *The Transmission of Schizophrenia.* Oxford, England: Pergamon Press; 1968:377-391.
4. Rosenthal D, Wender PH, Kety SS, Welner J, Schulsinger F. The adopted-away offspring of schizophrenics. *Am J Psychiatry.* 1971;128:307-311.
5. Heston LL. Psychiatric disorders in foster home reared children of schizophrenic mothers. *Br J Psychiatry.* 1966;112:819-825.
6. Karlsson JL. The rate of schizophrenia in foster-reared close relatives of schizophrenic index cases. *Biol Psychiatry.* 1970;2:285-290.
7. Tienari P, Sorri A, Lahti I, Naarala M, Wahlberg KE, Ronkko T, Pohjola J, Moring J. The Finnish adoptive family study of schizophrenia. *Yale J Biol Med.* 1985;58:227-237.
8. Tienari P. Interaction between genetic vulnerability and family environment: the Finnish adoptive family study of schizophrenia. *Acta Psychiatr Scand.* 1991; 84:460-465.
9. Bleuler E; Zinkin J, trans. *Dementia Praecox, or the Group of Schizophrenias: Monograph Series on Schizophrenia, No. 1.* New York, NY: International Universities Press; 1911/1950.
10. American Psychiatric Association, Committee on Nomenclature and Statistics. *Diagnostic and Statistical Manual of Mental Disorders, Second Edition.* Washington, DC: American Psychiatric Association Press; 1968.
11. Kendler KS. The super-normal control group in psychiatric genetics: possible artifactual evidence for coaggregation. *Psychiatr Genet.* 1990;1:45-53.
12. Cohen J. A coefficient of agreement for nominal scales. *Ed Psychol Meas.* 1960; 20:37-46.
13. Kety SS, Rosenthal D, Wender PH, Schulsinger F, Jacobsen B. The biologic and adoptive families of adopted individuals who became schizophrenic: prevalence of mental illness and other characteristics. In: Wynne LC, Cromwell RL, Matthysse S, eds. *The Nature of Schizophrenia.* New York, NY: John Wiley & Sons Inc; 1978:25-37.
14. Endicott J, Spitzer RL. A diagnostic interview: the Schedule for Affective Disorders and Schizophrenia. *Arch Gen Psychiatry.* 1978;35:837-844.
15. Kraepelin E. *Dementia Praecox and Paraphrenia.* Edinburgh, Scotland: E&S Livingstone; 1919.
16. Kendler KS, Gruenberg AM. An independent analysis of the Danish Adoption Study of schizophrenia, VI: the relationship between psychiatric disorders as defined by *DSM-III* in the relatives and adoptees. *Arch Gen Psychiatry.* 1984;41:555-564.
17. American Psychiatric Association, Committee on Nomenclature and Statistics. *Diagnostic and Statistical Manual of Mental Disorders, Third Edition.* Washington, DC: American Psychiatric Association; 1980.
18. Rosenthal D. *Genetic Theory and Abnormal Behavior.* New York, NY: McGraw-Hill International Book Co; 1970.
19. Squires-Wheeler E, Skodol AE, Friedman D, Erlenmeyer-Kimling L. The specificity of *DSM-III* schizotypal personality traits. *Psychol Med.* 1988;18:757-765.
20. Baron M, Gruen R, Asnis L, Kane J. Familial relatedness of schizophrenia and schizotypal states. *Am J Psychiatry.* 1983:140:1437-1442.
21. Torgersen S. Relationship of schizotypal personality disorder to schizophrenia: genetics. *Schizophr Bull.* 1985;11:554-563.
22. Siever LJ, Silverman JM, Horvath TB, Klar H, Coccaro E, Keefe RSE, Pinkham L, Rinaldi P, Mohs RC, Davis KL. Increased morbid risk for schizophrenia-related disorders in relatives of schizotypal personality disorder patients. *Arch Gen Psychiatry.* 1990;47:634-640.
23. Gottesman II. *Schizophrenia Genesis: The Origins of Madness.* New York, NY: WH Freeman & Co; 1991.
24. Roscoe JT. *Fundamental Research Statistics for the Behavioral Sciences.* New York, NY: Holt Rinehart & Winston; 1969.
25. Kety SS. Studies designed to disentangle genetic and environmental variables in schizophrenia: some epistemological questions and answers. *Am J Psychiatry.* 1976;133:1134-1137.
26. Kety SS, Rosenthal D, Wender PH, Schulsinger F. Studies based on a total sample of adopted individuals and their relatives: why they were necessary, what they demonstrated and failed to demonstrate. *Schizophr Bull.* 1976;2:413-428.
27. Kety SS. Mental illness in the biological and adoptive relatives of schizophrenic adoptees: findings relevant to genetic and environmental factors in etiology. *Am J Psychiatry.* 1983;140:720-727.
28. Wender PH, Rosenthal D, Kety SS, Schulsinger F, Welner J. Social class and psychopathology in adoptees. *Arch Gen Psychiatry.* 1973;28:318-325.
29. Plomin R, DeFries JC, McClearn GE. *Behavioral Genetics.* New York, NY: WH Freeman & Co; 1990:334-340.
30. Teasdale TW. Social class correlations among adoptees and their biological and adoptive parents. *Behav Genet.* 1979;9:103-114.

ORIGINAL ARTICLE

Independent Diagnoses of Adoptees and Relatives As Defined by *DSM-III* in the Provincial and National Samples of the Danish Adoption Study of Schizophrenia

Kenneth S. Kendler, MD; Alan M. Gruenberg, MD; Dennis K. Kinney, PhD

Background: This report describes the independent application of *DSM-III* criteria to the adoptees and relatives in the Provincial sample of the Danish Adoption Study of Schizophrenia of Kety and colleagues. We report these results and combine them with those reported previously for the Copenhagen sample to form the National sample.

Methods: Personal interviews and institutional record summaries of adoptees and biological and adoptive relatives were "blindly" diagnosed using *DSM-III* criteria. "Schizophrenia spectrum" was a priori defined as schizophrenia; schizoaffective disorder, mainly schizophrenic subtype; and schizotypal and paranoid personality disorders.

Results and Conclusion: In the Provincial sample, the prevalence of "spectrum" disorders was significantly greater in biological relatives of schizophrenia spectrum vs control adoptees. The results were also consistent with the genetic transmission of individual diagnoses within the spectrum. When combined into the National sample, the results provided strong evidence for (1) the genetic transmission of *DSM-III* schizophrenia; (2) a genetic relationship between *DSM-III* schizophrenia, mainly schizophrenic schizoaffective disorder, and schizotypal personality disorder; and (3) the absence of a significant genetic relationship between the schizophrenia spectrum and either psychotic nonspectrum disorders, major depression, or anxiety disorders. We found no evidence for the familial environment transmission of schizophrenia spectrum disorders. These results are consistent with the findings reported by Kety and coworkers from their diagnostic review.

(Arch Gen Psychiatry. 1994;51:456-468)

Of the numerous twin and adoption studies of schizophrenia performed during the past 60 years,[1,2] one of the most influential has been the investigation of biological and adoptive relatives of schizophrenic and control adoptees carried out in Denmark by Kety and coworkers.[3-7] This landmark study has gone through four phases. First, in 1968, Kety et al[3] reported results from blinded abstracts of hospital records on the biological and adoptive relatives of 34 pairs of matched schizophrenic and control individuals placed for adoption through the courts in the greater Copenhagen area. Second, in 1975, they published preliminary results of diagnoses based on a "blind" review of personal interviews with relatives from this "Copenhagen sample."[4] Third, in 1978, they published results of "blinded" abstracts of hospital records from relatives of 42 pairs of schizophrenic and control adoptees ascertained in the rest of Denmark, termed the "Provincial sample."[5] Combining the Copenhagen and Provincial samples produced the first results of a "National sample" of schizophrenic and matched control adoptees.[5] Finally, in the fourth phase, Kety and coworkers initially reported their blind diagnostic review of interviews with relatives in the Provincial and National samples in a preliminary form[6,8] and then, in the preceding article, more completely.[7]

Since this adoption study began in

From the Departments of Psychiatry and Human Genetics, Medical College of Virginia, Richmond (Dr Kendler); the Dave Garroway Laboratory, Pennsylvania Hospital, and the Department of Psychiatry, University of Pennsylvania School of Medicine, Philadelphia (Dr Gruenberg); and the Laboratories for Psychiatric Research, McLean Hospital, Belmont, Mass, and the Department of Psychiatry, Harvard Medical School, Boston, Mass (Dr Kinney).

See Materials and Methods on next page

MATERIALS AND METHODS

CONDUCTING THE INDEPENDENT REVIEW

We undertook a diagnostic review of interviews from the Provincial sample with the understanding that it would be completely independent from the review of these same interviews conducted by the original investigative team of Dr Kety and Paul Wender, MD. Therefore, aside from receiving copies of the same diagnostic material (interviews, institutional record summaries, and hospital abstracts), no conversation regarding the substance of the work took place between the two research groups until the first draft of manuscripts, including all results based respectively on final and independent diagnoses by the two groups, had been prepared. Thus, our diagnostic review, decisions about the sources of diagnostic information to be used, the inclusion vs exclusion of specific relatives, data analysis, and the initial written version of this article were conducted without knowing the specific decisions or results by Kety and Wender. A description of the method of the Provincial sample of the Danish Adoption Study has been described in a previous report.[7]

DIAGNOSTIC REVIEW

As in our review of the Copenhagen sample, blinded personal interviews and institutional record summaries with index adoptees were reviewed by one of two experienced psychiatric diagnosticians (K.S.K. or A.M.G.). The institutional record summaries, which are exhaustive abstracts of hospital records on index adoptees recorded on interview forms, were sufficiently different in format from the true interviews that we always knew that they were from an index adoptee. Otherwise, we were unaware whether personal interviews were from index or control adoptees or from their biological or adoptive relatives.

Individuals who had been personally contacted were placed into one of two categories: completed interviews and partial reports. Partial reports were prepared from those individual contacts in whom completed interviews could not be obtained. As with the Copenhagen sample, we reviewed these reports, which varied widely in the amount of information they contained, and classified them as adequate (n=9) or inadequate (n=20). Relatives with adequate partial reports were treated like relatives with completed interviews (and both are included when we refer to "interviewed relatives"), whereas relatives with inadequate reports were excluded from further analysis.

As in our analysis of the Copenhagen sample, the diagnoses presented here were based only on information from personal interviews and/or institutional record summaries in adoptees and interviews only from relatives. Hospital abstracts were not used and noninterviewed relatives were excluded from all analyses.

For two index adoptees, paternity could not be unambiguously assigned, as the biological mothers had indicated that there were two possible biological fathers. We chose to exclude their three possible paternal half siblings from analysis. In addition, one full sibling of an index adoptee was adopted together with the index adoptee into the same adoptive home. Again, we chose, a priori, to eliminate this individual (who was both a biological and adoptive relative) from all analyses.

Although we had the thorough interview from the Danish Adoption Study and the Schedule for Affective Disorders and Schizophrenia-Lifetime Version interview, information was not always available to rate each *DSM-III* criterion. Therefore, diagnoses were made nonhierarchically with three levels of certainty. *Definite* diagnoses were made when all diagnostic criteria could be met with a high degree of confidence. *Probable* diagnoses were given when we were confident of the diagnosis but, owing to a lack of information or ambiguity in the available information, we could not be certain that every single criterion was met. *Possible* diagnoses were made when we were reasonably confident of the clini-

Continued on next page

the 1960s, the approach to psychiatric diagnosis has moved from global descriptive criteria that characterized *DSM-II*[9] to the operationalized diagnostic criteria of *DSM-III*[10] and *DSM-III-R*.[11] The concept of schizophrenia has narrowed and a new diagnosis of possible relevance, schizotypal personality disorder (SPD), was created. To see whether the changes in diagnostic criteria would produce any substantial changes in the results of the Danish study, two of us (K.S.K. and A.M.G.), who had no previous role in the Danish Adoption Study, undertook in 1979, with the consent and support of the original investigative team, an independent review of all interviews with relatives and adoptees in the Copenhagen sample.

The *DSM-III* criteria for schizophrenia defined a narrower group of adoptees than those diagnosed as "chronic schizophrenia" by Kety and coworkers.[4,12] Compared with the "spectrum" diagnoses of Kety and coworkers of borderline and uncertain schizophrenia, the *DSM-III* criteria for SPD were more specific but less sensitive.[13] The substantive findings from this independent review confirmed the results of the original diagnostic review by Kety and coworkers.[4,12-17]

Interviews with probands and relatives from the Provincial sample were collected and edited by a team of colleagues in Denmark and the United States under the supervision of Seymour Kety, MD. When these interviews became available, it was decided that two of us (K.S.K. and A.M.G.), who had *no prior involvement* with the Provincial study, should complete an independent diagnostic review on this sample of interviews as had been done with the Copenhagen sample. In this

cal diagnosis but, owing to a lack of or ambiguity of available data, we could not be certain that diagnostic criteria were met. Diagnoses made at the probable or definite level were considered "narrow" diagnoses, whereas those made at the possible, probable, or definite level were considered "broad" diagnoses. As in our previous report,[14] the *DSM-III* diagnoses of generalized anxiety disorder and panic disorder were combined into a single category termed "anxiety disorder." Similarly, alcohol abuse and alcohol dependence were combined into a single category termed "alcoholism."

To assess interrater reliability, we diagnosed, "blind" each one to the other, 40 randomly chosen interviews. Using the broad diagnostic categories used in this report, diagnostic agreement was found in 38 (95%) of 40 cases ($\kappa[\pm SE]=.908\pm.047$).[18]

SCHIZOPHRENIA SPECTRUM

As in our previous report,[12] we defined, a priori, a schizophrenia spectrum consisting of the following *DSM-III* categories: schizophrenia, schizoaffective disorder (meeting Research Diagnostic Criteria[19] for the mainly schizophrenic subtype), SPD, and paranoid personality disorder. Although the Research Diagnostic Criteria provide two criteria with which to diagnose the mainly schizophrenic subtype of schizoaffective disorder, in this study, as in the Copenhagen sample, we only used the second criterion: the presence, for at least 1 week, of psychotic symptoms in the absence of prominent affective symptoms. This criterion is nearly identical with that found for schizoaffective disorder in *DSM-III-R*.[11]

DIAGNOSTIC HIERARCHIES AND THE CONTROL GROUP

Diagnostic hierarchies can complicate the interpretation of family/genetic studies.[20] Therefore, in the Provincial sample, multiple diagnoses were permitted and our analysis of nonschizophrenia spectrum diagnoses is initially presented without hierarchy. However, for schizophrenia spectrum disorders, there is an implicit hierarchy that is assumed in our analyses: schizophrenia, schizoaffective disorder, SPD, and paranoid personality disorder. Kendler and Gruenberg,[12] as well as Kety and colleagues[3,4,7] have previously reported results from this study using "supernormal" control adoptees—removing control adoptees with any major psychopathologic condition. However, this procedure is not without difficulty and can, by producing supernormal relatives of controls, give rise to spurious evidence for coaggregation.[21] Therefore, we take the conservative position and herein only report results for the unscreened control adoptees and their relatives.

STATISTICAL TESTS

For contingency tables where the expected values in all cells exceed 1 and the total number exceeds 20, an uncorrected χ^2 test is used[22,23]; otherwise, a modified Fisher's Exact Test is reported.[24] One-tailed *P* values are reported when there is a strong a priori prediction from our previous work[12-17] or from the literature.[1,2] Biological relatives in this sample are of two different types: first-degree relatives (parents and full siblings) and second-degree relatives (maternal and paternal half siblings). Because the percentage of first- and second-degree relatives is similar in the biological relatives of the index and control adoptees, collapsing the two together into a single contingency table for statistical analysis can be justified. As this approach is not ideal, we also performed logistic regression analyses in which proband status, relative type (first- vs second-degree), and their interaction could be separately tested, by a likelihood ratio χ^2 test (two-tailed *P* values), for their ability to predict diagnosis in relatives.[25]

article, we first report the results of that review and then combine those results with our earlier findings from the Copenhagen sample to present *DSM-III* diagnoses in adoptees and interviewed relatives from the national Danish Adoption Study.

RESULTS

THE PROVINCIAL SAMPLE

Index Adoptees

Adequate diagnostic information was available for all 42 index adoptees, who were assigned the following primary *DSM-III* diagnoses: schizophrenia in 19, schizoaffective disorder (mainly schizophrenic type) in two, SPD in 10, atypical psychosis in two, major depression in three (two with and one without psychotic features), atypical bipolar disorder in two, and obsessive-compulsive disorder, antisocial personality disorder, borderline personality disorder, and no psychiatric diagnosis in one each. By our a priori criteria, 31 of the index adoptees were in the schizophrenia spectrum and 11 were not.

Control Adoptees

The interview status of the 42 control adoptees was as follows: completed interview in 37, inadequate interview report in three, and no personal interview in two. Of the 37 control adoptees with adequate interview information, 25 had no psychiatric diagnosis, while the remaining 12 had the following primary diagnoses: major depression in six, anxiety disorder in five, and SPD in one.

Biological Relatives

The 42 index adoptees had 178 interviewed biological relatives of whom 38 were parents, 22 were full siblings, 63 were paternal half siblings, and 55 were maternal half siblings. The 42 control adoptees had 162 interviewed biological relatives of whom 42 were parents, 18 were full siblings, 51 were paternal half siblings, and 51 were maternal half siblings. Compared with the biological relatives of the control adoptees, the percentage of first- vs second-degree relatives did not differ significantly in the biological relatives of all index adoptees (χ^2=0.41) or in only the schizophrenia spectrum index adoptees (χ^2=0.01). The mean (±SD) age at interview of all biological relatives of control adoptees did not differ significantly from that for the biological relatives of index adoptees (43.9±15.4 vs 46.6±14.1 years, respectively; t=1.68).

Adoptive Relatives

The 42 index adoptees had 41 interviewed adoptive relatives of whom 26 were parents and 15 were siblings. The 42 control adoptees had 54 interviewed adoptive relatives of whom 34 were parents and 20 were siblings. The mean (±SD) age at interview of the adoptive relatives of the control adoptees did not differ significantly from that found for the adoptive relatives of all the index adoptees (62.7±19.2 vs 63.3±16.6 years, respectively; t=0.16).

Distribution of Schizophrenia Spectrum Disorders in Biological Relatives

The distribution of schizophrenia spectrum disorders in all biological relatives of the spectrum and nonspectrum *index* adoptees is seen in **Table 1**. At a trend level, the prevalence of schizophrenia spectrum disorders is higher in the biological relatives of spectrum adoptees than in the biological relatives of nonspectrum index adoptees (10.7% vs 2.6%, respectively; χ^2=2.39; P=.06; one-tailed). Of the nonspectrum adoptees, three had psychotic disorders, all diagnosed as atypical psychosis. No schizophrenia spectrum disorders were found in the 16 biological relatives of these "psychotic nonspectrum" index adoptees (vs biological relatives of spectrum adoptees; χ^2=1.90; P=.08; one-tailed).

The distribution of schizophrenia spectrum disorders in the biological relatives of the schizophrenic and spectrum index adoptees and the biological relatives of all control adoptees is compared in **Table 2**. A trend is seen toward a higher prevalence of schizophrenia spectrum disorders in the biological relatives of the schizophrenic adoptees vs in the biological relatives of all control adoptees (8.0% vs 3.7%, respectively; χ^2=2.09; P=.07; one-tailed). Although not shown, the prevalence of schizophrenia spectrum disorders in the biological relatives of the adoptees with schizoaffective disorder, mainly schizophrenic type, and SPD are both significantly greater than that found in the biological relatives of all control adoptees (χ^2=4.90, P=.01 and χ^2=7.03, P=.004, respectively, both one-tailed). Taken all together, the prevalence of schizophrenia spectrum disorders in the biological relatives of *all* the spectrum adoptees vs *all* control adoptees is highly significantly different (10.7% vs 3.7%, respectively; χ^2=5.70; P=.008; one-tailed).

The distribution of broadly defined schizophrenia spectrum disorders in only the first-degree and only the second-degree biological relatives of the schizophrenic and spectrum index adoptees and the biological relatives of all control adoptees is compared in **Table 3**. Several results are noteworthy. First, the prevalence of spectrum disorders is much greater in the first-degree than in the second-degree biological relatives of schizophrenic and of spectrum adoptees. For example, the rate of spectrum disorder in first-degree biological relatives of spectrum adoptees is 19.6% vs 5.6% in second-degree relatives (χ^2=6.63, P=.01, two-tailed). Unexpectedly, a

Table 1. Schizophrenia Spectrum Disorders in *All* Interviewed Biological Relatives of *Index* Adoptees From the *Provincial* Sample*

Adoptee's Diagnosis	No. of Subjects	Relative's Diagnosis, No. (%): Schizophrenia	SAD, MS	SPD	Schiz Spectrum
Schizophrenia Spectrum					
Schizophrenia	88	2 (2.3)	1 (1.1)	4 (4.5)	7 (8.0)
SAD, MS	11	1 (9.1)	0 (0)	1 (9.1)	2 (18.2)
SPD	41	0 (0)	1 (2.4)	5 (12.2)	6 (14.6)
Total	**140**	**3** (2.1)	**2** (1.4)	**10** (7.1)	**15** (10.7)
Nonspectrum					
Total	38	0 (0)	0 (0)	1 (2.6)	1 (2.6)

SAD, MS indicates schizoaffective disorder, mainly schizophenic subtype; SPD, schizotypal personality disorder; and schiz spectrum, schizophrenia spectrum.

Table 2. Schizophrenia Spectrum Disorders in *All* Interviewed Biological Relatives of Schizophrenic, Spectrum, and *All* Control Adoptees From the *Provincial* Sample*

Adoptee's Diagnosis	No. of Subjects	Relative's Diagnosis, No. (%): Schizophrenia	SAD, MS	SPD	Schiz Spectrum
Schizophrenia	88	2 (2.3)†	1 (1.1)	4 (4.5)‡	7 (8.0)§
Schiz spectrum	140	3 (2.1)‖	2 (1.4)	10 (7.1)¶	15 (10.7)#
Controls	162	1 (0.6)	0 (0)	5 (3.1)	6 (3.7)

Abbreviations are explained in the footnote to Table 1.
†*Versus controls,* χ^2=1.32; P=.13.
‡*Versus controls,* χ^2=0.34; P=.27.
§*Versus controls,* χ^2=2.09; P=.07.
‖*Versus controls,* χ^2=1.34; P=.12.
¶*Versus controls,* χ^2=2.62; P=.05.
#*Versus controls,* χ^2=5.70; P=.008.

Table 3. Schizophrenia Spectrum Disorders in Interviewed *First- and Second-Degree* Biological Relatives of Schizophrenic, Spectrum, and *All* Control Adoptees From the *Provincial* Sample*

Adoptee's Diagnosis	No. of Subjects	Degree of Relationship	Relative's Diagnosis, No. (%): Schizophrenia	SAD, MS	SPD	Schiz Spectrum
Schizophrenia	28	1st	2 (7.1)†	0 (0)	3 (10.7)‡	5 (17.9)§
	60	2nd	0 (0)	1 (1.7)	1 (1.7)‖	2 (3.3)¶
Schiz spectrum	51	1st	2 (3.9)#	1 (2.0)	7 (13.7)**	10 (19.6)††
	89	2nd	1 (1.1)	1 (1.1)	3 (3.4)‡‡	5 (5.6)§§
Controls	60	1st	1 (1.7)	0 (0)	3 (5.0)	4 (6.7)
	102	2nd	0 (0)	0 (0)	2 (2.0)	2 (2.0)

**Abbreviations are explained in the footnote to Table 1.*
†χ^2=1.74; *P*=.09, *vs relatives of controls within same degree of relationship.*
‡χ^2=0.98; *P*=.16, *vs relatives of controls within same degree of relationship.*
§χ^2=2.60; *P*=.05, *vs relatives of controls within same degree of relationship.*
‖χ^2=0.02, *P*=,89, *vs relatives of controls within same degree of relationship.*
¶χ^2=0.30; *P*=.29, *vs relatives of controls within same degree of relationship.*
#χ^2=0.53; *P*=.23, *vs relatives of controls within same degree of relationship.*
**χ^2=2.56; *P*=.05, *vs relatives of controls within same degree of relationship.*
††χ^2=4.19; *P*=.02, *vs relatives of controls within same degree of relationship.*
‡‡χ^2=0.37, *P*=.54, *vs relatives of controls within same degree of relationship.*
§§χ^2=1.80; *P*=.09, *vs relatives of controls within same degree of relationship.*

similar but nonsignificant trend is seen in the biological relatives of control adoptees.

Second, when examining only first-degree biological relatives, we find considerable evidence for the genetic transmission of spectrum disorders, in particular, (1) schizophrenia aggregates in relatives of schizophrenic adoptees (*P*=.09), (2) spectrum disorders aggregate in relatives of schizophrenic adoptees (*P*=.05), (3) SPD aggregates in relatives of spectrum adoptees (*P*=.05), and (4) spectrum disorders aggregate in relatives of spectrum adoptees (*P*=.02). A considerable portion of the evidence for genetic transmission of spectrum conditions is a result of the significant increased prevalence of SPD in the first-degree biological relatives of adoptees with a diagnosis of SPD (4 [19%] of 21) vs first-degree relatives of all controls (5.0%; χ^2=3.89, *P*=.02, one-tailed).

Third, there is only a weak and nonsignificant trend for increased rates for spectrum disorders in second-degree biological relatives of schizophrenic vs control adoptees and only modest evidence for an increased rate for spectrum disorders in second-degree biological relatives of all spectrum adoptees (*P*=.09, one-tailed).

It is of interest to compare the pattern of disorders in the two classes of first-degree relatives, parents, and full siblings because of the empirical finding, predicted by the decreased fitness of schizophrenic individuals, that schizophrenia is much less common in parents than in siblings of schizophrenic probands.[1,26] These results are replicated in the Provincial sample. Of the three cases of schizophrenia or schizoaffective disorder (mainly schizophrenic type) seen in the first-degree biological relatives of the spectrum adoptees, all three are in the 22 full siblings and none in the 29 parents (23.6% vs 0%, respectively; χ^2=4.20; *P*=.02; one-tailed).

The frequencies of spectrum disorders in the relatives of index and control probands were also analyzed by logistic regression. Examining schizophrenia spectrum disorders in the biological relatives of *schizophrenic* vs all control adoptees, we found a highly significant effect of "degree" (first vs second) (χ^2=7.54, *P*=.006), a marginal effect for proband status (schizophrenic vs control) (χ^2=2.65, *P*=.10), and no significant interaction (χ^2=0.21). Examining schizophrenia spectrum disorders in the biological relatives of *schizophrenia spectrum* vs all control adoptees, we found a highly significant effect of "degree" (first vs second) (χ^2=8.96, *P*=.003), a significant effect for proband status (schizophrenic vs control) (χ^2=5.97, *P*=.01), and no significant interaction (χ^2=0.02).

Narrowly Defined Diagnoses

Up until now, results were presented using broadly defined diagnoses. Using more narrowly defined diagnoses (ie, those made at only the definite or probable level), the prevalence of spectrum conditions in all biological relatives of schizophrenic, spectrum, and all control adoptees was five (5.7%) of 88, 10 (7.1%) of 140, and three (1.9%) of 162, respectively (relatives of schizophrenic vs control adoptees: χ^2=2.70, *P*=.05, one-tailed; relatives of spectrum vs control adoptees: χ^2=5.10, *P*=.01, one-tailed). Thus, the percentages of broadly defined schizophrenia spectrum disorders that met narrow criteria in the biological relatives of the schizophrenic, schizophrenic spectrum, and control adoptees were 71%, 67%, and 50%, respectively. In general, using narrower diagnostic criteria modestly increased the evidence for the genetic transmission of spectrum disorders.

Table 4. Nonschizophrenia Spectrum Disorder in *All* Interviewed Relatives of Schizophrenia Spectrum and *All* Control Adoptees From the *Provincial* Sample*

Adoptee's Diagnosis	No. of Subjects	Relative's Diagnosis, No. (%) Major Depression	Anxiety Disorder	Alcoholism
1st- and 2nd-Degree Relatives				
Schizophrenia	88	13 (14.8)	10 (11.4)	9 (10.2)†
Schizophrenia spectrum	140	15 (10.7)	18 (12.9)	11 (7.9)
Controls	162	18 (11.1)	19 (11.7)	6 (3.7)
1st-Degree Relatives				
Schizophrenia	28	7 (25.0)	5 (17.9)	3 (10.7)
Schizophrenia spectrum	51	9 (17.6)	10 (19.6)	4 (7.8)
Controls	60	6 (10.0)	11 (18.3)	2 (3.3)

**Diagnoses made nonhierarchically.*
†Significantly different at P<.05 from prevalence in the relatives of control adoptees.

Morbid Risk for Schizophrenia

Since schizophrenia has a variable age at onset, for many purposes lifetime prevalence is not as useful as morbid risk (MR). We present, calculated using the abridged Weinberg method (age of risk of 15 to 39 years), the MRs (±SE) for schizophrenia in all biological relatives of the following proband groups: all index adoptees—3 of 145=2.1%±1.2%; all control adoptees—1 of 120=0.8%±0.8%; schizophrenia spectrum adoptees—3 of 112.5=2.7%±1.5%; and schizophrenic adoptees—2 of 69.5=2.9%±2.0%. The MR (±SE) for schizophrenia in the first-degree biological relatives of the schizophrenia spectrum and schizophrenic adoptees was, respectively, 2 of 49.5=4.0%±2.8% and 2 of 26.5=7.5%±5.1%. In second-degree biological relatives of the schizophrenia spectrum adoptees, the MR for schizophrenia was 1 of 63=1.6%±1.6%.

Nonspectrum Diagnoses in Biological Relatives

The lifetime prevalence of major depression, anxiety disorder, and alcoholism diagnosed nonhierarchically in all relatives and in only first-degree relatives of the schizophrenic, schizophrenia spectrum, and all control adoptees is seen in **Table 4**. No significant differences are seen in the rates of either major depression or anxiety disorder in relatives of schizophrenic or schizophrenia spectrum vs control adoptees. However, the prevalence of alcoholism (alcohol abuse and alcohol dependence) is significantly greater in all biological relatives of schizophrenic adoptees (10.2%±3.2%) than in all biological relatives of controls (3.7%±1.5%) (χ^2=4.30, *df*=1, *P*=.04). A similar trend is seen in comparing all relatives of schizophrenia spectrum adoptees and controls or just first-degree relatives of schizophrenic and control adoptees, but these differences did not reach statistical significance.

Adoptive Relatives

No schizophrenia spectrum diagnosis was given to any interviewed adoptive relative in the Provincial sample. In the interviewed adoptive relatives of schizophrenic, schizophrenia spectrum, and control adoptees, no significant differences were seen in the prevalence rates of major depression (11.1%, 13.3%, and 7.4%, respectively), anxiety disorders (11.1%, 6.7%, and 5.6%, respectively) or alcoholism (5.6%, 3.3%, and 3.7%, respectively).

THE NATIONAL SAMPLE

Because our diagnostic reviews of the Copenhagen and Provincial samples were carried out by the same diagnosticians (K.S.K. and A.M.G.) using the same criteria (*DSM-III*), it is appropriate to combine results into a single National sample. Before this, however, it is of interest to examine the possible differences in the two samples.

The rates for schizophrenia, SPD, and total spectrum disorders were lower in the biological relatives of the schizophrenic and schizophrenia spectrum adoptees in the Provincial than in the Copenhagen sample. For the individual schizophrenia spectrum diagnoses, the only significant difference was a higher frequency of SPD in second-degree relatives of schizophrenic adoptees in the Copenhagen sample (χ^2=4.20, *df*=1, *P*=.04). However, examining together all the schizophrenia spectrum diagnoses produced significantly higher rates in the Copenhagen vs Provincial sample for all the biological relatives of the schizophrenic adoptees (χ^2=6.98, *df*=1, *P*=.01) and of the schizophrenia spectrum adoptees (χ^2=4.57, *df*=1, *P*=.03). Interestingly, no significant difference for total spectrum disorders was found in first-degree biological relatives in the two samples; but in second-degree relatives, all spectrum disorders were significantly more common in relatives of the schizophrenic (χ^2=6.49, *df*=1, *P*=.01) and the schizophrenia spectrum adoptees (χ^2=5.02, *df*=1, *P*=.03) in the Copenhagen vs Provincial sample.

Biological Relatives—Schizophrenia Spectrum Disorders

Table 5 presents the frequency of broadly defined schizophrenia spectrum disorders in all biological relatives of schizophrenic, schizophrenia spectrum, and control adoptees in the National sample. This table also reports traditional χ^2 analysis of differences in frequency of disorders in the various groups of relatives. In the National sample, the percentage of first- vs second-degree relatives is similar for control adoptees and schizophrenia spectrum adoptees (χ^2=0.58, not significant); therefore, combining results from both groups of relatives is probably appropriate.

Table 5. Schizophrenic Spectrum Disorders in *All* Interviewed Biological Relatives of Schizophrenic Spectrum and Control Adoptees From the *National* Sample*

Adoptee's Diagnosis	No. of Subjects	Relative's Diagnosis, No. (%) Schizophrenia	SAD, MS	SPD	PPD	Schiz Spectrum
Schizophrenia Spectrum						
Schizophrenia	123	4 (3.3)†	1 (0.8)	9 (7.3)†	2 (1.6)	16 (13.0)‡
SAD, MS	39	2 (5.1)†	0 (0)	3 (7.7)§	0 (0)	5 (12.8)†
SPD	47	0 (0)	1 (2.1)	7 (14.9)‡	1 (2.1)	9 (19.1)‡
Total	**209**	**6** (2.9)†	**2** (1.0)	**19** (9.1)‡	**3** (1.4)	**30** (14.4)‡
Controls						
Total	299	1 (0.3)	0 (0)	7 (2.3)	1 (0.3)	9 (3.0)

*Abbreviations are explained in the footnote to Table 1. In addition, PPD indicates paranoid personality disorder.
†P<.01, vs controls (one-tailed).
‡P<.0001, vs controls (one-tailed).
§P<.05, vs controls (one-tailed).

Because of the larger available sample size, we present results separately for relatives of index adoptees with schizophrenia, schizoaffective disorder (mainly schizophrenic type), and SPD, as well as for all of these together.

Compared with biological relatives of control adoptees, biological relatives of schizophrenic, schizoaffective disorder (mainly schizophrenic), and all schizophrenia spectrum adoptees have a significantly greater prevalence of schizophrenia (Table 5). Biological relatives of adoptees with schizophrenia, SPD, and all spectrum disorders also have, compared with biological relatives of controls, a significantly elevated risk for SPD. The prevalence of SPD is more than twice as high in biological relatives of schizotypal adoptees than in biological relatives of schizophrenic adoptees (14.9% vs 7.3%, respectively), although this difference is not statistically significant (χ^2=2.29, *df*=1).

In addition, logistic regression was used in the National sample to examine separately the impact of degree of relationship and adoptee status (index vs control) on risk for schizophrenia or schizophrenia spectrum in relatives (all *df*=1; all *P* values two-tailed). Predicting risk for schizophrenia in relatives of schizophrenic vs control adoptees, degree of relationship (χ^2=5.49, *P*=.02) and adoptee status (χ^2=7.26, *P*=.007) were significant, but their interaction was not (χ=0.24). A similar pattern was found in predicting spectrum disorders in these relatives: degree (χ^2=6.84, *P*=.009), adoptee status (χ^2=17.09, *P*<.0001), interaction (χ^2=0.22, not significant).

Examining relatives of schizophrenia spectrum vs control adoptees, the risk for schizophrenia was only predicted by adoptee status (χ^2=6.09, *P*=.01), as the effect of degree of relationship and the interaction were both nonsignificant (χ^2=1.89 and 0.76, respectively). The risk for schizophrenia spectrum in these relatives was significantly predicted by degree of relationship (χ^2=8.41, *P*=.04) and adoptee status (χ^2=23.65, *P*<.0001). Again, their interaction was nonsignificant (χ^2=0.06).

Results for only first-degree and only second-degree biological relatives in the National sample are seen in **Table 6**. Compared with relatives of controls, first-degree relatives of schizophrenic adoptees are at significantly increased risk for schizophrenia, SPD, and all spectrum disorders. First-degree relatives of schizotypal adoptees are at significantly increased risk for SPD and all spectrum disorders. The prevalence of spectrum disorders in first-degree relatives of all spectrum adoptees is highly significantly greater than in first-degree relatives of control adoptees (23.5% vs 4.7%, respectively; χ^2=15.00; *df*=1; *P*=.00005; one-tailed).

Compared with second-degree relatives of control adoptees, second-degree relatives of schizophrenic adoptees are at significantly increased risk only for all spectrum disorders. Second-degree relatives of adoptees with a diagnosis of schizoaffective disorder (mainly schizophrenic subtype) are, by contrast, at significantly increased risk for schizophrenia, SPD, and all spectrum disorders. Second-degree relatives of schizotypal adoptees are at significantly increased risk for SPD and all spectrum disorders. The prevalence of spectrum disorders in second-degree relatives of all spectrum adoptees is also highly significantly greater than in the second-degree relatives of control adoptees (9.9% vs 2.1%, respectively; χ^2=13.04; *df*=1; *P*=.0002; one-tailed).

Comparing the risk in maternal vs paternal half siblings may provide information regarding the possibility of intrauterine or early postnatal effects in the transmission of schizophrenia spectrum disorders. A modest trend was found for the prevalence of schizophrenia spectrum disorders to be greater in the maternal vs paternal half siblings of the schizophrenic adoptees (5 of 37 vs 2 of 48, respectively; χ^2=2.42; not significant). However, this trend disappeared when the sample was expanded to consider maternal vs paternal half siblings of all schizophrenia spectrum adoptees (8/65 vs 6/76, respectively; χ^2=0.76; not significant).

Table 6. Schizophrenia Spectrum Disorders in Interviewed *First- and Second-Degree* Biological Relatives of Schizophrenic, Spectrum, and *All* Control Adoptees From the *National* Sample*

Adoptee's Diagnosis	No. of Subjects	Degree of Relationship	Relatives Diagnosis, No. (%) Schizophrenia	SAD, MS	SPD	PPD	Schiz Spectrum
			Schizophrenia Spectrum				
Schizophrenia	38	1st	3 (7.9)	0 (0)	5 (13.2)	1 (2.6)	9 (23.7)‡
	85	2nd	1 (1.2)	1 (1.2)	4 (4.7)	1 (1.2)	7 (8.2)‡
SAD, MS	7	1st	0 (0)	0 (0)	0 (0)	0 (0)	0 (0)
	32	2nd	2 (6.3)	0 (0)	3 (9.4)‡	0 (0)	5 (15.6)†
SPD	23	1st	0 (0)	1 (4.3)	5 (21.7)‡	1 (4.3)	7 (30.4)§
	24	2nd	0 (0)	0 (0)	2 (8.3)‖	0 (0)	2 (8.3)‖
Totals	**68**	1st	**3** (4.4)	**1** (1.5)	**10** (14.7)‡	**2** (2.9)‖	**16** (23.5)§
	141	2nd	**3** (2.1)‖	**1** (0.7)	**9** (6.4)	**1** (0.7)	**14** (9.9)†
			Controls				
Totals	107	1st	1 (0.9)	0 (0)	4 (3.7)	0 (0)	5 (4.7)
	192	2nd	0 (0)	0 (0)	3 (1.6)	1 (0.5)	4 (2.1)

**Abbreviations are explained in the footnote to Table 1. In addition, PPD indicates paranoid personality disorder.*
†P<.001, vs relatives of controls within same degree of relationship (one-tailed).
‡P<.01, vs relatives of controls within same degree of relationship (one-tailed).
§P<.0001, vs relatives of controls within same degree of relationship (one-tailed).
‖P<.05, vs relatives of controls within same degree of relationship (one-tailed).

Using the abridged Weinberg method, the MRs (±SEs) for schizophrenia in the first- and second-degree relatives of the schizophrenic adoptees in the National sample equal, respectively, 3 of 36=8.3%±4.6% and 1 of 58=1.7%±1.7%. The MRs (±SEs) for schizophrenia in the first- and second-degree relatives of all spectrum adoptees in the National sample are, respectively, 3 of 65.5=4.6%±2.6% and 3 of 91.5=3.3%±1.9%.

Each index adoptee selected by Kety et al[4] was matched to a control adoptee. It can be argued that this matching should be used in the statistical analysis. The National sample contained 26 matched index-control biological families in which the index adoptee had a diagnosis of schizophrenia and in which at least one biological relative was interviewed. One or more cases of schizophrenia spectrum disorder were diagnosed in 10 of the index biological families vs in two of the control biological families (McNemar's χ^2=5.33, *df*=1, *P*=.01, one-tailed). There were 44 index-control pairs in which the index adoptee had a schizophrenia spectrum diagnosis. One or more cases of schizophrenia spectrum disorder were found in 20 of the index vs in six of the control biological families (McNemar's χ^2=8.91, *df*=1, *P*=.001, one-tailed).

In the National sample, there were 13 index adoptees with a nonaffective psychosis that did not meet criteria for a schizophrenia spectrum disorder (atypical psychosis in six; schizophreniform disorder in five; delusional disorder in one; schizoaffective disorder, other subtype in one). These "psychotic nonspectrum" adoptees had 47 biological relatives in whom only one (2.1%±2.1%) had a schizophrenia spectrum disorder. This prevalence is similar to that found in the biological relatives of controls and significantly lower than that found in the relatives of schizophrenia spectrum adoptees (χ^2=5.39, *P*=.01, one-tailed).

Biological Relatives—Nonschizophrenia Spectrum Disorders

Alcoholism was not recorded as a diagnosis in the Copenhagen sample, so our comparison is restricted to anxiety disorders and major depression. The prevalence rates (±SE) of major depression in all biological relatives of controls in the National sample (30 of 299=10.0%±1.7%) does not differ significantly from that found in all biological relatives of schizophrenic (15 of 123=12.2%±3.0%; χ^2=0.43) or schizophrenia spectrum adoptees (18 of 209=8.6%±1.9%; χ^2=0.30). The prevalence of major depression in the biological relatives of the mainly schizophrenic schizoaffective disorder adoptees (1 of 39=2.6%±2.6%) was nonsignificantly lower than that found in biological relatives of controls (χ^2=2.31).

For anxiety disorders, the rates were also quite similar in all biological relatives of controls (40 of 299=13.4%±2.0%) vs relatives of schizophrenic adoptees (14 of 123=11.4%±2.9%; χ^2=0.31, not significant) and schizophrenia spectrum adoptees (26 of 209=12.4%±2.3%; χ^2=0.10, not significant).

Adoptive Relatives

Only two cases of schizophrenia spectrum disorders were diagnosed in adoptive relatives in the National sample and

both of these were personality disorders (one paranoid and one schizotypal). The prevalence rates (±SE) of schizophrenia spectrum disorders in the adoptive relatives of all control adoptees (1 of 102=1.0%±1.0%) was not different from that found in the adoptive relatives of schizophrenic (0 of 30) or schizophrenia spectrum adoptees (1 of 51=2.0%±2.0%). There were 15 adoptive siblings of schizophrenia spectrum adoptees and eight adoptive siblings of schizophrenic adoptees in the National sample; none of them was given a schizophrenia spectrum diagnosis.

The prevalence rates (±SE) of major depression in the adoptive relatives of all control adoptees (8 of 102=7.8%±2.7%) did not differ significantly from that found in the adoptive relatives either of the schizophrenic (2 of 30=6.7%±4.6%; χ^2=0.05) or of the schizophrenia spectrum adoptees (4 of 51=7.8%±3.8%; χ^2=0.00). The prevalence rates (±SE) of anxiety disorder in the adoptive relatives of all control adoptees (13 of 102=12.7%±3.3%) did not differ significantly from that found in the adoptive relatives either of the schizophrenic (5 of 30=16.7%±6.8%; χ^2=0.30) or of the schizophrenia spectrum adoptees (8 of 51=15.7%±5.1%; χ^2=0.25).

COMMENT

In this study, we blindly applied *DSM-III* criteria to adoptees and their interviewed biological and adoptive relatives in the Provincial sample of the Danish Adoption Study of Schizohrenia conducted by Kety et al.[7] We reported these results and then, combining them with those reported previously for the Copenhagen sample, examined the results on *DSM-III* diagnoses in the adoptees and interviewed relatives in the National adoption sample.

THE SCHIZOPHRENIA SPECTRUM

Schizophrenia

In the Provincial sample, the frequency of schizophrenia was greater in the biological relatives of the schizophrenic and schizophrenia spectrum adoptees than in the biological relatives of the control adoptees, but these differences were not statistically significant. Power calculations suggest, however, that nonsignificant results are not unexpected. If the risks for schizophrenia in first- and second-degree relatives of the schizophrenic and control adoptees were 4.0% and 1.0%, respectively, the power of this sample to show a significant difference ($P<.05$, one-tailed) is only 48%.[27]

When the Provincial and Copenhagen samples are combined into the National sample, however, the frequency of *DSM-III* schizophrenia in the biological relatives of schizophrenic adoptees is significantly greater than in the biological relatives of the control adoptees. These results strongly support the hypothesis that the vulnerability to *DSM-III* schizophrenia is genetically transmitted. No significant difference was found in the risk of maternal and paternal half siblings of the schizophrenic or schizophrenia spectrum adoptees, although the statistical power to detect such a difference is modest in this sample. This result suggests that the transmission of *DSM-III* schizophrenia is due to genetic factors rather than shared maternal influences on the intrauterine or early postnatal environment.

Schizoaffective Disorder

In the Provincial sample, the prevalence of schizophrenia spectrum disorders in the biological relatives of the adoptees with schizoaffective disorder, mainly schizophrenic subtype, significantly exceeded that found in the biological relatives of control adoptees. Combining results to form the National sample, schizophrenia alone, as well as all schizophrenia spectrum disorders, but not major depression, were significantly more common in the biological relatives of adoptees with mainly schizophrenic schizoaffective disorder vs control adoptees.

Similar to *DSM-III-R*,[11] our diagnostic approach to schizoaffective disorder emphasizes the chronologic relationship between affective and psychotic features, this disorder being diagnosed only when psychotic symptoms are present for at least 1 week, when the patient is no longer suffering from prominent affective features. Our results, as well as those of a number of recent family studies,[26,28-32] suggest that, when so diagnosed, schizoaffective disorder has a close familial/genetic relationship with schizophrenia and the schizophrenia spectrum. In accord with some,[30] but not other recent family studies,[28,31,33] we failed to find evidence for a familial/genetic relationship between mainly schizophrenic schizoaffective disorder and unipolar affective illness.

Schizotypal Personality Disorder

The original Copenhagen Danish adoption studies were the first controlled blind investigation to report an excess of nonpsychotic schizophrenialike syndromes (termed "latent," "borderline," and/or "uncertain" schizophrenia) in the biological relatives of schizophrenic adoptees.[3,4] Based in large measure on these studies, and using criteria derived from interviews from the Copenhagen sample, Spitzer et al[34] proposed criteria for a new diagnostic entity: SPD.

Our analysis of the Copenhagen sample found, using *DSM-III* criteria, that SPD strongly aggregated in the biological relatives of schizophrenic and schizophrenia spectrum adoptees.[12,13] Most,[31,35-38] but not all,[39] family studies that have examined this question have also found evidence for a familial/genetic link between schizophrenia and SPD.

In the Provincial sample, we found higher rates for SPD in the biological relatives of schizophrenic and schizophrenia spectrum adoptees. However, this difference only

reached statistical significance for relatives of schizotypal and all schizophrenia spectrum adoptees. Interestingly, the excess risk for SPD in the relatives of the index adoptees in the Provincial sample was restricted to first-degree relatives. Only minor differences in risk for SPD were found in second-degree relatives.

While the results of the Provincial sample are consistent with previous studies suggesting a genetic relationship between SPD and schizophrenia, the findings are less striking than those of the Copenhagen sample or several recent family studies. Nonetheless, when the results of the Provincial and Copenhagen samples are combined into the National sample, the results show a highly significant increased risk for SPD in the relatives of the schizophrenic adoptees.

One unexpected result, seen in the Provincial and Copenhagen samples,[12] was the higher prevalence of SPD in the biological relatives of schizotypal adoptees than in the biological relatives of schizophrenic adoptees. This finding, although falling short of statistical significance, is contrary to the popular conceptual model in which SPD represents a "less severe" variant of schizophrenia. This model predicts that the rate for SPD should be *greater* in relatives of schizophrenic vs schizotypal probands. These results, consistent with findings from twin and family studies suggesting substantial heritability for schizotypal traits,[40-44] suggest that the genetic liability to schizotypal traits may in part be transmitted independently of the vulnerability to schizophrenia.

Schizophrenia Spectrum

Results from the application of *DSM-III* criteria to the Provincial and National samples provide strong support for the hypothesis of a genetic "schizophrenia spectrum." Specifically, these findings suggest that mainly schizophrenic schizoaffective disorder and SPD have a strong genetic relationship with schizophrenia. The results for paranoid personality disorder, although suggestive, are less clear. Our findings confirm, using a different diagnostic system, a key finding from the original analysis of the Copenhagen sample by Kety and coworkers[3,4] and support the wisdom of their sampling strategy for probands, in which they included a wide variety of schizophrenia-like syndromes.

NONSPECTRUM DISORDERS

Nonspectrum Psychotic Disorders

In the Copenhagen and Provincial samples, index adoptees were found with a nonaffective psychotic disorder that did not meet criteria for schizophrenia or schizoaffective disorder (mainly schizophrenic subtype). The rate of schizophrenia spectrum disorders in the biological relatives of these adoptees was similar to that found in relatives of controls and significantly lower than that found in relatives of the schizophrenia spectrum adoptees. This result suggests that these generally acute and good-prognosis psychotic disorders have little genetic relationship with the schizophrenia spectrum. This finding is not consistent with those of several recent large-sample family studies that suggest a familial relationship between schizophrenia and these nonschizophrenic, nonaffective psychoses.[26,31,32,45,46]

Depression

In the Provincial sample, a nonsignificant excess rate of major depression was found in the first-degree biological relatives of schizophrenic vs control adoptees. However, this trend was not found in the biological relatives of the schizophrenia spectrum adoptees. When results of the Provincial and Copenhagen samples were combined into the National sample, the rates of depression were very similar in the biological relatives of the control, schizophrenic, and schizophrenia spectrum adoptees. Overall, applying *DSM-III* criteria to this adoption sample, our results suggest, consistent with most,[33,36,37,39,45,47] but not all,[31,48,49] recent controlled studies using operationalized criteria, that schizophrenia and major depression have little or no familial/genetic relationship. Too few cases of bipolar disorder were found in the biological relatives in the National sample to provide useful information regarding the genetic relationship between schizophrenia and bipolar disorder.

Anxiety Disorder and Alcoholism

Applying *DSM-III* criteria to the Provincial sample, as in the Copenhagen sample, no significant difference was found in the prevalence of anxiety disorder in the biological relatives of the schizophrenic, schizophrenia spectrum, or control adoptees. Consistent with the results of all five recent controlled family studies,[31,33,36,37,45] these results indicate that schizophrenia and anxiety disorders have no substantial familial/genetic relationship.

In the Provincial adoption study, we found modest evidence of an increased risk for alcoholism in the biological relatives of schizophrenic vs control adoptees. This result just reached traditional levels of statistical significance when considering all cases. Examining either relatives of the schizophrenia spectrum adoptees or only cases in the nonschizophrenia spectrum relative, the result was no longer statistically significant.

An examination by Rimmer and Jacobsen[50] of interviewed relatives in the Copenhagen sample revealed nonsignificantly *lower* rates of alcoholism in the biological relatives of index vs control adoptees. Of the six recent controlled family or family history studies of schizophrenia reporting data on alcoholism in relatives, five found no significant difference in risk in the relatives of

schizophrenics vs controls,[31,33,35-37] whereas one found a significantly *lower* risk for alcoholism in the relatives of the schizophrenic vs control probands.[45] Clearly, further work is required to clarify the familial relationship between schizophrenia and alcoholism.

Adoptive Relatives

Consistent with results from the Copenhagen sample, the Provincial sample provided no evidence for the familial/environmental transmission of schizophrenia or schizophrenia spectrum disorders as defined by *DSM-III*. In the National sample, the rates of schizophrenia spectrum disorders were low and equal in the adoptive relatives of the schizophrenic and control adoptees. These results, which are consistent with those of previous adoption studies,[1,51] must be interpreted from the perspective of two potential limitations, both of which stem from the fact that more than 70% of the interviewed adoptive relatives were parents. First, adoptive parents are unlikely to suffer from early onset of severe forms of psychopathology because of the screening they undergo by adoptive agencies before child placement. While this bias should equally affect adoptive families of schizophrenic and control adoptees, it could lower the base rates of schizophrenia spectrum disorders sufficiently to give any test of differences in rates very low power.

SECOND, EXAMINING rates of schizophrenia spectrum disorders in adoptive parents only tests *direct* cultural transmission, which assumes that it is schizophrenia spectrum disorders in adoptive parents that would be schizophrenogenic. Another family of environmental models for *indirect* cultural transmission would postulate that the schizophrenogenic aspects of the familial environment are not captured by diagnoses in individual adoptive relatives of schizophrenia spectrum disorders.[52] However, models for *direct* and *indirect* cultural transmission of schizophrenia spectrum disorders would predict elevated rates of spectrum illness in adoptive siblings of schizophrenic or schizophrenia spectrum adoptees,[52] which were not seen in the modest number of such individuals contained in the National sample. Although our results provide no evidence for nongenetic familial transmission of schizophrenia, the power of these analyses, particularly for models of indirect cultural transmission, may be low.

DIFFERENCES BETWEEN THE COPENHAGEN AND PROVINCIAL SAMPLES

The risk for schizophrenia spectrum disorders by *DSM-III* was significantly lower in the biological relatives of the spectrum adoptees in the Provincial vs the Copenhagen sample. While this might be a true difference, for example resulting from the greater urbanization of the Copenhagen sample, three other explanations deserve consideration. First, criteria for SPD were developed in part from interviews of the Copenhagen sample.[34] It is possible that reapplying these criteria to the data set from which they were derived produced an artifactually elevated rate of illness in the biological relatives of the spectrum adoptees. Second, the diagnosticians (K.S.K. and A.M.G.) may have become more conservative in their application of criteria in the more than 10 years between reviews of the two samples. Third, the results could be due to sampling fluctuation. Most of the differences between the risk for spectrum disorders is found in the second-degree relatives of spectrum adoptees in the Provincial vs Copenhagen sample. This pattern is difficult to explain from any systematic effect.

COMPARISON OF OUR RESULTS WITH THOSE OF THE ORIGINAL INVESTIGATORS

An adverse effect of our independent approach to the diagnostic review and analysis of the Danish adoption studies is that it prevents any simple comparison between our findings and those of the original investigators.[7] Aside from differences in diagnosticians and diagnostic criteria, our studies differed in two other potentially important ways. First, the samples studied by the two teams were not exactly the same. The two groups did not agree on which relatives with partial information to include and we excluded a small number of relatives with uncertain paternity included by Kety et al.[7] We examined relatives of all control adoptees, while Kety et al[7] examined only those of screened control adoptees. Our sample was restricted to personally interviewed relatives, while Kety et al[7] included noninterviewed relatives.

Second, when examining the same subjects, the two teams did not always use the same sources of information. As in our review of the Copenhagen sample, results presented herein were based only on personal interviews in relatives. However, in their review, Kety et al[7] based diagnoses on personal interviews and, if available, hospital abstracts.

A complete examination of the sources of differences in the findings of our two groups is being prepared and is beyond the scope of this article. Preliminary analyses suggest that, controlling for differences in diagnostic information, our *DSM-III* criteria for schizophrenia and SPD defined a smaller group of adoptees and relatives than the categories of chronic and latent schizophrenia of Kety et al. Furthermore, consistent with previous findings,[45,53] the narrower syndromes defined by *DSM-III* may not have been optimal at identifying the biological relatives of schizophrenic adoptees.

LIMITATIONS OF THE SAMPLE

Two methodologic limitations of our diagnostic review of the Danish adoption studies warrant brief comment. First, because of format differences, we were not blind to the institutional record summaries and knew that these were prepared for index adoptees. Therefore, in assigning diagnoses to these cases, we always knew that they were index adoptees. However, as in the Copenhagen sample, we assigned a wide variety of diagnoses to these index probands and we always remained blind to the key independent variable: the relationship between relatives and adoptees.

Second, as in all family studies, in the Danish adoption studies, the interviewed relatives were almost certainly not a random sample of all relatives. It is probable that relatives who, either through refusal, out-migration, or premature death were unable to be interviewed, had higher rates of schizophrenia spectrum pathology than did interviewed relatives. Given the high completion rate of interviews in both the Provincial and Copenhagen samples, this bias is probably a modest one and, more likely than not, would diminish rather than enhance the observed aggregation of schizophrenia spectrum disorders in the biological relatives of spectrum adoptees.

Accepted for publication July 29, 1993.

This research was supported in part by grants MH-41953, MH-36088, and MH-31154 from the National Institute of Mental Health, Bethesda, Md, and grants 81-171 and BRSG-HIM (RR-05484) from the MacArthur Foundation, Chicago, Ill.

We thank Dr Seymour Kety; D. Rosenthal, PhD; F. Schulsinger, MD; and P. Wender, MD, for allowing us to review their data from the Danish Adoption Study of Schizophrenia, B. Jacobsen, MD; L. Jansson, MD; and B. Faber, MD, for conducting the personal interviews, and the adoptees and their families for their participation. We also thank J. Endicott, MD, for consultation on the training of the psychiatric interviewers, Dr Kety for advice on various aspects of the project, and Lisa L. Burkett, Tom Barnes, Michelle Chang, Sandra M. Cole, Anette Ganz, Elizabeth Gander, Kathleen Kelly, Juliet Regner, and Jennifer Restrepo for research assistance.

Reprint requests to Department of Psychiatry, Medical College of Virginia, Box 710, Richmond, VA 23298 (Dr Kendler).

REFERENCES

1. Gottesman II, Shields J. *Schizophrenia: The Epigenetic Puzzle.* New York, NY: Cambridge University Press; 1982.
2. Kendler KS, Diehl SR. The genetics of schizophrenia: a current, genetic-epidemiologic perspective. *Schizophr Bull.* 1993;19:261-285.
3. Kety SS, Rosenthal D, Wender PH, Schulsinger F. The types and prevalence of mental illness in the biological and adoptive families of adopted schizophrenics. *J Psychiatr Res.* 1968;6:345-362.
4. Kety SS, Rosenthal D, Wender PH, Schulsinger F, Jacobsen B. Mental illness in the biological and adoptive families of adopted individuals who have become schizophrenic: a preliminary report based on psychiatric interviews. In: Fieve R, Rosenthal D, Brill H, eds. *Genetic Research in Psychiatry.* Baltimore, Md: The Johns Hopkins Press; 1975:147-165.
5. Kety SS, Rosenthal D, Wender PH, Schulsinger F, Jacobsen B. The biological and adoptive families of adopted individuals who became schizophrenic: prevalence of mental illness and other characteristics. In: Wynne LC, Cromwell RL, Matthysse S, eds. *The Nature of Schizophrenia.* New York, NY: John Wiley & Sons Inc; 1978:25-37.
6. Kety SS. The significance of genetic factors in the etiology of schizophrenia: results from the National Study of Adoptees in Denmark. *J Psychiatr Res.* 1987; 21:423-429.
7. Kety SS, Wender P, Jacobsen B, Ingraham LJ, Jansson L, Faber B, Kinney DK. Mental illness in the biological and adoptive relatives of adopted individuals with schizophrenia: replication of the Copenhagen study in the rest of Denmark. *Arch Gen Psychiatry.* 1994;51:440-453.
8. Kety SS, Ingraham LJ. Genetic transmission and improved diagnosis of schizophrenia from pedigrees of adoptees. *J Psychiatr Res.* 1992;26:247-255.
9. American Psychiatric Association, Committee on Nomenclature and Statistics. *Diagnostic and Statistical Manual of Mental Disorders, Second Edition.* Washington, DC: American Psychiatric Association; 1968.
10. American Psychiatric Association, Committee on Nomenclature and Statistics. *Diagnostic and Statistical Manual of Mental Disorders, Third Edition.* Washington, DC: American Psychiatric Association; 1980.
11. American Psychiatric Association, Committee on Nomenclature and Statistics. *Diagnostic and Statistical Manual of Mental Disorders, Revised Third Edition.* Washington, DC: American Psychiatric Association; 1987.
12. Kendler KS, Gruenberg AM. An independent analysis of the Copenhagen sample of the Danish Adoption Study of Schizophrenia, VI: the relationship between psychiatric disorders as defined by *DSM-III* in the relatives and adoptees. *Arch Gen Psychiatry.* 1984;41:555-564.
13. Kendler KS, Gruenberg AM, Strauss JS. An independent analysis of the Copenhagen sample of the Danish Adoption Study of Schizophrenia, II: the relationship between schizotypal personality disorder and schizophrenia. *Arch Gen Psychiatry.* 1981;38:982-984.
14. Kendler KS, Gruenberg AM, Strauss JS. An independent analysis of the Copenhagen sample of the Danish Adoption Study of Schizophrenia, I: the relationship between anxiety disorder and schizophrenia. *Arch Gen Psychiatry.* 1981;38:973-977.
15. Kendler KS, Gruenberg AM, Strauss JS. An independent analysis of the Copenhagen sample of the Danish Adoption Study of Schizophrenia, III: the relationship between paranoid psychosis (delusional disorder) and the schizophrenia spectrum disorders. *Arch Gen Psychiatry.* 1981;38:985-987.
16. Kendler KS, Gruenberg AM, Strauss JS. An independent analysis of the Copenhagen sample of the Danish Adoption Study of Schizophrenia, IV: the relationship between major depressive disorder and schizophrenia. *Arch Gen Psychiatry.* 1982;39:639-642.
17. Kendler KS, Gruenberg AM. Genetic relationship between paranoid personality disorder and the 'schizophrenic spectrum' disorders. *Am J Psychiatry.* 1982; 139:1185-1186.
18. Cohen J. A coefficient of agreement for nominal scales. *Educ Psychol Measurement.* 1960;20:37-46.
19. Spitzer RL, Endicott J, Robins E. *Research Diagnostic Criteria for a Selected Group of Functional Disorders.* 2nd ed. New York: New York Psychiatric Institute; 1975.
20. Kendler KS. The impact of diagnostic hierarchies on prevalence estimates for psychiatric disorders. *Compr Psychiatry.* 1988;29:218-227.
21. Kendler KS. The super-normal control group in psychiatric genetics: possible artifactual evidence for coaggregation. *Psychiatr Genet.* 1990;1:45-53.
22. Camilli G, Hopkins KD. Applicability of chi-square to 2×2 contingency tables with small expected cell frequencies. *Psychol Bull.* 1978;85:163-167.
23. Bradley DR, Bradley TD, McGrath SG, Cutcomb SD. Type I error rate of the chi-square test of independence in R×C tables that have small expected frequencies. *Psychol Bull.* 1979;86:1290-1297.
24. Miettinen OS. Comment. *J Am Stat Assoc.* 1974;69:380-382.
25. *SUGI Supplemental Library User's Guide Version.* 5th ed. Cary, NC: SAS Institute Inc; 1986.
26. Kendler KS, McGuire M, Gruenberg AM, O'Hare A, Spellman M, Walsh D. The Roscommon Family Study, I: methods, diagnosis of probands, and risk of schizophrenia in relatives. *Arch Gen Psychiatry.* 1993;50:527-540.

27. Haynam GE, Govindarajulu Z, Leone FC. Tables of the cumulative non-central chi-square distribution. In: Harter HL, Owen DB, eds. *Selected Tables in Mathematical Statistics, I.* Providence, RI: American Mathematical Society; 1970:1-78.
28. Baron M, Gruen R, Asnis L, Kane J. Schizoaffective illness, schizophrenia and affective disorders: morbidity risk and genetic transmission. *Acta Psychiatr Scand.* 1982;65:253-262.
29. Kendler KS, Adler D. The pattern of psychotic illness in pairs of psychotic siblings. *Am J Psychiatry.* 1984;141:509-513.
30. Kendler KS, Gruenberg AM, Tsuang MT. A DSM-III family study of the nonschizophrenic psychotic disorders. *Am J Psychiatry.* 1986;143:1098-1105.
31. Gershon ES, DeLisi LE, Hamovit J, Nurnberger JI, Maxwell ME, Schreiber J, Dauphinais D, Dingman CW II, Guroff JJ. A controlled family study of chronic psychoses: schizophrenia and schizoaffective disorder. *Arch Gen Psychiatry.* 1988;45:328-336.
32. Kendler KS, McGuire M, Gruenberg AM, Spellman M, O'Hare A, Walsh D. The Roscommon Family Study, II: the risk of nonschizophrenic nonaffective psychoses in relatives. *Arch Gen Psychiatry.* 1993;50:645-652.
33. Kendler KS, McGuire M, Gruenberg AM, O'Hare A, Spellman M, Walsh D. The Roscommon Family Study, IV: affective illness, anxiety disorders, and alcoholism in relatives. *Arch Gen Psychiatry.* 1993;50:952-960.
34. Spitzer RL, Endicott J, Gibbon M. Crossing the border into borderline personality and borderline schizophrenia. *Arch Gen Psychiatry.* 1979;36:17-24.
35. Kendler KS, Masterson C, Ungaro R, Davis K. A family history study of schizophrenia-related personality disorder. *Am J Psychiatry.* 1984;141:424-427.
36. Baron M, Gruen R, Rainer JD, Kane J, Asnis L, Lord A. A family study of schizophrenia and normal control probands: implications for the spectrum concept of schizophrenia. *Am J Psychiatry.* 1985;142:447-455.
37. Frangos E, Athanassenas G, Tsitourides S, Katsanou N, Alexandrakou P. Prevalence of DSM-III schizophrenia among the first-degree relatives of schizophrenic probands. *Acta Psychiatr Scand.* 1985;72:382-386.
38. Kendler KS, McGuire M, Gruenberg AM, O'Hare A, Spellman M, Walsh D. The Roscommon Family Study, III: schizophrenia-related personality disorders in relatives. *Arch Gen Psychiatry.* 1993;50:781-788.
39. Coryell W, Zimmerman M. The heritability of schizophrenia and schizoaffective disorder: a family study. *Arch Gen Psychiatry.* 1988;45:323-327.
40. Torgersen S. Genetic and nosological aspects of schizotypal and borderline personality disorders: a twin study. *Arch Gen Psychiatry.* 1984;41:546-554.
41. Kendler KS, Heath AC, Martin NG. A genetic epidemiologic study of self-report suspiciousness. *Compr Psychiatry.* 1987;28:187-196.
42. Kendler KS, Hewitt JK. The structure of self-report schizotypy in twins. *J Pers Disord.* 1992;6:1-17.
43. Siever LJ, Silverman JM, Horvath TB, Klar H, Coccaro E, Keefe RSE, Pinkham L, Rinaldi P, Mohs RC, Davis KL. Increased morbid risk for schizophrenia-related disorders in relatives of schizotypal personality disordered patients. *Arch Gen Psychiatry.* 1990;47:634-640.
44. Claridge G, Hewitt JK. A biometrical study of schizotypy in a normal population. *Pers Individ Diff.* 1987;8:303-312.
45. Kendler KS, Gruenberg AM, Tsuang MT. Psychiatric illness in first-degree relatives of schizophrenic and surgical control patients: a family study using *DSM-III* criteria. *Arch Gen Psychiatry.* 1985;42:770-779.
46. Guze SB, Cloninger CR, Martin RL, Clayton PJ. A follow-up and family study of schizophrenia. *Arch Gen Psychiatry.* 1983;40:1273-1276.
47. Maj M, Starace F, Pirozzi R. A family study of DSM-III-R schizoaffective disorder, depressive type, compared with schizophrenia and psychotic and nonpsychotic major depression. *Am J Psychiatry.* 1991;148:612-616.
48. Maier W, Hallmayer J, Minges J, Lichtermann D. Affective and schizoaffective disorders: similarities and differences. In: Marneros A, Tsuang MT, eds. *Morbid Risks in Relatives of Affective Schizoaffective, and Schizophrenic Patients—Results of a Family Study.* New York: Springer-Verlag NY Inc; 1990:201-207.
49. Taylor MA, Berenbaum SA, Jampala VC, Cloninger CR. Are schizophrenia and affective disorder related? preliminary data from a family study. *Am J Psychiatry.* 1993;150:278-285.
50. Rimmer J, Jacobsen B. Alcoholism in schizophrenics and their relatives. *J Stud Alcohol.* 1977;38:1781-1784.
51. Kendler KS. The genetics of schizophrenia: an overview. In: Nasrallah HA, series ed.; Tsuang MT, Simpson JC, volume eds. *Handbook of Schizophrenia, III: Nosology, Epidemiology and Genetics.* Amsterdam, the Netherlands: Elsevier Science Publishers; 1988:437-462.
52. Kendler KS. Indirect vertical cultural transmission: a model for nongenetic parental influence on the liability to psychiatric illness. *Am J Psychiatry.* 1988; 145:657-665.
53. Kendler KS, Spitzer RL, Williams JB. Psychotic disorders in DSM-III-R. *Am J Psychiatry.* 1989;146:953-962.

ORIGINAL ARTICLE

Neuropsychological Deficits in Schizophrenics

Relationship to Age, Chronicity, and Dementia

Robert Heaton, PhD; Jane S. Paulsen, PhD; Lou Ann McAdams, PhD; Julie Kuck, MA; Sidney Zisook, MD; David Braff, MD; M. Jackuelyn Harris, MD; Dilip V. Jeste, MD

Background: We sought to determine whether neuropsychological impairment in schizophrenia is related to current age, age at onset, or duration of illness, and whether the pattern of such impairment can be distinguished from that caused by progressive dementias of Alzheimer's type. We administered a comprehensive neuropsychological test battery to a normal control group (n=38), a group of ambulatory patients with Alzheimer's disease (n=42), and three ambulatory schizophrenic groups: early onset–young (n=85), early onset–old (n=35), and late onset (n=22). Tests were grouped and analyzed according to eight major ability areas, and published procedures were used to remove the expected effects of normal aging.

Results: The three schizophrenic groups were found to be neuropsychologically similar to one another and different from normal controls and patients with Alzheimer's disease. There were no significant differences among the schizophrenic groups in level or pattern of neuropsychological functioning. Patients with Alzheimer's disease demonstrated less efficient learning and particularly more rapid forgetting than did the other groups.

Conclusions: These findings suggest that neuropsychological impairment in schizophrenia is unrelated to current age, age at onset, or duration of illness. The study further suggests that the encephalopathy associated with schizophrenia is essentially nonprogressive and produces a pattern of deficits that is different from that seen in progressive cortical dementias.

(Arch Gen Psychiatry. 1994;51:469-476)

From the Department of Psychiatry, University of California–San Diego.

Despite notable heterogeneity in the behavioral presentation of schizophrenia, there is general agreement regarding the presence of neuropsychological (NP) impairments that accompany the disorder. Impaired performance on standardized NP tests, especially those involving abstraction, attention, language, and memory, has frequently been reported,[1-4] and memory is likely to be impaired out of proportion to other NP functions.[3,5] There are indications, however, that the memory impairment is due to especially inefficient learning rather than to rapid forgetting of recently learned information.[6] Rapid forgetting of recently learned information, on the other hand, is a hallmark of progressive cortical dementias such as Alzheimer's disease (AD).

Relatively little is known about the potential interaction between the cognitive deficits associated with schizophrenia and aging.[7-9] The prevalence of schizophrenia among the elderly is estimated at 300 000, or 1% of the US population aged 65 and older.[10] Given the anticipated increases in life expectancy, this number is expected to grow. Research on late-life schizophrenia is essential to improved care of the aging population and also to our understanding of psychosis and the aging brain.

A number of long-term follow-up studies of schizophrenic patients have shown that the *clinical* prognosis of schizophrenia is better than that implied in Kraepelin's use of the term *dementia praecox*.[11] Bleuler, Huber, and Ciompi[12] all came to the same conclusion, ie, that schizophrenia is in no sense a "basically"

See Methods on next page

METHODS

SUBJECTS

A total of 222 subjects participated in this study: 38 NC subjects, 85 younger schizophrenic patients with disease onset before the age of 45 years (early-onset schizophrenia–young [EOS-Y]), 22 older schizophrenic patients with disease onset after the age of 45 years (LOS), 35 older patients with disease onset before the age of 45 years (early-onset schizophrenia–old [EOS-O]), and 42 patients with AD. Patients with schizophrenia were recruited for research purposes from the San Diego (Calif) Veterans Affairs Medical Center, the Mission Valley Veterans Affairs Outpatient Clinic, San Diego, the University of California, San Diego Medical Center and Psychiatry Outpatient Services, the San Diego County Mental Health Services, and private physicians. The AD subjects came from clinical referrals for testing in the University of Colorado Psychiatry Department Neuropsychology Laboratory, Denver. The NC subjects were obtained from the community in San Diego and were recruited to be comparable with the older patient groups in age and education. All the subjects were screened with a medical history questionnaire and physical examinations to exclude the following: history of moderate or severe head trauma (loss of consciousness [>30 minutes] or hospitalization for residual neurological findings) or other neurological disorder (except AD in the AD group), current alcohol or other substance abuse (no substance abuse for past 6 months), and systemic medical disease that was judged likely to affect central nervous system functions. For the patient groups, appropriate laboratory tests were performed, when indicated, to rule out other causes of cerebral dysfunction (eg, thyroid function tests, serum vitamin B_{12} levels, VDRL, and computed tomography or magnetic resonance imaging of the brain). The diagnosis of schizophrenia and subtype determination were assigned on the basis of a semistructured intake evaluation based on *DSM-III-R* criteria,[20] followed by research staffing where at least three board-certified psychiatrists agreed on the diagnosis of each schizophrenic patient. In addition, LOS subjects had to meet our own strict research criteria for LOS.[18]

Diagnostic evaluations for the AD sample have been described in detail by Filley et al.[21] Briefly, the diagnosis of AD was made by a senior staff neurologist according to the criteria developed by the National Institute of Neurological and Communicative Disorders and Stroke and the Alzheimer's Disease and Related Disorders Association.[22] The inclusion criteria were dementia documented by detailed clinical evaluation, deficits in at least two areas of cognition, and a progressive cognitive decline. To reduce the possibility of including multi-infarct dementias, patients with a score of 5 or greater on the Hachinski scale[23] were excluded from the AD group. All the AD patients were ambulatory and had a relatively recent onset of symptoms (mean duration of illness was 3.1 years).

CLINICAL EVALUATION

Structured neurological, medical, and socioeconomic histories were obtained, and physical examinations were performed by qualified physicians. To obtain as complete information as was possible from every available source, schizophrenic subjects' family members and significant others were interviewed, and all the available medical records from present and past treating physicians were acquired. The current daily neuroleptic dose was converted to milligrams of the chlorpromazine equivalent.[24(p3)] Age at illness onset was determined as the reported onset of prodromal symptoms in schizophrenia or the beginning of functional decline in AD.

The following rating scales were used with the NC and schizophrenic subjects: Brief Psychiatric Rating Scale,[25] Scales for the Assessment of Negative and Positive Symptoms,[26] and the Abnormal Involuntary Movement Scale.[27] All these assessments were performed by members of the research team who were not treating the schizophrenic patients, and the raters were kept "blind" to other clinical and NP information.

Table 1 summarizes the psychopathological and treatment characteristics of the schizophrenic groups. Three-group comparisons were significant on all of the rating scale scores of psychopathology (Brief Psychiatric Rating Scale and Scales for the Assessment of Negative and Positive Symptoms). Pairwise comparisons showed that the EOS-Y group had more severe global psychopathology and positive and negative symptoms than did the EOS-O group. Compared with the early-onset groups, a higher percentage of the LOS patients were classified as having the paranoid subtype. Finally, although there was an overall group difference in terms of the mean daily neuroleptic dose, pairwise differences were not significant with the Bonferroni correction. A three-group comparison of abnormal involuntary movements using the total Abnormal Involuntary Movement Scale score was significant, and pairwise comparisons demonstrated the least dyskinesia in the EOS-Y group. This finding is consistent with those findings in the previous literature suggesting an increased risk of tardive dyskinesia associated with aging.[28-31]

NP ASSESSMENT

All the subjects were administered an expanded Halstead-Reitan NP Test Battery in a standardized fashion by psychometrists. In selecting the NP tests, we began by defining the NP ability areas that we believed to be relevant in studies of aging, schizophrenia, and dementing disorders. Once the ability areas were defined (ie, verbal abilities, complex perceptual-motor skills, abstraction/flexibility of thinking, attention, learning, memory, sensory abilities, and motor skills), we chose tests that seemed to reflect these areas. The tests that were finally selected represented a balance between the need to be comprehensive and relevant, while at the same time recognizing limitations of time and the older subjects' physical ability to undergo prolonged testing.

In addition to the core Halstead-Reitan tests,[32] the bat-

tery included the Wechsler Adult Intelligence Scale–revised (WAIS-R[33]), the standard Wisconsin Card Sorting Test,[34] the Boston Naming Test,[35] the Grooved Pegboard Test,[36] the Reitan-Klove Sensory Perceptual Examination, a modified Aphasia Screening Test,[32] and the Story and Figure Memory Tests.[37] The total battery of tests usually took 8 hours to complete and was generally administered to an individual patient during 2 to 3 days. Rest breaks within sessions were arranged to accommodate the needs of each subject. The subjects were tested only when clinically and pharmacologically stable.

The individual test measures that contributed to the assessment of each of the eight major ability areas were as follows: (1) verbal—Aphasia Screening Test–Verbal, Boston Naming Test, WAIS-R Comprehension, WAIS-R Information, WAIS-R Similarities, and WAIS-R Vocabulary; (2) complex perceptual-motor skills—Aphasia Screening Test–Spatial Relations, Tactual Performance Test–total time, Trails A, WAIS-R Block Design, WAIS-R Digit Symbol, and WAIS-R Object Assembly; (3) abstraction and cognitive flexibility—Category Test, Trails B, and Wisconsin Card Sorting Test; (4) attention—Rhythm Test, Speech Sounds Perception Test, WAIS-R Arithmetic, and WAIS-R Digit Span; (5) learning—Figure Memory Test (Learning), Story Memory Test (Learning), Tactual Performance Test–location, and Tactual Performance Test–memory; (6) memory—Figure Memory (percent retention after 4-hour delay) and Story Memory (percent retention after 4-hour delay); (7) sensory abilities—Sensory Perceptual Examination (right and left errors) and Tactile Form Recognition Test (right and left times); and (8) motor skills—Finger Tapping Test (dominant and nondominant hands), Grooved Pegboard Test (dominant and nondominant hands), and Hand Dynamometer Test (dominant and nondominant hands).

All the raw scores on the NP tests were converted to age-, education-, and gender-corrected *T* scores.[37,38] These conversions were based on published data from large normative samples. In normal subjects, the *T* scores are normally distributed with a mean of 50 and an SD of 10. Two standard summary NP variables were considered from this battery: the WAIS-R Full-Scale IQ and the Average Impairment Rating from the Halstead-Reitan Battery.[32] To assist further in data reduction and in comparison of groups across ability areas, we computed summary scores called "deficit scores" for the entire test battery and for the eight major ability areas. To do this, the *T* score on each test was assigned a deficit rating based on the following scale: *T* scores equal to or greater than 40 represented no impairment (deficit score=0); 39 to 35 (mild impairment, deficit score=1); 34 to 30 (mild to moderate impairment, deficit score=2); 29 to 25 (moderate impairment, deficit score=3); 24 to 20 (moderate to severe impairment, deficit score=4); and below 20 (severe impairment, deficit score=5).

Deficit scores on each individual test were combined into deficit ratings for the eight major ability areas by using the following formula: sum of the individual deficit scores in a given ability area/number of tests in that ability area=ability deficit score. In addition, a Global Deficit Score was calculated (sum of all deficit scores/total number of tests administered) for each subject. If sufficient tests were not administered for deficit score calculations, the subjects were deleted from this analysis. For example, the Verbal Deficit Score was calculated when four of six tests were available, whereas the Memory Deficit Score could only be calculated if both tests (two of two) were available. Previous research has demonstrated the validity of the deficit score approach for detecting clinically significant impairment.[37] We have reported on some aspects of the NP performance of NC, EOS-Y,[6] LOS,[18] EOS-O, and AD[21] patients. This is, however, to our knowledge, the first comprehensive analysis comparing all these subject groups (including some additional subjects), and focusing on the overall NP impairment as well as on individual ability areas. We restricted our study to outpatients not only because a large majority of schizophrenic patients receive ambulatory care but also to obtain a comprehensive NP evaluation and to reduce possible confounds from neurological or other medical comorbidity.

STATISTICAL METHODS

Within each of the five subject groups (NC, EOS-Y, LOS, EOS-O, and AD), the mean and SD were calculated for each of the continuous demographical, clinical, and NP variables. When assumptions of normality or homogeneity of variance among the groups were violated for any variable, data were transformed by using square root, log, or reciprocal (inverse) transformations until parametric assumptions were met. After these assumptions were met with or without transformations, univariate analysis of variance (ANOVA) was conducted on demographic and clinical variables and the standard NP summary scores. An omnibus multivariate analysis of variance was conducted on the set of NP ability area deficit scores, and if significant, univariate ANOVAs were conducted on the individual ability area deficit scores. If an individual ANOVA was significant, post hoc comparisons were made between each pair of groups.

When achievement of normality and/or homogeneity by transformations was not possible, groups were compared by means of nonparametric statistics. For ordered variables, the Kruskal-Wallis ANOVA was used to compare medians among three or more groups. When the Kruskal-Wallis Test was significant, Mann-Whitney *U* tests were performed for pairs of the groups. Groups were compared on categorical variables by χ^2 tests. When an overall χ^2 was significant for multiple groups, χ^2 tests were performed on the distributions of pairs of the groups.

To reduce the risk of type I error due to multiple comparisons, we used Bonferroni corrections both for the overall number of ANOVA, Kruskal-Wallis, or χ^2 tests that were done and for the number of multiple comparison tests that were done on each variable.

Finally, a discriminant function analysis was performed to explore the degree to which NP ability area deficit scores could correctly classify individual subjects as being schizophrenic, AD, or NC.

Table 1. Psychopathological and Treatment Characteristics of Schizophrenic Groups*

Variable	EOS-Y (n=85)	LOS (n=22)	EOS-O (n=35)	*P*	Group Effects
Subtype, % paranoid	23.5	77.3	34.3	.0001†	LOS>EOS-O=EOS-Y
Neuroleptic dose (chlorpromazine)‡	805.2 (1392.2)	187.0 (203.8)	518.9 (781.2)	.0145	NS
BPRS score	36.6 (11.2)	33.2 (7.6)	30.8 (11.3)	.0078†	EOS-Y>EOS-O
SANS score	12.2 (5.0)	3.7 (3.2)	6.4 (4.5)	.0001†	EOS-Y>EOS-O=LOS
SAPS score	6.7 (4.3)	4.9 (3.7)	4.3 (4.0)	.0071†	EOS-Y>EOS-O
AIMS score	0.2 (0.5)	0.9 (1.3)	3.1 (3.9)	.0001†	EOS-O=LOS>EOS-Y

Values are means (SDs) or percentages. EOS-Y indicates early-onset schizophrenics–young; LOS, late-onset schizophrenics; EOS-O, early-onset schizophrenics–old; NS, nonsignificant with the Bonferroni correction; BPRS, Brief Psychiatric Rating Scale (total); SANS, Scale for the Assessment of Negative Symptoms (total global); SAPS, Scale for the Assessment of Positive Symptoms (total global); and AIMS, Abnormal Involuntary Movement Scale (total).

†P value significant with the Bonferroni correction. The statistical tests used for these analyses were as follows: F test for SAPS, Welch's F test for BPRS and SANS, Kruskal-Wallis for AIMS and chlorpromazine, and χ^2 for subtype.

‡Daily chlorpromazine neuroleptic dose in chlorpromazine equivalents (in milligrams).

or even "predominantly" unfavorable disease process that runs an inexorably deteriorating course. The proportions of patients with favorable outcomes (either recovery or mild end state) were 53% in the study by Bleuler, 57% in the study by Huber et al, and 59% in that by Ciompi.[12] Only 18% of the patients described by Ciompi[12] had "severe" end stage. These findings were corroborated in the 10 North American long-term follow-up studies of schizophrenia reviewed by McGlashan.[13] McGlashan concluded that the schizophrenia process appeared to plateau after 5 to 10 years of manifest illness. In contrast, Davidson and colleagues[14] noted that more than two thirds of 550 institutionalized elderly schizophrenic patients had Mental Status Examination scores consistent with a diagnosis of dementia. Results from these clinical studies emphasize the variations of outcome in schizophrenia. The NP abilities were not addressed in these studies, however, so the nature and degree of cognitive impairment in late-life schizophrenia remain unclear.

In a recent review addressing this issue, Heaton and Drexler[15] examined 100 cross-sectional studies and 10 longitudinal studies of NP functioning in schizophrenia. The results generally argued against the possibility of a progressive NP impairment and, in particular, suggested that schizophrenic patients probably do not have more rapid NP decline associated with the aging process. Heaton and Drexler[15] noted numerous methodological limitations of the available literature, however, qualifying the conclusions made. Given the paucity of systematic studies of cognitive changes in aging schizophrenic patients, further research in this area is warranted. Related, but separate, issues are whether age at disease onset or illness duration affects NP status. There have been very few NP studies of late-onset schizophrenia (LOS).[16-18] In terms of the relationship of NP impairment to chronicity, Goldberg et al[19] have suggested that schizophrenia is associated with a nonprogressive encephalopathy that originates during the developmental period.

The goals of the present study were (1) to examine NP abilities of carefully diagnosed samples of schizophrenic outpatients differing in current age and age at illness onset and (2) to compare the NP functioning of the schizophrenic groups with that of older normal control (NC) subjects and patients with AD. This study contributes to the available published literature in two ways. First, to our knowledge, this is the first NP study to compare well-characterized schizophrenic groups varying in age, age at onset, and illness duration. Second, the present study uses comprehensive standardized NP test instruments that have adequate normative standards available to correct for the expected effects of normal aging. The following hypotheses were proposed: (1) on measures of global cognitive functions that are corrected for normal aging, all the patient groups show impairment relative to NC subjects; (2) schizophrenic groups with longer illness duration do not demonstrate a greater level of impairment; (3) schizophrenic groups do not differ from one another with respect to pattern of NP functioning; and (4) on measures of specific cognitive deficits, AD patients demonstrate a different level and pattern of impairment than schizophrenic groups—more specifically, AD patients are more impaired overall and are particularly deficient in memory measures that rely on retention of information throughout a delay period.

RESULTS

Table 2 summarizes the demographic characteristics for the NC, EOS-Y, LOS, EOS-O, and AD groups, and the age at onset and illness duration data for the four patient groups. There were no significant group differences in education. The NC and AD groups were older than the LOS and EOS-O groups, and all of these were older than the EOS-Y group. The EOS-O group had a greater proportion of males, and the NC group had a greater proportion of females than the other groups. As noted above, the effects of normal aging and gender on NP measures were controlled in this study by using demographically

Table 2. Demographic and Global Cognitive Characteristics of the Five Subject Groups*

Variable	NC (n=38)	EOS-Y (n=85)	LOS (n=22)	EOS-O (n=35)	AD (n=42)	*P*	Group Effects
Age, y	65.7 (8.5); range, 46-84	30.4 (7.4); range, 18-49	59.0 (6.5); range, 47-87	55.9 (9.1); range, 43-72	65.6 (8.5); range, 48-86	.0001†	NC=AD>LOS=EOS-O>EOS-Y
Education, y	13.7 (2.2)	13.3 (1.8)	12.0 (3.2)	12.9 (2.4)	13.6 (3.7)	NS	NS
Gender, % M	34.2	62.4	63.6	88.6	57.1	.0001†	EOS-O>EOS-Y=AD=LOS>NC
Age at onset of illness, y	. . .	20.6 (6.7)	53.9 (6.1)	27.4 (8.4)	62.7 (7.9)	.0001†	AD>LOS>EOS-O>EOS-Y
Duration of illness, y	. . .	9.6 (6.7); range, 0-28	5.1 (5.4); range, 0-17	28.0 (12.1); range, 5-46	3.1 (1.9); range, 1-7	.0001†	EOS-O>EOS-Y>LOS=AD
Full-scale IQ	113.9 (10.6)	92.8 (13.2)	91.4 (12.0)	96.3 (13.2)	90.7 (15.9)	.0001	NC>EOS-O=LOS=EOS-Y=AD
Average impairment rating–T score	52.4 (8.6)	33.9 (11.7)	35.4 (7.4)	35.5 (10.6)	33.4 (7.5)	.0001	NC>EOS-O=LOS=EOS-Y=AD
GDS	0.22 (0.25)	0.82 (0.60)	0.74 (0.44)	0.86 (0.62)	1.51 (0.6)	.0001	AD>EOS-O=LOS=EOS-Y>NC

Values are means (SDs) or percentages. NC indicates normal controls; EOS-Y, early-onset schizophrenics–young; LOS, late-onset schizophrenics; EOS-O, early-onset schizophrenics–old; AD, Alzheimer's disease; NS, nonsignificant with the Bonferroni correction; GDS, Global Deficit Score.

†P value significant with the Bonferroni correction. The statistical tests used for these analyses were as follows: Welch's F test for all variables, except Kruskal-Wallis for duration of illness and χ^2 for gender.

corrected scores in all analyses. The LOS and AD groups were similar in terms of illness duration, although the EOS-Y group had a greater duration than the LOS and AD groups. As expected, the EOS-O group had a longer duration of illness than any other patient group.

Table 2 also summarizes the group comparisons on the three overall NP summary scores: the WAIS-R Full-Scale IQ, the Average Impairment Rating from the Halstead-Reitan Battery, and the Global Deficit Score that included tests from both of these batteries and the additional tests (most notably, those measuring learning and memory). All the subject groups had a mean Full-Scale IQ that was at least within the average range; yet, all the patient groups showed intellectual impairment relative to that of the NC group. Moreover, the patient groups did not differ significantly from each other in overall intellectual functioning. Similar findings were obtained on the Average Impairment Rating: all clinical groups were impaired relative to the NC group, but were not significantly different from one another. On the other hand, the Global Deficit Score (which included added tests of learning, memory, and other NP functions) revealed impairment that was significantly greater in the AD group than in schizophrenic groups. As with the other NP summary scores, the three schizophrenic groups showed comparable impairment on the Global Deficit Score.

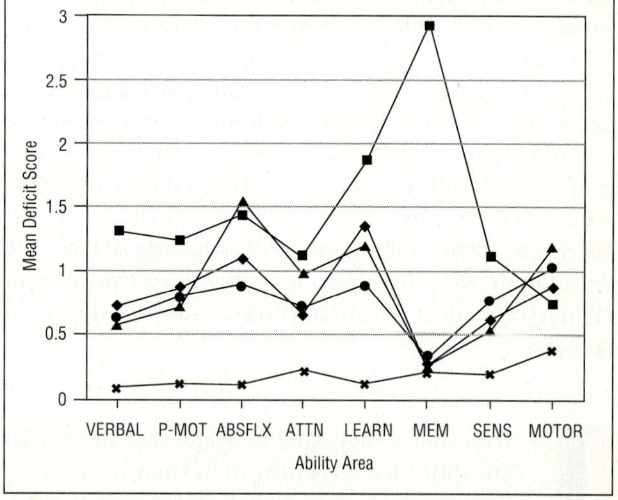

Ability area deficit scores for the five subject groups. Mean deficit scores on the eight neuropsychological ability areas for the five subject groups. Please see the text for statistical comparisons. VERBAL indicates verbal abilities; P-MOT, complex perceptual-motor skills; ABSFLX, abstraction and flexibility; ATTN, attention; LEARN, verbal and visual learning; MEM, verbal and visual memory (forgetting); SENS, sensory perceptual abilities; MOTOR, motor skills; squares, patients with Alzheimer's disease; triangles, early-onset schizophrenics–old; diamonds, early-onset schizophrenics–young; circles, late-onset schizophrenics; and X's, normal controls.

The **Figure** depicts the mean deficit scores for the five subject groups on the eight ability areas.

All schizophrenic groups were worse than the NC group on deficit scores for all the ability areas, except for memory; no schizophrenic group showed impairment on the Memory Deficit Score. By contrast, the AD group was worse than the NC group on memory ($P<.0001$), as well as on all other deficit scores.

An omnibus multivariate analysis of variance conducted on seven of the eight ability areas that were successfully transformed by using logs or reciprocals (ie, all except for memory) demonstrated a significant difference among the four patient groups on learning. The AD group demonstrated greater learning impairment than did the EOS-O and LOS groups; the three schizophrenic groups were not different from one another. The Memory Deficit Score was not included in the omnibus multivariate analysis of variance because the memory score distribution could not be corrected to permit parametric analyses (ie, the schizophrenic groups performed similarly to the NC group, showing no deficit, while the AD

group showed severe impairment on memory). Nonparametric analyses confirmed that the AD group had worse memory than all three schizophrenic groups that were not different from one another. Finally, although the patient groups showed verbal, complex perceptual-motor, abstraction, attention, sensory, and motor impairment relative to NC, with Bonferroni corrections, the patient groups did not differ significantly from one another.

We were interested in determining whether the above group differences in NP deficit scores were sufficiently robust to permit classification of individual subjects as schizophrenic, AD, or NC. Stepwise discriminant function analysis was used to explore this possibility, even though assumptions regarding normality of deficit score distributions were not met for all the variables. The discriminant analysis included a total of 191 subjects for whom all the necessary NP data were available. Two canonical functions were generated, and these used deficit scores from just three of the eight ability areas: learning, memory, and abstraction/flexibility of thinking. These functions were able to classify correctly 70.3% of the schizophrenic group, 88.2% of the AD group, and 89.7% of the NC group. A more conservative jackknifed classification performed equally well for the schizophrenic and AD groups, and correctly classified 86.2% of the NC group. The results further indicated that the NP discriminant functions rarely (ie, in less than 12% of cases) misclassified a schizophrenic subject as having AD, or vice versa; moreover, there was no tendency for this type of error to be made more often with LOS subjects than EOS subjects.

IT HAS BEEN suggested by some that the apparent abnormal forgetting in AD may actually reflect poor initial encoding; indeed, a few studies that have carefully matched groups on initial learning have found normal long-term forgetting in AD (see Kopelman,[39] for a review of this work). To explore further the nature of the memory disorders in AD and schizophrenia, we matched 23 pairs of AD patients and schizophrenic patients on initial levels of learning on the Story Memory Test (verbal learning), and 23 pairs on the learning component of the Figure Memory Test (nonverbal learning). Thus, for each pair of subjects, there was no difference in the amount of information recalled on the last learning trial. As predicted, when these carefully matched schizophrenic and AD subgroups were compared with respect to the percent of information retained during the delay period, the AD subgroup consistently showed much worse retention. This result was obtained for both the verbal and nonverbal memory tests, regardless of whether uncorrected raw scores or demographically corrected *T* scores were analyzed. Mean *T* scores on Story Memory were 48.9 for the schizophrenic group and 27.6 for the AD group ($t[22]=4.5$, $P<.001$). The respective means for the Figure Memory Test were 54.3 and 33.8 ($t[22]=7.7$, $P<.001$).

COMMENT

Consistent with previous NP studies of schizophrenia, our schizophrenic groups demonstrated mild to moderate impairments on measures of verbal ability, complex perceptual-motor speed, abstraction and flexibility of thinking, attention, learning, sensory abilities, and motor skills.[4,40,41] Moreover, when possible effects of normal aging were corrected, the NP profiles of the three schizophrenic groups were strikingly similar: there were no differences in either level or pattern of performance across the eight major ability areas. Thus, our results suggest that age at onset and duration of schizophrenic illnesses do not have a major impact on the associated NP impairment.

Although all the patient groups displayed significant levels of NP impairment, the pattern of deficits was quite different for the AD than for the schizophrenic groups. The fact that the same AD-schizophrenia differences occurred even in the LOS group is noteworthy, given the similarities of the LOS and AD groups with respect to age and duration of illness. This argues against the possibility that LOS patients have early AD with psychotic manifestations. The most marked AD-schizophrenia differences occurred on the deficit score that reflected rapid forgetting of new information throughout a delay period. By far, this was the most severe deficit for the AD patients, whereas none of the schizophrenic groups showed abnormal forgetting (Figure).

Our findings in this regard suggest an important distinction between efficiency with which new information is learned and the ability to recall such information after a delay. All of our schizophrenic groups were impaired on the former component of "memory" and normal on the latter component. This distinction is likely to be most apparent on memory tests that have a "savings" or "forgetting" score that reflects the percentage of initially learned information that is recalled after the delay period. Much of the previous research concerning memory in schizophrenia has analyzed a learning score and/or a delayed recall score that confounds initial learning with forgetting. A recent study by Gold and colleagues[5] calculated a memory score while controlling for the initial level of learning, and they also found impaired learning and a normal rate of forgetting in a schizophrenic group.

The preponderance of previous research suggests that cognitive decline occurs early in the course of schizophrenia with no evidence of progressive decline associated with age or duration of illness.[15,42] Although some investigators have suggested an increased incidence of AD in older schizophrenic patients,[43] other studies[14,44] have

failed to corroborate the clinical diagnosis of AD with neurohistological findings (eg, plaques, tangles). Ciompi,[12] too, had alluded to differences between schizophrenia deterioration and dementia; he concluded that "even in advanced age schizophrenia in no way assumes the character of a typical organic disease." Our findings are consistent with the postulated static encephalopathy of developmental origin in schizophrenia.[42] These results may not be generalizable to institutionalized patients. On the other hand, a large majority of the schizophrenic patients are ambulatory, community-dwelling outpatients, as in our study. Furthermore, the ambulatory setting avoids the effects of long-term institutionalization, and it also increases the likelihood that the observed cognitive impairment is not secondary to neurological or other medical comorbidity.

A possible limitation of the present schizophrenic group comparisons on NP variables relates to subtype differences among the groups. Our LOS group contained a preponderance of subjects with the paranoid subtype. While we did not find paranoid-nonparanoid differences among the eight ability deficit scores of the EOS-O group in this study, analyses of the EOS-Y deficit scores revealed that the nonparanoid group demonstrated greater impairment on the abstraction/flexibility of thinking deficit score (χ^2=9.7, $P<.002$). Previous findings from our laboratory also suggest that young schizophrenic patients with the paranoid subtype perform better than patients with the disorganized subtype on individual tests of abstraction, verbal ability, and psychomotor problem solving.[45] These mixed findings are consistent with the literature suggesting subtle NP differences among subtypes in young schizophrenic groups.[46,47] To our knowledge, subtype differences have not been documented or adequately studied in older schizophrenic patients. Additional longitudinal research is needed to determine the stability of subtype classifications across the life span and to determine whether any subtype differences in NP functioning represent state or trait phenomena.

It can be argued that some of the NP deficits in the schizophrenic group may be due to the effects of medication. Although there is evidence that anticholinergic drugs can interfere with cognitive functioning, especially learning and attention,[48] these medications are unlikely to account for the results of the present study. Typically, learning impairment is associated with higher anticholinergic dosage or a short-term change in anticholinergic medication regimen.[48,49] Not only was the average anticholinergic dosage low (2.26 mg/d of benztropine mesylate equivalent for EOS-O and LOS patients receiving anticholinergics) but also all the patients had been receiving stable doses of medications at the time of NP testing. Furthermore, follow-up analyses revealed no significant differences in any NP ability area between patients receiving vs those patients not receiving anticholinergic medication. Finally, a recent report demonstrated learning deficits in a never-medicated schizophrenic group.[3]

Much of the previous neurobehavioral research concerning late-life psychosis has used only single or a few NP measures. This practice limits the conclusions that can be made about the selectivity of particular deficits, as it fails to include a comprehensive assessment of varied cognitive abilities. The present results using an extensive test battery are consistent with our previous findings that NP impairment in schizophrenia is relatively diffuse.[6] The one exception to this has particular relevance to clinical neuropsychology: while inefficient learning is typical of schizophrenia, a finding of rapid forgetting in a schizophrenic patient may suggest an additional neuropathological process.

Accepted for publication November 3, 1993.

This work was supported in part by grants MH45131, MH43693, and MH49671-01 from the National Institute of Mental Health, Bethesda, Md, and by the Department of Veterans Affairs, Washington, DC.

Reprint requests to Department of Psychiatry, University of California, 3427 Fourth Ave, San Diego, CA 92103 (Dr Heaton).

REFERENCES

1. Green M, Walker E. Neuropsychological performance and positive and negative symptoms in schizophrenia. *J Abnorm Psychol.* 1985;94:460-469.
2. Green M, Walker E. Attentional performance in positive- and negative-symptom schizophrenia. *J Nerv Ment Dis.* 1986;174:208-213.
3. Saykin AJ, Gur RC, Gur RE, Mozley PD, Mozley LH, Resnick SM, Kester B, Stafiniak P. Neuropsychological function in schizophrenia: selective impairment in memory and learning. *Arch Gen Psychiatry.* 1991;48:618-624.
4. Levin S, Yurgelun-Todd D, Craft S. Contributions of clinical neuropsychology to the study of schizophrenia. *J Abnorm Psychol.* 1989;98:341-356.
5. Gold JM, Randolph C, Carpenter CJ, Goldberg TE, Weinberger DR. Forms of memory failure in schizophrenia. *J Abnorm Psychol.* 1992;101:487-494.
6. Braff DL, Heaton R, Kuck J, Cullum M, Moranville J, Grant I, Zisook S. The generalized pattern of neuropsychological deficits in outpatients with chronic schizophrenia with heterogeneous Wisconsin Card Sorting Test results. *Arch Gen Psychiatry.* 1991;48:891-898.
7. Cohen CI. Outcome of schizophrenia in later life: an overview. *Gerontologist.* 1990;30:790-797.
8. Harrow M, Marengo J, Pogue-Geile M, Pawelski TJ. Schizophrenic deficits in intelligence and abstract thinking: influence of aging and long-term institutionalization. In: Miller D, Cohen G, eds. *Schizophrenia, Paranoia, Schizophreniform Disorders in Later Life.* New Haven, Conn: Yale University Press; 1986: 133-144.
9. Niederehe G, Rusin MJ. Schizophrenia and aging: information processing patterns. In: Miller D, Cohen G, eds. *Schizophrenia, Paranoia, Schizophreniform Disorders in Later Life.* New Haven, Conn: Yale University Press; 1986:162-179.
10. Gurland BJ, Cross PS. Epidemiology of psychopathology in old age: some implications for clinical services. *Psychiatr Clin North Am.* 1982;5:11-26.
11. Kraepelin E; Barclay RM, trans-ed. *Dementia Praecox and Paraphrenia.* Edinburgh, Scotland: E & S Livingstone; 1919 (reprinted, Huntington, NY: Krieger; 1971).
12. Ciompi L. Catamnestic long-term study on the course of life and aging of schizophrenics. *Schizophr Bull.* 1980;6:606-618.
13. McGlashan TH. A selective review of recent North American long-term follow-up studies of schizophrenia. *Schizophr Bull.* 1988;14:515-542.
14. Davidson M, Powchik V, Haroutunian V, Harvey PD, Perl D, Losonczy MS,

Freske E, Bierer L, Mohs RC, Davis KL. Dementia-like symptoms in elderly schizophrenic patients. In: Program and abstracts of the 30th annual meeting of the American College of Neuropsychopharmacology; December 9-13, 1991; San Juan, Puerto Rico. Page 67.
15. Heaton RK, Drexler M. Clinical neuropsychological findings in schizophrenia and aging. In: Miller NE, Cohen GD, eds. *Schizophrenia and Aging.* New York, NY: Guilford Press; 1987:145-161.
16. Pearlson G, Rabins P. The late-onset psychoses: possible risk factors. In: Jeste DV, Zisook S, eds. *The Psychiatric Clinics of North America: Psychosis and Depression in the Elderly.* Philadelphia, Pa: WB Saunders Co; 1988:15-32.
17. Miller BL, Lesser IM, Boone KB, Hill E, Mehringer CM, Wong K. Brain lesions and cognitive function in late-life psychosis. *Br J Psychiatry.* 1991;158:76-82.
18. Jeste DV, Harris MJ, Pearlson GD, Rabins P, Lesser IM, Miller B, Coles C, Yassa R. Late onset schizophrenia: studying clinical validity. In: Jeste DV, Zisook S, eds. *The Psychiatric Clinics of North America: Psychosis and Depression in the Elderly.* Philadelphia, Pa: WB Saunders Co; 1988:1-13.
19. Goldberg TE, Hyde TM, Kleinman JE, Weinberger DR. The course of schizophrenia: neuropsychological evidence for a static encephalopathy. *Schizophr Bull.* In press.
20. Spitzer RL, Williams JBW, Gibbon M, First MB. *User's Guide for the Structured Clinical Interview for* DSM-III-R. Washington, DC: American Psychiatric Press; 1990.
21. Filley CM, Heaton RK, Nelson LM, Burks JS, Franklin GM. A comparison of dementia in Alzheimer's disease and multiple sclerosis. *Arch Neurol.* 1989;46: 157-161.
22. McKhann G, Drachman D, Folstein M, Katzman R, Price D, Stadlan EM. Clinical diagnosis of Alzheimer's disease: report of the NINCDS-ADRDA work group. *Neurology.* 1984;34:939-944.
23. Hachinski VC, Iliff LD, Zilhka E. Cerebral blood flow in dementia. *Arch Neurol.* 1975;32:632-637.
24. Jeste DV, Wyatt RJ. *Understanding and Treating Tardive Dyskinesia.* New York, NY: Guilford Press; 1982.
25. Overall JE. The Brief Psychiatric Rating Scale (BPRS): recent developments in ascertainment and scaling. *Psychopharmacol Bull.* 1988;24:97-99.
26. Andreasen NC, Olsen S. Negative versus positive schizophrenia: definition and validation. *Arch Gen Psychiatry.* 1982;39:789-794.
27. National Institute of Mental Health. Abnormal Involuntary Movement Scale (AIMS). *Early Clin Drug Eval Unit Intercom.* 1975;4:3-6.
28. Saltz BL, Kane JM, Woerner MG, Lieberman JA, Alvir JMJ, Blank K, Kahaner K, Foley C. Prospective study of tardive dyskinesia in the elderly. *Psychopharmacol Bull.* 1989;25:52-56.
29. Saltz BL, Woerner MG, Kane JM, Lieberman JA, Alvir JM, Bergmann KJ, Blank K, Koblenzer J, Kahaner K. Prospective study of tardive dyskinesia incidence in the elderly. *JAMA.* 1991;266:2402-2406.
30. Yassa R, Jeste DV. Gender differences in tardive dyskinesia: a critical review of the literature. *Schizophr Bull.* 1992;18:701-715.
31. Jeste DV, Caligiuri MP. Tardive dyskinesia 1993. *Schizophr Bull.* 1993;19:303-315.
32. Reitan RM, Wolfson D. *The Halstead-Reitan Neuropsychological Test Battery.* Tucson, Ariz: Neuropsychology Press; 1985.
33. Wechsler D. *Wechsler Adult Intelligence Scale–Revised.* Cleveland, Ohio: Psychological Corp; 1981.
34. Heaton RK. *A Manual for the Wisconsin Card Sorting Test.* Odessa, Fla: Psychological Assessment Resources Inc; 1981.
35. Kaplan EH, Goodglass H, Weintraub S. *The Boston Naming Test.* Boston, Mass: E Kaplan and H Goodglass; 1978.
36. Matthews CG, Klove N. *Instruction Manual for the Adult Neuropsychology Test Battery.* Madison, Wis: University of Wisconsin Medical School; 1964.
37. Heaton RK, Grant I, Mathews CG. *Comprehensive Norms for an Expanded Halstead-Reitan Battery: Demographic Corrections, Research Findings, and Clinical Applications.* Odessa, Fla: Psychological Assessment Resources Inc; 1991.
38. Thompson LL, Heaton RK. A comparison of the WAIS and WAIS-R using t-score conversions that correct for age, education, and sex. *J Clin Exp Neuropsychol.* 1989;11:478-488.
39. Kopelman MD. The 'new' and the 'old': components of the anterograde and retrograde memory loss in Korsakoff and Alzheimer patients. In: Squire LR, Butters N, eds. *Neuropsychology of Memory.* New York, NY: Guilford Press; 1992:130-146.
40. Goldstein G. The neuropsychology of schizophrenia. In: Grant I, Adams KM, eds. *Neuropsychological Assessment of Neuropsychiatric Disorders.* New York, NY: Oxford University Press Inc; 1986:147-171.
41. Seidman L. Schizophrenia and brain dysfunction: an integration of recent neurodiagnostic findings. *Psychol Bull.* 1983;94:195-238.
42. Goldberg TE, Hyde TM, Torrey F, Weinberger DR. Cognitive abilities across the life span in patients with schizophrenia. In: Program and abstracts of the 30th annual meeting of the American College of Neuropsychopharmacology; December 9-13, 1991; San Juan, Puerto Rico. Page 66.
43. Prohovnik I, Dwork A, Kaufman M, Willson N. Looking under the light: prevalence of Alzheimer's disease histopathology in a large schizophrenic autopsy series. In: Program and abstracts of the 30th annual meeting of the American College of Neuropsychopharmacology; December 9-13, 1991; San Juan, Puerto Rico. Page 67.
44. Davidson M, Powchik P, Haroutunian H, Purohit D, Perl D, Harvey P, Losonczy M, McCrystal J, Parella M, White L, Bierer L, Frecska E, Mohs RC, Davis KL. Dementia in elderly schizophrenic patients. *Biol Psychiatry.* 1992;31:193. Abstract.
45. Kuck J, Zisook S, Heaton RK, Moranville JT, McAdams LA, Braff DL. Neurocognitive heterogeneity in schizophrenia: an analysis of *DSM-III-R* clinical subtypes. In: Program and abstracts of the 10th annual meeting of the West Coast College of Biological Psychiatry; April 10-11, 1992; Santa Monica, Calif. Abstract.
46. Goldstein G, Halperin KM. Neuropsychological differences among subtypes of schizophrenia. *J Abnorm Psychol.* 1977;86:34-40.
47. Bornstein RA, Nasrallah HA, Olson SC, Coffman JA, Torello M, Schwarzkopf SB. Neuropsychological deficit in schizophrenic subtypes: paranoid, nonparanoid, and schizoaffective subgroups. *Psychiatry Res.* 1990;31:15-24.
48. Spohn HE, Strauss ME. Relation of neuroleptic and anticholinergic medication to cognitive functions in schizophrenia. *J Abnorm Psychol.* 1989;98:367-380.
49. Gold JM, Goldberg TE, Kleinman JE, Weinberger DR. The impact of symptomatic state and pharmacological treatment on cognitive functioning of patients with schizophrenia and mood disorders. In: Mohr E, Prouwers P, eds. *Handbook of Clinical Trials: The Neurobehavioral Approach.* Amsterdam, the Netherlands: Swets & Zeitlinger; 1991:185-214.

ORIGINAL ARTICLE

Myelination of a Key Relay Zone in the Hippocampal Formation Occurs in the Human Brain During Childhood, Adolescence, and Adulthood

Francine M. Benes, MD, PhD; Mary Turtle; Yusuf Khan; Peter Farol

Background: A previous study demonstrated that myelination of the superior medullary lamina along the surface of the parahippocampal gyrus is occurring in human brain during adolescence. To further investigate whether postnatal increases of myelination may continue during the second decade and possibly even longer, the extent of myelination in this region has been analyzed in 164 psychiatrically normal individuals aged newborn to 76 years.

Methods: Cross sections of the hippocampal formation with adjoining hippocampal gyrus were analyzed on a blinded basis using either a global rating scale or measurements of the area of myelin staining.

Results: A curvilinear increase in the extent of myelination between the first and sixth decades of life (r=.71 and r=.67, respectively) was observed. When the area of myelination was expressed relative to brain weight, there was a twofold increase between the first and second decades and an additional increase of 60% between the fourth and sixth decades. Female subjects showed a significantly greater degree of myelin staining than did male subjects during the interval of ages 6 to 29 years; however, after the third decade, there were no gender differences in the area of myelin staining.

Conclusions: The increased staining of myelin during the first and second decades principally occurred in the subicular region and adjacent portions of the presubiculum. During the fourth through sixth decades, however, it extended to progressively more lateral locations along the surface of the presubiculum. The precise origin(s) of the axons showing progressive myelination is unknown; however, the axons in the subiculum may include some perforant path fibers, while those found in the presubiculum may include cingulum bundle projections. Overall, our data are consistent with the idea that both early and late postnatal increases of myelination occur in a key corticolimbic relay area of the human brain and underscore the importance of applying a neurodevelopmental perspective to the study of psychopathology during childhood, adolescence, and even adulthood.

(Arch Gen Psychiatry. 1994;51:477-484)

IT HAS BEEN suggested by Yakovlev and Lecours[1] that associative neocortex of the human brain may continue to develop postnatally for up to 30 years and perhaps even longer. While the report of Yakovlev and Lecours is frequently cited, this concept has largely been a hypothetical one for which no empiric evidence had been reported until recently. A review of the normal developmental series in the Yakovlev Collection in Washington, DC, has suggested that the superior medullary lamina along the surface of the subiculum and presubiculum is actively myelinating during adolescence.[2] The study, however, reported only a small number of cases (N=11), and quantitative techniques were not employed. These results have made it imperative that additional cases, particularly ones from an independent source, be quantitatively investigated so that the precise interval during which such postnatal changes might be occurring can be identified. To further characterize postnatal increases of myelination in the hippocampal formation in humans, we collected 164 postmortem specimens from psychiatrically normal individuals encompassing eight de-

From the Department of Psychiatry (Dr Benes) and the Program in Neuroscience (Dr Benes), Harvard Medical School, Boston, Mass, and the Mailman Research Center, McLean Hospital, Belmont, Mass (Dr Benes, Ms Turtle, and Messrs Khan and Farol).

See Materials and Methods on next page

MATERIALS AND METHODS

TISSUE SPECIMENS

The postmortem specimens were from 146 cases from Boston (Mass) Children's Hospital (BCH) and 18 cases from the Massachusetts General Hospital (MGH), Boston, of subjects ranging in age from 0 to 33 years and 36 to 76 years, respectively. The cause of death for the BCH patients included congenital heart disease (n=22), cystic fibrosis (n=33), malignancy (n=50), and other miscellaneous disorders (n=41), including asthma, renal failure, sudden infant death, trauma, aplastic anemia, thalassemia, Marfan syndrome, inflammatory bowel disease, and varicella. Two patients from BCH had had neurologic complications, one with a seizure disorder and one with Arnold-Chiari malformation; however, in both cases a neuropathologist indicated that there were no abnormalities in the hippocampal formation. The MGH patients had died of a variety of causes, such as heart disease (n=8), liver failure (n=3), malignancy (n=2), pulmonary embolus (n=1), edema (n=1), perforated appendix (n=1), dissecting aneurysm (n=1), pneumonia (n=1), and postoperative complications (n=1). In samples from both BCH and MGH, patients with marked neurologic disease, inanition, or alcohol or other drug abuse were omitted from the sample. At the time of autopsy, the brains were removed and immediately weighed while still fresh.

TISSUE SECTIONS

Transverse 7-μm-thick sections of the hippocampal formation and adjoining entorhinal cortex taken approximately at the level of the lateral geniculate nucleus had been stained with Luxol fast blue and hematoxylin-eosin for routine neuropathologic examination. The specimens from BCH and MGH were matched for the level and orientation of cut as well as the overall quality of myelin staining and the absence of artifacts that would interfere with analysis. The slide for each case was codified and initially observed with a microscope (Leitz Laborlux 12) equipped with ×4 and ×10 objectives to evaluate the consistency of staining across the various specimens and to exclude any sections with gross artifacts that would interfere with the analyses described below.

ANALYTIC TECHNIQUES

With use of a projection microscope, specimens were blindly analyzed with three different methods. First, the degree of myelination was assessed with use of a global rating scale consisting of myelination scores of 0 (none), 1 (slight), 2 (mild-moderate), 3 (moderate), and 4 (heavy) that were based on both the overall intensity and the amount of staining. The intensity of the staining was quite faint in the first few years of life, but then reached a maximum at approximately 5 years of age. Beyond this point, while the intensity was relatively unchanged, the amount or area of staining showed discernible increases that were assessed by evaluating both the thickness of the myelin-stained zone as well as its length, ie, its lateral extension along the surface of the subiculum toward the presubiculum and eventually the parasubiculum. Before the actual analysis, the reliability of this instrument was established by two investigators (F.M.B. and M.T.) who independently rated a subset of 20 specimens, compared the respective scores, and repeated this process until an interrater reliability of at least 0.90 was attained. Thereafter, one of the investigators (M.T.) blindly rated the entire set of slides. The second method for analyzing the extent of myelin staining in the specimens consisted of measuring the area of myelin staining by tracing around the region of myelination along the surface of the subiculum, presubiculum, parasubiculum, and parahippocampal cortex (**Figure 1**) in an image obtained with a projecting microscope. The subregions of the hippocampal formation were corroborated by visualizing the sections with a bright field microscope and applying the distinctions established by Rosene and Van Hoesen.[3] A micrometric calibration slide was used to determine the correct magnification factor throughout the tracing and measurement process. An image analysis system (Bioquant System IV, R&M Biometrics, Nashville, Tenn) was then employed to determine the area of myelin staining (in square millimeters) within each tracing. For both the global rating scale and the area measurements, the data were expressed as a scatterplot with the area of myelin staining on the ordinate and age on the abscissa. The bivariate scatterplots were assessed with regression analysis, and a correlation coefficient was obtained for each data set. It was found that a second-order polynomial function best fit the data for both the global rating scale and the area measurements. The area of myelin staining was also expressed as a function of wet brain weight, and a mean and an SEM for this relative parameter was computed both separately for male and female subjects and in combination for the first through sixth decades. The data for the seventh and eighth decades were averaged together because the number of specimens free of pathologic changes that could be found for this period was small. The data within each decade showed a normal distribution, and a parametric Student *t* test was used to assess the significance of the differences between various decades and between the gender groups for each decade.

cades of life. With use of a computer-assisted quantitative technique, the extent of myelination has been measured along the surface of the hippocampal formation at the level of the subiculum, presubiculum, and parasubiculum. The data presented herein suggest that postnatal changes in the parahippocampal gyrus occur not only during childhood and adolescence but also much later.

RESULTS

Figure 1 shows several of the specimens employed in these studies. The blue-stained region along the surface of the subicular and presubicular regions of the parahippocampal gyrus is called the superior medullary lamina. Along the surface of the gyrus, there was a gradual increase in

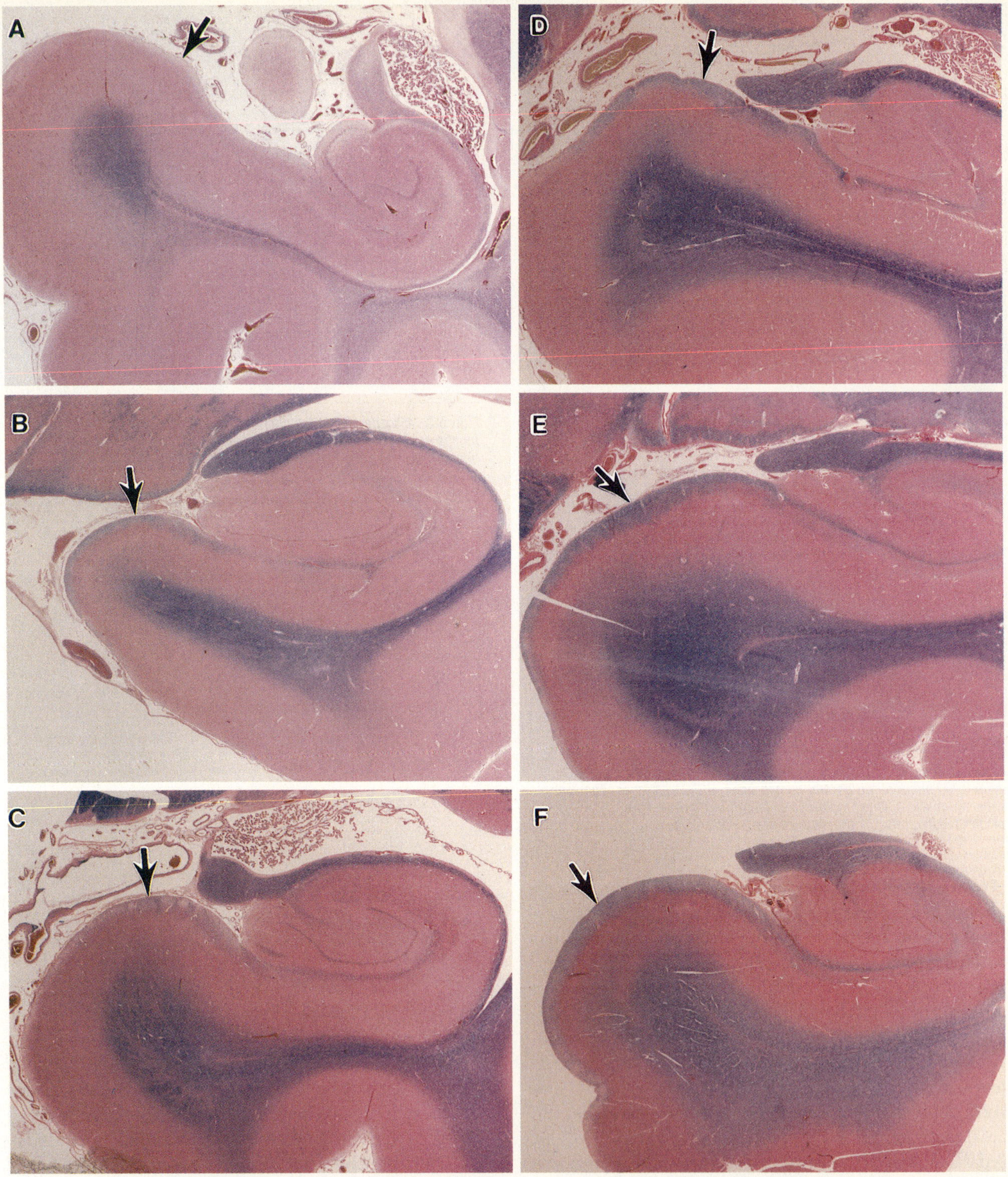

Figure 1. *Color photomicrographs showing cross sections of the hippocampal formation in the human brain at birth (A) and ages 8 years (B), 13 years (C), 24 years (D), 36 years (E), and 57 years (F). The arrows indicate the location of blue-stained myelinated fibers in the superior medullary lamina.*

the length of the myelinated zone that progressed in a medial-to-lateral direction (**Figure 2**). Specimens from the first through third decades showed staining principally along the surface of the subiculum and adjacent presubiculum (Figure 1, A through D), while those from approximately the fourth through sixth decades showed staining in progressively more lateral locations along the presubiculum and parasubiculum (Figure 1, E and F). According to the global rating scale, the degree of myelination shows a progressive increase ($r=.71$, $P\ll.0005$) between birth and approximately 35 to 40 years of age (**Figure 3**). When the area of myelination was obtained

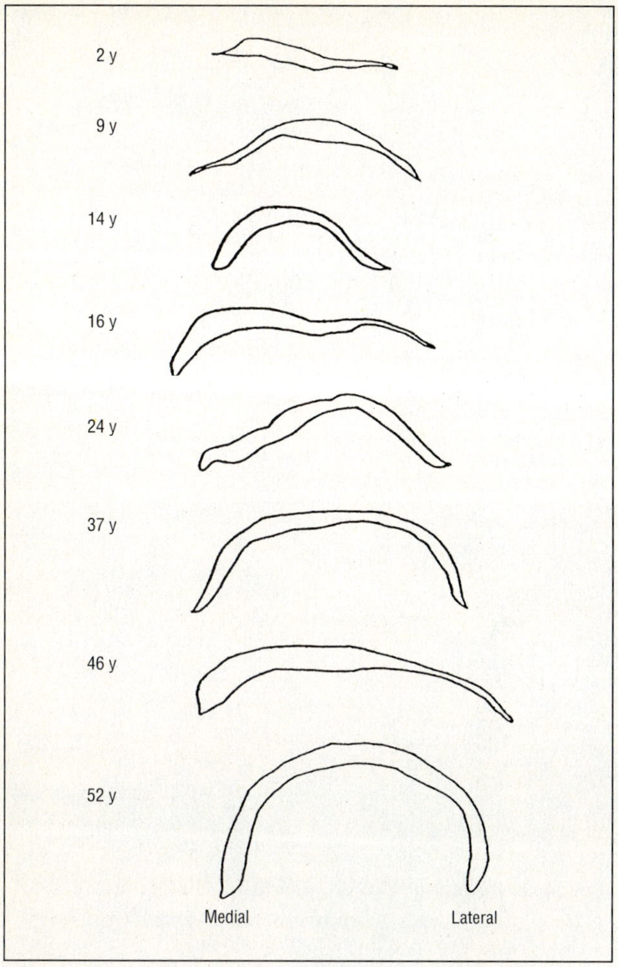

Figure 2. *A series of tracings around myelin staining in the superior medullary lamina of the normal human brain at different ages. The zone showing myelin staining increases in length in a progressive medial-to-lateral direction between ages 2 and 52 years.*

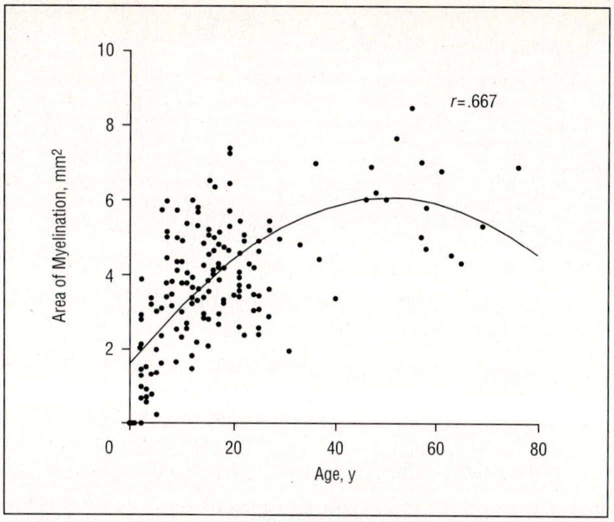

Figure 3. *A scatterplot of the area of myelin staining with respect to age for the superior medullary lamina of the hippocampal formation in the human brain. See the text for details.*

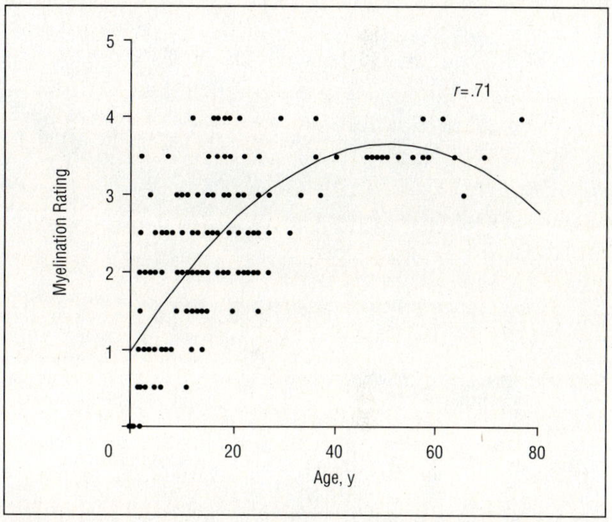

Figure 4. *A scatterplot of the global ratings of myelin staining with respect to age for the superior medullary lamina in the hippocampal formation of the human brain. See the text for details.*

(**Figure 4**), a similar progression occurred between birth and the fifth to sixth decades (r=.67, $P \leqslant .0005$). The average area of myelination in the first and second decades was increased 95%, from 2.2±0.3 mm² to 4.3±0.2 mm², respectively (t=6.9, $P<.0005$). The area of myelination in the fifth (5.6±0.8 mm²) and sixth (6.5±0.5 mm²) decades also increased by 33% and 55%, respectively, compared with that in the second decade, although the differences were only significant between the second and sixth decades (t=4.0, $P<.0005$). For both the global and areal measurements, the specimens from BCH were also separately analyzed according to diagnostic groupings that included cystic fibrosis, congenital heart disease, malignancy, or miscellaneous (infectious, inflammatory, genetic, or traumatic) causes of death. All such subgroups showed a pattern of findings similar to that for the whole group, although individuals with cystic fibrosis and congenital heart disease showed somewhat more variance in the myelination assessments.

The fresh brain weights (mean±SD) for several age ranges were similar to normative values described by other investigators[3] (**Table**). The brain weight showed the greatest change (41%) between 0 to 5 and 6 to 9 years of age. Thereafter, it was found to increase by an additional 5.4% by 10 to 19 years of age and then by only 2.2% during the third decade. When the area of myelination was expressed relative to brain weight according to various decades of age (**Figure 5**), this ratio increased by 92% between 0 to 9 and 10 to 19 years of age (F=45.5, P=.0001) but did not change appreciably until the fourth decade, when it increased by 43% (F=7.65, P=.0098). The ratio between the area of myelination and brain weight increased by an additional 23% during the fifth and sixth decades compared with the third decade (F=26.5, P=.0001).

The wet brain weights for female subjects were on average lower (approximately 8%) than those for men

Fresh Brain Weights*

Age, y	Mean±SD Brain Weight, g	Normative Brain Weights, g
0-4	915±321	752†
5-9	1291±173	1267,† 1316‡
10-19	1361±122	1334,† 1371‡
20-29	1391±110	1361,† 1389‡
30-79	1363±156	1373§

*Values shown are from Blinkov and Glezer.[4]
†From Table 113 from Blinkov and Glezer.[4]
‡From Table 111 from Blinkov and Glezer.[4]
§From Table 103 from Blinkov and Glezer.[4]

across all age groups (**Figure 6**), and this difference was similar to that reported in Blinkov and Glezer.[4] The relative number of male (n=87) and female (n=76) subjects was approximately the same, and the myelination data for each gender showed the same changes with respect to age as described above for the entire cohort. When the data were broken down according to gender (**Figure 7**), male and female subjects showed no differences between 0 and 5 years of age; however, for female subjects, the myelin ratio was 41% higher at 6 to 11 years of age (F=9.32, P=.005), 33% higher at 12 to 19 years of age (F=6.95, P=.01), and 23% higher at 20 to 29 years of age (F=4.66, P=.04). Thereafter, no significant difference was noted between the genders.

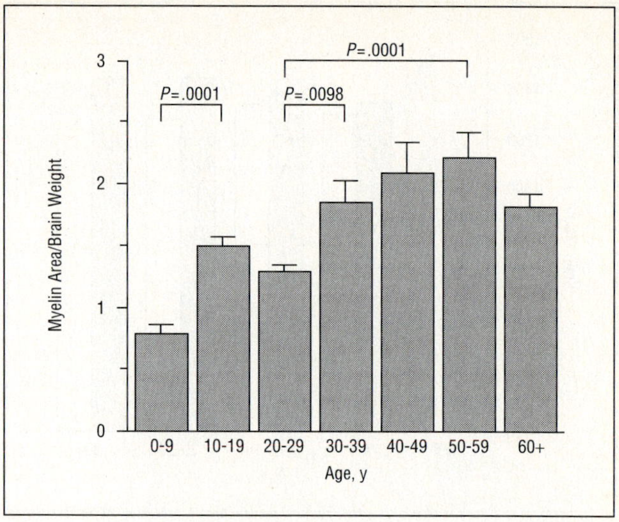

Figure 5. *A bar graph showing the average area of myelination (square millimeter) per gram wet weight of brain in the superior medullary lamina during several decades of life in the normal human brain. The data are expressed as the mean and SEM for each decade. The horizontal brackets indicate that there are significant differences between the two decades indicated. The probability that the differences are significant is indicated above the horizontal brackets.*

COMMENT

The results we obtained using both a global rating scale and measurements of the area of myelin staining have demonstrated a progressive increase in the myelination of the superior medullary lamina of the parahippocampal gyrus during childhood, adolescence, and adulthood. These changes are not due to shrinkage of the brain as a result of disease because the fresh brain weights for the subjects included in our study compare favorably with normative values reported in the literature (Table). In addition, these changes do not appear to be an artifact of combining cohorts from two different institutions, because specimens from patients from both BCH and MGH who died during the fourth decade were included, and the data for these cases overlapped. Also, it seems unlikely that differences in the quality of staining for the specimens from the respective institutions account for these findings, because specimens with either excessively light or heavy staining were not included in the study. Moreover, those that were included were carefully matched not only for the quality of staining but also for the level of cut through the hippocampal formation. The global rating scale that was intended to control for variances arising from inconsistencies of either staining or the level of cut yielded results similar to those obtained with the area measurements. An independent sample from the Yakovlev Collection, stained with an entirely different technique, the Weigert method, also showed similar late postnatal increases in the amount of myelination for the superior medullary lamina[2] when they were subsequently reanalyzed (F.M.B., unpublished data, 1991). In this latter post hoc analysis, the correlation coefficient for the area of myelination with respect to age was .75, a value that compares remarkably well with values of .71 and .67 that are reported herein for the global rating scale and the area of myelin staining, respectively.

Another point that must be raised with regard to our study is the question of whether the diseases from which the population from BCH suffered might have resulted in a retardation of normal cerebral maturation. If this were the case, a reduced rate of myelin formation could conceivably have made the myelination at later ages seem greater. To control for this possibility, the BCH specimens were examined separately according to diagnostic groups. The patients with congenital heart disease and cystic fibrosis tended to have chronic disorders that were often accompanied by hypoxemia, and this could have theoretically diminished the rate of myelination. The patients with cancer or miscellaneous disorders, on the other hand, often had a rather brief and less complicated course, and their cerebral maturation may have been closer to that of the general population. Consistent with this possibility, these latter two groups, accounting for a total of 91 cases, showed a sharp linear rise in the area of myelin staining between 0 and 25 years of age (r=.64 and r=.77, respectively) and, unlike the patients with cystic fibrosis and heart disease, showed little scatter around their respective linear function. Although it would be impossible to definitively control for the potential confound-

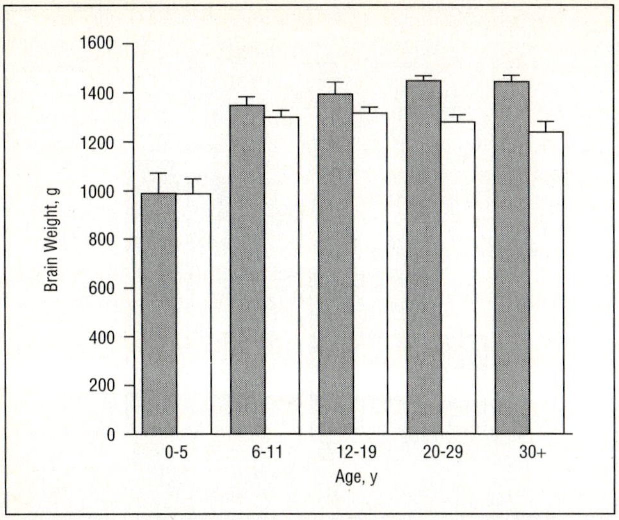

Figure 6. *A bar graph showing the average wet brain weight for male (shaded bars) and female (open bars) subjects at different intervals of postnatal life.*

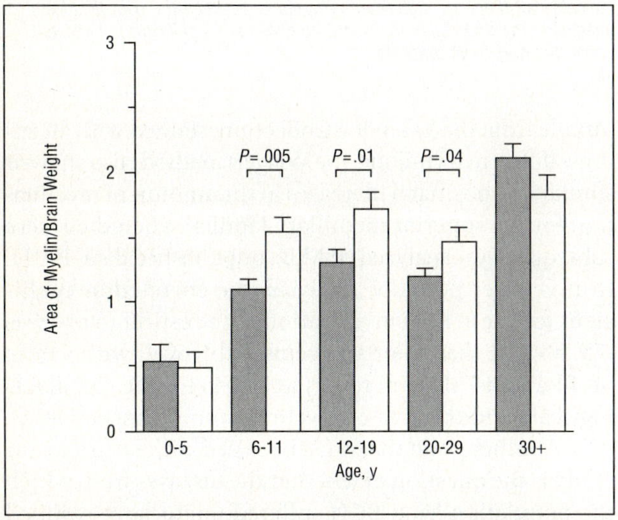

Figure 7. *A bar graph showing the average area of myelin staining (square millimeter) per gram wet weight of brain in the superior medullary lamina of normal male (shaded bars) and female (open bars) subjects as a function of fresh brain weight. Horizontal brackets indicate that the differences between adjoining decades are significant, and the value above is the probability of significance.*

ing effect of illness, the fact that the data for diagnostic subgroups from BCH overlapped argues against the findings reported herein being attributable to a general retardation of development in children with fatal illnesses. Moreover, the wide variations in both chronicity and basic pathophysiology for the BCH patients included in this study would not be expected to induce the same developmental perturbations.

A final consideration concerning our findings is whether differential shrinkage at different ages might somehow have contributed to the findings. As shown in Figure 1, the relative size of the hippocampal formation during the second half of the first decade and thereafter was similar. Moreover, if shrinkage during the first decade were greater, there would be a relative uniform decrease in size along the surface of the gyrus inward. In this setting, the area of myelin staining would decrease, but its subregional localization would not change appreciably. As described in the "Results" section, the myelin staining along the surface during the first decade was largely confined to the subiculum. During later decades, it was found in progressively more lateral locations over the presubiculum and eventually the parasubiculum. Based on the above discussion, it is unlikely that the findings described herein are artifactual or illusory. Accordingly, to our knowledge, our study provides the first quantitative evidence to support a long-held hypothesis that associative cortical regions of human brain continue myelinating well beyond childhood.[1]

It is worth considering why an increase in the amount of myelin visualized with Luxol fast blue staining may be indicative of an important developmental change. Both Luxol fast blue and Weigert's staining identify choline-containing phospholipids, particularly sphingolipids.[5] In rat brain, there is a progressive increase of sphingomyelin between postnatal days 3 and 330.[6-8] Between 15 days and 6 months of postnatal life, the total myelin content of rat brain increases by 1500%, while overall brain weight increases by only 50% to 60%.[9] When the sphingomyelin content is expressed with respect to the total amount of myelin lipid weight, it shows no change during the latter period.[9,10] Thus, the increased content of sphingomyelin occurring during development probably reflects an overall increase of myelin sheath. Accordingly, the increased myelin staining visualized with Luxol fast blue staining herein and with Weigert's staining in a previously published study[2] is probably indicative of new myelin sheath formation.

Visual inspection of the photomicrographs (Figure 1) reveals a progressive extension of myelin staining in a medial-to-lateral direction along the surface of the subicular-presubicular complex. Because the number of myelin lamellae increases with the caliber of an axon,[11] these accumulations could represent either de novo myelination of previously unmyelinated axons or increased numbers of myelin lamellae surrounding fibers that already have a myelin sheath. During myelinogenesis, oligodendroglial processes surrounding an axon shaft assume a mature myelin configuration in a relatively short period. In rat trigeminal nerve, myelination is associated with a marked increase of phospholipid synthesis between postnatal days 7 and 8, followed by a rapid decline toward baseline levels by day 15, as mature myelin sheath configurations appear.[12] Unless an axon shaft undergoes an additional increase in caliber,[11] no additional changes occur in the amount of myelin surrounding it. If an axon does increase in caliber, additional myelin lamellae form around preexisting ones and produce an increase in the cross-sectional size of the sheath. As with the de novo

formation of sheaths around unmyelinated axons, increased amounts of myelin lamellae would be expected to produce an increased area of staining, as noted herein.

In considering the functional implications for these late postnatal changes in the myelin content of the superior medullary lamina, it is pertinent to know what types of axon fibers might be present within this subregion of the parahippocampal gyrus. It was originally suggested that the fibers myelinating during adolescence might be those of the perforant path and distal portions of the cingulum bundle, two key links of the entorhinal and cingulate cortices, respectively, with the hippocampal formation.[2] Fibers of the perforant path originate from pyramidal cells in layers II and III of the entorhinal cortex[13] and pass through the pyramidal layer of the subiculum and the CA1 subfield before "penetrating" into the molecular layer of the area dentata. While active myelination in the subiculum was observed during the first and, to a lesser extent, second decades and might include perforant path axons, most of the fibers myelinating during adulthood were found considerably more lateral to where the latter fibers course toward the area dentata. Based on three-dimensional reconstructions, the cingulum bundle of the human brain sweeps in a ventral-to-rostral direction before merging with the superior medullary lamina within the presubiculum (F.M.B., unpublished data, 1987). As discussed above, the increasing myelin staining of the superior medullary lamina occurred in a medial-to-lateral direction, and, in individuals in the fourth decade of life and older, it occurred primarily along the surface of the presubiculum. Thus, at least some of the axons myelinating during adulthood may be from the cingulate gyrus, although subicular efferents to the posterior cingulate gyrus are also believed to course through superficial laminae.[3] Because both the subiculum and presubiculum are key relay areas of the hippocampal formation, axons in the superior medullary lamina, particularly those of the cingulum bundle, could play some role in the corticolimbic integration of emotional behaviors with cognitive processes.[2,14,15]

Cognitive development is generally believed to continue through approximately 12 to 16 years of age, a period during which the ability to abstract becomes integral to thinking.[16] Emotional development, on the other hand, is believed to continue beyond late adolescence and may be occurring as late as the fifth and sixth decades of life.[17] Although emotional maturity often seems to be an ill-defined construct,[18] it may involve changes, such as decreased anxiety, sociability,[18] and affect intensity,[19] that continue to occur through the midlife period. It is tantalizing to consider whether the increased amounts of myelin staining observed in the superior medullary lamina during the period of 10 to 19 years of age and later during the fourth through sixth decades could be directly or indirectly related to changes in emotional maturity believed to occur during these same periods. It is often said, although empiric data are lacking, that young girls attain emotional maturity before young boys. This idea probably emanates from the observation that girls are more likely than boys to show age-appropriate achievement in language skills, reading, and overall behavior at school.[20] Because female subjects between the ages of 6 and 29 years included herein had a significantly greater amount of myelin staining in the superior medullary lamina than did male subjects of the same ages, it is theoretically possible that this finding could be related, perhaps indirectly, to the greater degree of maturity noted in young female subjects. It is pertinent to this discussion to note that boys have a much higher incidence than girls of various types of childhood psychopathology, including Tourette's syndrome, attention-deficit disorder, encopresis and enuresis, autism, sleepwalking, and night terrors.[21] Is it plausible that delays in brain ontogeny in male subjects during childhood and adolescence might contribute, in some way, to their greater vulnerability for psychopathology?

THE SUPERIOR medullary lamina showing the late postnatal myelination described herein is involved in the relay of information among several brain regions implicated in the pathophysiology of schizophrenia. These regions include the hippocampal formation,[22,23] the parahippocampal gyrus,[23,24] and the anterior cingulate region.[25-28] It has been previously suggested that a disorder associated with a deterioration in both emotional experience and cognition[29] and one that also has a typical age at onset between 16 and 25 years[30] might involve pathophysiologic changes in these latter three corticolimbic areas and be "triggered" to appear in response to the late myelination seen in the subiculum and presubiculum.[2] In individuals "at risk" for schizophrenia, brain changes like those described herein during adolescence could be related to the activation of a latent trait[31] and the initiation of an excitotoxic injury in the various corticolimbic regions showing abnormalities in schizophrenics.[32] While male subjects with schizophrenia present at a younger age than female subjects with schizophrenia,[33,34] myelination of the superior medullary lamina occurs earlier in female compared with male subjects. Considering these latter two findings together, it seems unlikely that the increased amount of myelination in the superior medullary lamina observed during adolescence could in fact have a proximate relationship to the onset of schizophrenia. As discussed above for psychiatric disorders of childhood, delayed ontogenetic changes in male subjects could contribute to their vulnerability for an early onset of schizophrenia. Paradoxically, myelination in this region may be part of a protective, rather than a potentiating, framework for the appearance of symptoms in individuals at risk for this disorder.

A broader and more detailed understanding of postnatal brain ontogeny may provide important insights into the maturation of cognitive and emotional processes in healthy human subjects at different stages of life. In addition, essential information concerning the unique onset of psychopathology during childhood, adolescence, and perhaps even adulthood might also emerge from a neurodevelopmental approach to such investigations.[35,36]

Accepted for publication September 28, 1993.

This work was supported by grant MH00423 from the National Institute of Mental Health, Rockville, Md, and a gift from Anne Franchetti.

We would like to thank Hannah Kinney, MD, and the Neuropathology Department at BCH as well as Tessa Hedley-White, MD, and the Neuropathology Department at the MGH for their help in procuring the specimens used in this study.

Reprint requests to the Mailman Research Center, McLean Hospital, 115 Mill St, Belmont, MA 02178 (Dr Benes).

REFERENCES

1. Yakovlev P, Lecours A. The myelinogenetic cycles of regional maturation of the brain. In: Minkowski A, ed. *Regional Development of the Brain Early in Life.* Boston, Mass: Blackwell Scientific Publications Inc; 1967:3-70.
2. Benes FM. Myelination of cortical-hippocampal relays during late adolescence: anatomical correlates to the onset of schizophrenia. *Schizophr Bull.* 1989;15:585-594.
3. Rosene DL, Van Hoesen GW. The hippocampal formation of the primate brain: a review of some comparative aspects of cytoarchitecture and connections. In: Jones EG, Peters A, eds. *Cerebral Cortex.* New York, NY: Plenum Press; 1987; 6:345-456.
4. Blinkov SM, Glezer II. *The Human Brain in Figures and Tables: A Quantitative Handbook.* New York, NY: Plenum Press; 1968:123-136.
5. Adams CWM. *Neurohistochemistry.* Amsterdam, the Netherlands: Elsevier Science Publishers; 1965:20-22, 348-349.
6. Wells MA, Dittmer JC. A comprehensive study of the postnatal changes in the concentration of the lipids of developing rat brain. *Biochemistry.* 1967;6:3169-3175.
7. Cuzner ML, Davison AN. The lipid composition of rat brain myelin and subcellular fractions during development. *Biochem J.* 1968;106:29-34.
8. Davison AN. The biochemistry of the myelin sheath. In: Davison AN, Peters A, eds. *Myelination.* Springfield, Ill: Charles C Thomas Publisher; 1970:80-161.
9. Norton WT, Poduslo SE. Myelination in rat brain: changes in myelin composition during brain maturation. *J Neurochem.* 1973;21:759-773.
10. Horrocks LA. Composition of mouse brain myelin during development. *J Neurochem.* 1968;15:483-488.
11. Friede RL, Samorajski T. Relation between the number of myelin lamellae and axon circumference in fibers of vagus and sciatic nerves of mice. *J Comp Neurol.* 1967;130:223-231.
12. Benes FM, Higgins JA, Barrnett RJ. Ultrastructural localization of phospholipid synthesis in the rat trigeminal nerve during myelination. *J Cell Biol.* 1973;57:613-629.
13. Ruth RE, Collier TJ, Routtenberg A. Topography between the entorhinal cortex and the dentate septotemporal axis in rats, I: medial and intermediate entorhinal projecting cells. *J Comp Neurol.* 1982;209:69-78.
14. Papez JW. A proposed mechanism of emotion. *Arch Neurol Psychiatry.* 1937; 38:725-743.
15. Mesulam MM, Geschwind N. On the possible role of neocortex and its limbic connections in the process of attention and schizophrenia. *J Psychiatr Res.* 1978;14:249-259.
16. Piaget J. *The Origins of Intelligence in Children.* New York, NY: International Universities Press; 1952
17. Erikson EH. Identity and the life cycle. *Psychol Issues.* 1959;1:18-164.
18. Eysenck HJ. Personality and aging: an exploratory analysis. *J Soc Behav Pers.* 1988;3:11-21.
19. Diener E, Sandvik E, Larsen RF. Age and sex effects for affect intensity. *Dev Psychol.* 1985;21:542-546.
20. Jersild AT. *The Psychology of Adolescence.* 2nd ed. New York, NY: Macmillan Publishing Co Inc; 1963:136-140.
21. American Psychiatric Association, Committee on Nomenclature and Statistics. *Diagnostic and Statistical Manual of Mental Disorders, Third Edition.* Washington, DC: American Psychiatric Association; 1980.
22. Kovelman JA, Scheibel AB. A neurohistological correlate of schizophrenia. *Biol Psychiatry.* 1984;19:1601-1621.
23. Bogerts B, Meertz E, Schonfieldt-Bausch R. Basal ganglia and limbic system pathology in schizophrenia: a morphometric study of brain volume and shrinkage. *Arch Gen Psychiatry.* 1985;42:784-791.
24. Jakob H, Beckmann H. Prenatal development disturbances in the limbic allocortex in schizophrenics. *J Neural Transm.* 1986;65:303-326.
25. Benes FM, Bird ED. An analysis of the arrangement of neurons in the cingulate cortex of schizophrenic patients. *Arch Gen Psychiatry.* 1987;44:608-616.
26. Benes FM, Majocha R, Bird ED, Marrotta CA. Increased vertical axon numbers in cingulate cortex of schizophrenics. *Arch Gen Psychiatry.* 1987;44:1017-1021.
27. Benes FM, McSparren J, Bird ED, SanGiovanni JP, Vincent SL. Deficits in small interneurons in prefrontal and anterior cingulate cortex of schizophrenic and schizoaffective patients. *Arch Gen Psychiatry.* 1991;48:996-1001.
28. Benes FM, Vincent SL, Alsterberg G, Bird ED, SanGiovanni JP. Increased GABA receptor binding in supragranular layers of schizophrenic cingulate cortex. *J Neurosci.* 1992;11:925-947.
29. Bleuler E. *Dementia Praecox or the Group of Schizophrenias.* New York, NY: International Press; 1950.
30. Kraepelin E. *Dementia Praecox and Paraphrenia.* Edinburgh, Scotland: E & S Livingston; 1919
31. Weinberger DR. Implications of normal brain development for the pathogenesis of schizophrenia. *Arch Gen Psychiatry.* 1987;44:660-669.
32. Benes FM. Cingulate cortex in schizophrenia and other psychiatric disorders. In: Vogt BA, Gabriel M, eds. *The Neurobiology of Cingulate Cortex and Limbic Thalamus.* Boston, Mass: Birkhauser; 1993:581-605.
33. Lewine RR, Strauss JS, Gift TE. Sex differences in age at first hospital admission for schizophrenia: fact or artifact? *Am J Psychiatry.* 1981;138:440-444.
34. Seeman MV. Sex and schizophrenia. *Can J Psychiatry.* 1985;30:313-315.
35. Benes FM. Post-mortem structural analyses of schizophrenic brain: study designs and the interpretation of data. *Psychiatr Dev.* 1988;6:213-226.
36. Cicchetti D. *Risk and Protective Factors in the Development of Psychopathology.* New York, NY: Cambridge University Press; 1990.

ORIGINAL ARTICLE

The Panicogenic Effects of Cholecystokinin-Tetrapeptide Are Antagonized by L-365,260, a Central Cholecystokinin Receptor Antagonist, in Patients With Panic Disorder

Jacques Bradwejn, MD, FRCPC; Diana Koszycki, MA; Anne Couëtoux du Tertre, MD; Harold van Megen, MD; Johan den Boer, MD; Herman Westenberg, PhD; Lawrence Annable, DipStat

Background: We investigated whether the selective brain cholecystokinin (CCK_B) receptor antagonist, L-365,260, could antagonize the panicogenic effects of CCK-tetrapeptide (CCK-4) in patients with panic disorder.

Design: The study employed a double-blind, placebo-controlled, two-period crossover design. Patients (N=29) received a single oral dose of L-365,260 (10 or 50 mg) or placebo 90 minutes prior to injection of CCK-4. After a 1-week washout period, patients received a different dose of L-365,260 or placebo according to a balanced incomplete block design.

Results: The 50-mg dose of L-365,260 was superior to placebo in reducing the number ($P<.01$) and sum intensity ($P<.001$) of symptoms induced with CCK-4. Panic attack frequency following CCK-4 injection was 88% for patients receiving placebo, 33% for those receiving the 10-mg dose, and 0% for those receiving the 50-mg dose. The difference between the effects of the 50-mg dose and placebo was statistically significant ($P=.002$). Increases in heart rate following CCK-4 injection were markedly reduced with both the 50-mg ($P<.0001$) and 10-mg ($P<.01$) doses compared with placebo.

Conclusion: These data suggest that CCK_B receptors are an important site of action of exogenous CCK-4. It will be important to determine in future studies the efficacy of CCK_B receptor antagonists as antipanic agents.

(Arch Gen Psychiatry. 1994;51:486-493)

During the past decade, assessment of the neurochemical basis of panic disorder has focused on the potential dysfunction of norepinephrine, serotonin, γ-aminobutyric acid, and adenosine in particular.[1,2] More recent studies have sparked interest in the possible involvement of the cholecystokinin (CCK) system in the pathophysiology of panic disorder. Cholecystokinin is well characterized in the central nervous system[3-5] and is abundant in brain regions that have been postulated to be important in the promotion of panic symptoms, including the cortex, limbic area, and brain stem.[6] Exogenous administration of the tetrapeptide (CCK-4) and pentapeptide (pentagastrin) forms of CCK reliably produce a profile of symptoms reminiscent of spontaneous panic attacks in patients with panic disorder.[7-13] In addition, systematic studies of the behavioral effects of CCK-4 have revealed that this neuropeptide satisfies previously established criteria for an ideal panicogenic agent.[9-16]

Cholecystokinin exerts its effects via peripheral (CCK_A) receptors, which have a high affinity for the C-terminal octapeptide (CCK-8) in the sulfated form but low affinity for the unsulfated forms of CCK-8, CCK-4, or gastrin, and brain (CCK_B) receptors, which have a high affinity for all of these compounds.[17-19] The majority of CCK receptors in the central nervous system belong to the B subtype, although CCK_A receptors have been found in specific brain regions, including the area postrema, nucleus tractus solitarius, and interpeduncular nucleus, with some interspecies variation.[20]

See Subjects and Methods on next page

From the Department of Psychiatry, McGill University, Montreal, Quebec (Drs Bradwejn and Couëtoux du Tertre, Ms Koszycki, and Mr Annable), and the Department of Biological Psychiatry, University of Utrecht, the Netherlands (Drs van Megen, den Boer, and Westenberg).

SUBJECTS AND METHODS

SUBJECTS

Patients were recruited from the Anxiety Disorders Clinic of St Mary's Hospital, Montreal, Quebec (the Montreal site), a McGill University teaching hospital, and from the Department of Biological Psychiatry, the Academic Hospital, Utrecht, the Netherlands (the Utrecht site). Patients were invited to participate in the study if they had a current diagnosis of panic disorder (with or without agoraphobia) as defined by *DSM-III-R* criteria and experienced at least one panic attack a week for 4 weeks prior to the study. In addition, patients were required to be between 18 and 65 years of age, in good physical health as determined by physical examination, complete blood cell count, and blood chemistry profile which included thyroid function testing and electrocardiography, and able to discontinue prophylactic antipanic therapy. Women not using a reliable method of contraception were excluded from the study.

ETHICAL CONSIDERATIONS

The study was approved by the Health Protection Branch of Health and Welfare Canada, Ottawa, Ontario, and the Ethics Review Committees at both sites after submission of the protocol and the results of the analyses of the CCK-4 solutions. Patients who were eligible to participate in the study were provided with an informed consent form that contained a detailed description of the study and a description of the possible anxiogenic effects of CCK-4 and possible adverse events associated with L-365,260.

STUDY DESIGN

The study employed a double-blind, placebo-controlled, two-period crossover design. Patients received a single oral dose of L-365,260 (10 or 50 mg) or placebo 90 minutes prior to receiving an intravenous bolus injection of CCK-4. After a 1-week washout period, patients received a different dose of L-365,260 or placebo according to a balanced incomplete block design,[28] with each patient forming a block of size 2. The incomplete block design was used because, whereas the crossover design affords greater precision for treatment comparisons, it would have been undesirable to subject patients to more than two CCK-4 injections. The randomization scheme planned for each of 36 patients to receive two of the three possible treatment combinations (placebo and 10 mg of L-365,260; placebo and 50 mg of L-365,260; or 10 and 50 mg of L-365,260) in such a way that each combination was to be replicated an equal number of times in each order. Thus, under this plan, each treatment dose was to be received by 24 patients. However, because of early closure of the study and dropouts (see the "Results" section of the text), a total of 29 patients entered the study and the actual numbers of patients receiving placebo and 10 and 50 mg of L-365,260 were 17, 18, and 15, respectively.

INJECTION SOLUTION

The CCK-4 (30-33), consisting of an amino acid chain of Trp-Met-Asp-Phe-Nh_2, was synthesized by the Peptide Institute of Osaka, Japan. IAF Biochem of Montreal prepared the sterile solutions and performed the analysis for chemical content, sterility, and absence of pyrogenicity. An injected dose of 20 μg of CCK-4 in 0.9 mL of physiological saline solution was used in this study. Results from a previous dose-response study showed that this injection precipitated a panic attack in 75% of patients.[10] Thus, it was hypothesized that this dose would promote noticeable changes in behavior and other indexes of anxiety without being excessively potent to mask the effectiveness of L-365,260 to block the effects of CCK-4.

TREATMENT

The study medications consisted of two doses of L-365,260 (10 and 50 mg) and placebo. The medications were given orally in soft gelatin propylene glycol 600 capsules (0.5 mL).

Continued on next page

The use of CCK receptor agonists in clinical studies has been paralleled by the development of CCK antagonists with demonstrated ease of central penetration and selectivity for CCK_B and CCK_A receptor subtypes.[21-24] The first centrally acting antagonist to be developed was L-365,260, which is chemically known as (3R)-3(N'-[3-methylphenyl]ureido)-1, 3-dihydro-1-methyl-5-phenyl-2H-1,4-benzodiazepine-2-one.[25] This compound, a member of the 5-phenyl-1,4-benzodiazepine class of drugs, shows weak activity (IC_{50}=1.2 μmol/L) in vitro in displacing flunitrazepam from brain benzodiazepine receptors. Its affinity to more than 20 peptide and nonpeptide receptor systems is negligible (IC_{50}>10 μmol/L). In vitro, L-365,260 shows nanomolar affinity for CCK_B receptors of mouse, rat, guinea pig, dog, and human brains. Its affinity for CCK_A receptors is more than 100-fold weaker than that for CCK_B receptors.

Although capable of producing behavioral alterations consistent with the symptom profile of panic disorder, the mechanism by which CCK-4 exerts its pharmacological effects in humans is not well understood. Several investigations[26,27] using experimental animals have revealed that the anxiogenic effects of CCK-4 are blocked by selective CCK_B receptor antagonists, suggesting that CCK_B receptors are an important site of action of exogenous CCK-4. Accordingly, one objective of this study was to determine the contribution and role of CCK_B receptors in mediating behavioral and cardiovascular

ASSESSMENT

A Panic Symptom Scale (PSS)[12] derived from *DSM-III-R* was used to evaluate behavioral responses to CCK-4 injection. Each patient rated the intensity of panic symptoms on a scale of 0 (not present) to 4 (extremely severe). Symptoms not appearing on the PSS but spontaneously reported by patients were also rated. The following two variables were obtained from the PSS: a score reflecting the total number of symptoms (number of items that scored 1 or higher) and a sum intensity score (sum of the intensity ratings). A visual analog scale (VAS) was also used to measure subjective anxiety. Subjects were directed to indicate the severity of anxiety (most relaxed to most anxious) by transecting the 100-mm line with a vertical line. The length in millimeters, from the extreme 0 (most relaxed) to the vertical line made by the subject, was used to calculate VAS scores. Vital signs (blood pressure and heart rate) were recorded by a Dinamap vital signs monitor (Critikon, Tampa, Fla). A panic attack was defined according to patient self-report and global clinical impression.

PROCEDURE

The experiment took place in the Psychopharmacology Unit of the Montreal site and in the Department of Biological Psychiatry of the Utrecht site. Consumption of alcohol- or xanthine-containing beverages and foods was prohibited for 12 hours prior to the study. Treatment with a short-acting benzodiazepine was permitted as needed during the study. However, patients were required to remain drug free during the 48 hours immediately prior to each CCK-4 injection. Subjects sat on a reclining chair while an intravenous catheter was installed into the antecubital vein in the right arm, through which a 0.9% solution of sodium chloride was slowly dripped. A blood pressure cuff with a pulse monitor attached to the Dinamap vital signs monitor was installed on the left arm. The administration of CCK-4 was timed to occur 90 minutes after ingestion of the study treatments. One minute prior to administration of treatment and immediately prior to CCK-4 injection, subjects completed the VAS. Vital signs were collected at 20-second intervals until 120 seconds after the CCK-4 injection (at the Montreal site only). Subjects were instructed to describe fully any symptom they experienced since the CCK-4 injection. The onset, duration, and description of these symptoms were recorded. Onset of symptoms was defined as the latency for CCK-4 to produce the first symptom, and duration was defined as the time after onset of symptoms until the time that the subject indicated that the overall effects of CCK-4 had abated. Evaluation with the PSS and VAS was made once the overall effects of CCK-4 had diminished.

STATISTICAL ANALYSIS

Analysis of variance (ANOVA) appropriate for the incomplete block design was performed on all symptom measures. By using the general linear model approach, the data from patients who underwent two CCK-4 injections and from those who underwent one CCK-4 injection could be included. The model included terms for site (Montreal or Utrecht), patients nested within site, treatment (placebo, 10 or 50 mg of L-365-260), time of injection (first or second), treatment by site interaction, and treatment by time of injection interaction. The interaction terms were retained in the model only if significant ($P<.05$). The estimate of the difference between doses was adjusted for all other terms in the model by the least squares procedure. The program used was the SAS GLM procedure.[29] Pairwise differences between the three treatment means were of a priori interest and were tested without application of multiple comparison procedures. The frequency of panic attacks was analyzed by the weighted least squares means (linear model) approach for categorical data.[30] This analysis was carried out using the SAS CATMOD procedure.[29] Blood pressure and heart rate responses were submitted to analysis of covariance (ANCOVA) for the incomplete block design using the maximum change from baseline (peak value after injection minus time, −1 minute value) as the dependent variable and the baseline value as covariate. All data are presented as mean±SD. Statistical significance was assumed at $P<.05$ (two-tailed test).

changes during CCK-4 injection in patients with panic disorder. A second objective was to determine whether L-365,260 could produce a dose-dependent attenuation of CCK-4–induced panic symptoms. The data derived from this study could assist in the prediction of an effective and tolerable dose of L-365,260 for subsequent clinical trials of this agent in the treatment of panic disorder.

RESULTS

PATIENT CHARACTERISTICS

Twenty-nine patients entered the study; 19 were recruited from the Montreal site and 10 from the Utrecht site. Their age range was 19 to 49 years (median, 36 years of age); there were 10 men and 19 women. The duration of panic disorder ranged from 6 months to 30 years (median, 10 years). The median number of panic attacks was 3.0 (range, 1 to 11 attacks) during the week prior to intake and 13.0 (range, 4 to 45 attacks) during the month prior to intake. There were no statistically significant differences ($P>.05$) between sites for any of the patient characteristics. Nineteen patients were not using any psychotropic drugs in the 30 days prior to the study, and 10 patients were undergoing short-acting benzodiazepine therapy, which was discontinued 48 hours prior to each injection. Twenty-one patients received two treatments as planned: seven received placebo and 10 mg of

L-365,260; seven received placebo and 50 mg of L-365,260; and seven received 10 mg and 50 mg of L-365,260. Eight patients received one treatment only; three (two who received 10 mg of L-365,260 and one who received placebo) were withdrawn from the study after the first CCK-4 injection because of adverse events; five of the eight (two who received placebo, two who received 10 mg of L-365,260, and one who received 50 mg of L-365,260) received one CCK-4 injection only because the study was terminated by the study sponsor due to administrative reasons. All available data were included in the unbalanced incomplete block ANOVA.

Table 1. Effect of L-365,260 on Behavioral Responses to Cholecystokinin-Tetrapeptide Injection*

Variable	Treatment: Placebo (N=17)	L-365,260, 10 mg (N=18)	L-365,260, 50 mg (N=15)
No. of reported symptoms	12.2±3.6	9.0±4.1	5.7±4.2†
Sum intensity of symptoms	32.8±11.4	20.4±13.0	10.7±8.9‡§
Onset of symptoms, s	20.8±10.6	26.6±14.5	31.3±24.4
Duration of symptoms, s	254.6±417.0	311.9±511.2	130.0±66.3

*Values are expressed as the mean±SD.
†The 50-mg dose vs placebo ($t[18]=3.72$, $P<.01$; pairwise test).
‡The 50-mg dose vs placebo ($t[18]=4.18$, $P<.001$; pairwise test).
§The 50-mg dose vs 10-mg dose ($t[18]=2.32$, $P<.05$; pairwise test).

EFFECTS OF TREATMENT ON BEHAVIORAL RESPONSES TO CCK-4

Table 1 shows the mean (±SD) values for the number of reported symptoms, sum intensity of symptoms, and onset and duration of symptoms induced with CCK-4. No significant ($P>.05$) effect of time of injection, interaction of treatment and time of injection, or interaction of treatment and site occurred on any of these measures. A significant main effect of treatment emerged for the number of symptoms induced with CCK-4 ($F[2,18]=6.92$; $P<.01$) and the sum intensity of symptoms ($F[2,18]=8.76$; $P<.01$). Pairwise tests revealed that the 50-mg dose of L-365,260 produced significantly ($P<.01$) fewer symptoms than placebo. In addition, the sum intensity of symptoms score was significantly lower with the 50-mg dose than the 10-mg dose of L-365,260 ($P<.05$) and placebo ($P<.001$). No significant main effects of treatment were found for the onset ($F[2,11]=1.25$) and duration ($F[2,11]=0.27$) of symptoms.

Table 2. Effect of L-365,260 on *DSM-III-R* Panic Symptoms Induced With Cholecystokinin-Tetrapeptide

Symptoms*	Treatment, Mean±SD Symptom Score: Placebo (N=17)	L-365,260, 10 mg (N=18)	L-365,260, 50 mg (N=15)	Results of Comparison†: Placebo vs L-365,260, 10 mg	Placebo vs L-365,260, 50 mg	L-365,260, 10 mg vs L-365,260, 50 mg
Dyspnea	2.5±1.5	1.9±1.3	0.7±0.9	0.88	3.69‡	2.81§
Palpitations/rapid heartbeat	2.3±1.7	1.3±1.4	0.6±1.0	1.56	2.78§	1.21
Sweating	1.2±1.1	1.2±1.6	0.7±1.1	1.81	0.10	1.72
Faintness	1.7±1.4	0.5±1.0	0.4±0.6	2.29§	3.17‡	0.86
Unsteadiness‖	1.6±1.7	1.0±0.2	0.7±1.2	2.84§	2.99‡	0.29
Dizziness‖	2.3±1.4	1.2±1.0	0.7±1.0	2.73§	3.75‡	1.14
Shaking/trembling	1.2±1.3	0.6±1.0	0.6±1.0	1.95	2.33§	0.36
Nausea	1.1±1.4	0.9±1.4	0.4±0.9	0.42	1.21	0.80
Abdominal distress	2.3±1.4	1.3±1.5	0.9±1.1	1.97	2.50§	0.51
Choking	1.5±1.6	0.8±1.2	0.5±0.9	1.55	3.47‡	1.91
Chest pain/discomfort	2.1±1.5	1.2±1.3	0.5±0.9	2.89‡	5.35¶	2.45§
Paresthesia	2.2±1.5	0.9±1.4	0.5±0.8	1.29	1.98	0.68
Hot flushes/chills	2.3±1.2	1.9±1.6	0.6±1.0	0.26	2.68§	2.42§
Feeling unreal/detached	1.8±1.6	1.3±1.2	0.9±1.1	0.83	2.21§	1.37
Anxiety/fear/apprehension	3.1±1.0	2.1±1.5	1.0±1.4	1.48	3.72‡	2.22§
Fear of dying	1.1±1.3	0.4±0.9	0.0±0.0	1.11	3.18‡	2.06
Fear of losing control‖	1.0±1.3	0.9±1.4	0.9±1.4	1.09	1.47	0.43
Fear of going crazy	0.6±1.2	0.4±1.0	0.1±0.5	0.49	0.24	0.24

*Symptoms are rated on a scale of 0 (not present) to 4 (extremely severe).
†Pairwise comparisons between treatments were made without application of multiple comparisons.
‡$P<.01$ by pairwise test.
§$P<.05$ by pairwise test.
‖Indicates symptoms with significant treatment by site interactions ($P<.01$ to $P<.05$).
¶$P<.0001$ by pairwise test.

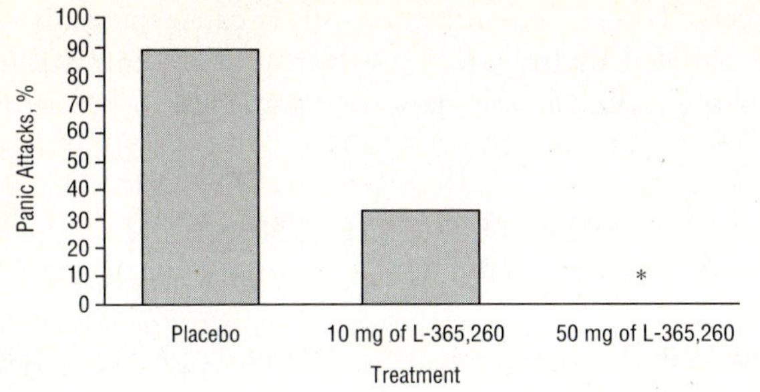

Figure 1. *Panic attack frequency following cholecystokinin-tetrapeptide injection. The actual numbers of patients who panicked when given placebo, the 10-mg dose of L-365,260, and the 50-mg dose of L-365,260 were 15 (88%) of 17, six (33%) of 18, and zero (0%) of 15, respectively. Asterisk indicates that the difference in panic frequency between the 50-mg dose and placebo was statistically significant (χ^2=9.85;* df=*1;* P<*.002).*

Table 2 displays the mean (±SD) intensity scores for the individual *DSM-III-R* panic symptoms elicited with CCK-4. No significant effects of time of injection or interactions of treatment and time of injection were found for any of the symptoms. Significant interactions of treatment by site occurred for dizziness (F[2,16]=4.72; *P*<.05), unsteadiness (F[2,16]=7.97; *P*<.01), and fear of losing control (F[2,16]=4.49; *P*<.05). When the treatments were compared within individual sites, significant treatment effects were found in the Utrecht sample only. The observed treatment differences favored the 10- and 50-mg doses over placebo for dizziness (*P*<.01) and unsteadiness (*P*<.001 and *P*<.05, respectively). In the Montreal sample, the effects were directionally the same for the 50-mg dose vs placebo, but weaker. By contrast, a reversal of effect for fear of losing control was found in the Utrecht sample, with placebo being superior to the 50-mg dose (*P*<.05). This reversal of effect was not evident in the Montreal sample, where the direction of the difference favored active treatment, but not significantly so.

Significant main effects of treatment without interactions were found for several PSS panic symptoms, including dyspnea (F[2,18]=7.45; *P*<.01), choking (F[2,18]=6.05; *P*<.01), chest pain/discomfort (F[2,18]=14.31; *P*<.001), faintness (F[2,18]=5.34; *P*<.05), palpitations/rapid heart rate (F[2,18]=3.87; *P*<.05), hot flushes/chills (F[2,18]=4.38; *P*<.05), anxiety/fear/apprehension (F[2,18]=7.01; *P*<.01), and fear of dying (F[2,18]=5.21; *P*<.05).

Main effects of treatment approached significance for shaking/trembling (F[2,18]=3.12; *P*<.07) and abdominal distress (F[2,18]=3.46; *P*<.06). The results of the pairwise tests for individual panic symptoms that did not display significant interactions of treatment by site are provided in Table 2. There were no significant main effects of treatment or interactions for symptoms that did not appear on the PSS but were spontaneously reported by patients.

Panic attack frequency following CCK-4 injection is shown in **Figure 1**. The weighted least squares means analysis revealed that the difference between treatments in panic frequency was statistically significant (χ^2=10.0; *df*=2; *P*=.007), but there was no significant difference in panic frequency between time of injection (χ^2=0.39; *df*=1; *P*=.53). Pairwise tests revealed that the difference in panic frequency between patients given 10 mg of L-365,260 and placebo was of borderline significance (χ^2=3.56; *df*=1; *P*=.06) and that between patients given 50 mg of L-365,260 and placebo was highly significant (χ^2=9.85; *df*=1; *P*=.002).

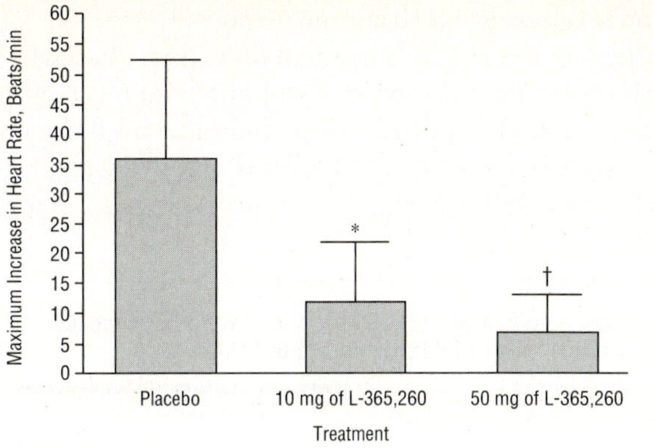

Figure 2. *Maximum increase in heart rate (mean±SD) following cholecystokinin-tetrapeptide injection, adjusted for baseline values. Asterisk indicates that the difference between the 10-mg dose of L-365,260 and placebo (t[11]=4.18;* P<*.01) was statistically significant; dagger, the difference between the 50-mg dose of L-365,260 and placebo (t[11]=6.24;* P≤*.0001) was statistically significant.*

EFFECTS OF TREATMENT ON CARDIOVASCULAR RESPONSES TO CCK-4

Cardiovascular responses to CCK-4 injection were obtained from the Montreal site only. For technical reasons, cardiovascular data were missing in one subject. No significant treatment by time of injection interactions occurred for mean peak changes from baseline in heart rate and blood pressure. The ANCOVA failed to reveal a significant main effect of treatment for the maximum increase in systolic (F[2,10]=0.64) and diastolic (F[2,10]=0.27) blood pressure. The mean (±SD) changes in systolic blood pressure adjusted for baseline differences for placebo, the 10-mg dose, and the 50-mg dose were 18.0±8.4, 5.8±6.9, and 10.7±8.4 mm Hg, respectively, and the adjusted mean changes in diastolic blood pressure were 12.5±10.6, 9.2±7.4, and 10.6±10.6 mm Hg, respectively.

By contrast, a highly significant main effect of treatment without interactions was detected for the maximum increase in heart rate (F[2,10]=14.34; *P*<.01). The adjusted mean peak change in heart rate from baseline after CCK-4 injection is displayed in **Figure 2**. Pairwise tests indicated that increases in heart rate following CCK-4 injection were considerably lower with both the 50-mg

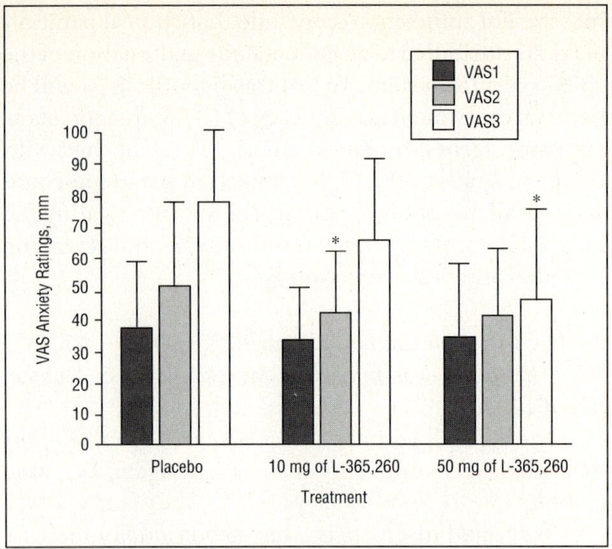

Figure 3. *Values for visual analog scale (VAS) ratings of anxiety (mean±SD) obtained before administration of treatment (VAS1), prior to cholecystokinin-tetrapeptide (CCK-4) injection (VAS2), and following CCK-4 injection (VAS3). Asterisk indicates pairwise tests showed significant (P<.05) differences between the 10-mg dose of L-365,260 and placebo for VAS2 ratings (t[18]=2.56) and between the 50-mg dose of L-365,260 and placebo for VAS3 ratings (t[18]= 2.32).*

($P \leq .0001$) and 10-mg ($P < .01$) doses of L-365,260 than with placebo. The analysis also revealed a significant main effect of time of injection ($F[1,11]=6.37$; $P < .05$), the average increase in heart rate being greater during the second relative to the first CCK-4 injection.

EFFECTS OF TREATMENT ON VAS RATINGS

Figure 3 displays the mean scores for VAS ratings of anxiety obtained before adminstration of the treatments (VAS1), immediately prior to CCK-4 injection (VAS2), and following CCK-4 injection (VAS3). No significant interactions of treatment and site or treatment and time of injection occurred on any of the VAS ratings. A significant main effect of time of injection for VAS2 ratings emerged ($F[1,18]=9.44$; $P < .01$), the average response being greater prior to the second CCK-4 injection.

The analysis revealed no significant differences between VAS scores obtained prior to administration of treatment ($F[2,18]=0.55$). However, a significant main effect of treatment was found for VAS scores obtained immediately prior to CCK-4 injection ($F[2,18]=3.61$; $P < .05$). Pairwise tests indicated that VAS2 scores were significantly lower with the 10-mg dose of L-365,260 than with placebo ($P < .05$). In addition, there was a trend toward a main effect of treatment for VAS3 scores ($F[2,18]=2.71$; $P < .10$). Subsequent analysis with pairwise tests revealed that VAS3 scores were significantly reduced with the 50-mg dose of the antagonist compared with placebo ($P < .05$).

COMMENT

The main finding of the present investigation is that pharmacological blockade of CCK_B receptors with a single oral dose of L-365,260, a selective and centrally acting CCK antagonist, attenuated the panicogenic effects of CCK-4 in patients with panic disorder. This effect, which was mainly observed with the highest dose administered (50 mg), suggests that CCK_B receptors are an important site of action of exogenous CCK-4 in humans. These clinical findings are paralleled by the data describing the effects of CCK_B receptor antagonists in experimental animals. In nonhuman primates, exogenous CCK-4 dose-dependently elicits a series of behavioral alterations (eg, increased vigilance, restlessness, immobility, and freezing) reminiscent of fear and defense posturing; these behavioral effects are fully antagonized by pretreatment with the CCK_B receptor antagonists LY262691 and LY247348.[31] In rodent-based tests of anxiety, pretreatment with selective CCK_B receptor antagonists markedly reduced anxiety produced by CCK receptor agonists.[26,27,32]

Although the results of the present study demonstrate that CCK_B receptor antagonists attenuate the panicogenic effects of CCK-4, such data do not establish that central CCK_B receptors are invariably the primary site of action of exogenous CCK-4. The extent to which CCK-4 crosses the blood-brain barrier has not been clarified. Moreover, CCK pathways, CCK_B binding sites, and CCK immunoreactivity have been identified in brainstem regions that are not completely shielded by the blood-brain barrier, including the nucleus tractus solitarius, medullary nuclei, and the parabrachial nucleus.[5,33,34] It is therefore conceivable that CCK-4 might act on these neuroanatomical sites in promoting symptoms of panic.[35]

It is reported here and elsewhere[9-12] that the latency to onset of panic symptoms with CCK-4 is rapid, and both the emotional (ie, anxiety, fear, and apprehension) and somatic (ie, dyspnea, tachycardia, and dizziness) symptoms of panic seem to occur quasi-simultaneously. Although a primary central action (in the limbic and/or cortical regions) of CCK-4 cannot be excluded, it is probable that lower brain regions are involved. These regions are interrelated by diverse neuronal projections and are connected to noradrenergic structures such as the locus coeruleus.[36-38] Neuronal projections also connect brainstem nuclei to limbic and cortical regions, and CCK is among the numerous networks connecting all of these regions. Stimulation of brain-stem neurons or an anomaly in their firing rate could easily result within milliseconds in a disruption of limbic and cortical neuronal networks, to which brain-stem neurons project. This process would manifest itself by the simultaneous appearance of emotional and somatic symptoms of panic. This neuroanatomical hypothesis of panic disorder is compatible with that proposed by Gorman et al,[6] in which a role for brainstem nuclei in the genesis of panic attacks is emphasized.

Congruous with previous data of Bradwejn et al,[10] we observed that exogenous CCK-4 had robust effects on heart rate and blood pressure. It is well documented that brain-stem mechanisms are involved in the control of respiration and cardiovascular function as well as other vital functions. Increases in breathing amplitude, respiration, blood pressure, and heart rate have been noted following electrical or pharmacological stimulation of the nucleus tractus solitarius,[39-41] the medullary nuclei,[37,42-46] and the parabrachial nucleus.[47] Further, there are experimental data to indicate that CCK interacts with these brain-stem mechanisms in modulating respiratory and cardiovascular functions. Microiontophoretic application of CCK-8S, a mixed CCK_A-CCK_B agonist, to neurons of the nucleus tractus solitarius has been reported to decrease both neuronal firing and respiratory frequency in cats, effects that were reversed by administration of CCK-4.[48] Taken together, it seems reasonable to conclude that exogenously administered CCK-4 produces respiratory and cardiovascular alterations in humans through a direct action on brain-stem mechanisms. It is also likely that the observed antagonism by L-365,260 of CCK-4–induced increases in heart rate is the result of CCK_B receptor blockade of these brain-stem nuclei.

An important question that remains to be addressed is whether the CCK system plays a pivotal role in pathological anxiety. Patients with panic disorder are hypersensitive to the panicogenic effects of CCK-4 and pentagastrin relative to normal control subjects.[7,8,13] It is also notable that naturally "uptight" monkeys exhibit an enhanced sensitivity to the anxiogenic effects of CCK-4 relative to "laid-back" monkeys.[49] Employing the elevated plus-maze paradigm, some investigators have determined that rats exhibiting low levels of exploratory behavior ("nervous" rats) have an increased density of CCK receptors in the frontal cortex relative to rats with high exploratory behavior ("nonanxious" rats).[50] Up-regulation of tritiated propiomylated CCK8 binding in the rat frontal cortex has also been observed following withdrawal from long-term diazepam administration.[51] Postmortem brain studies have revealed that CCK receptor binding is up-regulated in the frontal and cingulate cortex of suicide victims relative to matched controls.[52] Although the diagnostic characteristics of the suicide victims were unknown, it is likely that they experienced anxiety before death. An important step in testing the hypothesis of an endogenous anomaly of the CCK_B system in panic disorder will be pharmacological validation. If spontaneous panic attacks are indeed the result of increased activity of the CCK_B system, then CCK_B antagonists should have antipanic effects.

In conclusion, we have demonstrated that the panicogenic effects of CCK-4 can be significantly attenuated by pretreatment with the selective CCK_B antagonist, L-365,260. While these data suggest a role for CCK_B receptors in CCK-4–induced panic symptoms, the findings are not sufficient to conclude that clinical panic attacks are attributed to an endogenous malfunction of the CCK_B receptor system. To test this hypothesis, it will be necessary to evaluate the efficacy of CCK_B antagonists as antipanic agents. If clinical efficacy is established with these antagonists, the CCK-4 injection paradigm could serve as an important research tool for investigating the neurobiological substrate of panic attacks and screening potential antipanic compounds.

Accepted for publication February 25, 1994.

This study was funded by Merck, Sharp & Dohme, Blue Bell, Pa.

Presented in part at the 145th Annual Meeting of the American Psychiatric Association, Washington, DC, May 6, 1992.

We would like to extend our appreciation to Jeremy Haigh, Michael Traub, Scott Reines, and Chris Karkanias of Merck, Sharp & Dohme, Terlings Park, England (J.H. and M.T.), and United States (S.R. and C.K.), for their contribution to this study. We are also thankful to Natalie Audet, MSc, of McGill University for statistical analysis of the data and to Kim Anderson, BN, (St Mary's Hospital) for nursing assistance.

Reprint requests to Department of Psychiatry, St Mary's Hospital Center, 3830 Lacombe Ave, Montreal, Quebec, H3T 1M5 (Dr Bradwejn).

REFERENCES

1. Uhde TW, Tancer ME. Chemical models of panic: a review and critique. In: Tyer P, ed. *Pharmacology of Anxiety.* New York, NY: Oxford University Press; 1989: 109-131.
2. Nutt D, Lawson C. Panic attacks: a neurochemical overview of models and mechanisms. *Br J Psychiatry.* 1992;160:165-178.
3. Beinfeld MC. Cholecystokinin in the central nervous system: a mini-review. *Neuropeptide.* 1983;3:411-427.
4. Vanderhaegen J-J, Lofstra F, Vierendeels G, Gilles C, Deschepper C, Verbauck P. Cholecystokinin in the central nervous system and neurohypophysis. *Peptides.* 1981;2:81-88.
5. Rehfeld JF. Neuronal cholecystokinin: one or multiple neurotransmitters? *J Neurochem.* 1985;44:1-10.
6. Gorman JM, Liebowitz MR, Fyer AJ, Stein J. Neuro-anatomical hypothesis for panic disorder. *Am J Psychiatry.* 1989;146:148-161.
7. Abelson JL, Nesse RM. Cholecystokinin-4 and panic. *Arch Gen Psychiatry.* 1990; 47:395.
8. Van Megen HJGM, den Boer JA, Westenberg HGM, Haigh JRM, Traub M. Evidence of enhanced sensitivity for pentagastrin in panic disorder patients. *Clin Neuropharmacol.* 1992;15(suppl 1, part B):58B.
9. Bradwejn J, Koszycki D, Meterissian G. Cholecystokinin tetrapeptide induces panic attacks in patients with panic disorder. *Can J Psychiatry.* 1990;35:83-85.
10. Bradwejn J, Koszycki D. Comparison of CO_2-induced panic attacks with cholecystokinin-induced panic attacks in panic disorder. *Prog Neuropsychopharmacol Biol Psychiatry.* 1991;15:237-239.
11. Bradwejn J, Koszycki D, Annable L, Couëtoux du Tertre A, Reines S, Karkanias C. A dose-ranging study of the behavioral and cardiovascular effects of CCK-tetrapeptide in panic disorder. *Biol Psychiatry.* 1992;32:903-912.
12. Bradwejn J, Koszycki D, Payeur R, Bourin M, Borthwick H. Study of the replication of action of cholecystokinin in panic disorders. *Am J Psychiatry.* 1992; 149:962-964.
13. Bradwejn J, Koszycki D, Shriqui C. Enhanced sensitivity to cholecystokinin-

tetrapeptide in panic disorder: clinical and behavioral findings. *Arch Gen Psychiatry.* 1991;48:603-607.

14. Bradwejn J, Koszycki D. CCK_4 and panic attacks in man. In: Iversen S, Dourish C, Cooper F. eds. *Multiple Cholecystokinin Receptors in Man.* New York, NY: Oxford University Press; 1992:121-131.
15. Bradwejn J, Koszycki D, Bourin M. Dose ranging study of the effect of CCK_4 in healthy volunteers. *J Psychiatry Neurosci.* 1991;16:260-264.
16. Bradwejn J, Koszycki D. Imipramine antagonizes the panicogenic effects of CCK-4 in panic disorder patients. *Am J Psychiatry.* 1994;151:261-263.
17. Moran TH, Robinson PH, Goldrich MS, McHugh PR. Two brain cholecystokinin receptors: implications for behavioral actions. *Brain Res.* 1986;362:175-179.
18. Dourish CT, Hill DR. Classification and function of CCK receptors. *Trends Pharmacol Sci.* 1987;8:207-208.
19. Hill DR, Campbell NJ, Shaw TM, Woodruff GN. Autoradiographic localization and biochemical characterization of peripheral type CCK receptors in rat CNS using highly selective non-peptide CCK agonists. *J Neurosci.* 1987;7:2967-2976.
20. Zarbin MA, Innis RB, Wamsley JK, Snyder SH, Kuhar MJ. Autoradiographic localization of cholecystokinin receptors in rodent brain. *J Neurosci.* 1983;3: 877-906.
21. Martinez J, Rodriguez M, Lignon MF. Cholecystokinin receptor antagonist. In: Wang RY, Schoenfeld RC, eds. *Cholecystokinin Antagonists.* New York, NY: Alan R. Liss Inc; 1988:29-51.
22. Freidinger RM. Cholecystokinin and gastrin antagonists. *Med Res Rev.* 1989; 9:271-290.
23. Woodruff G, Hughes J. Cholecystokinin antagonists. *Ann Rev Pharmacol Toxicol.* 1991;31:469-501.
24. Howbert JJ, Lobb KL, Brown RF. A novel series of non-peptide CCK and gastrin antagonists: medicinal chemistry and electrophysiological demonstration of antagonism. In: Iversen S, Dourish C, Cooper F, eds. *Multiple Cholecystokinin Receptors in Man.* New York, NY: Oxford University Press; 1992:28-37.
25. Bock MG, DiPardo RM, Evans BE, Rittle KE, Whitter WL, Veber DF, Anderson PS, Freidinger RM. Benzodiazepine gastrin and brain cholecystokinin receptor ligands: L-365,260. *J Med Chem.* 1989;32:13-16.
26. Harro J, Vasar E. Evidence that CCK_B receptors mediate the regulation of exploratory behaviour in the rat. *Eur J Pharmacol.* 1991;193:379-381.
27. Singh L, Lewis AS, Field MJ, Hughes J, Woodruff GN. Evidence for an involvement of the brain cholecystokinin B receptor in anxiety. *Proc Natl Acad Sci U S A.* 1991;88:1130-1133.
28. Cockran WG, Cox GM. *Experimental Designs.* 2nd ed. New York, NY: John Wiley & Sons Inc; 1957.
29. SAS Institute Inc. *SAS/STAT Guide For Personal Computers, Version 6 Edition.* Cary, NC: SAS Institute Inc; 1987.
30. Grizzle JE, Starmer CF, Koch GG. Analysis of categorical data by linear models. *Biometrics.* 1969;25:489-504.
31. Palmour RE, Ervin FR, Bradwejn J, Howbert JJ. The anxiogenic and cardiovascular effects of CCK_A are blocked by the CCK_B antagonist LY262,691. *Abstracts of the 21th Annual Meeting of the Society for Neuroscience.* Washington, DC: Society for Neuroscience; 1991:1602.
32. Rataud J, Darche F, Piot O, Stutzmann JM, Bohme GA, Blanchard JC. "Anxiolytic" effect of CCK-antagonists on plus-maze behaviour in mice. *Brain Res.* 1991;548:315-317.
33. Takagi H, Kubota Y, Mori S, Tateishi K, Hamaoka T, Tohyama M. Fine structural studies of cholecystokinin-8–like immunoreactive neurons and axon terminals in the nucleus tractus solitarius of the rat. *J Comp Neurol.* 1984;227:369-379.
34. Mantyh PW, Hunt SP. Evidence for cholecystokinin-like immunoreactive neurons in the rat medulla oblongata which project to the spinal cord. *Brain Res.* 1984;291:49-54.
35. Harro J, Vasar E, Bradwejn J. Cholecystokinin in animal and human research on anxiety. *Trends Pharmacol Sci.* 1993;14:244-249.
36. Chan SHH, Chan JYH, Ong BG. Anatomic connections between nucleus reticularis rostroventrolateralis and some medullary cardiovascular sites in the rat. *Neurosci Lett.* 1986;71:277-282.
37. Dampney RAL, Goodchild AK, Robertson LG, Montgomery W. Role of ventrolateral medulla in vasomotor regulation: a correlative anatomical and physiological study. *Brain Res.* 1982;249:223-235.
38. Dampney RAL, Czachurski J, Dembowsky K, Goodchild AK, Seller H. Afferent connections and spinal projections of the pressor region in the rostral ventrolateral medulla of the cat. *J Auton Nerv Syst.* 1922;20:73-86.
39. Jordan D, Spyer KM. Brainstem integration of cardiovascular and pulmonary afferent activity. *Prog Brain Res.* 1986;67:295-314.
40. Kirchheim HR. Systematic arterial baroreceptor reflexes. *Physiol Rev.* 1976; 56:100-176.
41. Spyer KM. Neural organization and control of the baroreceptor reflex. *Rev Physiol Biochem Pharmacol.* 1981;88:23-124.
42. Ross CA, Ruggiero DA, Park DH, Joh TH, Sved AF, Fernandez-Pardal J, Saaverda JM, Reis DJ. Tonic vasomotor control by the rostral ventrolateral medulla: effect of electrical or chemical stimulation of the area containing C1 adrenaline neurons on arterial pressure, heart rate, and plasma catecholamines and vasopressin. *J Neurosci.* 1984;4:474-494.
43. Pilowsky R, West M, Chalmers J. Renal sympathetic nerve responses to stimulation, inhibition and destruction of the ventrolateral medulla in the rabbit. *Neurosci Lett.* 1985;60:51-55.
44. Gootman PR, Cohen MI. Evoked splanchnic potentials produced by electrical stimulation of medullary vasomotor regions. *Exp Brain Res.* 1971;13:1-14.
45. Adair JR, Hamilton BL, Scappaticci KA, Helke CJ, Gillis RA. Cardiovascular responses to electrical stimulation of the medullary raphe area of the cat. *Brain Res.* 1977;128:141-145.
46. Futuro-Neto HA, Coote JH. Desynchronized sleep-like pattern of sympathetic activity elicited by electrical stimulation of sites in the brainstem. *Brain Res.* 1982;252:269-276.
47. Marovitch S, Kumada M, Reis DJ. Role of parabrachialls in cardiovascular regulation in the cat. *Brain Res.* 1982;232:57-75.
48. Denavit-Saubié M, Hurlé MA, Morin-Surun MP, Foutz AS, Champagnat J. The effects of cholecystokinin-8 in the nucleus tractus solitarius. In: Vanderhaeghen JJ, Crawley JN, eds. *Neuronal Cholecystokinin.* New York: The New York Academy of Sciences; 1985:375-384.
49. Ervin F, Palmour R, Bradwejn J. A new primate model for PD. In:*American Psychiatric Association 144th Annual Meeting New Research Abstracts.* New Orleans, La: American Psychiatric Association; 1991:100.
50. Harro J, Kiivet RA, Lang A, Vasar E. Rats with anxious or non-anxious type of exploratory behaviour differ in their brain CCK-8 and benzodiazepine receptor characteristics. *Behav Brain Res.* 1990;39:63-71.
51. Harro J, Pold M, Vasar E. Anxiogenic-like action of caerulein, a CCK-8 receptor agonist, in the mouse: influence of acute and subchronic diazepam treatment. *Naunyn Schmidebergs Arch Pharmacol.* 1990;341:62-67.
52. Harro J, Marcusson J, Oreland L. Alterations in brain cholecystokinin receptors in suicide victims. *Eur Neuropsychopharmacol.* 1992;2:57-63.

ORIGINAL ARTICLE

Increased Density of Guanine Nucleotide–Binding Proteins in the Postmortem Brains of Heroin Addicts

Pablo V. Escriba, PhD; Magdalena Sastre, PhD; Jesús A. García-Sevilla, MD

Objective: To directly evaluate the guanine nucleotide–binding (G) protein subunits α, β, and γ, which are involved in the signal transduction of opioid receptors, in the postmortem brains of heroin addicts who had died of an opiate overdose.

Methods: Specimens of the frontal cortex (Brodmann's area 9) were collected from 11 heroin addicts and 10 control subjects without a history of drug abuse. The biochemical status of human brain G protein subunits during opiate dependence was studied by means of immunoblotting techniques. Solubilized G proteins were separated by gel electrophoresis, transferred to pyroxylin membranes (western blotting) labeled with specific antiserum samples, and quantitated by image analysis after enhanced chemoluminescence.

Results: In the frontal cortex, relevant increases in the immunoreactivities of $G\alpha i_{1/2}$ (19%±4%, $P<.005$), Gαo (29%±7%, $P<.005$), and Gαs (26%±5%, $P<.005$) but not of $G\alpha i_3$ were found in heroin addicts compared with age- and sex-matched controls. Moreover, the amount of G protein β-subunit immunoreactivity was also consistently increased (27%±8%, $P<.01$) compared with controls in the same brain region. These G protein changes in the brains of human opiate addicts paralleled (with the exception of Gαs) those obtained in the brains of morphine hydrochloride–dependent rats. The increase in Gαs immunoreactivity that was observed in the rat brain only after the short-term morphine administration (24%±3%, $P<.005$) suggests that the increase in Gαs immunoreactivity in the brains of human addicts could be the cellular response to a deadly overdose of heroin.

Conclusions: Alterations in the density of specific Gi and Go protein subunits that are coupled to μ-opioid and other opioid receptors may be of clinical relevance in opiate tolerance, dependence, and abstinence syndrome.

(Arch Gen Psychiatry. 1994;51:494-501)

GUANINE nucleotide–binding (G) proteins are heterotrimers composed of one α, one β, and one γ subunit. They are involved in the signal transduction of about 80% of the characterized receptors for hormones, neurotransmitters, and neuromodulators,[1,2] and they are mainly located in the plasma membrane but are also present in other subcellular compartments.[3,4] DNA cloning of several α subunits has shown that they belong to a gene family because they share a number of features such as binding sites for βγ subunits, guanosine triphosphate, and Mg^{2+}; guanosine triphosphatase activity; specific sites for ribosylation by some bacterial toxins (eg, pertussis and cholera toxins); and the capability to modulate an effector system. Although most G protein–coupled receptors exert their action in a given cell type through preferential G proteins, a single type of receptor can be coupled to several types of G proteins.[5] Thus, α_2-adrenergic receptors can inhibit or activate adenylyl cyclase by means of Gi or Gs proteins, respectively, under different experimental conditions.[6] In addition, there is further regulation of the activity of the G protein α subunit provided by βγ subunits.[7] On the other hand, a given type of G protein can be activated by different membrane receptors, which could be inter-

From the Laboratory of Neuropharmacology, the Department of Fundamental Biology and Health Sciences, the University of the Balearic Islands, Palma de Mallorca, Spain.

See Subjects and Methods on next page

SUBJECTS AND METHODS

SUBJECT SELECTION AND BRAIN SAMPLES

Human brains were obtained at autopsy from the Instituto Anatómico Forense, Palma de Mallorca, Spain. This study was approved by the research and ethical review board of the Fondo de Investigaciones Sanitarias, Madrid, Spain. Specimens of the frontal cortex (Brodmann's area 9) were collected from 11 subjects who had died of an opiate overdose as determined by the medical examiner, and they were immediately stored at −80°C. Detailed medical histories of these subjects were not available for this study, but based on the police reports that were made following interviews with family members, the medical examiner made the determination of a history of heroin addiction for these subjects. Morphine and other drug screening was carried out on blood and urine samples at the Instituto Nacional de Toxicología, Barcelona, Spain, using high-performance liquid or gas chromatography and/or mass spectrometry analyses or an enzymatic immunoassay (EMIT, Syva, Palo Alto, Calif) for qualitative determinations. Drug screening showed the presence of morphine in all opiate addicts in whom a heroin overdose was most probably the cause of death. Ethanol and/or other psychotropic drugs were also detected in most cases (**Table**). The control group consisted of similar brain specimens from 10 subjects without a history of neuropsychiatric disorders or drug abuse who died suddenly of various accidental causes. Toxicological screening in these control subjects gave negative results. Mean age, sex ratio, and postmortem delay (time from death to the storage of the brain specimens) were similar in control subjects and heroin addicts (Table). The influence of the postmortem delay (range, 24 to 72 hours) on G protein subunit immunoreactivities was assessed in preliminary studies. Tissue storage (time from freezing to immunoblot analysis; mean, 13±3 months) did not differ between controls and heroin addicts, and it did not influence G protein immunoreactivities (data not shown).

ADMINISTRATION OF MORPHINE TO ANIMALS

Male Sprague-Dawley rats (250 to 300 g) were used. The animals were housed under controlled environmental conditions (22°C, 70% humidity, and a 12-hour light/dark cycle) with free access to food and water. For the short-term administration of morphine hydrochloride, the rats received a single injection of the opiate (10 mg/kg, intraperitoneally). For the long-term administration of morphine hydrochloride, the rats were injected intraperitoneally three times daily (at 8 AM, 2 PM, and 8 PM) for 5 days with increasing doses of the opiate as follows: 10, 10, and 10 mg/kg on day 1; 10, 20, and 20 mg/kg on day 2; 20, 20, and 40 mg/kg on day 3; 40, 40, and 80 mg/kg on day 4; and 80 and 100 mg/kg on day 5. This protocol for long-term morphine administration has been shown to produce a high degree of tolerance and dependence in rats.[17] Thus, after morphine administration for 5 days, naloxone hydrochloride (2 mg/kg; intraperitoneally) precipitated a rapid and strong withdrawal reaction (data not shown). Two hours after the last drug injection, the animals were killed by decapitation, and specimens of the cerebral frontal cortex were dissected and stored at −80°C for no longer than 2 weeks until use. The G protein subunit immunoreactivities were quantitated in morphine-nondependent (short-term morphine administration) and morphine-dependent (long-term morphine administration) rats as well as after naloxone-precipitated withdrawal. The influence of various postmortem delays on G protein levels also was assessed in rats. For these experiments, the animals were killed by anoxia under argon and were maintained at either 4°C or room temperature (22°C). Brains were removed from the skull at various times (0, 12, 24, 48, and 72 hours after death) and were stored at −80°C until use. These experiments in rats were performed according to the guidelines of the University of the Balearic Islands, Palma de Mallorca.

IMMUNOBLOT ANALYSIS OF G PROTEINS AND α-TUBULIN AND QUANTITATION OF SPECIFIC IMMUNOREACTIVITY

Immunoblotting techniques with specific antiserum samples is the method of choice for the detection and quantitation of G protein subunits.[23] Twenty to sixty milligrams of cerebral frontal cortex was homogenized with a tissue blender (Ultra-Turrax, Janke & Kunkel, GMBH & Co KG, Staufen, Germany) in 2 mL of TRIS buffer (50 mmol/L, pH 7.5), containing ethylenediaminetetraacetic acid (1 mmol/L), magnesium chloride (2 mmol/L), and the protease inhibitors phenylmethylsulfonyl fluoride (1 mmol/L) and iodoacetamide (5 mmol/L). The samples were centrifuged at 17 000×g for 10 minutes at 4°C, and the resulting pellets were resuspended in 1 mL of the same buffer without protease inhibitors per 20 mg of original tissue (for the detection of $G\alpha i_{1/2}$ and Gβ) or per 60 mg of tissue (for the detection of $G\alpha i_3$, Gαs, and Gαo). The protein content in these samples was determined by the method of Lowry et al.[24]

Next, 15 μL of the tissue suspension was mixed with an equal volume of TRIS buffer (40 mmol/L, pH 6.8) and 2% sodium dodecyl sulfate and incubated at 75°C for 5 minutes. After cooling, 20 μL of *N*-ethylmaleimide (100 mmol/L) was added and the samples were incubated for 15 minutes at room temperature. Fifty microliters of electrophoresis loading buffer (TRIS buffer [62.5 mmol/L, pH 6.8], 3% sodium dodecyl sulfate, 20% glycerol, and 0.005% bromophenol blue) was added to the previous mixture, which was then boiled for 3 minutes. Five to twenty microliters of the resulting suspension was loaded in a 9% polyacrylamide gel (1 mm thickness) and submitted to electrophoresis (sodium dodecyl sulfate–polyacrylamide gel electrophoresis). Proteins were transferred to nitrocellulose membranes (immunoblotting or western blotting), which were incubated in phosphate-buffered saline solution (sodium chloride, 137 mmol/L; potassium chloride, 2.7 mmol/L; sodium phosphate, 12 mmol/L; and monobasic potassium phosphate, 1.38 mmol/L; pH 7.4) containing 5% nonfat dry milk, 0.5% bovine serum albumin, and 0.1% polyoxyeth-

Continued on next page

ylene-sorbitan monolaureate (Tween 20, Sigma Chemical Co, St Louis, Mo) (blocking solution)[25] for 1 hour at room temperature with gentle rocking. They were incubated overnight at 4°C in a blocking solution containing the appropriate amount of the primary antibody: dilutions of 1:7000 (anti-$G\alpha i_{1/2}$), 1:5000 (anti-Gβ), 1:4000 (anti-Gαo), and 1:3000 (anti-$G\alpha i_3$ and anti-Gαs). The secondary antibody, horseradish peroxidase–linked donkey antirabbit IgG, was incubated at a 1:5000 dilution in a blocking solution at room temperature for 2 hours.

α-Tubulin was separated and quantitated as described above using a monoclonal anti–α-tubulin (clone DM 1A) diluted at 1:3000 as the primary antibody. The secondary antibody, horseradish peroxidase–linked sheep antimouse IgG, was incubated at 1:5000 dilution as described above.

Immunoreactivity was detected with the Enhanced Chemiluminescence Western Blot Detection system (Amersham, Buckinghamshire, England) followed by exposure to film (Kodak X-AR, Eastman Kodak Co, Rochester, NY) for 1 to 10 minutes. Films were scanned in the transmittance mode with a resolution of 84 μm in an image analyzer (Bio Image, Millipore, Ann Arbor, Mich) using the software provided by the manufacturer.

For the quantitation of G proteins, duplicate problem samples were evaluated using standard curves (ie, total protein loaded vs integrated optical density [IOD]) consisting of at least four points of different protein content (usually 0.5 to 4 μg of protein) of either control subjects or naive rats, all loaded on the same gel. This quantitation procedure was repeated at least four times in different gels for a total of eight measurements for each human or rat brain and for each antiserum sample. The mean intra-assay and interassay coefficients of variation were 3% (same subject) and 13% (different subjects), respectively. A linear relationship between the amount of protein loaded into the gel well and the IOD was found over the entire range of protein content used. In a given gel, the amount of G proteins in the frontal cortex of two or three heroin addicts was compared with that of control subjects matched for age and postmortem delay as closely as possible. The same procedure was followed for the quantitation of G protein subunits in the brains of rats administered morphine.

The theoretical amount of protein (PT) loaded into the gel well was obtained by interpolation of the IOD value from a problem sample in the standard curve from controlsamples and was compared with the real amount of protein (PR) loaded into the gel well. The percentage increase in the G protein content was calculated as follows: Percentage increase over control = $[(PT/PR) \times 100] - 100$, where this value is zero for a control sample used as the standard. As described above, the immunoreactivity of the G proteins studied exhibited little variation within the experimental groups, with the exception of the 45-kd Gsα band as previously described.[8] For this reason, in the present study, the band corresponding to the Gsα subunit will be referred to as the 52-kd band. Relevant to this method, it was found that the values of IOD of the whole band were more reproducible than those obtained with conventional light beam photodensitometers, in which the values of absorbance were affected by the shape of the band. In the image analysis device used, each band is divided into over 2000 areas, and the sum of the absorbance of each one corresponds to the IOD value. Following this procedure and under the reported experimental conditions, the relationship between the amounts of protein loaded into a gel well and the IOD was linear in the range of protein content used in the experiments (**Figure 1**, top). The antiserum samples used labeled bands with molecular masses of 40 to 41 kd ($G\alpha i_{1/2}$ and $G\alpha i_3$), 45 and 52 kd (Gαs), 39 to 40 kd (Gαo), and 35 to 36 kd (Gβ) (Figure 1, bottom) in good agreement with previous studies.[8,9]

MATERIALS AND DRUGS

The following anti–G protein subunits polyclonal antisera raised against specific C-terminal peptides or the N-terminus (Gαo) were purchased from Dupont/New England Nuclear Corp, Homburg, Germany: anti-$G\alpha i_{1/2}$ (AS/7), anti-$G\alpha i_3$ (EC/2), anti-Gαo (GC/2), anti-Gαs (RM/1), and anti-Gβ (SW/1). The specificity of these antisera for the detection of human G protein subunits has been established in human platelet membranes[26] and in human postmortem brains.[8] Anti–α-tubulin monoclonal antibody (clone DM 1A) was purchased from Sigma Chemical Co. Horseradish peroxidase–linked donkey antirabbit and sheep antimouse IgG, as well as enhanced chemiluminescence reagents, were obtained from Amersham. Kodak XAR-2 film was used for autoradiography. Drugs used were morphine hydrochloride (Unión Químico-Farmacéutica SAE, Madrid) and naloxone hydrochloride (Endo Laboratories Inc, Garden City, NY). All other chemicals were obtained from Sigma Chemical Co.

STATISTICS

Results are expressed as means±SEM or SD. One-sample *t* test (identical in its implementation to the paired *t* test) was used for the statistical evaluations. The level of significance was chosen as $P=.05$.

preted as a mechanism of regulation of the convergence and divergence of neurotransmitter actions in the central nervous system, also referred to as receptor-receptor cross talk. Further evidence of the prominent role of G proteins in the regulation of the signaling pathways comes from the fact that abnormalities in the function and expression of various G proteins have been associated with various pathological processes.[2] In the context of neurochemical disorders of the human brain, abnormalities of G proteins appear to be present in endogenous depression[8,9] and other neuropsychiatric disorders.[10] Moreover, G proteins have also been found to be modulated by various psychotropic drug treatments such as antidepressants[11] and opiates.[12]

δ-Opioid and μ-opioid receptors inhibit adenylyl cyclase activity through G proteins that are sensitive to pertussis toxin in NG108-15 (neuroblastoma × glioma) cells[13]

Characteristics of Individual Heroin Addicts, the Heroin-Addict Group, and the Control Group*

	Sex	Age at Death, y	Drugs Other Than Morphine Detected†	Postmortem Delay, h
Individual heroin addicts				
1	M	24	ETH/BZD	46
2	M	42	COD/COC	24
3	M	23	BZD	22
4	F	15	None	60
5	F	25	COC/AMP	48
6	M	26	ETH/COC	48
7	M	26	ETH	26
8	M	22	ETH/BZD/CAN	34
9	M	21	COD/ETH	43
10	M	23	COC/CAN	36
11	M	30	BZD/CAN	48
Heroin-addict group (n=11)	9M/2F	25±2	...	39±4
Control group (n=10)	8M/2F	28±3	...	34±4

*Cause of death for all heroin addicts was an overdose. Group values are means±SEMs.

†Morphine was detected in all heroin addicts. Qualitative determinations of morphine and other drugs in plasma or urine were performed as indicated in the "Methods" section. Other opiates and drugs included codeine (COD), ethanol (ETH), cocaine (COC), benzodiazepines (BZD), amphetamines (AMP), and cannabinoids (CAN).

and in 7315c pituitary tumor cells.[14] Long-term exposure of 7315c cells to morphine leads to a loss in their ability to inhibit adenylyl cyclase, which parallels a marked decrease in the density of μ-opioid receptors.[15] In contrast, in vivo regulation of δ-opioid and μ-opioid receptors by long-term exposure to agonists has resulted in equivocal results with an increase, a decrease, or no alteration of the density of the receptors in the brain.[16] However, treatment with full agonists clearly induces opioid receptor downregulation, although this is not a necessary condition for the development of tolerance.[16] Thus, a reduction in the density of μ-opioid receptors in rodent brain membranes after long-term administration of morphine has been reported,[17,18] as well as a functional uncoupling of effector from receptor, expressed as a failure in guanylyl nucleotide regulation of μ-agonist binding.[18]

The long-term administration of opiates has been shown to result in a marked sensitization of the adenylyl cyclase–cyclic adenosine monophosphate (cAMP) system at every biochemical step between receptors and physiological responses.[19] This upregulation of the cAMP system appears to be a compensatory homeostatic response to the sustained inhibition of the opioid receptor system induced by long-term opiate administration (tolerant/dependent state).[19-21] In this context and as a relevant molecular mechanism, long-term opiate administration has been shown to cause, through a naltrexone-sensitive effect, an increase in the levels of pertussis toxin–mediated adenosine diphosphate–ribosylation of Gαi and Gαo proteins in the rat locus coeruleus.[12] This pioneer study[12] also demonstrated that the long-term use of morphine increased the amount of Gαo immunoreactivity in the locus coeruleus but not in the other brain regions (immunoreactive Gαi was not determined). Similar adaptive increases of various G proteins and enhanced coupling efficiency induced by long-term opiate administration have been observed in other systems.[22] Therefore, alterations in specific G protein subunits could be of relevance to the biochemical mechanisms that are associated with opiate tolerance, dependence, and withdrawal syndrome. However, there is no direct information on the status of G protein subunits in the human brain during chronic opiate addiction.

This study was designed to directly evaluate G protein subunits in postmortem brains of heroin addicts who had died of an opiate overdose. The results demonstrate the existence of relevant increases in the immunoreactivity of $G\alpha i_{1/2}$, Gαo, Gαs, and Gβ but not of $G\alpha i_3$ in the frontal cortex of heroin addicts. This high content of G proteins could compensate for the μ-opioid receptor downregulation and/or the functional receptor-effector uncoupling during the long-term use of opiates to maintain a certain level of signal transduction.

RESULTS

EFFECT OF POSTMORTEM DELAY ON G PROTEIN SUBUNITS IN HUMAN AND RAT BRAINS

Although there was no difference in the postmortem delay between the control (34±4 hours) and heroin addict (39±4 hours) groups (Table), the influence of the postmortem interval (24 to 72 hours) on G protein subunit immunoreactivities was first assessed to determine the pattern of degradation of these proteins in the human and the rat brains. In rats, postmortem delays of up to 72 hours at 4°C did not alter significantly the density of any of the G protein subunits ($G\alpha i_{1/2}$, $G\alpha i_3$, Gαo, Gαs, and Gβ) that were evaluated in the cerebral cortex. However, postmortem delays of 48 and 72 hours at room temperature (22°C) caused marked decreases in the levels of brain Gαs (26% and 43%, respectively) and $G\alpha i_3$ (28% and 55%, respectively; mean of two experiments). No significant changes were found for other G protein subunits ($G\alpha i_{1/2}$, Gαo, and Gβ) in the rat brain for up to 72 hours of postmortem delay at 22°C.

Human corpses usually spent a few hours at outdoor temperature (10°C to 20°C) until final storage at 4°C. In human control subjects, postmortem delays between 24 and 48 hours did not alter significantly the density of any of the G protein subunits measured in the frontal cortex (**Figure 2**). However, postmortem delays of 72 hours were associated with marked decreases in the

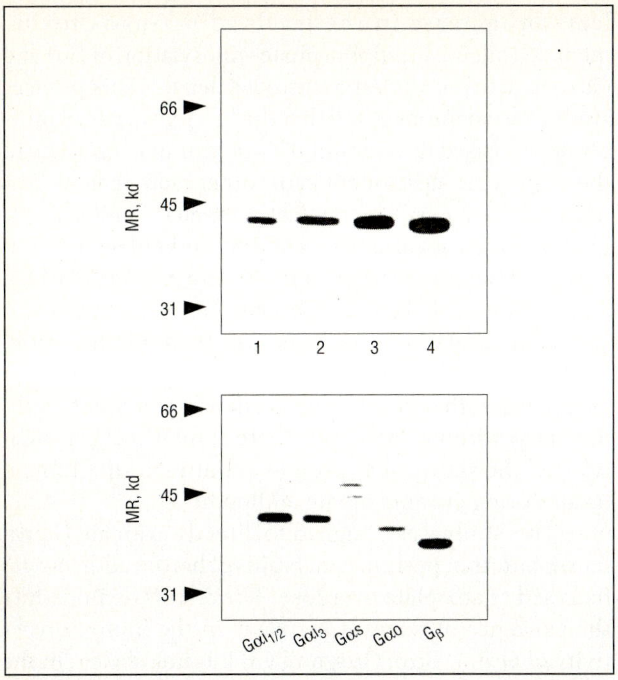

Figure 1. *Top, Human brain $\alpha i_{1/2}$ subunit guanine nucleotide–binding (G) protein signal intensity and protein content. The representative immunoblot of frontal cortex (Brodmann's area 9) membrane proteins was performed as described in the "Patients and Methods" section. The amount of total protein loaded per gel well was 0.8 μg (lane 1), 1.6 μg (lane 2), 2.0 μg (lane 3), and 2.4 μg (lane 4). The integrated optical density values measured by image analysis were 1.8, 3.6, 4.6, and 5.4, respectively. Bottom, Human brain G protein subunits. The representative immunoblot shows the relative mobility of $G\alpha i_{1/2}$, $G\alpha i_3$, Gαs, Gαo, and Gβ protein subunits in the frontal cortex. The two bands of Gαs correspond to 45- and 52-kd proteins. Molecular masses (MR) in kilodaltons estimated from referenced standards are shown.*

levels of $G\alpha i_{1/2}$ (42%), $G\alpha i_3$ (83%), and Gαs (47%). In contrast, no significant changes were observed in the immunoreactivity of Gαo and Gβ in the frontal cortex for postmortem delays of up to 72 hours (Figure 2). In control subjects and heroin addicts (n=21), specific G protein subunit immunoreactivities did not correlate with postmortem delays (range from 17 to 60 hours) (data not shown). These results indicated that at 4°C, human brain G proteins remain stable for a long period after death.

DENSITY OF G PROTEIN SUBUNITS AND α-TUBULIN IN THE POSTMORTEM BRAIN OF HEROIN ADDICTS

In heroin addicts who had morphine detected in their body fluids, the density of specific G protein α-subunits was significantly increased in the frontal cortex. Thus, relevant changes in the immunoreactivities of $G\alpha i_{1/2}$ (119%±4%, n=9, $P<.005$), Gαo (129%±7%, n=8, $P<.005$), and Gαs (126%±5%, n=8, $P<.005$) were found in heroin addicts compared with age- and sex-matched controls (**Figure 3**). Although the most abundant G protein in the brain is Go[27] and the frontal cortex is particularly enriched in this G protein,[28] the increases in α-subunit immunoreactivities for the various G proteins were of a similar magnitude. In contrast, the immunoreactivity of $G\alpha i_3$ was not increased significantly (102%±10%, n=9, $P>.05$) compared with that obtained in control-matched subjects. This 40- to 41-kd band had the greatest variability in immunoreactivity (interassay coefficient of variation, 29%), probably because of the low level of $G\alpha i_3$ in the brain.[29] On the other hand, the amount of G protein β-subunit immunoreactivity in the frontal cortex of heroin addicts was also consistently increased compared with that of controls (127%±8%, n=8, $P<.01$) (Figure 3). This β-subunit (35- to 36-kd band; Figure 1, bottom) and the βγ complex are involved in the high affinity coupling of G protein to receptors.

In a selected group of heroin addicts who showed the greatest increases in the immunoreactivity of $G\alpha i_{1/2}$ and Gαs, the levels of α-tubulin, a housekeeping control protein, were not increased significantly in the frontal cortex (103%±3%, n=5, $P>.05$) compared with those obtained in control-matched subjects. These negative results discounted possible unspecific effects of opiates on G protein levels.

EFFECT OF LONG-TERM MORPHINE ADMINISTRATION ON G PROTEIN SUBUNITS IN THE RAT BRAIN

Repeated administration of increasing doses of morphine hydrochloride (10 to 100 mg/kg, intraperitoneally) in rats for a period of 5 days resulted in the development of a high degree of opiate tolerance and dependence (see "Subjects and Methods" section). In these morphine-dependent rats, the density of specific G protein subunits was found to be increased in the brain, which was similar to the effect in heroin addicts. Thus, long-term morphine administration compared with saline solution administration induced significant changes in the immunoreactivities of $G\alpha i_{1/2}$ (130%±5%, n=5, $P<.005$), Gαo (128%±3%, n=5, $P<.005$), and Gβ (125%±4%, n=4, $P<.005$) but did not increase significantly those of $G\alpha i_3$ (106%±3%, n=5, $P>.05$) and Gαs (102%±5%, n=4, $P>.05$) in the rat cerebral cortex (**Figure 4**). These G protein changes in the brains of morphine-dependent rats, with the exception of Gαs, paralleled those observed in the postmortem brains of heroin addicts (Figure 3).

In marked contrast to the long-term administration, a single dose of morphine hydrochloride (10 mg/kg, intraperitoneally for 2 hours) increased significantly the immunoreactivity of Gαs (124%±3%, n=4, $P<.005$) but not those of the other G protein subunits (n=4) in the rat cerebral cortex (Figure 4). The increase in Gαs immunoreactivity that was observed in rats only after the administration of a single dose of morphine suggests that the increase in Gαs immunoreactivity in the brains of human addicts could be the cellular response to a single dose of heroin (a deadly overdose?) rather than to long-term exposure to the drug.

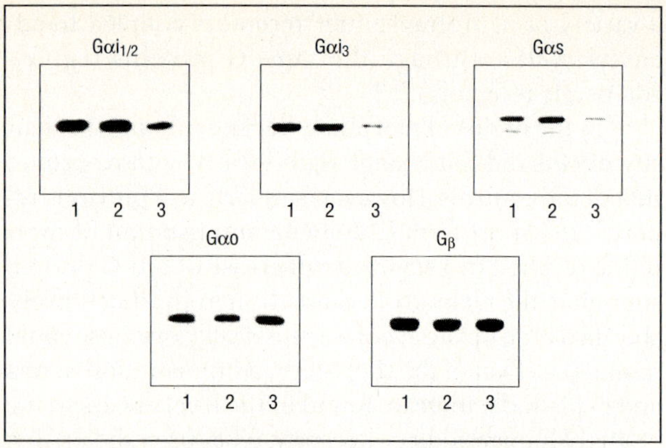

Figure 2. *The effect of postmortem delay on guanine nucleotide–binding (G) protein subunits in the human brain. Representative immunoblots for specific G protein subunits are shown for specimens of the frontal cortex (Brodmann's area 9) from three control subjects. Specimens were collected 24 hours (lane 1), 48 hours (lane 2), and 72 hours (lane 3) after death. Note that postmortem delays of up to 48 hours did not alter the immunoreactivity of any of the G protein subunits. Postmortem delays of 72 hours were associated with marked decreases in the immunoreactivity of* $G\alpha i_{1/2}$ *(42%),* $G\alpha i_3$ *(83%), and Gαs (47%) but not of Gαo and Gβ.*

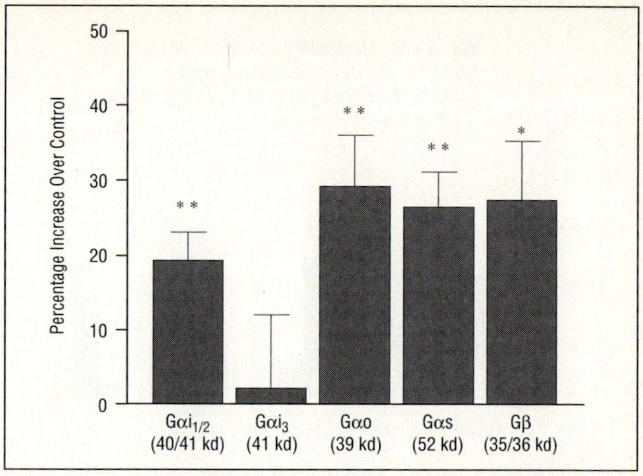

Figure 3. *Densities of guanine nucleotide–binding (G) protein subunits in the frontal cortex (Brodmann's area 9) of heroin addicts. Immunoblot analysis and quantitation of specific immunoreactivities were performed as described in the "Patients and Methods" section. Data are expressed as the mean±SEM percentage differences of the corresponding matched control group. Single asterisk indicates* $P<.01$*; double asterisks,* $P<.005$ *(one-sample* t *test).*

In morphine-dependent rats, naloxone hydrochloride–precipitated (2 mg/kg, intraperitoneally for 2 hours) withdrawal induced a rapid and strong behavioral reaction (data not shown) without any significant change in the pattern of G protein subunit immunoreactivities that is induced by long-term morphine use (n=2) (Figure 4). These results further suggested that the G protein adaptive changes that were observed in the postmortem brains of heroin addicts reflect those induced by morphine during the tolerant or dependent state.

COMMENT

The binding of opiate drugs to μ-opioid (and other opioid) receptors results in the inhibition of adenylyl cyclase activity through pertussis toxin–sensitive Gi and Go proteins. After long-term exposure to opiates, opiate addiction has been shown to be associated with a marked upregulation of the adenylyl cyclase–cAMP system, in which modulation of G proteins, as transducers of information, appears to be a relevant step.[19] However, studies on the effects of long-term exposure to opiates on G proteins in the brains of mammals are scarce,[12,30-32] and to our knowledge, this is the first report of increases in the density of G proteins in the postmortem brains of heroin addicts.

When neurochemical disorders of the human brain are investigated using autopsy samples, the influence of the postmortem delay should be considered. Because G protein subunits previously have not been studied extensively in the postmortem human brain, the effect of the postmortem delay on these proteins was first determined. It has been reported recently that postmortem delays at 4°C of less than 48 hours lead to the degradation of several G protein messenger RNAs (mRNAs) in the rat brain and that in the human brain, mRNA degradation was already evident for postmortem delays of less than 24 hours.[33] Messenger RNAs are, in general, more susceptible to enzyme degradation than are proteins because ribonucleases are ubiquitous and very stable enzymes, so G protein degradation was not expected to happen as rapidly as the degradation of the mRNA species encoding them. Thus, no significant changes were observed in the immunoreactivity of any of the G protein subunits ($G\alpha i_{1/2}$, $G\alpha i_3$, Gαo, Gαs, and Gβ) evaluated in the human and rat brains for postmortem delays of up to 48 hours at 4°C. Moreover, the density of Gαo and Gβ in the human frontal cortex remained unchanged for postmortem delays of up to 72 hours at 4°C. In the present study, human brains with postmortem delays of less than 50 hours (except one heroin addict and one matched control subject) were used. Therefore, these findings argue against confounding postmortem effects on the identified changes of G proteins in the brains of heroin addicts.

The results reported herein demonstrate the existence of relevant increases in the immunoreactivities of $G\alpha i_{1/2}$, Gαo, Gαs, and Gβ in the frontal cortices of heroin addicts. These G protein changes in the brains of human opiate addicts paralleled (with the exception of Gαs) those observed in the brains (cortices) of morphine-dependent rats, demonstrating biochemical adaptive mechanisms similar to the effects of opiates. These latter results are in line with and extend recent findings that report increases in the levels of Gαo and Gαs in the brains of morphine-dependent rats.[12,32] In the former study,[12] however, morphine-induced changes in the levels of Gαo and Gβ were not detected in the rat frontal cortex but were detected only in the locus coeruleus. This study[12] implicated the locus coeruleus as a unique target for the effects of opiates on G proteins. However, our results (increases in the levels of various G proteins in human and rat cerebral cortices) and

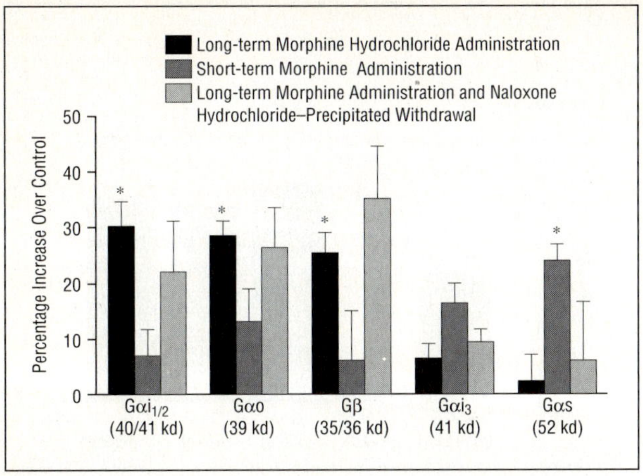

Figure 4. *The effect of morphine hydrochloride administration on guanine nucleotide–binding (G) protein subunits in the rat cerebral cortex. The long- and short-term administration of morphine and the long-term administration of morphine followed by naloxone hydrochloride–precipitated withdrawal, as well as the immunoblot analysis and quantitation of specific immunoreactivities, were performed as described in the "Patients and Methods" section. Data are expressed as the mean±SEM or SD (naloxone-precipitated withdrawal) percentage differences from the corresponding matched control group. Asterisks indicate* P<.005 *(one-sample* t *test).*

those of others[32] (increases in the levels of Gαs and Gαo as well as their mRNAs in the rat cerebral cortex, hypothalamus, and other brain regions) clearly indicate that long-term morphine administration induces increases in G protein subunits in brain regions other than the locus coeruleus. The discrepancies between studies might be due to the different degrees of tolerance and dependence induced by the different morphine administrations.[32]

Because Gαi and Gαo proteins have been associated with the signal transduction of opioid receptors,[12,13,19] an increase in the levels of these G proteins followed by upregulation of the adenylyl cyclase–cAMP system could compensate the μ-opioid receptor downregulation and/or functional receptor-effector uncoupling that are observed in cultured cells[15] and in rodent brain membranes[17,18] after long-term administration of morphine. Therefore, during the process of opiate addiction, the upregulation of the cAMP system observed in many experimental models is thought to be a relevant compensatory homeostatic response of the opioid system to maintain a certain level of signal transduction.[19-21] In line with this, specific G protein subunits ($G\alpha i_{1/2}$, Gαo, and Gβ) remained elevated in the rat brain 1 to 2 hours after the precipitation of morphine withdrawal with an opiate antagonist (our results) and returned to control levels by 6 to 72 hours, which paralleled the withdrawal syndrome.[30] In heroin addicts, the increased density of specific G proteins in the brain (our results) and the reported greater basal and colforsin-stimulated platelet adenylyl cyclase activities[34] also support the above hypothesis in human addicts. However, the phenomenon of supersensitive adenylyl cyclase is not exclusive of the opioid system; it should be considered a more general cellular adaptation to the long-term inhibition of the enzyme through a variety of neurotransmitter receptors coupled to adenylyl cyclase through the same G proteins (eg, α_2-adrenergic receptors).[35,36]

In the brains of morphine-dependent rats, the density of Gαs did not change significantly with respect to that of the controls. However, similarly to a previous report,[12] the short-term (2-hour) administration of morphine resulted in a significant increase of this G protein subunit in the rat brain. Because the heroin addicts probably died of an opiate overdose, this deadly overdose could mimic the effect of the short-term administration in rats and explain the increase found in the level of Gαs in the brains of human addicts. Recently, it has been shown that long-term morphine use induces an increase in the level of Gαs in primary cultures of rat striatal neurons[37] and that μ-opioid receptors are coupled to stimulatory G proteins in the rat olfactory bulb.[38] The increase in the levels of Gαs in the brains of heroin addicts and rats receiving short-term administrations of morphine could be explained as either a direct coupling of opioid receptors with stimulatory G proteins[38] or a mechanism of compensation to the overstimulated inhibitory pathway by opiate agonists.[39] It is of interest to note that the increase in the density of G protein β-subunit was similar to that observed for the various G protein α-subunits in the brains of both heroin addicts and morphine-dependent rats. It is reasonable to expect that the expression of the Gβ subunits was related to the expression of the Gα subunits to maintain the adequate stoichiometry of the heterotrimer. However, the Gβ subunit might play a more prominent role in the regulation of the signal transduction modulating the activity of the various Gα subunits and the effector systems.[7,40,41]

In the present study, most heroin addicts were polydrug abusers with mainly ethanol and cocaine detected in their body fluids, and these drugs could have altered the status of G proteins as they specifically relate to opiate addiction. However, using similar immunoblotting methods, long-term ethanol exposure in cultured cells has been shown to decrease the amount of Gαs but not that of Gαi,[42] and long-term administration of cocaine has been associated with decreases in the density of Gαi and Gαo and no alteration in the densities of Gαs and Gβ in the rat brain.[43] These findings argue against confounding drug effects on the identified changes of G proteins in the brains of heroin addicts because the G protein changes induced by ethanol and cocaine are opposite to those induced by morphine and heroin.

Our findings are the first direct evidence that specific G protein subunits are increased in the brains of heroin addicts and suggest that alterations in the density of G proteins may be of clinical relevance in opiate tolerance, dependence, and abstinence syndrome.

Accepted for publication February 25, 1994.

This study was supported by grant 6/1992 from the CITRAN Foundation, Barcelona, grant 93/0641 from the Fondo de Investigaciones Sanitarias, and grant PM 91/0069 from the Dirección General de Investigación Científica y Técnica and by a fellowship from the Ministerio de Educación y Ciencia, Madrid (Dr Sastre).

Read in part before a meeting of the British Pharmacological Society, Cambridge, England, January 5, 1993. Portions of this work have appeared in abstract form (Br J Pharmacol. *1993;108:30).*

The authors wish to thank the staff members of the Instituto Anatómico Forense for their cooperation, and Juan Luís Valverde, PhD, of the Instituto Nacional de Toxicología who supplied the toxicological data.

Reprint requests to Laboratori Neurofarmacologia, Departament de Biologia Fonamental i Ciències de la Salut, Universitat de les Illes Balears, Cra Valldemossa, Km 7.5, E-07071 Palma (Balears), Spain (Dr García-Sevilla).

REFERENCES

1. Birnbaumer L. G proteins in signal transduction. *Annu Rev Pharmacol Toxicol.* 1990;30:675-705.
2. Spiegel AM, Shenker A, Weinstein LS. Receptor-effector coupling by G proteins: implications for normal and abnormal signal transduction. *Endocr Rev.* 1992;13:536-565.
3. Lewis JM, Woolkalis MJ, Gerton GL, Smith RM, Jarret L, Manning DR. Subcellular distribution of the α subunit(s) of Gi: visualization by immunofluorescent and immunogold labeling. *Cell Regul.* 1991;2:1097-1113.
4. Gurich RW, Codina J, DuBose TD Jr. A potential role of guanine nucleotide-binding protein in the regulation of endosomal proton transport. *J Clin Invest.* 1991;87:1547-1552.
5. Gerhardt MA, Neubig RR. Multiple Gi protein subtypes regulate a single effector mechanism. *Mol Pharmacol.* 1991;40:707-711.
6. Eason MG, Kurose H, Holt BD, Raymond JR, Liggett SB. Simultaneous coupling of α_2-adrenergic receptors to two G-proteins with opposing effects. *J Biol Chem.* 1992;267:15795-15801.
7. Federman AD, Conklin BR, Schrader KA, Reed RR, Bourne HR. Hormonal stimulation of adenylyl cyclase through Gi-protein βγ subunits. *Nature.* 1992;356:159-161.
8. Young LT, Li PP, Kish SJ, Siu KP, Warsh JJ. Postmortem cerebral cortex Gsα-subunit levels are elevated in bipolar affective disorder. *Brain Res.* 1991;553:323-326.
9. Young LT, Li PP, Kish SJ, Siu KP, Kamble A, Hornykiewicz O, Warsh JJ. Cerebral cortex Gsα protein levels and forskolin-stimulated cyclic AMP formation are increased in bipolar affective disorders. *J Neurochem.* 1993;61:890-898.
10. Manji HK. G proteins: implications for psychiatry. *Am J Psychiatry.* 1992;149:746-760.
11. Lech K-P, Manji HK. Signal-transducing G proteins and antidepressant drugs: evidence for modulation of α subunit gene expression in the rat. *Biol Psychiatry.* 1992;32:549-579.
12. Nestler EJ, Erdos JJ, Terwilliger R, Duman RS, Tallman JF. Regulation of G proteins by chronic morphine in the rat locus coeruleus. *Brain Res.* 1989;476:230-239.
13. Kurose H, Katada T, Amano T, Ui M. Specific uncoupling by islet-activating protein, pertussis toxin, of negative signal transduction via α-adrenergic, cholinergic, and opiate receptors in neuroblastoma × glioma hybrid cells. *J Biol Chem.* 1983;258:4870-4875.
14. Puttfarcken PS, Werling LL, Cox BM. Effects of chronic morphine exposure on opioid inhibition of adenyl cyclase in 7315c cell membranes: a useful model for the study of tolerance at μ-opioid receptors. *Mol Pharmacol.* 1988;33:520-527.
15. Puttfarken PS, Cox BM. Morphine-induced desensitization and down-regulation at μ-receptors in 7315c pituitary tumor cells. *Life Sci.* 1989;45:1937-1942.
16. Yoburn BC, Billings B, Duttaroy A. Opioid receptor regulation in mice. *J Pharmacol Exp Ther.* 1993;265:314-320.
17. Ulibarri I, García-Sevilla JA, Ugedo L. Modulation of brain α_2-adrenoceptor and μ-opioid receptor densities during morphine dependence and spontaneous withdrawal in rats. *Naunyn-Schmiedebergs Arch Pharmacol.* 1987;336:530-537.
18. Werling LL, McMahon PN, Cox BM. Selective changes in μ-opioid receptor properties induced by chronic morphine induction. *Proc Natl Acad Sci U S A.* 1989;86:6393-6397.
19. Nestler EJ. Molecular mechanisms of drug addiction. *J Neurosci.* 1992;12:2439-2450.
20. Sharma SK, Klee WA, Niremberg M. Dual regulation of adenylate cyclase accounts for narcotic dependence and tolerance. *Proc Natl Acad Sci U S A.* 1975;72:3092-3096.
21. Collier HOJ. Cellular site of opiate dependence. *Nature.* 1980;283:625-629.
22. Ammer H, Schulz R. Coupling of prostaglandin E_1 receptors to the stimulatory GTP-binding protein Gs is enhanced in neuroblastoma × glioma (NG108-15) hybrid cells chronically exposed to an opioid. *Mol Pharmacol.* 1993;43:556-563.
23. Milligan G. Techniques used in the identification and analysis of function of pertussis toxin-sensitive guanine nucleotide binding proteins. *Biochem J.* 1988;255:1-13.
24. Lowry OH, Rosebrough NJ, Farr AL, Randall RJ. Protein measurement with the folin phenol reagent. *J Biol Chem.* 1951;193:265-275.
25. Harlow E, Lane D. *Antibodies: A Laboratory Manual.* Cold Spring Harbor, NY: Cold Spring Harbor Laboratory Press; 1988.
26. Simmonds WF, Goldsmith PK, Codina J, Unson CG, Spiegel AM. $G\alpha_{i2}$ mediates α_2-adrenergic inhibition of adenylyl cyclase in platelet membranes: in situ identification with Gα C-terminal antibodies. *Proc Natl Acad Sci U S A.* 1989;86:7809-7813.
27. Neer EJ. Structural and functional studies on Go protein. *Soc Gen Physiol Ser.* 1990;45:143-151.
28. Worley PF, Baraban JM, Snyder SH. Beyond receptors: multiple second-messenger systems in the brain. *Ann Neurol.* 1987;21:217-229.
29. Jones DT, Reed RR. Molecular cloning of five GTP-binding protein cDNA species from rat olfactory neuroepithelium. *J Biol Chem.* 1987;262:14241-14249.
30. Rasmunssen K, Beitner-Johnson DB, Krystal JH, Aghajanian GK, Nestler EJ. Opiate withdrawal and the rat locus coeruleus: behavioral, electrophysiological and biochemical correlates. *J Neurosci.* 1990;10:2308-2317.
31. Terwilliger RZ, Beitner-Johnson D, Sevarino KA, Crain SM, Nestler EJ. A general role for adaptations in G-proteins and the cyclic AMP system in mediating the chronic actions of morphine and cocaine on neuronal function. *Brain Res.* 1991;478:100-110.
32. Parolaro D, Rubino T, Gori E, Massi P, Bendotti C, Patrini G, Marcozzi C, Parenti M. In situ hybridization reveals specific increases in Gαs and Gαo mRNA in discrete brain regions of morphine-tolerant rats. *Eur J Pharmacol.* 1993;244:211-222.
33. Ross BM, Knowler JT, McCullock J. On the stability of messenger RNA and ribosomal RNA in the brains of control human subjects and patients with Alzheimer's disease. *J Neurochem.* 1992;58:1810-1819.
34. García-Sevilla JA, Ulibarri I, Ugedo L, Gutiérrez M. α_2-Adrenoceptor-mediated inhibition of platelet adenylate cyclase activity in heroin addicts in abstinence. *Psychopharmacology.* 1987;92:320-323.
35. Thomas JM, Hoffman BB. Adenylate cyclase supersensitivity: a general means of cellular adaptation to inhibitory agonists? *Trends Pharmacol Sci.* 1987;8:308-311.
36. Aghajanian GK, Wang YY. Common α_2- and opiate effector mechanisms in the locus coeruleus: intracellular studies in brain slices. *Neuropharmacology.* 1987;26:793-799.
37. Van Vliet BJ, Wardeh G, Mulder AH, Schoffelmeer ANM. Reciprocal effects of chronic morphine administration on stimulatory and inhibitory G-protein α subunits in primary cultures of rat striatal neurons. *Eur J Pharmacol.* 1991;208:341-342.
38. Olianas MC, Onali P. Characterization of opioid receptors mediating stimulation of adenyl cyclase activity in rat olfactory bulb. *Mol Pharmacol.* 1992;42:109-115.
39. Sánchez-Blázquez P, Garzón J. Intracerebroventricular injection of antibodies directed against Gsα enhances the supraspinal antinociception induced by morphine, β-endorphin and clonidine in mice. *Life Sci.* 1992;51:237-242.
40. Tang W-J, Gilman AG. Type-specific regulation of adenylyl cyclase by G protein βγ subunits. *Science.* 1991;254:1500-1503.
41. Schmidt CJ, Thomas TC, Levine MA, Neer NJ. Specificity of G protein β and γ subunit interactions. *J Biol Chem.* 1992;267:13807-13810.
42. Rabin RA. Ethanol-induced desensitization of adenylate cyclase: role of adenosine receptor and GTP-binding proteins. *J Pharmacol Exp Ther.* 1993;264:977-983.
43. Nestler EJ, Terwilliger RZ, Walker JR, Sevarino KA, Duman RS. Chronic cocaine treatment decreases levels of the G protein subunits Giα and Goα in discrete regions of rat brain. *J Neurochem.* 1990;55:1059-1082.

Lithium Prophylaxis in American Patients With Unipolar Disorder

A recent issue of *Current Opinion in Psychiatry* presented a section on mood disorders; two reviews by American authors dealt with long-term treatment. One[1] described maintenance treatment with antidepressants and electroconvulsive therapy (ECT) but did not mention prophylactic lithium treatment. The other[2] concluded that, in unipolar depressive disorder, "the routine use of lithium salts instead of, or in combination with, antidepressants does not appear well-justified as a first-line maintenance treatment." In the author's opinion, two studies had shown lithium treatment to be ineffective in patients with unipolar disorder: British psychiatrists[3] found no advantage of treatment with amitriptyline plus lithium over treatment with amitriptyline alone, and an American study[4] found treatment with lithium no better than placebo in patients whose index episode had been severe (although as effective as imipramine in those with an index episode of moderate intensity).

The former finding reveals, however, nothing about the value of lithium treatment alone, and it is difficult to see how the latter finding can outweigh the evidence of numerous studies published over the last 25 years. They show almost without exception that the prophylactic, recurrence-preventive action of lithium is as good in affective unipolar disorder as in bipolar.[5,6] In both disease forms, lithium maintenance treatment is associated with a low mortality.[7]

Should American experiences differ somewhat from European, the explanation may be that the American concept of unipolar affective illness is broader than the European and has come to encompass almost any mood disorder that is not bipolar.[5] It is therefore not surprising if some American researchers find lithium treatment less effective in unipolar affective illness that may include forms of depression never shown or claimed to respond to lithium prophylaxis.

In recent years, American research has proven that long-term treatment with antidepressants prophylactically is effective in recurrent depression.[8,9] Lithium prophylaxis is not mentioned in these reports; must one good thing necessarily oust another? Patients are entitled to all relevant therapeutic options, and those who suffer from recurrent depression without obvious psychosocial precipitating factors, have symptom-free intervals, and are without deviating character features might well be given a chance with lithium maintenance treatment, whether first or second line. The final choice may depend on how individual patients tolerate treatment with antidepressants and lithium, respectively.

Mogens Schou, MD
The Psychiatric Hospital
2 Skovagervej
Risskov, Denmark
DK-8240

1. Nobler MS, Sackeim HA. Pharmacotherapy and electroconvulsive therapy for mood disorders. *Curr Opin Psychiatry.* 1993;6:10-15.
2. Thase ME. Maintenance treatments of recurrent affective disorders. *Curr Opin Psychiatry.* 1993;6:16-21.
3. Johnstone EC, Owens DGC, Lambert MT, Crow TJ, Frith CD, Done DJ. Combination tricyclic antidepressant and lithium maintenance medication in unipolar and bipolar depressed patients. *J Affect Disord.* 1990;20:225-233.
4. Prien RF, Kupfer DJ, Mansky PA, Small JG, Tuason VB, Voss CB, Johnson WE. Drug therapy in the prevention of recurrences in unipolar and bipolar affective disorders. *Arch Gen Psychiatry.* 1984;41:1096-1104.
5. Goodwin FK, Jamison KR. *Manic-Depressive Illness.* New York, NY: Oxford University Press Inc; 1990.
6. Souza FGM, Goodwin GM. Lithium treatment and prophylaxis in unipolar depression: a meta-analysis. *Br J Psychiatry.* 1991;158:666-675.
7. Müller-Oerlinghausen B, Ahrens B, Grof E, Grof P, Lenz G, Schou M, Simhandl C, Thau K, Volk J, Wolf R, Wolf T. The effect of long-term lithium treatment on the mortality of patients with manic-depressive or schizo-affective illness. *Acta Psychiatr Scand.* 1992;86:218-222.
8. Frank E, Kupfer DJ, Perel JM, Cornes C, Jarrett DB, Mallinger AG, Thase ME, McEachran AB, Grochocinski VJ. Three-year outcomes for maintenance therapies in recurrent depression. *Arch Gen Psychiatry.* 1990;47:1093-1099.
9. Kupfer DJ, Frank E, Perel JM, Cornes C, Mallinger AG, Thase ME, McEachran AB, Grochocinski VJ. Five-year outcome for maintenance therapies in recurrent depression. *Arch Gen Psychiatry.* 1992:49:769-773.

In reply

Our recent review[1] of pharmacotherapy and ECT in the treatment of mood disorders covered new research during the period between August 1991 and August 1992. We are not aware of studies published during this period that examined the efficacy of lithium monotherapy as a continuation or maintenance treatment for unipolar depression. Dr Schou questions why lithium is not more frequently considered in the United States in this capacity. One explanation may be that current practice recommendations[2] are that patients receive as continuation and maintenance therapy the same medications to which they responded during the index episode. Indeed, there is some evidence that the dosage during maintenance treatment should be the same as that given during acute-phase treatment.[3] Since lithium monotherapy is rarely recommended in the acute-phase treatment of unipolar depression,[4] it would be unlikely that patients would receive such monotherapy as continuation or maintenance treatment.

With ECT, continuation and maintenance treatments are more complex. Electroconvulsive therapy is the only form of antidepressant therapy that is routinely discontinued following symptomatic response. Current guidelines are that patients receive antidepressants following successful treatment with ECT.[2,5] In practice, patients often receive the same class of medication following ECT that may have failed during the acute-phase treatment, prior to ECT. The wisdom of this practice has been questioned.[6] The only placebo-controlled trial of lithium monotherapy following remission of unipolar depression with ECT appeared over 10 years ago,[7] was limited by the small sample size, and failed to find a protective effect for lithium during the first 6 months following ECT, the period of the greatest risk for relapse.[6,8] Further out in time, lithium appeared to be of some value. Clearly, more research is needed to identify optimal strategies for continuation and maintenance treatment following ECT, including lithium monotherapy. Indeed, lithium, alone or in combination with other agents, may offer an alternative approach in preventing relapse in the ECT-responsive patient with unipolar depression.

Mitchell S. Nobler, MD
Harold A. Sackeim, PhD
Columbia University College of Physicians and Surgeons
722 W 168th St
New York, NY 10032

1. Nobler MS, Sackeim HA. Pharmacotherapy and electroconvulsive therapy for mood disorders. *Curr Opin Psychiatry.* 1993;6:10-15.
2. American Psychiatric Association Practice Guidelines for Major Depressive Disorder in Adults. *Am J Psychiatry.* 1993;150(suppl):1-26.
3. Frank E, Kupfer DJ, Perel JM, Cornes C, Jarrett DB, Mallinger AG, Thase ME, McEachran AB, Grochocinski VJ. Three-year outcomes for maintenance therapies in recurrent depression. *Arch Gen Psychiatry.* 1990;47:1093-1099.
4. Gelenberg AJ, Bassuk EL, Schoonover SC, eds. *The Practitioner's Guide to Psychoactive Drugs.* 3rd ed. New York, NY: Plenum Publishing Corp; 1991.
5. Abou-Saleh MT, Coppen AJ. Continuation therapy with antidepressants after electroconvulsive therapy. *Convulsive Ther.* 1988;4:263-268.
6. Sackeim HA, Prudic J, Devanand DP, Decina P, Kerr B, Malitz S. The impact of medication resistance and continuation pharmacotherapy on relapse following response to electroconvulsive therapy. *J Clin Psychopharmacol.* 1990;10:96-104.
7. Coppen AJ, Abou-Saleh MT, Milln P, Bailey J, Metcalfe M, Burns BH, Armond A. Lithium continuation therapy following electroconvulsive therapy. *Br J Psychiatry.* 1981;139:284-287.
8. Snaith RP. How much ECT does the depressed patient need? In: Palmer RL, ed. *Electroconvulsive Therapy: An Appraisal.* New York, NY: Oxford University Press; 1981.

Maintenance Therapy in Depression

The 5-year outcome study of recurrent depression by Kupfer et al[1] confirms the conclusion of the 1990 published 3-year outcome study by Frank et al in which they participated[2] that found high-dose antidepressant maintenance therapy was effective in preventing recurrence. The other conclusion drawn in this 1990 article, that there was "a modest prophylactic effect for monthly interpersonal therapy" is questionable. In that study, they attributed the differences in outcome to two factors: (1) imipramine hydrochloride (mainly) and (2) monthly interpersonal therapy (IPT) (a "modest effect").

Yearly Survival Rates*

Treatment Groups	Year, % (No. of Survivors/ No. of Patients) 1	2	3
Imipramine hydrochloride groups			
With IPT	84 (21/25)	76 (16/21)	94 (15/16)
Without IPT	61 (17/28)	76 (13/17)	100 (13/13)
Nonimipramine groups			
With IPT (combined IPT group and IPT with placebo group)	46 (12/26, 12/26)	63 (9/12, 6/12)	86 (8/9, 5/6)
Without IPT (placebo group)	22 (5/23)	60 (3/5)	67 (2/3)

**IPT indicates interpersonal therapy.*

We believe that a third factor could explain some of the results. Apart from imipramine, there were two variables, not one, that distinguished the non-IPT groups from the IPT groups: (1) lack of "maintenance IPT" and (2) severance of the relationship with the interpersonal therapist. This is a situation of loss that could cause depression, not because of any specific effects of IPT but owing to the nonspecific effect of the loss of a warm, confiding relationship that may occur in any supportive psychotherapy.

These two variables may be seen as mirror images, but the implications of attributing the observed results to one or the other are quite different. How does one decide which explanation is more likely? If maintenance IPT is the effective element, one would expect a lower recurrence rate in the IPT groups, not just in the first year but in later years as well. Conversely, if the loss of the relationship is the important factor, one might predict a higher recurrence rate in the non-IPT group soon after this loss in the first year, with perhaps less or no difference in the later years.

Reworking the data from Table 4 in the article by Frank et al[2] and allowing for imipramine's effect, we calculated the survival rates for each year (**Table**). Obviously, the major advantage of the IPT groups is in the first year. Our Table herein and the Figure on page 1097 in the article by Frank et al[2] suggest that a crucial assumption of the proportional hazards model, namely, that the hazard ratio does not change over time, has been violated. This assumption is usually checked by the use of time-dependent covariates in the survival model, although, in this case, the sample size may have been too small to detect the violation implied by our Table and

the Figure of Frank et al. As a simple proportional hazards model will not be appropriate if the time to peak hazard is earlier in some prognostic groups, for instance in those who discontinued IPT, then it is perhaps more appropriate to use a step-functioned proportional hazards model.[3] This is likely to support our conclusion that as non-IPT groups only fared worse in the first year, the likely cause was the loss of the therapist rather than any specific effect of IPT.

In their 5-year outcome study report, these authors state, "78% of the placebo survivors were continuing to receive monthly psychotherapy. For those patients not receiving either IPT or active medication, the proportion surviving was 11%."[1(p772)] Does this imply that IPT helped during the fourth and fifth years? It is difficult to see where these figures came from, or their significance. There were only nine patients in the placebo group of whom seven were receiving IPT and there were only three placebo survivors. How does one obtain 78% of three subjects or 11% of two subjects unless one is a vivisectionist? The gremlins may also have been at work in the 1990 article where they state, "almost 80% on active medication conditions survived 3 years without a recurrence."[2(p1098)] Our calculations from Table 4 on page 1097 of that article suggest that this figure should be 70% excluding noncompleters, or 53% if they are included.

Whether the initial pretrial intensive IPT helps to prevent recurrence is not addressed in this study[2] as all groups had this treatment. However, its effect is seen in its most uncontaminated form in the placebo-only group, which had pretrial IPT of approximately 20 sessions, which is more than that used in the NIMH (National Institute of Mental Health) Treatment of Depression Collaborative Research Program study.[4] The survival rates for this group (21% at 1 year, 13% at 2 years, and 8.7% at 3 years) are not encouraging.

Thus, we suggest the conclusion from these two studies is that in this group of patients with recurrent depression, monthly maintenance IPT may add little to the effect of imipramine. Whether a 20-session "burst" of IPT adds anything to the effectiveness of imipramine alone is not investigated here, but without continuing use of antidepressants, the prophylactic effect of IPT, if present, was clinically insufficient to prevent recurrence.

Gary J. Barnes, FRANZCP
Quentin Jones
39 E Esplanade
Manly, New South Wales
2095 Australia

1. Kupfer DJ, Frank E, Perel JM, Cornes C, Mallinger AG, Thase ME, McEachran AB, Grochocinski VJ. Five-year outcome for maintenance therapies in recurrent depression. *Arch Gen Psychiatry*. 1992;49:769-773.
2. Frank E, Kupfer DJ, Perel JM, Cornes C, Jarrett DB, Mallinger AG, Thase ME, McEachran AB, Grochocinski VJ. Three-year outcomes for maintenance therapies in recurrent depression. *Arch Gen Psychiatry*. 1990;47:1093-1099.
3. Gore SM, Pocock SJ, Kerr GR. Regression models and non-proportional hazards in the analysis of breast cancer survival. *Appl Statistics*. 1984;33:176-195.
4. Elkin I, Shea MT, Watkins JT, Imber SD, Sotsky SM, Collins F, Glass DR, Pilkonis PA, Leber WR, Docherty JP, Fiester SJ, Parloff MB. NIMH Treatment of Depression Collaborative Research Program: general effectiveness of treatments. *Arch Gen Psychiatry*. 1989;46:971-982.

In reply

We note with interest the letter of Drs Barnes and Jones. Although it may not be clear from reading our 1990 report,[1] the protocol required that even though IPT was discontinued in those patients assigned to the medication clinic visit condition, the relationship with their interpersonal therapist was not. Throughout the maintenance phase of this study, patients in the medication clinic visit condition continued to meet on a monthly basis with the same individual who had been their interpersonal therapist during the acute and continuation phases; however, the nature of the therapeutic interaction changed. Those assigned to the medication clinic visit condition spent approximately 20 minutes (vs the 45 minutes allotted for the maintenance IPT sessions) reviewing with their therapist any depressive or somatic symptoms they might have experienced in the previous month. Once this had been accomplished, the therapist was instructed to provide nonspecific support in a manner quite similar to that offered in the clinical management condition of the NIMH Treatment of Depression Collaborative Research Program.[2] Thus, while the focus was no longer on the patient's interpersonal concerns and the sessions were shorter, the personal relationship with the therapist was maintained. We consider this a rather stringent test of the efficacy of IPT.

Further evidence in support of the conclusion that there was a specific effect for maintenance IPT comes in our 1991 report[3] examining contributing factors to long-term survival in the maintenance IPT alone and maintenance IPT plus placebo conditions. In that article we demonstrate that while no demographic or clinical variables were related to long-term survival in the maintenance IPT conditions, specificity of IPT was related to long-term survival at the $P<.001$ *level. In other words, those patients whose maintenance treatment assignment changed nothing about the nature of the therapeutic interaction, but who were unable to focus consistently on interpersonal themes in that therapeutic interaction, received no more protection from the maintenance IPT treatment assignment than was afforded by the medication clinic visit assignment. Those patients who were able to maintain such a focus received very substantial protection, with a median survival time of 102 weeks (SE, 8 weeks).*

With respect to the appropriateness of the proportional hazards model for the analysis of these data, just as Barnes and Jones suspected, the test using a time-dependent covariate was not found to be significant ($P=.99$*, restricting data to the group who did not receive imipramine). While it is true that the sample size (*$n=75$ *for the*

group who did not receive imipramine during maintenance) may be too small to detect differences resulting from the nonproportionality of the hazards, there is no clear evidence that the assumption of the proportionality of the hazards does not exist. In fact, the hazard for recurrence remains greater throughout all 3 years for those subjects who did not receive IPT. It should also be noted that when the Kaplan-Meier product limit method was used to test for differences in the survival curves, a significant difference (P=.043 for the Mantel-Cox statistic) was found.

With respect to the language used and the exact proportion in our 1990 article, Barnes and Jones are correct in pointing out that we should more properly have said "cumulative probability of survival on active medication was almost 75% (estimated probability=.74, SE=.07)."

While we make no claim that monthly maintenance IPT adds to the effect of imipramine, we would argue that, taken together, the data from our 1990 and 1991 reports point to the potential of maintenance psychotherapy for significantly extending the well interval, if not providing complete prophylaxis. For those patients who cannot or will not take maintenance antidepressants, a well interval of almost 2 years seems greatly preferable to the roughly 20-week median survival time associated with the medication clinic visit and placebo conditions. We are currently working on methods to enhance the specificity of maintenance IPT and hope to be able to report on these methods in the near future.

Ellen Frank, PhD
David J. Kupfer, MD
Department of Psychiatry
University of Pittsburgh School of Medicine
West Psychiatric Center
3811 O'Hara St
Pittsburgh, PA 15213-2593

1. Frank E, Kupfer DJ, Perel JM, Cornes CL, Jarrett D, Mallinger A, Thase M, McEachran AB, Grochocinski VJ. Three-year outcomes for maintenance therapies in recurrent depression. *Arch Gen Psychiatry*. 1990;47:1093-1099.
2. Elkin I, Shea MT, Watkins JT, Imber SD, Sotsky SM, Collins JF, Glass DR, Pilkonis PA, Leber WR, Docherty JP, Fiester SJ, Parloff MB. NIMH Treatment of Depression Collaborative Research Program: general effectiveness of treatments. *Arch Gen Psychiatry*. 1989;46:971-982.
3. Frank E, Kupfer DJ, Wagner EF, McEachran A, Cornes C. Efficacy of interpersonal psychotherapy as a maintenance treatment for recurrent depression: contributing factors. *Arch Gen Psychiatry*. 1991;48:1053-1059.

Klein's Suffocation Theory of Panic

In a recent stimulating article, Dr Klein[1(p306)] boldly proposed that "many spontaneous panics occur when the brain's suffocation monitor erroneously signals a lack of useful air, thereby maladaptively triggering an evolved suffocation alarm system." Klein postulated that this is a physiological mechanism and that spontaneous panic attacks occur when the suffocation alarm threshold is pathologically lowered, or when psychosocial cues to suffocation are particularly salient. The theory spans a wide range of phenomena, although its primary focus is on spontaneous panic attacks.

We investigated the theory's main assumption that suffocation alarm hypersensitivity is a risk factor for panic disorder. Alarm hypersensitivity was operationalized by a recently developed measure of suffocation fear,[2] which we administered to a sample of 179 university students. The sample's mean age was 20 years and two thirds were women. We reasoned that people with hypersensitive alarms are more likely to have their alarms activated and hence likely to acquire a strong fear of suffocation. To test this assumption, we compared subjects with high suffocation fear (0.5 SD above the mean on the suffocation scale; n=49) with those with little or no suffocation fear (0.5 SD below the mean; n=68). Subjects completed a suffocation provocation test (breathing through a narrow straw for 2 minutes) that should activate the suffocation alarm in sensitive individuals. As predicted, subjects with high suffocation fear reported significantly more panic attacks than subjects with low suffocation fear (18.4% vs 1.5%; $\chi^2(1)=10.40$; $P<.003$). This supports the validity of our measure of suffocation fear as an index of the sensitivity of the putative suffocation alarm.

We administered a brief structured interview[2] that assessed whether subjects ever had panicked in enclosed spaces (ie, those situations likely to evoke suffocation) or in other situations. The interview also assessed whether subjects ever experienced spontaneous panic. Subjects with high suffocation fears reported a significantly greater incidence of panic in enclosed spaces (59.2% vs 16.2%; $\chi^2(1)=23.41$; $P<.001$) and in other situations (57.1% vs 20.6%; $\chi^2(1)=16.54$; $P<.001$). Subjects with high suffocation fears also reported a significantly greater incidence of spontaneous panic (32.7% vs 4.4%; $\chi^2(1)=16.70$; $P<.001$). These group differences were remarkably pronounced; compared with subjects with little or no suffocation fear, subjects with a high fear of suffocation were three times more likely to report situational panic and seven times more likely to report spontaneous panic.

These results support Klein's contention that suffocation alarm hypersensitivity is a risk factor for panic attacks. An important question for further investigation concerns the nature of this alarm. Klein asserts that the alarm is primarily biological in nature, whereas other theorists[3-5] propose that psychological factors play an important role. The significance of psychological factors is suggested by the fact that the fear of suffocation is readily reduced by psychological methods[6] and that panic attacks are readily eliminated by cognitive therapy.[7] Further progress in elucidating and evaluating Klein's theory will require precise definition of the postulated suffoca-

tion alarm mechanism and the validation of acceptable means of measuring its operation. Given the potential importance of the theory, such efforts are worthy of high priority.

Steven Taylor, PhD
Department of Psychiatry
University of British Columbia
2255 Westbrook Mall
Vancouver, British Columbia V6T 2A1
Canada

S. Rachman, PhD
Vancouver

1. Klein DF. False suffocation alarms, spontaneous panics, and related conditions: an integrative hypothesis. *Arch Gen Psychiatry.* 1993;50:306-317.
2. Rachman S, Taylor S. Analyses of claustrophobia. *J Anxiety Disord.* 1993;7: 281-291.
3. Clark DM. A cognitive approach to panic. *Behav Res Ther.* 1986;24:461-470.
4. Rachman S. *Fear and Courage.* 2nd ed. New York, NY: WH Freeman & Co; 1990.
5. Barlow DH. *Anxiety and its Disorders.* New York, NY: Guilford Press; 1988.
6. Booth R, Rachman S. The reduction of claustrophobia. *Behav Res Ther.* 1992; 30:207-221.
7. Margraf J, Barlow DH, Clark DM, Telch MJ. Psychological treatment of panic: Work in progress on outcome, active ingredients, and follow-up. *Behav Res Ther.* 1993;31;1-8.

In reply

Taylor and Rachman have provided valuable confirmation of my suffocation alarm theory of spontaneous panic. Null results on their part would have challenged the validity of this theory, so their supportive data is most welcome.

They propose that psychological factors play an important role; I do not deny this. My theory might be called physiocentric in that it makes a deranged physiological control system central to a broad range of symptomatic precipitants and manifestations. However, I emphasize that the kind of stimuli that elicit the suffocation false alarm are, at times, experiential. Further, my theory does not foreclose the possibility that the origin of the derangement may prove psychogenic, although I rather doubt it.

Taylor and Rachman have gone beyond the evidence by stating that panic attacks are readily eliminated by cognitive therapy. Proper controlled trials are still necessary in samples demonstrated to be medication-responsive by calibration against placebo. Also, much that has passed for behavioral treatment (eg, respiratory training) may actually be a physiological intervention. Appropriate experimentation will tell.

I would like to take this opportunity to acknowledge the enormous contributions of the late Dr Daniel X. Freedman to scientific psychiatry and to express my personal and professional loss. Danny told me quite clearly that he thought my study was an interesting hypothesis that he hoped would stimulate the field. Taylor and Rachman show that Danny was right once again.

Donald F. Klein, MD
Columbia University
College of Physicians and Surgeons
New York State Psychiatric Institute
Unit 22, 722 W 168th St
New York, NY 10032

The Prevalence of Schizophrenia in Ireland

The report by Kendler et al[1] on the risk of schizophrenia among relatives of Irish probands is an important genetic study. However, at the end of their report, they included a section on "The Prevalence of Schizophrenia in Ireland," which contains several inaccuracies.

First, they said that "our results do not support previous claims that the prevalence rate of schizophrenia is substantially elevated in the general population either in all of Ireland or in the West of Ireland." The work that they referenced[2] claimed that the schizophrenia rate in western Ireland was elevated only for individuals born prior to 1940. The study by Kendler et al[1] included only those individuals born in 1930 or later, so there was only a 10-year overlap in the year of birth of the individuals in the two studies. It is surprising that Kendler et al[1] did not note this difference because four of the authors on his article were also authors of the earlier study.

Second, Kendler et al[1] claimed that "the lifetime prevalence rates that we found for schizophrenia in our unselected control probands . . . [are not] outside the range reported in other populations." In fact, among these 143 unselected control probands, 11 had had a psychiatric hospitalization; schizophrenia was diagnosed in one; schizoaffective disorder, in one; schizophreniform disorder, in one; schizotypal personality disorder, in three; nonpsychotic bipolar disorder, in one; and psychotic major depression, in one. This is an impressive array of serious mental illnesses to be found among 143 unselected individuals anywhere. If only the two cases of schizophrenia and schizoaffective disorder are included, which would make it comparable to the other studies[3] referenced by Kendler et al,[1] the lifetime prevalence of these disorders in the unselected Irish population aged 18 years and older would be two in 143, or 14 per 1000. Among all prevalence studies done to date anywhere in the world, only the studies by Vaisanen[4] in Finland and Book[5] in northern Sweden have lifetime prevalence rates higher than those reported by Kendler et al.[1]

In view of these findings, it seems premature to conclude, as Kendler et al[1] do, that "the relatively high rates of schizophrenia found in the relatives of schizophrenic probands in the West of Ireland do not appear to result from high rates in the general population."

E. Fuller Torrey, MD
National Institute of Mental Health
Neuropsychiatric Center
St Elizabeth's Hospital
2700 Martin Luther King Ave SE
Washington, DC 20032

1. Kendler KS, McGuire M, Gruenberg AM, O'Hare A, Spellman M, Walsh D. The Roscommon family study, I: methods, diagnosis of probands, and risk of schizophrenia in relatives. *Arch Gen Psychiatry*. 1993;50:527-540.
2. Torrey EF, McGuire M, O'Hare A, Walsh D, Spellman MP. Endemic psychosis in Western Ireland. *Am J Psychiatry*. 1984;141:966-970.
3. Torrey EF. Prevalence studies in schizophrenia. *Br J Psychiatry*. 1987;150: 598-608.
4. Vaisanen E. Psychiatric disorders in Finland. *Acta Psychiatr Scand Suppl*. 1975; 263:22-33.
5. Book JA. A genetic and neuropsychiatric investigation of a North Swedish population. *Acta Genet Stat Med*. 1953;4:1-100.

In reply

Dr Torrey disagrees with one of the ancillary conclusions drawn from our analyses of the Roscommon Family Study.[1] We argued that our results are not consistent with earlier claims of an elevated rate of schizophrenia in Ireland generally or, more specifically, in the West of Ireland.

The question of high rates of schizophrenia in Ireland is an old issue that originated with reported high admission rates of Irish emigrants to New York State hospitals at the turn of the century.[2] These results were complemented both by early hospital data from Ireland, which also suggested increased rates of mental illness in general and schizophrenia in particular,[3] and more recently, by studies on the incidence of first hospitalization from the National Psychiatric In-Patient Reporting System, a nationwide register of admissions to and discharges from all Irish public and private psychiatric hospitals and units.[4] However, the use of these first-admission data to calculate incidence rates became less tenable when it was realized that despite efforts to the contrary, many hospitals in Ireland continued to use the category "first admission" to classify individuals with a first admission to that facility rather than a first admission in their lifetime. Thus, the same individual might have been counted several times as having a first onset of schizophrenia. Uncertainty was also raised about the reliability of the application of diagnostic categories such as schizophrenia in unsupervised hospital data.

Because of the limitation of these hospital data, psychiatric case registers were established in a number of locations throughout Ireland.[5] Using such a registry supplemented by a key informant survey in County Roscommon, Ireland, Torrey et al[6] investigated an area of this county that was suspected locally of having an unusually high prevalence of mental illness. The results confirmed the local impression, but no claim could be made from these data that these findings were representative of Ireland as a whole.

Community-based incidence and prevalence studies of schizophrenia in larger and more representative geographical regions in Ireland have since been carried out. Using careful, case-registry–based ascertainment that included reports from all inpatient and outpatient psychiatric facilities, these studies did not support either an increased incidence or an increased prevalence of schizophrenia in Ireland.[7,8] A further, multicenter World Health Organization–coordinated study in which identical case-finding and diagnostic techniques were used across 12 centers worldwide showed that the catchment area in Dublin, Ireland, had an incidence of schizophrenia in the midrange of that of the countries studied.[9]

Although it was not primarily designed with this in mind, the Roscommon Family Study does provide data to evaluate the claim for elevated lifetime prevalence (LTP) rates of schizophrenia in the West of Ireland. This study provides three independent measures of the LTP rates of schizophrenia diagnosed in an unselected Irish population by DSM-III-R *criteria[10]: unselected control probands aged 16 years or older (chosen from an electoral registry); their first-degree relatives, aged 16 years or older; and the entire catchment population of the Roscommon County Case Register. The first two of these samples were ascertained independent of treatment seeking, whereas the third estimates treated prevalence. However, these rates ought to be roughly comparable, as a high proportion of cases of schizophrenia in western countries have had psychiatric contact.[11]*

First, we found one case of schizophrenia in the 143 control probands, for an estimated LTP rate (±SE) of 1/143=0.7%±0.7%. Second, in 585 personally interviewed relatives of these unscreened controls, we found two cases of schizophrenia, for an estimated LTP rate (±SE) of 0.3%±0.2%. If relatives with only hospital records or family history evaluations were added, the results were the same: 3/878=0.3%±0.2%.

Third, in 1986, the catchment area for the Roscommon County Case Register contained 32 775 individuals born on or after 1930, of whom 20 686 were aged 15 years or older.[12] This registry contained 303 individuals with a registry diagnosis of schizophrenia who were born in or after 1930.[1] We were able to evaluate 282 of these individuals and found that 123 (43.6%) met DSM-III-R *criteria for schizophrenia. Assuming that this figure could be extrapolated to the 21 unevaluated probands, we would expect to diagnose 132 cases of* DSM-III-R *schizophrenia. In addition, we assessed 92 probands from the Roscommon County Case Register with a registry diagnosis of major affective illness and found three (3.2%) to meet* DSM-III-R *criteria for schizophrenia on follow-up. Because these 92 cases represented approximately 70% of all of the cases of major affective illness from the registry, had we evaluated all of them, we would have expected to ascertain approximately one additional case of schizophrenia. We can then estimate that the Roscommon County Case Register should contain 136 individuals born after 1930 with a* DSM-III-R *diagnosis of schizophrenia. It is possible that this is a slight underestimate because a few cases of schizophrenia might be in the registry only under other diagnoses, but this is unlikely to be a substantial number. The treated LTP rates (±SEs) of schizophrenia can then be calculated as 123/32 775=0.38%±0.04% in the total population and 136/20 686=0.66%±0.06% in those 15 years of age or older.*

These three independent estimates of LTP rates of schizophrenia in the population aged 15 years and older do not differ significantly from one another (χ^2=1.32, df=2, P=.52) and suggest that the LTP rate of DSM-III-R *schizophrenia in County Roscommon in individuals 15 years of age or older is probably between 0.6% and 0.7%. In the entire population, the parallel figure is probably about 0.4%. These figures are near the middle of the range for the LTP rates of schizophrenia reported in recent years, including those in the thorough review by Torrey.[13-15] Dohrenwend et al[16] calculated the median total population prevalence rate for schizophrenia from 35 studies at 0.38%. One recent report[17] based on personal interviews using* DSM-III *criteria[18] found LTP rates for schizophrenia of 0.64% in individuals aged 18 years or older in eastern Baltimore. It should also be noted that using data from the Roscommon County Case Register and expanding the definition of schizophrenia to include* DSM-III-R *schizoaffective disorder increases LTP rates by approximately 30%, resulting in estimates still within the range previously reported.*

We believe that this evidence justifies our conclusions that (1) the prevalence of schizophrenia is unlikely to be substantially increased in representative populations in Ireland or western Ireland and (2) the large increased risk for schizophrenia seen in relatives of schizophrenic probands in the Roscommon Family Study cannot be attributed to any general increased rate for this disorder in the Roscommon population.

Dermot Walsh, MB, FRCPI
Health Research Board
Dublin, Ireland
Kenneth S. Kendler, MD
Richmond, Va

Address correspondence to Department of Psychiatry, MCV, PO Box 980710, Richmond, VA 23298-0710 (Dr Kendler).

1. Kendler KS, McGuire M, Gruenberg AM, O'Hare A, Spellman M, Walsh D. The Roscommon Family Study, I: methods, diagnosis of probands, and risk of schizophrenia in relatives. *Arch Gen Psychiatry*. 1993;50:527-540.
2. Malzberg B, Lee E. *Migration and Mental Disease*. New York, NY: Social Science Research Council; 1956.
3. Walsh D. Mental illness in Ireland: some further observations. *J Ir Med Assoc*. 1971;64:404-409.
4. O'Hare A, Walsh D. *Activities of Irish Psychiatric Hospitals and Units, 1972*. Dublin, Ireland: The Medico-Social Research Board; 1974.
5. Walsh D, O'Hare A, Blake B, Halpenny JV, O'Brien PF. The treated prevalence of mental illness in the Republic of Ireland: the three-county case register study. *Psychol Med*. 1980;10:465-470.
6. Torrey EF, McGuire M, O'Hare A, Walsh D, Spellman MP. Endemic psychosis in Western Ireland. *Am J Psychiatry*. 1984;141:966-970.
7. Ni Nuallain M, O'Hare A, Walsh D. Incidence of schizophrenia in Ireland. *Psychol Med*. 1987;17:943-948.
8. Ni Nuallain M, O'Hare A, Walsh D. The prevalence of schizophrenia in three counties in Ireland. *Acta Psychiatr Scand*. 1990;82:136-140.
9. Sartorius N, Jablensky A, Korten A, Ernberg G, Anker M, Cooper JE, Day R. Early manifestations and first-contact incidence of schizophrenia in different cultures. *Psychol Med*. 1986;16:909-928.
10. American Psychiatric Association, Committee on Nomenclature and Statistics. *Diagnostic and Statistical Manual of Mental Disorders, Revised Third Edition*. Washington, DC: American Psychiatric Association; 1987.
11. Link B, Dohrenwend BP. Formulation of hypotheses about the ratio of untreated to treated cases in the true prevalence studies of functional psychiatric disorders in adults in the United States. In: Dohrenwend BP, Dohrenwend BS, Gould MS, Link B, Neugebauer R, Wunsch-Hitzig R, eds. *Mental Illness in the United States: Epidemiological Estimates*. New York, NY: Praeger; 1980:133-149.
12. *Census of Population of Ireland 1986*. Dublin, Ireland: Stationery Office; 1987:1.
13. Zerbin-Rüdin E. Endogene Psychosen. In: Becker PE, ed. *Humangenetik: ein kürzes Handbuch in fünf Banden*. Stuttgart, Germany: Thieme Medical Publishers Inc; 1967;2:446-577.
14. Eaton WW. Epidemiology of schizophrenia. *Epidemiol Rev*. 1985;7:105-126.
15. Torrey EF. Prevalence studies in schizophrenia. *Br J Psychiatry*. 1987;150: 598-608.
16. Dohrenwend BS, Dohrenwend BP, Gottesman II, Link B, Neugebauer R. Epidemiology and genetics of schizophrenia. *Soc Biol*. 1979;26:142-153.
17. Von Korff M, Nestadt G, Romanoski A, Anthony J, Eaton W, Merchant A, Chahal R, Kramer M, Folstein M, Gruenberg E. Prevalence of treated and untreated *DSM-III* schizophrenia: results of a two-stage community survey. *J Nerv Ment Dis*. 1985;173:577-581.
18. American Psychiatric Association, Committee on Nomenclature and Statistics. *Diagnostic and Statistical Manual of Mental Disorders, Third Edition*. Washington, DC: American Psychiatric Association; 1980.

Neural Circuits in Schizophrenia

The point made in the article by Carpenter et al[1] about the need for multiple assessment modalities in differentiating the neural circuits that are abnormal in subgroups of the schizophrenia syndrome is well taken. However, an important and well-documented neural circuit is omitted in their compilation of the "predicted pattern of neural circuit involvement" for subtypes of schizophrenia. There are strong data indicating that the neocortical superior temporal gyrus (STG) is a key circuit related to positive symptoms ("nondeficit schizophrenia," using the terminology of Carpenter et al[1]), with abnormalities being linked to auditory hallucinations, thought disorder, certain memory tasks, and altered metabolic and electrophysiological functional activity.

The presence of auditory hallucinations has been found to be associated with both structural and metabolic STG abnormalities. Barta et al[2] report correlations with magnetic resonance imaging volume reductions and Cleghorn et al[3] note correlations with abnormal regional metabolism in a fluorodeoxyglucose positron emission tomographic study. Our group has examined a clinically well-characterized group of subjects who met *DSM-III-R* criteria for schizophrenia and had predominantly positive symptoms (present in 11 of 15 subjects while four of 15 had a mixed symptom picture in the Andreasen classification). For these subjects, reductions in the magnetic resonance imaging volume of the posterior portion of the STG (predominantly on the left in this right-handed group) was associated with (1) clinically, an increase in thought disorder, measured by the Johnston-Holzman thought disorder index,[4] and an increase in Scale for the Assessment of Positive Symptoms–measured delusions (unpublished data, 1994); (2) poorer neuropsychological performance[5] on verbal paired-associates memory tasks (immediate recall, Wechsler Memory Scale–Revised); and (3) functionally, reduced amplitude of the P300 event-related potential over the left temporal scalp region.[6]

This neural circuit has thus been found to be a key variable in schizophrenia on the basis of the criteria of Carpenter et al of "simultaneous neurobehavioral assessment and structural and functional imaging assessments." In our opinion, it should be on all investigators' lists of items differentiating various subgroups of schizophrenia.

Robert W. McCarley, MD
Martha E. Shenton, PhD
Brian F. O'Donnell, PhD
Paul G. Nestor, PhD
Neuroscience Laboratory
Department of Psychiatry
Harvard Medical School and the Brockton/West Roxbury Veterans Affairs Medical Center
Brockton, MA 02401

1. Carpenter WT Jr, Buchanan RW, Kirkpatrick B, Tamminga C, Wood F. Strong inference, theory testing, and the neuroanatomy of schizophrenia. *Arch Gen Psychiatry*. 1993;50:825-831.
2. Barta PE, Pearlson GD, Powers RE, Richards SS, Tune LE. Auditory hallucinations and smaller superior temporal gyral volume in schizophrenia. *Am J Psychiatry*. 1990;147:1457-1462.
3. Cleghorn JM, Franco S, Szechtman B, Kaplan RD, Szechtman H, Brown GM, Nahmias C, Garnett ES. Toward a brain map of auditory hallucinations. *Am J Psychiatry*. 1992;149:1062-1069.
4. Shenton ME, Kikinis R, Jolesz FA, Pollak SD, LeMay M, Wible CG, Hokama H, Martin J, Metcalf D, Coleman M, McCarley RW. Abnormalities of the left temporal lobe and thought disorder in schizophrenia: a quantitative magnetic resonance imaging study. *N Engl J Med*. 1992;327:604-612.
5. Nestor PG, Shenton ME, McCarley RW, Haimson J, Smith RS, O'Donnell BF.

Neuropsychological correlates of MRI temporal lobe abnormalities in schizophrenia. *Am J Psychiatry*. 1993;150:190-197.
6. McCarley RW, Shenton ME, O'Donnell BF, Faux SF, Kikinis R, Nestor PG, Jolesz FA. Auditory P300 abnormalities and left posterior superior temporal gyrus volume reduction in schizophrenia. *Arch Gen Psychiatry*. 1993;50:190-197.

In reply

McCarley et al note the converging evidence for implicating the STG in the pathophysiology of schizophrenia and that STG findings correlate with positive psychotic symptoms. They assert that the STG should be on the list of neural circuits that we presented and on all investigators' lists of items differentiating subgroups of schizophrenia. We agree with the data but not with their conclusions. First, the neural circuits presented in the article were selected to illustrate the advantages of studying schizophrenia from a coherent theoretical framework and not to provide an exhaustive review of brain findings. Second, although the STG, as a single structure, may be very important in schizophrenia, we emphasized composite cortical-subcortical, parallel, segregated neural circuits subserving complex behavioral phenomenon such as psychosis. We do not agree that the STG defines a neural circuit, but we do include it as a cortical component of the anterior cingulate neural circuit already highlighted in our article as a possible substrate for positive psychotic symptoms. Third, McCarley and colleagues suggest that the STG should be on any list of items differentiating various subgroups of schizophrenia. But how so? All 15 of the subjects on whom they report had "prominent" positive psychotic symptoms, and neither this symptom complex nor the other clinical variables correlated with STG were used for heterogeneity reduction in the manner we advocated. If they are proposing that positive psychotic symptoms define the subgroup with STG abnormality, then it is also necessary to define the contrasting subgroup of schizophrenic patients who never had psychosis! In addition, we argued that it is important to distinguish state vs trait measures in hypothesis testing. Positive psychotic symptoms fluctuate markedly over time in most patients, but it is improbable that the magnetic resonance imaging volume of posterior STG changes with each shift in symptom status. Correlating state symptoms with state variables is quite valid, but it does not provide data for trait-based distinctions of pathophysiologically meaningful subgroups. For this reason, and others articulated in our essay, we emphasize the importance of using trait clinical variables to reduce heterogeneity in the investigation of schizophrenia etiology and pathophysiology.

William T. Carpenter, Jr, MD
Robert W. Buchanan, MD
Brian Kirkpatrick, MD
Carol Tamminga, MD
Frank Wood, PhD
Maryland Psychiatric Research Center
PO Box 21247
Baltimore, MD 21228

ONCE-DAILY

PAXIL 20 MG

PAROXETINE HCl

FOR DEPRESSION

PAXIL™ (brand of paroxetine hydrochloride)

See complete prescribing information in SmithKline Beecham Pharmaceuticals literature or *PDR*. The following is a brief summary.

INDICATIONS AND USAGE: *Paxil* is indicated for the treatment of depression.

CONTRAINDICATIONS: Concomitant use in patients taking monoamine oxidase inhibitors (MAOIs) is contraindicated. (See WARNINGS.)

WARNINGS: Interactions with MAOIs may occur. Given the fatal interactions reported with concomitant or immediately consecutive administration of MAOIs and other SSRIs, do not use *Paxil* in combination with a MAOI or within 2 weeks of discontinuing MAOI treatment. Allow at least 2 weeks after stopping *Paxil* before starting a MAOI.

PRECAUTIONS: As with all antidepressants, use *Paxil* cautiously in patients with a history of mania.

Use *Paxil* cautiously in patients with a history of seizures. Discontinue it in any patient who develops seizures.

The possibility of suicide attempt is inherent in depression and may persist until significant remission occurs. Close supervision of high-risk patients should accompany initial drug therapy. Write *Paxil* prescriptions for the smallest quantity of tablets consistent with good patient management in order to reduce the risk of overdose.

Reversible hyponatremia has been reported, mainly in elderly patients, patients taking diuretics or those who were otherwise volume depleted.

Clinical experience with *Paxil* in patients with concomitant systemic illness is limited. Use cautiously in patients with diseases or conditions that could affect metabolism or hemodynamic responses. Observe the usual cautions in cardiac patients. In patients with severe renal impairment (creatinine clearance <30 mL/min.) or severe hepatic impairment, a lower starting dose (10 mg) should be used.

Caution patients about operating hazardous machinery, including automobiles, until they are reasonably sure that *Paxil* therapy does not affect their ability to engage in such activities. Tell patients 1) to continue therapy as directed; 2) to inform physicians about other medications they are taking or plan to take; 3) to avoid alcohol while taking *Paxil*; 4) to notify their physicians if they become pregnant or intend to become pregnant during therapy, or if they're nursing.

Concomitant use of *Paxil* with tryptophan is not recommended. Use cautiously with warfarin. When administering *Paxil* with cimetidine, dosage adjustment of *Paxil* after the 20 mg starting dose should be guided by clinical effect. When co-administering *Paxil* with phenobarbital or phenytoin, no initial *Paxil* dosage adjustment is needed; base subsequent changes on clinical effect. Concomitant use of *Paxil* with drugs metabolized by cytochrome $P_{450}IID_6$ (antidepressants such as nortriptyline, amitriptyline, imipramine, desipramine and fluoxetine; phenothiazines such as thioridazine; Type 1C antiarrhythmics such as propafenone, flecainide and encainide) or with drugs that inhibit this enzyme (e.g., quinidine) may require lower doses than usually prescribed for either *Paxil* or the other drug; approach concomitant use cautiously. Administration of *Paxil* with another tightly protein-bound drug may shift plasma concentrations, resulting in adverse effects from either drug. Concomitant use of *Paxil* and alcohol in depressed patients is not advised. Undertake concomitant use of *Paxil* and lithium or digoxin cautiously. If adverse effects are seen when co-administering *Paxil* with procyclidine, reduce the procyclidine dose.

In 2-year studies, a significantly greater number of male rats in the 20 mg/kg/day group developed reticulum cell sarcomas vs. animals given doses of 1 or 5 mg/kg/day. There was also a significantly increased linear trend across dose groups for the occurrence of lymphoreticular tumors in male rats. Although there was a dose-related increase in the number of tumors in mice, there was no drug-related increase in the number of mice with tumors. The clinical significance of these findings is unknown. There is no evidence of mutagenicity with *Paxil*.

Serotonergic compounds are known to affect reproductive function in animals. Impaired reproductive function in rats (i.e., reduced pregnancy rate, increased pre- and post-implantation losses, decreased viability of pups) was found at *Paxil* doses 15 or more times the highest recommended human dose.

Pregnancy Category B. Reproduction studies performed in rats and rabbits at doses up to 50 and 6 times the maximum recommended human dose have revealed no evidence of teratogenic effects or of selective toxicity to the fetus. However, there are no adequate and well-controlled studies in pregnant women. *Paxil* should be used in pregnancy only if the benefits outweigh the risks. The effect of *Paxil* on labor and delivery in humans is unknown. Paroxetine is secreted in human milk; exercise caution when administering *Paxil* to a nursing woman.

Safety and effectiveness in children have not been established.

In worldwide *Paxil* clinical trials, 17% of *Paxil*-treated patients were ≥65 years of age. Pharmacokinetic studies revealed a decreased clearance in the elderly; however, there were no overall differences in the adverse event profile between older and younger patients.

ADVERSE REACTIONS: Incidence in Controlled Trials—*Commonly Observed Adverse Events in Controlled Clinical Trials:* The most commonly observed adverse events associated with the use of *Paxil* (incidence of 5% or greater and incidence for *Paxil* at least twice that for placebo): asthenia (15% vs. 6%), sweating (11% vs. 2%), nausea (26% vs. 9%), decreased appetite (6% vs. 2%), somnolence (23% vs. 9%), dizziness (13% vs. 6%), insomnia (13% vs. 6%), tremor (8% vs. 2%), nervousness (5% vs. 3%), ejaculatory disturbance (13% vs. 0%) and other male genital disorders (10% vs. 0%).

Twenty-one percent (881/4,126) of *Paxil* patients in worldwide clinical trials discontinued treatment due to an adverse event. The most common events (≥1%) associated with discontinuation and considered to be drug related include: somnolence, insomnia, agitation, tremor, anxiety, nausea, diarrhea, dry mouth, vomiting, asthenia, abnormal ejaculation, sweating. The following adverse events occurred in 6-week placebo-controlled trials of similar design at a frequency of 1% or more.

Body as a Whole: headache, asthenia, abdominal pain, fever, chest pain, trauma, back pain. **Cardiovascular:** palpitation, vasodilation, postural hypotension. **Dermatologic:** sweating, rash. **Gastrointestinal:** nausea, dry mouth, constipation, diarrhea, decreased appetite, flatulence, vomiting, oropharynx disorder, dyspepsia, increased appetite. **Musculoskeletal:** myopathy, myalgia, myasthenia. **Nervous System:** somnolence, dizziness, insomnia, tremor, nervousness, anxiety, paresthesia, libido decreased, agitation, drugged feeling, myoclonus, CNS stimulation, confusion. **Respiration:** respiratory disorder, yawn, pharyngitis. **Special Senses:** blurred vision, taste perversion. **Urogenital System:** ejaculatory disturbance, other male genital disorders, urinary frequency, urination disorder, female genital disorders.

Studies show a clear dose dependency for some of the more common adverse events associated with *Paxil* use. There was evidence of adaptation to some adverse events with continued *Paxil* therapy (e.g., nausea and dizziness). Significant weight loss may be an undesirable result of *Paxil* treatment for some patients but, on average, patients in controlled trials had minimal (about 1 lb) loss. In placebo-controlled clinical trials, *Paxil*-treated patients exhibited abnormal values on liver function tests no more frequently than placebo-treated patients.

Other Events Observed During the Premarketing Evaluation of *Paxil*: During premarketing assessment, multiple doses of *Paxil* were administered to 4,126 patients, and the following adverse events were reported. Note: "frequent" = events occurring in at least 1/100 patients; "infrequent" = 1/100 to 1/1000 patients; "rare" = less than 1/1000 patients. Events are classified within body system categories and enumerated in order of decreasing frequency using the following definitions. It is important to emphasize that although the events occurred during *Paxil* treatment, they were not necessarily caused by it.

Body as a Whole: *frequent:* chills, malaise; *infrequent:* allergic reaction, carcinoma, face edema, moniliasis, neck pain; *rare:* abscess, adrenergic syndrome, cellulitis, neck rigidity, pelvic pain, peritonitis, ulcer. **Cardiovascular System:** *frequent:* hypertension, syncope, tachycardia; *infrequent:* bradycardia, conduction abnormalities, electrocardiogram abnormal, hypotension, migraine, peripheral vascular disorder; *rare:* angina pectoris, arrhythmia, atrial fibrillation, bundle branch block, cerebral ischemia, cerebrovascular accident, congestive heart failure, low cardiac output, myocardial infarct, myocardial ischemia, pallor, phlebitis, pulmonary embolus, supraventricular extrasystoles, thrombosis, varicose vein, vascular headache, ventricular extrasystoles. **Digestive System:** *infrequent:* bruxism, dysphagia, eructation, glossitis, increased salivation, liver function tests abnormal, mouth ulceration, rectal hemorrhage; *rare:* aphthous stomatitis, bloody diarrhea, bulimia, colitis, duodenitis, esophagitis, fecal impactions, fecal incontinence, gastritis, gastroenteritis, gingivitis, hematemesis, hepatitis, ileus, jaundice, melena, peptic ulcer, salivary gland enlargement, stomach ulcer, stomatitis, tongue edema, tooth caries. **Endocrine System:** *rare:* diabetes mellitus, hyperthyroidism, hypothyroidism, thyroiditis. **Hemic and Lymphatic Systems:** *infrequent:* anemia, leukopenia, lymphadenopathy, purpura; *rare:* abnormal erythrocytes, eosinophilia, leukocytosis, lymphedema, abnormal lymphocytes, lymphocytosis, microcytic anemia, monocytosis, normocytic anemia. **Metabolic and Nutritional:** *frequent:* edema, weight gain, weight loss; *infrequent:* hyperglycemia, peripheral edema, thirst; *rare:* alkaline phosphatase increased, bilirubinemia, dehydration, gout, hypercholesteremia, hypocalcemia, hypoglycemia, hypokalemia, hyponatremia, SGOT increased, SGPT increased. **Musculoskeletal System:** *infrequent:* arthralgia, arthritis; *rare:* arthrosis, bursitis, myositis, osteoporosis, tetany. **Nervous System:** *frequent:* amnesia, CNS stimulation, concentration impaired, depression, emotional lability, vertigo; *infrequent:* abnormal thinking, akinesia, alcohol abuse, ataxia, convulsions, depersonalization, hallucinations, hyperkinesia, hypertonia, incoordination, lack of emotion, manic reaction, paranoid reaction; *rare:* abnormal electroencephalogram, abnormal gait, antisocial reaction, choreoathetosis, delirium, delusions, diplopia, drug dependence, dysarthria, dyskinesia, dystonia, euphoria, fasciculations, grand mal convulsion, hostility, hyperalgesia, hypokinesia, hysteria, libido increased, manic-depressive reaction, meningitis, myelitis, neuralgia, neuropathy, nystagmus, paralysis, psychosis, psychotic depression, reflexes increased, stupor, withdrawal syndrome. **Respiratory System:** *frequent:* cough increased, rhinitis; *infrequent:* asthma, bronchitis, dyspnea, epistaxis, hyperventilation, pneumonia, respiratory flu, sinusitis; *rare:* carcinoma of lung, hiccups, lung fibrosis, sputum increased. **Skin and Appendages:** *frequent:* pruritus; *infrequent:* acne, alopecia, dry skin, ecchymosis, eczema, furunculosis, urticaria; *rare:* angioedema, contact dermatitis, erythema nodosum, maculopapular rash, photosensitivity, skin discoloration, skin melanoma. **Special Senses:** *infrequent:* abnormality of accommodation, ear pain, eye pain, mydriasis, otitis media, taste loss, tinnitus; *rare:* amblyopia, cataract, conjunctivitis, corneal ulcer, exophthalmos, eye hemorrhage, glaucoma, hyperacusis, otitis externa, photophobia. **Urogenital System:** *infrequent:* abortion, amenorrhea, breast pain, cystitis, dysmenorrhea, dysuria, menorrhagia, nocturia, polyuria, urethritis, urinary incontinence, urinary retention, urinary urgency, vaginitis; *rare:* breast atrophy, breast carcinoma, breast neoplasm, female lactation, hematuria, kidney calculus, kidney function abnormal, kidney pain, mastitis, nephritis, oliguria, prostatic carcinoma, vaginal moniliasis.

Non-U.S. Postmarketing Reports

Voluntary reports of adverse events that have been received since market introduction and may have no causal relationship with *Paxil* include elevated liver function tests (the most severe case was a death due to liver necrosis, and one other case involving grossly elevated transaminases associated with severe liver dysfunction) and toxic epidermal necrolysis.

DRUG ABUSE AND DEPENDENCE: Controlled Substance Class: *Paxil* is not a controlled substance. Evaluate patients carefully for history of drug abuse and observe such patients closely for signs of *Paxil* misuse or abuse (e.g., development of tolerance, incrementations of dose, drug-seeking behavior).

BRS-PX:L5

SB SmithKline Beecham Pharmaceuticals

JANSSEN PHARMACEUTICA RESEARCH FOUNDATION

Philadelphia, PA 19101

It's your job to report an adverse reaction. Where do you turn?

To us.

1-800-FDA-1088.

FDA MEDWATCH

THE FDA MEDICAL PRODUCTS REPORTING PROGRAM

If it's serious, we need to know.

ORIGINAL ARTICLE

Life Events and the Research Diagnostic Criteria Endogenous Subtype

A Confirmation of the Distinction Using the Bedford College Methods

Ellen Frank, PhD; Barbara Anderson, MS; Charles F. Reynolds III, MD; Angela Ritenour; David J. Kupfer, MD

Background: Despite the advances in biological and psychosocial assessment methods, reliable distinction between depressed patients with endogenous presentations or melancholic symptom features and those with nonendogenous presentations has remained elusive.

Methods: Ninety patients with histories of frequent unipolar episodes classified as endogenous or nonendogenous by the Research Diagnostic Criteria were interviewed with the Bedford College Life Events and Difficulties Schedule regarding the 6 months before onset of their most recent episode of depression.

Results: Patients meeting the Research Diagnostic Criteria for definite endogenous subtype differed significantly from patients with nonendogenous features in terms of the proportion experiencing severe life stress in the 6 months before onset of their depressive episode ($P \leq .04$). Furthermore, survival analysis revealed a closer temporal association between severe event and depression onset among patients with nonendogenous features ($P < .02$).

Conclusion: Even among patients with a history of multiple recurrences of depression, psychological stress plays an important role in the timing of onset of episodes characterized by nonendogenous features.

(Arch Gen Psychiatry. 1994;51:519-524)

In the past 25 years, depressive disorders have been the focus of research efforts aimed at describing the phenomena and uncovering the causal factors associated with their expression. The heterogeneous nature of depression has, however, hindered the development of a coherent causal theory. Explicitly or implicitly, the search for the underlying cause(s) of depressive disorders has been driven by the notion that two broad categories of depression exist: psychologically based depression and biologically based depression.[1]

Substantial research on neurotransmitters, neuroendocrine function, and other putative biological markers has sought to identify correlates of a biological subtype.[2] Another subtype is thought to follow from external precipitating stressors. Psychosocial research has focused on causal factors such as life events, long-term stressors, and the lack of appropriate social support systems. However, uncertainty remains about how such factors relate to symptomatically defined subtypes of depression.[3-9]

While there is considerable agreement in the literature that antecedent life events may play a role in producing, triggering, or maintaining an episode of depression, the classic distinction between spontaneously occurring "endogenous" depressions and "reactive" depressions associated with precipitating life events has received inconsistent empirical support.[10-13] For a review of earlier efforts in this direction, see the accompanying article by Brown et al.[14]

In the present investigation, we have applied the life-event method, developed by Brown and Harris,[15] to a group of patients classified as having recurrent unipolar episodes of depressions according to the Re-

See also page 525

See Subjects and Methods on next page

From the Western Psychiatric Institute and Clinic, Department of Psychiatry, University of Pittsburgh (Pa).

SUBJECTS AND METHODS

SUBJECTS

The study population consisted of 90 depressed patients with a history of recurrent unipolar depression. At the life events interview, all subjects were remitted but continuing to participate in two ongoing research protocols of the Depression Prevention Program at Western Psychiatric Institute and Clinic (Pittsburgh, Pa). Fifty subjects, aged 60 to 80 years, participated in a study of maintenance therapies in late-life depression and the remaining 40, aged 20 to 40 years, participated in a study of biological and social rhythms in midlife. Subjects in both studies met nearly identical inclusion and exclusion criteria: they were required to be experiencing at least their second episode of unipolar depression according to the RDC, with the immediately preceding episode occurring no more than 2½ years before the onset of the index episode, and to have had a clear remission for at least 10 weeks before the onset of the index episode. A minimum Hamilton Rating Scale for Depression (HRS-D)[16] score of 15 was required for the midlife protocol and a minimum score of 17 was required for the late-life protocol. Patients for both protocols were recruited from medical referrals, self-referrals, and public information campaigns. All subjects gave informed consent.

After a 2-week drug-free washout, each subject was reevaluated for severity of depression and given a complete initial evaluation, including biological (all-night sleep electroencephalographic studies) and psychosocial (social adjustment, social support, etc) measures. However, because of the probable effect of acute illness on recall, life events were not evaluated at this time. Patients in the late-life maintenance therapies protocol were treated with a combination of nortriptyline hydrochloride and interpersonal psychotherapy.[17] The patients in the midlife protocol were treated first with interpersonal psychotherapy alone. If subjects failed to remit, imipramine hydrochloride or fluoxetine hydrochloride was added. At whatever point in these short-term treatment regimens the patient had maintained a Hamilton score of 7 or less (midlife protocol) or 10 or less (late-life protocol) for 3 weeks, a second biological and psychosocial evaluation was completed. At that time, the Bedford College (London, England) Life Events and Difficulties Schedule (LEDS)[15] was administered.

Before combining data from the two protocols into a single analysis, we examined the extent to which subjects differed on demographic and clinical characteristics, other than age or variables possibly associated with age or birth cohort. Since the midlife protocol stipulated a minimum HRS-D score of 15 and the late-life protocol, a score of 17 (reflecting the increased number of somatic complaints anticipated even in nondepressed elders), we expected and found higher mean depression severity ratings in subjects in the late-life protocol. There were slightly more males in the older group (**Table 1**). The groups did not differ in the proportion of black vs white subjects, the number of previous episodes, the duration of the index episode, or in the proportion of subjects experiencing their second vs third vs fourth or greater episode. Differences in marital status and education were consistent with expectations for the age and birth cohort of the two groups. While statistically the HRS-D scores were significantly higher ($P=.0004$) and the Global Assessment Scale scores were significantly lower ($P=.01$) in the late-life group, neither the three-point difference on the HRS-D nor the 3.5-point difference on the Global Assessment Scale represents a clinically meaningful difference between these two populations in terms of relative severity of illness. We thus concluded that it was legitimate to combine their data for analysis.

Once combined, the study population consisted of 90 subjects (70 women and 20 men) ranging in age from 22 to 82 years. The mean (±SD) age at onset of the first depressive episode was 37.9±17.9 years. Although only one previous episode was required, the mean (±SD) was 4.6±3.6. At entry, these patients reported an average index episode length of 24.8±26.4 weeks. All 40 of the younger subjects in the biological and social rhythms protocol were outpatients. Five (10%) of the 50 older subjects began treatment as inpatients and then completed their short-term treatment as outpatients. No differences were observed in their posthospital treatment course from that of the 45 older subjects beginning treatment as outpatients. The mean (±SD) HRS-D[16] and Global Assessment Scale[18] scores at the time of the entry into treatment were 21.5±4.2 and 56.0±6.2, respectively (Table 1).

DEPRESSIVE SYMPTOM FEATURES AND SUBTYPE

Diagnoses of major depression were determined by the Schedule for Affective Disorders and Schizophrenia—Lifetime version (SADS-L) interview.[19] The RDC[20] was applied to assign subjects to nonendogenous, probable endogenous, and definite endogenous subclassifications. According to the SADS-L and RDC, patients meet criteria for definite endogenous subtype if they demonstrate six of the following 10 symptoms: (1) distinct quality to depressed mood; (2) lack of reactivity to environmental changes; (3) mood regularly worse in morning; (4) pervasive loss of interest; (5) self-reproach or inappropriate guilt; (6) early morning awakening or middle insomnia; (7) retardation or agitation; (8) poor appetite; (9) substantial weight loss; and (10) loss of interest or pleasure that is not necessarily pervasive. At least one of the symptoms must be among the first four listed. Only four symptoms are required for probable endogenous subtype. In the Depression Prevention Program, SADS-L interviews are conducted by research nurse clinicians who maintain a minimum κ of 0.85 for diagnostic and subtype classification. As in previous reports,[21,22] we combined the probable and nonendogenous subgroups to create the most

homogeneous endogenous subgroup possible within the constraints of the SADS-L interviews. Thus, 56 subjects (62%) were classified as endogenous and 34 (38%) as nonendogenous. There was no difference between the younger and older subjects in the proportion of those whose episodes were classified as endogenous, and no differences between those subjects classified as endogenous and those classified as nonendogenous on any demographic or clinical characteristic.

LIFE EVENTS ASSESSMENTS

The LEDS[15] interviews were conducted and rated by interviewers with bachelor's or master's degrees who had participated in training workshops conducted by George Brown, PhD, and Tirril Harris, MA, at Bedford College or at our institution. Interviewers next participated in advanced training seminars at our institution with the Bedford College team. Life event ratings at our institution were supervised by the Bedford College researchers (via fax transmission) for the first 2 years of LEDS evaluation work.

The LEDS and SADS-L data were collected by different interviewers at different time intervals during the subject's participation in the research protocols. The life events interviewer was blind to the subject's subtype classification.

LIFE EVENTS AND DIFFICULTIES METHODS

The LEDS evaluation involves a semistructured interview aimed at events and difficulties in 10 domains: education, work, reproduction, money and/or possessions, housing, crime and/or legal, health, marital and/or partner relationships, other relationships, and death and miscellaneous. The events and difficulties are then rated with respect to contextual severity of threat and a variety of other dimensions. There is a comprehensive manual containing precedents of more than 2000 life events and difficulties. The rating approach is *contextual*, the interviewer attempting to specify the meaning of the event or difficulty for the individual, by considering biographical circumstances. Finally, interviewers bring their ratings to consensus meetings with other members of the research team who are blind to the subject's psychiatric status and timing of onset of illness. The primary variable of interest derived from the LEDS interviews is the categorization of events and difficulties as *provoking agents* in the onset of depression.

In the LEDS system, provoking agents are psychosocial stressors defined contextually, occurring in a designated period before illness onset, and thought to be causually related to the disorder.[15] Provoking agents are qualitatively defined to be of two types. *Severe events* are events with marked or moderate long-term contextual threat (ie, the top two points on a four-point scale) that are focused on the subject or jointly on the subject and a core person (defined in the context of the individual's circumstances and including, for example, first-degree family members, spouse, or confidants). Long-term contextual threat of events (ie, continuing threat at approximately 10 to 14 days after the event occurred) in contrast to short-term contextual threat (ie, day of the event or soon afterward) has been implicated as the critical aspect of life events in studies of depression onset. For example, if a subject's child is hit by an automobile but is uninjured and unaffected by the event 1 week later, the short-term threat would be rated as high; however, severe long-term threat would probably not be assigned even if there were some reason to believe the child was likely—perhaps because of a dangerous crossing on the way to school—to be hit again. Such a threat would only be mild because the chances of such disaster would still be low. *Major difficulties* are defined as problems rated at least 1, 2, or 3 on a six-point scale of severity, lasting at least 2 years, and not involving purely health problems, ie, health problems with no associated psychosocial consequences such as major change in role or caring responsibility or major embarrassment or stigma. While purely health problems have traditionally not been included as provoking agents in the Bedford College method, we were concerned that eliminating them in an assessment of the relationship of psychosocial stressors to depression onset in a population including elderly subjects might represent an oversight. We therefore examined our data with and without purely health difficulties.

Only those life events and difficulties assessed to be unrelated to the index episode of depression (ie, not "illness-related" according to the LEDS system) are eligible to qualify as provoking agents. Provoking agents form only a small minority of life events and difficulties recorded by the LEDS instrument. The LEDS system also permits categorizing life events as "independent" (ie, independent of any possible influence by the subject or "nonindependent," involving possible influence by the subject or focused jointly on the subject and a significant other). Both types of life events were analyzed.

DATA ANALYSIS

The χ^2 tests examined the proportion of subjects in each group experiencing a provoking agent in the 6 months before the onset of the index episode of depression. The temporal patterning of severely threatening life events in relation to episode onset was examined using an adaptation of the Kaplan-Meier estimate of the survival distribution.

The survival strategy we used is reversed relative to the way in which survival data are typically presented. Setting the date of episode onset as week 0 and working backward to the closest severely threatening life event, we would expect those patients whose episode was classified as endogenous according to RDC to demonstrate a longer survival time. Individuals experiencing no severely threatening life events in the 6 months before depression onset are represented as surviving the entire period in such a survival distribution.

Table 1. Demographic and Clinical Characteristics of Study Patients*

Variable	Younger Patients (n=40)	Older Patients (n=50)	Total Group (N=90)
Sex	5 M, 35 F	15 M, 35 F	20 M, 70 F
Age, y	36.7±8.5	67.8±5.9	54.0±17.1
Race, %			
B	2	4	6
W	38	46	84
Marital status, %			
Married	45	40.8	42.7
Divorced/separated	10	8.2	9.9
Single	45	12.2	27.0
Widowed	0	37.8	21.4
Education, %			
<High school	0	31.3	16.8
High school	12.5	40.8	28.1
Some college	27.5	20.4	23.6
College graduate	60.0	8.2	31.5
HRS-D score at entry (17 items)	19.8±3.9	22.9±3.9	21.5±4.2
GAS score at entry	57.9±6.7	54.5±5.4	56.0±6.2
Age at onset of first episode, y	24.5±7.6	48.0±16.8	37.9±17.9
No. of previous episodes	4.6±4.5	4.7±2.8	4.6±3.6
Duration of index episode, wk	25.5±23.4	24.2±28.9	24.8±26.4

Data are expressed as number of patients and mean±SD except where noted. HRS-D indicates Hamilton Rating Scale for Depression; GAS, Global Assessment Scale.

search Diagnostic Criteria (RDC) to examine the relationship between the endogenous or nonendogenous distinction and life stress. Specifically, we hypothesized that the proportion of subjects experiencing at least one provoking agent (severely threatening life event or major ongoing difficulty) in the 6 months before depression onset would be significantly greater in a nonendogenous group than in an endogenous group defined in symptomatic terms. We also hypothesized that the temporal patterning of severely stressful life events in the 6 months before depression onset would distinguish the two groups, with survival analysis revealing a closer temporal association of events to depression onset in the nonendogenous group.

RESULTS

The χ^2 analysis demonstrated that the presence of a provoking agent in the 6 months before depression onset was significantly associated with endogenous and nonendogenous group membership. When purely health difficulties were excluded, 65% (22/34) of the nonendogenous subtype group experienced at least one such provoking agent, compared with only 43% (24/56) of the endogenous subtype group (χ^2=4.04, *P*=.04). When purely health difficulties are included, the proportion of the two subtypes with a provoking agent were 71% (24/34) of the nonendogenous group and 46% (26/56) of the endogenous group (χ^2=5.00, *P*=.03). To confirm that our decision to combine patients in the midlife and late-life protocols was justified and that the relationship between subtype and provoking agent was similar in the two age groups, we next examined the proportion of the two subtypes with a provoking agent separately for the midlife and late-life groups. Among the midlife group, 69% (11/16) of the nonendogenous group and 46% (11/24) of the endogenous group had a provoking agent; among the late-life group, 61% (11/18) of the nonendogenous group and 41% (13/32) of the endogenous group had a provoking agent when purely health difficulties were excluded, and 72% (13/18) of the nonendogenous group and 47% (15/32) of the endogenous group had a provoking agent with the inclusion of purely health difficulties, suggesting a high degree of comparability between the midlife and late-life groups on these variables.

We believe that the relatively static χ^2 approach fails to describe the important temporal aspect of the relationship between stressful life events and episode onset. Therefore, we used the Kaplan-Meier estimate of the survival function to examine whether severely threatening life events occurred in closer proximity to the onset of depression for the nonendogenous group than for the endogenous group. As the **Figure** indicates, survival analysis revealed a significant difference (generalized Mantel-Cox, *P*<.02) between the two subtypes in terms of the temporal patterning of events in the period before episode onset. When we compared the groups in terms of median time from the occurrence of a severely threatening life event to onset of illness, the low proportion of subjects in the endogenous group experiencing severely threatening life events precluded the calculation of a median time for that group. However, when quartiles were examined, we found that 25% of the subjects in the nonendogenous subtype group had experienced episode onset within 1.14 weeks of the closest severely threatening life event in contrast to 16.57 weeks for the first quartile of the patients in the endogenous subtype group. Although we found no evidence of a differential relationship between provoking agents and the RDC endogenous subtype in midlife vs late-life groups, we examined the relationship among age, subtype, and proximity of a severely threatening life event to onset of the index episode of depression. Age was a nonsignificant covariate in the survival analysis of time from closest severely threatening life event to episode onset (*P*=.39).

Finally, we examined whether the two subtype groups differed on the proportion of events rated 1 to 4 on independence (ie, definitely or almost certainly independent of the subject's influence) vs those rated 5 to 11 on independence (ie, probably influenced by the subject's behavior), and whether these variables had a different temporal relationship to episode onset. The two groups did not differ with respect to the proportion of independent and nonindependent events (**Table 2**). A survival analysis examining independent events only revealed a similar temporal pattern to that found in the analysis of all severely threat-

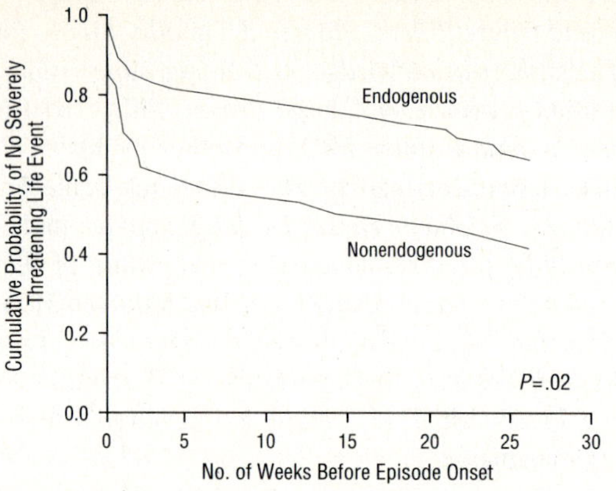

Cumulative proportion of 90 patients with recurrent unipolar episodes who had no severely threatening life event in the 6 months before episode onset.

ening life events but had insufficient power to reach conventional significance levels.

COMMENT

Our data point to a reasonably clear distinction between patients with recurrent unipolar episodes meeting the RDC for definite endogenous subtype and those whose episodes did not meet those criteria with respect to the probability of experiencing a provoking agent (severely threatening life event or major ongoing difficulty) in the 6 months before episode onset. Furthermore, analyses limited to severely threatening life events (excluding major ongoing difficulties) suggested a closer temporal relationship between severely threatening life events and depression onset among those patients whose episodes were classified as nonendogenous.

Obviously, there is substantial overlap between the first and second findings since the survival analysis takes account of the proportion in each group experiencing a severely threatening life event in the 6-month study period. Indeed, it is this difference in proportions that accounts for much of the statistical significance of the survival analysis of severely threatening life events. But we take note of the close temporal relationship (1.14 weeks) between the closest severely threatening life event and episode onset in the first quartile of the nonendogenous group, compared with the relatively long time (16.57 weeks) between the closest severely threatening life event and episode onset among the endogenous group. Equally interesting are the data presented in the accompanying article by Brown et al,[14] suggesting that the rate and patterning of severely threatening life events in the period before interview for a group of nondepressed community subjects does not differ from that observed in our patients whose episodes were classified as endogenous. This finding suggests that there may be a base rate of severely threatening life events unrelated to depression onset that is observed in nondepressed community-dwellers and in individuals whose episodes take the endogenous form.

Table 2. Independent and Nonindependent* Events in Endogenous and Nonendogenous Subtype Patients

	Endogenous (n=19)	Nonendogenous (n=19)	χ^2	*df*	*P*
Independent	9	8	0.11	1	.74
Nonindependent	10	11			

**Independent (events rated 1 to 4 on independence) and nonindependent (events rated 5 to 11).*

A potentially important factor in accounting for the results obtained herein and in the article by Brown et al is the relative role of life events in first, as opposed to subsequent, episodes of major depression among those classified with an endogenous symptom pattern. In both the Pittsburgh and Bedford College samples, it is only among patients with *recurrent* episodes characterized by an endogenous symptom pattern that a low rate of severely threatening life events is observed (34% in our report, 34% for the three studies averaged in the article by Brown et al, and 22% for the London study only). Among the patients with a first episode of depression characterized by an endogenous symptom pattern assessed by Brown et al, the rate of severely threatening life events and their proximity to episode onset was quite comparable with the rate observed in patients with a nonendogenous symptom pattern.

In contrast to earlier investigations of life stress and endogenous subtype, our study focused exclusively on a highly homogeneous population of outpatients with recurrent unipolar depression, with frequently occurring episodes. Somewhat paradoxically, our focus on such a restricted patient population (which might, theoretically, have been expected to have had the effect of reducing variability for examination of this question) may, in the light of the findings of Brown et al,[14] have actually eliminated some of the "noise" encountered in more mixed samples.

We wonder why (if the episodes under study are truly endogenous vs reactive in the literal sense) the difference between the endogenous and nonendogenous subtypes is not larger, either for the broader category of all provoking agents or the more restrictive analysis of severely threatening life events only. There are probably several factors that play into the relatively modest size of the difference between the two subgroups. As Klein[23] eloquently argued two decades ago, the symptomatic pattern of the nonprecipitated (literally, endogenous) depressive episode overlaps with that of precipitated episodes. He referred to such episodes as "endogenomorphic." Klein would argue that there will be a certain number of nonprecipitated episodes that do not have the endogenomorphic form in terms of manifest symptoms and vice versa. Furthermore, he states that it is early in the episode that one would expect to see the greatest concentration of endogenomorphic features. As the episode persists, one might expect to see the somatic complaints, dysphoric mood, and other features more generally associated with what he referred to as "chronic overreactive" and "acute"

dysphorias. It should be noted that the modal patient in this study had been ill for 5 months at the time of initial evaluation, a point at which these elaborations of the depressive syndrome may have made some "nonprecipitated" patients appear symptomatically more like the nonendogenous group. This could, perhaps, account for why 35% of the patients whose episodes were categorized as nonendogenous showed no evidence of a provoking agent in the 6 months before depression onset. It is also possible that some among our "probable endogenous" but categorized with the nonendogenous group, should more properly be considered endogenous. Finally, there is no question that the LEDS system does not consider all the possible factors that might precipitate depression. As we ourselves have earlier argued,[24] life events that are relatively benign with respect to threat as conceptualized by the LEDS system but that severely disrupt the pattern of daily life (eg, being transferred to a different plant an additional 2 hours' drive from home) might precipitate a depressive episode through disruption of circadian rhythms. But as yet, there is no evidence to substantiate this.

Our analysis does not address the question of the stability of the endogenous subtype, either from episode to episode within a recurrent population, or in the context of a single long episode within an individual patient. Unfortunately, insufficient data were gathered regarding the symptom patterns of previous episodes to make valid subtype determinations. With respect to shifts within the index episode, the RDC specifies that the episode should be subtyped based on the worst period during the episode. However, in the case of an episode that has gone on for 4 to 6 months, the patient is most likely to emphasize and the evaluator is most likely to be swayed by the current symptom presentation unless there is a profound disparity between the way the patient presents at the time of interview and the worst point of the episode.

Findings in the present study and in the accompanying article by Brown et al[14] suggest that careful assessment of psychosocial stressors may lead to significant distinctions between depressed patients with and without traditional endogenous symptom features and that further study may be worthwhile. Subsequent investigations of the relationship between provoking agents and endogenous or endogenomorphic symptom patterns would undoubtedly benefit from a focus on the stability of the endogenous subtype presentation over time. To fully understand the relationship between psychosocial factors and symptom patterning, it will also be necessary to study putative protective factors such as coping strategies and social support. Prospective studies of risks and protective factors in patients with previously well-established histories of recurrence may be especially valuable in this regard.

Accepted for publication February 25, 1994.

This study was supported by a grant from MacArthur Foundation Network 1 (Dr Frank), by grants 43832, 00295, 37869 (Dr Reynolds), and 30915 (Dr Kupfer) from the National Institute of Mental Health, Rockville, Md, as well as a MacArthur Foundation research grant (Drs Kupfer and Frank, and Cindy Ehlers, PhD, and Timothy Monk, PhD).

The authors acknowledge the training, supervision, and consultation provided by George Brown, PhD; Tirril Harris, MA; Antonia Bifulco, PhD; and other members of the Bedford College research group. They also thank Daniel Purdy, Renee Rhodes, Stephanie Helsel, Declan Patterson, and Sheri Johnson, PhD, for their conducting and rating of the life events interviews, and Anthony Mayo and Maureen McGuire for their management and analysis of the data reported herein.

Reprint requests to Department of Psychiatry, University of Pittsburgh, 3811 O'Hara St, Pittsburgh, PA 15213-2593 (Dr Kupfer).

REFERENCES

1. Free ML, Oei TPS. Biological and psychological processes in the treatment and maintenance of depression. *Clin Psychol Rev.* 1989;9:653-688.
2. Thase ME, Frank E, Kupfer DJK. Biological processes in major depression. In: Beckham EE, Leber WR, eds. *Handbook of Depression, Treatment, Assessment and Research.* Homewood, Ill: Dorsey Press; 1985:816-913.
3. Cooke DJ. The significance of life events as a cause of psychological and physical disorder. In: Cooper B, ed. *Psychiatric Epidemiology: Progress and Prospects.* Totowa, NJ: Croom Helm; 1987:67-80.
4. Brugha TS, Conway R. Categories of depression: reported life events in a controlled design. *Br J Psychiatry.* 1985;147:641-646.
5. Copeland JRM. Reactive and endogenous depressive illness and five-year outcome. *J Affect Disord.* 1984;6:153-162.
6. Cornell DG, Milden RS, Shrimp S. Stressful life events associated with endogenous depression. *J Nerv Ment Dis.* 1985;173:470-476.
7. Dolan RJ, Calloway SP, Fongay P, De Souza FVA, Wakeling A. Life events, depression and hypothalamic-pituitary-adrenal axis function. *Br J Psychiatry.* 1985;147:429-433.
8. Grove WM, Andreasen NC, Young M, Endicott J, Keller MB, Hirschfeld RMA, Reich T. Isolation and characterization of a nuclear depressive syndrome. *Psychol Med.* 1987;17:471-484.
9. Paykel ES, Rao BM, Taylor CN. Life stress and symptom pattern in out-patient depression. *Psychol Med.* 1984;14:559-568.
10. Winokur G, Black DW, Nasrallah A. Depressions secondary to other psychiatric disorders and medical illnesses. *Am J Psychiatry.* 1988;145:233-237.
11. Brown RP, Frances A, Kocsis JH, Mann JJ. Psychotic vs. nonpsychotic depression: comparison of treatment response. *J Nerv Ment Dis.* 1982;170:635-637.
12. Paykel ES. Recent life events and clinical depression. In: Gunderson EKE, Rahe HR, eds. *Life Stress and Illness.* Springfield, Ill: Charles C Thomas Publisher; 1974:134-163.
13. Paykel ES, Prusoff B, Klerman GL. The endogenous-neurotic continuum in depression. *J Psychiatr Res.* 1971;8:73-90.
14. Brown GW, Harris TO, Hepworth C. Life events and endogenous depression: a puzzle reexamined. *Arch Gen Psychiatry.* 1994;51:525-534.
15. Brown GW, Harris T. *Social Origins of Depression: A Study of Psychiatric Disorder in Women.* London, England: Tavistock Publishers; 1978.
16. Hamilton M. A rating scale for depression. *J Neurol Neurosurg Psychiatry.* 1960;23:56-62.
17. Klerman GL, Weissman MM, Rounsaville BJ, Chevron ES, eds. *Interpersonal Psychotherapy of Depression.* New York, NY: Basic Books Inc; 1984.
18. Endicott J, Spitzer RL, Fleiss JL, Cohen J. The Global Assessment Scale. *Arch Gen Psychiatry.* 1976;33:766-771.
19. Endicott J, Spitzer RL. A diagnostic interview: the Schedule for Affective Disorders and Schizophrenia. *Arch Gen Psychiatry.* 1978;35:837-844.
20. Spitzer RL, Endicott J, Robins E. *Research Diagnostic Criteria (RDC) for a Selected Group of Functional Disorders.* 3rd ed. New York: New York State Psychiatric Institute; 1985:1-40.
21. Frank E, Kupfer DJ, Perel JM, Cornes C, Jarrett DB, Mallinger AG, Thase ME, McEachran AB, Grochocinski VJ. Three-year outcomes for maintenance therapies in recurrent depression. *Arch Gen Psychiatry.* 1990;47:1093-1099.
22. Frank E, Kupfer DJ, Hamer T, Grochocinski VJ, McEachran AB. Maintenance treatment and psychobiologic correlates of endogenous subtypes. *J Affect Dis.* 1992;25:181-190.
23. Klein DF. Endogenomorphic depression: a conceptual and terminological revision. *Arch Gen Psychiatry.* 1974;31:447-454.
24. Ehlers CL, Frank E, Kupfer DJ. Social zeitgebers and biological rhythms. *Arch Gen Psychiatry.* 1988;45:948-952.

ORIGINAL ARTICLE

Life Events and Endogenous Depression

A Puzzle Reexamined

George William Brown, PhD; Tirril Olivia Harris, MA; Cathy Hepworth, MPhil

Background: Research has failed to find the expected clear-cut difference in the presence of events provoking onset in endogenous and nonendogenous depression.

Methods: A longitudinal study of 127 depressed female patients from two psychiatric departments were studied using the Present State Examination and the Life Event and Difficulty Schedule. Two earlier patient series using the same measures were employed to check findings, and two general population series were used to estimate the expected rate of life events.

Results: A large proportion of patients experienced a severely threatening event before onset, with the exception of a group defined by a British diagnostic category (a relatively small group of patients with melancholic/psychotic depression who were not experiencing their first episode). The results were broadly replicated in the two other patient series. The proportions of patients who experienced ongoing major difficulties did not differ between the groups.

Conclusions: The relative size of this melancholic/psychotic group of patients with a prior onset may well have varied markedly from study to study in previous research, and this may help to explain the puzzling variability in findings concerning the role of stressful events in endogenous depression.

(Arch Gen Psychiatry. 1994;51:525-534)

Systematic studies show a marked excess of certain stressors, particularly involving loss and disappointment, before the onset of clinical depression among both patient and nonpatient populations.[1] Along with this evidence, there is a common belief that some depressive conditions occur independently of external stressors, a view commonly linked to the concept of endogenous depression.[2-5] Many diagnostic schemes have been developed: on the one hand, there are reactive, psychogenic, situational, or neurotic conditions, and on the other hand, there are autonomous, endogenous, psychotic, or melancholic conditions. The latter set of conditions are conceived as having a basic biological susceptibility and as largely uninfluenced by life stress, although the use of these terms is notoriously variable, and the nature of the distinction is a source of doubt and debate.

It is often taken for granted that the endogenous group should display more biological markers, such as shortened rapid eye movement latency,[6] and a good deal of biological research has sought correlates of endogenous subtypes of depression. Although this has had some success, other research concludes that the presence or absence of a life event before onset has no clear-cut association with the type of depression.[7]

See also page 519

Research using the Life Event and Difficulty Schedule (LEDS) developed in London, England, has been typical. Initial analyses had no success in distinguishing patients with endogenous depression from patients with neurotic

From the Department of Social Policy and Social Science, Royal Holloway and Bedford New College, the University of London (England).

See Patients and Methods on next page

PATIENTS AND METHODS

SAMPLES

North London Depressed Psychiatric Patients

Initial Pool of Subjects. This project's aim, which will be detailed elsewhere (G.W.B., T.O.H., and C.H., unpublished data, 1994), was to obtain as representative a sample as possible of women aged 18 to 60 years who attended the psychiatric departments of two North London hospitals as either an inpatient, a day patient, or an outpatient with a diagnosis of primary depression of relatively recent onset (a maximum of 2 years before psychiatric contact) during a defined period in the mid 1980s. A total of 439 were identified.

Exclusion Criteria. Patients with a previous episode of schizophrenia or with an organic disorder that might give rise to depression type (either directly or through prescribed medications) were excluded; so too were patients with a history of substance abuse (but not axis II disorder) that predated the onset of their depressive episode. Abuse was defined according to the 10th edition of the Present State Examination [PSE]/Schedules for Clinical Assessment in Neuropsychiatry criteria that was already in the process of development.[28] Another exclusion criterion for this study was too long a course before admission for investigation of the effect of psychosocial factors on onset. Of the 282 eligible patients, 37 were found at interview to have features such as a history of drug abuse, which would exclude them, and 96 had disappeared or refused the interview. Thus, the final sample numbered only 149.

Representativeness of the Sample. A case-note comparison of the 96 patients with a recent onset who could not be interviewed suggested that there were no substantial differences between them and the 146 included in terms of 31 key demographic and clinical factors, with 47% being over age 40 years; about 30%, married or cohabitating; 40%, separated or divorced; and 47%, working class. As far as could be estimated from the case-note information on symptoms, the interviewed and untraced samples also closely resembled each other in terms of the proportion with a melancholic depression (about 21%) or agitated psychotic depression (about 8%), a reported family history of neurosis, psychosis, or alcoholism, and the numbers of previous episodes.

Sample Used in This Analysis. Only 127 of the 149 patients were included in this present analysis because 14 did not meet the criteria for major depression, three gave insufficient information, and five were found on later examination to have too gradual an onset for the purposes of this study. Thirty-five percent were inpatients; 47%, outpatients; 16%, day patients; and 2% only saw the psychiatrist in the emergency department and then defaulted on treatment. All had signed a paper giving informed consent.

In an attempt to provide a confirmation of the findings in the main sample, we had recourse to two other previously reported samples using the LEDS, both of which included men, although women were in the majority.

The Royal Free Hospital Sample

During 1979 and 1980, patients were selected from a variety of sources in Northwest London, including a district teaching hospital, a psychiatric hospital, a psychiatric day hospital, and a general practice.[29] Ages ranged from 20 to 70 years, and all met the Research Diagnostic Criteria (RDC) for primary depression.[30] Of 130 subjects considered, 72 were eligible according to the criteria of the PSE diagnostic CATEGO system in which classes of depression R and D were considered psychotic and N was considered neurotic.[29] Patients were excluded if they did not reach caseness depression, defined in terms of the Bedford College (London, England) scheme as having fewer than four of 10 core symptoms of depression in addition to depressed mood.

The Camberwell Patient Sample

A consecutive series of patients, aged 18 to 65 years, attending the Maudsley Hospital, South London, were interviewed during the years 1968 through 1970. The 111 female patients (71 inpatients and 40 outpatients) have been described extensively elsewhere[31] and were selected using the same exclusion criteria as were used for the main sample described above. A series of 35 male patients (26 inpatients and nine outpatients) was also collected.

General Population Samples

For comparative purposes, reference is also made to two general population inquiries. A random sample of 458 women living in Camberwell, South London, were interviewed in the early 1970s, and these women provide an estimate of the rate of events and difficulties in a nondepressed population once those suffering from caseness depression in the 12 months before the interview were excluded.[31] Another general population sample in Islington, an inner-city area in North London, of mothers with a child at home, which was collected in the early 1980s, provides similar data.[32] Both studies used the PSE and the LEDS.

MEASURES

Measurement of LEDS

The LEDS was used. This employs a semistructured interview and is based on a system of contextual measures that rely on precedents collected over a number of years. It has been found to have a low falloff in the reporting of events and difficulties over a period as long as 5 years before the

interview and a high agreement between the respondents and their relatives about the occurrence of the same events and difficulties. It has been extensively described elsewhere.[1,32-35]

The contextual method of rating deals with the likely meaning of events and difficulties. In assessing the threat of having a third child in an overcrowded apartment, for example, raters make a judgment of what most women in such circumstances would be likely to feel, taking into account what is known of the woman's plans and purposes as reflected in her biographical and current circumstances. By ignoring self-reports about responses to the event, various potential sources of bias stemming from the respondent can be ruled out. The method also guards equally against various biases principally stemming from the investigator.

Manuals that provide strict definitions of which incidents can be counted as events and directories that provide extensive examples of precedents of the various scale points of the ratings of contextual meaning (such as threat or loss) are designed to prevent the interviewers from allowing a knowledge of the respondent's symptoms or reported emotional responses to influence their ratings. Consensus meetings of the research team, which is blind to the subject's symptoms and reactions, provide a check on investigator bias.

The severity of threat in the LEDS is assessed in terms of both the immediate and the more long-term impact of events and the ongoing impact of difficulties. One type of event has proved so far to be of central etiological importance for depression: events that are severe, long-term contextual threats. They are defined by two rating scales. They must be rated as a 1 (marked) or a 2 (moderate) on a four-point scale of long-term threat judged in contextual terms at about 10 to 14 days after the event's occurrence and must also be focused on the subject, either alone or jointly with someone else.[31] Likewise, only a restricted class, termed major difficulties, appears to be of critical importance for depression. These must be marked at least 1 to 3 on a six-point scale of unpleasantness, involve nonhealth problems, and have lasted at least 2 years continuously.[31(pp130-137)] However, occasionally physical health difficulties are included if they restrict a subject's plans or activities in some critical way. The interrater reliability of the various ratings is high, typically exceeding an r of .85.[31]

The length of time before onset that is chosen to study life events has ranged from 3 to 12 months. However, the most general practice has been to take 6 months. Although the majority of severe events of etiological importance undoubtedly occur within 3 months, when the nature of the events and their excess relative to general population rates are taken into account, it appears highly likely that some events of etiological significance occur between 3 to 6 months before onset. Given the relative scarcity of severe events in the 6- to 12-month period (if there has not been one in the period up to 6 months), it is probably best not to extend the period beyond 6 months until a sufficiently large data set that is made up of a series of samples has been analyzed.

Severe events of which the threatening implication had been more or less neutralized before onset have been excluded, for example, in the case of a woman who planned to undergo a hysterectomy because of suspected cancer but who is told several weeks later that it was a false alarm. This type of resolution occurred for three women and, if anything, the exclusions go against the hypothesis (G.W.B., T.O.H., and C.H., unpublished data, 1994). Provoking agents are defined as either a severe event or a major difficulty.[31]

Measurement of Diagnostic Subtype

In the main North London patient sample, the diagnostic schedule employed was a shortened form of the PSE.[36,37] To form the Bedford College Clinical Interview and to allow a full comparison with the RDC approach,[38] this was supplemented by certain questions not routinely included in the PSE, such as whether the patient experienced excessive sleep, increased appetite, distinct quality of depressed mood, and a lack of reactivity. The Bedford College threshold for caseness has been found to be similar to if not a little more restrictive than that for probable major depression according to RDC criteria.[39,40] Because there were a number of results from the earlier work in Camberwell that required replication in North London, it was important to keep some degree of continuity in symptom measures. In the Camberwell patient sample (1968 through 1970), a related but more detailed schedule designed by John Copeland, MD, had been used to generate a distinction between endogenous and nonendogenous depression,[41] which, in those days, were termed psychotic and neurotic depression along the lines of the then current tradition in British psychiatry that used the terms psychotic and endogenous as if they were equivalent.[42-44] Herein, the more psychotic features such as delusions, which also figure in the definition of endogenous depression according to Feinberg and Carroll's scale,[45] were taken into account. Recently, these features are again being recognized as contributing to significant subgroupings of depression[46] and would be ignored by strict adherence to a twofold division of depression according to the endogenous criteria of the RDC and the melancholia rules of *DSM-III* or *DSM-III-R*.

As this account suggests, the range of diagnostic measures of relevance to the investigation of the hypothesis under consideration was considerable. However, we placed the most weight on a simple symptom score, ignoring other features that are often used for the dichotomy, such as prior personality and functioning. This symptom score emerged relatively late in the process of diagnostic diffentiation in the following manner. To approximate the earlier Camberwell dichotomy, a psychiatrist and a psychologist who were familiar with the previous data independently rated

Continued on next page

each patient as neurotic or endogenous. The rating was based on the presence and the severity of the following symptoms: diurnal variation, guilty ideas of reference, pathological guilt, delusions of guilt, hypochondriacal delusions, delusions of catastrophe, depressive hallucinations, delusions of reference, delusions of misinterpretation, delusions of persecution, appetite/weight loss, early waking, retardation, loss of libido, perceptual distortion, auditory hallucinations, visual hallucinations, distinct quality, lack of reactivity, and constipation coinciding with an episode. The psychotic symptoms in this list were mood congruent because any indication of schizophrenia at any point in the life span was an exclusion criterion. Interrater agreement was acceptable (Cohen's κ was 0.64).

The next stage involved the development of a melancholic/psychotic score based on these items. One point was allotted for each item, but because important information might be lost if the degree of vegetative disturbance was ignored and only its presence was counted, in four instances (weight loss, early waking, loss of libido, and retardation), a score of 2 was given if the PSE score was severe (ie, a PSE score of 2). The term psychotic has been added to melancholic to convey that more than traditional melancholic symptoms have been included in this endogenous group of episodes. This follows the practice of British psychiatry. A cutoff score of 6, based loosely on the earlier Camberwell results, was used to make the final distinction. A patient rated as endogenous by one rater and neurotic by the other and scoring a 6 or more was included in the endogenous group, whereas those with a similar interrater disagreement but a score of 5 or less were classified as neurotic. More details of this clinicians' rating of depressive morphologic characteristics will be presented in a future paper (T.O.H., G.W.B., T. J. K. Craig, MD, and C.H., unpublished data, 1994).

Other more familiar diagnostic ratings, such as RDC definite endogenous, are also used. However, the key analyses employ the melancholic/psychotic score in a straightforward fashion without consideration of any of the other clinical features that underlie the clinicians' dichotomy.

Previous Depressive Episode in Adulthood

In the North London series, previous episodes were investigated using the shortened PSE and the Bedford College caseness criteria.[39] This threshold aims to reflect current psychiatric practice. It is deliberately designed to identify case conditions that are comparable to those of women seen in outpatient psychiatric clinics. The Past History Schedule of the PSE had not yet been developed,[47] and we therefore adopted our own approach, which turned out to coincide closely with that of the Past History Schedule and of the Schedule for Affective Disorders and Schizophrenia lifetime measures. The approach was designed to minimize underreporting by also using past crises as staging points around which to use the PSE symptom probes. In this article, we are only concerned with the role of life events in the current episode, and because this had been identified in a different way (by the hospital admission lists), the increase in accuracy afforded by using the probe about crucial life experiences to identify past episodes introduces no corresponding disadvantage in terms of bias.

If answers about the key symptoms were affirmative, additional symptoms were covered; in other words, having identified an occasion in which key symptoms had occurred, the interviewer gave an abridged PSE, even though the occasion might have occurred as many as 20 years previously. Because information about symptoms as far back as this would likely be subject to error, episodes were grouped on a three-point scale as a probable case, a possible case, and a probable noncase, following the current Bedford College caseness criteria.[39] Finally, questions were asked about previous contact with the psychiatric services. In almost all instances, these episodes had also been described in the hospital case notes.

An earlier general population inquiry in Walthamstow, England, that used this approach gave encouraging results when family doctor surgery records were used as a check on validity.[48]

In the North London patient series, a comparison of case-note and interview-derived data for any episode prior to the index admission gave a κ of 0.68. However, for the purposes of this article, a final estimate of the number of patients who experienced a previous episode based on both sources of information probably resulted in greater accuracy overall. Only 5% of those who failed to mention episodes in response to the initial questions about key past symptoms reported episodes in response to probes about past crises.

In the other two samples used in this report as a check on the main sample, similar final estimates had been made based on both interview and case-note information. However, the interview information of these two samples was less detailed than that of the North London series and relied much more on items that concerned previous treatment by specialist and family doctor services than on the whole symptom picture. Furthermore, because information about childhood depression was not systematically recorded in these two samples, the measure used throughout this article involves only previous episodes that occurred in adulthood after age 17 years to permit comparisons of all three samples.

χ^2 Tests of significance with Yates' correction are used throughout. The survival analyses employ the SPSS/PC+ Advanced Statistics Package, which uses an algorithm of Lee and Desu[49] to calculate statistical significance.[50]

depression in terms of the presence of either severely threatening life events or ongoing major difficulties. The diagnosis was made by a research psychiatrist after a clinical interview using traditional British standards.[8,9] A discriminant function analysis of the symptoms was then used to obtain weights to characterize the endogenous and neurotic groups. As expected, the former were more retarded in movement, thought, and

emotion, and the latter, more active and emotional. To increase the chance of obtaining a difference, the weights obtained were used to differentiate the extreme and less extreme halves of each of the two original groups. This showed a nonsignificant tendency for the extreme half of the psychotic group to have had fewer negative experiences than the combination of the other half of the psychotic group and the whole neurotic group (eg, 48% vs 66% experienced a severe event). Moreover, even when a fifth of each group were reallocated to allow for possible diagnostic unreliability, no more than a modest, albeit significant, difference emerged.[10] This result is consistent with the negative findings of other reports, in which, at best, only small differences have been obtained.[11-15] Katschnig et al,[7] using the same life-event instrument, carried out a number of detailed analyses of depressed inpatients using different diagnostic schemes and reached the same conclusion. Bebbington et al[16] have been the exception in reporting a difference, but there were problems with their analysis,[17] and in a recent report based on a new series, they, too, have failed to find one.[18]

However, these results remain puzzling, and it is difficult to ignore the view of many that there are endogenous conditions that differ symptomatically from nonendogenous conditions and that are also more likely to develop in the absence of stress. There are many ways of categorizing depression,[19] but despite continued interest in improving diagnostic schemes,[20] it is difficult to believe that a clear-cut resolution will arise from diagnostic refinement alone.

There has been another set of interesting but conflicting findings concerning life events and depression. Some studies have found that events are more strongly linked to first episodes of depression.[21-24] These reports are echoed by an early exploration, where four or more episodes appeared to relate to a lowered rate of precipitating external events.[25] Such a falloff with episode number has been related to the course of bipolar conditions, and kindling and sensitization phenomena may play some part.[26] But other studies report, at best, small differences,[27] and our own LEDS research with nonbipolar depressive conditions has not found convincing evidence in either patient or nonpatient samples.

In the present report, using a new patient series, we have combined both issues in a single hypothesis that considers the diagnostic type and the ordinal number of the episode in light of each other, which, to our knowledge, has not been attempted. We test the hypothesis that only patients with an endogenous condition who have had a prior episode of depression will fail to show an increased rate of severely threatening events before onset. If so, some of the puzzling variability and inconsistency concerning the type of depression could be the result of samples that differ in the proportion of patients with a first onset of endogenous depression. A relatively low rate of such patients might be obtained in tertiary treatment centers, for example. The same kind of argument might also help to explain the inconsistency in results concerning the ordinal number of the episode and the presence of a life event. To reflect the two traditions underlying the hypothesis to be studied, life events on their own are the main focus; results for major difficulties are given briefly but will be discussed more fully elsewhere (G.W.B., T.O.H., and C.H., unpublished data, 1994).

Our use of several diagnostic schemes permits a more thorough investigation of the hypothesis.

RESULTS

Because we are concerned with differences in experiences between the diagnostic subgroups of patients, we will not deal in detail with the issue of the greater rate of severe events (or of difficulties) in the patient series compared with the general population. Numerous studies have now shown a substantial difference: roughly a threefold increase.[1]

DIAGNOSTIC TYPE AND PRESENCE OF AN EVENT

Research Diagnostic Criteria

Only 17 (13%) of the 127 women had definite endogenous depression and 43 (35%) had probable endogenous depression by RDC. Those classified as having definite endogenous depression by RDC did not experience significantly fewer severe events in the 6 months before onset than the other women: 47% (8/17) and 66% (73/110), respectively. When probable endogenous conditions were included, there was a similar negative result: 60% (36/60) of the overall RDC endogenous group experienced a severe event compared with 67% (45/67) of the rest.

Overall Neurotic vs Endogenous Distinction (Research Clinicians' Rating)

There was a tendency for the endogenous category to have fewer patients who experienced at least one severe life event within the 6 months than did the nonendogenous category, but the difference did not reach statistical significance (51% [20/39] compared with 69% [61/88], respectively; $\chi^2=3.06$, 1 *df*, $P<.10$).

Melancholic/Psychotic Score

If the simpler diagnostic procedure of employing a score of 6 or greater on the melancholic/psychotic index is used, a statistically significant difference does emerge with 40% (14/35) of the melancholic/psychotic group having ex-

perienced a severe event compared with 73% (67/92) of the rest (χ^2=10.72, 1 *df*, *P*<.01).

Figure 1 summarizes the results using this melancholic/psychotic score in a survival analysis for the 6-month period before onset. For comparative purposes, community women who were in the random sample of women in the Islington Population survey and who experienced onset of caseness depression are also included in the figure.[32] The distributions of depressed women in the general population, most of whom had not received psychiatric care, and of the patients in the nonmelancholic/nonpsychotic group were similar. The average time between a severe event and onset for those who experienced a severe event was 4.2 weeks in each. However, the distributions of these two groups were different from that of the patient high scorers, for whom the average time between the severe event and onset was 6.0 weeks (*P*<.01, 1 *df*, in each instance).

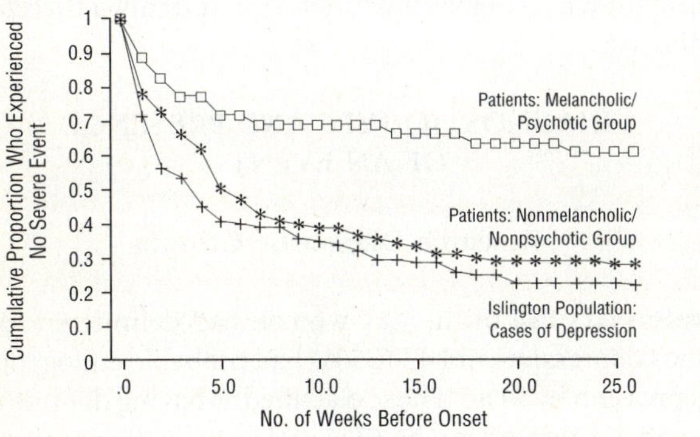

Figure 1. *Cumulative proportion of those who did not experience a severe event in the 6 months before onset among London patients and the general population.*

DIAGNOSTIC TYPE, ORDINAL NUMBER OF ADULT EPISODE, AND PRESENCE OF A SEVERE EVENT

RDC Endogenous Depression

Because only 17 patients showed definite RDC endogenous depression, little can be made of the fact that 71% (5/7) of the first episodes and 30% (3/10) of the subsequent episodes had been preceded by a severe event, but the trend was in the predicted direction. When the 43 probable RDC endogenous cases were combined, no trend was discernible.

Melancholic/Psychotic Score

When the melancholic/psychotic score is used with the number of adult episodes, the hypothesis concerning the unique status of those with a prior episode is confirmed: **Table 1** shows that only they experienced a low rate of severe events before onset. As predicted, the proportion of patients experiencing their first onset of melancholic/psychotic depression who experienced a severe event did not differ from the proportion of those in the nonmelancholic/nonpsychotic group who experienced a severe event, irrespective of episode. Moreover, the drop in the proportion who experienced a severe event among the melancholic/psychotic group occurred at the second episode. There is no suggestion of a more important difference in terms of the episode number after this; although the number of those with more than two episodes in the melancholic/psychotic group is small, there were 27 in the other groups and no evidence of any falloff. The difference in the proportions of those who experienced at least one severe event by diagnostic type and the first-episode–subsequent-episode division is highly significant (*P*<.001,

Table 1. Presence of a Severe Event by Ordinal Number of Adult Episodes of Depression in North London, England, Patients by Melancholic/Psychotic Score Within 6 Months of Onset

Melancholic/Psychotic Score	Percentage Who Experienced a Severe Event: Episode: First	Second	Third	Fourth	Fifth or Greater	Total
Low	71 (25/35)*	70 (21/30)	83 (10/12)	60 (3/5)	80 (8/10)	73 (**67/92**)
		Second–Fifth or Greater: 74 (**42/57**)†				
High	59 (10/17)*	15 (2/13)	33 (1/3)	100 (1/1)	0 (0/1)	40 (**14/35**)
		Second–Fifth or Greater: 22 (**4/18**)†				
Total	67 (**35/52**)	53 (**23/43**)	73 (**11/15**)	67 (**4/6**)	73 (**8/11**)	64 (**81/127**)

*Not significant.
†χ^2=13.18, 1 df, P<.001.

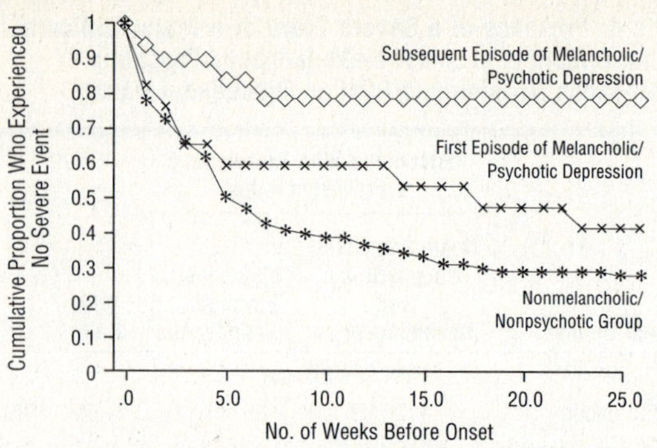

Figure 2. *Cumulative proportion of those who did not experience a severe event in the 6 months before onset among North London patients by diagnostic type and experience of a prior adult episode. Data for the nonmelancholic/nonpsychotic group included both first and subsequent episodes of depression.*

1 *df*). It is notable that there is no suggestion of a falloff when the total series is considered.

Figure 2 presents this last set of results in terms of a survival analysis. The results are clear-cut, although it needs to be borne in mind that only 35 patients were in the melancholic/psychotic group. Consistent with these results, the distribution of the patients with their first onset in the melancholic/psychotic group conforms closely to that of those in the nonmelancholic/nonpsychotic group as a whole (not significant). The comparisons that were significant in Table 1 are also significant here, ie, the comparisons of patients experiencing a subsequent onset of melancholic/psychotic depression with those experiencing their first onset of melancholic/psychotic depression ($P<.04$) and the comparison of patients experiencing a subsequent onset of melancholic/psychotic depression with those in the nonmelancholic/nonpsychotic group ($P<.003$). It can be added that the cumulative proportion of patients in the melancholic/psychotic group who experienced a severe event and who had a prior episode of depression approximates what would be expected on the basis of the nondepressed women in the Camberwell general population inquiry, in which, for the 419 women involved, there was a decrease of 18% in the 6 months, the proportion reducing steadily during this time.

The effects reported are unchanged when age is controlled, which is understandable given that age was unassociated with the presence of a severe event in the 6 months: 59% (41/69) of those younger than 40 years and 69% (40/58) of those older than 40 years had experienced such an event.

Because of the relatively small number of patients in the melancholic/psychotic group, we examined two other data sets, one from the Royal Free Hospital patient series and a second patient series studied in Camberwell in 1969. **Table 2** shows that the North London findings are repeated in the Royal Free Hospital series,

Table 2. Presence of a Severe Event in 6 Months of Onset by Melancholic/Psychotic or Endogenous Division and First or Subsequent Onset*

Patient Series	Percentage Who Experienced a Severe Event: Nonmelancholic/ Nonpsychotic and Nonendogenous	Melancholic/ Psychotic or Endogenous	Odds Ratio	*P*
First Adult Onset				
North London	71 (25/35)	59 (10/17)	1.75	NS
Royal Free Hospital	50 (5/10)	60 (6/10)	0.67	NS
Camberwell†	53 (24/45)	61 (20/33)	0.74	NS
Total	60 (**54/90**)	60 (**36/60**)	1.00	NS
Subsequent Adult Onset				
North London	74 (42/57)	22 (4/18)	9.80	.01
Royal Free Hospital	58 (7/12)	27 (7/26)	3.80	NS
Camberwell†	67 (16/24)	43 (19/44)	2.63	NS
Total	70 (**65/93**)	34 (**30/88**)	4.49	.001

**NS indicates not significant.*
†For the Camberwell general population, 18% (75/419) experienced a severe event.

but because of the numbers involved, the relevant difference does not reach statistical significance. Findings in the Camberwell series are again in the predicted direction but do not reach statistical significance. The overall findings for the three surveys shown in Table 2 are, however, clear: there is no difference by diagnostic type in the proportion of patients who experienced a severe event among those with a first onset (odds ratio, 0.97), but among those with a prior episode, there is a large difference in the proportion of patients who experienced such an event between those with melancholic/psychotic or endogenous depression and those with nonmelancholic/nonpsychotic and nonendogenous depression (odds ratio, 4.27; $P<.001$).

Finally, it should be noted that there was no relationship between the two clinical variables and the independence of the event (the degree to which it might depend on the patient's volition or behavior), and there were no sex differences in the results reported for the Royal Free Hospital and the Camberwell series, which involved some men.

MAJOR DIFFICULTIES AND THE HYPOTHESIS

When major difficulties are examined on their own, a similar distribution according to diagnosis and episode number does not emerge (**Table 3**).

Finally, when a combined index of provoking agent (either a severe event or a major difficulty) is employed, the patterning of results between the melancholic/psychotic, or endogenous, grouping and the first-episode–subsequent-episode grouping remains virtually un-

Table 3. Presence of a Major Difficulty in 6 Months of Onset by Melancholic/Psychotic or Endogenous Division and First or Subsequent Onset*

	Percentage Who Experienced a Major Difficulty		
Patient Series	Nonmelancholic/ Nonpsychotic and Nonendogenous	Melancholic/ Psychotic or Endogenous	Odds Ratio
	First Adult Onset		
North London	31 (11/35)	18 (3/17)	0.47
Royal Free Hospital	10 (1/10)	20 (2/10)	0.44
Camberwell	44 (20/45)	45 (15/33)	0.96
Total	36 (**32/90**)	33 (**20/60**)	1.10
	Subsequent Adult Onset		
North London	30 (17/57)	28 (5/18)	1.11
Royal Free Hospital	33 (4/12)	15 (4/26)	2.75
Camberwell	38 (9/24)	34 (15/44)	1.16
Total	32 (**30/93**)	27 (**24/88**)	1.27

*P *was not significant.*

Table 4. Presence of a Severe Event or a Major Difficulty Within 6 Months of Onset by Melancholic/Psychotic or Endogenous Division and First or Subsequent Onset*

	Percentage Who Experienced a Provoking Agent			
Patient Series	Nonmelancholic/ Nonpsychotic and Nonendogenous	Melancholic/ Psychotic or Endogenous	Odds Ratio	*P*
	First Adult Onset			
North London	74 (26/35)	65 (11/17)	1.56	NS
Royal Free Hospital	50 (5/10)	60 (6/10)	0.67	NS
Camberwell	69 (31/45)	76 (25/33)	0.71	NS
Total	69 (**62/90**)	70 (**42/60**)	0.95	NS
	Subsequent Adult Onset			
North London	79 (45/57)	39 (7/18)	5.89	.01
Royal Free Hospital	67 (8/12)	35 (9/26)	3.78	NS
Camberwell	75 (18/24)	59 (26/44)	2.08	NS
Total	76 (**71/93**)	48 (**42/88**)	3.53	.001

**NS indicates not significant.*

changed in the North London and Royal Free Hospital samples (**Table 4**). In the Camberwell sample, the difference between the endogenous group with a previous episode and the other groups is no longer approaching significance.

Unfortunately, the attempt to retest the hypothesis using the 2-year follow-up data was inconclusive. Of those with a melancholic/psychotic first episode at target intake, only four had a subsequent episode during the study period. Of these, none had melancholic/psychotic depression, so the fact that three experienced severe events is not relevant.

COMMENT

The focus of this investigation of life stress, diagnostic grouping of depression, and episode recurrence has been to illuminate one puzzling finding concerning life events using a type of event (severe within 6 months of onset) that has been widely found to provoke clinical depression. As predicted, the proportion of patients in North London who experienced a severe event was considerable. This held both for patients in the melancholic/psychotic group experiencing their first episode of depression in adulthood and for patients not in the melancholic/psychotic group irrespective of episode. These two groups formed the bulk of the patients, and the proportions of patients who experienced a severe event were similar to that found in women in the general population in whom depression had developed, none of whom was considered to be melancholic or psychotic. However, a much lower proportion of patients in the melancholic/psychotic group who were undergoing a subsequent onset had undergone a severe event, and this proportion was only slightly higher than that found in a comparison series of nondepressed women in the general population. The results were closely replicated in another recent series of London patients studied by another research group using the same life-event instrument. While the results for a series of patients studied 20 years earlier in Camberwell were less clear cut, the combined results for the three samples gave a highly significant overall result.

The findings may well supply one reason for the variability of results concerning the role of life events in studies of depressed patients. They suggest that the degree to which findings show a link will depend on the proportion of patients who are not experiencing a first episode of depression that an endogenous group happens to contain. The results would also explain why findings have been less variable in the general population, where cases are far less often melancholic or psychotic.[1] The findings are also entirely consistent with a study carried out in Pittsburgh, Pa, that used the LEDS with depressed patients, all of whom were experiencing a subsequent episode, in which there was a similar difference in the experience of severe events between endogenous and other patients.[51]

At present, the most plausible interpretation would appear to be as follows. First, that irrespective of clinical type, the great majority of first onsets of depression, whether treated by a psychiatrist or not, are provoked by a severe event. However, a relatively small proportion are almost certainly unprovoked, and this is compatible with a final common pathway view of depression. That is, a small proportion of first onsets will be found to be unprovoked irrespective of diagnostic type

or treatment status. In those cases, we suspect puerperal conditions are common.[5]

The same argument holds true for nonmelancholic/nonpsychotic depression in which there has been no prior episode. There is no hint in any of the three patient studies reviewed (nor in the general population series) that severe events are any less important in these patients than in those with a first onset.

However, in complete contrast, the results for the melancholic/psychotic group with a prior episode indicate that some kind of endogenous onset is likely. Indeed, the proportion who experienced a recent severe event may turn out to be not much greater than expected in a nondepressed general population sample. In the North London patient series, the fall in the proportion of patients in the melancholic/psychotic group who experienced a severe event occurred after just one episode. Unfortunately, because the numbers were small and because the other two series only collected systematic data about whether an episode was first or subsequent, this requires replication. This is particularly important because some of the published reports that were reviewed earlier suggest that the falloff in the proportion of patients who experienced an event increased with the number of episodes.

The somewhat serendipitous nature of the elaboration of the diagnostic measure that was employed in the North London patient sample (the melancholic/psychotic score) may provoke two contrasting interpretations. First, these results should not be taken as seriously as those obtained with better-known measures. Second, they deserve consideration and have implications for the need for refinement of the more widely used measures. For example, the key differences between the statistically significant results using the melancholic/psychotic score and those using the clinicians' dichotomous rating, which were not significant, probably reflect the fact that mildly endogenous conditions are not involved in the severe-event effect (that is, melancholic-seeming conditions with a score of less than 6). These results also have a bearing on the use of the RDC endogenous categories. The parallel results in the article by Frank and colleagues[51] were obtained with the definite, not the probable, RDC endogenous grouping. The sample discussed in that article had a much higher prevalence of RDC endogenous cases (62% compared with 13% herein), probably a result of the more particular treatment center from which it was recruited for a special study. This raises the distinct possibility that with a higher overall prevalence of RDC definite endogenous depression in our own sample, the trend in line with the hypothesis would have reached statistical significance, paralleling the result with the melancholic/psychotic score.

Finally, it is unlikely that the exclusion criteria employed could have contributed to a false-positive result. The omission of events that were dependent on psychiatric state (illness-related events in LEDS terms) means that the exclusion of patients with substance abuse probably made little difference. Furthermore, the exclusion of those whose onset preceded admission by too great a period for confident dating of life events and onset does not imply the exclusion of cases of chronic depression. Because the sample was followed up for an average of 3.8 years after target onset, we were able to report that 51% (65/127) of the episodes eventually lasted over 12 months at a caseness level, and 20% (25/127), over 2 years. These exclusions are therefore unlikely to have influenced the results, even if there were any grounds for suspecting that the chronicity of the melancholic/psychotic episodes could change the findings.

It is probably too early to conclude that psychosocial factors are unimportant for the patients in the melancholic/psychotic group who were experiencing a subsequent episode. There is some suggestion in Table 4 that major difficulties may be involved for these patients. The interpretation of this is complex and not crucial for the present article, which seeks only to throw light on the puzzling inconsistency of previous results involving events. We will explore the wider issue in another paper. Some effect by more minor events may still emerge, and in this other paper, we will discuss the possibility of provocation by severe events outside the 6 months and as far away as 1 year. We conclude that this cannot entirely be ruled out based on the present evidence. However, it does appear possible to conclude that as published studies have conceived the issue, the reactive-endogenous controversy may have arisen partly as a result of a failure to take account of the prior history of the disorder, and the inconsistent findings may have been partly a function of the patients who happened to have been studied. Insofar as tertiary centers have fewer patients with a first onset and more with particularly severe melancholic/psychotic conditions, evidence for differences concerning psychosocial provocation will have been more apparent. Perhaps the key message of this study is that there continues to be a place for consideration of stress in relation to psychiatric classification and that those preparing research reports concerning depression (and other conditions, for that matter) need to be more aware of the potential importance of nosocomial factors in the findings they obtain.

Accepted for publication February 25, 1994.

The research was supported by the Medical Research Council, London, and in part by Network I of the John D. and Catherine T. MacArthur Foundation, Chicago, Ill.

We are indebted to our colleagues Bernice Andrews, PhD; Antonia Bifulco, PhD; Linda Bridge; Rita Fichera, MSc; Patricia Garson; and Ruth Robinson, MSc, who par-

ticipated in the data collection; Laurie Letchford for work with the computer; and Tom Craig, MD, for his help with the diagnostic ratings. We are grateful to Paul Calloway, MD, and Ray Dolan, MD, for allowing us to use their data and to Scott Monroe, PhD, and Ellen Frank, PhD, for their valuable comments.

Reprint requests to 11 Bedford Sq, London, England WC1B 3RA (Dr Brown).

REFERENCES

1. Brown GW, Harris TO. Depression. In: Brown GW, Harris TO, eds. *Life Events and Illness.* New York, NY: Guilford Press; 1989:49-93.
2. Jackson SW. *Melancholia and Depression.* New Haven, Conn: Yale University Press; 1986:315-317.
3. Monroe SM, Depue RA. Life stress and depression. In: Becker J, Kleinman A, eds. *Psychosocial Aspects of Depression.* Hillsdale, NJ: Lawrence Erlbaum Associates Inc Publishers; 1991;101-130.
4. Askiskal HS, McKinney WRJ. Depressive disorders: towards a unified hypothesis. *Science.* 1973;182:20-29.
5. Martin CJ, Brown GW, Goldberg DP, Brockington IF. Psychosocial stress and puerperal depression. *J Affect Disord.* 1989;16:283-293.
6. Kupfer DJ. Biological markers of depression. In: Feighner JP, Boyer WF, eds. *Perspectives in Psychiatry: Diagnosis of Depression.* Chichester, England: John Wiley & Sons Ltd; 1991;2:79-98.
7. Katschnig H, Pakesch G, Egger-Zeidner E. Life stress and depressive subtypes: a review of present diagnostic criteria and recent research results. In: Katschnig H, ed. *Life Events and Psychiatric Disorders: Controversial Issues.* Cambridge, England: Cambridge University Press; 1986;201-245.
8. Ni Bhrolchain M. Psychotic and neurotic depression, I: some points of method. *Br J Psychiatry.* 1979;134:87-93.
9. Ni Bhrolchain M, Brown GW, Harris TO. Psychotic and neurotic depression, II: clinical characteristics. *Br J Psychiatry.* 1979;134:94-107.
10. Brown GW, Ni Bhrolchain M, Harris TO. Psychotic and neurotic depression, III: aetiological and background factors. *J Affect Disord.* 1979;1:195-211.
11. Paykel ES, Prusoff BA, Klerman GL. The endogenous-neurotic continuum in depression, rater independence and factor distributions. *J Psychiatr Res.* 1971; 8:73-90.
12. Thomson KC, Hendrie HC. Environmental stress in primary depressive illness. *Arch Gen Psychiatry.* 1972;26:130-132.
13. Leff MJ, Roatch JF, Bunney WE. Environmental factors preceding the onset of severe depressions. *Psychiatry.* 1970;33:293-311.
14. Roy A, Breier A, Doran AR, Picar D. Life events and depression: relation to subtypes. *J Affect Disord.* 1985;9:143-148.
15. Paykel ES, Rao BM, Taylor CN. Life stress and symptom pattern in out-patient depression. *Psychol Med.* 1984;14:559-568.
16. Bebbington P, Tennant C, Hurry J. Adversity and the nature of psychiatric disorder in the community. *J Affect Disord.* 1981;3:345-366.
17. Brown GW, Harris TO. Disease, distress and depression: a comment. *J Affect Disord.* 1982;4:1-8.
18. Bebbington P, McGuffin P. Interactive models of depression. In: Paykel E, Herbst K, eds. *Depression: An Integrative Approach.* London, England: Heinemann Medical Books; 1989:65-80.
19. Katschnig H. Discussion. In: Kringlen E, Lavik NJ, Torgersen S, eds. *Etiology of Mental Disorder.* Oslo, Norway: Dept of Psychiatry, University of Oslo. 1990; 123-147.
20. Parker G, Hadzi-Pavlovic D, Boyce P, Wilhelm K, Brodat YH, Mitchell P, Hickle I, Eyers K. Classifying depression by mental state signs. *Br J Psychiatry.* 1990; 157:55-65.
21. Ayuso Gutierrez JL, Fuentenebro de Diego F, Mendez Barroso R, Mateo Martin I. Analyse des facteurs declencheurs sur un echantillon de patients hospitalises pour depression endogene. *Ann Med Psychol (Paris).* 1981;139:759-769.
22. Dolan RJ, Calloway SP, Fonagy P, De Souza FVA, Wakeling A. Life events, depression and hypothalamic-pituitary-adrenal axis function. *Br J Psychiatry.* 1985;147:429-433.
23. Ezquiaga E, Gutierrez JLA, Lopez AG. Psychosocial factors and episode number in depression. *J Affect Disord.* 1987;12:135-138.
24. Ghaziuddin M, Ghaziuddin N, Stein G. The role of life events in the onset of depression: first versus recurrent episodes. *Can J Psychiatry.* 1990;35:239-242.
25. Angst J. *Atiologie und Nosologie Endogener Depressiver Psychosen.* Berlin, Germany: Springer-Verlag; 1966.
26. Post RM, Rubinow DR, Ballenger JC. Conditioning and sensitisation in the longitudinal course of affective illness. *Br J Psychiatry.* 1986;149:191-201.
27. Perris H. Life events and depression, III: relation to severity of the depressive syndrome. *J Affect Disord.* 1984;7:37-44.
28. Wing JK, Babor T, Brugha T, Burke J, Cooper JE, Giel R, Jablenski A, Regier D, Sartorius N. SCAN: schedules for clinical assessment in neuropsychiatry. *Arch Gen Psychiatry.* 1990;47:589-593.
29. Calloway SP, Dolan RJ, Fonagy P, De Souza VFA, Wakeling A. Endocrine changes and clinical profiles in depression. *Psychol Med.* 1984;14:749-765.
30. Spitzer RL, Endicott J, Robins E. Research diagnostic criteria: rationale and reliability. *Arch Gen Psychiatry.* 1978;35:773-782.
31. Brown GW, Harris TO. *Social Origins of Depression.* London, England: Tavistock Publications Ltd; 1978.
32. Brown GW, Craig TKJ, Harris TO. Depression: disease or distress? some epidemiological considerations. *Br J Psychiatry.* 1985;147:612-622.
33. Brown GW. Life events and the onset of depressive and schizophrenic conditions. In: Gunderson EKE, Rae RH, eds. *Life Stress and Illness.* Springfield, Ill: Charles C. Thomas Publisher; 1974:164-188.
34. Brown GW, Harris TO. Establishing causal links: the Bedford College Studies of Depression. In: Katschnig H, ed. *Life Events and Psychiatric Disorders.* Cambridge, England: Cambridge University Press; 1986:107-187.
35. Neilson E, Brown GW, Marmot M. Myocardial infarction. In: Brown GW, Harris TO, eds. *Life Events and Illness.* New York, NY: Guilford Press; 1989:313-342.
36. Wing JK, Cooper JE, Sartorious N. *The Measurement and Classification of Psychiatric Symptoms: An Instruction Manual for the Present State Examination and CATEGO Programme.* London, England: Cambridge University Press; 1974.
37. Wing JK, Nixon JM, Mann SA, Leff JP. Reliability of the PSE (ninth edition) used in a population study. *Psychol Med.* 1977;7:505-516.
38. Spitzer RL, Endicott J. *Schedule for Affective Disorders and Schizophrenia (SADS).* New York: Biometrics Research Division, New York State Psychiatry Institute; 1978.
39. Finlay-Jones R, Brown GW, Duncan-Jones P, Harris TO, Murphy E, Prudo R. Depression and anxiety in the community. *Psychol Med.* 1980;10:445-454.
40. Dean C, Surtees PG, Sashidharan SD. Comparison of research diagnostic systems in an Edinburgh community sample. *Br J Psychiatry.* 1986;142:247-256.
41. Copeland JRM. Psychotic and neurotic depression: discriminant function analysis and five-year outcome. *Psychol Med.* 1983;13:373-383.
42. Lewis AJ. Melancholia: a clinical survey of depressive states. *J Ment Sci.* 1934; 80:277-293.
43. Kendell RE. The classification of depressions: a review of contemporary confusion. *Br J Psychiatry.* 1976;129:15-28.
44. Garside RF, Kay DWK, Wilson IC, Deaton ID, Roth M. Depressive syndromes and the classification of patients. *Psychol Med.* 1971;1:333-338.
45. Feinberg M, Carroll BJ. Separation of subtypes of depression using discriminant analysis, I: separation of unipolar endogenous depression from nonendogenous depression. *Br J Psychiatry.* 1982;140:284-391.
46. Johnson J, Horworth E, Weissman MM. The validity of major depression with psychotic features based on a community study. *Arch Gen Psychiatry.* 1991; 48:1075-1081.
47. McGuffin P, Katz R, Aldrich J. Past and present state examination: the assessment of 'lifetime ever' psychopathology. *Psychol Med.* 1986;16:461-166.
48. Harris TO, Brown GW, Bifulco A. Loss of parent in childhood and adult psychiatric disorder: the Walthamstow Study 1: the role of lack of adequate parental care. *Psychol Med.* 1986;16:641-659.
49. Lee E, Desu M. A computer program for comparing κ samples with right-censored data. *Comput Programs Biomed.* 1972;2:315-321.
50. Norusis MJ/SPSS Inc. *SPSS/PC+ Advanced Statistics for the IBM PC/XT/AT and PS/2.* Chicago, Ill: SPSS International BV; 1990.
51. Frank E, Anderson B, Renolds III CF, Kupfer DJ, Ritenour A. Life events and the Research Diagnostic Criteria for endogenous subtype. *Arch Gen Psychiatry.* 1994;51:519-524.

ORIGINAL ARTICLE

A Controlled Prospective Study of *DSM-III* Adjustment Disorder in Childhood

Short-term Prognosis and Long-term Predictive Validity

Maria Kovacs, PhD; Constantine Gatsonis, PhD; Myrna Pollock, MSW; Phoebe Lucy Parrone, MS

Objectives: Using *DSM-III* criteria for adjustment disorder (AD), further operationalized by requiring at least three clinically significant symptoms, we sought to characterize this diagnosis in terms of presenting features, recovery, and predictive validity among juveniles.

Design: The samples included clinically referred, 8- to 13-year-old patients with the research diagnosis of AD (N=30) and a high rate of comorbid disorders and age- and comorbid disorder–matched psychopathologic controls (N=26). As part of a naturalistic, longitudinal, nosologic study, patients were repeatedly examined during an average follow-up interval of 7 to 8 years.

Results: Adjustment disorder was associated with six symptoms, on average, and 60% of the patients had other, specific psychiatric disorders. Adjustment disorder had a median episode length of 7 months and a 97% recovery rate. Comorbidity had no appreciable effect on recovery. Patients with adjustment disorder and controls had similar rates of new psychiatric disorders and other dysfunctional outcomes during the follow-up.

Conclusions: Among psychiatrically referred youths, the diagnosis of AD has clinical information value and identifies a syndromatic presentation that can be the focus of concern or treatment. It has a reasonably good short-term prognosis, in spite of the fact that patients with this diagnosis typically present with comorbid specific psychiatric disorders. Controlling for the effects of comorbidity, AD does not predict later dysfunction. To achieve a convergence of findings from research and clinical practice, it would be important to ensure a uniform application of specific, operational diagnostic criteria for AD.

(*Arch Gen Psychiatry.* 1994;51:535-541)

THE DIAGNOSTIC category of "adjustment disorder" (AD) was retained in the *DSM-III*[1] because of a belief that it serves a useful clinical purpose.[2] The category includes stress-induced maladaptive situational reactions that do not meet criteria for more specific disorders but do become the foci of treatment or concern. Individuals with an existing psychiatric illness may receive a diagnosis of AD as long as the "new" disturbance is not merely an exacerbation of the preexisting condition.[1,2] The stressor may be acute or chronic, the disorder must be evident within 3 months of the stressor, and the reaction does not have to be transient.[1] The description of AD has essentially remained the same in the *DSM-III-R*.[3]

Using extant records, Andreasen and Wasek[2] found support for several of the *DSM-III* criteria for AD. Since their article in 1980,[2] this diagnosis has remained a topic of clinical interest[4] but has attracted scant research attention. Concomitantly, little is known about the presenting features of AD. However, there are indications that an episode of AD probably lasts longer than 6 months.[2] Moreover, in a study of a large sample consisting mostly of adults, Fabrega and associates[5] found that *DSM-III* AD had concurrent and face validity. Patients with AD who presented to a psychiatric emergency service were characterized by levels of psychopathology or health that were intermediary to those of individuals who

From the Department of Psychiatry, University of Pittsburgh (Pa) School of Medicine (Dr Kovacs); the Western Psychiatric Institute and Clinic, Pittsburgh (Dr Kovacs and Mss Pollock and Parrone); and the Department of Health Care Policy, Harvard Medical School, Boston, Mass (Dr Gatsonis).

See Subjects and Methods on next page

SUBJECTS AND METHODS

SUBJECT ASCERTAINMENT

The potential subject pool consisted of participants in a longitudinal study of the nosology of childhood-onset depressive disorders. Criteria for study entry entailed the following: 8- to 13-years of age, no evidence of mental retardation or major systemic medical illness, ambulatory psychiatric status, and living with parents or legal guardians within commuting distance of greater Pittsburgh, Pa. Signed consents were obtained from parents and children for a 5-year follow-up period and then for subsequent follow-up intervals.

As described elsewhere,[14] children were recruited primarily through the child psychiatry outpatient service of the University of Pittsburgh and the general medical clinic of the Children's Hospital of Pittsburgh; a few were recruited through other avenues. Our research staff screened *consecutive* subjects who presented at our primary recruitment sites. Study inclusion was based on whether a child met our criteria; it was *not* based on referral reason or the service provider's diagnosis. The main investigation includes a group with a *DSM-III* diagnosis of some type of depression (19 patients with AD with depressed mood [ADDM], 23 with dysthymic disorder, 60 with major depressive disorder, and 32 with both major depressive and dysthymic disorders) and a psychiatric comparison group (N=49) with any *DSM-III* diagnosis but no current or past depression. In the main investigation, assignment to the depressed or comparison group was based on the primary research (index) diagnosis determined during the first 6 months of study entry.

ASSESSMENT SCHEDULE

The protocol stipulated three post-intake assessments in the first year of participation and semiannual assessments in later years. Owing to logistic problems ("no shows," staff shortage, families moving away, etc), the actual assessment intervals varied among the subjects. Families received monetary reimbursement at each assessment. The follow-up was naturalistic and we did not control treatment.

PSYCHIATRIC EVALUATION AND DIAGNOSIS

At each clinical assessment, first the parent was interviewed about the child, and then the child was interviewed separately by the same clinician. The interviewers were mental health professionals (master's and doctoral level) with prior experience in psychiatric settings, fully affiliated with this project and extensively trained in research interviews. The evaluations were conducted with the semistructured, comprehensive, symptom-oriented Interview Schedule for Children and Adolescents and its addenda. The interrater reliability of symptom ratings has been reported.[16]

After each interview, the clinician's final ratings of each symptom (according to the data supplied by parent and child) and historical information were reviewed by the group of research clinicians. Only symptoms at predefined levels of clinical severity (reflecting distress and/or functional impairment) counted toward a diagnosis. The diagnoses were consensually assigned, using *DSM-III* criteria.[1] Irrespective of the index disorder, if there were indications of other disorders, all pertinent diagnoses were assigned.

To diagnose an AD, we further operationalized *DSM-III* criteria by defining a "maladaptive reaction" as requiring *at least three* clinically significant symptoms in the pertinent symptom domain (reflecting distress and/or functional impairment). The report of the parent and/or child of the precipitating event was accepted, rather than the clinician judging whether an event was a stressor. An AD was *not* diagnosed if the patient met criteria for a specific disorder.[1(p299)] For example, *presenting complaints* of crying, moodiness, and sleep problems subsequent to the parents' divorce could lead to a diagnosis of major depressive disorder rather than ADDM if the child had a sufficient number of symptoms to meet criteria for the former. Similarly, if the presenting complaint for a child with an attention deficit disorder included school refusal and anxiety in response to a new school, AD with anxious mood would be diagnosed only if there were no other symptoms indicative of overanxious or separation anxiety disorder.

Structured questionnaires, including a life-event scale for children and adolescents, also were completed with parents to record anamnestic, demographic, and treatment information at each contact. The life-event scale, developed by Coddington,[17,18] is available in three age-normed versions and yields a quantified score. At intake, it was completed to reflect events in the prior year.

DEFINITION OF ONSET OF AND RECOVERY FROM A DISORDER

For history and onset and offset dates of disorders, we relied mostly on the parental report. Onset was dated to the time when the child had the full syndrome in question. For the specific psychiatric disorders, offset, or recovery, was defined as the absence of the relevant symptoms or at most one remaining clinically significant symptom and few, if any, subclinical symptoms of the pertinent syndrome, and the maintenance of the foregoing state for a minimum in-

were free of disorder and those who had specific psychiatric diagnoses.

According to other information, AD in childhood and adolescence portends poor outcome and significant psychiatric morbidity, undermining the belief that it is a benign condition.[6] In one sample of adolescents with AD,[7] major depression, substance use, and antisocial personality disorder were the most common diagnoses at a 5-year reevaluation; only 44% of the youths were completely well during the interim. Based on a 4-year reassessment of mostly young children with AD, Cantwell and Baker[8] reported a mere 26% recovery rate as well as high rates of new conditions.

terval of 2 months. If only three symptoms were present for an AD, recovery was considered if all the symptoms remitted. Subjects who recovered from an episode but then became symptomatic in less than 2 months were considered as still in the previous episode of illness.

To assist recall, informants drew a "lifeline," placed marker events (eg, holidays, birthdays) on it, and indicated the period of a disorder in relationship to the marker events. If an onset or offset date was uncertain, a calendar interval was delimited during which the symptoms emerged or remitted, respectively (eg, "between Christmas and Easter"). The date in question was then set at the midpoint of that interval. Onset and offset dates also were consensually assigned by the research clinicians.

SAMPLES AND MATCHING PROCEDURE

Two groups constitute the subjects for this article: (1) 30 children with a diagnosis of AD at study entry and (2) 26 diagnostically and demographically matched controls with no AD at study entry. The AD sample includes 19 subjects who entered the main study with the index diagnosis of ADDM, one who had an AD with disturbance of conduct (in addition to the index diagnosis of dysthymic disorder), and 10 who entered with an AD (other than ADDM) as part of the nondepressed group in the main study.

The control group was selected from among all the remaining subjects in the main investigation who did not have AD at intake. As documented later, 60% (N=18) of the youths with AD had *comorbid* psychiatric disorders. Therefore, the controls were selected so that the distribution of their diagnoses closely matched the comorbid conditions of the children with AD. In achieving a match, we controlled for gender as the next variable, followed by socioeconomic status (SES). The SES was dichotomized from Hollingshead's Two Factor Index of Social Position (August B. Hollingshead, unpublished copyrighted manuscript, New Haven, Conn, Yale University, 1957) as higher SES (classes I, II, and III) and lower SES (classes IV and V).

The characteristics of the groups at intake are depicted in **Table 1**. A fairly close match was achieved with respect to the distribution of psychiatric diagnoses, *not* counting the AD. The two groups had similar proportions of children with specific psychiatric disorders (Fisher's Exact Test, *P*=1.0), and externalizing disorders (Fisher's Exact Test, *P*=.578) that were the most prevalent specific *DSM-III* condition. In the comparison group, the 10 children with no diagnosis or V codes (38%) are accounted for by subjects who failed to meet *DSM-III* criteria for any disorder in spite of presenting complaints that may have included several symptoms. Typically, these youths had parent-child or family problems in the absence of a discrete stressor.

The two groups did not significantly differ on any of the demographic variables, according to χ^2 and *t* tests (*P* values between .28 and .94). These findings were reconfirmed by computations of exact *P* values.[19] Although we did *not* match for severity of life-events in the year prior to study entry (Coddington score), the groups did not significantly differ in that regard (*P*=.27). Therefore, the major distinguishing feature of the two groups was presence or absence of an AD at study entry.

FOLLOW-UP INTERVAL

Subjects were recruited during the period of April 1978 through March 1987. Before completing the first 5 years, five subjects with AD and one control dropped out or were lost to the study owing to geographic moves. The present analyses included data collected by September 1, 1990 (*the cutoff interview*). Because subjects were recruited sequentially, they had variable lengths of follow-up. However, the two groups had comparable lengths of follow-up (excepting one subject with AD who dropped out shortly after study entry): for patients with AD, mean follow-up was 7.45 years; for the controls, 7.87 years (*t*=0.52, *df*=53, *P*=.61). Unless otherwise noted, all subjects were included in all analyses.

STATISTICAL METHODS

Recovery from the AD was examined using survival analysis to accommodate censored observations.[20] Censored observations refer to the fact that, in a longitudinal study, some subjects drop out before the outcome of interest occurs, and others may not have experienced the outcome (in this case, recovery) by the last observation. By taking into account all information on all subjects, survival analysis provides a distribution of time to response (recovery) for the cohort.[20] The impact of covariates on time to recovery from AD was assessed via Cox regression analyses, also known as proportional hazards models.[20] The model yields an estimate of the regression coefficient and its SE for a covariate. A positive coefficient indicates that higher values of the covariate are associated with an increased hazard rate and a shorter time to criterion. In light of the small sample size, covariates of interest were examined in a series of univariate analyses, and significant findings were corroborated by computation of exact *P* values.[19] Finally, odds ratios were calculated to estimate the risk for selected outcomes during study observation for the AD group compared with the controls. These results also were verified by the computation of exact *P* values.[19]

However, the poor outcome reported for early-onset AD could have reflected methodologic confounds. For example, the accuracy of the diagnosis may have been affected by the age range and nature of the target population. In a study of children with speech and hearing impairments,[8] the youngest child with AD was 3 years old, and the sample's average age was 6.4 years. On 4-year follow-up, the most common new diagnosis was attention deficit disorder (11 of 19 cases), which must have an onset earlier than age 7.[1] Possibly, when first evaluated prior to age 7 years, the presentation of the children was not sufficiently crystallized to warrant the at-

Table 1. Demographic and Diagnostic Characteristics of Samples at Intake*

Variable	Subjects With AD (N=30)	Psychopathologic Controls (N=26)
Demographics†		
Male, %	60	65
Nonwhite, %	57	42
Lower (classes IV and V) SES, %	57	58
Age, y		
Mean	10.8	10.6
Range	8-13	8-13
Intact family of origin, %	20	27
Coddington score		
Mean	143	169
Range	27-280	0-377
DSM-III diagnosis, No. (%) of patients with		
AD	30 (100)	...
No specific disorder (or V code)	12 (40)‡	10 (38)
Conduct/attention deficit disorder§	9 (30)	10 (38)
Enuresis/encopresis§	3 (10)	3 (12)
Anxiety disorder§	4 (13)	2 (8)
Other chronic disorder§	2 (7)	1 (4)

*AD indicates adjustment disorder; SES, socioeconomic status. Coddington score and SES are explained in the "Subjects and Methods" section of the text.

†The two samples did not significantly differ on any of the demographic variables.

‡Two subjects had V codes. Specific disorder signifies any DSM-III diagnosis other than AD or V code.

§For subjects with AD, these represent comorbid disorders; for controls, primary disorders.

tention deficit diagnosis. The handicaps that characterized them also represented risk factors for eventual psychiatric disorder, even in the absence of AD.

Because AD is a nonpejorative psychiatric condition,[7] it also may have been overdiagnosed in youths. Indeed, Andreasen and Wasek[2] found that 25% of a sample of adolescents with AD had attempted suicide and that 17% probably "would have met *DSM-III* criteria for major depressive disorder" because they had the required symptoms. Suicide attempts among clinically referred youths occur mostly in the context of specific psychiatric disorders, including major depressive and dysthymic disorders, and rarely in the context of AD,[9] further suggesting that AD may have been incorrectly diagnosed in some cases. Reports that 5% to 12% of young inpatients with psychiatric disorders have AD[2,10] also raise the possibility of mislabeling.

Importantly, however, even if the AD was properly diagnosed, the negative prognosis that has been reported could have been due to comorbid disorders that were not recognized. Namely, because the comorbid diagnoses would be "specific" conditions such as depressive, anxiety, or conduct disorders, they could account for the eventual poor outcomes. Comorbidity would be expected based on evidence that over 40% of youths with a psychiatric diagnosis in epidemiologic investigations[11-13] and 70% or more of those in clinical settings have multiple concurrent disorders.[14,15]

The purpose of the present study was to examine AD in young patients and determine if, in a clinically referred population, long-term negative outcomes of this diagnosis are referable to the AD itself or comorbid conditions. Using extant research data on a sample of school-aged, clinically referred children who had AD and also had a high rate of comorbidity, we characterize AD in terms of presenting features, recovery, and predictive validity. To ensure diagnostic uniformity, we further operationalized the *DSM-III* criteria for AD by requiring at least three clinically significant symptoms. To examine the effects of comorbid psychiatric disorders on subsequent outcome, we used data from a psychopathologic control group, matched for age and types of specific *DSM-III* disorders, who did not have AD.

RESULTS

CHARACTERISTICS OF AD

An average of 5.7 symptoms constituted AD (mode, five symptoms; range, four to nine symptoms). Mean age at onset of AD was 10.3 years (range, 7 to 13 years). Of the 30 subjects with AD, 19 (63%) had ADDM, five (17%) had AD with mixed emotional features, three (10%) had AD with mixed disturbance of emotions and conduct, and three (10%) had AD with disturbance of conduct. For ADDM (N=19), the most common symptoms were feeling sad (95%), suicidal ideation (58%), reduced ability to experience pleasure (42%), self-deprecation (42%), and irritability (32%). For the other types of AD (N=11), the most common symptoms were disobedience (55%), irritability (45%), feeling sad (45%), anger, physical fighting, and anxiety (36% for each). The high rate of ADDM and the age at onset distribution were partly a function of the entry criteria for the main investigation. In the full AD sample, 60% (18/30) had comorbid psychiatric disorders (Table 1). Conduct and/or attention deficit disorders were the most frequent concurrent diagnoses.

The following stressors were identified in connection with AD (N=30): new school year/new school (30%), disrupted/changed family situation (23%), peer rejection/dislike/loss (13%), parental illness (10%), death of parent/grandparent (7%), move (7%), and other miscellaneous events (10%). For some children, multiple stressors were noted, but only the more inclusive was included in the foregoing tally. Note, however, that the AD group did not significantly differ from the controls in overall severity of life stress during the year prior to study entry (Coddington scores, Table 1).

RECOVERY FROM AD

During the follow-up, 29 of the 30 subjects recovered from the AD; the mean episode length was 8.87 months (range, 2.7 to 24.2 months). Using survival analysis (which includes data from the one child who discontinued participation while in the episode), median time to recovery was 7.42 months, and the cumulative probability of recovery was .97 by 24 months from onset. The rate of recovery was fairly rapid; by 6 months from AD onset, 38% of the subjects recovered and, by 12 months from onset, 76% of the subjects recovered.

The variables that were examined for their influence on time to recovery from AD included gender, SES, age at onset (in months), having a comorbid disorder, having an externalizing comorbid disorder, and the type of AD (whether with depressed mood). In univariate Cox regression analyses, only two variables were significant: age at onset (regression coefficient, .21, SE=0.11, P=.05) and having had ADDM (regression coefficient, .71, SE=0.42, P=.08). These results were reconfirmed by computation of exact P values (log-rank test for age dichotomized, P=.0229; for type of AD, P=.0653). Children who were older at the onset of AD recovered faster, and there was a trend for subjects with the depressed mood subtype to recover faster than subjects with other ADs.

PREDICTIVE VALIDITY: 'WELL TIME' DURING STUDY OBSERVATION

One index of the predictive validity of AD is subsequent wellness. If AD portends poor outcome, then children with AD should be well for shorter time periods than children who do not have the condition (controlling for comorbidity). We examined this issue by controlling for the fact that patients were observed for different time intervals. We computed the proportion of well time for each subject, from intake to the cutoff interview, defined as the number of days under observation that the patient was free of any *DSM-III* diagnosis (except V codes) divided by the number of days under observation. The results indicate that having AD has no appreciable negative impact on subsequent well time beyond the effects presumably due to the comorbid disorders (**Table 2**).

Both groups of patients were free of psychiatric disorder approximately 50% of the time while under observation (t=0.17, df=53, P=.87). *Median* well time indicates that half of both samples were disorder free between 60% and 70% of the time. Collapsing well time into arbitrary categories reveals that only about one third of both groups was almost always well (Table 2). This somewhat low rate appears to be a function of disorders *other* than the index AD and probably reflects the consequences of comorbid conditions, the distributions of which were matched across the two groups of patients.

Table 2. Proportions and Distributions of Well Time or Days Free of *DSM-III* Diagnosis During Study Observation*

Variable	Subjects With AD (N=29)†	Psychopathologic Controls (N=26)
Well time as continuous variable		
Mean (SE)	0.53 (0.07)	0.51 (0.08)
Median	0.66	0.65
Minimum	0.00	0.00
Maximum	1.00	1.00
Well time as categorical variable, % of time		
Almost always well (>80%)	27.6	34.6
Mostly well (50%-80%)	31.0	19.2
Sometimes well (10%-49%)	20.7	15.4
Rarely, if ever, well (<10%)	20.7	30.8

*Calculated by dividing number of days free of diagnosis (except V codes) by number of days of observation from intake to cutoff interview. AD indicates adjustment disorder.

†One subject who dropped out early is deleted.

PREDICTIVE VALIDITY: CLINICAL AND FUNCTIONAL OUTCOMES

As an alternative index of the predictive validity of AD, we examined whether the groups differed with respect to the *risk* for future disorders developing. It should be recalled that the two groups of patients had similar lengths of follow-up (one subject with AD who dropped out shortly after study entry was deleted from this analysis). In addition, at the cutoff interview, the patients with AD and controls were aged, on average, 18.2 years and 18.5 years, respectively (t=0.28, df=53, P=.78).

To examine clinical outcome, we ignored the *initial* or index diagnosis that was present at study entry and counted only subsequent disorders during the 7- to 8-year follow up. **Table 3** shows the relative odds of selected new disorders developing (first occurrence during the follow-up) and negative functional outcomes for the patients with AD vs the controls. None of the odds ratios was significant, indicating that both groups were similarly likely (or unlikely) to have new disorders and problems over time. For example, patients with AD and controls appeared to be similarly likely to have a future AD, eventual school problems, or psychiatric hospitalization. These findings were reconfirmed by computation of exact P values.

Odds ratios inform about the risk for outcomes in one group vs another, but not about the *rates* of the outcomes, the latter of which are presented in **Table 4**. As can be seen, for example, from among the youths with AD (N=29), a first episode of major depressive disorder developed in five patients (17%) compared with four

Table 3. Odds of Further Psychiatric Disorders and Dysfunctional Outcomes in the Sample With Initial Adjustment Disorder (AD) (N=29) Compared With the Sample of Psychopathologic Controls (N=26)*

Outcome	Odds Ratio	95% Confidence Intervals (Mantel-Haenszel Test)
New *DSM-III* diagnosis†		
AD	1.11	0.38-3.22
Anxiety disorder	0.88	0.16-4.82
Major depressive disorder	1.15	0.27-4.82
Substance use/abuse disorder	0.48	0.10-2.27
Dysfunctional outcome‡		
Failing a grade	0.30	0.08-1.14
Suspension from school	0.90	0.31-2.63
Psychiatric hospitalization	0.53	0.13-2.15

**One subject with AD who dropped out early is deleted.*
†First occurrence from intake to cutoff interview, excluding the index diagnosis.
‡From intake to cutoff interview.

Table 4. Rates of Further Psychiatric Disorders and Dysfunctional Outcomes After Study Entry

Outcome	Subjects With AD (N=29)*	Psychopathologic Controls (N=26)
New *DSM-III* diagnosis, %†		
AD	45	42
Anxiety disorder	10	12
Major depressive disorder	17	15
Substance use/abuse disorder	10	19
Dysfunctional outcome, %‡		
Failing a grade§	14	35
Suspension from school	55	58
Psychiatric hospitalization	14	23

**One subject with adjustment disorder (AD) who dropped out early is deleted.*
†First occurrence from intake to cutoff interview, excluding the index diagnosis.
‡From intake to cutoff interview.
§P=.08.

(15%) of the 26 controls. Later substance abuse was observed in three patients (10%) with AD and in five controls (19%). Four of the AD group (14%) compared with nine controls (35%) failed a grade at least once during the follow-up (subjects with AD were somewhat less likely to have this outcome, *P*=.08).

COMMENT

Using *DSM-III* criteria for AD further operationalized by requiring at least three clinically significant symptoms in the pertinent symptom domain, we sought to characterize this diagnosis with respect to presenting features, recovery, and predictive validity. Although our conclusions must be qualified by the nature and relatively small size of our sample of subjects with AD and the fact that AD was not a central focus of the main investigation, the data shed some light on several issues concerning this diagnosis in the preadult years. We found that among young, school-aged, clinic-based patients, the diagnosis has clinical information value, is associated with a good short-term prognosis, and often presents in the context of specific, comorbid psychiatric disorders. Controlling for the effects of comorbidity, we found no compelling evidence for a negative long-term prognosis during a follow-up period of 7 to 8 years specifically attributable to the earlier AD.

Our findings indicate that AD among school-aged youngsters is typically associated with five to six symptoms, *in excess* of those that characterize concurrent diagnoses. As a psychiatric label, AD therefore serves a useful purpose because it identifies a syndromatic presentation that can be the focus of treatment or concern. Concomitantly, the positive short-term prognosis supports the face validity of AD as a comparatively benign condition. In our sample, an AD from onset to recovery lasted 8 to 9 months, with a median time to recovery of 7 months and a cumulative probability of recovery close to 100% during a 2-year period.

According to the *DSM-III-R*,[3] AD should not last more than 6 months. Our findings suggest that this criterion may be unrealistic. In the present sample, it took about 7 months for 50% of the subjects to recover (median time to recovery). Andreasen and Wasek[2] similarly found persistent symptoms in adolescents with AD; at the time those young patients underwent evaluation, more than 60% already had been symptomatic for over 6 months. However, such symptom persistence may only be typical of psychiatrically referred youths. For example, there are indications that AD in response to the diagnosis of a medical disorder in school-aged children has a shorter duration.[21]

As noted by Rutter,[22] the events that precede ADs are mostly everyday disturbances. Indeed, our findings indicate that AD rarely was preceded by a major life crisis or traumatic event. Andreasen and Wasek[2] similarly concluded that, among clinically referred patients, few of the stressors associated with AD were overwhelming. It should be noted, however, that these data provide scant information about the role of life stress in the genesis of juvenile-onset psychiatric disorders. Recall that the children with AD and the controls were similar with regard to average levels of life stress during the year prior to study entry. According to *DSM-III*[1] and *DSM-III-R*,[3] even if a specific and presumably causal stressor is identified, if enough symptoms develop to meet diagnostic criteria for a more specific disorder, the latter label must be applied. Therefore, the presence of stressors does not automatically signify a diagnosis of AD, and, conversely, a diagnosis of a

specific disorder (eg, major depressive or anxiety disorder) does not imply the absence of causal stressful events.

The rate of psychiatric comorbidity in our sample with AD is convergent with evidence that, in clinically referred populations, multiple psychiatric disorders represent the rule. The finding that conduct and/or attention deficit disorders were the most frequent concurrent conditions probably reflects the comparatively high base rates of these diagnoses.[11-13] Interestingly, comorbid psychiatric disorders had no discernible effect on the speed of recovery from AD. The finding that younger children had longer episodes has to be cross-validated on larger samples.

The poor long-term outcome reported in the literature for early-onset AD suggests that this diagnosis in childhood is not benign. However, among both our patients with AD and the controls, we detected similar rates of dysfunction during the follow-up, probably attributable to the *specific* psychiatric conditions that were present initially. The rate of selected new-onset specific psychiatric disorders ranged from approximately 10% to 20%, and fewer than 40% of the patients became symptom free as the years passed. Controlling for the effects of initial comorbid disorders, early-onset AD made no discernible contribution to later psychiatric morbidity in the present study of clinically referred youths. However, our findings should not be interpreted to mean that early-onset AD has no negative sequelae at all. There may be some consequences of this condition, but if they exist, the effects were not sufficiently strong to be detected in our comparatively small sample.

According to Andreasen and Hoenk,[7] AD should predict "a relatively good outcome," and most patients should be "well at follow-up." The ideal test of this hypothesis would require samples with no (or low rates of) comorbid psychiatric disorders, all of whom have been exposed to the same stressor but in only some of whom AD developed: for instance, juveniles with a diagnosis of a specific medical disorder or exposed to the same familial or environmental stressor. Psychiatrically referred and nonreferred children also should be studied. Finally, to characterize AD more comprehensively, it would be important to ensure that in clinical practice, strict diagnostic guidelines are used. According to existing evidence,[2] clinical diagnoses may be applied unsystematically, making it difficult to achieve a convergence of findings from empirical research and clinical practice.

Accepted for publication January 3, 1994.

This research was supported by grant MH33990 from the National Institute of Mental Health, Health and Human Services Administration, Rockville, Md.

A previous version of this article was presented at the Annual Meeting of of the American Academy of Child and Adolescent Psychiatry, the Institute on Long-Term Outcome of Childhood Disorders, Washington, DC, 1992.

Appreciation is expressed to Lydia Voti, MS, who conducted statistical analyses, and the clinical interviewers who participated in this project over the years.

Address correspondence to Western Psychiatric Institute and Clinic, 3811 O'Hara St, Pittsburgh, PA 15213 (Dr Kovacs).

REFERENCES

1. American Psychiatric Association. *Diagnostic and Statistical Manual of Mental Disorders, Third Edition.* Washington, DC: American Psychiatric Association; 1980.
2. Andreasen NC, Wasek P. Adjustment disorders in adolescents and adults. *Arch Gen Psychiatry.* 1980;37:1166-1170.
3. American Psychiatric Association. *Diagnostic and Statistical Manual of Mental Disorders, Revised Third Edition.* Washington, DC: American Psychiatric Association; 1987.
4. Schatzberg AF. Anxiety and adjustment disorder: a treatment approach. *J Clin Psychiatry.* 1990;51:20-24.
5. Fabrega H, Mezzich JE, Mezzich AC. Adjustment disorder as a marginal or transitional illness category in *DSM-III. Arch Gen Psychiatry.* 1987;44:567-572.
6. Newcorn JH, Strain J. Adjustment disorder in children and adolescents. *J Am Acad Child Adolesc Psychiatry.* 1992;31:318-326.
7. Andreasen NC, Hoenk PR. The predictive value of adjustment disorders: a follow-up study. *Am J Psychiatry.* 1982;139:584-590.
8. Cantwell DP, Baker L. Stability and natural history of *DSM-III* childhood diagnoses. *J Am Acad Child Adolesc Psychiatry.* 1989;28:691-700.
9. Kovacs M, Goldston D, Gatsonis C. Suicidal behaviors and childhood-onset depressive disorders: a longitudinal investigation. *J Am Acad Child Adolesc Psychiatry.* 1993;32:8-20.
10. Faulstich ME, Moore JR, Carey MP, Ruggiero L, Gresham F. Prevalence of *DSM-III* conduct and adjustment disorders for adolescent psychiatric inpatients. *Adolescence.* 1986;21:333-337.
11. Bird HR, Canino G, Rubio-Stipec M, Gould MS, Ribera J, Sesman M, Woodbury M, Huertas-Goldman S, Pagan A, Sanchez-Lacay A, Moscoso M. Estimates of the prevalence of childhood maladjustment in a community survey in Puerto Rico. *Arch Gen Psychiatry.* 1988;45:1120-1126.
12. Bird HR, Gould MS, Yager T, Staghezza B, Canino G. Risk factors for maladjustment in Puerto Rican children. *J Am Acad Child Adolesc Psychiatry.* 1989; 28:847-850.
13. Anderson JC, Williams S, McGee R, Silva PA. *DSM-III* disorders in preadolescent children. *Arch Gen Psychiatry.* 1987;44:69-76.
14. Kovacs M, Feinberg TL, Crouse-Novak MA, Paulauskas SL, Finkelstein R. Depressive disorders in childhood, I: a longitudinal prospective study of characteristics and recovery. *Arch Gen Psychiatry.* 1984;41:229-237.
15. Last CG, Hersen M, Kazdin AE, Finkelstein R, Strauss CC. Comparison of *DSM-III* separation anxiety and overanxious disorders: demographic characteristics and patterns of comorbidity. *J Am Acad Child Adolesc Psychiatry.* 1987;26: 527-531.
16. Kovacs M. The interview schedule for children (ISC). *Psychopharmacol Bull.* 1985;21:991-994.
17. Coddington RD. The significance of life events as etiologic factors in the diseases of children, I: a survey of professional workers. *J Psychosom Res.* 1972; 16:7-18.
18. Coddington RD. The significance of life events as etiologic factors in the diseases of children, II: a study of a normal population. *J Psychosom Res.* 1972; 16:205-213.
19. CYTEL Software Corporation. *Statistical Software for Exact Nonparametric Inference, Version 2.* Cambridge, Mass: CYTEL Software Corporation; 1991.
20. Kalbfleisch JD, Prentice RL. *The Statistical Analysis of Failure Time Data.* New York, NY: John Wiley & Sons Inc; 1980.
21. Kovacs M, Feinberg TL, Paulauskas S, Finkelstein R, Pollock M, Crouse-Novak M. Initial coping responses and psychosocial characteristics of children with insulin-dependent diabetes mellitus. *J Pediatr.* 1985;106:827-834.
22. Rutter M. Stress, coping and development: some issues and some questions. *J Child Psychol Psychiatry.* 1981;22:323-356.

ORIGINAL ARTICLE

Minor Depression in a Cohort of Young Adults in Israel

Andrew E. Skodol, MD; Sharon Schwartz, PhD; Bruce P. Dohrenwend, PhD; Itzhak Levav, MD; Patrick E. Shrout, PhD

Background: A diagnosis of minor depression was considered for *DSM-IV*. Mild depression is thought to be common in primary care settings and in the community, but studies of the validity of minor depression as a separate diagnostic category are few.

Methods: Minor depression as defined by Research Diagnostic Criteria was assessed by psychiatrists using a modified Schedule for Affective Disorders and Schizophrenia–Lifetime version in a cohort of 5200 young adults in Israel. Subjects with year-prevalent minor depression were compared with subjects with major depression or generalized anxiety disorder and with controls on aspects of psychopathologic condition, psychosocial functioning, help-seeking behaviors, and demographic correlates.

Results: Symptomatically, minor depression appeared to be a mild version of major depression. Minor depression was associated with good teenage and general social functioning, but also with absence from work, separation or divorce, recent impairment in overall functioning, and help-seeking.

Conclusions: The results lend support for including minor depression or expanding severity modifiers in future classifications to better capture the phenomenon of subthreshold depression.

(Arch Gen Psychiatry. 1994;51:542-551)

From the Department of Psychiatry of the College of Physicians and Surgeons (Drs Skodol and Dohrenwend), Divisions of Epidemiology (Dr Schwartz) and Biostatistics (Dr Shrout) of the School of Public Health, Columbia University, and the New York State Psychiatric Institute (Drs Skodol and Dohrenwend), New York; and World Health Organization/Pan American Health Organization, Washington, DC (Dr Levav). Dr Shrout is now with the Department of Psychology, New York University, New York.

THE *DSM-IV* Task Force and its Mood Disorders Work Group considered the addition of a diagnostic category of minor depression to *DSM-IV*. According to *DSM-III* and *DSM-III-R*, patients who experience depressive symptoms too few in number for a diagnosis of major depression, too brief in duration for dysthymia, or not related to a psychosocial stressor as required by adjustment disorder can only have their conditions diagnosed in the residual category (depressive disorder, not otherwise specified). Since the problem of mild depression is thought to be common, particularly in primary care settings[1-6] and in the community,[7-11] its inclusion in a nonspecific, heterogeneous rubric is both unsatisfying and potentially detrimental to clinical care. A substantial proportion of people who are treated for symptoms of depression that do not meet criteria for a *DSM-III-R* diagnosis may be suffering from minor depression.[12]

In addition to its apparent prevalence, support for a diagnosis of minor depression in the official psychiatric nomenclature comes from studies suggesting that symptoms of depression that do not meet diagnostic criteria for major depression or dysthymia are associated with significant functional impairment and lead to substantial health care utilization.[10,11,13] For example, in the epidemiologic catchment area study in North Carolina, major depression was associated with a greater risk of disability than minor depression, but because minor depression was more common, people in the community with minor depression had 51% more disability days as a group than did people with major depression.[10] Minor depression was de-

See Methods on next page

METHODS

SAMPLE

The sampling frame consisted of first-generation Jewish Israelis born between 1949 and 1958 of either European or North African parents. Attention was restricted to this cohort to strengthen a test of social causation vs social selection as factors explaining inverse relations between certain psychiatric disorders and socioeconomic status, which was the principal aim of the epidemiologic study.[17] A stratified probability sample, equally balanced for gender, was extracted from the Israeli Population Register of the Ministry of Interior (N=19 000) in 1982. At that time, cohort members were between 24 and 33 years old.

The list of 19 000 was prescreened to firmly establish ethnicity (based on father's country of origin) and level of education. The completion rate for prescreening was 97.7%. A second stratified probability sample of 5200 persons living in Israel was obtained using gender, education, ethnicity, and year of birth as strata. Informed consent was obtained from all participants after the nature and possible consequences of the study were explained.

TWO-PHASE CASE IDENTIFICATION PROCEDURE

In the first phase of case identification, respondents were screened in their places of residence (including hospitals and prisons) by social workers, psychologists, and nurses. The screening phase was designed to identify possible cases for more extensive clinical evaluation. The screening instrument included symptom scales from the Psychiatric Epidemiology Research Interview (PERI)[18] and anamnestic questions suggestive of mental disorder. Shrout et al[19] had previously developed a discriminant function using seven PERI scales that had an overall sensitivity and specificity of 94% and 84%, respectively, for major mental disorders among Israelis. The anamnestic items included the following: current or past psychiatric treatment with mental health professionals, general practitioners, or religious or other counselors; illicit drug use; arrests; military psychiatric profile; and having been away without leave from the military. This composite instrument was administered to 4914 of the 5200 eligible respondents for a completion rate of 94.5%.

All respondents scoring above the preestablished cutpoint on the discriminant function rule or the 27-item PERI demoralization scale, answering any anamnestic question in the affirmative, or unable to complete the screening interview were referred for a clinical diagnostic interview (N=2643 screened positive). In addition, to determine the rate of false negatives using the screen, approximately 18% of the 2271 people who screened negative were randomly selected and referred for diagnostic interview. The total number of respondents selected for the second phase of case ascertainment was 3059. Of these, 39 were dead or had migrated after the first phase screening. Of the remainder, 2741 (90.8%) were successfully interviewed.

The second-phase psychiatric interview was based on a modified SADS-L.[20] The modifications primarily involved supplemental questions focused on obtaining additional history, more detailed symptom assessment akin to the full version of the SADS, and more detailed dating of episode onsets and offsets. The SADS-I (I for Israel) interviewing was conducted by 64 psychiatrists trained with the program for SADS/RDC developed at the New York State Psychiatric Institute, New York City.[21] The median number of interviews per clinician was 19. The majority of interviews were audiotaped and reviewed by SADS/RDC-trained staff psychologists. A preliminary reliability check of 64 interviews reviewed by staff indicated satisfactory overall agreement (κ=0.68). Final RDC diagnoses were established by staff supervised by one of us (I.L.). In some cases, additional information was obtained from respondents to finalize diagnostic assessments. Phase 2 of case identifica-

Continued on next page

fined as the presence of one or more symptoms of depression, one of which had to be depressed mood or anhedonia, without a diagnosis of major depression or dysthymia. In another epidemiologic catchment area study, Johnson et al[11] demonstrated that "from a population or 'service burden' perspective, more medical service utilization, suicide attempts, and other indicators of impairment result from [subthreshold] depressive symptoms than from cases more explicitly defined by the American Psychiatric Association's diagnostic manuals." In the Medical Outcomes Study, Wells et al[13] found that patients with current depressive symptoms in the absence of depressive disorder had significant impairment in physical, role, and social functioning; increased days spent in bed; poor perceived physical health; and increased bodily pain.

There are, nevertheless, arguments against a diagnosis of minor depression. First, the disturbance may be so prevalent as to be ubiquitous and trivial and thus may lead to unnecessary treatment. Second, cases may be inadequately assessed major depressions. Third, insufficient data exist on adequate treatments and the expected response.[14]

In the *DSM-IV Options Book*,[14] minor depression was one of two proposed possible categories for "subthreshold" or "subclinical" depression; the other was brief recurrent depression. The criteria for minor depression presented in the *DSM-IV Options Book* were very similar to those for minor depressive disorder in the Research Diagnostic Criteria (RDC).[15] According to the *DSM-IV Draft Criteria*,[16] minor depression was one of several examples of depressive disorder not otherwise specified and

tion was completed in August 1988. Respondents were between 25 and 39 years old at the time of diagnosis.

ANALYSES

Prevalence rates for RDC minor depressive disorder, major depressive disorder, and GAD were estimated for episodes meeting criteria at any time in the year prior to the SADS interview. Diagnoses were made at both the definite and probable levels using RDC rules.[15]

Research Diagnostic Criteria major depressive disorder is characterized by a distinct period of dysphoric mood or pervasive loss of interest or pleasure of 2 weeks' duration (for definite, 1 week for probable), coupled with at least five of eight (four for probable) associated symptoms (eg, poor appetite or weight loss, sleep difficulty) in the absence of signs or symptoms suggesting schizophrenia, which leads to impairment in functioning, taking medication, or seeking help. Research Diagnostic Criteria minor depressive disorder is characterized by a period of relatively persistent depressed mood of 2 weeks' duration (1 week for probable), coupled with two or more of 16 associated symptoms (the first eight of major depressive disorder plus others such as pessimistic attitude, brooding, and feelings of inadequacy), which results in impairment in functioning, taking medication, or seeking help. The episode of illness does not meet the criteria for major depressive disorder, intermittent depressive disorder (similar to *DSM-III-R* dysthymia), schizophrenia, schizoaffective disorder, or several other more pervasive disorders. Research Diagnostic Criteria GAD is a minor anxiety disorder characterized by relatively persistent generalized anxious mood of 2 weeks' duration, accompanied by at least one of five associated symptoms (eg, muscular tension, fidgeting), which also results in impairment in functioning, taking medication, or seeking help. The episode of illness does not meet criteria for panic disorder, major or minor depressive disorders, schizophrenia, or several other more pervasive disorders.

The sample data were weighted to estimate rates of disorders for the original cohort population. Weights were constructed to account for the sampling strata in the original sampling design, as well as for the oversampling of the screened positives.

Probable plus definite cases of each disorder were then compared with each other and with controls without any of the three target disorders. Variables related to severity of clinical course included types of symptoms, age at onset, episode length, recurrence rates, comorbidity, and history of suicide attempts. Functioning variables included marital status, history of military service, two measures of social adjustment, two measures of work functioning, and a measure of overall functioning. Social, work, and overall functioning were measured on the SADS-L[20] ordinal scales and were based on clinicians' judgments following suggested SADS-L probes. Respondents were asked if they had ever sought help for psychological problems from a variety of sources, including psychiatric hospitals and mental health professionals. Demographic variables included sex, ethnicity, age, and education.

Logistic regression analyses were conducted using a computer program (SUPERCARP)[22] that takes into account the complex sampling design. The log odds of disorder vs nondisorder were the outcomes, and the control and risk variables were explanatory factors in the analyses.[23] All logistic regression analyses included gender and ethnicity as control variables. For characteristics expected to be more common in controls than in cases, odds ratios with confidence intervals are presented for the odds of nondisorder vs disorder. For characteristics expected to be more common in cases than in controls, odds ratios are the odds of disorder vs nondisorder. All logistic regression analyses were repeated adding comorbidity, defined as any specific RDC diagnosis at the probable or definite level that was present within the year prior to the SADS-I interview, as a control variable.

was defined as a disorder with episodes of 2 weeks of depressive symptoms, but with fewer than the five symptoms required for major depressive disorder.

In this report, we present data on the diagnosis of minor depression from an epidemiologic study of a 10-year birth cohort of young adults in Israel. Cases were ascertained with a two-phase diagnostic procedure culminating in a face-to-face interview by a psychiatrist using a modified lifetime version of the Schedule for Affective Disorders and Schizophrenia (SADS-L), which included a section to assess minor depressive disorder according to RDC. In addition to having a focus on a definition of minor depression very similar to one proposed for *DSM-IV*, this study expands the existing database on associated morbidity and treatment utilization and extends into domains of premorbid adjustment and phenomenology.

Based on the discussion of pros and cons above, the strongest case for adding minor depression to official nomenclatures would be made if there were evidence of a syndrome of subthreshold depression related to dysfunction and help-seeking that (1) was not rare, but also not ubiquitous; (2) was not trivial; and (3) was related to, but was not merely misdiagnosed, major depression. We will organize our presentation around these three issues. First, compared with the potentially related diagnoses of major depressive disorder and generalized anxiety disorder (GAD), what is the 1-year prevalence of minor depressive disorder? Since RDC require either functional impairment and/or help-seeking for a diagnosis of minor depressive disorder, these rates are germane to the type of disorder with which proponents of the diagnosis are concerned. Second, compared with major depressive disorder and GAD, is minor depressive disorder trivial? This comparison is made with respect to

descriptive psychopathology (types of symptoms, age at onset, episode length, recurrence, comorbidity), premorbid and current psychosocial functioning, and help-seeking behaviors. Finally, does minor depressive disorder resemble major depressive disorder and/or GAD in terms of demographic correlates and overlap of lifetime diagnoses?

RESULTS

PREVALENCE OF MINOR DEPRESSION ASSOCIATED WITH FUNCTIONAL IMPAIRMENT OR HELP-SEEKING

Table 1 presents prevalence rates for major depressive disorder, minor depressive disorder, and GAD in the year prior to the SADS-I interview for young Israeli adults. Rates are given for the definite level of RDC diagnosis and for the definite and probable levels combined. Generalized anxiety disorder has the highest prevalence, followed by major depressive disorder, with minor depressive disorder least prevalent at each diagnostic level. In the results shown in Table 1, it was possible for a respondent to have an episode of more than one of these disorders, as an episode of a particular disorder ended and an episode of another began during the 1-year period. In subsequent comparisons, the following cases of definite or probable comorbid disorders were excluded: 15 persons with major depressive disorder and GAD in the year, four persons with major depressive disorder and minor depressive disorder, and three persons with minor depressive disorder and GAD.

See also pages 527 and 569

Table 1. One-Year Prevalence Rates per 100 of RDC Major Depressive Disorder, Minor Depressive Disorder, and Generalized Anxiety Disorder Among Young Israeli Adults*

Disorder	Rate	SE
Major depressive disorder		
Probable and definite	5.6	0.62
Definite only	4.0	0.52
Minor depressive disorder		
Probable and definite	2.6	0.40
Definite only†	2.2	0.38
Generalized anxiety disorder		
Probable and definite	7.9	1.16
Definite only	4.6	0.65

*RDC indicates Research Diagnostic Criteria.
†For minor depression, definite only, both probable and definite major depressive disorder are excluded.

SEVERITY OF MINOR DEPRESSION SYMPTOMS

Scores on the PERI symptom scales were compared for individuals with major and minor depressive disorder and GAD. As the results shown in **Table 2** indicate, except for antisocial history and problems due to drinking, those with major depressive disorder reported more severe symptoms than those with minor depressive disorder. Respondents with minor depressive disorder were similar to respondents with GAD except for more suicidal thoughts.

In keeping with the view that minor depressive disorder may be a symptomatically similar but less severe form of major depressive disorder, we compared the two groups on the eight symptoms of major depressive disorder, which are also the first eight of the 16 minor depressive symptoms in the RDC, as scored from the SADS-I diagnostic interviews. Those with major depressive disorder (probable plus definite) had a median number of 4.5 major symp-

Table 2. Comparison of Young Israeli Adults With Major Depressive Disorder, Minor Depressive Disorder, and Generalized Anxiety Disorder on Symptom Scales of the PERI*

	RDC Disorder				
				Planned Contrasts: *P*	
Symptom Scale	Major Depressive (A), Mean±SD	Minor Depressive (B), Mean±SD	Generalized Anxiety (C), Mean±SD	B vs A	B vs C
Demoralization	1.57±0.69	1.13±0.56	1.16±0.55	<.01	NS
Anxiety subscale	1.95±0.82	1.47±0.75	1.41±0.82	<.01	NS
Antisocial history	0.61±0.75	0.49±0.65	0.44±0.63	NS	NS
Problems due to drinking	0.07±0.24	0.05±0.26	0.04±0.19	NS	NS
False beliefs and perceptions	0.64±0.61	0.39±0.42	0.31±0.35	<.01	NS
Enervation	1.70±0.82	1.23±0.75	1.22±0.78	<.01	NS
Schizoid features	1.22±0.65	1.04±0.63	1.02±0.62	<.05	NS
Suicidal ideation	0.65±1.24	0.38±0.95	0.16±0.66	<.05	<.05

*PERI indicates Psychiatric Epidemiology Research Interview; RDC, Research Diagnostic Criteria; and NS, not significant.

toms compared with only 1.5 for those with minor depression (probable plus definite). However, substantial proportions of those with minor depressive disorder had reported symptoms of major depressive disorder. Overall, 68% of those with minor depression had one or two major symptoms and 24% had more than two. Only 8% had no symptom of major depressive disorder. Among those with minor depression, appetite change was rated as present by the psychiatrists for 47.8%, anhedonia for 42.2%, sleep change for 38.2%, and decreased concentration for 35.2%. Respondents with minor depressive disorder were scored as having low rates of suicidal ideation (3.0%), guilt (3.1%), psychomotor change (6.6%), and loss of energy (16.3%). The large majority (80%) of persons with definite minor depressive disorder who failed to meet criteria for probable major depressive disorder had one or two major symptoms less than required. The majority (61%) of persons with probable major depressive disorder had one symptom too few for definite. Virtually equal proportions of both groups (approximately 25%) were judged to have symptoms of anxiety.

Course

The median age at first onset of major depression (26 years) was significantly younger than for minor depres-

Table 3. Psychosocial Functioning Among Young Israeli Adults With Major Depressive Disorder, Minor Depressive Disorder, or Generalized Anxiety Disorder and Controls (N=2719)

	Diagnostic Groups									
	Major Depressive Disorder (n=212)*			Minor Depressive Disorder (n=98)			Generalized Anxiety Disorder (n=222)			
Variable	%†	OR‡	95% CI§	%	OR	95% CI	%	OR	95% CI	Controls, % (n=2187)
Quality of teenage social life										
Superior or very good	16.4	5.15	2.43-10.89‖	36.7	1.52	0.52-4.45	27.7	1.04	0.34-3.18	37.0
Good or fair	75.5	1.98	0.98-3.99	58.0	1.67	0.68-4.07	69.8	0.67	0.37-1.18	60.0
Poor and/or grossly inadequate	8.1	. . .		5.3	. . .		2.5	. . .		3.0
Personality disorder										
Antisocial	6.9	4.43	1.89-10.39‖	2.8	1.73	0.52-5.73	1.8	1.40	0.51-3.82	1.5
Schizotypal	13.7	2.53	1.41-4.56‖	8.1	1.48	0.67-3.26	9.8	1.93	0.96-3.89	5.4
Labile	13.6	2.62	1.45-4.75‖	1.4	0.25	0.05-1.17	5.6	1.12	0.55-2.29	5.1
Best level of social relations in past 5 y										
Superior or very good	25.2	3.60	1.61-8.05‖	41.9	1.05	0.20-5.50	28.3	1.19	0.40-3.55	43.7
Good or fair	64.9	1.77	0.85-3.68	53.2	1.06	0.22-5.07	68.5	0.55	0.19-1.60	51.4
Poor, very poor, or grossly inadequate	9.9	. . .		4.9	. . .		6.1	. . .		4.9
Work										
Working, student, housewife	65.7	. . .		79.2	. . .		87.9	. . .		90.2
Absence, past 5 y, <6 mo	17.1	3.74	2.04-6.86‖	13.9	2.61	1.12-6.10‖	10.1	1.85	0.92-3.75	5.9
Absence, past 5 y, >6 mo	17.2	5.10	2.68-9.71‖	6.9	1.83	0.81-4.17	2.0	0.58	0.25-1.37	4.0
Marital status										
Single	25.0	3.67	2.05-6.58‖	13.9	1.59	0.71-3.56	5.5	0.54	0.23-1.26	10.1
Married/widowed	58.0	. . .		71.6	. . .		88.4	. . .		84.7
Divorced/separated	17.0	4.53	2.34-8.75‖	14.6	3.32	1.51-7.27‖	6.1	1.13	0.51-2.48	5.2
Worst overall functioning past month										
No or few problems	13.0	. . .		17.4	. . .		18.7	. . .		58.3
Some problems	34.9	22.64	12.02-42.65‖	59.8	8.25	3.85-17.64‖	64.7	6.68	3.05-14.38‖	33.1
Significant decline in functioning	52.1	4.44	2.26-8.69‖	22.8	5.87	2.73-12.63‖	16.6	6.29	2.90-13.68‖	8.6
Ever made suicide attempt	13.2	3.06	1.64-5.73‖	3.8	1.08	0.36-3.27	2.6	0.82	0.39-1.70	3.4

**Unweighted Ns.*
†Percentages are uncontrolled.
‡OR indicates odds ratios, which for quality of teenage social life and best level of social relations in past 5 years are expressed as control:disorder. All other odds ratios are expressed as disorder:control. All odds ratios are adjusted for gender and ethnicity.
§CI indicates confidence interval.
‖P≤.05.

sive disorder (28 years) or GAD (28 years) (*P*<.001). There was no difference in median length of the longest episode (approximately 20 weeks). Only 7% of respondents diagnosed as having minor depression had an episode with a duration of greater than 2 years. The rate of recurrence was 50.1 among those with major depressive disorder compared with 31.4 among those with minor depressive disorder.

Functioning

Table 3 depicts the relationships between measures of psychosocial functioning in diverse areas at diverse times in the lives of the respondents and each of the three target disorders. Persons with minor depressive disorder or GAD and controls have distinctly better social functioning in early life than those with major depressive disorder. Few persons with major depressive disorder were judged by the research psychiatrists to have had superior or very good levels of quality of teenage social life, while approximately one third of each of the other diagnostic groups and of controls were rated as such. The odds for controls having superior or very good quality of teenage social life are more than five times higher than the odds for respondents with major depressive disorder. Research Diagnostic Criteria personality disorders with *DSM-III-R* counterparts (ie, labile, antisocial, and schizotypal) are more common among those with major depression; no rates differ between respondents with minor depression or GAD and controls. In terms of overall best level of social relations in the past 5 years, those with major depression, but not the other two disorders, report considerable social impairment. The odds for controls having superior or very good functioning in the past 5 years are 3.6 times higher than the odds for persons with major depression.

For work history, marital status, and overall functioning, impairment is very evident for respondents with major depression. Respondents with minor depression, however, also have significantly elevated rates of absence from work due to psychological problems for less than 6 months of the preceding 5 years, separation or divorce, and at least some problems and a significant decrease in functioning during the past month, compared with controls. The odds of persons with minor depression missing work for less than 6 months are 2.6 times higher, the odds of being divorced or separated are 3.2 times higher, and the odds of having a significant decline in functioning in the past month are almost six times higher than the odds for controls. Persons with GAD also have significant impairment in functioning in the past month. Only those with major depression have an increased rate of lifetime suicide attempts. There were no differences found in military history.

Help Seeking

Subjects with minor depression and those with major depression seek help from some professional (ie, medical doctor, clergy) more often than controls (**Table 4**). However, only those with major depression have elevated rates of psychiatric hospitalization and seek help from mental health professionals more than do controls.

DISTINCTIVENESS OF MINOR DEPRESSION FROM MAJOR DEPRESSION AND GAD DEMOGRAPHIC CORRELATES

Table 5 shows the demographic characteristics of persons in each diagnostic group and of the control group consisting of all persons in the sample other than those with one of these three diagnoses. Major depressive disorder and minor depressive disorder were more common among female subjects compared with the control population, but the strongest and only significant association was for major depressive disorder. Although subjects with major depression were younger than those with GAD or controls, people with minor depression fell in between and did not

Table 4. Help-Seeking by Young Israeli Adults With Major Depressive Disorder, Minor Depressive Disorder, or Generalized Anxiety Disorder and Controls (N=2719)

	Diagnostic Groups									
	Major Depressive Disorder (n=212)*			Minor Depressive Disorder (n=98)			Generalized Anxiety Disorder (n=222)			
Variable	%†	OR‡	95% CI§	%	OR	95% CI	%	OR	95% CI	Controls, % (n=2187)
Ever hospitalized	9.1	4.26	1.86-9.75‖	1.6	1.50	0.38-5.95	0.6	0.27	0.05-1.46	2.3
Sought help	36.1	1.63	1.07-2.48‖	43.6	2.25	1.22-4.15‖	33.2	1.45	0.82-2.54	25.6
Sought help from mental health professional	25.4	1.81	1.17-2.81‖	22.7	1.54	0.84-2.82	20.8	1.36	0.80-2.33	16.1

*Unweighted Ns.
†Percentages are uncontrolled.
‡OR indicates odds ratios, which are expressed as disorder:control. All odds ratios are adjusted for gender and ethnicity.
§CI indicates confidence interval.
‖$P \leq .05$.

Table 5. Demographic Characteristics of Young Israeli Adults With Major Depressive Disorder, Minor Depressive Disorder, or Generalized Anxiety Disorder at the Probable Plus Definite Levels and of Controls (N=2719)

	Diagnostic Groups									
	Major Depressive Disorder (n=212)*			Minor Depressive Disorder (n=98)			Generalized Anxiety Disorder (n=222)			
Characteristic	%†	OR‡	95% CI§	%	OR	95% CI	%	OR	95% CI	Controls, % (n=2187)
Sex										
Male	38.9	...		44.9	...		51.2	...		51.1
Female	61.1	1.65	1.05-2.60‖	55.1	1.29	0.69-2.42	48.8	0.99	0.52-1.89	48.9
Mean age, y	30.4	0.92	0.86-0.98‖	31.1	0.95	0.89-1.01	32.3	1.05	0.95-1.82	31.9
Ethnicity										
European	41.1	...		54.4	...		72.2	...		67.2
North African	58.9	2.94	1.88-4.60‖	45.6	1.72	0.90-3.29	27.8	0.79	0.47-1.30	32.8
Education										
Less than high school	30.9	2.17	0.95-4.94	36.6	1.73	0.58-5.12	23.1	2.00	0.63-6.40	23.5
High school graduate	63.2	2.64	1.26-5.56‖	49.4	1.07	0.41-2.84	65.2	2.01	0.65-6.21	57.4
College graduate	5.9	...		14.0	...		11.7	...		19.1

*Unweighted Ns.
†Percentages are uncontrolled.
‡OR indicates odds ratios, which are expressed as disorder:control. All odds ratios are adjusted for gender and ethnicity.
§CI indicates confidence interval.
‖$P \leq .05$.

differ significantly from those in the other diagnostic groups. Major depressive disorder was more common among Israelis of North African descent as opposed to European descent. Respondents with major depression were less likely to be college graduates than controls.

Lifetime Overlap

Lifetime overlap of disorders was examined in cases and controls. As noted earlier, case groups excluded persons who met criteria for more than one of the disorders of interest in the year prior to interview. Approximately 20% of respondents with year-prevalent minor depression or GAD and 17% of controls had lifetime major depression. Twelve percent of the case group with year-prevalent major depression, approximately 15% of the case group with GAD, and 11% of controls had lifetime diagnoses of minor depression. Approximately 6% of those with major depression, 7.5% with minor depression, and almost 12% of controls had lifetime GAD. The only significant difference between the case groups and controls was for the rate of lifetime GAD among those with year-prevalent major depression (5.8%) compared with controls (11.8%) (odds ratio=0.47, 95% confidence interval=0.24 to 0.89). Lifetime rates of major depression, minor depression, and GAD were not different among the relevant case groups.

EFFECT OF CORMORBIDITY

Only respondents with major depressive disorder had elevated rates of comorbid, year-prevalent RDC disorders compared with the base rates of other RDC disorders in the controls (47.0 vs 20.1; odds ratio=3.00; 95% confidence interval=1.89 to 4.76). Controlling for comorbidity reduced the size of the relationships between major depressive disorder and the functioning and help-seeking variables somewhat, but only two previously significant relationships became nonsignificant: general help-seeking and seeking help from a mental health professional. The overall effect of controlling for comorbidity was to reduce the differences between major depressive disorder and the other two case groups, but even with the added control, major depressive disorder remained more distinct from GAD than from minor depressive disorder. In fact, with comorbidity controlled, the only significant differences in functioning and help-seeking between the two depressed groups were that respondents with major depression had more often been in a psychiatric hospital and had more often made a suicide attempt than respondents with minor depresslon.

COMMENT

In the analyses in this report, we have focused on disorders present during the 1-year period prior to the SADS-I interview. From our prevalence rate comparisons, it is clear that minor depression, as defined by RDC, is not ubiquitous. Minor depressive disorder was found to be less prevalent than either RDC major depressive disorder or RDC GAD. Our 1-year prevalence rate of minor depressive disorder is somewhat lower than that found by Faravelli and Incerpi[24] across a representative age range of subjects in Florence, Italy, but it is similar to those de-

scribed by Merikangas et al,[12] which were obtained in later waves of the Zurich Cohort Study of Young Adults in a comparable age group. Elsewhere[25] we have shown that our rates of prevalence of disorder at the time of interview for major and minor depressive disorders do not differ substantially from those found in other community surveys conducted in the United States that have employed the SADS/RDC system.[26,27]

In contrast to our results, investigators using other diagnostic definitions have found that minor depression was more common than major.[10,11] This may in part be owing to the fact that RDC minor depressive disorder requires evidence of impairment or help-seeking (see also below). It is reasonable to expect that symptoms severe enough to meet criteria for major depressive disorder will be more likely to be associated with dysfunction than symptoms at the minor level. Relatively speaking, a greater proportion of persons with minor symptoms will be free of impairment than will those with major symptoms.

Minor depression, like GAD and in contrast to major depressive disorder, occurred in persons with relatively good early social adjustment. This relationship held true for quality of social life during the teen years, best overall level of social relations in the 5 years prior to interview, and absence of RDC personality disorder. Minor depressive disorder, major depressive disorder, and GAD are all associated with evidence of impairment in overall functioning. In contrast to GAD, however, minor and major depressive disorders were associated with specific impairment in marital functioning, as indicated by an association with divorce and with absence from work because of psychological problems. As might be expected, longer absences from work (ie, >6 months missed over the past 5 years) were associated only with the more severe major depressive disorder. These findings are consistent with those found by Broadhead et al[10] that subthreshold depressions may result in significant occupational disability.

In this study, we found that persons with minor depression and GAD were rarely hospitalized, compared with those with major depression, consistent with their less severe illnesses, at least to date. People with minor depression appeared to seek help for their disturbances at approximately the same rate as those with major depression, but they did not go as frequently to mental health professionals as those with major depression (although this difference was not significant). These findings are consistent with the general clinical and epidemiologic impressions that persons with minor depression are seen by caregivers other than psychiatrists and psychologists, most likely by primary care providers and nonmedical counselors and advisers.

In its differential associations with female gender and North African ethnicity, minor depressive disorder falls between major depressive disorder and GAD. Those with minor depression tend to be disproportionately female and North African, like those with major depression, but not to such a degree that they are significantly different from controls. The GAD group has the same proportion of females and North Africans as the controls.

Two additional points should be kept in mind in considering these results. First, the requirement by most RDC diagnoses that the disturbances result in impairment in functioning with family, at home, at school, at work, socially, in taking medication, or in seeking or being referred for help from someone may suggest a potential for circularity in a study using impairment or help-seeking variables to validate a diagnostic category. To minimize the potential for circular reasoning, we employed two comparison groups of patients with major depression and GAD, in addition to a control group. Since the diagnostic criteria for these two reference groups also require impairment or help-seeking, the relative impact of minor depressive disorder could still be assessed.

Second, in the logistic regression analyses presented in the tables, we controlled for gender and ethnicity, but not for comorbid mental disorder. Since not all RDC diagnoses are mutually exclusive, the possibility exists that an association with a variable measuring functioning may be influenced by a disorder that is comorbid with major or minor depressive disorder. Our control group, however, consists of all subjects in the sample other than those with major or minor depressive disorder or GAD.[28] Thus, comorbid diagnoses are distributed throughout the case and control samples. Also, to whatever extent comorbid diagnoses contribute to the relationships found, they contribute in their associations with the disorders under study.

FURTHERMORE, SINCE gender and ethnicity clearly precede disorder onset, relationships between diagnostic groups and functioning variables that were due to gender or ethnic differences would be confounded. Unlike gender and ethnicity, however, comorbid disorder may not lie outside the chain of causation between disorder and impact on functioning. Our analyses of the effects of comorbidity showed that associations between major depressive disorder and functioning and help-seeking variables become somewhat weaker. This suggests that comorbidity may be a proxy for severity and that controlling for comorbidity simply removed the impact of severity differentials among the case groups and between the case and control groups.

The results we have presented provide ammunition for those who advocated including minor depression in *DSM-IV* and for those who did not. An argument for including a diagnosis of minor depression may be mustered from the data that suggest that levels of impairment and help-seeking associated with minor depres-

sive disorder are comparable to those associated with GAD, a version of which will be in *DSM-IV*. Since the associations are considerably weaker for these two diagnoses compared with major depressive disorder, however, perhaps GAD should instead have been deleted.

As mentioned earlier, according to RDC, only anxious mood plus one other symptom (plus impairment or help-seeking) present for at least 2 weeks are required for a diagnosis of GAD, making it a mild disorder. And in fact, the evolution of the concept of GAD from RDC to *DSM-III* to *DSM-III-R* reveals a concern with redefining the criteria to increase the clinical significance of the disorder. In *DSM-III*, the number of symptoms required was increased to three and the minimum duration was set at 1 month. By *DSM-III-R*, the symptom level had risen to six and the duration had extended to 6 months. Similar concerns for clinical significance would have accompanied the addition of minor depression to *DSM-IV*. The number of symptoms required could have been set closer to the threshold of major depression (three or four symptoms, for example) or the duration extended to 1 month (or more) to eliminate time-limited disturbances that probably should be treated conservatively, if at all.

IT IS POSSIBLE, on the other hand, that minor depression represents a stage or phase of a generic depressive illness rather than a distinct category. This is suggested by its similarity to major depression in demographic correlates and in levels of functional impairment when comorbidity was controlled. Clinically, we also found that minor depression appeared to be a milder version of major depression with many of the same symptoms, but at a lesser frequency and severity. The clustering of major symptom counts around the diagnostic thresholds for definite minor, probable major, and definite major depressive disorders is consistent with a continuum of depressive psychopathology. The course data indicated some lifetime overlap between major and minor disorders. The degree of overlap may be greater than we found because persons with two or more major depressive episodes are not given a past diagnosis of minor depression (even if warranted) according to RDC. Thus, some earlier-onset, past minor depressions may have been missed. Broadhead et al[10] reported that almost 40% of persons in the North Carolina Epidemiologic Catchment Area study who had major depression on initial evaluation had remissions to the level of minor depression within a 1-year follow-up. Horwath et al[29] found that subclinical depressive symptoms were a strong predictor of the development of first-onset major depression over a 1-year period. Coryell et al[30] found that the presence of minor depression doubled the risk for relapse into a new episode of major depression over a 6-year period in a nonclinical population with a history of major depression. These data on course and our findings of symptom similarity suggest that at least for some persons, the syndromes of major and minor depression represent stages of a depressive illness that fluctuates in severity over time. Ormel et al[31] have recently documented the synchrony over time between the severity level of depressive (and anxiety) symptoms and the amount of disability experienced.

If major and minor symptom pictures are stages in a unitary illness, an option to adding a diagnosis of minor depression to *DSM-IV* would have been to expand the severity modifiers already present in *DSM-III-R* to capture more of the longitudinal variability in depressive disorders. As proposed by Mezzich and Sullivan,[32] a system of diagnostic modifiers referring to symptom severity at various stages of illness could have been made uniform across the diagnostic classification. Now in *DSM-III-R*, severity modifiers can be specified for any disorder to indicate that the disturbance is mild (but still above diagnostic threshold), moderate, severe, in partial remission or residual state, or in full remission. Some disorders, such as major depression, have slightly modified versions of the generic severity rating. Most notably absent is a designation for subthreshold or subclinical depressive disorder to capture early, potentially developing major depression. If, as Horwath et al[29] find, 50% of the attributable risk of first-episode major depression in the community is accounted for by depressive symptoms in the preceding year, early identification provides an opportunity for possible preventive intervention.

In the *DSM-IV Options Book*,[14] a proposal was made to differentiate three types of subthreshold cases: (1) persons in partial remission; (2) persons experiencing partial relapse after a period of full remission; and (3) persons in whom a condition was developing for the first time that was at a subsyndromal level of severity. These designations could have been integrated into the *DSM-IV* severity rating. Although familiarity and comfort with the use of diagnostic modifiers do not come easily to clinicians trained to think of disorders as concrete and specific entities, the use of a multiaxial designation for severity may depict more accurately the clinical reality of depressive illness than would the addition of yet another diagnostic category without sufficient distinctiveness.

The final decision for *DSM-IV* was to list minor depression as one of the examples of depressive disorder not otherwise specified. Suggested criteria appear in an appendix and are identical to criteria for major depressive episode except that only two to four depressive symptoms are present. Severity modifiers do not include a subthreshold designation and apply only to subjects who at some time have met full criteria for a major depressive episode.

Additional research is required to determine whether unipolar depression is a unitary illness, fluctuating in symptom severity and associated impairment, or whether it can be subdivided into discrete subtypes. For ex-

ample, demonstration that major and minor depression shared similar risk factors or long-term prognosis would weigh heavily on the side of a single disorder. Included in our future plans are analyses of life events, situational contexts, personality traits, and family history of mental disorders from an independent risk factor interview, in a case-control design. From these studies, we anticipate more evidence bearing on the validity of the diagnosis of minor depression.

Accepted for publication January 20, 1994.

This study was supported in part by grants MH30710 and MH30906-12 from the National Institute of Mental Health, Rockville, Md.

Read before the 144th Annual Meeting of the American Psychiatric Association, New Orleans, La, May 14, 1991.

Reprint requests to New York State Psychiatric Institute, 722 W 168th St, New York, NY 10032 (Dr Skodol).

REFERENCES

1. Shepherd M, Cooper B, Brown AC, Kalton GW. *Psychiatric Illness in General Practice.* London, England: Oxford University Press; 1966.
2. Hoeper EW, Nycz GR, Cleary PD, Regier DA, Goldberg ID. Estimated prevalence of RDC mental disorder in primary medical care. *Int J Ment Health.* 1979; 8:6-15.
3. Kessler LG, Cleary PD, Burke JD Jr. Psychiatric disorders in primary care: results of a follow-up study. *Arch Gen Psychiatry.* 1985;42:583-587.
4. Blacker CVR, Clare AW. Depressive disorder in primary care. *Br J Psychiatry.* 1987;150:737-751.
5. Barrett JE, Barrett JA, Oxman TE, Gerber PD. The prevalence of psychiatric disorders in a primary care practice. *Arch Gen Psychiatry.* 1988;45:1100-1106.
6. Ormel J, Koether MWJ, van den Brink W, van de Willige G. Recognition, management, and course of anxiety and depression in general practice. *Arch Gen Psychiatry.* 1991;48:700-706.
7. Boyd JH, Weissman MM. Epidemiology of affective disorders. *Arch Gen Psychiatry.* 1981;38:1039-1046.
8. Blazer D, Swartz M, Woodbury M, Manton KG, Hughes D, George LK. Depressive symptoms and depressive diagnoses in a community population: use of a new procedure for analysis of psychiatric classification. *Arch Gen Psychiatry.* 1988;45:1078-1084.
9. Bebbington P, Katz R, McGuffin P, Tennant C, Hurry J. The risk of minor depression before age 65: results from a community survey. *Psychol Med.* 1989; 19:393-400.
10. Broadhead WE, Blazer DG, George LK, Tse CK. Depression, disability days, and days lost from work in a prospective epidemiologic survey. *JAMA.* 1990; 264:2524-2528.
11. Johnson J, Weissman MM, Klerman GL. Service utilization and social morbidity associated with depressive symptoms in the community. *JAMA.* 1992; 267:1478-1483.
12. Merikangas KR, Ernst C, Maier W, Hoyer EB, Angst J. Minor depression: prospects for *DSM-IV.* In: Widiger TA, Frances A, Pincus H, First MB, Ross R, Davis WW, eds. *DSM-IV Source Book.* Washington, DC: American Psychiatric Press. In press.
13. Wells KB, Stewart A, Hayes RD. The functioning and well-being of depressed patients: results of the Medical Outcomes Study. *JAMA.* 1989;262:914-919.
14. American Psychiatric Association Task Force on *DSM-IV. DSM-IV Options Book.* Washington, DC: American Psychiatric Association; 1991.
15. Spitzer RL, Endicott J, Robins E. Research Diagnostic Criteria: rationale and reliability. *Arch Gen Psychiatry.* 1978;35:773-782.
16. American Psychiatric Association Task Force on *DSM-IV. DSM-IV Draft Criteria.* Washington, DC: American Psychiatric Association; 1993.
17. Dohrenwend BP, Levav I, Shrout PE, Schwartz S, Naveh G, Link BG, Skodol AE, Stueve A. Socioeconomic status and psychiatric disorders: the causation-selection issue. *Science.* 1992;255:946-952.
18. Dohrenwend BP, Shrout PE, Egri G, Mendelsohn FS. Measures of nonspecific psychological distress and other dimensions of psychopathology in the general population. *Arch Gen Psychiatry.* 1980;37:1229-1236.
19. Shrout PE, Dohrenwend BP, Levav I. A discriminant rule for screening cases of diverse diagnostic types: preliminary results. *J Consult Clin Psychol.* 1986; 54:314-319.
20. Endicott J, Spitzer RL. A diagnostic interview: the Schedule for Affective Disorders and Schizophrenia. *Arch Gen Psychiatry.* 1978;35:837-844.
21. Gibbon M, MacDonald-Scott P, Endicott J. Mastering the art of research interviewing: a model training procedure for diagnostic evaluation. *Arch Gen Psychiatry.* 1981;38:1259-1262.
22. Hidroglow MA, Fuller WA, Hickman R. *SUPERCARP.* 6th ed. Ames, Iowa: Iowa State University; 1975.
23. Schlesselman JJ. *Case Control Studies: Desiqn, Conduct, Analysis.* New York, NY: Oxford University Press Inc; 1982:267-269.
24. Faravelli G, Incerpi G. Epidemiology of affective disorders in Florence. *Acta Psychiatr Scand.* 1985;72:331-333.
25. Levav I, Kohn R, Dohrenwend BP, Shrout PE, Skodol AE, Schwartz S, Link BG, Naveh G. An epidemiologic study of mental disorders in a 10-year cohort of young adults in Israel. *Psychol Med.* 1993;23:691-707.
26. Weissman MM, Myers JK. Affective disorders in a US urban community: the use of Research Diagnostic Criteria in an epidemiological survey. *Arch Gen Psychiatry.* 1978;35:98-111.
27. Vernon SW, Roberts RE. Use of SADS-RDC in a tri-ethnic community survey. *Arch Gen Psychiatry.* 1982;39:47-52.
28. Schwartz S, Link BG. The 'well control' artifact in case/control studies of specific psychiatric disorders. *Psychol Med.* 1989;19:737-742.
29. Horwath E, Johnson J, Klerman GL, Weissman MM. Depressive symptoms as relative and attributable risk factors for first-onset major depression. *Arch Gen Psychiatry.* 1992;49:817-823.
30. Coryell W, Endicott J, Keller MB. Predictors of relapse into major depressive disorder in a nonclinical population. *Am J Psychiatry.* 1991;148:1353-1358.
31. Ormel J, Von Korff M, van den Brink W, Katon W, Brilman E, Oldehinkel T. Depression, anxiety and social disability in primary care show synchrony of change. *Am J Public Health.* 1993;83:385-390.
32. Mezzich JE, Sullivan PF. On measuring syndromic severity: a review paper for *DSM-IV.* In: Widiger TA, Frances A, Pincus H, First MB, Ross R, Davis WW, eds. *DSM-IV Source Book.* Washington, DC: American Psychiatric Press. In press.

Impaired Autonomic Nervous System Habituation in Those at Genetic Risk for Schizophrenia

J. Meggin Hollister, MA; Sarnoff A. Mednick, PhD, DrMed; Patricia Brennan, PhD; Tyrone D. Cannon, PhD

Background: Schizophrenia has been associated with habituation of skin conductance activity. Skin conductance data from the Copenhagen High Risk Project were analyzed. We hypothesized that genetic risk for schizophrenia and development of schizophrenia later in life are related to impaired habituation of autonomic nervous system activity.

Methods: Data were collected in 1962, when subjects averaged 15 years of age and had not yet qualified for a psychiatric diagnosis. Nonspecific fluctuations in electrodermal activity were monitored during a rest period free of sensory stimulation.

Results: We found that an increasing level of genetic risk for schizophrenia was related to impaired habituation of autonomic nervous system activity over time. Individuals with two schizophrenia-spectrum parents evidenced no habituation, those with one spectrum parent evidenced some habituation, and those with normal parents evidenced rapid habituation. Subjects who developed schizophrenia in adulthood evidenced significant deficits in habituation in adolescence.

Conclusions: These results suggest that impaired habituation of spontaneous autonomic nervous system activity may represent a behavioral marker of the genetic predisposition to schizophrenia.

(Arch Gen Psychiatry. 1994;51:552-558)

When schizophrenics describe how they experience their disability, they emphasize the difficulty they have in tuning out (habituating to) incidental, nontarget stimuli that nonschizophrenics can successfully ignore. This failure of habituation may contribute to the attentional disturbances of schizophrenia. In research settings, schizophrenics evidence impaired habituation in startle reflex[1-3] and skin conductance[4-8] paradigms. Autonomic conditioning studies of children with schizophrenic parents have also reported habituation deficits.[9,10] Twin studies have demonstrated that autonomic habituation (in humans) is strongly influenced by genetic factors.[11,12] It is possible that the habituation deficit is a part of the genetically transmitted predisposition to schizophrenia.

The precise determinants of impaired autonomic nervous system habituation have not been established. Neuroanatomic substrates implicated in studies of skin conductance orienting are the prefrontal,[13] pons, left temporal/amygdala regions,[14,15] and the hippocampus.[15-17] Other alternative mechanisms by which habituation may be affected include psychological factors, such as expressed emotion.

Using data collected as part of the Copenhagen High Risk Project, we examined habituation of autonomic nervous system activity in adolescents at three levels of genetic predisposition to schizophrenia: super high risk (SHR; both parents with schizophrenia-spectrum diagnoses), high risk (HR; one parent with a schizophrenia-spectrum diagnosis), and low risk (LR; neither parent with a schizophrenia-spectrum diagnosis). Electroder-

From the Social Science Research Institute, University of Southern California, Los Angeles (Ms Hollister and Drs Mednick and Brennan); and Department of Psychology, University of Pennsylvania, Philadelphia (Dr Cannon).

See Subjects and Methods on next page

SUBJECTS AND METHODS

SUBJECT SELECTION

Risk Group Classification

Mednick and Schulsinger[18,19] initiated the Copenhagen High Risk Project in 1962 to identify antecedents of schizophrenia. Subjects were classified by their genetic risk for schizophrenia. The study included 207 subjects in the HR group (offspring of schizophrenic mothers) and 104 subjects in the LR group (no history of hospitalization for mental illness in parents or grandparents) who were matched for sex, age, social class, and years of education (**Table 1**).[18,19] An HR mother was required to have a diagnosis of schizophrenia according to the *International Classification of Diseases, Eighth Revision,* and 5 years of psychiatric hospitalization or at least three separate hospitalizations of 3 months or more, or an extended hospitalization plus a State Invalid Pension for Schizophrenia.[18] Jorgensen et al[20] reexamined the HR mothers according to *DSM-III* criteria in 1987. They obtained hospital journals from all psychiatric admissions of the mothers up to 1975. Consequently, the rediagnoses included considerably more information than was available in 1962. After the rediagnosis, 92% of the HR mothers fulfilled *DSM-III-R* criteria for schizophrenia. (In the Jorgensen article [published before *DSM-III-R*], 10 women were diagnosed as having atypical psychosis [*DSM-III*]. They met the criteria for schizophenia except for their age at onset. By *DSM-III-R* criteria, these women were diagnosed as schizophrenic.) The remaining 8% of mothers had the following diagnoses: schizophreniform, three; schizoaffective, two; schizoaffective followed by major depression, one; paranoid, three; and obsessive-compulsive disorder followed by personality disorder, not otherwise specified, one. The original 1962 diagnoses were conservative; almost all mothers later met *DSM-III-R* diagnostic criteria. The children of the entire group of mothers diagnosed as schizophrenic in 1962 were retained for analyses to maintain comparability with previous reports on this sample.

A diagnostic study of the HR subjects' biologic fathers was conducted in 1980 through 1983.[21] Paternity was established by one or both of the following: the mother identified the father as the marital partner at time of conception, or the man was named on the child's birth certificate. Paternity was not verified through blood tests. Psychiatric hospital records were obtained on all fathers. Furthermore, all living fathers were asked to accept a home interview by a psychiatrist, which consisted of the Schedule for Affective Disorders and Schizophrenia–Lifetime Version,[22] characterologic items from the Current and Past Psychopathology Scales,[23] and the Schizophrenic Spectrum Schedule (developed by Ronald O. Rieder, MD). The paternal diagnosis was based on the interview and available case records according to Research Diagnostic Criteria /*DSM-III* criteria. If a father had a diagnosis in the schizophrenia spectrum (ie, schizophrenia, schizotypal personality disorder, or paranoid personality disorder), the children were assigned to the SHR group. Of the 207 HR subjects, 30 were found to have fathers with spectrum-disorder diagnoses, and 175 subjects were found to have fathers without spectrum-disorder diagnoses (two HR subjects were missing paternal psychiatric information). Therefore, the SHR group and the HR group consisted of 30 and 175 subjects, respectively. As indicated above, there were 104 subjects in the LR group.

Outcome Classification

Subjects were classified in one of three outcome groups: schizophrenia (SZ), other mental illness (OMI), and no mental illness (NMI). Recently, more than 90% of the original sample of SHR, HR, and LR subjects were reexamined by a psychiatrist.[24] The interviewer was unaware of the results of the previous psychiatric assessments and administered the Schedule for Affective Disorders and Schizophrenia–Lifetime Version,[22] the Present State Examination, the Present State Examination lifetime ratings of psychotic symptoms, the Present State Examination Syndrome Checklist[25] for current and lifetime psychopathology, the Scales for the Assessment of Positive and Negative Symptoms,[26,27] and the Personality Disorder Examination.[28] Diagnoses of the subjects were established according to *DSM-III-R* criteria.

A total of eight SHR, 23 HR, and two LR subjects received lifetime diagnoses of schizophrenia.[24] The SZ group was composed of the eight SHR subjects and the 23 HR subjects with lifetime diagnoses of schizophrenia. The two LR subjects who developed schizophrenia were not included in the analyses because they were not included in our "genetic risk" category. All subjects, regardless of risk group, who received a primary Axis I diagnosis of unipolar depression, bipolar depression, delusion disorder, schizophreniform disorder, atypical psychosis, alcohol abuse, drug

Continued on next page

mal activity was recorded for all the subjects in 1962. (Although much of the data from the electrodermal experimental sessions of the High Risk Project have been reported previously, data from a rest period preceding the experimental sessions were scored and analyzed for the first time for this study.) The first 15 minutes of the recording session was designated as a rest period in which the experimenter withdrew and no experimenter-controlled stimuli were presented. Under such conditions, spontaneous fluctuations in skin conductance, or nonspecific responses (NSRs), are usually observed.

The rate of NSRs has been shown to decline over time in normal subjects. This pattern of response can be interpreted as autonomic habituation to one's surrounding static environment or to one's internal stimuli. In this study, habituation of subjects was measured by a de-

abuse, and organic brain syndrome were combined into the OMI group. The NMI group was composed of all subjects, regardless of risk group, with no sign of psychopathology as assessed by the interviewing psychiatrist.

INSTRUMENTATION AND PROCEDURES

Electrodermal response measures were taken in 1962 when the children were at a mean age of 15.1 years (range, 10 to 19 years) in a 50-minute morning session that consisted of a rest period followed by an experimental period. The psychophysiology laboratory was located in a light- and sound-attenuated room in the Kommunehospitalet, Copenhagen, Denmark. After washing and alcohol swabbing at points of electrode placement, the subject was asked to relax in a reclining position on a hospital bed. Two zinc Beckman cup electrodes, 7 mm in diameter (with sponges soaked in a zinc sulfate solution), were attached to the left hand of each subject to record electrodermal activity by means of a polygraph.

Electrodermal recording commenced 5 to 10 minutes after electrode placement and was performed continuously until the conclusion of the session. The first 90 seconds of the rest period were used to establish calibration. Therefore, data collection for the rest period commenced after a 6.5- to 11.5-minute hydration period. The subject was permitted to relax for 13.5 minutes (rest period) before experimental procedures began.[18] The examiner remained still and out of sight of the subject. He noted any movement on the part of the subject and any noises that occurred in the laboratory. At the conclusion of the rest period, earphones were attached and the subject listened to instructions informing him or her of the procedure to follow. After a 70-second silent period after the instructions, eight presentations of a 1000-Hz, 54-dB tone occurred at intervals from 17 to 77 seconds to provide information about the subject's electrodermal orienting response. Any responses that occurred immediately after noises in the laboratory or movement on the part of the subject were noted by the examiner and not scored.

SCORING PROCEDURE

The rest period was divided into three blocks of 270 seconds each. An NSR was defined as a drop of 2.0% or more from the preceding resistance level.[29] The mean number of NSRs for each block was computed. The NSR frequency was calculated as the sum of the NSRs across the three blocks for each subject. After a training period, interrater reliability was investigated by having two independent individuals score 20 records selected at random. The intraclass correlation for the three blocks for the two scorers was computed. The correlations for blocks 1, 2, and 3 were .97, .94, and .97, respectively. The intercorrelation of the total NSR scores for the two scorers was $r(19)=.99$.

We also examined habituation during the orienting trials that followed the rest period. The subjects listened to eight 1000-Hz, 54-dB tones through headphones, and the speed of habituation was measured by the number of tones presented to a subject before he or she had three consecutive nonresponses to the orienting stimuli.

STATISTICAL PROCEDURES

Rest Period

One-way analyses of variance (ANOVAs) were conducted with the total frequency of NSRs and the number of NSRs per block used as the dependent variables, and with the risk group classification (SHR, HR, and LR) as the independent variable. Additional one-way ANOVAs were conducted with the total frequency of NSRs and the number of NSRs per block used as the dependent variables and the diagnostic group (SZ, OMI, and NMI) as the independent variable. Newman-Keuls tests were conducted to examine further the differences between the groups.

Repeated-measure ANOVAs (RM-ANOVAs) were subsequently conducted for each group to assess the effect of block number on nonspecific responding. The average number of NSRs per block was analyzed in these analyses. Huynh-Feldt ϵ correction was used in the RM-ANOVAs to obtain adjusted *df* when the Mauchly sphericity test was significant.[30] The Mauchly test of sphericity examines the hypothesis that the variance-covariance matrix of the transformed variables (block number) used to test the effect (time) has covariances of zero and equal variances.[31]

Orienting Trials

A correlation between the orienting habituation score and the third block score (the most sensitive indicant of habituation) was also computed. One-way ANOVAs were conducted with the orienting habituation score used as the dependent variable and genetic and diagnostic classification as the independent variables.

crease in the rate of NSRs during the rest period. In addition, habituation during orienting trials for these same subjects was assessed. We hypothesized that higher levels of genetic predisposition to schizophrenia would be associated with increasing impairment of habituation. Furthermore, development of schizophrenia later in life would be associated with habituation impairments in childhood.

RESULTS

GENETIC RISK AND HABITUATION

The three risk groups differed in nonspecific responding (**Figure 1**). We calculated the total number of NSRs (blocks 1+2+3) during the entire rest period for the SHR,

HR, and LR groups; the means and SDs for the SHR, HR, and LR groups were 13.68±13.28, 10.82±11.17, and 8.22±8.30 (mean±SD), respectively. The differences in NSR frequency were significant (F[2,299]=3.74, *P*=.02). Newman-Keuls tests disclosed significant differences between the LR and SHR groups (*P*=.05) Note that the differences in total NSR frequency mainly reflect differences that occurred in the second and third blocks.

An overall RM-ANOVA was used to probe the contribution of the block variable to the group NSR differences. Although the group×block interaction did not attain conventional α levels required for statistical significance (F[3.32,457]=.92), generally such omnibus tests of interactions lack statistical power,[32] and for this reason it has been recommended that focused contrasts be used to assess specific scientific hypotheses of interest.[32,33]

An RM-ANOVA that combined all subjects into a single sample demonstrated a significant effect of block (F[1.65,457]=9.08, *P*=.0004) that reflected habituation. However, when the sample was divided into the three risk groups and tested separately, a significant effect of block was *not* observed for the SHR group (F[2,56]=0.09), which reflected a lack of habituation. A significant effect of block was observed for the HR group (F[1.64,257]=5.00, *P*=.01), which reflected some habituation. A significant effect of block was observed for the LR group (F[1.41,127]=5.83, *P*=.009), which indicated habituation. Further evidence of habituation differences was demonstrated by paired *t* tests, which showed significant differences in the LR group between blocks 1 and 2 (*t*[92]=2.52, *P*=.013) and between blocks 1 and 3 (*t*[90]=2.58, *P*=.012). Significant differences were also revealed in the HR group between blocks 1 and 2 (*t*[159]=8.68, *P*=.001) and between blocks 1 and 3 (*t*[157]=5.84, *P*=.001). Thus, the LR and HR groups evidenced habituation. Nonsignificant differences between blocks were observed for the SHR group, indicating a lack of habituation.

Table 1. Sociodemographic Characteristics of the Super High-Risk, High-Risk, and Low-Risk Groups

	Risk Group		
	Super	High	Low
No. of subjects	30	175	104
Boys	15	101	59
Girls	15	74	45
Mean age in 1962*	15.3	15.0	15.1
Mean social class†	2.5	2.2	2.3
Mean years of education	7.2	6.8	7.3

**Age expressed in years.*
†On a scale of 0 (low) to 6 (high).

An alternative series of analyses was also informative in understanding the group differences in NSRs as a function of block. The three groups did not differ in mean number of NSRs during the first block of the rest period (F[2,280]=0.667, *P*=.51). Group differences almost reached significance for block 2 (F[2,296]=2.52, *P*=.08). A significant difference was observed among the three risk groups in block 3 (F[2,294]=5.93, *P*=.003).

The means and SDs corresponding to these group and block variables are shown in **Table 2**. By the third block, the LR group evidenced rapid habituation, the HR group evidenced an intermediate level of habituation, and the SHR group evidenced little or no habituation (Table 2, **Figure 1**). Newman-Keuls tests disclosed significant differences in block 3 between the LR and HR groups and between the LR and SHR groups (*P*=.05).

DIAGNOSTIC CLASSIFICATION AND HABITUATION

The SZ, OMI, and NMI groups did not differ in overall nonspecific responding (F[2,280]=1.74, *P*=.18). The means

Table 2. Nonspecific Responses in Blocks 1, 2, and 3 by Genetic Risk Groups and Diagnostic Groups

	No. of Nonspecific Responses					
	Block 1		Block 2		Block 3	
	Mean±SD	n*	Mean±SD	n*	Mean±SD	n*
Risk group						
Low	3.63±4.71	93	2.60±3.34	101	2.29±2.69	100
High	4.17±4.96	161	3.16±3.80	168	3.74±4.27	167
Super	4.71±3.59	29	4.40±5.79	30	4.53±4.95	30
Diagnostic group						
No mental illness	4.15±4.87	157	2.94±3.44	165	2.90±3.46	164
Other mental illness	3.59±3.98	79	3.33±3.93	84	3.72±4.10	85
Schizophrenia	4.66±5.83	29	3.90±6.30	31	5.06±5.72	31

**Numbers of subjects differ because of missing data. Only subjects with complete data across the three blocks were included in the repeated-measures analyses of variance. All subjects were included in other analyses.*

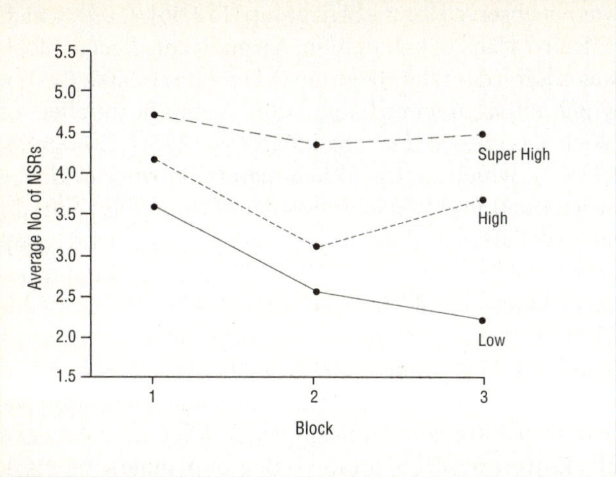

Figure 1. *Average number of nonspecific responses (NSRs) per block by risk group.*

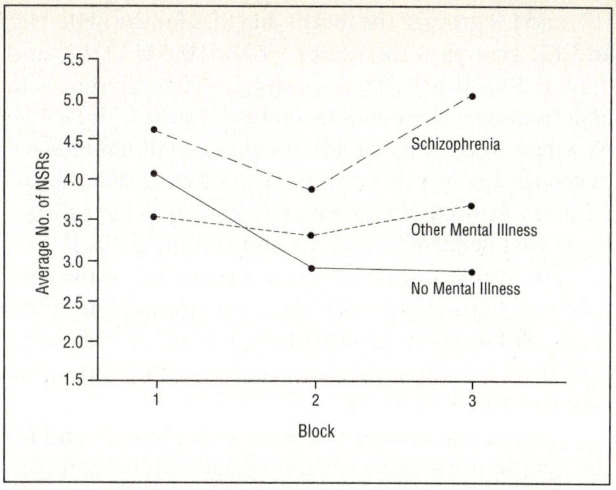

Figure 2. *Average number of nonspecific responses (NSRs) per block by diagnostic group.*

and SDs for the SZ, OMI, and NMI groups were 13.44±16.26, 10.83±10.92, and 9.61±9.44, respectively.

By RM-ANOVA, a nonsignificant group×block interaction was observed (F[3.35,352]=1.93, *P*=.12). However, a significant group×block interaction (F[1.65,297]=3.22, *P*=.05) and a significant main effect of block (F[1.65,297]=3.44, *P*=.04) were observed in a two-group RM-ANOVA that compared the SZ and NMI groups. The NMI group habituated during the rest period whereas the SZ group did not (**Figure 2**).

By RM-ANOVA, a nonsignificant effect of block was observed for the SZ group (F[2,56]=1.65). A nonsignificant effect of block was observed for the OMI group (F[2,156]=0.30). A significant effect of block was observed for the NMI group (F[1.58,242]=10.89, *P*=.0001), which reflected the general tendency of these subjects to habituate during the rest period.

The three groups (SZ, OMI, and NMI) did not differ in mean number of NSRs during the first block of the rest period (F[2,262]=0.638, *P*=.53). Group differences were not significant for block 2 (F[2,277]=0.87, *P*=.42). A significant difference was observed among the three groups in block 3 (F[2,277]=4.31, *P*=.01). Table 2 gives the means, SDs, and numbers of subjects. Newman-Keuls tests disclosed significant differences between the SZ and NMI groups (*P*=.05). Differences were not significant between the SZ and OMI groups, nor between the OMI and NMI groups. In Figure 2, the SZ group shows the least habituation, the OMI group shows a similar pattern, and the NMI group evidences habituation.

ORIENTING HABITUATION

The correlation between the orienting habituation score and the third block NSR score was *r*=.49, *P*<.05. Given the reliability of the two measures, this correlation indicates that the two measures are tapping similar habituation response tendencies. The mean (±SD) orienting scores for the risk groups, although not significantly different, were in the expected direction: SHR, 2.42±1.89; HR, 2.15±2.07; and LR, 2.0±1.77. The mean orienting scores for the diagnosis groups were not significantly different: SZ, 2.43±2.31; OMI, 2.03±2.05; and NMI, 2.23±1.88. Although the difference was not significant, the SZ group demonstrated poorer habituation than did the NMI group.

COMMENT

Our findings confirm the hypothesis that an increased level of genetic risk for schizophrenia is related to impaired ability to habituate autonomically to a relatively static environment. Poor habituation may be a part of the constellation of heritable factors that contribute to the cause of some types of schizophrenia.

Subjects in our sample who became schizophrenic in adulthood also evidenced significant deficits in habituation in adolescence; their rate of NSRs was higher at the end of a rest period than at the beginning. The large variance among the schizophrenics may reflect the genetic etiologic heterogeneity of the clinical condition of schizophrenia. A future study examining the symptoms and their relationship to habituation in childhood is planned. Children who developed schizophrenia in adulthood demonstrated significantly different patterns of habituation than children who were classified "not mentally ill" in adulthood. The habituation differences between those who became schizophrenic and those who developed other mental illnesses were not as striking. However, the habituation deficits in the SZ group were greater than those observed in the OMI group. Our findings suggest that habituation abnormalities in childhood may not be specific to those subjects who develop schizophrenia later in life.

OTHER FACTORS RELATING SCHIZOPHRENIA AND HABITUATION

The neuroanatomic substrates controlling the process of habituation are not established. However, the hippocampus has been shown to be important in the regulation of behavioral[34-37] and autonomic[16,17,38] habituation. Abnormality of the hippocampus is one of the most consistently replicated findings in neuropathology studies of schizophrenia.[39-44] The hippocampus develops rapidly during the second trimester.[45] The hippocampal anomalies observed in neuropathology studies of schizophrenics and the impairment of habituation may be a consequence of the *genetically triggered* second-trimester disruptions in neural development, hypothesized by Mednick et al.[46]

Psychological factors may also influence electrodermal activity habituation. Persistent and vivid thoughts and images may be more characteristic of the adolescent who will later be schizophrenic. Such thoughts may produce NSRs. Differential reaction to stress may affect electrodermal activity. Tarrier et al[47] examined differences in electrodermal activity between schizophrenics from families with high and low expressed emotion. They reported that both patient groups showed higher than normal rates of NSRs and were indistinguishable when only the experimenter was present. However, after a relative entered the room, the subjects from the low-expressed-emotion families showed a gradual decline in response frequency (habituation), whereas those from familes with high expressed emotion continued to exhibit elevated response frequency (failed habituation). These results suggest that being in a high-expressed-emotion family may be a source of impaired habituation in the schizophrenic relatives.

In addition to habituation deficits, attention and information processing abnormalities have been noted in patients with schizophrenia.[48,49] These deficits in attention and information processing may be related to habituation abnormalities. Habituation is critical for efficient information processing.[1-3] If an individual is unable to reduce responsiveness to repeated stimulation (ie, habituate), he or she may become overwhelmed by stimulation and become cognitively fragmented.[3] If the failure to habituate produces an inability to cease attending to irrelevant external or internal stimuli, then we should find that individuals with increased NSRs will evidence attentional deficits. In a study that used a selective attention task, Ohman et al[50] reported an increased number of both NSRs and attentional deficits in a group of schizophrenics. Perhaps poor habituation impaired the ability of their patient group to attend selectively to target stimuli or filter out nontarget stimuli. In a 1981 study, Zahn et al[6] suggested that slow habituation of the orienting response, increased nonspecific responding, and slower reaction time are related to fluctuations in attention for schizophrenic subjects.[6]

SUGGESTION FOR FUTURE RESEARCH

Typically, total NSR frequency is considered a measure of arousal.[51] If we had noted only total NSR frequency, we might have concluded that the SHR and HR groups were simply more aroused.[9] By examining responsiveness over time, we were able to conclude that the groups differed not only in number of responses but also in their pattern of responding. This finding should be considered in future studies that use NSRs as a dependent variable. A 15-minute examination period will probably show a different pattern of NSR production than a 5-minute period will. Such differences in the length of the period of measurement may explain why NSR findings in schizophrenia are sometimes conflicting.[52]

Accepted for publication February 25, 1994.

This research was supported by National Institute of Mental Health grants MH41469 and MH46014 and by National Institute of Mental Health Research Scientist Award MH00619 (Dr Mednick).

Special thanks are extended to Michael Dawson, PhD, and Adrian Raine, PhD, for their helpful suggestions.

Reprint requests to Social Science Research Institute, University of Southern California, Denney Research Bldg, Room 128, Los Angeles, CA 90089-1111 (Ms Hollister).

REFERENCES

1. Geyer MA, Braff DL. Startle habituation and sensorimotor gating in schizophrenia and related animal models. *Schizophr Bull.* 1987;13:643-668.
2. Braff DL, Geyer MA. Sensorimotor gating and schizophrenia. *Arch Gen Psychiatry.* 1990;47:181-188.
3. Braff DL, Grillon C, Geyer MA. Gating and habituation of the startle reflex in schizophrenic patients. *Arch Gen Psychiatry.* 1992;49:206-215.
4. Gruzelier J, Eves F, Connolly J, Hirsch S. Orienting, habituation, sensitization and dishabituation in the electrodermal system of consecutive, drug-free admissions for schizophrenia. *Biol Psychol.* 1981;12:187-209.
5. Zahn TP, Rosenthal D, Lawlor WG. Electrodermal and heart rate orienting reactions in chronic schizophrenia. *J Psychiatr Res.* 1968;6:117-134.
6. Zahn TP, Carpenter WT, McGlashan TH. Autonomic nervous system activity in acute schizophrenia, I: method and comparison with normal controls. *Arch Gen Psychiatry.* 1981;38:251-258.
7. Zahn TP, Carpenter WT, McGlashan TH. Autonomic nervous system activity in acute schizophrenia, II: relationships to short term prognosis and clinical state. *Arch Gen Psychiatry.* 1981;38:260-266.
8. Gruzelier JH, Connolly J, Eves F, et al. Effect of propranolol and phenothiazines on electrodermal orienting and habituation in schizophrenia. *Psychophysiol Med.* 1981;11:93-108.
9. Mednick SA, Schulsinger F. Studies of children at high risk for schizophrenia. In: Dean SR, ed. *Schizophrenia: The First Ten Dean Award Lectures.* New York, NY: MSS Information Corp; 1973.
10. Prentky RA, Salzman LF, Klein RH. Habituation and conditioning of skin conductance responses in children at high risk. *Schizophr Bull.* 1981;7:281-291.
11. Lykken DT, Iacono WG, Haroian K, McGue M, Bouchard JR. Habituation of the skin conductance response to strong stimuli: a twin study. *Psychophysiology.* 1988;25:4-15.
12. Lader MH, Wing L. *Physiological Measures, Sedative Drugs, and Morbid Anxiety.* London, England: Oxford University Press; 1966.
13. Dawson ME. Psychophysiology at the interface of clinical science, cognitive science, and neuroscience. *Psychophysiology.* 1990;27:243-255.
14. Raine A, Reynolds GP, Sheard C. Neuroanatomical correlates of skin conduc-

tance orienting in normal humans: a magnetic resonance imaging study. *Psychophysiology.* 1991;28:548-558.
15. Hazlett E, Dawson M, Buchsbaum MS, Nuechterlein KH. Reduced regional brain glucose metabolism assessed by PET in electrodermal nonresponder schizophrenics: a pilot study. *J Abnorm Psychol.* 1993;102:39-46.
16. Bagshaw MH, Kimble DP, Pribram KH. The GSR of monkeys during orienting and habituation and after ablation of the amygdala, hippocampus and inferotemporal cortex. *Neuropsychologia.* 1965;3:111-119.
17. Kaye H, Pearce JM. Hippocampal lesions attenuate latent inhibition and the decline of the orienting response in rats. *Q J Exp Psychol.* 1987;39B:107-126.
18. Mednick SA, Schulsinger F. A longitudinal study of children with a high risk for schizophrenia: a preliminary report. In: Vandenberg S, ed. *Methods and Goals in Human Behavior Genetics.* Orlando, Fla: Academic Press; 1965:255-296.
19. Mednick SA, Schulsinger F. Some premorbid characteristics related to breakdown in children with schizophrenic mothers. *J Psychiatr Res.* 1968;6: 267-291.
20. Jorgensen A, Teasdale TW, Parnas J, Schulsinger F, Schulsinger H, Mednick SA. The Copenhagen High-Risk Project: the diagnosis of maternal schizophrenia and its relation to offspring diagnosis. *Br J Psychiatry.* 1987;151:753-757.
21. Parnas J. Mates of schizophrenic mothers: a study of assortative mating from the American-Danish high risk study. *Br J Psychiatry.* 1985;146:490-497.
22. Spitzer RL, Endicott J. *Schedule for Affective Disorders and Schizophrenia–Lifetime Version (34th Ed).* New York, NY: New York Psychiatric Institute; 1978.
23. Endicott J, Spitzer RL. Current and Past Psychopathology Scales (CAPPS). *Arch Gen Psychiatry.* 1972;27:678-687.
24. Parnas J, Cannon T, Jacobsen B, Schulsinger H, Schulsinger F, Mednick SA. Lifetime *DSM-III-R* diagnostic outcomes of offspring of schizophrenic mothers. *Arch Gen Psychiatry.* 1993;50:707-714.
25. Wing JK, Cooper JE, Sartorius N. *The Measurement and Classification of Psychiatric Symptoms.* London, England: Cambridge University Press; 1974.
26. Andreasen NC. *The Scale for the Assessment of Negative Symptoms (SANS).* Iowa City, Iowa: University of Iowa; 1983.
27. Andreasen NC. *The Scale for the Assessment of Positive Symptoms (SAPS).* Iowa City, Iowa: University of Iowa; 1984.
28. Loranger AW, Sussman VL, Oldham JM, Russakoff LM. *Personality Disorder Examination: A Structured Interview for Making Diagnosis of* DSM-III-R *Personality Disorders.* White Plains, NY: Cornell Medical College; 1985.
29. Greenfield NS, Sternbach RA. *Handbook of Psychophysiology.* New York, NY: Holt Rinehart & Winston; 1972:395.
30. Huynh H, Feldt LS. Estimation of the Box correction for degrees of freedom from sample data in the randomized block and split-plot designs. *J Educ Stat.* 1976;1:69-82.
31. Norusis MJ. Storing memories: repeated measures analysis of variance. In: *SPSS-X Advanced Statistics Guide.* Chicago, Ill: SPSS Inc; 1988:257-293.
32. Cohen J. *Statistical Power Analysis for the Behavioral Sciences.* Hillsdale, NJ: Lawrence Erlbaum Assoc Publishers; 1988.
33. Rosenthal R, Rosnow RL. *Contrast Analysis: Focused Comparisons in the Analysis of Variance.* New York, NY: Cambridge University Press; 1985.
34. Kimble DP. Hippocampus and internal inhibition. *Psychol Bull.* 1968;70:285-295.
35. Vinogradova OS. Functional organization of the limbic system in the process of registration and information: facts and hypotheses. In: Isaacson RL, Pibram KH, eds. *The Hippocampus, Volume 2: Neurophysiology and Behavior.* New York, NY: Plenum Press; 1975:3-69.
36. Douglas RJ, Isaacson RL. Hippocampal lesions and activity. *Psychonomic Sci.* 1964;1:187-188.
37. Roberts WW, Dember WN, Brodwick M. Alternation and exploration in rats with hippocampal lesions. *J Comp Physiol Psychol.* 1962;55:695-700.
38. Teitlebaum H, Milner PM. Activity changes following partial hippocampal lesions in rats. *J Comp Physiol Psychol.* 1963;56:284-289.
39. McLardy T. Hippocampal zinc and structural deficit in brains from chronic alcoholics and some schizophrenics. *J Orthomol Psychiatry.* 1974;4:32-36.
40. Bogerts B. The neuropathology of schizophrenia: pathophysiological and neurodevelopmental implications. In: Mednick SA, Cannon TD, Barr CE, Lyon M, eds. *Fetal Neural Development and Adult Schizophrenia.* Cambridge, England: Cambridge University Press; 1991.
41. Jeste DV, Lohr JB. Hippocampal pathologic findings in schizophrenia. *Arch Gen Psychiatry.* 1989;46:1019-1024.
42. Kovelman JA, Scheibel AB. A neurohistological correlate of schizophrenia. *Biol Psychol.* 1984;19:1601-1621.
43. Falkai P, Bogerts B. Cell loss in the hippocampus of schizophrenics. *Eur Arch Psychiatry Neurol Sci.* 1986;236:154-161.
44. Akbarian S, Viñuela A, Kim JJ, Potkin S, Bunney WE, Jones EG. Distorted distribution of nicotinamide-adenine dinucleotide phosphate-diaphorase neurons in temporal lobe of schizophrenics implies anomalous cortical development. *Arch Gen Psychiatry.* 1993;50:178-187.
45. Mednick SA, Cannon TD, Barr CE, Lyon M, eds. *Fetal Neural Development and Adult Schizophrenia.* Cambridge, England: Cambridge University Press; 1991.
46. Mednick SA, Machon RA, Huttunen MO, Bonett D. Adult schizophrenia following prenatal exposure to an influenza epidemic. *Arch Gen Psychiatry.* 1988; 45:189-192.
47. Tarrier N, Vaughn CE, Lader MH, Leff JP. Bodily reactions to people and events in schizophrenia. *Arch Gen Psychiatry.* 1979;36:311-315.
48. Kraeplin E; Desfendorf AR (trans). *Clinical Psychiatry: A Textbook for Students and Physicians.* New York, NY: Macmillan Publishing Co Inc; 1921.
49. McGhie A, Chapman J. Disorders of attention and perception in early schizophrenia. *Br J Med Psychol.* 1961;34:103-115.
50. Ohman A, Nordby H, d'Elia G. Orienting and schizophrenia: stimulus significance, attention, and distraction in a signaled reaction time task. *J Abnorm Psychol.* 1986;95:326-334.
51. Ohman A. Electrodermal activity and vulnerability to schizophrenia: a review. *Biol Psychol.* 1981;12:87-145.
52. Dawson ME, Nuechterlein KH. Psychophysiological dysfunctions in the developmental course of schizophrenic disorders. *Schizophr Bull.* 1984;10: 204-232.

ORIGINAL ARTICLE

A Multicenter Investigation of Fixed-Dose Fluoxetine in the Treatment of Obsessive-compulsive Disorder

Gary D. Tollefson, MD, PhD; Alvin H. Rampey, Jr, PhD; Janet H. Potvin, PhD; Michael A. Jenike, MD; A. John Rush, MD; Roberto A. Dominguez, MD; Lorrin M. Koran, MD; M. Katherine Shear, MD; Wayne Goodman, MD; Laura A. Genduso, PharmD

Objectives: To determine the effectiveness of fluoxetine hydrochloride at fixed doses of 20 mg/d, 40 mg/d, and 60 mg/d in patients with obsessive-compulsive disorder (OCD) and to evaluate its safety.

Methods: Fixed-dose fluoxetine hydrochloride (20 mg/d, 40 mg/d, 60 mg/d) was compared with placebo in two randomized, double-blind, parallel, 13-week trials of identical design in 355 outpatients with OCD aged 15 to 70 years (*DSM-III-R* criteria; 1 year's duration or longer; depression secondary if present).

Results: Fluoxetine (all doses) was significantly ($P \leq .001$) superior to placebo on the Yale-Brown Obsessive Compulsive Scale (Y-BOCS) total score (mean baseline-to-end-point decrease, 4.6, 5.5, and 6.5 vs 0.9, respectively, studies pooled) and other efficacy measures ($P \leq .01$). A trend suggesting greater efficacy at 60 mg/d was observed. Most patients (79.2%) completed the study. Eight adverse events were statistically significantly more frequent with fluoxetine and one, with placebo. For some events, incidence tended to increase with increasing dosage; however, few patients discontinued treatment for any single event.

Conclusion: Fluoxetine was associated with a statistically significant reduction in OCD severity, including time engaged in obsessional and/or compulsive behaviors. Adverse events infrequently led to study discontinuation.

(Arch Gen Psychiatry. 1994;51:559-567)

From the Psychopharmacology Division, Eli Lilly and Company, Indianapolis, Ind (Drs Tollefson, Rampey, Potvin, and Genduso); the Departments of Psychiatry, Massachusetts General Hospital, Harvard Medical School, Boston (Dr Jenike), University of Texas Southwestern Medical School, Dallas (Dr Rush), University of Miami (Fla) School of Medicine, (Dr Dominguez); the Departments of Psychiatry and Behavioral Sciences, Stanford (Calif) University School of Medicine (Dr Koran); the Departments of Psychiatry, New York Hospital, Cornell University Medical College, Ithaca (Dr Shear); and Connecticut Mental Health Center, Yale University Medical School, New Haven (Dr Goodman). Dr Shear is currently with the University of Pittsburgh (Pa) Western Psychiatric Institute and Dr Goodman is currently with the University of Florida School of Medicine, Gainesville.

OBSESSIVE-COMPULSIVE disorder (OCD) occurs at a lifetime prevalence rate of 2% to 3% in the United States[1] and is characterized by recurrent ideas, impulses, or images (obsessions) and/or repetitive, seemingly purposeless behaviors (compulsions).[2] Because OCD impairs quality of life substantially in some patients, effective treatment alternatives are needed. While the cause of OCD remains unclear, increasing evidence suggests serotonergic (serotonin [5-HT]) involvement.[3-6] Agents that inhibit 5-HT reuptake (and perhaps inhibitors of monoamine oxidase) appear to exert more robust anti-obsessional effects than less 5-HT–selective medications such as desipramine hydrochloride and nortriptyline hydrochloride.[7,8] Neuroleptics, lithium, benzodiazepines, and monoamine oxidase inhibitors have not proven to be effective in the treatment of OCD.[9-12]

Clomipramine hydrochloride, a tricyclic compound active at the 5-HT transporter, has been the most extensively investigated agent in controlled trials of OCD.[13] The first reports of the efficacy of clomipramine in OCD appeared over 25 years ago[14] and, subsequently, the therapeutic value of clomipramine for the treatment of OCD has been well established.[15-23] However, like conventional tricyclic compounds, clomipramine lacks receptor selectivity and exhibits affinity for cholinergic, adrenergic, and histaminic receptors.[24] Pharmacological activity at these non–5-HT sites may result in adverse events that affect patient compliance and introduce undesirable side effects.[25] With clomipramine, such adverse events may require lowering the dose to levels that compromise efficacy.[13] Thus, there is an op-

See Patients and Methods on next page

PATIENTS AND METHODS

SELECTION OF PATIENTS

Three-hundred ninety-two ambulatory outpatients with a primary diagnosis of OCD from eight geographically distinct sites entered these trials. Of these patients, 355 were randomly allocated to double-blind therapy as follows: placebo (n=89) or fluoxetine hydrochloride at 20 mg/d (n=87), at 40 mg/d (n=89), and at 60 mg/d (n=90). All patients signed a written informed consent before entering the study. Eligible patients were between 14 and 70 years of age. Subjects satisfied the *DSM-III-R* criteria for OCD.[2] Obsessive-compulsive symptoms must have been of at least moderate severity, as defined by a rating of at least moderate or greater on the Clinical Global Impression (CGI)-Severity of OCD scale,[35] and a score on the Yale-Brown Obsessive Compulsive Scale (Y-BOCS)[36,37] of at least 16 (if both obsessions and compulsions were present) or at least 10 (if only obsessions or only compulsions were present).[36] Symptoms must have been present for at least 1 year prior to entering the study.

Comorbid nonbipolar depression, as defined by *DSM-III-R*, was permitted if judged clinically to be secondary to OCD and began after the onset of the OCD. However, other current Axis I diagnoses were exclusionary. All patients were required to be free of unstable or serious medical conditions. Patients could not have used psychotropic agents for 1 week prior to the placebo lead-in to the study. Concomitant psychotropic medications were not allowed during the study.

STUDY PROCEDURES

The trials consisted of a 1-week placebo lead-in followed by 13 weeks of double-blind treatment. A complete medical history and physical examination, laboratory tests, and electrocardiogram were obtained at study entrance. Following the 1-week, single-blind, placebo lead-in, patients exhibiting a 25% or greater reduction in Y-BOCS total score were discontinued from the study. Eligible patients were randomly assigned to one of four treatment groups: placebo or fluoxetine hydrochloride at doses of 20 mg, 40 mg, or 60 mg once daily; those assigned to the 60-mg/d treatment group received 40 mg/d for the first week.

Patients were examined by the treating clinicians (M.A.J., A.J.R., R.A.D., L.M.K., M.K.S., W.G., Robert Reichler, MD, Fred Reimherr, MD), who were blinded to the study medication. Assessments were conducted weekly for the first 2 weeks of the study and biweekly thereafter. The Y-BOCS served as the primary efficacy measure. Secondary measures included the Y-BOCS Compulsion and Obsession subscores, the total score on the first 17 items of the Hamilton Depression Rating Scale ($HAMD_{17}$),[38] the seven-point CGI-Severity and Improvement subscales,[35] a seven-point Patient Global Impression (PGI) scale,[35] and the eight-item OCD subscale from the Comprehensive Psychopathological Rating Scale (CPRS).[39]

Safety was assessed by the evaluation of the incidence of adverse events that first occurred or worsened during therapy (treatment-emergent adverse events), discontinuations for adverse events, clinical laboratory data, and vital signs. During the trials, adverse events were collected at each visit by nonprobing inquiry and by diary cards. All events were recorded without regard to causality. Vital signs were collected at every visit. The physical examination and baseline laboratory studies were repeated at study completion.

portunity to improve the risk-benefit profile in the pharmacotherapy of OCD.

Fluoxetine hydrochloride is a selective 5-HT uptake inhibitor with little direct activity at neurotransmitter binding sites.[26] Several recent pilot and open-label studies have reported its effectiveness in OCD.[27-34]

To further understand the role of fluoxetine in OCD, two large, parallel, multicenter, double-blind, fixed-dose, placebo-controlled trials of identical design were conducted. The primary objectives of the study were to determine whether fluoxetine hydrochloride at a fixed dose of 20 mg/d, 40 mg/d, or 60 mg/d would be statistically significantly more effective than placebo in treating the symptoms of OCD and to evaluate the safety profile of fluoxetine in OCD based on adverse drug-event incidence and discontinuations from the study. Additional objectives were to determine the relationship of dose and response, the role of secondary depressive comorbidity, and the effect of fluoxetine on obsessions and compulsions. This report presents data for the two trials combined.

RESULTS

PATIENT CHARACTERISTICS

Characteristics of the patient population at baseline are summarized in **Table 1** and **Table 2**. The population was predominantly white (90.7%) with a mean (±SD) age of 36.9±11.8 years (range, 15 to 70 years). The majority (94.4%) of patients had both obsessions and compulsions. Approximately half (54.9%) of the patients had a historical (18.0%) or secondary (36.9%) diagnosis of depression at baseline. Both baseline demographic (Table 1) and baseline clinical attributes (Table 2) were comparable across treatment groups.

STATISTICAL ANALYSES

All analyses were done using pooled data from both trials. Analysis of baseline comparability among treatment groups included evaluation of age, sex, race, presence of comorbid depression, and obsession vs compulsion subclassification. All randomly assigned patients (N=355) were included in the analyses of baseline demographics. Analyses of efficacy and safety (adverse events, vital signs, and clinical laboratory tests) included all randomly assigned patients who had at least one measurement after random assignment. All tests of hypotheses were carried out at a two-sided significance level of .05, unless otherwise indicated.

The primary efficacy analysis was the evaluation of the absolute change in the Y-BOCS total score from the baseline to the termination visit (last-visit-carried-forward analysis). Efficacy was also assessed by evaluating the mean Y-BOCS total scores at each follow-up visit (weekly analysis) for all patients with available data at that visit. A modified Bonferroni method[40] was used to adjust the significance level for the multiple hypothesis tests over time; significance criteria were adjusted at each week to maintain an overall significance level of .05.

A post hoc analysis was conducted on the Y-BOCS item 1 (length of time engaged in obsessional ideation) and item 6 (length of time engaged in compulsive behaviors) scores to determine the proportion of patients who experienced decreases in these scores. A decrease in score indicates less time spent in the pathological symptom and serves as a measure of functional improvement even though obsessive or compulsive symptoms still exist. A qualitative measure of improved patient function helps to interpret the benefit of treatment. For this analysis, improvement was defined as any decrease in an item 1 or item 6 score; substantial improvement was defined as a decrease in an item 1 or item 6 score from 3 or 4 at baseline to 0 or 1 at end point.

Response rates were determined for patients (n=311) who remained in therapy for at least 7 weeks after random assignment. A clinical response was defined as at least 35% improvement on the Y-BOCS total score from baseline to last recorded visit. Overall differences among treatment groups were assessed by a Pearson χ^2 test with 3 *df*. Pairwise treatment comparisons were also performed using Pearson's χ^2 test with 1 *df*. The Mantel-Haenszel χ^2 test was used to test for evidence of a linear association between categorical response rates and dose.[41]

Analysis of variance was performed on change from baseline for all continuous variables. For CGI-Improvement and PGI, analysis of variance was performed only on the end-point value. The complete design model for all continuous variables incorporated effects for treatment, investigator, and treatment-by-investigator interaction. Both the rank-transformed[42] and the raw data responses were evaluated. However, only the rank transformed analyses are provided because the data were generally nonnormal (Kolmogorov D statistic).[43] Treatment and investigator main effects were tested at a two-sided significance level of .05, while the treatment-by-investigator interaction was tested at a two-sided significance level of .15. The Jonckheere-Terpstra test[44] for ordered alternatives was used to test for a dose response for continuous outcome measures.

Categorical data, which included demographic variables, reasons for study discontinuation, and treatment-emergent adverse events, were evaluated using the Pearson and Mantel-Haenszel χ^2 tests. SAS procedures[43] were used to perform all statistical analyses.

EFFICACY

Change in Y-BOCS Total Score

The mean Y-BOCS total scores at each week are shown in **Figure 1**. The mean Y-BOCS total scores at each week and the corresponding range of scores are summarized in **Table 3**. Significant differences in the mean weekly scores (*P*<.001) favoring at least one dose level of fluoxetine were evident beginning with week 5 and continuing to study conclusion. Although the magnitude of the fluoxetine treatment effect relative to placebo varied across sites at weeks 11 and 13, all three fluoxetine treatment groups demonstrated numerically greater improvement in their Y-BOCS total scores than the placebo treatment group at all sites at both weeks.

Mean change in Y-BOCS total scores from baseline to end point (last-visit-carried-forward analysis) is shown in **Figure 2**. All three fluoxetine-treated groups experienced a statistically significantly greater improvement (*P*<.001) in mean Y-BOCS total scores than the placebo-treated group. However, end-point mean change was numerically greatest in the 60-mg/d fluoxetine hydrochloride treatment group. A statistically significant (*P*<.001) decreasing trend in change in Y-BOCS total score (ie, increasing improvement) was observed with increasing dosage of fluoxetine. Although the magnitude of the fluoxetine treatment effect relative to placebo varied across sites, the fluoxetine treatment groups demonstrated numerically greater improvement in Y-BOCS total score than the placebo treatment group at all sites.

Review of the baseline and end-point distributions of Y-BOCS total scores (data not shown) indicated that more than half of all fluoxetine-treated patients achieved an end-point Y-BOCS total score of 20 or less, which was greater than the number of placebo-treated patients who

Table 1. Baseline Demographic Characteristics*

Characteristic	All Patients (N=355)	Placebo Group (n=89)	Fluoxetine Hydrochloride Group, Dose 20 mg/d (n=87)	40 mg/d (n=89)	60 mg/d (n=90)
OCD classification					
Compulsive only	13 (3.7)	5 (5.6)	1 (1.1)	5 (5.6)	2 (2.2)
Obsessive only	7 (2.0)	2 (2.2)	2 (2.3)	2 (2.2)	1 (1.1)
Both	335 (94.4)	82 (92.1)	84 (96.6)	82 (92.1)	87 (96.7)
Sex					
F	196 (55.2)	46 (51.7)	46 (52.9)	49 (55.1)	55 (61.1)
M	159 (44.8)	43 (48.3)	41 (47.1)	40 (44.9)	35 (38.9)
Ethnicity					
White	322 (90.7)	81 (91.0)	82 (94.3)	79 (88.8)	80 (88.9)
Black	6 (1.7)	0 (0.0)	1 (1.1)	1 (1.1)	4 (4.4)
Other†	27 (7.6)	8 (9.0)	4 (4.6)	9 (10.1)	6 (6.7)
Age, y					
Mean±SD	36.9±11.8	37.2±12.3	38.0±12.7	37.0±10.8	35.4±11.3
Range	15-70	17-70	20-70	15-70	17-69
Comorbid depression					
$HAMD_{17}$ total score ≥12	124 (34.9)	26 (29.2)	31 (35.6)	31 (34.8)	36 (40.0)
$HAMD_{17}$ total score <12	231 (65.1)	63 (70.8)	56 (64.4)	58 (65.2)	54 (60.0)

**Data are presented as number (percent) unless otherwise indicated. OCD indicates obsessive-compulsive disorder; $HAMD_{17}$, first 17 items of Hamilton Depression Rating Scale.*

†Includes Asian, American Indian, Hispanic, and other.

Table 2. Baseline Efficacy Measurement Data by Treatment Group*

Measure	Placebo Group (n=89)	Fluoxetine Hydrochloride Group, Dose 20 mg/d (n=87)	40 mg/d (n=89)	60 mg/d (n=90)
Y-BOCS total score (score range, 0-40)	24.3 (5.7)	23.6 (5.7)	23.5 (5.6)	24.4 (5.1)
Y-BOCS compulsion subscore (score range, 0-20)	12.7 (3.0)	12.0 (3.6)	12.1 (3.1)	12.6 (2.8)
Y-BOCS obsession subscore (score range, 0-20)	11.6 (3.9)	11.6 (3.4)	11.4 (3.9)	11.8 (3.5)
$HAMD_{17}$ total score (score range, 0-52)	9.0 (5.9)	9.2 (5.9)	9.6 (5.2)	9.4 (5.9)
CGI-Severity†	5.0 (0.8)	5.0 (0.9)	5.1 (0.9)	5.1 (0.9)
CGI-Improvement‡	4.0 (0.4)	3.9 (0.4)	4.0 (0.6)	3.9 (0.4)
PGI-Improvement§	3.9 (0.5)	3.9 (0.5)	3.8 (0.7)	3.8 (0.6)
CPRS total score (score range, 0-24)	10.7 (3.5)	11.2 (3.8)	11.3 (3.7)	11.2 (3.6)

**Data are presented as mean (SD). Y-BOCS indicates Yale-Brown Obsessive Compulsive Scale; $HAMD_{17}$, first 17 items of Hamilton Depression Rating Scale; CGI, Clinical Global Impression; PGI, Patient Global Impression; and CPRS, Comprehensive Psychopathological Rating Scale. Analysis of variance of rank-transformed baseline scores indicated no statistically significant differences between groups at baseline.*

†Seven-point scale in which 1=normal and 7=extreme case of OCD.

‡Seven-point scale in which 1=very much improved and 7=very much worse.

§Seven-point scale in which 1=very much better and 7=very much worse.

achieved such a score (approximately one in three). Scores of 15 or less were twice as common with fluoxetine as placebo at end point.

Response Rates

At all three dose levels, a statistically significantly ($P<.001$) greater proportion of fluoxetine-treated than placebo-treated patients, who completed at least 7 weeks of treatment after random assignment, achieved a positive clinical response (at least 35% improvement in Y-BOCS total score from baseline to last visit). Response rates with placebo and fluoxetine hydrochloride doses of 20 mg/d, 40 mg/d, and 60 mg/d, respectively, were 8.5% (seven of 82 patients), 32.1% (25 of 78 patients), 32.4% (24 of 74 patients), and 35.1% (27 of 77 patients). There were no statistically significant differences in response rates among patients treated with fluoxetine hydrochloride at doses of 20 mg/d, 40 mg/d, or 60 mg/d. A statistically significant (Mantel-Haenszel χ^2 test, $P<.001$) linear association of increasing incidence of response with increasing fluoxetine dosage was observed.

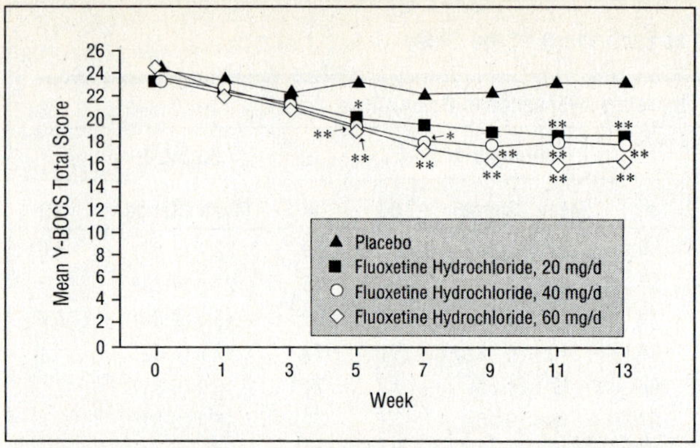

Figure 1. *Mean Yale-Brown Obsessive Compulsive Scale (Y-BOCS) total scores at each week of the study. Asterisks denote a statistically significant difference compared with placebo: single asterisk,* $P \leq .01$*; double asterisks,* $P \leq .001$.

Change in Secondary Efficacy Measures

Baseline-to-end-point change in Y-BOCS compulsion and obsession subscores, $HAMD_{17}$ total score, CGI-Severity score, CGI-Improvement and PGI-Improvement scores, and CPRS total score are shown in **Figure 3**. For all measures, all of the fluoxetine treatment groups experienced statistically significantly greater improvement at end point than did the placebo-treated group. Statistically significant treatment-by-investigator interactions were observed for all of these measures. Compared with placebo, numerically greater improvement was observed with at least two dose levels of fluoxetine at each site for all of these measures.

The baseline and end-point distributions of CGI-Improvement scores (data not shown) paralleled those of the Y-BOCS total scores. More than one third of fluoxetine-treated patients had an end-point CGI score of 1 or 2 vs one in 10 of those treated with placebo. While not statistically significant, the percentage of end-point scores of 1 or 2 numerically increased with dose. As a group, the mean end-point CGI-Improvement scores were comparable among the three fluoxetine arms and each was superior to the mean score with placebo.

Decrease in Y-BOCS Items 1 and 6 Scores

A statistically significantly ($P<.001$) greater proportion of patients in the 20-mg/d, 40-mg/d, and 60-mg/d fluoxetine hydrochloride groups than in the placebo group experienced improvement in time spent in obsessive and compulsive behaviors (item 1: 54.1%, 54.3%, and 48.3% vs 19.1%, respectively; item 6: 41.7%, 50.0%, and 55.7% vs 24.4%, respectively). Further, a statistically significantly ($P<.001$) greater proportion of patients in the 20-mg/d, 40-mg/d, and 60-mg/d fluoxetine hydrochloride groups than in the placebo group experienced substantial improvement in time spent in obsessive and compulsive behaviors (item 1: 7.3%, 17.0%, and 26.8% vs 1.6%, respectively; item 6: 15.4%, 20.8%, and 19.6% vs 3.6%, respectively).

SAFETY

The majority of patients (79.2%, 281/355) completed the study. Thirty-four patients (9.6%) were discontinued from the study because of an adverse event. The 20-mg/d fluoxetine hydrochloride group demonstrated statistically significantly ($P<.05$) fewer discontinuations for an adverse event (34.5%, 30/87) than either the 40-mg/d group (13.5%, 12/89) or the 60-mg/d group (18.9%, 17/90) and was not distinguished statistically from the placebo group (2.2%, 2/89). In contrast to early discontinuations in each of the three fluoxetine treatment groups, most early discontinuations in the placebo group were for lack of efficacy (7.9% [7/89] vs none of 87, 89, and 90, 0.0%, respectively, for each of the fluoxetine groups; $P<.01$).

The incidence of the most commonly reported treatment-emergent adverse events is shown in **Figure 4**. Statistically significant overall treatment differences in incidence were noted for three of these events (nausea, dry mouth, and tremor). Statistically significant overall treatment differences were also noted for yawn, sweating, vasodilatation, decreased libido, depression, and anorgasmia ($P<.05$). A statistically significant trend of increasing incidence with increasing fluoxetine dose was observed for some treatment-emergent adverse events. Discontinuation rates for specific adverse events were low (range, 1.1% to 2.3%). Fluoxetine was not associated with a statistically significant change in suicidality from baseline.[45] No seizures were reported during the 13 weeks of double-blind therapy.

With respect to laboratory findings, fluoxetine and placebo were comparable. No organ-system findings (eg, hepatomegaly) or persistent laboratory elevations (eg, liver function) were reported. Analysis of change in vital signs revealed no clinically meaningful differences. Among patients taking fluoxetine hydrochloride, six (7.0%) at 20 mg/d, 10 (11.4%) at 40 mg/d, and nine (10.1%) at 60 mg/d lost at least 4.5 kg vs six patients (6.8%) taking placebo ($P=.639$). Conversely, two patients (2.3%) taking placebo gained greater than 4.5 kg vs one patient (1.2%) taking 20 mg/d, three patients (3.4%) taking 40 mg/d, and one patient (1.1%) taking 60 mg/d of fluoxetine hydrochloride ($P=.663$).

COMMENT

Fluoxetine has been extensively studied and established as an effective treatment for depression.[46] Its safety profile represents a marked advantage over conventional antidepressants for many patients.[47] In the recent large multicenter trials, fluoxetine was found to be effective in treating the symptoms of OCD, extending the results of earlier open trials[27-33,48,49] and controlled trials[34,50] with small numbers of patients.

Table 3. Mean Yale-Brown Obsessive Compulsive Scale Total Scores at Each Week of the Study

	Placebo Group			Fluoxetine Hydrochloride Group, Dose: 20 mg/d			40 mg/d			60 mg/d		
Week	n	Mean (Range)	SD	n	Mean (Range)	SD	n	Mean (Range)	SD	n	Mean (Range)	SD
1	88	23.3 (10-36)	6.2	86	22.3 (7-36)	5.8	86	22.7 (7-36)	6.1	89	22.7 (3-33)	5.6
3	87	22.4 (8-37)	7.2	84	21.1 (6-34)	6.3	84	21.0 (3-37)	7.1	85	21.4 (4-35)	6.3
5	83	23.4 (7-37)	6.4	80	20.2 (4-34)	6.7	79	19.5 (0-36)	7.2	81	19.5 (2-34)	6.7
7	82	22.4 (7-40)	7.4	76	19.8 (4-36)	7.0	74	18.1 (4-34)	7.0	77	17.7 (1-32)	7.1
9	77	22.6 (6-40)	7.6	77	19.2 (0-39)	7.8	68	17.8 (1-35)	7.7	74	16.9 (0-31)	7.1
11	75	23.5 (4-38)	7.3	75	18.9 (0-36)	8.1	67	18.4 (0-35)	7.5	72	16.4 (0-31)	7.4
13	76	23.6 (3-40)	7.5	75	18.9 (0-37)	8.3	67	18.1 (0-35)	7.9	68	16.8 (0-31)	7.8

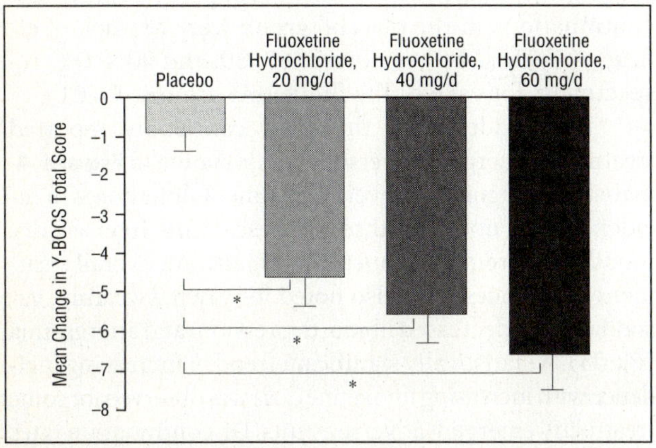

Figure 2. *Mean (±SEM) change in the Yale-Brown Obsessive Compulsive Scale (Y-BOCS) total score from baseline to end point. Asterisk denotes a statistically significant treatment difference compared with placebo (P≤.001). End-point Y-BOCS total scores for the placebo and 20-mg/d, 40-mg/d, and 60-mg/d fluoxetine hydrochloride groups were 23.5, 19.0, 18.3, and 17.9, respectively.*

The clinical trial experience during the initial development of fluoxetine hydrochloride as an antidepressant established that a 20-mg dose is typically effective in major depression.[46,51] However, this dose has not been extensively tested in OCD. Studies of fluoxetine in OCD to date[27-34] have used doses higher than the 20 mg typically used for depression.[46] For example, Fontaine and Chouinard[28] reported a beneficial clinical effect in five of seven patients treated with 60 to 80 mg of fluoxetine hydrochloride per day. Turner et al,[27] who studied doses of 80 mg/d, reported improvement in five of 10 fluoxetine hydrochloride–treated patients. In a 12-week, open-label trial of fluoxetine in 61 patients reported by Jenike et al,[30] a significant overall reduction from baseline in OCD symptoms was found. Both depressed and nondepressed patients with OCD exhibited an equal improvement. In their trial, patients received fluoxetine hydrochloride at 20 mg/d for 1 week, 40 mg/d for 3 weeks, 60 mg/d for 1 week, then 80 mg/d for 7 weeks. Liebowitz et al[31] described a 62% response rate in an open-label trial of 49 patients treated with up to 80 mg/d of fluoxetine hydrochloride for 12 weeks. Pigott et al[34] reported that five of 11 patients treated with fluoxetine hydrochloride at a gradually increasing dosage up to 80 mg/d in a double-blind crossover study experienced at least a 30% decrease in their OCD symptoms. In a second group, 18 of 21 patients who had been stabilized on clomipramine with at least partial success maintained a therapeutic benefit during a 10-week, double-blind, crossover to fluoxetine hydrochloride at a gradually increasing dose up to 80 mg/d. In contrast to those who used up to 80 mg/d, Kim and Dysken[32] found fluoxetine hydrochloride at 40 mg/d to be an effective dose.

In the present trial, three fixed doses (20 mg/d, 40 mg/d, and 60 mg/d) of fluoxetine hydrochloride were evaluated. Given the longer half-life of fluoxetine's principal metabolite, *N*-desmethylfluoxetine, a 13-week study was considered to be the minimum study duration to evaluate the effectiveness of the 20-mg/d dose. All three fluoxetine doses demonstrated statistically superior efficacy compared with placebo on the Y-BOCS total score ($P<.001$). It should be noted, however, that there was a trend for the 60-mg/d dose to be more effective than the 20-mg/d or 40-mg/d dose; therefore, for patients not responding to the lower doses, a trial of a higher dose may be warranted. Overall response at 60 mg/d might have been enhanced with a longer observational period. When titration above 20 mg/d is contemplated, a minimum of 5 treatment weeks should have passed. The additional benefit from a higher dose must be balanced against the greater likelihood of dose-related adverse events. Although compulsive behaviors have been considered more responsive to behavioral than to pharmacological therapy,[52] the present findings showed a statistically significant beneficial effect of fluoxetine on both compulsions and obsessions. These effects were independent of patients' antidepressant response. Placebo response was low, consistent with results of previous trials of OCD.[17,27,32] As in some other studies, symptoms of OCD demonstrated a response latency.[7,12,32] None of the fluoxetine treatment groups achieved statistically significantly greater improvement of symptoms than the placebo group until week 5. While the treatment differences were not statistically significant, 20 mg/d of fluoxetine hydrochloride appeared to have a somewhat slower onset of action as well

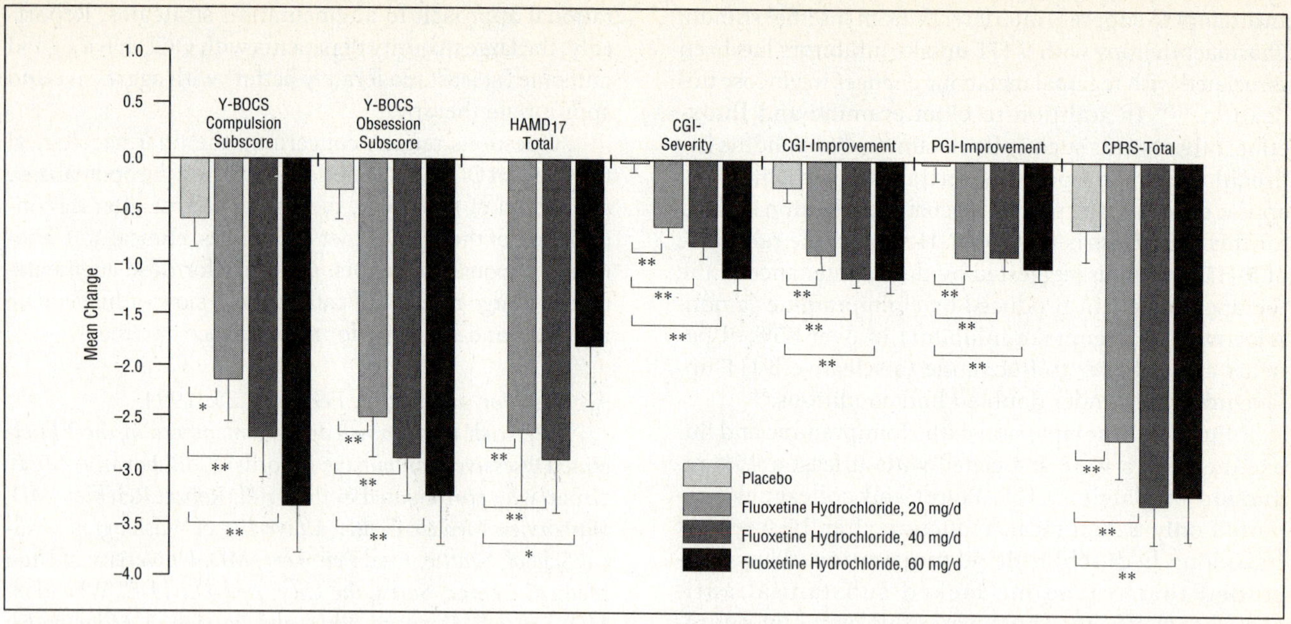

Figure 3. *Summary of the mean (±SEM) change in secondary efficacy measures from baseline to end point. Asterisks denote a statistically significant treatment difference: single asterisk,* P≤.01*; double asterisks,* P≤.001*; Y-BOCS, Yale-Brown Obsessive Compulsive Scale; $HAMD_{17}$, first 17 items of the Hamilton Depression Rating Scale; CGI, Clinical Global Impression scale; PGI, Patient Global Impression scale; and CPRS, Comprehensive Psychopathological Rating Scale.*

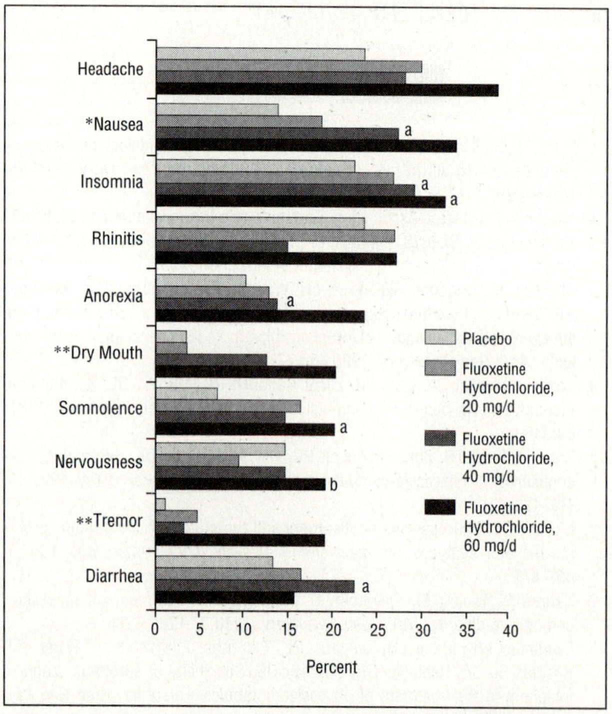

Figure 4. *Most commonly reported treatment-emergent adverse events. Asterisks denote a statistically significant overall treatment difference: single asterisk,* P≤.01*; double asterisks,* P≤.001*; a, one patient (1.1%) discontinued the study because of the event; b, two patients (2.3%) discontinued because of the event.*

as a less pronounced effect on symptoms than the two higher doses. The finding of effectiveness with all three fluoxetine doses lends support to the hypothesis that serotonin-based manipulation may be selectively helpful in controlling some of the symptoms of OCD.

In this patient population mean baseline $HAMD_{17}$ total scores were not high enough to suggest a high prevalence of comorbid mood disturbance. However, all three fluoxetine treatment groups exhibited a statistically significantly (*P*<.01) greater improvement on mood-related items than was experienced by placebo-treated patients. Patients with and without a concurrent mood disturbance ($HAMD_{17}$ total score ≥17 or HAMD item 1 ≥2) at baseline experienced a statistically significant anti-OCD treatment effect with fluoxetine.

Adverse events reported with fluoxetine were consistent with its known safety profile as has been reported in previous studies of fluoxetine in patients with OCD.[28,31] Overall treatment differences were statistically significant for three of the most commonly reported adverse events (nausea, dry mouth, and tremor). Discontinuation rates for specific adverse events were low, suggesting that events were well tolerated. For some adverse events, incidence was dose dependent. Discontinuations for adverse events were also dose dependent. Overall, it can be expected that the favorable side-effect profile of fluoxetine as well as a reduced need to titrate the dose may provide considerable advantages over other anti-OCD drug treatments. In turn, patient compliance in the short and long term may be enhanced.

No consistent 5-HT marker has emerged that reliably distinguishes patients with OCD from normal subjects.[53] However, the strongest neuropharmacological evidence for a 5-HT role in OCD stems from the efficacy of 5-HT uptake inhibitors in alleviating the symptoms of this disorder. The 5-HT projections are found in orbitofrontal cortex, cingulate cortex, and the head of the caudate. Several authors[54-56] have hypothesized that these centers form a circuit that is overactive in OCD, perhaps in

an attempt to suppress interference from internal stimuli. Pharmacotherapy with 5-HT uptake inhibitors has been associated with regional metabolic changes in glucose utilization.[57,58] In addition to clomipramine and fluoxetine, other agents such as fluvoxamine,[59] zimelidine hydrochloride,[60] and possibly sertraline hydrochloride[61] appear effective. The precise mechanism of action in OCD for this drug class is unknown. However, the relevance of 5-HT activity is suggested by the maintenance of the therapeutic benefit produced by clomipramine (a nonselective 5-HT reuptake inhibitor) in over 85% of patients crossed over to fluoxetine (a selective 5-HT uptake inhibitor) under double-blind conditions.[34]

Further, in comparison with clomipramine and fluoxetine, which were associated with at least a 95% reduction in platelet 5-HT, Pigott and colleagues[62] reported only a 26% mean reduction after 10 weeks of trazodone hydrochloride administration. They concluded that trazodone lacked substantial anti-obsessional effects. Thus, while this apparent neurochemical selectivity for anti-obsessional drugs points to a 5-HT mechanism, the locus is apparently not at the 5-HT_2 receptor.

Because the overall response rate to selective 5-HT uptake inhibitors is limited, the role of other neurotransmitters in OCD must be considered. In a preliminary meta-analytic comparison, it appeared a greater overall effect was associated with less 5-HT specificity.[59] While evidence is limited, a secondary reduction in noradrenergic or dopaminergic activity within certain brain regions where 5-HT is co-localized may also be contributing to drug efficacy.[63] In all likelihood, a variety of factors, eg, regional specificity, selective receptor subtype activity, and primary vs secondary adaptive changes, are operative. Any statement on the mechanism of selective serotonin uptake inhibitor pharmacotherapy in OCD is at best speculative.

Our findings confirm previous reports that 5-HT uptake inhibitors reduce the severity of OCD symptoms. In contrast to several previous reports of pharmacotherapy in OCD, this study examined a large sample of patients with rigorously diagnosed OCD, employed a fixed-dose design, used standardized outcome measures, and excluded patients with a concomitant primary depression.

Unlike conventional pharmacology trials of the affective disorders, patients with OCD tend to respond to drug treatment with less robust symptomatic improvements.[64] Across several blinded trials, approximately one third of patients with OCD achieved full response criteria. Some patients will remain chronically symptomatic to some degree despite optimal pharmacological intervention.[65] However limited, such improvements may be clinically significant, within the individual patient, in improving the quality of life (eg, the amount of time engaged in the pathological symptom). Evidence suggests that adjunctive behavioral therapies may substantially add to symptom relief.[66] In addition, Jenike[64] has outlined a rational approach to augmentation strategies. Reportedly, the large majority of patients with OCD have a good outcome (at least moderately better) with aggressive and appropriate therapy.[67]

Questions remain concerning the pharmacological treatment of OCD. Yet to be determined are the optimal dose and length of treatment, the risk of relapse after discontinuation of therapy, gender differences, clinical and laboratory response predictors, strategies for dose augmentation in a large number of patients with slow or inadequate response, and strategies for maintenance treatment.

Accepted for publication February 25, 1994.

We wish to acknowledge the members of the Fluoxetine Obsessive-Compulsive Disorder Collaborative Study Group who participated in this trial: Robert Reichler, MD, Harborview Medical Center, University of Washington Medical School, Seattle; Fred Reimherr, MD, University of Utah Medical Center, Salt Lake City; and David E. Wheadon, MD, Bruce E. Dornseif, PhD, and Patrick Q. Mooney, Eli Lilly and Company, Indianapolis, Ind.

Reprint requests to Psychopharmacology Division, Eli Lilly and Company, Lilly Corporate Center 2128, Indianapolis, IN 46285 (Dr Tollefson).

REFERENCES

1. Karno M, Golding JM, Sorenson SB, Burnam MA. The epidemiology of obsessive-compulsive disorder in five US communities. *Arch Gen Psychiatry.* 1988;45:1094-1099.
2. American Psychiatric Association, Committee on Nomenclature and Statistics. *Diagnostic and Statistical Manual of Mental Disorders, Revised Third Edition.* Washington, DC: American Psychiatric Association; 1987.
3. Charney DS, Goodman WK, Price LH, Woods SW, Rasmussen SA, Heninger GR. Serotonin function in obsessive-compulsive disorder: a comparison of the effects of tryptophan and *m*-chlorophenylpiperazine in patients and healthy subjects. *Arch Gen Psychiatry.* 1988;45:177-185.
4. Zohar J, Mueller EA, Insel TR, Zohar-Kadouch RC, Murphy DL. Serotonergic responsivity in obsessive-compulsive disorder. *Arch Gen Psychiatry.* 1987;44:946-951.
5. Zohar J, Insel TR, Zohar-Kadouch RC, Hill JL, Murphy DL. Serotonergic responsivity in obsessive-compulsive disorder. *Arch Gen Psychiatry.* 1988;45:167-172.
6. Murphy DL. Neuropsychiatric disorders and the multiple human brain serotonin receptor subtypes and subsystems. *Neuropsychopharmacology.* 1990;3:457-471.
7. Thoren P, Asberg M, Cronholm L. Clomipramine treatment of obsessive-compulsive disorder. *Arch Gen Psychiatry.* 1980;37:1281-1285.
8. Goodman WK, Price LH, Delgado PL, Palumbo J, Krystal JH, Nagy LM, Rasmussen SA, Heninger GR, Charney DS. Specificity of serotonin reuptake inhibitors in the treatment of obsessive-compulsive disorder. *Arch Gen Psychiatry.* 1990;47:577-585.
9. Trethowan JWH, Scott PAL. Chloropromazine in obsessive-compulsive and allied disorders. *Lancet.* 1955;268:781-785.
10. Rao AV. A controlled trial with 'Valium' in obsessive compulsive states. *J Indian Med Assoc.* 1964;42:564-567.
11. Orvin GH. Treatment of the phobic obsessive-compulsive patient with oxazepam, an improved benzodiazepine compound. *Psychomatics.* 1967;8:278-280.
12. Insel TR, Murphy DL, Cohen RM, Alterman I, Kitts C, Linnoila M. Obsessive-compulsive disorder: a double-blind trial of clomipramine and clorgyline. *Arch Gen Psychiatry.* 1983;40:605-612.
13. Clomipramine Collaborative Study Group. Clomipramine in the treatment of patients with obsessive-compulsive disorder. *Arch Gen Psychiatry.* 1991;48:730-738.
14. Fernandez-Cordoba E, Lopez-Ibor Alino J. La monoclorimipramina en enfer-

mos psiquiatricos resistentes a otros tratamientos. *Acta Luso-Esp Neurol Psiquiatr Ciene Afines.* 1967;26:119-147.

15. Amin MM, Ban TA, Pecknold JC, Klingner A. Clomipramine (Anafranil) and behavior therapy in obsessive-compulsive and phobic disorders. *J Int Med Res.* 1977;5(suppl 5):33-37.
16. Ananth J, Pecknold JC, Van Den Steen N, Engelsmann F. Double-blind comparative study of clomipramine and amitriptyline in obsessive neurosis. *Prog Neuropsychopharmacol Biol Psychiatry.* 1981;5:257-262.
17. DeVeaugh-Geiss J, Landau P, Katz R. Treatment of obsessive-compulsive disorder with clomipramine. *Psychiatr Ann.* 1989;19:97-101.
18. Capstick N. Clinical experience in the treatment of obsessional states. *J Int Med Res.* 1977;5(suppl 5):42-48.
19. Flament MF, Rapoport JL, Berg CJ, Sceery W, Kilts C, Mellstrom B, Linnoila M. Clomipramine treatment of childhood obsessive-compulsive disorder: a double-blind controlled study. *Arch Gen Psychiatry.* 1985;42:977-983.
20. Leonard HL, Swedo SE, Koby EV, Rapoport JL, Lenane MC, Cheslow DL, Hamburger SD. Treatment of obsessive-compulsive disorder with clomipramine and desmethylimipramine in children and adolescents: a double-blind crossover comparison. *Arch Gen Psychiatry.* 1989;46:1088-1092.
21. Marks IM, Stern RS, Mawson D, Cobb J, McDonald R. Clomipramine and exposure for obsessive-compulsive rituals, I. *Br J Psychiatry.* 1980;136:1-25.
22. Montgomery SA. Clomipramine in obsessional neurosis: a placebo-controlled trial. *Pharm Med.* 1990;1:189-192.
23. Thoren P, Asberg M, Cronholm B, Jornestedt L, Traskman L. Clomipramine treatment of obsessive-compulsive disorder, I: a controlled clinical trial. *Arch Gen Psychiatry.* 1980;37:1281-1285.
24. Rapoport J, Elkins R, Mikkelsen E. Clinical controlled trial of chlorimipramine in adolescents with obsessive-compulsive disorder. *Psychopharmacol Bull.* 1980; 16:61-65.
25. Montgomery SA. Which antidepressant? a review of the older treatments. In: Montgomery SA, ed. *Anxiety and Depression.* Hampshire, England: Wrightson Biomedical Publishing Ltd; 1990:31-44.
26. Thomas DR, Nelson DR, Johnson AM. Biochemical effects of the antidepressant paroxetine, a specific 5-hydroxytryptamine uptake inhibitor. *Psychopharmacology.* 1987;93:193-200.
27. Turner SM, Jacob RG, Beidel DC, Himmelhoch J. Fluoxetine treatment of obsessive-compulsive disorder. *J Clin Psychopharmacol.* 1985;5:207-212.
28. Fontaine R, Chouinard G. Fluoxetine in the treatment of obsessive-compulsive disorder. *Prog Neuropsychopharmacol Biol Psychiatry.* 1985;9:605-608.
29. Fontaine R, Chouinard G. Fluoxetine in the long-term maintenance treatment of obsessive-compulsive disorder. *Psychiatric Ann.* 1989;19:88-91.
30. Jenike MA, Buttolph L, Baer L, Ricciardi J, Holland A. Open trial of fluoxetine in obsessive-compulsive disorder. *Am J Psychiatry.* 1989;146:909-911.
31. Liebowitz MR, Hollander E, Schneier F, Campeas R, Hatterer J, Papp L, Fairbanks J, Sandberg D, Davies S, Stein M. Fluoxetine treatment of obsessive-compulsive disorder: an open clinical trial. *J Clin Psychopharmacol.* 1989;9:423-427.
32. Kim SW, Dysken MW. Open fixed dose trial of fluoxetine in the treatment of obsessive-compulsive disorder. *Drug Dev Res.* 1990;19:315-319.
33. Levine R, Hoffman JS, Day Knepple E, Kenin M. Long-term fluoxetine treatment of a large number of obsessive-compulsive patients. *J Clin Psychopharmacol.* 1989;9:281-283.
34. Pigott TA, Pato MT, Bernstein SE, Grover GN, Hill JL, Tolliver TJ, Murphy DL. Controlled comparisons of clomipramine and fluoxetine in the treatment of obsessive-compulsive disorder. *Arch Gen Psychiatry.* 1990;47:926-932.
35. Guy W. *ECDEU Assessment Manual for Psychopharmacology.* Washington, DC: US Dept of Health, Education, and Welfare; 1976:218-222.
36. Goodman WK, Price LH, Rasmussen SA, Mazure C, Fleischmann RL, Hill CL, Heninger GR, Charney DS. The Yale-Brown Obsessive Compulsive Scale, I: development, use, and reliability. *Arch Gen Psychiatry.* 1989;46:1006-1011.
37. Goodman WK, Price LH, Rasmussen SA, Mazure C, Delgado P, Heninger GR, Charney DS. The Yale-Brown Obsessive Compulsive Scale, II: validity. *Arch Gen Psychiatry.* 1989;46:1012-1016.
38. Hamilton M. Development of a rating scale for primary depressive illness. *Br J Soc Clin Psychol.* 1967;6:278-296.
39. Asberg M, Montgomery SA, Perris C, Shalling D, Sedvall G. A comprehensive psychopathological rating scale. *Acta Psychiatr Scand.* 1978;271(suppl):5-27.
40. Hommel G. A stagewise rejective multiple test procedure based on a modified Bonferroni test. *Biometrika.* 1988;75:383-386.
41. Mantel N, Haenszel W. Statistical aspects of the analysis of data from retrospective studies of disease. *J Natl Cancer Inst.* 1959;22:719-748.
42. Conover WJ, Iman RL. Rank transformations as a bridge between parametric and nonparametric statistics. *Am Statistician.* 1981;34:124-133.
43. SAS Institute Inc. *SAS Procedures Guide, Version 6.* 3rd ed. Cary, NC: SAS Institute Inc; 1990.
44. Hollander M, Wolfe DA. *Nonparametric Statistical Methods.* New York, NY: John Wiley & Sons Inc; 1973:120-123.
45. Beasley CM Jr, Potvin JH, Masica DN, Wheadon DE, Dornseif BE, Genduso LA. Fluoxetine: no association with suicidality in obsessive-compulsive disorder. *J Affect Disord.* 1992;24:1-10.
46. Boyer WF, Feighner JP. The efficacy of selective serotonin reuptake inhibitors in depression. In: Feighner JP, Boyer WF, eds. *Selective Serotonin Reuptake Inhibitors.* West Sussex, England: John Wiley & Sons Inc; 1991:92-94.
47. Cooper GL. The safety of fluoxetine—an update. *Br J Psychiatry.* 1988;153 (suppl 3):77-86.
48. Turner SM, Beidel DC, Stanley MA, Jacob RG. A comparison of fluoxetine, flooding and response prevention in the treatment of obsessive-compulsive disorder. *J Anxiety Disord.* 1988;2:219-225.
49. Fontaine R, Chouinard G. An open clinical trial of fluoxetine in the treatment of obsessive-compulsive disorder. *J Clin Psychopharmacol.* 1986;6:98-101.
50. Montgomery SA, McIntyre A, Osterheider M, Sarteschi P, Zitterl W, Zohar J, Birkett M, Wood AJ, the Lilly European OCD Study Group. A double-blind, placebo-controlled study of fluoxetine in patients with *DSM-III-R* obsessive-compulsive disorder. *Eur Neuropsychopharmacol.* 1993;3:143-152.
51. Altamura AC, Montgomery SA, Wernicke JF. The evidence for 20 mg a day of fluoxetine as the optimal dose in the treatment of depression. *Br J Psychiatry.* 1988;153(suppl 3):109-112.
52. Perse T. Obsessive-compulsive disorder: a treatment review. *J Clin Psychiatry.* 1988;49:48-55.
53. Insel TR, Winslow JT. Neurobiology of obsessive-compulsive disorder. *Psychiatr Clin North Am.* 1992;15:813-824.
54. Modell J, Mountz J, Curtis G, Greden J. Neurophysiologic dysfunction in basal ganglia/limbic striatal and thalamocortical circuits as a pathogenetic mechanism of obsessive-compulsive disorder. *J Neuropsychiatry.* 1989;1:27-36.
55. Rapoport J. Recent advances in obsessive-compulsive disorder. *Neuropsychopharmacology.* 1991;5:1-10.
56. Baxter L, Schwartz J, Guze B, Bergman K, Szuba M. Neuroimaging in obsessive-compulsive disorder: seeking the mediating neuroanatomy: In: Jenike M, Baer L, Minichiello W, eds. *Secondary Neuroimaging in Obsessive-Compulsive Disorder: Seeking the Mediating Neuroanatomy.* St Louis, Mo: Mosby–Year Book; 1990:167-188.
57. Baxter LR Jr, Schwartz JM, Bergman KS, Szuba MP, Guze BH, Mazziotta JC, Alazraki A, Selin CE, Ferng H-K, Munford P, Phelps ME. Caudate glucose metabolic rate changes with both drug and behavior therapy for obsessive-compulsive disorder. *Arch Gen Psychiatry.* 1992;49:681-689.
58. Benkelfat C, Nordahl TE, Semple WE, King C, Murphy DL, Cohen RM. Local cerebral glucose metabolic activity in obsessive-compulsive disorder: patients treated with clomipramine. *Arch Gen Psychiatry.* 1990;47:840-848.
59. Jenike MA, Hyman S, Baer L, Holland A, Minichiello WE, Buttolph L, Summergrad P, Seymour R, Ricciardi J. A controlled trial of fluvoxamine in obsessive-compulsive disorder: implications for a serotonergic theory. *Am J Psychiatry.* 1990;147:1209-1215.
60. Kahn RS, Westenberg HGM, Jolles J. Zimelidine treatment of obsessive-compulsive disorder. *Acta Psychiatr Scand.* 1984;69:259-261.
61. Chouinard G, Goodman W, Greist JH, Jenike M, Rasmussen S, White K, Hackett E, Gaffney M, Bick PA. Results of a double-blind placebo-controlled trial of a new serotonin uptake inhibitor, sertraline, in the treatment of obsessive-compulsive disorder. *Psychopharmacol Bull.* 1990;26:279-284.
62. Pigott TA, L'Heureux F, Rubenstein CS, Bernstein SE, Hill JI, Murphy DI. A double-blind, placebo-controlled study of trazodone in patients with obsessive-compulsive disorder. *J Clin Psychopharmacol.* 1992;12:156-162.
63. DeSimoni MG, DalToso G, Fodritto F, Sokola A, Algeri S. Modulation of striatal dopamine metabolism by the activity of dorsal raphe serotonergic afferences. *Brain Res.* 1987;411:81-88.
64. Jenike MA. Pharmacologic treatment of obsessive compulsive disorders. *Psychiatr Clin North Am.* 1992;15:895-919.
65. White K, Cole J. Pharmacotherapy. In: Bellack AS, Hersen M, eds. *Handbook of Comparative Treatments.* New York, NY: John Wiley & Sons Inc; 1990:266-284.
66. Jenike MA. Obsessive-compulsive and related disorders: a hidden epidemic. *N Engl J Med.* 1989;321:539-541.
67. Jenike MA, Baer L, Minichiello WE. *Obsessive-Compulsive Disorders: Theory and Management.* 2nd ed. St Louis, Mo: Mosby–Year Book; 1990.

ORIGINAL ARTICLE

Incentives Improve Outcome in Outpatient Behavioral Treatment of Cocaine Dependence

Stephen T. Higgins, PhD; Alan J. Budney, PhD; Warren K. Bickel, PhD; Florian E. Foerg; Robert Donham, MA; Gary J. Badger, MS

Objective: To assess whether incentives improved treatment outcome in ambulatory cocaine-dependent patients.

Method: Forty cocaine-dependent adults were randomly assigned to behavioral treatment with or without an added incentive program. The behavioral treatment was based on the Community Reinforcement Approach and was provided to both groups. Subjects in the group with incentives received vouchers exchangeable for retail items contingent on submitting cocaine-free urine specimens during weeks 1 through 12 of treatment, while the group without incentives received no vouchers during that period. The two groups were treated the same during weeks 13 through 24.

Results: Seventy-five percent of patients in the group with vouchers completed 24 weeks of treatment vs 40% in the group without vouchers (P=.03). Average durations of continuous cocaine abstinence documented via urinalysis during weeks 1 through 24 of treatment were 11.7±2.0 weeks in the group with vouchers vs 6.0±1.5 weeks in the group without vouchers (P=.03). At 24 weeks after treatment entry, the voucher group evidenced significantly greater improvement than the no-voucher group on the Drug scale of the Addiction Severity Index (ASI), and only the voucher group showed significant improvement on the ASI Psychiatric scale.

Conclusions: Incentives delivered contingent on submitting cocaine-free urine specimens significantly improve treatment outcome in ambulatory cocaine-dependent patients.

(Arch Gen Psychiatry. 1994;51:568-576)

COCAINE DEPENDENCE remains an intractable US public health problem that contributes to many of our most disturbing social crises, including the spread of infectious disease (eg, acquired immunodeficiency syndrome [AIDS], hepatitis, and tuberculosis), crime, violence, and neonatal drug exposure.[1-3] Although recreational cocaine use has decreased, regular use indicative of dependence and use by certain subgroups (eg, criminals) has remained stable or increased along with other disturbing trends like increases in cocaine-related emergency department visits, cocaine-related deaths, and the proportion of cocaine-related admissions to state-supported treatment facilities.[4-6]

There is no consensus regarding how to treat cocaine dependence. Considerable scientific effort has been directed at developing pharmacotherapies, and some encouraging initial studies suggested antidepressants were efficacious.[7,8] Subsequent studies have not supported the efficacy of antidepressants or any other psychotropic medications in the treatment of cocaine dependence,[9,10] although numerous potentially effective compounds are under investigation.

Even if effective pharmacotherapies are developed, combining them with effective psychosocial treatments will be necessary to address the multiple problems common in drug dependence.[11] In two controlled clinical trials conducted in our clinic,[12,13] a multicomponent behavioral treatment integrating contingency management proce-

From the Departments of Psychiatry (Drs Higgins, Budney, and Bickel and Messrs Foerg and Donham), Psychology (Drs Higgins, Budney, and Bickel), and Medical Biostatistics (Mr Badger), University of Vermont, Burlington.

See Subjects and Methods on next page

SUBJECTS AND METHODS

SUBJECTS

Forty subjects were recruited by advertisements in local newspapers, public service announcements on television and radio, notices mailed to local professionals, and posters located throughout the local community. Individuals had to be 18 years of age or older, meet *DSM-III-R* diagnostic criteria for active cocaine dependence, and have used cocaine within the past 30 days for inclusion. Opioid dependence, sedative dependence, psychosis, pregnancy, dementia, recent inpatient treatment for cocaine dependence, a medical condition precluding employment, or plans to leave the immediate geographical area within 6 months were exclusion criteria. Twelve individuals were thus excluded, the reasons being benzodiazepine and opiate dependence (seven individuals), pregnancy (one individual), active psychosis (one individual), plans to leave the area within 6 months (one individual), and recent inpatient hospitalizations (two individuals).

Minimum likelihood allocation[26] was used to randomize patients sequentially to one of two treatments: behavioral treatment with or without vouchers. The vouchers served as incentives. The purpose of this type of randomization was to achieve balance between the treatment groups for the following baseline characteristics that may influence outcome: gender, primary route of cocaine administration (intravenous vs other), whether the patient had a significant other who was not a drug abuser and was potentially willing to participate in treatment, legal matters pending, full-time employment status, and Psychiatric scale composite scores of 0.65 or greater on the Addiction Severity Index (ASI).[27] The ASI is a structured interview that assesses alcohol and drug use as well as important areas of functioning commonly affected by substance abuse (ie, Medical, Employment, Family/Social, Psychiatric, and Legal).[27,28] Composite scale scores can be calculated in each of the problem areas.[27] These composite scores are weighted combinations of individual items that provide reliable, valid, and sensitive measures of problem severity during the 30 days prior to the interview. The cutoff of 0.65 on the ASI Psychiatric scale used for stratification purposes in the present study was determined empirically in our clinic to identify patients with relatively high psychiatric severity ratings, which have been determined previously to predict poor outcome in substance abuse treatment.[28]

The stratification procedure succeeded in balancing the two groups on each of the following characteristics: the number of male patients in the voucher and no-voucher groups was 14 (70%) and 13 (65%), respectively; the number who indicated having a significant other who potentially could participate in treatment, 18 (90%) and 18 (90%), respectively; the number who reported legal matters pending, seven (35%) and five (25%), respectively; the number who reported full-time employment, seven (35%) and six (30%), respectively; the number who reported preference for the intravenous route of cocaine administration, six (30%) and four (20%), respectively; and the number scoring 0.65 or higher on the ASI Psychiatric composite scale, three (15%) and three (15%), respectively. The two groups did not differ significantly on any characteristic assessed at baseline (**Table 1**).

INTAKE

Informed consent was obtained, and the ASI, the Psychoactive Substance Abuse Disorder sections of the *DSM-III-R* checklist,[29] and questionnaires about demographics and history of drug use were completed at intake.

TREATMENT DURATION

Treatment duration for both groups was 24 weeks, with the initial 12 weeks representing the primary treatment period and the second 12 weeks, an aftercare period.

VOUCHER PROCEDURE

Urine specimens were collected from all subjects under staff observation on Mondays, Wednesdays, and Fridays during weeks 1 through 12 and Mondays and Thursdays during weeks 13 through 24. Specimens were screened immediately via an onsite Enzyme-Multiplied Immunoassay Technique (EMIT, Syva Corp, San Jose, Calif). All specimens were screened for benzoylecgonine, a cocaine metabolite, and one randomly selected specimen each week also was screened for the presence of other abused drugs. Breath alcohol levels were assessed at the time urine specimens were collected. Failure to submit a scheduled specimen was treated as a cocaine-positive result, and failure to submit scheduled specimens on five consecutive occasions resulted in termination from treatment in both treatment groups. Patients were informed of their urinalysis results immediately after submitting their specimens.

For those assigned to the voucher group, specimens collected during weeks 1 through 12 that were negative for benzoylecgonine earned points that were recorded on vouchers and given to subjects. Points were worth the equivalent of $0.25 each. Money was never provided directly to subjects. Instead, points were used to purchase retail items in the community. A staff member made all purchases. The first negative specimen was worth 10 points at $0.25 per point or $2.50. The value of vouchers for each subsequent consecutive negative specimen increased by five points (eg, 15 points for the second, 20 points for the third, etc). To further increase the likelihood of continuous cocaine abstinence, the equivalent of a $10 bonus was earned for each three consecutive negative specimens. Specimens that were cocaine positive or failure to submit a scheduled specimen reset the value of vouchers back to the initial $2.50 value from which they could escalate again according to the same schedule. Submission of five consecutive cocaine-negative specimens following submission of a positive specimen returned the value of points to where they were prior to the reset. Points could not be lost once earned.

Continued on next page

Patients and counselors jointly selected retail items to be purchased with the points. The items obtained were quite diverse and included YMCA passes, continuing education materials, fishing licenses, gift certificates to local restaurants, camera equipment, bicycle equipment, etc. Counselors retained veto power over all purchases. Purchases were only approved if counselors deemed them to be in concert with individual treatment goals of increasing drug-free prosocial activities.

Patients assigned to the no-voucher group received slips of paper after each urinalysis test. These slips of paper were physically comparable to those used as vouchers in the other treatment group. They indicated the outcome of the test but had no monetary value. This procedure was done to keep staff-patient interactions comparable across the two groups during urinalysis.

During weeks 13 through 24, urinalysis results were treated in the same manner across the two treatment groups. Subjects in both treatment groups received a single $1.00 Vermont State Lottery ticket per each cocaine-negative urinalysis result. Those assigned to the voucher group could earn the equivalent of $997.50 if they were continuously abstinent from cocaine during weeks 1 through 12 and $24 if they were abstinent during weeks 13 through 24.

COMMUNITY REINFORCEMENT APPROACH

The CRA was implemented with both treatment groups in 1-hour counseling sessions scheduled twice weekly for the initial 12 weeks and then once weekly during the final 12 weeks of treatment. Sessions focused on four general issues. First, subjects with a spouse, friend, or relative who was not a drug abuser and was willing to participate in treatment received reciprocal relationship counseling.[30] This is a validated procedure for instructing dyads how to negotiate positive changes in their relationship. To integrate CRA and contingency management procedures, significant others were telephoned immediately following each urinalysis test and informed of results. If the specimen was negative for cocaine, the significant other engaged in agreed-on activities with patients. If the result was positive for cocaine use, the significant other refrained from the activities but offered assistance to the patient in dealing with difficulties in achieving abstinence.

Second, subjects were instructed how to recognize antecedents and consequences of their cocaine use. They were counseled to restructure their daily activities to minimize contact with known antecedents, find alternatives for the positive consequences derived from cocaine use, and make explicit the negative consequences of cocaine use. Skills training was provided to those with specific deficits (eg, drug refusal, problem solving, and assertiveness). Counseling for AIDS prevention was provided to all patients in both treatment groups.

Third, unemployed patients were offered employment counseling,[31] and assistance also was provided for those interested in pursuing educational goals and job changes and those with miscellaneous practical needs such as financial counseling, alternative housing, and legal and social services.

Fourth, subjects were counseled to develop new recreational activities or to become reinvolved in those they pursued prior to beginning cocaine use. Counselors and subjects worked together to identify these activities. For those assigned to the voucher group, vouchers earned via cocaine-free urine specimens could be used to support the costs of initiating these activities.

The behavioral therapists were the same for both treatment groups and involved three master's level therapists (two women and one man [R.D.]) with 1 to 3 years of prior experience using this behavioral treatment for cocaine dependence.

All subjects who met *DSM-III-R* criteria for alcohol dependence or abuse were offered disulfiram therapy, which is an integral part of the CRA treatment for alcoholism. Forty percent (8/20) and 35% (7/20) of the voucher group and 65% (13/20) and 25% (5/20) of the no-voucher group received disulfiram therapy during weeks 1 through 12 and 13 through 24 of treatment, respectively. All subjects received a standard dose of 250 mg/d, except for one person in each group who received 500 mg/d after reporting being able to drink without a disulfiram reaction and one person in the voucher and two in the no-voucher groups who received 125 mg/d because of side effects at the standard dose. Disulfiram was ingested under clinic staff observation on urinalysis days, and, when possible, under the observation of a significant other on the other days.

END-OF-TREATMENT ASSESSMENT

End-of-treatment assessments were performed at 24 weeks after treatment entry, whether patients dropped out or completed treatment. Nineteen patients per group were inter-

dures (ie, incentives)[14] and the Community Reinforcement Approach (CRA)[15] was more efficacious than standard drug abuse counseling in retaining cocaine-dependent individuals in outpatient treatment and establishing clinically significant periods of continuous cocaine abstinence. The results obtained with this behavioral treatment were reliable and clinically meaningful, with approximately 85% of patients completing 12 weeks of treatment and 65% to 70% achieving 6 or more weeks of continuous cocaine abstinence across the two trials. By contrast, less than 45% of patients assigned to standard counseling completed 12 weeks of treatment, and we documented 6 or more weeks of continuous cocaine abstinence in only 5% to 10% of them.

While the positive initial results obtained with this treatment are encouraging, further assessment of its reliability and identification of its active components are essential for purposes of efficiency, cost-effectiveness, and dissemination. The primary goals of this intervention were to assemble a comprehensive treatment package that had a high likelihood of success and thereafter to conduct ex-

viewed; one patient per group was unavailable for follow-up. A urine specimen was collected under staff observation as part of that assessment, and the ASI was completed.

STATISTICAL METHODS

Comparisons between the treatment groups on baseline characteristics were performed using either two-sample t tests or Wilcoxon Rank Sum tests for continuous variables and χ^2 tests for nominal variables. The χ^2 tests also were used to compare treatment acceptability, treatment retention, and other drug use. For each subject, the longest documented period of continuous cocaine abstinence was computed separately for weeks 1 through 12, weeks 13 through 24, and the total treatment period (weeks 1 through 24). The distributions associated with continuous cocaine abstinence achieved during the 24 weeks in the two treatment groups were compared using a log-rank test. Treatment comparisons with respect to mean continuous cocaine abstinence and duration of treatment retention over the 24 weeks were performed using two-sample t tests. In addition, repeated measures analysis of variance (ANOVA) was used to compare treatment groups and study periods (weeks 1 through 12 vs 13 through 24) on abstinence achieved during the two 12-week periods. When results of the overall F test from this analysis indicated a significant difference between treatments, comparisons within each of the treatment periods were performed using Fisher's least significant difference (LSD) procedure. Missing urine specimens were treated as cocaine positive, which is a recommended method for dealing with missing data in substance abuse treatment research.[32] A Breslow-Day χ^2 test for homogeneity was used to determine if the treatment effect on retention was different for subjects whose specimens were cocaine negative vs those whose specimens were cocaine positive during week 1 of treatment. Variance component analysis was used to examine potential therapist effects on continuous cocaine abstinence, which was the primary outcome measure in this study. Repeated measures ANOVA was used to evaluate differences in changes observed between the pretreatment and posttreatment ASI assessments. Statistical analyses were performed using SAS Statistical Software,[33] and significance was determined at the 5% level.

Table 1. Subject Characteristics*

Characteristic	Voucher Group (N=20)	No-Voucher Group (N=20)
Demographics		
Mean age, y†	31.8±3.9	30.9±6.1
White, %	90	80
Male, %	70	65
Never married, %	45	35
≤12 y of education, %	70	85
Employed full time, %	35	55
Median weekly income (interquartile range), $‡	200 (113-350)	194 (122-280)
Cocaine use		
Preferred route, %		
Intranasal	55	45
Intravenous	30	20
Freebase	15	35
Median (interquartile range), g/wk	2.7 (1.5-5.2)	2.4 (1.5-3.2)
Other drug dependence, %		
Alcohol	45	65
Marijuana	10	15
Alcohol and marijuana	10	5
Addiction Severity Index composite scales, mean scores†		
Medical	0.11±0.22	0.13±0.30
Employment	0.54±0.31	0.65±0.28
Alcohol	0.29±0.28	0.40±0.31
Drug	0.25±0.06	0.23±0.08
Psychiatric	0.35±0.27	0.38±0.23
Legal	0.20±0.26	0.12±0.19
Family/Social	0.36±0.25	0.35±0.25
Beck Depression Inventory, mean score†	21.1±14.9	19.4±9.8
Michigan Alcoholism Screening Test, mean score†	16.8±15.1	19.8±13.5

*Treatment groups are described in the "Subjects and Methods" section of the text.
†Data are represented as mean±SD.
‡Data include employed and unemployed subjects.

periments that assessed which components were necessary to achieve a positive outcome. The present randomized trial evaluated the most novel component of this treatment: an incentive program wherein patients earn vouchers exchangeable for retail items contingent on documentation of cocaine abstinence via urinalysis.

Considering the widespread use of incentives in our society and their efficacy in the treatment of other forms of drug dependence,[16,17] investigating the systematic use of incentives to foster cocaine abstinence is warranted. An even more compelling rationale for investigating this question is the large body of basic scientific evidence documenting that the use of cocaine and other drugs is sensitive to systematically delivered consequences, both positive and negative.[18-23] We chose to investigate positive rather than negative consequences, because the former are more likely to be acceptable to patients and retain them in treatment. Using negative consequences for drug use may be effective for those patients who enter and remain in treatment. However, unless individuals are mandated to do so, most will either decline participation or drop out soon after experiencing the negative events.[24,25]

Finding treatments that are acceptable to cocaine abusers and thus increasing the number who enter and remain in treatment is essential to curtailing the public health and social problems enumerated above. The present study demonstrates that providing incentives in combination with a comprehensive behavioral intervention effectively retains cocaine-dependent individuals in treatment and engenders clinically significant periods of cocaine abstinence.

RESULTS

TREATMENT ACCEPTABILITY AND PATIENT RETENTION

Treatment acceptability was inferred from the number of subjects who attended more than one therapy session. All subjects in both treatment groups attended more than one therapy session, indicating high and comparable levels of initial patient acceptance.

With regard to treatment retention, 90% in the voucher group vs 65% in the no-voucher group completed 12 weeks of treatment ($\chi^2[1]=3.6$; $P=.06$), and 75% in the voucher group vs 40% in the no-voucher group completed 24 weeks ($\chi^2[1]=5.0$; $P=.03$). Average duration of retention in the voucher group was 21±1.5 (±SEM) weeks vs 15.7±2.0 weeks in the no-voucher group ($t[38]=2.1$; $P=.04$).

COCAINE ABSTINENCE

The voucher group consistently exceeded the no-voucher group in the percentages of patients who were documented via urinalysis to have achieved specific durations of continuous cocaine abstinence (log-rank $\chi^2[1]=4.4$; $P=.03$) (**Figure**). For example, 70%, 55%, and 30% of patients in the voucher group were documented to have achieved at least 5, 10, and 20 weeks of continuous cocaine abstinence, respectively, vs 50%, 15%, and 5%, respectively, in the no-voucher group.

With regard to average durations of continuous cocaine abstinence documented across the 24 weeks of treatment, the voucher group averaged 11.7±2.0 weeks vs 6.0±1.5 weeks in the no-voucher group ($t[38]=2.2$; $P=.03$) (Figure). The duration of continuous abstinence documented within each of the 12-week treatment periods was significantly longer in the voucher than the no-voucher groups ($F[1,38]=7.3$; $P=.01$). During weeks 1 through 12 of treatment when the voucher program was in effect, average duration of continuous cocaine abstinence documented in the voucher group was 7.2±1.1 weeks vs 3.9±0.9 weeks in the no-voucher group (Fisher's LSD, $P<.05$). Similarly, during weeks 13 through 24 when patients in both groups were treated the same, average duration of continuous cocaine abstinence documented in the voucher group was 6.1±1.0 weeks vs 2.7±0.8 weeks in the no-voucher group (Fisher's LSD, $P<.05$). The decrease in both treatment groups of approximately 1 week in average abstinence levels between weeks 1 through 12 and 13 through 24 was significant ($F[1,38]=5.5$; $P=.02$), but there was no evidence of greater decline in the voucher than the no-voucher group ($F[1,38]$, $P=.91$). This comparable decline in the two treatment groups indicates that the vouchers were successfully discontinued in the voucher group at the end of week 12 without producing

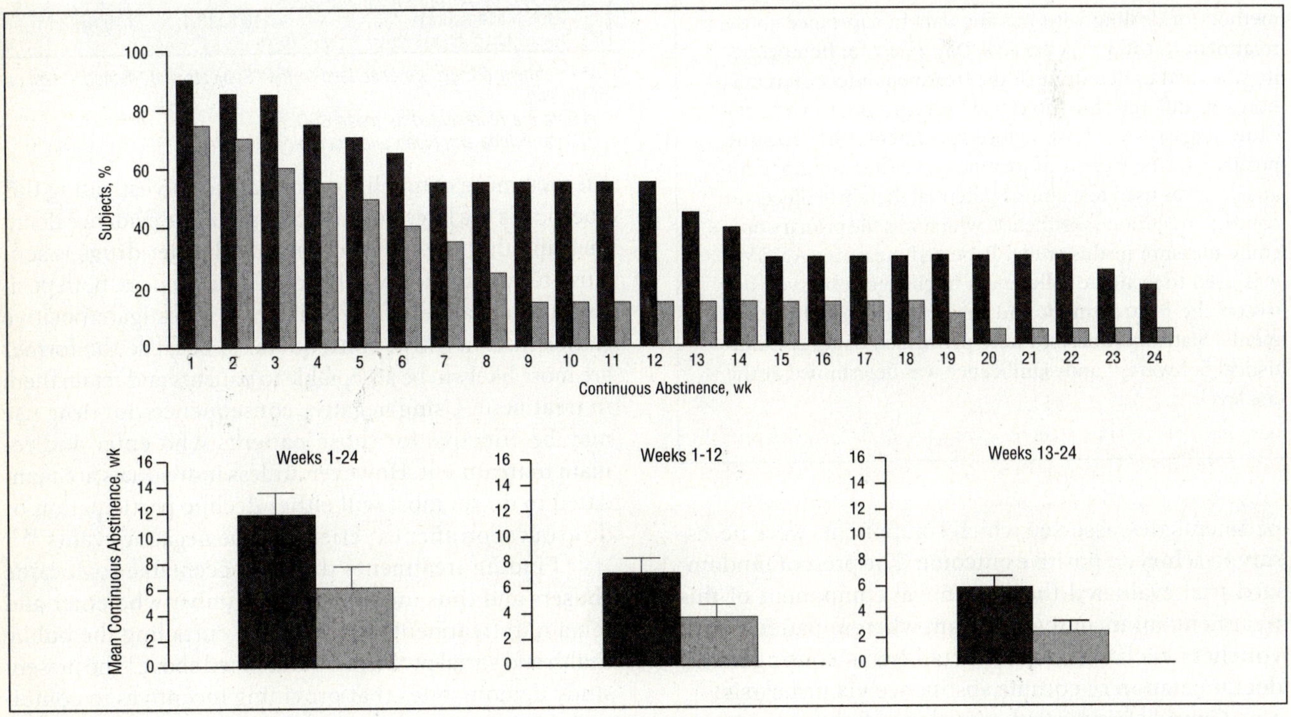

Top, Distributions of documented, continuous cocaine abstinence observed in each treatment group. The height of each bar represents the percentage of patients achieving a duration of abstinence greater than or equal to the number of weeks indicated. Note that the x-axis shows weeks of continuous abstinence and not consecutive treatment weeks. Bottom, Mean durations of continuous abstinence achieved in each treatment group during weeks 1 through 24, 1 through 12, and 13 through 24. Solid bars indicate the voucher group; shaded bars, the no-voucher group. Treatment groups are described in the "Subjects and Methods" section of the text.

any greater decrease in subsequent cocaine abstinence levels than would be expected had these subjects never received the vouchers.

As was noted above, patients in both treatment groups were treated by one of three therapists. Variance component analysis indicated that therapists accounted for less than 5% of the variability observed in continuous cocaine abstinence across subjects.

There were no significant differences between the two treatment groups in the percentages of subjects in whom cocaine abstinence was documented at the end-of-treatment assessment. Eighty percent in the voucher group and 75% in the no-voucher group provided cocaine-negative specimens at the 24-week assessment ($\chi^2[1]=0.14$; $P=.70$).

RELATIONSHIP OF EARLY IN-TREATMENT COCAINE USE TO OUTCOME

Drug use early in treatment has been noted previously to predict poor outcome in drug abuse treatment.[34] This analysis examined whether patients who exhibited difficulty achieving cocaine abstinence during week 1 of treatment benefited from the vouchers and also whether those who evidenced cocaine abstinence during that time did well without vouchers.

The treatment groups did not differ significantly in the number of patients with cocaine-positive specimens during week 1, with 10 (50%) and 12 (60%) such patients in the voucher and no-voucher groups, respectively ($\chi^2[1]=0.40$; $P=.52$). Among those patients, 70% (7/10) in the voucher group vs 17% (2/12) in the no-voucher group completed 24 weeks of treatment ($\chi^2[1]=6.4$; $P=.01$). Among patients with cocaine-negative specimens during week 1, both treatment groups did well; 80% (8/10) in the voucher group and 75% (6/8) in the no-voucher group completed 24 weeks of treatment ($\chi^2[1]=0.1$; $P=.80$). While the effects of vouchers on treatment retention were largely influenced by their effects in those patients who had difficulty early in treatment, the interaction between initial abstinence and treatment group was not statistically significant (Breslow-Day $\chi^2[1]=2.07$; $P=.15$).

Results of repeated measures ANOVA indicated that vouchers significantly increased continuous cocaine abstinence ($F[1,36]=5.02$; $P=.03$). Among patients with cocaine-positive specimens in week 1, those in the voucher group achieved an average of 6.9±2.2 weeks vs 2.4±0.8 weeks in the no-voucher group, demonstrating a positive effect of vouchers (Fisher's LSD procedure, $P<.05$). Among those with cocaine-negative specimens during week 1, the average duration of continuous cocaine abstinence was 16.4±2.7 weeks in the voucher group vs 11.3±2.8 weeks in the no-voucher group, indicating a similar positive effect of vouchers (Fisher's LSD, $P<.05$). There was no evidence of an interaction between treatment group and week 1 urinalysis results on continuous abstinence ($F[1,36]=0.01$; $P=.92$).

ADDICTION SEVERITY INDEX

The ASI assessments were completed prior to and at the end of treatment in 19 patients per group. The two treatment groups did not differ significantly on any of the ASI composite scores prior to treatment (**Table 2**). At the end of treatment, significant decreases from pretreatment scores were observed in both treatment groups on the ASI Family/Social ($F[1,36]=33.7$; $P<.001$), Alcohol ($F[1,36]=29.9$; $P<.001$), and Drug ($F[1,36]=154$; $P<.001$) composite scales (Table 2). The magnitude of change did not differ significantly between treatment groups on the Family/Social or Alcohol scales but was significantly greater in the voucher than the no-voucher group on the Drug scale ($F[1,36]=7.1$; $P=.01$). This difference was largely due to three items: (1) the mean number of days of cocaine use in the past 30 days decreased from 11.5±2.0 at pretreatment to 1.0±0.5 at 6 months in the voucher group vs 9.1±1.7 to 2.5±0.8 in the no-voucher group; (2) the mean number of days in the past 30 on which patients experienced drug problems decreased from 14.9±2.6 at pretreatment to 0.8±0.3 at 6 months in the voucher group vs 9.4±2.4 to 2.6±0.8 in the no-voucher group; and (3) how troubled or bothered patients were in the past 30 days by these drug problems (rated from 0 to 4, with

Table 2. Addiction Severity Index*

Composite Scale	Scores: Pretreatment	Scores: Posttreatment
Medical		
Voucher group	0.11±0.05	0.11±0.06
No-voucher group	0.14±0.07	0.13±0.06
Employment		
Voucher group	0.54±0.07	0.56±0.07
No-voucher group	0.68±0.06	0.64±0.06
Alcohol		
Voucher group	0.31±0.06	0.11±0.04†
No-voucher group	0.42±0.07	0.21±0.05†
Drug		
Voucher group	0.26±0.01	0.05±0.01†‡
No-voucher group	0.23±0.02	0.10±0.02†‡
Legal		
Voucher group	0.18±0.06	0.09±0.04
No-voucher group	0.12±0.05	0.14±0.05
Family/Social		
Voucher group	0.41±0.06	0.14±0.05†
No-voucher group	0.37±0.05	0.14±0.03†
Psychiatric		
Voucher group	0.37±0.06	0.13±0.03†
No-voucher group	0.39±0.05	0.31±0.05

*Scores are represented as mean±SEM. Voucher and no-voucher groups each consist of 19 subjects. Treatment groups are described in the "Subjects and Methods" section of the text.

†$P<.05$, a significant change from pretreatment scores.

‡$P<.05$, a significant difference between treatment groups.

higher scores indicating more problems) decreased from a pretreatment average of 3.6±0.1 to 0.9±0.3 in the voucher group vs 3.3±0.2 to 1.7±0.3 in the no-voucher group. Notably, on the first item concerning days of cocaine use in the past 30, 12 (63%) patients in the voucher group vs seven (37%) in the no-voucher group reported no use.

Differences between the treatment groups in the magnitude of change from pretreatment to follow-up on the ASI Psychiatric scale scores approached statistical significance ($F[1,36]=3.7$; $P=.06$). Scores decreased significantly from pretreatment levels in the voucher group (Fisher's LSD, $P<.05$) but not in the no-voucher group. The significant change in the voucher group was largely accounted for by (1) the percentage of patients who reported experiencing significant periods (3 or more consecutive days) of serious depression in the past 30 days that was not a direct result of drug/alcohol use decreased from 53% (10/19) prior to treatment to 21% (4/19) after treatment and (2) the percentage of people who reported significant periods of trouble understanding, concentrating, or remembering during the past 30 days that were not a direct result of drug/alcohol use decreased from 53% (10/19) prior to treatment to 10% (2/19) after treatment. Comparable changes for these two items in the no-voucher group were a change from 58% (11/19) prior to treatment to 79% (15/19) after treatment in the percentage of patients reporting periods of serious depression and a change from 58% (11/19) prior to treatment to 37% (7/19) after treatment in the percentage reporting trouble understanding, concentrating, or remembering.

OTHER DRUG USE

The most consistently detected form of other drug use was marijuana use, with 55% and 45% of the voucher and no-voucher groups, respectively, having positive test results at some point during the 24 weeks of treatment. However, the majority of urinalysis conducted for marijuana and other drugs had negative results in both groups, and none differed significantly across the two treatment groups. There was a trend toward more opioid use in the voucher than the no-voucher group ($\chi^2[1]=3.6$; $P=.06$), but that difference was largely explained by four patients in the voucher group who received prescription analgesics for other medical problems. Of the total specimens tested for opioids, 98% in the voucher group and 99% in the no-voucher group were negative, suggesting minimal use in either group.

COMMENT

There are six aspects of the present study on which we wish to comment.

First, the positive results achieved in the voucher group in this study provide a third replication demonstrating that this multicomponent, behavioral treatment is well accepted by cocaine-dependent patients, effectively retains them in outpatient treatment, and engenders clinically significant periods of cocaine abstinence in the majority of patients treated.[12,13] Considering the difficulties in reliably achieving positive results in controlled trials with cocaine-dependent patients, these are notable and encouraging characteristics of this treatment.[10] The positive results observed with this treatment and others[35-37] suggest that interventions based on behavioral and social-learning theories of drug abuse hold promise as effective treatments for cocaine dependence.

Second, the present results provide the first demonstration in a controlled trial that incentives improve outcome in patients enrolled in treatment for cocaine dependence. In our two prior trials conducted with this treatment, the effects of the vouchers could not be dissociated from the effects of the other treatment components.[12,13] The present results also are consistent with those from a prior study in patients receiving methadone maintenance, which demonstrated that providing medication take-home privileges contingent on submitting drug-free urine specimens increases cocaine abstinence.[38] Considered together, results from these studies provide compelling evidence that cocaine use in patient populations is sensitive to the systematic application of environmental consequences, as would be predicted based on the extensive basic science literature demonstrating the same in cocaine self-administration studies with nonhumans and humans.[18-22] Moreover, the present results suggest that patients with poor and good prognoses, based on early in-treatment cocaine use, benefit from the systematic delivery of positive consequences for cocaine abstinence. With regard to treatment retention, results observed in the present study suggest, but do not confirm, that patients with a poor prognosis may be especially helped by this voucher program.

Third, the present results suggest that incentives may reduce the high rates of psychiatric symptoms commonly observed in the cocaine-dependent population. Although the between-group differences on the ASI Psychiatric scale scores were not statistically significant at the .05 level, there was a clear trend ($P=.06$) in the direction of the voucher group showing greater improvement than the no-voucher group on this scale. Failure to detect a significant between-group difference is not surprising considering the relatively small sample size studied. The most parsimonious account of the improvement observed in the voucher group is that the incentives increased cocaine abstinence and treatment retention, which probably reduced some of the more notable adverse consequences of cocaine abuse (ie, depressed mood, impaired concentration, etc).[39] Also worth noting, however, is that the vouchers systematically increased the density of positive reinforcement, which is a goal of behavioral treatments for depression,[40] and that too may have improved patients' depressed mood.

Fourth, while the present results demonstrate that the voucher program is an active component of this treatment, they also suggest that other components may be active as

well. Sixty-five percent and 40% of those assigned to the no-voucher group completed 12 and 24 weeks of treatment, respectively, with an overall average of 6 weeks of continuous cocaine abstinence. Those levels of treatment retention and cocaine abstinence are encouraging considering the poor outcomes often reported in treating ambulatory cocaine-dependent patients with other psychosocial interventions.[41] The significant improvements observed in both treatment groups on the ASI Family/Social and Alcohol scale scores in the present study suggest that the CRA components addressing those problem areas may be active components of this multicomponent treatment, which is consistent with results from retrospective studies on this topic.[42,43] The failure to detect significant changes in either treatment group on the ASI Employment scale, by contrast, suggests that the CRA component on employment does not contribute to the positive outcomes observed with this treatment.

Fifth, the treatment outlined in this report may have the potential to help special populations like pregnant abusers. Several months of sustained abstinence in pregnant abusers could yield substantive long-term benefits. We have reported three replications, all conducted under controlled scientific conditions, demonstrating that this outpatient treatment is effective in establishing several months of continuous cocaine abstinence in the majority of patients treated. Although our studies were not conducted with pregnant abusers, and undoubtedly adjustments would be needed to accommodate their special needs, the main components of this treatment appear to have potential applicability to this population. Limitations on the use of pharmacotherapies in pregnant women further underscore the importance of identifying effective behavioral interventions for treating this population.

Sixth, there are at least two potential limitations of this study that merit comment. The first is a methodological limitation. The differences in continuous cocaine abstinence observed between the voucher and no-voucher groups in this study were not independent of the differential rates of treatment retention. That is, because the voucher group was retained in treatment for a significantly longer duration than the no-voucher group, there was greater opportunity to document cocaine abstinence in the former group. That is not to say that the differences in cocaine abstinence observed between the voucher and no-voucher groups in this study were merely an artifact of differential retention rates. Recall, for example, that when all patients except one in each group were assessed at the end of treatment, the voucher group evidenced significantly greater improvement on the ASI Drug scale than the no-voucher group, largely due to greater reductions in cocaine use and related problems. Nevertheless, it is a methodological limitation of the present study that precludes a thorough analysis of the mechanisms by which vouchers improved outcome. Future studies on this topic would be improved by inclusion of a third treatment group that receives vouchers contingent on clinic attendance but independent of urinalysis results. The addition of that group would effectively dissociate the effects of vouchers on cocaine abstinence and treatment retention, both of which are important outcome measures.

The second potential limitation pertains to the practical issue of cost. Subjects in the voucher group could have earned a maximum of $1022 in incentives, or $6.08 per treatment day, if they were continuously abstinent from cocaine throughout the 24 weeks of treatment. Because not all patients achieved the maximum, the actual average cost per patient for incentives in the voucher group was $601 total, or $3.58 per treatment day. Such costs may seem substantial at first blush, but they pale when considered against, for example, the tens of thousands of dollars often spent for inpatient hospitalizations for drug and alcohol abuse,[44] caring for persons who contract AIDS, tuberculosis, and other diseases common among drug abusers,[45] and caring for drug-exposed neonates.[46] Nevertheless, we recognize that an incentive program of even modest cost is likely to be impossible in many community clinics. Worth considering is whether community businesses might be willing to donate retail items for use as incentives, or whether special access to community recreation and other facilities (eg, swimming pools, quality basketball courts, and movie theaters) might prove to be effective incentives. Another possibility in patients with adequate resources is to have them submit a deposit at the start of treatment that could be earned back incrementally contingent on cocaine abstinence. Such contracts are effective in treating other forms of substance abuse as well as other types of behavioral disorders.[47,48] Through creative planning, community cooperation, and individualizing treatment plans, it may be possible to establish effective incentive programs for cocaine-dependent patients at minimal or no costs to clinics.

In closing, we believe it is important to recognize that incentives are used throughout western society for purposes ranging from improving performance in students and workers[49] to improving prenatal and newborn health care.[50] The basic principle that supports these diverse applications is reinforcement. Basic research has demonstrated the central role of reinforcement in the genesis and maintenance of cocaine and other forms of drug abuse.[51] The present study provides evidence that reinforcement is also important in treating cocaine dependence. An important clinical challenge is to devise strategies to further incorporate and evaluate that principle in prevention and treatment interventions. The voucher program and other features of the behavioral intervention outlined in this report illustrate just a few of the many possible ways that reinforcement may be effectively integrated into outpatient treatment for cocaine dependence.

Accepted for publication April 5, 1994.

Supported by Treatment Research Demonstration grants DA-06113 and DA-06969, Research Grant DA-08076, and

National Research Service Award DA-07242 from the National Institute on Drug Abuse, Rockville, Md.

Presented in part at the 1993 Annual Meeting of the College on Problems of Drug Dependence, Toronto, Ontario, June 13, 1993.

Reprint requests to Human Behavioral Pharmacology Laboratory, Department of Psychiatry, 38 Fletcher Pl, Ira Allen School, Burlington, VT 05401 (Dr Higgins).

REFERENCES

1. Chaisson RE, Bacchetti P, Osmond D, Brodie B, Sande MA, Moss AR. Cocaine use and HIV infection in intravenous drug users in San Francisco. *JAMA*. 1989; 261:561-565.
2. De La Rosa M, Lambert EY, Gropper B, eds. *Drugs and Violence: Causes, Correlates, and Consequences*. Washington, DC: US Government Printing Office; 1990. National Institute on Drug Abuse research monograph 103.
3. Kain ZN, Kain TS, Scarpelli EM. Cocaine exposure in utero: perinatal development and neonatal manifestations—review. *Clin Toxicol*. 1992;30:607-636.
4. *National Household Survey on Drug Abuse: Population Estimates 1991*. Rockville, Md: National Institute on Drug Abuse; 1991. Dept of Health and Human Services publication ADM 92-1887.
5. Harrison LD. Trends in illicit drug use in the United States: conflicting results from national surveys. *Int J Addict*. 1992;27:817-847.
6. Gfroerer JC, Brodsky MD. Frequent cocaine users and their use of treatment. *Am J Public Health*. 1993;83:1149-1154.
7. Gawin FH, Kleber HD. Cocaine abuse treatment: an open pilot trial with lithium and desipramine. *Arch Gen Psychiatry*. 1984;41:903-910.
8. Gawin FH, Kleber HD, Byck R, Rounsaville BJ, Kosten TR, Jatlow PI, Morgan C. Desipramine facilitation of initial cocaine abstinence. *Arch Gen Psychiatry*. 1989;46:117-121.
9. Weddington WW, Brown BS, Haertzen CA, Hess JM, Mahaffey JR, Kolar AF, Jaffe JH. Comparison of amantadine and desipramine combined with psychotherapy for treatment of cocaine dependence. *Am J Drug Alcohol Abuse*. 1991; 17:137-152.
10. Rawson RA, Obert JL, McCann MJ, Castro FG, Ling W. Cocaine abuse treatment: a review of current strategies. *J Subst Abuse*. 1991;3:457-491.
11. McLellan AT, Arndt IO, Metzger DS, Woody GE, O'Brien CP. The effects of psychosocial services in substance abuse treatment. *JAMA*. 1993;269:1953-1959.
12. Higgins ST, Delaney DD, Budney AJ, Bickel WK, Hughes JR, Foerg F, Fenwick JW. A behavioral approach to achieving initial cocaine abstinence. *Am J Psychiatry*. 1991;148:1218-1224.
13. Higgins ST, Budney AJ, Bickel WK, Hughes JR, Foerg F, Badger G. Achieving cocaine abstinence with a behavioral approach. *Am J Psychiatry*. 1993;150:763-769.
14. Bigelow GE, Stitzer ML, Griffiths RR, Liebson IA. Contingency management approaches to drug self-administration and drug abuse: efficacy and limitations. *Addict Behav*. 1981;6:241-252.
15. Sisson RW, Azrin NH. The Community Reinforcement Approach. In: Hester RK, Miller WR, eds. *Handbook of Alcoholism Treatment Approaches: Effective Alternatives*. New York, NY: Pergamon Press Inc; 1989:242-258.
16. Sorensen JL, Costantini MF, Wall TL, Gibson DR. Coupons attract high-risk untreated heroin users into detoxification. *Drug Alcohol Depend*. 1993;31:247-252.
17. Higgins ST, Stitzer ML, Bigelow GE, Liebson IA. Contingent methadone delivery: effects on illicit-opiate use. *Drug Alcohol Depend*. 1986;17:311-322.
18. Carroll ME, Lac ST, Nygaard SL. A concurrently available nondrug reinforcer prevents the acquisition or decreases the maintenance of cocaine-reinforced behavior. *Psychopharmacology*. 1989;97:23-29.
19. Nader NA, Woolverton WL. Effects of increasing the magnitude of an alternative reinforcer on drug choice in a discrete-trials choice procedure. *Psychopharmacology*. 1991;105:169-174.
20. Spealman RD. Behavior maintained by termination of a schedule of self-administered cocaine. *Science*. 1979;204:1231-1233.
21. Johanson CE. The effects of electric shock on responding maintained by cocaine injections in a choice procedure in the rhesus monkey. *Psychopharmacology*. 1977;53:277-282.
22. Higgins ST, Bickel WK, Hughes JR. Influence of an alternative reinforcer on human cocaine self-administration. *Life Sci*. In press.
23. Bickel WK, DeGrandpre RJ. Modeling drug abuse policy in the behavioral economics laboratory. In: Green L, Kagel JH, eds. *Advances in Behavioral Economics*. Norwood, NJ: Ablex Publishing Corp; 3. In press.
24. Anker AA, Crowley TJ. The use of contingency contracts in speciality clinics for cocaine abuse. In: Harris LS, ed. *Problems of Drug Dependence 1981*. Rockville, Md: National Institute on Drug Abuse; 1981:452-459. National Institute on Drug Abuse research monograph 41.
25. Stitzer ML, Bickel WK, Bigelow GE, Liebson IA. Effects of methadone dose contingencies on urinalysis test results of poly-abusing methadone-maintenance patients. *Drug Alcohol Depend*. 1986;18:341-348.
26. Aickin M. A program for balancing the allocation of subjects in a clinical trial. *Comput Biomed Res*. 1982;15:519-524.
27. McLellan AT, Luborsky L, Cacciola J, Griffith J, Evans F, Barr HL, O'Brien CP. New data from the Addiction Severity Index: reliability and validity in three centers. *J Nerv Ment Dis*. 1985;173:412-423.
28. McLellan AT, Luborsky L, Woody GE, O'Brien CP, Druley KA. Predicting response to alcohol and drug abuse treatments: role of psychiatric severity. *Arch Gen Psychiatry*. 1983;40;620-625.
29. Hudziak J, Helzer JE, Wetzel MW, Kessel KB, McGee B, Janca A, Przybeck P. The use of the *DSM-III-R* checklist for initial diagnostic assessments. *Compr Psychiatry*. 1993;34:375-383.
30. Azrin NH, Naster BJ, Jones R. Reciprocity counseling: a rapid learning-based procedure for marital counseling. *Behav Res Ther*. 1973;11:364-382.
31. Azrin NH, Besalel VA. *Job Club Counselor's Manual*. Baltimore, Md: University Park Press; 1980.
32. Nathan PE, Lansky D. Common methodological problems in research on the addictions. *J Consult Clin Psychol*. 1978;46:713-726.
33. SAS Institute Inc. *SAS User's Guide: Statistics, Version 5 Edition*. Cary, NC: SAS Institute Inc; 1985.
34. Iguchi MY, Stitzer ML. Predictors of opiate drug abuse during a 90-day methadone detoxification. *Am J Drug Alcohol Abuse*. 1991;17:279-294.
35. Carroll KM, Rounsaville BJ, Gawin FH. A comparative trial of psychotherapies for ambulatory cocaine abusers. *Am J Drug Alcohol Abuse*. 1991;17:229-247.
36. Childress AR, Hole AV, Ehrman RN, Robbins SJ, McLellan AT, O'Brien CP. Cue reactivity and cue reactivity interventions in drug dependence. In: Onken LS, Blaine JD, Boren JJ, eds. *Behavioral Treatments for Drug Abuse and Dependence*. Rockville, Md: National Institute on Drug Abuse; 1993:73-95. National Institutes of Health publication 93-3684. National Institute on Drug Abuse research monograph 137.
37. Rawson RA. Neurobehavioral treatment for cocaine dependency: a preliminary evaluation. In: Tims FM, Leukefeld CG, eds. *Cocaine Treatment: Research and Clinical Perspectives*. Rockville, Md: National Institute on Drug Abuse; 1993: 92-115. National Institutes of Health publication 93-3639. National Institute on Drug Abuse research monograph 135.
38. Stitzer ML, Iguchi MY, Felch LJ. Contingent take-home incentive. *J Consult Clin Psychol*. 1992;60:927-934.
39. Cottler LB, Shillington AM, Compton WM III, Mager D, Spitznagel EL. Subjective reports of withdrawal among cocaine users: recommendations for *DSM-IV*. *Drug Alcohol Depend*. 1993;33:97-104.
40. Lewinsohn PM. A behavioral approach to depression. In: Friedman R, Katz M, eds. *The Psychology of Depression: Contemporary Theory and Research*. Washington, DC: Winston; 1974:157-185.
41. Kang S-Y, Kleinman PH, Woody GE, Millman RB, Todd TC, Kemp J, Lipton DS. Outcomes for cocaine abusers after once-a-week psychosocial therapy. *Am J Psychiatry*. 1991;148:630-635.
42. Higgins ST, Budney AJ, Bickel WK, Hughes JR, Foerg F. Disulfiram therapy in patients abusing cocaine and alcohol. *Am J Psychiatry*. 1993;150:676-677.
43. Higgins ST, Budney AJ, Bickel WK, Badger GJ. Participation of significant others in outpatient behavioral treatment predicts greater cocaine abstinence. *Am J Drug Alcohol Abuse*. 1994;20:47-56.
44. Holder HD, Blose JO. Typical patterns and cost of alcoholism treatment across a variety of populations and providers. *Alcohol Clin Exp Res*. 1991;15:190-195.
45. Drucker E. AIDS and addiction in New York City. *Am J Drug Alcohol Abuse*. 1986;12:165-181.
46. Phibbs CS, Batemen DA, Schwartz RM. The neonatal costs of maternal cocaine use. *JAMA*. 1991;226:1521-1526.
47. Bigelow G, Strickler D, Liebson I, Griffiths R. Maintaining disulfiram ingestion among outpatient alcoholics. *Behav Res Ther*. 1976;14:378-381.
48. Epstein LH, Wing RR. Behavioral contracting: health behaviors. In: Franks C, ed. *New Developments in Behavior Therapy: From Research to Clinical Application*. New York, NY: The Haworth Press; 1984:409-449.
49. Damico M. Incentives in our schools. *Business Incentive Strategies*. 1992;51: 4-18.
50. *Caring for Tomorrow's Children*. Columbia, SC: Office of the Governor; 1993.
51. Goldberg SR, Stolerman IP. *Behavioral Analysis of Drug Dependence*. Orlando, Fla: Academic Press Inc; 1986.

ORIGINAL ARTICLE

Patterns of Risk in First-Degree Relatives of Patients With Alzheimer's Disease

Jeremy M. Silverman, PhD; Ge Li, MD, PhD; Michele L. Zaccario; Christopher J. Smith; James Schmeidler, PhD; Richard C. Mohs, PhD; Kenneth L. Davis, MD

Background: Although an increased cumulative risk for primary progressive dementia (PPD) has been repeatedly demonstrated in relatives of probands with Alzheimer's disease (AD), an examination of their rates of illness at different ages has not been previously undertaken. Such an examination might reveal possible age-related characteristics associated with a more familial variety of AD.

Methods: Using family history interviews and survival analysis, the cumulative risk for and 5-year age-specific hazard rates of PPD were assessed in the first-degree relatives of 200 probands with AD and two nondemented control groups—179 elderly ascertained through the Alzheimer's Disease Research Center (ADRC-derived controls) and 427 elderly ascertained from community senior centers (community controls).

Results: The PPD risk curve for the relatives of probands with AD rose to about 30% and was significantly higher than the curves for the relatives of the ADRC-derived and community controls, where comparable rates were observed (approximately 12%). The age-specific hazard rates of PPD were calculated in three groups of relatives for each 5-year interval from ages 45 to 49 years through ages 85 to 89 years. The age-specific relative risk (RR_i) for PPD in the relatives of probands with AD began to steadily diminish from the 75- to 79-year age interval (RR_i=13.49) through the 85- to 89-year age interval (RR_i=0.96) compared with the relatives of ADRC-derived controls and from the 60- to 64-year age interval (RR_i=16.15) through the 85- to 89-year age interval (RR_i=2.03) compared with the relatives of the community controls.

Conclusions: These data indicate that, for relatives of probands with AD, while the lifetime risk for PPD is greater than in relatives of controls, the familial contribution to the risk for PPD decreases with increasing age. The higher risk for PPD in relatives of probands with AD may be substantially diminished or even eliminated by the latter half of the ninth decade.

(Arch Gen Psychiatry. 1994;51:577-586)

ALTHOUGH A role for environmental factors in Alzheimer's disease (AD) is strongly suggested by the presence of long-lived monozygotic twins discordant for AD,[1,2] familial/genetic factors in this disease are also evident.[3] Several genetic markers have been linked to AD in small subgroups of unusual pedigrees with many affected family members.[4-7] The ϵ4 allele of the apolipoprotein E gene appears to have a dosage effect on the risk for AD,[8] and numerous case-control studies examining independent clinical series of patients with AD indicate the presence of familial although not definitely genetic factors in at least a significant proportion of more typical AD cases.[9-15] Furthermore, survival analysis studies of familial factors in AD have uniformly shown a significantly increased cumulative risk for an AD-like dementia—primary progressive dementia (PPD)—in first-degree relatives of probands with AD compared with those of nondemented controls.[16-25] Survival analysis uses the individual relative as the unit of analysis. Especially for late-onset disease, such an approach is preferable to treating the full family as a single

From the Psychiatry Service, Bronx (NY) Veterans Affairs Medical Center, and the Department of Psychiatry, Mt Sinai School of Medicine, New York, NY.

See Methods on next page

METHODS

PROBANDS

Consecutive patients with clinically diagnosed AD admitted to the psychogeriatric clinics associated with the Alzheimer's Disease Research Center (ADRC) at the Mt Sinai Medical Center, New York, NY, and the Bronx (NY) Veterans Affairs Medical Center are routinely referred for family history evaluation. Although no formal assessment was conducted regarding the proband's reason for coming to the psychogeriatric clinic, the probable motivation for most, if not all, families of the patients was the diagnosis and treatment of dementia. A proband's family history status was not a factor for entry into the psychogeriatric clinics or, in turn, inclusion in the study. The present proband sample consisted of 200 such patients with AD, a subset of which (N=79; mean±SE age at onset, 61.1±9.3 years) had been included in at least one prior family history study from this center.[20] The specific protocol used to establish the AD diagnosis has been described in detail elsewhere.[29] Briefly, all patients underwent evaluation by a psychiatrist trained in the assessment of dementia, with a clinical history, evaluation of mental status, and physical and laboratory examinations meeting National Institute of Neurological and Communicative Disorders and Stroke–Alzheimer's Disease and Related Disorders Association (NINCDS-ADRDA) criteria for probable AD.[33]

CONTROLS

Two control groups were used. For neither group was family history status a determinant for inclusion. The first group, the ADRC-derived controls, consisted of 179 nondemented elderly controls ascertained through their prior association with the ADRC either through marriage to a proband with AD seen in our clinic (N=94) or as volunteers or spouses of volunteers participating in biological, longitudinal, or other studies of AD conducted by the ADRC (N=85). About one third (N=57) of the present series had been included in at least one earlier report from this center.[20]

A second control group was ascertained through a community rather than a clinical setting. These index subjects were 215 Italian and 212 Jewish nondemented elderly (aged 65 years or older) who had participated in a previously published epidemiological investigation of AD and who were ascertained through senior centers for medically well elderly in New York City's Lower East Side.[34] Their first-degree relatives were assessed by the same methods as those used for the proband and the ADRC-derived control groups. As described in the earlier report, both the Italian and Jewish relatives of nondemented elderly index subjects showed significantly higher risk for PPD than those observed in two groups of nondemented index subjects of non-European origin—Puerto Rican and Chinese. Since well over 90% of the proband group were white and of European ancestry, the Italian and Jewish groups were deemed appropriate as controls. As previously described,[34] the observed cumulative risk curves for the Italian and Jewish groups were similar to one another in shape and estimated cumulative risk. Thus, in the present study, we combined these two groups into one group of community controls (N=427).

FAMILY HISTORY ASSESSMENT

Family informants were interviewed with the AD Risk Questionnaire[18] to enumerate first-degree relatives of an index subject and systematically assess basic demographic information and the presence of any cognitive deficits in each of them. When a relative was reported to have had even a slight memory problem or other cognitive impairments during this screen, the Dementia Questionnaire (DQ)[27] was administered. The DQ assesses, through informants, the symptoms, course, and features of the dementia in family members, permitting a family history diagnostic classification for the presence and likely type of dementia. It is also used to estimate the age at onset of a dementia, defined as the reported age at which the first definite symptom emerged. Since the absence of a direct examination precludes a diagnosis of probable AD by NINCDS-ADRDA criteria, the DQ collects information enabling the categorization of dementing illness in relatives into three groups: (1) PPD (*DSM-III* criteria for primary degenerative dementia[35] modified for family history data) that is aimed at identifying individuals with an AD-like dementia but may include some with multi-infarct and other types of progressive dementias not readily attributable to other identifiable causes such as diabetes, alcohol, or a major stroke; (2) stroke-related dementia; and (3) other central nervous system dis-

unit, as in traditional case-control methodology, to avoid effects due to family size and age structure and to derive direct estimates of the risk for illness.

While the presence of familial factors in AD is clear, a precise delineation of the familial risk for PPD in relatives of probands with AD has been more difficult to determine.[3] Estimates of the cumulative risk in relatives of probands with AD have ranged from 23%[26] to 67%.[21] This wide range is probably due in part to methodological differences[23,25,27-30] and small samples—typically less than 100 probands[17-22]—yielding unstable risk estimates. In addition, little attention has been given to the pattern of illness across the late life span in this group. For example, there has been no published investigation of the levels of risk in relatives of probands with AD at specific age intervals. It would be useful, however, to establish whether changes in these levels over different age intervals follow patterns similar to those observed in the general population.[31,32] That is, while presumably at higher levels overall, it remains to be determined whether rates increase through the ninth decade and beyond in relatives of probands with AD. Such an investigation might reveal specific characteristics of a more famil-

ease. The DQ has previously demonstrated good interinformant and interrater agreement in probands with AD and normal elderly control populations for detecting the presence or absence, the type, and the age at onset of a dementia.[27,28] In addition, in a study of the validity of the DQ in a series of elderly subjects ranging broadly in the severity of cognitive symptoms, the agreement between diagnoses determined entirely by a DQ interview with an informant and an independent clinical examination was good, with 90% specificity and 100% sensitivity.[36]

In the case of the community controls, the index subject served as the sole family informant. For the proband group and ADRC-derived controls, two family informants were sought for each index subject but, for 69 (34.5%) families of probands with AD and 62 (34.6%) families of ADRC-derived controls, only one informant was obtained. First informants were usually the spouse or primary caregiver for the probands and the index subjects themselves for the controls. Second informants were identified usually by asking the first informant for the individual best informed about the family (usually siblings). Although the proband and ADRC-derived control groups differed from the community control group with respect to the usual number of informants, there was no significant difference between families assessed by one vs two family informants among either probands or ADRC-derived controls in the frequency of PPD (for probands, $\chi^2=0.06$; $df=1$; differences were not significant; for ADRC-derived controls, $\chi^2=0.90$; $df=1$; differences were not significant).

STATISTICS

The actuarial life-table method[37] using 1-year intervals after age 45 years was used to estimate the cumulative risk for PPD. The cumulative risk was obtained by subtracting the estimated cumulative probability of survival from unity. This procedure allows for the comparison of cumulative risk curves while taking censored data into account, ie, the fact that unaffected relatives contribute information regarding the risk for disease only through their current age or age at death. The 1-year interval used for constructing the actuarial life table was the smallest possible measurable unit that was reasonable considering the constraints of family history methodology and the insidious onset of PPD. In the actuarial method, the number of incident subjects (relatives of index subjects with PPD) within an interval is divided by the number of unaffected relatives who are alive and at risk of the disorder at the start of the interval minus one half the number of relatives who are censored during the interval. This method, when used with the smallest measured time unit available on the relatives, ie, a year, was thus likely to be slightly more accurate compared with the Kaplan-Meier product limit estimation procedure, which uses a very similar formula but assumes no censorship within the time unit. The Mantel-Cox (MC) log-rank χ^2 test was used to test the null hypothesis that relatives of probands and controls had the same cumulative risk curves. The test of the difference between two estimated proportions, based on their respective estimated SDs, was used to test the null hypothesis that the relatives of the probands vs those of the controls had the same cumulative risk estimates.

The estimated hazard rate at the midpoint of each 5-year interval, $\hbar(t_{mi})$, was determined by dividing the number of cases occurring within the age interval, d_i, by the number of risk years of the relatives at risk during the interval, using a correction factor for age and incident subjects during the interval:

$$\hbar(t_{mi})=d_i/\{[n_i-(0.5\times d_i)]b_i\}$$

where n_i equals the sum of one half of the relatives alive at the beginning of the interval, but censored during the interval, plus all the relatives who had incident cases of PPD during the interval or lived beyond the interval unaffected, and b_i equals the number of time units included in the interval (ie, 5 years).[37]

Group differences between absolute age-specific hazard rate values, the age-specific risk difference (RD_i), were tested using the test of the difference between two proportions. In addition, the age-specific relative risks (RR_is), calculated by dividing the age-specific hazard rate in the relatives of the probands by the equivalent in the relatives of the controls, were derived to assess the relative degree of increased risk at a specific age interval associated with being a relative of a proband. An RR_i was considered significant when the upper and lower boundaries of the 95% confidence intervals excluded 1.00. The age-specific attributable risk, ie, the proportion of incident subjects with PPD in the interval attributable to a first-degree relationship with a proband, was calculated by subtracting one from the RR_i and dividing the result by the RR_i: $(RR_i-1)/RR_i$.[38]

ial variety of AD. The assessment of cumulative risk does not directly show whether the risk for PPD remains constant, increases, or diminishes over different age ranges, since this statistic incorporates the rate at a given age along with the full cumulative rate prior to that age. The patterns of illness at different ages could be more directly examined by investigating the age-specific hazard rate, ie, the probability per time unit (eg, 1 year) of developing a disease over a specified age interval (eg, 65 to 69 years) in a group of subjects alive and at risk of the disease within that interval. Such an examination might reveal possible age-related characteristics associated with a more familial variety of AD that are otherwise obscured using only cumulative risk curves. If such an association is apparent, the onset characteristics of the sample of probands with AD, which have previously been reported to be associated with age at onset in their affected relatives,[16] might then be further investigated in terms of the patterns of risk in the relatives of probands with AD distinguished by proband age at onset. Toward this end, in the present study, in addition to calculating the cumulative risk in the relatives of the largest published series of probands with AD so analyzed, we also examined the 5-year

Table 1. Characteristics of Probands With AD, ADRC-Derived Controls, and Community Controls and Their First-Degree Relatives*

	Index Subjects				First-Degree Relatives ≥45 Years of Age						
					Total Relatives		Sex, No. (%)		Generation, No.		
Index Group	No.	Mean (SD) Age, y	Male, No. (%)	FHx+,† No. (%)	No.	Mean (SD) Age, y	M	F	Parent	Sibling	Child
Probands	200	69.1 (8.9)	110 (55)	68 (34.0)	1001	67.5 (12.0)	481 (48)	520 (52)	343	579	79
ADRC-derived controls	179	67.9 (8.9)	97 (54)	14 (12.8)	761	69.2 (12.0)	376 (49)	385 (51)	318	409	34‡
Community controls	427	74.0 (5.6)	90 (21)	54 (12.6)	2656	68.1 (12.2)	1354 (51)	1302 (49)	774	1485	397

*AD indicates Alzheimer's disease; ADRC, Alzheimer's Disease Research Center.
†FHx+ indicates family history–positive, or index subjects with at least one first-degree relative with primary progressive dementia.
‡Children of the nondemented spouses of probands with AD were categorized only as relatives of probands.

age-specific hazard rates from ages 45 to 90 years in relatives of probands with AD and compared them with the rates in the relatives of two control groups.

RESULTS

The demographic characteristics and family history status of the proband and the two control groups are provided in **Table 1**. The mean age (t=1.13; df=377; differences were not significant) and distribution by gender (χ^2=0.00; df=1; differences were not significant) among the probands and the ADRC-derived controls were similar, but the community controls were predominantly female (χ^2=71.09; df=1; P<.0001) and were significantly older (t=12.67; df=624; P<.001). The mean age at onset among the probands was 64.6±9.6 years. There was a significant association between the age at onset in the probands and their affected relatives (r=.30; P<.01). The families of probands were significantly more likely to have at least one first-degree relative with PPD by age 90 years than families of the ADRC-derived controls (χ^2=38.18; df=1; P<.0001) or community controls (χ^2=25.26; df=1; P<.0001). Also shown in Table 1 are the demographic characteristics of the first-degree relatives of the three index-subject groups. The gender distribution (χ^2=2.25; df=2; differences were not significant) and mean age (F=2.63 [2, 4415]; differences were not significant) of the first-degree relatives were similar across the three groups.

Figure 1 shows the cumulative risk curve for the relatives of the probands, the ADRC-derived controls, and the community controls. In the first-degree relatives of the probands, the cumulative risk for PPD rose to 29.57%±3.71% by age 88 years in the relatives of the probands. In the relatives of the ADRC-derived controls, the cumulative risk for PPD rose to 12.44%±3.35% by age 87 years. The risk curve of this control group was significantly different than that for the relatives of the probands (MC log-rank, χ^2=31.78; df=1; P<.0001), and the cumulative risk estimates were significantly different (z=3.42; P<.001). Similar to the ADRC-derived control group, the cumulative risk for PPD rose to 11.7%±1.98% by age 89 years in the relatives of the community control group, and both the risk curve and the cumulative risk were significantly different from those for the relatives of the probands (MC log-rank, χ^2=67.32; df=1; P<.0001; z=4.24; P<.0001).

Figure 2 shows the hazard rates over the 45-year age range from 45 through 89 years for each of the nine age intervals. The number of subjects with PPD and age-corrected exposed relatives in each group at each interval are included in **Table 2**. The hazard rates of PPD among at-risk relatives of the probands showed continuous increases until the 80- to 84-year age interval. In the 85- to 89-year age interval, however, the hazard rate dropped by 35% from the previous interval. In the relatives of the ADRC-derived controls, the hazard rate for PPD remained at zero in the first four age intervals, then rose continuously until the last assessed age interval. Finally, in the relatives of the community controls, the hazard rate of PPD was above zero but extremely low in the 45- to 49-year age interval, fell to zero in the next two intervals, increased from the 55- to 59-year age interval through the 80- to 84-year age interval, and finally dropped by 23% in the last age interval (85- to 89-year age interval).

Table 2 shows the age-corrected relatives at risk and the cases of PPD in the three groups for each 5-year age interval, as well as the statistical comparisons of the age-specific RD_is and RR_is for PPD between the proband group and the two control groups. In the first eight age intervals, the RD_i, ie, the *absolute* difference in hazard rates, between relatives of the probands and of the two control groups was significant and consistently increased from one interval to the next. In the 85- to 89-year age interval, however, the RD_i between the relatives of the probands and those of ADRC-derived controls, although close to zero and not significant, was slightly negative, indicating a trivially higher rate in the relatives of the controls. The RD_i between the relatives of the probands and the relatives of community controls at this last age interval was also not significant. Although still comparatively large, the RD_i in this latter comparison was smaller than for the two previous age intervals.

The age-specific RR_i, ie, the *relative* difference in age-specific hazard rates, between the relatives of the pro-

bands and controls, were also assessed. Included in Table 2 are the RR_is for PPD, when calculable, for the relatives of the probands compared with those of the two control groups for each of the nine age intervals assessed. Compared with the ADRC-derived controls, the RR_i for PPD in the relatives of the probands rose from the fifth to the seventh age interval, dropped in the eighth age interval, and finally fell slightly and nonsignificantly below 1.00 in the last age interval. In comparison to the community controls, the RR_i for the relatives of the probands was not significant in the first age interval, not calculable in the next two age intervals (due to a zero denominator), peaked in the 60- to 64-year age interval, and then declined steadily through the last age interval, which was not significant.

The probands were then dichotomized into early-onset (<70 years; N=137) and late-onset (≥70 years; N=63) groups. **Figure 3** shows the age-specific hazard rates in the relatives of these two proband subgroups for each of the 5-year age intervals from 45 through 89 years. The similarity in risk characteristics between the relatives of the two control groups led us to combine them into a single group of relatives of nondemented controls (Figure 3). In the relatives of the early-onset group, the RD_is increased steadily and were significantly greater than those of the relatives of the control group from the 65- to 69-year age interval through the 80- to 84-year age interval. In the 85- to 89-year age interval, however, the RD_i declined from the preceding interval and was not significant (**Table 3**).

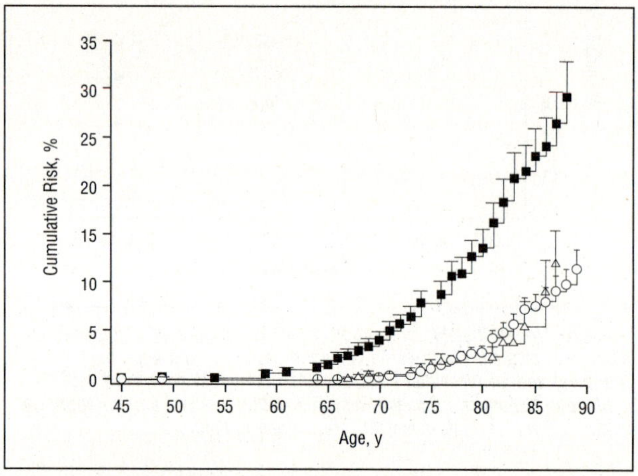

Figure 1. *Cumulative risk curves of primary progressive dementia in the first-degree relatives of probands with Alzheimer's disease (AD) (squares), Alzheimer's Disease Research Center–derived controls (triangles), and community controls (circles).*

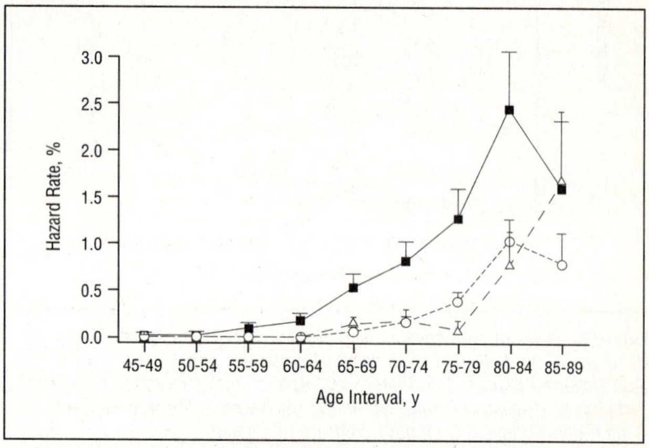

Figure 2. *Five-year age-specific hazard rates, $\hat{h}(t_{mi})$, of primary progressive dementia in the first-degree relatives of probands with Alzheimer's disease (AD) (squares), Alzheimer's Disease Research Center–derived controls (triangles), and community controls (circles).*

Table 2. Age-Specific Subjects With PPD, Age-Corrected Relatives at Risk, Risk Difference (RD_i), and Relative Risk (RR_i) for PPD in Relatives of Probands With AD, ADRC-Derived Controls (ADRCC), and Community Controls (CC)*

	Subjects With PPD (d_i) and Relatives at Risk (n_i)†						Relatives of Probands vs Relatives of Controls									
	Probands		ADRCC		CC		ADRCC					CC				
Age Internal, y	d_i	n_i	d_i	n_i	d_i	n_i	RD_i, %‡	z	P	RR_i §	95% CI‖	RD_i, %‡	z	P	RR_i §	95% CI‖
45-49	1	958.5	0	739.0	1	2496.0	0.02	NA	. . .	∞	NA	0.01	0.58	NS	2.61	0.18-37.58
50-54	1	877.5	0	692.5	0	2271.5	0.02	NA	. . .	∞	NA	0.02	NA	. . .	∞	NA
55-59	4	784.0	0	631.0	0	2051.0	0.10	NA	. . .	∞	NA	0.10	NA	. . .	∞	NA
60-64	6	671.5	0	547.0	1	1799.5	0.18	NA	. . .	∞	NA	0.17	2.27	<.05	16.15	3.38-77.10
65-69	14	533.0	3	442.0	5	1448.5	0.39	2.44	.01	3.91	1.22-12.43	0.46	3.18	<.001	7.70	3.24-18.28
70-74	15	380.0	3	322.0	9	1052.0	0.62	2.64	<.01	4.30	1.38-13.44	0.64	2.93	<.005	4.69	2.21-9.95
75-79	15	245.5	1	214.5	13	690.5	1.26	3.45	<.001	13.49	2.85-63.67	0.97	2.57	<.01	3.32	1.64-6.70
80-84	16	139.0	5	131.0	19	380.5	1.52	2.37	<.05	3.13	1.20-8.14	1.28	2.17	<.05	2.38	1.24-4.57
85-89	5	65.0	5	62.5	6	155.5	–0.07	–0.65	NS	0.96	0.27-3.35	0.82	1.04	NS	2.03	0.63-6.55

**PPD indicates primary progressive dementia; AD, Alzheimer's disease; ADRC, Alzheimer's Disease Research Center; NA, not applicable; NS, not significant; and CI, confidence intervals.*

†n_i *(Age-specific relatives at risk)=($\frac{1}{2}\times c_i+d_i+j_i$), where c_i is the number of unaffected n_i with a current age or age at death within the interval (ie, censored); d_i, the number affected within the interval; and j_i, the number unaffected during the interval who lived through the interval.*

‡*The RD_i is calculated by subtracting the age-specific hazard rate in the relatives of the controls from the equivalent in the relatives of the probands.*

§*The RR_i is calculated by dividing the age-specific hazard rate in the relatives of the probands by the equivalent in the relatives of the controls.*

‖*The 95% confidence interval is $RR_i^{1\pm(1.96/x)}$.*

In the relatives of the late-onset group, the RD_is showed a more modest increasing trend from the 70- to 74-year age interval through the 80- to 84-year age interval to a decline in the last age interval; none of these RD_is were significant. The relatives of both the early- and late-onset groups showed a peak age-specific hazard rate at the penultimate age interval examined. Examination of the RR_i of PPD in the family members of the early-onset group compared with those of the control group (Table 3) revealed an essentially downward trend (although the RR_i in the 75- to 79-year age interval was slightly higher than in the preceding age interval) from a 14-fold increase in the 60- to 64-year age interval to less than a twofold increase in the 85- to 89-year age interval. The RR_i for PPD in the relatives of the late-onset group also showed a downward trend from the 70- to 74-year age interval through the last age

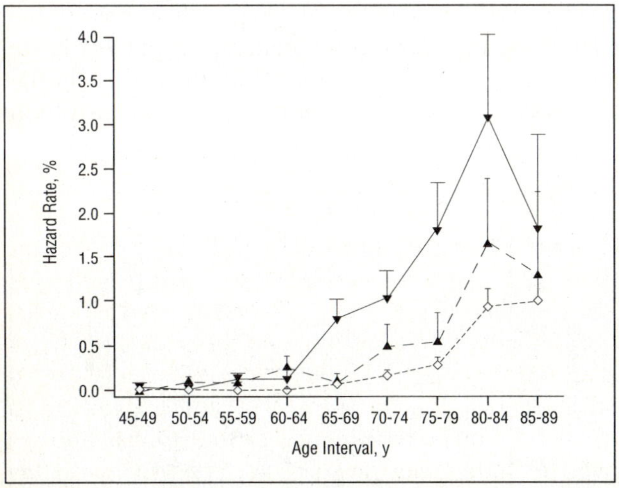

Figure 3. *Five-year age-specific hazard rates, $\hat{h}(t_{mi})$, of primary progressive dementia in the first-degree relatives of probands with early (<70 years of age) (inverted triangles) and late(≥70 years of age) (triangles) onset of Alzheimer's disease (AD) and combined (Alzheimer's Disease Research Center–derived and community) controls (diamonds).*

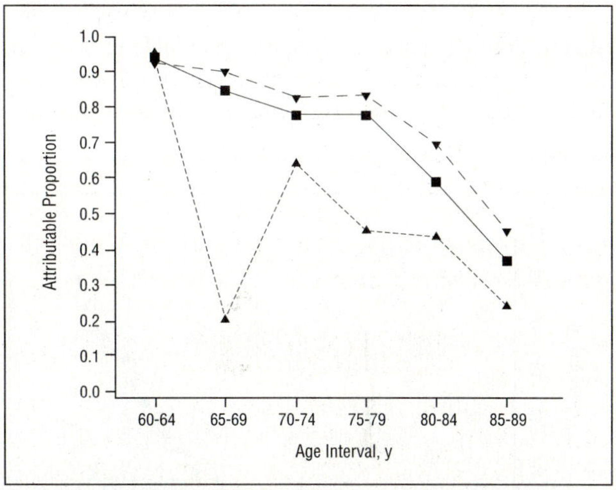

Figure 4. *The attributable proportion of primary progressive dementia in relatives of probands with early- (inverted triangles) and late-onset (triangles) and all Alzheimer's disease (AD) (squares) compared with the combined (Alzheimer's Disease Research Center–derived and community) controls. Early- and late-onset AD are defined in Figure 3.*

Table 3. Age-Specific Subjects With PPD, Age-Corrected Relatives at Risk, Risk Difference (RD_i), and Relative Risk (RR_i) for PPD in Relatives of Probands With Early- and Late-Onset AD and Combined ADRC-Derived and Community Controls*

	Subjects With PPD (d_i) and Relatives at Risk (n_i)†						Relatives of Probands vs Relatives of Combined Controls									
	Probands With Early-Onset AD‡		Probands With Late-Onset AD§		Combined Controls‖		Relatives of Probands With Early-Onset AD					Relatives of Probands With Late-Onset AD				
Age Interval, y	d_i	n_i	d_i	n_i	d_i	n_i	RD_i, %	z	P	RR_i #	95% CI**	RD_i, %	z	P	RR_i #	95% CI**
45-49	1	642.5	0	315.5	1	3236.0	0.02	0.63	NS	5.04	0.42-60.89	−0.01	NA	. . .	0.00	. . .
50-54	0	590.0	1	287.0	0	2965.0	0.00	NA	. . .	NA	. . .	0.07	NA	. . .	∞	. . .
55-59	3	520.5	1	263.5	0	2683.0	0.12	1.71	NS	∞	. . .	0.08	NA	. . .	∞	. . .
60-64	3	430.0	3	240.5	1	2347.5	0.13	1.61	NS	16.43	3.11-86.86	0.24	1.71	NS	29.46	6.83-127.09
65-69	13	326.0	1	206.0	8	1890.5	0.74	3.15	<.01	9.59	4.67-19.72	0.02	0.19	NS	1.14	0.14-9.17
70-74	11	217.0	4	162.5	12	1374.5	0.87	2.74	<.01	5.93	2.88-12.23	0.32	1.26	NS	2.84	0.96-8.04
75-79	13	136.5	3	108.5	14	906.0	1.71	3.04	<.01	6.42	3.12-12.45	0.25	0.75	NS	1.80	0.52-6.17
80-84	10	75.5	5	62.5	24	512.5	1.88	2.06	<.05	2.95	1.45-6.03	0.71	0.93	NS	1.74	0.67-4.53
85-89	3	34.0	2	31.0	11	219.0	.82	0.74	NS	1.79	0.50-6.38	0.30	0.30	NS	1.29	0.28-5.87

PPD indicates primary progressive dementia; AD, Alzheimer's disease; ADRC, Alzheimer's Disease Research Center; NA, not applicable; NS, not significant; and CI, confidence intervals.

†n_i *(Age-specific relatives at risk)=(½×c_i+d_i+j_i), where c_i is the number of unaffected n_i with a current age or age at death within the interval (ie, censored);* d_i*, the number affected within the interval; and* j_i*, the number unaffected during the interval who lived through the interval.*

‡*Early-onset AD is defined as age at onset of less than 70 years (N=137).*

§*Late-onset AD is defined as age at onset of 70 years or greater (N=63).*

‖*Combined controls are composed of the ADRC-derived and community controls (N=606).*

¶*The RD_i is calculated by subtracting the age-specific hazard rate in the relatives of the controls from the equivalent in the relatives of the probands.*

#*The RR_i is calculated by dividing the age-specific hazard rate in the relatives of the probands by the equivalent in the relatives of the controls.*

***The 95% confidence interval is $RR_i^{1\pm(1.96/x)}$.*

interval, but here the increased RR_is were far less pronounced, even in most of the earlier age intervals, and differed from 1.0 only in the 60- to 64-year age interval. Very similar results were obtained when the relatives of the two control groups were analyzed separately.

Finally, **Figure 4** shows the age-specific attributable proportion of cases of PPD in the relatives of the early-onset and late-onset groups and all probands compared with the relatives of the combined controls in the intervals where continuities between adjacent age intervals could be assessed, the 60- to 64-year age interval through the 85- to 89-year age interval. With one exception (the late-onset group, in which the 65- to 69-year age interval through the 70- to 74-year age interval was assessed), the attributable proportion dropped continuously from above 0.9 in both proband groups at the 60- to 64-year age interval to 0.44 in the early-onset group, 0.23 in the late-onset group, and 0.36 in the full proband group.

COMMENT

Consistent with virtually all previous family history studies of AD using survival analysis,[16-25] the observed cumulative risk for PPD among the first-degree relatives of the probands was significantly greater than that observed among the relatives of both the ADRC-derived and community controls, further supporting the presence of familial aggregation in AD. In addition, the significantly higher PPD age-specific hazard rates in the relatives of the probands through the 80- to 84-year age interval and peaking rates at that age interval indicate that, before the last half of the ninth decade, as yet unaffected relatives of probands with AD are at greater risk of PPD than relatives of controls at the same ages. In the latter half of that decade, however, the absolute hazard rate in the relatives of the probands dropped by a third and did not significantly differ from rates in either control group. In contrast to the peak absolute excess risk, the relative familial contribution to the hazard rate of PPD, estimated by the age-specific RR_i for relatives of the probands compared with those of the controls, peaked earlier—at the 75- to 79-year age interval in the ADRC-derived controls and at the 60- to 64-year age interval in the community controls—and thereafter decreased sharply. Finally, the proportion of PPD attributable to a first-degree relationship to a proband compared with relationships to the combined controls diminished from the early 60s to the late 70s and then dropped more precipitously in the ninth decade. Such a trend suggests that the impact of familial factors on the risk for PPD may begin to decline in the seventh or eighth decade relative to other causes. Furthermore, in comparisons with both control groups, the RR_i for PPD during the 85- to 89-year age interval did not significantly differ from 1.00. Although a failure to detect significant differences is not the same as showing that these hazard rates are truly the same in all three groups, these results suggest that the proportion of risk for PPD attributable to a first-degree relationship to a proband with AD is substantially reduced by the late 80s and raise the possibility that at such ages the excess risk in this group of relatives may be fully expended. Thus, these data support the frequently hypothesized but inconsistently supported[16,20,22,23,25,39] inverse relationship between the familial factors in AD and age at onset; late-onset AD may identify a less familial form of this disease.

Previous studies addressing this issue have generally dichotomized groups of probands with AD at an onset cutoff point (eg, age 65 years) and compared the cumulative risk estimates in relatives of probands with early-onset AD with those of probands with late-onset AD. Two studies found significantly increased risk for AD in relatives of probands with early-onset disease,[16,39] but several others did not.[20,22,23,25] Taken together, the preponderance of evidence from these earlier studies have not supported the hypothesis that familial factors in AD are more likely in early-onset cases. However, the singular division of a proband sample into early- and late-onset groups at an arbitrary cutoff point to compare a summarized estimate of risk in relatives reduces statistical power and fails to use much of the available onset information in the relatives. In contrast, the primary analyses of the present study rely on longer-term trends, indicating declining RR_is in the relatives of the probands with AD compared with those of controls. Thus, the major analyses in this study avoid both the subdivision of the proband sample and a reliance on the comparison of a single lifetime risk estimate. Furthermore, these estimates are typically derived largely from the very late ages when only a small number of relatives are uncensored and hence still contributing risk information. Our alternative methodology uses the full range of onset characteristics in the relatives of probands with AD, providing a more comprehensive analysis of the relationship between onset and familial aggregation in AD.

Although the number of relatives living to a given age range will affect the extent of possible error of the hazard estimate, it is important to note that the decline in the RR_is or age-specific attributable proportion (a derivative of the former) with increased age cannot be explained by possible differences in age structure between the different groups of relatives, and the decline in the hazard rate in the last age interval among the relatives of the probands cannot be ascribed to the reduced number of family members living to that age range relative to earlier age intervals. For each group, the calculation of the age-specific hazard rates depends on only those relatives who entered the specific risk period assessed.

The lifetime cumulative risk observed among the probands, about 30% by age 88 years, is substantially lower than that observed in several earlier reports,[19-22,24] including two studies using much smaller subsets of the current series[19,20] (in which estimates were approximately 45% to 50%). One explanation for this reduction is the possibility of changing proportions of heteroge-

neous subgroups in this sample. In particular, the mean onset age among probands increased by 3.5 years, raising the possibility that the lower cumulative risk in the present greatly enlarged sample may be the result of the increased number of probands with later-onset disease. In addition, most,[16,23,25,26] but not all,[24] studies using samples of 100 or more probands have reported estimates of the cumulative risk for PPD similar to that observed in the present study. A large sample of probands is crucial for survival analytic studies of AD because the sample of relatives under investigation rapidly diminishes with increasing age. In most previous studies, the numbers of relatives at risk in the ninth decade have been very small (frequently less than 25) and, as a result, the SEs of the cumulative risk estimates have been quite large.[18-25] In the present investigation constituting the largest published survival analysis family history study of AD, there were still 65 age-corrected relatives at risk of PPD by the end of the ninth decade, and the SE of the cumulative risk estimate by age 88 years was 3.7%.

The background risk for PPD, as measured by the age-specific hazard rates in the two control groups, predominantly emerges after age 65 years, and by the late 80s appears to either diminish slightly, as in the community control group, or rise still further, as in the ADRC-derived control group. Overall, there was a striking similarity in the age-related risk characteristics between the relatives of the two control groups despite the rather different methods employed to ascertain the controls themselves. Thus, the differing levels of risk in the last age interval may merely reflect random variation rather than a true divergence between groups, as these levels did not significantly differ and, overall, the age-specific hazard rates between the two control groups were generally quite similar. Nevertheless, the pattern of continuously rising risk in the ADRC-derived control group is more consistent with observations in population-based incidence studies of AD.[31,32] Comparing the relatives of probands with AD with both these groups suggests that, even if the risk for PPD attributable to specifically familial factors has been eliminated by the end of the ninth decade, the long-lived relatives of probands with AD have not escaped the risk for disease. Instead, this risk is now comparable to that of other late octogenarians.

The relative decline with increasing age of the familial contribution to the hazard rate might indicate shifting proportions across the lifespan of incident familial vs sporadic cases among the relatives of the probands. Familial cases may tend to emerge at earlier onset times, with increasing proportions of sporadic cases emerging at later age intervals. Thus, these data provide indirect but intriguing evidence for the possibility that, with increasing age, there may be an increased likelihood that an incident case of AD emerges unrelated to familial factors, *even among the affected relatives of probands with AD.*

A reduced likelihood of familially associated AD with increasing age has implications for studies attempting to identify biological and clinical correlates of familial AD. Family history status has frequently been used to divide subjects with AD into more and less familial groups to examine other variables that may be associated with familial factors of AD.[40-42] Making family history status distinctions, however, might not only suffer from the well-known problem of misclassifying some subjects with a negative family history as nonfamilial when familial factors are actually present but not evident due to small family size and censored data (false negatives). In addition, such distinctions may also misclassify some subjects with a positive family history as familial because of the presence of a relative with PPD that in fact emerges unrelated to familial factors (false positives). The diminishing RR_i with increasing age in the relatives of the probands suggests that the likelihood of including false positives may increase with the onset age of an identified secondary case.

It is also possible that the familial factor present in relatives of probands with AD is associated with a tendency for earlier expression of disease rather than liability (although for most practical purposes, expression delayed long enough renders vacuous the notion of liability). Under this possibility, groups in which the familial factor is present might have similarly *shaped* patterns of hazard as nonfamilial groups with comparable liability, but the risk for disease expression in the familial group may be shifted leftward to earlier ages. Hazard rates in controls, under this possibility, would be expected to rise to similar levels but at later ages, and the theoretical peak might exceed the normal human lifespan and hence remain unobserved. Thus, presuming truncated distributions, both the patterns of hazard rates observed in the relatives of the ADRC-derived control group and the consistent increases in the age-specific incidence observed in the general population[31,32] (but not the community control group's decrease in the rate in the 85- to 89-year age interval) could be interpreted as consistent with this possibility.

In a similar vein, the significant correlation in age at onset between probands and their affected relatives observed here and elsewhere[16] might suggest specificity of familial transmission of age at onset. Under this possibility, while vulnerable relatives of probands with earlier-onset AD might show earlier expression of disease, vulnerable relatives of probands with later-onset AD might manifest disease only if they lived to very late ages. As discussed above in relation to the controls, if the liability is comparable between the relatives of probands with early- and late-onset AD, then the pattern of rates between the two groups should be similar but shifted apart; the peak age-specific hazard rate of the early-onset group would be expected to appear earlier than the peak of the late-onset group. However, our comparison of the pattern of age-

specific hazard rates in the relatives of the early- and late-onset groups does not support this possibility. Not only were the age-specific hazard rates in the late-onset group consistently lower than in the early-onset group after the 55- to 59-year age interval, but they did not continue to increase in the 85- to 89-year age interval, the same interval in which rates in the early-onset group began to decline. Among relatives of the late-onset group, none of the RD_is were significantly different from those of the controls. Furthermore, in contrast to what would be expected with specificity of familial transmission of age at onset, the RR_i of PPD in the relatives of probands with late-onset AD compared with controls and in turn the attributable proportion declined in the later age intervals, and only one RR_i associated with a comparatively *early* age interval differed from 1.0. Such results do not support the aforementioned hypothesis. Instead they are consistent with the diminishing role of familial factors in AD with increasing age relative to other causes.

The pattern of hazard rates in the relatives of probands with early- and late-onset AD raise questions about the meaning of the significant but still modest (r=.30) age-at-onset correlation between probands and affected relatives. Such correlations only employ those probands with identified secondary cases, leaving out probands without secondary cases as well as all unaffected relatives. In so doing, the correlations fail to incorporate the overall age-related risk in the populations from which the identified cases derive. A comparable level of correlation derived under these conditions would be expected if, rather than specificity of familial transmission of age at onset across all age ranges, familial factors in AD were most important at earlier ages and less so at later ones when the incidence of AD overall was far higher. Not only would early-onset cases obviously tend to cluster together in families with familial AD, but the occasional sporadic secondary cases (ie, those not arising from the presence of familial factors) that might emerge among the relatives of probands with late-onset nonfamilial AD—at rates not significantly greater than those of controls—would be more likely to also have a late onset.

OUR CHOICE OF age 70 years as the cutoff for defining early- and late-onset AD had the advantage of best balancing the number of relatives living to late age intervals, providing optimally contrasting hazard rate estimates. Although at earlier age intervals the two groups are less evenly balanced, the number of relatives available even in the smaller of the two groups—more than 200—makes the need for comparable sample sizes far less important. Nevertheless, the numbers of age-corrected at-risk relatives in this last observed age interval in both the early- (N=34) and late-onset (N=31) groups were modest. A larger data set with more long-lived relatives will be needed to better delineate the effect of onset in probands on the pattern of the hazard rate of PPD.

Several more general methodological issues require consideration. First, similar to most family history studies of AD,[17,19-26] the ascertainment of probands in this study was clinic based, leading to a sample of relatively younger probands with earlier onset of AD than population-based methods. The familial characteristics of probands with onset of AD in the ages of peak incidence of this disease (in the ninth and 10th decades) remain essentially unexamined. Second, as in all analyses of familial risk, the characteristics of relatives within families, while treated as independent observations, are in fact correlated to some extent, leading to a probable underestimation of the P values.[43] However, the significance of the comparisons of *cumulative* risk and early age-specific hazard rates between groups are very robust. Furthermore, while at later age ranges there is a reduction in the levels of significance for hazard rate comparisons, the major focus of this study is on the patterns of risk over different age intervals and the *decreasing* significance of familial factors with increasing age. Third, in contrast to the probands and the ADRC-derived controls, who had large and equivalent proportions of family histories collected with two informants, the community controls were uniformly collected from only the index subject, perhaps leading to reduced sensitivity for detecting cases of dementia in this group. This concern is mitigated, however, both by the similarity in risk curves for PPD between the two control groups and the failure to detect even marginally significant differences in rates of PPD according to the number of family informants in the other two groups. Fourth, the reliance on family informants in all groups to provide information on relatives,[44] however rigorously collected, will lead to greater diagnostic uncertainty than a procedure including a direct assessment. Informants may be unaware or reluctant to acknowledge the presence of dementia in a relative, and it is possible that such factors might operate differentially between groups, with, for example, informants searching harder to identify dementia in relatives of probands than controls.[24] In late-onset diseases, the use of informants is difficult to avoid since mortality usually proscribes the direct examination of those relatives of greatest interest. To enhance the comprehensiveness and uniformity of the data collection, standardized instruments were used with demonstrated reliability[27,28] and validity[36] and with questions on concrete behaviors that do not require informants to acknowledge the presence of a "disease" in their relatives. Furthermore, the observation of differing *patterns* of risk across time between relatives of probands and controls is not readily attributable to recall bias. Nevertheless, accumulation of still larger samples with very long-lived relatives might further clarify the hazard patterns of relatives of probands with AD at more finely demarcated and even later age intervals.

Accepted for publication March 22, 1994.

This study was supported by grants AG-02219 and AG-05138 from the National Institute of Aging, Bethesda, Md, and the New York (NY) Community Trust.

Address correspondence to Psychiatry Service, 116A, Bronx VA Medical Center, 130 W Kingsbridge Rd, Bronx, NY 10468 (Dr Silverman).

REFERENCES

1. Nee LE, Eldrigge R, Sunderland T, Thomas CB, Katz D, Thomson KE. Dementia of the Alzheimer type: clinical and family study of 22 twin pairs. *Neurology.* 1986;37:359-363.
2. Rapoport SI, Pettigrew KD, Schapiro MB. Discordance and concordance of dementia of the Alzheimer type (DAT) in monozygotic twins indicate heritable and sporadic forms of Alzheimer's disease. *Neurology.* 1991;41:1549-1553.
3. Li G, Silverman JM, Mohs RC. Clinical genetic studies of Alzheimer's disease. *Psychiatr Clin North Am.* 1991;14:267-285.
4. St George-Hyslop P, Tanzi RE, Polinsky RJ, Haines JL, Nee L, Watkins PC, Myers RH, Feldman RG, Pollen D, Drachman D, Growton J, Bruni A, Foncin JF, Salmon D, Frommelt P, Amaducci L, Sorbi S, Placentini S, Steward JD, Hobbs WJ, Conneally PM, Gusella JF. The genetic defect causing familial Alzheimer's disease maps on chromosome 21. *Science.* 1987;235:885-890.
5. Goate A, Chartier-Harlin M-C, Mullan M, Brown J, Crawford F, Fidani L, Giuffra L, Haynes A, Irving N, James L, Mant R, Newton P, Rooke K, Roques P, Talbot C, Pericak-Vance M, Roses A, Williamson R, Rossor M, Owen M, Hardy J. Segregation of a missense mutation in the amyloid precursor protein gene with familial Alzheimer's diease. *Nature.* 1991;349:704-706.
6. Pericak-Vance MA, Bebout JL, Gaskell PC Jr, Yamaoka LH, Hung W-Y, Earl NL, Heyman A, Clark CM, Roses AM. Linkage studies in familial Alzheimer disease: evidence for chromosome 19 linkage. *Am J Hum Genet.* 1991;48:1034-1050.
7. Schellenberg GD, Bird TD, Wijsman EM, Orr HT, Anderson L, Nemens E, White JA, Bonnycastle L, Weber JL, Alonso ME, Potter H, Heston LL, Martin GM. Genetic linkage evidence for a familial Alzheimer's disease locus on chromosome 14. *Science.* 1992;258:668-671.
8. Corder EH, Saunders AM, Strittmatter WJ, Schmechel DE, Gaskell PC, Small GW, Roses AD, Haines JL, Pericak-Vance MA. Gene dose of apolipoprotein E type 4 allele and the risk of Alzheimer's disease in late onset families. *Science.* 1993;261:921-923.
9. Heyman A, Wilkinson WE, Stafford JA, Helms MJ, Sigmon AH, Weinberg T. Alzheimer's disease: a study of epidemiological aspects. *Ann Neurol.* 1984; 15:335-341.
10. Shalat SL, Seltzer B, Pidcock C, Baker ELJ. Risk factors for Alzheimer's disease: a case-control study. *Neurology.* 1987;37:1630-1633.
11. Amaducci LA, Fratiglioni L, Rocca WA, Fieschi C, Livmen P, Pedone D, Bracco L, Lippa A, Gandolfo C, Bino G, Prencipe M, Bonatti ML, Girotti F, Carella F, Tavotta B, Ferla S, Lenzi GL, Carole A, Gambi A, Grigoletto F, Schoenberge BS. Risk factors for clinically diagnosed Alzheimer's disease: a case-control study of an Italian population. *Neurology.* 1986;36:922-931.
12. Graves AB, White E, Koepell TD, Reifler BV, van Belle G, Larson EB, Raskind M. A case-control study of Alzheimer's disease. *Ann Neurol.* 1990;28:766-774.
13. Broe GA, Henderson AS, Creasey H, McCusker E, Korten AE, Jorm AD, Longley W, Anthony JC. A case-control study of Alzheimer's disease in Australia. *Neurology.* 1990;40:1698-1707.
14. Mendez MF, Underwood KL, Zander BA, Mastri AR, Sung JH, Frey WH. Risk factors in Alzheimer's disease: a clinicopathologic study. *Neurology.* 1992;42:770-775.
15. Li G, Shen YC, Li YT, Chen CH, Zhau YW, Silverman JM. A case-control study of Alzheimer's disease in China. *Neurology.* 1992;42:1481-1488.
16. Heston LL, Mastri AR, Anderson VE, White J. Dementia of the Alzheimer type: clinical genetics, natural history, and associated conditions. *Arch Gen Psychiatry.* 1981;38:976-981.
17. Heyman A, Wilkenson WE, Hurwitz BJ, Schmechel D, Sigmon AH, Weinberg T, Helms J, Swift M. Alzheimer's disease: genetic aspects and associated clinical disorders. *Ann Neurol.* 1983;14:507-515.
18. Breitner JCS, Folstein MF. Familial Alzheimer's disease: a prevalent disorder with specific clinical features. *Psychol Med.* 1984;14:63-80.
19. Mohs RC, Breitner JCS, Silverman JM, Davis KL. Alzheimer's disease: morbid risk among first-degree relatives approximates 50% by 90 years of age. *Arch Gen Psychiatry.* 1987;44:405-408.
20. Breitner JCS, Silverman JM, Mohs RC, Davis KL. Familial aggregation in Alzheimer's disease: comparison of risk among relatives of early- and late-onset cases, and among male and female relatives in successive generations. *Neurology.* 1988;38:207-212.
21. Martin RL, Gerteis G, Gabrielli WF. A family genetic study of dementia of Alzheimer type. *Arch Gen Psychiatry.* 1988;45:894-900.
22. Huff FJ, Auerbach J, Chakravarti A, Boller F. Risk of dementia in relatives of patients with Alzheimer's disease. *Neurology.* 1988;38:786-790.
23. Farrer LA, O'Sullivan DM, Cupples LA, Growden JH, Myers RH. Assessment of genetic risk for Alzheimer's disease among first-degree relatives. *Ann Neurol.* 1989;25:485-493.
24. Mayeux R, Sano M, Chen J, Tattemichi T, Stern Y. Risk of dementia in first-degree relatives of patients with Alzheimer's disease and related disorders. *Arch Neurol.* 1991;48:268-273.
25. Silverman JM, Raiford K, Edland S, Fillenbaum G, Morris JC, Clark C, Kukall W, Heyman A. The Consortium to Establish a Registry for Alzheimer's Disease (CERAD), VI: family history assessment: a multi-center study of first-degree relatives of Alzheimer's disease probands and nondemented spouse controls. *Neurology.* In press.
26. Sadovnick AD, Irwin ME, Baird PA, Beattie L. Genetic studies on an Alzheimer clinical population. *Genet Epidemiol.* 1989;6:633-643.
27. Silverman JM, Breitner JCS, Mohs RC, Davis KL. Reliability of the family history method in genetic studies of Alzheimer's disease and related dementias. *Am J Psychiatry.* 1986;43:1279-1282.
28. Silverman JM, Keefe RSE, Mohs RC, Davis KL. A study of the reliability of the family history method in genetic studies of Alzheimer's disease. *Alzheimer Dis Assoc Disord.* 1990;3:218-223.
29. Bierer LM, Silverman JM, Mohs RC, Haroutunian V, Li G, Purohit D, Breitner JCS, Perl D, Davis KL. Morbid risk to first-degree relatives of neuropathologically confirmed cases of Alzheimer's disease. *Dementia.* 1992;3:134-139.
30. Breitner JCS, Magruder-Habib KM. Criteria for onset critically influence the estimation of familial risk in Alzheimer's disease. *Genet Epidemiol.* 1989;6: 663-669.
31. Kokmen E, Chandra V, Schoenberg BS. Trend in incidence of dementing illness in Rochester, Minnesota, in three quinquennial periods, 1960-1974. *Neurology.* 1988;38:975-980.
32. Copeland JRM, Davidson IA, Dewey ME, Gilmore C, Larkin BA, McWilliam C, Saunders PA, Scott A, Sharma V, Sullivan C. Alzheimer's disease, other dementias, depression and pseudo-dementia: prevalence, incidence and three year outcome in Liverpool. *Br J Psychiatry.* 1992;161:230-239.
33. McKhann G, Drachman D, Folstein MF, Katzman R, Price D, Stadlen E. Clinical diagnosis of Alzheimer's disease: report of the NINCDS-ADRDA work group under the auspices of the Department of Health and Human Services Task Force on Alzheimer's Disease. *Neurology.* 1984;34:939-944.
34. Silverman JM, Li G, Schear S, Wang ZX, Sotolongo C, Somary K, Mohs RC. A cross-cultural family history study of primary progressive dementia in relatives of nondemented elderly Chinese, Italians, Jews, and Puerto Ricans. *Acta Psychiatr Scand.* 1992;85:211-217.
35. American Psychiatric Association. *Diagnostic and Statistical Manual of Mental Disorders, Third Edition.* Washington, DC: American Psychiatric Association; 1980.
36. Kawas C, Segal J, Stewart WF, Corrada-Bravo, Thal L. A validation of the "Dementia Questionnaire." *Arch Neurol.* In press.
37. Lee ET. *Statistical Methods for Survival Data Analysis.* 2nd ed. New York, NY: John Wiley & Sons Inc; 1992.
38. Rothman KJ. *Modern Epidemiology.* Boston, Mass: Little Brown & Co Inc; 1986.
39. Mayeux R, Ottman R, Tang M-X, Noboa-Bauza L, Marder K, Gurland B, Stern Y. Genetic susceptibility and head injury as risk factors for Alzheimer's disease among community-dwelling elderly persons and their first-degree relatives. *Ann Neurol.* 1993;33:494-501.
40. Knesevich JW, Toro FR, Morris JC, LaBarge E. Aphasia, family history, and the longitudinal course of senile dementia of the Alzheimer's type. *Psychiatry Res.* 1985;14:255-263.
41. Stern RG, Mohs RC, Bierer LM, Silverman JM, Schmeidler J, Davidson M, Davis KL. Deterioration on the Blessed test in Alzheimer's disease: longitudinal data and their implications for clinical trials and identification of subtypes. *Psychiatry Res.* 1992;42:101-110.
42. Luchins DJ, Cohen D, Hanrahan P, Eisdorfer C, Paveza G, Ashfor JW, Gorelick P, Hirschman R, Freels S, Levy P, Semla T, Shaw H. Are there clinical differences between familial and nonfamilial Alzheimer's disease? *Am J Psychiatry.* 1992;149:1023-1027.
43. Mack W, Langholz B, Thomas DC. Survival models of familial aggregation of cancer. *Environ Health Perspect.* 1990;87:27-35.
44. Kukall WA, Larson EB. Distinguishing Alzheimer's disease from other dementia: questionnaire responses of close relatives and autopsy results. *J Am Geriatr Soc.* 1989;37:521-527.

Interpersonal Psychotherapy

Current Status

Myrna M. Weissman, PhD, John C. Markowitz, MD

Interpersonal psychotherapy (IPT), a time-limited treatment for major depression, was developed, defined in a manual,[1] and tested in randomized clinical trials by the late Gerald L. Klerman, MD, and collaborators. It has subsequently been modified for different age groups and types of mood and nonmood disorders and for use as a long-term treatment.[2] Having begun as a research intervention, IPT has yet to be well disseminated among clinicians or in residency training programs. The publication of efficacy data, the recent appearance of two practice guidelines that include IPT among treatments for depression,[3-5] and the interest in defined treatments for managed care have led to increasing requests for information and training.

This article will briefly describe the concepts and techniques of IPT and the current status of adaptation, efficacy data, and training. Our purpose is to provide a quick guide to recent developments and a reference list but not a comprehensive review. While our focus is on major depression, the adaptation of IPT for mild and chronic depressions and nonmood disorders is included because of their relevance to or, in some cases, comorbidity with major depression.

THE PRACTICE GUIDELINES

In 1993, two practice guidelines for mental health professionals[3] and primary care practitioners[4-7] appeared. The two sets of guidelines differ considerably in scope, audience, and level of scientific certainty required as a basic recommendation. Neither claims to define the standard of care for any individual patient. Both discuss IPT as an acute and maintenance treatment for depression, used alone or in combination with medication.

American Psychiatric Association (APA) Practice Guidelines

The APA practice guidelines for major depression in adults include psychotherapeutic management, psychodynamic psychotherapy and psychoanalysis, brief therapy, behavior therapy (BT), cognitive behavior therapy (CBT), marital, family, and group therapies, and IPT, stating that their "specific categorizations are primarily useful for heuristic or research purposes."[3(p4)] The APA practice guidelines do not require efficacy data from controlled clinical trials as a criterion for inclusion. Interpersonal psychotherapy is described as being useful for patients in the "midst of recent conflicts with significant others and for those having difficulty adjusting to an altered career or social role or other life transition."[3(p6)]

Primary Care Guidelines

The clinical practice guidelines for the treatment of depression in primary care settings are more extensive, consisting of two detailed volumes for the clinician,[4,5]

From the Department of Epidemiology in Psychiatry, College of Physicians and Surgeons of Columbia University (Dr Weissman), the Division of Clinical and Genetic Epidemiology, New York State Psychiatric Institute (Dr Weissman), and the Department of Psychiatry, Cornell University Medical College (Dr Markowitz), New York, NY.

a quick reference guide,[6] and a patient volume.[7]

Both the physician and the patient guides list IPT as well as CBT, BT, and brief dynamic and marital therapies as treatments for depression. The primary care guides do not recommend psychotherapy as sole treatment for patients with severe or psychotic depression and note that "treatments with established efficacy are preferred initially over less tested or untested interventions."[5(p38)] Interpersonal psychotherapy is recommended as an acute treatment for symptom removal, prevention of relapse and recurrence, correction of causal psychological problems with secondary symptom resolution, and correction of secondary consequences of depression. For the continuation and maintenance phases of treatment, the guidelines state that medication alone may be sufficient to prevent relapse or recurrence and to maintain remission of recurrent depression.[8]

The guidelines describe IPT, CBT, and BT as "effective in most cases of mild-to-moderate depression,"[6(p12)] but indications "for continuation phase psychotherapy are unclear,"[6(p18)] even though "two studies are suggestive that continuation psychotherapy may reduce the relapse rate."[6(p18)] The patient guidelines list BT, cognitive therapy, and IPT as being the "most well-studied for their effectiveness in reducing symptoms of major depressive disorder."[7(p23)] Regarding continuation psychotherapy, the patient is advised, "If your depression gets better with psychotherapy, you and your health provider can decide if your therapy should continue and for how long."[7(p24)]

> In general maintenance (long-term) psychotherapy by itself is not recommended unless there are reasons, such as pregnancy or severe side effects that keep you from taking medicine. While maintenance psychotherapy does not prevent another episode of depression, some research suggests that it can delay a recurrence.[7(p24-25)]

The patient is advised that, with combined medication and psychotherapy,

> More than half of patients feel better after 6 to 8 weeks. Combined treatment may be most helpful for longer lasting depression, for those with symptoms between episodes or for those who do not respond fully to medication or psychotherapy alone.[7(p24)]

OVERVIEW OF IPT

Detailed discussion of the concepts, strategies,[1] and new modifications of IPT have been published.[2] Efficacy studies of psychotherapy for the treatment of depression and in general have been reviewed in several publications[9-13] and by R. B. Jarrett, PhD, and A. J. Rush, MD (unpublished data, 1993).

Interpersonal psychotherapy was initially formulated as a time-limited, weekly outpatient treatment of depressed patients.[1] Based on the ideas of the interpersonal school,[14] IPT makes no assumptions about origin but uses the connection between onset of depressive symptoms and current interpersonal problems as a treatment focus. Interpersonal psychotherapy generally deals with current rather than past interpersonal relationships, focusing on the patient's immediate social context, and attempts to intervene in symptom formation and social dysfunction associated with depression rather than enduring aspects of personality.

Interpersonal psychotherapy as an acute treatment has three phases. The first, usually constituting the first one to three sessions, includes diagnostic evaluation and psychiatric history and sets the framework for the treatment. The therapist reviews symptoms, diagnoses depression by standard criteria,[15] and gives the patient the sick role.[16] The sick role may excuse the patient from overwhelming social obligations but requires the patient to work in treatment to recover full function. During the initial session, the psychiatric history includes a review of the patient's current social functioning and current close relationships, their patterns, and mutual expectations. Changes in relationships proximal to the onset of symptoms are elucidated (eg, death of a loved one, children leaving home, worsening marital strife, or isolation from a confidant). This review provides a framework for understanding the social and interpersonal context of the onset of depressive symptoms and defines the focus of treatment.

The therapist assesses the need for medication based on symptom severity, history, response to treatment, and patient preference and then educates the patient about depression by explicitly discussing the diagnosis, including the constellation of symptoms that define the diagnosis and what the patient might expect from treatment. The therapist then links the depressive syndrome to the patient's interpersonal situation within the framework of one of four interpersonal problem areas: grief, interpersonal role disputes, role transitions, or interpersonal deficits.

In the middle phase, the therapist pursues strategies defined in the manual[1] that are specific to the chosen interpersonal problem area. For grief, defined as complicated bereavement following the death of a loved one, the therapist facilitates mourning and gradually helps the patient to find new activities and relationships to compensate for the loss. Role disputes are conflicts with a significant other: a spouse or other family members, coworker, or close friend. The therapist helps the patient explore the relationship and the nature of the dispute. They consider options to resolve it. Failing this, they may conclude that the relationship has reached an impasse and consider ways to end and replace it with better alternatives. Role transition includes changed life sta-

tus: the beginning or end of a relationship or career, a move, promotion, retirement, graduation, diagnosis of a medical illness, or loss of a treasured ideal. The patient is helped to deal with the change by recognizing positive and negative aspects of the new role he or she is assuming and assets and liabilities of the old role this replaces. Interpersonal deficits, the residual fourth IPT problem area, define the patient as significantly lacking in social skills, including initiating or sustaining relationships.

Interpersonal psychotherapy sessions address present "here-and-now" problems rather than childhood or developmental issues. Sessions open with the question "How have things been since we last met?" This focuses the patient on recent interpersonal events and recent mood, which the therapist attempts to link. Therapists take an active, nonneutral, supportive, and hopeful stance.

The final phase of IPT, typically the last few weeks of treatment, encourages the patient to recognize and consolidate therapeutic gains and to develop ways of identifying and countering depressive symptoms should they arise in the future.

USE OF IPT IN MOOD DISORDER

Acute Treatment of Major Depression

The efficacy of IPT as a treatment for acute depression was first demonstrated in a four-cell, 16-week randomized trial of IPT and amitriptyline therapy alone and in combination, with nonscheduled treatment as a control, for 81 outpatients with major depression.[17,18] There were no significant differences between IPT and amitriptyline therapy in symptom reduction by the end of treatment. However, the effects of amitriptyline were apparent 1 to 2 weeks earlier. Each active treatment more effectively reduced symptoms than did a nonscheduled control, and combined amitriptyline therapy and IPT was more effective overall than either active treatment alone. A 1-year naturalistic follow-up found many patients had sustained benefits from the brief IPT intervention. Significantly better psychosocial functioning developed in patients who received IPT, whether or not they received medication; this effect on social function had not been evident at the end of the 16-week trial in any treatment group.[19] Many patients from all treatment groups, however, required additional treatment by the time of the 1-year follow-up.

The most ambitious acute treatment study to date was the multisite National Institute of Mental Health Treatment of Depression Collaborative Research Program (NIMH TDCRP),[20] which randomly assigned 250 depressed outpatients to 16 weeks of imipramine therapy, IPT, CBT, or placebo. Most subjects completed at least 15 weeks or 12 treatment sessions. Less symptomatic patients (Hamilton Depression Score, <20) improved with all treatments, including placebo. Imipramine induced the most rapid response and was most consistently superior to placebo. Interpersonal psychotherapy was comparable with imipramine therapy on several outcome measures and showed a mean outcome superior to placebo for the more severely depressed patients (Hamilton Depression Score, ≥20), whereas CBT was not superior to placebo for this group. The study did not include a combined medication/psychotherapy cell.

Klein and Ross[21] recently reanalyzed the efficacy data from the NIMH TDCRP. They argued that inappropriately stringent levels for statistical significance in testing heterogeneity of slope and pairwise group differences had lowered the power to detect treatment differences and yielded the unwarranted conclusion that the active treatments were indistinguishable (ie, a type II statistical error). Reanalysis using the Johnson-Neyman technique produced an ordering for treatment efficacy with "medication superior to psychotherapy, [and] the psychotherapies somewhat superior to placebo . . . particularly among the symptomatic and impaired patients."[21(p241)] The authors found "CBT relatively inferior to IPT for patients with BDI [Beck Depression Inventory] scores greater than approximately 30, generally considered the boundary between moderate and severe depression."[21(p247)] In summary, the findings of the reanalysis are fairly consistent with results reported by Elkin et al,[20] but differences among treatments were sharpened by the reanalysis.

Continuation/Maintenance Treatment

Interpersonal psychotherapy was first developed and tested in an 8-month, six-cell trial[22,23] that today would be considered continuation rather than maintenance treatment. One hundred fifty acutely depressed outpatient women who responded (symptom reduction rated by a clinical interviewer, ≥50%) to 4 to 6 weeks of amitriptyline therapy were randomized to receive 8 months of treatment with *weekly* IPT alone, amitriptyline therapy alone, combined amitriptyline therapy and IPT, IPT and placebo, placebo alone, or no pill. Randomization to IPT or a low-contact condition occurred at entry into the continuation phase, whereas randomization to medication, placebo, or no pill occurred at the end of the second month of continuation. Maintenance pharmacotherapy was found to prevent relapse and symptom exacerbation,[24] whereas IPT improved social functioning.[23] The effects of psychotherapy on social functioning were not apparent for 6 to 8 months. No negative treatment interactions were found, and, because of differential effects of the treatments, combined psychotherapy-pharmacotherapy was considered the best outcome.

In the longest maintenance trial, Frank et al[25,26] studied 128 outpatients with recurrent depression (ie, histories of at least three acute major depressive episodes) who responded to 12 weeks of continuation treatment for the acute episode and 20 weeks of continuation treatment with imipramine and IPT. Interpersonal psychotherapy was modified (IPT-M) for this maintenance trial primarily by emphasizing those problems that persist or develop as a consequence of remission. Owing to the length of treatment, multiple problem areas were addressed.[25]

Patients were randomly assigned to receive 3 years of maintenance therapy in one of five cells: monthly maintenance IPT-M (1) alone, (2) combined with imipramine therapy, or (3) combined with placebo or medication clinic visits for either (4) continuing high-dose imipramine therapy or (5) placebo without further psychotherapy.[8,26,27] This study was unique in using the *highest* dose of medication ever in a maintenance trial (mean dose, 200 mg/d) and the *lowest* dose of IPT ever (monthly).

Findings showed the highest significant effect for maintenance imipramine therapy in preventing recurrence (survival time), a modest but significant effect for IPT-M, and a trend for superiority of combined treatment.[26] After 1 year, major depression had recurred in 65% of patients receiving placebo, 46% receiving IPT-M without imipramine, 17.9% receiving imipramine alone, and only 8% receiving imipramine and IPT-M. At 3 years, mean survival without recurrence of depression was 45 weeks for placebo, 74 weeks for IPT-M plus placebo, 82 weeks for IPT-M alone, 124 weeks for imipramine therapy alone, and 131 weeks for imipramine therapy and IPT-M. Patients in whom IPT-M maintained a strong interpersonal focus in treatment had longer lengths of survival without symptomatic recurrence.[26,27] The 82-week survival time without recurrence with IPT-M alone for patients with a history of recurrence would suffice to protect many women with recurrent depression through pregnancy and nursing without medication. The effects of more frequent maintenance IPT-M (eg, fortnightly) require testing. A study of differing doses of IPT-M is under way by researchers at the Western Psychiatric Institute, Pittsburgh, Pa (the Pittsburgh group).

Geriatric Depressed Patients

One 6-week pilot study comparing IPT with nortriptyline therapy in 30 geriatric depressed patients showed some advantages for IPT, largely owing to medication side effects that produced higher attrition.[28] Interpersonal psychotherapy was not modified for this study.

A 3-year maintenance study[2] for geriatric patients with recurrent depression is under way using a similar design to the study by Frank et al. Interpersonal psychotherapy was modified for geriatric patients as IPT-late-life maintenance treatment (IPT-LLM). This study compares IPT-LLM alone, nortriptyline therapy alone, IPT-LLM plus nortriptyline therapy, IPT-LLM plus placebo, and placebo alone in a randomized discontinuation maintenance study.[29] The manual has been modified to allow more flexible length of session, as elderly patients may not be able to sustain 50-minute sessions. Special interpersonal problems of an elderly population have been identified (eg, older patients may want to address early-life relationships in their psychotherapy), which distinguishes IPT-LLM from the typical here-and-now focus of IPT.[2]

Depressed Adolescents

Mufson et al[30] have modified IPT to incorporate adolescent developmental issues (IPT-A), adding as a fifth problem area the single-parent family, an interpersonal situation found frequently among their adolescent patients.[29,30] In a recently completed open study, 14 patients were significantly less depressed after a 12-week trial than at intake. A controlled clinical trial comparing IPT-A with case management is under way.

Depressed Patients With Human Immunodeficiency Virus (HIV)

Markowitz et al[31] have modified IPT for depressed patients with HIV (IPT-HIV), emphasizing the common issues among this population, which include concern about illness, death, grief, and role transitions. In a pilot open trial, 21 of 24 patients responded with a reduction of depression. Most patients felt that brief therapy was suitable for their situation, in which time is precious and quick results are needed. A 16-week randomized clinical trial is being conducted by Markowitz et al (with the late Samuel W. Perry, MD),[32] comparing IPT-HIV with CBT, supportive psychotherapy, and imipramine therapy plus supportive psychotherapy.

Patients With Dysthymia

In the modification of IPT for dysthymia (IPT-D), patients are encouraged to reconceptualize what they had seen as their character flaws as ego-dystonic chronic mood-dependent symptoms.[2] Contrary to expectation, two open trials found that dysthymic patients with lifelong chronicity had a reduction of depressive symptoms in 16 weekly IPT-D sessions. Markowitz[33] and Kocsis et al[34] have treated a total of 16 pilot subjects. None worsened, and 11 experienced remission. Medication benefits roughly half of dysthymic patients,[34] but nonresponders may need psychotherapy, and even medication responders may benefit from combined treatment.[35] Based on the positive pilot results, a comparative study of IPT-D, medication therapy, and placebo is planned.

Depressed Primary Care Patients

A clinical trial comparing IPT with pharmacotherapy for depressed ambulatory medical patients in a primary care setting is under way by Schulberg et al.[36] The IPT manual is unchanged. However, IPT is designed to conform with the practices of the primary care center, eg, nurses take vital signs and blood pressure prior to each session. If a patient is hospitalized for medical reasons, IPT continues in the hospital when possible.

Patients With Bipolar Disorder

Ehlers and colleagues[37] are assessing the benefits of IPT modified by social zeitgeber theory, ie, behavioral management of daily schedule and sleep patterns, as a maintenance treatment in an ongoing study of patients with lithium-stabilized bipolar disorder (IPT-BP), comparing IPT-BP with medication therapy.[38] The 3-year maintenance treatment will initially include biweekly IPT-BP visits that taper to monthly sessions in the final 2 years.

Depressed Patients With Marital Disputes

Since marital conflict, separation, and divorce have been associated with the onset and course of depressive episodes,[39] and individual psychotherapy for depressed patients in marital disputes may lead to premature termination of some marriages,[40] a manual was developed for a conjoint IPT for depressed patients with marital disputes (IPT-CM).[2] Conjoint marital IPT focuses on the current marital dispute and involves the spouse in all sessions. Eighteen patients with major depression linked to the onset or exacerbation of marital disputes were randomly assigned to 16 weeks of individual IPT or IPT-CM. Patients receiving both treatments showed the same reduction in depressive symptoms. However, patients receiving IPT-CM had significantly better marital adjustment, greater marital affection, and better sexual relations than did patients receiving IPT alone.[41] These preliminary findings require replication with a larger sample and other control groups.

USE WITH OTHER PSYCHIATRIC DISORDERS

Interpersonal Counseling (IPC) for Distress

Many patients presenting to primary care practices have symptoms but do not meet criteria for a specific psychiatric disorder. These symptoms can be debilitating and result in high utilization of medical procedures.[42] Interpersonal counseling, based on IPT, was designed for patients who are in distress but who do not have serious concurrent psychiatric disorders.[2] It is administered by health care professionals, usually a nurse practitioner without psychiatric training, for a maximum of six sessions. The first session can be as long as 30 minutes, and subsequent sessions are briefer.

Interpersonal counseling therapists assess the patient's current functioning, recent life events, occupational and familial stress, and changes in interpersonal relationships and assume that such events may provide the context in which emotional and bodily symptoms occur. One hundred twenty-eight patients coming to a primary care clinic and scoring 6 or higher on the Goldberg General Health Questionnaire (GHQ) were randomized either to IPC or usual care without psychological treatment.[43] Over an average of 3 months, often involving only one to two sessions, patients receiving IPC had significantly greater symptom relief than controls as assessed by the GHQ, particularly an improvement of depressed mood. Interpersonal counseling led to *greater* rather than *less* use of mental health care services by patients newly attuned to the psychological source of their symptoms.

IPC in Hospitalized Elderly Patients

Mossey and others[44] have initiated a clinical trial of IPC with elderly hospitalized medically ill patients who have some depressive symptoms. Hospitalized patients over 60 years of age who do not meet criteria for major depression but have depressive symptoms on two consecutive assessments are randomized to either IPC or usual care. A nondepressed control group is also being followed up. Results for the first 37 patients indicate that IPC is feasible and acceptable. Assessments at 3 months show a reduction in depressive symptoms among the IPC group and a slight increase in symptoms among the controls. Rehospitalization in the IPC and the nondepressed groups was similar (11% and 15%, respectively) and significantly less than in the depressed control group receiving usual care (50%). This study is ongoing.

Drug Abuse

Interpersonal therapy has not been shown to be effective in two clinical trials with substance abusers. In the first study, complicated by high attrition, Rounsaville et al[45] found no benefit for adjunctive IPT added to standard treatment compared with the standard program alone for 72 opiate abusers undergoing methadone maintenance therapy. The same team in a separate trial found 12 weeks of IPT ineffective with marginally worse results than BT for 42 cocaine abusers attempting to achieve abstinence.[46]

Bulimia

Fairburn et al[47] have made some changes in IPT for two studies of bu-

limic patients. They use fewer, differently scheduled sessions, primarily to be compatible with CBT, with which it was being compared. Other than during the assessment phase, when a history of the eating problem is obtained, the content of the IPT approach is similar to that for depression: little reference is made to the patient's eating disorder during the course of treatment.[2]

Seventy-five patients with bulimia nervosa were randomly assigned to CBT, IPT, or BT for 19 sessions over 18 weeks, with a 12-month follow-up. Few patients receiving BT ceased binge eating and purging. Patients receiving CBT and IPT made equivalent and substantial changes across all areas of symptoms, with IPT taking longer to achieve effects.[47,48] A multisite replication of this study comparing CBT and IPT in bulimia is under way at Stanford (Calif) University and Columbia University, New York, NY, in collaboration with investigators at Oxford (England) University and Rutgers–The State University, New Brunswick, NJ.

Group Format for Bulimia

Drawing on the experience of Fairburn et al,[47,48] Wilfley et al[49] developed a modification of IPT in a group format (IPT-G) of 16 weekly sessions and tested it in comparison with group CBT and a waiting list (WL) control treatment in 56 women with nonpurging bulimia. Both IPT-G and CBT significantly reduced binge eating, but WL treatment did not.

IPT ADAPTATIONS UNDER DEVELOPMENT

Adaptations of IPT are currently being planned or are under development for panic disorder (K. Shear, MD, Western Psychiatric Institute), borderline personality disorder (L. Gilles, PhD, Clark Institute of Psychiatry–Toronto, Ontario), depressed caregivers of patients with traumatic brain injuries (L. Pessar, MD, Buffalo, NY), depressed newly abstinent alcoholics (J. Markowitz, MD, and J. Mahler, MD, Cornell University Medical College, New York, NY), depressed pregnant women (M. Spinelli, MD, Columbia University), posttraumatic stress disorder as a sequelae of breast cancer in young women (D. Pelcovitz, North Shore University Hospital, Cornell University Medical College), and protracted bereavement (M. D. Miller, PhD, Western Psychiatric Institute, Pittsburgh, Pa).

TRAINING IN IPT

Until recently, the number of IPT practitioners has been quite small and almost exclusively limited to participants in research studies. Interpersonal psychotherapy is now being included at professional workshops and conferences (eg, training courses have been conducted at university centers in Switzerland and Iceland), and the IPT manual[1] has been translated into Italian and Japanese. A training videotape has been produced and is available through Kingsley Communications, Houston, Tex. The tape contains an overall description of IPT and demonstrates the initial assessment phase of treatment. An IPT training program for licensed mental health care professionals is being developed by David Barlow, PhD, Albany, NY. Residents at Columbia University and Cornell University are currently receiving training in IPT.

Although the principles of IPT are straightforward, we think that training beyond reading the manual is required.[50,51] We recommend that candidates have a graduate clinical degree (MD, PhD, MSW, or RN) and several years of experience conducting psychotherapy. Training programs for IPT are designed to help experienced therapists refocus their treatment to learn a new technique and are not designed to teach novices to be therapists. The training used in the NIMH TDCRP has become a model for subsequent research studies. This includes a brief didactic phase in which the manual is read and reviewed and a longer supervised practicum during which the therapist treats patients under supervision, monitored by actual videotapes of the session.[52] Rounsaville et al[53] have demonstrated that therapists who performed well on their first supervised case did not require further intensive supervision and that experienced therapists committed to the approach required less supervision.[51]

CONCLUSION

Evidence from controlled clinical trials suggests that IPT is a reasonable alternative or adjunct to medication as an acute, continuation, and/or maintenance treatment for patients with major depression. It is a promising but still not fully tested treatment for depressed adolescents and geriatric patients, HIV-positive depressed patients, patients with dysthymia or bulimia, patients with mild depression seen in primary care, and depressed patients and their spouses with marital disputes. More efficacy data are needed in these areas before any claims can be made clearly. Claims based on open trials only cannot be considered evidence of efficacy. Interpersonal psychotherapy is not effective, compared with standard drug programs, for patients addicted to opiates and cocaine. Several IPT clinical trials are under way or in planning stages, based on manual modification, and several manuals are being developed. The manuals differ in the depth of their modifications, and some modifications for different disorders have not been formalized. There is little agreement on what a manual of an IPT adaptation should include.

We view the development of psychotherapy manuals as positive, as they will meet the growing request from third-party payers, managed care professionals, and patients for accountability and speci-

fication of treatment. Manuals are also a necessary first step for testing efficacy. However, there should be clarification and basic guidelines developed for the content of manuals. We believe that psychiatric residency and other mental health care treatment training programs should include clinical instruction in the new time-limited psychotherapies described in the manuals, in addition to providing exposure to long-term psychotherapy. To our knowledge, there is no accepted model psychotherapy curriculum.

Even for experienced therapists, training programs in IPT are still not widely available, but wider dissemination is planned. The established training criteria for research have produced reliable therapists for clinical trials. However, the educational process for IPT in clinical practice requires further study. For example, what educational level and experience is required to learn IPT? Does an experienced therapist require supervision? Will reading the manual suffice? Specific research on the components of IPT, often termed "dismantling studies," might be useful. For example, we view the initial diagnostic and assessment phase of IPT as essential to the clinical treatment of all depressed patients. The efficacy of using the initial IPT phase only vs the full treatment in which the interpersonal context of the depression is managed might be tested. Further research on how long to extend IPT before discarding it for another treatment in patients who do not respond is necessary. Data from the study by Ehlers et al[37] showed the value of monthly maintenance IPT for patients with recurrent depression. There needs to be a series of studies of IPT dosage (eg, weekly, biweekly, or monthly). These studies would be comparable to phase 1 or 2 drug trials.

It is unclear how efficacy data for psychotherapies like IPT will be used in health care reform. Will standardization of treatment be required? What type of education, credentials, and training will be required? What type of evidence of effectiveness and/or cost offsetting will be required? Will untested psychotherapies be reimbursed? Will psychotherapy be reimbursed at all? Will limits be placed on the amount, length, or duration of treatment? We believe that strict caps on psychotherapy reimbursement for certain patients will not be in the best interests of those patients (eg, for patients with recurrent depression who cannot take or fail to respond to medication or depressed women during pregnancy and nursing). The efficacy of antidepressant pharmacotherapy is unequivocal. However, medicating depressed patients without psychological management or monitoring is likely to lead to poor compliance and missed suicide risk. At a minimum, clinical management of depression should entail the tasks defined by the initial phase of IPT: explaining the diagnosis and its spectrum of symptoms, the expected clinical course, side effects, range of treatment alternatives, and linkage between the onset of symptoms and social and interpersonal problems. The role of evidence (ie, controlled clinical trials) in shaping policy on reimbursement needs to be evaluated. Time limits on treatment such as IPT are a necessary part of research protocols. Moreover, clinical trials usually exclude the complicated patients with comorbidity seen in clinical practice. Reimbursement policy when based on data extracted from clinical trials should allow for these contingencies. We need to know how the efficacy of IPT in clinical research translates into effectiveness when used by general clinicians for ordinary cases.

We believe that the best interests of all depressed patients are ensured by the availability of a range of treatment modalities whose efficacy has been established in controlled clinical trials. However, psychotherapy research is a cottage industry. There is no analogue to the Food and Drug Administration for psychotherapy to evaluate claims of efficacy and no corporate industry to develop new treatments and take these treatments through the phases of testing. It is no surprise that there are considerable gaps in empirically based guides for the use of psychotherapy.

Accepted for publication April 5, 1994.

Reprint requests to College of Physicians and Surgeons of Columbia University, New York State Psychiatric Institute, 722 W 168th St, Unit 14, New York, NY 10032 (Dr Weissman).

REFERENCES

1. Klerman GL, Weissman MM, Rounsaville BJ, Chevron ES. *Interpersonal Psychotherapy of Depression.* New York, NY: Basic Books Inc Publishers; 1984.
2. Klerman GL, Weissman MM. *New Applications of Interpersonal Psychotherapy.* Washington, DC: American Psychiatric Press Inc; 1993.
3. Karasu TB, Docherty JP, Gelenberg A, Kupfer DJ, Merriam AE, Shadoan R. Practice guideline for major depressive disorder in adults. *Am J Psychiatry.* 1993;150(suppl):1-26.
4. Depression Guideline Panel. *Clinical Practice Guideline: Depression in Primary Care: Detection and Diagnosis.* Rockville, Md: US Dept of Health and Human Services, Agency for Health Care Policy and Research; 1993;1. Agency for Health Care Policy and Research publication 93-0550.
5. Depression Guideline Panel. *Clinical Practice Guideline: Depression in Primary Care: Treatment of Major Depression.* Rockville, Md: US Dept of Health and Human Services, Agency for Health Care Policy and Research; 1993;2. Agency for Health Care Policy and Research publication 93-0551.
6. Depression Guideline Panel. *Clinical Practice Guideline: Quick Reference Guide for Clinicians: Depression in Primary Care: Detection, Diagnosis, and Treatment.* Rockville, Md: US Dept of Health and Human Services, Agency for Health Care Policy and Research; 1993. Agency for Health Care Policy and Research publication 93-0552.
7. Depression Guideline Panel. *Clinical Practice Guideline: Depression Is a Treatable Illness: A Patient's Guide.* Rockville, Md: US Dept of Health and Human Services, Agency for Health Care Policy and Research; 1993. Agency for Health Care Policy and Research publication 93-0553.
8. Frank E, Kupfer DJ, Perel JM. Early recurrence in unipolar depression. *Arch Gen Psychiatry.* 1989; 46:397-400.
9. Klerman GL, Weissman MM, Markowitz JC, Glick I, Wilner PJ, Mason B, Shear MK. Medication and psychotherapy. In: Bergin AE, Garfield SB, eds. *Handbook of Psychotherapy and Behavior Change.* 4th ed. New York, NY: John Wiley & Sons Inc; 1994:734-782.

10. Weissman MM. The psychological treatment of depression: an update of clinical trials. In: Williams JBW, Spitzer RL, eds. *Psychotherapy Research: Where Are We and Where Should We Go?* New York, NY: Guilford Press; 1984.
11. Weissman MM, Jarrett RB, Rush JA. Psychotherapy and its relevance to the pharmacotherapy of major depression: a decade later (1976-1985). In: DiMascio A, Killam KF, eds. *Psychopharmacology: The Third Generation of Progress.* New York, NY: Raven Press; 1987: 1059-1069.
12. Conte HR, Plutchik R, Wild KV, Karasu TB. Combined psychotherapy and pharmacotherapy for depression. *Arch Gen Psychiatry.* 1986;43:471-479.
13. Hollon SD, Beck AT. Psychotherapy and drug therapy: comparison and combinations. In: Garfield SL, Bergin AE, eds. *Handbook of Psychotherapy and Behavior Change: An Empirical Analysis.* 2nd ed. New York, NY: John Wiley & Sons Inc; 1978.
14. Sullivan HS, ed. *The Interpersonal Theory of Psychiatry.* New York, NY: WW Norton; 1953.
15. American Psychiatric Association. *Diagnostic and Statistical Manual of Mental Disorders, Revised Third Edition.* Washington, DC: American Psychiatric Association; 1987.
16. Parsons T. Illness and the role of the physician: a sociological perspective. *Am J Orthopsychiatry.* 1951;21:452-460.
17. DiMascio A, Weissman MM, Prusoff BA, Neu C, Zwilling M, Klerman GL. Differential symptom reduction by drugs and psychotherapy in acute depression. *Arch Gen Psychiatry.* 1979;36:1450-1456.
18. Weissman MM, Prusoff BA, DiMascio A, Neu C, Goklaney M, Klerman GL. The efficacy of drugs and psychotherapy in the treatment of acute depressive episodes. *Am J Psychiatry.* 1979;136: 555-558.
19. Weissman MM, Klerman GL, Prusoff BA, Sholomskas D, Padian N. Depressed outpatients: results one year after treatment with drugs and/or interpersonal psychotherapy. *Arch Gen Psychiatry.* 1981;38:51-55.
20. Elkin I, Shea MT, Watkins JT, Imber SD, Sotsky SM, Collins JF, Glass DR, Pilkonis PA, Leber WR, Docherty JP, Fiester SJ, Parloff MB. National Institute of Mental Health Treatment of Depression Collaborative Research Program: general effectiveness of treatments. *Arch Gen Psychiatry.* 1989;46:971-982.
21. Klein DF, Ross DC. Reanalysis of the National Institute of Mental Health Treatment of Depression Collaborative Research Program general effectiveness report. *Neuropsychopharmacology.* 1993;8:241-251.
22. Klerman GL, DiMascio A, Weissman MM, Prusoff BA, Paykel ES. Treatment of depression by drugs and psychotherapy. *Am J Psychiatry.* 1974; 131:186-191.
23. Paykel ES, DiMascio A, Haskell D, Prusoff BA. Effects of maintenance amitriptyline and psychotherapy on symptoms of depression. *Psychol Med.* 1975;5:67-77.
24. Weissman MM, Klerman GL, Paykel ES, Prusoff BA, Hanson B. Treatment effects on the social adjustment of depressed patients. *Arch Gen Psychiatry.* 1974;30:771-778.
25. Frank E. Interpersonal psychotherapy as a maintenance treatment for patients with recurrent depression. *Psychotherapy.* 1991;28:259-266.
26. Frank E, Kupfer DJ, Perel JM, Cornes C, Jarrett DB, Mallinger AG, Thase ME, McEachran AB, Grochociniski VJ. Three-year outcomes for maintenance therapies in recurrent depression. *Arch Gen Psychiatry.* 1990;47:1093-1099.
27. Frank E, Kupfer DJ, Wagner EF, McEachran AB, Cornes C. Efficacy of interpersonal psychotherapy as a maintenance treatment of recurrent depression: contributing factors. *Arch Gen Psychiatry.* 1991;48:1053-1059.
28. Sloane RB, Stapes FR, Schneider LS. Interpersonal therapy versus nortriptyline for depression in the elderly. In: Burrows GD, Norman TR, Dennerstein L, eds. *Clinical and Pharmacological Studies in Psychiatric Disorders.* London, England: John Libbey; 1985:344-346.
29. Reynolds CF, Frank E, Perel JM, Imber SD, Cornes C, Morycz RK, Mazumdar S, Miller M, Pollock BG, Rifai AH, Stack JA, George CJ, Houck PR, Kupfer DJ. Combined pharmacotherapy and psychotherapy in the acute and continuation treatment of elderly patients with recurrent major depression: a preliminary report. *Am J Psychiatry.* 1992;149:1687-1692.
30. Mufson L, Moreau D, Weissman MM, Klerman GL, eds. *Interpersonal Therapy for Depressed Adolescents.* New York, NY: Guilford Press; 1993.
31. Markowitz JC, Klerman GL, Perry SW. Interpersonal psychotherapy of depressed HIV-seropositive patients. *Hosp Community Psychiatry.* 1992;43:885-890.
32. Markowitz JC, Klerman GL, Perry SW, Clougherty KF, Mayers A. Interpersonal therapy of depressed HIV-positive patients. Presented at the 146th Annual Meeting of the American Psychiatric Association; May 1993; San Francisco, Calif.
33. Markowitz JC. Dysthymia: psychosocial treatment strategies. Presented at the 146th Annual Meeting of the American Psychiatric Association; May 1993; San Francisco, Calif.
34. Kocsis JH, Frances AJ, Voss C, Mann JJ, Mason BJ, Sweeney J. Imipramine treatment for chronic depression. *Arch Gen Psychiatry.* 1988; 45:253-257.
35. Markowitz JC. Psychotherapy of the post-dysthymic patient. *J Psychother Pract Res.* 1993; 2:157-163.
36. Schulberg HC, Scott CP, Madonia MJ, Imber SD. Applications of interpersonal psychotherapy to depression in primary care practice. In: Klerman GL, Weissman MM, eds. *New Applications of Interpersonal Psychotherapy.* Washington, DC: American Psychiatric Press; 1993.
37. Ehlers CL, Frank E, Kupfer DJ. Social zeitgebers and biological rhythms: a unified approach to understanding the etiology of depression. *Arch Gen Psychiatry.* 1988;45:948-952.
38. Frank E. Biological order and disorder. Presented at the Meeting of the American Psychosomatic Society; March 1991; Santa Fe, NM.
39. Rounsaville BJ, Weissman MM, Prusoff BA, Herceg-Baron RL. Marital disputes and treatment outcome in depressed women. *Compr Psychiatry.* 1979;20:483-490.
40. Gurman AS, Kniskern DP. Research on marital and family therapy: progress, perspective, and prospect. In: Garfield SB, Bergen AB, eds. *Handbook of Psychotherapy and Behavior Change.* New York, NY: John Wiley & Sons Inc; 1978:817-902.
41. Foley SH, Rounsaville BJ, Weissman MM, Sholomskas D, Chevron E. Individual versus conjoint interpersonal psychotherapy for depressed patients with marital disputes. *Int J Fam Psychiatry.* 1989;10:29-42.
42. Wells KB, Stewart A, Hays RD, Burnam A, Rogers W, Daniels M, Berry S, Greenfield S, Ware J. The functioning and well-being of depressed patients: results from the Medical Outcomes Study. *JAMA.* 1989;262:914-919.
43. Klerman GL, Budman S, Berwick D, et al. Efficacy of brief psychosocial intervention for symptoms of stress and distress among patients in primary care. *Med Care.* 1987;25:1078-1088.
44. Mossey JM, Knott KA, Katz IR. Treatment of subsyndromal depressive symptoms in hospitalized medically ill elderly. Presented at the Annual Scientific Meetings of the Gerontological Society of America; November 1992; Washington, DC.
45. Rounsaville BJ, Glazer W, Wilber CH, et al. Short-term interpersonal psychotherapy in methadone-maintained opiate addicts. *Arch Gen Psychiatry.* 1983;40:629-636.
46. Carroll KM, Rounsaville BJ, Gawin FH. A comparative trial of psychotherapies for ambulatory cocaine abusers: relapse prevention and interpersonal psychotherapy. *Am J Drug Alcohol Abuse.* 1991;17:229-247.
47. Fairburn CG, Jones R, Peveler RC, Carr SJ, Solomon RA, O'Connor ME, Burton J, Hope RA. Three psychological treatments for bulimia nervosa: a comparative trial. *Arch Gen Psychiatry.* 1991;48:463-469.
48. Fairburn CG, Jones R, Peveler RC, Hope RA, O'Connor M. Psychotherapy and bulimia nervosa: longer-term effects of interpersonal psychotherapy, behavior therapy, and cognitive behavior therapy. *Arch Gen Psychiatry.* 1993;50:419-428.
49. Wilfley DE, Agras WS, Telch CF, Rossiter E, Schneider J, Cole AC, Sifford L, Raeburn S. Group cognitive-behavioral therapy and group interpersonal psychotherapy for the nonpurging bulimic individual: a controlled comparison. *J Consult Clin Psychol.* 1993;61:296-305.
50. Weissman MM, Rounsaville BJ, Chevron ES. Training psychotherapists to participate in psychotherapy outcome studies: identifying and dealing with the research requirement. *Am J Psychiatry.* 1982;139:1442-1446.
51. Rounsaville BJ, O'Malley SS, Foley SH, Weissman MM. The role of manual-guided training in the conduct and efficacy of interpersonal psychotherapy for depression. *J Consult Clin Psychol.* 1988;56:681-688.
52. Chevron ES, Rounsaville BJ. Evaluating the clinical skills of psychotherapists: a comparison of techniques. *Arch Gen Psychiatry.* 1983;40:1129-1132.
53. Rounsaville BJ, Chevron ES, Weissman MM, Prusoff BA, Frank E. Training therapists to perform interpersonal psychotherapy in clinical trials. *Compr Psychiatry.* 1986;27:364-371.

ORIGINAL ARTICLE

High-Dose Selegiline in Treatment-Resistant Older Depressive Patients

Trey Sunderland, MD; Robert M. Cohen, MD, PhD; Susan Molchan, MD; Brian A. Lawlor, MD; Alan M. Mellow, MD, PhD; Paul A. Newhouse, MD; Pierre N. Tariot, MD; Edward A. Mueller, MD; Dennis L. Murphy, MD

Background: We examined the effect of high-dose selegiline in 16 treatment-resistant older depressive patients. We hypothesized that selegiline, at a dosage of 60 mg/d, would be at least partially effective but that the higher doses would not maintain the monoamine oxidase B selectivity observed with the lower doses of selegiline.

Methods: Sixteen treatment-resistant subjects (mean [±SD] age, 65.6±9.3 years) entered a double-blind, randomized, crossover study of placebo vs 3 weeks of selegiline at a dosage of 60 mg/d. Objective measures of mood and behavior were obtained in all subjects, and 10 of the subjects underwent repeated lumbar punctures for analysis of monoamine metabolites in the cerebrospinal fluid.

Results: Objective measures of mood and behavior revealed significant improvement in the Hamilton Depression Rating Scale score (37.4% decrease), the Global Depression score (22.7% decrease), and the Brief Psychiatric Rating Scale score (19.3% decrease); subjective behavioral measures, however, did not show significant improvement during the 3-week medication trial. Cerebrospinal fluid values revealed a statistically significant drop in 3-methoxy-4-hydroxyphenylglycol (51%) and 5-hydroxyindoleacetic acid (17%) levels, and there was a significant lowering of systolic blood pressure on standing (15%), but these changes were not accompanied by clinical side effects.

Conclusions: Our results suggest that high-dose selegiline can be an effective antidepressant in treatment-resistant older depressive patients. While the selegiline dose required has nonselective monoamine oxidase effects and thus would not be free of possible tyramine interactions, other advantages suggest that further investigations with selegiline are warranted in this population.

(Arch Gen Psychiatry. 1994;51:607-615)

From the Section on Geriatric Psychiatry, Laboratory of Clinical Science (Drs Sunderland, Molchan, and Murphy), and the Laboratory of Cerebral Metabolism (Dr Cohen), the National Institute of Mental Health, Bethesda, Md; the Department of Psychiatry, St James Hospital, Dublin, Ireland (Dr Lawlor); the Department of Psychiatry, University of Michigan, School of Medicine, Ann Arbor (Dr Mellow); the Department of Psychiatry, University of Vermont School of Medicine, Burlington (Dr Newhouse); the Department of Psychiatry, University of Rochester (NY) Medical Center (Dr Tariot); and Rutland (Vt) Community Mental Health Center (Dr Mueller).

TREATMENT-RESISTANT depression is generally defined as the lack of therapeutic response to previous antidepressant trials. While there is not yet complete consensus on the specifics of the "treatment-resistant" diagnosis, proposed operational criteria center on the number of adequate previous therapeutic trials.[1-4] Currently, to our knowledge, there are no double-blind, placebo-controlled studies of treatment-resistant depression in the elderly, even though up to one third are considered to be refractory to treatment.[5-7]

Because the elderly are generally considered to be sensitive to the cardiovascular and anticholinergic effects of traditional tricyclic drugs, the monoamine oxidase inhibitors (MAOIs), particularly selegiline (formerly L-deprenyl), are of interest for treatment-resistant subjects.[8-10] Selegiline was reportedly effective in younger depressed adults[11] and safe in low doses in various neuropsychiatric populations.[12-14] When initially introduced,[15-17] it was believed that selegiline was a selective monoamine oxidase B (MAO-B) inhibitor without the complicating tyramine interaction of nonselective MAOIs; however, we have since documented that selegiline is associated with increased tyramine pressor sensitivity at long-term doses above 20 to 30 mg/d.[18] Despite the lack of MAO-B specificity, it is

See Subjects and Methods on next page

SUBJECTS AND METHODS

SUBJECTS

Sixteen treatment-resistant older subjects (four men and 12 women) with *DSM-III-R* major depression participated in this study (mean [±SD] age, 65.6±9.3 years; range, 55 to 78 years). The subjects had a mean of 12.6±2.4 years of education, a mean Wechsler Memory Scale score of 98±9, and a mean 17-item Hamilton Depression Rating Scale (HDRS-17) score of 24.6±6.6. Subjects had undergone at least two clinical trials of antidepressants without success before referral to the National Institute of Mental Health (NIMH) as having "treatment-resistant" depression. In fact, the subjects had been treated with an average of 4.2±1.5 clinically available antidepressants before being admitted to the NIMH. Six of the subjects had previously received electroconvulsive therapy, and in 10 subjects treatment with at least one MAOI had failed. In addition to their standard antidepressant regimens, 13 of the 16 subjects had received augmentation treatment with lithium, liothyronine sodium (Cytomel), and/or stimulants. For inclusion in the study, all subjects had an HDRS-17 score of 18 or higher, and none showed evidence of severe cognitive impairments or had a history of bipolar disorders.

METHODS

Before entering into the trial, a complete medical reevaluation was performed to rule out thyroid disease, cerebrovascular accident, metabolic abnormality, severe cardiovascular disease, and chronic pulmonary disease. All subjects were without serious medical illness at the time of entry into our trial and were free of any psychoactive medication for at least 3 weeks. There was no evidence of improvement during the 3-week inpatient observation period before entry into the study. All subjects were maintained on a strict MAOI diet (foods containing monoamines such as histamine, serotonin, and dopamine were also limited).[19]

Medication trials were conducted in a placebo-controlled, double-blind, random fashion while subjects remained inpatients at the NIMH. Selegiline (60 mg/d) and placebo were each administered for at least 21 days. The dose was chosen after preliminary experience with low-dose selegiline (10 mg/d) in 11 adult subjects with treatment-resistant depression (mean age, 55.1±13.5 years) and middle-dose selegiline (30 mg/d) in six subjects (mean age, 52.5±12.4 years) failed to reveal marked clinical effects (T.S., R.M.C., P.A.N., E.A.M., D.L.M., unpublished data, 1989). Our pilot experience revealed no improvement on any of the behavioral ratings in the 11 subjects with selegiline (10 mg/d) for an average of 21 days, nor were there serious side effects. For the six subjects who received selegiline at a dosage of 30 mg/d, there was a trend on the HDRS-17 for some improvement; however, there was no improvement seen on the other objective scales or on any subjective scales. This preliminary experience served as a rationale for testing the 60-mg/d dose; more complete data on these pilot studies are available on request.

Five of the 16 subjects in our study had previously participated in a pharmacologic study involving intravenous tyramine during treatment with lower-dose selegiline.[18] In each case, the double-blind trial of selegiline was preceded by a placebo wash-out period of at least 3 weeks. The other 11 subjects had never received selegiline and were randomly assigned to receive placebo or selegiline as the first treatment in the crossover trial. In addition, these 11 subjects underwent limited cognitive testing while receiv-

still possible that higher-dose selegiline would have clinical advantages, such as a reduced side-effect profile or increased efficacy in patients with depression that is refractory to treatment. Thus, we tested whether high-dose selegiline would be a safe and effective antidepressant drug in a group of treatment-resistant elderly depressive patients.

RESULTS

BEHAVIORAL CHANGES

As can be seen in **Table 1**, the older depressive patients (N=16) showed significant improvement as a group while receiving 60 mg/d of selegiline compared with placebo treatment. These improvements were most obvious in the HDRS-17 scores (24.6±6.4 to 15.4±9.2, $P<.01$) and BPRS scores (40.3±12.4 to 34.9±11.5, $P<.01$) but were also evident in the global measures of depression ($P<.05$) and anxiety ($P<.05$) and several subscales of the BPRS, including the Anxiety-Depression ($P<.01$), Activation ($P<.01$), Hostility ($P<.05$), and Depression ($P<.01$) subscales. The placebo end-point values for the depressive patients were not statistically different from the non-blind ratings performed before entry into the study, supporting the clinical impression that there was no significant placebo response in this group of patients with treatment-resistant depression. Overall, there were no significant changes in self-ratings during this 3-week period, as measured by the Profile of Mood States, NIMH Self-Rating Scale, Beck Depression Inventory, and a global visual analog scale for depression. However, the responder subgroup did show some evidence of improvement by self-report on the Profile of Mood States Anxiety ($P<.05$) and Depression ($P<.05$) subscales by the end of 3 weeks of receiving selegiline.

ing and not receiving the drug based on previous results with patients with Alzheimer's disease.[12]

Baseline testing included various cognitive and behavioral measures. The cognitive tests for depressed patients involved measures of episodic memory (Buschke Selective Reminding Task),[20] attention (Vigilance Task),[21] and semantic memory (Category Retrieval).[22] Most subjects were also assessed at baseline with the Wechsler Memory Scale[23]; none of the patients showed evidence of pseudodementia (Wechsler Memory Scale mean score, 98±9). Blind behavioral ratings for all 16 subjects were obtained by trained observers (physicians and nurses) and subjective (patient) reports. To establish and maintain interrater reliability, the research staff participates in ongoing weekly consensus training. The behavioral scales used included the HDRS,[24] the Brief Psychiatric Rating Scale (BPRS),[25,26] the Profile of Mood States,[27] the Beck Depression Inventory,[28] the NIMH Self-Rating Scale,[26] and global measures of mood.[29] The BPRS was included because of reports that selegiline was partially metabolized to amphetamine, which might contribute to an activating effect.[30-32]

Blood samples were obtained for the determination of platelet MAO activity and platelet counts during drug and placebo conditions after at least 21 days of the current regimen and were processed as previously described.[33] Platelet carbon 14–benzylamine determination was expressed as benzylaldehyde produced per 10^8 platelets per hour. Each morning, after at least 15 minutes of equilibration while lying down, subjects were asked to stand quietly for 5 minutes, at which time orthostatic blood pressure measurements were recorded by an automated blood pressure instrument (Dynamap, Critikon Corp, Tampa, Fla).

Lumbar punctures were performed once for each treatment condition in 10 patients who underwent repeated lumbar punctures after receiving placebo and selegiline for approximately 3 weeks. Subjects fasted overnight and were kept at bed rest before the procedure, except for early morning voiding; cerebrospinal fluid (CSF) was obtained following lumbar puncture in the lateral decubitus position between 8 and 9 AM. The samples were immediately frozen without preservative on dry ice and then stored at −70°C for subsequent measurements of the norepinephrine metabolite 3-methoxy-4-hydroxyphenylglycol (MHPG), the serotonin metabolite 5-hydroxyindoleacetic acid (5-HIAA), and the dopamine metabolite homovanillic acid (HVA). The assays were performed by high-pressure liquid chromatography with electrochemical detection[34] on samples from the 5- to 8-mL aliquot of CSF collection. Somatostatinlike immunoreactivity (SLI) was measured from the 26th-mL aliquot, as described elsewhere.[35]

DATA ANALYSIS

Statistical analysis was performed by paired comparisons between drug and placebo end-point conditions for the behavioral measures and biologic variables. When overall test scores were found to be significantly different, subscale values were then compared where appropriate. For purposes of further analysis, the 16 subjects were divided into "responders" and "nonresponders" based on the end-point HDRS-17 score while receiving selegiline. Specifically, an HDRS-17 score of 11 or lower at the end of the 60-mg/d selegiline phase indicated responders, whereas a postselegiline HDRS-17 score of 12 or higher indicated nonresponders. This designation was adapted from that used by Mann and colleagues[11] in a previous study of selegiline in depressive patients. Differences between responders and nonresponders were assessed across behavioral, cognitive, and biologic variables. Data in the text and tables are presented as mean±SD, unless otherwise specified.

RESPONDERS VS NONRESPONDERS

When the 16 subjects were divided into responders and nonresponders, several differences emerged. Responders were somewhat older (70.1±6.2 vs 61.0±10.1 years, $P<.05$), less depressed (HDRS-17 score, 21.1±3.5 vs 28.0±7.4, $P<.04$), and less anxious (Global Anxiety score, 6.3±0.7 vs 8.3±0.9, $P<.01$) at baseline than the nonresponder cohort (**Table 2**). Because the responder group was significantly less depressed than the nonresponder cohort at baseline, group differences across drug conditions were also calculated in absolute HDRS score changes and percent HDRS score changes. As with the total HDRS scores, the responders demonstrated a greater mean absolute and mean percentage drop than the nonresponders on the HDRS-17 (14.1±5.4 vs 5.3±7.3, t=2.757, $P<.02$, and 65.0%±16.2% vs 15.4%±22.5%, t=5.063, $P<.01$). Owing to the similarity of findings across all definitions of responders vs nonresponders, further comparisons of these groups were made with the absolute cut-off criteria of a total score of 11 or less on the HDRS-17.

The responders did better at baseline than the nonresponders on most of the cognitive tests performed (eg, Buschke Free Recall: 6.0±1.3 vs 4.0±1.3 for total words recalled, t=5.86, $P<.05$). Nonetheless, there were no significant changes in cognitive tests for either the responders or nonresponders while receiving selegiline. Baseline biologic markers, including platelet MAO levels and CSF measures, did not differentiate between the responders and nonresponders. Furthermore, there were no distinctions between responders and nonresponders in their platelet MAO levels while receiving selegiline (Table 2). In fact, platelet MAO levels were significantly reduced in both groups by more than 95% while patients were receiving selegiline compared with placebo levels (0.8±0.6 vs 16.9±5.7 nmol/10^8 platelets per hour, t=10.43, $P<.001$). This effect was generally seen as soon as 1 day after selegiline therapy

Table 1. Results of Objective Rating Instruments in 16 Older Treatment-Resistant Depressed Subjects Following Placebo and High-Dose Selegiline (60 mg/d) Treatment*

	Placebo Group (n=16)	Selegiline Group (n=16)	Paired *t*	*P*
17-item Hamilton Depression Rating Scale	24.6±6.4	15.4±9.2	5.02	.001
Global scales (range, 1-15)				
Impairment	6.5±2.5	5.3±2.4	3.32	.01
Depression	7.5±2.3	5.8±2.7	2.26	.05
Mania	1.0±0.0	1.0±0.0	...	...
Psychosis	1.7±1.3	1.9±1.8	...	...
Anxiety	7.2±1.3	5.2±2.2	2.83	.02
BPRS totals				
18-item	40.3±12.4	34.9±11.5	3.16	.01
24-item	54.8±15.4	44.2±15.3	3.79	.01
BPRS subscales				
Anxiety-Depression	3.5±1.0	2.7±1.0	3.63	.01
Anergia	2.1±1.0	1.9±0.8	...	...
Thought Disorder	1.2±0.5	1.2±0.4	...	...
Activation	2.0±0.6	1.5±0.4	4.27	.001
Hostility	2.2±1.2	1.6±0.9	2.40	.05
Depression	3.7±1.1	2.7±1.3	3.73	.01
Mania	1.6±0.3	1.3±0.2	4.72	.001

**BPRS indicates Brief Psychiatric Rating Scale.*

was begun. There were no significant changes in liver enzyme values for any subject receiving selegiline.

VITAL SIGNS

In the overall group (N=16), selegiline treatment was associated with a higher supine pulse (81±13/min vs 71±13/min, $P<.02$), a lower standing diastolic blood pressure (75±11 vs 84±11 mm Hg, $P<.05$), and a lower standing systolic blood pressure (115±15 vs 136±20 mm Hg, $P<.01$) than placebo treatment (**Table 3**). Under the stress of an orthostatic challenge, there were larger discrepancies between drug and placebo conditions for the diastolic blood pressure changes (−4±11 vs 9±9 mm Hg, $P<.01$) and systolic blood pressure changes (−22±25 vs 1±15 mm Hg, $P<.01$). Using the responder vs nonresponder dichotomy, the nonresponders tended to have a lower systolic blood pressure in the supine position and a higher pulse when standing while receiving placebo, whereas the responders had a smaller pulse increase on standing than nonresponders (13±9/min vs 25±12/min, t=2.31, $P<.05$) (Table 2). While receiving selegiline, the responders had a lower diastolic blood pressure on standing than the nonresponders (69±13 vs 81±6 mm Hg, t=2.361, $P<.05$), and there was a trend for the responders to demonstrate a greater fall in systolic (−32±22 vs −13±25 mm Hg) and diastolic (−8±9 vs 0±11 mm Hg) blood pressures.

CSF VARIABLES

In the subgroup of patients who underwent repeated lumbar punctures (N=10), selegiline resulted in significant reductions in the CSF MHPG level (53±15 to 26±18 pmol/mL, t=7.63, df=9, $P<.01$) and CSF 5-HIAA level (103±25 to 86±19 pmol/mL, t=2.29, df=9, $P<.05$) compared with placebo values (**Figure**). The CSF HVA level fell 21% during selegiline treatment (169±67 to 134±54 pmol/mL), but this change was not statistically significant with this small group of subjects. There were no significant differences in monoamine metabolite values across drug conditions between subjects who received placebo first and those who received selegiline first. Finally, CSF SLI, which we have previously shown to be reduced in elderly depressive patients compared with controls,[36] tended to go lower still with selegiline treatment in both responders (41.4±8.2 to 35.2±25.4 pg/mL) and nonresponders (48.5±23.8 to 30.5±6.0 pg/mL).

SIDE EFFECTS

No serious side effects were noted during our study. Some subjects reported occasional episodes of dizziness or lightheadedness. Insomnia was noted in two individuals, drowsiness in four individuals, and dry mouth in six individuals, but these numbers were not significantly greater than those reporting these side effects during the placebo phase. The only significant change in side effects

Table 2. Selegiline Responders and Nonresponders Are Compared at Baseline for Demographic, Behavioral, Cognitive, and Biologic Variables*

Variable	Responders (n=8)	Non-responders (n=8)	Paired t	P
Demographic				
Gender, M/F	3/5	1/7	...	...
Age, y	70.1±6.2	61.0±10.1	2.19	.0462
Education, y	12.4±2.7	12.8±2.3	...	...
Behavioral				
HDRS-17	21.1±3.5	28.0±7.4	−2.38	.0323
Anxiety (range, 1-15)	6.3±0.7	8.3±0.9	−4.99	.0002
Cognitive†				
Buschke FR (range, 0-12)	6.0±1.3	4.0±1.3	5.86	.0385
Buschke Con (range, 0-1)	0.49±0.18	0.28±0.31	4.73	.0577
Biologic‡				
Platelet MAO, nmol/10^8 platelets per hour	15.9±5.3	17.7±6.3	...	...
CSF MHPG, pmol/mL	48±11	60±18	1.50	.1589
CSF SLI, pg/mL	45±13	50±21	...	...
Vital signs				
Lying systolic BP, mm Hg	140±13	125±18	1.99	.0671
Standing pulse, beats/min	83±11	96±16	1.92	.0761
Orthostatic pulse change, beats/min	13±9	25±12	2.31	.0365

*HDRS-17 indicates 17-item Hamilton Depression Rating Scale; Anxiety, Bunney-Hamburg Global Anxiety Rating Scale; Buschke FR, Buschke Selection Reminding Task–Free Recall; Buschke Con, Buschke Selective Reminding Task–Consistency Score; MAO, monoamine oxidase; CSF, cerebrospinal fluid, MHPG, 3-methoxy-4-hydroxyphenylglycol; SLI, somatostatinlike immunoreactivity; and BP, blood pressure.

†Cognitive variables are available for only 11 subjects (seven responders and four nonresponders).

‡The CSF measures are available for only 14 subjects at baseline (eight responders and six nonresponders).

on the NIMH Self-Rating Scale was a decrease in the rating for irritability while receiving selegiline ($P<.05$).

CLINICAL FOLLOW-UP

The eight responders showed sustained clinical benefit when switched to a clinically available MAOI while still in the hospital, despite the fact that five of the eight previously had not shown a response to MAOIs. Informal clinical review with the patients' families over the telephone revealed no substantial relapses for at least 6 months after discharge. The remaining eight subjects who failed to show a response to selegiline were subsequently treated clinically with either electroconvulsive therapy or other standard antidepressant regimens.

COMMENT

Previous studies of selegiline as an antidepressant have concentrated on lower doses and younger populations.[11,17,37] To our knowledge, ours is the first study to test selegiline in older depressive patients and uses higher doses than previous treatment studies. We observed evidence of behavioral improvement in 50% of patients with treatment-resistant depression with 60 mg/d of selegiline compared with placebo. Eight of the subjects met criteria to be considered responders, even after a mean time of only 3 weeks of receiving the high dose. In another three subjects, there was evidence of behavioral improvement but not of sufficient magnitude to reach our objective criteria for success. These significant objective changes while receiving selegiline were not reflected in equivalent subjective improvements in the group at large, although the responder subgroup did show modest evidence of subjective improvement, even after just 3 weeks of receiving selegiline. Had the clinical trial been extended, the objective and particularly the subjective behavioral changes might have been even greater, as elderly and younger depressive patients alike have continued to show improvement while receiving MAOIs up to week 6 in other treatment studies.[10,11]

Table 3. Blood Pressure and Pulse Results Before and After (5 Minutes) Orthostatic Challenge in 16 Subjects Who Received Placebo and Selegiline (60 mg/d) for 3 Weeks

Vital Sign*	Selegiline Dose, mg/d	Supine	Standing	% Orthostatic Change
Systolic BP, mm Hg	0	134±15	136±20	1
	60	132±18	112±15†	−15
Diastolic BP, mm Hg	0	76±13	84±11	11
	60	79±8	75±11‡	−5
Pulse, beats/min	0	71±13	91±15	28
	60	81±13‡	95±18	17

*BP indicates blood pressure.
†$P<.01$ compared with baseline value.
‡$P<.05$ compared with baseline value.

RESPONDERS VS NONRESPONDERS

When responders were directly compared with nonresponders to identify baseline predictors of success, the responders were more likely to be older, less depressed, less anxious, and more intact cognitively than nonresponders (Table 1). The anxiety rating was particularly useful; no subject with a Global Anxiety score of 8 or higher at baseline was a responder. Because platelet counts and brain MAO-B levels increase with age,[38,39] we expected that the platelet MAO level might be of predictive value, especially because the responders were significantly older than the nonresponders. While we do not have data on brain MAO-B levels in these subjects, we can say that platelet MAO levels were not predictive of

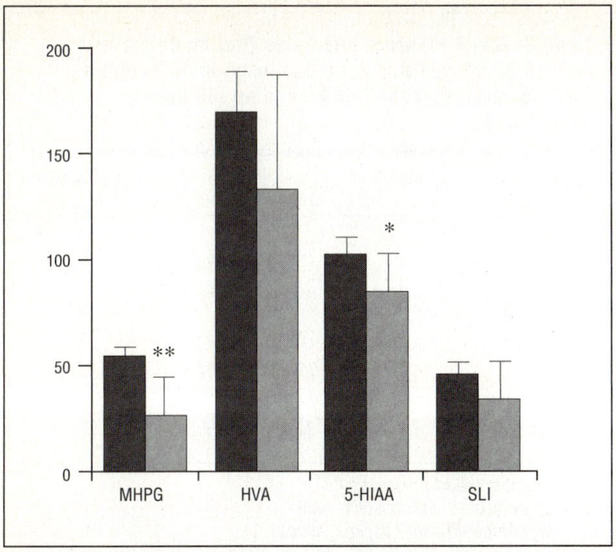

Cerebrospinal fluid levels of monoamine metabolites and somatostatinlike immunoreactivity (SLI) in 10 older depressive patients who underwent lumbar punctures before and after 3 weeks of treatment with 60 mg/d of selegiline (light-shaded bars) or placebo (black bars). MHPG indicates 3-methoxy-4-hydroxyphenylglycol; HVA, homovanillic acid; and 5-HIAA, 5-hydroxyindoleacetic acid. Data are expressed as mean±SD in picomoles per milliliter for monoamine metabolites and picograms per milliliter for SLI. Single asterisk indicates P<.05; *double asterisk,* P<.01, *compared with placebo values.*

therapeutic response; in fact, responders actually had nonsignificantly lower baseline platelet MAO levels.

Of the biologic variables collected, only the blood pressure levels significantly distinguished the nonresponders from the responders. For instance, while receiving placebo, the responders tended to have a higher systolic blood pressure when supine and a lower pulse rate when standing. When the patients were challenged to stand for 5 minutes at baseline, the pulse rate increase of the responders was approximately half that of the nonresponders. Other orthostatic markers did not differ between groups. Earlier reports had suggested that pretreatment orthostatic hypotension was predictive of therapeutic response to tricyclic antidepressants in the elderly,[40-42] although a recent report has failed to replicate this finding.[43] In our study, there was no evidence of baseline orthostatic hypotension in the responders.

Under treatment conditions, the overall selegiline group showed a significant elevation of lying pulse and significant drops in systolic and diastolic blood pressure levels on standing. The orthostatic fall in systolic blood pressure while receiving selegiline approaches that found previously with imipramine in elderly depressive patients.[44] Despite the fact that the cardiovascular changes with high-dose selegiline are greater than those noted in younger depressive patients receiving lower doses of selegiline,[11] clorgyline,[45,46] or phenelzine,[47] no falls secondary to orthostatic hypotension were observed in these 16 elderly depressive patients. Furthermore, no patients dropped out of our study because of dizziness, a somewhat surprising finding given that dizziness is frequently noted with standard MAOI and tricyclic treatment of the elderly.[44,48-51] The responders tended to have a higher resting systolic blood pressure and demonstrated less of a pulse change to orthostatic challenge than did the nonresponders receiving placebo, and it is possible that the responders had more of a cardiovascular reserve at baseline. More in-depth study of the sympathetic nervous system of these depressed subjects with concomitant adrenergic markers, such as plasma norepinephrine and epinephrine levels, would be useful in future studies.

MECHANISM OF ACTION

One mechanistic issue commonly raised about selegiline is the fact that it is metabolized to amphetamine in the brain[30,31] and that this conversion might account for a stimulant effect.[32] In our study, however, there was no evidence of amphetaminelike effects in subjects receiving dosages of 60 mg/d for 3 weeks. On the contrary, there were significant decreases in Activation and Mania subscale scores on the BPRS, an overall reduction in anxiety, and a decrease in self-reported irritability. Insomnia was occasionally reported as a side effect, but it occurred no more often than with placebo and did not result in any substantial objective loss of sleep. Selegiline is rapidly absorbed by the gastrointestinal tract and distributed into the tissues and is metabolized mainly by the liver to the stereospecific metabolites L-desmethyl selegiline, L-amphetamine, and L-methamphetamine before being excreted mostly in urine. These metabolites have been found in equal concentrations in the plasma and CSF of patients receiving long-term selegiline treatment,[52] but they do not appear to generate a stimulant effect[53] both because of their relatively low concentrations and, more importantly, because they are the less active L-isomers of amphetamine. This lack of stimulant effect with selegiline is further supported by a recent study of selegiline in sleep-deprived healthy subjects that revealed no significant effects on sleep latency.[54]

The obvious mechanism of action of selegiline as an antidepressant is that of MAO inhibition. In human brain, the B form of the enzyme is known to account for more than 60% of the MAO.[55,56] Important MAO-B substrates include the monoamines dopamine and phenylethylamine, but nonhuman primate studies have also documented that MAO-B is frequently localized in serotonin-containing neurons in the brain,[57] suggesting a possible regulatory or neuroprotective role for this enzyme. At MAO-B selective doses in rodents, selegiline treatment has been associated with small increases in α_1-adrenoceptor agonist affinity and an increase in dopamine uptake sites but not with changes in density, binding affinity, or apomorphine sensitivity of dopaminergic receptors (D_1 and D_2 subtypes).[58-60] These animal find-

ings are supported by a lack of change in the dopamine metabolite 3,4-dihydroxyphenylacetic acid in the plasma of patients with Parkinson's disease receiving long-term treatment with 10 mg/d of selegiline.[61] However, at the higher doses expected to inhibit MAO-A as well as MAO-B activity, selegiline reduced the concentration of dopamine metabolites in animal striatal brain microdialysate in much the same way as the selective MAO-A inhibitor clorgyline.[53] The pattern of CSF monoamine metabolite changes in our study was consistent with the action of a mixed MAO-A and MAO-B inhibitor. These findings are similar to the results found previously in a group of patients with Alzheimer's disease[36] but are of a smaller magnitude than those reported with clorgyline and pargyline.[62] In any case, it is clear that the higher doses of selegiline are associated with mixed MAO inhibition.

CLINICAL UTILITY OF SELEGILINE

If, as these preclinical and laboratory studies suggest, higher doses of selegiline simply convert its MAO-B selective profile to that of a nonselective MAOI, are there any advantages to selegiline as a clinical antidepressant over those currently available? There are several points for consideration. First, high-dose selegiline was well tolerated cardiovascularly by all subjects tested in our study. Given that these subjects were older depressive patients who are especially vulnerable to the blood pressure effects of most antidepressant regimens,[63] the relative lack of individual cardiovascular toxic effects is intriguing. Nonetheless, the drug was associated with statistically significant lowering of systolic and diastolic blood pressure measurements, which might still be clinically important in some individuals, especially in longer trials. Second, selegiline has been associated with evidence of sharply reduced oxidant stress, reduced 1-methyl-4-phenyl-1,2,5,6 tetrahydropyridine (MPTP) toxicity, or a prolonged life expectancy.[64-67] Whether this possible neuroprotective effect is lost when the drug is administered to humans in nonselective doses is unknown, but this information would be important in planning long-term treatment for neuropsychiatric populations, including patients with Parkinson's disease and Alzheimer's disease and in older depressive patients.[12-14,68-75] Third, selegiline was associated with little or no evidence of anticholinergic effects in this population and no evidence whatsoever of cognitive impairment. Because the elderly are particularly prone to anticholinergic effects,[36] this is an important advantage, although not unique to selegiline. Finally, high-dose selegiline was not associated with the bothersome side effects frequently encountered with clinically available MAOIs, such as sudden weight gain, insomnia, and edema. Given the brevity of the trial and the relatively small number of depressed subjects, this side-effect information should be interpreted cautiously, but it does suggest that further study is warranted.

CONCLUSION

Selegiline appears to be an effective antidepressant in older patients with treatment-resistant depression. While low-dose selegiline (10 mg/d) may have some mood-lifting effects in nondepressed subjects, such as patients with Parkinson's disease or Alzheimer's disease,[12,76] or when low-dose selegiline is given in combination with phenylalanine,[17] our data suggest that higher, non–MAO-B selective doses of selegiline may be required to reverse moderate to severe depression in the elderly. In fact, the data from our study of high-dose selegiline (60 mg/d) support earlier data from our laboratory indicating that MAO-A inhibition and the subsequent consequences of this inhibition rather than MAO-B inhibition alone may be required for antidepressant efficacy.[77,78] Data from our study combined with those from a previous study involving younger adults[11] suggest that nonselective MAOI dosages of selegiline between 30 and 60 mg/d are required for adequate antidepressant response, much more than the 5- to 10-mg doses of selegiline recently suggested in the American Psychiatric Association's practice guideline for major depressive disorder in adults.[79] In fact, because the CSF MHPG values were reduced only by 50% with selegiline compared with previous reports of 80% to 95% reduction with clorgyline and other mixed MAO inhibitors,[62] it is possible that selegiline doses higher than 60 mg/d would provide even better antidepressant responses. Further studies comparing high-dose selegiline treatment with other nonselective or MAO-A–selective MAOIs are required to determine whether selegiline provides any unique antidepressant, clinical side-effect profile or neuroprotective advantages or if certain subpopulations of adult and elderly depressive patients are especially responsive to selegiline.

Accepted for publication December 15, 1993.

The authors would especially like to thank Karen Putnam for her organizational and statistical expertise in the preparation of the manuscript and David R. Rubinow, MD, Candy Davis, and Teresa Tolliver, PhD, for their efforts with the CSF somatostatin and platelet monoamine oxidase assays. We also thank Marcia Minichiello, MS, for the recording of the clinical data and Wilma Davis for her help in the preparation of the manuscript.

Reprint requests to the Section on Geriatric Psychiatry, Laboratory of Clinical Science, NIH Clinical Center, Bldg 10, Room 3D41, 9000 Rockville Pike, Bethesda, MD 20892 (Dr Sunderland).

REFERENCES

1. Ayd FJ. Treatment resistant depression. *Int Drug Ther Newslett.* 1983;18:25-27.
2. Fawcett J, Kravitz HM. Treatment refractory depression. In: Schatzberg AF, ed. *Common Treatment Problems in Depression.* Washington, DC: American Psychiatric Association; 1985:2-27.

3. Schatzberg AF, Cole JO, Elliott GR. Recent view on treatment-resistant depression. In: Halbreich U, Feinberg SS, ed. *Psychosocial Aspects of Nonresponse to Antidepressant Drugs.* Washington, DC: American Psychiatric Press; 1986:95-109.
4. Nierenberg AA, Keck PEJ, Samson J, Rothschild AJ, Schatzberg AF. Methodological considerations for the study of treatment-resistant depression. In: Amsterdam JD, ed. *Advances in Neuropsychiatry and Psychopharmacology.* New York, NY: Raven Press; 1991:1-12.
5. Goff DC, Jenike MA. Treatment-resistant depression in the elderly. *J Am Genet Soc.* 1986;34:63-70.
6. Post F. The management and nature of depressive illness in late life: a follow through study. *Br J Psychiatry.* 1972;121:393-404.
7. Murphy E. The prognosis of depression in old age. *Br J Psychiatry.* 1983;121: 393-404.
8. Knoll J. Selective inhibition of B type monoamine oxidase in the brain: a drug strategy to improve the quality of life in senescence. In: Weverling JA, ed. *Strategy in Drug Research.* Amsterdam, the Netherlands: Elsevier Science Publishers; 1982:107-135.
9. Murphy DL, Cohen RM, Sunderland T, Mueller E. Selective monoamine oxidase inhibitors in treatment-resistant depression. In: Zohar J, Belmaker RH, eds. *Treating Resistant Depression.* New York, NY: Spectrum Press; 1987:257-268.
10. Georgotas A, Friedman E, McCarthy M, Mann J, Krakowski M, Siegel R, Ferris S. Resistant geriatric depressions and therapeutic response to monoamine oxidase inhibitors. *Biol Psychiatry.* 1983;18:195-205.
11. Mann JJ, Aarons SF, Wilner PJ, Keilp JG, Sweeney JA, Pearlstein T, Frances AJ, Kocsis JH, Brown RP. A controlled study of the antidepressant efficacy and side effects of (−)-deprenyl: a selective monoamine oxidase inhibitor. *Arch Gen Psychiatry.* 1989;46:45-50.
12. Tariot PN, Cohen RM, Sunderland T, Newhouse PA, Yount D, Mellow AM, Weingartner H, Mueller EA, Murphy DL. L-deprenyl in Alzheimer's disease: preliminary evidence for behavioral change with monoamine oxidase B inhibition. *Arch Gen Psychiatry.* 1987;44:427-433.
13. Shoulson I. Deprenyl and tocopherol antioxidative therapy of parkinsonism (DATATOP): Parkinson Study Group. *Acta Neurol Scand.* 1989;126:171-175.
14. Langston JW. Selegiline as neuroprotective therapy in Parkinson's disease: concepts and controversies. *Neurology.* 1990;40:61-69.
15. Knoll J, Ecseri Z, Kelemen K, Nievel J, Knoll B. Phenylisopropinylamine (E-250): a new spectrum psychic energizer. *Arch Int Pharmacodyn Ther.* 1965; 155:154-164.
16. Elsworth JD, Glover V, Reynolds GP, Sandler M, Lees AJ, Puapradit P, Shaw KM, Stern KM, Kumar P. Deprenyl administration in man: a selective monoamine oxidase B inhibitor without the 'cheese effect.' *Psychopharmacology.* 1978;57:33-38.
17. Birkmayer W, Riederer P, Linauer W, Knoll J. L-Deprenyl plus L-phenylalanine in the treatment of depression. *J Neural Transm.* 1984;59:81-87.
18. Sunderland T, Mueller EA, Cohen RM, Jimerson DC, Pickar D, Murphy DL. Tyramine pressor sensitivity changes during deprenyl treatment. *Psychopharmacology.* 1985;86:432-437.
19. Murphy DT, Sunderland T, Cohen RM. Monoamine oxidase-inhibiting antidepressants: a clinical update. *Psychiatr Clin North Am.* 1984;7:549-562.
20. Buschke H. Selective reminding for analysis of memory and learning. *J Verbal Learning Verbal Behav.* 1973;12:543-550.
21. Cohen RM, Cohen MR, Weingartner H, Pickar D, Murphy DL. Naloxone affects task performance in normal subjects. *Psychiatry Res.* 1983;8:127-136.
22. Palermo DS, Jenkins JJ. *Word association Norms: Grade School Through College.* Minneapolis, Minn: University of Minnesota Press; 1964.
23. Wechsler D. *Wechsler Memory Scale, Revised.* New York, NY: Psychological Corp; 1987.
24. Hamilton M. A rating scale for depression. *J Neurol Neurosurg Psychiatry.* 1960;23:56-61.
25. Overall JE, Gorham DR. The Brief Psychiatric Rating Scale. *Psychol Rep.* 1962; 10:799-812.
26. Murphy DL, Pickar D, Alterman IS. Methods for the quantitative assessment of depressive and manic behavior. In: Burdock EI, Sudilovsky A, Gershon S, eds. *Quantitative Techniques for the Evaluation of the Behavior of Psychiatric Patients.* New York, NY: Marcel Dekker Inc; 1982:355-392.
27. McNair DM, Lorr M, Droppleman LF. *Manual for the Profile of Mood States.* San Diego, Calif: Educational and Industrial Testing Service; 1971.
28. Beck AT, Ward CH, Mendelson M, Mock J, Erbaugh J. An inventory for measuring depression. *Arch Gen Psychiatry.* 1961;4:561-571.
29. Bunney WE, Hamburg DA. Methods for reliable longitudinal observation of behavior. *Arch Gen Psychiatry.* 1963;9:280-284.
30. Reynolds GP, Riederer P, Sandler M, Jellinger K, Seemann D. Amphetamine and 2-phenylethylamine in post-mortem parkinsonian brain after (−)deprenyl administration. *J Neural Transm.* 1978;43:272-277.
31. Karoum DF, Wyatt RJ. Metabolism of (−)deprenyl's therapeutic benefit: a biochemical assessment. *Neurology.* 1982;32:503-509.
32. Roselaar SE, Langdon N, Lock CB, Jenner P, Parkes JD. Selegiline in narcolepsy. *Sleep.* 1987;10:491-495.
33. Murphy DL, Wright C, Buchsbaum M, Costa J, Nichols A, Wyatt R. Platelet and plasma amine activities in 650 normals: sex and age differences and stability over time. *Biochem Med.* 1976;16:254-265.
34. Scheinin M, Chang W-H, Kirk KL, Linnoila M. Simultaneous determination of 3-methoxy-4-hydroxyphenylglycol, 5-hydroxyindoleacetic acid and homovanillic acid in cerebrospinal fluid with high performance liquid chromatography using electrochemical detection. *Anal Biochem.* 1983;131:246-253.
35. Patel Y, Rao K, Reichlin S. Somatostatin in human cerebrospinal fluid. *N Engl J Med.* 1977;296:529-533.
36. Sunderland T, Tariot PN, Cohen RM, Newhouse PA, Mellow AM, Mueller EA, Murphy DL. Dose-dependent effects of deprenyl on CSF monoamine metabolites in patients with Alzheimer's disease. *Psychopharmacology.* 1987;91:293-296.
37. Quitkin FM, Liebowitz MR, Stewart JW, McGrath PJ, Harrison W, Rabkin JG, Markowitz J, Davies SO. L-deprenyl in atypical depressives. *Arch Gen Psychiatry.* 1984;41:777-781.
38. Sparks DL, Woeltz VM, Markesbery WR. Alterations in brain monoamine oxidase activity in aging, Alzheimer's disease, and Pick's disease. *Arch Neurol.* 1991;48:718-721.
39. Robinson DS, Davis JM, Nies A, Ravaris CL, Sylvester D. Relation of sex and aging to monoamine oxidase activity of human brain, plasma, and platelets. *Arch Gen Psychiatry.* 1971;24:536-539.
40. Jarvik LF, Read SL, Mintz J, Neshkes RE. Pretreatment orthostatic hypotension in geriatric depression: predictor of response to imipramine and doxepin. *J Clin Psychopharmacol.* 1983;3:368-372.
41. Schneider LS, Sloane RB, Staples FR, Bender M. Pretreatment orthostatic hypotension as a predictor of response to nortriptyline in geriatric depression. *J Clin Psychopharmacol.* 1986;6:172-176.
42. Stack JA, Reynolds CF, Perel JM, Houck PR, Hoch CC, Kupfer DJ. Pretreatment systolic orthostatic blood pressure (PSOP) and treatment response in elderly depressed patients. *J Clin Psychopharmacol.* 1988;8:116-120.
43. Diehl DJ, Houck PR, Paradis C, Miller M, Reynolds CF III. Pretreatment systolic orthostatic blood pressure and treatment response in geriatric depression: a revisit. *J Clin Psychopharmacol.* 1993;13:189-193.
44. Neshkes RE, Gerner R, Jarvik LF, Mintz J, Joseph J, Linde S, Aldrich J, Conolly ME, Rosen R, Hill M. Orthostatic effect of imipramine and doxepin in depressed geriatric outpatients. *J Clin Psychopharmacol.* 1985;5:102-106.
45. Murphy DL, Roy B, Pickar D, Lipper S, Cohen RM, Jimerson D, Lake CR, Muscettola G, Saavedra J, Kopin IJ. Cardiovascular changes accompanying MAO inhibition in man. In: Usdin E, Weiner N, Youdim MBH, eds. *Function and Regulation of Monoamine Enzymes: Basic and Clinical Aspects.* New York, NY: Macmillan Publishing Co Inc; 1981:549-560.
46. Murphy DL, Lipper S, Slater S, Shiling D. Selectivity of clorgyline and pargyline as inhibitors of monamine oxidases A and B in vivo in man. *Psychopharmacology.* 1979;62:129-132.
47. Kronig MH, Roose SP, Walsh BT, Woodring S, Glassman AH. Blood pressure effects of phenelzine. *J Clin Psychopharmacol.* 1983;3:307-310.
48. Rockwell E, Lam RW, Zisook S. Antidepressant drug studies in the elderly. *Psychiatr Clin North Am.* 1988;11:215-233.
49. Georgotas A, McCue RE, Hapworth W, Friedman E, Kim OM, Welkowitz J, Chang I, Cooper TB. Comparative efficacy and safety of MAOIs versus TCAs in treating depression in the elderly. *Biol Psychiatry.* 1986;21:1155-1166.
50. Rabkin JG, Quitin FM, McGrath P, Harrison W, Tricamo E. Adverse reactions to monoamine oxidase inhibitors, II: treatment correlates and clinical management. *J Clin Psychopharmacol.* 1985;5:2-9.
51. Thayssen P, Bjerre M, Kragh-Sorensen P, Moller M, Petersen OL, Kristensen CB, Gram LF. Cardiovascular effects of imipramine and nortriptyline in elderly patients. *Psychopharmacology.* 1981;74:360-364.
52. Heinonen EH, Myllyla V, Sotaniemi K, Lammintausta R, Saloonen JS, Anttial M, Savijarvi M, Kotila M, Rinne UK. Pharmacokinetics and metabolism of selegiline. *Acta Neurol Scand.* 1989;126:93-99.
53. Butcher SP, Fairbrother IS, Kelly JS, Arbuthnott GW. Effects of selective mono-

amine oxidase inhibitors on the in vivo release and metabolism of dopamine in the rat striatum. *J Neurochem.* 1990;55:981-988.

54. Newhouse PA, Penetar DM, Fertig JB, Thorne DR, Sing HC, Thomas ML, Cochran JC, Belenkey GL. Stimulant drug effects on performance and behavior after prolonged sleep deprivation: a comparison of amphetamine, nicotine, and deprenyl. *Milit Psychol.* 1992;4:207-233.
55. Jossan SS, d'Argy R, Gillberg PG, Aquilonius SM, Langstrom B, Halldin C, Bjurling P, Stalnacke CG, Fowler J, MacGregor R, Oreland L. Localization of monoamine oxidase B in human brain by autoradiographical use of 11C-labelled L-deprenyl. *J Neural Transm.* 1989;77:55-64.
56. Fowler JS, MacGregor RR, Wolf AP, Arnett CD, Dewey SL, Schlyer D, Christman D, Logan J, Smith M, Sachs H, Aquilonius SM, Bjurling P, Halldin C, Hartvig P, Leenders KL, Lundqvist H, Oreland L, Stalnacke C-G, Langstrom B. Mapping human brain monoamine oxidase A and B with 11C-labeled suicide inactivators and PET. *Science.* 1987;235:481-485.
57. Westlund KN, Denney RM, Kochersperger LM, Rose RM, Abell CW. Distinct monoamine oxidase A and B populations in primate brain. *Science.* 1985;230: 181-183.
58. Klimek V, Nowak G, Zak J, Maj J. The effect of repeated treatment with brofaromine, moclobemide and deprenyl on α_1-adrenergic and dopaminergic receptors in the rat brain. *Neurosci Lett.* 1990;108:189-194.
59. Timar J, Knoll B, Knoll J. Long-term administration of (−)deprenyl (selegiline), a compound which facilitates dopaminergic tone in the brain, leaves the sensitivity of dopamine receptors to apomorphine unchanged. *Arch Int Pharmacodyn Ther.* 1986;284:255-266.
60. Wiener HL, Hashim A, Lajtha A, Sershen H. Chronic L-deprenyl–induced up-regulation of the dopamine uptake carrier. *Eur J Pharmacol.* 1989;163:191-194.
61. Cedarbaum JM, Silvestri M, Clark M, Harts A, Kutt H. L-deprenyl, levodopa pharmocokinetics, and response fluctuations in Parkinson's disease. *Clin Neuropharmacol.* 1990;13:29-35.
62. Major LF, Murphy DL, Lipper S, Gordon E. Effects of clorgyline and pargyline on deaminated metabolites of norepinephrine, dopamine and serotonin in human cerebrospinal fluid. *J Neurochem.* 1978;32:229-231.
63. Ray WA, Griffin MR, Schaffner W, Baugh DK, Melton LJI. Psychotropic drug use and the risk of hip fracture. *N Engl J Med.* 1987;316:363-369.
64. Cohen G, Spina MB. Deprenyl suppresses the oxidant stress associated with increased dopamine turnover. *Ann Neurol.* 1989;26:689-690.
65. Hess A. The effects of monoamine oxidase inhibition and dopamine uptake blockade on MPTP-induced increase of 2-[^{3}H] deoxyglucose uptake in specific mesencephalic catecholaminergic nuclei. *Neurosci Lett.* 1990;112:7-13.
66. Milgram NW, Racine RJ, Nellis P, Mendonca A, Ivy GO. Maintenance on L-deprenyl prolongs life in aged male rats. *Life Sci.* 1990;47:415-420.
67. Knoll J. The striatal dopamine dependency of life span in male rats: longevity study with (−)deprenyl. *Mech Ageing Dev.* 1988;46:237-262.
68. Reding M, Haycox J, Blass J. Depression in patients referred to a dementia clinic: a 3-year prospective study. *Arch Neurol.* 1985;42:894-896.
69. Parkinson Study Group. DATATOP: a multicenter controlled clinical trial in early Parkinson's disease. *Arch Neurol.* 1989;46:1052-1060.
70. Sivertsen B, Dupont E, Mikkelsen B, Mogensen P, Rasmussen C, Boesen F, Heinonen E. Selegiline and levodopa in early or moderately advanced Parkinson's disease: a double-blind controlled short- and long-term study. *Acta Neurol Scand Suppl.* 1989;126:147-152.
71. Elizan TS, Yahr MD, Moros DA, Mendoza MR, Pang S, Bodian CA. Selegiline as an adjunct to conventional levodopa therapy in Parkinson's disease: experience with this type B monoamine oxidase inhibitor in 200 patients. *Arch Neurol.* 1989;46:1280-1283.
72. Campi N, Todeschini GP, Scarzella L. Selegiline versus L-acetylcarnitine in the treatment of Alzheimer-type dementia. *Clin Ther.* 1990;12:306-314.
73. Monteverde A, Gnemmi P, Rossi F, Monteverde A, Finall GC. Selegiline in the treatment of mild to moderate Alzheimer-type dementia. *Clin Ther.* 1990;12: 315-322.
74. Martignoni E, Bono G, Blandini F, Sinforiani E, Merlo P, Nappi G. Monoamines and related metabolite levels in the cerebrospinal fluid of patients with dementia of Alzheimer type: influence of treatment with L-deprenyl. *J Neural Transm.* 1991;3:15-25.
75. Parkinson Study Group. Effects of tocopherol and deprenyl on the progression of disability in early Parkinson's disease. *N Engl J Med.* 1993;328:176-183.
76. Koller WC, Giron LT. Selegiline HCL: selective MAO-type B inhibitor. *Neurology.* 1990;40:58-60.
77. Lipper S, Murphy DL, Slater S, Buchsbaum MS. Comparative behavioral effects of clorgyline and pargyline in man: a preliminary evaluation. *Psychopharmacology.* 1979;62:123-128.
78. Murphy DL, Aulakh CS, Garrick NA, Sunderland T. Monoamine oxidase inhibitors as antidepressants: implications for the mechanism of action of antidepressants and the psychobiology of the affective disorders and some related disorders. In: Meltzer HY, ed. *Psychopharmacology: The Third Generation of Progress.* New York, NY: Raven Press; 1987:545-552.
79. Work Group on Major Depressive Disorder. Practice guidelines for major depressive disorder in adults. *Am J Psychiatry.* 1993;150(suppl):1-26.

The 24-Hour Profiles of Cortisol, Prolactin, and Growth Hormone Secretion in Mania

Paul Linkowski, MD, PhD; Myriam Kerkhofs, PhD; Anne Van Onderbergen, MD; Philippe Hubain, MD; Georges Copinschi, MD, PhD; Mireille L'Hermite-Balériaux, MS; Raoul Leclercq, MD; Michele Brasseur, MD; Julien Mendlewicz, MD, PhD; Eve Van Cauter, PhD

Objective: To characterize sleep and the 24-hour profiles of cortisol, prolactin (PRL), and growth hormone (GH) secretion in mania.

Methods: Blood was sampled at 15-minute intervals, and sleep was polygraphically recorded in eight unmedicated male patients with pure mania and the results compared with those from a group of 14 healthy age-matched controls. The circadian, sleep-related, and pulsatile hormonal variations were quantitatively characterized using specially designed computer algorithms.

Results: The manic state was associated with alterations of corticotropic activity and circadian rhythmicity partially overlapping those previously observed in acute endogenous depression, consisting of an elevation of nocturnal cortisol levels and an early timing of the nadir of the circadian variation. Sleep onset was delayed and the sleep period was reduced. A trend for short rapid eye movement latencies was apparent in the adult patients. Both the amount and the temporal organization of PRL and GH secretion were normal.

Conclusion: The manic state seems to be characterized by similar but less severe neuroendocrine and circadian abnormalities, compared with major depression.

(Arch Gen Psychiatry. 1994;51:616-624)

From the School of Medicine, Université Libre de Bruxelles, Brussels, Belgium (Drs Linkowski, Kerkhofs, Van Onderbergen, Hubain, Copinschi, L'Hermite-Balériaux, Leclercq, Brasseur, and Mendlewicz), and the Department of Medicine, University of Chicago, Ill (Dr Van Cauter).

THE HYPOTHESIS that a disorder of biological rhythms may be implicated in the origin of manic depression has been proposed and discussed for several decades.[1,2] The cyclical nature of the illness and the observations in the depressed state of an advance in the morning awakening, a reduced rapid eye movement (REM) latency, and a pronounced diurnal variation in mood have initially provided support for the concept of abnormal circadian timing in manic depression. Mechanistic models implying a disturbance in the central circadian clock in the origin and the cyclicity of the illness have been developed and have provided testable working hypotheses regarding alterations of timing and amplitude of circadian rhythms in the depressed and manic states.[1,2] In the depressed state, the 24-hour secretory profiles of pituitary and pituitary-dependent hormones have been characterized in detail in a number of chronobiological studies.[3-15] Most of these studies have shown the existence of a hyperactivity of the corticotropic axis, resulting in elevated plasma cortisol levels.[3,4,11,14,15] Growth hormone (GH) secretion during wakefulness may be increased or normal.[6,7] Sleep-related release appears to be either normal or diminished.[6,7,10] Prolactin (PRL) concentrations are normal throughout the 24-hour cycle.[5,13] In a subset of endogenously depressed patients, a disorder of circadian timekeeping was demonstrated, consisting of an earlier occurrence of some hormonal events that are controlled by the central circadian pacemaker.[3,8,11,13,14] This advance of circadian rhythms was consistently observed in patients with unipolar rather than bipolar illness.[11,13] While clinical remission following antidepressant treatment is generally associated with a normalization of the amount and the temporal organization of pituitary-dependent secretions,[12] it is not

See Subjects and Methods on next page

SUBJECTS AND METHODS

PATIENTS AND CONTROLS

Eight men with a definite diagnosis of mania who were hospitalized for an acute relapse of bipolar illness were studied. The mean (±SD) age was 41±19 years (range, 14 to 62 years). Each patient met the research diagnostic criteria[20] for mania, according to the Schedule for Affective Disorders and Schizophrenia.[21] None of the patients presented with a marked admixture of manic and depressive symptoms. Only one patient (patient 4) had psychotic symptoms, and they were of moderate severity. All patients were in good physical health, and none had evidence of neurologic disease. Patients known to have taken any neuroleptic drug during a 6-week period before admission were excluded from the study. The patients were studied after a drug washout period of at least 8 days in the hospital. None of the patients had received regular lithium treatment during the 3-month period preceding admission. Despite the fact that the Department of Psychiatry at Hôpital Erasme, Université Libre de Bruxelles, Brussels, Belgium, admits approximately 50 patients per year with a diagnosis of mania, the present study of eight drug-free manic patients required 4 years to complete, owing to the restrictions on recruitment and the demanding nature of the protocol. Particular care was taken not to include patients with a history of drug abuse. Two of the eight patients comsumed moderate amounts of alcohol. No patient had a history of primary sleep disorder. None had ever been treated with depot neuroleptic preparations.

The Beigel-Murphy Manic Scale[22] was used to assess the patient's condition on the day of the study. **Table 1** gives the age, REM latency during the night with blood sampling, score on the Beigel-Murphy Manic Scale, and duration of drug washout in the hospital and prior to admission for each patient.

The controls were 14 healthy men in the same age range as the manic patients, without present or past mental illness and without a family history of psychiatric disorders. Their mean (±SD) age was 39±17 years (range, 15 to 62 years). After giving informed consent, all patients and controls underwent a physical examination and routine laboratory tests.

EXPERIMENTAL PROTOCOL

All subjects were studied in the Sleep Laboratory of the Department of Psychiatry, Hôpital Erasme. Polygraphic recordings of sleep were, whenever possible, obtained on four consecutive nights, after one night of habituation to laboratory conditions. On the day preceding the last night of recording, a catheter was inserted into a forearm vein between noon and 1 PM. Blood sampling at 15-minute intervals started 1 hour later and lasted 25 hours. Data collected during the first hour of sampling were discarded to avoid possible artifactual effects related to the venipuncture stress. During the night, the catheter was connected to plastic tubing extending into the adjacent room. All subjects were ambulatory during daytime and had breakfast (8 AM), lunch (12:30 PM), and dinner (7 PM). No snacks were allowed between meals. Bedtime was self-selected. During bedtime hours, the subjects were recumbent and the lights were turned off. Daytime naps were not allowed.

HORMONAL ASSAYS

Blood samples were immediately centrifuged at 4°C, and plasma was frozen at −20°C until assayed. All hormonal determinations were performed in duplicate. Plasma PRL levels were measured by a homologous radioimmunoassay (RIA). The lower limit of sensitivity of the assay was 0.6 μg/L, and the intra-assay coefficient of variation averaged 10% throughout the physiologic range. The interassay of variation was below 20%. Plasma GH levels were measured by an RIA with a lower limit of sensitivity of 0.4 μg/L.[23] The mean intra-assay coefficient of variation was 9% in the range of 0.4 to 2.0 μg/L, 6% in the range of 2 to 5 μg/L, and 5% for values greater than 5 μg/L. The interassay coefficient of variation averaged 15%. Plasma cortisol levels were determined by a radiocompetition assay[24] with a lower limit of sensitivity of 10 nmol/L, an intra-assay coefficient of variation of 5%, and an interassay coefficient of variation of less than 10%. For all hormones, all samples from a given 24-hour study were analyzed in the same assay.

SLEEP ANALYSIS

The polygraphic recordings of sleep were scored visually at 20-second intervals in stages wake, I, II, III, IV, and REM, based on standardized criteria.[25] Sleep onset was defined as

Continued on next page

known whether the alterations observed during the depressed state are specific to this condition. In particular, in bipolar illness, it is not known whether the switch to the manic state is associated with persistent advanced-, normal-, or delayed-phase circadian rhythms. Indeed, data on circadian rhythm abnormalities and neuroendocrine function in mania are very scarce. Difficulties in obtaining a valid set of hormonal samples comcomitantly with polygraphic sleep recordings in manic or hypomanic patients who are not receiving medication are obviously responsible for the paucity of data. A pioneer study of three manic patients by Sachar[16] described elevated cortisol levels in two of the patients but normal levels in the third one. Akesode et al[17] have also reported data on the 24-hour cortisol secretion profiles in three manic patients, showing high cortisol concentrations in one of them. A number of studies that used either 24-hour urinary excretion, single blood samples, or a combination of both did not find cortisol abnormalities in manic patients.[18] Chronobiological studies have been essentially limited to longitudinal studies of rap-

the timing of occurrence of the first 20-second intervals scored as stages II, III, IV, or REM. Morning awakening was defined as the timing of occurrence of the last 20-second epoch scored stage II, III, IV, or REM, preceding the behavioral decision to get out of bed. Sleep latency was defined as the time interval between bedtime (coinciding with the beginning of recording and lights off) and sleep onset. The sleep period time was defined as the interval separating sleep onset from final morning awakening. The total sleep time was calculated as the sleep period time minus the total duration of awakenings. Sleep efficiency was defined as the ratio of total sleep time to total time of recording. The total duration of each stage was expressed in minutes. The duration of slow-wave sleep was defined as the sum of the durations of stages III and IV, and REM latency was defined as the interval separating sleep onset from the first 20-second interval scored as REM.

QUANTITATIVE ANALYSIS OF THE CORTISOL AND PRL SECRETION PROFILES

Mean hormonal concentrations were calculated over the 24-hour span as well as over the following two complementary time intervals: 10 PM to 10 AM (nocturnal), which included the sleep periods of all patients and controls, and 10 AM to 10 PM (daytime), during which all patients and controls were awake at all times. The circadian variations of cortisol and PRL levels were evaluated by building a best-fit curve obtained by repeated periodogram calculations.[26] The acrophases and nadirs were defined as the timing of occurrence of maxima and minima, respectively, in the best-fit curve. The amplitude of the best-fit curve was defined as 50% of the difference between its maximum and its minimum and was expressed in absolute concentration units (absolute amplitude) as well as in the percentage of the 24-hour mean level (relative amplitude). Confidence intervals at a minimum level of 95% were calculated for the amplitude, the acrophases, and the nadirs. Significant pulses of cortisol and PRL concentrations were identified and characterized using a previously described computerized algorithm (ULTRA).[27] A pulse was considered significant if both its increment and its decline exceeded, in relative terms, twice the intra-assay coefficient of variation in the relevant range of concentration. The durations of the ascending and declining limbs were defined as the time intervals separating the maximum (peak) from the preceding and the following troughs, respectively. The increment of the pulse was defined as the difference between the level at the peak and the level at the preceding trough. For each subject, the data on pulse increments were summarized by the median pulse increment because of the non-Gaussian nature of their distribution.

QUANTITATIVE ANALYSIS OF THE GH SECRETION PROFILES

Because the 24-hour profile of plasma GH secretion is characterized by consistently low levels abruptly interrupted by secretory pulses with no detectable baseline variation, no best-fit curve was calculated for the GH secretion profiles. Significant pulses of GH secretion were identified with the same computer program as described above for cortisol and PRL secretion, with the same threshold criteria. However, increases or decreases in the GH level ranging from 0.4 to 1.0 μg/L were not considered significant. The amount of GH secreted in each pulse during both its ascending and declining portions was estimated as described previously by integrating the differential equation $dC/dt=S-kC$. This equation describes the time evolution of the plasma concentration (C) resulting from secretion at rate S and disappearance at rate kC, where k is related to the half-life of the hormone ($t\times\frac{1}{2}$) through the equation $k=(\ln^2)/(t\times\frac{1}{2})$.[28] A half-life of 19 minutes and a volume of distribution of 7% of body weight were used in these calculations. The total amounts of GH secreted during the 24-hour span, during wake and during sleep, and during the daytime and nocturnal periods were determined by summing the amounts of GH secreted in each pulse identified in the corresponding time period.

GROUP STATISTICS

Group data were compared by *t* test. Correlations were estimated with the Pearson coefficient of correlation. Unless otherwise indicated, all group values are expressed as the mean±SD.

idly cycling patients[19] who may not be representative of bipolar illness in general.

The present study represents an attempt to define neuroendocrine function and to establish the status of the circadian system in the manic state, using well-characterized hormonal secretion profiles as markers of phase and amplitude. The 24-hour profiles of cortisol, PRL, and GH secretions in mania were studied in eight manic men and 14 controls, using our previously validated method involving blood sampling at 15-minute intervals, polygraphic sleep recordings, and detailed quantitative analysis of the hormonal variations.

RESULTS

SLEEP

Due to variable compliance to the protocol in relationship with a very severe clinical state in some patients, as well as technical difficulties, a total of 19 nights of polygraphic sleep recordings were obtained in the eight manic patients. All patients had at least one habituation night and a night with blood sampling. In addition to the habituation night, the two adult patients who were most severely

Table 1. Clinical Characteristics of the Manic Men

Patient No.	Age, y	REM Latency, min*	Beigel-Murphy Manic Scale Score	Age at Onset of Bipolar Illness, y	Duration of Drug Washout: Out of Hospital	Duration of Drug Washout: In Hospital, d
1	14	137	293	13	0†	8
2	15	73	193	14	6 wk	8
3	26	82	114	21	4 wk	10
4	49	60	171	25	2 y	9
5	50	‡	187	34	0§	11
6	56	25	355	24	1 y	8
7	57	44	119	22	1 wk	9
8	61	0	121	31	2 wk	9

**REM indicates rapid eye movement.*
†Patient was drug naive.
‡No REM stage was recorded during the night with blood sampling.
§Patient was treated with benzodiazepines.

affected (patients 5 and 6) had only one night of recording. One patient had two nights of recording, and five patients and all controls underwent the complete protocol (one habituation night and three recording nights). Sleep results obtained in a subsample of six manic patients and six controls during nights of recording without blood sampling have been reported previously.[29]

Table 2 reports mean sleep variables during the night with blood sampling in manic patients and controls. On average, sleep onset occurred 44 minutes earlier in controls than in manic patients. This result reflected a preference for a later bedtime in the manic patients, since sleep latency was similar in both groups of subjects. The mean sleep period time was 80 minutes shorter in manic patients than in controls. A similar difference (ie, 70 minutes) was observed for the total sleep time. The younger subjects of the manic group (patients 1 and 2, 14 and 16 years of age, respectively) had substantially longer total sleep times (ie, 458 minutes and 440 minutes, respectively) than the older patients (who averaged 269±96 minutes). When the comparison of total sleep time between manic patients and controls is limited to subjects over 20 years of age, the difference is statistically significant (269±96 minutes vs 367±71 minutes; $P<.03$). Sleep efficiency, the number and the total duration of nocturnal awakenings, and total amounts of stages I, II, IV, and REM were similar in both groups. However, the manic patients had significantly shorter stage III times than the controls. The REM latencies during the night with blood sampling ranged between 0 and 137 minutes in manic patients (60±44 minutes) and 2 and 140 minutes in controls (75±35 minutes), a nonstatistically significant difference. However, when subjects under 20 years of age are excluded from this comparison, the mean REM latency in the manic group is 42±32 minutes (n=6) vs 79±33 minutes in controls (n=11; $P<.05$). For purposes of comparison with previous studies of REM distribution in manic patients,[30,31] **Figure 1** shows the REM latencies observed in both groups of subjects during the nights of recording without blood sampling. Nights without any epoch-scored REM are not represented. When the entire age range was considered, there was a wide overlap in the values of REM latencies in the two groups. When the mean REM latency from all nights of recording was considered for each patient and control, the group mean latencies were 73±50 minutes for the patients and 84±31 minutes for the controls. When subjects under 20 years of age are excluded from this comparison, a trend toward shorter REM latencies in manic patients becomes apparent (manic patients, 52±37 minutes; controls, 80±30 minutes; $P<.15$). Three of the eight manic patients, but none of the controls, had a mean REM latency below 50 minutes.

Table 2. Sleep Variables in Manic Patients and in Normal Controls During the Night With Blood Sampling*

	Manic Patients (N=8)	Healthy Controls (N=14)	P†
Time of sleep onset, h (±min)	12:34 AM±38	11:50 PM±35	.02
Sleep latency, min	34±19	33±23	.91
Sleep period, min	378±115	457±63	.05
Total sleep time, min	314±117	384±68	.09
Sleep efficiency, %	69±22	76±11	.32
No. of awakenings	23±9	33±18	.15
Time awake, min	65±58	73±46	.73
Duration of sleep stages, min			
I	37±24	52±28	.22
II	180±95	203±41	.45
III	15±10	32±17	.02
IV	35±47	30±38	.81
REM‡ sleep, min	46±31	67±22	.81
REM latency, min	60±44	75±33	.39

**Data are given as mean±SD.*
†P<.05 indicates significance.
‡REM indicates rapid eye movement.

24-HOUR CORTISOL SECRETION PROFILES

The classic circadian variation of cortisol levels with early morning acrophase and progressive decline throughout the

afternoon followed by a quiescent period was found in all manic patients and controls. **Figure 2** illustrates typical cortisol secretion profiles obtained in one control and in two manic patients. The mean cortisol secretion profiles obtained in the two groups are shown in **Figure 3**. In the left panel, the data are referenced to clock time, whereas in the right panel, sleep onset is used as the reference time point. Both representations clearly show that the manic patients had higher cortisol levels than controls during the evening and the night. Mean cortisol levels during the daytime period were similar in both groups of subjects, but during the nocturnal period cortisolemia was significantly higher in the patients with mania than in the controls (**Table 3**). When examined in relation to the time of sleep onset (Figure 3, right), mean cortisol levels were elevated in the manic patients compared with the controls during the 2-hour interval preceding sleep (220±146 vs 132±69 nmol/L; $P<.07$) as well as throughout the sleep period (334±69 vs 256±50 nmol/L; $P<.05$). The mean cortisol concentration during sleep was not correlated with the amount of wake or the amount of any other sleep stage. Table 3 gives the mean characteristics of the circadian and ultradian variations of cortisol secretion for the two groups. The amplitude of the circadian variation and the timing of the morning acrophase were similar in both groups of subjects. However, the nadir occurred significantly earlier in the manic patients than in the controls, and this advance averaged 97 minutes. The individual values for the timing of the circadian nadirs are shown for each patient and control in **Figure 4**. Confirming our previous observations, there was a significant correlation between age and timing of occurrence of the nocturnal nadir in controls ($r=-.72$; $P<.01$), the nadir occurring earlier in older subjects. The difference in timing of cortisol nadir between the manic patients and the controls was not primarily related to the older subjects of both groups, since it remained significant ($P<.05$) when subjects over 50 years of age were excluded from the test. This finding was confirmed by analysis of covariance, with the effects of both age and group being significant ($P<.01$ and $P=.01$, respectively). In the manic group, the correlation between the timing of the nocturnal nadir and age failed to reach significance ($r=.49$). The number of significant cortisol pulses was higher in manic patients than in controls. Median pulse increments did not differ between the two groups.

24-HOUR PRL SECRETION PROFILES

Figure 2 shows representative PRL secretion profiles of one control and two manic patients. **Figure 5** illustrates the mean 24-hour profiles of PRL secretion in manic patients compared with controls. The normal 24-hour variation of plasma PRL secretion, consisting of a nocturnal secretory increase culminating in a midsleep acrophase and a progressive decline until a minimum was reached around noon, was observed in all patients and controls. Mean 24-hour concentrations did not differ between the two groups. Daytime concentrations were elevated but well within the physiologic range in two of the manic patients (patients 2 and 3, with concentrations of 11.1 and 10.7 μg/L, respectively, compared with a mean concentration of 5.6±1.4 μg/L for the other manic patients), so that the mean profile observed in the manic group was higher than in the controls, but this difference was not statistically significant at the group level ($P=.34$). Table 3 reports the mean characteristics of the 24-hour PRL secretion profiles in the two groups. The timing and the magnitude of the nocturnal elevation were similar in both groups. However, manic patients had on average more PRL pulses during the 24-hour span than controls, but the median pulse increments were similar in both groups (Table 3).

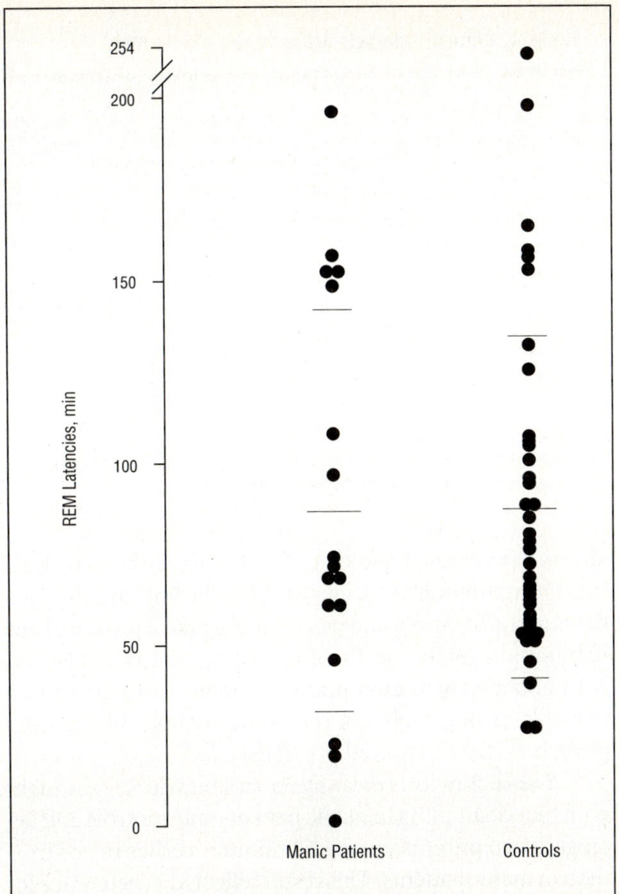

Figure 1. *Values of the rapid eye movement (REM) latency observed during the nights of recording in the eight manic patients (of a total of 19 nights of recording, no REM stages were recorded for two nights; these nights are thus not represented) and in the 14 healthy controls (total of 42 nights of recording). For each group, the horizontal lines show the mean±1 SD. In the manic group, but not in the control group, all REM latencies above 120 minutes were observed in the two adolescent patients.*

24-HOUR GH SECRETION PROFILES

The mean 24-hour profiles of plasma GH secretion in manic patients compared with controls are shown in **Figure 6**. Individual 24-hour GH secretion profiles are presented in Figure 2. The elevation of GH levels following sleep onset is apparent. Indeed, in 12 of the 14 controls and in five of

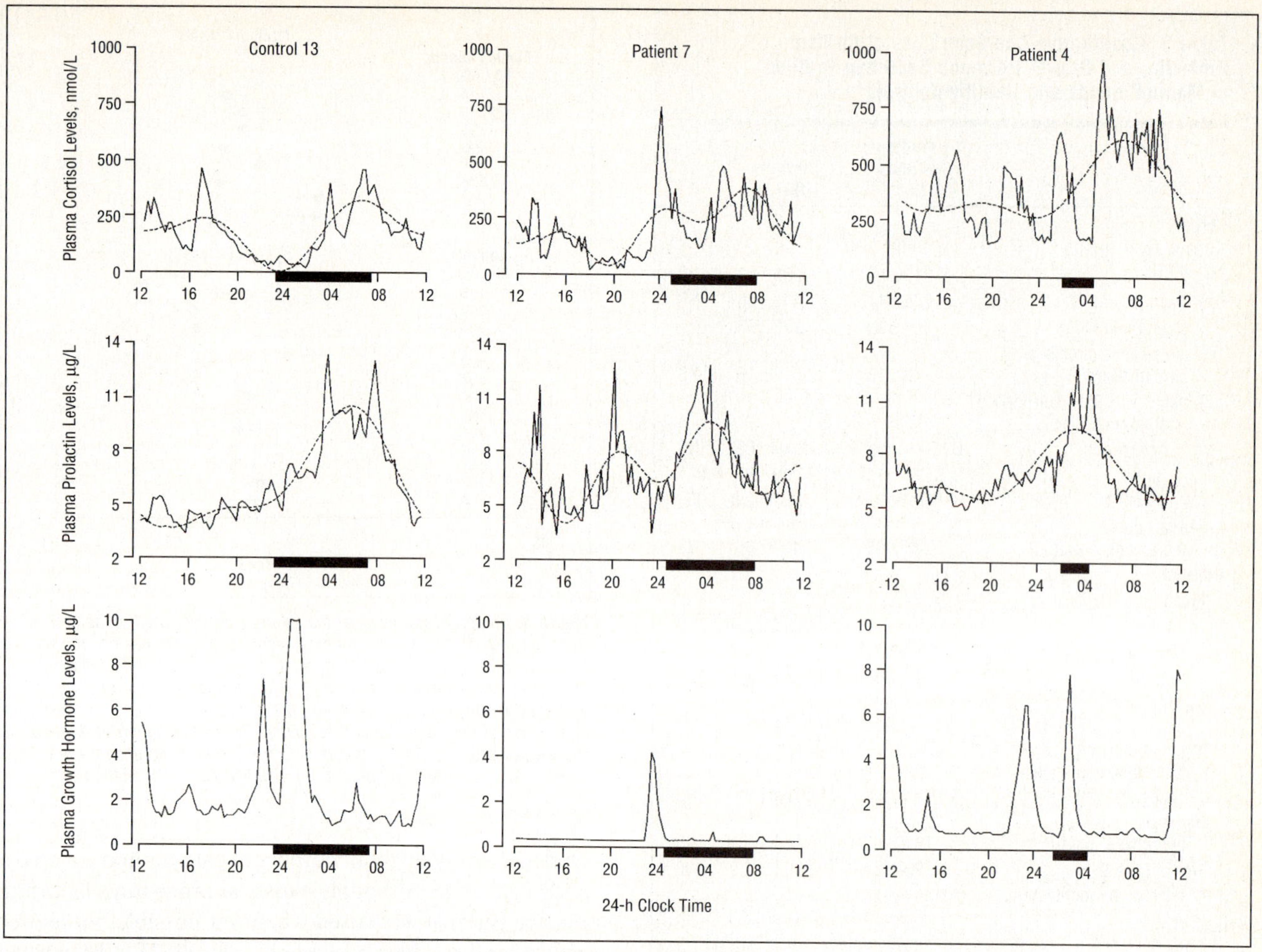

Figure 2. *Representative 24-hour profiles of plasma cortisol, prolactin, and growth hormone secretions in one healthy control (control 13, 60 years of age) and two manic patients (patient 7, 57 years of age, and patient 4, 49 years of age). The broken lines represent the best-fit curve obtained by periodogram calculation. The black bars correspond to the individual sleep period.*

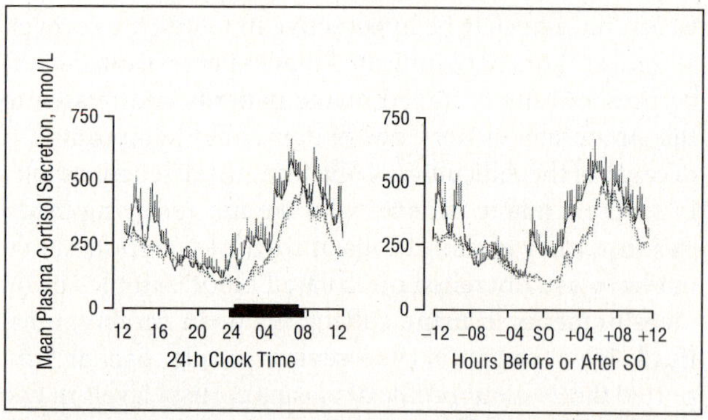

Figure 3. *Mean 24-hour profiles of plasma cortisol secretion in manic patients (solid lines) and healthy controls (broken lines). At each time point, the vertical lines represent the SE of the group mean. Left, Clock time is used as the reference for the time axis. The black bars above and below the x-axis represent the mean sleep periods of the manic and control groups, respectively. Right, Data are referenced with respect to the timing of sleep onset (SO). Note that, on average, the manic patients have elevated cortisol levels throughout the nocturnal period.*

the eight manic patients, a GH pulse with a maximum plasma level occurring within 2 hours after sleep onset could be observed. This difference in proportion of subjects presenting a sleep-onset pulse is not statistically significant $\chi^2=1.56$). In five of the eight manic patients and nine of the 14 controls, a significant GH pulse also occurred before sleep onset. The amount of hormone secreted in this pulse at sleep onset was similar in the manic patients and in the controls. As shown in Table 3, differences in the total amount of GH secretion, daytime secretion, and nocturnal secretion between the two groups were nonsignificant. Similarly, the number of significant GH pulses per 24-hour cycle and the median pulse increment were similar in both groups.

COMMENT

The present study has examined in detail the spontaneous variations of cortisol, PRL, and GH secretions and their modulation by sleep and circadian rhythmicity in carefully screened men with pure mania and in age-matched controls. The major finding of the study is that, in this population, the manic state was associated with alterations of corticotropic activity and circadian rhythmicity partially overlapping those previously observed in acutely de-

Table 3. Quantitative Characteristics of Cortisol, Prolactin, and Growth Hormone Secretion Profiles in Manic Patients and Healthy Controls*

	Manic Patients (N=8)	Controls (N=14)	*P*
Cortisol			
Mean level, nmol/L			
24-h	317±99	256±47	NS
Daytime	275±116	240±55	NS
Nocturnal	364±93	273±55	.01
Mean relative circadian amplitude, %	63±18	71±16	NS
Timing, h (±95% confidence interval, min)			
Acrophase	6:56 AM±111	7:28 AM±62	NS
Nadir	9:52 PM±117	11:29 PM±81	.04
No. of pulses	17.4±2.9	14.7±2.8	.05
Median pulse increment, nmol/L	141±63	124±65	NS
Prolactin†			
Mean level, μg/L			
24-h	8.4±1.3	7.5±2.4	NS
Daytime	7.1±2.8	6.0±1.8	NS
Nocturnal	9.7±4.5	9.4±3.4	NS
Mean relative circadian amplitude, %	42±16	52±22	NS
Timing of acrophase, h (±95% confidence interval, min)	4:19 AM±65	4:30 AM±84	NS
Value of nocturnal acrophase, μg/L	12.8±6.2	12.5±5.5	NS
No. of pulses	9.4±2.8	6.5±2.2	.003
Median pulse increment μg/L	3.9±1.9	4.8±2.5	NS
Growth hormone			
Secretion, μg			
24-h	379±329	539±438	NS
Daytime	99±121	147±166	NS
Nocturnal	281±226	392±43	NS
At sleep onset	152±120	188±144	NS
Timing of sleep onset pulse, h (±min)	1:54 AM±31‡	12:48 AM±29§	.001
Timing from sleep onset to sleep onset pulse, min	73±25‡	57±24§	NS
No. of pulses	4.0±2.8	4.8±3.0	NS
Median pulse increment, μg/L	5.2±3.4	5.9±4.1	NS

*Data are given as mean±SD. NS indicates not significant.
†Profiles were obtained in seven manic patients.
‡Sleep onset pulse was observed in five manic patients.
§Sleep onset pulse was observed in 12 controls.*

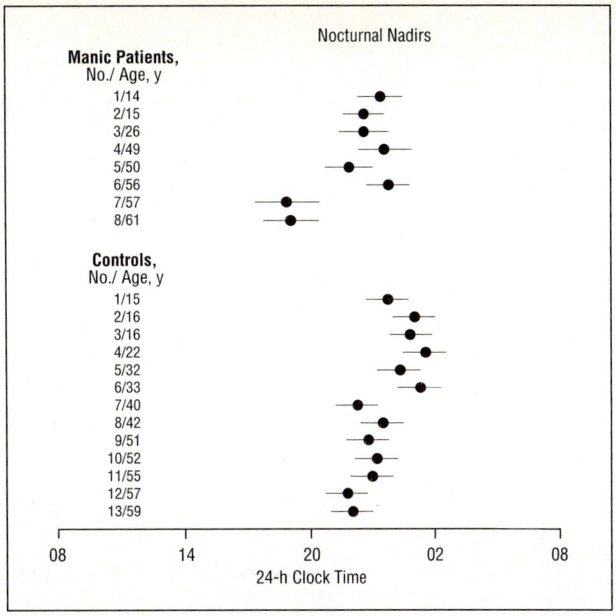

Figure 4. *Timing of the nadir of the 24-hour cortisol rhythm, as derived from the best-fit curve in the manic patients and in the healthy controls. For each individual value, the horizontal lines represent ±1 confidence interval at the minimum level of 95%. The patients and controls are arranged in advancing age, revealing the negative correlation between age and timing of the nocturnal cortisol nadir. The earlier timing of the nadir in the manic group compared with the control group is significant even when subjects over 50 years of age are not included in the calculation.*

pressed subjects, consisting of an elevation of nocturnal cortisol levels and an early timing of the nadir of the circadian variation. In addition, in our adult manic patients, a trend for a reduction of REM latency, a classic finding in depression, was also present. Both the amount and the temporal organization of PRL and GH secretion were normal.

Our study has several limitations inherent to the difficulties of recruiting manic subjects who can be treated for weeks without medication and can comply with a demanding protocol, and therefore the conclusions need to be considered as preliminary. In particular, our sample included a relatively small number of patients and covered a wide age range. Although statistical procedures factoring the age variable were used whenever possible, these procedures may not have adequately controlled for the marked alterations in sleep and neuroendocrine rhythms that occur throughout maturation and senescence.

Previous studies had already suggested that the corticotropic axis may be hyperactive in mania.[18] However, several authors have indicated that hypercortisolism may be present only in mixed manic patients and related to the simultaneous presence of depressive symptoms.[32,33] Because of the difficulties of obtaining serial blood samples in severely manic patients who are not receiving medication, earlier investigations of cortisol secretion in mania have usually relied on isolated blood samples or on measurements in urine collections or in cerebrospinal fluid. However, in a 1975 review article, Sachar[16] reported the 24-hour profile of plasma cortisol levels in two manic subjects and showed the existence of hypercortisolemia in the more severely affected patient. In a recent study of hypothalamic-adrenocortical function in mixed and pure mania,[33] plasma cortisol levels in the morning and in the afternoon did not differ from normal. In contrast, in another study,[18] plasma cortisol levels were found to be raised during the daytime in about half of the manic patients and at midnight in nearly all patients. The present study shows unequivocally that plasma cortisol concentrations are normal during the daytime but elevated during the evening and nighttime in

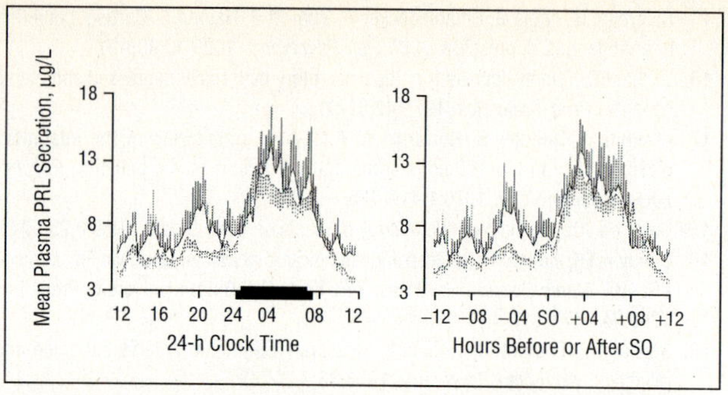

Figure 5. *Mean 24-hour profiles of plasma prolactin (PRL) secretion in manic patients (solid lines) and healthy controls (broken lines). At each time point, the vertical lines represent the SE of the group mean. Left, Clock time is used as the reference for the time axis. The black bars above and below the x-axis represent the mean sleep periods of the manic and control groups, respectively. The PRL levels rise after sleep onset (SO) in both groups, and the rise occurs later in manic patients, who have a later bedtime. Right, Data are referenced with respect to the timing of SO. In this representation, the timing of the nocturnal elevation of PRL levels is similar in both groups. The apparently higher daytime PRL levels in the manic group compared with the control group are not statistically significant.*

male patients with pure mania. Thus, the manic state seems to be associated with a failure to adequately suppress adrenocortical activity at the normal time of nocturnal quiescence. This abnormality is associated with an advance of the nadir of the 24-hour variation, an event that signals the beginning of the rise toward the early morning maximum and is believed to be timed by the central circadian clock. The concomitant trend toward a reduction in REM latency, another process modulated by circadian rhythmicity, is consistent with the hypothesis of a chronobiological alteration of central nervous system origin. It is noteworthy that, in our manic patients, sleep onset was delayed compared with controls, and thus sleep did not exert masking effects on the timing of the cortisol nadir.[34]

In acutely depressed bipolar patients, several studies[3,4,11,14,15] have shown that cortisol levels are elevated throughout the 24-hour cycle rather than during the evening and nighttime only, as was the case in our sample of manic men. An early timing of the cortisol nadir, of the same order of magnitude as observed here in manic subjects, may occur in the depressed state but is more consistently observed in unipolar, rather than bipolar, depression.[11,14,15] This early occurrence of the cortisol nadir is often associated with a reduced REM latency and has therefore been interpreted as reflecting an alteration of the circadian phase. Further studies, using several simultaneous markers, will be necessary to determine whether the manic state is associated with abnormal circadian timing.

Our observation of a tendency for shorter REM latencies in our adult patients is consistent with a recent report[31] showing reduced REM latencies in mania and suggesting that common mechanisms may underlie the sleep disturbances in mania and in depression. In agreement with previous observations,[30,31] sleep onset was delayed and the

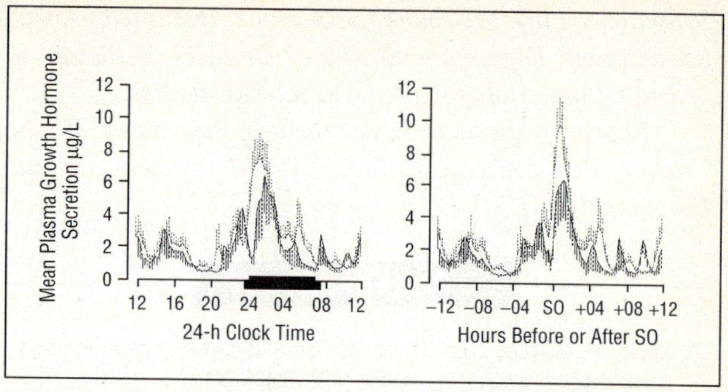

Figure 6. *Mean 24-hour profiles of plasma growth hormone secretion in manic patients (solid lines) and healthy controls (broken lines). At each time point, the vertical lines represent the SE of the group mean. Left, Clock time is used as the reference for the time axis. The black bars above and below the x-axis represent the mean sleep periods of the manic and control groups, respectively. Right, Data are referenced with respect to the timing of sleep onset (SO).*

sleep period was reduced in our manic patients compared with the controls.

Limited evidence had indicated the absence of major abnormalities of the lactotropic and somatotropic axes in mania.[18,35] The present findings confirm and extend these data by showing that the 24-hour patterns of PRL and GH secretions in pure manic patients are essentially superimposable to those observed in age-matched controls, even during the sleep period. While the somatotropic and lactotropic axes may be reactive to certain types of stress, such as pain or intense physical exercise, the condition of prolonged psychological stress that characterizes both the depressed and the manic states does not seem to have detectable effects on peripheral levels of PRL and GH. Thus, in mania, some of the modifications in peptidergic and neurotransmitter activity that have been implicated in other forms of affective illness either are not present or their expression is prevented by homeostatic mechanisms.

Our observations suggest that the pure manic state is associated with a hyperactivity of the hypothalamopituitary-adrenal axis during the nocturnal period concomitant with a trend for shortened REM latencies. The amounts and temporal patterns of PRL and GH secretion are normal.

Accepted for publication February 25, 1994.

This work was supported in part by grant DK-41814 from the National Institutes of Health, Bethesda, Md; a grant from the MacArthur Foundation (Mental Health Network II), Chicago, Ill; grant AFOSR 90-022 from the Air Force Office of Scientific Research, Washington, DC; a grant from the Belgian Fonds National de la Recherche Scientifique Médicale, Brussels; and the Association Nationale d'Aide aux Handicapés, Rotary Club, Brussels.

We thank Bernard Jacques, Nadia Haverals, Michéle Coppens, and Monique Zanen for excellent technical assistance, Etienne Stanus, PhD, for invaluable help with software development, and Rachel Leproult for preparing the figures. Calculations for the GH radioimmunoassay were performed with the use of a computer program developed by

S. Swillens, PhD. We thank the National Institute of Arthritis, Diabetes, Digestive and Kidney Diseases, Bethesda, for providing materials for the GH and PRL assays.

Reprint requests to Department of Psychiatry, Hôpital Erasme, 808 route de Lennik, B-1070 Brussels, Belgium (Dr Linkowski).

REFERENCES

1. Kripke DF, Mullaney DJ, Atkinson M, Wolf S. Circadian rhythm disorders in manic depressives. *Biol Psychiatry.* 1978;13:335-341.
2. Wehr TA, Goodwin FK, eds. *Circadian Rhythms in Psychiatry.* Pacific Grove, Calif: Boxwood Press; 1983:129-184.
3. Sachar EO, Hellman L, Roffwarg H, Halpern F, Fukushima D, Gallagher T. Disrupted 24-hour patterns of cortisol secretion in psychotic depression. *Arch Gen Psychiatry.* 1973;28:19-24.
4. Rubin RT, Poland RE, Lesser IM, Winston RA, Blodgett ALN. Neuroendocrine aspects of primary endogenous depression, I: cortisol secretory dynamics in patients and matched controls. *Arch Gen Psychiatry.* 1987;44:328-336.
5. Rubin RT, Poland RE, Lesser IM, Martin DJ. Neuroendocrine aspects of primary endogenous depression, V: serum prolactin measures in patients and matched control subjects. *Biol Psychiatry.* 1989;25:4-21.
6. Rubin RT, Poland RE, Lesser IM. Neuroendocrine aspects of primary endogenous depression, X: serum growth hormone measures in patients and matched control subjects. *Biol Psychiatry.* 1990;27:1065-1082.
7. Mendlewicz J, Linkowski P, Kerkhofs M, Desmedt D, Golstein J, Copinschi G, Van Cauter E. Diurnal hypersecretion of growth hormone in depression. *J Clin Endocrinol Metab.* 1985;60:505-512.
8. Jarrett DB, Coble PA, Kupfer DJ. Reduced cortisol latency in depressive illness. *Arch Gen Psychiatry.* 1983;40:506-511.
9. Jarrett DB, Miewald JM, Fedorka IB, Coble P, Kupfer DJ, Greenhouse JB. Prolactin secretion during sleep: a comparison between depressed patients and healthy control subjects. *Biol Psychiatry.* 1987;22:1216-1226.
10. Jarrett DB, Miewald JM, Kupfer DJ. Recurrent depression is associated with a persistent reduction in sleep-related growth hormone secretion. *Arch Gen Psychiatry.* 1990;47:113-118.
11. Linkowski P, Mendlewicz J, Leclercq R, Brasseur H, Hubain P, Golstein J, Copinschi G, Van Cauter E. The 24-hour profile of adrenocorticotropin and cortisol in major depressive illness. *J Clin Endocrinol Metab.* 1985;61:429-438.
12. Linkowski P, Mendlewicz J, Kerkhofs M, Leclercq R, Golstein J, Brasseur M, Copinschi G, Van Cauter E. 24-hour profiles of adrenocorticotropin, cortisol, and growth hormone in major depressive illness: effect of antidepressant treatment. *J Clin Endocrinol Metab.* 1987;65:141-152.
13. Linkowski P, Van Cauter E, L'Hermite-Balériaux M, Kerkhofs, M, Hubain P, L'Hermite M, Mendlewicz J. The 24-hour profile of plasma prolactin in men with major endogenous depressive illness. *Arch Gen Psychiatry.* 1989;46:813-819.
14. Pfohl B, Sherman B, Schlechte J, Stone R. Pituitary-adrenal axis rhythm disturbances in psychiatric depression. *Arch Gen Psychiatry.* 1985;42:897-903.
15. Halbreich U, Asnis G, Shindledecker R, Zumoff B, Nathan S. Cortisol secretion in endogenous depression. *Arch Gen Psychiatry.* 1985;42:909-914.
16. Sachar ED. Twenty-four-hour cortisol secretory patterns in depressed and manic patients. *Prog Brain Res.* 1975;42:81-91.
17. Akesode A, Hendler N, Kowarski A. A 24-hour monitoring of the integrated plasma concentration of aldosterone and cortisol in manic patients. *Psychoneuroendocrinology.* 1976;1:419-426.
18. Cookson JC. The neuroendocrinology of mania. *J Affect Disord.* 1985;8:233-241.
19. Goodwin FK, Jamison KR. Sleep and biological rhythms. In: Goodwin FK, Jamison KR, eds. *Manic Depressive Illness.* New York, NY: Oxford University Press Inc; 1990:541-574.
20. Spitzer RL, Endicott J, Robins E. Research diagnostic criteria: rationale and reliability. *Arch Gen Psychiatry.* 1978;35:773-782.
21. Endicott J, Spitzer RL. A diagnostic interview: the Schedule for Affective Disorders and Schizophrenia. *Arch Gen Psychiatry.* 1978;35:837-849.
22. Beigel A, Murphy D, Bunney W. The manic state rating scale: scale construction, reliability and validity. *Arch Gen Psychiatry.* 1971;25:225-262.
23. Virasoro E, Copinschi G, Bruno OD, Leclercq R. Radioimmunoassay of human growth hormone using a charcoal-dextran separation procedure. *Clin Chim Acta.* 1971;31:294-297.
24. Leclercq R, Leclercq-Meyer V. Methode radioimmunologique simple et rapide du dosage du cortisol plasmatique. *Ann Biol Clin (Paris).* 1979;37:118-125.
25. Rechtschaffen A, Kales A. *A Manual of Standardized Terminology, Techniques and Scoring System for Sleep Stages of Human Subjects.* Washington, DC: Government Printing Office: 1968.
26. Van Cauter E. Method for characterization of 24-h temporal variation of blood constituents. *Am J Physiol.* 1979;237:E255-E264.
27. Van Cauter E. Estimating false-positive and false-negative errors in analyses of hormonal pulsatility. *Am J Physiol.* 1988;254:E786-E794.
28. Van Cauter E, Kerkhofs M, Caufriez A, Van Onderbergen A, Thorner MO, Copinschi G. A quantitative estimation of GH secretion in normal man: reproducibility and relation to sleep and time of day. *J Clin Endocrinol Metab.* 1992; 74:1441-1450.
29. Linkowski P, Kerkhofs M, Rielaert C, Mendlewicz J. Sleep during mania in manic-depressive males. *Eur Arch Psychiatr Neurol Sci.* 1986;235:339-341.
30. Hudson JI, Lipinski JF, Frankenburg FR, Grochocinski VJ, Kupfer DJ. Electroencephalographic sleep in mania. *Arch Gen Psychiatry.* 1988;45:267-273.
31. Hudson JI, Lipinski JF, Keck PE, Aizley HG, Lukas SE, Rothschild AJ, Waternaux CM, Kupfer DJ. Polysomnographic characteristics of young manic patients: comparison with unipolar depressed and normal control subjects. *Arch Gen Psychiatry.* 1992;49:378-383.
32. Carroll BJ. Neuroendocrine function in mania. In: Shopsin B, ed. *Manic Illness.* New York, NY: Raven Press; 1979.
33. Swann AC, Stokes PE, Casper R, Secunda SK, Bowden CLI, Berman N, Katz MM, Robins E. Hypothalamic-pituitary-adrenocortical function in mixed and pure mania. *Acta Psychiatr Scand.* 1992;85:270-274.
34. Weitzman ED, Zimmerman JC, Czeisler CA, Ronda JM. Cortisol secretion is inhibited during sleep in normal man. *J Clin Endocrinol Metab.* 1983;56:352-358.
35. Kuruvilla A, Srikrishna G, Peedicayil J, Kuruvilla K, Kanagasabapathy AS. Serum prolactin levels in manic patients. *Biol Psychiatry.* 1991;30:421-423.

Conversions From Système International (SI) Units to Conventional Units (Modified From *The SI Manual in Health Care*)

System*	Component	SI Reference Interval†	SI Unit	Conversion Factor (Divide by)	Conventional Reference Interval†	Conventional Unit
S	Cortisol					
	8 AM	110-520	nmol/L	27.59	4-19	µg/dL
	4 PM	50-410	nmol/L	27.59	2-15	µg/dL
	Midnight	<140	nmol/L	27.59	<5	µg/dL
P, S	Growth hormone					
	Male (fasting)	0-5	µg/L	1.00	0-5	ng/mL
P	Prolactin	<20	µg/L	1.00	<20	ng/mL

*P represents plasma; S, serum.

†These reference values are not intended to be definitive since each laboratory determines its own values. They are provided for illustration only.

ORIGINAL ARTICLE

Carbamazepine Increases Cerebrospinal Fluid Thyrotropin-Releasing Hormone Levels in Affectively Ill Patients

Lauren B. Marangell, MD; Mark S. George, MD; Garth Bissette, PhD; Peggy Pazzaglia, MD; Teresa Huggins, PhD; Robert M. Post, MD

Background: Thyrotropin-releasing hormone is an endogenous tripeptide with endocrine-independent neurophysiologic properties that may be relevant to affective or seizure disorders. We studied the effect of carbamazepine, which has both mood-stabilizing and anticonvulsant properties, on cerebrospinal fluid thyrotropin-releasing hormone levels in affectively ill patients.

Method: Paired cerebrospinal fluid samples were collected from nine inpatients with mood disorders, both while medication free and while taking carbamazepine for an average of longer than 1 month at 950 mg/d, achieving blood levels of 8.8 mg/L.

Results: Carbamazepine treatment was consistently and significantly associated with increased cerebrospinal fluid thyrotropin-releasing hormone levels ($P<.0001$).

Conclusion: As carbamazepine-induced increases in thyrotropin-releasing hormone levels could be relevant to either its psychotropic or anticonvulsant properties, further clinical and preclinical investigation of this finding appears indicated.

(Arch Gen Psychiatry. 1994;51:625-628)

IT HAS LONG BEEN recognized that a complex relationship exists between thyroid hormones and affective disorders.[1-4] Thyrotropin-releasing hormone (TRH) is a tripeptide named and predominantly known for its role in the hypothalamic-pituitary-thyroid axis, maintaining homeostatic levels of peripheral thyroid hormones. As with other peptides, TRH has also been found to function directly as a neuromodulatory substance.[5] As reviewed elsewhere,[6,7] the neurobehavioral effects of TRH are generally stimulatory, such as arousal from sleep, hibernation, or drug-induced sedation. However, when TRH is microinjected into the hypothalamus of active squirrels, motor activity decreases, as opposed to the arousing effect of TRH on sleeping squirrels, indicating state-dependent properties.[8] This ability to temper both hyperactive and hypoactive states could be particularly relevant to the treatment of bipolar mood disorders. Additionally, high-affinity TRH receptors are found in humans, with the highest concentration in the amygdala and hippocampus,[9] further suggesting its possible importance in modulating limbic system function.

Previous studies have found increased cerebrospinal fluid (CSF) TRH levels in depressed patients compared with controls[10,11]; however, further study is needed to determine if this relative increase represents a natural compensatory mechanism or a pathologic process.[12] Direct assessment of TRH as a treatment modality in affective disorders has been hindered by its short serum half-life and its relative inability to cross the blood-brain barrier in humans.[13] The effects of medication on CSF TRH levels in humans may provide an avenue to assess further the potential role of TRH in affective disorders. Carbamazepine is an anticonvulsant that has also been shown to be

See Patients and Methods on next page

From the Biological Psychiatry Branch, National Institute of Mental Health, Bethesda, Md (Drs Marangell, George, Pazzaglia, Huggins, and Post); and Department of Psychiatry, Duke University Medical Center, Durham, NC (Dr Bissette). Dr Marangell is now with the Department of Psychiatry, Baylor College of Medicine, Houston, Tex.

PATIENTS AND METHODS

All subjects were inpatients at the National Institutes of Health Clinical Center, Bethesda, Md, between 1982 and 1992 as participants in affective disorders protocols of the National Institute of Mental Health Biological Psychiatry Branch, and all gave oral and written informed consent for a double-blind clinical trial with carbamazepine and the lumbar puncture procedures involved. Subjects included four women and five men with a mean age of 36 years (range, 25 to 55 years). All patients met criteria for major affective disorder by *DSM-III-R* criteria (two had bipolar disorder type 1, five had bipolar disorder type 2, and two had unipolar depression) confirmed by a research psychiatrist using the Life Charting method.[17] Patient characteristics are summarized in the **Table**. All patients were free of comorbid medical problems by history, physical examination, thorough laboratory screening, and brain imaging.

All lumbar punctures were performed with the patient in the lateral decubitus position between 8 AM and 10 AM after overnight fasting and bed rest and after at least 2 weeks on a low-monoamine diet. Patients were free of all psychotropic medications for at least 2 weeks before the medication-free samples were collected. For the carbamazepine sample, patients had been receiving carbamazepine monotherapy for an average of 37 days (range, 23 to 69 days), at an average dose of 956 mg/d (range, 600 to 1600 mg/d), with the last dose given the previous evening. An average of 2.7 months elapsed between conditions, without consistent seasonal changes. A total of 30 mL of CSF was withdrawn, clinical specimens were immediately sent for analysis, and research samples were allocated from two tubes of 10 mL each and then immediately frozen at −70°C. An aliquot from the 15th to 25th mL was used for this assay.

Mood was rated daily using the Bunney-Hamburg Rating Scale[18] by trained research nurses who were unaware of the medication status of the patient. The order of treatment (placebo vs carbamazepine) was determined by clinical consideration; seven patients received the placebo condition first, two the carbamazepine condition. At the time of the medication-free lumbar punctures, one patient was severely depressed, four were mildly depressed, and three were rated within the normal range of mood variation as defined by the Bunney-Hamburg score. No subject exhibited manic symptoms (Table). The decision to participate in a carbamazepine protocol for either acute treatment or prophylaxis was based on the longitudinal course of illness, independent of the severity of depression at the time of CSF evaluation.

The radioimmunoassay for TRH was prepared as previously described.[11] The radioimmunoassay for TRH uses an antibody developed in rabbits. It recognizes TRH and 3-methyl-His-TRH but does not recognize any other fragment of the TRH molecule or any other known neuropeptides. This antiserum is used in a double-antibody, displacement radioimmunoassay at a final dilution of 1:80 000, has an inhibition concentration (50%) of 20 pg, and can reliably detect 0.625 pg of TRH per tube. The intra-assay variation is 12%. All of the samples in this study were measured by one of us (G.B.) in a single assay. The samples were measured in duplicate with their identity unknown.

Comparisons of CSF TRH concentration between medication-free and carbamazepine samples were analyzed by means of paired Student's *t* tests. Additionally, multiple regression analyses or *t* tests, as appropriate for the given variable, were performed to determine if significant correlations existed between clinical and biochemical variables, such as depression scores and peripheral thyroid measures and CSF TRH concentration.

effective in some depressed[14] and manic[15,16] patients. We report that carbamazepine significantly increased TRH levels in the CSF of nine patients with major affective disorder.

RESULTS

All nine patients demonstrated an increased CSF TRH level in response to carbamazepine treatment. The mean (±SE) CSF TRH level in the medication-free state was 1.50±0.15 pg/mL, compared with 4.45±0.35 pg/mL in the carbamazepine-treated group (t=7.69, P<.0001; **Figure**). Although there was no significant correlation between the change in CSF TRH level and the change in depression scores (r=.22), this data set included only one patient who exhibited a marked mood change across study conditions.

There was not a statistically significant relationship between CSF TRH level and diagnosis, patient age, or gender. There was no relationship between years in storage and CSF TRH level in the carbamazepine condition (r=−.037). In the placebo condition, a higher CSF TRH level was associated with a longer time in storage (r=.73, P=.02), which is the opposite of what would occur with degradation over time. There was not a statistically significant relationship between CSF TRH level and carbamazepine dose (r=.23), the duration of carbamazepine treatment (r=.37), or carbamazepine plasma level (r=.49, P=.18).

Carbamazepine decreased levels of thyroxine, free thyroxine, and triiodothyronine, as reported in larger samples[19-23]; however, decrements in these indexes were not related to the increases in CSF TRH level. On the contrary, the relationships were in the opposite direction; the less the serum triiodothyronine level decreased, the more the CSF TRH level increased (r=.70, P<.05). There was also a trend for lesser decreases in serum thyroxine level (r=.48) and greater increases in thyrotropin level (r=.34) to be associated with larger increases in CSF TRH level.

Demographic Characteristics and CSF TRH Measure*

Patient/ Sex/Age, y	Diagnosis	Bunney-Hamburg Depression Rating		CSF TRH, pg/mL		CBZ Dose, mg	CBZ Level, mg/L	Days of CBZ Therapy
		Placebo	CBZ	Placebo	CBZ			
1/F/39	BP2	10	2	2.25	3.41	600	6.2	28
2/F/50	BP1	4	8	2.00	4.57	1600	8.3	42
3/F/37	UP	4	4	1.35	3.80	600	7.6	37
4/M/30	UP	4	6	1.61	4.98	1200	13.3	34
5/M/29	BP1	3	2	1.67	6.54	1000	9.6	49
6/F/32	BP2	4	3	1.24	3.67	800	7.6	24
7/F/55	BP2	6	4	0.85	5.39	800	8.9	28
8/M/28	BP2	3	6	0.90	3.38	1200	9.2	23
9/M/25	BP2	1	2	1.69	4.30	800	8.3	69
Means/. . . /36	. . .	4.3	4.1	1.50	4.45	956	8.8	37

**CSF indicates cerebrospinal fluid; TRH, thyrotropin-releasing hormone; CBZ, carbamazepine; BP2, bipolar depression type 2; BP1, bipolar depression type 1; and UP, unipolar depression.*

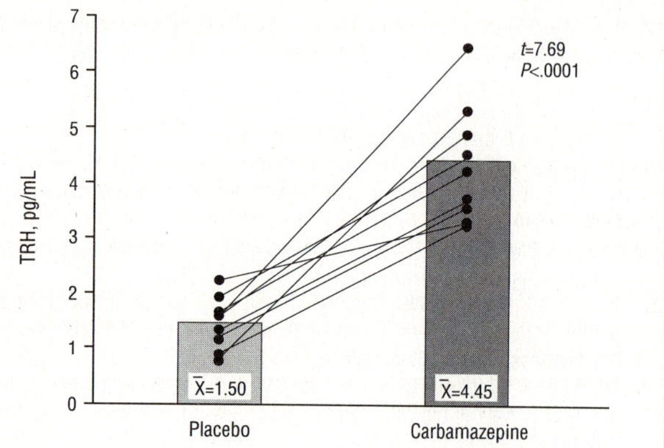

Increases in cerebrospinal fluid thyrotropin-releasing hormone (TRH) levels during carbamazepine treatment.

COMMENT

Affectively ill patients taking carbamazepine had consistently and significantly higher CSF TRH concentrations compared to their medication-free state. Several methodologic issues deserve comment. The TRH values reported herein are below those previously reported in the literature,[10] including other older studies that used the same antisera.[11,24] This may be because the primary antisera used in the assay had been frozen and thawed on several occasions before the current study, which is known to lower sensitivity. As such, the absolute values are less reliable than those previously reported, but proportional changes remain valid. All samples reported herein were run in one batch, and all values were above the reliable detection limit of 0.625 pg of TRH per tube. The assay's inhibiting concentration (50%) remained unchanged, but since our samples were at the low end of the curve, the intra-assay variation was 12%. This intra-assay variation was higher than usual but not sufficient to account for the relative changes we report. There is no known gradient for CSF TRH level in first 30 mL; therefore, our use of an aliquot from the 15th to the 25th mL, as opposed to Banki and coworkers'[11] use of an earlier sample, should not account for the differences in absolute values. Taken together, it appears that the relative increase in CSF TRH level observed during carbamazepine treatment is valid, but absolute values of CSF TRH across studies should be compared with reservation.

Although the samples were collected during a 10-year period, each pair was collected in a shorter time span (average, 2.7 months), without a consistent seasonal shift (ie, no one season predominated in either condition). The stability of TRH levels over time has not been formally studied or established, largely because of technical problems, as the assay requires 1.5 to 2.0 mL of CSF. However, serial measures up to 3 years have found no significant change over time (G.B., unpublished observations, 1988), and in this study, no relationship was found between TRH values during carbamazepine treatment and duration of storage time. Longer freezer time was associated with higher TRH levels in the medication-free group, making degradation over time unlikely.

Our current finding could be consistent with previous observations of a blunted thyrotropin response to intravenous protirelin challenge reported to occur with carbamazepine.[22,25] A blunted TRH response may occur secondary to relatively high levels of endogenous TRH-producing receptor down-regulation, which renders the pituitary less responsive to exogenous stimulation.[26] Classically, peripheral thyroid hormones provide feedback to the hypothalamus, so that decreased levels of thyroid hormones provide a signal that more output is required, and TRH level is increased. Although carbamazepine decreases levels of serum thyroid hormones,[21,22,27] this is not likely to account for the present finding, since greater dec-

rements in thyroid indexes were associated with smaller increases in CSF TRH levels.

It is possible that the concentration of TRH, which has stimulatory properties, increases as a compensation for the sedative effects sometimes associated with carbamazepine, although this is unlikely, as sedation is uncommon at this point of long-term administration. Although there was no correlation between changes in CSF TRH level and depression or its degree of improvement, this relationship should be further explored in a larger sample of more acutely depressed patients who show a larger range of clinical responses.

Other mechanisms that could account for the increases in TRH level with carbamazepine treatment include a multitude of endocrine and neurotransmitter systems affected by carbamazepine[28]; further clinical and preclinical investigations are required to identify the critical systems involved. It is of interest, however, that carbamazepine's anticonvulsant effect on amygdala-kindled seizures may require an increase in levels of TRH or some other endogenous adaptation after seizures.[12] Amygdala-kindled seizures increase TRH levels[29] and induce the expression of TRH messenger RNA.[30,31] Carbamazepine is an effective anticonvulsant when administered after a series of amygdala-kindled seizures, but when animals are given sufficient time off from seizures (>4 days), carbamazepine is no longer an effective anticonvulsant[12] and levels of TRH messenger RNA are no longer increased; moreover, when animals lose responsiveness to carbamazepine via tolerance, seizure-induced increases in TRH mRNA no longer occur.[32,33] The potential role of increases in TRH levels in carbamazepine's anticonvulsant or psychotropic effects now deserves further preclinical and clinical study.

Accepted for publication March 22, 1994.

This study was supported in part by National Institute of Mental Health grant MH-45975 (Dr Bissette).

Reprint requests to National Institutes of Health, Bldg 10, Room 3N212, 9000 Rockville Pike, Bethesda, MD 20892 (Dr Post).

REFERENCES

1. Kirkegaard C, Faber J. Altered serum levels of thyroxine, triiodothyronines and diiodothyronines in endogenous depression. *Acta Endocrinol.* 1981;96:199-207.
2. Joffe RT, Roy-Byrne PP, Uhde TW, Post RM. Thyroid function and affective illness: a reappraisal. *Biol Psychiatry.* 1984;19:1685-1691.
3. Bauer MS, Whybrow PC. Thyroid hormones and the central nervous system in affective illness: interactions that may have clinical significance. *Integr Psychiatry.* 1988;6:75-100.
4. Prange AJ Jr, Loosen PT, Wilson IC, Lipton MA. The therapeutic use of hormones of the thyroid axis in depression. In: Post RM, Ballenger JC, eds. *Neurobiology of Mood Disorders.* Baltimore, Md: Williams & Wilkins; 1984:311-322.
5. Plotnikoff NP, Prange AJ, Breese GR, Anderson MS. Enhancement of DOPA activity by a hypothalamic hormone, thyrotropin releasing hormone, TRH. *Science.* 1972;178:417-418.
6. Reichlin S. Neural functions of TRH. *Acta Endocrinol.* 1986;S276:21-33.
7. Winokur A. The relevance of thyrotropin-releasing hormone to psychiatric disorders. In: Nemeroff CB, ed. *Neuropeptides in Psychiatric Disorders.* Washington, DC: APA Press; 1991:13-28.
8. Stanton TL, Beckman AL, Winokur A. Thyrotropin-releasing hormone effects in the central nervous system: dependence on arousal state. *Science.* 1981;214:678-681.
9. Manaker S, Eichen A, Winokur A, Rhodes CH, Rainbow TC. Autoradiographic localization of thyrotropin releasing hormone receptors in human brain. *Neurology.* 1986;36:641-646.
10. Kirkegaard C, Faber J, Hummer L, Rogowski P. Increased levels of TRH in cerebrospinal fluid from patients with endogenous depression. *Psychoneuroendocrinology.* 1979;4:227-235.
11. Banki CM, Bissette G, Arato M, Nemeroff CB. Elevation of immunoreactive CSF TRH in depressed patients. *Am J Psychiatry.* 1988;145:1526-1531.
12. Post RM, Weiss SRB. Endogenous biochemical abnormalities in affective illness: therapeutic vs. pathogenic. *Biol Psychiatry.* 1992;32:469-484.
13. Brooks BR, Kalin N, Beaulieu DA, Barksdale C, Sufit RL, Dills DG. Thyrotropin releasing hormone uptake into serum and cerebrospinal fluid following intravenous or subcutaneous administration. *Neurol Res.* 1988;10:236-238.
14. Post RM, Uhde TW, Roy-Byrne PP, Joffe RT. Antidepressant effects of carbamazepine. *Am J Psychiatry.* 1986;143:29-34.
15. Post RM, Uhde TW, Roy-Byrne PP, Joffe RT. Correlates of antimanic response to carbamazepine. *Psychiatry Res.* 1987;21:71-83.
16. Post RM, Altshuler LL, Ketter T, Denicoff K, Weiss SRB. Antiepileptic drugs in affective illness: clinical and theoretical implications. *Adv Neurol.* 1991;55:239-277.
17. Post RM, Roy-Byrne PP, Uhde TW. Graphic representation of the life course of illness in patients with affective disorder. *Am J Psychiatry.* 1988;145:844-848.
18. Bunney WE Jr, Hamburg DA. Methods for reliable longitudinal observation of behavior. *Arch Gen Psychiatry.* 1963;9:280-294.
19. Tanaka K, Kodama S, Yokoyama S, Komatsu M, Konishi H, Momota K, Matsuo T. Thyroid function in children with long-term anticonvulsant treatment. *Pediatr Neurosci.* 1987;13:90-94.
20. Isojarvi JI, Pakarinen AJ, Myllyla VV. Thyroid function in epileptic patients treated with carbamazepine. *Arch Neurol.* 1989;46:1175-1178.
21. Connell JMC, Rapeport WG, Gordon S, Brodie MJ. Changes in circulating thyroid hormones during short-term hepatic induction with carbamazepine. *Eur J Clin Pharmacol.* 1984;26:453-456.
22. Roy-Byrne PP, Joffe RT, Uhde TW, Post RM. Carbamazepine and thyroid function in affectively ill patients: clinical and theoretical implications. *Arch Gen Psychiatry.* 1984;41:1150-1153.
23. Roy-Byrne PP, Joffe RT, Uhde TW. Effects of carbamazepine on thyroid function in affectively ill patients: clinical and theoretical implications. *Arch Gen Psychiatry.* 1984;41:1150-1153.
24. Banki CM, Karmacsi L, Bissette G, Nemeroff CB. Cerebrospinal fluid neuropeptides in dementia. *Biol Psychiatry.* 1992;32:452-456.
25. Joffe RT, Post RM, Ballenger JC, Rebar R, Gold PW. The neuroendocrine effects of carbamazepine in patients with affective illness. *Epilepsia.* 1986;27:156-160.
26. Ormston BJ, Garry R, Cryer RJ, Besser GM, Hall R. Thyrotropin-releasing hormone as a thyroid function test. *Lancet.* 1971;2:10.
27. Post RM, Weiss SRB, Chuang D-M. Mechanisms of action of anticonvulsants in affective disorders: comparisons with lithium. *J Clin Psychopharmacol.* 1992;12:23S-35S.
28. Post RM, Weiss SRB. Sensitization, kindling, and carbamazepine: an update on their implications for the course of affective illness. *Pharmacopsychiatry.* 1992;25:41-44.
29. Meyerhoff JL, Bates VE, Kubek MJ. Elevated TRH levels in pyriform cortex after partial and fully generalized kindled seizures. *Brain Res.* 1990;525:144-148.
30. Kubek MJ, Fuson KS, Aydelotte MR, Knoblach SM. Kindling increases neuronal production of thyrotropin-releasing hormone mRNA in seizure foci as determined by in situ hybridization histochemistry. *Epilepsia.* 1990;31:633.
31. Rosen JB, Cain CJ, Weiss SRB, Post RM. Alterations in mRNA of enkephalin, dynorphin and thyrotropin-releasing hormone during amygdala kindling: an in situ hybridization study. *Mol Brain Res.* 1992;15:247-255.
32. Rosen JB, Weiss SRB, Post RM. Contingent tolerance to carbamazepine: alteration in TRH mRNA and TRH receptor binding in limbic structures. *Brain Res.* In press.
33. Rosen JB, Kim S-Y, Post RM. Differential regional and time course increases in thyrotropin-releasing hormone, neuropeptide Y, and enkephalin mRNAs following an amygdala-kindled siezure. *Mol Brain Res.* In press.

ORIGINAL ARTICLE

Elevation of Serum Free Triiodothyronine, Total Triiodothyronine, Thyroxine-Binding Globulin, and Total Thyroxine Levels in Combat-Related Posttraumatic Stress Disorder

John Mason, MD; Steven Southwick, MD; Rachel Yehuda, PhD; Sheila Wang, PhD; Sherry Riney; Douglas Bremner, MD; David Johnson, PhD; Hadar Lubin, MD; Dudley Blake, PhD; Gang Zhou; Fred Gusman, MSW; Dennis Charney, MD

Background: This study was designed to assess both central and peripheral aspects of thyroid function in combat-related posttraumatic stress disorder (PTSD), with the particular purpose of finding a mechanistic explanation for an imbalance between serum levels of free thyroxine (T_4) and total T_4 previously observed in pilot work.

Methods: A total of 96 male combat veterans with PTSD diagnosed by *DSM-III-R* (72 from the West Haven, Conn, Veterans Affairs Medical Center and 24 from the Menlo Park, Calif, Veterans Affairs Medical Center) were compared with 24 male control subjects. One or more serum samples were analyzed by radioimmunoassays for levels of total T_4, free T_4, total triiodothyronine (T_3), free T_3, T_4-binding globulin, and thyrotropin.

Results: The pilot observation of moderately elevated total T_4 levels with no elevation in free T_4 levels in patients with PTSD was confirmed, suggesting the hypotheses that (1) there may be an increased peripheral conversion of free T_4 by deiodination to T_3 or (2) there may be an increased binding of T_4 secondary to elevated T_4-binding globulin levels. Our findings support both hypotheses. The PTSD groups all showed a marked and sustained elevation in levels of both total T_3 and free T_3, as well as elevated T_3/T_4 ratios, supporting the increased T_3 conversion hypothesis. The PTSD groups also showed a marked and sustained increase in T_4-binding globulin levels, supporting the increased binding hypothesis. Thyrotropin levels did not differ between PTSD and control groups.

Conclusions: These findings demonstrate an unusual pattern of thyroid alterations, featuring substantial elevations in total T_3, free T_3, and T_4-binding globulin levels, in combat-related PTSD that differs from established endocrinopathies, such as classic hyperthyroidism, T_3 thyrotoxicosis, or chronic T_4-binding globulin elevation.

(Arch Gen Psychiatry. 1994;51:629-641)

From the National Center for Posttraumatic Stress Disorder, Clinical Neuroscience Division, Veterans Affairs Medical Center, West Haven, Conn, and Department of Psychiatry, Yale University School of Medicine, New Haven, Conn (Drs Mason, Southwick, Wang, Bremner, Johnson, Lubin, and Charney and Mr Zhou); Department of Psychiatry, Mount Sinai Medical School, New York, NY (Dr Yehuda); and Clinical and Educational Division, Veterans Affairs Medical Center, Menlo Park, Calif (Ms Riney, Dr Blake, and Mr Gusman).

EVIDENCE OF an important relationship between traumatic stress and thyroid function has a long history.[1] The original clinical report of hyperthyroidism by Parry[2] in 1825 described the onset of symptoms in a woman 4 months after a terrifying experience in which she was accidentally thrown down the stairs in a wheelchair. This classic observation has since been extensively confirmed, as reviewed in 1927 by Bram,[3] who reported that a clear history of traumatic stress was found in 85% of more than 3000 cases of thyrotoxicosis. The precipitating conditions largely involved severe life-threatening crises, now commonly referred to as "traumatic stress," such as fires, shipwrecks, earthquakes, combat experiences, and narrow escapes from accidents, as well as various types of object loss. Extreme fear concerning biologic survival appeared to be the most striking common feature associated with these stressful experiences. Recent research continues to confirm the observation that more patients with hyperthyroidism give a history of major traumatic stress than do members of a control population.[4] Important relationships between the thyroid system and stress have also been

See Subjects and Methods on next page

demonstrated in many preclinical studies in both normal humans and animals that have shown alterations in thyroid hormone secretion in response to a variety of psychologically stressful situations.[1] More generally, a substantial number of clinical psychoendocrine studies have examined the role of the hypothalamic-pituitary-thyroid (HPT) axis in relation to a wide variety of psychiatric illnesses, including both affective and schizophrenic disorders.[5-7] There is strong support, therefore, for considering the thyroid hormones as fully qualified "stress hormones" to be included in psychoendocrine studies, even though they have so far received much less attention than has cortisol or the catecholamines in this regard.

With this background in mind, we included free thyroxine (FT_4) and total thyroxine (TT_4) assays, as part of a profile of stress-responsive hormonal measures, in a pilot psychoendocrine study of posttraumatic stress disorder (PTSD) in combat veteran inpatients at the West Haven (Conn) Veterans Affairs Medical Center.[8] Although many years have elapsed since the actual military combat experience of Vietnam veterans with PTSD,

SUBJECTS AND METHODS

Because the conditions of patient recruitment and ward milieu may differ widely from one study to another, and because hormonal systems are so sensitive to even relatively subtle psychosocial influences, our experience has indicated that it is important to describe these factors in some detail in characterizing PTSD patient samples.

RECRUITMENT OF PATIENTS WITH PTSD

Four samples of male combat veterans with PTSD were studied by the National Center for PTSD, including three successive samples, each composed of 24 patients, admitted to the West Haven Veterans Affairs Medical Center inpatient treatment program, along with one sample of 24 patients admitted to the Menlo Park (Calif) Veterans Affairs Medical Center inpatient treatment program. As a comparison group, 24 normal control subjects were studied. Informed consent was obtained from all patients and control subjects.

The diagnosis of PTSD was established by means of *DSM-III-R* criteria on the basis of the Structured Clinical Interview for *DSM-III-R*.[17] Other clinical assessments included the Mississippi Scale for Combat-Related PTSD,[18] the Clinician-Administered PTSD Scale,[19] and the Combat Exposure Scale.[20] Overall mean scores relating to the severity of PTSD were 132 for the Mississippi Scale, 30 for the Combat Exposure Scale, 41 for the Clinician-Administered PTSD Scale frequency sum, and 34 for the Clinician-Administered PTSD Scale intensity sum. There were no significant differences in these scores between the three West Haven groups, but the Menlo Park values were generally slightly lower (Mississippi Scale, 94%; Combat Exposure Scale, 84%; Clinician-Administered PTSD Scale frequency sum, 73%; and the Clinician-Administered PTSD Scale intensity sum, 87%) than those for the West Haven groups, perhaps because of minor differences in the approach to patient selection. With regard to the comorbid rate of other psychiatric illnesses in the overall patient sample, diagnostic criteria were met by 79% for previous alcohol abuse, 40% for major depressive disorder, 25% for polysubstance abuse, and 19% for anxiety disorder.

Exclusion criteria included psychotic disorders, major medical illnesses, hormonal medication, organic brain syndrome, and current drug or alcohol abuse less than 3 months before the study. Urine toxicologic screening for substance abuse was done on admission and at intervals during the hospitalization period. About 50% of the patients had been taking some psychiatric medication previously, mostly antidepressants or benzodiazepines, and the 72 patients in the West Haven sample were required to begin withdrawal 3 weeks before entering the protocol and to remain without medication during the study. The Menlo Park group was permitted to continue medication at the time of the study, but they showed no significant differences in thyroid hormone levels from the West Haven sample.

All the patients with PTSD were recruited for participation in research-oriented inpatient treatment programs of about 3 months' duration in the Veterans Affairs National Center for PTSD. None of the patients was admitted in an acute crisis stage, and all were screened for scheduled admission with a requirement that there was some current level of stability in their life.

SELECTION FACTORS AND WARD MILIEU

Selection factors included favoring patients who were judged not likely to create serious ward management problems and who were judged likely to be able to tolerate and complete the lengthy and demanding treatment program. The West Haven treatment program was designed to deal intensively with both the primary trauma in combat and the secondary trauma connected with the return home. All patients knew ahead of time that they would be required to be free of medication, in some cases for the first time in many years. They knew that they would be involved in community activities and in close and continuing interaction with other patients within groups, as a member of a 12-patient cohort. They anticipated that they would be expected to disclose traumatic experiences and feelings related to Vietnam, in many cases things they had seldom confided to anyone in the past. They also knew that they would be expected to express their feelings concerning traumatic experiences through writing, drawing, drama, and art. The dropout rate, however, was relatively low, about 13%, and mostly involved patients who lapsed into drug

use early in the program. Throughout hospitalization, there was an intensive schedule of 32 hours per week of individual and group therapy, as well as substantial demands on patient time for participation in a variety of biologic or psychological research projects, so that the setting did not facilitate the use of avoidant coping strategies. The program at Menlo Park was generally similar to that at West Haven, but the milieu was perhaps less intensive in certain respects.

CONTROL SUBJECTS AND DEMOGRAPHIC FACTORS

Most of the control subjects were recruited by advertisement as participants in a concurrent challenge test research project at the West Haven Center, and baseline blood samples were obtained on an outpatient basis in the same location and by the same staff personnel as were the patient samples. Most control subjects were veterans; 13 had a negative history and 11 a positive history of combat exposure. None met *DSM-III-R* criteria for PTSD. Mississippi Scale scores ranged up to only 81, which, although possibly indicating partial PTSD in a few subjects, was well below the lower limit of the range of patient values, which was 105. All control subjects were screened to exclude both psychiatric and medical illnesses. The control group was demographically similar to the patient groups in all respects, except for a younger mean age of 38 years. However, there were no significant correlations between age and any of the hormonal measures used in this study, and statistical adjustments to correct for the age difference disclosed that this variable did not affect the significance of any of the reported hormonal differences between the patient and control groups.

The total sample of 96 patients was predominantly white (78%), with an average age of 42.5 years, weight of 84 kg, and height of 178 cm. All four samples were closely similar demographically except in race. The Menlo Park sample was 46% white, 42% Hispanic, and 8% black, but no significant differences were observed in any of the hormones measured in this study between the white and Hispanic subgroups. The total West Haven sample (n=72) was 88% white and 11% black, with all but one black patient included in the first subgroup of 24 patients.

HORMONAL MEASUREMENTS

Blood samples (10 mL) for thyroid hormone assays were collected at 8 to 9 AM in all subjects, and, after setting of the clot and centrifugation, the serum was divided into three 1.5-mL aliquots in small glass vials and frozen at −70°C until assayed. Because six different hormonal assays were to be performed on each sample, the three aliquots minimized freezing and rethawing cycles as a potential source of hormonal instability and analytic error, especially since two different hormonal assays were usually done concurrently when each aliquot was thawed for the first time. In the three West Haven groups, blood samples were obtained during the admission period from all 72 patients, during the discharge period about 12 weeks later from 63 patients, and during the midcourse period from 47 patients, while the single sample obtained from the Menlo Park group represented variable points for different individuals during the course of hospitalization, since the collections were done during a single calendar week by a visiting research team from the West Haven unit. As detailed earlier, the West Haven patients were free of medication during the period when the initial sample was obtained.

Serum TT_4, FT_4, and TT_3 concentrations were measured by RIA procedures, with the use of kits (Incstar Corp, Stillwater, Minn). The interassay coefficient of variation in our laboratory was 3.7% for TT_4, 4.2% for FT_4, and 6.0% for TT_3.

Serum FT_3 concentrations were measured by an RIA kit procedure (Diagnostic Products Corp, Los Angeles, Calif). The interassay coefficient of variation in our laboratory for FT_3 was 2.7%.

Serum thyrotropin concentrations were measured by means of a sensitive third-generation RIA kit (Incstar Corp), and the interassay coefficient of variation was 4.0% in our laboratory. The serum TBG procedure also used an RIA kit (Incstar Corp) with an interassay coefficient of variation of 3.0% in our laboratory.

Statistical comparisons were made between the control group and multiple PTSD groups by means of a one-way analysis of variance with Duncan's Multiple Range Test. Matched sample *t* tests were used for within-subject comparisons of first vs last samples, and unpaired *t* tests were used for other group comparisons. Correlational analyses were made with Pearson product-moment correlations.

it seemed reasonable to examine the possibility that PTSD, as a disorder that involves the chronic, relentless memory and reexperiencing of severely traumatic combat events, might on a long-term basis be associated with a clinically significant degree of thyroid hyperactivity even though flagrant classic thyrotoxicosis was not evident. There is an increasing body of evidence that relatively modest changes in thyroid hormone levels may have important clinical significance in relation to psychiatric disorders, even though the hormonal values remain within the "normal range," as specified for the diagnosis of glandular disease in the field of clinical endocrinology.[6] It was also of interest that the presenting clinical picture of hyperthyroidism includes such psychiatric symptoms as anxiety, irritability, explosive anger, jumpiness or exaggerated startle, restlessness, insomnia, difficulty in concentration, and other cognitive and affective disturbances commonly seen in patients with PTSD.[9] The pilot study confirmed the expectation that the patients with PTSD would have relatively high TT_4 mean levels in comparison with other diagnostic subgroups of psychiatric patients, but also yielded the unexpected and intriguing

finding that FT_4 levels were not comparably elevated.[8] It was this observation of an altered FT_4/TT_4 ratio that raised the questions leading to the present study and indicated that a more detailed assessment of thyroid function and a comparison with normal control subjects was needed to determine the pathophysiologic basis for the apparent discordance between TT_4 and FT_4 levels in PTSD.

To help visualize the rather complex physiologic issues involved in evaluating thyroid function, **Figure 1** presents a diagrammatic simplification of the secretory pathways of the HPT axis. The articulation of the thyroid system with the central nervous system through hypothalamic thyrotropin-releasing hormone (TRH), which stimulates secretion of anterior pituitary thyrotropin, which in turn stimulates the thyroid gland to release thyroxine (T_4), is well known. Less widely known, however, are the pathways from this point on that involve the fate and disposition of the large amounts of FT_4 secreted by the thyroid gland. Nearly all of the T_4 secreted is soon bound to T_4-binding globulin (TBG) in the circulating blood, whereas only a tiny percentage (0.03%) remains in free or unbound form.[10] The TT_4 value, therefore, can be viewed as essentially a measure of the level of T_4 in the bound form.

One possible explanation, then, for the discordance between the relatively high TT_4 and the relatively low FT_4 levels in PTSD might be an increase in TBG level leading to a larger overall concentration of circulating T_4 in the bound form.

A second possible explanation is provided by the fact that a substantial portion of the T_4 secreted daily, perhaps as much as one third to one half, is converted peripherally by enzymatic monodeiodination in extrathyroidal tissues to triiodothyronine (T_3), which is metabolically two to four times more powerful than T_4 and is apparently the primary agent exerting the influence of the thyroid system at the cellular level throughout the body. It is important to realize that by far the greatest source of the production of T_3, probably about 80%, is from this peripheral conversion process, so that only about 20% of T_3 is produced by central TRH-thyrotropin stimulation of the thyroid gland.[11] In fact, estimates of the percentage of T_3 produced by conversion from T_4 range as high as 90%, and Chopra[12] stated that "the generation of T_3 from T_4 peripherally accounts for most, if not nearly all, of T_3 production in normal humans." It is possible, then, that an increase in the rate of peripheral conversion of FT_4 to T_3 might explain the finding of the relatively low FT_4 levels in PTSD, if the latter hormone was being "used up" excessively to produce increased amounts of T_3. It is also of special interest that one of the factors that appears to be capable of increasing T_3 conversion is elevation of peripheral catecholamine levels,[13,14] a condition known to be present on a long-term basis in PTSD.[8]

The line of reasoning inspired by these pilot findings suggests the need to develop a methodologic approach that will deal more fully with the unusual complexity of the functional organization of the HPT system than has been possible until very recently. During the past 20 years, a substantial effort has been devoted to the study of the role of the HPT axis in the pathogenesis and treatment of affective disorders, particularly depression, with a focus largely on the central aspects of HPT organization involving TRH function. Yet some key findings in this field, such as the abnormal thyrotropin response to TRH in some depressed patients, still remain mechanistically unexplained.[7,15] Until recently, highly refined methods for thyroid hormone measurement have been limited to TT_4, with only relatively indirect methods, such as the FT_4 index or T_3 uptake measure, otherwise available for the estimate of T_4 binding, and with no sufficiently specific and sensitive methods available for the evaluation of other crucial components of the HPT system, especially for T_3. As suggested by Lipton,[16] the relatively slow rate at which we are so far "unraveling the mysteries of the HPT axis" may be in part, at least, because of the rate-limiting factor of the lack of suitable micromethods, so that the radioimmunoassay (RIA) procedures that have recently become commercially available for the measurement of FT_4, free T_3 (FT_3), total T_3 (TT_3), TBG, and thyrotropin offer considerable hope for new insights in future psychoendocrine research with this complex system. These revolutionary methodologic advances, in fact, provided a major incentive for us to pursue the present follow-up study of our earlier pilot findings in PTSD with an enlarged battery of hormonal assays, for the purposes of replication and obtaining insight into the pathophysiologic mechanisms underlying the imbalance between FT_4 vs TT_4 levels in this disorder.

RESULTS

REPLICATION OF PILOT STUDY SERUM T_4 FINDINGS

TT_4 Levels

As shown in the bar graph portion of **Figure 2**, comparison of the mean initial TT_4 level of all 96 patients (110 ± 2.4 nmol/L) with that of the 24 control subjects (87 ± 3.6 nmol/L) showed a significant elevation in the overall PTSD sample ($t=4.46$, $P<.00001$). With regard to replication of this finding in the four successive 24-patient PTSD groups, Figure 2 also presents a scatterplot of all the raw individual and group TT_4 data (1-MP represents the Menlo Park group; and 2-WH, 3-WH, and 4-WH, the three West Haven groups), showing the consistency with which these large, inde-

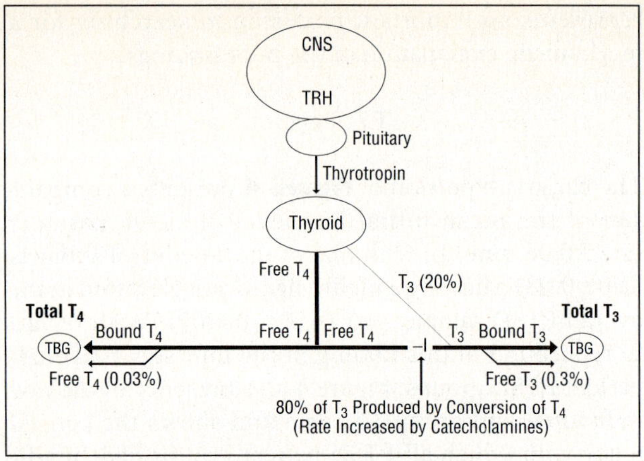

Figure 1. *Organization of the hypothalamic-pituitary-thyroid system. CNS indicates central nervous system; TRH, thyrotropin-releasing hormone; T_4, thyroxine; T_3, triiodothyronine; and TBG, thyroxine-binding globulin.*

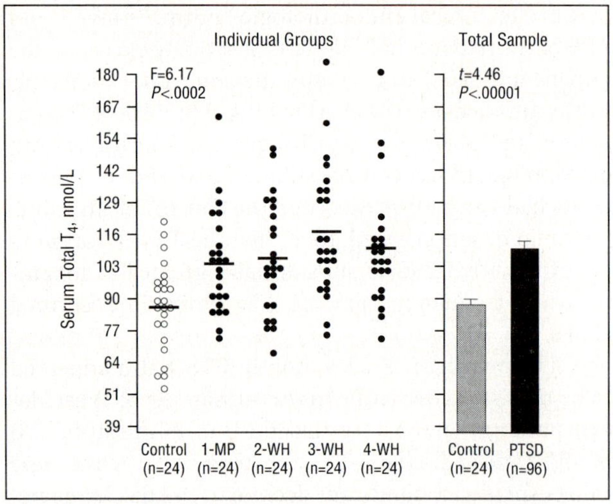

Figure 2. *Total thyroxine (T_4) elevations in four samples of patients with posttraumatic stress disorder (PTSD). 1-MP indicates first Menlo Park (Calif) Veterans Affairs Medical Center group; and 2-WH, 3-WH, and 4-WH, second, third, and fourth West Haven (Conn) Veterans Affairs Medical Center groups. Horizontal lines indicate group mean values.*

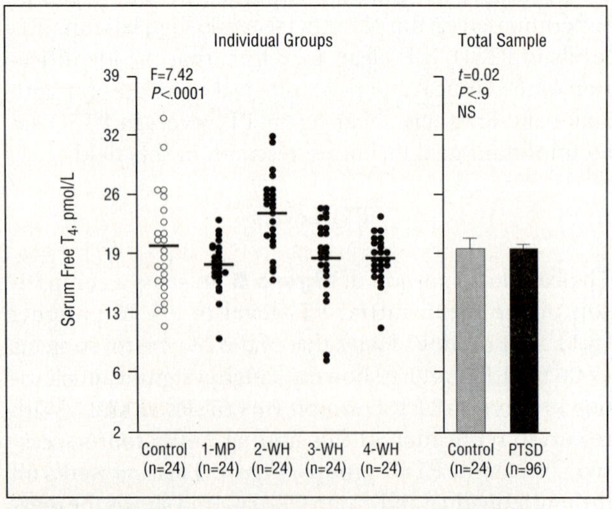

Figure 3. *Free thyroxine (T_4) levels in four samples of patients with posttraumatic stress disorder (PTSD). See Figure 2 for explanation of groups. NS indicates not significant.*

pendent PTSD patient samples had significantly higher mean levels than the control group ($F[4,119]=6.17$, $P<.0002$; controls<1-MP=2-WH=3-WH=4-WH).

The mean TT_4 levels of the PTSD groups were in the upper middle part of the clinical endocrinologic "normal range," and only 5% of the patients exceeded the upper limit of 152 nmol/L, into the zone that may indicate the presence of glandular disease. The upper limit of the control group range, however, was exceeded by 27% of the patients, and the control mean value was exceeded by 83% of the patients.

While the Menlo Park sample involved study at only a single point in time, an additional TT_4 measurement was obtained during the discharge period in a subsample (n=63) of the West Haven patients for comparison with the admission sample. The mean values for the admission period (112±2.8 nmol/L) and discharge period (110±3.1 nmol/L) showed no significant difference over time, and the discharge sample remained significantly elevated above the control mean of 87±3.6 nmol/L ($t=3.66$, $P<.0004$). Against this background of persistent moderate elevation of TT_4 levels, however, episodic fluctuations were at certain times superimposed in individual patients and in individual groups, so that future studies should search for the clinical and psychological correlates of altered TT_4 levels in PTSD within both an acute and a chronic perspective.

The present findings are similar to those in the original pilot study[8] of nine patients with PTSD, whose mean TT_4 level of 119±6.9 nmol/L does not differ significantly from the 110±2.4 nmol/L level of the present PTSD sample, while values of both of these PTSD groups are significantly higher than the control level of 87±3.6 nmol/L ($F[2,128]=11.73$, $P<.0001$). The slightly higher values in the earlier study might be accounted for by the greater symptom severity in the patients in the pilot study, who were admitted through the emergency department to a general admissions and evaluation ward for treatment during a period of acute decompensation and crisis and who generally had more functional impairment than the present patients volunteering for an elective, cohort-oriented treatment program.

FT_4 Levels

The bar graph portion of **Figure 3** presents a comparison of the mean initial FT_4 level in all 96 patients (20±0.4 pmol/L) with that of the 24 control subjects (20±1.0 pmol/L), showing no significant difference ($t=0.02$, $P<.9$); both groups had virtually identical values. With regard to replication of this finding in the four successive 24-patient PTSD groups, Figure 3 also presents all the raw individual and group FT_4 data, indicating that three of the four patient groups showed a trend to be lower than the control group, but that the first West Haven sample of 24

patients (2-WH) had a significantly elevated mean FT_4 level of 24±0.8 pmol/L ($F[4,119]=7.42$, $P<.0001$; 2-WH>control=1-MP=3-WH=4-WH). This atypically high initial level in the first West Haven group appears to represent a temporary episodic or phase elevation, since a second sample from the same group 6 weeks later showed a mean value of 19±0.9 pmol/L, similar to the initial values of the other three PTSD groups. There were no changes in study design or known situational factors related to the initial period of sample collection in the first West Haven group that might explain the finding, and the reason for this atypically high initial level remains to be determined. We did observe that most of the individual patients with the highest initial FT_4 levels in this group also tended concurrently to have the highest levels of the other thyroid measures, so that relationships between T_3 and T_4 levels, as will be discussed later, were relatively similar in all four patient groups. The generally lower levels for FT_4 in comparison with TT_4 in PTSD are further evidenced by the fact, as shown in Figure 3, that the upper limit of the control subject FT_4 range was exceeded by 0% of the patients (vs 27% for TT_4) and only 41% of the patients were above the control mean FT_4 value (vs 83% for TT_4).

With regard to change in FT_4 levels over time in the West Haven patients with PTSD (n=63) studied with both admission and discharge samples, the mean values at admission (21±0.5 pmol/L) and at discharge (20±0.5 pmol/L) indicated a significant decline in levels ($t=2.59$, $P<.01$) between the two points, but the discharge level was still not significantly different from the control mean value of 20±1.0 pmol/L ($t=0.89$, $P<.4$). While there was evidence of episodic fluctuations in FT_4 levels on occasion, these appeared generally to be not as marked or common as those observed in TT_4 levels.

These FT_4 findings appear to replicate those of the pilot study,[8] in which the mean FT_4 level for nine patients with PTSD of 19±0.8 pmol/L did not differ significantly from the 20±0.4 pmol/L of the present PTSD group or the 20±1.0 pmol/L of the control group ($F[2,128]=0.10$, $P<.9$). If the findings of elevation of TT_4 levels, but no elevation of FT_4 levels, in PTSD are viewed together and expressed quantitatively in terms of the FT_4/TT_4 ratio, the mean ratio values of 0.166±0.01 in the pilot group and of 0.188±0.01 in the present overall sample are significantly lower than the mean value of 0.233±0.01 in the control group ($F[2,128]=9.26$, $P<.0002$), indicating an imbalance characterized by *less* FT_4 vs *more* TT_4 in PTSD.

EXTENSION OF THE STUDY TO SERUM T_3 LEVELS

As indicated in the discussion of Figure 1, one possible explanation for the lowered FT_4/TT_4 ratio in PTSD might be an increased rate of conversion of FT_4 to T_3 in peripheral extrathyroidal tissues, where about 80% of circulating T_3 is produced, so that the measurement of T_3 levels represents an important next step in searching for a mechanistic explanation of the pilot findings.

TT_3 Levels

The bar graph portion of **Figure 4** presents a comparison of the mean initial TT_3 level of all 96 patients (2.7±0.06 nmol/L) with that of the 24 control subjects (2.0±0.08), showing a highly significant elevation in the overall PTSD sample ($t=6.14$, $P<.00001$). With regard to replication of this finding in the four successive 24-patient PTSD groups, Figure 4 also presents all the raw individual and group TT_3 data and shows the consistency with which all PTSD patient groups had significantly higher mean levels than the control group ($F[4,119]=13.28$, $P<.0001$; controls<1-MP=2-WH=3-WH=4-WH). The mean TT_3 levels were in the upper part of the clinical endocrinologic "normal range," and 21% of the patients had values that actually exceeded the upper limit of 3.1 nmol/L into the zone associated with T_3 thyrotoxicosis. It is also striking that 64% of the patients with PTSD had values that exceeded the upper limit of the range of the control subjects and 98% of the patients had values that exceeded the control mean value. It should be emphasized, then, that the TT_3 elevation in patients with PTSD is substantially greater in magnitude and frequency than the TT_4 elevation described above.

This marked TT_3 elevation in PTSD also appeared to be persistent over time in the subsample of West Haven patients (n=63) studied both at admission (2.8 nmol/L) and at discharge (2.5±0.06 nmol/L). While these values showed a significant decline in the discharge period ($t=3.38$, $P<.001$), the discharge level remained significantly higher than the control mean value of 2.0±0.06 nmol/L ($t=5.78$, $P<.00001$). Some individual patients and individual groups showed considerable change in levels over time, so that episodic or phase fluctuation can be superimposed on top of the persistently high baseline TT_3 levels in PTSD. It is clear, therefore, that the identification of the clinical and psychological correlates for both acute and long-term changes in TT_3 levels in PTSD are an important goal for future research in this field.

FT_3 Levels

The bar graph portion of **Figure 5** presents a comparison of the mean initial FT_3 level of all 96 patients (5.11±0.11 pmol/L) with that of the 24 control subjects (4.06±0.15 pmol/L), showing a highly significant elevation in the overall PTSD sample ($t=4.67$, $P<.00001$). With regard to replication of this finding in the four successive 24-patient PTSD groups, Figure 5 also presents all the raw individual and group FT_3 data and shows the great consistency with which all the PTSD patient groups had significantly higher mean FT_3 levels than the control group

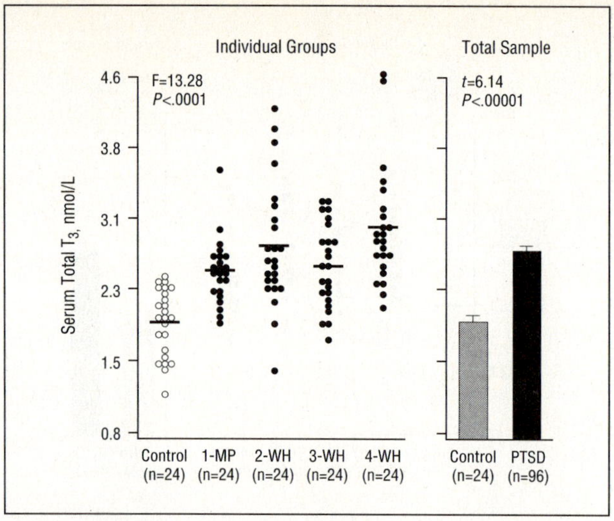

Figure 4. *Total triiodothyronine (T_3) elevations in four samples of patients with posttraumatic stress disorder (PTSD). See Figure 2 for explanation of groups.*

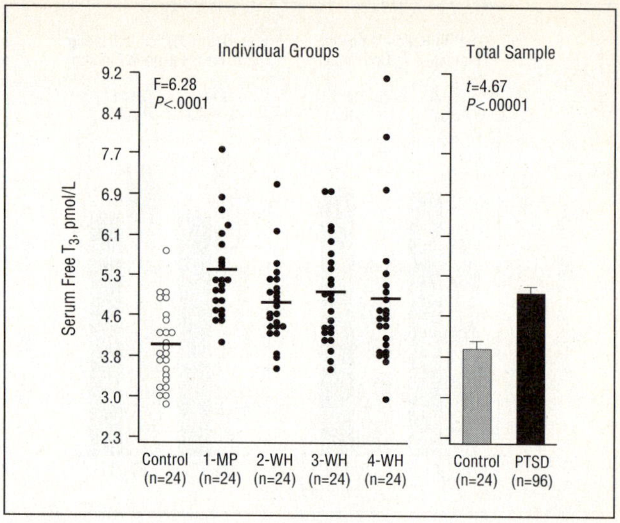

Figure 5. *Free triiodothyronine (T_3) elevations in four samples of patients with posttraumatic stress disorder (PTSD). See Figure 2 for explanation of groups.*

($F[4,119]=6.28$, $P<.0001$; controls<1-MP=2-WH=3-WH=4-WH). The mean FT_3 levels of the PTSD groups are in the upper middle part of the clinical endocrinologic "normal range," and only 8% of the patients had values that exceeded the upper limit of 6.76 pmol/L. The preponderance of patient values above the control values, however, was again evident, with 45% of the patients having levels above the values of all but one of the control subjects, and 87% of the patients had values exceeding the control mean value.

Persistence of the elevation in FT_3 levels is supported by the data from the West Haven patients (n=63) studied at two points in time, the mean value at discharge (5.15±0.12 pmol/L) being significantly higher than both the admission value (4.99±0.12 pmol/L) ($t=2.17$, $P<.03$) and the mean control value (4.06±0.15 pmol/L) ($t=4.97$, $P<.00001$). There was moderate fluctuation in FT_3 levels at times in both individual patients and individual groups, but in general there was considerably less episodic or phase fluctuation than was observed for TT_3 levels.

EVALUATION OF THE INCREASED T_3 CONVERSION HYPOTHESIS

The finding of marked and sustained elevations of both TT_3 and FT_3 levels, in the face of only a moderate elevation of TT_4 level and no significant change in FT_4 level, appears to indicate that serious consideration should be given to the hypothesis that there may be an increased rate of peripheral extrathyroidal conversion of T_3 from deiodination of T_4 in PTSD, as postulated earlier in relation to the thyroid hormonal interactions outlined in Figure 1. The marked FT_3 increase alone appears to argue strongly for this hypothesis, since about 80% of T_3 is produced by this conversion process, and it would appear difficult to explain such a disproportionately large, selective increase in FT_3 levels without the principal source of T_3 production, the conversion process, being prominently involved.

A useful strategy for testing this hypothesis is the quantitative examination of the alterations in the relationships between the T_4 and T_3 measurements, as expressed in terms of various ratios. If the FT_4 level is relatively low because it is being "used up" peripherally more rapidly to produce T_3, then the most obvious expectations might be for increases in both the TT_3/FT_4 ratio and the FT_3/FT_4 ratio, indicating that levels of both TT_3 and FT_3 are disproportionately elevated in relation to the FT_4 level.

FT_3/FT_4 Ratio

As shown in the left side of **Figure 6**, there was a significant elevation in the FT_3/FT_4 ratio ($t=2.56$, $P<.01$) in the PTSD group, reflecting the degree to which FT_3 levels are disproportionately high in relation to FT_4 levels in PTSD. This finding, along with the significant elevation of FT_3 levels emphasized above, is of crucial importance in the evaluation of our hypotheses, since the FT_3 elevation cannot be explained by the increased binding hypothesis, but could most likely be explained as the result of increased peripheral conversion of T_3, although the possibility should be considered that it might also, in part, be related to an increased central stimulation of T_3 secretion from the thyroid through elevation of thyrotropin secretion.

TT_3/FT_4 Ratio

Since FT_4 is the immediate precursor of T_3 and since TT_3 represents most fully the overall pool of circulating T_3, of which about 80% is derived from peripheral conversion of FT_4, the TT_3/FT_4 ratio logically should

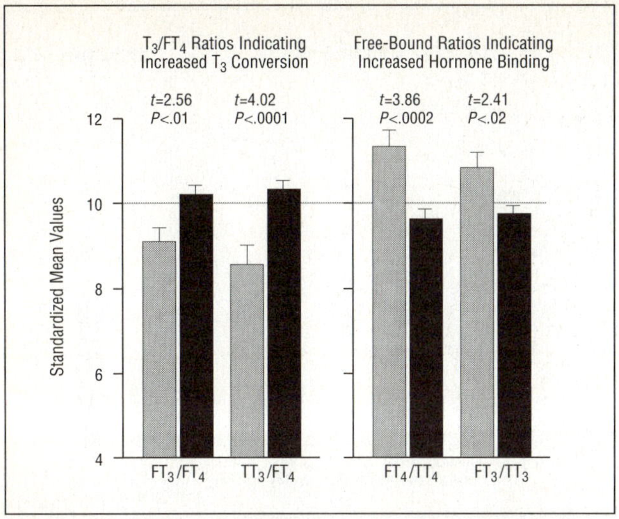

Figure 6. *Summary of alterations in thyroid hormone ratios in patients with posttraumatic stress disorder (dark-shaded bars; n=96) and values in controls (light-shaded bars; n=24). Horizontal dotted line indicates standardized mean. T_3 indicates triiodothyronine; FT_4, free thyroxine; FT_3, free T_3; TT_3, total T_3; and TT_4, total thyroxine.*

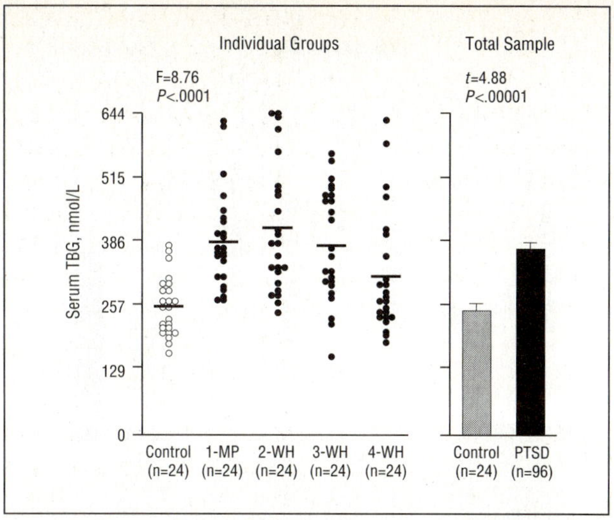

Figure 7. *Thyroxine-binding globulin (TBG) elevations in four samples of patients with posttraumatic stress disorder (PTSD). See Figure 2 for explanation of groups.*

be the single most useful quantitative index of the degree to which T_3 conversion from T_4 may be increased in PTSD. Figure 6 confirms accordingly that the TT_3/FT_4 ratio is the most significantly elevated of the various ratios in our PTSD sample ($t=4.02$, $P<.0001$); along with the elevated FT_3/FT_4 ratio and elevated FT_3 levels, this finding appears to provide important further support for the increased T_3 conversion hypothesis in PTSD. These findings certainly do not, however, rule out the possibility that there may also be a concurrent alteration in hormonal binding, so that at least two pathophysiologic mechanisms may be operating as an underlying basis for the altered thyroid hormone profile in PTSD, including increased TBG production as well as increased T_3 conversion. For this reason, it is important to proceed next to a direct evaluation of the increased binding hypothesis.

EVALUATION OF THE INCREASED BINDING HYPOTHESIS

The finding of elevated TT_3 and, especially, elevated TT_4 levels in the face of lower FT_4 levels raises the possibility that there may be increased binding of thyroid hormone in PTSD. As a preliminary step in considering this hypothesis, it is useful to examine the ratios between the free and total (bound) fractions for both T_4 and T_3.

FT_4/TT_4 Ratio

As shown in the right side of Figure 6, the FT_4/TT_4 ratio was significantly lower in the overall PTSD group than in the control group ($t=3.86$, $P<.0002$). This finding, reflecting disproportionately less FT_4 and more bound T_4 in PTSD, could readily be explained by an underlying primary elevation in the binding protein, a possibility that can be directly evaluated by the measurement of TBG in the same samples. This hypothesis would also predict a decrease in the FT_3/TT_3 ratio, if a greater proportion of T_3 is shifted to the bound form from the free form because of excessive TBG.

FT_3/TT_3 Ratio

Figure 6 confirms that there was also a significant decrease in the FT_3/TT_3 ratio ($t=2.41$, $P<.02$) in the PTSD group, indicating that an increased proportion of T_3 is in the bound form. Along with the FT_4/TT_4 decrease described above, this finding builds further support for the hypothesis that there might be increased thyroid hormone binding in PTSD and indicates the need to measure directly the levels of the main binding protein, TBG, in our samples.

TBG Levels

The bar graph portion of **Figure 7** presents a comparison of the mean initial TBG level of all 96 patients (376±13 nmol/L) with that of the 24 control subjects (252±13 nmol/L), showing a highly significant elevation in the overall PTSD sample ($t=4.88$, $P<.0001$). With regard to replication of this finding in the four successive 24-patient PTSD groups, Figure 7 also presents all the raw individual and group TBG data, showing the great consistency with which all the patient groups had significantly higher mean levels than the control group ($F[4,119]=8.76$, $P<.0001$; controls<1-MP=2-WH=3-WH=4-WH). The mean TBG levels of the PTSD groups

were generally in the uppermost part of the clinical endocrinologic "normal range," and values in 42% of the patients exceeded the upper limit of 386 nmol/L, which was also the upper limit of the range of the control subjects, while values in 86% of the patients exceeded the control mean value.

With regard to the persistence of this elevation in TBG levels in the West Haven patients (n=63) studied at two points in time, the mean values at admission (372±15 nmol/L) and at discharge (377±15 nmol/L) showed no significant difference (t=0.67, P<.5), and the values in the discharge sample remained significantly higher (t=3.76, P<.0003) than the control mean of 252±13 nmol/L. While these findings indicate that the TBG elevation in PTSD is generally sustained, appreciable superimposed fluctuations were observed at times in individual patients and in individual groups, indicating the need for further studies of the clinical factors related to episodic or phase variations in TBG levels in PTSD.

The substantial and sustained elevations in TBG clearly provide strong support for the hypothesis that TBG may play an important role in the elevations in TT_4 and TT_3 levels in our PTSD sample, but they also raise for further consideration the question of the nature of the underlying mechanisms producing the TBG elevations.

Possible Reasons for the TBG Elevation

Since one of the known causes for TBG elevation is liver disease, which is often present in connection with alcohol and other drug abuse in patients with PTSD, the levels of serum alanine aminotransferase, perhaps the most specific available index of active hepatocellular damage, were studied in our patients in relation to TBG and the various thyroid hormone measures. An interesting pattern of relationships was discovered. First, serum alanine aminotransferase levels showed significant positive correlations with TBG (r=.384, P<.0001) and TT_4 (r=.214, P<.04) levels, a significant negative correlation with FT_4 level (r=−.352, P<.0005), *but no significant correlations* with either TT_3 (r=.035, P<.7) or FT_3 (r=.093, P<.4). This pattern suggests the possibility that, while TBG elevation may play an important role in relation to T_4, it is not a major factor in relation to the T_3 changes in PTSD. This conclusion also appears to receive support from the comparison of a subsample of 51 patients with PTSD who have normal alanine aminotransferase levels with the control group. This analysis showed highly significant elevations in both TT_3 (t=6.70, P<.00001) and FT_3 (t=4.31, P<.00001) levels in the PTSD subgroup without active liver damage, as indicated by alanine aminotransferase levels. This PTSD subsample also showed significant elevations in the levels of TT_4 (t=3.88, P<.0002) and TBG (t=3.64, P<.0005), but no significant difference from the controls in FT_4 (P<.4) or thyrotropin (P<.9) levels, so that the overall thyroid profile is the same as in the total PTSD sample.

Table 1. Hormonal Intercorrelations in Overall PTSD Patient Sample*

	FT_3	TT_3	FT_4	TT_4	TBG	Thyrotropin
FT_3	...	.593†	.043	.652†	.577†	−.173
TT_3	...	...	.134	.576†	.438†	−.044
FT_4	...	...	...	.181	−.099	−.226‡
TT_4	...	...	...	...	.653†	−.128
TBG	...	...	...	...	...	.082

*PTSD indicates posttraumatic stress disorder; FT_3, free triiodothyronine; TT_3, total triiodothyronine; FT_4, free thyroxine; TT_4, total thyroxine; and TBG, thyroxine-binding globulin.
†P<.0001.
‡P<.03.

Since another known cause of TBG elevation is an increase in estrogen levels, serum estradiol was measured in the West Haven subsample of 72 patients with PTSD, with the use of an RIA kit (Diagnostic Products Corp). The mean estradiol level was 133±7 pmol/L, which is well below the normal upper limit of 202 pmol/L. When TBG values in patients with PTSD were split into two subgroups according to the median, there was no significant difference (t=0.65, P<.5) in the mean estrogen level (138±12 pmol/L) in the top-half subgroup (n=36) vs that (129±7 pmol/L) in the bottom-half subgroup (n=36). Estrogen levels do not appear to have a major role in the elevation of TBG levels in our PTSD sample.

Sustained FT_3 elevations were also examined as a possible TBG stimulus. In studying the intercorrelations between TBG levels and the various thyroid hormone measurements in the patients with PTSD, as shown in **Table 1**, we observed the expected significant positive correlations between TBG and both TT_4 (P<.0001) and TT_3 (P<.0001) levels, as well as the lack of any significant correlation with FT_4 levels.

Of note, however, was the unexpected, highly significant *positive* correlation between FT_3 and TBG (P<.0001) in terms of its mechanistic implications. If, from a pathophysiologic standpoint, TBG were the primary moving force in the relationship with FT_3, one would not predict any elevation in FT_3 levels, but would logically expect either no significant correlation or a negative correlation between TBG and FT_3. On the other hand, this unexpected finding could be logically explained if the FT_3 elevation were the primary moving force, representing a metabolically powerful agent acting in a feedback fashion to evoke a compensatory TBG elevation, for the purpose of binding and inactivating T_3 to maintain a euthyroid state in the face of persistently excessive FT_3 production. The same explanation was supported by a t test analysis of high-TBG vs low-TBG halves of the patient sample, by means of a median split, which showed that the mean FT_3 level was significantly higher in the

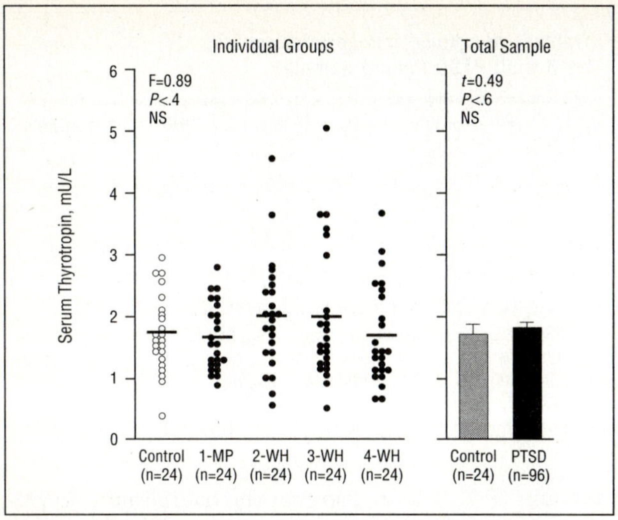

Figure 8. *Thyrotropin levels in four samples of patients with posttraumatic stress disorder (PTSD). See Figure 2 for explanation of groups. NS indicates not significant.*

high-TBG subgroup (t=5.16, P<.00001). It is also important to note that the subgroup of 51 patients with PTSD with alanine aminotransferase levels in the normal range showed a significant elevation of TBG levels, indicating some basis other than liver damage for the TBG increase. However, this suggestion that the FT_3 elevation may play a role in stimulating TBG elevation in PTSD is largely hypothetical and apparently without precedent in the literature. Nonetheless, it appears to present an intriguing possibility for further evaluation of this unexpected finding.

STUDY OF SERUM THYROTROPIN AND THE CENTRAL-STIMULATION HYPOTHESIS

Since an increase in centrally induced pituitary thyrotropin secretion leading to an increased supply of thyroid hormone might also contribute to the elevated thyroid hormone levels in PTSD, we included the measurement of serum thyrotropin levels in our assay battery. However, because thyrotropin stimulation of the thyroid gland normally contributes only a small portion (20%) to the total production of T_3, the central-stimulation hypothesis seems considerably less likely to explain the marked T_3 elevations in PTSD than does the increased T_3 conversion hypothesis.

The bar graph portion of **Figure 8** presents a comparison of the mean initial thyrotropin level of all 96 patients (1.84±0.08 mU/L) with that of the 24 control subjects (1.75±0.14 mU/L), showing no significant difference between the two groups (t=0.49, P<.6). With regard to replication of this finding in the four successive 24-patient PTSD groups, Figure 8 also presents all the raw individual and group thyrotropin data and shows the consistency with which the patient group mean levels were only slightly higher or slightly lower than that of the control group. The upper limit of the control subjects was exceeded by only 10% of the patients, and the patient group mean values varied only between 1.38±0.20 mU/L and 2.01±0.18 mU/L. Thus, thyrotropin levels generally fluctuated relatively little, remained in the middle to lower part of the clinical endocrinologic "normal range," and apparently do not have a prominent role in determining the thyroid hormone alterations in PTSD. Despite the relatively narrow range in thyrotropin levels, however, Table 1 shows a significant negative correlation between thyrotropin and FT_4 levels, which may indicate some negative feedback stimulation of thyrotropin in patients with low FT_4 levels.

STUDY OF REVERSE T_3 LEVELS

Since the levels of reverse T_3 have been useful in the characterization of some HPT axis syndromes, serum reverse T_3 levels were determined on a subsample of 20 patients with PTSD and 20 control subjects, by means of an RIA kit (Wien Laboratories Inc, Succasunna, NJ). The mean level for the patients with PTSD (0.40±0.02 nmol/L) was not significantly different (t=0.49, P<0.6) from that of the control group (0.41±0.02 nmol/L), and the values are well within the normal range of 0.28 to 0.54 nmol/L. This is an interesting finding in that TBG elevations are known to promote reverse T_3 elevations because of the strong binding affinity of the latter. In contrast, the levels of reverse T_3 are often reciprocally low when regular T_3 levels are high, so that one might speculate that in our present PTSD sample such a lowering effect may be counterbalanced by the elevating effect of the concurrent TBG elevation, with the net effect of little difference from normal.

COMMENT

The principal findings in this study are the marked and sustained elevations of FT_3 and TT_3 levels and of TBG levels in male patients with PTSD related to combat experience in Vietnam. These findings from a sample of 96 patients appear to be robust in terms of both the degree of statistical significance and the replicability in three successive 24-patient samples from the same inpatient ward, as well as in two regionally different patient samples from the East and West Coasts. In the West Haven sample studied at two points in time, the T_3 levels were significantly elevated in both the admission and discharge periods. With regard to the question of whether the T_3 changes are related to PTSD or simply to combat exposure, we found that those control subjects who were veterans with combat experience did show mean T_3 levels somewhat higher than those of subjects with no com-

bat experience, but the levels in both control subgroups were significantly lower than those in the PTSD group, so that combat exposure alone cannot explain our findings.[21]

The discovery of marked elevations in both FT_3 and TT_3 levels in PTSD appears to have some especially important practical and theoretical implications. From a purely endocrinologic standpoint, the pattern of thyroid hormone alterations in PTSD appears to be unusual, if not unique, and apparently has escaped attention up to this point largely because of the limitations of the routine clinical laboratory thyroid tests, which focus on T_4 measures to screen for the most common or classic thyroid glandular disorders. As shown in **Table 2**, the thyroid profile in PTSD is not that of classic hyperthyroidism, in which the FT_4 level is elevated and the TBG level is unchanged or decreased slightly, or that of T_3 thyrotoxicosis, in which the FT_4 level is moderately elevated and the TBG level unchanged, or that of a primary TBG increase, from liver disease or other causes, in which the FT_3 level would not be elevated. There appears to be no previously reported common or clearly recognized clinical endocrinopathy that provides an exact precedent for the unusual thyroid profile alterations in PTSD, so that we must to a large extent generate our own hypotheses about the possible mechanisms involved in the pathophysiology of this disorder.

Perhaps the pattern most closely similar to that of PTSD is that of primary TBG elevation, but while the observed elevation in TBG levels in our sample could explain part of the pattern, especially that involving high TT_4 and low FT_4 levels, the marked elevation in FT_3 levels becomes an extremely important discriminant in ruling out TBG elevation as a sole mechanistic basis for our findings. The likelihood that an additional mechanism beyond TBG elevation is operating in PTSD is supported by the finding of increases in the TT_3/FT_4 and FT_3/FT_4 ratios, which indicate that the T_3 elevations are most likely the result of increased peripheral conversion of T_4 to T_3, the process that accounts for 80% or more of the production of T_3 in the body. Of the various factors reported to be capable of increasing the rate of T_3 conversion, the elevation of peripheral catecholamine levels[13,14] appears to be the most likely underlying basis for the T_3 elevations. We have found chronic urinary catecholamine elevations to be an especially characteristic feature of the overall hormonal profile in PTSD both in our pilot study[8] and in our present large sample of patients. If it turns out ultimately that the T_3 findings are properly explained on this basis, then the uniqueness of the thyroid profile in PTSD would become understandable as a natural consequence of the chronic, marked, sustained elevations in peripheral catecholamine levels that are likewise associated with this disorder in an unusual, if not unique, fashion.[8,22] If the catecholamine-conversion hypothesis proves not to explain fully the elevated T_3 levels, then it may be necessary to consider other hypothetical mechanisms, perhaps even the possibility of direct neural stimulation of T_3 from the thyroid gland itself in relation to traumatic stress.

THE IMPRESSIVE elevation of TBG levels in PTSD also deserves some emphasis and raises some interesting questions concerning underlying mechanisms. The liver damage, commonly linked with alcohol or other drug abuse in patients with PTSD, may account for this change in some cases; however, the fact that the TBG level is elevated in many patients without active liver damage, as judged by alanine aminotransferase levels, raises the possibility that a second underlying mechanism may also be involved. In this connection, one of the most puzzling and intriguing findings in this study is the highly significant, *positive* correlation between FT_3 levels and TBG levels. If the TBG elevation were the primary driving force in this relationship, one would, of course, expect the diametrically opposite finding of a *negative* correlation between TBG and FT_3. By contrast, the actual finding appears to suggest the possibility that T_3 may be acting as the primary driving force and is stimulating a compensatory increase in TBG, perhaps in an attempt to maintain a euthyroid state in the face of chronically elevated T_3 production. In any event, this finding appears worthy of further study and may provide an important key to help in the understanding of the unusual thyroid alterations in PTSD.

The question of the clinical significance of the altered thyroid profile in PTSD, especially the T_3 elevations, is clearly important to pursue in further studies. As our work has progressed, we have been able to include an increasingly large battery of psychometric measurements of symptoms and both state and trait psychological factors that we are currently beginning to evaluate in relation to the thyroid findings.[21] As one example, in a subsample of our patients with PTSD

Table 2. Comparison of PTSD and Some Clinical Endocrinopathies*

	TT_4	FT_4	TT_3	FT_3	TBG
Hyperthyroidism	LI	LI	LI	LI	0
T_3 thyrotoxicosis	MI	MI	LI	LI	0
TBG elevation	MI	0	MI	0	LI
PTSD	MI	0	LI	MI	LI

**PTSD indicates posttraumatic stress disorder; TT_4, total thyroxine; FT_4, free thyroxine; TT_3, total triiodothyronine; FT_3, free triiodothyronine; TBG, thyroxine-binding globulin; LI, large increase; MI, moderate increase; and 0, little or no change.*

with repeated measures over time, we found some preliminary evidence of a significant relationship between T_3 levels and core PTSD symptoms, particularly "hyperarousal," as measured by the Clinician-Administered PTSD Scale rating.[21] There is a special need for further studies to determine more conclusively whether the T_3 elevations have a close relationship to such symptoms as sleep disturbances, restlessness, irritability, explosive anger, increased startle, difficulty in concentrating, anxiety, or other common features of PTSD that have also been traditionally linked with hyperthyroidism. If such relationships are found, they might strengthen the rationale for future pilot studies of various treatment approaches based on the use of such medications as propranolol and propylthiouracil, which are known to decrease the rate of the peripheral conversion of T_4 to T_3. A study by Kolb et al[23] of propranolol treatment of patients with PTSD, based on a rationale connected with the elevated sympathetic nervous system activity in this disorder, reported numerous symptom improvements, such as better sleep, fewer nightmares, less explosive anger, fewer intrusive thoughts, decreased startle response, and better psychosocial adaptation in 11 of 12 patients.

The issue of comorbidity in PTSD studies[24] is clearly important, but it is also proving to be unusually difficult to assess because of the high percentage rates and the multiplicity of the comorbid diagnoses commonly observed in Vietnam veterans with PTSD. A variety of research strategies may ultimately be required, including standard statistical analyses based on the distribution of diagnostic categories within a given patient sample, correlational analyses of hormones in relation to ratings of specific symptoms that help to discriminate between diagnostic categories, and longitudinal studies of patients with PTSD in which the time relationships between phases of hormonal change and phases of change in diagnosis-related symptoms or symptom clusters are closely examined. It will also be necessary, of course, to compare PTSD groups with groups of patients meeting diagnostic criteria for each of the major comorbid diagnoses, such as major depressive disorder, panic disorder, drug abuse, alcoholism, or borderline character disorder, but not meeting criteria for PTSD. Our work along these lines has so far not yielded any indication of important confounding diagnostic factors in relation to the T_3 elevations, but because of the large sample required for this task, we regard our current evaluation as preliminary and are continuing to enlarge our PTSD patient sample for subgroup analyses and conducting new studies with the various comparison diagnostic groups listed above.

The full implications of our findings from a clinical diagnostic standpoint remain to be determined with the future application of the present battery of thyroid measures not only to the study of comorbidity in PTSD, but also to other major psychiatric diagnostic subgroups, including psychotic disorders. In related work, we have reported that such multivariate procedures as stepwise discriminant analysis and multidimensional scaling applied to profiles of three or more hormonal measures (involving only T_4 as a thyroid measure) can yield diagnostic classification accuracy above 90% in discriminating between two psychiatric diagnostic subgroups.[25] The more complex thyroid profile used in the present study should add further discriminating power to the multidimensional approach for developing hormonal criteria to aid in the diagnosis of PTSD in future work in this field. It should also be pointed out that the hormonal profile may be especially useful in helping to discriminate between subgroups within a primary diagnostic category[8] and appears to provide a promising approach in the search for subtypes of patients with PTSD, to help evaluate the extent to which heterogeneity in patient samples is presently a confounding problem, for both clinical and research purposes.

Finally, the present study provides encouragement that the recent availability of refined new RIA micromethods from commercial sources permits a more complete assessment and "unraveling" of thyroid pathophysiology in psychiatric disorders, as foreseen by Lipton.[16] It appears that PTSD provides an example to emphasize that, although it is certainly logical to think primarily of the central aspects of HPT function in the field of stress and psychoendocrine research, it is also important to include assessment of peripheral as well as central mechanisms as fully as possible, especially in view of the unusual role of extrathyroidal mechanisms in T_3 production. While our present findings point to the special importance of a secondary peripheral mechanism in PTSD and revealed no detectable alteration in pituitary thyrotropin levels, the possible role of central HPT mechanisms in PTSD remains to be studied more fully. In an earlier pilot study, we noticed a possible tendency toward augmentation of the thyrotropin response to protirelin in some patients with PTSD,[26] but a much larger sample of patients and possibly the use of graded doses of protirelin will be required before more broad and firm conclusions can be drawn about the central level of HPT function in PTSD.

Accepted for publication March 22, 1994.

Read in part before the Annual Convention of the International Society for Traumatic Stress Studies, Washington, DC, October 27, 1991.

Reprint requests to VA Medical Center/116A, West Haven, CT 06516 (Dr Mason).

REFERENCES

1. Mason JW. A review of psychoendocrine research on the pituitary-thyroid system. *Psychosom Med.* 1968;30:666-681.
2. Parry CH. *Collections From the Unpublished Writings of the Late C. H. Parry.* London, England: Underwoods; 1825;2.
3. Bram I. Psychic trauma and pathogenesis of exophthalmic goiter. *Endocrinology.* 1927;11:106-116.
4. Leclerc J, Germain M, Weryla G, Duquenne M, Hartemann P. Role of stressful life events in the onset of Grave's disease. Read before the 10th International Thyroid Conference; 1991; the Hague, the Netherlands.
5. Whybrow P, Ferrell R. Thyroid state and human behavior: contributions from a clinical perspective. In: Prange AJ, ed. *The Thyroid Axis, Drugs, and Behavior.* New York, NY: Raven Press; 1974:5-28.
6. Mason JW, Kennedy JL, Kosten TR, Giller EL. Serum thyroxine levels in schizophrenic and affective disorder diagnostic subgroups. *J Nerv Ment Dis.* 1989; 177:351-358.
7. Nemeroff CB. Clinical significance of psychoneuroendocrinology in psychiatry: focus on the thyroid and adrenal. *J Clin Psychiatry.* 1989;50:13-22.
8. Mason JW, Kosten TR, Southwick SM, Giller EL. The use of psychoendocrine strategies in post-traumatic stress disorder. *J Appl Soc Psychol.* 1990;20:1822-1846.
9. Whybrow PC. Behavioral and psychiatric aspects of thyrotoxicosis. In: Utiger RD, Braverman LE, eds. *The Thyroid.* Philadelphia, Pa: JB Lippincott Co; 1991: 863-870.
10. Woeber KA. Tests of thyroid hormone transport. In: Ingbar SH, Braverman LE, eds. *The Thyroid.* Philadelphia, Pa: JB Lippincott Co; 1986:502-510.
11. Borst GC, Eil C, Burman KD. Euthyroid hyperthyroxinemia. *Ann Intern Med.* 1983;98:366-378.
12. Chopra IJ. Nature, sources, and relative biological significance of thyroid circulating hormones. In: Ingbar SH, Braverman LE, eds. *The Thyroid.* Philadelphia, Pa: JB Lippincott Co; 1986:136-153.
13. Galton VA. Thyroid hormone-catecholamine interrelationships. *Endocrinology.* 1965;77:278-284.
14. Lumholtz IB, Siersbaik K, Nielsen K, Faber J, Kirkegaard C, Friis TH. Effects of propranolol on extrathyroidal metabolism of thyroxine and 3,3′,5-triiodothyronine evaluated by noncompartmental kinetics. *J Clin Endocrinol Metab.* 1978;47:587-589.
15. Nemeroff CB, Evans DL. Thyrotropin-releasing hormone (TRH), the thyroid axis, and affective disorder. *Ann N Y Acad Sci.* 1989;553:304-310.
16. Lipton MA. Introduction. In: Prange AJ, ed. *The Thyroid Axis, Drugs, and Behavior.* New York, NY: Raven Press; 1979:1-4.
17. Spitzer RL, Williams JB, Gibbon M, First MB. *Structured Clinical Interview for* DSM-III-R*: Patient Version SCID-P, Version 1.0.* Washington, DC: American Psychiatric Press; 1990.
18. Keane TM, Caddell JM, Taylor KL. Mississippi scale for combat-related post-traumatic stress disorder: three studies in reliability and validity. *J Consult Clin Psychol.* 1988;56:85-90.
19. Blake DD, Weathers FW, Nagy LM, Kaloupek DG, Klauminzer G, Charney DS, Keane TM. A clinician rating scale for assessing current and lifetime PTSD: the CAPS-1. *Behav Therapist.* 1990;13:187-188.
20. Keane TM, Fairbank JA, Caddell JM, Zimering RT, Taylor KL, Mora CA. Clinical evaluation of a measure to assess combat exposure. *Psychol Assess J Consult Clin Psychol.* 1989;1:53-55.
21. Mason J, Wang S, Southwick S, Yehuda R, Bremner D, Riney S, Lubin H, Johnson D, Charney D. Clinical implications of thyroid alterations in post-traumatic stress disorder: some current research strategies. In: Friedman M, Charney D, Deutch A, eds. *Neurobiological and Clinical Consequences of Stress: From Normal Adaptation to PTSD.* New York, NY: Raven Press. In press.
22. Kosten TR, Mason JW, Giller EL, Ostroff RB, Harkness L. Sustained urinary norepinephrine and epinephrine elevation in post-traumatic stress disorder. *Psychoneuroendocrinology.* 1987;12:13-20.
23. Kolb LC, Burris BC, Griffiths S. Propranolol and clonidine in the treatment of posttraumatic stress disorders of war. In: VanderKolk BA, ed. *Posttraumatic Stress Disorder: Psychological and Biological Sequelae.* Washington, DC: American Psychiatric Press; 1984:97-105.
24. Keane TM, Wolfe J. Comorbidity in post-traumatic stress disorder: an analysis of community and clinical studies. *J Appl Soc Psychol.* 1990;20:1776-1788.
25. Mason JW, Kosten TR, Giller EL. Multidimensional hormonal discrimination of paranoid schizophrenic from bipolar manic patients. *Biol Psychiatry.* 1991;29: 457-466.
26. Kosten TR, Wahby V, Giller E, Mason J. The dexamethasone suppression test and thyrotropin-releasing hormone stimulation test in posttraumatic stress disorder. *Biol Psychiatry.* 1990;28:657-664.

Theme Issues on Cancer and Health Promotion and Disease Prevention

The *Journal of the American Medical Association* is planning to publish a theme issue on cancer in February 1995 and another theme issue on health promotion and disease prevention in April 1995. The *Archives of General Psychiatry* will also consider papers on these topics for its concurrent issues.

The purpose of these theme issues is to expose *JAMA*'s and the *ARCHIVES*' broad readerships to the latest high-quality research and critical thinking in these areas.

Original research contributions, special communications, and review articles dealing with any aspect of the above issues will be considered. All submissions will be subject to *JAMA*'s or the *ARCHIVES*' rigorous review process.

Papers submitted by September 1 will have the best chance for acceptance.

ORIGINAL ARTICLE

Risk Factors for Spontaneous Dyskinesia in Schizophrenia

Wayne S. Fenton, MD; Richard Jed Wyatt, MD; Thomas H. McGlashan, MD

Objective: We describe the prevalence, clinical correlates, and prognostic significance of spontaneous dyskinesias among 100 patients with schizophrenia from the Chestnut Lodge Follow-up Study who had never received treatment with neuroleptic agents up to and including the baseline assessment.

Design: Extensive case records were screened and descriptions of abnormal movements were recorded verbatim for blind rating. Neuroleptic-naive patients with and without abnormal oral-facial movements were compared across sign and symptom, schizophrenia subtype, and illness natural history variables.

Results: Excluding three patients with motor symptoms who had a history of neurologic illness or injury and three who had received prochlorperazine maleate therapy (Compazine), 23% of patient records documented some form of movement disorder; 15% documented oral-facial dyskinesias with sufficient detail so that their presence was considered nearly certain. Compared with patients with schizophrenia without oral-facial movements, patients with oral-facial dyskinesias were more likely to demonstrate a lower IQ score, had more negative symptoms at index admission, and were more symptomatic at follow-up an average of 23 years later. Both the classic hebephrenic schizophrenia subtype and Carpenter's Criteria for the Deficit Syndrome defined high-risk groups for spontaneous oral-facial dyskinesia.

Conclusions: In previous studies, intellectual impairment and negative symptoms have been described as risk factors for neuroleptic-induced tardive dyskinesia. The present data, however, suggest that in many cases oral-facial dyskinesias in patients with intellectual impairment and negative symptoms may actually represent spontaneous movement disorders associated with hebephrenic or deficit forms of schizophrenia.

(Arch Gen Psychiatry. 1994;51:643-650)

From the Chestnut Lodge Research Institute, Rockville, Md (Dr Fenton); the Department of Psychiatry and Behavioral Science, George Washington University School of Medicine, Washington, DC (Dr Fenton); the Neuropsychiatry Branch, National Institute of Mental Health Neuroscience Center at St Elizabeth's, Washington, DC (Dr Wyatt); and the Yale Psychiatric Institute, New Haven, Conn (Dr McGlashan).

SPONTANEOUS dyskinesias among patients with schizophrenia were described long before the introduction of neuroleptic medications,[1-4] but in recent years they have been studied primarily as a condition confounding our ability to estimate the true risk of neuroleptic-induced tardive dyskinesias.[5-9] It is now recognized that to accurately estimate the risk of neuroleptic-induced dyskinesia, the expected rate of spontaneous dyskinesia must be subtracted from the observed prevalence of movement disorders in the clinical population under study.[6-8,10]

In an effort to understand why, despite comparable neuroleptic exposure, some patients have involuntary movements while others do not, a substantial research effort has been directed toward identifying risk factors for neuroleptic-induced tardive dyskinesia.[10] In addition to advancing age,[10,11] intellectual impairment and negative symptoms appear to be the risk factors most consistently associated with tardive dyskinesia.[12-17] Efforts to identify risk factors for the development of neuroleptic-induced tardive dyskinesia, however, must also account for the possibility of an association between these putative risk factors and spontaneous dyskinesia. Because of the difficulty (for ethi-

See Methods on next page

cal reasons) of obtaining non–neuroleptic-treated control populations, very little is known of the risk factors for spontaneous dyskinesia within schizophrenia. As a result, considerable uncertainty remains about the extent to which movement disorders among neuroleptic-treated patients represent an effect of treatment, a manifestation of the illness for which the treatment was prescribed, or an interaction between illness-based vulnerability and medication exposure.[5,9,12-22] Knowledge of an association between spontaneous dyskinesia and specific psychopathologic domains within schizophrenia would allow a better understanding both of the risk factors for tardive dyskinesia and of the heterogeneity of schizophrenia per se.

The availability of an unusually rich clinical database, including long-term follow-up data on a group of patients treated largely in the preneuroleptic era, allowed us to estimate the prevalence and investigate the clinical and natural history of illness correlates and long-term prognostic significance of spontaneous dyskinesias in schizophrenia.

METHODS

Detailed methodologic outlines of the Chestnut Lodge Follow-up Study and Schizophrenia Subtype Project have been described previously.[23-26] The original follow-up study included all patients (N=532) without an organic brain syndrome treated for at least 90 days and discharged from Chestnut Lodge Hospital, Rockville, Md, between 1950 and 1975. Medical records were summarized onto 25-page abstracts, and a battery of baseline demographic, predictor, and sign and symptom variables, including the criteria of several diagnostic systems, were coded. Outcome data for patients in the cohort were collected "blind" to baseline data via interviews with the subjects and/or significant others an average of 19 years (range, 2 to 32 years) after index admission.

The subtype project was conducted blind to both the medical record abstract and outcome data. One of us (W.S.F.) used original medical records to rate all patients who met research (*DSM-III* or Feighner) criteria for schizophrenia (N=187). These patients were rated on additional illness natural history variables and on positive and negative symptom severity, and retrospective rediagnosis was performed using several schizophrenia subtype criteria. In addition to ratings obtained at index admission to Chestnut Lodge Hospital, sufficiently detailed records were available in the charts of 125 patients (67%) to allow ratings of symptoms at an earlier (usually the first) hospital admission that occurred an average of 4.5 years prior to index admission. The interrater reliability of all measures used in these studies has been reported previously.[23-26] The current study includes patients with schizophrenia from the original follow-up cohort who had never received treatment with neuroleptic medications (N=100).

MEDICATION STATUS

Based on all available records, patients' past exposure to psychotropic medications and current medication status were rated at both first and index admissions. At first admission (average year, 1954), 98% of patients (123 of 125) were receiving no psychotropic medication. By the time of index admission (average year, 1959) 53% (100 of 187) had never received treatment with neuroleptic agents.

RATINGS OF ABNORMAL MOVEMENTS

Original medical records for all patients with schizophrenia (N=187) were used to identify patients with motor abnormalities. These records were extensive (averaging more than 100 pages per patient) and contained the reports of multiple informants, including the treating psychiatrist, internist, psychologist, social worker, nursing staff, and family members. In addition, verbatim transcripts of one or more 2-hour clinical case conferences were available for about 90% of patients. All clinical material referencing each patient's condition up to and including the third month of the index hospitalization was carefully screened (by W.S.F. and Beth Lee, RN) for descriptions of abnormal movements, defined broadly as any movements noted by an observer to be unusual or out of the ordinary. These descriptions were copied verbatim and transcribed to forms that allowed rating at a later date blind to all clinical information, including history of neuroleptic exposure. After defining rules for rating movements as abnormal, two of us (W.S.F. and R.J.W.) independently rated all blinded transcriptions, categorizing abnormal movements as present or absent in eight body areas: face, mouth, eyes and periorbital areas, neck, upper extremities, lower extremities, gait, and body/trunk. Overall agreement on the

RESULTS

The mean age of illness onset for lifetime neuroleptic-naive patients was 21 years (range, 2 to 42 years; mean year, 1947); mean age at first admission, 24 years (range, 11 to 44 years; mean year, 1950); and mean age at index admission, 28 years (range, 16 to 55 years; mean year, 1954). Fifty-two percent of patients were female. At index admission, two thirds (67%) of patients were age 30 years or younger, 92% were age 40 years or younger, and 98% were age 50 years or younger. Fifty-eight percent of patients had electroconvulsive therapy and 58% percent had insulin coma treatment prior to index admission. Follow-up interviews for this sample were conducted an average of 23 years following index admission (mean age, 52 years; range, 28 to 76 years).

presence of movement disorder was adequate (κ=.69), and disagreements were resolved by consensus judgment prior to final data coding.

A review of the clinical material revealed that descriptions of oral and facial dyskinesias were often quite detailed, while description of movements in other body areas were frequently more ambiguous. To minimize type I error (the inclusion of false positives), we decided a priori to study clinical and illness natural history correlates only among a narrowly defined group of patients whose records documented an oral-facial dyskinesia in sufficient detail to allow determination of its presence with near certainty. Patients whose records referenced "grimaces" or "abnormal movements" were not included in this narrowly defined group unless these references were accompanied by additional explicit clinical descriptions of the abnormal oral or facial movements. Spontaneous dyskinesia was considered "definite" if abnormal oral and/or facial movements were noted along with a specific clinical description.

PREDICTORS AND CLINICAL CORRELATES

As described previously,[25] 26 clinical elements grouped into eight domains were selected as key components of illness natural history. These domains and variables include genetic predisposition (family history of schizophrenia, affective disorder, any hospitalization), developmental predisposition (neonatal trauma, childhood behavior problems, asociality in childhood), premorbid functioning (social functioning, marital status, work, skills and interests, and IQ score [Wechsler Bellevue Intelligence Scale {WBIS} or Wechsler Adult Intelligence Scale {WAIS}]), illness onset features (age of onset, first hospitalization, index hospitalization, type of onset, and distinctiveness of illness), early illness course (intermittent vs continuous, reactivity to life events), subtype stability, long-term outcome (social functioning, work functioning, symptom severity, hospitalization, and sum and clinical global outcome and living situation), and suicide mortality. In addition to these illness natural history variables, two schizophrenia subtype systems were applied to test their ability to define a group of patients at high risk for spontaneous oral-facial dyskinesia. These included our research diagnosis for the classic (paranoid, hebephrenic, and undifferentiated—designed to approximate *DSM-III-R*) subtypes[25] and Carpenter's criteria for the deficit syndrome.[27] Carpenter's 1987 criteria for the deficit syndrome,[28] which differ slightly from more recent criteria, were used in this study.

We report the overall prevalence of broadly defined (any) and narrowly defined (definite oral-facial) movement disorders for our sample of 100 lifetime neuroleptic-naive patients with schizophrenia. Patients with and without spontaneous oral-facial dyskinesia are then compared across variables within each illness natural history domain and across subtype systems using χ^2 analysis for categorical variables and the t test for dimensional/dependent variables. To offset the probability of chance findings, individual α levels were set for variables in each domain by dividing .05 by the number of variables in the domain.[29] All tests were two-tailed. Finally, to explore symptomatic correlates of spontaneous dyskinesias, the severity of individual positive and negative symptoms rated retrospectively at index admission using the Positive and Negative Symptom Scale (PANSS)[30] was compared for patients with and without oral-facial dyskinesias. Archival information referencing the patient's condition during a 9-month window of observation (6 months before admission and the first 3 months of the index hospitalization) was used to assign ratings on the Positive and Negative Symptom Scale.[26]

PREVALENCE OF BROADLY DEFINED MOVEMENT DISORDERS

Overall, 28% (28 of 100) of patient records documented some form of movement disorder. **Table 1** gives clinical descriptions of abnormal movements in different body areas among these patients.

A review of the medical and developmental histories of patients with movement disorders revealed that three patients had a history of neurologic illness or injury (one with Jacksonian and grand mal seizures as an adult, one with two head injuries with loss of consciousness at ages 10 and 12 years, and one with febrile delirium at age 2½ years). The records of three other patients documented previous exposure to prochlorperazine maleate (Compazine) (used as a tranquilizer in the 1950s around the time chlorpromazine was introduced). Since it is possible that movement disorders in these patients could represent the sequelae of neurologic processes other than schizophrenia or a drug effect, they were excluded from further analysis. Excluding these six individuals, the percentages of neuroleptic-naive patients with abnormal movements described in various body areas were face or mouth, 19% (18 of 94); eyes and periorbital areas, 7% (seven of 94); neck, 3% (three of 94); arm, 11% (10 of 94); leg, 2% (two of 94); gait, 6% (six of 94); and trunk, 3% (three of 94).

PREVALENCE OF NARROWLY DEFINED ORAL-FACIAL DYSKINESIA

Fifteen percent of records (14 of 94) documented oral-facial dyskinesias with sufficient detail to be considered definite. These clinical descriptions are outlined in **Table 2**. The mean±SD age at index admission for patients with spontaneous oral-facial dyskinesia was 28±8 years. Eight (57%) of these 14 patients were male. Among neuroleptic-naive patients in this sample, neither age, nor

Table 1. Abnormal Movements Noted Among Lifetime Neuroleptic-Naive Patients With Schizophrenia

Face	**Mouth**
Made faces	Abnormal movements
Myoclonic twitches	Tongue movements
Grimaces	Chewing, sucking, pouting
Mannerisms	Protruding tongue
Tics	Opening and closing to make "pop"
Twitching	Hissing
Neck	**Eyes and Periorbital Areas**
Tics	Tics
Jerking head	Rapid blinking
Dystonic movements	Continuous squinting
Twitch	Fluttering eyelids
Head tilted	Flicking eyelids
	Raising eyebrows
Hands	Bizarre or special movements
Compulsive-like activity	Tics of eyelid
Athetoid movements	
Extraneous movements	**Arms**
Feminine gestures	Twitching
Rhythmical movements	Extraneous movements
Flexed hands, or flexed fingers	Athetoid movements
Jerky movements	Dystonic movements
Mannerisms	Shaking
Tic	Gestures
	Manneristic motion
Feet	Compulsive-like activity
Compulsive-like activity	Loss of associated movements in walking
Extraneous movements	
	Legs
Body	Rhythmical movements
Twitching	Twitching
Jerking	
Stooped/unusual posture (camptocormic)	**Gait**
	Feminine gait
	Bizarre/unusual gait

Table 2. Verbatim Descriptions of Oral-Facial Dyskinesia in Lifetime Neuroleptic-Naive Patients With Schizophrenia

Peculiar facial grimacing, especially of the mouth . . . twisting her mouth when talking . . . sometimes makes pouting motions with lips.
She was twitching her body about, and making aimless jerking motions with her arms and hands, some looking in a strange manner at whatever she was seeing. She was sucking her lips in and out, and making a hissing sound.
There were a fair number of mannerisms and facial movement, the most noticeable one being flipping of his upper lip. He had another mannerism of winding his arm around his head, and stroking his brow, as though from behind.
Facial mannerisms such a flicking eyelids and raising eyebrows.
Manifests bizarre eye movements . . . showed some facial mannerisms while talking; . . . facial tics.
Compulsive-like activity in the movement of her hands and feet . . . facial twitching, rigidity of limbs, some movement of the hands and feet.
Had some tic-like facial movements.
Nervous movements of her head . . . extraneous hand and body movements . . . gestures and grimaces . . . deeply preoccupied with thoughts accompanied by gestures, facial grimaces and posturing . . . makes a "smack" whispering sound, as if she is about to spit . . . sucking sound . . . the eye would turn in and there were facial twitches and the whole body would be jerking in movement as if she were being pinched or shocked . . . the hands would move in athetoid movement.
He kept his right hand flexed and the middle finger seemed larger than the others . . . another pattern consisted of great preoccupation and withdrawal, accompanied by facial grimacing, sucking, and licking his fingers . . . at other times he is quite withdrawn, has special eye movements, and facial movements.
There was much facial grimacing, frowning, jutting the lower jaw forward and forming his mouth in the shape of a snout . . . many grimacing expressions of the face.
Grimacing . . . there was considerable grimacing, with sucking and protruding of her lips.
Facial tics, would blink and grimace . . . eye tics.
Constant myoclonic twitches of right side of face.
Goes through ritualistic gestures with feet prior to speaking . . . holds lips in an exaggerated pout.

gender, nor previous exposure to electroconvulsive therapy or insulin therapy was associated with spontaneous oral-facial dyskinesia.

CLINICAL CORRELATES

Natural History of Illness

No variables from the domains of genetic or developmental predisposition were associated with spontaneous oral-facial dyskinesia at the requisite α levels. Among the premorbid functioning indices studied, a lower early morbid IQ score was significantly associated with spontaneous oral-facial dyskinesia (mean±SD, 104±15 vs 115±13, t=3.11, df=92, P<.002). No illness onset or early course variables were significant at the requisite α levels. At follow-up, patients with spontaneous oral-facial dyskinesia were rated as symptomatic for a significantly greater portion of the follow-up period than patients who had no dyskinesia (rated on a 5-point scale, where 0 indicates symptomatic the entire time and 4 indicates no symptomatic periods; 0.3±0.6 vs 1.1±1.3, t=3.47, df=33.95, P<.001).

Positive and Negative Symptoms

At index admission, patients with spontaneous oral-facial dyskinesia received significantly (P<.05) greater ratings on five negative symptoms: emotional withdrawal, poor rapport, passive/apathy/social withdrawal, lack of spontaneity and flow of conversation, and stereotyped thinking. Overall negative symptom severity was significantly greater (23.6±9.0 vs 16.4±8.6, t=−2.87, df=92, P<.005). Compared with those who had no movement disorder, patients with spontaneous oral-facial dyskinesia demonstrated a significantly greater degree of conceptual disorganization. The two groups did not differ on any other posi-

tive symptoms or on overall positive symptom severity (**Table 3**).

SCHIZOPHRENIA SUBTYPES

Twenty-eight patients (30%) met criteria for the deficit syndrome. Using classic subtype criteria, 38 (40%), 13 (14%), and 43 (46%) patients, respectively, met the criteria for paranoid, hebephrenic, and undifferentiated schizophrenia. Patients with hebephrenia were a subset of patients with the deficit syndrome; nearly all (12 of 13) patients assigned a diagnosis of hebephrenic subtype also met criteria for the deficit syndrome. Both the deficit syndrome and the hebephrenia/disorganized classic schizophrenia subtype criteria defined high-risk groups for spontaneous oral-facial dyskinesia. Nine (32%) of 28 patients with the deficit syndrome but only five (8%) of 66 patients without the deficit syndrome demonstrated spontaneous oral-facial dyskinesia (χ^2=7.52, *df*=1, *P*<.006). The percentages of patients with paranoid, hebephrenic, and undifferentiated schizophrenia who had spontaneous oral-facial dyskinesia were 11% (four of 38), 46% (six of 13), and 9% (four of 43), respectively (χ^2=11.65, *df*=2, *P*<.003). The broader deficit syndrome "captured" two thirds of patients (nine of 14) with spontaneous oral-facial dyskinesia; 46% (six of 14) met criteria for hebephrenia.

COMMENT

Our findings must be considered in light of this study's methodologic strengths and weaknesses. Patients treated at Chestnut Lodge Hospital during the period of this study were unusual in at least two respects: most had demonstrated considerable chronicity by the time of index admission (80% had been ill for 2 years or longer) and all were from upper socioeconomic strata. Thus, for example, the mean IQ score (104) reported here as indicative of cognitive dysfunction is meaningful only in our population consisting of offspring of highly accomplished and/or affluent parents, where premorbid intelligence is expected to be considerably higher.[31] Although the socioeconomic status of the sample may limit generalizability, this also renders generic causes of neurological dysfunction (eg, poverty, poor nutrition, birth trauma, or undiagnosed neurologic disease) less likely and thus yields a more rigorous test of the prevalence and correlates of spontaneous dyskinesia in schizophrenia.

In addition to sample limitations, our reliance on archival material to obtain descriptions and rate movement disorders is far from ideal. Because clinicians working in the 1940s, 1950s, and 1960s did not systematically search for or describe abnormal movements, selection bias is a possibility. For example, it is possible that clinicians were more likely to notice or document movement disorders among inactive patients with negative symptoms. In addition, the absence of systematic description raises uncertainty concerning the nature and significance of the abnormal movements described. The broad list of movements outlined in Table 1 is clearly heterogeneous and may include tics, compulsions, mannerisms, stereotypies, dystonias, myoclonus, tremors, and other abnormal movements. Many of these movements fall outside of descriptions of tardive dyskinesia as it is currently conceptualized.[11] In contrast, the more restrictive list of oral-facial movements enumerated in Table 2 appears to us to overlap substantially with modern descriptions of the phenomenologic characteristics of tardive dyskinesia as described by Klawans et al,[32] Granacher,[33] Kane et al,[11] and others and as operationalized in the Abnormal Involuntary Movement Scale (AIMS).[34]

Clarification of the relationship between spontaneous movement disorders associated with schizophrenia and neuroleptic-induced tardive dyskinesias has considerable clinical, theoretical, and medicolegal significance. A rigorous exploration of this area would require repeated longitudinal assessments of a large non–neuroleptic-treated cohort of patients with schizophrenia. Given current treatment standards, it is extremely unlikely that such a study could or should be conducted. Similarly, the likelihood that a large sample of neuroleptic-naive patients several years into their ill-

Table 3. Positive and Negative Symptoms Among Patients With Schizophrenia With (N=14) and Without (N=80) Spontaneous Oral-Facial Dyskinesia

	Mean Rating*			
Symptom	Patients With Dyskinesia (n=14)	Patients Without Dyskinesia (n=80)	*t*	*P*†
Negative				
Blunted affect	2.6	2.2	−1.00	NS
Emotional withdrawal	3.9	2.7	−2.22	.03
Poor rapport	4.0	2.7	−2.42	.017
Social withdrawal	4.2	2.7	−3.14	.002
Abstract thinking	3.0	2.1	−1.83	NS
Lack spontaneity	3.5	2.4	−2.02	.046
Stereotyped thinking	2.4	1.6	−2.05	.044
Global negative	23.6	16.4	−2.87	.005
Positive				
Delusions	3.9	3.9	0.11	NS
Conceptual disorganization	3.1	2.1	−2.29	.024
Hallucinations	3.3	2.5	−1.41	NS
Excitement	3.2	2.7	−0.96	NS
Grandiosity	2.1	2.1	−0.22	NS
Suspiciousness	2.4	2.5	0.10	NS
Hostility	3.4	2.8	−1.21	NS
Global positive	21.5	18.6	−1.56	NS

**The Positive and Negative Symptom Scale was used, with individual symptom severity rated on a scale of 1 to 7.*
†NS indicates not significant.

ness will be found for concurrent cross-sectional study is small. For these reasons, while fraught with uncertainty, reliance on detailed archival data is likely the only means of gaining access to information about spontaneous dyskinesia in schizophrenia.

To compensate in part for the uncertainty inherent in relying on records for descriptions of movement disorders, our analysis of predictors and clinical correlates focused on the narrowly defined group of patients with clearly described abnormal oral-facial movements with no overt history of neurologic illness, injury, or drug exposure that could explain the abnormal movements. If examined today blind to history of medication exposure, would these lifetime neuroleptic-naive patients with schizophrenia, be assessed as having tardive dyskinesia? This question cannot be answered decisively, but based on data presented here and other descriptions of movement disorders from the preneuroleptic era,[1-4] we believe in many cases the answer would be yes. Those who do not find the similarity between these clinical descriptions and tardive dyskinesia compelling will necessarily draw different conclusions than those who do.

Estimates of the prevalence of spontaneous movement disorders currently used to correct the risk of neuroleptic-induced dyskinesias derive largely from studies of diagnostically heterogeneous, institutionalized, and elderly individuals never treated with neuroleptic agents.[3,6,7] In these populations, advancing age, long institutionalization, and organic mental syndromes are associated with spontaneous dyskinesia.[3,7] The decisive control group for neuroleptic-treated patients with schizophrenia, however, is patients with schizophrenia who have not been treated with neuroleptic agents.[14]

Available data on patients with a specific diagnosis of schizophrenia are sparse and contradictory. Owens et al[35] reported a prevalence of spontaneous dyskinesia (a rating ≥2 on one or more items of the Abnormal Involuntary Movement Scale [AIMS]) of 53% (n=25) among a unique group of 47 long-institutionalized but lifetime neuroleptic-naive patients with a diagnosis of schizophrenia according to the Feighner criteria (mean age, 67 years) who were treated in a psychosocially oriented inpatient setting by a clinician who eschewed biological therapies. This surprisingly high prevalence was nevertheless lower than that observed (67% [243 of 364]) among a comparable but younger group (mean age, 57 years) of long-institutionalized neuroleptic-treated patients in the same setting; the observed incremental elevation in prevalence among neuroleptic-treated patients increased slightly when the samples were corrected for age differences.[18] In contrast, studying a group of young patients (mean age, 24 years) with schizophrenia by the *DSM-III* criteria early in their illness (duration, 6 to 12 months), Chorfi and Moussaoui[37] found a 14% prevalence (seven of 50) of abnormal movements among patients who had received medication but no abnormal movements in either neuroleptic-naive patients with schizophrenia or normal controls.

Data derived from our current sample of lifetime neuroleptic-naive patients with schizophrenia (diagnosed in most according to the *DSM-III* criteria) (mean age, 28 years) who had been ill an average of 7 years suggest a prevalence of abnormal movements between 15% (14 of 94) and 23% (22 of 94), depending on the stringency of definition. This figure is roughly in line with that reported by Turner,[2] who, in a retrospective review of case records of patients (age unreported) treated at the Ticehurst House Asylum in Sussex, England, between 1850 and 1889, found descriptions of broadly defined movement disorders akin to tardive dyskinesia in the records of 28% of patients with a retrospective diagnosis of schizophrenia according to the Research Diagnostic Criteria.[38] In Turner's sample, a substantially lower prevalence of movement disorders was found among patients with diagnoses other than schizophrenia. Considered together, the available data point to a specific association between spontaneous movement disorder and schizophrenia, with increasing prevalence linked to age and/or chronicity.

To our knowledge, with the possible exception of age or chronicity,[6,22] risk factors for spontaneous dyskinesia within schizophrenia have not been reported. Our data suggest that among domains of schizophrenic psychopathology, spontaneous movement disorders are most linked to negative symptoms, cognitive deterioration, and a chronic course. Perhaps because our sample included few patients over age 40 years, age per se was not associated with spontaneous dyskinesia. Studies of the natural history of schizophrenia subtypes indicate that patients with enduring negative symptoms are likely to suffer from a progressive and unremitting disorder that in most instances results in lifelong disability.[26,39] The sample of Owens et al,[35] substantially skewed toward severe and unremitting schizophrenia, suggests a base rate of spontaneous dyskinesia above 50% by the time such patients reach their mid-60s.

These findings have clear implications for understanding risk factors for neuroleptic-induced tardive dyskinesia. While there is compelling evidence that, compared with neuroleptic-treated patients without tardive dyskinesia, neuroleptic-treated patients with tardive dyskinesia are likely to demonstrate a greater degree of "organicity" as evidenced by negative symptoms, cognitive dysfunction, neurologic soft signs, and perhaps enlarged cerebral ventricles,[12-13,21,22,40-41] in many such patients the emergence of movement disorders may represent spontaneous dyskinesia associated with progression of illness. Waddington[40,41] has suggested that neurolep-

tic therapy may hasten the appearance of dyskinetic movements in individuals who have the greatest likelihood of developing such movements spontaneously as a result of a deteriorating form of schizophrenia.

Our data indicate that the risk of spontaneous dyskinesia among patients in their late 20s is four times greater for those with the deficit syndrome than for those without the deficit syndrome (32% [nine of 28] vs 8% [five of 66]). The relatively high risk of spontaneous movement disorders among patients with deficit supports the emerging evidence for the validity of this syndrome[28,42-47] and raises the possibility that enduring negative symptoms, cognitive dysfunction, and movement disorders represent a triad of signs that share a common or related underlying pathophysiology. In contrast to these findings for deficit schizophrenia, in a recent study of neuroleptic-naive patients, most of whom (22 of 24) had paranoid schizophrenia, a significant prevalence of signs of parkinsonism (tremor, rigidity, and bradykinesia) was found.[48]

The co-occurrence of negative/deficit symptoms, lower IQ score, and spontaneous dyskinesias in neuroleptic-naive patients with schizophrenia is consistent with recent formulations that the pathophysiology of this disorder may include increased mesolimbic dopamine activity coupled with decreased mesocortical dopamine activity.[49] Several positron emission tomography studies have found associations between negative and/or deficit symptoms and reduced cerebral blood flow or metabolic activity in general[50] or in specific frontal or prefrontal cortical regions.[46,51-53] According to the updated dopamine hypothesis,[49] such "hypofrontality" may be associated with or even trigger increased dopamine activity in the striatal circuits of the mesolimbic system. The hypofrontal state is associated with deficit symptoms and inferior cognitive performance, and the hyperdopaminergic mesolimbic state is associated with positive psychotic symptoms and spontaneous dyskinetic movements (extrapyramidal hyperfunction). Such formulations will of course remain speculative pending further empirical support or disconfirmation.

MEDICOLEGAL CAUTION

Tardive dyskinesia is increasingly an area of medicolegal concern.[54] Available data regarding spontaneous dyskinesia in schizophrenia point to the inherent impossibility of determining the specific cause of a movement disorder in any particular instance. The administration of any treatment must occur within the framework of informed consent, which often includes a discussion of diagnosis, the potential risks and benefits of treatment, alternative treatments, and prognosis.[55] In this context, those clinicians who find the case for a significant prevalence of spontaneous dyskinesia in schizophrenia compelling may find it prudent to inform patients and families that the progression of schizophrenia (particularly the deficit and disorganized forms of schizophrenia) may be accompanied by the emergence of movement disorders. Treatment with neuroleptic agents may add incrementally to the risk of abnormal movements inherent in the illness or may hasten the appearance of such movements, but to an extent that has not been fully determined.

Accepted for publication April 27, 1994.

This study was supported in part by a Young Investigator Award (Dr Fenton) from the National Alliance for Research on Schizophrenia and Affective Disorders, Chicago, Ill.

The authors thank Rebecca Hecht-Lewis, PhD, Keith de la Cruz, and Stacey Link for data entry and verification; Karen K. Bardenstein, PhD, for reliability testing; Beth Lee, RN, for assistance with chart reviews; and Dexter M. Bullard, Jr, MD, for general and institutional support.

Reprint requests to Chestnut Lodge Research Institute, 500 W Montgomery Ave, Rockville, MD 20850 (Dr Fenton).

REFERENCES

1. Kraepelin EL. *Textbook of Psychiatry: Dementia Praecox.* London, England: McMillan Publishers Ltd; 1919;3.
2. Turner T. Rich and mad in Victorian England. *Psychol Med.* 1989;19:29-44.
3. Casey DE, Hansen TE. Spontaneous dyskinesias. In: Jeste DV, Wyatt RJ, eds. *Neuropsychiatric Movement Disorders.* Washington, DC: American Psychiatric Press Inc; 1984:67-96.
4. Waddington JL, Crow TJ. Abnormal involuntary movements and psychosis in the preneuroleptic era and in unmedicated patients: implications for the concept of tardive dyskinesia. In: Wolf ME, Mosniam AD, eds. *Tardive Dyskinesia: Biological Mechanisms and Clinical Aspects.* Washington, DC: American Psychiatric Press Inc; 1988:51-66.
5. Rogers D. The motor disorders of severe psychiatric illness: a conflict of paradigms. *Br J Psychiatry.* 1985;147:221-232.
6. Khot V, Wyatt RJ. Not all that moves is tardive dyskinesia. *Am J Psychiatry.* 1991;148:661-666.
7. Morganstern H, Glazer WM, Niedzwiecki D, Nourjah P. The impact of neuroleptic medication on tardive dyskinesia: a meta-analysis of published studies. *Am J Public Health.* 1987;77:717-724.
8. Casey DE. Spontaneous and tardive dyskinesias: clinical and laboratory studies. *J Clin Psychiatry.* 1985;46:42-47.
9. Crow TJ, Cross AJ, Johnstone EC, Owen F, Owens DGC, Waddington JL. Abnormal involuntary movements in schizophrenia: are they related to the disease process or its treatment? are they associated with changes in dopamine receptors? *J Clin Psychopharmacol.* 1982;2:336-340.
10. Kane JM, Smith JM. Tardive dyskinesia: Prevalence and risk factors, 1959 to 1979. *Arch General Psychiatry.* 1982;39:473-481.
11. Kane JM, Woerner M, Lieberman J, Kinon B. Tardive dyskinesia. In: *Neuropsychiatric Movement Disorders.* Washington, DC: American Psychiatric Press Inc; 1984:97-118.
12. Waddington JL, Youssef HA, Dolphin C, Kinsella A. Cognitive dysfunction, negative symptoms, and tardive dyskinesia in schizophrenia. *Arch Gen Psychiatry.* 1987;44:907-912.
13. Waddington JL, Youssef HA. Late onset involuntary movements in chronic schizophrenia: relationship of tardive dyskinesia to intellectual impairment and negative symptoms. *Br J Psychiatry.* 1986;149:616-620.
14. Waddington JL, Youssef HA. The lifetime outcome and involuntary movements of schizophrenia never treated with neuroleptic drugs. *Br J Psychiatry.* 1990;156:106-108.

15. Owens DGC, Johnstone EC. The disabilities of chronic schizophrenia: their nature and factors contributing to their development. *Br J Psychiatry.* 1980;136: 384-395.
16. Manschreck TC, Keuthen NJ, Schneyer ML, Celada MT, Laughery J, Collins P. Abnormal involuntary movements and chronic schizophrenic disorders. *Biol Psychiatry.* 1990;7:150-158.
17. McGlashan TH, Fenton WS. The positive-negative distinction in schizophrenia: review of natural history validators. *Arch Gen Psychiatry.* 1992;49:63-73.
18. Owens DGC. Involuntary disorders of movement in chronic schizophrenia: the role of illness and its treatment. In: Casey DE, Chase TN, Christensen AV, Gerlach J, eds. *Dyskinesia: Research and Treatment.* Berlin, Germany: Springer-Verlag; 1985:79-87.
19. Turek IS. Drug-induced dyskinesia: reality or myth? *Dis Nerv Syst.* 1975:36; 397-399.
20. McKenna PJ, Lund CE, Mortimer AM, Biggins CA. Motor, volitional and behavioral disorders in schizophrenia, II: the 'conflict of paradigms' hypothesis. *Br J Psychiatry.* 1991;158:328-336.
21. Waddington JL. Tardive dyskinesia in schizophrenia and other disorders: associations with ageing, cognitive dysfunction and structural brain pathology in relation to neuroleptic exposure. *Hum Psychopharmacol.* 1987;2:11-22.
22. Waddington JL. Schizophrenia, affective psychosis, and other disorders treated with neuroleptic drugs: the enigma of tardive dyskinesia, its neurobiological determinants, and the conflict of paradigms. *Int Rev Neurobiol.* 1989;31:297-353.
23. McGlashan TH. The Chestnut Lodge Follow-up Study, I: follow-up methodology and study sample. *Arch Gen Psychiatry.* 1984;41:573-585.
24. McGlashan TH. The Chestnut Lodge Follow-up Study, II: long-term outcome of schizophrenia and affective disorders. *Arch Gen Psychiatry.* 1984;41:586-601.
25. Fenton WS, McGlashan TH. Natural history of schizophrenia subtypes, I: longitudinal study of paranoid, hebephrenic, and undifferentiated schizophrenia. *Arch Gen Psychiatry.* 1991;48:969-977.
26. Fenton WS, McGlashan TH. Natural history of schizophrenia subtypes, II: positive and negative symptoms and long-term course. *Arch Gen Psychiatry.* 1991; 48:978-986.
27. Carpenter WT, Heinrichs DW, Wagman AMI. Deficit and non-deficit forms of schizophrenia: the concept. *Am J Psychiatry.* 1988;145:578-583.
28. Wagman AMI, Heinrichs DW, Carpenter WT. Deficit and non-deficit forms of schizophrenia: neuropsychological evaluation. *Psychiatry Res.* 1987;22:319-330.
29. Grove WM, Andreasen NC. Simultaneous tests of multiple hypotheses in exploratory research. *J Nerv Ment Dis.* 1982;170:3-8.
30. Kay SR, Opler LA, Fishbein A. *Positive And Negative Syndrome Scale (PANSS) Rating Manual.* Toronto, Ontario: Multihealth Systems Inc; 1992.
31. Fenton WS, McGlashan TH, Heinssen RK. DSM-III versus DSM-III-R criteria for schizophrenia. *Am J Psychiatry.* 1989;146:686.
32. Klawans HL, Goetz CG, Perlick S. Tardive dyskinesia: review and update. *Am J Psychiatry.* 1980;137:900-908.
33. Granacher RP. Differential diagnosis of tardive dyskinesia: an overview. *Am J Psychiatry.* 1981;138:1288-1297.
34. Guy W, ed. Abnormal Involuntary Movement Scale (AIMS). In: *ECDEU Assessment Manual for Psychopharmacology, Revised, 1976.* Rockville, Md: Alcohol, Drug Abuse, and Mental Health Administration; 1976:534-537. US Dept of Health, Education, and Welfare publication ADM 76-338.
35. Owen DGC, Johnstone EC, Frith CD. Spontaneous involuntary disorders of movement: their prevalence, severity, and distribution in chronic schizophrenics with and without treatment with neuroleptics. *Arch Gen Psychiatry.* 1982;39:452-461.
36. Feighner JP, Robins E, Guze SB, Woodruff RA. Diagnostic criteria for use in psychiatric research. *Arch Gen Psychiatry.* 1972:26:57-63.
37. Chorfi M, Moussaoui D. Lack of dyskinesias in unmedicated schizophrenics. *Psychopharmacology.* 1989;97:423.
38. Spitzer RL, Endicott J, Robins E. *Research Diagnostic Criteria (RDC) for a Selected Group of Functional Disorders.* 3rd ed. New York, NY: New York State Psychiatric Institute; 1975.
39. McGlashan TH, Fenton WS. Subtype progression and pathophysiologic deterioration in early schizophrenia. *Schizophr Bull.* 1993;19:71-84.
40. Waddington JL. Spontaneous orofacial movements induced in rodents by very long-term neuroleptic drug administration: phenomenology, pathophysiology and putative relationship to tardive dyskinesia. *Psychopharmacology.* 1990; 101:431-447.
41. Waddington JL. Tardive dyskinesia in schizophrenia and other disorders: association with aging, cognitive dysfunction and structural brain pathology in relation to neuroleptic exposure. *Human Psychopharmacol.* 1987;2:11-22.
42. Buchanan RW, Kirkpatrick B, Heinrichs DW, Carpenter WT. Clinical correlates of the deficit syndrome in schizophrenia. *Am J Psychiatry.* 1990;147:290-294.
43. Kirkpatrick B, Buchanan RW. Anhedonia and the deficit syndrome of schizophrenia. *Psychiatr Res.* 1989;31:25-30.
44. Thaker GK, Kirkpatrick B, Buchanan RW, Ellsberry R. Oculomotor abnormalities and their clinical cocorrelates in schizophrenia. *Psychopharmacol Bull.* 1989; 25:491-497.
45. Buchanan RW, Kirkpatrick B, Tamminga CA. Differential patterns of glucose metabolism in deficit and non-deficit schizophrenia. *Biol Psychiatry.* 1989;25:99A.
46. Tamminga CA, Thaker GK, Buchanan RW, Kirkpatrick B. Limbic system abnormalities identified in schizophrenia using positron emission tomography with fluorodeoxyglucose and neocortical alterations with the deficit syndrome. *Arch Gen Psychiatry.* 1992;49:522-530.
47. Buchanan RW, Breier A, Kirkpatrick B, Elkashef A, Munson RC, Gellad F, Carpenter WT. Structural abnormalities in deficit and non-deficit schizophrenia. *Am J Psychiatry.* 1993;150:59-65.
48. Caligiuri MP, Lohr JB, Jeste DV. Parkinsonism in neuroleptic-naive schizophrenic patients. *Am J Psychiatry.* 1993;150:1343-1348.
49. Davis KL, Kahn RS, Ko G, Davidson M. Dopamine in schizophrenia: a review and reconceptualization. *Am J Psychiatry.* 1991;148:1474-1486.
50. Volkow ND, Wolf AP, Van Gelder P, Brodie JD, Overall JE, Cancro R, Gomez-Mont F. Phenomenological correlates of metabolic activity in 18 patients with chronic schizophrenia. *Am J Psychiatry.* 1987;114:151-158.
51. Liddle PF, Friston KJ, Frith CD, Hirsch SR, Jones T, Frackowiack RSJ. Patterns of cerebral blood flow in schizophrenia. *Br J Psychiatry.* 1992:160;179-186.
52. Andreasen NC, Rezai K, Alliger R, Swayze VS, Flaum M, Kirchner P, Cohen G, O'Leary DS. Hypofrontality in neuroleptic-naive patients and in patients with chronic schizophrenia. *Arch Gen Psychiatry.* 1992:49:943-958.
53. Wolkin A, Sanfilipo M, Wolf AP, Angrist B, Brokie JD, Rotrosen J. Negative symptoms and hypofrontality in chronic schizophrenia. *Arch Gen Psychiatry.* 1992;49:959-965.
54. Simon RI. Ethical and legal issues in neuropsychiatry. In: Yudofsky SC, Hales RE, eds. *Textbook of Neuropsychiatry.* Washington, DC: American Psychiatric Press Inc; 1992:773-805.
55. Simon RI. *Clinical Psychiatry and the Law.* 2nd ed. Washington, DC: American Psychiatric Press Inc; 1992.

ORIGINAL ARTICLE

Neuropsychological Functioning in Siblings Discordant for Schizophrenia and Healthy Volunteers

Tyrone D. Cannon, PhD; Lisa Eyler Zorrilla, MA; Derri Shtasel, MD; Raquel E. Gur, MD, PhD; Ruben C. Gur, PhD; Elysa J. Marco; Paul Moberg, PhD; R. Arlen Price, PhD

Objective: To determine whether schizophrenics and their nonschizophrenic siblings have a similar pattern of neuropsychological deficit when compared with normal controls.

Design and Participants: Fifteen probands with schizophrenia, 16 of their nonschizophrenic siblings, and 31 unrelated, demographically balanced, normal individuals underwent evaluation with a comprehensive neuropsychological test battery. All subjects were screened for history of head injury, neurologic illness, major medical conditions, substance use, and axis I psychiatric disorders other than schizophrenia. Probands underwent evaluation twice: once at intake when half had never received neuroleptic medication and the other half had received none for a minimum of 2 weeks, and again at the 2- to 4-week follow-up, after stabilization with neuroleptic medications.

Results: Both schizophrenics and their nonschizophrenic siblings were impaired neuropsychologically compared with normal controls, with the nonschizophrenic siblings' performance intermediate between that of the schizophrenic siblings and the normal controls on all measures of functioning. The shapes of the deficit profiles of schizophrenic patients and their siblings were similar; in patients, verbal memory, abstraction, attention, and language functions were significantly more affected compared with spatial abilities, spatial memory, and sensory-motor functions, with a nonsignificant trend in the same direction in siblings. Cognitive functioning in patients was found to be stable across changes in medication status and clinical state. Four fifths of patients obtained more deviant scores than their nonschizophrenic siblings. Among the sibling group, those with probable and certain diagnoses of schizotypal personality disorder were more impaired compared with those without schizophrenia-spectrum symptoms.

Conclusion: These results support the hypothesis that impaired information processing aggregates in the family members of schizophrenics and may serve as an indicator of genetic vulnerability to the disorder. Further work is needed to establish whether particular areas of functioning are selectively impaired in relatives and to determine whether the performance deficits are mediated by structural and/or metabolic disturbances in specific brain regions.

(Arch Gen Psychiatry. 1994;51:651-661)

TWIN, FAMILY, and adoption studies of schizophrenia have demonstrated a substantial genetic component to the transmission of the disorder,[1-7] but the nature of the genetic diathesis and the mode of inheritance remain to be identified.[8] A major consequence of this uncertainty is that it cannot be determined if a given individual carries a predisposing genotype. One approach to resolving this issue is to search for biological or behavioral characteristics that mark the presence (or degree) of genetic predisposition to the disorder.[9,10] Such "endophenotypic" markers are likely to be closer to the mechanism of gene action than the clinical phenotype. The ultimate promise of such marker variables is to facilitate linkage analyses aimed at identifying the genetic locus/loci involved and to permit isolation of environmental contributors to illness ex-

From the Departments of Psychology (Dr Cannon and Ms Zorrilla) and Psychiatry (Drs Cannon, Shtasel, R. E. Gur, R. C. Gur, Moberg, and Price and Mss Zorrilla and Marco), University of Pennsylvania, Philadelphia.

See Subjects and Methods on next page

SUBJECTS AND METHODS

SUBJECTS

The sample consisted of 15 probands, 16 of their full siblings, and 31 unrelated, normal controls, all of whom were recruited and underwent evaluation by the Mental Health Clinical Research Center (MHCRC) in the Department of Psychiatry at the University of Pennsylvania, Philadelphia. All subjects received a psychiatric interview (ie, Structured Clinical Interview for *DSM-III-R*, Patient or Nonpatient Edition)[49] and physical examination, including routine laboratory tests. Probands were rated on standard scales of positive and negative symptoms (Scale for the Assessment of Positive Symptoms [SAPS][50] and Scale for the Assessment of Negative Symptoms [SANS][51]). Siblings received a structured interview for assessment of axis II psychopathology.[52] Exclusion criteria were any major medical illness that could affect brain function (including hypertension and cardiac, endocrine, renal, and pulmonary disease), current or past substance disorder (according to *DSM-III-R* criteria[53] assessed by history from proband and family, review of records, and screening for toxic substances), neurologic condition (eg, migraine headaches), history of head injury with loss of consciousness, and age of less than 18 or greater than 45 years. All probands had to meet *DSM-III-R* criteria for schizophrenia, with no other concurrent diagnoses. Siblings had to be within 5 years of age of their proband and free of any axis I syndrome. Normal controls had to be free of any axis I disorder and without a family history of schizophrenia.

The 15 probands used in our study represent those MHCRC probands with siblings who met the eligibility criteria summarized above and who agreed to participate. The probands had a mean (±SD) age at onset of 24.4±6 years and a mean (±SD) duration of illness of 4.4±5 years. Seven probands were first-episode patients who had never been previously hospitalized and had never received neuroleptic medication at the time of the intake assessment. These seven probands have been followed up for a minimum of 1 year and the diagnosis of schizophrenia confirmed in each case. The remaining eight probands had a mean number of 3.5 previous psychiatric hospitalizations and had not received neuroleptic medication at least 2 weeks prior to the intake assessment (range, 2 to 364 weeks). Each proband had at least one full sibling who also underwent evaluation. Twelve siblings were of the same gender as their schizophrenic sibling; four siblings (two male and two female) were of the opposite gender of their schizophrenic sibling. Three of the siblings met *DSM-III-R* criteria for schizotypal personality disorder (SPD); three others were rated positively on two or more of the nine SPD criteria and were given diagnoses of probable SPD. The normal controls were drawn from the larger pool of MHCRC controls. Each proband and each sibling were matched to one normal control on the following variables: age (within 5 years), gender, race, handedness, educational level (within 2 years), and parental educational level (ie, level of the mother and father combined, within 4 years).

Table 1 summarizes demographic characteristics of the three groups. Nearly perfect matching was achieved on all the variables except handedness. Too few left-handed controls were sampled to achieve perfect matching on this variable; however, there was not a significant difference in handedness distribution (or in terms of any of the other demographic variables) between probands, siblings, and controls.

NEUROPSYCHOLOGICAL EVALUATION

A comprehensive neuropsychological test battery was administered to each subject by predoctoral (including L.E.Z.) and postdoctoral examiners who worked under the supervision of neuropsychology faculty and who had extensive training with the battery prior to the assessments. A second examiner independently rescored each protocol to eliminate errors and to permit establishment of interrater reliability for scoring.

Probands were examined twice, first at intake assessment when they had received no medication for a minimum of 2 weeks and again at the 2- to 4-week follow-up, after stabilization with clinically determined doses of neuroleptic medication. All subjects received the same battery of tests in a fixed order, with the exception of probands, who received an abbreviated version of the battery at intake to avoid contamination effects due to fatigue or florid psychosis. Total time for the test battery was about 4 hours. However, subjects were allowed to take breaks as needed, and in many cases the battery was broken into two sessions over a span of 2 days. Examiners attempted to obtain maximal performance at all times. Occasionally a proband was unable to complete a test, in which case his or her score for that test was coded as missing. One proband had not yet undergone evaluation at follow-up and is used only in the analyses involving intake measures. The intake data for two of the probands and 11 of the controls were used in our previous report on patient-control differences.[13] The neuropsychological test data of siblings and all of the probands at follow-up have not been used in previous publications.

The test battery[14,45-48,54-63] is presented in **Table 2**. In addition to the published tests referenced, we employed a modified, microprocessor-controlled version of the vigilance and distractibility tasks of the Continuous Performance Test (Gordan Diagnostic Systems, DeWitt, NY).[56] The vigilance condition requires subjects to monitor a three-digit display that presents a random series of single digits in the middle position. The subject is instructed to press the response button only when a specified sequence occurs (eg, 9 after a 1). In the distractibility condition, random digits are presented as distracters in the left and right positions of the display. Both tasks are 6 minutes in duration. Performance was measured as the total number of targets detected (of 30) in each condition.

The raw test scores were rescaled to standard equivalents (ie, z scores), using the means and SDs of the normal control group. There is a trade-off in advantages and disadvantages according to whether z scores are based on data from within-study controls or the published normative data available for these tests. The primary advantage of within-study norms is that the level of cognitive functioning in the proband and sibling groups can be interpreted with respect to the performance of a normal control group that is well-matched in terms of sociodemographic factors that influence variability in cognitive performance (eg, age, gender, parental social class, education, and handedness). The major advantage of using published norms is that these are generally based on much larger sample sizes of normal subjects than the control group in our study (N=31). However, the latter approach has two major disadvantages in that such groups are generally not well matched to the population of schizophrenics on the relevant sociodemographic variables, and rarely are such normative data stratified according to levels of these sociodemographic dimensions (which would be necessary to ascertain the appropriate values from which to calculate deviation scores for the probands). It is important to note that, in either case, the interpretation of deviance from normal is typically based on z scores or on an analogous measure such as percentiles. In clinical settings, a score of 1 to 2 SDs below normal (which translates to a z score of -1 to -2) is generally interpreted to be deviant.

Test data were reduced into seven summary measures by averaging each subject's z scores on tests assessing the same functional domain. Summary measures were formed for the following domains: abstraction (ABS), attention (ATT), spatial abilities (SPT), verbal memory (VME), spatial memory (SME), language abilities (LNG), and sensory-motor functions (SMO). This organization represents a minor modification of our previously published 10-domain profile in that (1) measures of verbal learning are collapsed with measures of verbal recall into a single VME factor; (2) measures of verbal ability and language functions are collapsed into a single LNG factor; and (3) measures of visual attention and auditory attention are collapsed into a single ATT factor. This set of variable definitions is consistent with the results of several factor analyses of comparable batteries in the published literature (see Saykin et al[13]) and is now the standard for publications emanating from this laboratory.

Probands' domain scores at follow-up assessment using only those tests available in the intake version of the test battery were not significantly different from their domain scores at follow-up assessment using all of the tests in the battery. Thus, the abbreviated (intake) version of the test battery appears to provide information equivalent to the full battery.

STATISTICAL ANALYSES

The seven summary neuropsychological measures were used as dependent variables in multivariate analyses of variance (MANOVAs),[64] with the study group (ie, probands, siblings, and controls) serving as the between-subject variable and domain of functioning (ie, ABS, ATT, etc) serving as the within-subject factor. One analysis used probands' intake (while receiving no neuroleptic medication) performance measures, and another analysis used probands' follow-up (while receiving medication) performance measures. These analyses were used to test for overall group differences in degree of deficit and profile shape. Selectivity of deficits was examined using within-group domain-wise contrasts in which the mean scores on the ABS, ATT, LNG, and VME functions were contrasted with the mean scores on the remaining functions in the profile (ie, SAS PROC GLM contrast procedure).[64] To examine the stability of probands' deficits across medication status, a separate MANOVA was conducted on probands' intake and follow-up performance measures, treating neuroleptic medication status (ie, not receiving vs receiving) and domain as within-subject variables.

Significant multivariate effects were followed by univariate analyses examining group differences on each of the summary neuropsychological measures. The matched-pair t statistic was used for the proband vs sibling comparisons, and the t statistic for independent samples was used for the proband vs control and sibling vs control comparisons. An advantage of the MANOVA approach used here is that univariate tests are examined only in the presence of significant multivariate effects, a practice that controls for the type I error rate and reduces the total number of tests conducted.

To determine the sensitivity of each index as an indicator of schizophrenia, we computed the percentage of cases in which the proband had a more deviant score than his or her sibling on each of the seven summary measures (ie, pair-wise or within-family sensitivity) and compared this index to the percentages of cases whose values on each measure fell outside of the ranges of the sibling and control groups (ie, outlier or between-family sensitivity). Minimums were used to define sensitivity in the outlier analyses (rather than another distributional measure, such as 1 or 2 SDs below the relevant group mean) since this provides a measure of sensitivity that is comparable to that obtained in the pair-wise analyses. That is, in the pair-wise analyses, the proband is being compared with his or her sibling in terms of absolute performance on a person-by-person basis rather than on the basis of a distributional deviation. Since we sampled only one sibling and one proband per family, there is no within-family distribution available on which to compute SDs. Thus, if we used 1 or 2 SDs below the control group mean to define outlier status, there would be no corresponding definition to use for the siblings when calculating pair-wise sensitivity rates.

To assess for the possibility of a bimodal distribution of performance in the sibling group, we also calculated the percentages of siblings whose scores on each measure were 1 SD or more below the control group mean and below the control group minimum.

Table 1. Demographic Characteristics of Schizophrenic Probands, Siblings, and Normal Controls

Characteristic	Probands (N=15)	Siblings (N=16)	Controls (N=31)
Gender, %			
Female	33	44	39
Male	67	56	61
Race, %			
African American	60	63	61
White	40	37	39
Handedness, %			
Right	73	87	87
Left	27	13	13
Mean (±SD) age, y	28.7 (8.6)	31.6 (10.3)	28.3 (6.5)
Mean (±SD) education, y	13.2 (2.0)	14.2 (2.8)	14.5 (1.9)
Mean (±SD) parental education, y	12.1 (2.3)	12.1 (2.3)	12.0 (2.7)

pression among genotypic carriers, possibly leading to prevention or treatment strategies.

Several lines of evidence implicate disturbances in certain information-processing domains as candidate indicators of predisposition to schizophrenia. Specific cognitive deficits have been observed during both active and remitted phases of the illness.[10-12] We have previously reported on a comprehensive neuropsychological examination of 36 schizophrenic patients while not receiving medication and 36 demographically balanced normal controls.[13] Against a background of global impairment, the patients were most impaired on tests of learning and memory functions. We have recently conducted a similar analysis using an expanded sample of 68 patients and 68 controls and found that memory, attention, abstraction, and language functions were more severely affected compared with spatial and sensory-motor functions in the patients.[14] We have also found that patients' performance is independent of current or prior treatment with neuroleptic medication.[15] Together, these findings argue against the interpretation that the cognitive deficits observed in schizophrenia are secondary to active psychotic symptoms, neuroleptic treatment, or other illness factors and suggest instead that the deficits mark the presence of a stable underlying vulnerability to the disorder. Studies that examine the same patients over time do not, however, address the issue of whether the deficits are genetically mediated.

Studies of affected and unaffected first-degree relatives permit examination of the putative heritability of cognitive disturbances in schizophrenia. Several studies have compared neuropsychological test performance of children of schizophrenic parents with that of children of normal parents.[16-32] A consistent finding of these studies is that a subgroup of the schizophrenic parents' offspring performs relatively poorly on tests of attention,[16-22] learning,[23-25] verbal ability,[26-29] and neuromotor functions,[30-32] supporting the notion that some offspring inherit a liability to schizophrenia that is reflected during childhood in the form of cognitive and motor impairments. A major advantage of these studies is that cognitive and motor functioning were assessed prospectively, before schizophrenia developed in any of the offspring or they received psychiatric treatment. It remains to be determined, however, if impaired functioning in these areas does in fact predict an eventual diagnosis in the schizophrenia spectrum.

Table 2. Neuropsychological Test Battery by Functional Domain*

Abstraction
Categories and perseverative responses, Wisconsin Card Sorting Test (Heaton[47])†
Stroop Color and Word Test (Golden[54])†
Trail-Making Test B, HRB (Reitan and Wolfson[46])†
Attention
Stroop Color and Word Test[54]†
Trail-Making Test A, HRB[46]†
Digit Span and Digit Symbol, WAIS-R (Wechsler[55])
Vigilance and Distractibility, Continuous Performance Test (Gordan[56])†
Spatial ability
Benton Line Orientation Test (Benton et al[57])†
Block Design, WAIS-R[55]
Rosen Drawing Test (Kareken et al[14])
Verbal memory
Logical Memory Passages (immediate and 30-min delay), WMS (Wechsler[45] and Russell[58])
Learning trials 1 through 5, California Verbal Learning Test (Delis et al[59])†
Paired Associate Learning Test, WMS[45,58]
Spatial memory
Design Reproduction (immediate and 30-min delay), WMS[45,58]†
Facial Recognition Test (immediate and 30-min delay) (Gur et al[60])
Language
Controlled Oral Word Association (letters C, F, and L), MAE (Benton and Hamsher[61])
Animal Naming and Boston Naming Tests, BDAE (Goodglass and Kaplan[62])
Comprehension of Complex Ideational Material, BDAE[62]
Sentence Repetition, MAE[61]
Reading Recognition, WRAT-R (Jastrak and Wilkinson[48])
Vocabulary, WAIS-R[55]
Token Test, MAE[61]†
Sensory-motor
Reitan-Klove Sensory-Perceptual Exam, HRB[46]
Thumb-Finger Sequential Touch (right and left hands), LNNB[63]†
Finger Tapping (right and left hands), HRB[46]

**HRB indicates Halstead-Reitan Battery; WAIS-R, Wechsler Adult Intelligence Scale–Revised; WMS, Wechsler Memory Scale; MAE, Multilingual Aphasia Examination; BDAE, Boston Diagnostic Aphasia Examination; WRAT-R, Wide Range Achievement Test–Revised; and LNNB, Luria Nebraska Neuropsychological Battery.*

†Included in the abbreviated (intake) version of the battery.

Another group of studies has examined nonschizophrenic siblings (and in some cases parents) of schizophrenic probands.[33-41] Siblings share on average 50% of their genes with the probands and are therefore expected to manifest endophenotypic markers of genetic predisposition to schizophrenia more frequently (and to a greater degree) than unrelated, normal individuals from the general population. In addition, because siblings control for a share of the (nonschizophrenia-related) between-family genetic and environmental variability in brain function, they provide a better estimate of the baseline level of functioning of a proband than do unrelated normal individuals. It is thus possible to assess the sensitivity of particular cognitive deficits as indicators of schizophrenia within families. In general, both schizophrenics and their nonschizophrenic siblings have been found to be impaired neuropsychologically compared with normal controls, particularly on tests of sustained attention,[33-39] abstraction (ie, perseverative tendencies),[37-40] and language functions.[37-39,41] These studies are also consistent in demonstrating that all or nearly all schizophrenics are more impaired on these measures than the well individuals in their own families, which represents a substantial improvement over the 50% to 60% sensitivity estimates obtained in group comparisons with unrelated, normal controls. None of these studies, however, employed a comprehensive test battery that would permit one to determine if these areas of deficit are selectively associated with familial risk for schizophrenia.

A recent study examined 16 sets of identical twins discordant for schizophrenia and seven sets of normal identical twins with a battery of 26 neuropsychological tests.[42] The schizophrenic twins performed more poorly on all of the tests relative to their unaffected co-twins, and significantly so on tests of verbal memory, abstraction, attention, and verbal fluency. Using a Bonferroni adjusted significance level of .002, the unaffected co-twins of schizophrenics did not differ significantly from the normal twin pairs on any of the tests. However, their mean scores were in the deviant direction on 20 of the 24 comparisons, and without the Bonferroni correction, their mean scores were significantly different from those of the normal twins on tests of attention and verbal memory, with trends toward differences on tests of abstraction and language functions. This study has been criticized as having insufficient power to detect differences between the unaffected co-twins and the normal twins.[43,44] In fact, the unaffected co-twins of schizophrenics differed from the normal twins by a factor of about 1 SD on tests of verbal memory, attention, abstraction, and language (ie, Δ=0.82, 1.30, 1.14, and 0.74 for the Logical Prose subtest of the Wechsler Memory Scale,[45] Trail Making Test A of the Halstead-Reitan Battery,[46] number of categories obtained on the Wisconsin Card Sorting Test,[47] and Reading score on the Wide Range Achievement Test–Revised,[48] respectively). These substantial effect sizes would have been apparent if the unaffected co-twins' data had been converted to *z* scores, using the means and SDs of the normal twin-pair group. It is critical to note that, given the magnitude of these differences, the failure of the probability values to fall below the authors' criterion for significance is primarily a reflection of the sample sizes involved. (The significance level of a *t* test is governed by the magnitude of the mean difference, the variances, and the sample sizes.) Another limitation of this study (and most of the other investigations involving adult relatives of schizophrenics) is that neither probands nor relatives were excluded on the basis of secondary factors that could affect brain function, such as somatic or neurologic illness, substance abuse disorder, other psychiatric disorders, history of head injury, and, in the case of the probands, current or prior treatment with neuroleptic medication.

In the present study, we performed a comprehensive neuropsychological examination of schizophrenic probands, their nonschizophrenic siblings, and a large sample of demographically balanced normal controls. Each group was carefully screened to exclude individuals with a history of head injury, substance use, axis I psychiatric disorder other than schizophrenia, or major medical illness. Patients underwent evaluation twice, once at intake when half had never received neuroleptic medication and the other half had received none for a minimum of 2 weeks, and again at a 2- to 4-week follow-up, after stabilization with neuroleptic medication. Test data for the probands and siblings were converted to *z* scores (using the means and SDs of the normal control group), and summary measures were formed for seven functional domains: abstraction, attention, spatial reasoning, verbal memory, visual memory, language, and sensory-motor functions. This procedure permitted evaluation of group differences in magnitude of deficit as well as in shape of deficit profile.

Based on the work reviewed above, we predicted that (1) both probands and their nonschizophrenic siblings would be deviant neuropsychologically compared with normal controls, with siblings' performance intermediate between that of probands and controls; (2) the shapes of the deficit profiles of probands and siblings would be similar, such that in both groups, attention, abstraction, language, and verbal memory functions would be more severely affected relative to other functions; and (3) most or all probands would be deviant in these areas compared with their well siblings.

RESULTS

PROFILE ANALYSIS

The *z* score profile on the neuropsychological battery of the sibling pairs discordant for schizophrenia and the normal controls is shown in the **Figure**. Separate lines are

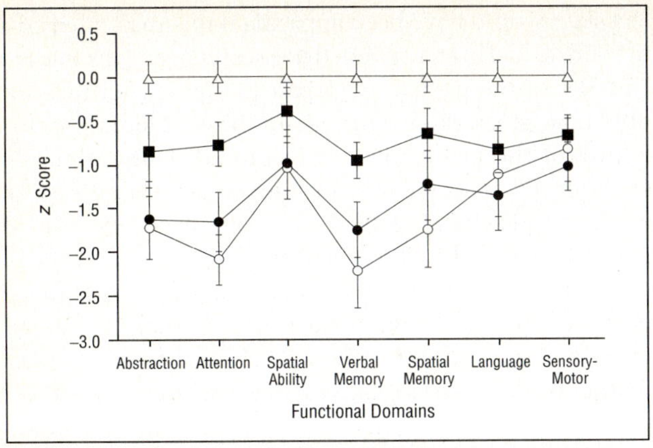

Neuropsychological profiles (mean z scores [±SEMs]) of schizophrenic probands while not receiving neuroleptic medication (open circles) and after stabilization with neuroleptic medication (solid circles), nonschizophrenic siblings of probands (squares), and demographically balanced normal controls (triangles). Probands differed significantly from controls on all domains, regardless of medication status. Siblings differed significantly from controls on all domains except for spatial ability. The results of the proband vs sibling comparisons are given in Table 3. Domains are defined in Table 2 and the "Subjects and Methods" section of the text.

Table 3. *t* Statistics and Significance Levels for Pair-wise Contrasts on Seven Functional Domains*

	Probands Receiving No Medication		Probands Receiving Medication		
Domain	P vs C	P vs S	P vs C	P vs S	S vs C
Asbtraction	−4.6†	−5.3†	−3.9†	−1.6	−2.2‡
Attention	−7.5†	−3.4§	−5.7†	−2.9§	−2.7§
Spatial ability	−2.5§	−1.1	−3.5†	−1.4	−1.4
Verbal memory	−6.7†	−4.9†	−6.1†	−5.3†	−3.5†
Spatial memory	−4.7†	−4.2†	−3.7†	−1.9	−2.0‡
Language	−2.9§	−0.1	−4.2†	−2.6§	−2.7§
Sensory-motor	−2.1‡	−1.8	−4.2†	−1.1	−2.9§

**P vs C indicates probands vs controls (t's for independent samples); P vs S, probands vs siblings (matched-pair t's); and S vs C, siblings vs controls (t's for independent samples).*
†P<.001.
‡P<.05.
§P<.01.

used to plot probands' performance measures while not receiving and while receiving neuroleptic medication. By definition, the normal control group has a mean of 0, an SD of 1, and an SEM of 0.18 (ie, $1/\sqrt{31}$) on each measure.

There were no differences between the results of the analyses using probands' data while not receiving and while receiving medication. In view of this, and for ease of reporting, only the multivariate analysis involving probands' follow-up measures will be described. There was a significant overall main effect of group ($F[2,58]=16.4$; $P<.0001$) and significant overall differences between probands and controls ($F[1,58]=31.0$; $P<.0001$) and between siblings and controls ($F[1,58]=9.5$; $P<.003$). These results indicate that both schizophrenics and their nonschizophrenic siblings are neuropsychologically impaired compared with normal individuals from the general population. In addition, there was a significant overall difference between probands and siblings ($F[1,58]=5.4$; $P<.05$). This finding, combined with the lack of a significant interaction of this group contrast with domain of functioning ($F[1,58]=0.6$ [not significant]), indicates that there is a quantitative but not qualitative difference in cognitive functioning between probands and their siblings (ie, the shape of their deficit profiles is the same). By multivariate contrast analysis, it was determined that the mean scores on the ABS, ATT, VME, and LNG measures were significantly lower compared with those of the SPT, VME, and SMO measures in probands ($F[1,58]=7.1$; $P<.01$), with a nonsignificant trend in the same direction in siblings ($F[1,58]=2.4$; $P<.15$).

The results of the univariate analyses are shown in **Table 3**. Probands obtained significantly lower mean scores on every measure compared with normal controls, regardless of medication status. Probands' mean scores were also lower than those of the siblings on every measure, and significantly so on ABS (while not receiving medication), ATT (while not receiving and while receiving medication), VME (while not receiving and while receiving medication), LNG (while not receiving medication), and SPT (while receiving medication). Siblings scored significantly lower than normal controls on all measures except SPT.

STABILITY OF COGNITIVE DEFICITS ACROSS CHANGES IN MEDICATION STATUS AND CLINICAL STATE

In the multivariate analysis of probands' performance measures while not receiving and while receiving medication, neither the overall main effect of medication status nor the interaction of medication status with domain was significant ($F[1,14]=0.0$ [not significant] and $F[6,78]=0.6$ [not significant], respectively). Thus, probands' cognitive deficits were robust with respect to the presence or absence of neuroleptic treatment.

To determine whether the stability of probands' cognitive deficits was independent of changes in clinical state, we examined change in the severity of positive and negative symptoms from the intake assessment to the time of the follow-up cognitive testing. Probands' overall positive symptom scores (ie, the average of all SAPS items) declined significantly from intake assessment to follow-up (mean[±SD] at intake, 1.27±.43; mean[±SD] at follow-up, 0.47±.33; $t(14)=4.76$; $P<.001$). Each of the SAPS subscales (ie, Hallucinations, Delusions, Bizarre Behavior, and Formal Thought Disorder) followed this pattern. With the exception of SPT, probands' neuropsychological domain scores at either assessment were not significantly correlated with their SAPS scores at intake

Table 4. Outlier and Pair-wise Hit Rates on Seven Functional Domains*

	% of Scores of Probands When Receiving No Medication			% of Scores of Probands When Receiving Medication			% of Scores of Siblings	
	<C Min	<S Min	<Sib	<C Min	<S Min	<Sib	<C1	<C Min
Domain								
Abstraction	31	25	100	33	33	67	56	6
Attention	63	0	81	60	0	73	31	25
Spatial ability	33	0	75	27	0	60	38	19
Verbal memory	40	13	86	67	27	93	44	6
Spatial memory	47	42	92	47	33	60	44	38
Language	0	23	46	60	27	80	44	31
Sensory-motor	29	50	71	47	7	53	44	44
Means	35	22	79	49	18	69	43	24

For probands, <C min indicates scores that were below the normal control group minimum; <S min, below the sibling group minimum; and <Sib, below those of their own siblings. For siblings, <C1 indicates scores that were 1 SD or more below the control group mean; <C min, below the control group minimum.

or follow-up assessment or with their degree of improvement in positive symptoms across assessments (ρ's ranged from −.47 to .23 [not significant]). Probands' SPT scores correlated negatively with their SAPS scores at the initial assessment (ρ=−.67; $P<.05$) and positively with their SAPS scores at the follow-up assessment (ρ=.52; $P<.06$). Their degree of improvement in positive symptoms across assessments was significantly negatively correlated with their SPT scores at both assessments (ρ=−.83 and −.76, respectively; $P<.01$). Thus, with the exception of SPT, probands' neuropsychological performance appears to be independent of positive psychotic symptoms and of changes in positive psychotic symptoms over time.

Probands' overall negative symptoms scores (ie, average of all SANS items) did not change significantly from intake assessment to follow-up (mean[±SD] at intake, 2.12±.92; mean[±SD] at follow-up, 1.86±.83; $t[14]=0.25$ [not significant]). Each of the SANS subscales (ie, Flat Affect, Alogia, Apathy, Anhedonia, and Attentional Impairment) followed this pattern. Although probands' overall level of negative symptoms paralleled their cognitive deficits in terms of stability across measurement points, negative symptoms are not likely to explain the probands' impaired neuropsychological performance, since there were no significant correlations between any of the probands' neuropsychological domain scores at either assessment and their SANS scores at intake or follow-up assessment or their degree of improvement in negative symptoms across assessments (ρ's ranged from −.35 to .25 [not significant]).

SENSITIVITY ANALYSES

Table 4 gives the sensitivities of each neuropsychological summary measure as an indicator of schizophrenia using both outlier (between-family) and matched-pair (within-family) approaches. While not receiving medication, from 0% to 63% of probands scored below the control group minima on these measures (cross-domain average, 35%), and from 0% to 50% scored below the sibling group minima (average, 22%). In contrast, from 46% to 100% of probands scored below the values obtained by the nonschizophrenic siblings in their own families (average, 79%). Similar results were obtained using probands' measures while receiving medication. The highest within-family sensitivity rates were for ABS while not receiving medication (100%) and for VME while receiving medication (93%).

Table 4 also gives the percentages of siblings who were classified as deviant on each summary measure based on their degree of difference from the normal control group. From 31% to 56% of the sibling sample scored 1 SD or below the control group mean on the seven summary measures (cross-domain average, 43%), and from 6% to 44% scored below the control group minima (average, 24%). Of the 11 siblings who had one or more summary scores that were 1 SD or more below the control group mean, six had diagnoses of probable or definite SPD, compared with zero of five siblings whose summary scores were in the normal range ($P<.058$, Fisher's Exact Test).

COMMENT

Schizophrenics and their nonschizophrenic siblings were found to be impaired neuropsychologically compared with a demographically balanced sample of normal individuals from the general population. The shapes of the deficit profiles of probands and siblings were similar, with the nonschizophrenic siblings' performance intermediate between that of the schizophrenic siblings and the normal controls on all measures of functioning. Cognitive functioning in probands was found to be independent of medication status and clinical state. Among the

sibling group, those with probable and certain diagnoses of SPD were more impaired compared with those without schizophrenia-spectrum diagnoses.

Together, these findings support the hypothesis that impairments in selected areas of information processing are markers of genetic vulnerability to schizophrenia. There are several advantages of our study over prior investigations in substantiating this hypothesis.

FIRST, WE EXCLUDED any individual with a history of substance abuse, axis I disorder other than schizophrenia, neurologic condition, head injury with loss of consciousness, or medical illness. The application of these exclusion criteria, together with the use of a case-control matching procedure that balanced the groups on all major demographic characteristics, ensures that the differences in cognitive functioning between probands, siblings, and controls are not confounded with any known nonschizophrenia-related acquired or inherited brain disorder.

Second, our study had sufficient statistical power to detect differences between nonschizophrenic siblings of schizophrenic probands and normal controls. In particular, our ability to detect differences was greater than that of the study by Goldberg et al[42] discussed above, despite the fact that there were 16 discordant relatives in each study. Power was increased in our study in three ways: (1) the use of a larger group of normal individuals reduced the amount of error associated with the performance measures in the controls; (2) the use of a multivariate rather than exclusively univariate approach to data analysis necessitated a less severe adjustment of the significance level since significant overall differences were required before examining univariate effects; and (3) the use of summary measures rather than individual test scores reduced the chance of type I error since fewer comparisons were conducted.

Third, our study employed a repeated-measures design to examine the effects of medication status on cognitive functioning in the probands. The lack of significant differences between probands' intake and follow-up performance measures, combined with the finding that probands' levels of positive symptoms were reduced to the mild range at the follow-up assessment, allows us to rule out neuroleptic treatment and the effects of acute psychosis as explanations of the probands' cognitive deficits. In addition, with the exception of spatial reasoning, none of the neuropsychological functions were significantly correlated with levels of positive symptoms at intake or follow-up assessment or with degree of improvement in positive symptoms across assessments. While probands' levels of negative symptoms paralleled their cognitive deficits in terms of stability across measurement points, negative symptoms are also not a likely explanation for their impaired cognitive performance since we could detect no significant relationships between neuropsychological functioning and severity of negative symptoms at intake or follow-up assessment or degree of improvement in negative symptoms across assessments. It is of course possible that two influences were operating with opposite effect across measurement points, ie, practice effects operating to improve performance and neuroleptic effects operating to reduce performance. This explanation seems unlikely, however, since it is difficult to imagine how such a complex interaction of effects would produce precisely the same profile of deficits as observed at intake.

Fourth, we were able to address the issue of selectivity of deficits by employing a comprehensive test battery and expressing the data as standard equivalents in seven major functional domains. In probands, ABS, ATT, VME, and LNG functions were significantly more impaired relative to SPT, SME, and SMO functions. A trend in this direction was also observed in siblings but was not significant. A larger sample size will thus be needed to investigate the issue of selectivity of deficits in siblings. In addition, future efforts should ensure that the tests used in the different domains of functioning are similar in terms of reliability and degree of difficulty.[65,66] Although the reliabilities of the instruments used in our study are comparable across domains, the tests were not specifically calibrated to the same degree of difficulty.

Fifth, the use of siblings controlled for a share of the nonschizophrenia-related, between-family variability in cognitive performance and allowed us to examine the sensitivity of neuropsychological deficits as indicators of schizophrenia in families. On average, 80% of probands were found to be more impaired than the nonschizophrenic siblings from their own families, compared with only 20% of probands whose values were below the range of the sibling group and 35% of probands whose values were below the range of unrelated normal controls.

Our study also has some limitations. Siblings typically share many environmental characteristics in addition to sharing, on average, 50% of their genes. Thus, the effects of environment and heredity are confounded in the sibling design. However, shared environmental factors are not a likely explanation for the observed similarities in cognitive functioning in probands and their siblings, for the following three major reasons: (1) adoption studies have demonstrated that shared environment makes a negligible contribution to schizophrenia[5-7]; (2) in records-based studies conducted in Scandinavia, there is no evidence that perinatal complications and other environmental sources of brain lesions run in the families of schizophrenics[67,68]; and (3) in our study, we excluded individuals on the basis of all major postnatal environmental causes of brain injury. On the other hand, there is very good reason to suspect that the differences observed between the probands and siblings in our study

are environmental. In studies of monozygotic (MZ) twins discordant for schizophrenia, the schizophrenic twin has consistently been found to have suffered more complications during delivery.[67,69] In addition, in the Copenhagen schizophrenia high-risk project, offspring of schizophrenic mothers in whom schizophrenia developed had significantly more pregnancy and birth complications than those who remained healthy or in whom SPD developed.[70,71]

It is also important to note that the design typically used to investigate genetic vs environmental effects, ie, discordant MZ twin pairs, is superior to the discordant sibling design only with respect to the interpretation of intrapair differences, which in the case of MZ twins can be confidently attributed to environmental sources. The discordant MZ twin design is no more definitive than the discordant sibling design in its ability to separate genetic and environmental sources of differences between nonschizophrenic relatives and normal controls. In fact, discordant MZ twins may be less advantageous in this context than discordant siblings. That is, because a much larger percentage of the siblings of schizophrenic probands are expected not to be schizophrenic than are co-twins (ie, 90% vs 40%), selection on the basis of discordancy in twins may bias the sample composition toward a less genetic form of the disorder than selection on the basis of discordancy in siblings. On other hand, it is important to emphasize that in the only published study examining neuropsychological functioning in MZ twins discordant for schizophrenia,[42] the effect sizes for the differences between the nonschizophrenic twins and normal controls were quite similar to those observed in the present study (ie, on the order of 1 SD).

In view of the large body of evidence indicating a genetic relationship between schizophrenia and SPD,[72-78] the finding that the subgroup of siblings with deviant neuropsychological test scores were more likely to have schizotypal features than those without deviant test scores provides further support for the hypothesis that the deficits observed in our study are associated with genetic predisposition to schizophrenia. The present findings also raise the possibility that neuropsychological deficits may be more sensitive and reliable indicators of the schizotypal phenotype than the *DSM-III-R* criteria for SPD.

The results of our study are consistent with those of numerous prior investigations[14-42] that have examined co-twins, siblings, offspring, and parents of schizophrenics in indicating that a subgroup of these relatives is impaired neuropsychologically, possibly more so in the domains of ABS, ATT, VME, and LNG functions than those of SPT, SME, and SMO functions.

This pattern of results tentatively suggests the hypothesis that temporal and frontal lobe dysfunctions are part of an inherited neurobiological substrate of schizophrenia. Medial temporal lobe structures (including the hippocampus, entorhinal cortex, and parahippocampal gyrus) have been shown to play important roles in explicit or declarative memory, such as recall of word lists and other semantic material.[79,80] Using the xenon-133 clearance method to measure cerebral blood flow during neurobehavioral challenge tasks, we have demonstrated that schizophrenics show abnormal regional activation in the temporal lobes during recall testing and that this anomalous activation pattern is correlated with poorer memory performance.[81] It is also interesting to note that abnormalities of medial temporal lobe structures are the most consistent findings of postmortem and MRI studies of schizophrenics and that some of the postmortem findings have been attributed to genetic or teratogenic disturbances of brain development during gestation, further supporting the notion of the temporal lobes as sites of vulnerability in this disorder.[82,83] The frontal lobes have also been shown to mediate some aspects of memory (eg, memory for temporal order)[84] as well as other higher cognitive functions that have been found to be deviant in schizophrenics and their first-degree relatives, including abstract reasoning, mental control, and attention.[85,86] While structural abnormalities and resting metabolic deficits in the frontal region of schizophrenics remain controversial,[87,88] prefrontal functional deficits during neurobehavioral challenge tests appear to be reliable.[89,90] Finally, there is a large body of evidence indicating that language functions are left-hemisphere lateralized in most right-handed individuals.[91] Some studies have suggested that structural and functional abnormalities may be more pronounced in the left compared with the right hemisphere of schizophrenics.[92] In view of the tendency noted in our study for siblings to have greater deficits on verbal compared with spatial functions, the left hemisphere may also be compromised to a greater degree in relatives.

IF SCHIZOPHRENICS and their nonschizophrenic relatives share a common underlying neurobiological vulnerability to schizophrenia as our results suggest, it will be necessary to isolate factors that are responsible for expression of psychosis in some individuals with this vulnerability but not others. One possibility is suggested by a diathesis-stress framework of schizophrenia-spectrum disorders.[66,93,94] According to this model, schizophrenia and SPD are unified by a common genetic diathesis, one expression of which is cellular migratory failure and other signs of dysgenesis in various regions of the cerebral cortex. Among individuals with this genetic diathesis, subcortical abnormalities in addition to the genetically mediated cortical abnormalities develop in those who experience severe delivery complications; the subcortical abnormalities then contribute to the development of overt schizophrenia.

Further work is also needed to address the selectiv-

ity of the association of deficits in verbal memory, attention, language, and executive functions with familial risk for schizophrenia and to investigate whether deficits in these areas of functioning are mediated by structural and/or metabolic disturbances in specific brain regions.

Accepted for publication April 5, 1994.

This research was supported by grants MH48207 (Dr Cannon) and MH43880 (Dr R. E. Gur) from the National Institute of Mental Health, Rockville, Md.

Address correspondence to Department of Psychology, University of Pennsylvania, 3815 Walnut St, Philadelphia, PA 19104 (Dr Cannon).

REFERENCES

1. Gottesman II, Shields J. *Schizophrenia: The Epigenetic Puzzle.* New York, NY: Cambridge University Press; 1982.
2. Fisher M. Psychoses in the offspring of schizophrenic monozygotic twins and their normal co-twins. *Br J Psychiatry.* 1971;118:43-52.
3. Kendler KS. Overview: a current perspective on twin studies of schizophrenia. *Am J Psychiatry.* 1983;140:1413-1425.
4. Stephens DA, Atkinson MW, Kay DWK, Roth M, Garside RF. Psychiatric morbidity in parents and sibs of schizophrenics and non-schizophrenics. *Br J Psychiatry.* 1975;127:97-108.
5. Kety SS. The significance of genetic factors in the etiology of schizophrenia: results from the national study of adoptees in Denmark. *J Psychiatr Res.* 1987; 4:423-429.
6. Kety SS, Rosenthal D, Wender PH, Schulsinger F, Jacobsen B. The biological and adoptive families of adopted individuals who become schizophrenic: prevalance of mental illness and other characteristics. In: Wynne LC, Cromwell RL, Mytthysse S, eds. *The Nature of Schizophrenia: New Approaches to Research and Treatment.* New York, NY: John Wiley & Sons Inc; 1978:25-37.
7. Heston LL. Psychiatric disorders in foster home reared children of schizophrenics. *Br J Psychiatry.* 1966;112:819-825.
8. Gottesman II, McGuffin P, Farmer AE. Clinical genetics as clues to the "real" genetics of schizophrenia (a decade of modest gains while playing for time). *Schizophr Bull.* 1987;13:23-47.
9. DeLisi LE, Goldin LR, Gershon ES. Studies of biological factors associated with the inheritance of schizophrenia: a selective review. *J Psychiatr Res.* 1987;21: 507-513.
10. Spring BJ, Zubin J. Attention and information processing as indicators of vulnerability to schizophrenic episodes. In: Wynne LC, Cromwell RL, Matthysse S, eds. *The Nature of Schizophrenia: Approaches to Research and Treatment.* New York, NY: John Wiley & Sons Inc; 1978:366-375.
11. Nuechterlein KH, Dawson ME. Information processing dysfunctions in the developmental course of schizophrenic disorders. *Schizophr Bull.* 1984;10:160-203.
12. Asarnow RF, MacCrimmon DJ. Residual performance deficit in clinically remitted schizophrenia: a marker of schizophrenia? *J Abnorm Psychol.* 1978; 87:597-608.
13. Saykin AJ, Gur RC, Gur RE, Mozley PD, Mozley LH, Resnick SM, Kester B, Stafiniak P. Neuropsychological function in schizophrenia: selective impairment in memory and learning. *Arch Gen Psychiatry.* 1991;48:618-624.
14. Kareken DA, Gur RE, Gur RC, Resnick SM, Mozley PD, Mozley LH, Saykin AJ. Cognitive functioning and ventricular brain ratio in schizophrenia. *Neuropsychology.* In press.
15. Saykin AJ, Shtasel DL, Gur RE, Kester DB, Mozley LH, Stafiniak P, Gur RC. Neuropsychological deficits in neuroleptic naive, first-episode schizophrenia. *Arch Gen Psychiatry.* 1994;51:124-131.
16. Asarnow RF, Steffy RA, MacCrimmon DJ, Cleghorn JM. An attentional assessment of foster children at risk for schizophrenia. *J Abnorm Psychol.* 1977;86: 267-275.
17. Cohler B, Grunebaum H, Weiss J, Gamer E, Gallant D. Disturbances of attention among schizophrenic, depressed, and well mothers and their young children. *J Child Psychol Psychiatry.* 1977;18:115-135.
18. Erlenmeyer-Kimling L, Cornblatt BA. A summary of attentional findings in the New York High-Risk Project. *J Psychiatr Res.* 1992;26:405-426.
19. Erlenmeyer-Kimling L, Golden RR, Cornblatt BA. A taxometric analysis of cognitive and neuromotor variables in children at risk for schizophrenia. *J Abnorm Psychol.* 1989;98:203-208.
20. Gamer E, Gallant D, Grunebaum HU, Cohler BJ. Children of psychotic mothers: performance of 3-year-old children on tests of attention. *Arch Gen Psychiatry.* 1977;34:592-597.
21. Nuechterlein KH. Signal detection in vigilance tasks and behavioral attitudes among offspring of schizophrenic mothers and among hyperactive children. *J Abnorm Psychol.* 1983;92:4-28.
22. Rutschmann J, Cornblatt B, Erlenmeyer-Kimling L. Sustained attention in children at risk for schizophrenia: findings with two visual continuous performance tests in a new sample. *J Abnorm Child Psychol.* 1986;14:365-385.
23. Driscoll RM. Intentional and incidental learning in children vulnerable to psychopathology. In: Watt NF, Anthony EJ, Wynne LC, Rolf JE, eds. *Children at Risk for Schizophrenia: A Longitudinal Perspective.* New York, NY: Cambridge University Press; 1984:320-326.
24. Klein RH, Salzman LF. Response-contingent learning in children at risk. In: Watt NF, Anthony EJ, Wynne LC, Rolf JE, eds. *Children at Risk for Schizophrenia: A Longitudinal Perspective.* New York, NY: Cambridge University Press; 1984:371-375.
25. Rutschmann J, Cornblatt B, Erlenmeyer-Kimling L. Auditory recognition memory in children at risk for schizophrenia: report on a verbal continuous recognition task. *Psychiatr Res.* 1980;3:151-161.
26. Gruzelier J, Mednick S, Schulsinger F. Lateralized impairments in the WISC profile of children at risk for psychopathology. In: Gruzelier J, Flor-Henry P, eds. *Hemispheric Asymmetries in Function of Psychopathology.* Amsterdam, the Netherlands: Elsevier Science Publishing; 1979:105-110.
27. Harvey P, Weintraub S, Neal J. Speech competence of children vulnerable to psychopathology. *J Abnorm Child Psychol.* 1982;10:373-388.
28. Worland J, Hesselbrock V. The intelligence of children and their parents with schizophrenia and related illness. *J Child Psychol Psychiatr.* 1980;21:191-201.
29. Vachon RA. Neuropsychological and intellectual functioning of children at genetic risk for major mental disorder. *Dissert Abstracts Int.* 1989;50:2638.
30. Fish B. Neurobiologic antecedents of schizophrenia in children: evidence for an inherited, congenital, neurointegrative defect. *Arch Gen Psychiatry.* 1977; 34:1297-1313.
31. Marcus J, Hans SL, Mednick SA, Schulsinger F, Michelsen N. Neurological dysfunctioning in offspring of schizophrenics in Israel and Denmark: a replication analysis. *Arch Gen Psychiatry.* 1985;42:753-761.
32. Fish B, Marcus J, Hans SL, Auerbach JG. Infants at risk for schizophrenia: sequelae of a neurointegrative defect: a review and replication analysis of pandysmaturation in the Jerusalem Infant Development Study. *Arch Gen Psychiatry.* 1992;49:221-235.
33. DeAmicis LA, Cromwell RL. Reaction time crossover in process schizophrenic patients, their relatives, and control subjects. *J Nerv Ment Dis.* 1979;167:593-600.
34. Wood RL, Cook M. Attentional deficit in the siblings of schizophrenics. *Psychol Med.* 1979;9:465-467.
35. Maier W, Franke P, Hain C, Kopp B, Rist F. Neuropsychological indicators of the vulnerability to schizophrenia. *Prog Neuropsychopharmacol Biol Psychiatry.* 1992;16:703-715.
36. Mirsky AF, Lochhead SJ, Jones BP, Kugelmass S, Walsh D, Kender KS. On familial factors in the attentional deficit in schizophrenia: a review and report of two new subject samples. *J Psychiatr Res.* 1992;26:383-403.
37. Steinhauer SR, Zubin J, Condray R, Shaw DB, Peters JL, Vankamen DP. Electrophysiological and behavioral signs of attention disturbance in schizophrenics and their siblings. In: Tamminga CA, Schultz SC, eds. *Advances in Neuropsychiatry and Psychopharmacology: Schizophrenia Research.* New York, NY: Raven Press; 1990;1:169-178.
38. Watson JR. Neuropsychological impairment among schizophrenic probands and their siblings. *Dissert Abstracts Int.* 1989;49:5535.
39. Pogue-Geile M. Siblings of schizophrenic probands: presence of neuropsychological impairments. *Schizophr Res.* 1990;3:62.
40. Franke P, Maier W, Hain C, Klingler T. Wisconsin Card Sorting Test: an indicator of vulnerability to schizophrenia? *Schizophr Res.* 1992;6:243-249.
41. Condray R, Steinhauer SR, Goldstein G. Language comprehension in schizophrenics and their brothers. *Biol Psychiatry.* 1992;32:790-802.

42. Goldberg TD, Ragland JD, Torrey EF, Gold JM. Neuropsychological assessment of monozygotic twins discordant for schizophrenia. *Arch Gen Psychiatry.* 1990;47:1066-1072.
43. Green MF. Neuropsychological performance in the unaffected twin. *Arch Gen Psychiatry.* 1992;49:247.
44. Goldberg TD, Torrey EF, Weinberger DR. In reply. *Arch Gen Psychiatry.* 1992; 49:247.
45. Wechsler D. A standardized memory scale for clinical use. *J Psychol.* 1945; 19:87-95.
46. Reitan RM, Wolfson D. *The Halstead-Reitan Neuropsychological Test Battery: Theory and Clinical Interpretation.* Tucson, Ariz: Neuropsychology Press; 1985.
47. Heaton RK. *Wisconsin Card Sorting Test Manual.* Odessa, Fla: Psychological Assessment Resources; 1981.
48. Jastak S, Wilkinson GS. *Wide Range Achievement Test-Revised, Manual.* Wilmington, Del: Jastak Associates Inc; 1984.
49. Spitzer RL, Williams JB, Gibbon M. *Instruction Manual for the Structured Clinical Interview for* DSM-III-R *(SCID).* New York: Biometrics Research Department, New York State Psychiatric Institute; 1987.
50. Andreasen NC. *The Scale for the Assessment of Positive Symptoms (SAPS).* Iowa City: The University of Iowa; 1984.
51. Andreasen NC. *The Scale for the Assessment of Negative Symptoms (SANS).* Iowa City: The University of Iowa; 1983.
52. Spitzer RL, Williams JB, Gibbon M, First MB. *Structured Clinical Interview for DSM-III-R Personality Disorders (SCID-II).* New York: Biometrics Research Department, New York State Psychiatric Institute; 1987.
53. American Psychiatric Association. *Diagnostic and Statistical Manual of Mental Disorders, Revised Third Edition.* Washington, DC: American Psychiatric Association; 1987.
54. Golden CJ. *Stroop Color and Word Test: A Manual for Clinical and Experimental Uses.* Chicago, Ill: Stoelting Co; 1978.
55. Wechsler D. *Wechsler Adult Intelligence Scale–Revised (WAIS-R), Manual.* Cleveland, Ohio: The Psychological Corp; 1981.
56. Gordan M. *Manual, Gordan Diagnostic System.* New York, NY: Gordan Diagnostic Systems Inc; 1986.
57. Benton AL, Hannay HJ, Varney NR. Visual perception of line direction in patients with unilateral brain disease. *Neurology.* 1975;25:907-910.
58. Russell EW. A multiple scoring method for assessment of complex memory functions. *J Consult Clin Psychol.* 1975;43:800-809.
59. Delis DC, Kramer JH, Kaplan E, Ober BA. *California Verbal Learning Test, Research Edition.* Cleveland, Ohio: The Psychological Corp; 1983.
60. Gur RC, Saykin AJ, Benton A, Kaplan E, Levin H, Kester B, Gur RE. 'Behavioral Imaging,' III: interexpert agreement and reliability of weightings. *Neuropsychiatry Neuropsychol Behav Neurol.* 1990;3:113-124.
61. Benton AL, Hamsher K. *Multilingual Aphasia Examination.* Iowa City: University of Iowa; 1976.
62. Goodglass H, Kaplan E. *The Assessment of Aphasia and Related Disorders.* 2nd ed. Philadelphia, Pa: Lea & Febiger; 1983.
63. Golden CJ, Hammeke TA, Purisch AD. *Luria-Nebraska Neuropsychological Battery, Manual.* Los Angeles, Calif: Western Psychological Services; 1980.
64. SAS Institute. *SAS/STAT User's Guide.* Cary, NC: SAS Institute; 1988.
65. Chapman LJ, Chapman JP. The measurement of differential deficits. *J Psychiatr Res.* 1978;14:303-311.
66. Chapman LJ, Chapman JP. Strategies for resolving the heterogeneity of schizophrenics and their relatives using cognitive measures. *J Abnorm Psychol.* 1989; 98:357-366.
67. McNeil TF, Kaij L. Obstetric factors and perinatal injuries. In: Tsuang MT, Simpson JC, eds. *Handbook of Schizophrenia: Nosology, Epidemiology and Genetics.* New York, NY: Elsevier Science Publishing Co; 1988;3:319-344.
68. Cannon TD, Mednick SA, Parnas J, Schulsinger F, Praestholm J, Vestergaard A. Developmental brain abnormalities in the offspring of schizophrenic mothers, I: contributions of genetic and perinatal contributions. *Arch Gen Psychiatry.* 1993;50:551-564.
69. Pollin W, Stabeneau JR. Biological, psychological and historical differences in a series of monozygotic twins discordant for schizophrenia. In: Rosenthal D, Kety SS, eds. *The Transmission of Schizophrenia.* Elmsford, NY: Pergamon Press Inc; 1968:317-332.
70. Parnas J, Schulsinger F, Teasdale TW, Schulsinger H, Feldman PM, Mednick SA. Perinatal complications and clinical outcome within the schizophrenia spectrum. *Br J Psychiatry.* 1982;140:416-420.
71. Cannon TD, Mednick SA, Parnas J. Antecedents of predominantly negative- and predominantly positive-symptom schizophrenia in a high-risk population. *Arch Gen Psychiatry.* 1990;47:622-632.
72. Parnas J, Cannon TD, Jacobsen B, Schulsinger H, Schulsinger F, Mednick SA. Lifetime *DSM-III-R* diagnostic outcomes in offspring of schizophrenic mothers: results from the Copenhagen High-Risk Study. *Arch Gen Psychiatry.* 1993; 50:707-714.
73. Kety SS. The significance of genetic factors in the etiology of schizophrenia: results from the national study of adoptees in Denmark. *J Psychiatr Res.* 1987; 4:423-429.
74. Farmer AE, McGuffin P, Gottesman II. Twin concordance for *DSM-III* schizophrenia. *Arch Gen Psychiatry.* 1987;44:634-641.
75. Kendler KS, Gruenberg AM, Strauss JS. An independent analysis of the Copenhagen sample of the Danish adoption study of schiozphrenia, II: the relationship between schizotypal personality disorder and schizophrenia. *Arch Gen Psychiatry.* 1981;38:982-984.
76. Baron M, Gruen R, Asnis L, Kane J. Familial relatedness of schizophrenia and schizotypal states. *Am J Psychiatry.* 1983;140:1437-1442.
77. Siever LJ, Silverman JM, Horvath TB, Klar H, Coccaro E, Keefe RSE, Pinkham L, Rinaldi P, Mohs RC, Davis KL. Increased morbid risk for schizophrenia-related disorders in relatives of schizotypal personality disordered patients. *Arch Gen Psychiatry.* 1990;47:634-640.
78. Thaker G, Adami H, Moran M, Lahti A, Cassady S. Psychiatric illnesses in families of subjects with schizophrenia-spectrum personality disorders: high morbidity risks for unspecified functional psychoses and schizophrenia. *Am J Psychiatry.* 1993;150:66-71.
79. Milner B. Psychological aspects of focal epilepsy and its neurosurgical management. *Adv Neurol.* 1975;8:299-321.
80. Squire LR, Butters N. *Neuropsychology of Memory.* New York, NY: Guilford Press; 1984.
81. Gur RE, Jaggi JL, Shtasel DL, Ragland JD, Gur RC. Cerebral blood flow in schizophrenia: effects of memory processing on regional activation. *Psychiatry Res.* In press.
82. Cannon TD, Marco E. Structural brain abnormalities as indicators of vulnerability to schizophrenia. *Schizophr Bull.* In press.
83. Bogerts B. The neuropathology of schizophrenia: pathophysiological and neurodevelopmental implications. In: Mednick SA, Cannon TD, Barr CE, Lyon M, eds. *Fetal Neural Development and Adult Schizophrenia.* New York, NY: Cambridge University Press; 1991:153-173.
84. Stuss DT, Kaplan EF, Benson DF, Weir WS, Chiulli S, Sarazin FF. Evidence for the involvement of orbitofrontal cortex in memory functions: an interference effect. *J Comp Physiol Psychol.* 1982;96:913-925.
85. Teuber H-L. Neuropsychology: effects of focal brain lesions. *Neuropsychol Res Prog Bull.* 1972;10:381-384.
86. Stuss DT, Benson DF, Kaplan EF, Weir WS, Naeser MA, Lieberman I, Ferrill D. The involvement of orbito-frontal cerebrum in cognitive tasks. *Neuropsychologia.* 1983;21:235-249.
87. Andreasen NC, Ehrhardt JC, Swayze VW II, Alliger RJ, Yuh WT, Cohen G, Ziebell S. Magnetic resonance imaging of the brain in schizophrenia: the pathophysiologic significance of structural abnormalities. *Arch Gen Psychiatry.* 1990; 47:35-44.
88. Buchsbaum MS. Positron emission tomography in schizophrenia. In: Meltzer HY, ed. *Psychopharmacology: The Third Generation of Progress.* New York, NY: Raven Press; 1987:783-792.
89. Weinberger DR, Berman KF, Zec RF. Physiologic dysfunction of dorsolateral prefrontal cortex in schizophrenia, I: regional cerebral blood flow evidence. *Arch Gen Psychiatry.* 1986;43:114-124.
90. Rubin P, Holm S, Friberg L, Videbech P, Andersen HS, Bendsen BB, Stromso N, Larsen JK, Lassen NA, Hemmingsen R. Altered modulation of prefrontal and subcortical brain activity in newly diagnosed schizophrenia and schizophreniform disorder: a regional cerebral blood flow study. *Arch Gen Psychiatry.* 1991;48:987-995.
91. Kolb B, Whishaw IQ. *Fundamentals of Human Neuropsychology.* New York, NY: WH Freeman; 1990.
92. Crow TJ. Temporal lobe asymmetries as the key to the etiology of schizophrenia. *Schizophr Bull.* 1990;16:433-443.
93. Cannon TD, Mednick SA, Parnas J. Genetic and perinatal determinants of structural brain deficits in schizophrenia. *Arch Gen Psychiatry.* 1989;46:883-889.
94. Cannon TD, Mednick SA. The schizophrenia high-risk project in Copenhagen: three decades of progress. *Acta Psychiatr Scand.* 1993;370:33-47.

Retrocallosal White Matter Abnormalities in Patients With Obsessive-compulsive Disorder

Many studies have implicated the orbital gyrus and caudate nucleus as factors in obsessive-compulsive disorder (OCD).[1] However, several recent neuropsychological and positron emission tomographic imaging studies have suggested that posterior parts of the brain may also be involved.[2-6] Based on these findings, it is possible that OCD symptoms might result from a problem with higher-level perceptual processing in the retrocallosal region, which could have an underlying structural substrate.

To study this hypothesis, using morphometric volume analysis of the retrocallosal region, we performed magnetic resonance imaging (MRI) scans of six female patients with OCD and eight female controls matched for age (mean±SD age of patients: 30.8±5.7 years; range, 20 to 37 years; mean age of controls: 27.3±5.3 years; range, 17 to 33 years), handedness, and education (five of six OCD patients had a college or graduate education; all controls had a college or graduate education). The patients had been moderately ill for over 3 years, had met *DSM-III-R* criteria for OCD as determined by the Structured Clinical Interview for Diagnosis, and had typical cleaning compulsions with one also having hoarding compulsions. One patient was not taking medication, two were taking clomipramine hydrochloride, two were receiving fluoxetine hydrochloride, and one was taking the combination of haloperidol decanoate, propantheline bromide, and alprazolam. Two patients also had major depression that developed after the onset of OCD, two patients had social phobia, and one patient had a history of an eating disorder. No control subjects were taking psychotropic medication and none had a history of psychiatric illness.

Coronal three-dimensional T_1-weighted spoiled gradient echo MRI scans were performed with a standard pulse sequence adapted for this purpose.[7] Analyses were performed blindly in a random sequence. To allow for reproducible comparisons across subjects, a three-dimensional coordinate transformation and positional normalization was performed.[8] Anatomic segmentation was performed on the normalized T_1-weighted images using intensity contour mapping and differential intensity contour algorithms.[7,9] Volumes were calculated by summing the total voxels from the structure outlines in all planes where a structure appeared.[9] Structures extracted from each scan included retrocallosal (defined as those slices posterior to and not including the corpus callosum) white and gray matter along with the regional lateral ventricle.[8] Corpus callosum length and total area were determined on the reformatted normalized midsagittal slice by adaptation of the method of Witelson.[10]

Retrocallosal Volume and Corpus Callosum Area and Length Comparisons Between OCD and Control Groups*

Region of Interest	OCD Group (n=6)	Control Group (n=8)	*t* (*df*=12)	*P*
Retrocallosal cortex, cm³				
R	88.2±9.9	98.2±8.9	2.0	.07
L	98.1±17.0	102.3±8.3	0.6	.55
Retrocallosal white matter, cm³				
R	55.4±7.2	64.2±6.5	2.4	.03
L	59.3±5.1	66.0±5.2	2.4	.03
Retrocallosal lateral ventricles, cm³				
R	0.41±0.24	1.23±0.99	2.0	.07
L	0.96±0.77	1.76±1.19	1.4	.18
Corpus callosum				
Total area cm²	7.25±0.52	7.37±0.61	.36	.72
Length, cm	7.52±0.34	7.52±0.44	0.0	.99

**OCD indicates obsessive-compulsive disorder. Values are mean±SD.*

The **Table** shows the results of the group comparisons. All retrocallosal volume measures showed right-sided decreases in the patient group compared with the control group (all *P* values ≤.07). Also, there was a left-sided decrease in retrocallosal white matter (*P*=.03) in the patient group. The corpus callosum had a similar area and anterior-posterior length between patients and controls, indicating that altered landmarks for the retrocallosal region did not account for cortex or white matter volume differences.

The ratios of cortex or white matter to ipsilateral retrocallosal total volume were similar between patients and controls. Given that white matter accounts for approximately one third of the total volume, a 10% to 15% change would not alter the ratios. The retrocallosal region includes the parieto-occipital area, which has been implicated bilaterally in multimodal sensory integration,[11] and on the right side it is associated with visuospatial memory.[2]

This pilot study showed no evidence of ventricular enlargement and a cortical volume less than normal on the right side but not on the left, which is more compatible with a neurodevelopmental process than with a neurodegenerative one.[12] The principal determinant of vol-

ume increase during the postnatal years is myelination and glial proliferation rather than cytogenesis and formation of new axonal pathways.[13] Impairment in the development of myelination might produce the observed differences, particularly as myelination continues into the third generation of life,[14] when OCD symptoms often appear. These findings are consistent with previous orbital gyrus and basal ganglia abnormalities[6,15] given the extensive connections between these regions and the retrocallosal region. A blindly analyzed morphometric study of complete brains in a larger cohort of OCD subjects and controls with tighter educational matching has just been completed and it has confirmed these preliminary findings.

Hans C. Breiter, MD
OCD Clinic-CNY-9
Massachusetts General Hospital
Charlestown, MA 02129
Pauline A. Filipek, MD
David N. Kennedy, PhD
Lee Baer, PhD
Dawn A. Pitcher
Michael J. Olivares
Boston, Mass
Perry F. Renshaw, MD, PhD
Belmont, Mass
Verne S. Caviness, Jr, MD, DPhil
Michael A. Jenike, MD
Boston, Mass

1. Baxter LR, Schwartz JM, Guze BH, Bergman K, Szuba MP. Neuroimaging in obsessive-compulsive disorder: seeking the mediating neuroanatomy. In: Jenike MA, Baer L, Minichiello WE, eds. *Obsessive-Compulsive Disorders: Theory and Management*. 2nd ed. Chicago, Ill: Year Book Medical Publishers Inc; 1990.
2. Boone KB, Ananth J, Philpott L, Kaur A, Djenderedjian A. Neuropsychological characteristics of nondepressed adults with obsessive-compulsive disorder. *Neuropsychiatry Neuropsychol Behav Neurol*. 1991;4:96-109.
3. Brown H, Kosslyn SM, Breiter HC, Baer L, Jenike MA. Can obsessive-compulsive patients discriminate between percepts and mental images? a signal detection analysis. *J Abnorm Psychol*. In press.
4. Nordahl TE, Benkelfat D, Semple WE, Gross M, King AC, Cohen RM. Cerebral glucose metabolic rates in obsessive-compulsive disorder. *Neuropsychopharmacology*. 1989;2:23-28.
5. Benkelfat C, Nordahl TE, Semple WE, King AC, Murphy DL, Cohen RM. Local cerebral glucose metabolic rates in obsessive-compulsive disorder. *Arch Gen Psychiatry*. 1990;47:840-848.
6. Rauch SL, Jenike MA, Alpert NM, Baer L, Breiter HCR, Savage CR, Fischman AJ. Regional cerebral blood flow measured during symptom provocation in obsessive-compulsive disorder using 15-labeled carbon dioxide and positron emission tomography. *Arch Gen Psychiatry*. 1994;51:62-70.
7. Filipek PA, Kennedy DN, Caviness VS, Rossnick SL, Spraggins TA, Starewicz PM. MRI-based morphometry: development and application to normal controls. *Ann Neurol*. 1989;25:61-67.
8. Filipek PA, Kennedy DN, Caviness VS. Neuroimaging. In: Boller F, Grafman J, eds. *Handbook of Neuropsychology*. Amsterdam, the Netherlands: Elsevier Science Publishers; 1992;6:301-329.
9. Kennedy DN, Filipek PA, Caviness VS. Anatomic segmentation and volumetric calculation in nuclear magnetic resonance imaging. *IEEE Trans Med Imaging*. 1989;8:1-7.
10. Witelson SE. Age and sex differences in the isthmus and genu of the human corpus callosum: a postmortem morphological study. *Brain*. 1989;112:799-835.
11. Mesulam M-M. Patterns in behavioral neuroanatomy: association areas, the limbic system, and hemispheric specialization. In: Mesulam M-M, ed. *Principles of Behavioral Neurology*. Philadelphia, Pa: FA Davis Co Publishers; 1985:259-288.
12. Adams RD, Victor M. *Principles of Neurology*. New York, NY: McGraw-Hill International Book Co; 1985:859-937.
13. Innocenti GM. The development of projections from cerebral cortex. *Progress in Sensory Physiology*. Heidelberg, Germany: Springer-Verlag; 1991;12.
14. Yakovlev PI, Lecours AR. The myelogenetic cycles of neuronal maturation of the brain. *Histopathology of the Nervous System*. Springfield, Ill: Charles C Thomas Publisher; 1982:3-70.
15. Luxenberg JS, Swedo SE, Flament AF, Friedland RP, Rapaport JL, Rapaport SI. Neuroanatomical abnormalities in obsessive-compulsive disorder detected with quantitative x-ray computed tomography. *Am J Psychiatry*. 1988; 145:1089-1093.

Mania Induced by Citalopram

Citalopram is an antidepressant that acts by inhibiting the reuptake of serotonin and that has been recently introduced into Switzerland. An investigation has shown that about 10% of the depressed patients who were treated using tricyclics or monoamine oxidase inhibitors have antidepressant-associated hypomanic or manic episodes.[1] Some authors[2-5] propose that such patients suffer from misdiagnosed bipolar disorder. Three serotonin reuptake inhibitors (fluoxetine,[6,7] fluvoxamine,[8,9] and paroxetine[10]) have been implicated in the appearance of manic and hypomanic episodes when used in therapeutic doses. This letter describes a manic episode induced by citalopram.

A major depressive episode of moderate intensity (296.32 of the *DSM-III-R*) associated with alcohol abuse (305.00 of the *DSM-III-R*) developed in a 52-year-old man with no personal or family history of depression or bipolar disorder. He required psychiatric hospitalization because of a high suicide risk. He was given febarbamate (a sedative commonly used in Europe) at a dosage of 600 mg/d for 5 days in association with citalopram (20 mg/d). A clear improvement in the depressive symptoms was observed after 4 weeks, with mood normalization after 6 weeks.

During the seventh week of treatment, a manic episode with insomnia, euphoria, psychomotor agitation, logorrhea, flight of ideas, disinhibition, injudicious spending, and delusional ideas of megalomania and persecution developed. This resulted in the extension of his hospitalization. Citalopram administration was discontinued and replaced by the administration of haloperidol (6 mg/d). The result was an improvement in the manic symptoms and mood normalization within 1 week. The patient left the hospital euthymic and with no further medication.

Although citalopram remains the most selective of the serotonin reuptake inhibitors, this case, which, to our knowledge, is the first case reported in the literature, demonstrates that a change toward a manic state can be induced by citalopram. Furthermore, the manic episode ends rapidly once citalopram administration is replaced by the administration of small doses of haloperidol. This rapid reaction to the treatment may suggest that secondary manic episodes caused by changes in antidepressant treatment are less severe and easier to manage than manic episodes that occur in bipolar type 1 cases.

This observation may invalidate the hypothesis that a change to mania requires an increase in central catecholamine transmission but does not exclude the possibility that serotonin reuptake inhibitors may have indirect effects on the central noradrenergic system.

Christian Bryois, MD
François Ferrero, MD
University Psychiatric Hospital CH
1008 Prilly-Lausanne
Switzerland

Reprint requests to University Psychiatric Hospital CH, 1008 Prilly-Lausanne, Switzerland (Dr Bryois).

1. Bunney WE Jr. Psychopharmacology of the switch process in affective illness. In: Lipton MA, DiMascio A, Killam KF, eds. *Psychopharmacology: A Generation of Progress.* New York, NY: Raven Press; 1978:1249-1259.
2. Akiskal HS, Walker P, Puzantian UR. Bipolar outcome in the course of depressive illness. *J Affect Disord.* 1983;51:15-28.
3. Pickar D, Murphy DL, Cohen RM, Campbell IC, Lipper S. Selective and nonselective monoamine oxidase inhibitors: behavioral disturbances during their administration to depressed patients. *Arch Gen Psychiatry.* 1982;39:535-540.
4. Wehr TA, Goodwin FK. Can antidepressants cause mania and worsen the course of affective illness? *Am J Psychiatry.* 1987;144:1403-1411.
5. Zis AP, Cowdry RW, Wehr TA, Muscettola G, Goodwin FK. Tricyclic-induced mania and MHPG excretion. *Psychiatry Res.* 1979;1:93-99.
6. Hon D, Preskhorn SH. Mania during fluoxetine treatment for recurrent depression. *Am J Psychiatry.* 1989;146:1638-1639.
7. Lensgraf SJ, Favazza AR. Antidepressant-induced mania. *Am J Psychiatry.* 1990;147:1569.
8. Burrai C, Bocchetta A, DelZompo M. Mania and fluvoxamine. *Am J Psychiatry.* 1991;148:1263-1264.
9. Peyre F, Verdoux H, Bourgeois M. Fluvoxamine: etude de l'effet du traitement sur un groupe de 189 déprimés hospitalisés. *Encephale.* 1992;18:73-74.
10. Dunbar G. Aspects of tolerability and safety for paroxetine. *Nord J Psychiatry.* 1992;46(suppl 27):41-46.

Arachidonic Acid: A Common Link in the Biology of Schizophrenia?

There is evidence of abnormalities of prostaglandin synthesis and action in schizophrenia; thus, there are reports of increased activity of phospholipase A_2,[1] increased plasma levels of prostaglandin E_2,[2] and subsensitivity of platelet prostaglandin receptors.[3] The main precursor for prostaglandin synthesis is arachidonic acid, which is released from membrane phospholipid by phospholipase A_2. One possible consequence of increased phospholipase A_2 activity would be the depletion of arachidonic acid.

In the course of a study of membrane fatty acids, we measured[4] red blood cell membrane arachidonic acid in a group of 23 hospitalized neuroleptic-treated schizophrenic patients (16 men and 7 women) aged 28 to 75 years (mean age, 55 years) and 16 control subjects matched for age and sex. We also measured the plasma levels of thiobarbituric acid reactive substances (TBARS) in the same blood samples. Thiobarbituric acid reactive substances are a measure of lipid peroxidation products and can be increased by endoperoxides produced enzymatically from prostaglandin synthesis.[5]

Red blood cell membrane arachidonic acid concentration was significantly ($P<.01$, Student's t test) reduced in schizophrenic patients (11.9±6.2 [mean±SD] mg/100 mg total membrane phospholipid) relative to the control subjects (17.3±3.6 [mean±SD] mg/100 mg). There appears to be a bimodal distribution in the schizophrenic patients, with one subgroup having markedly lower concentrations than the control group (**Figure**). Furthermore, there was a significant ($P<.01$) negative correlation (Pearson's $r=-.5$) between TBARS and membrane arachidonic acid concentration in the schizophrenic group. No statistically significant correlation was found between neuroleptic dosage, as chlorpromazine hydrochloride equivalents, and TBARS or arachidonic acid concentration, nor was there any relationship with neuroleptic class. We cannot be certain that changes in red blood cell membranes are reflected in the brain, but it is noteworthy that arachidonic acid is particularly concentrated in brain phospholipids and that a recent study using magnetic resonance spectroscopy showed evidence of an increased breakdown of membrane phospholipids in the prefrontal cortex of drug-naive, first-episode schizophrenics.[6]

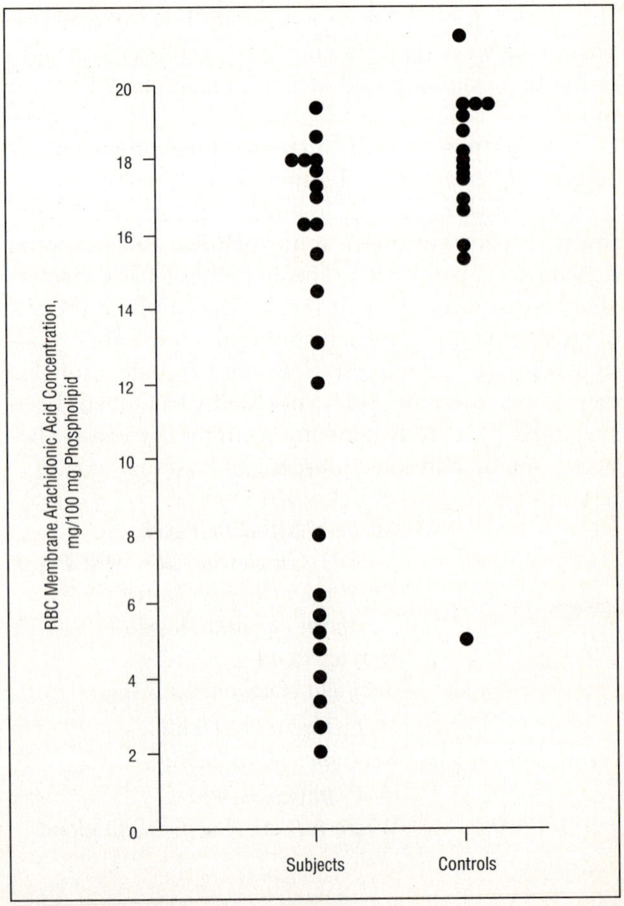

Red blood cell (RBC) membrane arachidonic acid concentrations in schizophrenic patients and normal controls.

Arachidonic acid is a second messenger that is involved in glutamatergic neurotransmission.[7] Activation of *N*-methyl-D-aspartate receptors by glutamate stimulates phospholipase A_2 to release arachidonic acid, and this in turn facilitates long-term potentiation of glutamate synapses in the hippocampus, probably by blocking glutamate uptake. Reduced availability of arachidonic acid would therefore impair glutamatergic neurotransmission. There is evidence from postmortem studies that glutamate neurotransmitter systems are impaired in schizophrenia and it has been proposed that schizophrenia is due to a dopamine-glutamate imbalance.[8] Blockade of dopamine receptors with neuroleptic drugs would thus enhance glutamatergic neurotransmission. In addition, plasma arachidonic acid has been shown to correlate with infant neurodevelopmental performance,[9] which is notable in the light of recent interest in schizophrenia as a neurodevelopmental disorder.

The generation of free radical activity during increased arachidonic acid metabolism provides a plausible hypothesis for the causation of neuronal deficits and other morphological abnormalities that have been identified in the brains of schizophrenic patients.[10] Free radicals are known to mediate peroxidative damage in hippocampal and other neurons.[11] Involvement of free radical activity in neuronal deficits leading to ventricular enlargement in schizophrenia is suggested by a reported correlation between depletion of the protective enzyme glutathione peroxidase and an increased ventricle-brain ratio.[12]

We propose that the increased breakdown and resulting depletion of arachidonic acid is a common factor that integrates biologic findings on prostaglandin synthesis, neurotransmitter abnormalities, and neuronal deficits in schizophrenia. This hypothesis has considerable heuristic value for further studies on both the etiology and treatment of schizophrenia. If the abnormality is a metabolic one, this does not preclude a role for dietary manipulation. Such a possibility has already been suggested by a study showing a strong correlation between outcome in schizophrenia and national diet.[13]

M. Peet, MB, FRCPsych
J. D. E. Laugharne, MB, MRCPsych
Department of Psychiatry
Northern General Hospital
Herries Road
Sheffield, England S5 7AU
D. F. Horrobin, DPhil
Kentville, Nova Scotia
G. P. Reynolds, PhD
Western Bank, Sheffield, England

1. Gattaz WF, Hubner CK, Nevalainan TJ, Thuren T, Kinnunen PKJ. Increased serum phospholipase A_2 activity in schizophrenia: a replication study. *Biol Psychiatry*. 1990;28:495-501.
2. Kaiya H, Vematsu M, Ofuji M, Nishida A, Takeuchi K, Nozaki M, Indaka E. Elevated plasma prostaglandin E_2 levels in schizophrenia. *J Neural Transm Gen Sect*. 1989;77:39-46.
3. Kanof PD, Davidson M, Johns CA, Mohs RC, Davis KL. Clinical correlates of platelet prostaglandin receptor subsensitivity in schizophrenia. *Am J Psychiatry*. 1987;144:1556-1560.
4. Manku MS, Horrobin DF, Huang Y-S, Morse N. Fatty acids in plasma and red cell membranes. *Lipids*. 1983;18:906-908.
5. Halliwell B, Gutteridge JMC. The thiobarbituric (TBA) test. In: *Free Radicals in Biology and Medicine*. Oxford, England: Clarendon Press; 1989:228-233.
6. Pettegrew JW, Keshaven MS, Panchalingam K, Strychor S, Kaplan DB, Tretta M, Allen M. Alterations in brain high-energy phosphate and membrane phospholipid metabolism in first episode drug-naive schizophrenics. *Arch Gen Psychiatry*. 1991;48:563-568.
7. Barbour B, Szatkowski M, Ingledew N, Attwell D. Arachidonic acid induces a prolonged inhibition of glutamate uptake into glial cells. *Nature*. 1989;342:918-920.
8. Carlsson M, Carlsson A. Schizophrenia: a subcortical neurotransmitter imbalance syndrome? *Schizophr Bull*. 1990;16:425-432.
9. Carlsson SE, Werkman SH, Peeples JM, Cooke RJ, Wilson WM. Plasma phospholipid arachidonic acid and growth and development of pre-term infants. In: Koletzko B, Okken A, Rey J, Salle B, Van Biervielt JP, eds. *Recent Advances in Infant Feeding*. Stuttgart, Germany: Georg Thieme Verlag; 1992.
10. Royston MC, Lewis SW. Brain pathology in schizophrenia: developmental or degenerative? *Curr Opin Psychiatry*. 1993;6:70-73.
11. Pellmar TC, Neel KL, Lee KH. Free radicals mediate peroxidative damage in guinea pig hippocampus in vitro. *J Neurosci Res*. 1989;24:437-444.
12. Buckman TD, Kling AS, Eiduson S, Sutphin MS, Steinberg A. Glutathione peroxidase and CT-scan abnormalities in schizophrenia. *Biol Psychiatry*. 1987;22:1349-1356.
13. Christinsen O, Christinsen E. Fat consumption and schizophrenia. *Acta Psychiatr Scand*. 1988;78:587-591.

Interactions of Serotonin Reuptake Inhibitors With Tricyclic Antidepressants

Clinically significant antagonistic interactions of the serotonin reuptake inhibitor (SRI) fluoxetine with the metabolic clearance of other drugs are well known.[1-4] They include increases in circulating concentrations of tricyclic antidepressants (TCAs) by 100% to 500%.[1,5] Whether such interactions also occur clinically to a similar degree with other SRIs is less clear. Crewe and colleagues[6] found that several SRIs can interfere with the activity of a major drug-metabolizing pathway, the human hepatic microsomal cytochrome P-450-2D6 isozyme, in vitro. Paroxetine was most potent against the oxidation of a test agent, sparteine; fluoxetine and sertraline were slightly less active, whereas the experimental agents citalopram and fluvoxamine were weaker (inhibition constants of 0.15, 0.6, 0.7, 5.1, and 8.2 μmol/L, respectively). Although these laboratory data are suggestive, clinical studies of the effects of SRIs other than fluoxetine on TCA metabolism are very limited.

Despite an in vitro action of sertraline against the cytochrome P-450-2D6 oxidase, Preskorn and colleagues[7] found limited clinical effects of this SRI on circulating levels of desipramine in human subjects. However, recent case reports describe clinically significant

interactions of sertraline and desipramine, with elevations of serum levels of the TCA by 60%[8] to 150%.[9] Consistent with its potent in vitro inhibition of microsomal oxidation,[6] paroxetine markedly decreased the clearance of desipramine in human subjects,[10] whereas citalopram, a weak inhibitor in vitro,[6] had no effect on the serum levels of amitriptyline or nortriptyline in five patients.[11] Nevertheless, in vitro effects may not necessarily predict clinical drug interactions: fluvoxamine was 55 times weaker than paroxetine against microsomal drug oxidation in vitro[6] but had a clinically toxic TCA-elevating effect in at least four patients.[12]

These findings indicate that SRIs vary in their interactions with hepatic enzymes and in their ability to increase circulating concentrations of TCAs or other drugs. Additional variance can arise from genetically based individual or ethnic differences, as well as from developmental changes, in the efficiency of microsomal oxidase pathways, which tend to be consistent within individuals for various agents.[4,10,13] The genetically determined low efficiency of the cytochrome P-450-2D6 oxidase and related metabolic pathways occurs in a small minority (≤10%) of whites, blacks, and Asians.[4,13] However, even within the genetic majority, drug metabolism can vary between individuals by up to 100-fold,[14] and children are more efficient in the oxidative metabolic clearance of TCAs than are adults and the elderly.[15] Relatively rapid clearance of a TCA can be suspected clinically from a relatively low ratio of serum TCA concentration to daily dose, particularly dose corrected for body weight (nanograms per milliliter per milligram per kilogram, a crude measure of drug clearance). Such persons may be at risk for a relatively large increase in TCA level when an SRI is added.[10]

Accordingly, interference by paroxetine with the clearance of desipramine in human subjects was five times greater in persons who were heavily dependent on drug metabolism via cytochrome P-450-2D6 than in those who were not, as evaluated by in vivo clearance of a standard test agent, sparteine.[10] There also is a suggestive predictive association between a lower ratio of circulating drug concentration to daily dose during TCA treatment alone and its larger increase during cotreatment with fluoxetine ($r=-.62$ in four cases).[1] In another suggestive case with a relatively low basal ratio of desipramine level to dose, there also was a marked increase (2.5-fold) when sertraline was added.[9] That is, patients who require relatively high daily doses of a TCA to obtain a nominally therapeutic blood level may be at an increased risk for interactive effects when an SRI is added.

Based on these findings, we propose the following for further experimental testing. Currently available SRIs should be suspected of being able to increase circulating concentrations of TCAs or other agents to potentially toxic levels in some patients. This risk may be especially great in children and in adults who normally clear drugs through hepatic oxidative pathways rapidly, as may be indicated by their having relatively low ratios of serum drug concentration to daily dose.

Anand P. Popli, MD
Ross J. Baldessarini, MD
Jonathan O. Cole, MD
Department of Psychiatry
McLean Hospital
Harvard Medical School
115 Mill St
Belmont, MA 02178

Supported in part by grants MH-31154 and MH-47370 from the National Institute of Mental Health of the US Public Health Service, Bethesda, Md, and a McLean Hospital Fellowship in Psychopharmacology.

Address correspondence to Bipolar and Psychotic Disorders and Psychopharmacology Programs, McLean Hospital, 115 Mill St, Belmont, MA 02178 (Dr Baldessarini).

1. Aranow RB, Hudson JI, Pope HG Jr, Grady TA, Laage RA, Bell IR, Cole JO. Elevated antidepressant plasma levels after addition of fluoxetine. *Am J Psychiatry.* 1989;146:911-913.
2. Van Harten J. Clinical pharmacokinetics of selective serotonin reuptake inhibitors. *Clin Pharmacokinet.* 1993;24:203-220.
3. Centorrino F, Baldessarini RJ, Kando J, Frankenburg FR, Volpicelli SA, Puopolo PR, Flood JG. Serum concentrations of clozapine and its major metabolites: effects of cotreatment with clozapine, fluoxetine or valproate. *Am J Psychiatry.* 1994;151:123-125.
4. von Moltke LL, Greenblatt DJ, Harmatz JS, Shader RI. Cytochromes in psychopharmacology. *J Clin Psychopharmacol.* 1994;14:1-4.
5. Goodnick PJ. Influence of fluoxetine on plasma levels of desipramine. *Am J Psychiatry.* 1989;146:552.
6. Crewe HK, Lennard MS, Tucker GT, Woods FR, Haddock RE. The effect of selective serotonin reuptake inhibitors on cytochrome P_{450}-2D6 activity in human liver microsomes. *Br J Clin Pharmacol.* 1992;34:262-265.
7. Preskorn SH, Alderman J, Harris S, Chung M, Harison W, Messig M. Pharmacokinetics of desipramine coadministered with sertraline or fluoxetine. *J Clin Psychopharmacol.* 1994;14:90-98.
8. Lydiard RB, Anton RF, Cunningham T. Interaction between sertraline and tricyclic antidepressants. *Am J Psychiatry.* 1993;150:1125-1126.
9. Barros J, Asnis G. An interaction of sertraline and desipramine. *Am J Psychiatry.* 1994;151:300.
10. Brøsen K, Hansen JG, Nielsen KK, Sindrup SH, Gram LF. Inhibition by paroxetine of desipramine metabolism in extensive but not in poor metabolizers of sparteine. *Eur J Clin Pharmacol.* 1993;44:349-355.
11. Baettig D, Bondolfi G, Montaldi S, Amey M, Baumann P. Tricyclic antidepressant plasma levels after augmentation with citalopram: a case study. *Eur J Clin Pharmacol.* 1993;44:403-405.
12. Spina E, Campo GM, Avenoso A, Pollicino MA, Caputi AP. Interaction between fluvoxamine and imipramine/desipramine in four patients. *Ther Drug Monit.* 1992;14:194-196.
13. Gibaldi M. Ethnic differences in the assessment and treatment of disease. *Pharmacotherapy.* 1993;13:170-176.
14. Bertilsson L, Dahl M-L, Ekqvist B, Jerling M, Llerena A. Genetic regulation of the disposition of psychotropic drugs. In: Meltzer HY, Nerozzi D, eds. *Current Practices and Future Developments in the Pharmacotherapy of Mental Disorders.* Amsterdam, the Netherlands: Elsevier Scientific Publications Inc; 1991:73-80.
15. Wilens TE, Biederman J, Baldessarini RJ, Puopolo PR, Flood JG. Developmental changes in serum concentrations of desipramine and 2-hydroxydesipramine during treatment with desipramine. *J Am Acad Child Adolesc Psychiatry.* 1992;31:691-698.

Professional Opportunities

Archives of General Psychiatry is an exceptional journal that provides physicians with the latest medical and technological information in the psychiatric field. It is an excellent source for recruiting, reaching over 30,220 psychiatrists each month.

All advertising orders must be submitted in writing by mail or fax. Although the American Medical Association believes the classified advertisements in these pages to be from reputable sources, the Association does not assume liability concerning them. Acceptance of advertising is restricted to physician recruitment opportunities, practices for sale, medical office space for sale or rent, and medical equipment for sale.

For information on rates, deadlines, and policies for *Archives of General Psychiatry* Classifieds, contact your classified service representative at 800-AMA-2260 or 312-464-2475/2490/2491/4485.

Nationwide
PSYCHIATRY
&
NEUROLOGY
Positions

We know how busy you are.
Let us do the mundane busy work.

1 (800) 428-4406

Dunhill Professional Search

Psychiatry

BELOIT MEMORIAL HOSPITAL IS RECRUITING FOR A BE/BC psychiatrist for solo practice in an ambulatory setting. Located in South Central Wisconsin. Beloit is an ideal place to raise a family with an excellent school system and a private, highly rated liberal arts college. Very attractive and reasonable real estate. Located within 90 minutes of three major metropolitan areas: Madison, Milwaukee, and Chicago. Financial package includes a production-based income guarantee and excellent benefit options. Contact: Jacquelyn Degenhardt, Physician Recruitment, Beloit Memorial Hospital, 1969 W Hart Road, Beloit, WI 53511, or 800-637-2641 ext 5757.

Also see ads "Nationwide PSYCHIATRY & NEUROLOGY" and "VA PSYCHIATRIST" on this page.

Academic/Faculty

RESEARCHER IN TRAUMATIC STRESS DISORDERS OF CHILdren and Adolescents: Assistant Professor/Associate Professor/Professor, Department of Psychiatry, University of California, San Francisco, San Francisco General Hospital. The Department of Psychiatry at the University of California, San Francisco (UCSF), seeks a board-eligible or board-certified research psychiatrist or licensed clinical psychologist with demonstrated research expertise in treatment outcome research in the field of traumatic stress disorders, or other disorders associated with exposure of children or adolescents to trauma, or in the fields of anxiety or mood disorders of children or adolescents. This position will be located at San Francisco General Hospital (SFGH), a major teaching hospital of UCSF. Responsibilities include organizing and carrying out treatment outcome research in Trauma with predominantly low-income and minority children or adolescents, and research mentorship of faculty and trainees. The position is supported by monies from the UCSF/city budget and carries Academic Senate membership. Experience in the conduct of research with a multiethnic population is preferred. Eligibility for California licensure is required. Applications must be received by November 15, 1994. Please send a letter describing your research experience and a CV to Search Committee Chair, c/o David Bell, UCSF, 401 Parnassus Avenue, Box CAS-0984, San Francisco, CA 94143-0984. UCSF is an Equal Opportunity/Affirmative Action Employer. Women and minorities are strongly encouraged to apply.

RESEARCHER IN ADULT TRAUMATIC STRESS DISORDERS: Assistant Professor/Associate Professor/Professor, Department of Psychiatry, University of California, San Francisco, San Francisco General Hospital. The Department of Psychiatry at the University of California, San Francisco (UCSF), seeks a board-eligible or board-certified research psychiatrist or a licensed clinical psychologist with research expertise in traumatic stress disorders. This position will be located at San Francisco General Hospital, a major teaching hospital of UCSF. Responsibilities include organizing and carrying out treatment outcome research in trauma with predominantly low-income and minority adult populations, and research mentorship of faculty and trainees. The position is supported by a state-funded salary line and carries Academic Senate membership. Requirements include demonstrated expertise as a grant-funded investigator in treatment outcome research in the field of traumatic stress or in other anxiety or mood disorders; candidates must show commitment to focus on trauma treatment outcome research. Experience in the conduct of psychiatric or psychological research with women or minority populations is preferred. Eligibility for California licensure is required. Applications must be received by October 17, 1994. Please send letter of interest and curriculum vitae to Search Committee Chair, c/o Rita Emelia-McLinn, SFVAMC (116A), 4150 Clement Street, San Francisco, CA 94121. UCSF is an Equal Opportunity/Affirmative Action Employer. Women and minorities are strongly encouraged to apply.

Also see ad "GEROPSYCHIATRY FACULTY" on this page.

Locum Tenens Wanted

HKA LOCUM TENENS is looking for quality general psychiatry physicians to do Locum Tenens. We have opportunities coast-to-coast. We furnish Occurrence Malpractice Insurance (no tail necessary). Please call **HKA LOCUM TENENS at (800)226-6347, Extension AM7.1.**

VA PSYCHIATRIST

We seek an academically oriented psychiatrist to develop clinical and research programs in adult psychiatry or substance abuse. This position would include clinical work in inpatient or outpatient adult psychiatry, or an appointment in ambulatory substance abuse.
Faculty appointment available.
Salary range to $119,589 according to qualifications; many fringe benefits.

For additional information please phone (201) 676-1000 ext. 1421 or write to:

Paul Schneck, M.D., Chief, Psychiatry Service, DVA Medical Center, East Orange, New Jersey 07018-1095

Department of Veterans Affairs Medical Center

East Orange VA Medical Center ★ 385 Tremont Avenue, East Orange, NJ 07018 -1095

The VA is an Equal Opportunity Employer M/F/V/H

GEROPSYCHIATRY FACULTY
University of Michigan

Academic geropsychiatrist wanted for tenure-track position (Assistant Professor) at the Ann Arbor VA Medical Center and University of Michigan in Ann Arbor, MI. Position involves participation in clinical care, education, and research in a developing geropsychiatry division with an active fellowship training program. Successful candidate will have adequate "protected time" and should have demonstrated potential for developing an independent research program in a clinical or preclinical area related to geriatric psychiatry. MD or MD-PhD applicants with clinical and/or laboratory-based research interests are appropriate. Candidates should be fellowship-trained in geriatric psychiatry and hold the ABPN Certificate of Added Qualifications in Geriatric Psychiatry. The Medical Center and University provide an extraordinarily rich academic environment, fostering collaborations among faculty both within Psychiatry and in other departments. University has NIA-funded Alzheimer's Disease Research Center and Geriatric Research and Training Center, as well as NIAAA-funded Alcohol Research Center, specializing in aging. VAMC has a Geriatric Research, Educational, and Clinical Center (GRECC). Successful applicant must be eligible for full-time faculty appointment in University of Michigan Medical School. The Ann Arbor VAMC and The University of Michigan are equal opportunity employers. Please send CV to Alan M. Mellow, MD, PhD, Chief, Psychiatry Service (116A), Ann Arbor VA Medical Center, 2215 Fuller Road, Ann Arbor, MI 48105.

Reduction of Cerebral Blood Flow in Older Depressed Patients

Ira M. Lesser, MD; Ismael Mena, MD; Kyle B. Boone, PhD; Bruce L. Miller, MD; C. Mark Mehringer, MD; Marcy Wohl, RN

Background: We investigated regional cerebral blood flow in older, drug-free depressed patients and examined factors that might be related to rCBF.

Methods: We studied 39 physically healthy depressed patients over the age of 50 years and 20 psychiatrically healthy control subjects. Regional cerebral blood flow was measured with single photon emission computed tomography, using both xenon 133 (to quantify regional cerebral blood flow) and ^{99m}Tc-hexamethylpropylene amine oxime (to make regional comparisons). From magnetic resonance imaging, we derived a semiquantitative measure of areas of white matter hyperintensity and a ventricle-to-brain ratio.

Results: Patients exhibited a global reduction in regional cerebral blood flow compared with controls, with the orbital frontal and inferior temporal areas affected bilaterally. Regional cerebral blood flow was also reduced in higher brain slices in the right but not the left hemisphere. Significant predictors of lowered regional cerebral blood flow were being depressed, being male, and having a greater ventricle-to-brain ratio. There appeared to be a subgroup of patients who demonstrated large areas of white matter hyperintensity and low regional cerebral blood flow.

Conclusions: Cerebral blood flow was lower in older, medication-free depressed patients than in age-matched control subjects, involved the orbital frontal and anterior temporal regions, and was more reduced in the right hemisphere.

(Arch Gen Psychiatry. 1994;51:677-686)

DEPRESSIVE ILLNESS in the elderly is a major health problem, with high rates of chronicity, suicide, and, according to some, relative treatment resistance.[1] Many studies suggest that older depressed patients demonstrate more structural brain abnormalities (eg, areas of white matter hyperintensity [WMH]) than age-matched control subjects. It also has been reported that patients with late-onset depression have greater areas of WMH than age-matched elderly depressed patients who had early onset of depression.[2-8]

Studies of cerebral blood flow and cerebral metabolism provide information about the functional integrity of the brain, and these functional data can complement studies of brain structure obtained with magnetic resonance imaging (MRI). Single photon emission computed tomography (SPECT) allows the determination of whole-brain and regional cerebral blood flow (rCBF), and recently SPECT has been used to investigate brain function in a variety of psychiatric disorders.[9-14] Although both SPECT and positron emission tomography (PET) have been utilized for patients with mood disorders, few studies have specifically targeted older patients with depression.

The results of SPECT studies in depression have been variable. Some investigators have described decreases in whole-brain rCBF in depressed patients,[15-19] while others have reported no difference in rCBF compared with controls.[20-23] In addition, some have reported lower rCBF in the right

From the Departments of Psychiatry (Drs Lesser and Boone and Ms Wohl), Radiology (Drs Mena and Mehringer), and Neurology (Dr Miller), Harbor-UCLA Medical Center, Torrance, Calif.

See Methods on next page

anterior hemisphere,[22] others have reported lowered rCBF in the left hemisphere,[15,24] and others have reported more widespread regional differences throughout the cortex.[18] The one study that exclusively comprised older depressed patients showed globally decreased uptake of the radiotracer ^{99m}Tc-hexamethylpropylene amine oxime (^{99m}Tc-HMPAO) compared with that of controls.[19]

Studies using PET have also yielded variable results. The most consistently replicated findings have been decreases in the left, and to a lesser extent the right, dorsal anterolateral prefrontal cortex.[25-29] In one study of older depressed patients, the cerebral metabolism was reported to be globally decreased compared with that of controls.[30]

The variability in these results may reflect a number of factors: inclusion/exclusion criteria, sample size, age, cognitive status, medical and neurological status of the subjects, type of control subjects, medication status of subjects, choice of radiotracer, and statistical method for data analyses. The present study was undertaken to assess rCBF in a relatively homogeneous group of nondemented, medication-free older depressed patients and in healthy, age-matched controls. Unique to this study, we utilized both xenon 133 to quantitatively assess rCBF and ^{99m}Tc-HMPAO (which provides much greater resolution) to study regional differences in uptake; we also collected semiquantitative MRI data regarding WMH and ventricle-to-brain ratio (VBR) in each patient.

METHODS

Depressed patients were recruited from inpatient wards, outpatient clinics, and community referrals. Potential subjects had a telephone screening interview, and if they seemed to meet criteria, they were scheduled for a diagnostic interview with the Structured Clinical Interview for *DSM-III-R* (SCID).[31] To be eligible, patients had to meet the *DSM-III-R*[32] criteria for a current major depressive episode, with the modification that symptoms must have been present for at least 1 month. Only unipolar depressed patients were studied. For the depression to be classified as late-onset depression, it had to have begun after age 50 years; patients with late-onset depression could have had several distinct episodes, but the first one must have occurred after age 50 years. We also included a group with recurrent depression, defined as patients over 50 years old who had at least one other separate major depressive episode prior to age 35 years. Psychiatric exclusion criteria included a hypomanic or manic episode, alcohol or substance dependence disorder in the past 5 years, and any history of psychosis. Subjects with a history of head trauma severe enough to have caused loss of consciousness were excluded. All patients had to have a baseline Hamilton Depression Scale (HAM-D)[33] score of 15 or greater and a Mini–Mental State examination (MMSE)[34] score greater than 24.

Controls were recruited from hospital personnel, newspaper advertising, and local retirement groups. They were interviewed with the Structured Clinical Interview for *DSM-III-R* (nonpatient version). To be included, controls must not have met the criteria for a lifetime diagnosis of major depressive episode, dysthymic disorder, hypomanic or manic episode, alcohol or substance dependence in the past 5 years, or psychotic symptoms.

All subjects underwent screening medical, neurological, and laboratory examinations that included complete blood cell count, a blood chemistry panel, and thyroid function tests. Those with focal neurological findings or with systemic neurologic illness (eg, Parkinson's disease, seizure disorder), those taking medications with potential central nervous system side effects (eg, β-blockers, α-methyldopa, corticosteroids, narcotic analgesics), and those with significant abnormal findings on laboratory examination, particularly those indicating possible alcohol abuse, were excluded. Urine toxicology screens were performed to exclude those covertly using illegal substances. We obtained histories regarding treatment for hypertension and recorded at least two resting blood pressures.

All subjects were studied off psychoactive medications. For those who were receiving antidepressant therapy, a minimum of 2 weeks off medications was required (none had been receiving fluoxetine or monoamine oxidase inhibitors). For those who had been receiving benzodiazepine therapy, their medication was withdrawn slowly, and they were drug-free for a minimum of 1 week prior to study. We obtained written informed consent from all participants in the study. The MRI but not the SPECT results of some patients and some controls have previously been reported.[6,35]

SINGLE PHOTON EMISSION COMPUTED TOMOGRAPHY

Subjects were studied awake with their eyes open; subjects were in a supine position, with low ambient light and noise. Xenon 133 SPECT scans were done after patients inhaled 1100 MBq of ^{133}Xe gas, using high-sensitivity collimation with a brain-dedicated unit (Headtome II, Shimadzu, Kyoto, Japan). The resolution using ^{133}Xe was approximately 20 mm. Two brain slices were acquired simultaneously. Patients were positioned in the gantry using as the reference plane the line from the orbit to the external auditory meatus, the orbitomeatal (OM) line. The slices obtained were 2 and 6 cm parallel to this reference line (OM+2 cm and OM+6 cm). The acquisition had three phases: (1) background, 1 minute; (2) inhalation of 1100 MBq of ^{133}Xe and oxygen from a closed system, 1 minute; and (3) washout phase, when the patient inhaled room air and exhaled into a trap system, 6 minutes. The end-tidal carbon dioxide level and respiratory rate were monitored continuously (model 78354A, Hewlett-Packard Co, Palo Alto, Calif). Xenon 133 activity in exhaled air was monitored, and a ^{133}Xe time activity curve was constructed on a

pixel-by-pixel basis in the washout images of the brain. A single exponential model was used that assumed that SPECT images separated gray from white matter. Only the first exponential (gray matter flow) was used for calculation.[36] The resulting images represent cerebral blood flow (CBF) and were displayed using a color scale coded to milliliters per 100 g of tissue per minute.

Cerebral blood flow quantification was achieved by using adjacent regions of interest (ROIs) drawn manually that covered the entire cortex, without blind regions (**Figure 1**). All ROIs were circular and were 1.9 cm in diameter. For each subject, 11 ROIs in the OM+2-cm slice and 16 ROIs in the OM+6-cm slice were analyzed. The midline ROI in the OM+2-cm slice was excluded because this area is close to the ethmoid cells and is likely to have high concentrations of ^{133}Xe, causing potential artifacts.

After each subject received 1100 MBq of ^{99m}Tc-HMPAO (Ceretec, Amersham, Arlington Heights, Ill) injected intravenously, HMPAO SPECT scans were done. Scanning started 2 hours after injection to clear soft tissue background activity. The same brain-dedicated imaging device, equipped with a high-resolution collimator, was used for ^{99m}Tc-HMPAO imaging as for ^{133}Xe imaging. The resolution using ^{99m}Tc-HMPAO was approximately 8 mm. The first acquisitions were completed in 10 minutes, followed by three body shifts of 16 mm each that imaged the 32 mm of blind interslice space. In 40 minutes we acquired 12 transaxial cuts, each 16 mm thick, covering the whole brain, without blind regions. Transaxial scans were parallel, starting at the OM line, and four adjacent slices were analyzed. The ROIs were drawn manually, ranging from 150 to 250 pixels, covering the entire cortex, without blind regions (**Figure 2**). The reproducibility of generating the ROIs was good (interobserver variability, defined as the SE of the estimate, was 7.2.%). A total of 84 ROIs per subject were analyzed, 12 in slice 2 and 24 each in slices 3, 4, and 5. For data analysis, data from the ROIs in slices 3, 4, and 5 were collapsed so that there were 12 ROIs in each slice.

The data from the brain-dedicated imaging device were analyzed in a fast-processing computer (Sophy, Sopha Medical, Columbia, Mass). The counts per pixel were obtained and used to calculate the mean uptake in each ROI.

MAGNETIC RESONANCE IMAGING

The procedures used in the MRI examination and the quantification of WMH have been described in detail previously[6,37] and will only be briefly reported here. A Picker MRI device with a 1.5-T superconducting magnet was utilized (Picker International, Cleveland, Ohio), and scans were performed in multiple planes. Axial scans were done along the canthomeatal line from the skull base to the vertex in 10-mm sections. A repetition time of 2000 ms was employed, and echo times of 20 and 100 ms were used to give relative T1- and T2-weighted scans, respectively. The scans were transferred to magnetic tape, and specific measurements were made at a viewing console. A cursor under control of a joystick was used to outline the periphery of any ROI. The area was automatically calculated (to within 0.01 cm^2) once the region was delineated. Areas of WMH were defined as areas in the white matter, separate from the ventricles, that demonstrated prolonged T2 relaxation times, appearing as areas of hyperintensity. All T2 axial sections were examined for lesions: the area of WMH on each slice was summed to provide an overall estimate the extent of white matter involvement. Coronal and sagittal images were used to corroborate and better define the location of abnormalities. All measurements were made independently by one of two raters who were blind to diagnosis. Reliability in the measurement of WMH was assessed by calculating intraclass correlations between the two raters (r=.83).[6]

A VBR was calculated by having raters outline the lateral ventricles and the total brain area measured on a proton density–weighted axial section through the image containing the largest extent of the bodies of the lateral ventricles. The T2 scan was not utilized because in some instances it was difficult to differentiate ventricle from WMH. The ventricular area was subtracted from the total brain area, and the resulting number was divided into the ventricular area and then multiplied by 100. Two independent observers, a neuroradiologist and a neurologist, each read MRIs from 15 randomly selected cases, blind to subject status. Intraclass correlation for their VBR measurements was excellent (r=.97).[6]

RESULTS

SUBJECTS

Thirty-nine depressed subjects with a mean (SD) age of 60.9 (8.1) years were studied. The mean age of the 22 men was 62.5 (8.4) years and of the 17 women was 58.8 (7.3) years, a nonsignificant difference (t=1.47, P<.15, df=37). Thirty-seven patients were white and two were Hispanic. Eleven patients (seven women and four men, mean age of 55.9 [5.2] years) were considered to have recurrent depression, and the remaining 28 had their first episode after 50 years of age. The patients had a mean HAM-D score of 20.1 (5.7) and had been depressed for a mean of 22.8 (19.1) months. Only a few patients were initially evaluated as inpatients; the greater part of their testing was completed on an outpatient basis. The mean level of education was 15.0 (2.4) years, and the mean MMSE score was 28.7 (1.5). There were no significant differences between patients with late-onset and recurrent depression for HAM-D score, length (in months) of present episode, education, or MMSE score.

Twenty control subjects with a mean age of 69.1 (6.5) years were studied. The mean age of the eight men was 66.5 (6.3) years and of the 12 women was 70.8 (6.3) years, a nonsignificant difference (t=1.49, P<.15, df=18). Seventeen controls were white, two were African American, and one was Asian. Their mean level of education

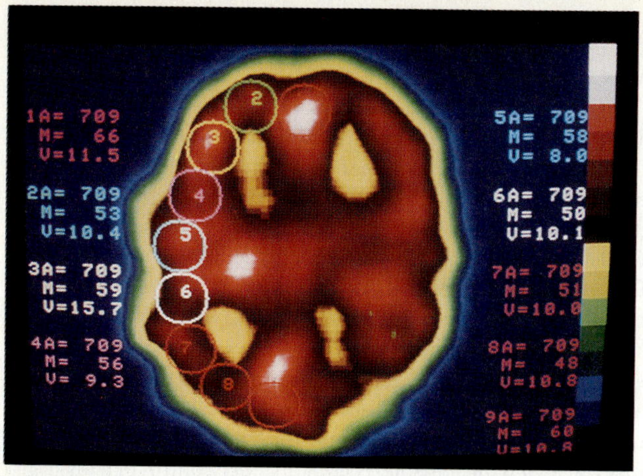

Figure 1. *Xenon 133 blood flow tomogram taken 6 cm above the orbitomeatal line. The numbered circles represent the regions of interest (diameter, 1.9 cm), shown for the right hemisphere.*

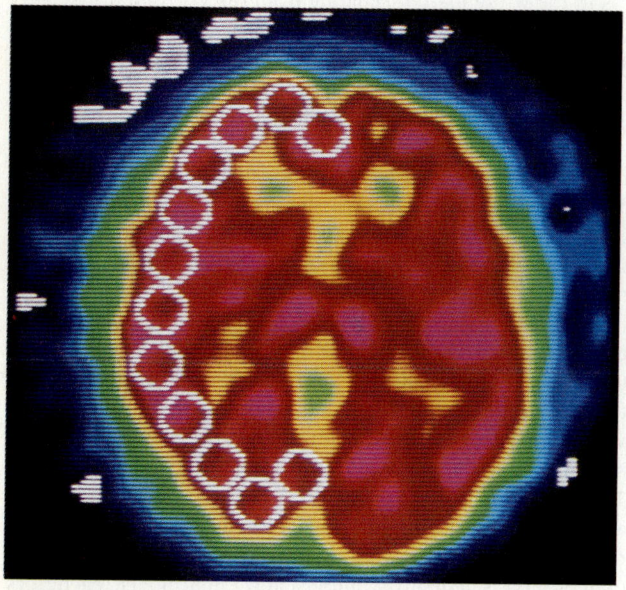

Figure 2. *^{99m}Tc-hexamethylpropylene amine oxime uptake tomogram, with circles representing regions of interest, shown for the right hemisphere.*

was 14.5 (2.1) years, and their mean MMSE score was 29.2 (1.2).

The patient group was significantly younger than the control group (*t*=3.91, *P*<.002, *df*=57). The proportion of men and women in both groups was not significantly different (χ^2=1.45, *P*<.2, *df*=1). There was no significant difference in education (*t*=.85, *P*<.4, *df*=57) or MMSE score (*t*=1.12, *P*<.3, *df*=57) between groups.

MAGNETIC RESONANCE IMAGING

Twenty-eight patients (72%) had a total area of WMH less than 1 cm^2, five patients (13%) between 1 and 10 cm^2, and six patients (15%) greater than 10 cm^2. Thirteen controls (65%) had a total area of WMH less than 1 cm^2, six controls (30%) between 1 and 10 cm^2, and one control (5%) greater than 10 cm^2. Although a threefold higher percentage of patients had a total area of WMH greater than 10 cm^2 (5% vs 16%), Kruskal-Wallis analysis (for non-normally distributed data) showed that there was no overall significant difference in WMH between patients and controls (Kruskal-Wallis analysis, 0.17; *P*<.7). Compared with subjects who had no or a small area of WMH (17% [seven of 41 subjects]), a higher percentage of subjects with a large area of WMH (57% [four of seven subjects]) were hypertensive. Comparison of male and female patients showed a trend for men to have greater areas of WMH (Kruskal-Wallis analysis, 2.74; *P*<.1). Five of the six patients with the largest areas of WMH were men. None of the patients with recurrent depression had a total area of WMH greater than 1.2 cm^2.

The VBR was not significantly different between patients and controls (9.6 vs 10.0, *t*=.38, *P*<.7, *df*=55). Male patients had larger VBRs than female patients, but the difference was not significant (9.9 vs 8.6, *t*=1.16, *P*<.3, *df*=35). Patients with late-onset depression had larger VBRs than patients with recurrent depression, but this was not a significant difference (10.1 [3.9] vs 8.3 [3.0], *t*=1.32, *P*<.19, *df*=36).

^{133}Xe rCBF VALUES

We calculated whole-brain as well as right- and left-hemisphere rCBF by averaging the rCBF values for the circular ROIs in each of the two ^{133}Xe slices. For the OM+2 slice, ROI 1 was not analyzed, as noted above.

An analysis of variance of whole-brain rCBF using depression status and sex as the independent variables showed that there was a main effect for depression (F=18.58, *P*<.0001), a strong trend for sex having a main effect (F=3.92, *P*<.052), with the men having a lower rCBF, and a significant interaction of depression×sex (F=6.33, *P*<.02). Whole-brain rCBF was 37.9 (5.3) mL/100 g per minute for patients vs 43.8 (4.9) mL/100 g per minute for controls, an average of 13.5% lower. Only three controls had an rCBF below the mean of the patient group. Similar differences were seen in patients in both the right (37.6 [5.4] vs 43.2 [5.0] mL/100 g per minute, *t*=3.81, *P*<.003, *df*=57) and left (37.6 [5.2] vs 43.3 [4.9] mL/100 g per minute, *t*=4.06, *P*<.0001, *df*=57) hemispheres. The late-onset group had a lower rCBF than the recurrent group, although the difference was not significant (37.4 [4.5] vs 39.4 [7.2] mL/100 g per minute, *t*=1.01, *P*>.3, *df*=37). The HAM-D score in the patients was not significantly correlated with whole-brain rCBF (*r*=.09).

The interaction between whole-brain rCBF and sex is shown in **Figure 3**. Pairwise tests showed that male patients had lower whole-brain rCBF than female patients (35.3 [4.7] vs 41.4 [3.7] mL/100 g per minute, *t*=4.31, *P*<.0001, *df*=37) and male controls (35.3 [4.7] vs 44.3 [4.5] mL/100 g per minute, *t*=4.43, *P*<.0001, *df*=28). There was no significant difference between male and female controls (44.3 [4.5] vs 43.5 [5.3] mL/100 g

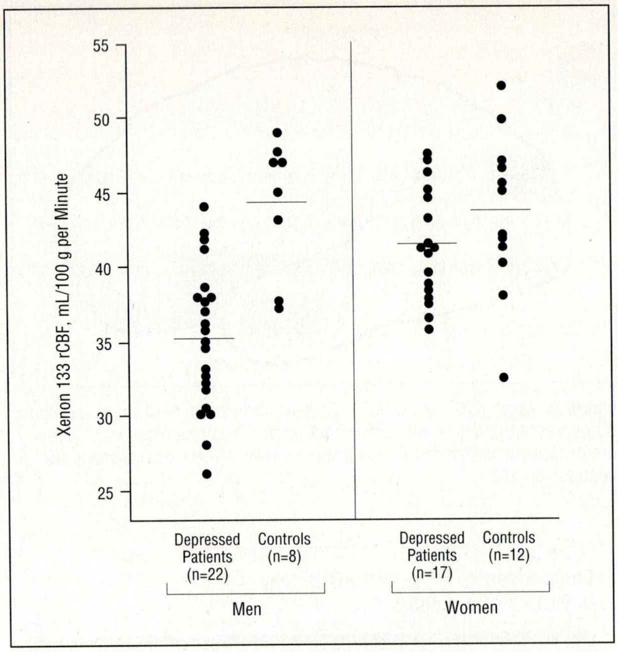

Figure 3. *Whole-brain regional cerebral blood flow (rCBF) obtained with ^{133}Xe single photon emission computed tomography for individual subjects as a function of depression status and sex. Horizontal bars indicate subgroup means.*

per minute, t=.16, P>.8, df=18), and although female patients had lower rCBF than female controls, this difference was not significant (41.4 [3.7] vs 43.5 [5.3] mL/100 g per minute, t=1.40, P<.2, df=27). As shown, the depressed men had the lowest rCBF of all groups. Neither severity of depression nor length of illness differed between the male and female patients (HAM-D score, 20.8 for men and 19.2 for women, t=.8, P>.4, df=37; length of illness, 22.5 months for men and 23.1 months for women, t=.09, P>.9, df=37).

Because there was a difference in age between the patients and controls, we chose a subset of both patients and controls who could be matched for age and sex. Fourteen such pairs were obtained. Patients who were not included were mostly those under 60 years old; controls not included were mostly older (>70 years) women. This new sample consisted of eight men and six women; both groups had a mean age of 66.6 years. There was no significant difference in VBR between the groups. Whole-brain rCBF was significantly lower in the patients (37.6 vs 44.1 mL/100 g per minute, P<.005). Similar differences were noted in the right (P<.004) and left (P<.006) hemispheres.

The Spearman rank correlation between WMH and whole-brain rCBF was −.27, a nonsignificant correlation. When this was calculated separately for male and female patients, neither correlation was significant (−.27 and .01, respectively). However, four of the five male patients with the largest total area of WMH had a whole-brain rCBF equal to or below the mean of the male patients, and the one woman with a total area of WMH greater than 10 cm^2 had the lowest rCBF of all the female patients. On the other hand, seven of the 12 men with the lowest rCBF had no or minimal areas of WMH.

The VBR was significantly (negatively) correlated with whole-brain rCBF for all patients (r=−.6, P<.01) as well as for male (r=−.46, P<.05) and female (r=−.63, P<.01) patients considered separately.

To assess what variable or combination of variables contributed to whole-brain rCBF, we used a stepwise linear regression analysis first on the total sample of 59 subjects and then on the depressed patients alone. For the combined sample we used age, sex, depression status, VBR, and WMH (using dummy variables to compare <1, 1 to 10, and >10 cm^2) as predictor variables. The presence of depression and VBR were significant contributors, accounting for 35% of whole-brain rCBF variance (for depression: regression coefficient [SE], 6.46 [1.42]; for VBR: regression coefficient [SE], −0.49 [0.19]). We next did a regression analysis of the depressed patients, using age, sex, HAM-D score, VBR, and WMH as independent variables. Sex and VBR were significant predictors, accounting for 41% of rCBF variance (for sex: regression coefficient [SE], 4.63 [1.37]; for VBR: regression coefficient [SE], −0.50 [0.18]).

REGIONAL CEREBRAL ^{99M}TC-HMPAO UPTAKE

Comparisons between the uptake of ^{99m}Tc-HMPAO in patients and controls, expressed as percentage of uptake (converted to decimal equivalents) normalized to the maximal uptake of the brain, are shown in **Figure 4** (right hemisphere) and **Figure 5** (left hemisphere). These figures represent schematic sagittal sections of the brain so that the ROIs can be approximated to neuroanatomic regions. Because there were many separate comparisons between patients and controls, we chose to consider P<.01 as representing real differences between groups. In addition, when differences extended across adjacent regions of interest in the same slice or vertically across slices, this was taken as further evidence of a significant difference.[13]

Compared with controls, patients demonstrated highly significant reductions in uptake of ^{99m}Tc-HMPAO in multiple areas across the four slices. Particularly striking were the reductions in the frontal, temporal, and parietal regions in all four slices of the right hemisphere (Figure 4). For the left hemisphere, reductions were most evident in the frontal, temporal and parietal regions of the two lower slices, but there were few significant reductions in the left hemisphere of depressed patients in slices 4 and 5 (Figure 5).

The **Table** shows paired t test comparisons of the ^{99m}Tc-HMPAO uptake of corresponding ROIs from each hemisphere for the depressed patients. The most consistent differences were reduced uptake in the upper two slices of the right hemisphere, particularly in the more anterior regions, compared with the left hemisphere. There was no lateralization of uptake in the lower slices, in-

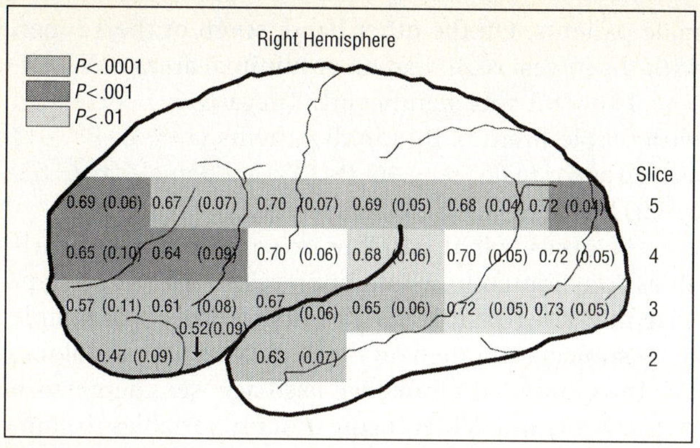

Figure 4. *Mean (SD) uptake of* ^{99m}*Tc-hexamethylpropylene amine oxime in 39 depressed patients in four brain slices in the right hemisphere. Values are expressed as decimal equivalents.* P *values are for comparisons with controls (n=20).*

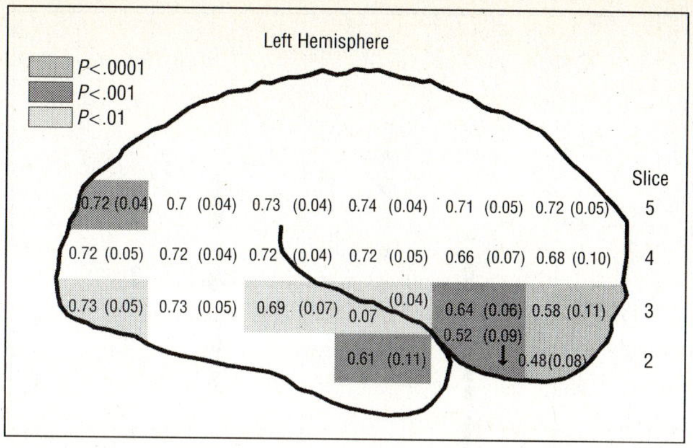

Figure 5. *Mean (SD) uptake of* ^{99m}*Tc-hexamethylpropylene amine oxime in 39 depressed patients in four brain slices in the left hemisphere. Values are expressed as decimal equivalents.* P *values are for comparisons with controls (n=20).*

cluding the orbital frontal areas. For further analyses, we grouped data into right anterior, left anterior, right posterior, and left posterior brain regions. These were calculated by collapsing the three most anterior ROIs and the three most posterior ROIs in each hemisphere, excluding the midline frontal and occipital regions.

To further assess what factor(s) or interactions of factors affected uptake of ^{99m}Tc-HMPAO, we calculated a series of repeated-measures analyses of variance, with ^{99m}Tc-HMPAO uptake as the dependent variable; hemisphere, slice, and region as three within-subject factors; and sex and diagnosis as grouping variables. When the factors were considered individually, brain slice was significant (F=82.0, $P<.00001$), with lower slices showing reduced uptake; diagnosis was significant (F=47.2, $P<.00001$), with depressed subjects showing reduced uptake; sex was significant (F=4.88, $P<.03$), with men having reduced uptake; and hemisphere and region were not significant.

There were significant interactions of slice×diagnosis (F=9.38, $P<.00001$), slice×sex (F=7.14, $P<.0002$), and slice×diagnosis×sex (F=3.71, $P<.01$). When hemisphere was considered in concert with other factors, there were significant interactions of hemisphere×diagnosis (F=10.47, $P<.002$) and of slice×hemisphere×diagnosis (F=4.89, $P<.003$) but not of hemisphere×sex or of hemisphere×diagnosis×sex. Similarly, when region was considered, we found significant interactions of hemisphere×region (F=51.1, $P<.00001$) and of hemisphere×region×diagnosis (F=13.63, $P<.0005$) but not of hemisphere×region×sex. Finally, there were significant interactions of slice×hemisphere×region (F=23.64, $P<.00001$) and of slice×hemisphere×region×sex (F=3.52, $P<.02$).

Correlations between total HAM-D score and uptake of ^{99m}Tc-HMPAO in individual ROIs were of small magnitude. None accounted for more than 9% of the variance, there was no clear-cut pattern of significant correlations, and given the large number of comparisons, the few significant ones may have occurred by chance alone.

Comparison of ^{99m}Tc-HMPAO Uptake in ROIs by Hemisphere*

	^{99m}Tc-HMPAO Uptake†			
	Right Hemisphere	Left Hemisphere	*t*‡	*P*
Slice 2				
Anterior	.47	.48	1.31	.20
↓	.52	.52	0.64	.52
Posterior	.63	.61	1.18	.24
Slice 3				
Anterior	.57	.58	1.50	.14
↓	.61	.64	2.97	.005
↓	.67	.70	3.65	.008
↓	.65	.69	3.58	.001
Posterior	.72	.73	1.13	.27
Slice 4				
Anterior	.65	.68	3.20	.003
↓	.64	.66	1.93	.06
↓	.70	.72	3.21	.003
↓	.68	.72	4.72	<.0001
Posterior	.70	.72	3.04	.004
Slice 5				
Anterior	.69	.72	4.39	.0001
↓	.67	.71	3.34	.002
↓	.70	.74	3.81	.0005
↓	.69	.73	5.52	<.0001
Posterior	.68	.70	3.89	.0004

**HMPAO indicates hexamethylpropylene amine oxime; ROIs, regions of interest.*

†Values are expressed as decimal equivalents.

‡Matched-pair tests.

Using the subset of 14 matched pairs described above, uptake of ^{99m}Tc-HMPAO followed much the same pattern as seen in the entire sample. Patients demonstrated significant reductions in uptake in the lower two slices, particularly in the anterior areas and more pronounced in the right hemisphere. There were only a few significant differences in regional uptake in the upper two slices.

COMMENT

These were the major findings in this study of medication-free, nondemented, moderately depressed patients over the age of 50 years: (1) Compared with controls, patients had significant reductions in whole-brain and right- and left-hemisphere rCBF measured by ^{133}Xe SPECT and reduced uptake of ^{99m}Tc-HMPAO bilaterally in the orbital frontal, inferotemporal, and parietal areas. In the high frontal, superotemporal, and parietal areas, rCBF was decreased in the right but not the left hemisphere. (2) Uptake of ^{99m}Tc-HMPAO was reduced more extensively in the right hemisphere. (3) Of the variables studied, the major contributors to reduced rCBF in all subjects were being depressed and having a larger VBR. For the patients, the major contributors were being male and having a larger VBR. When VBR was matched in patients and controls, the blood-flow differences remained. (4) Severity of depression, as measured by HAM-D, was not correlated with whole-brain rCBF or ^{99m}Tc-HMPAO uptake. The absence of the more severely depressed patients might be an important factor in our finding no correlation between severity of depression and blood flow; thus, these results may not be generalizable to more severely depressed patients.

The repeated-measures analyses of variance indicated that not only are individual factors related to blood flow but interactions of factors are also important to consider. Having a diagnosis of depression, being male, and lower brain slices were all associated with lower uptake of ^{99m}Tc-HMPAO. However, although there was not an overall difference in ^{99m}Tc-HMPAO uptake when hemisphere or region was considered by itself, there were significant interactions of hemisphere×diagnosis, hemisphere×region×diagnosis, and region×hemisphere×diagnosis. The results of these analyses underscore the need to consider multivariate approaches to the data; the fact that many previous studies did not analyze data in this way may account for many of the differences in results reported in the literature.

A number of considerations add to the strength of these findings. Our depressed patients were otherwise healthy and none were taking medications with central nervous system effects. The percentage of patients with hypertension (controlled) was similar to that of controls (regarding both history and duration of hypertension treatment as well as current resting blood pressure), and there was no difference between groups in the frequency of smoking. Similarly, no gender differences in smoking or hypertension history were present. Although there was a statistically significant difference in age, the patients (60.9 years) were younger than the controls (69.1 years). If rCBF decreases with age (and in this age group, this is not well established), then the fact that our patients who were younger than controls had decreased rCBF enhances the strength of this finding. Additionally, when we matched patients and controls for age and sex, which also eliminated the difference in VBR between groups, the findings were essentially the same.

These results are in agreement with those of several previous studies but at variance with others. However, to our knowledge, the present study is the only one in which rCBF was assessed by SPECT using both ^{133}Xe (to quantitate rCBF) and ^{99m}Tc-HMPAO (to perform regional assessments) and in which WMH and VBR were quantified in the same (drug-free) patients.

COMPARISON WITH OTHER STUDIES

The two studies in older depressed patients that most closely resembled ours reported reductions in rCBF. Upadhyaya et al[19] studied 18 patients with major depressive episode who had a mean age of 77 years using ^{99m}Tc-HMPAO SPECT. The depressed patients had significantly decreased ^{99m}Tc-HMPAO uptake globally and a trend toward decreased uptake in all regions of interest compared with control subjects. Only four of the 18 patients were men, while six of the 12 controls were men. The HAM-D scores were not significantly correlated with uptake in any regions.

Sackheim et al[18] used ^{133}Xe SPECT to study 41 drug-free (except for low-dose benzodiazepine therapy) patients with a mean age of 62 years (range, 35 to 80 years) who met the Research Diagnostic Criteria[38] for major depressive disorder, endogenous type. The depressed patients had lower rCBF globally (averaging 12% lower than controls) and also demonstrated abnormal regional distribution compared with controls. Topographic analyses indicated blood-flow reductions in the prefrontal, frontal, central, superotemporal, and anteroparietal regions. The average reduction in blood flow in the depressed patients was similar to that reported in the present study, as was the finding that, as a group, depressed men had the lowest rCBF.

Other studies also support the major findings noted here, although differing methods make comparisons more difficult. For example, Schlegel et al,[17] using the short-lived radiotracer gold Au 195m, reported global reductions in rCBF, with more involvement of the right hemisphere, in 21 depressed patients with a mean age of 45 years. Kanaya and Yonekawa[23] reported decreases in rCBF in all cerebral regions, with, however, more involvement in the left hemisphere. Austin et al,[39] using ^{99m}Tc-exametazime, reported that 40 depressed patients (mean age, 47 years) demonstrated reduced uptake in most cortical (particularly in the temporal, inferofrontal, and parietal areas) and subcortical regions.

On the other hand, several reports show no difference between patient and control groups, although these studies were not performed exclusively in older patients and used ^{133}Xe, which has poorer resolution than ^{99m}Tc-HMPAO. Silfverskiold and Risberg[21] measured rCBF by ^{133}Xe inhalation in 15 unipolar depressed patients with a mean age of 56 years. Both mean rCBF and regional distribution were similar in the patient group and a well-matched control group. Using ^{133}Xe SPECT, Delvenne et al[22] found no differences

in whole-brain, right-, and left-hemisphere rCBF in 38 younger depressed patients (mean age, 39 years). However cortical blood flow, measured in the outer cerebral rim of one slice, was decreased in the left hemisphere in endogenously depressed patients. Gur et al,[20] using ^{133}Xe with a multiprobe method, found no difference in resting rCBF between controls and 14 unipolar medicated depressed patients with a mean age of 31 years.

Studies using PET have reported on cerebral metabolism rather than rCBF. Baxter et al[26] found decreased glucose metabolism in the anterolateral prefrontal cortex in unipolar depressed, bipolar depressed, and obsessive-compulsive patients with depression (mean ages in the mid-30s). Although this group and others[25,28] had previously reported that metabolism was lower in the left anterolateral prefrontal cortex, Baxter et al[26] later noted that this decrease was relatively symmetric. Other PET studies showed decreased rCBF in the left anterior cingulate and left dorsolateral prefrontal area in 23 subjects with a mean age of 57 years[29]; significant reductions in frontal metabolism, most apparent in the anterior and right frontal cortex, in six younger depressed patients compared with controls[27]; and significant reductions in glucose metabolism in the right temporal lobes in moderately depressed patients, with a trend toward reduction in the left temporal lobes, compared with controls (ages were not given).[40] One study of eight older depressed patients (mean age, 72 years) reported decreased whole brain cerebral metabolic rates as well as regional decreases in all neocortical and subcortical areas in patients compared with controls.[30]

Despite some conflicting data, the majority of SPECT and PET studies show significant reductions in blood flow or metabolism in depressed patients compared with controls. This is particularly true in studies in which older and unmedicated patients have been evaluated. In those studies in which reductions have been found, there is agreement that frontal areas are involved most extensively. However, some suggest involvement of the right hemisphere while others suggest involvement of the left hemisphere. Given the wide range of methodological approaches, statistical analyses, and demographic characteristics among patients and controls, this variability is understandable.

LOCALIZATION OF REDUCED rCBF

Patients exhibited more extensive reductions compared with controls in ^{133}Xe rCBF and ^{99m}Tc-HMPAO uptake in the right hemisphere than in the left hemisphere. Although both right- and left-hemisphere rCBF decreases were found in the orbital frontal, inferotemporal, and inferoparietal lobes, only right-hemisphere reductions were seen in slices 4 and 5, which included the dorsolateral frontal, cingulum, and midparietal regions. Comparisons between corresponding ROIs in the right and left hemispheres provided further support for a greater reduction in the right hemisphere. There were no right-left differences in the most inferior slice (slice 2), including the orbital frontal cortex, or in the most frontal or most posterior region in slice 3. However, there were consistent differences in the high frontal and parietal slices in all regions studied.

It is simplistic to try to localize depression to a particular brain region or even to a hemisphere. Although we found more hypoperfusion of the right hemisphere, there was extensive involvement in orbital frontal and anterior temporal structures bilaterally, similar to what was reported by Baxter et al[26] with PET. These regions are part of the limbic system, which is an important neuroanantomic circuit involved in mood and motivation. Dysfunction in this area has been known to be associated with depression.[41]

Although Robinson and colleagues suggested that poststroke depression was most likely to occur when the stroke was in the left hemisphere and close to the frontal pole,[42,43] further data from this group[44] and others[45-47] have cast doubt on the strength of this finding. When additional factors were considered (eg, dorsal-ventral and frontal-nonfrontal interactions, history of depression), the predominance of left-sided lesions waned. Furthermore, it is not clear that the mechanism(s) by which depression follows discrete brain injury is the same as the mechanism(s) of depression that develops in the absence of brain trauma.

Our finding of more hypoperfusion in the higher cuts of the right hemisphere is interesting but difficult to understand in a neuroanatomic framework related to mood. There is support in the literature, however, for a predominant right-hemisphere deficit in depression.[48,49] Data from neuropsychological studies in depressed patients, including our own data on elderly patients, have been interpreted to indicate relatively selective right-hemisphere defects.[48,50-53] Using data from a variety of studies, Coffey[49] reviewed cerebral laterality and depression and concluded that right-hemisphere involvement may be more important for the perception, experience, and expression of emotion. His conclusion included a proposed right-hemisphere dominance model of depression.

SIGNIFICANCE OF THESE FINDINGS

This study does not answer why blood flow is reduced in older depressed patients, but several possibilities exist: (1) A preexisting gross structural defect or, possibly, a neuronal loss in the brain predisposes individuals to depression and lowered blood flow. (2) The findings are relevant only to older depressed patients and reflect cerebrovascular disease or early degenerative dementia. (3) The depression in some way leads to lowered blood flow. (4) This association is an epiphenomenon.

Although the area of WMH in patients and controls was not statistically different, there did appear to be a subgroup of patients with large areas of WMH who

also had low rCBF. Given that brain injury is known to cause depression[42-47] and that areas of WMH are associated with depression in older patients,[2-8] WMH may have been a predisposing factor for both depression and lowered blood flow in some subjects.[54] However, this did not appear to be the mechanism for the majority of patients.

The comparison of imaging findings in the patients with late-onset and recurrent depression is interesting and leads to several testable hypotheses. Similar to reports by others,[4] we found that patients with recurrent depression had smaller areas of WMH than patients with late-onset depression, suggesting that WMH and, perhaps, associated vascular disease are more related to depression that begins late in life. On the other hand, although there was a trend for late-onset patients to have lower rCBF, this was not significant. If this finding is replicated in a larger sample (and one better matched for age and sex than the sample in the present study), it might imply that the rCBF changes in patients with recurrent depression are not associated with structural changes but could be state dependent. On the other hand, the rCBF decreases seen in patients with large areas of WMH may be more linked to structural changes and thus a trait finding. Prospective studies such as those described below could help answer this question.

Few studies have measured both cortical atrophy and rCBF. Similar to our findings, Waldemar et al[55] reported that cortical atrophy but not age was the only significant determinant of global rCBF in normal subjects with an age range of 20 to 90 years. It is unclear what relationship atrophy has with lowered blood flow and depression and whether this relationship holds in younger depressed patients. It is interesting that increased VBR, albeit only an approximate marker for cortical atrophy, was associated with lowered rCBF. One possible explanation is that these patients have decreased neuronal activity, which results in decreased blood flow. A model for this would be Alzheimer's or Pick's disease, in which there is clear reduction in rCBF in those areas most affected by neuronal loss.[56] This neuronal dysfunction in turn could lead to behavioral changes that constitute depression. Indeed, it has been shown that in some older patients depression may be an early marker for degenerative dementia.[57] Also, tentative support for an association of neuronal loss and depression comes from Bowen et al,[58] who reported data from a postmortem study of seven depressed patients with a mean age of 60 years. The gray matter of each lobe and the cingulate gyrus were equal in weight to those from matched controls. However, the pars opercularis, temporal pole, and parahippocampal gyrus weighed less in the depressed patients, and, according to histological and radioimmunoassay analyses, there was peptide loss (somatostatin) in the temporal pole in depressed patients. These data suggested that the corticocortical connections between the temporal pole and frontal lobe had degenerated in patients with depression. The areas found to be abnormal in this postmortem study were similar to those found to have reduced blood flow or reduced uptake in the present investigation.

With the data presented here, there is no way to know whether the depression caused the blood-flow changes. If this were true, it would imply that brain structure was not necessarily affected and would constitute the strongest case for the blood-flow changes as a state phenomenon. The few studies that have reported on blood flow during depression and in remission have indicated that blood flow does improve with resolution of depression.[20,59] These repeated measurements of rCBF were made while patients were receiving medications, and it was not reported whether these patients had WMH or other structural brain changes.

Larger-scale prospective studies in which rCBF is assessed when the patient is depressed and then in remission (and off medications) are necessary to help elucidate the mechanism(s) involved with reduced rCBF. At the same time, MRI data should be collected to assess structural and functional abnormalities in the same brain regions. These studies should be conducted among patients with a wide range of ages to assess whether the changes found in our study are unique to older patients. An additional strategy would be to use another measure of brain function, such as neuropsychological testing, to help assess whether the blood-flow changes seen in depression affect cognition and to determine whether these cognitive changes reflect the location where the blood flow is most reduced. Finally, prospective treatment studies could test the intriguing hypothesis that reduced blood flow, perhaps in conjunction with WMH and/or cortical atrophy, leads to poorer treatment response.

Accepted for publication June 7, 1994.

This study was supported by grant MH04360 from the National Institute of Mental Health (Dr Lesser) and by contract 90-70042 from the Department of Mental Health, State of California (Dr Lesser).

The authors thank Francisca Alamos for technical help and Nancy Berman, PhD, for statistical advice.

Reprint requests to Department of Psychiatry, Harbor-UCLA Medical Center, Box 498, 1000 Carson St, Torrance, CA 90509 (Dr Lesser).

REFERENCES

1. NIMH Panel. NIH Consensus Development Conference: The Diagnosis and Treatment of Depression in Late Life; November 4-6, 1991; Washington, DC.
2. Alexopoulos GS, Meyers BS, Young RC, Abrams RC, Shamolan CA. Brain changes in geriatric depression. *Int J Geriatr Psychiatry.* 1988;3:157-161.
3. Coffey CE, Figiel GS, Djang WT, Weiner RD. Subcortical hyperintensity on magnetic resonance imaging: a comparison of normal and depressed elderly subjects. *Am J Psychiatry.* 1990;147:187-189.
4. Figiel GS, Krishnan KRR, Doraiswamy PM, Rao VP, Nemeroff CB, Boyko OB. Subcortical hyperintensities on brain magnetic resonance imaging: a comparison between late age onset and early onset elderly depressed subjects. *Neurobiol Aging.* 1991;26:245-247.

5. Krishnan KRR. Organic bases of depression in the elderly. *Annu Rev Med.* 1991;42:261-266.
6. Lesser IM, Miller BL, Boone KB, Hill-Gutierrez E, Mehringer CM, Wong K, Mena I. Brain injury and cognitive function in late-onset depression. *J Neuropsychiatry Clin Neurosci.* 1991;3:33-40.
7. Rabins PV, Pearlson GD, Aylward E, Kumar AJ, Dowell K. Cortical magnetic resonance imaging changes in elderly inpatients with major depression. *Am J Psychiatry.* 1991;148:617-620.
8. Baldwin RC. Late life depression and structural brain changes: a review of recent magnetic resonance imaging research. *Int J Geriatr Psychiatry.* 1993;8:115-123.
9. Andreasen NC. Brain imaging: applications in psychiatry. *Science.* 1988;239:1381-1388.
10. Van Heertum RL. Brain SPECT imaging and psychiatry. *J Clin Psychiatry.* 1992;53(suppl):7-12. [Supplement in Clinical Applications of NeuroSPECT in Psychiatry.]
11. Volkow ND, Tancredi L. Current and future applications of SPECT in clinical psychiatry. *J Clin Psychiatry.* 1992;53(suppl):26-28. [Supplement in Clinical Applications of NeuroSPECT in Psychiatry.]
12. Berman KF, Torrey EF, Daniel DG, Weinberger DR. Regional cerebral blood flow in monozygotic twins discordant for schizophrenia. *Arch Gen Psychiatry.* 1992;49:927-924.
13. Rubin RT, Villanueva JM, Ananth J, Trajmar PG, Mena I. Regional xenon 133 cerebral blood flow and cerebral technetium ^{99m}HMPAO uptake in unmedicated patients with obsessive-compulsive disorder and matched normal control subjects. *Arch Gen Psychiatry.* 1992;49:695-702.
14. Zilbovicius M, Garreau B, Tzourio N, Mazoyer B, Bruck B, Martinot JL, Raynaud C, Samson Y, Syrota A, Gilbert L. Regional cerebral blood flow in childhood autism: a SPECT study. *Am J Psychiatry.* 1992;149:924-930.
15. Mathew RJ, Meyer JS, Francis DJ, Semchuk KM, Mortel K, Claghorn JL. Cerebral blood flow in depression. *Am J Psychiatry.* 1980;137:1449-1450.
16. Gustafson L, Risberg J, Silfverskiold P. Regional cerebral blood flow in organic dementia and affective disorders. *Adv Biol Psychiatry.* 1981;6:109-116.
17. Schlegel S, Aldenhoff JB, Eissner D, Linder P, Nickel O. Regional cerebral blood flow in depression: associations with psychopathology. *J Affective Disord.* 1989;17:211-218.
18. Sackheim HA, Prohovnik I, Moeller JR, Brown RP, Apter S, Prudic J, Devanand DP, Mukherjee S. Regional cerebral blood flow in mood disorders. *Arch Gen Psychiatry.* 1990;47:60-69.
19. Upadhyaya AK, Abou-Saleh MT, Wilson K, Grime SJ, Critchley M. A study of depression in old age using single-photon emission computerised tomography. *Br J Psychiatry.* 1990;157(suppl 9):76-81.
20. Gur RE, Skolnick B, Gur RC, Caroff S, Rieger W, Obrist WD, Younkin D, Reivich M. Brain function in psychiatric disorders, II: regional cerebral blood flow in medicated unipolar depressives. *Arch Gen Psychiatry.* 1984;41:695-699.
21. Silfverskiold P, Risberg J. Regional cerebral blood flow in depression and mania. *Arch Gen Psychiatry.* 1989;46:253-259.
22. Delvenne V, Delecluse F, Hubain P, Schoutens A, DeMaertelaer V, Mendlewicz J. Regional cerebral blood flow in patients with affective disorders. *Br J Psychiatry.* 1990;157:359-365.
23. Kanaya T, Yonekawa M. Regional cerebral blood flow in depression. *Jpn J Psychiatry.* 1990;44:571-576.
24. Mayberg HS, Jeffery PJ, Wagner HN, Simpson SG. Regional cerebral blood flow in patients with refractory unipolar depression measured with TC-99m HMPAO SPECT. *J Nucl Med.* 1991;32:951.
25. Baxter LR, Phelps ME, Mazziotta JC, Schwartz JM, Gerner RH, Selin CE, Sumida RM. Cerebral metabolic rates for glucose in mood disorders: studies with positron emission tomography and fluorodeoxyglucose F18. *Arch Gen Psychiatry.* 1985;42:441-447.
26. Baxter LR, Schwartz JM, Phelps ME, Mazziota JC, Guze BH, Selin CE, Gerner RH, Sumida RM. Reduction of prefrontal cortex glucose metabolism common to three types of depression. *Arch Gen Psychiatry.* 1989;46:243-250.
27. Hurwitz TA, Clark C, Murphy E, Klonoff H, Martin WRW, Pate BD. Regional cerebral glucose metabolism in major depressive disorder. *Can J Psychiatry.* 1990;35:684-688.
28. Martinot JL, Hardy P, Feline A, Huret JD, Mazoyer B, Attar-Levy D, Pappata S, Syrota A. Left prefrontal glucose hypometabolism in the depressed state: a confirmation. *Am J Psychiatry.* 1990;147:1313-1317.
29. Bench CJ, Friston KJ, Brown RG, Scott LC, Frackowiak RSJ, Dolan R. The anatomy of melancholia: focal abnormalities of cerebral blood flow in major depression. *Psychol Med.* 1992;22:607-615.
30. Kumar A, Nadel DM, Alavi A, Smith RJ, Reivich M. High resolution 18 FDG PET studies in late-life depression. *J Nucl Med.* 1992;33:1013.
31. Spitzer RL, Williams JB. *Structured Clinical Interview for DSM-III-R.* New York, NY: New York State Psychiatric Institute; 1986.
32. American Psychiatric Association, Committee on Nomenclature and Statistics. *Diagnostic and Statistical Manual of Mental Disorders, Revised Third Edition.* Washington, DC: American Psychiatric Association; 1987.
33. Hamilton M. Development of a rating scale for primary depressive illness. *Br J Soc Psychol.* 1967;6:278-296.
34. Folstein MF, Folstein SE, McHugh PR. 'Mini-Mental State': a practical method for grading the cognitive state of patients for the clinician. *J Psychiatr Res.* 1975;12:185-198.
35. Boone KB, Miller BL, Lesser IM, Mehringer CM, Hill-Gutierrez E, Goldberg M, Berman NG. Neuropsychological correlates of white matter lesions in health elderly subjects. *Arch Neurol.* 1992;49:549-554.
36. Kanno I, Lassen NA. Two methods for calculating regional cerebral blood flow from emission computed tomography of inert gas concentrations. *J Comput Assist Tomogr.* 1979;3:71-76.
37. Miller BL, Lesser IM, Boone KB, Hill E, Mehringer CM, Wong K. Brain injury and cognitive function in late-life psychosis. *Br J Psychiatry.* 1991;158:76-82.
38. Spitzer RL, Endicott J, Robins E. *Research Diagnostic Criteria for a Selected Group of Functional Disorders.* New York, NY: Biometrics Research Division, New York State Psychiatric Institute, 1977.
39. Austin M-P, Dougall N, Ross M, Murray C, O'Carrol RE, Moffoot A, Ebmeier KP, Goodwin GM. Single photon emission tomography with ^{99m}Tc-exametazime in major depression and the pattern of brain activity underlying the psychotic/neurotic continuum. *J Affective Disord.* 1992;26:31-44.
40. Post RM, DeLisi LE, Holcomb HH, Uhde TW, Cohen R, Buchsbaum MS. Glucose utilization in the temporal cortex of affectively ill patients: positron emission tomography. *Biol Psychiatry.* 1987;22:545-553.
41. MacLean PD. Some psychiatric implications of physiological studies on frontotemporal portion of limbic system (visceral brain). *Electroencephalogr Clin Neurophysiol.* 1952;4:407-421.
42. Robinson RG, Kubos KL, Starr LB, Rao K, Price TR. Mood disorders in stroke patients: importance of location of lesion. *Brain.* 1984;107:81-93.
43. Robinson RG, Starr LB, Kubos KL, Price TR. A two year longitudinal study of post-stroke mood disorders: findings during the initial evaluation. *Stroke.* 1983;14:736-741.
44. Starkstein SE, Bryer JB, Berthier ML, Cohen B, Price TR, Robinson RG. Depression after stroke: the importance of cerebral hemisphere asymmetries. *J Neuropsychiatry Clin Neurosci.* 1991;3:276-285.
45. Sinyor D, Jacques P, Kaloukpeg G, Becker R, Goldenberg M, Coopersmith H. Post-stroke depression and lesion location: an attempted replication. *Brain.* 1986;109:537-546.
46. Stern RA, Bachman DL. Depressive symptoms following stroke. *Am J Psychiatry.* 1991;148:351-356.
47. Eastwood MR, Rifat SL, Nobbs H, Ruderman J. Mood disorder following cerebrovascular accident. *Br J Psychiatry.* 1989;154:195-200.
48. Flor-Henry P. On certain aspects of the localization of the cerebral systems regulating and determining emotion. *Biol Psychiatry.* 1979;14:677-698.
49. Coffey CE. Cerebral laterality and emotion: the neurology of depression. *Compr Psychiatry.* 1987;28:197-219.
50. Abrams R, Taylor MA. Cognitive dysfunction in melancholia. *Psychol Med.* 1987;17:359-362.
51. Deptula D, Manevitz A, Yozawitz A. Asymmetry of recall in depression. *J Clin Exp Neuropsychol.* 1991;13:854-870.
52. Fromm D, Schopflocher D. Neuropsychological test performance in depressed patients before and after drug therapy. *Biol Psychiatry.* 1984;19:55-72.
53. Boone KB, Lesser IM, Miller BL, Mena I. Cognition and rCBF in late-onset depression. *J Clin Exp Neuropsychol.* 1993;15:72.
54. Lesser IM, Hill-Gutierrez E, Miller BL, Boone KB. Late-onset depression with white matter lesions. *Psychosomatics.* 1993;34:364-367.
55. Waldemar G, Hasselbach SG, Anderson AR, Delecluse F, Petersen P, Johnsen A, Paulson OB. ^{99}Tc-d,l-HMPAO and SPECT of the brain in normal aging. *J Cereb Blood Flow Metab.* 1991;11:508-521.
56. Jagust WJ, Reed BR, Seab JP, Kramer JH, Budinger TF. Clinical-physiological correlates of Alzheimer's disease and frontal lobe dementia. *Am J Physiol Imaging.* 1989;4:89-96.
57. Miller BL, Cummings JL, Villanueva-Meyer, Boone KB, Mehringer CM, Lesser IM, Mena I. Frontal lobe degeneration: clinical, neuropsychological, and SPECT characteristics. *Neurology.* 1991;41:1374-1382.
58. Bowen DM, Najlerahim A, Procter AW, Francis PT, Murphy E. Circumscribed changes of the cerebral cortex in neuropsychiatric disorders of later life. *Proc Natl Acad Sci U S A.* 1989;86:9504-9508.
59. Kumar A, Mozley D, Dunham C, Velchik M, Reilley J, Gottlieb G, Alavi A. Semi-quantitative I-123 IMP SPECT studies in late onset depression before and after treatment. *Int J Geriatr Psychiatry.* 1991;6:775-777.

ORIGINAL ARTICLE

Mood-Lowering Effect of Tryptophan Depletion

Enhanced Susceptibility in Young Men at Genetic Risk for Major Affective Disorders

Chawki Benkelfat, MD; Mark A. Ellenbogen; Peggy Dean, RN; Roberta M. Palmour, PhD; Simon N. Young, PhD

Methods: A double-blind placebo-controlled cross-over study in which plasma tryptophan was manipulated by administration of a tryptophan-deficient amino acid mixture. In the placebo condition, all subjects received a nutritionally balanced amino acid mixture that contained tryptophan. To further standardize baseline amino acids, each subject was provided with a low-protein diet the day before amino acid challenges. Subjects were euthymic, healthy men aged 18 to 30 years with either a multigenerational family history of affective illness or no family history of psychiatric illness in the present or in the two previous generations. Each subject was screened with a structured clinical interview to rule out a personal history of psychiatric illness.

Results: Plasma tryptophan was reduced by 89% 5 hours after the administration of the tryptophan-deficient amino acid mixture. Six of 20 subjects with a family history of affective illness and none of 19 subjects without a family history of psychiatric illness showed a lowering of mood of 10 or more points on the Profile of Mood States depression scale (P=.012, Fisher's Exact Test) 5 hours after tryptophan depletion. No significant mood changes were observed following the control treatment (balanced amino acid mixture) in either group.

Conclusions: Our data support the hypothesis that subjects with no prior depressive episodes but with a multigenerational family history of major affective disorder show a greater reduction in mood after tryptophan depletion. They are also consistent with theories that implicate deficient serotonergic function as one possible etiological factor in major depressive disorders.

(Arch Gen Psychiatry. 1994;51:687-697)

The possibility that dysfunctional serotonergic neurotransmission may contribute to the cause of depression is still considered by many to be a useful working hypothesis.[1] Because of the limitations of research on humans, support for the serotonin hypothesis remains largely correlational or indirect. For example, although studies on cerebrospinal fluid (CSF) 5-hydroxyindoleacetic acid (5-HIAA) suggest that low serotonin levels are often associated with depression,[2] this does not necessarily imply that low serotonin is responsible for the depressed mood. Also, evidence suggesting that the blockade or potentiation of serotonergic function causes relapse[3] or enhances antidepressant action,[4] respectively, indicates something about the therapy of depression but not necessarily about its cause. Tryptophan depletion is a research strategy that theoretically provides data about the functional consequences of lowering brain serotonin levels in humans and in animals. In this technique, subjects are given a mixture of amino acids devoid of tryptophan. This induces protein synthesis, and the resulting incorporation of tryptophan into protein leads to a rapid (5-hour) and substantial (80% to 90%) lowering of tryptophan in plasma and tissues.[5-8] Because tryptophan hydroxylase, the rate-limiting enzyme for serotonin synthesis, is normally about half saturated in the human brain,[9] this decline in tryptophan availability is thought to reduce the rate of brain serotonin synthesis. The advantage of this paradigm is that any resulting change in mood or behavior is a consequence of the effects of the

See Subjects and Methods on next page

From the Department of Psychiatry, McGill University, Montreal, Quebec, Canada.

SUBJECTS AND METHODS

SELECTION OF SUBJECTS

Male subjects aged 18 to 30 years were recruited for this study through local newspaper advertisements between March 1991 and July 1992. Inclusion criteria for all subjects included the willingness to participate, good physical health, and an informed knowledge of the medical and psychiatric health of their relatives. Exclusion criteria included adoption, evidence of past or present MAD, evidence of any present Axis I *DSM-III-R* diagnosis, and significant medical illness. Psychiatric evaluations were conducted for all subjects by a trained psychiatric research nurse (P.D.) in consultation with the project psychiatrist (C.B.), using the nonpatient version of the Structured Clinical Interview for *DSM-III-R*.[30]

The inclusion criterion for subjects at genetic risk for MAD was a multigenerational family history of MAD (FH+) as defined by the presence of at least three documented cases of MAD in a minimum of two generations, including at least one affected first-degree relative. In the case of small families, subjects with two documented cases of MAD in first-degree relatives in two generations (ie, parent and sibling) were also included in this study. Subjects who had a single first-degree relative with MAD or who had only second-degree relatives with MAD were excluded from this study. We defined MAD as including both bipolar disorder and recurrent major depression. The inclusion criterion for subjects at no genetic risk for MAD was the absence of documented cases of MAD in all known first, second, and third-degree relatives (FH−). The FH− subjects with multigenerational family histories of any other Axis I disorder were excluded from the study. The FH− subjects were used as the comparison group.

Family history information was obtained in two or three distinct stages of direct interviews with each subject (and/or with a person designated by the subject as knowledgeable about the family history). In stage 1, subjects were interviewed by telephone concerning their personal psychiatric and medical history, and initial family history information was gathered. If a subject appeared to meet our inclusion criteria, he was asked to contact other knowledgeable family members to acquire more precise family history information, and a formal family history interview by a research assistant (M.A.E.) trained in genetic psychiatric interviews was scheduled (stage 2). A detailed family history, including first-, second-, and third-degree relatives, was then elicited systematically. Questions pertaining to hospitalization or medical treatment of MAD, alcohol and other drug abuse, and other physical disorders were emphasized. If there were still issues of uncertainty regarding any relative following this interview, subjects were once again instructed to contact knowledgeable family members and obtain detailed information on the relative(s) of interest, or with the permission of the subject, a knowledgeable relative was contacted directly by the interviewer (stage 3). No family member was considered to be affected unless there was objective evidence supporting a retrospective diagnosis of MAD as well as evidence of chronicity according to Family History Research Diagnostic Criteria.[31,32] Exemplary data included a history of hospitalization for depression and/or mania, a history of attempted or successful suicide, and maintenance treatment with lithium carbonate and/or antidepressant medications, for example. These methods have been shown to identify diagnoses of MAD with high specificity and stability but with reduced sensitivity compared with true diagnoses.[33-35] Genetic histories were obtained to the third degree from FH− subjects with the same rigor used in obtaining information about FH+ subjects and their relatives.

DESIGN OF THE STUDY

Overview

The experiment was a double-blind placebo-controlled cross-over study. The order of treatments was randomized in blocks of six. All subjects participated in a tryptophan-depletion experimental session and a nutritionally balanced amino acid control session, which were at least 1 week apart. Each session consisted of two consecutive days. On day 1, each subject ate a low-protein diet. On day 2, subjects consumed either a tryptophan-free amino acid drink or a similar amino acid drink that also contained the appropriate amount of L-tryptophan for a nutritionally balanced protein source. Behavioral measurements and a venous blood sample were collected before and 5 hours after ingestion of the amino acid drink.

Details of the Procedure

One or two subjects were scheduled per test day. When two subjects were tested on the same day, both FH+ and FH− subjects were included. Prepacked, precooked meals were delivered to the subject's home by a research assistant. These meals were similar in tryptophan (160 mg/24 h), protein (22.6 g/24 h), and caloric (9290 kJ/24 h) content to the low-protein diet used by Delgado et al.[6] The same diet was provided before both treatment days to help maintain blindness for both subjects and investigators and to standardize baseline behavior. Subjects were instructed to eat at regular hours and were allowed ad libitum water and up to 3 cups of coffee or tea per day.

Subjects who had given informed consent were asked to arrive for day 2 experimental sessions at 9 AM after having fasted since midnight the previous night. Observer-based and subjective rating scales of mood states were completed, and a 10-mL venous blood sample was taken for measurement of baseline total and free (non–albumin-bound) plasma tryptophan. Each subject was then given either a tryptophan-free amino acid drink or a nutritionally balanced amino acid drink containing 2.3 g of L-tryptophan, as well as other amino acids. For the next 5 hours, subjects stayed in a single room and were entertained by being shown one or two of three movies (*Diner*, *Star Trek IV*, and *The Right Stuff*) and by being allowed to read magazines. The movies and reading material were cho-

sen to be relatively affectively neutral. Five hours after the ingestion of amino acids, rating scales were again administered, and a second blood sample was drawn. At the completion of the testing session, each subject was given a high-protein snack and received a 1-g L-tryptophan tablet. Subjects in the tryptophan-depletion session were given tryptophan to restore their tryptophan levels, whereas subjects following the balanced-mixture session were given tryptophan to maintain the double-blind status of the study. The tryptophan preparation used is available by prescription in Canada and has not been associated with any cases of eosinophilia myalgia syndrome.[36] Clinical supervision was offered for at least 1 hour after the termination of the experiment, with contact maintained by phone when necessary in the evening and during the day following the experimental session. All subjects resumed their normal diet between the two experimental sessions.

The research assistant who administered the rating scales (M.E.) was blind to the nature of the amino acid mixture administered.

Amino Acid Drinks

The tryptophan-deficient amino acid mixture was the same as that used by Young et al[5] and consisted of 15 amino acids: L-alanine, 5.5 g; L-arginine, 4.9 g; L-cysteine, 2.7 g; glycine, 3.2 g; L-histidine, 3.2 g; L-isoleucine, 8 g; L-leucine, 13.5 g; L-lysine monohydrochloride, 11 g; L-methionine, 3 g; L-phenylalanine, 5.7 g; L-proline, 12.2 g; L-serine, 6.9 g; L-threonine, 6.9 g; L-tyrosine, 6.9 g; and L-valine, 8.9 g. The balanced amino acid mixture contained the same amino acids plus 2.3 g of L-tryptophan. The amino acids were given in the same proportion as they occur in human milk, which is presumably close to the optimum amino acid composition for humans except that glutamate and aspartate were excluded because of concerns about their toxicity. This would not affect the ability of the tryptophan-deficient mixture to lower tryptophan availability because glutamate and aspartate are not essential amino acids. For the tryptophan-deficient mixture, 100 g of amino acids were ingested. This is approximately the amount of amino acids in a 500-g steak. Because of the unpleasant taste of methionine, cysteine, and arginine, these amino acids were put into capsules and administered separately while the subjects were ingesting the rest of the amino acids, which were suspended in water. The amino acid mixture was prepared within a few minutes of oral administration by mixing the powdered amino acids with 150 mL of water, 100 mL of chocolate syrup, and 1.1 g of sodium cyclamate. Subjects were asked to swallow the suspension in as short a time as possible because of its somewhat unpalatable taste.

MEASUREMENT OF MOOD AND OTHER BEHAVIORAL CHANGES

Mood changes were evaluated with objective and subjective rating scales. The Hamilton Depression Rating Scale (HDRS)[37] was administered by a psychiatric nurse at the times noted above. Subjective scales included the Bipolar Profile of Mood States (POMS),[38,39] the Visual Analogue Mood Scale (VAMS),[40] the state part of the State-Trait Anxiety Inventory,[41] the Hopkins Symptom Checklist (SCL-90),[42] and the Beck Depression Inventory (BDI).[43] The bipolar form of the POMS, the principal measure used in these studies, is composed of six bipolar scales: agreeable-hostile, composed-anxious, elated-depressed, confident-unsure, energetic-tired, and clearheaded-confused, and it is highly sensitive to nonclinical changes in mood states. The VAMS consists of sixteen 100-mm horizontal lines, each representing a bipolar dimension of a mood state, on which the subject is instructed to place a perpendicular mark in the location that best describes his mood state.

DETERMINATION OF PLASMA TRYPTOPHAN CONCENTRATIONS

Plasma tryptophan was measured in all blood samples as an index of the extent of tryptophan depletion. The free (non–albumin bound) plasma tryptophan concentration was assumed to be the concentration of tryptophan found in an ultrafiltrate of plasma prepared at 25°C under an atmosphere containing 5% carbon dioxide in a centrifugal ultrafilter (MPS-1, Amicon Inc, Beverly, Mass) using YMT membranes (Millipore Waters, Bedford, Mass). Tryptophan in the ultrafiltrate and in the plasma was measured by high-performance liquid chromatography on a reverse-phase column (μBondapak C_{18}, Millipore Waters) with fluorometric detection.

DATA ANALYSIS

Demographic characteristics of FH+ and FH− subjects were compared by a one-way analysis of variance (ANOVA). All behavioral and blood data were analyzed using a four-way mixed-design ANOVA (order by group by treatment by time). Order (balanced mixture first, tryptophan-deficient mixture first) and group (FH+, FH−) were independent factors; treatment and time were within-subject repeated measures. Planned comparisons were performed for statistically significant factor effects or factor interactions. Fisher's Exact Test (one-tailed) was used to compare the declines in POMS depression (POMS-D) score of FH+ and FH− subjects. A decline of 10 points (one SD in the distribution of standardized POMS-D scores in the general population) was the planned criterion for discrimination between responders and nonresponders. The relationship between mood changes and the degree of change in plasma tryptophan level was assessed using Pearson's correlations.

ETHICS

All subjects who participated in the study gave written informed consent. The study was approved by the Research Ethics Board of the Department of Psychiatry, McGill University, Montreal, Quebec, Canada. All subjects were paid $80 for their participation in the study.

tryptophan-deficient amino acid mixture, and, by implication, of a lowering of central nervous system serotonin.

In humans, tryptophan depletion often results in a lowering of mood, the magnitude of which may be related to the baseline state of the subjects. Delgado et al[6] studied depressed patients who had been treated successfully with antidepressants. The patients continued to receive antidepressants at the time of the study, and their mood, although improved from their original depressed state, was considerably lower than the population means. In the majority of these subjects, the manipulation resulted in a temporary reappearance of the full syndrome of clinical depression within 5 hours. Earlier, Young et al[5] had studied normal male subjects whose depression scale scores were in the high normal range. In these subjects, there was a moderate lowering of mood but no appearance of clinically relevant depressive symptoms. Recently, Abbott et al[10] studied normal men with below average depression scale scores (ie, euthymic subjects). In this population, tryptophan depletion did not result in any lowering of mood. A plausible interpretation of the results of these three studies is that the degree of mood lowering depends on the susceptibility of the subject to lowered mood or depression. One way to test this hypothesis is to study normal subjects who have never been depressed but who are at risk for depression. Young adults with a significant family history for major affective disorders (MADs) may have a genetic predisposition for depression and fulfill this criterion.

Over the past 50 years, research in genetic epidemiology has provided strong evidence of a heritable component in MAD. The frequency of MAD among first-degree relatives of affected probands is 20% to 37%[11-14] compared with a population prevalence of 6% to 10%.[15,16] Concordance in monozygotic twins is 2 to 3 times as high as concordance in dizygotic twins,[17-19] in accord with the findings of contemporary segregation studies demonstrating that MAD is not inherited in a simple mendelian fashion.[20,21] Adoption studies of MAD, although few in number, consistently support the concept that risk is transmitted biologically and that shared intrafamilial environment contributes little to the risk of the development of MAD.[22-25] A contribution of independent environmental factors, however, is posited in all published segregation studies of MAD.[20,21]

Although conclusive proof is lacking, there is general agreement that MAD is clinically and genetically heterogenous.[21,26-28] Of particular relevance to this report is the distinction between familial and sporadic cases of MAD. Both in the research literature and in the clinic,[29] kindreds with multiple affected individuals in each of several generations contrast sharply with families in which only one or two, perhaps distantly related, persons are affected. Although neither group alone constitutes the population of MAD, this distinction is important in designing studies that compare subjects with and without a family history of psychiatric disease. In the present study, we recruited index subjects from multiplex, multigenerational families with strictly defined MAD and control subjects with no family history of MAD. We predicted that tryptophan depletion would lower mood to a greater extent in subjects with a family history of MAD.

RESULTS

DEMOGRAPHIC CHARACTERISTICS AND BASELINE MEASURES OF THE STUDY SAMPLE

Demographic characteristics of the study sample are displayed in **Table 1**. In total, 143 potential FH+ subjects and 60 potential FH− subjects were evaluated in person and over the telephone for participation in the study. Thirty-eight FH+ and six FH− subjects were excluded on the basis of a personal *DSM-III-R* Axis I diagnosis and/or a medical ailment; 75 FH+ and 10 FH− subjects were excluded on the basis of inadequate family history, and seven FH+ and 20 FH− subjects either did not show up for our interviews or dropped out before beginning the study. Furthermore, three FH+ and five FH− subjects chose not to complete the study. Reasons for dropouts included the following: vomiting (FH+, n=2; FH−, n=3), severe headache and/or prolonged nausea (FH−, n=2), and noncompliance (FH+, n=1). These subjects were not included because it would be impossible to interpret their data. The final sample consisted of 20 unrelated FH+ and 19 unrelated FH− subjects.

Demographic and baseline mood measures between FH+ and FH− subjects did not differ significantly, with the exception of there being greater anxiety scores and number of alcoholic drinks consumed per week in FH+ subjects (Table 1). Using the average of baseline scores in the tryptophan-depletion and balanced-mixture condition, FH+ subjects had significantly higher HDRS scores (mean±SD for FH+ subjects, 2.7±1.8; mean±SD for FH− subjects, 1.3±1.4; $F[1,37]=8.1$, $P<.007$). In no case did HDRS baseline scores come close to reaching a level of clinical significance, suggesting that both FH+ and FH− subjects were euthymic at the time of the study. Furthermore, analysis of individual HDRS items at baseline revealed that group differences were due to higher ratings of anxiety in the FH+ group, specifically on the psychic anxiety ($F[1,37]=5.6$, $P<.03$) and somatic anxiety ($F[1,37]=3.6$, $P<.07$) items. This is consistent with the fact that FH+ subjects had significantly higher baseline anxiety levels compared with controls on both the POMS anxiety subscale ($F[1,37]=8.9$, $P<.005$) and the State-Trait Anxiety Inventory ($F[1,36]=4.4$, $P<.05$). However, as with the HDRS differences, these differences were not clinically significant. There were no significant baseline differences in depression scores on the POMS, SCL-90, VAMS, or BDI or on the items of the HDRS that related directly to lowered mood. Subjects differed by definition with respect to family history of affective disorders but also with respect to a family history of alcoholism.

CHANGES IN PLASMA TRYPTOPHAN CONCENTRATIONS

The tryptophan-deficient amino acid mixture resulted in a marked decline in plasma free and total tryptophan concentrations (**Table 2**), whereas the balanced-mixture treatment caused almost a 50% increase in plasma tryptophan concentration. Repeated measures ANOVA for plasma free tryptophan concentrations showed highly significant condition (tryptophan depletion vs balanced mixture) ($F[1,36]=279$, $P<.001$) and time effects (baseline vs posttreatment) ($F[1,36]=28$, $P<.001$), with a significant condition by time interaction ($F[1,36]=224$, $P<.001$). There was no order effect (balanced or tryptophan-deficient mixture first) and no difference between FH+ and FH− subjects. For both groups, the decline in total plasma tryptophan levels was almost 90%.

Table 1. Demographic and Family History Characteristics of Subjects at Risk for MAD and of Normal Controls*

	FH+	FH−
Demographic Characteristics		
Number	20	19
Age, y	24.1±2.8	22.3±3.4
Education, y	13.65±1.76	13.6±2.1
No. of drinks per week	5.15±3.7	2.9±3.5
Weight, kg	73.2±9.3	71.3±11.4
Height, cm	178.2±6.1	176.0±7.9
Mean no. affected relatives per subject	3.45±1.1	0
Psychiatric Disorders in Relatives		
MAD		
First-degree relatives, No. (%)	30 (39)	0
Second-degree relatives, No. (%)	32 (28)	0
Third-degree relatives, No. (%)	7 (ND)	0 (ND)
Alcohol and other drug abuse		
First-degree relatives, No. (%)	4 (5)	2 (3)
Second-degree relatives, No. (%)	9 (7)	2 (1)
Third-degree relatives, No. (%)	0 (ND)	3 (ND)

*MAD indicates major affective disorder; FH+, subjects at risk for MAD; FH−, normal controls; and ND, not determined.

†Percentages of affected relatives were calculated individually for each family, using the total number of affected relatives as the numerator and the total number of relatives at risk as the denominator. Proportions for third-degree relatives could not be generated due to the lack of information regarding the total number of these relatives.

CHANGES IN MOOD

The change in the depression subscale of the POMS after the administration of balanced and tryptophan-deficient drinks to FH+ and FH− subjects is shown in the **Figure**. The effect of the tryptophan-deficient amino acid mixtures on FH+ and FH− subjects was studied using two different statistical techniques. Using the Fisher's Exact Test (one-tailed), we compared the number of subjects in each group who reached a threshold decline in mood after receiving the tryptophan-deficient mixture (**Table 3**). Six of 20 FH+ subjects but none of 19 FH− subjects attained a predetermined 10-point decline in the POMS-D scale (Fisher's Exact Test, $P=.012$). The difference between FH+ and FH− subjects reached the highest level of significance using a nine-point decline in the POMS-D score as the threshold criterion (seven of 20 FH+ vs none of 19 FH− subjects, $P=.005$) but was statistically significant for every decline between four and 11 points.

The second method used for differentiating the effect of tryptophan-depletion treatments on FH+ and FH− subjects was a four-way mixed design ANOVA (group and order, with treatment and time as repeated measures). An analysis of the data showed that order effects (tryptophan-deficient mixture then balanced mixture vs balanced mixture then tryptophan-deficient mixture) were not significant for any dependent measure, so all analyses reported below were collapsed over order. For the POMS depression subscale (**Table 4**), there were trends for the main effect of family history ($F[1,37]=3.4$, $P<.08$) and for the

Table 2. Changes in Total and Free Plasma Tryptophan Levels Following the Ingestion of a Balanced and Tryptophan-Depleted Amino Acid Load*

	Balanced Mixture		Tryptophan-Depleted Mixture	
Time of Administration	FH+ (n=20)	FH− (n=19)	FH+ (n=20)	FH− (n=18)
Total Plasma Tryptophan				
Pretreatment, µg/mL	11.6±2.8	11.6±1.5	11.6±3.1	11.3±2.0
Posttreatment (+5 h), µg/mL	17.0±5.2	16.9±6.6	1.3±0.6	1.22±0.5
Percentage change	50.30	45.40	−88.50	−89
Free Plasma Tryptophan				
Pretreatment, µg/mL	1.3±0.2	1.4±0.3†	1.4±0.2	1.4±0.2
Posttreatment (+5 h), µg/mL	2.1±0.7	2.3±0.8	0.3±0.2	0.3±0.4
Percentage change	64.80	64.10†	−88.50	−89

*FH+ indicates subjects at risk for major affective disorder; FH−, normal controls. Values are expressed as mean±SD.
†n=18.

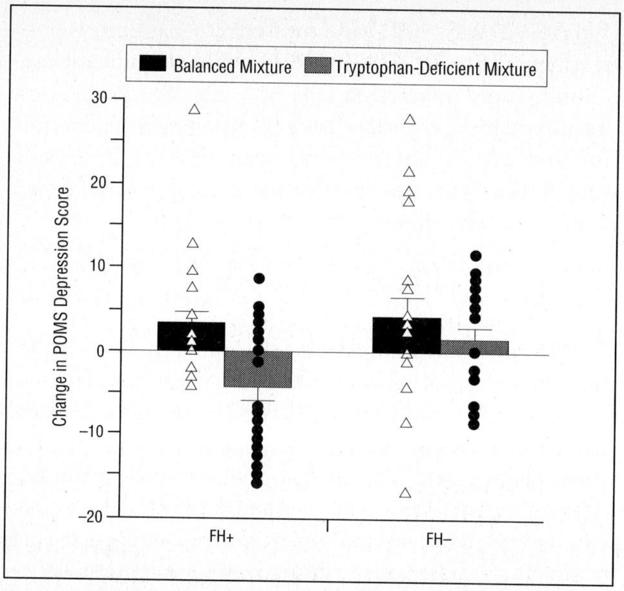

Individual and mean (±SE) change in scores on the Bipolar Profile of Mood States (POMS) depression-elation scale of subjects at genetic risk for major affective disorder (FH+) (n=20) and of normal controls (FH−) (n=19) following the ingestion of a balanced and tryptophan-deficient amino acid load. The FH+ subjects experienced a significant lowering of mood compared with FH− subjects in the tryptophan-depletion condition (P<.02); no significant differences between groups occurred in the balanced condition.

Table 3. Changes in POMS-D Score During Tryptophan Depletion: Sensitivity and Criterion Threshold for Distinguishing Subjects at Genetic Risk for MAD From Normal Controls*

	No. of Subjects Experiencing a Lowering of Mood		
Change in POMS-D Score†	FH+ (n=20)	FH− (n=19)	*P*‡
−2	10	5	NS
−3	10	5	NS
−4	10	4	.047
−5	10	4	.047
−6	10	4	.047
−7	9	2	.017
−8	8	1	.01
−9	7	0	.005
−10	6	0	.012
−11	5	0	.027
−12	4	0	.059
−13	3	0	NS
−14	2	0	NS

**POMS-D indicates the bipolar Profile of Mood States depression scale; MAD, major affective disorder; FH+, subjects at risk for MAD; FH−, normal controls; NS, not significant.*

†Difference from pretreatment to posttreatment administration. A change in score of −10 was the original criteria for defining a lowering of mood.

‡Probability values indicate significance of Fisher's Exact Test (one-tailed), comparing the respective proportions of FH+ and FH− subjects who satisfied the criteria of a decline of POMS-D subscore of the corresponding number of points.

family history by time interaction ($F[1,37]=3.7$, $P<.07$), and there was a significant treatment by time interaction ($F[1,37]=7.6$, $P<.01$). A significant lowering of mood took place only in the FH+ subjects and only as a result of tryptophan depletion ($F[1,37]=7.2$, $P<.02$). Further analysis of the treatment by time interaction demonstrated that there was an overall elevation of mood following the balanced (control) amino acid mixture ($F[1,37]=7.3$, $P<.02$); this effect was similar for the FH− and FH+ groups.

An ANOVA for the sad-happy item of the VAMS (**Table 5**) revealed significant treatment by time ($F[1,37]=8.4$, $P<0.006$) and treatment by time by family history ($F[1,37]=4.6$, $P<.04$) interactions; no significant main effects were found. As was found on the POMS, there was a significant lowering of mood following the tryptophan-depletion treatment in the FH+ group only ($F[1,37]=4.4$, $P<.05$) and a significant increase in mood following the balanced-mixture treatment independent of group ($F[1,37]=5.2$, $P<.03$).

Analysis of the three clinical rating scales for depression (SCL-90, HDRS, and BDI) administered in this study yielded few significant results besides the baseline differences discussed previously. Mean BDI and HDRS scores in either group or after either treatment did not indicate even subclinical levels of depression, and no changes occurred after tryptophan depletion. The mean BDI score in the FH− subjects was 1.2 before the tryptophan-deficient mixture and 0.9 5 hours later, whereas in the FH+ group, the corresponding means were 1.3 and 1.7. On the SCL-90 depression scale, there was a significant condition by time interaction ($F[1,36]=9.3$, $P<.005$), which was largely due to a significant elevation of mood after the balanced-mixture treatment in both groups ($F[1,36]=11.6$, $P<.003$); no changes were found in the tryptophan-depletion treatment.

OTHER SUBJECTIVE CHANGES

Anxiety ratings on the POMS differed significantly between treatments ($F[1,37]=13.1$, $P<.001$) in the direction of higher relative anxiety levels as a result of tryptophan depletion. There were also significant condition by time ($F[1,37]=4.3$, $P<.05$) and group by time interactions ($F[1,37]=5.2$, $P<.03$). Comparisons of the cell means demonstrated that the FH+ group had a significant decrease in anxiety during the balanced-mixture treatment compared with the FH− group ($F[1,37]=4.7$, $P<.04$). Thus, higher baseline anxiety scores in the FH+ group fell to a level similar to that in the FH− group after the balanced-mixture treatment. No differences between groups occurred after the tryptophan-depletion treatment. On the State-Trait Anxiety Inventory, there was a treatment by time interaction ($F[1,36]=10.5$, $P<.004$) that resulted from a significant decrease in anxiety following the balanced-mixture treatment ($F[1,36]=10.4$, $P<.004$), and there was a slight, nonsig-

Table 4. Changes on the POMS Following the Ingestion of a Balanced and Tryptophan-Depleted Amino Acid Load in Subjects at Risk for MAD and in Normal Controls*

		Balanced Amino Acid Load Scores				Tryptophan-Depleted Amino Acid Load Scores			
POMS Scale	Group	Before Treatment	After Treatment	Change in Score†	P‡	Before Treatment	After Treatment	Change in Score†	P‡
Elation-depression	FH−	56.3±2.6	60.6±2.1	4.3±2.3	NS	57.2±2.0	58.9±2.0	1.7±1.4	<.02
	FH+	54.0±1.6	57.3±1.1	3.3±1.6		55.2±1.7	51.2±1.6	−4.0±1.6	
Composed-anxious	FH−	65.6±1.3	63.8±2.1	−1.8±1.6	<.04	63.6±1.5	59.0±2.1	−4.6±2.3	NS
	FH+	59.2±2.0	62.9±2.0	3.7±1.9		58.2±1.7	57.8±1.8	−0.4±1.7	
Energetic-tired	FH−	54.4±2.6	58.0±2.5	3.6±2.1	NS	57.1±2.7	56.3±2.0	−0.8±2.9	NS
	FH+	49.5±2.3	57.8±1.5	8.3±2.3		52.9±2.0	48.4±1.6	−4.5±2.7	
Agreeable-hostile	FH−	56.2±2.0	59.1±2.0	2.9±1.6	NS	57.6±1.9	57.2±2.2	−0.4±1.4	NS
	FH+	53.0±2.3	56.2±1.9	3.2±2.1		53.2±2.1	51.4±1.7	−1.8±1.8	
Confident-unsure	FH−	57.7±2.1	59.9±1.6	2.2±1.8	NS	58.7±2.1	60.1±1.8	1.4±1.3	<.04
	FH+	56.8±1.9	61.1±1.4	4.3±1.6		58.3±1.7	54.7±1.6	−3.6±1.9	
Clearheaded-confused	FH−	59.4±1.9	60.7±1.9	1.3±1.9	NS	59.9±1.5	59.1±1.7	−0.8±0.9	NS
	FH+	58.0±1.9	63.4±1.7	5.4±2.1		58.4±1.8	55.6±1.7	−2.8±1.7	

Profile of Mood States (POMS) scores (mean±SE) are given in normative t scores. MAD indicates major affective disorder; FH−, normal controls; FH+, subjects at risk for MAD; NS, not significant.

†A positive change in score represents a heightening of the mood state (ie, toward "elation" in the first scale), and a negative change in score represents a lowering of the mood state (ie, toward "depression").

‡Probabilities refer to group by time planned comparisons (one-way analysis of variance) performed in each treatment.

nificant increase in the tryptophan-depletion treatment ($F[1,36]=3.0$, $P<.095$).

The POMS confident-unsure scale and the proficient-incompetent item of the VAMS exhibited significant treatment by time interactions (POMS: $F[1,37]=8.5$, $P<.007$; VAMS: $F[1,37]=6.8$, $P<.02$), and there was a significant group by treatment by time interaction on the POMS, as well as a trend for significance on the VAMS (POMS: $F[1,37]=5.7$, $P<.03$; VAMS: $F[1,37]=3.1$, $P<.09$). Planned comparisons of these two scales revealed a significant decrease in confidence (POMS) and proficiency (VAMS) in the FH+ group compared with controls; this occurred only after the tryptophan-depletion treatment (POMS: $F[1,37]=4.8$, $P<.04$; VAMS: $F[1,37]=7.9$, $P<.008$).

RELATIONSHIP BETWEEN RATING SCALE SCORES AND OTHER VARIABLES

The magnitude of changes within a treatment group was not correlated with either the absolute levels of plasma tryptophan or with the changes in plasma tryptophan levels for any of the rating scales used. In the FH+ group, there was no significant correlation between the number of relatives with MAD and the change in POMS mood scores after tryptophan depletion.

COMMENT

SUMMARY OF FINDINGS

In the present study, we attempted an initial examination of the intersection between neurochemistry, behavior, and genetics. Normal male subjects with a multigenerational family history of MAD showed greater mood-lowering effects of tryptophan depletion than did age-matched subjects with no family history of psychiatric illness as measured by the depression scale of the POMS and the happy-sad scale of the VAMS. Six (30%) of 20 FH+ subjects and none of 19 FH− subjects showed a decline of 10 points or greater on the POMS depression scale. As in previous studies of normal men,[5,44] the lowering of mood was not of the same magnitude as that seen in clinical depression. The positive effects were not the consequence of group differences in baseline mood scores or of a differential reduction of plasma tryptophan in FH+ subjects. These data provide a rationale for testing the hypothesis that tryptophan depletion might reveal a vulnerability to depression in some subjects with a multigenerational family history of MAD.

METHODOLOGICAL CONSIDERATIONS

The present study has a number of potential limitations that must be considered in evaluating its strengths and weaknesses. First, pedigree information was collected by the family history method rather than from a personal interview of each family member. Personal interviews would have allowed us to have more detailed information on each family member, especially with regard to anxiety disorders or diagnoses that cannot be made reliably with the family history method. In addition, it would have increased the reliability of ascertainment for FH− subjects. For MAD, the family history method is known to have a high specificity but a low sensitivity: multigen-

Table 5. Changes on the VAMS Following the Ingestion of a Balanced and a Tryptophan-Depleted Amino Acid Load in Subjects at Risk for MAD and in Normal Controls*

		Balanced Amino Acid Load Scores				Tryptophan-Depleted Amino Acid Load Scores			
VAMS Item	Group	Before Treatment	After Treatment	Change in Score†	P‡	Before Treatment	After Treatment	Change in Score†	P‡
Happy-sad	FH−	22.2±5.9	17.9±5.1	−4.3±4.4	NS	22.9±5.9	21.1±5.3	−1.8±4.0	<.05
	FH+	26.8±3.4	19.4±2.6	−7.4±2.7		23.0±3.4	31.4±3.7	8.4±2.8	
Calm-excited	FH−	15.4±3.9	19.4±5.3	4.0±6.0	NS	17.7±4.3	24.9±4.8	7.2±4.9	
	FH+	25.6±4.1	26.2±4.4	0.6±5.6		19.8±2.7	25.5±3.4	5.7±3.5	
Strong-feeble	FH−	33.2±6.5	34.8±6.8	1.6±4.5	<.02	33.7±5.3	29.4±4.9	−4.3±5.1	NS
	FH+	38.6±3.7	23.8±2.8	−14.8±4.7		39.0±5.1	43.8±4.2	4.8±5.1	
Amicable-antagonistic	FH−	30.3±6.2	22.4±5.9	−7.9±3.0	<.04	28.1±6.1	28.6±6.7	0.5±2.7	NS
	FH+	21.9±3.3	21.8±3.2	−0.1±2.1		21.3±3.7	26.4±3.5	5.1±2.4	
Proficient-incompetent	FH−	31.8±6.1	25.3±5.7	−6.5±5.5	NS	26.1±5.5	22.8±5.6	−3.3±3.7	<.01
	FH+	29.2±3.7	21.6±3.0	−7.6±3.9		22.4±3.4	31.8±3.8	9.4±2.7	
Gregarious-withdrawn	FH−	34.5±6.1	26.6±5.5	−7.9±4.5	NS	33.5±5.7	30.4±5.3	−3.1±4.0	(<.09)
	FH+	37.7±3.5	32.6±3.3	−5.1±3.8		36.5±4.6	45.2±4.5	8.7±5.3	
Clearheaded-muzzy	FH−	29.8±6.3	31.1±6.7	1.3±5.3	NS	30.5±5.8	27.1±5.1	−3.4±4.6	(<.07)
	FH+	33.8±5.0	22.5±2.6	−11.3±6.3		27.3±4.5	35.9±4.0	8.6±4.5	
Content-discontent	FH−	17.2±3.9	13.3±3.7	−3.9±3.4	NS	21.4±3.8	23.5±5.0	2.1±4.9	NS
	FH+	24.6±3.3	18.7±2.3	−5.9±3.0		24.8±3.7	35.8±4.1	11.0±3.6	

*VAMS indicates Visual Analogue Mood Scale; MAD, major affective disorder; FH−, normal controls; FH+, subjects at risk for MAD; NS, not significant.
†A positive change in score represents a lowering of the mood state (ie, toward "sad" in the first item), and a negative change in score represents a heightening of mood state (ie, toward "happy").
‡Probabilities refer to group by time planned comparisons (one-way analysis of variance) performed in each treatment. Parentheses indicate trend.

erational kindreds are likely to be correctly classified, but there might well be isolated cases of MAD in FH− kindreds. As no responders (those with a change of 10 or more points on the POMS depression scale) were seen in the FH− group, misclassification would have no effect on the basic finding.

Second, it is possible that FH+ subjects might have experienced a greater change in mood as a consequence of being told in the informed consent that ingestion of amino acid mixtures might have an effect on mood. If this effect was pronounced, FH+ subjects would have been expected to show a decline in mood scores after the ingestion of the balanced mixture as well as after the tryptophan-deficient amino acid mixture, and this was not the case. Nonetheless, we cannot rule out the possibility that FH+ subjects paid more attention to their negative symptoms than did FH− subjects.

In this study, the FH+ subjects showed a greater occurrence of alcoholism in their relatives than did normal controls. Helzer and Winokur[45] reported a greater incidence of alcoholism in relatives of male bipolar probands than in relatives of controls, suggesting that MADs and alcoholism may be part of the same disease spectrum. Hence, comorbidity with alcoholism may be a possible confounding variable in this study. However, most recent studies investigating the patterns of cotransmission of depression and alcoholism in families contradict the spectrum concept[46]: although there is an increased statistical risk for depression in first-degree relatives of alcoholics and vice versa, mathematical modeling of cotransmission suggests that this is not the consequence of shared, transmitted etiological factors of either genetic or environmental origin. If these conclusions hold true, the increased vulnerability of the FH+ subjects to the mood-lowering effect of tryptophan depletion cannot be simplistically accounted for by an increased incidence of alcoholism in their families.

A fourth factor that must be considered when interpreting the results is the biochemical consequence of tryptophan depletion. Whereas the effects of tryptophan depletion on brain serotonin levels in rodents and monkeys are well characterized, the extent to which tryptophan depletion lowers brain serotonin levels in humans is not yet known. In this study, as in previous studies,[5,6,8,10,44,47-51] the tryptophan-deficient amino acid mixture caused a substantial lowering of plasma tryptophan levels. Because human brain tryptophan hydroxylase is about half saturated with tryptophan,[9] a decrease in tryptophan availability would be expected to lower brain serotonin levels, and indeed, in monkeys, lowering plasma tryptophan levels by administering a tryptophan-deficient amino acid mixture lowers CSF 5-HIAA concentrations by approximately 25% to 30%.[47] It is also possible that lowering brain tryptophan levels may lower the level of other psychoactive tryptophan metabolites such as melatonin, tryptamine, quinolinic acid, and ky-

nurenic acid or that it may lower brain nicotinamide-adenine dinucleotide or protein synthesis or influence neuroendocrine regulation or overall neurotransmitter balance. However, in one study, short-term tryptophan depletion did not alter plasma prolactin levels, although overall there was a significant positive correlation between plasma tryptophan and plasma prolactin levels.[52] Finally, the administration of a protein load may have important endocrine effects, particularly in association with tryptophan depletion.

EFFECTS OF TRYPTOPHAN DEPLETION ON MOOD: ADDITIONAL EVIDENCE SUPPORTING THE SEROTONERGIC HYPOTHESIS OF DEPRESSION

Tryptophan depletion was associated with a definite decline in mood, which was significantly greater in FH+ subjects than in FH− subjects. As in previous studies of normal men,[5,44] the reduction of mood was not of the same magnitude as that seen in clinical depression. Nonetheless, the lack of mood change after tryptophan depletion in the FH− subjects contrasts with the original finding of lowered mood in normal male subjects.[5,44] In these previous studies, there was only a cursory screening of subjects; some might well have met the criteria for a positive family history. Although baseline depression scale scores in these earlier subjects were normal, they clustered toward the high end of the normal distribution (ie, in the direction of "sad"). Control subjects in the present study were similar to a recently studied group of well-screened subjects with depression scale scores in the low normal range.[10] These subjects showed no lowering of mood after tryptophan depletion. The failure of tryptophan depletion to lower mood in untreated depressed patients[53] requires further investigation. In this study, baseline scores were near the upper end of the scale, suggesting that a ceiling effect may pertain. Also patients were studied using clinical scales such as the HDRS rather than a scale designed to measure rapid changes in mood such as the POMS.

While definite effects were seen on the POMS depression scale and the VAMS happy-sad scale, other scales also revealed significant effects of tryptophan depletion in FH+ subjects. These included the POMS confident-unsure scale and the VAMS proficient-incompetent scale. The changes seen in these other scales could well be secondary to the decline in mood. Thus, a previous study[5] showed that normal men who received a tryptophan-deficient amino acid mixture paid selective attention to dysphoric stimuli. This could lead the subjects to rate themselves as more unsure and incompetent.

The data reviewed so far support the hypothesis that serotonin is involved directly in the control of mood. This is consistent with the fact that studies of serotonin and serotonin receptors in postmortem brains of depressed patients and studies of the serotonin metabolite 5-HIAA in the CSF of depressed patients show that brain serotonin metabolism is low in some but not all depressed patients.[1] Furthermore, depressed patients with low CSF 5-HIAA continue to exhibit low levels on follow-up, despite clinical recovery.[54-56] Patients with low serotonin levels show more frequent relapses than do patients with normal serotonin levels, suggesting that low serotonin levels may predispose some patients to depression.[57] In normal subjects, low CSF 5-HIAA levels tend to be associated with a family history of depression.[58] Various studies in the literature involving the measurement of plasma amino acid levels report decreased availability of tryptophan in depressed patients.[59-61] However, the magnitude of the decline in plasma tryptophan availability reported in depressed patients is considerably less than that seen in our subjects after ingestion of the tryptophan-deficient amino acid mixture. Thus, low serotonin levels are probably one factor contributing to MAD in a condition that is most likely heterogeneous and complex in its cause, but low tryptophan availability is unlikely to be the basis for depression except in rare cases.

THE AFFECTIVE RESPONSE TO TRYPTOPHAN DEPLETION: A PUTATIVE PHENOTYPIC MARKER IN AFFECTIVE ILLNESS?

The affective response to tryptophan depletion is heuristically attractive as a potential biological marker of MAD because it combines the experimental manipulation of a neurotransmitter system that is widely thought to be implicated in depression with the behavioral changes related to the symptoms seen in patients. Much work remains to be done, however, before this phenotypic response pattern can be proffered as a biological marker. Tests of stability, specificity, and sensitivity will all be necessary. In patients who are successfully treated with antidepressant medications (especially selective inhibitors of serotonin reuptake), Delgado et al[6] have shown that tryptophan depletion induces clinical signs of depression that are qualitatively different from the worsening of mood seen in normal volunteers.[5,10,44] By contrast, patients with bipolar disorders who are stable on lithium therapy (C.B., B. Selette, R.M.P., M.A.E., P.D., S.N.Y., unpublished data, 1993) and depressed patients who are not receiving medication[53] do not display mood changes of a clinical magnitude in response to tryptophan depletion. As discussed above, this latter finding might reflect a ceiling effect or the lack of sensitivity of the rating scale used rather than complete insensitivity to tryptophan depletion. There has been no test as yet of the effects of tryptophan depletion in patients with MAD who are not receiving medication and are in remission.

It is perhaps worth noting that the successful validation of a phenotypic marker, such as the affective response to tryptophan depletion, would be useful both

clinically and in genetic linkage studies because the penetrance of the marker is likely to be higher than the penetrance of the overt illness. It would then theoretically be possible to test the cosegregation between highly polymorphic DNA markers and the affective response to tryptophan depletion rather than the cosegregation between linkage markers and MAD.

CONCLUSION

One of the methods available for studying the role of brain serotonin in MADs is the tryptophan depletion paradigm. Subjects receive an amino acid mixture that dramatically lowers their plasma tryptophan levels and, thus, presumably, their brain serotonin levels. We applied this research strategy to the study of subjects at risk for MAD to further elucidate the role of putative serotonergic abnormalities in the neurobiology of depression. We demonstrated that these FH+ subjects showed a greater lowering of mood after tryptophan depletion compared with subjects with no family history of MAD. Our findings provide a rationale for testing the hypothesis that a lowering of mood after tryptophan depletion might reveal a vulnerability to depression in patients with MAD and in some of their first-degree relatives and that it may thus have value as a neurobiological probe in genetic research. The validation of such a marker would have implications in mental health, in particular with respect to genetic counseling and prophylaxis for the affective illness.

Accepted for publication June 13, 1994.

This work was supported by the Fonds de la Recherche en Santé du Quebec, Montreal (Drs Benkelfat, Palmour, and Young) and the Medical Research Council of Canada, Ottawa, Ontario (Drs Young and Palmour). Dr Benkelfat is the recipient of a joint Medical Research Council of Canada and Pharmaceutical Manufacturers Association of Canada (Ottawa) Scholarship and a Health Research Foundation–Pharmaceutical Manufacturers Association of Canada–Medical Research Council Career Award in Medicine.

We thank Franceen Lenoff for technical assistance, Liz Rusnak for editorial assistance, and Pierre Blier, MD, for medical consultations.

Reprint requests to the Department of Psychiatry, McGill University, 1033 Pine Ave W, Montreal, Quebec, Canada, H3A 1A1 (Dr Palmour).

REFERENCES

1. Meltzer HY, Lowy MT. The serotonin hypothesis of depression. In: Meltzer HY, ed. *Psychopharmacology: The Third Generation of Progress.* New York, NY: Raven Press; 1987:513-526.
2. Meltzer HY. Serotonergic dysfunction in depression. *Br J Psychiatry.* 1989; 155:25-31.
3. Shopsin B, Friedman E, Gershon S. Parachlorophenylalanine reversal of tranylcypromine effects in depressed patients. *Arch Gen Psychiatry.* 1976;33:811-822.
4. Blier P, de Montigny C, Chaput Y. A role for serotonin in the mechanism of action of antidepressant drugs: preclinical data. *J Clin Psychiatry.* 1990;51 (suppl):14-20.
5. Young SN, Smith SE, Pihl RO, Ervin FR. Tryptophan depletion causes a rapid lowering of mood in normal males. *Psychopharmacology.* 1985;87:173-177.
6. Delgado PL, Charney DS, Price LH, Aghajanian GK, Landis H, Heninger GR. Serotonin function and the mechanism of antidepressant action: reversal of antidepressant-induced remission by rapid depletion of plasma tryptophan. *Arch Gen Psychiatry.* 1990;47:411-418.
7. Gessa GL, Biggio G, Fadda F, Corsini GV, Tagliamonte A. Effect of oral administration of tryptophan-free amino acid mixtures on serum tryptophan, brain tryptophan and serotonin metabolism. *J Neurochem.* 1974;22:869-870.
8. Moja EA, Antinoro E, Cesa-Bianchi M, Gessa GL. Increases in stage 4 sleep after ingestion of a tryptophan-free diet in humans. *Pharmacol Res Commun.* 1984;16:909-914.
9. Young SN, Gauthier S. Effect of tryptophan administration on tryptophan, 5-hydroxyindoleacetic acid, and indoleacetic acid in human lumbar and cisternal cerebrospinal fluid. *J Neurol Neurosurg Psychiatry.* 1981;44:323-327.
10. Abbott FV, Etienne P, Franklin KBJ, Morgan MJ, Sewitch MJ, Young SN. Acute tryptophan depletion blocks morphine analgesia in the cold-pressor test in humans. *Psychopharmacology.* 1992;108:60-66.
11. Angst J, Frey R, Lohmeyer B, Zerbin-Rudin E. Bipolar manic-depressive psychoses: results of a genetic investigation. *Hum Genet.* 1980;55:237-254.
12. Gershon ES, Hamovit J, Guroff JJ, Dibble E, Leckman JF, Sceery W, Targum SD, Nurnberger JI, Goldin LR, Bunney WE. A family study of schizoaffective, bipolar I, bipolar II, unipolar, and normal control probands. *Arch Gen Psychiatry.* 1982;39:1157-1167.
13. Andreasson NC, Rice J, Endicott J, Reich T, Coryell W, Grove WM. Familial rates of affective disorder: a report from the NIMH Collaborative Study. *Arch Gen Psychiatry.* 1987;44:461-469.
14. Weissman MM, Gershon ES, Kidd KK, Prusoff BA, Leckman JF, Dibble E, Hamovit J, Thompson WD, Pauls DL, Guroff JJ. Psychiatric disorders in the relatives of probands with affective disorders: the Yale University-National Institute of Mental Health collaborative study. *Arch Gen Psychiatry.* 1984;41: 13-21.
15. Bland RC. Long-term mental illness in Canada: an epidemiological perspective on schizophrenia and affective disorders. *Can J Psychiatry.* 1979;29:242-246.
16. Prusoff BA, Merikangas KR, Weissman MM. Lifetime prevalence and age of onset of psychiatric disorders: recall 4 years later. *J Psychiatr Res.* 1988;22: 107-117.
17. Bertelsen A, Harvald B, Hauge M. A Danish twin study of manic-depressive disorder. *Br J Psychiatry.* 1977;130:330-351.
18. Bertelsen A. A Danish twin study of manic-depressive disorders. In: Schou M, Strömgren E, eds. *Origin, Prevention and Treatment of Affective Disorders.* Orlando, Fla: Academic Press Inc, 1979;227-239.
19. Price J. Neurotic and endogenous depression: a phylogenetic view. *Br J Psychiatry.* 1968;114:119-120.
20. Goldin LR, Gershon ES, Targum SD, Sparkes RS, McGinniss M. Segregation and linkage analyses in families of patients with bipolar, unipolar and schizoaffective mood disorders. *Am J Hum Genet.* 1983;35:1274-1287.
21. Cox N, Reich T, Rice J, Elston R, Schober J, Keats B. Segregation and linkage analyses of bipolar and major depressive illness in multigenerational pedigrees. *J Psychiatr Res.* 1989;23:109-123.
22. Mendlewicz J, Rainer JD. Adoption study supporting genetic transmission of manic-depressive illness. *Nature.* 1977;268:327-329.
23. Wender PH, Kety SS, Rosenthal D, Schulsinger F, Ortmann J, Lunde I. Psychiatric disorders in the biological and adoptive families of adopted individuals with affective disorders. *Arch Gen Psychiatry.* 1986;43:923-929.
24. Cadoret RM. Evidence for genetic inheritance of primary affective disorder in adoptees. *Am J Psychiatry.* 1978;135:463-486.
25. Kendler KS, Neale MC, Kessler RC, Heath AC, Eaves LJ. A population-based twin study of major depression in women: the impact of varying definitions of illness. *Arch Gen Psychiatry.* 1992;49:257-266.
26. Gershon ES, Berrettini W, Nurnberger I, Goldin LR. Genetics of affective disorders. In: Meltzer HY, ed. *Psychopharmacology: The Third Generation of Progress.* New York, NY: Raven Press; 1987:481-491.
27. Blehar MC, Weissman MM, Gershon ES, Hirschfield RMA. Family and genetic studies of affective disorders. *Arch Gen Psychiatry.* 1988;45:269-292.

28. Baron M. Molecular genetics of affective psychoses. In: Mendlewicz J, Hippius H, eds. *Genetic Research in Psychiatry.* Berlin, Germany: Springer-Verlag; 1992: 1-17.
29. Palmour RM. Genetic counselling for affective illness. *Psychiatr J Univ Ottawa.* 1989;14:323-327.
30. Spitzer RL. *Structured Clinical Interview for DSM-IIIR.* New York, NY: New York State Psychiatric Institute Biometrics Research Department; 1987.
31. Spitzer RL, Endicott J, Robins E. Research Diagnostic Criteria. *Arch Gen Psychiatry.* 1978;35:773-782.
32. Andreasson NC, Endicott J, Spitzer L, Winokur G. The family history method using diagnostic criteria: reliability and validity. *Arch Gen Psychiatry.* 1977; 34:1229-1235.
33. Andreasson NC, Rice J, Endicott J, Reich T, Coryell W. The family history approach to diagnosis: how useful is it? *Arch Gen Psychiatry.* 1986;43:421-429.
34. Thompson WD, Orvaschel H, Prusoff BA, Kidd KK. An evaluation of the family history method for ascertaining psychiatric disorders. *Arch Gen Psychiatry.* 1982;39:53-58.
35. Rice JP, Rochberg N, Endicott J, Lavori PW, Miller C. Stability of psychiatric diagnoses: an application to the affective disorders. *Arch Gen Psychiatry.* 1992; 49:824-830.
36. Wilkins K. Eosinophilia-myalgia syndrome. *Can Med Assoc J.* 1990;142:1265-1266.
37. Hamilton M. Rating depressive patients. *J Clin Psychiatry.* 1960;41:21-24.
38. McNair DM, Lorr M, Droppleman LF. *Manual for the Profile of Mood States.* San Diego, Calif: Educational and Industrial Testing Service; 1988.
39. Lorr M, McNair DM, Fisher S. Evidence for bipolar mood states. *J Pers Assess.* 1982;46:432-436.
40. Bond A, Lader M. The use of analogue scales in rating subjective feelings. *Br J Med Psychol.* 1974;47:211-218.
41. Spielberger C, Gorsuch R, Lushene R. *Manual for the State-Trait Anxiety Inventory.* Palo Alto, CA: Consulting Psychologists Press; 1970.
42. Derogatis L. *SCL-90-R Manual-II.* Towson, Md: Clinical Psychometric Research; 1983.
43. Beck AT, Ward CH, Mendelson M, Mock JE, Erbaugh JK. An inventory for measuring depression. *Arch Gen Psychiatry.* 1961;4:561-571.
44. Smith SE, Pihl RO, Young SN, Ervin FR. A test of possible cognitive and environmental influences on the mood-lowering effect of tryptophan depletion in normal males. *Psychopharmacology.* 1987;91:451-457.
45. Helzer JE, Winokur G. A family interview study of male manic-depressives. *Arch Gen Psychiatry.* 1974;31:73-77.
46. Maier W, Merikangas KR. Cotransmission and comorbidity of affective disorders, anxiety disorders, and alcoholism in families. In: Mendlewicz J, Hippius H, eds. *Genetic Research in Psychiatry.* Berlin, Germany: Springer-Verlag; 1992: 207-217.
47. Young SN, Ervin FR, Pihl RO, Finn P. Biochemical aspects of tryptophan depletion in primates. *Psychopharmacology.* 1989;98:508-511.
48. Young SN, Tourjman SV, Teff KL, Pihl RO, Anderson GH. The effect of lowering plasma tryptophan on food selection in normal males. *Pharmacol Biochem Behav.* 1988;31:149-152.
49. Smith SE, Pihl RO, Young SN, Ervin FR. Elevation and reduction of plasma tryptophan and their effects on aggression and perceptual sensitivity in normal males. *Aggressive Behav.* 1986;12:393-407.
50. Zacchia C, Pihl RO, Young SN, Ervin FR. The influence of altered tryptophan availability on ethanol intoxication in normal men. *J Stud Alcohol.* 1987;48: 535-540.
51. Pihl RO, Young SN, Ervin FR, Plotnick S. The influence of tryptophan availability on selection of alcohol and water by men. *J Stud Alcohol.* 1987;48: 260-264.
52. Danjou P, Hamon M, Lacomblez L, Warot D, Kecskemeti S, Puech AJ. Psychomotor, subjective and neuroendocrine effects of acute tryptophan depletion in the healthy volunteer. *Psychiatr Psychobiol.* 1990;5:31-38.
53. Miller HL, Delgado PL, Salomon RM, Licinio J, Barr LC, Charney DS. Acute tryptophan depletion: a method of studying antidepressant action. *J Clin Psychiatry.* 1992;53:28-35.
54. Coppen A, Prange AJ, Whybrow PC, Noguera R. Abnormalities of indoleamines in affective disorders. *Arch Gen Psychiatry.* 1972;26:474-478.
55. van Praag HM. Significance of biochemical parameters in the diagnosis, treatment and prevention of depressive disorders. *Biol Psychiatry.* 1977;12:101-131.
56. Träskman-Bendz L, Asberg M, Bertilsson L, Thoren P. CSF monoamine metabolites of depressed patients during illness and after recovery. *Acta Psychiatr Scand.* 1984;69:333-342.
57. van Praag HM, de Haan S. Central serotonin metabolism and frequency of depression. *Psychiatry Res.* 1979;1:219-224.
58. Sedvall G, Fryö B, Gullberg B, Nybäack H, Wiesel FA, Wode-Helgodt B. Relationship in normal volunteers between concentrations of monoamine metabolites in cerebrospinal fluid and family history of psychiatric morbidity. *Br J Psychiatry.* 1980;136:366-247.
59. Maes M, Vandewoude M, Schotte C, Martin M, D'Hondt P, Scharpe S, Blockx P. The decreased availability of L-tryptophan in depressed females: clinical and biological correlates. *Prog Neuropsychopharmacol Biol Psychiatry.* 1990;14: 903-919.
60. DeMeyer MK, Shea PA, Hendrie HC, Yoshimura NN. Plasma tryptophan and five other amino acids in depressed and normal subjects. *Arch Gen Psychiatry.* 1981;38:642-646.
61. Dunlop SR, Hendrie HC, Shea PA, Brittain HM. Ratio of plasma tryptophan to five other amino acids in depressed subjects: a follow-up. *Arch Gen Psychiatry.* 1983;40:1033-1034.

Increased Evening Activation of the Hypothalamic-Pituitary-Adrenal Axis in Depressed Patients

Elizabeth A. Young, MD; Roger F. Haskett, MD; Leon Grunhaus, MD; Atul Pande, MD; Virginia Murphy Weinberg, RN; Stanley J. Watson, MD, PhD; Huda Akil, PhD

Objective: To determine whether depressed patients demonstrate hypothalamic-pituitary-adrenal (HPA) axis activation during the late afternoon and evening, a time when the HPA axis is usually quiescent in normal subjects.

Methods: We administered metyrapone, an 11-β-hydroxylase inhibitor of cortisol synthesis, to normal controls and depressed patients between 4 and 10 PM. Metyrapone blockade of cortisol secretion would amplify any HPA axis secretion.

Results: In 10 normal control subjects, administration of metyrapone lowered plasma cortisol levels to a mean of 36 nmol/L. No rebound corticotropin or β-endorphin secretion was seen in these normal controls between 4 and 10 PM, supporting the existence of a period of minimal endogenous corticotropin releasing factor drive. Compared with a group of placebo-treated depressed patients (n=10), metyrapone-treated depressed subjects (n=17) had significantly decreased plasma cortisol concentrations. However, in contrast to normal controls treated with metyrapone, metyrapone-treated depressed patients demonstrated rebound corticotroph secretion, particularly between 7:30 and 10 PM (P=.036 for patients vs normal controls for β-endorphin secretion from 4:30 to 10 PM).

Conclusion: These data support the hypothesis of increased corticotropin releasing factor drive in the evening in depressed subjects and are in agreement with the longstanding observation of "early escape" from dexamethasone suppression between 4 and 11 PM in depressed patients.

(Arch Gen Psychiatry. 1994;51:701-707)

IN DEPRESSION, hypothalamic-pituitary-adrenal (HPA) axis overactivity, as assessed by cortisol hypersecretion, has been repeatedly demonstrated.[1-6] A number of studies have suggested that cortisol hypersecretion is most obvious in the late afternoon or evening, when circadian activation of the HPA axis should be minimal. Work by Halbreich and colleagues[4] suggested that a single cortisol sample drawn in the afternoon could discriminate depressed from nondepressed subjects. Work by Carroll and collaborators[7,8] demonstrated that late afternoon and evening was the best period to distinguish "escape" from dexamethasone suppression. Similarly, we found that late afternoon was the best time to detect nonsuppression of corticotroph secretion following the administration of dexamethasone.[9] While the dexamethasone suppression test has proved useful in demonstrating the existence of HPA axis abnormalities in depression, the underlying physiological abnormality is less clear. Although the dexamethasone suppression test is viewed as a test of the sensitivity of the HPA axis to negative feedback, an alternative explanation is possible. The dexamethasone suppression test evaluates the balance between endogenous HPA axis activation (corticotropin releasing factor [CRF]) and negative feedback (dexamethasone). Following the administration of dexamethasone at 11:30 PM, normal control subjects have sup-

From the Department of Psychiatry and the Mental Health Research Institute, University of Michigan Medical Center, Ann Arbor. Dr Haskett is now with the Department of Psychiatry, Western Psychiatric Institute, Pittsburgh, Pa. Dr Grunhaus is now with the Department of Psychiatry, Sheba Hospital, Tel Hashomer, Israel. Dr Pande is now with Eli Lilly Pharmaceuticals, Indianapolis, Ind.

See Methods on next page

METHODS

SUBJECT SELECTION

All patients presented to the University of Michigan Depression Research Program, Ann Arbor, which consists of both inpatient and outpatient treatment facilities. Thirteen of the 27 patients were inpatients; the remainder were outpatients. All patients met the Research Diagnostic Criteria for major depressive disorder as assessed by the structured interview of the Schedule for Affective Disorders and Schizophrenia (SADS).[14] Twenty-five of the 27 patients also met the criteria for probable or definite endogenous subtype of depression. All patients had been free of significant drug and alcohol abuse for at least 3 years; in cases where past alcohol and drug abuse had occurred, the first episode of depression preceded the onset of alcohol or drug abuse. The 17-item Hamilton Depression Rating Scale (HDRS) was filled out by the treating psychiatrist within 5 days of the study. This rating was always a pretreatment rating; however, if two HDRS scores were available for the patient, one before and one after the study day, the HDRS score for the date closest to the study date was used. Patients were free of all drugs for a minimum of 10 days, except for aspirin and acetaminophen, which are not known to affect the HPA axis. Inpatients were studied a minimum of 5 days following inpatient hospitalization. Patients with known medical illnesses were excluded. Normal controls were recruited by public advertising and were screened for family history of psychiatric disorders and alcoholism.

All controls were screened with the Schedule for Affective Disorders and Schizophrenia–Lifetime version and fulfilled the criteria for never mentally ill. Routine screening blood work and physical examination excluded subjects with medical illness. Normal controls were matched by age and sex with the initial group of metyrapone-treated depressed patients. Because all the normal controls demonstrated similar patterns of hormone secretion following metyrapone treatment, fewer normal controls than depressed patients were studied. All patients and controls had normal thyroid hormone values (thyroxine and thyrotropin). Female patients and controls had a negative pregnancy test result. All subjects gave informed consent for these studies, and the protocol was approved by the University of Michigan Institutional Review Board.

STUDY DESIGN

All patients and normal controls were studied in one of two identical "study rooms" that were designed to minimize stress and outside stimulation for patient studies. These rooms are located adjacent to the inpatient unit. Outpatients and controls presented between 3:30 and 4 PM, while inpatients were brought to these rooms from the inpatient unit. An intravenous catheter for blood drawing was inserted at 4 PM, followed by the administration of metyrapone (750 mg) or placebo (ascorbic acid). Because the amount of blood drawn for this study was equivalent to 1 U, we were unable to study the same subject both at baseline and following metyrapone challenge. Thus, independent groups of patients were entered into the placebo and metyrapone groups. A second dose of metyrapone or placebo was given at 7:30 PM. All subjects ate dinner between 5:30 and 6:15 PM. Blood for β-LPH/β-endorphin, corticotropin, and cortisol determinations was drawn every 30 minutes between 4 and 10 PM. Blood for corticotropin and β-LPH/β-endorphin determinations was drawn into potassium ethylenediaminetetraacetic acid tubes; blood for cortisol determinations was drawn into heparin-containing Vacutainer tubes. All samples were drawn on ice and centrifuged immediately; the plasma was separated and then frozen on dry ice. Plasma for peptide assays was acidified at the time of collection and stored at −70°C until extraction.

HORMONAL ASSAYS

Plasma for β-LPH/β-endorphin and corticotropin determinations was extracted with Sep Pak C_{18} cartridges, then lyophilized. The β-endorphin radioimmunoassay utilizes an antibody raised to β-endorphin (human sequence) and demonstrates 100% cross-reactivity with β-LPH and proopiomelanocortin (POMC), the precursor protein of β-LPH and β-endorphin. The optimal conditions for this assay for human plasma have been previously described.[15] The corticotropin radioimmunoassay utilizes an antibody raised to $ACTH_{11-24}$ (human sequence) that recognizes $ACTH_{1-39}$, glycosylated $ACTH_{1-39}$ and proopiomelanocortin. However, the antibody does not recognize α–melanocyte-stimulating hormone (N-acetyl $ACTH_{1-13}$ amide). The assay procedure for plasma has been previously described.[16] Cortisol was assayed by a high-performance liquid chromatography procedure that discriminates cortisol from 11-deoxycortisol. Before injection of the high-performance liquid chromatography column, metyrapone was separated from cortisol and 11-deoxycortisol by an organic extraction with a 1-to-1 ratio of methylene chloride and a 1N solution of hydrochloric acid. These high-performance liquid chromatography steroid measures were further validated by comparison with values of combined cortisol plus 11-deoxycortisol measured by the corticosteroid binding globulin assay; disagreement between measures by the two methods was not more than 10%.

DATA ANALYSIS

Data were analyzed by a repeated-measure analysis of variance examining the effects of treatment over time (single-factor analysis of variance) as well as by a two-way analysis of variance comparing normal controls with depressed patients. The 4 PM values were excluded from data analyses because these values, obtained immediately following intravenous insertion, demonstrated substantial effects of intravenous insertion on plasma concentrations of both peptides and cortisol.

pressed plasma cortisol concentrations throughout the day and evening[8,10] despite waning plasma dexamethasone concentrations.[1-13] This suggests that diminished endogenous HPA axis activation in the late afternoon and evening may contribute to suppression of plasma cortisol in normal control subjects. In contrast, rather than abnormal feedback in response to dexamethasone, depressed patients may demonstrate increased activation of the HPA axis during the late afternoon and evening. Consequently, a significant part of the HPA axis abnormalities in depression may result from the continued activation of HPA axis secretion in the late afternoon and evening, a period when the system is normally quiescent.

To uncover and amplify this hypothesized increased activation of the HPA axis in depressed patients in the late afternoon and evening, we administered metyrapone, an inhibitor of cortisol synthesis, between 4 and 10 PM and monitored corticotroph secretion by measurement of β-lipotropin (β-LPH)/β-endorphin and corticotropin levels. We hypothesized that (1) if activation of the HPA axis is normally absent during the evening, then blockade of cortisol synthesis would not lead to rebound corticotroph secretion in normal controls, and (2) if depression were accompanied by HPA axis activation in the evening, then blockade of cortisol production would lead to an amplification of corticotroph secretion in these patients. The studies presented here characterize the hormonal response of depressed patients as a group and compare their hormonal profiles with those of a group of age- and sex-matched normal control subjects.

RESULTS

The study population is described in **Table 1**. The three groups demonstrated similar sex ratios (1:1). The metyrapone-treated patients were significantly older than the placebo-treated patients (P=.018, Student's t test). The mean HDRS score did not differ significantly between metyrapone- and placebo-treated patients. The only side effect of metyrapone administration was mild nausea in a few control subjects who had not eaten lunch. Thereafter, we instructed all subjects to eat lunch at noon the day of the study, and no additional problems were encountered. Patients did not complain of distress or anxiety during the course of the study.

EFFECT OF METYRAPONE ON HORMONAL MEASURES IN NORMAL CONTROLS

The effect of metyrapone on hormone measures will be presented in two ways, as figures showing the actual profile of hormone secretion (mean±SE) and in table form presenting the mean hormone concentrations over the two halves of the study.

Because the HPA axis is quiescent in the late afternoon and evening in normal subjects, we hypothesized that the administration of metyrapone would lower the plasma cortisol concentration in normal subjects without stimulating rebound secretion of corticotropin or β-LPH/β-endorphin. The effect of metyrapone administration on the plasma cortisol profile of the normal controls is shown in **Figure 1**. As can be observed, following metyrapone treatment, cortisol concentrations fell to less than 55 nmol/L and remained low throughout the study. The fall in plasma cortisol concentrations was not accompanied by rebound β-LPH/β-endorphin secretion.

Table 2 summarizes hormone values by time period for the normal controls. These values were obtained by averaging the plasma hormone concentrations for all time points between 4:30 and 7 PM and then between 7:30 and 10 PM, providing an index of mean hormone secretion over these periods. Following metyra-

Table 1. Demographic Characteristics of Normal Controls and Depressed Patients

		Depressed Patients	
	Normal Controls	Placebo Group	Metyrapone Group
No. of subjects	10	10	17
M	5	5	8
F	5	5	9
Age, y*	41.8±10	33.8±9.6	46.8±14.6
Hamilton Depression Rating Scale score*	. . .	21±5	18.2±6

**Values are mean± SD.*

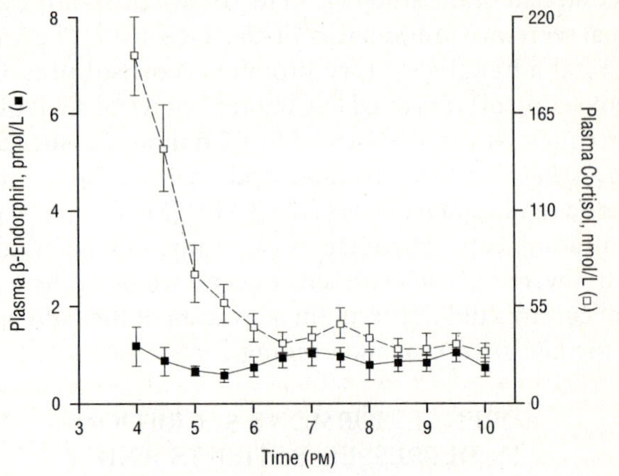

Figure 1. *Plasma cortisol and β-endorphin responses to the administration of metyrapone in normal control subjects. Metyrapone was administered at 4 PM, after the baseline sample was drawn, and at 7:30 PM. Following the initial dose of metyrapone, plasma cortisol concentrations declined to low levels and remained below 55 nmol/L. This decrease in plasma cortisol concentrations was not accompanied by an increase in β-endorphin secretion.*

Table 2. Hormone Measurements After Metyrapone Administration*

	Normal Controls		Depressed Patients	
	4:30-7 PM	7:30-10 PM	4:30-7 PM	7:30-10 PM
Cortisol, nmol/L	66±17	36±22	74±19	52±14
β-Lipotropin/β-endorphin, pmol/L	0.9±0.1	0.9±0.1	1.5±0.1	2.4±0.2
11-Deoxycortisol, nmol/L	28±9	40±5	29±9	69±6
Total adrenal (cortisol plus 11-deoxycortisol), nmol/L	88±14	72±6	107±14	121±6
β-Lipotropin/β-endorphin (corticotropin subset), pmol/L	0.6±0.1	0.6±0.1	1.1±0.2	1.7±0.2
Corticotropin, pmol/L	0.4±0.2	0.4±0.1	1.1±0.5	1.4±0.8

Values are mean±SD.

pone administration, plasma cortisol concentrations declined, and the inactive precursor, 11-deoxycortisol, was secreted by the adrenal gland instead of cortisol. By the second half of the study (7:30 to 10 PM), 50% of the adrenal secretory product was 11-deoxycortisol. The level of total adrenal secretory products (cortisol plus 11-deoxycortisol) remained low but relatively constant over the course of the study (83.2 vs 67.6 nmol/L), suggesting a steady but low activation of adrenal secretion. There was no significant increase of the β-LPH/β-endorphin concentration over the course of the study, demonstrating that lowered plasma cortisol concentrations in the normal controls did not result in activation of the HPA axis in the late afternoon and evening.

ADRENAL HORMONE SECRETION IN DEPRESSED PATIENTS AND NORMAL CONTROLS

The effect of metyrapone administration on plasma cortisol concentrations in depressed patients is shown in **Figure 2**, top. Although both the placebo and metyrapone groups demonstrated a decline in plasma cortisol concentrations, the patients who received metyrapone had a faster decline and had relatively steady but low concentrations of plasma cortisol during the last half of the study (7:30 to 10 PM). Metyrapone treatment was associated with significantly decreased plasma cortisol concentrations in the depressed patients. Plasma cortisol concentrations were similar in the metyrapone-treated depressed patients and normal controls (Figure 2, bottom), with a significant decrease in both groups over the course of the study. This decrease occurred during the initial phase of the study, since there were no significant effects (group, repeated measure, or interaction) between 7:30 and 10 PM.

As with the normal controls, the blockade of cortisol production resulted in significantly increased plasma concentrations of 11-deoxycortisol in the depressed patients (**Figure 3**). However, the effect was amplified in the patient population compared with the controls. Following the second dose of metyrapone (7:30 PM), total adrenal steroid production (cortisol plus 11-deoxycortisol) demonstrated a trend toward increased adrenal steroid production ($P=.05$) in the depressed patients compared with normal controls. Thus, although the depressed patients had increased adrenal secretory activity over the course of the study, metyrapone adequately blocked cortisol production in the depressed pa-

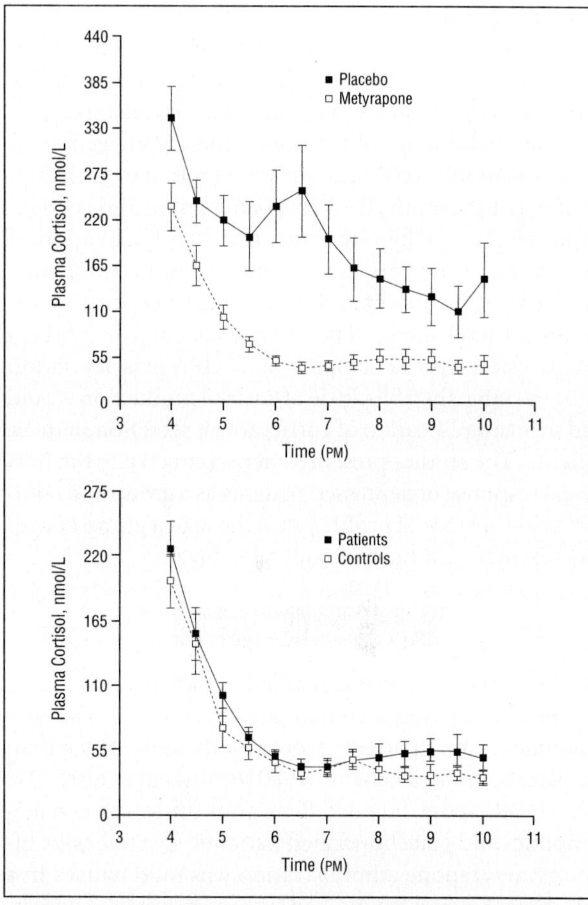

Figure 2. *Top, Plasma cortisol concentrations in depressed patients given either metyrapone or placebo. Although plasma cortisol concentrations decreased in both groups of depressed patients, administration of metyrapone resulted in a faster decline and lower absolute concentrations of plasma cortisol in depressed subjects (significant treatment effect of metyrapone by analysis of variance: F=30.2, df=1, P=.0001; significant interaction between time and treatment by analysis of variance: F=12.2, df=1, P=.0007). Bottom, Metyrapone-treated depressed patients had declines in plasma cortisol levels similar to those of metyrapone-treated normal control subjects.*

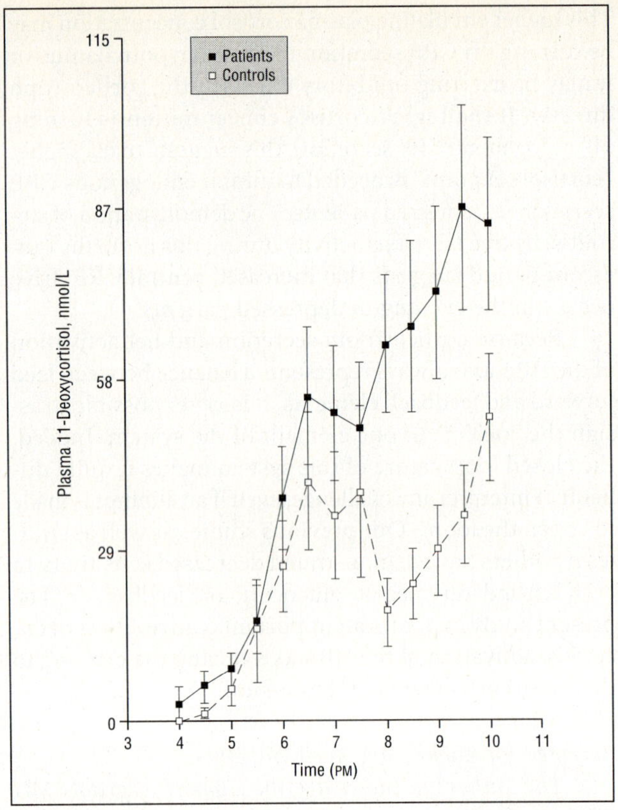

Figure 3. *Plasma 11-deoxycortisol secretion in normal controls and depressed patients. Metyrapone blockade of 11-β-hydroxylase results in the secretion of the inactive precursor, 11-deoxycortisol, from the adrenal gland. At baseline, 11-deoxycortisol concentrations were undetectable in all subjects, but they increased over time in both normal controls and depressed patients, with significantly higher concentrations in depressed patients (significant treatment effect of metyrapone by analysis of variance: F=14.63,* P*=.0001; significant interaction between group and time by analysis of variance: F=1.9,* P*=.039).*

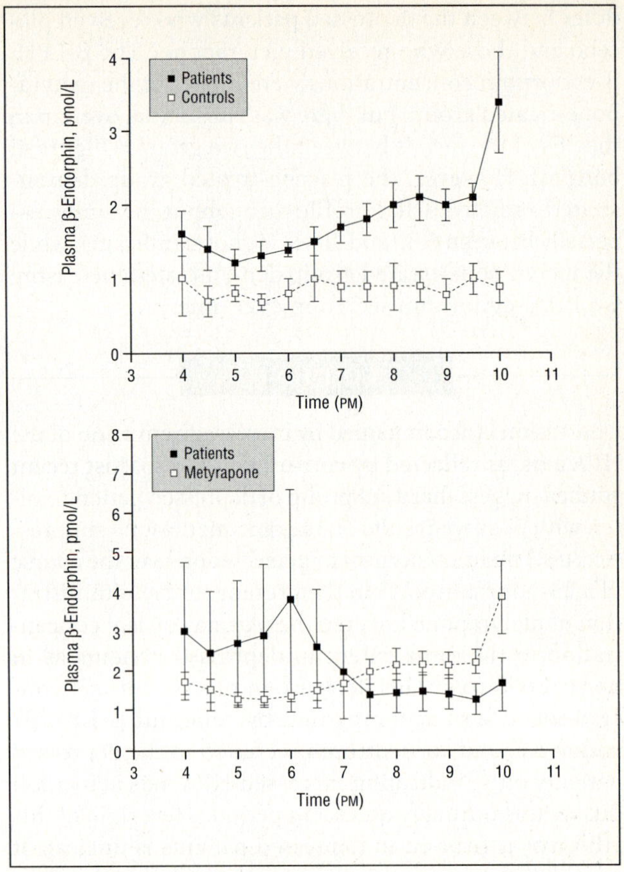

Figure 4. *Top, Plasma β-endorphin secretion in normal controls and depressed patients given metyrapone. While the normal controls demonstrated a flat profile of β-endorphin concentrations over the course of the evening, the depressed patients demonstrated progressive activation (significant treatment effect of metyrapone by analysis of variance: F=2.7,* df*=1,* P*=.0021; significant difference between patients and controls by analysis of variance: F=4.9,* df*=1,* P*=.036). Bottom, Depressed patients given placebo demonstrated a flat profile of plasma β-endorphin concentrations over the course of the evening, while metyrapone-treated patients demonstrated a progressive increase in β-endorphin concentrations.*

tients, and we can compare corticotroph activity between patients and normal controls.

CORTICOTROPH SECRETION IN DEPRESSED PATIENTS AND NORMAL CONTROLS

Our hypothesis was that the metyrapone-induced decrease in cortisol concentrations would result in rebound corticotropin and β-LPH/β-endorphin secretion in depressed patients. Was this the case? The peptide secretion data shown in **Figure 4**, top, demonstrate a significant difference between depressed patients and normal controls in plasma β-LPH/β-endorphin concentrations following metyrapone treatment. The depressed patients clearly demonstrate rebound β-LPH/β-endorphin secretion following metyrapone treatment, while the profile of plasma β-LPH/β-endorphin secretion in normal controls is flat. In no case did a normal control demonstrate activation of β-LPH/β-endorphin secretion following metyrapone administration. In contrast, among patients, the degree of activation of β-LPH/β-endorphin secretion following metyrapone administration varied, without clear differences in the clinical picture. However, we had no objective criteria to define any patient as normal or abnormal so that we could determine what clinical variables might influence the response to metyrapone. In a subset of normal controls and depressed patients, both β-LPH/β-endorphin and corticotropin concentrations were measured. The β-LPH/β-endorphin data and corticotropin data for this subset are shown in Table 2. Both hormones demonstrated increased corticotroph secretory activity in the depressed patients, although the greater sensitivity of the β-LPH/β-endorphin radioimmunoassay yielded more reliable data (a smaller SD). Of note, the increased corticotropin secretory activity began before the second dose of metyrapone was administered (7:30 PM). The baseline level for corticotropin for 4:30 to 6 PM was 0.8±0.4 pmol/L (data not shown). Compared with baseline, both hormones demonstrated increased secretion in depressed patients during the second half of the study.

Finally, did β-LPH/β-endorphin secretory activity

differ between the depressed patients who received placebo and those who received metyrapone? The β-LPH/β-endorphin concentrations were higher in the metyrapone-treated group, but there was substantial overlap in the SEs of the means between the two groups (Figure 4, bottom). However, the placebo-treated group demonstrated a relatively flat profile throughout the study, especially between 6:30 and 10 PM (*P*, not significant), while the metyrapone-treated group demonstrated increasing β-LPH/β-endorphin secretion over time.

COMMENT

Depression is accompanied by increased activation of the HPA axis, as reflected by cortisol measures. Most recent studies suggest that a subgroup of depressed patients (often with positive results on the dexamethasone suppression test) manifest cortisol hypersecretion over the course of a 24-hour period.[1-6] In the present study, administration of metyrapone lowered the plasma cortisol concentration to the same extent in depressed patients as in normal controls. This decrease in plasma cortisol concentration was accompanied by rebound β-LPH/β-endorphin and corticotropin secretion in the depressed patients only, indicating increased HPA axis activation during this normally quiescent period. The origin of this HPA axis activation in depressed patients is unclear. It may represent a nonspecific stress response to the challenge study, a circadian phase difference between depressed patients and normal controls, or excessive activation of the axis by depression itself.

THE EXISTENCE of spontaneous secretory activity of the anterior pituitary corticotroph can be demonstrated in vitro; anterior pituitary corticotrophs secrete corticotropin without stimulation by secretagogues, such as CRF or arginine vasopressin. The addition of glucocorticoids has no effect on this baseline secretion, but glucocorticoids are able to inhibit the secretory response to CRF.[17,18] The results from the metyrapone-treated normal subjects clearly support the data from rodents indicating that there are periods when the HPA axis does not appear to be activated and that lowering the plasma cortisol concentration during these periods has no effect on corticotropin secretion. This is also in agreement with the findings of Iranmanesh et al[19] demonstrating the existence of corticotropin secretory pulses during the nadir of the circadian rhythm that appear to be intrinsic to the pituitary.

The difference in β-LPH/β-endorphin concentrations between the placebo-treated and metyrapone-treated depressed patients suggests that under normal circumstances, the higher evening cortisol concentration of the depressed patients restrains corticotroph secretion. This higher circulating plasma cortisol concentration may be turning off CRF secretion from the hypothalamus or it may be exerting inhibitory effects at the corticotroph directly. If the higher cortisol concentration is turning off endogenous CRF secretion, this suggests that a higher "cortisol set point" is needed to inhibit endogenous CRF secretion in depressed patients. The demonstration of steroid-sensitive HPA axis activity during this normally quiescent period suggests that increased central CRF drive occurs in the evening in depressed patients.

Because corticotropin secretion and net activation of the HPA axis always represents a balance between feed forward and feedback elements, it is never possible to assign the "defect" to one element of the system. Indeed, the closed loop nature of this system makes it quite difficult to interpret any challenge, even if an attempt is made to "open the loop." Our previous studies as well as studies by others have demonstrated decreased sensitivity to both fast and intermediate glucocorticoid feedback.[7,20] The present study supports an important contribution of excessive activation of the HPA axis during the evening to the hypercortisolemia of depression.

Accepted for publication April 27, 1994.

The authors acknowledge the support of grants MH 00427 to Dr Young and MH 42251 to Drs Akil and Watson from the National Institute of Mental Health, Rockville, Md, and grant MO1 RR00042 (general clinical research center grant) from the National Institutes of Health, Bethesda, Md.

Presented in part at the 45th Annual Meeting of the Society of Biological Psychiatry, May 10, 1990, New York, NY.

Reprint requests to Mental Health Research Unit, 205 Zina Pitcher Pl, Ann Arbor, MI 48109 (Dr Young).

REFERENCES

1. Carroll BJ, Curtis GC, Mendels J: Neuroendocrine regulation in depression, I: limbic system-adrenocortical dysfunction. *Arch Gen Psychiatry.* 1976;33:1039-1044.
2. Rubin RT, Poland RE, Lesser IM, Winston RA, Blodgett N. Neuroendocrine aspects of primary endogenous depression, I: cortisol secretory dynamics in patients and matched controls. *Arch Gen Psychiatry.* 1987;44:328-336.
3. Sachar EJ, Hellman L, Roffwarg HP, Halpern FS, Fukush DK, Gallagher TF. Disrupted 24 hour patterns of cortisol secretion in psychotic depressives. *Arch Gen Psychiatry.* 1973;28:19-24.
4. Halbreich U, Asnis GM, Schindledecker R, Zurnoff B, Nathan RS. Cortisol secretion in endogenous depression, I: basal plasma levels. *Arch Gen Psychiatry.* 1985;42:909-914.
5. Pfohl R, Sherman B, Schlecter J, Stone R. Pituitary/adrenal axis rhythm disturbances in psychiatric patients. *Arch Gen Psychiatry.* 1985;42:897-903.
6. Linkowski P, Mendelwicz J, Kerkhofs M, LeClercq R, Goldstein J, Brasseur M, Copinschi G, van Cauter E. 24 hour profiles of ACTH, cortisol and growth hormone in major depressive illness: effect of antidepressant treatment. *J Clin Endocrinol Metab.* 1987;65:141-152.
7. Carroll BJ, Feinberg M, Greden JF, Tarika J, Albala AA, Haskett RF, James N, Kronfol Z, Lohr N, Steiner M, DeVigne JP, Young EA. A specific laboratory test for the diagnosis of melancholia: standardization, validation, and clinical utility. *Arch Gen Psychiatry.* 1981;38:15-22.

8. Carroll BJ, Curtis GC, Mendels J. Neuroendocrine regulation in depression, II: discrimination of depressed from nondepressed patients. *Arch Gen Psychiatry.* 1976;33:1051-1058.
9. Young EA, Haskett RF, Kotun J, Grunhaus L, Greden JF, Watson SJ, Akil H. Dissociation between corticotroph and adrenal response to dexamethasone. *Arch Gen Psychiatry.* 1993;50:395-403.
10. Stokes PE, Stoll PM, Koslow SH, Maas JW, Davis JM, Swann AC, Robins E. Pretreatment DST and hypothalamic-pituitary-adrenocortical function in depressed patients and comparison groups: a multicenter study. *Arch Gen Psychiatry.* 1984;41:257-267.
11. Meikle AW. Dexamethasone suppression tests: usefulness of simultaneous measurements of plasma cortisol and dexamethasone. *Clin Endocrinol.* 1982;16:401-408.
12. Maguire KP, Schweitzer I, Biddle N, Bridge S, Tiller JWG. The dexamethasone suppression test: importance of dexamethasone concentrations. *Biol Psychiatry.* 1987;22:957-967.
13. O'Sullivan BT, Hunt GE, Johnson GF, Caterson ID. The plasma dexamethasone window: evidence supporting its usefulness to validate dexamethasone suppression test results. *Biol Psychiatry.* 1989;25:739-754.
14. Endicott I, Spitzer RL. A diagnostic interview: Schedule for Affective Disorders and Schizophrenia. *Arch Gen Psychiatry.* 1978;35:837-844.
15. Cahill CA, Matthews JD, Akil H. Human plasma beta-endorphin-like peptides: a rapid high recovery extraction technique and validation of radioimmunoassay. *J Clin Endocrinol Metab.* 1983;56:992-997.
16. Young EA, Akil H. CRF stimulation of ACTH/beta-endorphin release: effect of acute and chronic stress. *Endocrinology.* 1985;117:23-30.
17. Young EA, Akil H. Paradoxical effect of corticosteroids on pituitary ACTH/β-endorphin release in stressed animals. *Psychoneuroendocrinology.* 1988;13:317-321.
18. Dallman MF, Akana SF, Cascio ES, Darlington DN, Jacobson L, Levin N. Regulation of ACTH secretion: variations on a theme of B. *Recent Prog Horm Res.* 1987;43:113-173.
19. Iranmanesh A, Lizzalde G, Short D, Veldhuis JD. Intensive venous sampling paradigms disclose high frequency adrenocorticotropin release episodes in normal men. *J Clin Endocrinol Metab.* 1990;71:1276-1283.
20. Young EA, Haskett RF, Watson SJ, Akil H. Loss of glucocorticoid fast feedback in depression. *Arch Gen Psychiatry.* 1991;48:693-699.

Conversions From Système International (SI) Units to Traditional Units (Modified From *The SI Manual in Health Care*)

System	Component	SI Reference Interval*	SI Unit	Conversion Factor (Divide by)	Traditional Reference Interval*	Traditional Unit
Plasma	Corticotropin (ACTH)	4-22	pmol/L	0.2202	20-100	pg/mL
Serum	Cortisol					
	8 AM	110-520	nmol/L	27.59	4-19	μg/dL
	4 PM	50-410	nmol/L	27.59	2-15	μg/dL
	Midnight	<140	nmol/L	27.59	<5	μg/dL
Serum	11-Deoxycortisol	0-60	nmol/L	28.86	0-2	μg/dL

These reference values are not intended to be definitive since each laboratory determines its own values. They are provided for illustration only.

Suicide and Mortality Patterns in Anxiety Neurosis and Depressive Neurosis

Christer Allgulander, MD

Background: The diverging views on suicide risk in patients with morbid anxiety called for a sufficiently large study to estimate the suicide risk in patients with anxiety neurosis and depressive neurosis.

Methods: The identities of all 9912 patients with anxiety neurosis and all 38 529 patients with depressive neurosis in the national Psychiatric Case Register in Sweden between 1973 and 1983, without any other psychiatric diagnoses, were matched with the national Cause-of-Death Register. The observed causes of death among the 9910 patients who died in 1990 or earlier were compared with those expected in the general population.

Results: There were 1481 determined and 265 undetermined suicides among the patients; ie, 18% of all deaths. The standardized mortality ratio of suicide before the age of 45 years among men and women with anxiety neurosis was 6.7 and 4.9, respectively; for depressive neurosis, 12.6 and 15.7, respectively. The suicide risk was much higher within 3 months of leaving the hospital. Standardized mortality ratios of death caused by ischemic heart disease and traumatic injury were marginally elevated among men in both diagnostic groups. Women in both categories were at increased risk for death caused by alcohol abuse and cirrhosis of the liver. Obstructive pulmonary disease was another notable cause of death, reflecting the aggravation of anxiety-depressive symptoms by airway obstruction or the effects of tobacco smoking.

Conclusions: The risk of completed suicide among former inpatients with primary anxiety neurosis was higher than in previous, smaller studies and higher yet in patients with depressive neurosis. This hazard may hopefully be reduced by optimizing immediate and long-term treatment for the severely affected.

(Arch Gen Psychiatry. 1994;51:708-712)

THE EXCESS mortality in psychiatric patients is thought to have biological and psychosocial determinants but also to be confounded by selection bias in inpatient studies.[1] Suicide, accounting for the largest number of lost years among death causes, ought to be preventable by treatment of the preexisting mental disorder in many instances.[2] Suicide often occurs soon after hospital discharge in patients characterized by hopelessness or interpersonal disruptions, regardless of the type of diagnosis.[3-5] This calls for continued preventive efforts directed at high-risk patients.

A genetic contribution to mortality patterns has been reported for adoptees in the general population and for twins with psychiatric disorders.[6-9] This pertains both to suicide and to disease-related causes of death. There is some support for the hypothesis that heritability for suicide may exist, independent of a concurrent symptom diagnosis.[10,11] Furthermore, it has been proposed that individuals with the same genetic substrate and personality traits may present with predominantly anxious or depressive symptoms, depending on circumstances.[12,13] Three prospective studies of community samples support this possibility by showing diagnostic instability in anxiety disorders.[14]

In the new nosology, panic disorder has been associated with suicidal ideation and attempts.[15] Whether these are conducive to

See Methods on next page

From the Karolinska Institute, Stockholm, Sweden; the Department of Clinical Neuroscience and Family Medicine, Section of Psychiatry, Huddinge (Sweden) University Hospital; and the Department of Psychiatry, Washington University School of Medicine, St Louis, Mo.

METHODS

All discharge diagnoses from all psychiatric inpatient facilities in Sweden (mean population, 8.2 million) were cumulatively filed on computer between 1973 and 1983. Of a total of 1 328 766 admissions, 1 243 152 (94%) were attributable to 366 003 identifiable patients. Their identities were matched with the national Cause-of-Death Register, which is a cumulative database of all death certificates. This yielded 122 245 patients who had died by 1990. A copy of the file without patient names was created for this study. It included diagnoses and death causes according to the World Health Organization's 1966 *International Classification of Diseases, Eighth Revision* (*ICD-8*), as well as demographic data. The Data Inspection Board, the National Board of Health and Welfare, and Statistics Sweden all consented to the study.

In the study file, all probands were located who had been discharged from the hospital with at least one diagnosis of anxiety neurosis (*ICD-8* 300.00), phobic neurosis (*ICD-8* 300.20), neurasthenic neurosis (*ICD-8* 300.50), or combinations of these but with no other psychiatric diagnoses. Patients could have obtained one or more of these diagnoses during repeated inpatient stays since 1973. All patients with additional psychiatric diagnoses were excluded. This selection was considered to best approximate the *DSM-III-R* diagnoses of panic disorder, phobic disorder, and generalized anxiety disorder, hence called *anxiety neurosis*.[27] Similarly, all probands with *depressive neurosis* were targeted (*ICD-8* 300.40, 300.41), with no other psychiatric diagnoses on record. This category is similar to dysthymic disorder in *DSM-III-R*. The causes of death were divided into relevant categories, including determined (*ICD-8* E950-E959) and undetermined (*ICD-8* E980-E989) suicides. The latter code is used "when it is stated that an investigation by a medical or legal authority has not determined whether the injuries are accidental, suicidal or homicidal."

Descriptive tabulations were made with the use of software (SAS Institute, Cary, NC). Excess mortality among the probands was analyzed using standardized mortality ratios (SMRs), the number of deaths occurring among the probands divided by the number of deaths expected if the age-specific death rate were the same as in the general population. These ratios were calculated using mortality statistics for 1973 to 1989 from the general population by sex and 5-year age groups. The time of entry into the group at risk was the time of first hospital discharge. The time of departure was the time of death or the end of the follow-up period. The life-table technique was used to describe the hazard of suicide by time from hospital discharge in three age groups: 15 to 44, 45 to 64, and 65 to 94 years.

completed suicide has been questioned.[16,17] About 20% of the deaths among previously hospitalized patients with anxiety disorders are suicides, a proportion similar to that in depressive disorders.[18,19] One prospective community study showed the highest rate of suicide attempts, 30%, in those with both panic and depressive symptoms.[20] Suicides have also been overlooked in the past, as was the case in a follow-up study of 126 neurotic patients treated in the 1930s; four of nine deaths were suicides.[21]

Whether cardiovascular disease is more common in anxiety or depressive disorders and whether there is a preventive effect of treatment are being discussed.[22-26] This study aimed at exploring a large and representative group of patients to estimate the risk for suicide and disease-related deaths in patients with anxiety or depressive neurosis, uncontaminated by other psychiatric diagnoses. It built on two smaller studies that showed an excess of suicide among patients with anxiety or depressive neuroses.[27,28]

RESULTS

A total of 9911 probands were categorized as having pure anxiety neurosis, of whom 58% had an *ICD-8* diagnosis of anxiety neurosis, 29% had neurasthenic neurosis, 7% had phobic neurosis, and 7% had at least two of the above. A total of 38 529 probands had a diagnosis of pure depressive neurosis. There were 1481 determined and 265 undetermined suicides among them.

DESCRIPTIVE DATA

Among the probands with a diagnosis of anxiety neurosis, the median age at the time of first admission to a psychiatric unit was 39 years (range, 15 to 89 years), while those with depressive neurosis were older, with a median age of 48 years (range, 15 to 93 years). The median total number of inpatient days during the 11-year period was 16 days (mean, 38 days) among those with anxiety neurosis, with 90% having a total of 83 days or less. For those with depressive neurosis, the median number was 14 days (mean, 36 days), with 90% having a total of 78 days or less. With the caution that recorded marital status was missing for 34% of the probands in both categories, 35% of those anxious or depressed were married at the time of first index admission, and 12% and 17% of those anxious and depressed, respectively, were divorced or widowed. Only 2.9% of those with anxiety neurosis and 3.4% of those with depressive neurosis had a somatic diagnosis recorded at the time of first admission (**Table 1**).

MORTALITY PATTERN

Among the men, 24% died; among the women, 19% died. Eighteen percent of all 9910 deaths were determined or undetermined suicides (**Table 2**). There were 74 deaths (0.75%) caused by alcohol or drug abuse or alcohol he-

patic cirrhosis, and there were 14 homicides. Among the men in both categories, there were 1159 deaths (30%) caused by ischemic heart disease, while the proportion was lower among the women, with 1468 deaths (25%).

RISK ESTIMATES

Focusing on suicide, women with depressive neurosis were at highest risk, declining slightly with increasing age (**Table 3**). The suicide SMR in both men and women with anxiety neurosis was also substantially increased, with no decline with increasing age.

The risk of nontraumatic death (excluding suicide, homicide, and traumatic injury) was somewhat reduced among women in both categories (SMR, 0.7; 95% confidence interval [CI], 0.6 to 0.7) and slightly elevated among men with anxiety neurosis (SMR, 1.3; 95% CI, 1.2 to 1.4; $P<.001$) and depressive neurosis (SMR, 1.2; 95% CI, 1.1 to 1.2; $P<.001$). As these deaths were broken down into categories, alcohol abuse conferred an SMR of 3.3 (95% CI, 1.1 to 7.7; $P=.04$) in women with anxiety neurosis and of 2.8 (95% CI, 1.4 to 4.1; $P<.001$) in women with depressive neurosis. There were also 12 deaths of alcoholic hepatic cirrhosis among women with depressive neurosis (SMR, 2.2; 95% CI, 2.9 to 3.8; $P=.02$). Men with anxiety neurosis were also at risk for death caused by obstructive pulmonary disease (SMR, 2.8; 95% CI, 1.3 to 4.6; $P=.008$), as were both men (SMR, 2.6; 95% CI, 2.1 to 3.0; $P<.001$) and women (SMR, 2.2; 95% CI, 1.8 to 2.6; $P<.001$) with depressive neurosis. Traumatic injury was marginally more common than expected in men with depressive neurosis (SMR, 1.5; 95% CI, 1.2 to 1.8; $P<.001$). Men with anxiety neurosis were also at marginally increased risk of death caused by ischemic heart disease (SMR, 1.4; 95% CI, 1.2 to 1.6; $P<.001$), as were men with depressive neurosis (SMR, 1.3; 95% CI, 1.2 to 1.3; $P<.001$).

Among patients 15 through 44 years old, the suicide hazard after leaving the hospital declined with time in all groups, faster among men than among women (**Figure**). Suicide SMRs during the first 3 months after leaving the hospital were much higher than later during follow-up in the combined age groups, among both men (SMR, 105; 95% CI, 80 to 130; $P<.001$) and women (SMR, 124; 95% CI, 92 to 156; $P<.001$) with depressive neurosis and among both men (SMR, 55; 95% CI, 29 to 96; $P<.001$) and women (SMR, 38; 95% CI, 14 to 82; $P<.001$) with anxiety neurosis. Even after 8 years of observation, the suicide SMRs remained elevated (data available on request from the author).

Table 1. Somatic Diagnoses Recorded at the First Psychiatric Unit Admission, by Sex and Diagnosis

	Men, No.		Women, No.	
Prior Somatic Diagnoses	Anxiety Neurosis (n=3256)	Depressive Neurosis (n=12 781)	Anxiety Neurosis (n=6655)	Depressive Neurosis (n=25 748)
Malignant neoplasm	9	71	18	79
Thyroid disease	2	10	28	91
Central nervous system disease	41	183	72	284
Ischemic heart disease	34	114	30	157
Cerebrovascular disease	9	50	19	106
Obstructive pulmonary disease	7	68	22	80
Hepatic cirrhosis	0	3	0	1
Traumatic injury	14	125	19	133
Drug adverse events	10	165	37	385

Table 2. Deaths Before Age 95 Years by Cause, Sex, and Diagnosis

	Men, No. (%)		Women, No. (%)	
Cause	Anxiety Neurosis	Depressive Neurosis	Anxiety Neurosis	Depressive Neurosis
Suicide				
Determined	86 (16.1)	640 (19.0)	65 (7.9)	690 (13.4)
Undetermined	14 (2.6)	93 (2.8)	21 (2.6)	137 (2.7)
Homicide	0 (0.0)	4 (0.1)	3 (0.4)	7 (0.1)
Traumatic injury	24 (4.5)	114 (3.4)	26 (3.2)	146 (2.8)
Alcohol or drug abuse	7 (1.3)	14 (0.4)	6 (0.7)	19 (0.4)
Hepatic cirrhosis	3 (0.6)	10 (0.3)	3 (0.4)	12 (0.2)
Obstructive pulmonary disease	10 (1.9)	88 (2.6)	25 (3.0)	126 (2.4)
Malignant neoplasm	97 (18.2)	492 (14.6)	204 (24.8)	963 (18.7)
Ischemic heart disease	171 (32.0)	988 (29.3)	186 (22.6)	1282 (24.9)
Cerebrovascular disease	26 (4.9)	241 (7.1)	83 (10.1)	512 (9.9)
Other	96 (18.0)	691 (20.5)	200 (24.3)	1253 (24.3)
Total*	**534** (100.1)	**3375** (100.1)	**822** (100.0)	**5147** (99.8)

Percentages may not add to 100% because of rounding.

COMMENT

The principal finding of this study was a suicide risk of 5.7 compared with the general population among 9911 men and women in Sweden with an inpatient diagnosis of pure anxiety neurosis. A suicide risk was also found among 38 529 inpatients with depressive neurosis (SMR, 11.3 in men and 14.5 in women). The hazard of suicide was much higher within 3 months of hospital discharge but remained elevated throughout the entire period of observation.

Alcohol abuse may have aggravated the anxiety dis-

Table 3. Determined and Undetermined Suicides Observed and Expected During the 17 Years of Observation, by Diagnosis, Age, Sex, and Standardized Mortality Ratios (SMRs)*

	Men		Women	
	Anxiety Neurosis (n=3256)	Depressive Neurosis (n=12 781)	Anxiety Neurosis (n=6655)	Depressive Neurosis (n=25 748)
Age 15-44 y				
No. Observed	55	286	32	276
No. Expected	8.3	22.7	6.6	17.6
SMR (95% CI)	6.7 (4.9-8.4)	12.6 (11.2-14.1)	4.9 (3.2-6.6)	15.7 (13.9-17.6)
Age 45-64 y				
No. Observed	34	281	39	361
No. Expected	7.0	27.8	6.2	24.3
SMR (95% CI)	4.8 (3.2-6.5)	10.1 (8.9-11.3)	6.3 (4.3-8.2)	14.9 (13.3-16.4)
Age 65-94 y				
No. Observed	11	166	15	192
No. Expected	2.1	14.6	2.4	15.5
SMR (95% CI)	5.2 (2.6-9.2)	11.4 (9.6-13.1)	6.3 (3.5-10.3)	12.4 (10.7-14.2)

**P*<.001 for all SMRs by χ^2 analysis of the null hypothesis of no excess mortality. The SMR is the number of deaths occuring among the probands divided by the number of deaths expected if the age-specific death rate were the same as in the general population. Ninety-five percent confidence intervals (CIs) were calculated with normal approximations unless there were fewer than 20 deaths, in which case the Poisson distribution was used.*

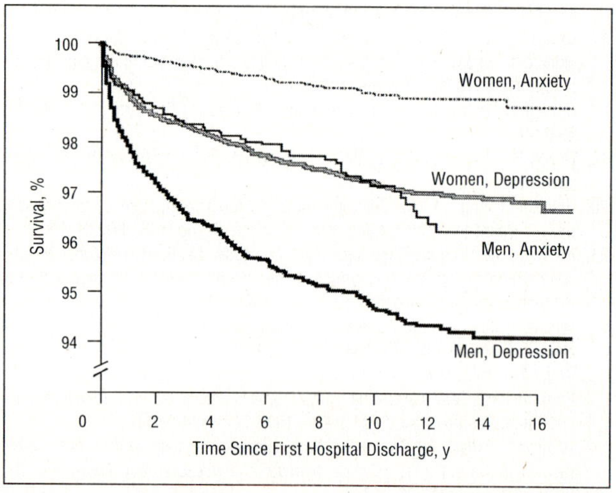

Suicide hazard (Kaplan-Meier survival function) among patients 15 through 44 years of age with anxiety neurosis or depressive neurosis, from the first discharge from a psychiatric unit.

order or may have become apparent only at the time of death, causing some excess deaths among women. Alcohol abuse is more often overlooked in women; in one psychiatric chart study, a diagnosis of alcohol abuse was missing in 20% of the women and 10% of the men.[29] Obstructive pulmonary disease caused some premature deaths, in keeping with findings of airway obstruction in patients with anxiety and depression.[30] Whether such conditions aggravate mental symptoms or are caused by smoking requires further study.

The probands were not sampled. They were all identifiable inpatients in all Swedish psychiatric units during 11 years. They were part of an ethnically homogeneous population with equal access to public health care, regardless of financial status. Diagnoses were uniformly made by the *ICD-8* glossary, but operationalized criteria were lacking. There is little reason to believe that diagnostic procedures changed during the study period. Diagnoses were confirmed by a psychiatrist at the time of hospital discharge. Treatments were generally voluntary and supportive and included exposure to agoraphobic situations, brief psychotherapy, and in most instances pharmacotherapy with anxiolytic agents, low doses of tricyclic antidepressant or phenothiazine agents, or hypnotic agents.

In 1979 and 1982, 6% of all male inpatients and 10% of all female inpatients in Sweden had diagnoses of neuroses. The proportion of all such people affected in Sweden cannot be estimated. One must assume that those who qualified as inpatients had the most maladaptive behavior or the most stressors. With the removal of every third hospital bed when the system was reformed in 1984 and harder admission criteria, neurotic patients were less likely to be admitted.

Despite the uniformity of patients and procedures, the data quality cannot match that of patients with prospective, multiaxial diagnoses. The psychiatric morbidity of the probands prior to 1973 is unknown. In the years between hospital treatment and death, life events and health problems may have influenced mortality. Diagnoses were not quite reliable and complete, in light of the deaths caused by substance abuse among women and the fact that the personality dimension is often overlooked in studies of symptom diagnoses. The instability of diagnoses over time in other studies underscores the importance of longitudinal studies in validating nosology.[31] Identity matching between the two registers might have incorporated some negligible errors that, if corrected, would enhance statistical significance. Inclusion

of the undetermined suicide category is customary, since about one third of these deaths are rated as intentional suicide on closer scrutiny. We therefore erred on the conservative side.

Despite the proliferation of psychiatric services in Sweden, most suicides occur among persons who have not sought treatment, and while the risk increases many times with hospitalization, the type of inpatient diagnosis has less to do with the magnitude of the risk than generally believed.[5] The findings of this study imply that suicide prevention must be pursued vigorously in patients with morbid anxiety and impaired functioning. The much higher risk soon after leaving the hospital suggests that preventive monitoring should be instituted immediately.

From a public health perspective, efforts should be made to identify cases in the community and to educate care providers in diagnosing and treating patients with anxiety and depressive disorders.[32] Prospective, replicable, controlled treatment studies of representative community cases will be required to assess the cost-effectiveness of treatment intervention, both immediate and long-term. Based on current wisdom, such studies should compare behavioral therapy with cognitive therapy and pharmacotherapy and with various combinations of these, pending further etiological research. The public (and health economists) may assess our performance to determine whether the expense is justified.

Accepted for publication June 24, 1994.

This study was supported by grants from the Swedish Council on Technology Assessment in Health Care and from the SALUS Fund, Stockholm, Sweden, and from the Upjohn Co, Kalamazoo, Mich.

Lena Brandt, BSc, Karolinska Institute, Stockholm, performed the statistical analyses. Curt-Lennart Spetz, the National Board of Health and Welfare, Stockholm, created the data set. George E. Murphy, MD, and Philip W. Lavori, PhD, gave advice.

Reprint requests to Section of Psychiatry, Huddinge Hospital, R63, Huddinge, S-141 86, Sweden (Dr Allgulander).

REFERENCES

1. Black DW, Winokur G, Nasrallah A. Is death from natural causes still excessive in psychiatric patients? *J Nerv Ment Dis.* 1987;175:674-680.
2. Conwell Y, Caine ED. Rational suicide and the right to die: reality and myth. *N Engl J Med.* 1991;325:1100-1102.
3. Fawcett J, Scheftner W, Clark D, Hedeker D, Gibbons R, Coryell W. Clinical predictors of suicide in patients with major affective disorders: a controlled prospective study. *Am J Psychiatry.* 1987;144:35-40.
4. Murphy GE. Suicide and substance abuse. *Arch Gen Psychiatry.* 1988;45:593-594.
5. Allgulander C, Allebeck P, Przybeck TR, Rice JP. Risk of suicide by psychiatric diagnosis in Stockholm County: a longitudinal study of 80,970 psychiatric inpatients. *Eur Arch Psychiatry Clin Neurosci.* 1992;241:323-326.
6. Roy A, Segal NL, Centerwall BS, Robinette D. Suicide in twins. *Arch Gen Psychiatry.* 1991;48:29-32.
7. Mitterauer B. A contribution to the discussion of the role of the genetic factor in suicide, based on five studies in an epidemiologically defined area (province of Salzburg, Austria). *Compr Psychiatry.* 1990;31:557-65.
8. Sörensen TIA, Nielsen GG, Andersen PK, Teasdale TW. Genetic and environmental influences on premature death in adult adoptees. *N Engl J Med.* 1988; 318:727-732.
9. Kendler KS. A twin study of mortality in schizophrenia and neurosis. *Arch Gen Psychiatry.* 1986;43:643-649.
10. Sherif F, Marcusson J, Oreland L. Brain gamma-aminobutyrate transaminase and monoamine oxidase: activities in suicide victims. *Eur Arch Psychiatry Clin Neurosci.* 1991;241:139-144.
11. Apter A, van Praag HM, Plutchik R, Sevy S, Korn M, Brown S-L. Interrelationships among anxiety, aggression, impulsivity, and mood: a serotonergically linked cluster? *Psychiatry Res.* 1990;32:191-199.
12. Kendler KS, Neale MC, Kessler RC, Heath AC, Eaves LJ. Major depression and generalized anxiety disorder: same genes, (partly) different environments? *Arch Gen Psychiatry.* 1992;49:716-722.
13. Tyrer P, Seivewright N, Ferguson B, Tyrer J. The general neurotic syndrome: a coaxial diagnosis of anxiety, depression and personality disorder. *Acta Psychiatr Scand.* 1992;85:201-206.
14. Angst J, Vollrath M. The natural history of anxiety disorders. *Acta Psychiatr Scand.* 1991;84:446-452.
15. Weissman MM, Klerman GL, Markowitz JS, Oullette R. Suicidal ideation and suicide attempts in panic disorder and attacks. *N Engl J Med.* 1989;321:1209-1214.
16. Friedman S, Jones JC, Chernen L, Barlow DH. Suicidal ideation and suicide attempts among patients with panic disorder: a survey of two outpatient clinics. *Am J Psychiatry.* 1992;149:680-685.
17. Beck AT, Steer RA, Sanderson WC, Madland Skeie T. Panic disorder and suicidal ideation and behavior: discrepant findings in psychiatric outpatients. *Am J Psychiatry.* 1991;148:1195-1199.
18. Coryell W. Panic disorder and mortality. *Psychiatr Clin North Am.* 1988;11: 433-440.
19. Noyes R Jr. Suicide and panic disorder: a review. *J Affective Disord.* 1991; 22:1-11.
20. Vollrath M, Angst J. Outcome of panic and depression in a seven-year follow-up: results of the Zurich study. *Acta Psychiatr Scand.* 1989;80:591-596.
21. Ernst K. Die Prognose der Neurosen. In: Müller M, Spatz H, Vogel P, eds. *Monographien aus dem Gesamtgebiete der Neurologie und Psychiatrie.* Berlin, Germany: Springer-Verlag; 1959:1-140. [No. 85.]
22. Weeke A, Juel K, Vaeth M. Cardiovascular death and manic-depressive psychosis. *J Affective Disord.* 1987;13:287-92.
23. Weissman MM, Markowitz JS, Oullette R, Greenwald S, Kahn MA, Kahn JP. Panic disorder and cardiovascular/cerebrovascular problems: results from a community survey. *Am J Psychiatry.* 1990;147:1504-1508.
24. Hayward C, Clark DB, Taylor BC. Panic disorder, anxiety, and cardiovascular risk. In: Ballenger J, ed. *Clinical Aspects of Panic Disorder.* New York, NY: Wiley-Liss Inc; 1990:99-110.
25. Nutzinger DO. Herz und Angst: Herzbezogene Ängste und kardiovaskuläres Morbiditätsrisiko bei Patienten mit einer Angststörung. *Nervenarzt.* 1992;63: 187-193.
26. Angst J. Verlauf der affektiven Psychosen. In: Kisker KP, Lauter H, Meyer JE, Muller C, Strömgren E, eds. *Psychiatrie der Gegenwart, 5: Affektive Psychosen.* 3rd ed. Berlin, Germany: Springer-Verlag; 1987:115-123.
27. Allgulander C, Lavori PW. Excess mortality among 3302 patients with 'pure' anxiety neurosis. *Arch Gen Psychiatry.* 1991;48:599-602.
28. Allgulander C, Lavori PW. Causes of death among 936 elderly patients with 'pure' anxiety neurosis in Stockholm County, Sweden, and in patients with depressive neurosis or both diagnoses. *Compr Psychiatry.* 1993;34:299-302.
29. Allgulander C, Borg S. Sedative-hypnotic and alcohol dependence among psychiatric inpatients. *Br J Addict.* 1978;73:123-128.
30. Wells KB, Golding JM, Burnam MA. Affective, substance use, and anxiety disorders in persons with arthritis, diabetes, heart disease, high blood pressure, or chronic lung conditions. *Gen Hosp Psychiatry.* 1992;11:320-327.
31. Stanton MW, Joyce PR. Stability of psychiatric diagnoses in New Zealand psychiatric hospitals. *Aust N Z J Psychiatry.* 1993;27:2-8.
32. Rutz W, von Knorring L, Wålinder J. Long-term effects of an educational program for general practitioners given by the Swedish Committee for the Prevention and Treatment of Depression. *Acta Psychiatr Scand.* 1992;85:83-88.

ORIGINAL ARTICLE

Noradrenergic Dysregulation During Discontinuation of Cocaine Use in Addicts

Christopher J. McDougle, MD; Jed E. Black, MD; Robert T. Malison, MD; Ralf C. Zimmermann, MD; Thomas R. Kosten, MD; George R. Heninger, MD; Lawrence H. Price, MD

Background: The primary objective of the study was to prospectively determine possible noradrenergic dysregulation in cocaine addicts by assessing biochemical, behavioral, and cardiovascular responses to intravenous yohimbine hydrochloride during early and late discontinuation of cocaine use.

Methods: Twelve male and two female hospitalized cocaine-dependent subjects (mean±SD age, 30.9±7.3 years) who were not seeking primary treatment for addiction participated voluntarily for monetary remuneration. Following an initial test dose of intranasal cocaine, 2 mg/kg, cocaine addicts received single-blind, monitored cocaine insufflation, 2 mg/kg three times each day, for 3 consecutive days. One to two days (early discontinuation) and 15 to 16 days (late discontinuation) after the last dose of cocaine, subjects received double-blind, randomized intravenous infusions of yohimbine hydrochloride, 0.4 mg/kg, or placebo. Plasma 3-methoxy-4-hydroxyphenylethylene glycol (MHPG) and plasma cortisol levels, anxiety-related symptoms on clinician- and subject-rated scales, blood pressure, and heart rate were measured throughout each test day. Ten of 14 subjects completed the entire study.

Results: Subjects had a significantly greater placebo-corrected MHPG response to yohimbine during early compared with late discontinuation. Subjects rated themselves significantly more nervous following yohimbine administration during early compared with late discontinuation. Seventy-one percent of subjects experienced a yohimbine-induced panic attack during early discontinuation compared with none during late discontinuation.

Conclusions: The results of this study provide evidence of an underlying dysregulation in noradrenergic function and a vulnerability to panic anxiety during early discontinuation of cocaine use in addicts. Additional investigations of noradrenergic function appear warranted to further clarify derangements associated with cocaine addiction.

(Arch Gen Psychiatry. 1994;51:713-719)

COCAINE ABUSE remains a major public health problem in the United States.[1,2] Recurrent use is due to cocaine's potent reinforcing properties,[3] combined with the drug's ability to transiently reduce symptoms of anxiety, dysphoria, and craving that can emerge during discontinuation of use.[4] A better delineation of the neurobiological determinants of cocaine abstinence symptoms might lead to the development of pharmacological treatment strategies targeted at interrupting the cocaine abuse cycle.

The clinical signs and symptoms that emerge in chronic cocaine abusers on abrupt discontinuation of use of the drug appear to vary, depending on the context of the treatment setting. For example, outpatient chronic cocaine abusers described experiencing fatigue, depressed mood, agitation, diaphoresis, nausea, sleep disturbance, paranoia, and drug craving. Gawin and Kleber[4] organized a three-phase sequence of cocaine abstinence symptoms that could last 10 weeks or longer. In contrast, Weddington et al[5] and Satel et al[6] found that inpatient cocaine-dependent subjects' ratings of craving, physical discom-

From the Department of Psychiatry, the Clinical Neuroscience Research Unit of the Abraham Ribicoff Research Facilities, Connecticut Mental Health Center, Yale University School of Medicine, New Haven.

See Subjects and Methods on next page

SUBJECTS AND METHODS

SUBJECTS

The sample consisted of 12 male and two female inpatient subjects, aged 21 to 46 years (mean±SD age, 30.9±7.3 years) who had given voluntary written informed consent to participate in the study at the Clinical Neuroscience Research Unit of the Connecticut Mental Health Center, New Haven. All subjects met *DSM-III-R*[26] criteria for a current diagnosis of cocaine dependence, based on a direct clinical interview by one of us (C.J.M.). The primary method of administration for all 14 subjects was smoking the freebase form of cocaine. A minimum "street" use of cocaine, by history, of 14 g during the proceeding 3 months, with (1) at least one previous episode of using at least 3 g within a 5-day period and (2) use of at least 1 g/wk for the 2 weeks prior to admission, was required. Urine samples positive for cocaine during the 2 weeks prior to entry and on admission were also required.

Subjects were excluded from the study if they (1) were currently using other drugs (including opioids, sedatives and hypnotics, antidepressants, antipsychotics, or other stimulants), except for marijuana or alcohol, more than twice weekly (based on history and plasma and urine toxicological screenings); (2) had met *DSM-III-R* criteria for dependence on other drugs, including marijuana or alcohol, within the past year; (3) had a history of intravenous use of drugs other than cocaine; (4) presented with a history of serious medical or neurological illness; or (5) met *DSM-III-R* criteria for schizophrenia, schizoaffective disorder, bipolar disorder, major depression, panic disorder with or without agoraphobia, mental retardation, or organic mental disorder unrelated to cocaine use.

Subjects who met the inclusion criteria and were not excluded from the study by the additional criteria underwent a complete physical and neurological evaluation, including electrocardiography and laboratory tests of renal, hepatic, pancreatic, hematopoietic, and thyroid functions. In addition, screenings for hepatitis and human immunodeficiency virus were performed. Plasma cholinesterase activity was also determined to exclude individuals who might be at risk of toxic effects of cocaine by virtue of a deficiency. Subjects determined to be medically ill were excluded from the study. Subjects were not primarily seeking treatment for addiction but participated voluntarily for monetary remuneration. Subjects were paid for completed portions of the study.

PROCEDURE

On admission, subjects started a caffeine-free, vanillylmandelic acid–free diet to eliminate foods that might alter measures of catecholamine function. On the day of admission, subjects received an intranasal test dose of cocaine, 2 mg/kg, insufflated through a straw under nursing supervision, to screen for individuals with unusual or idiosyncratic sensitivity to cocaine. Subjects and ward staff were blinded to the active or placebo nature of the drug. Three days after the test dose, subjects began receiving single-blind active doses of cocaine, 2 mg/kg intranasally, under the direct supervision of the medication nurse, at 9 AM, 1 PM, and 5 PM for 3 consecutive days (**Figure 1**). The purpose of this stabilization period was to ensure that all subjects would be withdrawn from a fixed daily dose of cocaine. On the day of the cocaine test dose and during the 3 days of cocaine administration, electrocardiograms were obtained twice daily to assess any unusual cardiovascular response. To minimize the possibility of covert ingestion of unauthorized drugs during the study, subjects were confined to the locked research unit and visitors were restricted to immediate family members, with staff monitoring of visits if indicated. To ensure that nonstudy drugs were not covertly used by subjects during the protocol, supervised urine specimens were obtained three times a week for toxicological analysis. From the time of admission to the time of completion of the study, no psychotropic medication was administered.

Each subject received four challenge tests (two active drug and two placebo) of the NE system with intravenous yohimbine hydrochloride, 0.4 mg/kg, or placebo, infused over 10 minutes. The first set of challenge test days occurred during early discontination of cocaine use, and the second set occurred 2 weeks later, during late discontination. These time points were 1 to 2 and 15 to 16 days, respectively, after the last dose of cocaine. Each set of challenge test days included random assignment to one active yohimbine test day and one placebo (0.45% saline solution) test day (Figure 1). Subjects, research nurses, and laboratory staff were blinded to the composition and sequence of administration of the test agent.

On each challenge test day, the same procedure was used. Subjects fasted overnight for 10 hours and throughout the 4-hour test, which began at 8:30 AM. They were supine, with the head elevated, throughout the test, except for standing to void and to permit measurement of standing vital signs by a research nurse who was in constant attendance. They were not allowed to sleep. Blood samples, behavioral ratings, and vital signs were obtained frequently throughout each challenge test day.

fort, anxiety, and depression decreased in a nonphasic, linear fashion during a 3- to 4-week hospitalization.

Numerous clinical reports have described the onset of anxiety and panic attacks during cocaine intoxication, as well as during abstinence.[7-14] Occasionally, autonomous panic disorder develops and persists despite no further drug use. Consistent with these findings, preclinical studies have shown cocaine to be anxiogenic during administration[15-17] and on discontinuation of use.[18,19] In view of the considerable evidence that norepinephrine (NE) con-

BIOCHEMICAL VARIABLES

Blood was sampled from an intravenous cannula in a forearm vein that was kept patent with normal saline solution. Beginning 1 hour after insertion of the intravenous catheter and throughout each test day, blood samples were obtained for measurement of plasma MHPG and cortisol levels. Samples were obtained for MHPG at 15 and 5 minutes before (baseline) and at 60, 90, 120, 180, and 240 minutes after the yohimbine or placebo test dose. Cortisol sampling occurred at baseline and 30, 45, 60, 75, 90, 120, 180, and 240 minutes after the test dose.

BEHAVIORAL RATINGS

Visual analog scales (VASs) completed by the subject were used to evaluate the change of 10 different mood states (angry, calm, depressed, energetic, fearful, high, irritable, mellow, nervous, and tired).[20,25] The VAS was scored in millimeters from the left side of a 100-mm line to a perpendicular mark made by the subject at the point corresponding to his or her mood state at that time. The score could range from 0 (not at all) to 100 mm (most ever). Subjects also completed the Panic Attack Symptom Scale (PASS), a self-rated symptom checklist for the cognitive and somatic symptoms of panic listed in *DSM-III-R*.[26] Each item was rated on a six-point scale from zero (none) to five (extreme).

The VAS and the PASS were administered at baseline and 15, 30, 45, 60, 75, 90, 120, and 240 minutes after the test dose. Each subject underwent assessment by one of us (C.J.M.) a research psychiatrist blinded to the test dose to determine whether he or she had a panic attack during each test session. This determination was based on direct clinical observation and the subject's self-report. Two criteria were used to determine whether a subject had a panic attack after the test dose: (1) a crescendo increase in subjective nervousness, reflected by a rise of at least 25 mm on the VAS measure of nervousness, and (2) an increase over baseline on four or more items of the *DSM-III-R* symptoms of a panic attack as recorded on the PASS.[22]

PHYSIOLOGICAL ASSESSMENT

Sitting and standing blood pressure and pulse were determined in the usual clinical fashion with a mercury sphygmomanometer at baseline and 15, 30, 45, 60, 75, 90, 120, and 240 minutes after the test dose. Following the 240-minute time point, subjects were provided with food and underwent medical assessment, including electrocardiography. No medical complications occurred during the test procedures.

BIOCHEMICAL METHODS

Blood samples were kept on ice for no more than 2 hours prior to separation of plasma in a refrigerated centrifuge. Plasma was stored at −70°C until assay. For determination of plasma-free MHPG levels, 0.5 mg of sodium metabisulfite and 200 ng of deuterated MHPG were added to each plasma aliquot before freezing. Sample preparation followed a modified version of the method of Dekirmenjian and Maas.[27] Measurement of plasma-free MHPG was carried out by selected ion monitoring, using a quadripolar mass spectrometer with gas chromatographic inlet system. The intra-assay and interassay coefficients of variation of this method were 6% and 11%, respectively. Plasma cortisol levels were measured using a radioimmunoassay kit with intra-assay and interassay coefficients of variation of 3.2% and 5.0%, respectively. All specimens were assayed in duplicate to reduce variance, with resulting values averaged to yield the reported individual value.

DATA ANALYSIS

During the course of the study, four subjects withdrew from participation. All these subjects made the decision to stop participating following the first set of challenges (early discontinuation). Two of the subjects declined further participation owing to the intensity of the panic attack they experienced during the first set of challenges, while the other two subjects left owing to the desire to be discharged from the hospital. Because the purpose of the study was to compare biochemical, behavioral, and cardiovascular responsivity in cocaine addicts during early and late discontinuation of cocaine use, only data from the 10 subjects who completed both sets of challenges were included in the full data analysis.

The baseline measures for each variable did not differ between test days within each phase of discontinuation (early and late). These measures were averaged to yield a single baseline for each variable at each phase of discontinuation, with baselines between phases compared using the paired *t* test.

Analysis of variance (ANOVA) with repeated measures was used to determine the main effects of the test drug (yohimbine vs placebo), phase of discontinuation (early vs late), and time of sampling (after administration of the test dose) for each of the biochemical, behavioral, and physiological variables. The differential effects of yohimbine and placebo were reflected in the interactions of the test drug with time and, most directly, the test drug with time and phase of discontinuation. All statistical tests were two tailed, with significance set at $P<.05$. Data analysis used SPSS[28] and SAS[29] programs.

tributes to the pathophysiological features of panic disorder[20-22] and of cocaine's ability to potently block central NE synaptic uptake,[23] it is conceivable that cocaine-related anxiety and panic attacks are the result of an underlying dysregulation in NE function.

The primary objectives of the current study were to prospectively investigate NE function, anxiety symptoms, and cardiovascular reactivity during early and late discontination of regular cocaine ingestion in chronic cocaine abusers under controlled, inpatient conditions. Yohimbine hy-

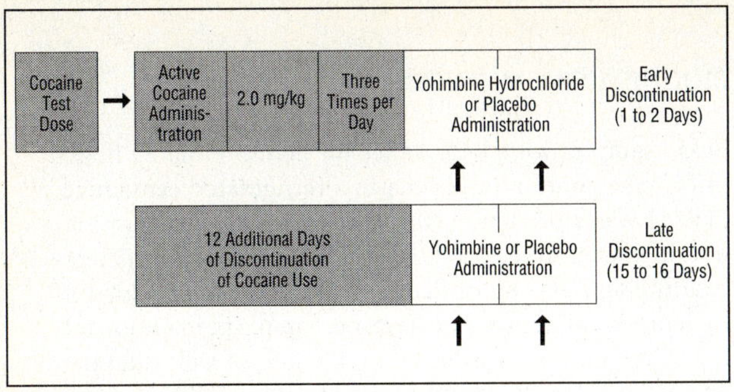

Figure 1. *Study design.*

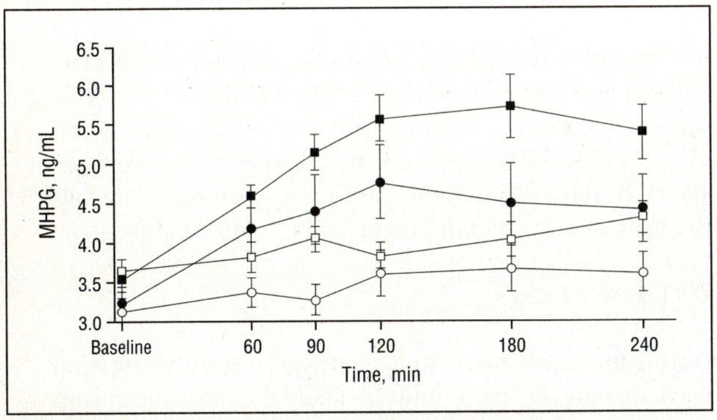

Figure 2. *Effects of intravenous yohimbine hydrochloride (solid symbols) and placebo (open symbols) on plasma 3-methoxy-4-hydroxyphenylethylene glycol (MHPG) levels in subjects addicted to cocaine during early (squares) or late discontinuation of cocaine use (circles).*

drochloride, an α_2-adrenergic receptor antagonist that has been shown to increase NE turnover in laboratory animals[24] and humans,[25] was used as a pharmacological challenge agent to investigate these variables. Levels of plasma 3-methoxy-4-hydroxyphenylethylene glycol (MHPG), the principal metabolite of brain NE, and plasma cortisol, an indirect neurohormonal index of NE function, were the neurochemical measures used to assess NE responsivity in this study. Structured rating scales were used to assess behavioral effects, and vital signs were obtained to monitor cardiovascular response. To our knowledge, this is the first investigation of NE function during discontinuation of cocaine use following the controlled administration of cocaine in humans.

RESULTS

BIOCHEMICAL VARIABLES

There was a trend for subjects to have higher baseline plasma MHPG levels during early compared with late discontinuation (3.6±0.5 ng/mL vs 3.2±0.6 ng/mL, respectively; t=1.9; df=9; P<.09). The ANOVA of the plasma MHPG response to yohimbine showed a significant interaction effect of yohimbine with time during both early (F=13.2; df=9,81; P<.0001) and late discontinuation (F=9.8; df=9,81; P<.0001) (**Figure 2**). There was also a significant interaction effect of yohimbine with phase of discontinuation and time (F=2.7; df=9,81; P<.05) (Figure 2), indicating a greater MHPG response during early compared with late discontinuation.

No significant difference was identified for baseline measures of plasma cortisol levels between early and late discontinuation (295.2±99.3 nmol/L vs 295.2±135.2 nmol/L, respectively; t=0.0; df=9; differences were not significant). The ANOVA of the plasma cortisol response to yohimbine did not show a significant interaction effect of yohimbine with time during early discontinuation (F=1.8; df=9,81; P<.15), but the interaction effect was significant during late discontinuation (F=4.8; df=9,81; P<.001). Comparison of the cortisol response during early and late discontinuation, however, did not show a significant interaction effect of yohimbine with phase of discontinuation and time (F=0.5; df=9,81; differences were not significant).

BEHAVIORAL VARIABLES

Subjects were significantly more fearful (8.1±16.0 vs 2.4±8.3; t=2.2; df=9; P<.05) and nervous (16.2±17.1 vs 4.4±10.4; t=4.2; df=9; P<.002) at baseline during early compared with late discontinuation, respectively. No other significant differences in baseline measures of behavioral variables were identified between discontinuation phases.

During early discontinuation, the ANOVA of behavioral responses to yohimbine showed that subjects became significantly less calm (F=2.9; df=8,72; P<.008) and mellow (F=2.1; df=8,72; P<.04) and significantly more energetic (F=2.6; df=8,72; P<.01), high (F=2.1; df=8,72; P<.05), and nervous (F=4.4; df=8,72; P<.0002) (**Figure 3**). During late discontinuation, subjects became significantly more energetic (F=2.6; df=8,72; P<.02) and nervous (F=2.5; df=8,72; P<.02) (Figure 3). Significant interaction effects of yohimbine with phase of discontinuation and time indicated lower ratings for mellowness (F=2.1; df=8,72; P<.05) and higher ratings for nervousness (F=2.3; df=8,72; P<.03) (Figure 3) during early vs late discontinuation.

During early discontinuation, yohimbine administration produced a behavioral state meeting *DSM-III-R* and study criteria for a panic attack in 8 of 10 subjects who completed both sets of challenge test days, and in two of four subjects who completed only the first set of challenges (total of 71%). None of the 14 subjects had a panic attack following placebo administration (**Figure 4**). During late discontinuation, none of the 10 subjects who completed both sets of challenges had a panic attack following yohimbine or placebo administration (Figure 4) (P<.0005, Fisher's Exact Test).

PHYSIOLOGICAL VARIABLES

No significant differences were found for baseline measures of blood pressure or pulse between discontinuation phases. The ANOVA of physiological responses to yohimbine showed significant interaction effects of yo-

himbine with time for sitting systolic blood pressure during both early (F=7.1; *df*=8,72; *P*<.0001) and late discontinuation (F=2.7; *df*=8,72; *P*<.01). Similar increases in standing systolic blood pressure were also seen during early (F=4.4; *df*=8,72; *P*<.0002) and late discontinuation (F=5.1; *df*=8,72; *P*<.0001). No significant interaction effects were found for diastolic blood pressure or pulse. There were no significant interaction effects of yohimbine with phase of discontinuation and time for any of the physiological measures.

COMMENT

The results of this study suggest that acute discontinuation of the repeated insufflation of cocaine in chronic abusers is associated with increased NE responsivity and heightened states of yohimbine-induced panic anxiety. This functional increase in NE tone during early compared with late discontinuation of cocaine use is reflected by the significantly increased MHPG response to yohimbine, which may be consistent with increased NE turnover,[25] the significantly increased ratings of nervousness, and the marked increase in the number of panic attacks. The percentage of subjects experiencing a yohimbine-induced panic attack during early discontinuation (71%) was similar to that of patients with panic disorder who have experienced panic attacks (63%) while undergoing an identical testing procedure, using the same criteria to define a panic attack, in the same research setting.[22] As Gorman and colleagues[30] point out, clear definition of the criteria for a panic attack is critical to allow for comparison of rates of panic across studies. The decreased MHPG response 2 weeks after the last dose of cocaine suggests that NE metabolism may equilibrate during the course of continued cocaine abstinence. Similarly, the lower ratings of nervousness and absence of yohimbine-induced panic attacks during late discontinuation indicate that the associated behavioral sequelae may also be reduced.

The increased MHPG response to yohimbine that occurred during early discontinuation of cocaine use in this study may represent a compensatory response of presynaptic NE neurons to an acute deficiency of synaptic NE. A similar compensatory response has been demonstrated in preclinical studies, in which the activity of tyrosine hydroxylase, the rate-limiting enzyme for NE synthesis, was found to be increased after exposure to cocaine.[31] Although a significant amount of plasma MHPG is derived from peripheral sources,[32] the plasma MHPG level has been shown to correlate with more direct measures of brain NE turnover,[33] suggesting that it may, under certain conditions, be a valid measure of central NE metabolism.[34] However, it is entirely possible that cocaine may have directly or indirectly affected the responsiveness of the peripheral sympathetic nervous system, as manifested by the response of systolic blood pressure to yohimbine, thus accounting for the increased MHPG response. The direct mea-

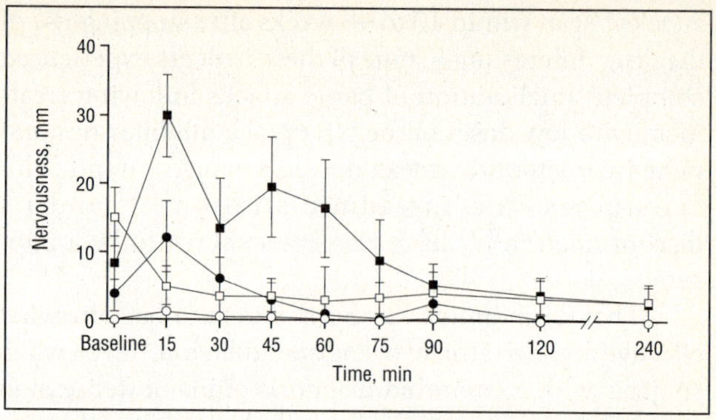

Figure 3. *Effects of intravenous yohimbine hydrochloride (solid symbols) and placebo (open symbols) on ratings of nervousness in subjects addicted to cocaine during early (squares) or late discontinuation of cocaine use (circles). Measurement of nervousness is described in the "Behavioral Ratings" subsection of the "Subjects and Methods" section of the text.*

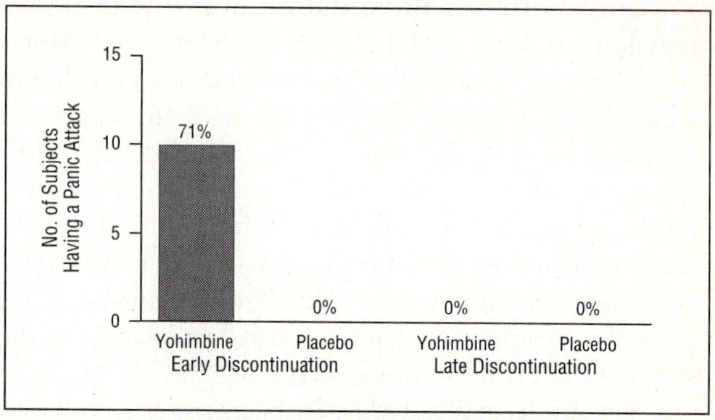

Figure 4. *Rate of yohimbine hydrochloride or placebo-induced panic attacks in subjects addicted to cocaine during early and late discontinuation of cocaine use (*P*<.0005, Fisher's Exact Test).*

surement of NE rather than MHPG levels and an assessment of NE peripheral kinetics would have been useful in more clearly delineating central from peripheral effects of discontinuation of cocaine use on NE responsivity in this study.

There have been numerous reports of cocaine-precipitated panic attacks, as well as panic disorder that developed following the discontinuation of cocaine use.[7-14] Aronson and Craig[9] described three patients whose panic disorder began during recreational intranasal cocaine use and persisted autonomously after the drug use was stopped. Similarly, Price and Giannini[11] and Pohl et al[10] described the onset and persistence of panic disorder in patients who had been abusing crack and freebase cocaine, respectively. Geracioti and Post[14] suggested that cocaine-induced panic disorder can develop even after the inhalation of only a small amount of the drug. In an analysis of data obtained on 5896 subjects who were part of the Epidemiologic Catchment Area study,[35] users of cocaine were more than 14 times as likely to have had a panic attack than a control group. Finally, 13 of 68 patients enrolled in the UCLA Anxiety Disorders Program during a 1-year period had cocaine-related panic disorder.[13] In four patients, panic attacks began during drug use, and, in the others, panic

attacks began within 10 to 48 weeks after stopping use of the drug. Interestingly, nine of these patients experienced complete amelioration of panic attacks following treatment with low doses of the NE uptake inhibitor desipramine hydrochloride (mean dose, 28.9 mg/d). In preclinical studies, cocaine administration[15-17] and its discontinuation[18,19] have also been shown to be anxiogenic.

That desipramine has been shown to be somewhat effective in the treatment of cocaine addiction,[36] even when subjects with a comorbid diagnosis of major depression are excluded,[37] provides indirect evidence that a dysregulation in NE function may contribute to the pathophysiological features of cocaine addiction and abstinence states. Furthermore, repeated desipramine treatment significantly down-regulated β-adrenergic receptors and shortened the duration of postwithdrawal anhedonia in a rat model of cocaine abstinence.[38] Moreover, the magnitude of the β-adrenergic receptor down-regulation correlated significantly with the degree of effectiveness of desipramine in reversing the postwithdrawal anhedonia.[38] In contrast, two recently published controlled studies showed desipramine to have few benefits with respect to reducing cocaine use in methadone-maintained cocaine abusers,[39,40] and other investigators have found that desipramine is no different from placebo in the treatment of primary cocaine addicts.[41,42]

The results of this study must be interpreted with caution with regard to yohimbine's effects on NE function. Although clinical responses to yohimbine are consistent with α_2-adrenergic receptor blockade,[20-22,25,43] yohimbine also binds with lower affinity to other receptors, including the α_1-adrenergic,[44] dopamine-2,[24] serotonin,[45] and imidazoline-preferring[46] receptors. Recently, however, it was shown that yohimbine produces a pattern of behavioral and neuroendocrine responses in healthy human subjects similar to that of idazoxan,[43] an α_2-adrenergic antagonist with greater α_2- than α_1-adrenergic receptor selectivity[44] that does not appear to block dopamine or serotonin receptors with high affinity.[47-49]

It should be acknowledged that relatively low and infrequent doses of cocaine were administered in this study compared with naturalistic street use of cocaine. However, significant neurobiological changes were found following discontinuation of cocaine use. The occurrence of these alterations in NE function in a controlled, inpatient clinical environment strongly suggests that neurobiological changes of similar or greater magnitude would be present in a naturalistic setting, where higher and more frequent doses of cocaine are used.

CONCLUSIONS

While other neurotransmitter systems, including dopamine[50] and serotonin,[51] have been shown to contribute to the pathophysiological features of cocaine abstinence symptoms, the results of this study implicate NE function in the mediation of cocaine-related panic anxiety and some of the biochemical effects of acute discontinuation of cocaine use in addicts. This NE dysregulation may underlie the symptoms of anxiety, panic, and dysphoria that frequently dominate states of euphoria in chronic cocaine use. Some individuals may continue to use cocaine not to attain a feeling of well-being but rather in a futile attempt to transiently ameliorate discontinuation-related anxiety and panic. Others often use cocaine and ethanol together, a combination associated with increased morbidity and mortality, in an effort to reduce the "jitters" induced by cocaine.[52] Additional controlled studies of NE function, possibly in combination with brain imaging techniques, appear warranted to further clarify derangements associated with cocaine addiction.

Accepted for publication May 6, 1994.

This study was supported in part by grant DA04060 from the National Institute of Drug Abuse, Rockville, Md, grants MH25642 and MH30929 from the National Institute of Mental Health, Rockville, the State of Connecticut, and a 1990-to-1992 National Alliance for Research on Schizophrenia and Affective Disorders Young Investigator Award (Dr McDougle).

We thank Beth Ruff and Betsy Kyle of the research and clerical staff at the Clinical Neuroscience Research Unit for their expert assistance.

Reprint requests to Clinical Neuroscience Research Unit of the Abraham Ribicoff Research Facilities, Connecticut Mental Health Center, 34 Park St, New Haven, CT 06519 (Dr McDougle).

REFERENCES

1. Substance Abuse and Mental Health Services Administration. *National Household Survey on Drug Abuse: Population Estimates, 1993.* Washington, DC: US Dept of Health and Human Services; 1993. Dept of Health and Human Services publication SMA93-2053.
2. Closser MH. Cocaine epidemiology. In: Kosten TR, Kleber HD, eds. *Clinician's Guide to Cocaine Addiction: Theory, Research, and Treatment.* New York, NY: The Guilford Press; 1992:225-240.
3. Ritz MC, Lamb RJ, Goldberg SR, Kuhar MJ. Cocaine receptors on dopamine transporters are related to self-administration of cocaine. *Science.* 1987;237: 1219-1223.
4. Gawin FH, Kleber HD. Abstinence symptomatology and psychiatric diagnosis in cocaine abusers: clinical observations. *Arch Gen Psychiatry.* 1986;43:107-133.
5. Weddington WW, Brown BS, Haertzen CA, Cone EJ, Dax EM, Herning RI, Michaelson BS. Changes in mood, craving, and sleep during acute short-term abstinence reported by male cocaine addicts: a controlled, residential study. *Arch Gen Psychiatry.* 1990;47:861-868.
6. Satel SL, Price LH, Palumbo JM, McDougle CJ, Krystal JH, Gawin F, Charney DS, Heninger GR, Kleber HD. Clinical phenomenology and neurobiology of cocaine cessation: a prospective inpatient study. *Am J Psychiatry.* 1991;148: 1712-1716.
7. Jeri FR, Sanchez CC, del Pozo T, Fernandez M, Carbajal C. Further experience with the syndromes produced by coca paste smoking. *Bull Narc.* 1978;3:1-11.
8. Washton AM, Gold MS. Chronic cocaine abuse: evidence for adverse effects on health and functioning. *Psychiatry Ann.* 1984;14:733-739.
9. Aronson T, Craig T. Cocaine precipitation of panic disorder. *Am J Psychiatry.* 1986;143:643-645.

10. Pohl R, Balon R, Yeragani V. More on cocaine and panic disorder. *Am J Psychiatry.* 1987;144:1363.
11. Price WA, Giannini AJ. Phencyclidine and 'crack'-precipitated panic disorder. *Am J Psychiatry.* 1987;144:686-687.
12. Louie AK, Lannon RA, Ketter TA. Treatment of cocaine-induced panic disorder. *Am J Psychiatry.* 1989;146:40-44.
13. Bystritsky A, Ackerman D, Pasnau R. Low-dose desipramine treatment of cocaine-related panic attacks. *J Nerv Ment Dis.* 1991;179:755-758.
14. Geracioti TJ, Post R. Onset of panic disorder associated with rare use of cocaine. *Biol Psychiatry.* 1991;29:403-406.
15. Shearman GT, Lal H. Discriminative stimulus properties of cocaine related to an anxiogenic action. *Prog Neuropsychopharmacol Biol Psychiatry.* 1981;5:57-63.
16. Ettenberg A, Geist TD. Animal model for investigating the anxiogenic effects of self-administered cocaine. *Psychopharmacology.* 1991;103:455-461.
17. Yang X-M, Gorman AL, Dunn AJ, Goeders NE. Anxiogenic effects of acute and chronic cocaine administration: neurochemical and behavioral studies. *Pharmacol Biochem Behav.* 1992;41:643-650.
18. Wood D, Lal H. Anxiogenic properties of cocaine withdrawal. *Life Sci.* 1987; 41:1431-1436.
19. Wood DM, Laraby PR, Lal H. A pentylenetetrazol-like stimulus during cocaine withdrawal: blockade by diazepam but not haloperidol. *Drug Dev Res.* 1989; 16:269-276.
20. Charney DS, Heninger GR, Breier A. Noradrenergic function in panic anxiety: effects of yohimbine in healthy subjects and patients with agoraphobia and panic disorder. *Arch Gen Psychiatry.* 1984;41:751-763.
21. Charney DS, Woods SW, Goodman WK, Heninger GR. Neurobiological mechanisms of panic anxiety: biochemical and behavioral correlates of yohimbine-induced panic attacks. *Am J Psychiatry.* 1987;1447:1030-1036.
22. Charney DS, Woods SW, Krystal JH, Nagy LM, Heninger GR. Noradrenergic neuronal dysregulation in panic disorder: the effects of intravenous yohimbine and clonidine in panic disorder patients. *Acta Psychiatr Scand.* 1992;86:273-282.
23. Iverson LL. *Handbook of Psychopharmacology: Biochemistry of Biogenic Amines.* 1975;3:381-442.
24. Scatton B, Zivkivic B, Dedek J. Antidopaminergic properties of yohimbine. *J Pharmacol Exp Ther.* 1980;215:494-499.
25. Charney DS, Heninger GR, Sternberg DE. Assessment of α_2 adrenergic autoreceptor function in humans: effects of oral yohimbine. *Life Sci.* 1982;30:2033-2041.
26. American Psychiatric Association. *Diagnostic and Statistical Manual of Mental Disorders, Revised Third Edition.* Washington, DC: American Psychiatric Association; 1987.
27. Dekirmenjian H, Maas JW. MHPG in plasma. *Clin Chim Acta.* 1974;52:203-208.
28. *SPSS User's Guide.* 2nd ed. Chicago, Ill: SPSS Inc; 1986.
29. *SAS User's Guide: Statistics, 1982 Edition.* Cary, NC: SAS Institute Inc; 1982.
30. Gorman JM, Fyer MR, Liebowitz MR, Klein DF. *Psychopharmacology: The Third Generation of Progress.* New York, NY: Raven Press; 1987:985-993.
31. Patrick RL, Barchas JD. Potentiation by cocaine of the stimulus-induced increase in dopamine synthesis in rat brain striatal synaptosomes. *Neuropharmacology.* 1977;16:327.
32. Blombery PA, Kopin IJ, Gordon EK, Markey SP, Ebert MH. Conversion of MHPG to vanillylmandelic acid: implications for the importance of urinary MHPG. *Arch Gen Psychiatry.* 1980;37:1095-1098.
33. Karoum F, Mayer-Schwing J, Potkin SG, Wyatt RJ. Presence of free sulfate and glucuronide-conjugated MHPG in human brain, cerebrospinal fluid and plasma. *Brain Res.* 1977;125:333-339.
34. Leckman JF, Maas JW. Plasma MHPG: relationship to brain noradrenergic systems and emerging clinical applications. In: Post RM, Ballenger JC, eds. *Neurobiology of Mood Disorders.* Baltimore, Md: Williams & Wilkins; 1984:529-538.
35. Anthony J, Tien A, Petronis K. Epidemiologic evidence on cocaine use and panic attacks. *Am J Epidemiol.* 1989;129:543-549.
36. Gawin FH, Kleber HD. Cocaine abuse treatment: open pilot trial with desipramine and lithium carbonate. *Arch Gen Psychiatry.* 1984;41:903-910.
37. Gawin FH, Kleber HD, Byck R, Rounsaville BJ, Kosten TR, Jatlow PI, Morgan C. Desipramine facilitation of initial cocaine abstinence. *Arch Gen Psychiatry.* 1989;46:117-121.
38. Markou A, Hauger RL, Koob GF. Desmethylimipramine attenuates cocaine withdrawal in rats. *Psychopharmacology.* 1992;109:305-314.
39. Arndt IO, Dorozynsky L, Woody GE, McLellan AT, O'Brien CP. Desipramine treatment of cocaine dependence in methadone-maintained patients. *Arch Gen Psychiatry.* 1992;49:888-893.
40. Kosten TR, Morgan CM, Falcione J, Schottenfeld RS. Pharmacotherapy for cocaine-abusing methadone-maintained patients using amantadine or desipramine. *Arch Gen Psychiatry.* 1992;49:894-898.
41. Tennant FS, Tarver AL. *Double-Blind Comparison of Desipramine and Placebo in Withdrawal From Cocaine Dependence.* Washington, DC: National Institute on Drug Abuse; 1984:159-163. National Institute on Drug Abuse research monograph 55.
42. Weddington WW, Brown BS, Haertzen CA, Hess Jm, Mahaffey JR, Kolar AF, Jaffe JH. Comparison of amantadine and desipramine combined with psychotherapy for treatment of cocaine dependence. *Am J Drug Alcohol Abuse.* 1991; 17:137-152.
43. Krystal JH, McDougle CJ, Woods SW, Price LH, Heninger GR, Charney DS. Dose-response relationship for oral idazoxan effects in healthy human subjects: comparison with oral yohimbine. *Psychopharmacology.* 1992;108:313-319.
44. Doxey JC, Lane AC, Roach AG, Virdee NK. Comparison of the α-adrenoceptor antagonist profiles of idazoxan (RX 781094), yohimbine, rauwolscine, and corynanthine. *Naunyn Schmiedebergs Arch Pharmacol.* 1984;325:136-144.
45. Dwoskin LP, Neal BS, Sparber SB. Evidence for anti-serotonergic properties of yohimbine. *Pharmacol Biochem Behav.* 1988;31:321-326.
46. Ernsberger P, Giuliano R, Willette RN, Reis DJ. Role of imidazole receptors in the vasodepressor response to clonidine analogs in the rostral ventrolateral medulla. *J Pharmacol Exp Ther.* 1990;253:408-418.
47. Doxey JC, Roach AG, Smith CFC. Studies on RX 781094: a selective, potent and specific antagonist of α_2-adrenoceptors. *Br J Pharmacol.* 1983;78:489-505.
48. Scatton B, Dedek J, Zivkovic B. Lack of involvement of α_2-adrenoceptors in the regulation of striatal dopaminergic transmission. *Eur J Pharmacol.* 1983; 86:427-433.
49. Pettibone DJ, Pfleuger AB, Totaro JA. Comparison of the effects of recently developed α_2-adrenergic antagonists with yohimbine and rauwolscine on monoamine synthesis in rat brain. *Biochem Pharmacol.* 1985;34:1093-1097.
50. McDougle CJ, Price LH, Palumbo JM, Kosten TR, Kleber HD, Heninger GR. Dopaminergic responsivity during cocaine cessation: a pilot study. *Psychiatry Res.* 1992;43:77-85.
51. Van de Kar LD, Rittenhouse PA, O'Connor P, Palionis T, Brownfield MS, Lent SJ, Carnes M, Bethea CL. Effect of cocaine injections on the neuroendocrine response to the serotonin agonist MK-212. *Biol Psychiatry.* 1992;32:258-269.
52. McCance-Katz EF, Price LH, McDougle CJ, Kosten TR, Black JE, Jatlow PI. Concurrent cocaine-ethanol ingestion in humans: pharmacology, physiology, behavior, and the role of cocaethylene. *Psychopharmacology.* 1993;111:39-46.

Conversions From Système International (SI) Units to Traditional Units (Modified From *The SI Manual in Health Care*)

System	Component	SI Reference Interval*	SI Unit	Conversion Factor (Divide by)	Traditional Reference Interval*	Traditional Unit
Serum	Cortisol					
	8 AM	110-520	nmol/L	27.59	4-19	μg/dL
	4 PM	50-410	nmol/L	27.59	2-15	μg/dL
	Midnight	<140	nmol/L	27.59	<5	μg/dL

**These reference values are not intended to be definitive since each laboratory determines its own values. They are provided for illustration only.*

Buspirone Treatment of Anxious Alcoholics

A Placebo-Controlled Trial

Henry R. Kranzler, MD; Joseph A. Burleson, PhD; Frances K. Del Boca, PhD; Thomas F. Babor, PhD; Patricia Korner, RN; Joseph Brown, PhD; Michael J. Bohn, MD

Background: Symptoms of anxiety are common in alcoholics and may contribute to relapse following initiation of abstinence. Buspirone hydrochloride, a serotonin$_{1A}$ partial agonist, has a pharmacologic profile that may be particularly suited to the treatment of anxious alcoholics.

Methods: We conducted a randomized, 12-week, placebo-controlled trial of buspirone in 61 anxious alcoholics, all of whom also received weekly relapse prevention psychotherapy. Outcomes were measured at the end of treatment and at a 6-month follow-up evaluation.

Results: Buspirone therapy was associated with greater retention in the 12-week treatment trial, reduced anxiety, a slower return to heavy alcohol consumption, and fewer drinking days during the follow-up period.

Conclusions: Buspirone appears to have a useful role in the treatment of anxious alcoholics. Further research is needed to clarify which patient characteristics and concomitant treatments result in optimal response to buspirone therapy.

(Arch Gen Psychiatry. 1994;51:720-731)

SYMPTOMS OF anxiety are common among alcoholics both in the community[1] and clinical settings.[2,3] The relationship between anxiety and heavy alcohol consumption appears to be reciprocal, insofar as anxiety has been shown to be both a cause and a consequence of heavy alcohol consumption.[4] Specifically, long-term administration of ethanol to alcoholics in a research setting has been shown to produce increased levels of anxiety.[5] Furthermore, the anxiety level was found to be inversely related to the duration of abstinence from alcohol.[6] At the same time, heavy alcohol consumption is common among patients seeking treatment for anxiety disorders, the majority of whom report having begun heavy alcohol consumption in an effort to reduce anxiety symptoms.[7] Anxiety symptoms have also been implicated as a cause of relapse to heavy alcohol consumption among abstinent alcoholics.[8] Finally, treatment of an anxiety disorder may result in improvement in the substance use disorder.[9]

Abnormalities in serotonin (5-HT) neurotransmission may help to explain the association between alcohol consumption and anxiety.[10] Alcoholics have a variety of abnormalities in 5-HT neurotransmission, including low cerebrospinal fluid levels of 5-hydroxyindoleacetic acid, the major metabolite of 5-HT.[11,12] These findings suggest that alcoholics have diminished 5-HT neurotransmission.[13] Furthermore, research on alcoholics shows an inverse relationship between 5-hydroxyindoleacetic acid levels in cerebrospinal fluid and the time elapsed since alcohol was last consumed.[14] One possible explanation for this finding is that in alcoholics, 5-HT release following acute ethanol administration may normalize low levels of 5-HT in the brain.[13]

A wide variety of 5-HT agonists (eg, precursors and reuptake inhibitors) reduce alcohol consumption by animals.[15] A number of selective serotonin uptake in-

See Subjects and Methods on next page

From the Alcohol Research Center, Department of Psychiatry, University of Connecticut Health Center, Farmington.

SUBJECTS AND METHODS

RECRUITMENT PROCEDURES

Subjects were primarily recruited through advertisements inviting them to participate in a study of a medication for use by anxious persons who drink heavily. The recruitment procedure and the study protocol were approved by the Institutional Review Board of the University of Connecticut Health Center, Farmington. All subjects gave written, informed consent prior to participation. Following a telephone screening interview, potential subjects were interviewed in person by one of us (P.K.) who took a general medical and psychiatric history and administered the HAM-A.[46] Eligible subjects were then interviewed by two of us (H.R.K. and M.J.B.) who administered the Psychoactive Substance Use Disorders section of the Structured Clinical Interview for *DSM-III-R*.[52] Comorbid anxiety and mood disorder diagnoses were made using the computerized Diagnostic Interview Schedule, which yields *DSM-III* diagnoses[53] with acceptable reliability and validity.[54,55] These interviews were followed by a clinical laboratory evaluation (complete blood cell count, urinalysis, blood chemistry profile, and, for women, a serum pregnancy test) and physical examination.

Subjects were included in the study if they currently met *DSM-III-R* criteria for alcohol dependence,[56] expressed a desire to maintain abstinence for the 12-week treatment phase of the study, were willing to be randomly assigned to treatment with buspirone or placebo, and were willing to participate in weekly cognitive-behavioral psychotherapy. Subjects were required to maintain abstinence from alcohol for a minimum of 7 days before randomization to treatment. At the end of that time, they were included only if they had a score of 15 or higher on the HAM-A. Although the decision to require an initial period of abstinence limits the severity of alcohol dependence in the sample (and consequently, the ability to generalize the findings to other samples of alcoholics), it has two advantages. First, it helps to reduce the confounding effects of anxiety symptoms attributable to persistent alcohol withdrawal.[57] Second, it more accurately reflects standard clinical practice, in which a period of abstinence generally precedes efforts at rehabilitation of ambulatory alcoholics.

Subjects were excluded if they currently met criteria for another *DSM-III-R* psychoactive substance use (other than nicotine) disorder; reported heavy use of a psychoactive drug in the week prior to screening; were without a stable residence; or showed evidence of psychosis, melancholic depression, bipolar disorder, significant cognitive impairment, or suicidal ideation. Subjects were also excluded if there was clinical or laboratory evidence of a serious medical illness (eg, unstable angina pectoris, lupus erythematosus, chronic obstructive pulmonary disease, or infectious hepatitis) or pregnancy. Subjects with a history of moderate-to-severe alcohol withdrawal and who were not recently abstinent from alcohol were excluded to minimize the confounding of anxiety symptoms with symptoms of acute alcohol withdrawal.

SUBJECTS

Following the initial telephone interview, a total of 162 subjects (80.9% men) were interviewed in person by one of us (P.K.). Four subjects were recruited following inpatient alcoholism rehabilitation. Otherwise eligible subjects (n=101) were excluded for the following reasons: decision by the subject not to participate after the requirements of the study were explained in detail (n=30), HAM-A score of less than 15 (n=27), moderate-to-severe alcohol withdrawal (n=17), medical illness (n=14), failure to meet current alcohol dependence criteria (n=6), comorbid psychiatric illness that required treatment in excess of that provided in the study protocol (n=4), recent psychoactive drug use (n=2), and homelessness (n=1). A total of 61 subjects were, therefore, randomly assigned to receive either buspirone (n=31) or placebo (n=30). There were no significant between-group differences on a variety of demographic variables (**Table 1**). Of the four subjects enrolled in the study following inpatient rehabilitation, two were assigned to each treatment group to maintain comparability between groups with respect to severity of alcoholism.

TREATMENT PROCEDURES

Medication was provided in opaque capsules containing either one or two tablets of buspirone hydrochloride, 5 mg, or matched placebo. Twenty-five milligrams of riboflavin was included in each capsule to facilitate compliance monitoring (Frances Del Boca, PhD, Henry R. Kranzler, MD, Joseph Brown, PhD, Patricia Korner, RN, unpublished data, 1992). Subjects were also given a daily multivitamin formulation containing a negligible amount of riboflavin in place of any vitamins they were currently using. This procedure removed a potential source of exogenous riboflavin that might confound assessment of compliance by detection of urinary riboflavin levels.

Subjects initially received one single-dose capsule (ie, buspirone hydrochloride, 5 mg, or placebo) three times daily (TID). If tolerated, the doses were then increased every 3 to 4 days by one additional capsule TID to a maximum dosage of buspirone hydrochloride, 20 mg TID, or an equivalent number of placebo capsules. The maximal dose was generally reached by the end of the second week of treatment. The mean maximal daily dose was 10.5 (±2.7) tablets (52.5 [±13.5] mg) for buspirone hydrochloride–treated subjects and 10.2 (±3.3) tablets for placebo-treated subjects. This difference was not statistically significant ($F[1,58]=0.12$; $P=.72$). At the end of the 12-week treatment period, the medication therapy was tapered over a 3-day period and then discontinued.

Continued on next page

In addition to weekly medication monitoring, subjects in both the buspirone and placebo groups received weekly, individual, cognitive-behavioral psychotherapy administered by masters'- or doctoral-level psychologists (including one of us [J.B.]) experienced in the provision of such treatment to alcohol-dependent subjects. This therapy was conducted using a 12-session treatment manual that focused on relapse prevention[58] and skills training.[59] Both have been shown to help in the maintenance of abstinence and or reduction of consumption in alcoholics.[59,60] Each 1-hour session focused on relapse prevention skills. Topics covered included high risk and trigger identification, cognitive approaches to intense negative emotions, craving management, relaxation training, leisure skills, problem solving, decision making, anger management, assertiveness, drink refusal, family issues, and anxiety management.

A typical session began with the measurement of vital signs and the collection of weekly reports of anxiety and adverse effects of the medication. This part was followed by a brief review of the past week's activities, which focused specifically on any lapses in sobriety or difficult times. If a lapse had occurred in the intervening week, the therapist had the option of postponing the didactic topic scheduled for that week and proceeding instead with a special lapse analysis session. If this option was exercised, the therapist would then choose a subsequent session to be excluded, based on his or her knowledge of the subject's personal strengths and weaknesses. Additional sessions were not added in the event that a lapse occurred. Subjects were required to miss no more than three therapy sessions during the 12-week treatment period. Subjects were encouraged, but not required, to attend meetings of Alcoholics Anonymous (AA). Although not encouraged, subjects were allowed to attend ambulatory therapy sessions, in addition to the therapy sessions provided in the study, as long as psychoactive medications were not used.

ASSESSMENTS

Parallel assessments were conducted at baseline, at the end of the 12-week treatment phase, and 6 months following the end of treatment. All assessments were performed by staff who were blinded to treatment status. The Time-Line Follow-Back Assessment method (TLFB)[61] was used to estimate daily alcohol consumption before, during, and following treatment. A self-reported questionnaire[62] was used to evaluate histories of lifetime alcohol consumption and alcoholism treatment. Other assessments included the Beck Depression Inventory[63] and the Michigan Alcoholism Screening Test.[64]

Assessments repeated weekly during the 12-week treatment period included breath alcohol testing, a questionnaire on the use of alcohol and other drugs that inquired about the use of all psychoactive substances during the week preceding the visit and treatment received outside of the study protocol (including attendance at AA meetings); a side-effects questionnaire; and the HAM-A. Urine samples were collected weekly and examined for the presence of riboflavin, which provided an objective measure of compliance with the medication regimen (Frances Del Boca, PhD, Henry R. Kranzler, MD, Joseph Brown, PhD, Patricia Korner, RN, unpublished data, 1992). At three times during the treatment period (ie, at weeks 4, 8, and 12), urine was also tested for the presence of other drugs. Although in the consent form subjects were told that urine would be tested for the presence of other drugs, they did not know which samples were being sent for drug testing.

At the end of active treatment (ie, after 12 weeks for most subjects and at the time of study discontinuation for those subjects who did not complete the study), a research assessment was repeated. This measure consisted of the TLFB and a questionnaire asking subjects whether they thought they had received buspirone or placebo. Of the 61 subjects enrolled in the study, 58 (95.1%) were interviewed at the end of treatment. At this time, a repeated laboratory evaluation was conducted, including testing for γ-glutamyl transpeptidase (γ-GTP) and aspartate aminotransferase (AST) levels. A telephone interview was also conducted with a collateral informant nominated previously by the subject to provide concurrent validation of alcohol use (ie, the number of days on which alcohol was consumed [drinking days] and the number of days on which the subject was intoxicated) and signs of anxiety during the preceding 30 days. Frequency ratings (one indicated almost never; two, sometimes; three, often; and four, almost always) of the subject's sleep problems, nervousness, and tension were combined into a single continuous measure of general anxiety.

A follow-up assessment (ie, the TLFB) was conducted 9 months after the initiation of treatment (ie, 6 months after the active treatment phase was completed or, for those who did not complete the study, the scheduled time of completion). Of the 61 subjects enrolled in the study, 50 (82.0%) were interviewed at follow-up. Eleven subjects (six of whom were in the buspirone group) were not available for follow-up. Informant interviews were also conducted at this time.

VALIDATION OF SELF-REPORTS AND COMPLIANCE WITH TREATMENT

Correlations between self-reported measures and reports from collateral informants revealed a relatively high degree of association. Reports by the informant of subjects'

hibitors attenuate alcohol consumption in human subjects who drink heavily.[16-20] Direct 5-HT agonists, such as buspirone (a 5-HT_{1A} partial agonist) reduce alcohol intake by alcohol-preferring rodents[21,22] and monkeys.[23] Engel and colleagues[24] and Svensson and colleagues[25] showed that the selective 5-HT_{1A} agonists 8-hydroxy-2 (di-n-propylamino) tetralin and ipsapirone hydrochloride reduced both ethanol intake and the preference for

anxiety symptoms during the treatment period were significantly correlated with HAM-A scores (r=.49; P=.002). The number of drinking days during the treatment period was significantly correlated with informants' reports of both the number of drinking days (r=.73; P<.001) and the number of days on which the subject drank to intoxication (r=.67; P<.001). The number of drinks consumed per day during the treatment period was also significantly correlated with the informants' reports of the number of drinking days (r=.68; P<.001) and the number of days of intoxication (r=.65; P<.001). Similar associations were observed between self-reported alcohol consumption and informants' reports at the 6-month follow-up. The self-reported number of drinking days was associated with informants' reports of both the number of drinking days (r=.68; P=.001) and the number of days of intoxication (r=.48; P=.03). The number of drinks consumed per day during the 6-month follow-up period was also significantly correlated with the informants' reports: the number of drinking days (r=.80; P=.001) and the number of days of intoxication (r=.56; P=.01).

As described above, serum levels of γ-GTP and AST were also measured at the end of treatment and at the 6-month follow-up to validate self-reported alcohol consumption. At the end of treatment, the number of drinking days correlated with both γ-GTP (r=.40; P=.003) and AST (r=.32; P=.01) levels. Similarly, number of drinks consumed per day correlated with levels of both hepatic enzymes (γ-GTP, r=.47 and P<.001; AST, r=.47 and P<.001). At the time of the 6-month follow-up, the number of drinking days correlated with both γ-GTP (r=.63; P=.002) and AST (r=.44; P=.03) levels. At that time point, the number of drinks consumed per day also correlated with levels of both enzymes (GGTP, r=.56 and P=.008; AST, r=.59 and P=.005).

Buspirone-treated subjects underwent riboflavin testing an average of 7.5 (±4.2) times during the study, compared with 8.1 (±3.3) times for placebo-treated subjects, a nonsignificant difference ($F[1,50]$=0.30; P=.59). Riboflavin testing revealed a high rate of medication compliance in both groups. Of the total number of urine samples collected, buspirone-treated subjects had an average of 93% (±12%) that were rated as positive for riboflavin, while placebo-treated subjects had an average of 96% (±7%) that were rated as positive for riboflavin. This difference was also not significant ($F[1,49]$=0.74; P=.39).

Only one urine sample from one subject was positive for a drug other than alcohol or the study medication (ie, cocaine). On no occasion did breath testing reveal a blood alcohol level in excess of 0.05 mg/dL, with the highest value obtained being 0.004 mg/dL, well below a level suggestive of recent heavy alcohol consumption.

The results of these analyses indicate that subjects were providing relatively accurate self-reported information. Subjects in both groups also appear to have been taking their medication with sufficient regularity to provide an adequate test of the study hypotheses.

STATISTICAL ANALYSES

Survival Analysis

Follow-up life-table (survival) analyses were performed on two alcohol consumption measures: the number of weeks to first drinking day and the first heavy drinking day (ie, five or more standard drinks consumed in a day) following randomization to treatment. The Wilcoxon (Gehan) test[65] was used to test the null hypothesis that the survival distributions of the buspirone-treated group were the same as those of the placebo-treated group. An average survival score was calculated for each group by an algorithm that compared each case in the data set to all others. The group having the longer average time to the terminal event received a positive score, while the group having the shorter average time received a negative score.

Multiple Regression

Various baseline assessments were used to predict changes in anxiety and alcohol consumption. Multiple linear regression was used hierarchically to step in each predictor in a logical sequence. The effects of baseline measures of both anxiety and alcohol consumption on end-point and 6-month follow-up measures of anxiety and alcohol consumption were the first to be accounted. This effort controlled for initial severity of both anxiety and alcohol consumption. The effects of the groups were then assessed, followed by the effects of differential lengths of treatment. Finally, interactions between treatment group and other selected predictors (ie, covariates), viz, treatment group by baseline HAM-A score and treatment group by the number of weeks of treatment, were assessed. The Johnson-Neyman technique[66] was used to specify the form of any interaction between treatment group and covariates. This procedure identifies the value of the covariate beyond which one treatment group differs significantly from the other on a given dependent measure.

Initial analyses of gender as a predictor showed no significant main or interactive effects on subsequent anxiety or alcohol consumption measures. Gender was, therefore, excluded from subsequent analyses. Analysis of end of treatment values employed the last observation carried forward. Effect size (f) statistics were calculated for those analyses that yielded significant medication group effects.[67]

ethanol in a free-choice situation. Similarly, in rats, the $5\text{-}HT_{1A}$ agonist gepirone hydrochloride has been shown to reduce alcohol consumption by up to 47% without disrupting motor behavior.[26]

Serotonergic abnormalities have also been observed in both animal models of anxiety[27,28] and patients with anxiety disorders.[29-31] A variety of serotonergic medications, including buspirone hydrochloride and

the selective serotonin uptake inhibitor fluvoxamine, are effective for the treatment of anxiety disorders.[32-34]

Given evidence that heavy alcohol consumption represents an effort on the part of some alcoholics to treat their anxiety symptoms, one strategy for preventing relapse in these patients is the treatment of comorbid anxiety disorders.[35] Kissin[36] listed three optimal qualities for an anxiolytic in the treatment of chronic alcoholism. It should (1) be effective in maintaining individuals in treatment, (2) have a low abuse potential, and (3) not potentiate the effects of alcohol. He reviewed a number of studies that showed chlordiazepoxide hydrochloride to be effective in retaining alcoholics in long-term outpatient treatment. While benzodiazepines are the most studied and widely prescribed anxiolytics, their potential for both overdose in combination with alcohol and abuse by alcoholics[37] may contraindicate their prolonged use in this patient population.[35] Although not all benzodiazepines have equal potential for abuse,[38,39] a nonbenzodiazepine anxiolytic such as buspirone[40] may be preferable in the treatment of comorbid anxiety and alcoholism. In contrast with benzodiazepines, buspirone does not enhance alcohol-induced impairment of psychomotor skills,[41,42] nor is it known to have abuse liability.[43-45]

Based on its anxiolytic efficacy and its comparatively benign side-effect profile, a number of studies of buspirone have been conducted in alcohol-dependent patients. In an open trial of buspirone in alcoholics, anxious patients (ie, with a Hamilton Anxiety Rating Scale [HAM-A][46] score of 15 or higher) reported a decrease in both anxiety and the desire to drink.[47] Olivera and colleagues[48] conducted an open trial of buspirone in patients with comorbid anxiety and a variety of comorbid substance use disorders. They observed a significant reduction in anxiety during treatment, but they did not report measures of alcohol or drug use. In a double-blind, placebo-controlled trial in alcoholics, treatment with buspirone produced significantly greater retention in treatment and greater decreases in alcohol craving, anxiety, and depression.[49] Both groups showed significant declines in alcohol consumption, with no differential effect of buspirone on this measure. Tollefson and colleagues[50] recently reported an advantage of buspirone over placebo in abstinent alcoholics with comorbid generalized anxiety disorder. Compared with placebo-treated subjects, buspirone-treated subjects were less likely to discontinue therapy prematurely, had greater reductions in anxiety levels, and showed greater improvement on a subjective, global rating of alcohol consumption. Unfortunately, actual alcohol consumption was not measured directly in this study. In contrast with these two reports, a recent study by Malcolm and colleagues[51] of alcoholic veterans in aftercare showed no differences between groups of patients treated with buspirone or placebo on measures of either anxiety or alcohol consumption.

We conducted a double-blind, placebo-controlled trial of buspirone as an adjunct therapy to cognitive-behavioral psychotherapy in anxious, ambulatory alcoholics. We hypothesized that buspirone would provide an anxiolytic advantage over placebo in these newly abstinent subjects, thereby enhancing their retention in treatment. Further, we predicted that this reduction in anxiety would, together with a direct effect on the motivation to drink, result in decreased alcohol consumption in the buspirone-treated group. We chose to use medication therapy as an adjunct to relapse prevention therapy, because it is in combination with psychotherapy that medication therapy is most likely to be successful in the treatment of alcoholism. We also expected that any enduring effects of the medication would be enhanced by a learning-based treatment. Consequently, we hypothesized that the beneficial effects of buspirone on alcohol consumption would persist 6 months after therapy was discontinued.

RESULTS

MEASURES OF ANXIETY AND ALCOHOL CONSUMPTION

Pretreatment measures of anxiety and alcohol consumption for both the buspirone and placebo groups are shown in **Table 2**. There were no significant between-group differences for baseline HAM-A score, the number of drinking days during the pretreatment period, or the number of drinks consumed per drinking day (drinking intensity) during the pretreatment period. The number of drinks consumed per day during the pretreatment period, however, differed significantly as a function of treatment group, with placebo-treated subjects reporting significantly more drinks consumed per day. The pretreatment measure was entered first as a predictor in multiple regression, thereby controling for this difference in subsequent analyses in which the number of drinks consumed per day was the dependent measure.

Table 1. Demographic Characteristics

Variable	Treatment Group: Buspirone Hydrochloride (N=31)	Treatment Group: Placebo (N=30)	Difference Between Groups: Test Statistic	Difference Between Groups: P
Male, %	74.2	80	χ^2=0.29	.59
Mean (±SD) age, y	38.5 (9.1)	40.4 (9.6)	F=0.62	.44
White, %	100	90	χ^2=3.26	.07
Married or cohabitating, %	53.3	60.0	χ^2=0.27	.60
Mean (±SD) education, y	14.2 (2.2)	14.5 (2.7)	F=0.27	.60
Employed, %	83.9	80.0	χ^2=0.15	.69

ADVERSE EFFECTS OF MEDICATION TREATMENT

The most commonly reported adverse effects during medication treatment were dizziness or lightheadedness (buspirone-treated subjects, 48.4%; placebo-treated subjects, 30.0%), sedation (buspirone-treated subjects, 35.5%; placebo-treated subjects, 30.0%), headache (buspirone-treated subjects, 25.8%; placebo-treated subjects, 33.3%), changes in sexual interest or performance (buspirone-treated subjects, 25.8%; placebo-treated subjects, 26.7%), changes in appetite (buspirone-treated subjects, 19.4%; placebo-treated subjects, 23.3%), and a sensation of impaired mentation (buspirone-treated subjects, 25.8%; placebo-treated subjects, 16.7%). Results of χ^2 analysis revealed no significant differences in the frequency of these adverse effects between buspirone and placebo groups. Despite the effort to maintain double-blind conditions, 73% (19/26) buspirone-treated subjects and 67% (12/18) placebo-treated subjects were able to identify correctly the treatment they received ($\chi^2[1]=6.85$; $P<.01$).

TREATMENT RETENTION

Forty-two subjects (68.9%) completed the 12-week active treatment phase of the study. This number includes 26 buspirone- (83.9%) and 16 placebo-treated subjects (53.3%), as shown in **Figure 1**. Of the subjects who did not complete the 12-week treatment period, six (including two buspirone-treated subjects) identified side effects as the basis for their decision to withdraw. Relapse to heavy consumption of alcohol led five subjects (including two buspirone-treated subjects) to discontinue study participation.

The number of weeks of study participation was not significantly associated with either the baseline HAM-A score or three pretreatment measures of alcohol consumption ($P>.10$). There was, however, a significant difference in attrition between treatment groups ($\beta=-0.317$; $F[1,55]=6.05$; $P=.02$). Placebo-treated subjects spent significantly fewer weeks in the study (n=30, mean number of weeks, 8.17; SD=4.53) than buspirone-treated subjects (n=31; mean number of weeks, 10.94; SD=2.66). The very large effect size ($f=0.535$) related to buspirone's advantage in maintaining subjects in treatment provides strong support for the first major hypothesis of the study. There was no significant interaction between baseline HAM-A score and treatment group ($P>.10$), suggesting that buspirone treatment did not differentially enhance treatment retention among subjects with greater anxiety.

As might be expected, there was a high correlation between the number of weeks subjects used medication and the number of psychotherapy sessions in which they participated ($r=.95$; $P<.001$). Placebo-treated subjects (n=30; mean number of sessions, 7.06; SD=4.32) participated in significantly fewer relapse prevention psychotherapy sessions than buspirone-treated subjects (n=31; mean number of sessions, 9.74; SD=2.82) ($F[1,59]=8.23$; $P=.006$).

In addition to the treatment provided in the study protocol, some subjects attended AA meetings (22.6% [7/31] of buspirone- and 23.3% [7/30] of placebo-treated subjects; $\chi^2[1]=.005$; $P=.94$). The mean number of AA meetings attended during the treatment period was 4.88 (±13.93). During the posttreatment period, subjects attended a mean of 13.52 (±32.17) AA meetings. There was no between-group difference for the number of AA meetings attended during the treatment or follow-up periods ($P>.10$). During the treatment period, some subjects also participated in other ambulatory treatments (16.1% [5/31] of buspirone- and 13.3% [4/30] of placebo-treated subjects; $\chi^2[1]=.09$; $P=.76$). The mean number of additional sessions during the treatment period was 3.26 (±12.80), whereas during the posttreatment period, it was 9.40 (±25.87). There was no between-group difference for the number of therapy sessions attended during the treatment or follow-up periods ($P>.10$).

Table 2. Severity of Pretreatment Alcoholism and Comorbid Psychiatric Features

	Treatment Group*		Difference Between Groups	
Variable	Buspirone Hydrochloride (N=31)	Placebo (N=30)	Test Statistic	*P*
Heavy alcohol consumption, y	13.5 (8.0)	12.4 (8.7)	F=0.24	.63
MAST score†	25.6 (11.5)	25.7 (12.5)	F=0.001	.98
No. of prior treatments for alcoholism	2.0 (3.2)	1.7 (2.4)	F=0.14	.71
No. of drinking days‡	37.5 (16.1)	42.5 (12.2)	F=2.07	.16
No. of drinks consumed per day‡	6.1 (4.2)	9.0 (5.6)	F=4.98	.03
Drinking intensity, No. of drinks‡	11.1 (7.0)	13.4 (8.2)	F=1.18	.28
No. of prior treatments for psychiatric problems	0.9 (0.1)	1.0 (0.1)	F=0.38	.54
Current generalized anxiety disorder, % of patients	46.4	36.7	χ^2=0.56	.45
Current anxiety disorder, % of patients§	51.6	50.0	χ^2=0.30	.59
Current major depression, % of patients	25.0	26.6	χ^2=0.02	.88
Beck Depression Inventory score	16.2 (7.8)	15.7 (6.7)	F=0.05	.82
Baseline HAM-A score∥	20.4 (5.1)	20.9 (6.1)	F=0.10	.76

*Data are presented as mean (±SD), unless otherwise specified.
†MAST indicates Michigan Alcoholism Screening Test.[64]
‡Indicates during the 60 days prior to study enrollment. Drinking days are defined as days on which alcohol was consumed. Drinking intensity is defined as the number of drinks consumed per drinking day.
§Includes generalized anxiety disorder, panic disorder, simple phobia, social phobia, agoraphobia, and obsessive-compulsive disorder.
∥HAM-A indicates Hamilton Anxiety Rating Scale.[46]

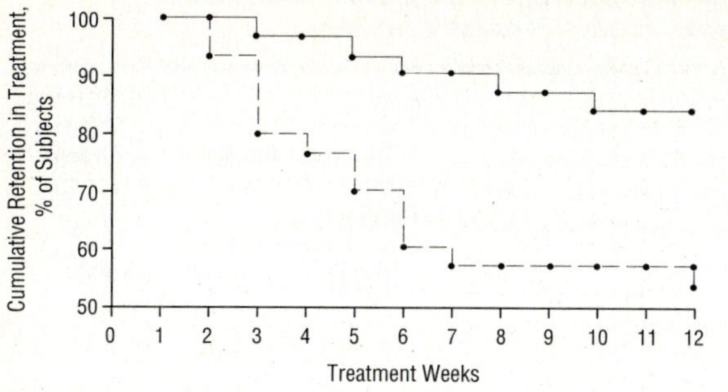

Figure 1. *Life-table (survival) analysis of retention of subjects in treatment. Dashed line indicates placebo-treated subjects (n=30); solid line, buspirone hydrochloride–treated subjects (n=31).*

EFFECT OF TREATMENT ON ANXIETY

There was a trend for placebo-treated subjects to have higher HAM-A scores at the end of treatment (buspirone-treated subjects, mean score=5.8 and SD=5.4; placebo-treated subjects, mean score=8.3; SD=5.9; β=0.222; F[1,54]=2.84; *P*<.10). There was a significant interaction between treatment group and baseline HAM-A score (β=0.241, F[1,52]=4.40; *P*=.04), reflecting a medium-sized effect (*f*=0.291). Application of the Johnson-Neyman technique[66] revealed that, among subjects with a baseline HAM-A score of 27 or higher, treatment with buspirone (n=4) resulted in significantly lower end-point HAM-A scores than did treatment with placebo (n=5). For those subjects with a baseline HAM-A score of 26 or higher, there was no significant effect of medication on end-point HAM-A score. The longer subjects remained in treatment, the lower their mean HAM-A scores were at the end of treatment (β=−0.542; F[1,53]=19.16; *P*<.001). Finally, the interaction between treatment group and the number of weeks of treatment also approached significance (β=0.209; F(1,51)=2.80; *P*=.10).

EFFECT OF TREATMENT ON ALCOHOL CONSUMPTION DURING THE TREATMENT PERIOD

Figure 2 illustrates the second main study hypothesis that there was a significant difference in the interval to first heavy drinking day following randomization (Wilcoxon [Gehan] statistic, 4.64; *df*=1; *P*=.03). However, the groups did not differ on the number of weeks to first alcohol consumption following randomization (mean survival, 0.42 for buspirone-treated subjects and −0.48 for placebo-treated subjects; Wilcoxon [Gehan] statistic, .01; *df*=1; *P*=.91).

Table 3 shows means and SDs for alcohol consumption measures during the treatment and 6-month follow-up periods, while **Table 4** shows standardized β coefficients from the multiple regression analyses conducted using the three consumption measures as dependent variables.

Drinking Days

There was a trend for buspirone-treated subjects to have fewer drinking days during the treatment period than placebo-treated subjects (F[1,54]=3.04; *P*=.09). The number of drinking days did not differ as a function of the interaction between treatment group and baseline HAM-A score (*P*>.10). The number of drinking days during treatment was negatively correlated with the number of weeks of treatment (F[1,53]=24.27; *P*<.001), ie, the longer the period of treatment, the fewer the number of drinking days were. There was also a significant interaction between treatment group and the number of weeks of treatment (*F*[1,51]=4.83; *P*=.03). Application of the Johnson-Neyman technique[66] revealed that, for those subjects who stayed in the study for 2 weeks or less, buspirone treatment (n=1) was associated with significantly more drinking days than placebo treatment (n=4). For those subjects who stayed in the study for 3 weeks or more, there was no difference between treatment groups. This finding reflects a medium-sized effect (*f*=0.308) of the interaction on the number of drinking days, although its clinical significance appears limited, insofar as it involves so few subjects.

Drinks per Day

The number of drinks consumed per day during treatment correlated significantly with the number of drinks consumed per day during the pretreatment period (F[1,56]=10.55; *P*=.002). As was true for the number of drinking days during treatment, there was a significant negative correlation between the number of drinks consumed per day and the number of weeks of treatment (F[1,53]=20.97; *P*<.001), ie, the longer the treatment, the fewer the number of drinks consumed per day were. The number of drinks consumed per day did not differ as a function of treatment group or the interactions between treatment group and baseline HAM-A score or the number of weeks of treatment (*P*>.10).

Drinking Intensity

Drinking intensity during treatment correlated significantly with drinking intensity during the pretreatment period (*F*[1,56]=20.71; *P*<.001). Drinking intensity during treatment also showed a significant negative correlation with the number of weeks of treatment, such that the more weeks of treatment, the lower the drinking intensity was (F[1,53]=12.61; *P*=.001). Drinking intensity during treatment did not differ as a function of treat-

ment group or the interactions between treatment group and baseline HAM-A score or the number of weeks of treatment (*P*>.10).

EFFECT OF TREATMENT ON ALCOHOL CONSUMPTION AT 6-MONTH FOLLOW-UP

Drinking Days

As hypothesized, at follow-up, placebo-treated subjects reported significantly more drinking days than buspirone-treated subjects ($F[1,46]=7.84$; $P=.007$), which represents a large-sized effect ($f=0.413$). The interaction of treatment group and baseline HAM-A score approached significance ($F[1,44]=2.96$; $P<.10$), such that at higher levels of baseline anxiety, the positive effects of the buspirone relative to the placebo treatment tended to be stronger. The interaction between treatment group and the number of weeks of treatment was not a significant predictor of drinking days at follow-up.

Drinks per Day

The number of drinks consumed per day at follow-up was significantly correlated with the number of drinks consumed per day during the pretreatment period ($F[1,48]=12.58$; $P=.001$). At follow-up, there was also a significant correlation between the number of drinks consumed per day and baseline HAM-A score ($F[1,47]=7.83$; $P=.007$), such that the higher the level of baseline anxiety, the greater the number of drinks consumed per day at follow-up was. There was a trend for placebo-treated subjects to report more drinks consumed per day than buspirone-treated subjects ($F[1,46]=2.99$; $P<.10$). There was also a significant interaction of treatment group and baseline HAM-A score on the number of drinks consumed per day ($F[1,44]=3.99$; $P=.05$), which represents a medium-sized effect ($f=0.301$). Specifically, application of the Johnson-Neyman technique[66] revealed that, for subjects with baseline HAM-A scores of 21 or higher, buspirone treatment (n=11) resulted in significantly fewer drinks consumed per day at follow-up than did placebo treatment (n=9). However, for those subjects with baseline HAM-A scores of 20 or lower, there was no effect of medication on the number of drinks consumed per day at follow-up. The interaction of treatment group with the number of weeks of treatment was not a significant predictor of the number of drinks consumed per day at follow-up (*P*>.10).

Drinking Intensity

Drinking intensity at follow-up was significantly correlated with drinking intensity during the pretreatment period ($F[1,48]=29.18$; $P<.001$). Drinking intensity at follow-up was also significantly correlated with baseline HAM-A score, such that the higher the baseline anxiety level, the greater the drinking intensity at follow-up was ($F[1,47]=5.44$; $P=.02$). Drinking intensity at follow-up did not, however, differ significantly as a function of treatment group, nor were any of the interactions significant predictors (*P*>.10).

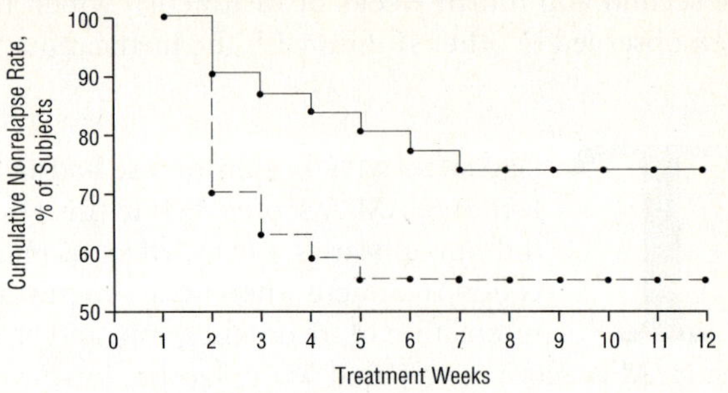

Figure 2. *Life-table (survival) analysis of relapse to heavy alcohol consumption. Dashed line indicates placebo-treated subjects (n=27); solid line, buspirone hydrochloride–treated subjects (n=31).*

COMMENT

Buspirone-treated subjects were significantly more likely to remain in treatment than were placebo-treated subjects (Figure 1). The enhanced retention, a very large treatment effect, appears to have been a function of the medication, insofar as pretreatment alcohol consumption and baseline anxiety levels did not significantly predict duration of treatment. The finding of reduced attrition among buspirone-treated patients is consistent with the results of two other placebo-controlled studies of buspirone treatment in alcoholics.[49,50] The 1992 study by Malcolm et al[51] differs from both the two previously published studies[49,50] and the present study in that Malcolm et al found no difference in treatment retention between buspirone- and placebo-treated groups. The absence of an effect of medication on treatment retention in the study by Malcolm et al[51] may be related to both the greater severity of alcohol dependence among their subjects and the less structured psychosocial treatment provided in that study.

Treatment with buspirone for fewer than 3 weeks was associated with greater frequency of alcohol consumption during treatment. It would appear, however, that this effect has limited clinical importance, in that it was significant for only one buspirone-treated subject. Furthermore, this effect may be an artifact of carrying forward the last observation in that, for subjects who completed only 1 or 2 weeks of treatment, the last observation may not have been an accurate estimate of their alcohol consumption during the entire treatment period. Nonetheless, it is consistent with a delayed thera-

peutic effect of buspirone (ie, maximum effect between the second and fourth weeks of treatment), which has been observed in other studies with the medication.[68]

TREATMENT WITH buspirone also had an effect on HAM-A scores. While this effect did not appear as a main effect of medication treatment, there was a significant interaction of treatment group and baseline HAM-A score. Compared with placebo, buspirone was significantly more effective as an anxiolytic among subjects with high pretreatment levels of anxiety. The evidence that buspirone has greater anxiolytic efficacy in subjects with high levels of anxiety is consistent with the results of an earlier uncontrolled study.[47] Whereas in the present study we excluded subjects with clear evidence of acute alcohol withdrawal, we may not have adequately accounted for protracted withdrawal.[57,69] The findings reported herein may, therefore, reflect the fact that only persistent anxiety symptoms (ie, those symptoms that persist beyond the resolution of acute alcohol withdrawal[70]) respond to treatment with buspirone. Such an effect is consistent with the pharmacologic effects of the medication, which has been shown to have minimal activity at the γ-aminobutyric acid–benzodiazepine receptor complex.[71] There was also a trend for buspirone-treated subjects to have lower mean end-of-treatment HAM-A scores when treated for a longer period of time. As with the effect on frequency of alcohol consumption, this trend is consistent with the delayed therapeutic effect of buspirone.[68]

Although subjects were selected on the basis of their score on the HAM-A rather than the presence of a comorbid anxiety disorder, approximately half of the subjects met current diagnostic criteria for an anxiety disorder (Table 2), the most prevalent of which was generalized anxiety disorder. To compare the predictive power of these diagnostic groupings on treatment outcome, analyses were conducted that included anxiety disorder diagnoses (ie, the presence or absence of a current or lifetime diagnosis of generalized anxiety disorder and the presence or absence of a current or lifetime diagnosis of any anxiety disorder). These analyses were conducted in parallel fashion with those described above for HAM-A, except that the anxiety disorder diagnoses replaced the HAM-A score as a predictor variable in the multiple regression analysis. The analyses resulted in only one significant main effect: current generalized anxiety disorder predicted the HAM-A score at the end of treatment. This finding suggests that a continuous measure of anxiety symptoms (ie, the HAM-A) is a better predictor of response to buspirone treatment than dichotomous anxiety disorder diagnoses. While the computerized Diagnostic Interview Schedule has been shown to have acceptable reliability and validity,[54,55] a clinician-administered diagnostic interview might have provided a better basis on which to evaluate the predictive power of categorical anxiety disorder diagnoses. Nonetheless, the data presented here are consistent with the distinction drawn between transient and enduring anxiety symptoms in patients with substance abuse disorder.[4] Recent work[72] has yielded little support for the distinction between substance-induced and independent anxiety disorders, suggesting that it may be profitable to rethink traditional distinctions based on the temporal sequence of onset of anxiety and substance abuse symptoms (eg, primary and secondary).[73]

Buspirone treatment resulted in a longer time to relapse to heavy consumption of alcohol during the treatment period (Figure 2). Although during the treatment period there was only a trend for buspirone to reduce the frequency of alcohol consumption, during the 6-month follow-up period buspirone-treated subjects had significantly fewer drinking days than did placebo-treated subjects. Reduced consumption was not associated with increased use of other drugs, at least as evidenced by results of urine toxicologic tests, the vast majority of which were negative for the presence of other drugs. There was also a trend for buspirone-treated subjects to consume fewer drinks per day during the 6-month follow-up period. During this time there was a significant interaction between buspirone and baseline HAM-A scores such that, at high levels of anxiety, buspirone-treated subjects consumed fewer drinks per day, while at low levels of anxiety there was no difference between treatment groups. Together with its effect to reduce anxiety during treatment, these findings provide support for the hypotheses that buspirone reduces alcohol consumption as a consequence of its anxiolytic effects and that, in combination with skills training, the effect may endure beyond the active treatment period.

Table 3. End of Treatment and Posttreatment Measures of Alcohol Consumption

Variable*	Treatment Group: Buspirone Hydrochloride	Treatment Group: Placebo
Treatment period		
No. of drinking days	3.6 (11.0)	9.6 (13.3)†
No. of drinks consumed per day	0.7 (2.9)	2.1 (4.6)
Drinking intensity, No. of drinks	3.3 (6.0)	6.6 (8.2)
Posttreatment period		
No. of drinking days	9.5 (14.4)	24.8 (21.8)‡
No. of drinks consumed per day	0.9 (1.9)	4.8 (7.2)†
Drinking intensity, No. of drinks	2.4 (4.5)	7.0 (9.2)

*Data are presented as mean±SD. Drinking days and drinking intensity are defined in Table 2.
†P<.10.
‡P<.01.

Table 4. Predictors of Alcohol Consumption During Treatment and at Posttreatment Follow-up

	Standardized β Coefficents					
Dependent Variable*	Pretreatment Drinking Measure	Baseline HAM-A Score†	Treatment Group	Interaction of Treatment Group and HAM-A Score†	No. of Weeks of Treatment	Interaction of Treatment Group and No. of Weeks of Treatment
Treatment period						
Drinking days	0.090	0.133	0.232‡	0.070	−0.589§	0.274‖
Drinks consumed per day	0.398¶	0.097	0.063	−0.030	−0.540§	0.156
Drinking intensity	0.520§	−0.100	0.112	−0.121	−0.410§	0.086
Posttreatment period						
Drinking days	0.010	0.102	0.380¶	0.247‡	−0.071	−0.173
Drinks consumed per day	0.456§	0.338¶	0.217‡	0.252‖	−0.106	−0.098
Drinking intensity	0.615§	0.262‖	0.155	0.112	−0.111	0.024

*Drinking days and drinking intensity are defined in Table 2.
†HAM-A indicates Hamilton Anxiety Rating Scale.[46]
‡$P \leq .10$.
§$P < .001$.
‖$P \leq .05$.
¶$P < .01$.

The duration of subjects' treatment participation also had effects independent of the specific medication they received. During the treatment period, there was an inverse relationship between this measure and both the number of drinks consumed per day and drinking intensity. Independent of the treatment condition, the longer subjects remained in treatment, the fewer drinks they consumed. These findings are consistent with studies of anxiolytic medications showing that a longer duration of treatment is associated with better treatment outcomes in alcoholics.[36] In the present study, enhanced retention and improved outcomes appear to represent an effect of treatment insofar as both baseline anxiety level and pretreatment measures of alcohol consumption did not predict duration of treatment. It should be noted, however, that the treatment provided included both medication and weekly cognitive-behavioral psychotherapy. A limited number of subjects also participated in AA and/or other ambulatory treatments in addition to that provided in the study protocol, although there were no between-group differences in such participation during either the treatment or posttreatment periods. Given the absence of a control for the effects of relapse prevention training, no firm conclusions can be drawn from these results regarding the efficacy of the psychotherapy.

Many of the effects of buspirone were only evident with a longer duration of treatment and among subjects with higher levels of anxiety. These findings are consistent with the pharmacologic profile of the drug.[68,71] Reports by collateral informants and hepatic enzyme levels provide support for the validity of both self-reported alcohol consumption and anxiety symptoms.

Based on the findings reported herein, we recommend the use of buspirone for the treatment of anxious alcoholics, both to enhance treatment retention and delay relapse to heavy alcohol consumption. Furthermore, in alcoholics with moderate-to-severe anxiety, the medication appears to reduce anxiety, as well as the frequency and quantity of alcohol consumption. Without attempting to diminish the importance of psychiatric diagnosis as a basis for therapeutic decision making, the data presented herein suggest that a continuous measure of anxiety (ie, the HAM-A) may be more useful in identifying patients for whom treatment with buspirone is most likely to be beneficial as an adjunct to psychosocial treatment. For such an approach to be efficacious, it would be advantageous to maintain therapy at a substantial dosage of the medication (eg, 40 to 60 mg/d) for a minimum of 4 to 6 weeks (Figure 1).

The results of the present study should, however, be interpreted in light of several limitations. First, while differential attrition is an outcome in and of itself, the large rate of dropping out from the study limits to some extent the conclusions that can be drawn from it. This effect would seemingly lead to an underestimation of the efficacy of buspirone by limiting the period of risk for placebo-treated subjects. That is, given the high correlation in the present study between the number of weeks of treatment and alcohol consumption outcomes during the treatment period, greater attrition among the placebo-treated group may have resulted in an underestimation of their alcohol consumption. Such an effect would result from carrying the last observation forward. Furthermore, limited statistical power resulting from the comparatively small sample sizes, combined with attrition, may also have obscured some treatment effects. A second limitation was that the double blind was penetrated. Insofar as subjects were able to identify cor-

rectly the treatment they received, the observed effects may have been due to expectancy rather than being pharmacologic. A third limitation of the present study is the absence of the HAM-A measure at the 6-month follow-up. This lack makes it impossible to examine the enduring effects of treatment on anxiety and the association of changes in anxiety level with changes in alcohol consumption. Furthermore, we employed a 60-day time frame for each of the research assessments. This had a minimal effect on estimates of alcohol consumption during the treatment period, since subjects reported their alcohol consumption weekly during this period. However, during the 6-month follow-up, the final 60 days of the period represented only one third of the elapsed time and as such may have been an inaccurate representation of the entire period. Despite these limitations, there was evidence that subjects' reports were accurate, to the extent that hepatic enzyme levels and reports by collateral informants provided adequate validation of self-reported anxiety and alcohol consumption.

While further studies of buspirone are needed to define more clearly the role of this medication in the treatment of alcoholism, it would appear that such studies are best conducted as adjuncts to psychosocial treatment. We chose to employ weekly relapse prevention psychotherapy in this sample of mild to moderately severe alcoholics. In severely dependent patient groups, more intensive psychosocial treatment would appear to be warranted. As this research suggests, the variable findings that have been reported to date in studies of buspirone treatment of alcoholics may, in large measure, be related to differences among studies in both the severity of the patients' alcoholism and intensity and degree of structure of the concomitant psychosocial care that was provided.

Accepted for publication June 13, 1994.

Supported by grants P50-AA03510, T32-AA07290, and K20-AA00143 (Dr Kranzler) from the National Institute on Alcohol Abuse and Alcoholism, Rockville, Md. Buspirone and matched placebo were generously donated by Mead-Johnson Pharmaceuticals, Evansville, Ind.

The authors wish to acknowledge the contributions of Roger E. Meyer, MD, and Bruce Rounsaville, MD, in the design of the study and Neil Liebowitz, MD, Linda Berger, MA, Laura Ginther, PsyD, Gail Myers, and Katherine Wilson in the conduct of the research.

Reprint requests to Department of Psychiatry, University of Connecticut Health Center, 263 Farmington Ave, Farmington, CT 06030-2103 (Dr Kranzler).

REFERENCES

1. Helzer J, Pryzbeck T. The co-occurrence of alcoholism with other psychiatric disorders in the general population and its impact on treatment. *J Stud Alcohol.* 1988;49:210-224.
2. Hesselbrock MN, Meyer RE, Keener JJ. Psychopathology in hospitalized alcoholics. *Arch Gen Psychiatry.* 1985;42:1050-1055.
3. Ross HE, Glaser FB, Germanson T. The prevalence of psychiatric disorders in patients with alcohol and other drug problems. *Arch Gen Psychiatry.* 1988; 45:1023-1031.
4. Kranzler HR, Liebowitz N. Anxiety and depression in substance abuse: clinical implications. In: Frazier S, ed. *Anxiety and Depression: Medical Clinics of North America.* Philadelphia, Pa: Williams & Wilkins; 1988;72:867-885.
5. Nathan PE, O'Brien JS. An experimental analysis of the behavior of alcoholics and nonalcoholics during prolonged experimental drinking: a necessary precursor of behavior therapy? *Behav Ther.* 1971;2:455-476.
6. Brown SA, Irwin M, Schuckit MA. Changes in anxiety among abstinent male alcoholics. *J Stud Alcohol.* 1991;52:55-61.
7. Bibb JL, Chambless CL. Alcohol use and abuse among diagnosed agoraphobics. *Behav Res Ther.* 1986;24:49-58.
8. Pickens RW, Hatsukami DK, Spicer JW, Svikis DS. Relapse by alcohol abusers. *Alcohol Clin Exp Res.* 1985;9:244-247.
9. Quitkin FM, Rifkin A, Kaplan J, Klein DF. Phobic anxiety syndrome complicated by drug dependence and addiction: a treatable form of drug abuse. *Arch Gen Psychiatry.* 1972;27:159-162.
10. Tollefson GD. Serotonin and alcohol: interrelationships. *Psychopathology.* 1989; 22(suppl 1):37-48.
11. Gorelick DA. Serotonin uptake blockers and the treatment of alcoholism. In: Galanter M, ed. *Recent Developments in Alcoholism.* New York, NY: Plenum Press; 1989;7:267-281.
12. Roy A, Virkkunen M, Linnoila M. Serotonin in suicide, violence, and alcoholism. In: Coccaro EF, Murphy DL, eds. *Serotonin in Major Psychiatric Disorders.* Washington, DC: American Psychiatric Press; 1990.
13. Ballenger JC, Goodwin FK, Major LF, Brown GL. Alcohol and central serotonin metabolism in man. *Arch Gen Psychiatry.* 1979;36:224-227.
14. Banki CJ. Factors influencing monamine metabolites and tryptophan in patients with alcohol dependence. *J Neural Transm.* 1981;50:98-101.
15. Naranjo CA, Sellers EM, Lawrin MO. Modulation of ethanol intake by serotonin uptake inhibitors. *J Clin Psychiatry.* 1986;47(suppl):16-22.
16. Naranjo CA, Sellers EM, Roach CA, Woodley DV, Sanchez-Craig M, Sykora K. Zimelidine-induced variations in alcohol intake by nondepressed heavy drinkers. *Clin Pharmacol Ther.* 1984;35:374-381.
17. Naranjo CA, Sellers EM, Sullivan JT, Woodley DV, Kadlec K, Sykora K. The serotonin uptake inhibitor citalopram attenuates ethanol intake. *Clin Pharmacol Ther.* 1987;41:266-274.
18. Naranjo CA, Sullivan JT, Kadlec KE, Woodley-Remus DV, Kennedy G, Sellers EM. Differential effects of viqualine on alcohol intake and other consummatory behaviors. *Clin Pharmacol Ther.* 1989;46:301-309.
19. Naranjo CA, Kadlec KE, Sanhueza P, Woodley-Remus D, Sellers EM. Fluoxetine differentially alters alcohol intake and other consummatory behaviors in problem drinkers. *Clin Pharmacol Ther.* 1990;47:490-498.
20. Gorelick DA, Paredes A. Effect of fluoxetine on alcohol consumption in male alcoholics. *Alcohol Clin Exp Res.* 1992;16:261-265.
21. Kostowski W, Dyr W. Effects of the 5-HT-1A receptor agonists on ethanol preference in the rat. *Alcohol.* 1992;9:283-286.
22. Privette TH, Hornsby RI, Myers RD. Buspirone alters alcohol drinking induced in rats by tetrahydropapaveroline injected into brain monoaminergic pathways. *Alcohol.* 1988;5:147-152.
23. Collins DM, Myers RD. Buspirone attenuates volitional alcohol intake in the chronically drinking monkey. *Alcohol.* 1987;4:49-56.
24. Engel JA, Fahlke C, Hard E, Johannessen K, SvenssonI, Soderpalm P. Serotonergic and dopaminergic involvement in ethanol intake. *Clin Neuropharmacol.* 1992;15(suppl 1):64A-65A.
25. Svensson L, Fahlke C, Hard E, Engel JA. Involvement of the serotonergic system in ethanol intake in the rat. *Alcohol.* 1993;10:219-224.
26. Knapp DJ, Benjamin D, Pohorecky LA. Effects of gepirone on ethanol consumption, exploratory behavior, and motor performance in rats. *Drug Dev Res.* 1992;26:319-341.
27. Gardner CR. Recent developments in 5HT-related pharmacology of animal models of anxiety. *Pharmacol Biochem Behav.* 1986;24:1479-1485.
28. Chopin PH, Briley M. Animal models of anxiety: the effect of compounds that modify 5-HT neurotransmission. *Trends Pharmacol Sci.* 1987;8:383-388.
29. Charney DS, Woods SW, Goodman WK, Heninger GR. Serotonin function in anxiety, II: effects of the serotonin agonist m-CPP in panic disorder patients and healthy subjects. *Psychopharmacology (Berl).* 1987;92:14-24.

30. Charney DS, Goodman WK, Price LH, Woods SW, Rasmussen SA, Heninger GR. Serotonin function in obsessive-compulsive disorder: comparison of the effects of trytophan and *m*-chlorophenylpiperarine in patients and healthy subjects. *Arch Gen Psychiatry.* 1988;45:177-185.
31. Zohar J, Insel TR, Zohar-Kadouch RC, Hill JL, Murphy DL. Serotonergic responsivity in obsessive-compulsive disorder: effects of chronic clomipramine treatment. *Arch Gen Psychiatry.* 1988;45:167-172.
32. Feighner JP, Merideth CH, Hendrickson GA. A double-blind comparison of buspirone and diazepam in outpatients with generalized anxiety disorder. *J Clin Psychiatry.* 1982;43(section 2 of No. 12):103-107.
33. Goodman WK, Price LH, Rasmussen SA, Delgado PL, Heninger GR, Charney DS. Efficacy of fluvoxamine in obsessive-compulsive disorder. *Arch Gen Psychiatry.* 1989;46:36-44.
34. Rickels K, Weisman K, Norstad N, Singer M, Stoltz D, Brown A, Danton J. Buspirone and diazepam in anxiety: a controlled study. *J Clin Psychiatry.* 1982; 43(section 2 of No. 12):81-86.
35. Meyer RE. Anxiolytics and the alcoholic patient. *J Stud Alcohol.* 1986;47:269-273.
36. Kissin B. The use of psychoactive drugs in the long-term treatment of chronic alcoholics. *Ann N Y Acad Sci.* 1975;252:385-395.
37. Ciraulo DA, Barnhill JG, Greenblatt DJ, Shader RI, Ciraulo AM, Tarmey MF, Molloy MA, Foti ME. Abuse liability and clinical pharmacokinetics of alprazolam in alcoholic men. *J Clin Psychiatry.* 1988;49:333-337.
38. Jaffe JH, Ciraulo DA, Nies A, Dixon RB, Monroe LL. Abuse potential of halazepam and of diazepam in patients recently treated for acute alcohol withdrawal. *Clin Pharmacol Ther.* 1983;34:623-630.
39. Griffiths RR, McLeod DR, Bigelow GE, Liebson IA, Roache JD, Nowowieski P. Comparison of diazepam and oxazepam: preference, liking and extent of abuse. *J Pharmacol Exp Ther.* 1984;229:501-508.
40. Taylor DP, Eison MS, Riblet LA, Vandermaelen CP. Pharmacological and clinical effects of buspirone. *Pharmacol Biochem Behav.* 1985;23:687-694.
41. Mattila MJ, Aranko K, Seppala T. Acute effects of buspirone and alcohol on psychomotor skills. *J Clin Psychiatry.* 1982;43:56-60.
42. Seppala T, Aranko K, Mattila MJ, Shrotriya RC. Effects of alcohol on buspirone and lorazepam actions. *Clin Pharmacol Ther.* 1982;32:201-207.
43. Balster RL. Abuse potential of buspirone and related drugs. *J Clin Psychopharmacol.* 1990;10(suppl):31S-37S.
44. Cole JO, Orzack MH, Beake B, Bird M, Bar Tel Y. Assessment of abuse liability of buspirone in recreational sedative users. *J Clin Psychiatry.* 1982;43:69-74.
45. Griffith JD, Jasinski DR, Casten GP, McKinney GR. Investigation of the abuse liability of buspirone in alcohol-dependent patients. *Am J Med.* 1986;80(suppl 3B):30-35.
46. Hamilton M. The assessment of anxiety states by rating. *Br J Med Psychol.* 1959;32:50-55.
47. Kranzler HR, Meyer RE. Open trial of buspirone in alcoholics. *J Clin Psychopharmacol.* 1989;9:379-380.
48. Olivera AA, Sarvis S, Heard C. Anxiety disorders coexisting with substance dependence: treatment with buspirone. *Curr Ther Res.* 1990;47:52-61.
49. Bruno F. Buspirone in the treatment of alcoholic patients. *Psychopathology.* 1989;22(suppl):49-59.
50. Tollefson GD, Montague-Clouse J, Tollefson SL. Treatment of comorbid generalized anxiety in a recently detoxified alcohol population with a selective serotonergic drug (buspirone). *J Clin Psychopharmacol.* 1992;12:19-26.
51. Malcolm R, Anton RF, Randall CL, Johnston A, Brady K, Thevos A. A placebo-controlled trial of buspirone in anxious inpatient alcoholics. *Alcohol Clin Exp Res.* 1992;16:1007-1013.
52. Spitzer RL, Williams JBW, Gibbon M, First MB. The Structured Clinical Interview for *DSM-III-R* (SCID), I: history, rationale and description. *Arch Gen Psychiatry.* 1992;49:624-629.
53. American Psychiatric Association. *Diagnostic and Statistical Manual of Mental Disorders, Third Edition.* Washington DC: American Psychiatric Association; 1980.
54. Blouin AG, Perez EL, Blouin JH. Computerized administration of the Diagnostic Interview Schedule. *Psychiatry Res.* 1988;23:335-344.
55. Levitan RD, Blouin AG, Navarro JR, Hill J. Validity of the computerized DIS for diagnosing psychiatric inpatients. *Can J Psychiatry.* 1991;36:728-731.
56. American Psychiatric Association. *Diagnostic and Statistical Manual of Mental Disorders, Revised Third Edition.* Washington, DC: American Psychiatric Association; 1987.
57. Roelofs S. Hyperventilation, anxiety, craving for alcohol: a subacute alcohol withdrawal syndrome. *Alcohol.* 1985;2:501-505.
58. Marlatt GA, Gordon JR. *Relapse Prevention.* New York, NY: Guilford; 1985.
59. Chaney EF. Social skills training. In: Hester RK, Miller WR, eds. *Handbook of Alcoholism Treatment Approaches: Effective Alternatives.* New York, NY: Pergamon Press Inc; 1989;206-221.
60. Annis HM, Davis CS. Relapse prevention. In: Hester RK, Miller WR, eds. *Handbook of Alcoholism Treatment Approaches: Effective Alternatives.* New York, NY: Pergamon Press Inc; 1989;170-182.
61. Sobell MB, Maisto SA, Sobell LC, Cooper AM, Cooper TC, Sanders B. Developing a prototype for evaluating alcohol treatment effectiveness. In: Sobell LC, Sobell MB, Ward E, eds. *Evaluating Alcohol and Drug Abuse Treatment Effectiveness: Recent Advances.* New York, NY: Pergamon Press Inc; 1980.
62. Hesselbrock M, Babor TF, Hesselbrock V, Meyer RE, Workman K. 'Never believe an alcoholic?' on the validity of self-report measures of alcohol dependence and related constructs. *Int J Addict.* 1983;18:593-609.
63. Beck AT, Ward CH, Mendelson M, Mock J, Erbaugh J. An inventory for measuring depression. *Arch Gen Psychiatry.* 1961;4:561-571.
64. Selzer ML. The Michigan Alcoholism Screening Test: the quest for a new diagnostic instrument. *Am J Psychiatry.* 1971;127:1653-1658.
65. Lee ET. *Statistical Methods for Survival Analysis.* New York, NY: John Wiley & Sons Inc; 1992.
66. Johnson PO, Neyman J. Tests of certain linear hypotheses and their application to some educational problems. *Stat Res Memoirs.* 1936;1:57-93.
67. Cohen J. *Statistical Power for the Behavioral Sciences.* 2nd ed. Hillsdale, NJ; Lawrence Erlbaum Associates Inc; 1988.
68. Schuckit MA. Clinical studies of buspirone. *Psychopathology.* 1984;17(suppl 3):61-68.
69. Begleiter H, Porjesz B. Persistence of a 'subacute withdrawal syndrome': following chronic ethanol intake. *Drug Alcohol Depend.* 1979;4:353-357.
70. Thevos AK, Johnston AL, Latham PK, Randall CL, Adinoff B, Malcolm R. Symptoms of anxiety in inpatient alcoholics with and without *DSM-III-R* anxiety diagnoses. *Alcohol Clin Exp Res.* 1991;15:102-105.
71. Riblet LA, Taylor DP, Eison MS, Stanton HC. Pharmacology and neurochemistry of buspirone. *J Clin Psychiatry.* 1982;43(12, section 2):11-16.
72. Kadden RM, Kranzler HR, Rounsaville BJ. Validity of the distinction between 'substance-induced' and 'independent' depression and anxiety disorders. *Am J Addictions.* In press.
73. Schuckit MA. The clinical implications of primary diagnostic groups among alcoholics. *Arch Gen Psychiatry.* 1985;42:1043-1049.

Predicting Early Onset of Male Antisocial Behavior From Preschool Behavior

Richard E. Tremblay, PhD; Robert O. Pihl, PhD; Frank Vitaro, PhD; Patricia L. Dobkin, PhD

Methods: Data from a large longitudinal study of boys who were between kindergarten and age 13 years were used to (1) test whether Gray's and Cloninger's personality dimensions measured in kindergarten predicted the early onset of stable, highly delinquent behavior; (2) test whether 1, 2, or 3 dimensions were needed; and (3) test the predictive value of a categorical approach.

Results: The impulsivity dimension was the best predictor of the early onset of stable, highly delinquent behavior. Anxiety and reward dependence made significant but weaker contributions. The categorical approach corroborated Cloninger's suggestion that boys who are high in impulsivity, low in anxiety, and low in reward dependence would be more at risk for delinquent involvement. Boys who were high in impulsivity and low in anxiety but high in reward dependence were much less at risk for delinquency. Differences in antisocial behavior among extreme kindergarten personality groups were stable from ages 11 to 13 years.

Conclusions: The behavioral activating system appears to be the major dimension underlying the propensity toward early onset of antisocial behavior, but both the behavioral inhibition system and the need for social rewards play important roles. The behavioral style (personality) that results from the interplay of these systems is clearly in place by the kindergarten year. Preventive efforts should target preschool children with at-risk behavior profiles. However, longitudinal-experimental studies with at least yearly assessments between birth and school-entry age are needed to understand the extent to which the behavioral styles are antecedent to preschool disruptive behavior disorders.

(Arch Gen Psychiatry. 1994;51:732-739)

THE IDEA THAT childhood behavior can predict later social behavior is not new. In *The Republic*, Plato argued that the guardians of the state needed to be chosen early in life because of the impact of early education. The 19th century social reformers were convinced that children from the "perishing and dangerous classes" would lead a criminal way of life if they did not receive a proper education.[1,2] The original contribution of the 20th century probably has been the systematic conduction of longitudinal studies in different cultures to verify prospectively the precise value of childhood predictors for later antisocial behavior.[3-11]

In Loeber and Stouthamer-Loeber's review of prospective longitudinal studies,[12] the best predictors of future delinquency were early conduct problems such as aggression, stealing, truancy, lying, and drug use. These behaviors can be considered early forms of delinquent behavior. Recognizing the stability of deviant behaviors, some[13-15] concluded that childhood conduct problems and delinquency are the expression of the same underlying continuum. The latter could be genetically inherited, the result of a perinatal physiological trauma, acquired in infancy, or the result of interactions between these different causal factors.[14,16-19]

Because most subjects in the studies reviewed by Loeber and Stouthamer-Loeber were between 10 and 15 years of age when the studies started, the results can be re-

From the Research Unit of Children's Psycho-Social Maladjustment (Drs Tremblay, Pihl, Vitaro, and Dobkin), the University of Montréal (Drs Tremblay and Vitaro), and McGill University (Drs Pihl and Dobkin), Montreal, Quebec.

See Subjects and Methods on next page

SUBJECTS AND METHODS

SUBJECTS

The subjects were boys who had been participating in a longitudinal study since their kindergarten year in 1984. They attended half-day kindergarten classes at French public schools in Montreal, Quebec. To obtain a high base rate of boys at risk for delinquent behavior, the 53 schools with the lowest socioeconomic index were chosen. Teachers were asked to rate each boy in their classes. Teachers normally had a morning and an afternoon group, each containing approximately eight boys and eight girls. Ratings were returned by 87% of the teachers, and 1161 boys were rated. To control for cultural effects, the boys were included in the study only if both of their biological parents were born in Canada and their mother tongue was French. These criteria created a homogeneous low socioeconomic status, white, French-speaking sample. After applying these criteria and eliminating boys whose families refused to participate further in the study or could not be traced after the initial assessment, 1034 boys (89%) remained. The number of boys with self-reported delinquent behavior between 10 and 13 years of age was 915 (88% of the original 1034 subjects). In kindergarten, the majority of the boys lived with both biological parents (67%), 24% lived alone with their mothers, and 5% lived with their mothers and a man who was not the boy's father; the rest (4%) lived in other family arrangements (eg, with grandparents or with father and stepmother). Parents' mean age at the birth of their son was 25.4 years (SD, 4.8 years) for mothers and 28.4 years (SD, 5.6 years) for fathers. This varied from 15 to 45 years for mothers and from 16 to 56 years for fathers. The mean number of years of school completed was 10.5 years (SD, 2.8 years) for mothers and 10.7 years (SD, 3.2 years) for fathers. The majority of the parents were unskilled workers. When in kindergarten, the majority of the boys were thus living with parents who had not completed high school and whose residence was in the poorest areas of a large metropolitan city. The mean and median family income at age 10 years (1988) was between $25 000 and $30 000 (Canadian dollars) ($19 000 to $23 000 in US dollars) compared with a median income of $44 000 (Canadian dollars) for couples with children in Canada in 1987.[45]

INSTRUMENTS AND PROCEDURE

Personality Dimensions and Categories

The boys' kindergarten behaviors were rated by teachers using 28 items from the Preschool Behavior Questionnaire[46] and 10 items from the Prosocial Behavior Questionnaire.[47] Items were selected to measure Gray's[24,26,48] and Cloninger's[33] impulsivity and anxiety dimensions Cloninger's reward-dependence dimension. Items referring to aggressive, oppositional, or antisocial behaviors were not included. For anxiety or harm avoidance, defined by Cloninger as cautious, apprehensive, inhibited behavior, three items were selected: is worried, worries about many things; tends to be fearful or afraid of new things or new situations; and cries easily. The α value for internal consistency was .72. Test-retest reliability with a 1-month interval from a similar sample was .63. For impulsivity or novelty seeking, defined by Cloninger as impulsive, excitable, and exploratory behaviors, two items were selected: restless, runs about or jumps up and down, and does not keep still, squirmy, fidgety child. The α value for internal consistency was .89; the test-retest reliability was .69. For reward dependence, defined by Cloninger as warm, sympathetic, sentimental behavior, 10 items were selected: praises others, shows sympathy, helps sick child, helps hurt child, helps child with a difficult task, helps clean up mess, invites bystander, stops quarrels, helps pick up objects, and comforts upset child. The α value for internal consistency was .91; the test-retest reliability was .70. The correlations between the three dimensions were low (r=.12 for

Continued on next page

garded as a demonstration that the early onset of frequent delinquent behavior (ie, in preadolescence or early adolescence) is a good predictor of the maintenance of such behavior. Investigators are now encouraged to study the links between preschool behavior and the early onset of delinquent behavior in preadolescence.[20,21] In one of the few longitudinal studies that have clearly addressed this issue, White and colleagues[22] analyzed data from the Dunedin Multidisciplinary Health and Developmental Study; assessments at ages 3 and 5 years were used to predict delinquent status at the age of 11 years. It was shown that motor problems and parent-rated behavior problems at ages 3 and 5 years discriminated the children who were rated most delinquent at age 11 years (9.4% of the boys and 2.6% of the girls). The best predictor was parent-rated behavior problems at age 5 years, followed by the mother reporting the child to be "difficult to manage" at 3 years of age and composite ratings of externalizing behaviors at age 3 years. These results support the hypothesis that very early disruptive behavior is relatively stable and often translates into delinquent behavior in preadolescence.[20,23]

It is hard to believe, however, that children are born with antisocial behavior problems. We need a theory that will explain how infant behaviors are transformed into stable, socially deviant behaviors. Because most of the longitudinal predictive studies of delinquency were looking at the stability of deviant behavior, their theoretical background has generally been limited to the stability hypothesis. A wide range of deviant behaviors were chosen as possible predictors. This shotgun approach was probably used because of the high cost of longitudinal studies and the lack of a clear consensus vis-à-vis a domi-

anxiety and impulsivity, r=.10 for anxiety and reward dependence, and r=−.13 for impulsivity and social dependence; N=1034). In labeling the three dimensions (anxiety, impulsivity, and reward dependence), an effort was made to use terms that reflected the theories being tested. Other labels could be used; the impulsivity dimension might be labeled "overactivity," and the reward dependence scale, "prosociality."

Cut-off points for the low and high ends of the dimensions had to be chosen to create Cloninger's eight extreme personality categories. The anxiety and impulsivity dimensions had skewed distributions. For both dimensions, approximately 40% of the subjects had a score of 0. This score was chosen as the low-end cut-off score for both dimensions. The 40th percentile was also used as the low-end cut-off point for the reward dependence dimension. The high-end cut-off point was chosen at the 60th percentile to obtain a similar number of subjects from both ends of the scales. **Table 1** presents the expected and observed distribution of subjects in the eight personality categories. The distribution was marginally similar to chance expectation (likelihood ratio, χ^2=29.2, P=.08). The largest deviation from the expected distribution was for the cyclothymic group; 10% of the boys were classified as such, compared with the expected 7%. The "others" group included all of the subjects (n=396; 43.2%) who were not at the extreme on at least one of the three dimensions. The number of subjects in each extreme personality category was large enough for statistical analyses (n, 53 to 91). It can be seen that a large number of subjects are needed to use this approach with a general population–based sample.

Self-reported Delinquency

At ages 10 to 13 years, the boys were tested in small groups at their schools between March and May; they answered 27 self-reported delinquency items distributed in a questionnaire about school, family, friends, and leisure activities. The items were as follows: steal from school, from store, from home; keep object worth less than $10; steal bicycle; sell stolen goods; keep object worth between $10 and $100; steal objects worth more than $100; breaking and entering; enter without paying; trespassing; take drugs, alcohol; get drunk; destroy school material, other material; vandalism at school; destroy objects at home; vandalize car; set a fire; strong-arm; gang fights; use weapon in a fight; fist fight; beat up someone; carry a weapon; and throw objects at persons. The 27 items were scored on a scale of 1 to 4 (never, once or twice, often, and very often) and were summed to obtain a total delinquency score (mean α=.88; mean 1-year test-retest reliability, .68). At ages 11 to 13 years, the boys were asked how often they had committed the delinquent behaviors in the past 12 months. At age 10 years, they were asked whether they had ever committed the delinquent behaviors and how often. **Table 2** presents the correlations among the self-reported delinquency scores from ages 10 to 13 years.

To select the boys who had early onset of frequent delinquent behaviors between ages 10 and 13 years, the total delinquency score was first computed for each year. Those above the 80th percentile on that score for a given year were considered to have high delinquency involvement for that year. Those who were found to be among the highly delinquent group for at least two thirds of their ratings were retained as the early-onset frequently delinquent group (n=92; 10.6% of the total sample). Of these boys, 80% (n=74) reported having ever beaten someone who had not done anything to them compared with 23% for the rest of the sample ($\chi^2[1]$=130.8; P<<.001); 90% (n=83) compared with 33% reported ever shoplifting ($\chi^2[1]$=109.0; P<<.001); 89% (n=82) compared with 32% reported ever using a weapon in a fight ($\chi^2[1]$=114.1; P<<.001); 71% (n=65) compared with 16% reported ever breaking or stealing part of a car ($\chi^2[1]$=146.1; P<<.001); and 71% (n=65) compared with 25% reported ever having been drunk ($\chi^2[1]$=85.4; P<<.001).

nant theory.[20,21] Launching a large-scale longitudinal study based on one theoretical perspective would be a risky enterprise. However, we need to go beyond the simple demonstration that from a long list of predictors, some will predict delinquent behavior and that these predictors are those that are most similar to the outcome criteria.

Personality theorists have regularly generated theories of antisocial behavior, but few have been tested from a developmental perspective with longitudinal data from early childhood onward. Two recent formulations have been the object of some empirical assessment in youths. Gray's model[24-26] has been used recently to explain children's conduct disorder,[27-29] whereas Cloninger's model[30-32] has been tested with reference to children's risk for alcohol abuse.[33]

Gray[24,34] proposed that the neurotic and extroverted dimensions of Eysenck[35] be replaced by anxiety and impulsivity dimensions. Using studies of drug therapies to reduce anxiety, Gray[25] showed that there is a well-defined physiological locus for behavioral inhibition, ie, the septohippocampal system. In a two-dimensional space, Eysenck[35] placed anxiety in the middle of the quadrant formed by high introversion and high neuroticism. He also placed impulsivity in the middle of the quadrant formed by high extroversion and high neuroticism. Gray's model simply rotated Eysenck's dimensions at a 30° angle. Gray[24,25] argues that this model provides a more parsimonious representation of reality because one dimension (anxiety) is needed instead of two (introversion and neuroticism) to represent a behavioral system (behavioral inhibition system) that has a clear physiological locus (the septohippocampal system) and responds to conditioned stimuli for punishment and the lack of a reward. Impulsivity is linked to a behavioral activation system that controls active approach and avoidance of conditioned stimuli for reward and the lack of punishment, whereas

Table 1. Distribution of Subjects in the Personality Profiles*

	Dimensions				
Profiles	Impulsivity	Anxiety	Reward Dependence	Expected, No. (%)	Observed, No. (%)
Antisocial	High	Low	Low	63 (6.9)	54 (5.9)
Histrionic	High	Low	High	68 (7.4)	59 (6.5)
Explosive-schizoid	High	High	Low	68 (7.4)	74 (8.1)
Passive-aggressive	High	High	High	73 (8.0)	69 (7.6)
Schizoid	Low	Low	Low	59 (6.5)	59 (6.5)
Cyclothymic	Low	Low	High	64 (7.0)	91 (10.0)
Obsessive	Low	High	Low	64 (7.0)	58 (6.4)
Passive-dependent	Low	High	High	69 (7.5)	56 (6.1)
Others	NA	NA	NA	386 (42.3)	394 (42.9)

**Likelihood ratio, χ^2=28.9, P=.09. NA indicates not applicable.*

a third system, the fight/flight system, controls escape and defensive behavior in response to unconditioned signals of punishment and lack of reward.[36,37] Gray's work has focused more on the anxiety dimension than on the impulsivity and fight/flight dimensions. Using Gray's model, Quay[28] suggested that conduct disorder was related to an oversensitive behavioral activation system (see also Newman[38]). On the other hand, Lahey and colleagues[27] used the same model to suggest subtypes of antisocial children, ie, children with conduct disorder with and without anxiety. They thus stressed the importance of taking into account the strength of both the behavioral inhibition system and the behavioral activation system to explain conduct disorder. Quay[29] recently called for studies that would help clarify the separate and joint actions of these systems in cases of conduct disorder.

Cloninger[30,31] proposed a three-dimensional personality model that includes Gray's anxiety and impulsivity dimensions plus aspects of Eysenck's "psychotism" dimension. He labeled the anxiety dimension "harm avoidance." Those high in harm avoidance are cautious, apprehensive, and inhibited; those who are low in this dimension are fearless, carefree, and uninhibited. The impulsivity dimension was labeled "novelty seeking." Exploratory behavior, excitability, and impulsivity typify persons high in this dimension; those low in novelty seeking are described as reflexive, rigid, and stoic. The third dimension was labeled "reward dependence." Highly reward-dependent individuals are described as warm, sentimental, and persistent; those low in reward dependence, as tough-minded, detached, and emotionally cool.

An important difference between Gray's and Cloninger's models is that Gray links impulsivity to reward dependence, whereas Cloninger differentiates these two dimensions by relying on the hypothesis that they are associated with two different neuromodulators: dopamine regulates impulsive behavior, whereas norepinephrine regulates reward dependence.[30] The outcome of interactions between the three postulated dimensions is also an important characteristic of Cloninger's model.[30,31] He suggests that each dimension is controlled by separate brain systems and neuromodulators that interact in such a way that the response based on one system will vary depending on the responses from the other systems. For example, highly harm-avoidant individuals will behave differently depending on whether they are low or high in reward dependence and low or high in novelty seeking. Eight extreme personality patterns (disorders) are generated from the interaction of the three dimensions when the two extremes of the continuum are used. For example, individuals high in novelty seeking, low in harm avoidance, and low in reward dependence would be classified as "antisocial" in the tradition of primary psychopathy,[39,40] whereas individuals with the same pattern except for the reward dependence dimension would be classified as "histrionic," ie, attention seeking, charming, and craving excitement.[31]

It is of interest to note that such an approach is similar to the suggestions made by Hinde and Dennis,[41] Cairns et al,[42] and Magnusson and Bergman[43] to study profiles (a person approach) and not only associations between variables (a variable approach). Cloninger[30] stresses the importance of distinguishing the underlying biogenetic dimensions from the phenotypic structure of personality.

This article addresses three questions concerning Gray's and Cloninger's personality models. First, we wanted to verify to what extent they could be used to characterize kindergarten boys' behavior and predict early onset of delinquency, ie, stable, highly delinquent behavior from preadolescence to early adolescence. An effort was made to assess the three personality dimensions with kindergarten behaviors that did not depict antisocial behavior so that the prediction of later delinquency would not be an assessment of the stability of antisocial behavior. Second, we wanted to address a parsimony issue by testing to what extent 1, 2, or 3 personality dimensions were needed to predict early onset of delinquency. Quay,[28] Gottfredson and Hirschi,[13] and Rowe and Osgood[19] argued for one dimension to explain antisocial behavior (impulsivity), Lahey et al[27] argued for two dimensions (impulsivity and anxiety),

Table 2. Correlations Between Self-reported Delinquency Scores From Ages 10 to 13 Years

	11 y	12 y	13 y
10 y	.45	.33	.33
11 y	. . .	.54	.50
12 y	. . .	. . .	.58

and Cloninger[31] and Eysenck and Gudjonsson,[44] argued for three dimensions. Finally, we wanted to verify whether, as suggested by Cloninger,[30,31] a categorical approach could correctly classify boys with early onset of high delinquency and how stable was this phenomenon between ages 11 and 13 years.

RESULTS

A logistic regression analysis was used to predict the delinquent–not delinquent classification from the three personality dimensions measured on a continuous scale in kindergarten. A backward procedure was used in which the three variables were first entered and then removed if their contribution to the equation was $P>.15$. The best predictive model of delinquent behavior (goodness of fit, $\chi^2[910]=894.62$, $P=.64$) included high impulsivity as the strongest predictor (Wald's $\chi^2[1]=20.1$, $P<.0001$), low anxiety as the second-strongest predictor (Wald's $\chi^2[1]=5.9$, $P<.016$), and low reward dependence as a third predictor (Wald's $\chi^2[1]=4.8$, $P<.029$). To check for the contribution of interactions between the three dimensions, a stepwise forward procedure was then used. The three variables were forced in the first step, and the interactions were left free to enter in the next step. No interactions were added to the equation, indicating that no interaction term made a significant contribution after the main effects were accounted for.

The analyses were then performed to check the distribution of delinquents within Cloninger's eight personality categories. **Figure 1** presents the distribution of the 92 frequently delinquent boys among the eight extreme personality categories and the rest of the sample (labeled "others" in the figure). It can be seen that, as predicted, the boys from the antisocial personality group were at highest risk of being classified as frequently delinquent (28%). The passive-aggressive and explosive schizoid groups followed with 15% and 12%, respectively, of their members classified as frequently delinquent. The percentages for each of the other personality categories were all below the base-rate level (10%); the percentage of frequently delinquent boys in the others category was identical to the base rate. The comparison of the proportion of delinquents in the antisocial group with each of the other groups, with a logistic regression model (goodness of fit, $\chi^2[905]=913.87$, $P=.41$), indicated significant differences for each comparison except for the contrast between the antisocial and the passive-aggressive groups. These results also clearly showed that the boys with high impulsivity ratings in kindergarten were more at risk for early onset of frequent delinquent behavior than were those with low impulsivity ratings, with the exception of those who were also low in anxiety and high in reward dependence, ie, the histrionic group. The difference in the percentage of delinquent boys in the antisocial and the histrionic groups (odds ratio, 4.2) was particularly striking, considering that in kindergarten, they were different in only one dimension, ie, reward dependence. Similar significant differences between personality categories that had identical levels for two of three dimensions could be observed for the antisocial group compared with the schizoid group (odds ratio, 4.2) and for the passive-aggressive group compared with the passive-dependent group (odds ratio, 9.3). These results underline the relative risk for each kindergarten group of being identified among the frequently delinquent group between the ages of 10 and 13 years. It is, however, important to note that 42% (39/92) of the frequently delinquent boys originated from the kindergarten group without an extreme personality profile (ie, the "others" group in Figure 1).

A final set of analyses was conducted to assess the extent to which the association between kindergarten personality categories and early onset of frequent delinquent behavior was a stable phenomenon between the ages of 11 and 13 years.[48] The age of 11 years rather than 10 years was used because the questions for delinquent behavior for 10-year-olds asked if they had ever done the deviant behavior and how often, whereas the questions at ages 11 through 13 years asked if they had done the deviant behavior, and how often, in the past 12 months. The frequency of delinquent behavior was expected to increase from age 11 to 13 years because of the general increase in antisocial behavior during adolescence. The important question was to what extent would the differences among kindergarten personality categories that were observed for the dichotomous variable used in the preceeding analysis (stable delinquent vs not stable delinquent between the ages of 10 and 13 years) hold true for two nonaggregated continuous measures taken 2 years apart? **Figure 2** represents the mean total self-reported delinquency score for each of the nine personality categories at ages 11 and 13 years. First, a repeated measures analysis of variance (nine personality categories by two ages) was performed to test the effect of kindergarten personality category and ages on self-reported delinquency. The personality category effect and the age effect were significant ($F[8,877]=5.42$, $P<.0001$; $F[1,877]=7.78$, $P<.005$, respectively). The interaction between both factors was not significant ($F[8,877]=0.58$; $P>.05$). Self-reported delinquency increased from age 11 to 13 years for each personality category except for the passive-aggressive category (Figure 2). The antisocial kindergarten category had the highest score, and the passive-dependent category had the lowest score at both ages 11 and 13. To verify the extent to which each personality category had the same relative level of delinquency at both

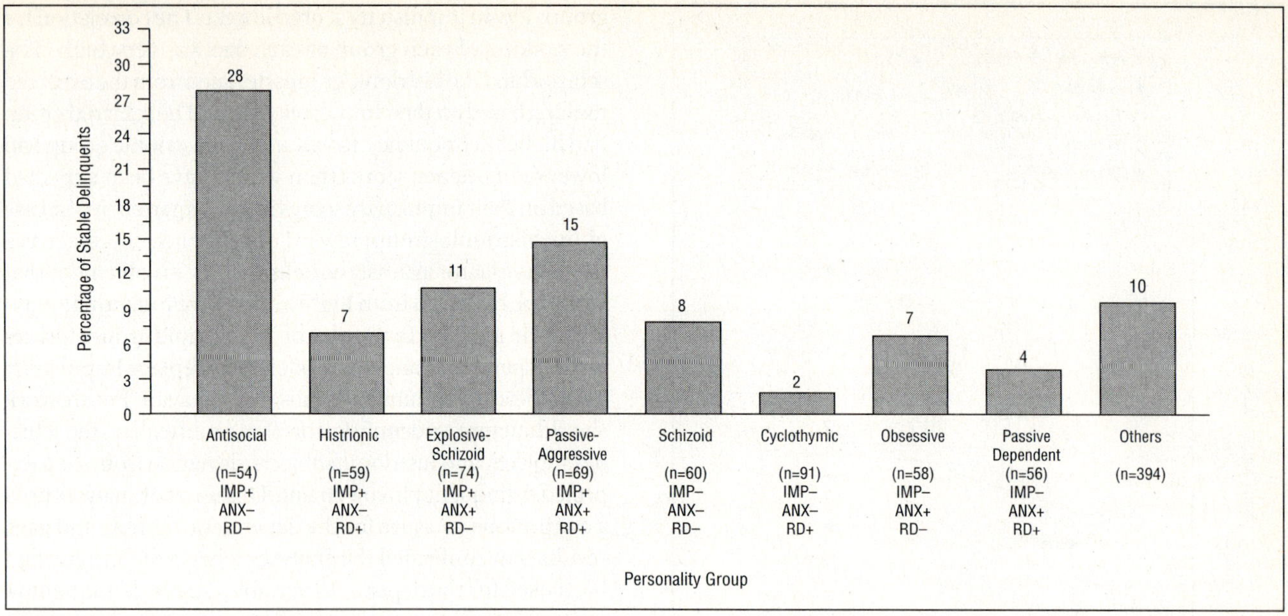

Figure 1. *Percentage of stable delinquents between the ages 10 and 13 years for the eight extreme kindergarten personality groups and all other subjects (others). IMP indicates impulsive; ANX, anxious; RD, reward dependent; plus sign, high on the given dimension; and minus sign, low on the given dimension.*

ages, two correlation analyses were performed. A Spearman Rank Correlation Coefficient (ρ=.90, P<.0001, n=9) and a Pearson correlation coefficient (r=.94, P<.0001, n=9) using the personality categories' mean delinquency score indicated that at ages 11 and 13, the relative level of delinquency among groups based on kindergarten personality measures was stable.

COMMENT

This article reports on a longitudinal study of inner-city boys from kindergarten to age 13 years, which was used to test the predictive value of kindergarten personality manifestations for early onset of delinquent behavior. Based on Gray's[25,26] and Cloninger's[30,31] models, three personality dimensions were extracted from kindergarten teacher ratings: impulsivity, anxiety, and reward dependence. The results of a logistic regression analysis showed that high impulsivity rated by kindergarten teachers was the personality dimension that best predicted which boys would have the highest self-reported delinquency scores from ages 10 to 13 years. Anxiety and reward dependence also made small independent contributions to the prediction. Thus, the three personality dimensions as rated by kindergarten teachers did contribute to explaining the early onset of delinquent behavior, but impulsivity made the major contribution. As suggested by Quay[28] and Newman,[38] these results confirm that Gray's behavioral activating system may be the major dimension underlying the propensity toward antisocial behavior (see also Gottfredson and Hirschi[13]). As suggested by Lahey and colleagues,[27] the significant anxiety effect, albeit weak, indicates that the behavioral inhibition system can play a role in both preventing and fostering antisocial behavior. Reward dependence made the smallest contribution but had a meaningful impact when a categorical approach was taken.

The measure of impulsivity in this study was based on items that are generally used to assess hyperactivity. The boys most at risk for antisocial behavior were thus rated overactive in kindergarten. These results corroborate a number of studies that have shown that hyperactivity increases the risk of later antisocial behavior.[49-51] The impulsivity and novelty seeking personality dimensions of Gray and Cloninger clearly overlap with the impulsivity and overactivity of the attention-deficit hyperactivity disorder.[52,53] Longitudinal studies from birth to school-entry age should attempt to sort out the developmental sequence of impulsivity, overactivity, attention-deficit hyperactivity disorder, and antisocial behavior by frequent monitoring of these dimensions for large samples of at-risk subjects.

Using Cloninger's[31] classification of extreme personality types, we verified to what extent boys with stable early onset of delinquent behavior were found in specific personality categories. Results confirmed Cloninger's prediction that subjects who are high in impulsivity, low in anxiety, and low in reward dependence would be the most at risk for antisocial behavior. The proportion of delinquent boys was highest in the antisocial category when compared with all other categories except the passive-aggressive category. It should be noted that the antisocial and passive-aggressive categories shared only the high impulsivity dimension. These results appear to reflect the interaction between impulsivity and anxiety that was predicted by Lahey and colleagues.[27] However, it must be noted that these two categories of boys also differed in the reward dependence dimension. In contrast, the antisocial and histrionic categories shared both the high impulsivity and low anxiety dimensions but had significantly different proportions of highly delinquent boys.

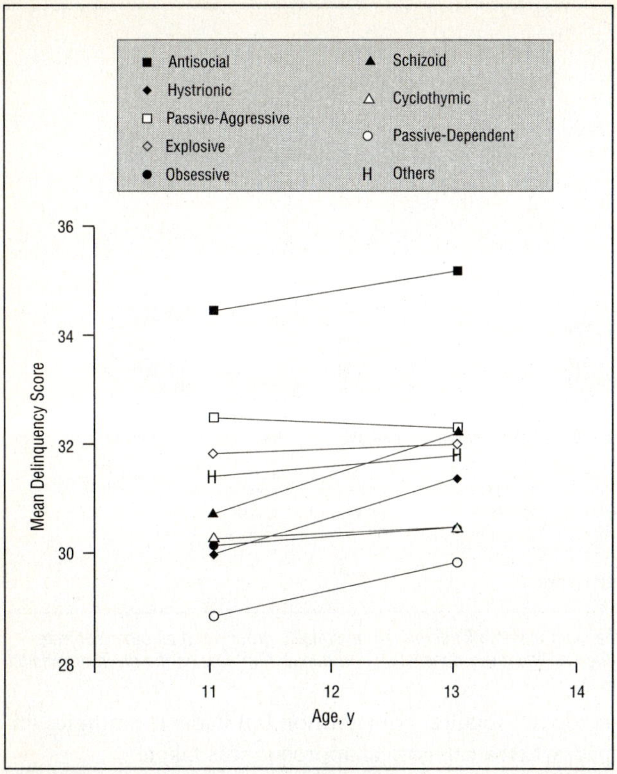

Figure 2. *Mean self-reported delinquent behavior score at ages 11 and 13 years for the eight extreme kindergarten personality groups and all other subjects (others).*

Reward dependence of the histrionic boys did appear to protect them from high involvement in delinquency, although they were highly impulsive and low in anxiety. Thus, the analyses of differences between categories show the important role of the three personality dimensions when extreme personality categories are associated with an extreme behavior such as stable, highly antisocial behavior. Although the logistic regression, which used the whole continuum of each personality dimension, showed only modest predictive values for anxiety and reward dependence and no significant interaction effects, it can be seen that the categorical analyses revealed statistically significant and theoretically meaningful differences between categories of subjects who shared two of three dimensions, including impulsivity. The difference between the antisocial and histrionic groups was remarkable in this respect. This result confirms the usefulness of the person approach in data analysis.[41-43]

The longitudinal data on delinquent behavior were also used to check the extent to which kindergarten personality dimensions were associated with delinquent behavior at the start of puberty (age, 11 years) and during puberty (age, 13 years). Results showed that this association was generally stable at a time when boys go through one of life's most important transitional periods. The increase in reported delinquent behaviors was significant from ages 11 to 13 years, but at both ages, the antisocial group scored highest and the passive-dependent group scored lowest; three of the four highly impulsive groups scored highest, and three of the four groups low in impulsivity scored lowest. The correlation for the ranking of each group at each age was very high. The schizoid and the histrionic groups deviated from the expected ranking based on their impulsivity score. The schizoid group had higher delinquency scores and the histrionic group had lower delinquency scores than would have been expected based on their impulsivity scores in kindergarten. In the case of the histrionic group, reward dependence could act as a protective factor against the delinquency involvement that would be expected from highly impulsive individuals who are low in anxiety. In the case of the schizoid group, low reward dependence and low anxiety may replace impulsivity as a sufficient disinhibitor of antisocial behavior. Future work should attempt to identify factors that could explain the schizoid subjects' and histrionic subjects' deviation from their expected delinquency involvement. This series of analyses used a continuous measure for the dependent variable and gave results that confirmed the analyses when a dichotomy had been used for the dependent variable (stable delinquent vs not stable delinquent).

The kindergarten teacher ratings used in this study were not the optimum measures of the three personality dimensions. It will be important to replicate this study with behavioral assessments designed to assess these specific personality models. Replications are also needed to determine to what extent the results can be generalized to girls and boys raised in different circumstances. Results, however, confirmed the theoretical basis of the personality dimensions to predict antisocial behavior and showed substantial stability over a long period when boys undergo important developmental changes. Predictive studies of antisocial behavior have shown that antisocial behavior is relatively stable from early childhood to adolescence.[10,22] This study demonstrates that personality dimensions that do not include antisocial behavior were good predictors of later antisocial behavior. One would expect that the personality dimensions and antisocial behavior at age 6 years would be highly correlated. To understand to what extent these personality dimensions are the basis on which antisocial behavior develops, studies are needed in which both the personality dimensions and antisocial behavior are monitored with independent measures from birth to school entry. Alternatively, if the modification of young children's basic personality dimensions could be achieved through early intervention, this would help clarify the extent to which changes in antisocial behavior follow.

Accepted for publication June 13, 1994.

This study was supported by grants from the government of Quebec's Conseil Québćois de la Recherche Sociale (CQRS) and Fonds pour la Formation de Chercheurs et l'Aide à la Recherce (FCAR), Quebec city, the Social Sciences and Humanities Research Council of Canada, Ottawa, Ontario, and the University of Montréal.

We thank Pierre Charlebois, PhD, Claude Gagnon, PhD, Serge Larivée, PhD, and Marc LeBlanc, PhD, for par-

ticipating in the planning and execution of the longitudinal study; Hélène Beauchesne, MSc, and Lucille David, MSc, for coordinating the data collection; Hélène Boileau; Lyse Desmarais-Gervais, MSc; Diane Héroux; and Maria Rosa for creating the data banks and performing the statistical analyses; Mihn T. Trinh, MSc, for providing the documentation; Bernard Boulerice, MSc, for providing the statistical expertise; and Chantal Bruneau and Francine Ploude, for secretarial assistance. We thank three anonymous reviewers for their suggestions.

Reprint requests to Research Unit on Children's Psycho-Social Maladjustment, University of Montreal, 750 E Gouin Blvd, Montreal, Quebec, Canada H2C 1A6 (Dr Tremblay).

REFERENCES

1. Carpenter M. *Reformatory Schools for the Children of the Perishing and Dangerous Classes and for Juvenile Offenders.* London, England: The Woburn Press; 1968:1851.
2. Platt AM. *The Child Savers.* Chicago, Ill: University of Chicago Press; 1977.
3. Robins LN. *Deviant Children Grown Up.* Baltimore, Md: Williams & Wilkins; 1966.
4. Eron LD, Huesmann LR, Zelli A. The role of parental variables in the learning of aggression. In: Pepler DJ, Rubin KH, eds. *The Development and Treatment of Childhood Aggression.* Hillsdale, NJ: Lawrence Erlbaum Associates Inc; 1991:169-188.
5. Farrington DP. Childhood aggression and adult violence: early precursors and life outcomes. In: Pepler DJ, Rubin KH, eds. *The Development and Treatment of Childhood Aggression.* Hillsdale, NJ: Laurence Erlbaum; 1991:5-29.
6. McCord J. Family relationships, juvenile delinquency, and adult criminality. *Criminology.* 1991;29:397-417.
7. Moffitt TE. Juvenile delinquency and attention deficit disorder: developmental trajectories from age 3 to age 15. *Child Dev.* 1990;61;893-910.
8. Pulkkinen L, Tremblay RE. Patterns of boys' social adjustment in two cultures and at different ages. *Int J Behav Dev.* 1992;15:527-553.
9. Stattin H, Magnusson D. The role of early aggressive behavior in the frequency, seriousness and types of later crime. *J Consult Clin Psychol.* 1989; 57:710-718.
10. Tremblay RE, Masse B, Perron D, LeBlanc M, Schwartzman AE, Ledingham JE. Early disruptive behavior, poor school achievement, delinquent behavior and delinquent personality. *J Consult Clin Psychol.* 1992;60:64-72.
11. Werner EE, Smith RS. *Kauai's Children Come of Age.* Honolulu, Hawaii: The University Press of Hawaii; 1977.
12. Loeber R, Stouthamer-Loeber M. Prediction. In: Quay HC, ed. *Handbook of Juvenile Delinquency.* New York, NY: John Wiley & Sons; 1987:325-382.
13. Gottfredson MR, Hirschi T. *A General Theory of Crime.* Stanford, Calif: Stanford University Press; 1990.
14. Reiss AJ, Roth JA. *Understanding and Preventing Violence.* Washington, DC: National Academy Press; 1993.
15. Rowe DC. Inherited dispositions toward learning delinquent and criminal behavior: new evidence. In: Ellis L, Hoffman H, eds. *Crime in Biological, Social, and Moral Contexts.* New York, NY: Praeger Publishers; 1990:121-133.
16. Dodge KA. Nature versus nurture in childhood conduct disorder: it is time to ask a different question. *Dev Psychol.* 1990;26:698-701.
17. Lytton H. Child and parent effects in boys' conduct disorder: a reinterpretation. *Dev Psychol.* 1990;26:683-697.
18. Mednick SA, Kandel E. Genetic and perinatal factors in violence. In: Mednick SA, Moffitt TE, eds. *Biological Contributions to Crime Causation.* Drodrecht, the Netherlands: Martinus Nijhoff; 1988:121-134.
19. Rowe DC, Osgood DW. A latent trait approach to unifying criminal careers. *Criminology.* 1990;28:237-270.
20. Farrington DP, Loeber R, Elliott DS, Hawkins D, Kandel DB, Klein MW, McCord J, Rowe DC, Tremblay RE. Advancing knowledge about the onset of delinquency and crime. In: Lahey BB, Kazdin AE, eds. *Advances in Clinical Child Psychology.* New York, NY: Plenum Publishing Corp; 1990:283-342.
21. Tonry M, Ohlin LE, Farrington DP, Adams K, Earls F, Rowe DC, Sampson RJ, Tremblay RE. *Human Development and Criminal Behavior: New Ways of Advancing Knowledge.* New York, NY: Springer-Verlag; 1991.
22. White JL, Moffitt TE, Earls F, Robins L, Silva PA. How early can we tell? *Criminology.* 1990;28:507-533.
23. Loeber R. Development and risk factors of juvenile antisocial behavior and delinquency. *Clin Psychol Rev.* 1990;10:1-41.
24. Gray JA. A critique of Eysenck's theory of personality. In: Eysenck HJ, ed. *A Model for Personality.* New York, NY: Springer-Verlag; 1981:246-276.
25. Gray JA. *The Neuropsychology of Anxiety.* New York, NY: Oxford University Press; 1982.
26. Gray JA. Where should we search for biologically based dimensions of personality. *Z Differentielle Diagnostische Psychol.* 1983;4:163-174.
27. Lahey BB, McBurnett K, Loeber R, Hart EL. Psychobiology of conduct disorder. In: Sholevar GP, ed. *Conduct Disorders in Children and Adolescents: Assessments and Interventions.* Washington, DC: American Psychiatric Press. In press.
28. Quay HC. The behavioral reward and inhibition system in childhood behavior disorder. In: Bloomingdal LM, eds. *Attention Deficit Disorder.* Oxford, England: Pergamon Press In; 1988;3:176-186.
29. Quay HC.The psychobiology of undersocial aggressive conduct disorder: a theoretical perspective. *Dev Psychopathology.* 1993;5:165-180.
30. Cloninger CR. A unified biosocial theory of personality and its role in the development of anxiety states. *Psychiatr Dev.* 1986;3:167-226.
31. Cloninger CR. A systematic method for clinical description and classification of personality variants: a proposal. *Arch Gen Psychiatry.* 1987;44:573-588.
32. Cloninger CR. Neurogenetic adaptive mechanisms in alcoholism. *Science.* 1987; 236:410-416.
33. Cloninger CR, Sigvardson S, Bohman M. Childhood personality predicts alcohol abuse in young adults. *Alcohol Clin Exp Res.* 1988;12:494-505.
34. Gray JA. The psychophysiological basis of introversion-extraversion. *Behav Res Ther.* 1970;8:249-266.
35. Eysenck HJ. *The Stucture of Human Personality.* London, England: Methuen & Co; 1970.
36. Gray JA. The structure of the emotions and the limbic system. In: Porter R, Knight J, eds. *Physiology, Emotion and Psychosomatic Illness.* Amsterdam, the Netherlands; Elsevier Science Publishers; 1972.
37. Gray JA. Brain systems that mediate both emotion and cognition. *Cogn Emotion.* 1990;4:269-288.
38. Newman JP. Reaction to punishment in extraverts and psychopaths. *J Res Pers.* 1987;21:464-480.
39. Cleckley H. *The Mask of Sanity.* St Louis, Mo: Mosby–Year Book; 1976.
40. Hare RD, Cox DN. Clinical and empirical conceptions of psychopathy, and the selection of subjects for research. In: Hare RD, Schalling D, eds. *Psychopathic Behavior: Approaches to Research.* Toronto, Ontario: John Wiley & Sons; 1987:1-21.
41. Hinde RA, Dennis A. Categorizing individuals: an alternative to linear analysis. *Int J Behav Dev.* 1986;9:105-119.
42. Cairns RB, Cairns BD, Neckerman HJ. Early school dropout: configurations and determinants. *Child Dev.* 1988;60:1437-1452.
43. Magnusson D, Bergman LR. A pattern approach to the study of pathways from childhood to adulthood. In: Robins LN, Rutter M, eds. *Straight and Devious Pathways From Childhood to Adulthood.* New York, NY: Cambridge University Press; 1990:101-116.
44. Eysenck HJ, Gudjonsson GH. *The Causes and Cures of Criminality.* New York, NY: Plenum Publishing Corp; 1989.
45. Mitchell A. The economic circumstances of Ontario's families and children. In: Barnhorst R, Johnson LC, eds. *The State of the Child in Ontario.* Toronto, Ontario: Oxford University Press; 22-47.
46. Behar LB, Stringfield S. A behavior rating scale for the preschool child. *Dev Psychol.* 1974;10:601-610.
47. Weir K, Duveen G. Further development and validation of the prosocial behaviour questionnaire for use by teachers. *J Child Psychol Psychiatry.* 1981;22:357-374.
48. Gray JA, Owens S, Davis N, Tsaltas E. Psychological and physiological relations between anxiety and impulsivity. In: Zuckerman M, ed. *Biological Bases of Sensation Seeking, Impulsivity and Anxiety.* Hillsdale, NJ: Lawrence Erlbaum Associates Inc; 1983:189-218.
49. Farrington D, Loeber R, Van Kammen WB. The long term criminal outcomes of conduct problem boys with or without impulsive-inattentive behavior. In: Robins LN, Rutter M, eds. *Straight and Devious Pathways From Childhood to Adulthood.* New York, NY: Cambridge University Press; 1990:62-81.
50. Satterfield JH. Childhood diagnostic and neurophysiological predictors of teenage arrest rates. In: Mednick SA, Moffitt TE, Stack SH, eds. *The Causes of Crime.* New York, NY: Cambridge University Press; 1987;9:146-167.
51. Weiss G, Hechtman LT. *Hyperactive Children Grown Up: ADHD in Children, Adolescents, and Adults.* New York, NY: Guilford Press; 1993.
52. Barkley RA. *Attention Deficit Hyperactivity Disorder: A Handbook for Diagnosis and Treatment.* New York, NY: Guilford Press; 1990.
53. Douglas VI. Stop, look, and listen: the problem of sustained attention and impulse control in hyperactive and normal children. *Can J Behav Sci.* 1972;4:259-292.

Untreated Anxiety Among Adult Primary Care Patients in a Health Maintenance Organization

Sheila K. Fifer, PhD; Susan D. Mathias, MPH; Donald L. Patrick, PhD, MSPH; Peter D. Mazonson, MD, MBA; Deborah P. Lubeck, PhD; Don P. Buesching, PhD

Background: Untreated anxiety may be particularly difficult for primary care physicians to recognize and diagnose because there are no reliable demographic or medical profiles for patients with this condition and because these patients present with a high rate of comorbid psychological conditions that complicate selection of treatment.

Method: A prospective assessment of untreated anxiety symptoms and disorders among primary care patients.

Results: Approximately 10% of eligible patients screened in clinic waiting rooms of a mixed-model health maintenance organization reported elevated symptoms and/or disorders of anxiety that were unrecognized and untreated. These patients with untreated anxiety reported significantly worse functioning on both physical and emotional measures than "not anxious" comparison patients; in fact these patients reported reduced functioning levels within ranges that would be expected for patients with chronic physical diseases, such as diabetes and congestive heart failure. The most severe reductions in functioning were reported by untreated patients whose anxiety was mixed with depression symptoms or disorders.

Conclusion: Primary care physicians may benefit from screening tools and consultations by mental health specialists to assist in recognition and diagnosis of anxiety symptoms and disorders alone and mixed with depression.

(Arch Gen Psychiatry. 1994;51:740-750)

PREVIOUS RESEARCH has confirmed that individuals with mental health problems are heavy users of the primary care health services system, where they continue to be underdiagnosed and undertreated.[1,2] The present study offers specific estimates of the frequency of untreated anxiety symptoms and disorders in a health maintenance organization and also characterizes the health burden and psychological comorbidity associated with untreated anxiety in primary care.

Many patients seen by primary care physicians present with not only medical but also emotional problems, yet these emotional problems frequently go untreated. Although 27% to 48% of patients presenting to primary care providers may have emotional problems,[3-7] it is believed that fewer than half are detected or treated.[8,9] Untreated emotional problems affect both the quality and the costs of primary health care.[10-12] Patients with undetected emotional problems have been found to be high users of medical services and to receive repeated diagnosis and treatment for medical conditions while their emotional problems remain untreated.[11-13] Untreated emotional symptoms and problems are not self-limiting but may persist for years and may be associated with continuing return visits.[3,14,15]

Emotional problems are among the most difficult conditions for primary care physicians to detect, diagnose, and treat. Impediments to improved care include physicians' lack of time to recognize and diagnose or to refer, patients' resistance to diagnosis and treatment, and inadequate insurance reimbursement for psychological care. Equally important, however, is the lack of information available to primary care

From the Technology Assessment Group Inc, San Francisco, Calif (Drs Fifer, Mazonson, and Lubeck and Ms Mathias); the Department of Health Services, University of Washington School of Public Health, Seattle (Dr Patrick); the Department of Medicine, Stanford University, Palo Alto, Calif (Dr Lubeck); and the Upjohn Co, Kalamazoo, Mich (Dr Buesching).
Dr Buesching is now with Eli Lilly & Co, Indianapolis, Ind.
Dr Buesching is a former employee of the Upjohn Co but owns no stock or options to purchase further stock in that company. The other authors own no stock or options in the Upjohn Co.

See Methods on next page

METHODS

STUDY POPULATION AND SITE

The study population consisted of 637 eligible patients from a total population of 10 190 adult primary care patients who presented during a 4-month period to the clinics of 75 participating primary care physicians. Physicians' practices ranged in size from one practitioner to a group practice of 12. All physicians were under contract to the TakeCare/Lincoln National Health Plan (now named the FHP/TakeCare National Health Plan), a mixed-model health maintenance organization (HMO) in a region of central Colorado that included urban (Denver), suburban, and rural communities. The HMO maintained a total enrollment of approximately 112 000 patients who could select from 285 contracted primary care physicians. Enrollees' benefits included coverage for care given by primary care physicians and/or by a capitated mental health provider organization offering counseling by psychologists, psychiatrists, psychiatric social workers, and other mental health specialists. Benefit coverage included both counseling and pharmacotherapy, with complete coverage for visits and no allocated ceilings. Patients could be referred to the mental health provider by their physician, by self-referral, or by their employer.

PROCEDURES AND MEASURES

To identify patients with unrecognized and untreated anxiety, a three-step screening process was used: an initial waiting room screening questionnaire, a medical records review, and a baseline interview. To be eligible for the study, patients had to meet four criteria: between 21 and 65 years of age, enrolled in the HMO for a minimum of 6 months, no dual benefits, and presented to one of the participating primary care physicians during the study period. Also, since patients were screened only once, return patients were excluded. Waiting room staff briefly described the study to patients. After completing the informed consent and medical release forms, patients were offered a screening questionnaire and a cash honorarium.

Waiting Room Screen

A self-administered three-part questionnaire completed in the waiting room (a synopsis of all measures used, their validation, and scoring is available to interested readers on request from the authors) measured the following:

Symptoms of Anxiety and Depression. It is generally recognized that self-rated scales contain a nonspecific psychological distress component as well as specific factors that distinguish anxiety (hyperarousal) from depression (anhedonia).[23] A 52-item abbreviated checklist for symptoms of anxiety and depression, referred to here as the Symptom Checklist 52 (SCL-52), is a selection of five scales taken in full from the longer Symptom Checklist 90–Revised (SCL-90-R). The SCL-90 was designed to assess symptoms of multiple dimensions and is capable of identifying and discriminating between clinical groups with overlapping diagnoses.[31] In the screening questionnaire, we used the four subscales that measure symptoms of types of anxiety (general, phobic, somatic, and obsessive-compulsive) and the scale for depressive symptoms.[32,33] Possible scores for each subscale range between 30 and 81, with 54 representing the symptom level of nonpatients in normative cohort validation studies.[34] A baseline cutoff point of 61 on any one of these four subscales was used for this study. The Global Anxiety Score (GAS) indicates the overall anxiety symptom level based on the mean scores of all four anxiety subscales.[35]

Functioning and Well-being. The Medical Outcomes Study (MOS) Short-Form Health Survey (SF-36) (also known as the RAND 36-Item Health Survey) included eight domains: physical functioning, social functioning, limitations in daily activity caused by physical health (role—physical), emotional problems (role—emotional), mental health, energy, pain, and general health perceptions.[36] These subscales are scored from 0 to 100, with 100 representing optimal health status.

Mental Health Treatment. Items developed for this study asked whether, during the past 6 months, the patient had had mental health problems recognized or had been treated for mental health problems or stress. If care had been received, the items asked whether that care was given by a general physician, a medical specialist, or a counselor, and whether drug therapy had been given.

To be included in the study, respondents could not have received treatment for an emotional condition during the previous 6 months, and they had to score 63 or higher on at least one of the four anxiety symptom subscales of the SCL-52. The screening cutoff point was set two points higher than the baseline cutoff point of 61 to compensate for an anticipated decrease in score on subsequent administration of the SCL-90-R because of regression to the mean or measurement error. A score of 60 places an individual in the 84th percentile of the normative sample. These cutoff points were selected based on the results of two pretests and in conjunction with experts in the area of psychiatric screens and diagnostic instruments.

Medical Record Review

Medical records of all respondents selected during the initial screen were examined for evidence of prior diagnosis

Continued on next page

physicians concerning specific psychological symptoms and disorders that are prevalent among their patients and the relative health burden associated with these symptoms and disorders. Such information would help primary care physicians assess which of the many conditions constituting emotional problems—such as depression, anxiety, substance abuse, adjustment, and personality problems—are both prevalent among their patients and carry a suf-

or treatment of an emotional disorder. Given the difficulty other researchers have had distinguishing recognition and treatment,[14] no such distinction was attempted. Patients whose clinical records showed no evidence of recognition, diagnosis, or treatment for an emotional disorder requiring counseling, psychotropic drug therapy, or any other type of treatment for stress or psychological distress and who had not been referred to or received care from the HMO's mental health provider during the preceding 6 months were considered "unrecognized and untreated." Medical records were reviewed by a mental health therapist and a nurse-practitioner under supervision by two general internists. Records of the mental health provider were reviewed by the staff of that organization.

Follow-up Interview

Eligible patients were invited to a follow-up interview. Time between the waiting room screen and the follow-up interview averaged slightly over 5 weeks, sufficient to exclude patients whose elevated responses to the initial waiting room screen may have reflected transitory anxiety. The follow-up interviews were composed of two parts, a longer version of the self-administered screening questionnaire and a diagnostic evaluation. There were four measurements: (1) for symptoms, the complete version of the SCL-90-R[32]; (2) for functioning and well-being, the SF-36 (identical to the screening survey); (3) for comorbid physical conditions, a self-reported checklist from the National Health Interview Survey[37]; and (4) for diagnostic evaluation, selected sections of the computerized version of the Diagnostic Interview Schedule (DIS) of the National Institute of Mental Health.[1] The Quick Diagnostic Interview Schedule III-R (Q-DIS-III-R)[38,39] interviews were conducted for eight anxiety disorders as well as for depression and alcohol/substance use and were administered by trained lay interviewers. Interviews were conducted at appointments reserved solely for that purpose, to preclude the effects of additional stress associated with a medical visit.

Patients who scored 61 or higher on at least one of the four SCL-90-R anxiety subscales were considered likely to have clinically significant symptoms.[33] Patients who scored above this cutoff point constituted the study group of patients with unrecognized and untreated anxiety.

STATISTICAL ANALYSES AND TEST FOR BIAS

For comparisons between the patients who were not anxious and the patients with untreated and treated anxiety, an analysis of covariance model was used, controlling for differences in age and sex. Similarly, other outcome measures were compared using an analysis of covariance model, controlling for differences in age and sex between the study groups and subgroups. Adjusted mean scores for each group are reported. A *t* test adjusted for multiple comparisons was used to evaluate paired-group differences. Adjustments were made using $P<.05$ and dividing by the number of comparisons. For example, if six panel comparisons are made, the level of significance was .008 (.05/6). Data were analyzed using the SAS General Linear Models (GLM) procedure (version 6.04 for the personal computer, SAS Institute, Cary, NC) for the personal computer. All variables were evaluated for the presence and absence of missing data and were found to be consistent across all groups.

Two additional surveys of the waiting room patient population were conducted to test for biases in the sampling process. First, we questioned a random sample of 45 waiting room patients, stratified by practice group, who declined to take the screening questionnaire (nonresponders). The SCL-52 and the SF-36 were administered to nonresponders over the telephone to determine whether they differed from responders in levels of anxiety, functioning, and well-being or in demographic characteristics. The group of 45 nonresponders showed no statistically significant differences from responders using χ^2 analysis of the dichotomous variable of sex and the ordinal variable of age. Scores on the SF-36, the SCL-52 anxiety and depression subscales, and the Global Anxiety Scale were each evaluated using a two-sample *t* test that treated the scores as interval measurements. Nonresponders differed from responders on one of the eight SF-36 subscales, reporting lower levels of physical functioning (mean [SD] score, 76.6 [24.6] for nonresponders and 85.2 [21.2] for responders; $P=.006$).

A second stratified random sample of 56 patients who met all the study criteria but had lower levels of anxiety symptoms, up to 0.75 SD below the initial screening cutoff point, were given identical follow-up questionnaires and interviews approximately 5 weeks after the initial screen to determine the false-negative rate of the SCL-52 questionnaire. The SCL-52 had comparable false-positive and false-negative error rates of 28% (288 of 1027) and 30% (17 of 56), respectively. The false-negative rate was based on a comparison of this control group's scores on the SCL-52 and their scores on the same anxiety subscale sections of the SCL-90-R administered at baseline.

In addition to the patient self-report survey for comorbid physical conditions, a record review was conducted for comorbid physical conditions. The rate of agreement between the two indicators of comorbidity was .90 or higher (ie, 90% or more of records agreed with patient self-reports) for seven conditions (diabetes, kidney disease, stroke or other neurologic condition, cancer, blood disease, heart disease, and lung disease) and between .88 and .76 for the remaining four conditions (hypertension, urinary or gynecological disorder, stomach or intestinal disorder, and arthritis, rheumatism, or other bone or joint disease).

ficient functioning burden to warrant additional efforts to detect and treat.

The emotional condition for which such information is available is depression. Recent research has established that depressive symptoms and disorders are common and debilitating conditions among primary care patients. The prevalence of depressive symptoms and disorders among primary care patients ranges as high as 48%.[6,16]

Between 12% and 51% of these cases are detected by physicians, with detection rates lower among patients in prepaid plans than among fee-for-service patients.[6,8,17] Depression has been shown to reduce patients' functioning and well-being, and this reduction is equivalent to or more severe than the disability levels associated with chronic medical conditions such as diabetes and arthritis.[18] Patients with subsyndromal depression report reduced functioning and well-being, as do those patients with depression sufficiently severe to be diagnosed as a disorder.[18,19]

The aim of this study was to determine whether anxiety is common among primary care patients and whether it is associated with reduced functioning and well-being. While few studies have examined anxiety in the US primary care population, epidemiological studies in the general population have reported anxiety symptoms and disorders at prevalences of 6.6% to 14.9%,[20] higher than those estimated for depression.[1,2] An examination of the association between psychiatric disorders and chronic medical conditions in the general population found that only anxiety disorders, not depression or substance use disorders, were uniquely associated with chronic medical conditions.[11] Whereas there have been few studies that specifically examine anxiety symptoms and disorders among US primary care patients,[4,21] Dutch researchers observed a higher prevalence, lower recognition rate, and longer episode duration for anxiety than for depression among primary care patients.[3]

A related aim was to assess the frequency with which untreated anxiety is mixed with depression and whether patients with anxiety who report coexisting depression experience further reductions in functioning and well-being. The relationship between anxiety and depression—whether they constitute one disease or two or combine to form a third, distinct condition—is a subject of considerable unresolved debate.[22-29] Previous research has established that the overlap of anxiety and depression is more common at the subsyndromal level than in more severe cases that meet diagnostic criteria; thus, this overlap may be more common among primary care patients than among the patients with more severe cases seen in psychiatric care.[24,26] Other research has suggested that patients with more severe cases who have both anxiety and depression disorders have higher rates of health care utilization and greater impairment in social functioning than patients with pure anxiety or pure depression disorders.[26] In addition to constituting a large subgroup of primary care patients with anxiety who are in need of care, patients with both anxiety and depression may constitute a subgroup that primary care physicians should recognize and treat differently from patients with pure anxiety disorders. Patients whose anxiety coexists with depression may present with different symptoms than patients with anxiety alone and may require distinct treatment plans.[22,23,30] The primary purpose of this study was not to address that debate but to document the frequency and burden of depression among patients with untreated anxiety.

The present study addressed the following questions: (1) How common are untreated anxiety symptoms and disorders among primary care patients for whom mental health care is both accessible and covered by insurance? (2) To what degree is untreated anxiety associated with reduced functioning and well-being? (3) Is coexisting depression associated with further reductions in functioning among patients with untreated anxiety? (4) Are there demographic variables or comorbid physical conditions that can help identify patients with untreated anxiety who are likely to have the greatest reductions in functioning and well-being?

RESULTS

THE SCREENING PROCESS

The screening process is illustrated in **Figure 1**. During the 4-month study period, 10 190 patients were offered the waiting room screening questionnaire. Of the 78% (n=7914) who chose to respond, 20% (n=1607) were ineligible for the study because they (1) did not sign the consent forms (n=778), (2) did not have 6-month enrollment in the HMO or had dual benefits (n=548), (3) furnished incomplete responses (n=421), or (4) were not within the correct age range (n=209). Some respondents had multiple exclusions. Of the 6307 respondents eligible for further evaluation, 33%

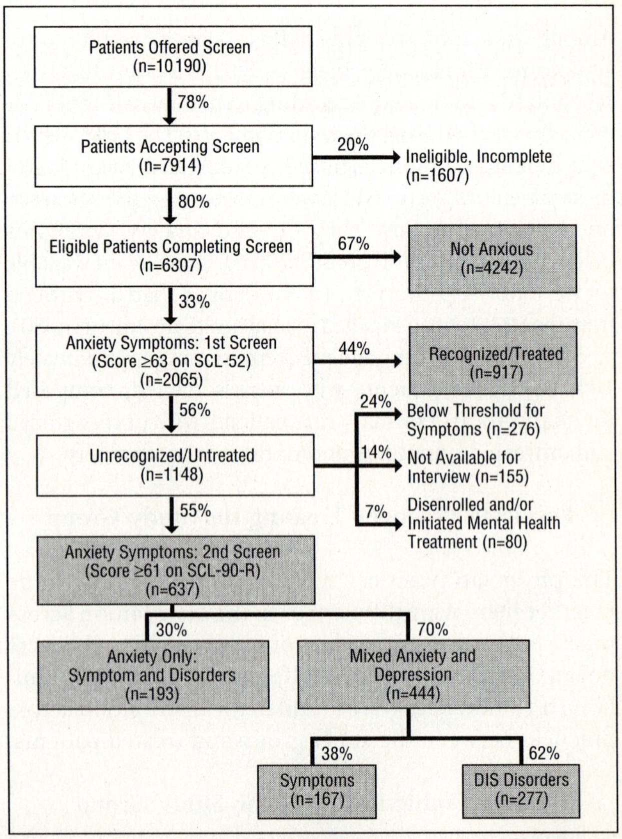

Figure 1. *Flow chart of sampling procedure. SCL-52 indicates Symptom Checklist 52; SCL-90-R, Symptom Checklist 90–Revised; and DIS, the Diagnostic Interview Schedule of the National Institute of Mental Health.*

Table 1. Demographic Characteristics and Symptoms

	Patients Who Were Not Anxious (n=4242)	Patients With Untreated Anxiety (n=637)	Patients With Treated Anxiety (n=917)
Gender, % (No.)*			
M	34 (1429)	44 (281)	30 (273)
F	66 (2813)	56 (356)	70 (644)
Age, y†	39.6‡ (10.8)	41.7‡§ (11.2)	40.4§ (10.3)
Anxiety symptoms (SCL-52)‖			
Highest anxiety subscale score†	54.4‡¶ (6.3)	68.4‡§ (5.7)	70.4§¶ (5.9)
Global Anxiety Score†	48.1‡¶ (5.8)	60.4‡§ (5.3)	62.0§¶ (5.4)
Symptomatic on 1 or more anxiety subscales, % (No.)*	...	71 (452)	77 (702)
Depression symptoms (SCL-52)‖			
Depression subscale score†	50.0‡¶ (9.3)	63.0‡§ (8.5)	64.4§¶ (8.7)

*$P<.05$ by χ^2 analysis.
†Values are mean (SD).
‡$P<.05$ by t test, adjusted for multiple comparisons, for the difference between patients who were not anxious and patients with untreated anxiety.
§$P<.05$ by t test, adjusted for multiple comparisons, for the difference between patients with untreated and treated anxiety.
‖Scores are adjusted for age and sex. The range is 31 to 81, with higher scores indicating worse symptoms. SCL-52 indicates Symptom Checklist 52.
¶$P<.05$ by t test, adjusted for multiple comparisons, for the difference between patients who were not anxious and patients with treated anxiety.

(n=2065) reported anxiety levels at or above the screening cutoff point (a score of 63). The remaining 4242 respondents, whose anxiety symptoms were below the cutoff point, constituted the "not anxious" comparison group.

Defining the Study Group

Among the 2065 patients whose screen results were symptomatic for anxiety, in 44% (n=917) anxiety had been recognized and treated, according to patient self-report or record review. Among the remaining 56% (n=1148), anxiety symptoms were unrecognized and untreated. Nearly half of these patients (45% [n=511]) were disqualified after the baseline interview because they (1) had anxiety symptoms below the second cutoff point (n=276), (2) were unavailable for the follow-up interview (n=155), or (3) had disenrolled from the HMO or had initiated mental health treatment (n=80). The remaining 637 respondents, representing approximately 10% of eligible patients who were screened, composed the study group of primary care patients with unrecognized and untreated symptoms and/or disorders of anxiety.

Physician Practices Treating the Study Group

The physician practices were examined to determine whether there were differences in the distribution across practices between the study group and patients who were not anxious. No significant differences were found. Similarly, no differences were found in the distribution across practices between the study group and treated patients.

Demographic Profile of the Study Group

The untreated anxiety study group was compared for gender and age with the 4242 patients who were not anxious who scored below the screening cutoff point of 63, as shown in **Table 1**. A χ^2 analysis indicated that the untreated anxiety group had a higher proportion of males and was slightly older than the not anxious group ($P<.001$ by t test).

CHARACTERISTICS OF THE STUDY GROUP

Anxiety Symptoms

The anxiety levels measured by the SCL-52 were substantially higher in the study group (mean score, 68.4) than in the not anxious control group (mean score, 54.4; $P<.001$) (Table 1). Patients with untreated anxiety also had a significantly higher Global Anxiety Score than the not anxious group ($P<.001$). This high Global Anxiety Score reflects the fact that 71% of the study group had elevated scores on multiple anxiety symptom subscales. Patients with untreated anxiety, however, had less severe symptoms than patients with treated anxiety (n=917) both on the highest anxiety subscale score and on the Global Anxiety Score ($P<.001$).

Depression Symptoms

The level of depression was significantly higher in the study group (mean score, 63.0) than in the not anxious control group (mean score, 50.0; $P<.01$) (Table 1).

Functioning and Well-being

Figure 2 shows that the levels of functioning and well-being were significantly lower on each of the eight SF-36 measures for the study group than for the not anxious control group ($P<.001$ by t test). The numerical differ-

ences in scores between the two groups of patients for each 100-point subscale ranged from 11.5 for physical functioning to 28.5 for role—emotional. The study group scored 77.2 and 60.0, respectively, for these two measures, and the not anxious control group scored 88.7 and 88.5, respectively. These values suggest markedly worse functional status among patients with untreated anxiety compared with patients who were not anxious.

Comorbid Physical Conditions

As shown in **Table 2**, comorbid physical conditions for the study group were within the ranges expected for primary care patients. While 68% of these patients reported some medical comorbidity, the mean (SD) number of comorbid physical conditions for the study group was only 1.3 (1.2) and ranged from 0 to 7. The most commonly reported conditions were arthritis (30%), hypertension (23%), and stomach diseases (16%). The presence of comorbidity was related to reduced health status as measured by the SF-36 subscales for physical functioning, pain, and general health perceptions. There was no association, however, between comorbid physical conditions and scores on the SF-36 subscales for mental health, social functioning, role functioning, or energy.

ACCOMPANYING PSYCHOLOGICAL SYMPTOMS AND DISORDERS

Most patients with untreated anxiety also reported additional psychological problems (Table 2). The mean score on the Global Severity Index, a measure of overall psychological distress,[40] was significantly higher (64.2±7.1, $P<.001$) than the normative mean for the general population (50±10).[33] This elevated Global Severity Index score is indicative of multiple severe symptoms associated with anxiety and depression.

Mixed Anxiety and Depression Symptoms

A high proportion (70%) of patients with untreated anxiety also reported elevated symptoms of depression, scoring 61 or above on the depression subscale of the SCL-90-R (Table 2). This score is equivalent to the cutoff point selected for clinically significant levels of anxiety and was chosen after reviewing normative and pretest data. These patients had a mean depression subscale score of 67.1, well above scores commonly used to identify levels of depression appropriate for treatment.[32,33]

Depression, Anxiety, and Substance Use Disorders

Over half of the study group patients (52%), included initially for symptoms of anxiety, were found to have diagnosable disorders of anxiety, depression, or substance use by Q-DIS-III-R evaluation (Table 2). Among these patients, more than half had multiple disorders. The most prevalent disorder, depression, was found in 25% of patients in the study group. Posttraumatic stress disorder was the most common anxiety disorder, diagnosed in 17% of the study group. Other anxiety disor-

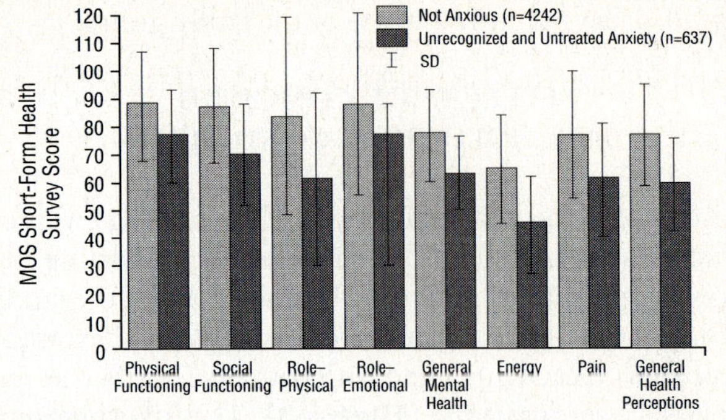

Figure 2. *Baseline adjusted mean scores for functioning and well-being on the Medical Outcomes Study Short-Form Health Survey (SF-36) for patients who were not anxious and patients with unrecognized and untreated anxiety. The scale runs from 0 to 100, and 100 is the optimal score. Scores are adjusted for sex and age.* $P<.001$ *by* t *test for all subscales.*

Table 2. Psychological and Comorbid Physical Conditions of Patients With Untreated Anxiety (n=637)

Comorbid physical conditions	
Patients, % (No.)	68 (436)
No. reported*	1.3 (1.2)
Mental distress (SCL-90-R)†	
Global Severity Index score*‡	64.2 (7.1)
Depression symptoms (SCL-90-R)†	
Depression subscale score ≥61, % (No.)	70 (444)
Depression subscale score*§	67.1 (5.3)
DIS disorders, % (No.)‖	
≥1 disorder	52 (335)
1 disorder only	24 (153)
Multiple disorders	28 (182)
Disorders reported, % (No.)	
Depression	25 (158)
Posttraumatic stress	17 (110)
Simple phobia	15 (94)
Social phobia	14 (89)
Agoraphobia	13 (83)
Generalized anxiety	9 (55)
Panic	5 (31)
Obsession	3 (17)
Compulsion	1 (7)
Alcohol/substance use	6 (42)

**Values are mean (SD).*
†SCL-90-R indicates Symptom Checklist 90–Revised.
‡Range, 44.75 to 81.0; higher scores indicate worse symptoms.
§This mean value is for patients who scored above the cutoff point of 61.0. Range, 61.0 to 81.0; higher scores indicate worse symptoms.
‖DIS indicates the Diagnostic Interview Schedule of the National Institute of Mental Health.

ders common in the study group were simple phobia, social phobia, and agoraphobia. Alcohol/substance use disorders occurred in 6% of the study group.

EFFECTS OF COMORBID PSYCHOLOGICAL CONDITIONS

To compare the relative impact on functioning levels of anxiety symptoms and disorders and of coexisting depressive symptoms and disorders, we divided the study group into three subgroups and compared these subgroups with each other and with patients classified as not anxious after screening (**Figure 3**). The first subgroup comprised patients with pure anxiety, those who reported symptoms and/or disorders of anxiety without coexisting depression. Both anxiety symptoms and disorders are included in this subgroup because no significant difference in SF-36 scores was reported by patients with pure anxiety symptoms and disorders. These patients with anxiety reported significantly lower functioning levels on six of eight subscales than patients who were not anxious. While they reported lower scores in all measures of physical and social functioning, patients with anxiety reported mental health and emotional functioning scores equivalent to those of the not anxious control group.

The second subgroup comprised patients who reported symptoms of both anxiety and depression but no DIS disorders. This subgroup is of interest because other research has found such patients to have impairment in social and work functioning despite their failure to meet criteria for disorder.[22,24] This subgroup is also of interest because it *roughly corresponds* to a category, mixed anxiety/depression, considered and declined as a new *DSM-IV* category.[41] Although it was declined, criteria were set to guide further research into the utility of this definition as a new official category. Our second subgroup met these *DSM-IV* criteria in having symptoms of dysphoric mood that persisted for over 1 month (our two screenings were over 1 month apart) and in not having any other mood, mental, or substance abuse disorder. While we do not know what proportion of this second subgroup also met the *DSM-IV* research criteria for no previous disorder or for various persistent accompanying symptoms, we do know that these patients as a group met the *DSM-IV* research criteria for significant distress or impairment in social, occupational, or other important areas of functioning.[19] Specifically, patients in this subgroup reported lower functioning levels than patients with pure anxiety on the five subscales measuring emotional functioning and well-being.

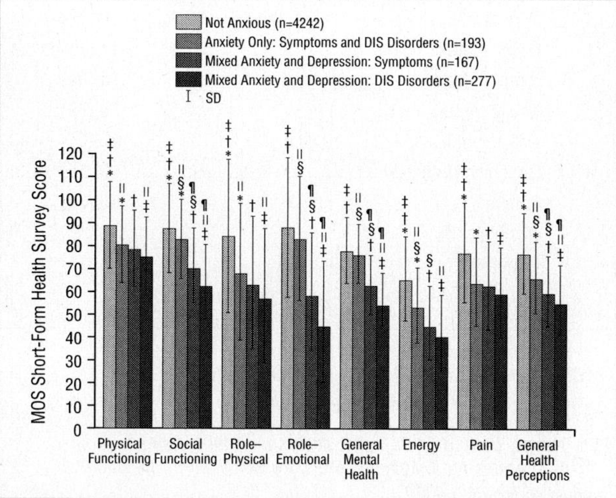

Figure 3. *Baseline adjusted mean scores for functioning and well-being on the Medical Outcomes Study Short-Form Health Survey (SF-36) for patients who were not anxious and three subgroups of patients with unrecognized and untreated anxiety. The scale runs from 0 to 100, and 100 is the optimal score. Scores are adjusted for sex and age. DIS indicates the Diagnostic Interview Schedule of the National Institute of Mental Health. Footnote symbols indicate significant differences (*P<.05*) by* t *test, adjusted for multiple comparisons, within each subscale.*

The third subgroup was symptoms of anxiety and depression with DIS disorders. This subgroup comprised all remaining patients with anxiety and coexisting depression who were found to meet the criteria for at least one DIS disorder and who would not, therefore, be considered part of the new diagnostic category for mixed anxiety and depression.[23,24] The most common combination (43% [n=119]) within this subgroup was anxiety disorders combined with depression symptoms. Patients in this third subgroup of anxiety and depression with a DIS disorder reported lower levels of functioning than patients in the anxiety and depressive symptoms subgroup on the four subscales measuring emotional and social functioning and energy.

As shown in **Table 3**, these three subgroups were similar in characteristics that often affect functional status, such as education, income, marital status, rates of self-reported medical comorbidities, and rates of debilitating illness, such as cancer, arthritis, and heart disease. The three subgroups were also similar in the mix of physician practice groups from which they received care. Findings for SF-36 functioning levels were controlled for differences in age and gender. Despite this, as shown in Figure 3, the three patient subgroups reported a clear pattern of progressively worse functioning levels. This progression of lower functioning levels was statistically significant on four subscales: social functioning, role—emotional, general mental health, and general health perceptions ($P<.008$ by t test). In the four remaining subscales, the same trend was observable but not statistically significant.

COMMENT

The purpose of this study was to determine whether untreated anxiety, alone or coexisting with depression, is common among primary care patients and whether it is associated with reduced functioning and well-being. Our

Table 3. Demographic Characteristics and Symptoms of Patients Who Were Not Anxious and of Three Subgroups of Patients With Untreated Anxiety

		Patients With Untreated Anxiety†		
	Patients Who Were Not Anxious (n=4242)*	Anxiety Only: Symptoms and DIS Disorders (n=193)	Mixed Anxiety and Depression: Symptoms Only (n=167)	Mixed Anxiety and Depression: DIS Disorders (n=277)
Gender, % (No.)‡				
M	34 (1429)	40 (77)	55 (92)	40 (112)
F	66 (2813)	60 (116)	45 (75)	60 (165)
Age, y§	39.6‖ ¶ (10.8)	42.9‖ # ** (11.4)	44.3¶ # †† (11.4)	39.2** †† (10.2)
Race, % (No.)				
W	NA	81 (156)	82 (138)	77 (214)
B	NA	1 (3)	1 (1)	5 (14)
Hispanic	NA	16 (31)	14 (23)	15 (41)
Other	NA	1 (3)	3 (5)	3 (8)
Education, % (No.)				
≤12 y	NA	34 (66)	28 (47)	32 (88)
13-15 y	NA	34 (66)	37 (62)	42 (118)
College (16 y)	NA	21 (41)	21 (35)	17 (46)
Graduate school	NA	10 (20)	14 (23)	9 (25)
Marital status, % (No.)				
Single, never married	NA	8 (16)	7 (11)	7 (20)
Married/living with partner	NA	79 (153)	80 (132)	75 (207)
Separated/divorced/widowed	NA	12 (24)	14 (23)	18 (50)
Family income (1990), $/y, % (No.)				
<20 000	NA	22 (43)	20 (34)	24 (67)
20 000-29 999	NA	17 (34)	22 (36)	18 (51)
30 000-39 999	NA	24 (47)	23 (39)	21 (57)
40 000-49 999	NA	9 (17)	12 (21)	16 (44)
≥50 000	NA	27 (52)	22 (37)	20 (56)
Comorbid physical conditions				
None, % (No.)	NA	30 (59)	30 (50)	33 (92)
≥1, % (No.)	NA	70 (134)	70 (117)	67 (185)
No. reported§	NA	1.2 (1.1)	1.4 (1.4)	1.2 (1.3)
Anxiety symptoms (SCL-52)‡‡				
Highest Anxiety Subscale score§	54.2 ‖ ¶ (5.6)	64.7 ‖ # ** (3.4)	68.4 ¶ # †† (5.2)	70.8** †† (6.3)
Global Anxiety Score§	47.9 ‖¶ (4.2)	55.8 ‖ # ** (4.2)	60.8 ¶ # †† (5.1)	63.3** †† (6.0)
Depression symptoms (SCL-52)‡‡				
Depression subscale score§	50.1‖ ¶ §§ (8.6)	54.7‖#** (4.5)	66.4 ¶ # (4.6)	67.2** §§ (6.2)
Mental distress (SCL-52)‡‡				
Global Severity Index score§	NA	57.5 #** (4.3)	65.5 # †† (4.8)	68.2** †† (6.4)

*NA indicates data not available.
†DIS indicates the Diagnostic Interview Schedule of the National Institute of Mental Health.
‡$P<.05$ by χ^2 analysis.
§Values are mean (SD).
‖$P<.05$ by t test, adjusted for multiple comparisons, for the difference between patients who were not anxious and patients with anxiety only.
¶$P<.05$ by t test, adjusted for multiple comparisons, for the difference between patients who were not anxious and patients with mixed anxiety and depression: symptoms only.
#$P<.05$ by t test, adjusted for multiple comparisons, for the difference between patients with anxiety only and patients with mixed anxiety and depression: symptoms only.
**$P<.05$ by t test, adjusted for multiple comparisons, for the difference between patients with anxiety only and patients with mixed anxiety and depression: DIS disorders.
††$P<.05$ by t test, adjusted for multiple comparisons, for the difference between patients with mixed anxiety and depression: symptoms only vs DIS disorders.
‡‡SCL-52 indicates Symptom Checklist 52.
§§$P<.05$ by t test, adjusted for multiple comparisons, for the difference between patients who were not anxious and patients with mixed anxiety and depression: DIS disorders.

results confirm both these suggestions and offer estimates regarding the frequency and functioning burden associated with untreated anxiety alone and anxiety coexisting with depression in primary care.

LIMITATIONS

Our findings are necessarily limited by the design of our study and also by the measurements we employed. To screen and

interview large numbers of patients, rather than clinician ratings, we employed a patient self-report survey to measure anxiety and depression symptoms and the DIS to assess disorders. We also relied on patient self-reports of comorbidities without measurement of severity of illness. Because the data presented here come only from screening and baseline assessments, we cannot comment on whether untreated anxiety among primary care patients and the reduced functioning status we associate with it are progressive or self-limiting or whether they tend to respond to or resist treatment. Longitudinal research is needed to determine the consequences of these patients remaining untreated vs receiving care. We studied only a working-age population within an HMO that offered benefits and coverage for mental health care. We are not able, therefore, to comment on the frequency of untreated anxiety or its associated health burden in several important populations for whom findings may be quite different: children, adolescents, and the elderly. The studied HMO appeared to offer broad mental health benefits, giving its beneficiaries unusually good access to mental health care, thus representing a provider system in which untreated anxiety should be unusually low. However, this HMO may present informal barriers to care (of which we are unaware) that may have discouraged physicians from treating mental health problems and may have discouraged patients from compliance with mental health interventions. Given the capitated nature of the HMO's contract with the mental health provider, however, the HMO had little incentive to discourage referrals.

FREQUENCY OF UNTREATED ANXIETY

We found that 10% of the adult primary care patients we studied had untreated anxiety. Despite this HMO's advantages in mental health care coverage and accessibility, in only 44% of anxious patients was anxiety recognized and treated. These treated patients were more likely to be female and were likely to have higher levels of anxiety than patients whose anxiety was unrecognized. These rates and profiles are similar to those reported for primary care patients with depressive symptoms and disorders.[6,11,16] This relatively low level of recognition and treatment suggests that affordability and access are not the only impediments to the treatment of psychological distress.[7] Other considerations not assessed here, such as physician skills or attitudes and patient acceptance, may also influence treatment rates.

In fact, our estimates of untreated anxiety in this HMO may be lower than the prevalence of untreated anxiety in primary care in general. First, we excluded from our study newly enrolled patients, who have been demonstrated to have unusually high rates of untreated emotional problems.[3,5] Second, our study site offered unusually good access to and reimbursement for mental health care and thus may have less untreated anxiety than providers in general. Although this site was a prepaid health plan and other studies have suggested that prepaid plans are less likely to recognize and treat for depression than a fee-for-service model,[17] these studies did not control for the extent of insurance coverage or for accessibility of mental health care. Thus, it seems likely that despite their prepaid status, our patients faced substantially fewer formal barriers to access and affordability than most primary care patients.

FUNCTIONING STATUS

In comparing patients who had untreated anxiety with patients who were not anxious, we found evidence that patients with untreated anxiety are not merely the "worried well" but have substantially reduced functioning and well-being and may have as much need for treatment as patients who present with chronic medical conditions. Our study group of patients with untreated anxiety reported functioning and well-being scores within ranges characteristic of patients who have chronic physical diseases.[42] These patients with untreated anxiety reported worse functioning and well-being across all measures than patients without anxiety, who themselves reported lower functioning status than a general population.[43] The dramatic difference between scores reported by patients with untreated anxiety and patients without anxiety suggests a clear impact of untreated anxiety—with and without depression—on health status. On the measure of general health perceptions, patients with untreated anxiety reported a score 18 points lower (60.3) than that of patients who did not report anxiety symptoms (77.9). A smaller difference of 13 points on this measure has been reported to be equivalent to the effect on a healthy person of developing diabetes or congestive heart failure.[44]

Marked differences in health status between the anxious and not anxious groups were found not only in emotional functioning and well-being but also in physical functioning. On the physical functioning scale, which assesses capacities to perform physical activities, patients with untreated anxiety reported a score 11.4 points lower than that of the patients without anxiety. A nine-point difference in a similar physical functioning measure has been shown to be equivalent to the effect of a healthy person developing arthritis or back problems.[42]

ANXIETY SYMPTOMS AND DIS DISORDERS

Our findings parallel reports on depression among primary care patients showing that patients with symptoms and disorders exhibit similar functioning burdens.[19,20] While the subgroup of patients reporting pure anxiety (unmixed with depression) had lower functioning levels than patients who were not anxious on scales measuring physical and social functioning, role—physical, energy, bodily pain, and general health perceptions ($P<.008$ by t test), there was no difference in functioning levels between patients with pure anxiety who

reported symptoms and those who reported DIS disorders. This finding suggests that, as with depressed patients, it is appropriate to evaluate anxious patients for treatment whether their condition is "only symptomatic" or is diagnosed as a disorder.

COEXISTING DEPRESSION

Patients who reported symptoms of both anxiety and depression were found to have significantly lower functioning levels than patients with pure anxiety. This subgroup corresponds to the category of mixed anxiety and depression, under consideration as a new diagnostic category. Our findings, then, support the position that in subsyndromal patients, mixed anxiety and depression carries sufficient impairment to warrant treatment, supporting the findings by other researchers of disability among such patients.[24] In measures of emotional functioning and well-being, these patients with subsyndromal anxiety and depression reported lower functioning than patients with anxiety disorders.

Greater reductions in functioning, however, were found in a third subgroup of patients who reported coexisting anxiety and depression with one or both conditions sufficiently severe to be recognized as a DIS disorder. These further reductions were reported in emotional and social functioning and in energy. Thus, if depression disorders are a common complication of long-term anxiety,[25,27] patients with untreated anxiety who develop these complications may be at risk for further impairment. It has also been suggested that depressive symptoms are a common and often unrecognized complication in anxiety disorders.[25] Our findings support this suggestion and indicate that such depressive symptoms are associated with reductions in health status beyond those associated with pure anxiety symptoms or disorders.

SCREENING FOR ANXIETY IN PRIMARY CARE

Our findings support the potential value of screening tools for both anxiety and depression in primary care. Although we screened only for anxiety, 70% of patients with untreated anxiety also had symptoms and/or disorders of depression. This prevalence of depression in patients with anxiety is higher than previously estimated[3] but resembles estimates for the prevalence both of depression among patients with panic disorder[45] and of anxiety among patients with depression.[22] This finding suggests that coexisting anxiety and depression may be more prevalent among primary care patients than anxiety alone. Even though a depression screen would presumably identify many of these patients with anxiety, our findings support the position that patients who report both conditions sustain an additional health burden and should be identified as having coexisting conditions. While the system used here, a double screen, would not be practical for use in primary care, more pragmatic screens are now being tested in clinical settings.[46,47] Recent work has validated a three-item screen for depression and suggests that similar brief surveys for anxiety and mixed anxiety and depression may also be feasible.[48] There are several new screening products, such as the Symptom Driven Diagnostic Screen–Primary Care (SDSS-PC)[46] and Primary Care Evaluation of Mental Disorders (PRIME-MD),[49] designed to alert physicians to patients at risk for anxiety with or without coexisting depression. Contrary to earlier studies in the general population,[50] we found that anxious patients have no distinct demographic or medical profile. Because of this lack of an identifying profile and the high rate of complicating psychological comorbid conditions, clinicians need assistance in both identifying and diagnosing anxiety in patients who commonly remain untreated despite their reduced functioning status.

Accepted for publication April 5, 1994.

This study was supported by a grant from the Upjohn Co, Kalamazoo, Mich.

This study was presented in a preliminary and incomplete form at the Sixth Annual National Institute of Mental Health Research Conference on Primary Care Mental Health Research, Washington, DC, October 20, 1992, and at the Third Primary Care Research Conference on Challenges in Practice-Based Research of the Agency for Health Care Policy and Research, Atlanta, Ga, January 12, 1993.

The authors acknowledge the helpful advice and comments of Meryl Brod, PhD, San Francisco Institute on Aging at Mount Zion Medical Center; Curtis J. Henke, PhD, University of California at San Francisco; Wayne Katon, MD, University of Washington at Seattle; Kathryn M. Magruder, MPH, PhD, National Institute of Mental Health, Rockville, Md; Anita Stewart, PhD, Institute on Health and Aging, University of California at San Francisco; Janet Williams, DSW, New York State Psychiatric Institute, New York; and Ed Yelin, PhD, University of California at San Francisco.

We also thank Ruth Calucin, MPH, who conducted the data analysis; Claudia Seastrum, MA, who coordinated data collection with primary care sites; Suzanne LeClaire, RN, who managed record reviews; Pierre Malek, MD, who assisted in recruiting sites for participation and in liaison with study arm physicians; and Suzanne Lessard and Megeen Egan, who prepared the manuscript.

Reprint requests to Technology Assessment Group Inc, Suite 201, 490 Second St, San Francisco, CA 94107 (Dr Fifer).

REFERENCES

1. Regier DA, Hirschfeld RM, Goodwin FK, Burke JD Jr, Lazar JB, Judd LL. The NIMH Depression Awareness, Recognition, and Treatment Program: structure, aims, and scientific basis. *Am J Psychiatry.* 1988;145:1351-1357.

2. Regier DA, Narrow WE, Rae DS, Manderscheid RW, Locke BZ, Goodwin FK. The de facto US mental and addictive disorders service system: Epidemiologic Catchment Area prospective 1-year prevalence rates of disorders and services. *Arch Gen Psychiatry.* 1993;50:85-94.
3. Ormel J, Koeter MWJ, van den Brink W, van de Willige G. Recognition, management, and course of anxiety and depression in general practice. *Arch Gen Psychiatry.* 1991;48:700-706.
4. Kessler LG, Cleary PD, Burke JD Jr. Psychiatric disorders in primary care: results of a follow-up study. *Arch Gen Psychiatry.* 1985;42:583-587.
5. Klerman GL, Budman S, Berwick D, Weissman MM, Damico-White J, Demby A, Feldstein M. Efficacy of a brief psychosocial intervention for symptoms of stress and distress among patients in primary care. *Med Care.* 1987;25:1078-1088.
6. Zung WWK, Magill M, Moore JT, George DT. Recognition and treatment of depression in a family medicine practice. *J Clin Psychiatry.* 1983;44:3-6.
7. DelVecchio Good MJ, Good BJ, Cleary PD. Do patient attitudes influence physician recognition of psychosocial problems in primary care? *J Fam Pract.* 1987;25:53-59.
8. Magruder-Habib K, Zung WWK, Feussner JR. Improving physicians' recognition and treatment of depression in general medical care: results from a randomized clinical trial. *Med Care.* 1990;28:239-250.
9. Shapiro S, Skinner EA, Kessler LG, Von Korff M, German PS, Tischler GL, Leaf PJ, Benham L, Cottler L, Regier DA. Utilization of health and mental health services: three Epidemiologic Catchment Area sites. *Arch Gen Psychiatry.* 1984; 41:971-978.
10. Wells KB, Golding JM, Burnam MA. Chronic medical conditions in a sample of the general population with anxiety, affective, and substance use disorders. *Am J Psychiatry.* 1989;146:1440-1446.
11. Hankin JR, Steinwachs DM, Regier DA, Burns BJ, Goldberg ID, Hoeper EW. Use of general medical care services by persons with mental disorders. *Arch Gen Psychiatry.* 1982;39:225-231.
12. Manning WG, Wells KB. The effects of psychological distress and psychological well-being on use of medical services. *Med Care.* 1992;30:541-553.
13. Katon W, Von Korff M, Lin E, Lipscomb P, Russo J, Wagner E, Polk E. Distressed high utilizers of medical care: *DSM-III-R* diagnoses and treatment needs. *Gen Hosp Psychiatry.* 1990;12:335-362.
14. Van den Brink W, Leenstra A, Ormel J, van de Willige G. Mental health intervention programs in primary care: their scientific basis. *J Affect Disord.* 1991; 21:273-284.
15. Wells KB, Burnam MA, Rogers W, Hays R, Camp P. The course of depression in adult outpatients: results from the Medical Outcomes Study. *Arch Gen Psychiatry.* 1992;49:788-794.
16. Magill MK, Zung WWK. Clinical decisions about diagnosis and treatment for depression identified by screening. *J Fam Pract.* 1982;14:1144-1149.
17. Wells KB, Hays RD, Burnam MA, Rogers W, Greenfield S, Ware JE. Detection of depressive disorder for patients receiving prepaid or fee-for-service care: results from the Medical Outcomes Study. *JAMA.* 1989;262:3298-3302.
18. Wells KB, Stewart A, Hays RD, Burnam MA, Rogers W, Daniels M, Berry S, Greenfield S, Ware J. The functioning and well-being of depressed patients: results from the Medical Outcomes Study. *JAMA.* 1989;262:914-919.
19. Broadhead WE, Tse CKJ, Sigmon A, Yarnall KSH, Burns B. *Services Outcomes of Minor Depression in Primary Care.* Presented as an abstract at the Sixth Annual National Institute of Mental Health International Research Conference on Primary Care Mental Health Research: Concepts, Methods, and Obstacles; October 19, 1992; Tysons Corner, Va.
20. Myers JK, Weissman MM, Tischler GL, Holzer CE III, Leaf PJ, Orvaschel H, Anthony JC, Boyd JH, Burke JD Jr, Kramer M, Stoltzman R. Six-month prevalence of psychiatric disorders in three communities: 1980 to 1982. *Arch Gen Psychiatry.* 1984;41:959-967.
21. Hoeper EW, Nycz GR, Kessler LG, Burke JD Jr, Pierce WD. The usefulness of screening for mental illness. *Lancet.* 1984;1:33-35.
22. Lydiard RB. Coexisting depression and anxiety: special diagnostic and treatment issues. *J Clin Psychiatry.* 1991;51(suppl):48-54.
23. Clark LA, Watson D. Tripartite model of anxiety and depression: psychometric evidence and taxonomic implications. *J Abnorm Psychol.* 1991;100:316-336.
24. Katon W, Roy-Byrne PP. Mixed anxiety and depression. *J Abnorm Psychol.* 1991;100:337-345.
25. Boulenger JP, Lavallie YJ. Mixed anxiety and depression: diagnostic issues. *J Clin Psychiatry.* 1993;54(suppl 1):3-8.
26. Wittchen HU, Essau CA. Comorbidity and mixed anxiety-depressive disorders: is there epidemiologic evidence? *J Clin Psychiatry.* 1993;54(suppl 1): 9-15.
27. Frances A, Manning D, Marin D, Kocsis J, McKinney K, Hall W, Kline M. Relationship of anxiety and depression. *Psychopharmacology.* 1992;106:S82-S86.
28. Wetzler S, Katz MM. Problems with the differentiation of anxiety and depression. *J Psychiatr Res.* 1989;23:1-12.
29. Zung WWK. The differentiation of anxiety and depressive disorders: a biometric approach. *Psychosomatics.* 1971;12:380-384.
30. Michels R, Marzuk PM. Medical progress: progress in psychiatry. *N Engl J Med.* 1993;329:628-638.
31. Derogatis LR, Lipman RS, Rickels K, Uhlenhuth EH, Covi L. The Hopkins Symptom Checklist (HSCL): a self-report symptom inventory. *Behav Sci.* 1974;19: 1-15.
32. Derogatis LR, Lipman RS, Covi L. SCL-90: an outpatient psychiatric rating scale—preliminary report. *Psychopharmacol Bull.* 1973;9:13-27.
33. Derogatis LR. *SCL-90-R: Administration, Scoring and Procedures Manual II.* Towson, Md: Clinical Psychometric Research; 1983.
34. Derogatis LR, Rickels K, Rock A. The SCL-90 and the MMPI: a step in the validation of a new self-report scale. *Br J Psychiatry.* 1976;128:280-289.
35. Mathias SD, Fifer SK, Mazonson PD, Lubeck DP, Patrick DL. The measurement of anxiety among adult primary care patients in a health maintenance organization using a newly developed global anxiety score. Presented as an abstract at the Sixth Annual National Institute of Mental Health International Research Conference on Primary Care Mental Health Research: Concepts, Methods, and Obstacles; October 20, 1992; Tysons Corner, Va.
36. Stewart AL, Sherbourne CD, Hays RD, Wells KB, Nelson EC, Kamberg CJ, Rogers WH, Berry SH, Ware JE. Summary and discussion of MOS measures. In: Stewart AL, Ware JE, eds. *Measuring Functioning and Well-being: The Medical Outcomes Study Approach.* Durham, NC: Duke University Press; 1992: 345-371.
37. Kovar M, Poe G. The National Health Interview Survey Design 1973-1984 and Procedures 1975-1983. *Vital Health Stat 1.* 1985:No. 18.
38. Marcus S, Robins LN, Bucholz K. *Quick Diagnostic Interview Schedule III-R: Version 1.0.* St Louis, Mo: Steven Msrcus; 1991. [Computer program.]
39. Robins LN, Helzer JE, Croughan J, Ratcliff KS. National Institute of Mental Health Diagnostic Interview Schedule: its history, characteristics, and validity. *Arch Gen Psychiatry.* 1981;38:381-389.
40. Wiggins S, Whyte P, Huggins M, Adam S, Theilmann J, Bloch M, Sheps SB, Schechter MT, Hayden MR. The psychological consequences of predictive testing for Huntington's disease. *N Engl J Med.* 1992;327:1401-1405.
41. American Psychiatric Association, Committee on Nomenclature and Statistics. *Diagnostic and Statistical Manual of Mental Disorders, Fourth Edition.* Washington, DC: American Psychiatric Association; 1994.
42. Stewart AL, Greenfield S, Hays RD, Wells K, Rogers WH, Berry SD, McGlynn EA, Ware JE. Functional status and well-being of patients with chronic conditions: results from the Medical Outcomes Study. *JAMA.* 1989;262:907-913.
43. Wetzler HP, Radosevich DM. *Health Status Questionnaire (SF-36) Technical Report.* Bloomington, Minn: InterStudy; 1992.
44. Kravitz RL, Greenfield S, Rogers W, Manning WG Jr, Zubkoff M, Nelson EC, Tarlov AR, Ware JE Jr. Differences in the mix of patients among medical specialties and systems of care: results from the Medical Outcomes Study. *JAMA.* 1992;267:1617-1623.
45. Katon W, Vitaliano PP, Russo J, Cormier L, Anderson K, Jones M. Panic disorder: epidemiology in primary care. *J Fam Pract.* 1986;23:233-239.
46. Blacklow R, Broadhead WE, Weissman M, Klerman G, Barrett J, Gross G, Coleman J. Symptom Driven Diagnostic System–Primary Care (SDDS-PC): a report of work in progress. Presented as an abstract at the Sixth Annual National Institute of Mental Health International Research Conference on Primary Care, Mental Health Research: Concepts, Methods, and Obstacles; October 18, 1992; Tysons Corner, Va.
47. Williams JBW, Spitzer RL. Prime-MD: a new system for the evaluation of mental disorders in primary care. Presented as an abstract at the Sixth Annual National Institute of Mental Health International Research Conference on Primary Care, Mental Health Research: Concepts, Methods, and Obstacles; October 18, 1992; Tysons Corner, Va.
48. Rost K, Burnam MA, Smith GR. Development of screeners for depressive disorders and substance disorder history. *Med Care.* 1993;31:189-200.
49. Spitzer RL, Williams JB, Kroenke K, Linzer M, de Gruy FV III, Hahn SR, Brody D, Johnson JG. Utility of a new procedure for diagnosing mental disorders in primary care: the PRIME-MD 1000 Study. *JAMA.* In press.
50. Murphy JM, Olivier DC, Monson RR, Sobol AM, Federman EB, Leighton AH. Depression and anxiety in relation to social status: a prospective epidemiologic study. *Arch Gen Psychiatry.* 1991;48:223-229.

Effects of the Menstrual Cycle on Dependent Variables in Mood Disorder Research

Ellen Leibenluft, MD; Patricia L. Fiero, MA; David R. Rubinow, MD

The purpose of this article is to review the literature on the effects of the menstrual cycle on dependent variables in mood disorder research to inform investigators which physiological measures are likely to be significantly affected by menstrual cycle fluctuations and precisely how they might be affected. The following variables are discussed: prolactin; growth hormone; the hypothalamic-pituitary-thyroid axis (including thyrotropin, triiodothyronine, and thyroxine); the hypothalamic-pituitary-adrenal axis (cortisol, corticotropin, and β-endorphin); melatonin; sleep; body temperature; and neurotransmitter activity (serotonergic and adrenergic systems). Body temperature and plasma and urinary norepinephrine vary predictably over the menstrual cycle. Prolactin and β-endorphin may have peaks in the periovulatory phase, whereas serotonin levels in platelet-poor plasma may reach a nadir at that time. Triiodothyronine, thyroxine, cortisol, and melatonin do not appear to vary systematically over the course of the menstrual cycle, whereas the data for growth hormone, thyrotropin, corticotropin, and sleep are inconclusive.

(*Arch Gen Psychiatry. 1994;51:761-781*)

Of all age groups, women between menarche and menopause are at the highest risk for affective illness.[1] In addition, one form of mood disorder, late luteal phase dysphoric disorder, is regularly associated with a specific phase of the menstrual cycle.[2] These observations indicate that the hormonal fluctuations of the menstrual cycle may contribute to the pathophysiology of mood disorders and that an understanding of the effects of the menstrual cycle on dependent variables in mood disorder research could help to elucidate the underlying neurobiology of affective illnesses. Furthermore, because most psychiatric investigators do not control for menstrual cycle phase, cyclic changes that occur in biological variables might explain some of the equivocal results that are so often encountered in the literature.

From the Clinical Psychobiology Branch (Dr Leibenluft and Ms Fiero) and the Section on Behavioral Endocrinology, Biological Psychiatry Branch (Dr Rubinow), the National Institute of Mental Health, Bethesda, Md. Ms Fiero is currently affiliated with the Department of Psychology, University of Virginia, Charlottesville.

Controlling for menstrual cycle phase in all clinical research studies would be prohibitively laborious and expensive. Therefore, it is important for investigators to know which physiological measures are likely to be significantly affected by menstrual cycle fluctuations and precisely how they are affected. This information can then be used to make informed decisions about whether and how menstrual cycle phase should be taken into account in study design. This article is intended to further this end by reviewing the existing literature on the variability over the menstrual cycle of commonly used dependent variables in mood disorder research. Although we acknowledge that the precise role of any of these variables in the etiology of depression remains unclear, we have selected them because they are frequently studied by mood disorder researchers. The variables that we will review are as follows: prolactin (PRL) levels; growth hormone (GH) levels; the hypothalamic-pituitary-thyroid axis (thyrotro-

pin [TSH], triiodothyronine [T_3], and thyroxine [T_4] levels); the hypothalamic-pituitary-adrenal (HPA) axis (cortisol, corticotropin [ACTH], and β-endorphin levels); melatonin levels; sleep; body temperature; and neurotransmitter activity (serotonergic and adrenergic systems). After reviewing the literature, we will discuss its methodological implications for mood disorder research and suggest appropriate research strategies.

METHODOLOGICAL ISSUES

Many studies have attempted to elucidate the effects of the menstrual cycle on the biological measures that are commonly examined in mood disorder research. However, these studies employ a variety of methods to select and study subjects and have produced inconsistent results. These inconsistencies limit our ability to generalize from the data obtained and highlight the importance of carefully evaluating the methods of each study. The following are specific issues that require attention.

Determination of Ovulation

Although most investigators attempt to establish the presence of ovulation in subjects prior to study entry, surprisingly few investigators attempt to establish when and even if ovulation occurs once the study is initiated. Instead, blood samples are identified in relation to the number of days since the onset of menstruation. This is problematic because, to accurately determine menstrual cycle phase, one must know not only when menses occurred but also whether and when ovulation occurred.

The menstrual cycle can be divided into three phases (follicular, ovulatory, and luteal), each of which has its own characteristic endocrine profile. The follicular phase begins on the first day of menses and ends roughly 36 hours before ovulation, with the onset of the luteinizing hormone (LH) surge. During the follicular phase, under the control of follicle-stimulating hormone, ovarian follicles develop and secrete ever increasing levels of estrogen. Progesterone levels during this phase are minimal (<4 nmol/L). At the end of the follicular phase, there is a sudden sharp increase in estrogen, which lasts for 1 day and initiates the subsequent surge in LH levels, which triggers ovulation. The ovulation phase then occurs over 2 to 3 days and includes the LH surge and the release of the mature egg from the ovarian follicle. Following ovulation, the remaining part of the follicle, the corpus luteum, secretes high levels of both estrogen and progesterone until it atrophies and estrogen and progesterone levels drop, the latter providing the signal for menstruation. Whereas the luteal phase duration is fairly consistent (mean, approximately 14 days), the follicular phase may be highly variable in length. Thus, without knowing whether and when ovulation occurred, one cannot know whether a blood sample obtained 15 days prior to menses is in the follicular, ovulatory, or luteal phase.

The timing of ovulation can most conveniently be determined by employing kits that use monoclonal antibodies to detect the high urinary levels of LH that occur during the LH surge. Subsequent blood samples can then be indexed to the day of the LH surge. An alternative method for detecting ovulation involves monitoring basal body temperature (BBT) because progesterone is thermogenic and causes an increase in BBT. However, compared with urinary LH monitoring, BBT monitoring is less convenient and less accurate because ovulation may occur without an increase in BBT and BBT readings must be obtained before the patient arises in the morning. The occurrence of ovulation (in contrast to its timing) can most easily be confirmed by obtaining plasma progesterone levels, which should be greater than 6 nmol/L during the luteal phase.

Interindividual Variation

As noted above, there is wide interindividual variation in the duration of the follicular phase and, therefore, in the total length of the cycle.[3] For this reason, studies that use a longitudinal research design and compare the same subjects at multiple time points are superior to those that compare different groups of women sampled at different phases in the cycle. Furthermore, investigators seldom evaluate more than 10 subjects per group in a given study. Given the interindividual variation both in the characteristics of the menstrual cycle and in the dependent variables, such small sample sizes may not provide adequate statistical power to detect even clinically meaningful differences at the significance levels reported.[4]

Circadian and Seasonal Rhythmicity

The time of day at which sampling occurs also demands particular attention because many of the dependent variables considered herein exhibit marked circadian rhythmicity. The timing of sample collection varies from study to study, and many investigators obtain only a single daily sample of the relevant dependent variable. Once-a-day samples may be inadequate for estimating mean plasma levels, given the episodic and pulsatile nature of hormonal secretion.

In addition to circadian rhythmicity, some hormones, such as PRL,[5] thyroid hormones,[6] and melatonin,[5] exhibit a seasonal variability that prevents direct comparisons between the results of studies occurring at different times of year. Except for a subset of those studying melatonin,[5,7-9] few reports disclose the season during which samples were collected. Other un-

controlled factors that may obscure the relationship between the menstrual cycle and the various dependent variables include the timing and length of sleep, the timing of meals and their macronutrient content, stress, and the intake of nicotine, alcohol, caffeine, or other substances.[10]

Inclusion Criteria

Although all studies considered herein use normal, healthy women, many studies do not elaborate further on their inclusion criteria; those that do, differ in the nature and stringency of their criteria for normalcy. Relatively few studies[11-17] screened out subjects with a history of psychiatric illness, and fewer still used standardized diagnostic interviews to make this determination.[13-16]

Given these methodological considerations, we included studies in our review if they met the following criteria:

1. Subjects were normal, healthy, spontaneously menstruating women who were studied in two or more menstrual phases. To obtain an adequate survey of the literature, we included studies that took samples from different women in different phases of the menstrual cycle, even though, as noted above, this study design has limitations.
2. Except where otherwise noted, ovulation was determined by observing the appropriate changes in BBT, levels of ovarian steroids (estrogen and progesterone), and/or LH levels.
3. Circadian variation was at least partially accounted for either by sampling during the same time period each day or by sampling at regular intervals over a 24-hour period.

In addition, studies were excluded from our review if they did not substantiate their inferences with statistical analyses or if they did not report when blood samples were drawn with respect to the menstrual cycle. These criteria were established as a minimal level of methodological soundness, but all of the factors mentioned in the preceding paragraphs should be considered when comparing the relative merits of the studies meeting these minimal criteria.

PROLACTIN

Baseline Secretion

Estrogen is thought to be a releasing factor for PRL,[18,19] acting at multiple sites to control the secretion of PRL from the anterior pituitary. Specifically, an estrogen response element on the PRL gene prompts transcription,[20,21] and estrogen can impair the ability of dopamine (DA) agonists to inhibit PRL synthesis.[22] Furthermore, estrogen increases the number of PRL-secreting cells in the pituitary gland[18] and inhibits the normal short feedback loop on PRL by suppressing hypothalamic DA secretion, thereby allowing sustained PRL secretion.[23] At least one study[24] shows that administration of estradiol to healthy men results in increased mean daily levels of PRL. Therefore, there is reason to suspect that PRL secretion may fluctuate with estrogen levels over the course of the menstrual cycle. In addition, a number of studies have demonstrated a close correlation between LH and PRL levels around the time of ovulation, so that the preovulatory LH surge is accompanied by a transient, twofold to fivefold increase in PRL levels.[25-29]

The circatrigintan, or monthly, variation of PRL is particularly difficult to evaluate for several reasons. First, because the highest levels of PRL are secreted during sleep,[30] it is optimal for studies to include blood samples drawn when patients are asleep. However, only eight of the 16 studies reviewed herein did so. Second, normal levels of PRL vary widely between individuals, introducing another source of variance into the data. Third, PRL secretion is highly responsive to environmental stimuli, such as exercise,[31,32] meals (especially those high in fat and protein),[33,34] stress,[31,35] sexual intercourse,[31,35] and possibly environmental light.[36] The studies reviewed herein varied in how they dealt with these potential confounds. Some, but not all, studies restricted patient activity,[25,37-41] standardized the 24-hour light-dark period[5,37,42] and mealtimes,[25,40,41] and attempted to standardize the timing and duration of sleep.[5,42]

Despite these methodological complexities, several generalizations can be made based on the studies listed in **Table 1**.[5,25,37,38,40-51] Of the 10 studies that measured mean levels of PRL in at least three phases (follicular, ovulatory, and luteal), five[41,47,49-51] found that PRL levels increased at midcycle. The magnitude of the increase varied from approximately 35%[49,50] to approximately 200%.[41,51] The other five studies[5,42,45,46] that measured mean levels of PRL in at least three phases found no significant differences between any two phases. These results are consistent with the studies cited above, which indicate that a short-lived peak in PRL levels occurs around ovulation, but this peak escapes detection unless the experimental conditions are optimal. In fact, two of the five studies that found no significant phase differences used only menstrual dates to determine menstrual phase and, therefore, may not have sampled at ovulation.[5,42] Three other studies[45,46] that found no significant phase differences and that used a physiological measure of ovulation found higher levels of PRL at ovulation, but the difference was not statistically significant. Furthermore, studies that did find significant phase differences grouped the data by phase before performing statistical analyses, whereas the two studies that did not find significant phase differences simply compared levels of PRL on each day of the cycle with every other day. Again, this suggests that there is a transient increase in PRL at ovulation.

The seven remaining studies[25,37,38,40,43,44,48] in Table 1 did not include a measure at midcycle and compared PRL levels in only the fol-

Table 1. Studies Comparing Baseline PRL Levels Across the Menstrual Cycle*

Source, y	No. of Subjects	Method of Determining Ovulation†	Phases of the Cycle Compared‡	Time of Day Sampled	Standardized Conditions	Results†§
			Multiple Samples Over 24 h			
Tennekoon and Lenton,[40] 1985	12	BBT, progesterone, menstrual dates	F (3 to 10)‖ L (17 to 27)‖	Every hour for 24 h in each phase	No daytime naps; standard mealtimes; restricted to bed	Evening rise in L > in F
Armeanu et al,[43] 1986	10	Urinary LH surge	F (−12 to −8)¶ L (5 to 11)¶	Every 2 h for 26 h in each phase	None stated	Mean levels for evening peak in L > in F; nocturnal and morning levels: no significant change
Brzezinski et al,[42] 1988	14	BBT, progesterone, menstrual dates	EF (1 to 7)‖ PO (13 to 16)‖ ML (21 to 25)‖	Every 2 h for 24 hr in each phase	Standard light-dark period, meal content, sleep period	No significant change (area under the curve; cosinor analysis)
Clifton et al,[38] 1988	5	BBT, progesterone for 1 cycle preceding study	EF (1 to 4)‖ LF (9 to 12)‖ ML (21 to 24)‖	Every 20 min for 24 h in each phase	Restricted to bed, no caffeine, no smoking	No significant change
Kivela et al,[5] 1988	12	Menstrual dates; LH measured but unclear if it was used to determine ovulation	EF (2)‖ LF (10)‖ PO (14)‖ LL (25)‖	Every 6 h for 24 h in each phase	Standard light-dark period, sleep period	No significant change
Tennekoon and Lenton,[41] 1988	17	BBT, progesterone LH, estradiol, menstrual dates	EF (−14 to −11)¶ MF(−10 to −6)¶ LF (−5 to −2)¶ PO (−1 to 1)¶ EL (6 to 9)¶ LL (10 to 14)¶	Every hour for 24 h in each phase	No daytime naps; standard mealtimes; restricted to bed	Daytime and 24 h means highest in PO
Caradente et al,[44] 1989	15	BBT, progesterone, menstrual dates	EF, LF, EL, LL	Every 2 h for 24 h in each phase	None stated	Mesor and afternoon rise higher in EL and LL than in EF; cosinor analysis
			Multiple Samples Over <24 h			
McNeilly and Chard[45] (study B), 1974	6	LH, FSH, estradiol, progesterone	F (6 to 8)‖ PO (14 to 16)‖ L (26 to 28)‖	Every 15 min for 9.5 h (9 AM-4:30 PM) in each phase	None stated	No significant change
Besset,[37] 1980	6	BBT and menstrual dates for previous 2 cycles	F (7)‖ L (21)‖	Every 20 min for 10 h (10 PM-8 AM) in each phase	Standard light-dark period, sleep period, constant temperature; restricted to bed	Mean F levels > L levels
Backstrom et al,[25] 1982	11 (6 F, 7 L)	Urinary pregnanediol (for subjects studied in L phase only)	EF (1 to 4)‖ MF (5 to 9)‖ LF (10 to 14)‖ EL (1 to 4)¶ ML (4 to 10)¶ LL (≥10)¶	Every 15 min for 6 h (9 AM-3 PM)	Restricted to bed during sampling period; standard mealtime for breakfast and lunch	Mean F levels > L levels

licular and luteal phases. Results of these studies were inconsistent. Two reported greater PRL levels in the follicular phase than in the luteal phase,[25,37] and one reported the reverse,[44] whereas other investigators found no significant difference between the two phases for 24-hour levels[38,43,48] or for the nocturnal surge.[40] One of the studies[37] that found higher mean PRL levels in the follicular phase than in the luteal phase also found that total sleep time was greater in the follicular phase; because sleep enhances PRL secretion,[30] these findings may be causally related.

In addition to the nocturnal peak in PRL secretion, a second, smaller surge has been observed in the late afternoon or early evening.[52] Three studies[40,43,44] in Table 1 sampled frequently enough to evaluate possible changes in this secondary peak in PRL secretion and reported the circadian rhythm that they observed. All three studies found no difference over the menstrual cycle in the height of the nocturnal peak or in the level of the nadir but did find an increase in the evening peak during the luteal phase. These results are particularly interesting in light of the fact that Linkowski et al[53] found that depressed men were more likely to demonstrate an early-evening peak in PRL

Table 1. Studies Comparing Baseline PRL Levels Across the Menstrual Cycle* (cont)

Source, y	No. of Subjects	Method of Determining Ovulation†	Phases of the Cycle Compared‡	Time of Day Sampled	Standardized Conditions	Results†§
One Sample Per 24 h						
Ehara et al,[46] 1973	11	LH, progesterone	All days	8 AM-12 PM, daily for 1 cycle	None stated	PO rise not significant
McNeilly and Chard[45] (study A), 1974	8	LH, FSH, estradiol, progesterone	All days of cycle	8 AM-10:30 AM, daily for 1 cycle	None stated	PO rise not significant
Franchimont et al,[47] 1976	14	BBT, FSH, LH, estradiol, progesterone during study cycle	PO (−2 to 2)¶ F (≤−3)¶ L (≥3)¶	8 AM-10 AM, daily for 1 cyclo	None stated	Mean levels highest in PO; L lcvcl>F lcvcl
Reymond and Lemarchand-Beraud,[48] 1976	10	LH, FSH	EF (4 to 6)‖ PO (14 to 15)‖ L (22 to 26)‖	9 AM-9:30 AM, once each phase	No OCs	No significant change
Vekemans et al,[49] 1977	51	LH	F (−11 to −2)¶ PO (−1 to 1)¶ L (2 to 11)¶	10 AM-4 PM, daily for 1 cycle	None stated	Mean levels highest in PO; L level>F level
Dada et al,[50] 1981	17	BBT from previous cycle, LH surge	F (−6)¶ PO (0)¶ L (6)¶	9 AM-11 AM, daily (except on alternate days for first 8 days) for 1 cycle	None stated	Mean levels highest in PO; LF level>EL level
Shi-Fan et al,[51] 1986	100	LH, FSH, estradiol, progesterone	EF (<−7)¶ LF (−7 to −3)¶ PO (0)¶ EL (3 to 7)¶ LL (>7)¶	4 PM-6 PM, daily for 1 cycle	None stated	Mean levels highest in PO

*PRL indicates prolactin; BBT, basal body temperature; F, follicular phase; L, luteal phase; LH, luteinizing hormone; EF, early follicular phase; PO, periovulatory phase; ML, midluteal phase; LF, late follicular phase; LL, late luteal phase; MF, midfollicular phase; EL, early luteal phase; and FSH, follicle-stimulating hormone.

†Gonadal steroids, gonadotropins, and dependent variables were measured in blood unless otherwise noted.

‡Numbers in parentheses refer to the day of the menstrual cycle when no attempt was made to synchronize cycles to ovulation, (see parallels footnote below) and to number of days from ovulation when cycles were synchronized to ovulation (see paragraph symbol footnote below).

§Analysis of variance or Student's t test was used to analyze data except where otherwise indicated. All results are statistically significant at the .05 level of significance unless otherwise indicated in the "Results" or "Phases of the Cycle Compared" column.

‖No attempt was made to synchronize cycles to ovulation; day 1 indicates the first day of menses.

¶Cycles were synchronized to ovulation such that day 0 corresponds to the estimated day of ovulation.

secretion than were male controls. Obviously, investigators attempting to replicate this finding in depressed women should control for the phase of the menstrual cycle.

Challenge Studies

Studies examining the PRL response to challenge across the menstrual cycle have yielded results that are consistent with those of the baseline studies in that those studies that looked for a difference at midcycle generally found it, in the direction of increased secretion. Thus, O'Keane and colleagues[54] reported a midcycle enhancement of the PRL response to D-fenfluramine, De Marinis et al[55] found a midcycle augmentation of the PRL response to GH-releasing hormone, and Reymond and Lemarchand-Beraud[48] found an increased PRL response to thyrotropin-releasing hormone (TRH) in the periovulatory phase. Holst et al[56] found that secretin infusions were capable of suppressing PRL but only during the follicular and luteal phases and not during midcycle. Hoehe[12] reported an increased PRL response to the opiate receptor agonist fentanyl during ovulation compared with that during menstruation; in a sample of five women, these differences were substantial but not significant, introducing the possibility of a type II error. The only exception to the general rule of midcycle enhancement is the study by Espinosa de los Monteros et al,[57] which used metoclopramide as a challenge agent and found no difference across the menstrual cycle.

Again, as with the baseline studies, those studies that do not include a measure around the time of ovulation generally have inconsistent results. Thus, one study reported an increase in the PRL response to melatonin during the follicular phase,[58] whereas another reported an increase during the luteal phase.[59] Infusion of either buspirone hydrochloride[60] or TRH[61] has been reported to cause an increased PRL response during the luteal phase compared with the follicular phase, whereas one study[62] found an increase in the PRL response to L-tryptophan infusion during the follicular phase compared with the luteal phase. Studies evalu-

ating the PRL response to haloperidol,[63] histamine,[64] and *m*-chlorophenyl piperazine[65] found no change across the cycle.

GROWTH HORMONE

Baseline Studies

Growth hormone is closely related to PRL structurally and phylogenically, and the two hormones exhibit many similar qualities. Like PRL, GH responds to a wide variety of influences, including exercise, physical and emotional stress, high-protein meals, hypoglycemia, changes in temperature, and sleep.[31,32,66,67] Also like PRL, the majority of GH is secreted during sleep, plasma concentrations are generally higher in premenopausal women than in men,[68] and estrogen levels influence the secretory pattern. For example, estrogen levels appear to correlate positively with both the peak level of GH and the area under the GH response curve following the administration of GH-releasing hormone.[69] Growth hormone has also been shown to increase in response to short- and long-term administration of estradiol.[24]

Our literature search revealed only six studies[37,70-74] of GH secretion over the menstrual cycle that met our minimal methodological criteria. Frequent sampling is particularly important for the accurate measurement of GH, which may be undetectable between secretory pulses. As outlined in **Table 2**,[37,70-74] only the study by Besset[37] performed frequent sampling. This study, which found that mean GH levels were higher in the follicular phase than in the luteal phase, is also the only one that sampled during sleep, when the majority of GH is released. In addition, these investigators screened out individuals who were more than 10% over their ideal body weight (GH levels are suppressed in obese patients[75]) or who were receiving medications, provided a standard light-dark period and constant temperature, and kept subjects in bed during the 10-hour nocturnal sampling period. However, this study is limited by its small sample size (n=6) and by the investigators' failure to correct for multiple comparisons.

Table 2. Studies Comparing Baseline GH Levels Across the Menstrual Cycle*

Source, y	No. of Subjects	Method of Determining Ovulation†	Phases of the Cycle Compared‡	Time of Day Sampled	Standardized Conditions	Results†§
			Multiple Samples Over ≤24 h			
Besset,[37] 1980	6	BBT and menstrual dates for previous 2 cycles	F (7)‖ L (21)‖	Every 20 min for 10 h (10 PM-8 AM) in each phase	Standard sleep period, light-dark period, constant temperature; restricted to bed	Mean F levels >L levels
Holst et al,[70] 1989	8	Progesterone, LH	F (≤−4)¶ PO (−1 to 1)¶ L (progesterone >25 nmol/L)	9 AM-10 AM, 2 samples 15 min apart on 9 d during 1 cycle	Supine position during sampling; overnight fast	No significant change
			One Sample Per 24 h			
Saxena et al,[71] 1974	6	LH, estradiol, progesterone	F (−11 to −1)¶ L (1 to 11)¶	7 AM-8:30 AM, daily in each phase	Overnight fast	No significant change
Genazzani et al,[72] 1975	5	LH, FSH for 2 prior cycles	EF (−11 to −6)¶ F (−3 to −2)¶ PO (−3 to 3)¶ L (5 to 14)¶	9 AM, daily for 2 cycles	Breakfast time	Mean level highest in PO; L vs F not significant
Guidoux et al,[73] 1986	6	LH, FSH, estrogen, progesterone	EF (1 to 6)‖ MF (7 to 10)‖ LF (11 to 13)‖ PO (14 to 15)‖ L (16 to 28)‖	Morning, daily for 1 cycle	None stated	Mean EF level < L level
Stone and Marrs,[74] 1991	9	LH, FSH, estradiol, progesterone	All days of cycle	8 AM-10 AM, daily for cycle	No intercourse during study cycle; no food or exercise in morning before blood was drawn	No significant change

*GH indicates growth hormone; BBT, basal body temperature; F, follicular phase; L, luteal phase; LH, luteinizing hormone; PO, periovulatory phase; EF, early follicular phase; FSH, follicle-stimulating hormone; LF, late follicular phase; and MF, midfollicular phase.

†Gonadal steroids, gonadotropins, and dependent variables were measured in blood unless otherwise noted.

‡Numbers in parentheses refer to the day of the menstrual cycle when no attempt was made to synchronize cycles to ovulation (see parallels footnote below) and to number of days from ovulation when cycles were synchronized to ovulation (see paragraph symbol footnote below).

§Analysis of variance or Student's *t* test was used to analyze data except where otherwise indicated. All results are statistically significant at the .05 level of significance unless otherwise indicated in the "Results" or "Phases of the Cycle Compared" column.

‖No attempt was made to synchronize cycles to ovulation; day 1 indicates the first day of menses.

¶Cycles were synchronized to ovulation such that day 0 corresponds to the estimated day of ovulation.

Four other studies[70,72-74] compared mean levels of GH in the periovulatory, luteal, and follicular phases. Two[70,74] of these found no significant differences in mean GH levels across the cycle, whereas the third study[72] found a peak in mean GH values at midcycle. The fourth study[73] found GH levels in the early follicular phase to be significantly lower than levels in the luteal phase. The remaining study compared mean levels of GH in only the luteal and follicular phases and found no significant difference between phases.[71]

Challenge Studies

Eleven GH challenge studies[12,55,76-83] met our criteria for review. Two studies evaluated the response of GH to GH-releasing hormone; both found no significant difference in the mean responsiveness of GH over two[76] or three[55] phases of the menstrual cycle. Using a high dose of the challenge agent, Evans et al[77] found no change in mean levels or in peak levels of GH response to GH-releasing factor 40 (a 40–amino acid fragment of GH- releasing factor) between the follicular and luteal phases. Similarly, Penalva et al[78] found no differences in the GH response to GH-releasing peptide 6, a synthetic compound that stimulates GH release on days 5, 12, and 20 of the menstrual cycle. Hinz et al[76] found no significant difference in desipramine hydrochloride–stimulated GH levels between the follicular and luteal phases in normal subjects, and Bancroft et al[62] found no significant difference in the GH response to L-tryptophan infusion in the follicular phase compared with that in the luteal phase.

Five studies[12,79-81,83] do show a circatrigintan variation in the GH response to challenge. Specifically, Knigge et al[83] showed an enhanced response of GH to TRH and gonadotropin-releasing hormone following histamine administration during the luteal phase compared with that during the follicular phase. Three studies, one each using clonidine,[79] an opiate agonist,[12] and arginine,[80] reported an increased GH response during ovulation compared with that during menstruation. O'Keane and Dinan[81] found that the GH response to pyridostigmine, a cholinesterase inhibitor that inhibits somatostatin release, increased steadily from the follicular phase to ovulation and the luteal phase. Taken together, these studies may indicate that the GH response to at least some challenge agents varies across the menstrual cycle, with the most robust response occurring in the luteal phase, followed by the ovulatory period, and with the lowest response occurring in the follicular phase and during menses. Clearly, many questions remain about the variability of GH baseline levels and the GH response to challenge over the menstrual cycle.

HYPOTHALAMIC-PITUITARY-THYROID AXIS

Baseline Studies

In addition to influencing the secretion of PRL and GH, estrogen also appears to modify the function of the hypothalamic-pituitary-thyroid axis.[10] Thyroid function is frequently altered during puberty, pregnancy, and menopause, and women show a greater TSH response to TRH than do men.[82] Estrogen appears to mediate these effects, perhaps by enhancing the response of TRH receptors in the pituitary thyrotrophs.[82,84] Estrogen also increases circulating levels of T_4-binding globulin, resulting in increased concentrations of total thyronines without a significant change in the unbound levels of these hormones.[10,82]

Only two studies obtained from the literature review met our criteria.[11,48] Therefore, to present a sufficiently comprehensive review of the literature, four studies that did not verify ovulation but instead used dates to estimate the phases of the menstrual cycle were included,[16,85-87] as was one study that did not state the time of day that blood samples were drawn[88] (**Table 3**).

The first study considered[86] was expressly designed to determine whether thyroid-related hormones exhibited a circatrigintan rhythm. These authors measured levels of T_3, T_4, and TSH between 7 AM and 11 AM daily for one menstrual cycle in 11 women and found no significant change across the cycle. Similarly, Sawin et al[88] found no difference in levels of T_3, T_4, and TSH measured in the follicular, periovulatory, and luteal phases of 10 women. Three other studies[11,16,85] also found no significant difference in the basal levels of TSH when they compared the luteal phase with the follicular phase, although two other groups[48,87] did report significantly higher TSH levels during the luteal phase compared with the follicular phase in 10 women. Thus, the preponderance of evidence on basal levels of T_3, T_4, and TSH suggests that the levels of these hormones remain relatively constant during the normal menstrual cycle. However, it should be noted that none of these studies included sampling of TSH at night, when the majority of TSH secretion occurs. Therefore, to our knowledge, a definitive study of TSH secretion across the menstrual cycle has not yet been conducted.

Several other thyroid-related variables have been evaluated for the presence of a circatrigintan rhythm. Rasmussen et al[87] have reported a significant increase in levels of serum thyroglobulin during the luteal phase compared with that during the follicular phase, whereas another study[89] found no significant change in T_4-binding globulin levels over the course of the cycle. Finally, three studies[87,89,90] observed systematic fluctuation in thyroid volume over the course of the menstrual cycle, but the pattern of the fluctuation differed from study to study.

Table 3. Studies Comparing Baseline HPT Variables Across the Menstrual Cycle*

Source, y	No. of Subjects	Method of Determining Ovulation†	Phases of the Cycle Compared‡	Time of Day Sampled	Standardized Conditions	Results†§
Weeke,[85] 1974	6	None	F (7 to 9)‖ L (19 to 21)‖	7 AM-9 AM, 2 samples 15 min apart	No OCs; subjects in supine position; fasting	No significant change in TSH level
Weeke and Hansen,[86] 1975	11	LH	All days of cycle	7 AM-11 AM, daily for 1 cycle	No medication	No significant change in TSH, T_3, or T_4 levels
Reymond and Lemarchand-Beraud,[48] 1976	10	LH, FSH	EF (4 to 6)‖ PO (14 to 15)‖ L (22 to 26)‖	9 AM-9:30 AM, 2 samples 15 min apart	No OCs	TSH level lower in L than in F
Sawin et al,[88] 1978	10	Estradiol, progesterone, LH	F (4 to 6)‖ PO (13 to 15 d before onset of next menses) L (5 to 7 d before onset of next menses)	Not stated	No OCs	No significant change in TSH, T_3, or T_4 levels
Roy-Byrne et al,[16] 1987	9	None	F (15 to 25 d before menses) L (3 to 7 d before menses)	8 AM-9 AM, 2 samples 15 min apart	No psychiatric or medical illness; no medication; fasting	No significant change in TSH level
Casper et al,[11] 1989	19	Progesterone	F (7 to 12)‖ L (20 to 27)‖	8 AM-4 PM, 1 sample	No history of psychiatric illness; no medications; no eating, drinking, or smoking on study days	No significant change in TSH level
Rasmussen et al,[87] 1989	11	None	Definition of phases not stated; measurements taken on cycle days 2, 9, 16, and 23 and on day 2 of next cycle	Morning, weekly for 1 cycle	No medication	TSH levels on day 2 < on day 23

*One or two samples per 24 h. HPT indicates hypothalamic-pituitary-thyroid; F, follicular phase; L, luteal phase; OC, oral contraceptives; TSH, thyrotropin; LH, luteinizing hormone; T_3, triiodothyronine; T_4, thyroxine; FSH, follicle-stimulating hormone; EF, early follicular phase; and PO, periovulatory phase.

†Gonadal steroids, gonadotropins, and dependent variables were measured in blood unless otherwise noted.

‡Numbers in parentheses refer to the day of the menstrual cycle.

§Analysis of variance or Student's *t* test was used to analyze data except where otherwise indicated. All results are statistically significant at the .05 level of significance unless otherwise indicated in the "Results" or "Phases of the Cycle Compared" column.

‖No attempt was made to synchronize cycles to ovulation; day 1 indicates the first day of menses.

Challenge Studies

Several investigators[11,16,48,85,88,91] have examined the TSH response to the infusion of TRH, looking for evidence of a circatrigintan rhythm (**Table 4**). Two groups[16,88] who measured TSH response to an infusion of 500 μg of TRH found no differences in stimulated TSH levels across the menstrual cycle. Four other studies[11,48,85,91] compared TSH levels following a 200-μg infusion of TRH. Two of these studies found no significant difference between the follicular and luteal phases when comparing peak TSH values in the 90-minute[11] and 120-minute[85] intervals following TRH administration. However, the other two studies[48,91] found an augmented TSH response in the follicular phase compared with that in the luteal phase. These contradictory results may be attributable to differences in the operational definition of TSH response. Groups that compared average TSH levels after the administration of TRH found significantly higher TSH levels in the follicular phase,[48,91] whereas investigators who used either maximum TSH values after the administration of TRH[11,85,88] or maximum incremental change in TSH concentrations[16,48] found no significant differences between menstrual phases. Interestingly, none of the studies analyzed differences in the area under the curve between cycle phases, a method that would take full advantage of the data.[92]

Two studies[93,94] observed TSH response to TRH following the administration of dopaminergic agents. The first study[93] considered the effects of DA agonists (bromocriptine and pergolide) on basal TSH levels and on TSH response to TRH in seven normally cycling women. The effect of the DA agonists was to suppress baseline levels of TSH in all phases (follicular, preovulatory, and luteal), and the degree of inhibi-

Table 4. Studies Comparing TRH Stimulation Test Across the Menstrual Cycle*

Source, y	No. of Subjects	Method of Determining Ovulation†	Phases of the Cycle Compared‡	Time of TRH (Sampling Intervals)§	Statistical Analysis	Results†¶
			200 μg of TRH			
Sanchez-Franco et al,[91] 1973	20 (10 F, 10 L)	LH	F (7 to 8)‖ L (21 to 22)‖	8 AM-10 AM, (−15, 0, 5, 10, 15, 30, 45, 60)	Student's *t* test on mean TSH values	F level>L level
Weeke,[85] 1974	6	None	F (7 to 9)‖ L (19 to 21)‖	7 AM-9 AM (−15, 0, 5, 10, 15, 20, 25, 30, 45, 60, 120)	Student's *t* test on peak TSH values	No significant change
Reymond and Lemarchand-Beraud,[48] 1976	10	LH, FSH	EF (4 to 6)‖ PO (14 to 15)‖ L (22 to 26)‖	9 AM-9:30 AM (−15, 0, 10, 20, 30, 45, 60, 120)	Student's *t* test on maximal increase in TSH and on the sum of TSH increments over all time points	No significant change in maximal increase in TSH level; for sum of TSH increments over all time points, EF level>PO level
			500 μg of TRH			
Sawin et al,[88] 1978	10	Estradiol, progesterone, LH	EF (4 to 6)‖ PO (13 to 15)‖ ML (5 to 7 d before expected onset of next menses)	Time of day not stated (−15, 0, 15, 30, 45, 60); two cycles	Student's *t* test on peak TSH values	No significant change
Roy-Byrne et al,[16] 1987	9	None	F (15 to 25 d before menses) L (3 to 7 d before menses)	9 AM (−30, −15, 30, 45)	Student's *t* test on maximal increase in TSH values	No significant change
Casper et al,[11] 1989	19	Progesterone	F (7 to 12)‖ L (20 to 27)‖	8 AM-4 PM (0, 15, 30, 45, 60, 90)	ANOVA and Tukey's test on peak TSH values	No significant change

**TRH indicates thyrotropin-releasing hormone; LH, luteinizing hormone; F, follicular phase; L, luteal phase; TSH, thyrotropin; FSH, follicle-stimulating hormone; EF, early follicular phase; PO, periovulatory phase; ML, midluteal phase; and ANOVA, analysis of variance.*

†Gonadal steroids, gonadotropins, and dependent variables were measured in blood unless otherwise noted.

‡Numbers in parentheses refer to the day of the menstrual cycle.

§Initial time is time of TRH injection. Numbers in parentheses indicate minutes before (represented by a negative sign) or after the TRH injection that blood was sampled for TSH levels.

‖No attempt was made to synchronize cycles to ovulation; day 1 indicates the first day of menses.

¶Analysis of variance or Student's t *test was used to analyze data except where otherwise indicated. All results are statistically significant at the .05 level of significance unless otherwise indicated in the "Results" or "Phases of the Cycle Compared" column.*

tion was significantly greater in the luteal phase than in the follicular phase. The TSH response to TRH was inhibited to the same degree in all three phases. In the converse paradigm, Seki and Nagata[94] infused metoclopramide, a DA antagonist, in seven normal women during the follicular and luteal phases of the menstrual cycle. Basal TSH levels were enhanced in all menstrual cycle phases, but the degree of enhancement was greater in the follicular phase than in the luteal phase. The results of both of these studies suggest either increased sensitivity to DA in the luteal phase or increased dopaminergic tone in the follicular phase.

HPA AXIS

Baseline Studies

A relatively large number of studies meeting our criteria examined HPA function across the menstrual cycle (**Table 5**).[12,14,15,71,72,95-101] For basal cortisol levels, the results were generally in agreement, with most studies finding no significant difference between cortisol levels in the luteal and follicular phases,[14,44,71,97,98] even in the one study that sampled nocturnally.[95] Similarly, most studies that examined basal cortisol levels in the menstrual and periovulatory phases[12] or in three phases (luteal, follicular, and periovulatory or luteal, follicular, and during menses)[15,99,101,102] found nonsignificant differences between phases. However, two studies[72,100] did find basal cortisol levels to be higher in the luteal phase than in the follicular phase, and one of these[72] found basal cortisol levels to be highest at midcycle.

The synthesis of ACTH, β-endorphin, and α-melanocyte–stimulating hormone results from the expression of the pro-opiomelanocortin gene.[103] The two studies[72,104] measuring basal levels of ACTH across the cycle have yielded conflicting results; Genazzani et al[72] reported the highest levels at midcycle compared with those during the follicular and luteal phases,

Table 5. Studies Comparing Baseline HPA Variables Across the Menstrual Cycle*

Source, y	No. of Subjects	Method of Determining Ovulation†	Phases of the Cycle Compared‡	Time of Day Sampled	Standardized Conditions	Results†§
Multiple Samples Over 24 h						
Steiner et al,[95] 1984	2	BBT during study cycle and previous cycle	F (9)‖ LL (26)‖	Every 30 min for 24 h in each phase	No premenstrual syndrome	No significant change in cortisol level
Caradente et al,[96] 1990	15	Progesterone, menstrual dates	EF, LF, EL, LL	Every 2 h for 24 h in each phase	None stated	No significant change in cortisol or DHEA-S level; cosinor analysis
Multiple Samples Over <24 h						
Graf et al,[97] 1989	6	BBT	F (3 and 4)‖ L (6 and 7)¶	Every 2 h for 16 h each night (6 PM-10 AM) of each phase	No OCs, standardized sleep period	No significant change in cortisol
One Sample per 24 h or Multiple Samples in 60 min						
Saxena et al,[71] 1974	6	LH, estradiol, progesterone	F (−11 to −1)¶ L (1 to 11)¶	7 AM-8:30 AM, daily in each phase	Overnight fast	No significant change in cortisol
Genazzani et al,[72] 1975	5	LH, FSH for study cycle and prior cycle	F (−7 to −4)¶ PO (−2 to 0)¶ EL (1 to 10)¶ LL (11 to 14)¶	9 AM, daily for 1 cycle	Breakfast time	Cortisol level highest at PO, L level>F level; for ACTH, PO level>L level, PO level>F level
Schoneshofer and Wagner,[98] 1977	28 (14F,14L)	Progesterone	F (progesterone <2 nmol/L) L (progesterone >10 nmol/L)	8 AM-9 AM in each phase	No OCs	No significant change in glucocorticoids or mineralocorticoids
Parker et al,[99] 1981	6	BBT, progesterone, LH	All days	8 AM-10 AM, daily for 1 cycle	None stated	No significant change in cortisol or DHEA-S levels
Hoehe,[12] 1988	5	BBT for 2 prior cycles	F (2)‖ PO (1)¶	8:30 AM-9:30 AM, every 30 min for 1 h in each phase	No medical or psychiatric history of illness; within 5% of ideal weight; no medications; no alcohol; standard sleep time; fasting blood sample	No significant change in cortisol levels
Rubinow et al,[15] 1988	9	Progesterone	F (M onset to ovulation) L (from ovulation to M onset)	7 AM-8 AM, on days 1, 5, 10, 15, 18, 21, 23, 25, 27 after menses onset	No psychiatric illness, fasting blood sample; no medications	No significant change in cortisol or DHEA-S levels
Rabin et al,[14] 1990	7	Progesterone	F (2 to 8)‖ L (21 to 27)‖	6 PM-9 PM in each phase	No premenstrual syndrome or other psychiatric disorder	No significant change in urinary free cortisol
Tersman et al,[100] 1991	15	Progesterone	F (5 to 7)‖ L (24 to 26)‖	8 AM-12 PM in each phase	No medication; no smoking in morning	Cortisol level in L greater than in F
Heitkemper et al,[101] 1991	18	Progesterone, estradiol	M (1 to 2) F (7 to 9)‖ L (−10 to −8)‖	Morning, in each phase	No IUD or OCs; no cardiovascular, gynecologic, gastrointestinal or renal abnormalities	No significant change in cortisol

**HPA indicates hypothalamic-pituitary-adrenal; BBT, basal body temperature; F, follicular phase; LL, late luteal phase; EF, early follicular phase; LF, late follicular phase; EL, early luteal phase; DHEA-S, dihydroepiandrosterone sulfate; L, luteal phase; LH, luteinizing hormone; FSH, follicle-stimulating hormone; PO, periovulatory phase; ACTH, corticotropin; M, menses; IUD, intrauterine device; and OC, oral contraceptive.*

†Gonadal steroids, gonadotropins, and dependent variables were measured in blood unless otherwise noted.

‡Numbers in parentheses refer to the day of the menstrual cycle when no attempt was made to synchronize cycles to ovulation (see the parallels footnote below) and to number of days from ovulation when cycles were synchronized to ovulation (see the paragraph symbol footnote below).

§Analysis of variance or Student's t *test was used to analyze data except where otherwise indicated. All results are statistically significant at the .05 level of significance unless otherwise indicated in the "Results" or "Phases of the Cycle Compared" column.*

‖No attempt was made to synchronize cycles to ovulation; day 1 indicates the first day of menses.

¶Cycles were synchronized to ovulation such that day 0 corresponds to the estimated day of ovulation.

whereas a more recent study by Mauri et al[104] found no difference in basal ACTH levels across the menstrual cycle. However, Mauri et al[104] did find that α-melanocyte–stimulating hormone levels were highest in the late follicular phase compared with those in the early follicular or early luteal phases. Circatrigintan variation in β-endorphin has been extensively studied because the opioid system inhibits hypothalamic gonadotropin-releasing hormone secretion and thus plays an important role in the regulation of the menstrual cycle.[105] Three studies[106-108] have documented a significant increase in plasma levels of β-endorphin around the time of the ovulatory LH peak. Two other studies that did not find a significant difference across the cycle nevertheless documented higher mean levels, as well as the greatest variance, during the periovulatory phase.[109,110] Tulenheimo et al[111] also did not find a significant difference across the cycle but sampled at considerably wider intervals than the other studies. Therefore, a number of studies suggest that plasma β-endorphin levels are increased in the period from approximately 3 days before to 1 day after ovulation. It is also interesting to note that Graf et al[97] found that β-endorphin secretion had a diurnal rhythm, with a peak from 6 AM to 10 AM, in the luteal phase only.

Challenge Studies

Like the baseline studies reported above, studies that examined the response of the HPA axis to challenge generally have not found differences in responsiveness over the course of the menstrual cycle. Two studies[112,113] found no differences in postchallenge dexamethasone cortisol levels in normal women who were studied in the follicular and luteal phases. However, one study[114] of women with major depressive disorder did report significant changes in the maximal postchallenge dexamethasone cortisol levels over the course of the menstrual cycle, with lower levels during menses and the follicular phase than during the ovulatory and luteal phases. Patient report of the onset of menses was used to date menstrual phase; the study did not include a normal control group and, to our knowledge, has not been replicated.

Other studies have examined the cortisol response to stress,[115] fentanyl,[12] L-tryptophan,[62] and exercise,[116] and the ACTH and cortisol responses to corticotropin-releasing hormone[14] across the menstrual cycle. None of these studies found significant differences between the follicular and luteal phases[12,14,62] or between follicular, periovulatory, and luteal phases.[115] One study[117] did find that 2-hour mean plasma cortisol and ACTH levels were higher in the luteal phase than in the follicular phase following a 10-mg morning dose of metoclopramide in 15 normal women.

MELATONIN

Baseline Studies

In seasonally breeding animals, the photoperiod regulates reproductive function. The photoperiodic signal is transduced by pineal melatonin secretion; because melatonin secretion is suppressed by light, levels of the hormone increase when the animal is exposed to a short photoperiod.[118] Thus, in summer-breeding mammals such as the hamster and rat, melatonin has been viewed as an antigonadotropic hormone, whereas in winter-breeding animals such as sheep and rhesus monkeys, melatonin stimulates activity of the hypothalamic-pituitary-gonadal axis.[119,120] There is some evidence that melatonin may modulate reproductive function in humans. Melatonin concentrations are higher in ovarian follicular fluid than in the surrounding serum, and in Finnish women, these concentrations are higher in winter (when the conception rate is relatively low) than in summer.[121,122] Melatonin levels are also elevated in amenorrheic women and in those receiving oral contraceptives,[9,42,123-125] and melatonin administration can inhibit ovulation.[126] Finally, there is evidence that melatonin can stimulate progesterone secretion by in vitro preparations of human ovary.[127,128]

A number of studies have examined variations in melatonin secretion over the course of the menstrual cycle (**Table 6**).[5,7-9,42,121,129-134] Studies that sampled once a day have yielded variable results,[8,133,134] but daily samples are insufficient to describe the important characteristics of the melatonin secretory profile (namely, onset time, offset time, and amplitude). Nearly all studies that sampled more than once in 24 hours found no change in melatonin levels across the menstrual cycle.[5,7,42,123,129,131,132] Of these, the study by Parry et al[131] is particularly notable because the patients were placed in dim light at 6 AM, thereby allowing measurement of the entire nocturnal melatonin curve. Only one study using multiple samples across 24 hours found a significant difference between phases: Webley and Leidenberger[130] reported that the area under the melatonin curve was significantly greater in the luteal phase than in the follicular phase and that the administration of exogenous progestins increased the melatonin secretion. Using a daily urinary sample of melatonin, Brun et al[9] also reported increased melatonin secretion in the luteal phase.

Several authors[7,135] have noted that the preovulatory LH surge tends to occur in the early morning, when melatonin levels are falling rapidly. However, a causal relationship between these events has not been established.[7,135,136] Our literature search was unable to locate any challenge studies for melatonin that met our methodological criteria.

Table 6. Studies Comparing Baseline Melatonin Levels Across the Menstrual Cycle*

Source, y	No. of Subjects	Method of Determining Ovulation†	Phases of the Cycle Compared‡	Time of Day Sampled	Standardized Conditions	Results†§
Multiple Samples Over 24 h						
Fellenberg et al,[129] 1982	2	Pregnanediol, estrone	F, PO, L; phases not defined	Twice daily between 7:30 AM and 9:00 AM and again at bedtime	No medications	No significant change in urinary melatonin levels
Webley and Leidenberger,[130] 1986	10	LH, progesterone, BBT	F, L; phases not defined	Every 4 h for 24 h in each phase	"Nightime" light 100-400 lux; sleep period: 12 AM-8 AM	For area under the curve, L level>F level
Kivela et al,[5] 1988	12	FSH, LH	(2, 10, 14, 25) in 2 cycles, 1 winter, 1 summer‖	Every 6 h for 24 h in each phase beginning at 6 AM	In dim room: 10 PM-8 AM; awakened for sampling	No significant change in mean melatonin levels
Brzezinski et al,[42] 1988	14	BBT, progesterone	EF (1 to 7)‖ PO (13 to 16)‖ ML (21 to 25)‖	Every 2 h for 24 h in each phase, starting at 1 PM	No medications; no IUDs; in dark room: 11 PM-7 AM; mealtimes standardized	No significant change in mean melatonin levels
Berga and Yen,[123] 1990	8	LH, FSH, progesterone, estradiol, ultrasonogram in LF	EF (−12 to −6)¶ LF (−5 to 0)¶ ML (4 to 9)¶ LL (10 to 13)¶	Every hour from 10 AM-5 PM and every 30 min from 5 PM-10 AM in each phase	No medications; in dark: 11 PM-7 AM; sleep period and mealtimes standardized	No significant change in timing, duration, height of peak, or area under the curve
Zimmerman et al,[7] 1990	8	LH, ultrasonogram in LF	EF (4)‖ PO (−1 and 0)¶	Every 4 h for 24 h in EF; every 4 h for 72 h in PO	No medications; "nightime" light <50 lux; sleep period: 12 AM-7 AM	No significant change in area under the curve
Parry et al,[131] 1990	8	LH, progesterone, estradiol	F (6 to 10) LF (10 to 14) ML (5 to 9 d after LH surge) LL (10 to 14 d after LH surge)	Every 30 min from 6 PM-9 AM, once in each phase	No recent history of medical or psychiatric illness; dim light <100 lux; eyeshades: 11 PM-7 AM	No significant change in melatonin for area under the curve, onset, offset, peak, or duration
Ito et al,[132] 1993	4	BBT	M LF (not defined) EL (not defined) LL (not defined)	Every hour for 24 h on third day in each phase	Constant temperature (20°C-24°C) and humidity (50%-70%); no daytime naps	No significant change in plasma melatonin levels
Single Sample per 24 h						
Wetterberg et al,[8] 1976	5	Progesterone, LH	3-day segments; synchronized to ovulation	Morning, daily for 1 cycle	No OCs	Peak melatonin levels were reached 12 days prior to ovulation
Brun et al,[9] 1987	9	LH, progesterone, estradiol	F, L; phases not defined	7 PM-7 AM, daily	No medications	For urinary melatonin, L level>F level
Cecchettin et al,[133] 1987	10	Progesterone, estradiol	Phases not defined	9 AM daily	None stated	Acrophase in EF (−98°)# by cosinor analysis
Fernandez et al,[134] 1990	20	FSH, LH, estradiol, progesterone	F, L; phases not defined	8 AM-9 AM, daily in each phase	None stated	F level>L level

**F indicates follicular phase; PO, periovulatory phase; L, luteal phase; LH, luteinizing hormone; BBT, basal body temperature; FSH, follicle-stimulating hormone; EF, early follicular phase; ML, midluteal phase; IUD, intrauterine device; LF, late follicular phase; LL, late luteal phase; M, menses; EL, early luteal phase; and OC, oral contraceptive.*

†Gonadal steroids, gonadotropins, and dependent variables were measured in blood unless otherwise noted.

‡Numbers in parentheses refer to the day of the menstrual cycle when no attempt was made to synchronize cycles to ovulation (see the parallels footnote below) and to number of days from ovulation when cycles were synchronized to ovulation (see the paragraph symbol footnote below).

§Analysis of variance or Student's t test was used to analyze data except where otherwise indicated. All results are statistically significant at the .05 level of significance unless otherwise indicated in the "Results" or "Phases of the Cycle Compared" column.

‖No attempt was made to synchronize cycles to ovulation; day 1 indicates the first day of menses.

¶Cycles were synchronized to ovulation such that day 0 corresponds to the estimated day of ovulation.

#Time of the menstrual cycle based on a 360° plot.

Table 7. Studies Comparing Sleep Variables Across the Menstrual Cycle*

Source, y	No. of Subjects	Method of Determining Ovulation†	Phases of the Cycle Compared‡	Time of Day Sampled	Standardized Conditions	Results†§
Ho,[144] 1972	3	LH, FSH	M F (7 to 9)‖ L (2 to 6 d before onset of next M)	EEG on 2 consecutive nights in each phase for 3 cycles	No illness; no medication	No significant change in REM sleep across the cycle; for total amount of stage 3 and stage 4 sleep, L level>F level, L level>M level
Patkai et al,[145] 1974	6	BBT	F (6 to 10)‖ PO (12 to 16)‖ EL (1 to 5)¶ LL (5 d prior to M onset)	Subjects self-rated quality and duration of sleep for 5 d/wk for 2 cycles	No OCs	Hours of sleep greatest in L and subjective quality of sleep lowest during L
Williams and MacLean,[17] 1980	9	BBT	Not defined	EEG on every third night for 1 cycle	No medication or psychiatric disturbance	No significant changes in sleep patterns
Parry et al,[13] 1989	8	Progesterone, BBT	Each cycle divided equally into EF, LF, EL, LL	EEG on 2 nights/wk for 1 cycle	No medical or psychiatric illness	Significant change in percentage of stage 3 sleep, minutes of stage 3 sleep, and No. of intermittent awakenings; no post hoc differences between phases
Lee et al,[146] 1990	13	Progesterone, BBT	F (3 to 10)‖ L (3 to 12 d before onset of next M)	EEG on 2 nights in each phase	No medications	REM latency shorter during L than F; no significant differences in latency to sleep onset or percentage of REM sleep
Ito et al,[132] 1993	7	BBT	M LF (not defined) EL (not defined) LL (not defined)	EEG on 2 nights in each phase	Constant temperature (20°C-24°C) and humidity (50%-70%); no daytime naps	Significant differences in amount of time in stage 3 and stage 4 sleep across phases

**LH indicates luteinizing hormone; FSH, follicle-stimulating hormone; F, follicular phase; L, luteal phase; EEG, electroencephalography; REM, rapid eye movement; BBT, basal body temperature; PO, periovulatory phase; EL, early luteal phase; EF, early follicular phase; LL, late luteal phase; OC, oral contraceptive; LF, late follicular phase; and M, menses.*

†Gonadal steroids, gonadotropins, and dependent variables were measured in blood unless otherwise noted.

‡Numbers in parentheses refer to the day of the menstrual cycle when no attempt was made to synchronize cycles to ovulation (see the parallels footnote below) and to number of days from ovulation when cycles were synchronized to ovulation (see the paragraph symbol footnote below).

§Analysis of variance or Student's t test was used to analyze data except where otherwise indicated. All results are statistically significant at the .05 level of significance unless otherwise indicated in the "Results" or "Phases of the Cycle Compared" column.

‖No attempt was made to synchronize cycles to ovulation; day 1 indicates the first day of menses.

¶Cycles were synchronized to ovulation such that day 0 corresponds to the estimated day of ovulation.

SLEEP

Several lines of evidence suggest that gonadal steroids may play a role in sleep regulation. For example, progesterone has been demonstrated to have soporific effects.[137,138] Menopause is frequently associated with a dramatic increase in sleep disturbance,[139] and exogenous estrogen replacement in menopausal women has been associated with increased sleep duration,[139] decreased sleep latency, and increased rapid eye movement (REM) sleep.[140] However, it is unclear whether these perimenopausal sleep disturbances are simply the result of awakenings caused by hot flashes. The one study[141] that addressed this question found that women awoke before the occurrence of the skin temperature changes caused by the hot flash, indicating that the thermoregulatory change and the awakening may be two distinct, centrally mediated events.

Given the possible etiologic links between sleep and affective illness[142] and between gonadal steroids and affective illness,[143] it is surprising that so little research has been devoted to the effects of gonadal steroids on the human sleep-activity cycle. Only six studies, which included a total of 46 patients, met our criteria for inclusion in this review (**Table 7**).[13,17,132,144-146] Two early studies[144,145] presented evidence that sleep disturbance and total sleep time are greater in the luteal phase than in the follicular phase. Specifically, Ho[144] reported more stage 3 and stage 4 sleep in the late luteal phase than in the menstrual or follicular phases

in three women, whereas Patkai et al[145] reported a greater average number of hours of sleep and greater subjective sleep disturbance during the late luteal phase than during the early luteal and early and late follicular phases in six women.[145] Two more recent studies,[13,132] however, supported the finding of increased awakenings in the second half of the menstrual cycle but found that stage 3 and stage 4 sleep was decreased at that time. Thus, Parry et al[13] monitored electroencephalographic sleep recordings of eight normal women two nights a week throughout one menstrual cycle. Analysis of variance showed that the percentage of stage 3 sleep, the minutes of stage 3 sleep, and the number of intermittent awakenings changed significantly over the four phases (early follicular, late follicular, early luteal, and late luteal). Although post hoc *t* tests revealed no differences in the pairwise comparisons, the direction of change was such that the number of awakenings increased in the luteal phase, whereas stage 3 sleep decreased in the luteal phase. Similarly, Ito et al[132] noted a significant decrease in stage 3 and stage 4 sleep in the ovulatory and luteal phases compared with that in the menstrual and follicular phases, along with a nonsignificant increase in the number of awakenings in the luteal phase.

Lee et al[146] reported decreased REM latency during the luteal phase compared with that during the follicular phase; to our knowledge, these results have not been replicated. Lee et al did not find a difference in sleep efficiency (total sleep time divided by time in bed) between the follicular and luteal phases, but the number of awakenings was not reported. In the study by Lee et al[146] and in other studies,[17,144] no significant differences were found across the cycle for the amount of REM sleep, the total sleep time, the sleep onset latency to stage 1 or stage 2 sleep, or the percentage of sleep time spent in the various stages of REM and non-REM sleep.

All of these studies were limited by small sample size and by the fact that the artificial conditions of the sleep laboratory may have distorted the subjects' normal sleep patterns. Nevertheless, few or no changes across the menstrual cycle were reported.

TEMPERATURE

In healthy individuals, body temperature fluctuates predictably over the course of a 24-hour period, with peak temperatures in the middle of the day and the nadir a few hours before waking. Temperature fluctuation as a function of ovarian cyclicity was demonstrated nearly 100 years ago, when Giles[147] showed that BBT was higher in the luteal phase than in the follicular phase in premenopausal women. As a likely mechanism for this phenomenon, progesterone administration increases body temperature in animals,[148-151] whereas estrogen administration has the opposite effect.[148,151,152]

Recent studies have documented clearly the relationship between the circadian temperature rhythm and the menstrual cycle. The results of the studies meeting our criteria (summarized in **Table 8**[153-159]) indicate that the 24-hour temperature minimum,[154,156,158] the 24-hour temperature maximum,[154,158] and the 24-hour temperature mean[154,155] are all higher in the luteal phase than in the follicular phase. Thus, both the nocturnal nadir and the daytime peak are higher in the luteal phase than in the follicular phase. However, because the increase in nocturnal nadir during the luteal phase is greater than the increase in the diurnal peak that also occurs in that phase, the amplitude of the temperature waveform is lower during the luteal phase than during the follicular phase.[155,158] Recent studies[157,159] performed under conditions that control for the effects of light, activity, and food intake on temperature demonstrate that the temperature rhythm is phase delayed (shifted later) in the luteal phase compared with that in the follicular phase.

Given the association between the luteal phase and increased temperature on the one hand and between depression and the luteal phase on the other, it is interesting that several studies[160] indicate that depressed patients may have higher nocturnal temperature nadirs than do normal controls. However, most of these studies do not control for phase of the menstrual cycle or for menopausal status.[161,162] In a study by Severino et al[158] that examined the relationship between nocturnal temperature, mood disorder, and menstrual cycle phase, women with late luteal phase dysphoric disorder had higher nocturnal body temperatures than did normal women in all phases of the menstrual cycle, but women with noncyclic dysphoria differed from normal controls only during the follicular phase of the cycle. As Severino et al note, these results demonstrate the importance of documenting menstrual status in studies of the relationship between nocturnal body temperature and mood in women.

NEUROTRANSMITTER ACTIVITY

Because each of the dependent variables discussed above is regulated by one or more neurotransmitter systems, all of the studies reviewed thus far indirectly reflect neurotransmitter activity over the menstrual cycle. In addition, a more limited number of studies attempt to examine directly whether the activity of individual neurotransmitter systems varies according to menstrual cycle phase. In particular, the serotonergic and adrenergic systems have received some study.

In animals, the effects of estrogen on the serotonergic system have been well documented and include modulation of serotonin (5-HT) synthesis, turnover, uptake, content, and

binding sites, as well as regulation (usually amplification) of responses to 5-HT (particularly 5-HT_{1A}) agonists.[163-166] In humans, a number of studies have assessed the serotoninergic system. Blum et al[167] demonstrated a decrease in 5-HT levels in platelet-poor plasma during ovulation compared with values during the follicular or luteal phases. Tam et al[39] compared platelet 5-HT uptake on days 1, 10, and 24 of three consecutive cycles and found increased uptake and decreased affinity on day 24. Ashby et al[168] reported that the inhibitory activity of an aqueous plasma fraction on platelet 5-HT uptake was greater when the fraction was derived from blood drawn in the premenstrual phase than in the postmenstrual phase in women with premenstrual syndrome but not in controls. However, the difference between phases in patients was significant only when the largest volume of plasma fraction (60 mL) was used, and each group contained only five patients. Furthermore, the inhibitory effect of the aqueous plasma fraction on 5-HT uptake in rat prosencephalon synaptosomes was greater postmenstrually in controls than in patients with premenstrual syndrome, for whom no effect of cycle was observed. Three studies of platelet imipramine binding[169-171] found no menstrual cycle phase effect on the number of binding sites or their affinity. In addition to the absence of consistency across studies, interpretation of the above noted findings is complicated by the uncertain relationship that exists between imipramine binding, platelet 5-HT uptake, and brain 5-HT regulation.

Estrogen inhibits monoamine oxidase activity in the hypothalamus and the limbic system of rats, an effect that is reversed by progesterone.[172,173] Consistent with these observations, two groups of investigators[174,175] reported that plasma monoamine oxidase activity was decreased during the time of the cycle when estrogen levels were high. In contrast, Belmaker et al[176] reported that peak platelet monoamine oxidase activity occurred during ovulation, with a nadir 5 to 11 days later. However, Belmaker et al note that

Table 8. Studies Comparing Temperature Variables Across the Menstrual Cycle*

Source, y	No. of Subjects	Method of Determining Ovulation†	Phases of the Cycle Compared‡	Time of Day Sampled	Standardized Conditions	Results†§
Caradente et al,[53] 1987	10	Progesterone, BBT, LH, FSH	EF, LF, EL, LL; phases not defined	Every 10 min for 24 h a day for 2 cycles except for menses	None stated	Circatrigintan rhythm identified (cosinor analysis)
Rogacz et al,[154] 1987	6	Progesterone, BBT, LH, estradiol	F, L; phases not defined	Continuous monitoring for minimum of 40 d	None stated	Maximum, minimum, and height of 24-h temperature wave, L level>F level (waveform analysis)
Lee,[155] 1988	13	BBT, progesterone	MF (3 to 10)‖ ML (4 to 12 before onset of next menses)	33 consecutive hours in each phase for 1 cycle	No medical or psychiatric illness	Higher mesor and lower amplitude in L than in F (cosinor analysis)
Rogacz et al,[156,157] 1988	10	Progesterone, BBT, LH, estradiol	F (3 to 6)‖ L (7 to 9)¶	Every hour for 40 h in each phase	Semirecumbent position in constant indoor light during monitoring	Average minimum 24-h temperature, L level>F level; rhythm phase delayed in luteal phase
Severino et al,[158] 1991	6	BBT, LH	EF (3 to 8)‖ LF (−3 to 0)¶ ML (−10 to −7)¶ LL (1 to 3 days prior to menses onset)	Every minute for 3 d in each of 4 consecutive weeks of 1 cycle	No medical or psychiatric illness; no medications	Maximum and minimum 24-h temperatures, L level>F level; amplitude, L level<F level
Veith et al,[159] 1993	8	BBT	F, L; phases not defined	Continuous monitoring for 7-10 d in each phase	Semirecumbent position in constant indoor light during monitoring for 2-3 days in each phase	Rhythm phase delayed in luteal phase

*BBT indicates basal body temperature; LH, luteinizing hormone; FSH, follicle-stimulating hormone; EF, early follicular phase; LF, late follicular phase; EL, early luteal phase; LL, late luteal phase; F, follicular phase; L, luteal phase; MF, midfollicular phase; and ML, midluteal phase.

†Gonadal steroids, gonadotropins, and dependent variables were measured in blood unless otherwise noted.

‡Numbers in parentheses refer to the day of the menstrual cycle when no attempt was made to synchronize cycles to ovulation (see the parallels footnote below) and to number of days from ovulation when cycles were synchronized to ovulation (see the paragraph symbol footnote below).

§Analysis of variance or Student's t test was used to analyze data except where otherwise indicated. All results are statistically significant at the .05 level of significance unless otherwise indicated in the "Results" or "Phases of the Cycle Compared" column.

‖No attempt was made to synchronize cycles to ovulation; day 1 indicates the first day of menses.

¶Cycles were synchronized to ovulation such that day 0 corresponds to the estimated day of ovulation.

platelet monoamine oxidase activity may reflect the hormonal milieu that existed up to 10 days earlier when the platelets were in the megakaryocyte stage.

Several studies of the adrenergic system show an increase in norepinephrine activity that begins shortly before ovulation and continues throughout the luteal phase. Of the eight studies that examined changes in urinary catecholamine levels over the menstrual cycle,[101,145,177-182] all but two[101,145] found that urinary excretion of norepinephrine was greater in the luteal phase than in the follicular phase. Five investigators[167,177,180,183,184] have demonstrated a similar pattern in plasma norepinephrine levels. In contrast, Santala et al[185] sampled only four times during the cycle and did not find variation in plasma norepinephrine levels. Several investigators[101,177,178,180,181] who also studied urine epinephrine levels found little or no consistent change across the menstrual cycle.

In contrast to the generally positive findings concerning levels of urine and plasma norepinephrine, studies of adrenergic receptor changes over the menstrual cycle have generally been negative. Five studies that examined platelet α_2-adrenergic binding [169,170,184,186,187] and two that examined β_2-adrenergic binding in lymphocytes and platelets[184,185] reported negative results. Two studies were positive: Stowell et al[170] reported a significantly higher number of lymphocyte β_2-adrenergic receptors in the follicular phase, whereas Jones et al[188] reported that the number of platelet α_2-adrenergic receptors was highest at the beginning of menstruation and decreased at midcycle.

Studies in animals suggest that gonadal steroids can modulate DA, γ-aminobutyric acid (GABA), and acetylcholine receptor function. Both inhibitory and stimulatory effects of estrogen on DA receptors in rodents have been described.[189,190] Ring A–reduced metabolites of progesterone are more powerful positive modulators of the $GABA_A$ receptor chloride ion channel complex than are the hypnotic barbiturates; progesterone also reverses the decrease in the number of $GABA_A$ receptors induced by estrogen in several estrogen-sensitive brain regions.[191,192] Finally, estradiol increases the number of muscarinic receptors in the hypothalamus.[193] However, to our knowledge, alterations in the characteristics of these receptor systems over the menstrual cycle have not been studied in humans.

SUMMARY AND CONCLUSIONS

Based on the literature summarized above and acknowledging that any conclusions must be viewed as preliminary, we would make the following methodological recommendations. These recommendations are particularly germane to studies with small numbers of subjects because investigators studying large samples of women might expect menstrual cycle phase to be randomly distributed in their sample. In the case of protocols for which the dependent variables are T_3, T_4, cortisol, or melatonin, the bulk of the literature indicates that menstrual cycle phase is unlikely to affect the results. On the other hand, investigators studying core body temperature or plasma norepinephrine levels should be aware that these variables have predictable and relatively well-described fluctuations across the menstrual cycle. When the dependent variable is PRL or β-endorphin, investigators who wish to eliminate menstrual cycle effects might do so if they avoid studying women in the periovulatory phase of the cycle because studies indicate that these hormones may have a peak in activity at that time. In addition, one study[167] shows that 5-HT levels in platelet-poor plasma may reach a nadir around ovulation, so, again, investigators of this variable may wish to avoid obtaining values at that time. Investigators measuring PRL levels in the late afternoon or early evening should be aware that PRL secretion during that time is probably somewhat higher in the luteal phase than in other phases of the cycle.

In the case of several other variables, the literature is either too limited or too contradictory to permit even preliminary recommendations. Growth hormone in particular requires more study. The available data indicate that both baseline GH levels and GH response to challenge may vary across the menstrual cycle. Studies also indicate that GH levels vary in relation to estrogen levels. Thus, it is difficult to justify ignoring menstrual cycle phase in studies of GH, yet the available data do not clearly identify fluctuations related to the menstrual cycle. Similarly, the literature leaves several important questions unanswered concerning TSH. There are indications that TSH response to TRH stimulation may be somewhat higher in the follicular phase than in the luteal phase. But the pattern of TSH secretion across the menstrual cycle both at baseline and in response to stimulation has not been well studied using highly sensitive assays and bearing in mind the circadian rhythm of TSH secretion. Also, as noted above, there have been surprisingly few studies of the effects of the menstrual cycle on the sleep-activity cycle.

Documenting menstrual cycle effects on any variable, including those related to receptor activity, is laborious work that requires frequent blood samples to be taken. Carefully designed studies are needed to further describe variations in the 5-HT, GABA, acetylcholine, and other neurotransmitter systems. Although there is extensive literature on HPA abnormalities in depressed patients, there has been little study of how gender, the menstrual cycle, or menopausal status may affect the incidence or physiological implica-

tions of these abnormalities. Such studies may be particularly important in clarifying the role of the HPA axis in affective illness because glucocorticoids and gonadal steroids can bind to the same receptors.[194] For example, Young et al[195] have demonstrated that luteal-phase progesterone levels can have antiglucocorticoid effects in normal women and that in depressed subjects, gender and menopausal status affect the degree of hypercortisolemia and dexamethasone resistance.

Certainly, mood disorder research is arduous enough without the added burden of having to schedule procedures at a particular time in a woman's menstrual cycle. In certain circumstances, however, accepting this added burden may ultimately lead to more conclusive and informative results. At the very least, all researchers should document whether female subjects are premenopausal and, if so, the cycle day on which procedures were performed. Investigators would then be able to do post hoc analyses of possible effects of the menstrual cycle on their data. In addition, subsequent literature reviews could pool data across studies and perform meta-analyses that would greatly increase our understanding of how the menstrual cycle affects the dependent variables in mood disorder research. Indeed, such analyses might contribute significantly to our understanding of the neurobiology of mood disorders.

Accepted for publication August 1, 1994.

We thank Thomas A. Wehr, MD, and Peter J. Schmidt, MD, for their comments on an earlier draft of the manuscript and Jason A. Seidel for assistance with manuscript preparation.

Reprint requests to Clinical Psychobiology Branch, National Institute of Mental Health, Bldg 10, Room 4S-239, 10 Center Dr MSC 1390, Bethesda, MD 20892-1390 (Dr Leibenluft).

REFERENCES

1. Robins LN, Regier DA. *Psychiatric Disorders in America: The Epidemiologic Catchment Area Study.* New York, NY: Free Press; 1991.
2. American Psychiatric Association. *Diagnostic and Statistical Manual of Mental Disorders, Revised Third Edition.* Washington, DC: American Psychiatric Association; 1987.
3. Treloar AE, Boynton FE, Benn BU, Brown BW. Variation of human menstrual cycle through reproductive life. *Int J Fertil.* 1967;12:77-126.
4. Cohen J. A power primer. *Psychol Bull.* 1992; 112:155-159.
5. Kivela A, Kauppila P, Ylostalo O, Vakkuri O, Leppaluoto J. Seasonal, menstrual and circadian secretion of melatonin, gonadotropins and prolactin in women. *Acta Physiol Scand.* 1988; 132:321-327.
6. Smals AGH, Ross HA, Kloppenborg PWC. Seasonal variation in serum T3 and T4 levels in man. *J Clin Endocrinol Metab.* 1977;44:998-1001.
7. Zimmerman RC, Schroder S, Baars S, Schumacher M, Weise H-C. Melatonin and the ovulatory luteinizing hormone surge. *Fertil Steril.* 1990;54:612-618.
8. Wetterberg L, Arendt J, Paunier L, Sizonenko PC, van Donselaar W, Heyden T. Human serum melatonin changes during the menstrual cycle. *J Clin Endocrinol Metab.* 1976;42:185-188.
9. Brun J, Claustrat B, David M. Urinary melatonin, LH, oestradiol, and progesterone excretion during the menstrual cycle or in women taking oral contraceptives. *Acta Endocrinol (Copenh).* 1987;116:145-149.
10. Yen SSC, Jaffe RB. *Reproductive Endocrinology.* Philadelphia, Pa: WB Saunders Co; 1991.
11. Casper RF, Patel-Christopher A, Powell A. Thyrotropin and prolactin responses to thyrotropin-releasing hormone in premenstrual syndrome. *J Clin Endocrinol Metab.* 1989;68:608-612.
12. Hoehe M. Influence of the menstrual cycle on neuroendocrine and behavioral responses to an opiate agonist in humans: preliminary results. *Psychoneuroendocrinology.* 1988;13:339-344.
13. Parry BL, Mendelson WB, Duncan WC, Sack DA, Wehr TA. Longitudinal sleep EEG, temperature, and activity measurements across the menstrual cycle in patients with premenstrual depression and in age-matched controls. *Psychiatr Res.* 1989;30:285-303.
14. Rabin DS, Schmidt PJ, Campbell G, Gold PW, Jensvold M, Rubinow DR, Chrousos GP. Hypothalamic-pituitary-adrenal function in patients with the premenstrual syndrome. *J Clin Endocrinol Metab.* 1990;71:1158-1162.
15. Rubinow DR, Hoban MC, Grover GN, Galloway DS, Roy-Byrne P, Andersen R, Merriam GR. Changes in plasma hormones across the menstrual cycle in patients with menstrually related mood disorder and in control subjects. *Am J Obstet Gynecol.* 1988;158:5-11.
16. Roy-Byrne PP, Rubinow DR, Hoban MC, Grover GN, Blank D. TSH and prolactin responses to TRH in patients with premenstrual syndrome. *Am J Psychiatry.* 1987;144:480-484.
17. Williams DL, MacLean A. Relationship between the menstrual cycle and the sleep of young women. *Sleep Res.* 1980;9:129. Abstract.
18. Cooke NE. Prolactin: normal synthesis, regulation, and actins. In: DeGroot LJ, Besser GM, Cahill GF Jr, Marshall JC, Nelson DH, Odell WD, Potts JT Jr, Rubenstein AH, Steinberger E, eds. *Endocrinology.* 2nd ed. Philadelphia, Pa: WB Saunders Co; 1989;1:384-407.
19. Goodman HM. *Basic Medical Endocrinology.* New York, NY: Raven Press; 1988.
20. Maurer R, Notides A. Identification of an estrogen-responsive element from the 5′ flanking region of the rat. *Mol Cell Biol.* 1987; 7:4247-4254.
21. Waterman M, Adler S, Nelson C, Greene G, Evans R, Rosenfeld M. A single domain of the estrogen receptor confers deoxyribonucleic acid binding and transcriptional activation of the rat prolactin gene. *Mol Endocrinol.* 1988;2:14-21.
22. Maurer R. Relationship between estradiol, ergocryptine, and thyroid hormone: effects on prolactin synthesis and prolactin mRNA levels. *Endocrinology.* 1982;110:1515-1520.
23. Cramer O, Parker C, Porter J. Estrogen inhibition of dopamine release into hypophyseal portal blood. *Endocrinology.* 1979;104:419-422.
24. Wiedemann E, Schwartz E, Frantz AG. Acute and chronic estrogen effects upon serum somatomedin activity, growth hormone, and prolactin in man. *J Clin Endocrinol Metab.* 1976;42:942-952.
25. Backstrom CT, McNeilly AS, Leask RM, Baird DT. Pulsatile secretion of LH, FSH, prolactin, oestradiol and progesterone during the human menstrual cycle. *Clin Endocrinol (Oxf).* 1982; 17:29-42.
26. Djahnbakhch O, McNeilly AS, Warner PM, Swanston IA, Baird DT. Changes in plasma levels of prolactin in relation to those of FSH, oestradiol, androstenedione and progesterone around the preovulatory surge of LH in women. *Clin Endocrinol (Oxf).* 1984;20:463-472.
27. Gonen Y, Casper RF. Transient hyperprolactinemia is associated with a midcycle luteinizing hormone surge. *Fertil Steril.* 1990;54:936-938.
28. Inaudi P, Reymond MJ, Rey F, Genazzani AD, Lemarchand-Beraud T. Pulsatile secretion of gonadotropins and prolactin during the follicular and luteal phases of the menstrual cycle: analysis of instantaneous secretion rate and secretory concomitance. *Fertil Steril.* 1992;58:51-59.
29. Tennekoon KH, Lenton EA. Synchronous secretion of LH and prolactin during the normal menstrual cycle. *Asia Oceania J Obstet Gynaecol.* 1993;19:101-107.
30. Sassin JF, Frantz AG, Kapen S, Weitzman ED. The nocturnal rise of human prolactin is dependent on sleep. *J Clin Endocrinol Metab.* 1973; 37:436-442.
31. Noel GL, Suh HK, Stone G, Frantz AG. Human prolactin growth hormone release during surgery and other conditions of stress. *J Clin Endocrinol Metab.* 1972;35:840-851.
32. Frewin DB, Frantz AG, Downey JA. The effect of ambient temperature on the growth hormone and prolactin response to exercise. *Aust*

J Exp Biol Med Sci. 1976;54:97-101.

33. Ishizuka B, Quigley ME, Yen SSC. Pituitary hormone release in response to food ingestion: evidence for neuroendocrine signals from gut to brain. *J Clin Endocrinol Metab.* 1983;57:1111-1116.
34. Quigley E, Ropert JF, Yen SSC. Acute prolactin release triggered by feeding. *J Clin Endocrinol Metab.* 1981;52:1043-1045.
35. Baulieu EE, Kelly P. *Hormones: From Molecules to Disease.* Paris, France: Hermann Publishers in Arts and Science; 1990.
36. Bispink G, Zimmerman R, Weise HC, Leidenberger F. Influence of melatonin on the sleep-independent component of prolactin secretion. *J Pineal Res.* 1990;8:97-106.
37. Besset A. Sleep-related GH and PRL secretion during the menstrual cycle in normal women. In: Tigu-Mures, ed. *Sleep 1978.* Basel, Switzerland: S Karger; 1980:189-199.
38. Clifton DK, Aksel S, Bremner WJ, Steiner RA, Soules MR. Statistical evaluation of coincident prolactin and luteinizing hormone pulses during the normal menstrual cycle. *J Clin Endocrinol Metab.* 1988;67:832-838.
39. Tam WYK, Chan M-Y, Lee PHK. The menstrual cycle and platelet 5-HT uptake. *Psychosom Med.* 1985;47:352-362.
40. Tennekoon KH, Lenton EA. Early evening prolactin rise in women with regular cycles. *J Reprod Fertil.* 1985;73:523-527.
41. Tennekoon KH, Lenton EA. Circatrigintan rhythm of prolactin. *Ceylon Med J.* 1988;33:57-61.
42. Brzezinski A, Lynch HJ, Seibel MM, Deng MH, Nader TM, Wurtman RJ. The circadian rhythm of plasma melatonin during the normal menstrual cycle and in amenorrheic women. *J Clin Endocrinol Metab.* 1988;66:891-895.
43. Armeanu MC, Frolich M, Lequin RM. Circadian rhythm of prolactin during the menstrual cycle. *Fertil Steril.* 1986;46:315-316.
44. Caradente F, Angeli A, Candiani G. Rhythms in the ovulatory cycle, I: prolactin. *Chronobiologia.* 1989;16:35-44.
45. McNeilly AS, Chard T. Circulating levels of prolactin during the menstrual cycle. *Clin Endocrinol (Oxf).* 1974;3:105-112.
46. Ehara Y, Siler T, VandenBerg G, Sinha YN, Yen SSC. Circulating prolactin levels during the menstrual cycle: episodic release and diurnal variation. *Am J Obstet Gynecol.* 1973;117:962-970.
47. Franchimont P, Dourcy C, Legros J, Reuter A, Vrindts-Gevaert Y, Van Cauwenberge JR, Gaspard U. Prolactin levels during the menstrual cycle. *Clin Endocrinol (Oxf).* 1976;5:643-650.
48. Reymond M, Lemarchand-Beraud TH. Effects of oestrogens on prolactin and thyrotrophin responses to TRH in women during the menstrual cycle and under oral contraceptive treatment. *Clin Endocrinol (Oxf).* 1976;5:429-437.
49. Vekemans M, Delvoye M, L'Hermite M, Robyn C. Serum prolactin levels during the menstrual cycle. *J Clin Endocrinol Metab.* 1977;44:989-993.
50. Dada OA, Ladipo OA, Osinusi BO, Osotimehin BO, Nduka EU. Circulating blood levels of gonadotropins and prolactin in the normal menstrual cycle. *Int J Gynaecol Obstet.* 1981;19:291-294.
51. Shi-Fan L, Zhong-Xing W, Yao-E Y, Sheng-Min B, Bei-Zhu Z, Jin-Zhi W, Yi-E W, Xin-Ying P. Hormone changes during the menstrual cycle of Chinese women. *J Reprod Fertil.* 1986;76:43-52.
52. Nokin WA, Vekemans M, L'Hermite M, Robyn C. Circadian periodicity of serum prolactin concentrations in man. *BMJ.* 1972;3:561-572.
53. Linkowski P, Van Cauter E, L'Hermite-Baleriaux M, Kerkhofs M, Hubaln P, L'Hermite M, Mendlewicz J. The 24-hour profile of plasma prolactin in men with major endogenous depressive illness. *Arch Gen Psychiatry.* 1989;46:813-819.
54. O'Keane V, O'Hanlon M, Webb M, Dinan T. d-Fenfluramine/prolactin response throughout the menstrual cycle: evidence for an oestrogen-induced alteration. *Clin Endocrinol (Oxf).* 1991;34:289-292.
55. De Marinis L, Mancini A, D'Amico C, Sambo P, Tofani A, Calabro F, La Brocca A, Barbarino A. Periovulatory plasma prolactin response to synthetic growth hormone-releasing hormone in normal women. *Metabolism.* 1989;38:275-277.
56. Holst N, Jenssen TG, Burhol PG, Haug E. Prolactin response to secretin during the spontaneous menstrual cycle in women. *Gynecol Obstet Invest.* 1991;31:37-41.
57. Espinosa de los Monteros A, Cornejo J, Parra A. Differential prolactin response to oral metoclopramide in nulliparous versus parous women throughout the menstrual cycle. *Fertil Steril.* 1991;55:885-889.
58. Terzolo M, Piovesan A, Osella G, Torta M, Buniva T, Paccotti P, Wierdis T, Angeli A. Exogenous melatonin enhances the TRH-induced prolactin release in normally cycling women: a sex-specific effect. *Gynecol Endocrinol.* 1991;5:83-84.
59. Webley GE, Lenton EA. The temporal relationship between melatonin and prolactin in women. *Fertil Steril.* 1987;48:218-222.
60. Dinan T, Siobhan B, Yatham L, Mobayed M, O'Hanlon M. The reproducibility of the prolactin response to buspirone: relationship to the menstrual cycle. *Int Clin Psychopharmacol.* 1990;5:119-123.
61. Boyd AE III, Sanchez-Franco F. Changes in prolactin response to thyrotropin-releasing-hormone (TRH) during the menstrual cycle of normal women. *J Clin Endocrinol Metab.* 1976;44:985-989.
62. Bancroft J, Cook A, Davidson D, Bennie J, Goodwin G. Blunting of neuroendocrine responses to infusion of L-tryptophan in women with perimenstrual mood change. *Psychol Med.* 1991;21:305-312.
63. Asnis GM, Sachar DJ, Langer G, Tabrizi MA, Nathan RS, Halpern FS, Halbreich U. Prolactin responses to haloperidol in normal young women. *Psychoneuroendocrinology.* 1988;13:515-520.
64. Knigge U, Benedikte T, Flemming W, Svenstrup B, Christiansen P. Effect of histamine on basal and TRH/LH-RH-stimulated PRL and LH secretion during different phases of the menstrual cycle in normal women. *Neuroendocrinology.* 1985;41:337-341.
65. Su T. Effects of m-CPP in PMS. In: New research program and abstracts of the meeting of the American Psychiatric Association; May 22-27, 1993; San Francisco, Calif. Abstract NR514.
66. Friesen H, Hwang P, Guyda H, Tolis G, Tyson J, Meyers R. A radioimmunoassay for human prolactin. In: Boyns AR, Griffiths K, eds. *Prolactin and Carcinogenesis.* Cardiff, Wales: Alpha Omega Alpha; 1972:64-80.
67. Martin JB. Brain regulation of growth hormone secretion. In: Martini L, Ganong WF, eds. *Frontiers in Neuroendocrinology.* New York, NY: Raven Press; 1976;4:129-168.
68. Ho KY, Evans WS, Blizzard RM, Veldhuis JD, Merriam GR, Samojlik E, Furlanetto R, Rogol AD, Kaiser DL, Thorner MO. Effects of sex and age on the 24-hour profile of growth hormone secretion in man: importance of endogenous estradiol concentrations. *J Clin Endocrinol Metab.* 1987;64:51-58.
69. Lang I, Schernthaner G, Pietschmann P, Kurz R, Stephenson JM, Templ H. Effects of sex and age on growth hormone response to growth hormone-releasing hormone in healthy individuals. *J Clin Endocrinol Metab.* 1987;65:535-540.
70. Holst N, Jenssen TG, Burhol PG, Haug E, Forsdahl F. Plasma gastrointestinal hormones during spontaneous and induced menstrual cycles. *J Clin Endocrinol Metab.* 1989;68:1160-1166.
71. Saxena BN, Dusitsin N, Lazarus L. Human growth hormone (HGH), thyroid stimulating hormone (TSH) and cortisol levels in the serum of menstruating Thai women. *J Obstet Gynaecol Br Commonwealth.* 1974;81:563-567.
72. Genazzani AR, Lemarchand-Beraud TH, Aubert ML, Felber JP. Pattern of plasma ACTH, hGH, and cortisol during menstrual cycle. *J Clin Endocrinol Metab.* 1975;41:431-437.
73. Guidoux S, Garnier PIE, Schimpff RM. Effect of the variations of female sex hormones during the menstrual cycle upon serum somatomedin and growth-promoting activity. *Horm Res.* 1986;23:31-37.
74. Stone BA, Marrs RP. Growth hormone in serum of women during the menstrual cycle and during controlled ovarian hyperstimulation. *Fertil Steril.* 1991;56:52-58.
75. Daughaday W. Growth hormone: normal synthesis, secretion, control, and mechanisms of action. In: de Groot L, ed. *Endocrinology.* Philadelphia, Pa: WB Saunders Co; 1989:318-329.
76. Hinz A, Laakmann G, Kropp F, Dick G. Influence of growth hormone releasing hormone (GHRH) on the growth hormone (GH) secretion in healthy female and male subjects. *Pharmacopsychiatry.* 1988;21:445-446.
77. Evans WS, Borges JLC, Vance ML, Kaiser D, Rogol AD, Furlanetto R, Rivier J, Vale W, Thorner M. Effects of human pancreatic growth hormone-releasing factor-40 on serum growth hormone, prolactin, luteinizing hormone, follicle-stimulating hormone, and somatomedin-C concentrations in normal women throughout the menstrual cycle. *J Clin Endocrinol Metab.* 1984;59:1006-1010.
78. Penalva A, Pombo M, Carballo A, Barreiro J, Casanueva FF, Dieguez C. Influence of sex, age and adrenergic pathways on the growth hor-

mone response to GHRP-6. *Clin Endocrinol (Oxf)* 1993;38:87-91.

79. Matussek N, Ackenheil M, Herz M. The dependence of the clonidine growth hormone test on alcohol drinking habits and the menstrual cycle. *Psychoneuroendocrinology*. 1984;9:173-177.
80. Merimee TJ, Fineberg SE. Studies of the sex-based variation of human growth hormone secretion. *J Clin Endocrinol.* 1971;33:896-902.
81. O'Keane V, Dinan TG. Sex steroid priming effects on growth hormone response to pyridostigmine throughout the menstrual cycle. *J Clin Endocrinol Metab.* 1992;75:11-14.
82. Larsen PR, Ingbar SH. The thyroid gland. In: Wilson JD, Foster DW, eds. *Williams Textbook of Endocrinology*. Philadelphia, Pa: WB Saunders Co; 1992:357-487.
83. Knigge U, Thuesen B, Dejgaard A, Svenstrup B, Bennett P. Histamine-induced paradoxical GH response to TRH/GnRH in men and women: dependence on gonadal steroid hormones. *Acta Endocrinol (Copenh)*. 1990;122:354-360.
84. De Lean A, Ferland L, Drouin J, Kelly PA, Labrie F. Modulation of pituitary thyrotropin releasing hormone receptor levels by estrogens and thyroid hormones. *Endocrinology.* 1977; 100:1496-1504.
85. Weeke J. Thyrotropin response to thyrotropin releasing hormone in normal subjects. *Eur J Clin Invest.* 1974;4:29-32.
86. Weeke J, Hansen AP. Serum TSH and serum T3 levels during normal menstrual cycles and during cycles on oral contraceptives. *Acta Endocrinol (Copenh).* 1975;79:431-438.
87. Rasmussen NG, Hornnes PJ, Hegedus L, Feldt-Rasmussen U. Serum thyroglobulin during the menstrual cycle, during pregnancy, and post partum. *Acta Endocrinol (Copenh).* 1989;121: 168-173.
88. Sawin CT, Hershinan JM, Boyd AE, Longcope C, Bacharach P. The relationship of changes in serum estradiol and progesterone during the menstrual cycle to the thyrotropin and prolactin responses to thryotropin-releasing hormone. *J Clin Endocrinol Metab.* 1978;47:1296-1302.
89. Hegedus L, Karstrup S, Rasmussen N. Evidence of cyclic alterations of thyroid size during the menstrual cycle in healthy women. *J Obstet Gynecol.* 1986;155:142-145.
90. De Remigis P, Raggiunti B, Nepa A, Giandonato S, Faraone G, Sensi S. Thyroid volume variation during the menstrual cycle in healthy subjects. In: International Society for Chronobiology, ed. *Chronobiology: Its Role in Clinical Medicine, General Biology, and Agriculture.* New York, NY: Wiley-Liss Inc; 1990:169-173.
91. Sanchez-Franco F, Garcia MD, Cacicedo L, Martin-Zurro A, Escobar Del Rey F. Influence of sex phase of the menstrual cycle on thyrotropin (TSH) response to thyrotropin-releasing hormone (TRH). *J Clin Endocrinol Metab.* 1973; 37:736-740.
92. de Mendonca Lirna CA, Vandel S, Bizouard P. The thyrotropin-releasing hormone test: some statistical considerations. *Eur Psychiatry.* 1992; 7:39-42.
93. Kletzky OA, Shangold GA. Variability and selectivity of anterior pituitary response to dopamine agonists throughout the normal menstrual cycle. *Am J Obstet Gynecol.* 1986;154: 362-367.
94. Seki K, Nagata I. Effects of a dopamine antagonist (metoclopramide) on the release of LH, FSH, TSH and PRL in normal women throughout the menstrual cycle. *Acta Endocrinol (Copenh).*
95. Steiner M, Haskett RF, Carroll BJ. Circadian hormone secretory profiles in women with severe premenstrual tension syndrome. *Br J Obstet Gynaecol.* 1984;91:466-471. 1990;122:211-216.
96. Caradente F, Angeli A, Candiani GB, Crosignani PG, Dammacco F, DeCecco L, Marrama P, Massobrio M, Martini L. Rhythms in the ovulatory cycle, III: cortisol and dehydroepiandrosterone sulfate (DHEA-S). *Chronobiologia.* 1990; 17:209-217.
97. Graf M, Distler W, Flecken A. Diurnal rhythm of plasma B-endorphin related to the menstrual cycle. *Geburtshilfe Frauenheilkd.* 1989; 49:121-124.
98. Schoneshofer M, Wagner GG. Sex differences in corticosteroids in man. *J Clin Endocrinol Metab.* 1977;45:814-817.
99. Parker CR Jr, Winkel CA, Rush M Jr, Porter JC, MacDonald PC. Plasma concentrations of 11-deoxycorticosterone in women during the menstrual cycle. *Obstet Gynecol.* 1981;58:26-30.
100. Tersman Z, Collins A, Eneroth P. Cardiovascular responses to psychological and physiological stressors during the menstrual cycle. *Psychosom Med.* 1991;53:185-197.
101. Heitkemper M, Jarrett M, Bond EF, Turner P. GI symptoms, function, and psychophysiological arousal in dysmenorrheic women. *Nurs Res.* 1991;40:20-26.
102. Aubert ML, Lemarchand-Beraud TH, Degualllaume R, Desaulles PA. Cortisol secretion during the normal menstrual cycle. *Eighth Acta Endocrinol Congr.* 1971;55(suppl):78.
103. Bloom FE. The endorphins: a growing family of pharmacologically pertinent peptides. *Ann Rev Pharmacol Toxicol.* 1983;23:151-160.
104. Mauri A, Martellotta MC, Melis MR, Caminiti F, Serri F, Fratta W. Plasma alpha-melanocyte-stimulating hormone during the menstrual cycle in women. *Horm Res.* 1990;34:66-70.
105. Ferin M, Van Vugt D, Wardlaw S. The hypothalamic control of the menstrual cycle and the role of endogenous opioid peptides. *Recent Prog Horm Res.* 1984;39:441-450.
106. Laatikainen T, Raisanen I, Tulenheimo A, Salminen K. Plasma β-endorphin and the menstrual cycle. *Fertil Steril.* 1985;38:701-706.
107. Vribcky KW, Baumstark JS, Wells IC, Hilgers TW, Kable WT, Elias CJ. Evidence for the involvement of β-endorphin in the human menstrual cycle. *Fertil Steril.* 1982;38:701-704.
108. Petraglia F, DiMeo G, DeLeo V, Nappi C, Facchinetti F, Genazzani AR. Plasma β-endorphin levels in anovulatory states: changes after treatments for the induction of ovulation. *Fertil Steril.* 1986;45:185-190.
109. Hamilton JA, Gallant S. Premenstrual symptom changes and plasma β-endorphin β-lipotropin throughout the menstrual cycle. *Psychoneuroendocrinology.* 1988;13:505-514.
110. Veith JL, Anderson J, Slade SA, Thompson P, Laugel GR, Getzlaf S. Plasma β-endorphin, pain thresholds and anxiety levels across the human menstrual cycle. *Physiol Behav.* 1984;32: 31-35.
111. Tulenheimo A, Laatikainen T, Salminen K. Plasma β-endorphin immunoreactivity in premenstrual tension. *Br J Obstet Gynaecol.* 1987;94: 26-29.
112. Parker CR Jr, Rush M, MacDonald PC. Serum concentrations of deoxycorticosterone in women during the luteal phase of the ovarian cycle are not suppressed by dexamethasone treatment. *J Steroid Biochem.* 1983;19:1313-1317.
113. Roy-Byrne PP, Rubinow DR, Gwirtsman H, Hoban C, Grover GN. Cortisol response to dexamethasone in women with premenstrual syndrome. *Neuropsychobiology.* 1986;16:61-63.
114. Tandon R, Haskett RF, Cardona D, Alcser K, Greden JF. Menstrual cycle effects on the dexamethasone suppression test in major depression. *Biol Psychiatry.* 1991;29:485-488.
115. Collins A, Eneroth P, Landgren B. Psychoneuroendocrine stress responses and mood as related to the menstrual cycle. *Psychosom Med.* 1985;47:512-527.
116. Kanaley JA, Boileau RA, Bahr JM, Misner JE, Nelson RA. Cortisol levels during prolonged exercise: the influence of menstrual phase and menstrual status. *Int J Sports Med.* 1992;13: 332-336.
117. Seki K. Variability of cortisol and adrenocorticotropic hormone responses to metoclopramide during the menstrual cycle. *Gynecol Obstet Invest.* 1989;27:201-203.
118. Cardinali DP. Melatonin: a mammalian pineal hormone. *Endocr Rev.* 1981;2:327-346.
119. Johnson LY, Reiter RI. The pineal gland and its effects on mammalian reproduction. *Prog Reprod Biol.* 1971;4:116-122.
120. Tamarkin L, Barird CJ, Almeida OFX. Melatonin: a coordinating signal for mammalian reproduction? *Science.* 1985;227:714-720.
121. Brzezinski A, Seibel MM, Lynch HJ, Deng M-H, Wurtman RI. Melatonin in human preovulatory follicular fluid. *J Clin Endocrinol Metab.* 1987;64:865-867.
122. Ronnberg L, Kauppila A, Leppaluoto J, Martikainen H, Vakkuri O. Circadian and seasonal variation in human preovulatory follicular fluid melatonin concentration. *J Clin Endocrinol Metab.* 1990;71:493-496.
123. Berga SL, Yen SSC. Circadian pattern of plasma melatonin concentrations during four phases of the human menstrual cycle. *Metabolism.* 1990; 51:1606-1612.
124. Laughlin G, Loucks A, Yen S. Marked augmentation of nocturnal melatonin secretion in amenorrheic athletes, but not in cycling athletes: unaltered by opoidergic or dopaminergic blockade. *J Clin Endocrinol Metab.* 1991;73:1321-1326.
125. Tortosa F, Puig-Domingo M, Peinado M-A, Oriola J, Webb SM, de Levia A. Enhanced circadian rhythm of melatonin in anorexia nervosa. *Acta Endocrinol (Copenh).* 1989;120:574-578.
126. Voordouw BCG, Euser R, Verdonk RER, Alberda BT, De Jong FH, Drogendijk AC, Fauser BCJM, Cohen M. Melatonin and melatonin-progestin combinations alter pituitary-ovarian function in women and can inhibit ovulation. *J Clin Endocrinol Metab.* 1992;74:108-117.
127. MacPhee AA, Cole FE, Rice BF. The effect of melatonin on steroidgenesis by the human ovary

in vitro. *J Clin Endocrinol Metab.* 1975;40:688-696.

128. Webley GE, Luck MR. Melatonin directly stimulates the secretion of progesterone by human and bovine granulosa cells in vitro. *J Reprod Fertil.* 1986;78:711-717.
129. Fellenberg M, Phillipou G, Seamark RF. Urinary 6-sulphatoxy melatonin excretion during the human menstrual cycle. *Clin Endocrinol (Oxf).* 1982;17:71-75.
130. Webley G, Leidenberger F. The circadian pattern of melatonin and its positive relationship with progesterone in women. *J Clin Endocrinol Metab.* 1986;63:323-328.
131. Parry BL, Berga SL, Kripke DF, Klauber MR, Laughlin GA, Yen SSC, Gillin JC. Altered waveform of plasma nocturnal melatonin secretion in premenstrual depression. *Arch Gen Psychiatry.* 1990;47:1139-1146.
132. Ito M, Kohsaka M, Fukuda N, Honma K, Honma S, Katsuno Y, Honma H, Kawai I, Morita N, Miyamoto T. Effects of menstrual cycle on plasma melatonin level and sleep characteristics. *Jpn J Psychiatry Neurol.* 1993;47:478-479.
133. Cecchettin M, Marzagalli G, Marchesi L, Cariddi A, Sorcie V, Tarquini B. Serum melatonin during menstrual cycle. *Chronobiologia.* 1987;14:163. Abstract.
134. Fernandez B, Malde JL, Montero A, Acuna D. Relationship between adenohypophyseal and steroid hormones and variations in serum and urinary melatonin levels during the ovarian cycle, perimenopause and menopause in healthy women. *J Steroid Biochem.* 1990;35:257-262.
135. Brzezinski A, Lynch HJ, Wurtman RI, Seibel MM. Possible contribution of melatonin to the timing of the luteinizing hormone surge. *N Engl J Med.* 1987;316:1550-1551.
136. de Leiva A, Tortosa F, Peinado MA, Serrano J, Rodriguez-Espinosa J, Puig-Domingo M. Episodic nyctohemeral secretion of melatonin in adult humans: lack of relation with LH pulsatile pattern. *Acta Endocrinol (Copenh).* 1990;122:76-82.
137. Merryman W, Boiman R, Barnes L, Rothchild I. Progesterone "anaesthesia" in human subjects. *J Clin Endocrinol.* 1954;14:1567-1569.
138. Herrmann WM, Beach RC. Experimental and clinical data indicating the psychotropic properties of progestogens. *Postgrad Med J.* 1978;54 (suppl 2):82-87.
139. Brugge KL, Kripke F, Ancoli-Israel S, Gaifinkel L. The association of menopausal status and age with sleep disorders. *Sleep Res.* 1989;18:208. Abstract.
140. Regestein QR, Schiff I, Tulchinsky D, Ryan KG. Relationships among estrogen-induced psychophysiological changes in hypogonadal women. *Psychosom Med.* 1981;43:147-155.
141. Erlik Y, Tataryn IV, Meldrum DR, Lomax P, Bajorek JG, Judd HL. Association of waking episodes with menopausal hot flashes. *JAMA.* 1981;245:1741-1744.
142. Wehr TA, Sack DA. The relevance of sleep research to affective illness. In: Koella WP, Obal F, Schulz H, Visser P, eds. *Sleep '86.* Stuttgart, Germany: Gustav Fisher; 1988:207-211.
143. Dennerstein L, Abraham SF. Affective changes and the menstrual cycle. In: Beumont PJV, Burrows GD, eds. *Handbook of Psychiatry and Endocrinology.* Amsterdam, the Netherlands: Elsevier Science Publishers; 1982:367-400.
144. Ho MA. Sex hormones and the sleep of women. *Sleep Res.* 1972;1:184. Abstract.
145. Patkai P, Johansson G, Post B. Mood, alertness and sympathetic-adrenal medullary activity during the menstrual cycle. *Psychosom Med.* 1974;36:503-512.
146. Lee KA, Shaver JF, Giblin EC, Woods NF. Sleep patterns related to menstrual cycle phase and premenstrual affective symptoms. *Sleep.* 1990;13:403-409.
147. Giles AE. The cyclical or wave theory of menstruation, with observations on the variations in pulse and temperature in relation to menstruation. *Trans Obstet Soc Lond.* 1897;39:115-124.
148. Israel SL, Schneller O. The thermogenic property of progesterone. *Fertil Steril.* 1950;1:53-65.
149. Gianaroli L, Moggian G. Die temperatursteigernde Wirkung der weiblichen Sexualsteroide. *Gynaecologia.* 1953;136:129-136.
150. Marrone BL, Gentry RT, Wade GN. Gonadal hormones and body temperature in rats: effects of estrous cycles, castration and steroid replacement. *Physiol Behav.* 1976;17:419-425.
151. Wrenn TR, Bitman J, Sykes JF. The thermogenic influence of progesterone in ovariectomized cows. *Endocrinology.* 1959;65:317-321.
152. Brown RE, Gander GW, Goodale F. Estrogen and cortisone: effects on thermoregulation in the female rabbit. *Proc Soc Exp Biol Med.* 1970;134:83-86.
153. Caradente F, Angeli A, Crosignani P, Dammacco F, De Cecco L, Ferrario VF, Halberg F, Marrama P, Martini L, Massobrio M, Vizzotto L. Circatrigintan rectal temperature and endocrine rhythms of clinically healthy, menstrually cycling women. *Adv Chronobiol.* 1987(Part B):533-548.
154. Rogacz S, Duffy J, Czeisler CA. Ambulatory body temperature monitoring in ovulating women throughout the MC. *Sleep Res.* 1987;16:633. Abstract.
155. Lee KA. Circadian temperature rhythms in relation to menstrual cycle phase. *J Biol Rhythms.* 1988;3:255-263.
156. Rogacz S, Duffy JF, Ronda JM, Czeisler CA. The increase in body temperature during the luteal phase of the menstrual cycle is only observed during the subjective night and is independent of sleep. *Sleep Res.* 1988;17:395. Abstract.
157. Rogacz S, Duffy J, Ronda J, Czeisler C. Endogenous cricadian temperature amplitude is reduced and phase is delayed in the luteal phase of the menstrual cycle in ovulating women. In: Program and abstracts from the 1988 meeting of the Society for Research on Biological Rhythms; Amelia Island, Fla.
158. Severino SK, Wagner DR, Moline ML, Hurt SW, Pollak CP, Zendell S. High nocturnal body temperature in premenstrual syndrome and late luteal phase dysphoric disorder. *Am J Psychiatry.* 1991;148:1329-1335.
159. Veith S, Kohler W, Fey P, Schmidt K, Fleissner G, Pflug B. The influence of the menstrual cycle on the female circadian system. In: Program and abstracts from the 1993 meeting of the Society for Light Treatment and Biological Rhythms; June 19-20, 1993; San Diego, Calif.
160. Wehr TA. Seasonal vulnerability to depression: implications for etiology and treatment. *L'Encephale.* 1992;18:479-483.
161. Souetre E, Salavati E, Wehr TA, Sack DA, Krebs B, Darcourt G. Twenty-four-hour profiles of body temperature and plasma TSH in bipolar patients during depression and during remission and in normal control subjects. *Am J Psychiatry.* 1988;145:1133-1137.
162. Pflug B, Erikson R, Johnsson A. Depression and daily temperature: a long-term study. *Acta Psychiatr Scand.* 1976;54:254-266.
163. Biegon A, Fischette CT, Rainbow TC, McEwen BS. Serotonin receptor modulation by estrogen in discrete brain nuclei. *Neuroendocrinology.* 1982;287-291.
164. Cohen I, Wise P. Effects of estradiol on the diurnal rhythm of serotonin activity in microdissected areas of ovariectomized rats. *Endocrinology.* 1988;122:2619-2625.
165. Fischette CT, Biegon A, McEwen BS. Sex differences in serotonin receptor binding in rat brain. *Science.* 1983;222:333-335.
166. Rehavi M, Sepcuti H, Weizman A. Upregulation of imipramine binding and serotonin uptake by estradiol in female rat brain. *Brain Res.* 1987;410:135-139.
167. Blum I, Nessiel L, David A, Graff E, Harsat A, Weissglas L, Gabbay U, Sulkes J, Yerushalmy Y, Vered Y. Plasma neurotransmitter profile during different phases of the ovulatory cycle. *J Clin Endocrinol Metab.* 1992;75:924-929.
168. Ashby CR, Carr LA, Cook CL, Steptoe MM, Franks DD. Alteration of 5-HT uptake by plasma fractions in the premenstrual syndrome. *J Neural Transm Gen Sect.* 1990;79:41-50.
169. Peters JR, Elliott JM, Grahame-Smith DO. The effect of oral contraceptives on platelet noradrenaline and 5-hydroxytryptamine receptors and aggregation. In: Turner P, ed. *Clinical Pharmacology and Therapeutics.* London, England: MacMillan Publishing Co Inc; 1980:165-174.
170. Stowell LI, McIntosh CJ, Cooke R, Ellis PM. Adrenoceptor and imipramine receptor binding during the menstrual cycle. *Acta Psychiatr Scand.* 1988;78:366-368.
171. Poirier M-F, Benkelfat C, Galzin A-M, Langer SZ. Platelet 3H-imipramine binding and steroid hormones serum concentrations during the menstrual cycle. *Psychopharmacology.* 1986;88:86-89.
172. Luine VN, Rhodes J. Gonadal hormone regulation of MAO and other enzymes in hypothalamic areas. *Neuroendocrinology.* 1983;36:235-241.
173. Luine VN, Khylchevskaya RI, McEwen BS. Effect of gonadal steroids on activities of monoamine oxidase and choline acetylase in rat brain. *Brain Res.* 1975;86:293-306.
174. Briggs M, Briggs M. Relationship between monoamine oxidase activity and sex hormone concentration in human blood plasma. *J Reprod Fertil.* 1972;29:447-450.
175. Klaiber EL, Kobayashi Y, Broverman DM, Hall F. Plasma monoamine oxidase activity in regularly menstruating women and in amenorrheic women receiving cyclic treatment with estrogens and a progestin. *J Clin Endocrinol Metab.*

1971;33:630-638.

176. Belmaker RH, Murphy DL, Wyatt RI, Loriaux DL. Human platelet monoamine oxidase changes during the menstrual cycle. *Arch Gen Psychiatry.* 1974;31:553-556.

177. Zuspan FP, Zuspan KJ. Ovulatory plasma amine (epinephrine and norepinephrine) surge in the woman. *Am J Obstet Gynecol.* 1973;117:654-661.

178. Zuspan FP, Rao P. Thermogenic alterations in the woman, I: interaction of amines, ovulation, and basal body temperature. *Am J Obstet Gynecol.* 1974;118:671-678.

179. Kobus E, Wasilewska E, Bargiel Z. Urinary excretion of catecholamines (CA) and vanilmandelic acid (VMA) during a normal menstrual cycle. *Bull Acad Polonaise Sci Biol.* 1979;27:71-74.

180. Goldstein DS, Levinson P, Keiser HR. Plasma and urinary catecholamines during the human ovulatory cycle. *Am J Obstet Gynecol.* 1983;146:824-829.

181. Feichtinger W, Kemeter P, Salzer H, Euller A, Kom A, Fuolmek R, Friedrich F. Daily epinephrine and norepinepherine excretion in urine of normal cyclic women compared with prolactin, LH, FSH, estradiol, progesterone, testosterone and cortisol. In: Zichella L, Pancheri P, eds. *Psychoneuroendocrinology in Reproduction.* Amsterdam, the Netherlands: Elsevier Science Publishers; 1979:215-223.

182. DeLeon-Jones FA, Steinberg J, Dekirmejian H, Garver D. MHPG excretion during the menstrual cycle of women. *Commun Psychopharmacol.* 1978;2:267-274.

183. Feichtinger W, Kemeter P, Salzer H, Euller A, Korn A, Friedrich F. Urinary catecholamine excretion in women with a normal menstrual cycle. *Wien Klin Wochenschr.* 1980;92:365-368.

184. Rosen SG, Berk MA, Popp DA, Serusclat P, Smith EB, Shah SD, Ginsberg AM, Clutter WE, Cryer PE. β_2 and α_2-adrenergic receptors and receptor coupling adenylate cyclase in human monoculear leukocytes and platelets in response to physiological variations of sex steroids. *J Clin Endocrinol Metab.* 1984;58:1068-1076.

185. Santala M, Vilska S, Saarikosi S, Castern O. Lymphocyte β_2-adrenoceptor density during enstrual cycle and pregnancy, in delivery and puerperium. *Eur J Obstet Gynecol Reprod Biol.* 1990;34:79-87.

186. Sundaresan PR, Madan MK, Kelvie SL, Weintraub M. Platelet alpha-2 adrenoceptors and menstrual cycle. *Clin Pharmacol Ther.* 1985;37:337-342.

187. Theodorou AE, Mistry H, Davies SL, Yamaguchi Y, Horton RW. Platelet β_2-adrenoceptor binding and function during the menstrual cycle. *J Psychiatr Res.* 1987;21:163-169.

188. Jones SB, Bylund DB, Rieser CA, Shekim WO, Byer JA, Carr GW. α_2-adrenergic receptor binding in human platelets: alterations during the menstrual cycle. *Clin Pharmacol Ther.* 1983;34:90-96.

189. Nausieda PA, Koiller WC, Weiner WJ, Klawans HL. Modification of postsynaptic dopaminergic sensitivity by female sex hormones. *Life Sci.* 1979;25:521-526.

190. Dipaola T, Carmichael R, Labrie F, Raynaud JP. Effects of estrogen on the characteristics of [3H] spiroperidol and [3H] Ru 24213 binding in rat anterior pituitary gland and brain. *Mol Cell Endocrinol.* 1979;16:99-112.

191. Harrison NL, Majewska MD, Harrington JW, Barker JL. Structure-activity relationships or steroid interaction with the γ-aminobutyric acids receptor complex. *J Pharmacol Exp Ther.* 1987;41:346-353.

192. Majewska MD. Actions of steroids on neuron: role in personality, mood, stress, and disease. *Integr Psychiatry.* 1987;5:258-273.

193. Rainbow TC, Degroff V, Luine VN, McEwen BS. Estradiol 17B increases the number of uscarinic receptors in hypothalamic nuclei. *Brain Res.* 1980;198:239-243.

194. Green S, Chambon P. Oestradiol induction of a glucocorticoid-responsive gene by a chimeric receptor. *Nature.* 1987;325:75-78.

195. Young EA, Haskett RF, Akil H, Watson SJ. Influence of gonadal steroids and menopausal status on HPA axis regulation in depression. *Biol Psychiatry.* 1992;31:132A. Abstract.

Conversions From Système International (SI) Units to Traditional Units (Modified From *The SI Manual in Health Care*)

System	Component	SI Reference Interval*	SI Unit	Conversion Factor (Divide by)	Traditional Reference Interval*	Traditional Unit
Plasma	Progesterone					
	Follicular phase	<6	nmol/L	3.180	<2	ng/mL
	Luteal phase	6-64	nmol/L	3.180	2-20	ng/mL

**These reference values are not intended to be definitive since each laboratory determines its own values. They are provided for illustration only.*

ORIGINAL ARTICLE

Elevated Cerebrospinal Fluid Levels of Oxytocin in Obsessive-compulsive Disorder

Comparison With Tourette's Syndrome and Healthy Controls

James F. Leckman, MD; Wayne K. Goodman, MD; William G. North, PhD; Phillip B. Chappell, MD; Lawrence H. Price, MD; David L. Pauls, PhD; George M. Anderson, PhD; Mark A. Riddle, MD; Maureen McSwiggan-Hardin, MSN; Christopher J. McDougle, MD; Linda C. Barr, MD; Donald J. Cohen, MD

Background: Limited neurobiological data have implicated central arginine vasopressin in the pathobiology of obsessive-compulsive disorder (OCD). Based on twin, family genetic, and pharmacological studies, some forms of OCD are etiologically related to Tourette's syndrome. The role of arginine vasopressin and related compounds such as oxytocin in Tourette's syndrome has not been previously explored.

Methods: To compare cerebrospinal fluid (CSF) levels of arginine vasopressin and oxytocin, we collected CSF at midday in a standardized fashion from a total of 83 individuals (29 patients with OCD, 23 patients with Tourette's syndrome, and 31 normal controls). We also collected family study data on each subject to determine which subjects had a family history positive for Tourette's syndrome, OCD, or related syndromes.

Results: In contrast to previous reports, we report similar concentrations of arginine vasopressin for all three groups but increased oxytocin levels in patients with OCD. Remarkably, this increase was observed only in a subset of patients with OCD (n=22) independently identified as being *without* a personal or family history of tic disorders (P=.0003). In this subgroup of patients, the CSF oxytocin level was correlated with current severity of OCD (n=19, r=.47, $P<.05$).

Conclusions: A possible role for oxytocin in the neurobiology of a subtype of OCD is suggested by the elevated CSF levels of oxytocin and by the correlation between CSF oxytocin levels and OCD severity. These findings reinforce the value of family genetic data in identifying biologically homogeneous (and perhaps more etiologically homogeneous) groups of patients with OCD. Together with emerging pharmacological data showing differential responsiveness to treatment of tic-related OCD vs non–tic-related OCD, these data also argue strongly for the incorporation of tic-relatedness as a variable in biological and behavioral studies of patients with OCD.

(Arch Gen Psychiatry. 1994;51:782-792)

From Child Study Center (Drs Leckman, Chappell, Pauls, Anderson, and Cohen) and General Clinical Research Centers (Dr Leckman), Depts of Psychiatry (Drs Leckman, Price, McDougle, Barr, and Cohen), Pediatrics (Drs Leckman and Cohen), and Genetics (Dr Pauls), and Abraham Ribicoff Research Facilities, Connecticut Mental Health Center (Drs Price and McDougle), Yale University School of Medicine, New Haven, Conn; Dept of Psychiatry, University of Florida College of Medicine, Gainesville (Dr Goodman); Dept of Physiology, Dartmouth Medical School, Hanover, NH (Dr North); Dept of Psychiatry and Behavioral Science, Johns Hopkins Medical Institutions, Baltimore, Md (Dr Riddle); and Dept of Psychiatry, Medical College of Georgia, Augusta (Ms McSwiggan-Hardin).

OBSESSIVE-compulsive disorder (OCD) is characterized by sudden, recurrent upsetting thoughts or images that intrude into consciousness (obsessions) and rule governed acts that the person feels driven to perform (compulsions). Based on family genetic data, OCD is likely to be an etiologically heterogeneous set of conditions. Some forms of OCD are familial and may be associated with a specific genetic vulnerability.[1,2] Others present as sporadic cases. Among the familial cases, a portion appear to be etiologically related to Tourette's syndrome and other tic disorders.[3,4] Data from clinical drug trials offer additional support for the distinction between Tourette's syndrome–related OCD and other forms of the disorder.[5,6]

Neurobiological and pharmacological data have implicated central monoaminergic and neuropeptidergic systems in the pathophysiology of OCD, Tourette's syndrome, and related disorders.[7-9] Based on their cognitive and behavioral effects and their neuroanatomic distributions,[10-13] recent interest has focused on the role of two closely related neurosecretory nonapeptides, arginine vasopressin and oxytocin. Hypothesized relationships have emphasized the role of arginine vasopressin in promoting repetitive grooming behav-

See Subjects and Procedures on next page

SUBJECTS AND PROCEDURES

SUBJECTS

During the course of this study, we obtained CSF in a standardized fashion from a total of 116 individuals (39 patients with OCD, 33 patients with Tourette's syndrome, and 44 normal controls). Most of the patients with OCD and normal control subjects were recruited locally within the state of Connecticut. The patients with Tourette's syndrome were recruited from a wider geographic area with the help of the national Tourette Syndrome Association and local chapters in Connecticut, New York, Massachusetts, Rhode Island, New Jersey, and Pennsylvania. Members of the state Tourette Syndrome Association organizations were contacted by letter and invited to participate in a range of ongoing studies. Each medication-free member who expressed an interest in participating in a research study was contacted. Preliminary reports concerning this data set have appeared elsewhere.[23,24] Additional reports concerning other CSF neurochemical measures (biogenic amines) will be published elsewhere.[25]

The initial diagnosis was made clinically using *DSM-III-R* criteria.[26] Patients and controls and, if available, their first-degree relatives (parents and siblings) and spouses also completed a semistructured diagnostic interview based on the Diagnostic Interview Schedule, as previously described.[27] The final diagnoses were made independently by two diagnosticians (J.F.L. and D.L.P.) using all available information.[28] When diagnostic disagreements arose, a joint review of all materials was performed, and a "best estimate" consensus diagnosis was made. In comorbid cases in which an individual received diagnoses of both OCD and a tic disorder, a "principal diagnosis" was assigned based on the individual's clinical presentation and the level of disability associated with each set of symptoms. Based on these diagnostic estimates, five patients were dropped from the study because they were not judged to have a principal diagnosis of either Tourette's syndrome or OCD. Seven normal control subjects were found to have a positive family history of either OCD or a tic disorder and were excluded from this sample. Twenty-one of the remaining 104 subjects had insufficient CSF to permit determination of arginine vasopressin and oxytocin levels, yielding a final sample size of 83.

PROCEDURES

Subjects gave informed consent before participating in the study. Subjects were medication-free for a minimum of 4 weeks (2 months in the case of neuroleptic agents) prior to the lumbar puncture. Approximately half of the lumbar punctures were performed at the Abraham Ribicoff Research Facilities of the Connecticut Mental Health Center, New Haven (most subjects with a principal diagnosis of OCD and half of the control subjects). The other lumbar punctures were performed at the General Clinical Research Center of Yale–New Haven Medical Center (most patients with Tourette's syndrome and half of the control subjects). All subjects were in good health and underwent a physical examination, standard hematologic and clinical chemistry studies, urinalysis, and electrocardiogram to screen for medical disorders. Height and weight were recorded at the time of admission. The ideal body weight percentage (for height and sex) was transcribed from actuarial tables.[29]

Subjects were asked to adhere to a low-monoamine diet for 1 day prior to the lumbar puncture. After a carbohydrate breakfast, subjects were placed at bed rest between 7 and 8 AM for 4 to 5 hours prior to the procedure. At 12:30 PM the lumbar puncture was performed using the L4-5 interspace with the patient in the lateral decubitus position. A total of 11 to 21 mL of CSF was collected. Aliquots were frozen at −70°C to −80°C until they were assayed.

CLINICAL RATINGS

Patients and controls also underwent an extensive psychiatric evaluation immediately prior to the lumbar puncture, including clinician ratings of severity of obsessive-compulsive and tic symptoms using the Yale-Brown Obsessive-Compulsive Scale (Y-BOCS)[30,31] and the Yale Global Tic Severity Scale (YGTSS).[32] Depression and anxiety were also evaluated using the clinician-rated Hamilton Depression and Anxiety Scales (HAM-D and HAM-A, re-

Continued on next page

iors, possibly analogous to hand washing and cleaning compulsions, and in maintaining conditioned responses to aversive stimuli in experimental animals.[10-14] Elevated levels of cerebrospinal fluid (CSF) arginine vasopressin in patients with OCD[15] and anecdotal clinical reports of OCD among patients with diabetes insipidus, in which central arginine vasopressin levels are increased,[16,17] are also consistent with this hypothesis. Other speculations have focused on the possible role of the sexually dimorphic extrahypothalamic arginine vasopressin projections in mediating tic symptoms.[18]

The empirical evidence indicating a role for oxytocin in the pathogenesis of OCD is meager and has mostly focused on the potential role of oxytocin as a therapeutic agent.[19-21] In addition, one study reported that the CSF arginine vasopressin–oxytocin ratio was negatively correlated with obsessive-compulsive symptom severity.[22]

We have measured arginine vasopressin and oxytocin levels in the CSF of patients with OCD, patients with Tourette's syndrome, and psychiatrically healthy controls. In contrast to previous reports, we report similar arginine vasopressin concentrations for all three groups but increased oxytocin levels in patients with OCD who had no personal or family history of tic disorders.

spectively).[33,34] The 21-item version of the HAM-D scale was modified by omitting the last item on obsessive-compulsive symptoms, with scores potentially ranging from 0 to 61. The 14-item HAM-A scale was used, with scores potentially ranging from 0 to 56.

NEUROPEPTIDE ASSAYS

Radioimmunoassays for arginine vasopressin and oxytocin levels in CSF were performed in duplicate at two dilutions under equilibrium conditions.[35,36] The antiserum used in the assay for arginine vasopressin is chiefly directed against the ring moiety of this molecule and was employed at a final dilution of 1:12 000. The antiserum used in the assay for oxytocin is directed against the C-terminal tail of oxytocin and was employed in the assay at a final dilution of 1:80 000. A reverse-phase high-performance liquid chromatography characterization of the immunoreactivity of oxytocin and arginine vasopressin in CSF was performed, using a column (46×250 mm) of 10 μm of C_{18} micron Bondapak (Waters Associates, Milford, Mass). Peptide elution from this column was achieved with a linear gradient (0 to 80% over 60 minutes) of acetonitrile in 0.05% trichloroacetic acid at a flow rate of 1 mL/min. Immunoreactive arginine vasopressin and oxytocin from CSF were eluted as single large peaks at 21 and 25 minutes, respectively. In a separate run, standard preparations of synthetic arginine vasopressin and oxytocin were eluted in identical fractions from this column. The interassay variation, intra-assay variation, and cross-reactivity of these assays procedures are presented in **Table 1**.

In reviewing the CSF data, one outlier was identified, a 26-year-old female patient with non–tic-related OCD. Both her CSF arginine vasopressin (81.7 pmol/L) and oxytocin (41.2 pmol/L) levels were markedly elevated and greater than 2 SDs from their respective overall means.

Cerebrospinal fluid dynorphin A (1-8) was measured in a single batch in a duplicate 100-μL sample using a radioimmunoassay kit from Peninsula Laboratories (Belmont, Calif). The rabbit antiserum provided was reported not to crossreact (<0.01%) with other forms of dynorphin or dynorphin A. Standard and sample counts were determined, with average coefficients of variation of 3.0% and 3.1%, respectively.

All of the neuropeptide assays were performed blind to the diagnostic and clinical status of the subjects.

ASSAYS FOR BIOGENIC AMINES

The concentrations of tyrosine, homovanillic acid, tryptophan, and 5-hydroxyindoleacetic acid in the CSF were determined using a previously described sensitive and specific high-performance liquid chromatography assay with interassay coefficients of variation of 5% to 9%.[23,37] Levels of norepinephrine were determined by high-performance liquid chromatography following alumina extraction of 0.5 to 2.0 mL of CSF.[25,38] An interassay coefficient of variation for the CSF norepinephrine assay of 7.5% (n=15) was observed for replicate samples, with a detectability limit of less than 0.15 nmol/L (25 pg/mL). The concentration of 3-methoxy-4-hydroxyphenylethylene glycol in the CSF was determined by high-performance liquid chromatography, with an interassay coefficient of variation of 6.7% (n=12) and a limit of detectability of less than 5.43 nmol/L (1 ng/mL).[25,39] Diagnostic group differences for these CSF biogenic amines will be reported elsewhere.[25] As with the neuropeptides, all assays for biogenic amines were performed blind to the diagnostic and clinical status of the subjects.

STATISTICAL ANALYSIS

Results are reported as means±1 SD. Chi-square analysis, Student's unpaired *t* test (two-tailed), and general linear models procedures (followed by Duncan's Multiple Range Tests to account for multiple comparisons) were performed to compare the neuropeptide levels and other variables across groups. The principal models used to evaluate diagnostic status (an independent class variable) were a three-group model (normal controls vs patients with OCD vs patients with Tourette's syndrome) and a four-group model (normal controls vs patients with non–tic-related OCD vs patients with tic-related OCD vs patients with Tourette's syndrome). Pearson correlation coefficients were calculated to test for possible associations among variables. All analyses were performed both with and without the outlier included.

RESULTS

SAMPLE CHARACTERISTICS

Demographic and clinical data on the final sample of 83 subjects (47 males and 36 females, aged 13 to 60 years) are presented in **Table 2**. As noted, no significant differences were found with regard to sex, current age, height, weight, or percentage of ideal body weight.[29]

As expected, the overall comparisons across the three diagnostic groups were highly significant for symptoms of both depression ($F[2,78]=37.9$, $P=.0001$) and anxiety ($F[2,70]=42.5$, $P=.0001$). Post hoc testing revealed that patients with OCD were significantly more depressed and anxious than patients with Tourette's syndrome ($P<.001$), and patients with Tourette's syndrome, in turn, were significantly more depressed and anxious than normal controls ($P<.001$) (Table 2).

Table 3 presents the frequency of lifetime comorbid psychiatric diagnoses in the two patient groups. For some analyses, patients with Tourette's syndrome who had a comorbid diagnosis of OCD (n=14) were combined with patients with OCD who had a personal or family history of a tic disorder (n=8) to form a new category

of tic-related OCD (n=22). In other exploratory analyses, all subjects were restratified by the comorbid diagnosis of major depression (current, lifetime but not current, and never) and by the diagnosis of generalized anxiety disorder (current, lifetime but not current, and never).

CSF MEASURES

The overall comparison of CSF oxytocin levels across the three diagnostic groups was significant ($F[2,80]=7.66$, $P=.0009$). Post hoc testing revealed that the OCD group had significantly ($P<.01$) higher CSF oxytocin levels than either the Tourette's syndrome group or the normal control group (**Figure 1**). When the outlier was removed, the significant difference across the groups was strengthened ($F[2,79]=8.22$, $P=.0006$). The overall four-group (comparison (normal controls vs patients with) Tourette's syndrome vs patients with tic-related OCD vs patients with non–tic-related OCD) was also significant ($F[3,79]=6.95$, $P=.0003$); patients with tic-related OCD had a mean CSF oxytocin level (6.2±5.5 pmol/L) similar to those of both patients with Tourette's syndrome (4.6±2.2 pmol/L) and normal controls (5.0±2.7 pmol/L) but markedly less than that of patients with non–tic-related OCD (10.8±8.7 pmol/L).

In contrast, no significant differences were observed in CSF arginine vasopressin measures using either the three- or four-group comparisons (Figure 1).

Table 1. Radioimmunoassay Characteristics of Vasopressin and Oxytocin

Substance	Range for Measurement	Intra-assay Variation, %	Interassay Variation, %	Cross-reactivity
Arginine vasopressin	0.1 to 8 pmol (0.1 to 16 pg)	6	8	1:14 000*
Oxytocin	0.2 to 16 pmol (0.2 to 16 pg)	8	10	1:1000†

*With oxytocin.
†With arginine vasopressin.

CSF MEASURES VS DEMOGRAPHIC VARIABLES

In univariate analyses of the entire data set, females were found to have significantly higher CSF oxytocin levels than males (7.4±4.4 vs 5.1±3.6 pmol/L, $F[1,81]=6.73$, $P=.01$). When sex was entered as a class variable along with diagnostic group (patients with OCD, patients with Tourette's syndrome, and normal controls), diagnosis remained an important variable ($F[1,2,2]=6.40$, $P<.003$), while, in contrast, sex was no longer significant once diagnosis was placed in the model. There was no sex-by-diagnosis interaction. There were no sex differences observed in the CSF arginine vasopressin data.

Table 2. Demographic and Clinical Characteristics*

	Normal Controls (N=31)	Patients With Obsessive-compulsive Disorder (N=29)	Patients With Tourette's Syndrome (N=23)
Sex, M/F	19/12	12/17	16/7
Age, y	33.0±11.0 (19.1-58.2)	33.7±12.6 (18.5-60.7)	29.6±8.5 (13.1-43.6)
Height, cm	172±11 (142-189)	170±11 (131-188)	174±9 (157-188)
% of ideal body weight†	102±12 (82-137)‡	102±13 (79-129)§	101±16 (81-137)
Age at obsessive-compulsive symptom onset, y	...	19.3±7.5 (2.0-30.0)	9.4±6.5 (2.0-26.0)‖
Severity of obsessive-compulsive symptoms (total Y-BOCS score)¶	...	24.1±7.4 (12.0-36.0)#	12.2±11.1 (0.0-34.0)
Age at tic onset, y	...	5.5±4.9 (2.0-9.0)**	6.4±2.1 (3.0-10.0)
Tic severity (YGTSS score)††	...	5.0±7.3 (0.0-16.0)	47.6±10.0 (8.0-84.0)§
Severity of anxiety (HAM-A score)‡‡	0.8±1.6 (0.0-8.0)§§	14.3±7.4 (1.0-29.0)‖‖	8.9±6.0 (0.0-21.0)§
Severity of depression (HAM-D score)¶¶	0.6±1.4 (0.0-5.0)	7.0±9.5 (4.0-38.0)#	10.0±8.8 (0.0-34.0)##

*Values are mean±SD (range).
†Based on age, sex, and height.[29]
‡n=30.
§n=20.
‖n=13.
¶Y-BOCS indicates Yale-Brown Obsessive-Compulsive Scale (range, 0 to 40).[30,31]
#n=28.
**n=2.
††YGTSS indicates Yale Global Tic Severity Scale (range, 0 to 100).[32]
‡‡HAM-A indicates Hamilton Anxiety Scale (the 14-item version) (range, 0 to 56).[34]
§§n=29.
‖‖n=24.
¶¶HAM-D indicates Hamilton Depression Scale (the 21-item version, modified to exclude the last item on obsessive-compulsive symptoms) (range, 0 to 61).[33]
##n=22.

Table 3. Current and Lifetime Comorbid *DSM-III-R* Psychiatric Diagnoses for the Obsessive-compulsive Disorder and Tourette's Syndrome Groups

	Primary Diagnosis*	
Comorbid Diagnosis	Obsessive-compulsive Disorder (N=29)	Tourette's Syndrome (N=23)
Obsessive-compulsive disorder	NA	14 (61)
Tourette's syndrome	0 (0)	NA
Chronic motor tic disorder	4 (14)	NA
Major depression		
Current	12 (50)†	4 (22)‡
Lifetime	24 (86)§	15 (68)‖
Generalized anxiety disorder		
Current	9 (38)†	1 (6)‡
Lifetime	20 (71)§	10 (45)‖
Panic disorder, lifetime	10 (36)§	7 (32)‖
Any other anxiety disorder, lifetime	15 (54)§	7 (32)‖
Attention-deficit hyperactivity disorder	4 (14)§	9 (41)‖

*NA indicates not applicable.
†n=24.
‡n=18.
§n=28.
‖n=22.

When the outlier was removed from the data set, height was inversely correlated with CSF oxytocin level (n=82, $r=-.31$, $P=.004$). When height was entered in the general linear model as a continuous covariate, both height ($P<.02$) and diagnostic group ($P<.002$) remained significantly related to CSF oxytocin level. When both height and sex were included in the model, height ($P<.04$) and diagnostic group ($P<.002$) but not sex were significantly related to CSF oxytocin level. This suggests that the observed sex effect is explained by the height differences between males and females and not by other gender-related factors. This was confirmed in a separate analysis of height and sex (with diagnostic group excluded from the model), in which height ($P<.005$) but not sex was related to CSF oxytocin concentration. No other relationships were detected between any demographic variables, including age, and CSF arginine vasopressin or oxytocin level ($P>.25$ for all comparisons).

CSF MEASURES VS CLINICAL VARIABLES

Across all groups that participated in the study, a significant correlation was observed between the total Y-BOCS score and CSF oxytocin level (n=82, $r=.27$, $P=.02$). As shown in **Figure 2**, when patients with OCD (either a principal or comorbid diagnosis of OCD) were restratified into tic-related (n=22) vs non–tic-related OCD (n=21), the relationship between CSF oxytocin level and Y-BOCS score was strengthened in the group with non–tic-related OCD (n=19, $r=.47$, $P<.05$) and disappeared in the group with tic-related OCD. The relationship was strongest (n=19, $r=.49$, $P<.05$) between Y-BOCS compulsion subscore and CSF oxytocin level in the group with non–tic-related OCD.

No significant correlations were observed between ratings of tic severity, depression, or anxiety and CSF arginine vasopressin or oxytocin level. Including either the HAM-D or HAM-A scores in a general linear model with diagnostic groups as continuous covariates did not alter the significance of the relationship between CSF oxytocin level and diagnostic group. Similarly, when the data were restratified by either comorbid major depression (current, lifetime but not current, and never) or comorbid generalized anxiety disorder (current, lifetime but not current, and never), the resulting overall comparisons (in which CSF arginine vasopressin or oxytocin level was included as the dependent measure) were not significant.

RELATIONSHIP TO OTHER CSF MEASURES

Based on data collected in this study concerning other CSF measures, reported elsewhere,[25] no significant correlations were observed between either CSF arginine vasopressin or oxytocin level and other CSF measures (tyrosine, norepinephrine, homovanillic acid, tryptophan, 5-hydroxyindoleacetic acid, or dynorphin A [1-8] level) (with or without the outlier included). Remarkably, a subgroup analysis revealed that, when the outlier was removed, CSF oxytocin level was significantly related to CSF tryptophan level (n=20, $r=.47$, $P<.04$), 5-hydroxylindoleacetic acid level (n=20, $r=.66$, $P=.001$), norepinephrine level (n=19, $r=.67$, $P<.002$), and dynorphin A (1-8) level (n=20, $r=-.52$, $P<.02$) in the non–tic-related OCD group (**Figure 3**). With the outlier included in the data set, only the correlations between CSF oxytocin level and CSF 5-hydroxyindoleacetic acid level and CSF norepinephrine level remained significant. No other associations of CSF oxytocin or arginine vasopressin level with other CSF measures were observed.

COMMENT

We report a marked elevation of CSF oxytocin level in patients with OCD. This finding is confined to a subset of patients with OCD who had no personal or family history of a tic disorder. Within this subgroup, the current severity of obsessive-compulsive symptoms, particularly compulsive behaviors, was correlated with CSF oxytocin level. If confirmed, these findings open a new chapter in our understanding of the neurobiological substrate that underlies some but not all forms of OCD. They also reinforce the value of family genetic data in identifying more biologically, and perhaps etiologically, homogeneous groups of patients.

Together with emerging pharmacological data show-

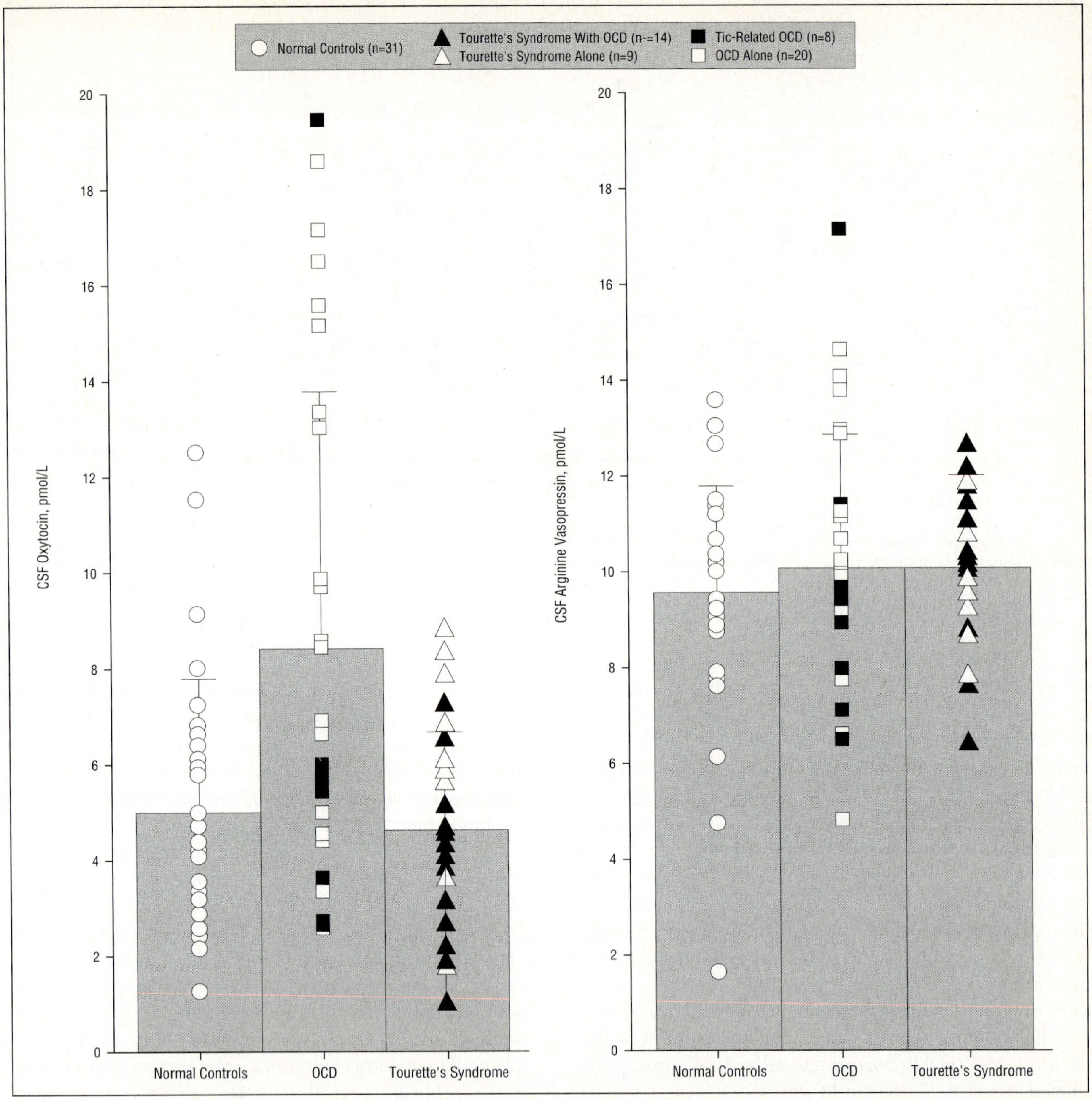

Figure 1. *Cerebrospinal fluid (CSF) oxytocin (left) and arginine vasopressin (right) levels in patients with obsessive-compulsive disorder (OCD), patients with Tourette's syndrome, and normal control subjects. The OCD group had significantly higher CSF levels of oxytocin (*P*<.01) than either the normal control group or the Tourette's syndrome group. No mean differences in CSF arginine vasopressin levels were found among the three major diagnostic groups.*

ing differential responsiveness of tic-related OCD vs non–tic-related OCD,[5,6] these data argue strongly for incorporation of tic-relatedness as a variable in biological and behavioral studies of patients with OCD. Failure to assess this variable may lead to biological heterogeneity and inconclusive or misleading results.

Some caution is warranted in the interpretation of these results. Potentially confounding factors include the fact that this sample was composed of two cohorts studied at two separate sites at the same institution (see above). Despite our best efforts, it is possible that subtle differences in the handling of these two cohorts (routine care, diet) influenced the outcome. Future studies should also include patients with other anxiety disorders to establish the specificity of this finding for other anxiety disorders.

Oxytocin is synthesized in hypothalamic cells, primarily within the paraventricular and supraoptic nuclei, which in rodents project to the neurohypophysis and to sites throughout the neural axis, including the limbic forebrain, the caudal brain stem, and the spinal cord.[40-43] Oxytocin is secreted in a pulsatile fashion directly into

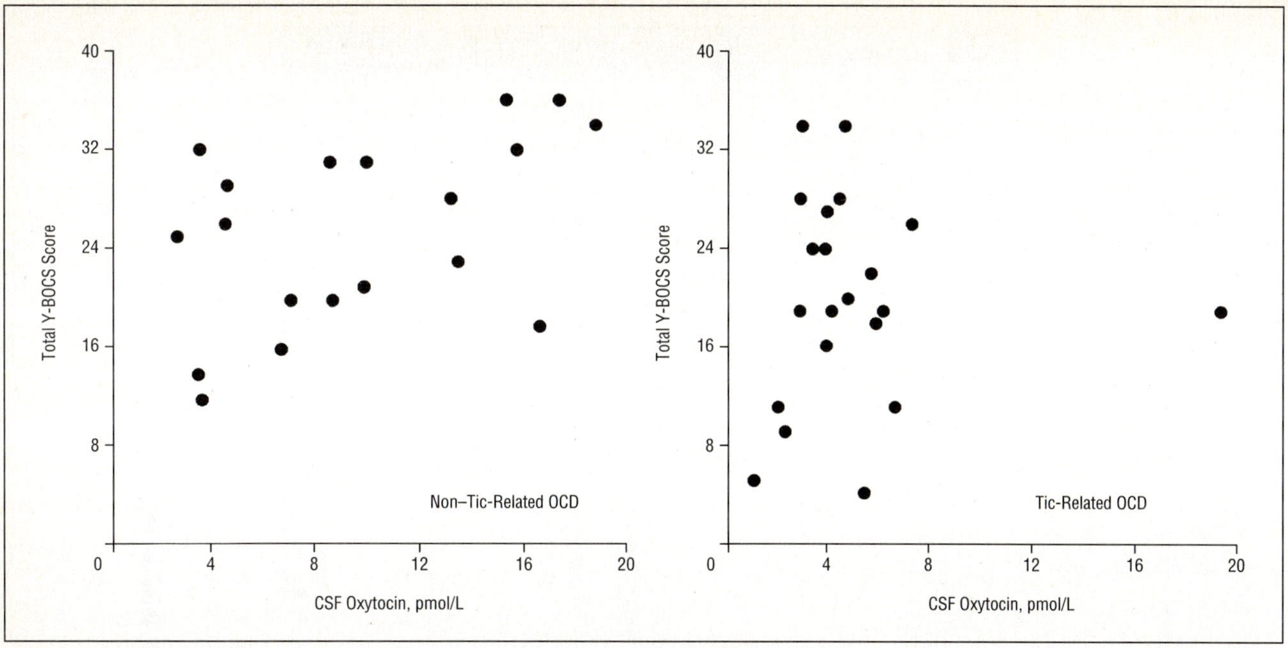

Figure 2. *Relationship of cerebrospinal fluid (CSF) oxytocin level and total Yale-Brown Obesessive-Compulsive Scale (Y-BOCS) score among subjects with a diagnosis of obsessive-compulsive disorder (OCD) stratified by tic-related status. The CSF oxytocin level was significantly correlated (n=19,* r*=.47,* P*<.05) with the total Y-BOCS score among patients with OCD who had no personal or family history of tics (left). No correlation was observed in the patients with tic-related OCD (right).*

the peripheral circulation as well as from sites immediately adjacent to the third ventricle in conjunction with its carrier protein, oxytocin-neurophysin.[43-45] The half-life of centrally or peripherally administered oxytocin is species specific. In humans, the plasma half-life of oxytocin is between 1 and 6 minutes, while its CSF half-life is approximately 20 minutes.[46] There is a circadian rhythm of CSF oxytocin but not plasma oxytocin, with peak values reported at midday.[47] Oxytocin does not pass easily through the blood-brain barrier, although some bidirectional transport may occur. This suggests that the oxytocin measured in this study was likely from the central nervous system rather than from the neurohypophysis. It is also possible that the skewed distribution of oxytocin levels observed in the non–tic-related OCD group was caused either by the pulsatile nature of oxytocin release or by the ability of oxytocin to stimulate its own release or by both.[48-50] In addition, the measurement of oxytocin in lumbar CSF may be insensitive to oxytocin changes occurring in the telencephalon. This may be consistent with the finding of caudal-rostral oxytocin gradients in the CSF of rhesus and cynomolgus monkeys[51] and with the observation that the paraventricular nuclei spinal projections arise largely from the posteriorly positioned lateral parvocellular paraventricular subnuclei.[52] If the five major subdivisions of parvocellular neurons in the paraventricular nuclei are to some extent functionally independent, this might suggest that overactivity in one or more of the remaining parvicellular subdivisions is key to the development of OCD.

Putative oxytocin receptors have been identified in a variety of forebrain sites, including the ventromedial hypothalamus, lateral segment of the bed nucleus of the stria terminalis, central amygdala, anterior olfactory nucleus, lateral septum, dorsal-medial aspects of the caudate nucleus, taenia tectae, and ventral subiculum of the hippocampus.[13,53-55] Although the distribution of oxytocin receptors is similar in male and female rodent brains, the distribution of these receptors varies markedly over the course of development. For example, in the rat, oxytocin binding in the cingulate cortex, globus pallidus, and intralaminar thalamic nuclei is intense only during infancy.[56,57] The significance of this developmental change vis-à-vis the neurobiologic characteristics of OCD is not understood. However, many of these sites have been implicated in previous functional brain imaging studies and reports of neurosurgical procedures that affect obsessive-compulsive symptoms.[58]

The observed positive correlations between CSF oxytocin level and CSF 5-hydroxyindoleacetic acid and norepinephrine levels in a subgroup of patients with OCD are intriguing given reports that the administration of serotonergic agonists and norepinephrine increases oxytocin secretion.[59,60] Related clinical observations include the findings of Thorén and coworkers[61] that OCD with high CSF levels of 5-hydroxyindoleacetic acid responds favorably to clomipramine therapy and that there was a significant association between the magnitude of improvement of obsessive-compulsive symptoms and the extent of the fall in CSF 5-hydroxyindolacetic acid levels.

Similarly, the reported κ-mediated tonic opioid inhibition of oxytocin release is consistent with the sig-

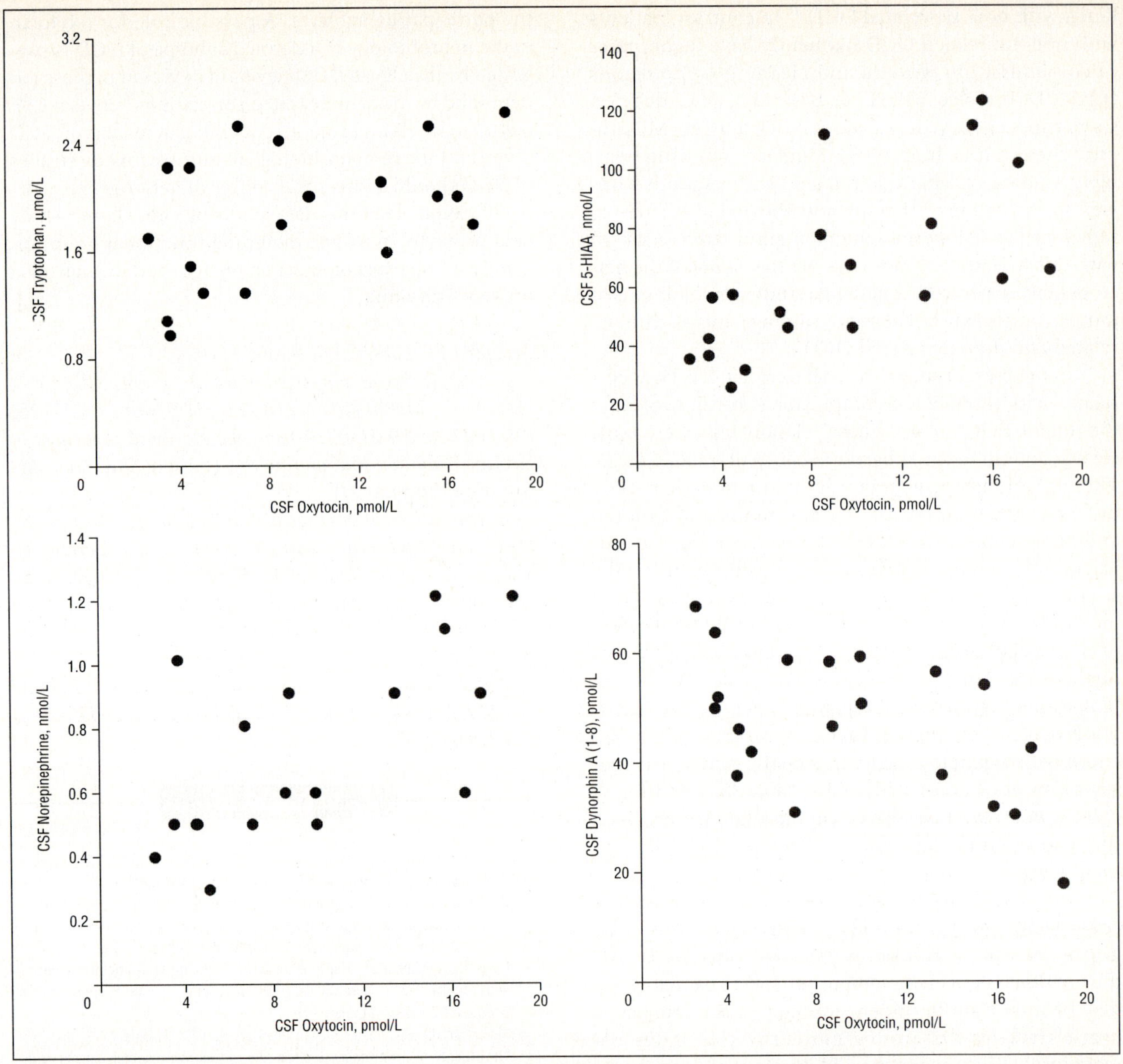

Figure 3. *Association of cerebrospinal fluid (CSF) oxytocin level and CSF tryptophan (top left), 5-hydroxyindoleacetic acid (5-HIAA) (top right), norepinephrine (bottom left), and dynorphin A (1-8) (bottom right) levels among patients with OCD who had no personal or family history of tics. The CSF oxytocin level was significantly related to the CSF tryptophan (n=20, r=.47, P<.04), 5-HIAA (n=20, r=.66, P=.001), norepinephrine (n=19, r=.67, P<.002), and dynorphin A (1-8) (n=20, r=−.52, P<.02) levels.*

nificant inverse relationship between CSF oxytocin level and dynorphin A (1-8) level in the present report.[62,63] This observation may also be consistent with the report by Insel and Pickar[64] that high doses of naloxone, sufficient to block κ as well as μ and δ opiate receptors, exacerbate obsessive-compulsive symptoms.

Although these data require replication, it is tempting to speculate about the emerging picture of central oxytocin and its apparent role in a range of cognitive,[10,65] grooming,[66] affiliative,[13] and sexual[67] behaviors and about how these behaviors are disrupted in some forms of OCD.[68] Consistent with previous reports,[69,70] the group with non–tic-related OCD had a significantly earlier age of onset. This group also had a significantly higher score on the Y-BOCS than the group with tic-related OCD. We predict that more complete characterization of this subgroup of patients with OCD will reveal further differences in symptom profiles, responses to challenge agents (particularly those that can dramatically increase or decrease oxytocin secretion), responses to behavioral and pharmacological treatments, and patterns of brain activation during functional brain imaging studies. Limited data already support many aspects of this hypothesis. Phenomenological studies have reported higher rates of certain compulsive behaviors, such as touching rituals, among patients with tic-related OCD than among pa-

tients with non–tic-related OCD.[71] In contrast, patients with non–tic-related OCD frequently have higher rates of contamination worries and cleaning compulsions (J.F.L., D. E. Grice, MD, L. C. Barr, MD, A. C. deVries, C. Martin, D.J.C., W.K.G., and S. A. Rasmussen, MD, unpublished results, June 1994). Similarly, our drug treatment studies, in which tic-related OCD responded less well to fluvoxamine therapy and showed a differential sensitivity to haloperidol augmentation, are consistent with this hypothesis.[5] It is possible that some of the heterogeneity observed in challenge studies involving serotonin agonists may be caused by mixing patients with tic-related and non–tic-related OCD.[72,73]

In the present study, the CSF oxytocin level was correlated with the Y-BOCS compulsion subscale score and the total Y-BOCS score. These relationships were most clearly present in the subgroup of non–tic-related OCD. These relationships were not found in an earlier study by Swedo and coworkers[22] of a large number of children and adolescents with OCD. However, Swedo and colleagues did report an inverse relationship between the arginine vasopressin-oxytocin ratio and a number of OCD measures. In addition, we did not replicate their finding of an association between CSF oxytocin level and scores on the HAM-D and another depression scale. Possible explanations for these discrepancies include the likelihood that Swedo and colleagues' sample was heterogenous with regard to tic status, given the generally earlier age of onset of tic-related OCD (Table 1). The time of collection of CSF may also be an important factor, given the reported time-dependent midday peak of CSF oxytocin levels.

In contrast to an earlier report by Altemus and coworkers,[15] we did not find increased CSF levels of arginine vasopressin among patients with OCD. Although differences in the composition of the patient group may be important in understanding this discrepancy, a more striking difference concerns the order-of-magnitude difference in the CSF levels of arginine vasopressin in the present report and elsewhere[36] compared with the levels in the report by Altemus and colleagues as well as in a number of earlier reports concerning CSF arginine vasopressin levels in psychiatric and neurologic patients.[74-78] Differences in the antibodies used may account for these differences. However, the immunoreactivity of the various antibodies to different preparations of arginine vasopressin and arginine vasopressin analogues suggests that many assays are highly specific and are to some extent directed against similar portions of the arginine vasopressin molecule.[35,79] Failure to correct for arginine vasopressin lost in the extraction procedures used in many of these reports may also be an important source of variability.[75-78] Further work is needed to reconcile these differences.

In summary, this is the first large-scale CSF study of OCD to ascertain rigorously the tic-related status of the participating subjects. A possible role for oxytocin in the neurobiology of a defined subtype of OCD is suggested by the elevated CSF levels of oxytocin in these patients and by the demonstrated correlations between CSF oxytocin levels and concurrent clinician ratings of OCD severity. Future neurobiological and treatment studies of OCD should address this source of heterogeneity. Restratification of existing data sets using either family study data or oxytocin status, including functional brain imaging and pharmacological challenge studies, may also prove worthwhile.

Accepted for publication May 13, 1994.

This work was supported in part by grants MH44843, MH49351, MH00508, NS16648, HD03008, RR00125, RR06022, and MH30929 from the National Institutes of Health, Bethesda, Md, and by the Tourette Syndrome Association, Bayside, NY.

The authors thank Susan Gagnon, Sharon I. Ort, RN, MPH, Lawrence Scahill, MSN, MPH, Paul J. Lombroso, MD, Robert A. Makuch, PhD, Bradley S. Peterson, MD, and Yanki Yazgan, MD, for their assistance in completing the project and for their comments on an early draft of this report.

Reprint requests to Yale Child Study Center, PO Box 207900, 230 S Frontage Rd, New Haven, CT 06520-7900 (Dr Leckman).

REFERENCES

1. Lewis A. Problems of obsessional illness. *Proc R Soc Med.* 1935;28:325-336.
2. Brown FW. Heredity in the psychoneuroses. *Proc R Soc Med.* 1942;35:785-790.
3. Pauls DL, Towbin KE, Leckman JF, Zahner GEP, Cohen DJ. Gilles de la Tourette's syndrome and obsessive compulsive disorder: evidence supporting a genetic relationship. *Arch Gen Psychiatry.* 1986;43:1180-1182.
4. Pauls DL, Leckman JF. The inheritance of Gilles de la Tourette's syndrome and associated behaviors: evidence for autosomal dominant transmission. *N Engl J Med.* 1986;315:993-997.
5. McDougle CJ, Goodman WK, Leckman JF, Barr LC, Heninger GR, Price LH. The efficacy of fluvoxamine in obsessive compulsive disorder: effects of comorbid chronic tic disorder. *J Clin Psychopharmacol.* 1993;13:354-358.
6. McDougle CJ, Goodman WK, Leckman JF, Lee NC, Heninger GR, Price LH. Haloperidol addition in fluvoxamine-refractory obsessive-compulsive disorder: a double-blind, placebo-controlled study in patients with and without tics. *Arch Gen Psychiatry.* 1994;51:302-308.
7. Yaryura-Tobias JA, Neziroglu F, Bergman L. Chlorimipramine, for obsessive-compulsive neurosis: an organic approach. *Curr Ther Res.* 1976;20:541-548.
8. Insel TR, Mueller EA, Alterman I, Linnoila M, Murphy DL. Obsessive-compulsive disorder and serotonin: is there a connection? *Biol Psychiatry.* 1985; 20:1174-1188.
9. Goodman WR, McDougle CJ, Price LH, Riddle MA, Pauls DL, Leckman JF. Beyond the serotonin hypothesis: a role for dopamine in some forms of obsessive compulsive disorder? *J Clin Psychiatry.* 1990;51:36-43.
10. De Wied D, Joels M, Burbach JPH, De Jong W, De Kloet ER, Gaffori WJ, Urban IJA, Van Ree JM, Van Wimersma Greidanus TB, Veldhuis HD, Versteeg DHG, Wiegant VM. *Peptide Hormones: Effects and Mechanisms of Action.* Boca Raton, Florida: CRC Press Inc; 1988;1:97-140.
11. Sahgal A. A critique of the vasopressin-memory hypothesis. *Psychopharmacology.* 1984;83:215-228.
12. De Vries GJ, Buijs RM, Van Leeuwen FW, Caffe AR, Swaab DF. The vasopressinergic innervation of the brain in normal and castrated rats. *J Comp Neurol.* 1985;233:236-254.

13. Insel TR. Oxytocin—a neuropeptide for affiliation: evidence from behavioral, receptor autoradiographic, and comparative studies. *Psychoneuroendocrinology.* 1992;17:1-35.
14. Delanoy RL, Dunn AJ, Tintner R. Behavioral responses to intracerebroventricularly administered neurohypophyseal peptides in mice. *Horm Behav.* 1978; 11:348-362.
15. Altemus M, Pigott T, Kalogeras KT, Demitrack M, Dubbert B, Murphy DL, Gold PW. Abnormalities in the regulation of vasopressin and corticotropin releasing factor secretion in obsessive-compulsive disorder. *Arch Gen Psychiatry.* 1992; 49:9-20.
16. Barton R. Diabetes insipidus and obsessional neurosis. *Adv Biochem Psychopharmacol.* 1987;43:347-349.
17. Barton R. Diabetes insipidus and obsessional neurosis: a syndrome. *Lancet.* 1965;1:133-135.
18. Peterson BP, Leckman JF, Scahill L, Naftolin F, Keefe D, Charest NJ, Cohen DJ. Steroid hormones and CNS sexual dimorphisms modulate symptom expression in Tourette's syndrome. *Psychoneuroendocrinology.* 1992;17:553-563.
19. Ansseau M, Legros JJ, Mormont C, Cerfontaine JL, Papart P, Geenen V, Adam F, Franck G. Intranasal oxytocin in obsessive-compulsive disorder. *Psychoneuroendocrinology.* 1987;12:231-236.
20. Charles G, Guillaume R, Schittecatte M, Pholien P, Van Wettere JP, Wilmotte J. Oxytocin in the treatment of obsessive-compulsive disorder: a report of two cases. *Psychiatr Psychobiol.* 1989;4:111-116.
21. den Boer JA, Westenberg GM. Oxytocin in obsessive compulsive disorder. *Peptides.* 1992;13:1083-1085.
22. Swedo SE, Leonard HL, Kruesi MJ, Rettew DC, Listwak SJ, Berrettini W, Stipetic M, Hamburger S, Gold PW, Potter WZ, Rapoport JL. Cerebrospinal fluid neurochemistry in children and adolescents with obsessive-compulsive disorder. *Arch Gen Psychiatry.* 1992;49:29-36.
23. Leckman JF, Riddle MA, Berrettini WH, Anderson GM, Hardin MT, Chappell P, Bissette G, Nemeoff CB, Goodman WK, Cohen DJ. Elevated CSF dynorphin A (1-8) in Tourette's syndrome. *Life Sci.* 1988;43:2015-2023.
24. Leckman JF, Goodman WK, Riddle MA, Hardin MT, Anderson GM. Low CSF 5HIAA and obsessions of violence: report of two cases. *Psychiatry Res.* 1990; 33:95-99.
25. Leckman JF, Goodman WK, Anderson GM, Riddle MA, Chappell PB, McSwiggan-Hardin MT, McDougle CJ, Scahill LD, Ort SI, Pauls DL, Cohen DJ, Price LH. CSF biogenic amines in obsessive compulsive disorder, Tourette's syndrome, and healthy controls. *Neuropsychopharmacology.* In press.
26. American Psychiatric Association, Committee on Nomenclature and Statistics. *Diagnostic and Statistical Manual of Mental Disorders, Revised Third Edition.* Washington, DC: American Psychiatric Association; 1987.
27. Pauls DL, Hurst CR. *Schedule for Tourette's Syndrome and Other Behavioral Syndromes.* New Haven, Conn: Yale University Child Study Center; 1987.
28. Leckman JF, Sholomskas D, Thompson WD, Belanger A, Weissman MM. Best estimate of lifetime psychiatric diagnosis: a methodologic study. *Arch Gen Psychiatry.* 1982;39:879-883.
29. Society of Actuaries. *Build and Blood Pressure Study.* Chicago: Society of Actuaries; 1959:16.
30. Goodman WK, Price LH, Rasmussen SA, Mazure C, Fleischmann RL, Hill CL, Heninger GR, Charney DS. The Yale-Brown Obsessive-Compulsive Scale (Y-BOCS), I: development, use, and reliability. *Arch Gen Psychiatry.* 1989;46: 1006-1011.
31. Goodman WK, Price LH, Rasmussen SA, Mazure C, Delgado P, Heninger GR, Charney DS. The Yale-Brown Obsessive-Compulsive Scale (Y-BOCS), II: validity. *Arch Gen Psychiatry.* 1989;46:1012-1016.
32. Leckman JF, Riddle MA, Hardin MT, Ort SI, Swartz KL, Stevenson J, Cohen DJ. The Yale Global Tic Severity Scale (YGTSS): initial testing of a clinical-rated scale of tic severity. *J Am Acad Child Adolesc Psychiatry.* 1989;28:566-573.
33. Hamilton M. Development of a rating scale for primary depressive illness. *Br J Soc Clin Psychol.* 1967;6:278-296.
34. Hamilton M. The assessment of anxiety states by rating. *Br J Psychol.* 1959; 32:50-55.
35. North WG, LaRochelle FT Jr, Haldar J, Sawyer WH, Valtin H. Characterization of an antiserum used in a radioimmunoassay for arginine-vasopressin: implications for reference standards. *Endocrinology.* 1978;103:1976-1984.
36. North WG, Harbaugh R, Reeder T. An evaluation of human neurophysin production in Alzheimer's disease: preliminary observations. *Neurobiol Aging.*1992; 13:261-265.
37. Anderson GM, Young JG, Cohen DJ. A rapid liquid chromatographic method for the determination of tyrosine, tryptophan, 5-hydroxyindoleacetic acid and homovanillic acid in cerebrospinal fluid. *J Chromatography.* 1979:142:501-505.
38. Anderson GM, Durkin TA, Morton JB, Cohen DJ. Liquid chromatographic determination of urinary catecholamines after one-step alumina extraction. *J Chromatography.* 1988;424:373-377.
39. Anderson GM, Young JG, Batter DK, Young SN, Cohen DJ, Shaywitz BA. Determination of indoles and catechols in rat brain and pineal using liquid chromatography with fluorometric and amperometric detection. *J Chromatography.* 1981;223:315-320.
40. Nieuwenhuys R. *Chemoarchitecture of the Brain.* New York, NY: Springer-Verlag NY Inc; 1985:84-86.
41. Buijs RM, DeVries GJ, Van Leeuwen RW, Swaab DF. Vasopressin and oxytocin: distribution and putative functions in the brain. *Prog Brain Res.* 1983;60: 115-122.
42. Sawchenko PE, Swanson LW. The organization and biochemical specificity of afferent projections to the paraventricular and supraoptic nuclei. *Prog Brain Res.* 1983;60:19-29.
43. Swanson LW, Sawchenko PE. Hypothalamic integration: organization of the paraventricular and supraoptic nuclei. *Annu Rev Neurosci.* 1983;6:269-324.
44. Bargmann W, Scharrer E. The origin of the posterior pituitary hormones. *Am Sci.* 1951;39:255-249.
45. Gainer H, Altstein M, Whitnall WS. The biosynthesis and secretion of oxytocin and vasopressin. In: Knobil E, Neill J, eds. *The Physiology of Reproduction.* New York, NY: Raven Press; 1988:2265-2281.
46. Mens WBJ, Witter A, Van Wimersma Greidanus TB. Penetration of neurohypophyseal hormones from plasma into cerebrospinal fluid (CSF): half-times of disappearance of these neuropeptides from CSF. *Brain Res.* 1983;262:143-149.
47. Amico JA, Tenicela R, Johnston J, Robinson AG. A time dependent peak of oxytocin exists in cerebrospinal fluid but not plasma of humans. *J Clin Endocrinol Metab.* 1983;57:947-951.
48. Falke N. Oxytocin stimulates oxytocin release from isolated nerve terminals of rat neural lobes. *Neuropeptides.* 1989;14:269-274.
49. Moos F, Freund-Mercier JM, Guerne Y, Guerne JM, Stoeckel ME, Richard P. Release of oxytocin and vasopressin by magnocellular nuclei in vitro: specific facilitatory effect of oxytocin on its own release. *J Endocrinol.* 1984;102:63-72.
50. Theodosis DT. Oxytocin-immunoreactive terminals synapse on oxytocin neurones in the supraoptic nucleus. *Nature.* 1985;313:682-684.
51. Amico JA, Levin SC, Cameron JL. Circadian rhythm of oxytocin in the cerebrospinal fluid of rhesus and cynomolgus monkeys: effects of castration and adrenalectomy and presence of a caudal-rostral gradient. *Neuroendocrinology.* 1989;50:624-632.
52. Wagner CK, Clemens LG. Neurophysin-containing pathway from the paraventricular nucleus of the hypothalamus to a sexually dimorphic motor nucleus in the lumbar spinal cord. *J Comp Neurol.* 1993;336:106-116.
53. Freund-Mercier MJ, Stoeckel ME, Palacios JM, Pazos A, Reichhart JM, Porte A, Richard PH. Pharmacological characteristics and anatomical distribution of [^{3}H]oxytocin-binding sites in the Wistar rat brain studied by autoradiography. *Neuroscience.* 1987;20:599-614.
54. De Kloet ER, Rotteveel F, Voorhuis TAM, Terlou M. Topography of binding sites for neurohypophyseal hormones in rat brain. *Eur J Pharmacol.* 1985; 110:113-119.
55. Tribollet E, Barberis C, Jard S, Dubois-Dauphin M, Dreifuss JJ. Localization and pharmacological characterization of high affinity binding sites for vasopressin and oxytocin in the rat brain by light microscopic autoradiography. *Brain Res.* 1988;442:105-118.
56. Shapiro LE, Insel TR. Ontogeny of oxytocin receptors in the rat forebrain: a quantitative study. *Synapse.* 1989;4:259-266.
57. Tribollet E, Charpak S, Schmidt A, Dubois-Dauphin M, Dreifuss JJ. Appearance and transient expression of oxytocin receptors in fetal, infant, and peripubertal rat brain studied by autoradiography and electrophysiology. *J Neurosci.* 1989;9:1764-1778.
58. Insel TR. Toward a neuroanatomy of obsessive-compulsive disorder. *Arch Gen Psychiatry.* 1992;49:739-744.
59. Van de Kar LD. Neuroendocrine pharmacology of serotonergic neurons. *Annu Rev Pharmacol Toxicol.* 1991;31:289-320.
60. Crowley WR, O'Donahue TL, George JM, Jacobowitz DM. Changes in pituitary

oxytocin and vasopressin during the estrous cycle and after ovarian hormones: evidence for the mediation of norepinephrine. *Life Sci.* 1987;23:2579-2586.

61. Thorén P, Asberg M, Bertilsson L, Mellström B, Sjöqvist F, Träskman L. Clomipramine treatment of obsessive-compulsive disorder. *Arch Gen Psychiatry.* 1980;37:1289-1294.
62. Leng G, Russell JA. Opioid control of oxytocin secretion. In: Yoshida S, Share L, eds. *Recent Progress in Posterior Pituitary Hormones 1988.* Amsterdam, the Netherlands: Excerpta Medica; 1988:89-96. [International Congress Series 797.]
63. Neumann I, Russell JA, Wolff B, Landgraf R. Naloxone increases the release of oxytocin, but not vasopressin, within limbic brain areas of conscious parturient rats: a push-pull perfusion study. *Neuroendocrinology.* 1991;54:545-551.
64. Insel TR, Pickar D. Naloxone administration in obsessive-compulsive disorder: report of two cases. *Am J Psychiatry.* 1983;140:1219-1220.
65. de Wied D, Diamant M, Fodor M. Central nervous system effects of neurohypophyseal hormones and related peptides. *Front Neuroendocrinol.* 1993;14:251-302.
66. Winslow JT, Insel TR. Social status in pairs of male squirrel monkeys determines the behavioral response to central oxytocin administration. *J Neurosci.* 1991;11:2032-2038.
67. Carter CS. Oxytocin and sexual behavior. *Neurosci Biobehav Rev.* 1992;16:131-144.
68. Leckman JF, Goodman WK, North WG, Chappell PB, Price LH, Pauls DL, Anderson GM, Riddle MA, McSwiggan-Hardin MT, McDougle CJ, Barr LC, Cohen DJ. The role of central oxytocin in obsessive compulsive disorder and related normal behavior. *Psychoneuroendocrinology.* In press.
69. Swedo SE, Rapoport JL, Leonard HL, Lenane M, Cheslow D. Obsessive-compulsive disorder in children and adolescents: clinical phenomenology of 70 consecutive cases. *Arch Gen Psychiatry.* 1989;46:335-341.
70. Riddle MA, Scahill L, King R, Hardin MT, Towbin KE, Ort SI, Leckman JF, Cohen DJ. Obsessive compulsive disorder in children and adolescents: phenomenology and family history. *J Am Acad Child Adolesc Psychiatry.* 1990;29:766-772.
71. Holzer JC, Goodman WK, McDougle CJ, Baer L, Boyarsky BK, Leckman JF, Price LH. Obsessive compulsive disorder with and without a chronic tic disorder: a comparison of symptoms in 70 patients. *Br J Psychiatry.* 1994;164:469-473.
72. Charney DS, Goodman WK, Price LH, Woods SW, Rasmussen SA, Heninger GR. Serotonin function in obsessive-compulsive disorder. *Arch Gen Psychiatry.* 1988;45:177-185.
73. Hollander E, DeCaria CM, Nitescu A, Gully R, Suckow RF, Cooper TB, Gorman JM, Klein DF, Liebowitz MR. Serotonergic function in obsessive-compulsive disorder. *Arch Gen Psychiatry.* 1992;49:21-28.
74. Jenkins JS, Mather HM, Ang V. Vasopressin in human cerebrospinal fluid. *J Clin Endocrinol Metab.* 1980;50:364-367.
75. Reid AC, Morton JJ. Arginine vasopressin levels in cerebrospinal fluid in neurological disease. *J Neurol Sci.* 1982;54:295-301.
76. Beckmann H, Lang RF, Gattaz WF. Vasopressin-oxytocin in cerebrospinal fluid of schizophrenic patients and normal controls. *Psychoneuroendocrinology.* 1985;10:187-191.
77. Sørensen PS, Gjerris A, Hammer M. Cerebrospinal fluid vasopressin in neurological and psychiatric disease. *J Neurol Neurosurg Psychiatry.* 1985:48:50-57.
78. Demitrack MA, Kalogeras KT, Altemus M, Pigott TA, Listwak SJ, Gold PW. Plasma and cerebrospinal fluid measures of arginine vasopressin secretion in patients with bulimia nervosa and in healthy subjects. *J Clin Endocrinol Metab.* 1992;74:1277-1283.
79. Hammer M. Radioimmunoassay of 8-arginine-vasopressin (antidiuretic hormone) in human plasma. *Scand J Clin Lab Invest.* 1978;38:707-716.

Conversions From Système International (SI) Units to Traditional Units (Modified From *The SI Manual in Health Care*)

System	Component	SI Reference Interval*	SI Unit	Conversion Factor (Divide by)	Traditional Reference Interval*	Traditional Unit
Plasma	Amino acid fractionation					
	Tryptophan	25-125	μmol/L	48.97	0.5-2.5	mg/dL
Urine	5-Hydroxyindoleacetate (as 5-hydroxyindoleacetic acid [5-HIAA])	10-40	μmol/d	5.230	2.8	mg/24 hr
Plasma	Norepinephrine (radioenzymatic procedure)	1.27-2.81 (at rest for 15 min)	nmol/L	0.005911	215-475 (at rest for 15 min)	pg/mL

These reference values are not intended to be definitive since each laboratory determines its own values. They are provided for illustration only.

Changes in Cerebrospinal Fluid Neurochemistry During Treatment of Obsessive-compulsive Disorder With Clomipramine

Margaret Altemus, MD; Susan E. Swedo, MD; Henrietta L. Leonard, MD; Dan Richter; David R. Rubinow, MD; William Z. Potter, MD; Judith L. Rapoport, MD

Background: This study examined the effect of long-term (mean, 19 months) treatment with clomipramine hydrochloride on cerebrospinal fluid (CSF) levels of several neuropeptides and monoamine metabolites in children and adolescents with obsessive-compulsive disorder.

Methods: The CSF levels of corticotropin-releasing hormone, vasopressin, somatostatin, and oxytocin and of the monoamine metabolites 5-hydroxyindolacetic acid, homovanillic acid, and 3-methoxy-4-hydroxyphenylglycol were measured in 17 children and adolescents with obsessive-compulsive disorder before and after long-term treatment with clomipramine.

Results: Treatment resulted in significant decreases in CSF levels of corticotropin-releasing hormone (mean±SD, 175±32 vs 152±25 pmol/L, $P<.03$) and vasopressin (mean±SD, 1.30±0.57 vs 0.86±0.54 pmol/L, $P<.02$) and a trend toward a decrease in somatostatin levels (mean±SD, 21.3±8.5 vs 15.3±9.8 pmol/L, $P<.06$). Treatment also significantly increased CSF oxytocin levels (mean±SD, 6.05±1.60 vs 6.70±1.44 pmol/L, $P<.01$). Significant changes in CSF monoamine metabolite levels with treatment included significant decreases in CSF levels of 5-hydroxyindolacetic acid (mean±SD, 109±31 vs 77±23 pmol/mL, $P<.001$), CSF homovanillic acid (mean±SD, 273±111 vs 237±101 pmol/mL, $P<.04$), and 3-methoxy-4-hydroxyphenylglycol (mean±SD, 42.4±10.2 vs 36.1±4.8 pmol/L, $P<.02$) and a significant increase in the homovanillic acid–5-hydroxyindolacetic acid ratio (mean±SD, 2.44±0.46 vs 3.42±0.84, $P<.0001$).

Conclusions: These neuropeptide results coupled with evidence that central administration of corticotropin-releasing hormone, vasopressin, and somatostatin to laboratory animals increases arousal and acquisition of conditioned behaviors whereas central administration of oxytocin has opposite behavioral effects are consistent with a role for these neuropeptides in the pathophysiologic processes and pharmacologic treatment of obsessive-compulsive disorder.

(Arch Gen Psychiatry. 1994;51:794-803)

RECENT REPORTS[1,2] have suggested that abnormalities in cerebrospinal fluid (CSF) levels of corticotropin-releasing hormone (CRH), vasopressin, and somatostatin may be present in adult patients with obsessive-compulsive disorder (OCD). In pediatric subjects with OCD, significant correlations have been noted between CSF levels of oxytocin and vasopressin and scores on OCD, anxiety, and depression symptom rating scales.[3] Evidence that central administration of CRH, vasopressin, somatostatin, and oxytocin to laboratory animals is associated with the modulation of arousal and conditioned behaviors[4-8] suggests that these peptides may play a role in the pathophysiologic processes of OCD. The peptidergic systems that produce hyperarousal and delayed extinction of conditioned behaviors in experimental animals may contribute to the anxiety and preservative thoughts and behaviors characteristic of OCD in humans. To further investigate the role of CRH, vasopressin, somatostatin, and oxytocin in OCD, we measured CSF levels of these peptides in 17 children and adolescents before and during long-term (8.5 to 34 months)

From the Laboratory of Clinical Science (Dr Altemus), the Child Psychiatry Branch (Drs Swedo, Leonard, Rapoport, and Mr Richter), the Biological Psychiatry Branch (Dr Rubinow), and the Experimental Therapeutics Branch of the Division of Intramural Research Programs (Dr Potter), National Institute of Mental Health, Bethesda, Md.

See Subjects and Methods on next page

SUBJECTS AND METHODS

SUBJECTS

Seventeen children and adolescents with severe, primary OCD who had pretreatment and posttreatment lumbar punctures were included in this study. All members of a group of 48 previously described[22] consecutive patients who were admitted to a clomipramine treatment trial were asked to have pretreatment and posttreatment lumbar punctures. All who consented were included in this study. Subjects were included in the original clomipramine treatment study if they had egodystonic compulsions and/or obsessions that were of a sufficient severity to cause substantial interference in daily functioning (*DSM-III* diagnostic criteria[23]) and that had been present for at least 1 year. The exclusion criteria were as follows: an IQ less than 70, a neurologic disorder (including Gilles de la Tourette's syndrome), psychosis, primary affective disorder, and primary eating disorder. Secondary depression or a history of affective disorder was not an exclusionary criterion. Psychiatric diagnoses were made on the basis of clinical interviews conducted by at least two psychiatrists from the Child Psychiatry Branch of the National Institute of Mental Health (NIMH), Bethesda, Md, and by structured interviews, including the Diagnostic Interview for Children and Adolescents,[24] administered by another trained clinician.

Pretreatment CSF neuropeptide and monoamine measures from the 43 patients who had pretreatment lumbar punctures were included in a prior report.[3]

All 17 subjects included in this report had both pretreatment and posttreatment lumbar punctures and were medication free for a minimum of 4 weeks (6 weeks for neuroleptics) before the pretreatment lumbar puncture, except one patient who continued to receive theophylline and albuterol sulfate and one patient who received tetracycline hydrochloride. Four to six weeks prior to entering the study, three patients discontinued treatment with a tricyclic antidepressant, two discontinued treatment with a tricyclic antidepressant and a benzodiazepine, and one discontinued treatment with a neuroleptic drug. Eleven of these subjects had not received any psychotropic drugs during the 5 months preceding the pretreatment lumbar puncture. None of the subjects had previously received clomipramine or a selective serotonin-reuptake blocker.

The mean±SD age of the 10 boys and seven girls in this report was 14.0±3.0 years (range, 7.3 to 17.1 years) at the pretreatment lumbar puncture and 15.7±3.1 years (range, 8.8 to 19.0 years) at the posttreatment lumbar puncture. Four subjects were prepubertal at the time of the pretreatment lumbar puncture. Two remained prepubertal (Tanner stage 1) at the posttreatment lumbar puncture, and two had entered puberty (Tanner stage 3 and Tanner stage 4).

All 17 subjects included in this report had experienced improvement in OCD symptoms over the course of treatment with clomipramine. All 17 patients were receiving clomipramine openly at the time of the second lumbar puncture, except one who had discontinued treatment with clomipramine 8 months prior to his second lumbar puncture and had maintained a reduction in OCD, anxiety, and depression symptoms. Mean±SD duration of treatment with clomipramine was 19.8±7.0 months (range, 8.5 to 34.0 months). Mean±SD clomipramine hydrochloride dose at the posttreatment lumbar puncture was 154±72 mg (range, 0 to 250 mg). Mean±SD plasma level of clomipramine at the posttreatment lumbar puncture was 380±190 nmol/L (range, 70 to 790 nmol/L). At the time of the posttreatment lumbar puncture, two subjects were receiving 1000 mg of L-tryptophan daily in addition to clomipramine.

Comorbid Axis I diagnoses at the time of the pretreatment lumbar puncture included attention-deficit disorder (four subjects), oppositional disorder (four subjects), major depression (five subjects), overanxious disorder (three subjects), adjustment disorder (two subjects), phobias (two subjects), and separation anxiety disorder (one subject). Two subjects met the criteria for OCD alone. Comorbid Axis I diagnoses at the time of the posttreatment lumbar puncture included attention-deficit disorder (four subjects), oppositional disorder (two subjects), major depression (two subjects), overanxious disorder (four subjects), and dysthymia (one subject).

Five subjects had a lifetime history of tic disorder, and one of these subjects met the criteria for Gilles de la Tourette's syndrome at the time of his posttreatment lumbar puncture.

LUMBAR PUNCTURE

All subjects adhered to a low-monoamine diet for 3 days preceding each lumbar puncture. The diet excluded foods that contain significant amounts of monoamines, such as cheese, nuts, chocolate, aged or smoked meat or sauces, and several fruits. Except for getting up once briefly to void, the subjects remained at bed rest from midnight the night before and were at continuous bed rest for a minimum of 1 hour before the lumbar puncture, which was conducted between 9 and 10:30 AM. Lumbar punctures were performed in the L4-5 interspace, with the patient in the lateral decubitus position. The study was approved by the NIMH Institutional Review Board. Parental informed consent and the patient's informed assent were obtained before each lumbar puncture.

The first 3 mL of CSF collected was used for routine clinical tests (cell count, electrolyte analysis, and immunoglobulin quantification). The next 6 mL of CSF was collected as a pool on ice, divided into 1 mL aliquots, frozen on dry ice within 15 minutes, and then stored at −70°C until assayed. Aliquots from the 6-mL pool that did not contain additives were used for peptide assays, aliquots containing a few grains of ascorbic acid were used for monoamine metabolite assays, and an aliquot containing 100 μL of 1N acetic acid was used for somatostatin assays.

Continued on next page

PEPTIDE ASSAYS

All pretreatment and posttreatment CSF somatostatin samples were measured in one radioimmunoassay using an unextracted sample and a modification of a previously described technique[25] that included the delayed addition of a carbon 18–purified (Sep-Pak, Millipore, Milford, Mass) label (iodide 125–tyrosine 1 somatotropin-release–inhibiting factor) (New England Nuclear, Wilmington, Del), synthetic cyclic somatostatin standards, rabbit antisomatostatin antibody (Incstar, Stillwater, Minn), and charcoal separation. The detection limit of this assay was 0.78 pmol/L, and the mean intraassay coefficient of variation was 4.3%.

A single 2 mL of extracted CSF sample was used for the measurement of vasopressin, CRH, and oxytocin for each subject at each time point. Recovery of all three peptides was greater than 90%. The CSF vasopressin assay was performed as previously described[1] except that CSF was extracted using the procedure described for plasma samples and a different antibody was used (Arnel, New York, NY). The detection limit of the vasopressin assay was 0.48 pmol/L, and the mean intraassay coefficient of variation for all samples was 2.0%. The CSF CRH[26] and oxytocin[27] assays were performed as previously described. The detection limits were 99 pmol/L and 1.4 pmol/L and the mean intra-assay coefficients of variation for all samples were 2.4% and 2.5%, respectively.

Because pretreatment CSF samples from these patients had been assayed for CRH, vasopressin, oxytocin, and other substances previously,[3] in some patients, inadequate amounts of pretreatment CSF were available to measure pretreatment and posttreatment samples together in the current assays for vasopressin, CRH, and oxytocin. In these cases (n=8), pretreatment values were obtained from the single earlier assay for each peptide using the same methods and performed in the same laboratory. To correct for differences in standards between the earlier assay and the current assay, pretreatment values from the current assay for each peptide were compared with pretreatment values for the same subjects from the earlier assay for each peptide. Linear regression was used to calculate the correlation between the two assays and to determine a linear transformation for the values from the earlier assay for each peptide (for vasopressin, n=9, r=.82; for CRH, n=5, r=.87; and for oxytocin, n=11, r=.89).

Values that fell below the detection limit of any peptide assay (90% binding) were entered as the detection limit value for statistical analysis. Because of laboratory error or an insufficient sample volume, eight subjects did not have paired somatostatin data, one subject did not have paired CSF vasopressin and CRH values, two additional subjects had missing CSF CRH data, and one subject had missing CSF oxytocin data.

MONOAMINE ASSAYS

Levels of the monoamine metabolites homovanillic acid (HVA), 3-methoxy-4-hydroxyphenylglycol (MHPG), and 5-HIAA in CSF were assayed by high-pressure liquid chromatography with electrochemical detection[28] on unextracted samples. All pretreatment and posttreatment samples were measured in one assay. Intra-assay coefficients of variation for HVA, MHPG, and 5-HIAA were 3.8%, 3.3%, and 8.0%, respectively. The sensitivity of the method was 1 pmol/mL for all three metabolites.

CLINICAL ASSESSMENT

Baseline and posttreatment ratings of OCD symptom severity, depression, and anxiety were measured with the Leyton Obsessional Inventory–Child Version,[29] the Ward and Insel Obsessive-compulsive Ratings for OCD,[22,30] the Hamilton Depression Rating Scale,[31] and the NIMH Global Scales for OCD, depression, anxiety, and overall functioning.[32]

STATISTICS

All results are reported as mean±SD. Changes in symptom ratings and CSF neurochemistries following treatment were determined using paired, two-tailed t tests. Relationships between variables were determined by Pearson Product-Moment Correlation Coefficient analyses. Bonferroni corrections were made for multiple comparisons among the neurochemistry t tests and among the correlational comparisons.

Because CSF 5-HIAA, HVA, and oxytocin levels have been correlated with age during childhood and adolescence,[3,33-36] CSF values for these substances were age corrected using regression equations that were obtained from the larger group of 43 child and adolescent patients with OCD on whom pretreatment lumbar punctures had been performed.[3] Previous analyses of the pretreatment CSF values from the larger group of 43 subjects revealed that when the effect of age was removed, pubertal stage, height, and weight did not contribute significantly to the variance.[3]

treatment with clomipramine hydrochloride. All subjects included in the study had responded to various degrees to treatment with clomipramine.

In addition, because pretreatment CSF levels of 5-hydroxyindoleacetic acid (5-HIAA) in patients with OCD have been positively correlated with measures of improvement following treatment with clomipramine,[3,9] we also compared CSF monoamine metabolite levels before and after long-term treatment. Moreover, possible relationships between changes in CSF monoamine metabolites and CSF neuropeptides were assessed in light of preclinical evidence that central CRH, vasopressin, somatostatin, and oxytocin activity are modulated by monoaminergic systems.[10-15] Finally, the unusually long du-

ration of treatment in this study, together with a relatively large sample size, allowed us to determine whether the changes noted in CSF monoamines after short-term treatment with serotonin-reuptake blockers and other antidepressants in prior studies[16-21] are maintained over a longer course of treatment.

RESULTS

CLINICAL RATINGS

As expected, because all patients were clomipramine responders, there was a significant mean decrease in all measures of OCD, depression, and anxiety symptoms from the pretreatment to the posttreatment time points. Values are shown in the **Table**. The mean symptoms ratings for the group decreased from moderately severe OCD to the subclinical range.

CSF NEUROPEPTIDES

After treatment with clomipramine, there was a significant decrease in CSF levels of CRH and vasopressin and a trend toward reduction of CSF somatostatin levels. The CSF CRH values decreased from 175±32 to 152±25 pmol/L (n=14, t=2.6, P<.03) (**Figure 1**). The CSF vasopressin values decreased from 1.30±0.57 to 0.86±0.54 pmol/L (n=16, t=2.8, P<.02) (**Figure 2**). Five posttreatment and no pretreatment CSF vasopressin values were below the detection limit of the assay. The CSF somatostatin level decreased from 21.3±8.5 to 15.3±9.8 pmol/L (n=9, t=2.2, P<.06) (**Figure 3**). There was a nonsignificant increase in CSF oxytocin values with treatment from 6.0±1.7 to 6.3±1.4 pmol/L (n=16, t=−1.5, P=.16). When oxytocin values were age-corrected, this increase with treatment reached statistical significance (6.05±1.60 pmol/L vs 6.70±1.44 pmol/L; t=3.0, P<.01) (**Figure 4**).

Similar changes were found when the analyses were performed on the subgroup of subjects who had pretreatment and posttreatment CSF CRH, vasopressin, and oxytocin levels measured in the same assay. Levels of CRH decreased from 170±18 to 152±21 pmol/L (t=3.6, P<.03), vasopressin levels decreased from 1.56±0.78 to 0.79±0.48 pmol/L (t=2.5, P<.05), and oxytocin levels did not change significantly (6.92±1.58 vs 6.92±1.36 pmol/L, t=0.01, P=.99).

None of the changes in CSF neuropeptides in the full set of patients was significant when corrected for multiple comparisons.

CSF MONOAMINE METABOLITES

There were significant decreases in CSF levels of 5-HIAA, MHPG, and HVA with treatment. Uncorrected CSF 5-HIAA levels decreased from 110±40 to 64±23 pmol/mL (n=17, t=7.1, P<.001), and age-adjusted CSF 5-HIAA decreased from 109±31 to 77±23 pmol/mL (n=17, t=4.8, P<.001) (**Figure 5**). The CSF MHPG levels decreased from 42.4±10.2 to 36.1±4.8 pmol/mL (t=2.3, P<.03) (**Figure 6**). Uncorrected CSF HVA levels decreased from 269±125 to 224±117 pmol/mL (t=3.1, P<.001), and age-adjusted CSF HVA levels decreased from 273±111 to 237±101 pmol/mL (t=2.2, P<.04) (**Figure 7**). The ratio of CSF HVA–5-HIAA increased from 2.44±0.46 to 3.42±0.84 (t=−6.9, P<.0001) (**Figure 8**), reflecting the steeper decrease in the 5-HIAA level than in the HVA level after treatment (23.3% vs 13.2%).

Only the changes in CSF 5-HIAA levels (raw and age-corrected) and raw HVA levels and the ratio of HVA–5-HIAA remained statistically significant after correction for multiple comparisons.

RELATIONSHIPS AMONG VARIABLES

Correlations were performed among the changes with treatment (pretreatment to posttreatment values) in the eight CSF measures and the 10 clinical ratings, as well as among the length of treatment, the clomipramine dose, and the

Change in Clinical Ratings With Treatment With Clomiprimine*

Rating Scale	Clinical Rating: Pretreatment	Clinical Rating: Posttreatment	Percentage of Change±SD (Range)
NIMH Global Scale for OCD	8.9±1.5	4.9±1.9†	−45±22 (−75.0 to 0)
Ward Rating	15.2±1.9	9.6±3.2†	−37±17 (−60.0 to −6.3)
Insel Rating	30.8±6.8	14.2±8.4†	−55±24 (−82.0 to −6.6)
Leyton-Y	21.7±7.6	7.4±8.2†	−67±30 (−100.0 to −13.6)
Leyton-R	35.4±13.9	10.2±10.7†	−66±32 (−100.0 to −12.5)
Leyton-I	41.7±23.6	9.5±17.0†	−78±30 (−100.0 to 0)
Hamilton Depression Rating Scale	6.4±4.2	3.0±3.4†	−13±54 (−100.0 to 33.0)
NIMH Global Scale for Depression	4.2±2.1	1.7±1.3†	−51±33 (−85.7 to 0)
NIMH Global Scale for Anxiety	5.3±2.1	2.2±1.4†	−52±28 (−86.0 to 0)
NIMH Global Scale for Functioning	7.7±1.9	4.1±2.0†	−42±29 (−83.3 to −16.6)

**NIMH indicates National Institute of Mental Health, Bethesda, Md; OCD, obsessive-compulsive disorder.*
†Reduced compared with pretreatment values; P<.001.

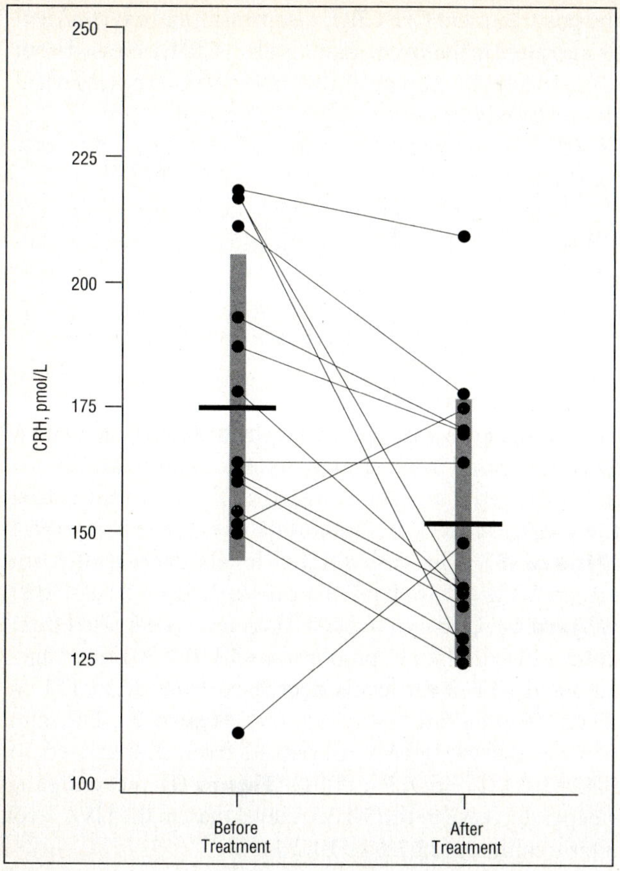

Figure 1. *Cerebrospinal fluid levels of corticotropin-releasing hormone (CRH) before and after treatment with clomipramine. The gray vertical bars and the intersecting solid horizontal bars represent mean±SD.*

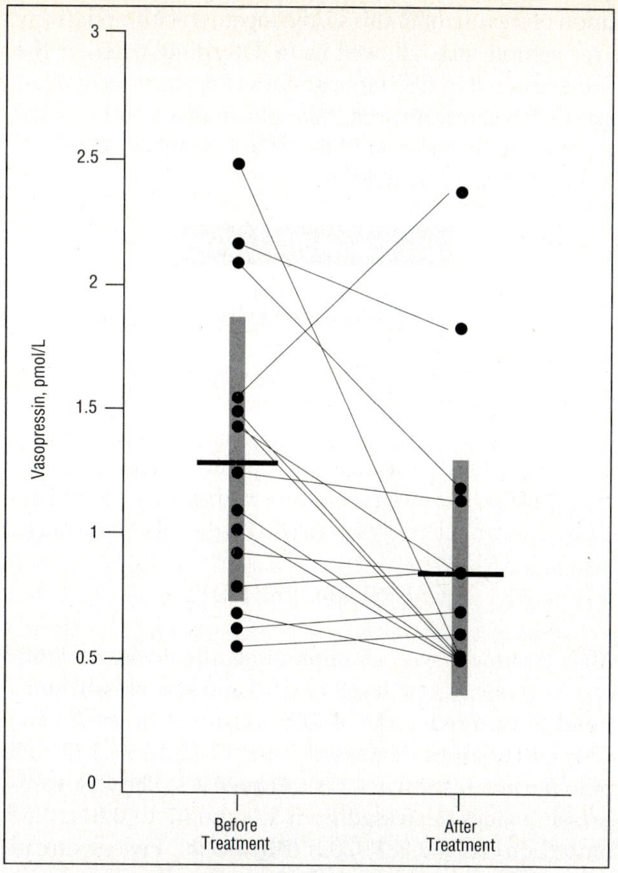

Figure 2. *Cerebrospinal fluid levels of vasopressin before and after treatment with clomipramine. The gray vertical bars and the intersecting solid horizontal bars represent mean±SD.*

plasma level of clomipramine.

Correlations among the changes in CSF measures that were significant or approached significance included changes in age-corrected 5-HIAA and age-corrected HVA levels (n=17, r=.71, P<.01), changes in CRH and age-corrected HVA levels (n=14, r=.57, P=.03), changes in MHPG and somatostatin levels (n=9, r=.60, P<.03), and changes in CRH and vasopressin levels (n=14, r=.45, P<.09). However, after correction for multiple comparisons, only the HVA–5-HIAA correlation met the criteria for statistical significance.

There was a significant positive correlation between the length of treatment and the degree of decrease in CSF vasopressin level (n=16, r=.49, P<.05). There was also a positive correlation between the dose of clomipramine and the degree of reduction of CSF MHPG level (n=17, r=.54, P<.02). However, higher blood levels of clomipramine were associated with a lesser decrease in the CSF HVA level (n=16, r=−.55, P<.03) and in the CSF 5-HIAA level (n=15, r=−5.2, P<.04). Higher blood levels of clomipramine were also associated with less of a change on one of the Leyton subscales (Leyton-Y; n=15, r=−5.2, P<.05).

Greater improvement in one OCD rating scale was associated with a lesser increase in the CSF oxytocin level (NIMH Global OCD, n=16, r=−.53, P<.04).

After correction for multiple comparisons, however, none of the correlations between changes in neurochemical measures from pretreatment to posttreatment and between treatment, clomipramine dosage, or change in clinical variables remained statistically significant.

Subjects with and without comorbid major depression had similar changes in CSF monoamine metabolite and peptide levels.

Three subjects with a lifetime history of tic disorder and six without a lifetime history of tic disorder had CSF somatostatin measurements. There was a significantly greater reduction in somatostatin level with treatment in the subjects with a history of tic disorder compared with those without (14.01±8.71 vs. 2.01±4.01 pmol/L, t=3.0, P<.03). Otherwise, subjects with and without a lifetime history of tic disorder had similar changes during treatment in clinical ratings and in CSF monoamine metabolite and peptide levels.

COMMENT

In a group of children and adolescents with primary OCD, long-term treatment with clomipramine was associated with significant reductions in CSF CRH and vasopressin levels,

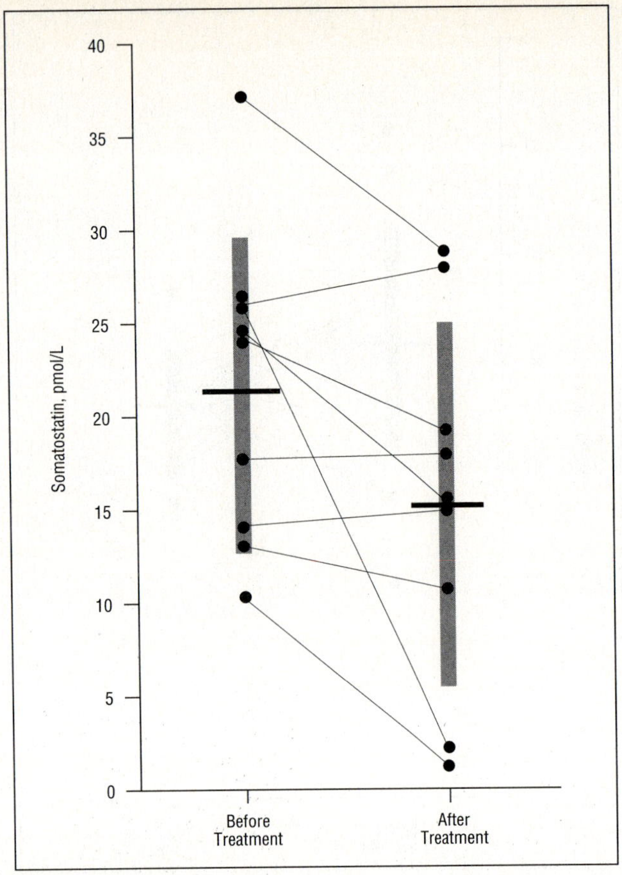

Figure 3. *Cerebrospinal fluid levels of somatostatin before and after treatment with clomipramine. The gray vertical bars and the intersecting solid horizontal bars represent mean±SD.*

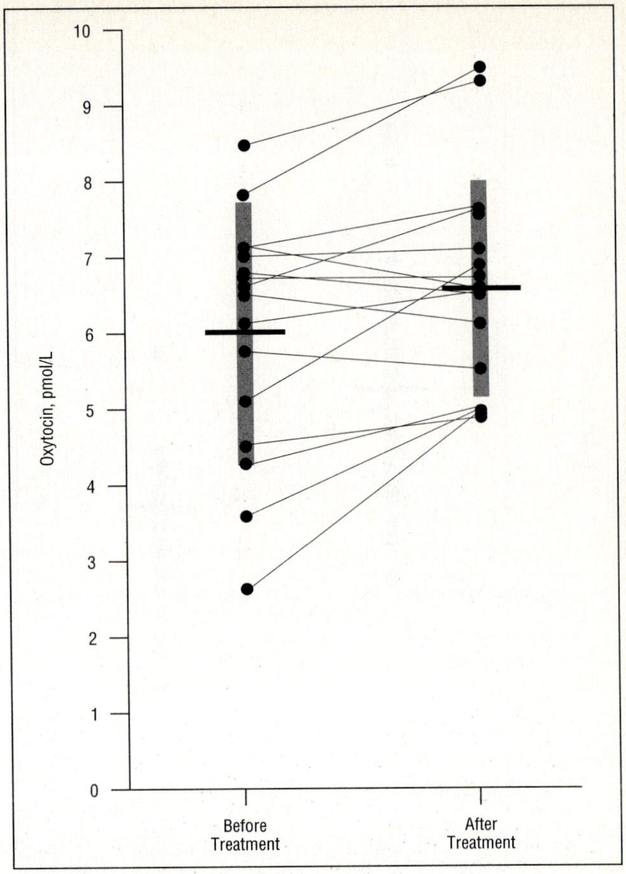

Figure 4. *Age-corrected cerebrospinal fluid levels of oxytocin before and after treatment with clomipramine. The gray vertical bars and the intersecting solid horizontal bars represent mean±SD.*

a trend toward reduction in CSF somatostatin levels, a significant increase in CSF oxytocin levels, and significant reductions in the CSF monoamine metabolites 5-HIAA, MHPG, and HVA. To our knowledge, this is the largest series to date of paired pretreatment and posttreatment CSF measures of neuropeptides in any age group and the largest series to date of paired pretreatment and posttreatment CSF monoamine metabolite measures in adolescents. In addition, to our knowledge, this is the only study to examine CSF monoamine metabolites before and after more than 8 months of treatment with antidepressants.

Because we had only 17 subjects in this study and all were treatment responders, we had limited power to examine the relationship of these neurochemical changes to symptomatic improvement. Although the CSF 5-HIAA level had been correlated with symptom severity and degree of improvement after treatment in an earlier larger study of pretreatment CSF measures in children and adolescents with OCD,[3] in this smaller group consisting of responders only, these correlations were not evident.

It is also difficult to reconcile the negative correlation between pretreatment CSF vasopressin levels and OCD symptom severity found in the larger study[3] with the significant decrease in CSF vasopressin levels after treatment reported herein. Similarly, despite a strong, positive correlation between pretreatment CSF oxytocin levels and depression symptom severity in the earlier study, in this study, CSF oxytocin levels actually increased further with treatment. Finally, the negative correlation between symptom improvement and the degree of increase in CSF oxytocin levels in the current study is difficult to understand in the context of a significant group increase in CSF oxytocin levels with treatment. Thus, these results should be interpreted cautiously. These findings of the current study are consistent, however, with other studies of the effects of antidepressants on central neuropeptide activity.

Our finding of reduced CSF levels of CRH and vasopressin after clomipramine treatment agrees with results from a prior, smaller study of depressed adults treated with fluoxetine, another serotonin-reuptake–blocking antidepressant.[37] The decrease in CSF levels of CRH, vasopressin, and somatostatin in the patients with OCD after successful treatment with clomipramine also parallels reports that in adults with OCD, CSF levels of these three peptides are elevated[1,2] and that CSF somatostatin levels may also be elevated in children and adolescents with OCD.[38]

Because at this time there is little known about the anatomical sources of the neuropeptides measured in CSF, the specific neural subsystems underlying these neuropeptide changes remain to be determined. However, the selective

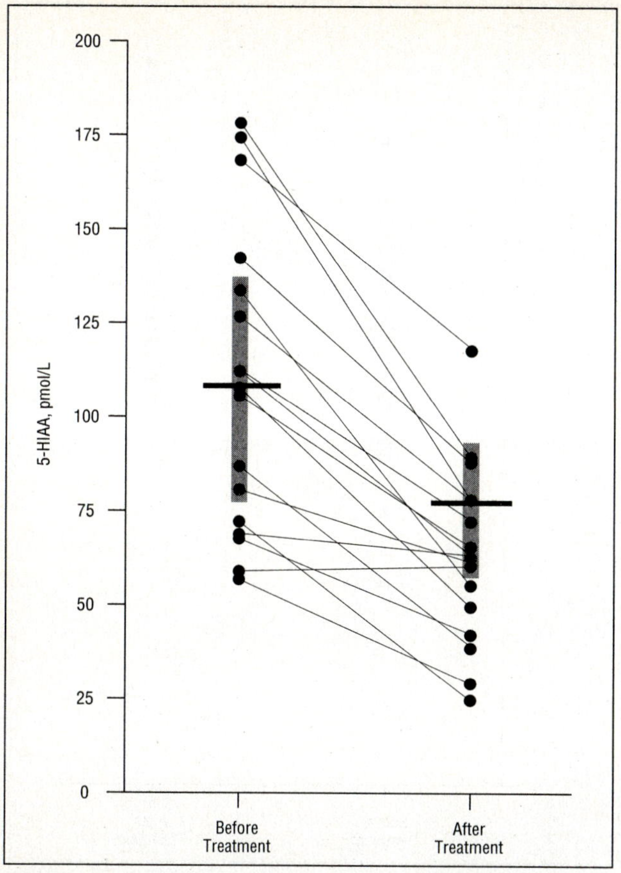

Figure 5. *Age-corrected cerebrospinal fluid levels of 5-hydroxyindoleacetic acid (5-HIAA) before and after treatment with clomipramine. The gray vertical bars and the intersecting solid horizontal bars represent mean± SD.*

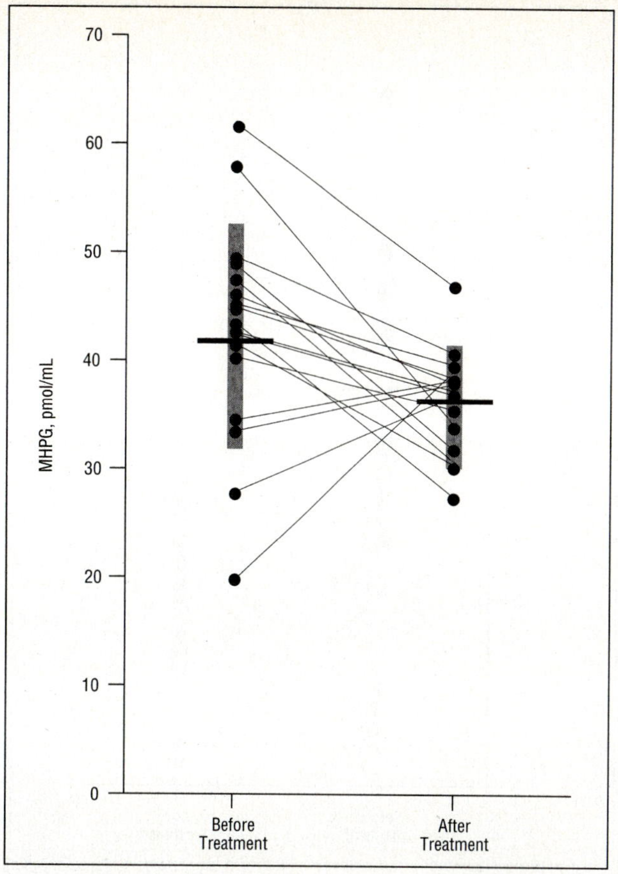

Figure 6. *Cerebrospinal fluid levels of 3-methoxy-4-hydroxyphenylglycol (MHPG) before and after treatment with clomipramine. The gray vertical bars and the intersecting solid horizontal bars represent mean± SD.*

elevations in CSF levels of CRH, vasopressin, and somatostatin in the ill state and the reduction of CSF levels of these peptides with successful treatment may point to a possible pathophysiological role for these peptides in the illness. Because of their wide distribution in the central nervous system and their likely paracrine and endocrine modes of action,[39] neuropeptides have the potential to coordinate diverse systems that are associated with particular behavioral responses. Specifically, the enhanced arousal and delay in extinction of conditioned behaviors observed after central administration of CRH, vasopressin, and somatostatin in animals may be analogous to the hyperarousal and overlearned ritualistic responses to anxiety seen in patients with OCD. Reduction of CSF levels of these peptides after clomipramine treatment and concomitant elevation of CSF oxytocin levels, a peptide that enhances the extinction of conditioned behaviors,[2,4] suggests that the modulation of neuropeptide activity might contribute to the effect of clomipramine during the treatment of OCD.

Elevated CSF levels of CRH, vasopressin, and somatostatin in OCD also may be related to the selective response of this illness to serotonin-reuptake–blocking antidepressants. The decrease in CSF vasopressin levels after clomipramine treatment in the current study and after fluoxetine treatment in the study of DeBellis et al[37] contrasts with a recent report of no change in CSF vasopressin levels after the treatment of normal subjects with amitriptyline hydrochloride,[40] a non–serotonin-selective antidepressant that is not an effective treatment for OCD. Similarly, the trend toward a decrease in CSF somatostatin levels that was observed in this study after treatment with clomipramine was not evident in groups of depressed adults treated with electroconvulsive therapy[41] or a non–serotonin-selective antidepressant.[42,43] In contrast, CSF CRH levels seem to decrease in response to successful treatment with both serotonin-selective[37] and non–serotonin-selective[40,43] antidepressants as well as possibly in response to electroconvulsive therapy.[41,44,45]

These proposed unique effects of serotonin-reuptake–blocking agents to lower CSF levels of vasopressin and somatostatin are supported by data from studies of long-term antidepressant treatment in rats. Whereas long-term treatment with a wide variety of antidepressants lowers CRH messenger RNA (mRNA) expression in the hypothalamus,[46] only long-term treatment with a serotonin-reuptake–blocking agent was effective in reducing vasopressin secretion from the hypothalamus.[14] There is also evidence that long-term treatment with 5-hydroxytryptophan or serotonin-reuptake blockers but not other antidepressants may reduce brain somatostatin content.[13,47]

This report of changes in CSF levels of monoamine

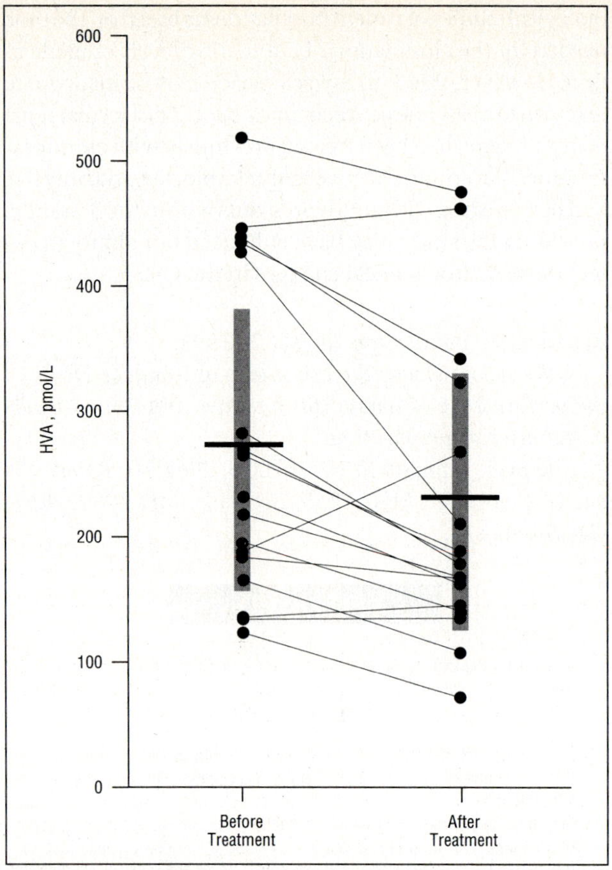

Figure 7. *Age-corrected cerebrospinal fluid levels of homovanillic acid (HVA) before and after treatment with clomipramine. The gray vertical bars and the intersecting solid horizontal bars represent mean±SD.*

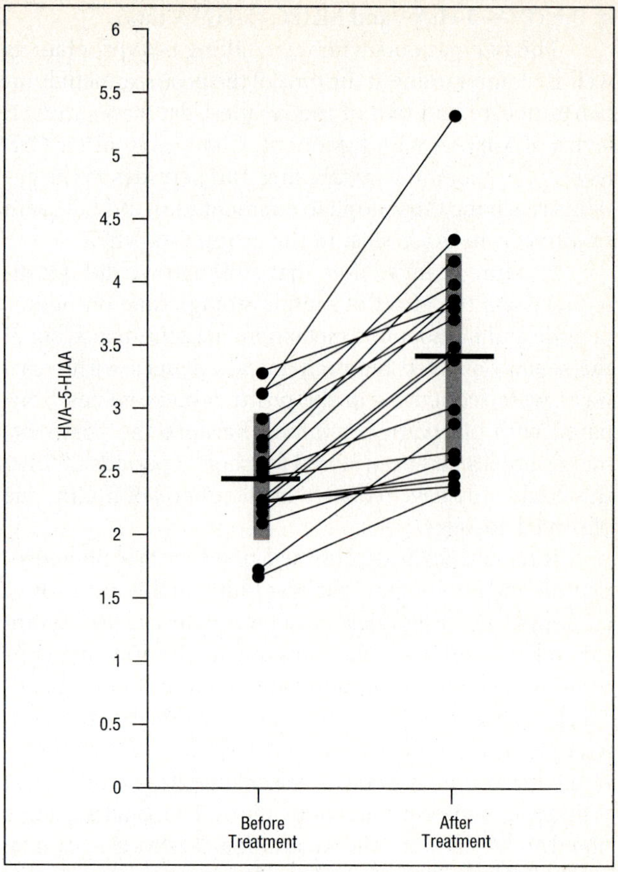

Figure 8. *Cerebrospinal fluid homovanillic acid–hydroxyindoleacetic acid (HVA–5-HIAA) ratio before and after treatment with clomipramine. The gray vertical bars and the intersecting solid horizontal bars represent mean±SD.*

metabolites after long-term treatment points out that changes in central monoamine levels that were noted in earlier studies[16-21] of 3 to 6 weeks' duration persist during treatment averaging 19 months in duration.

The present finding of significant decreases in CSF levels of 5-HIAA and MHPG after long-term treatment are consistent with previous studies[16-21] of the effects of shorter-term antidepressant treatment. In numerous investigations,[17-21,48-50] both serotonin-selective and norepinephrine-selective reuptake inhibitors seem to reduce CSF levels of 5-HIAA and MHPG reliably.

Reported changes in CSF levels of HVA have been more variable, even among non–serotonin-selective tricyclic antidepressant drugs.[16,17,48,51] Previous shorter-term treatment studies with serotonin-reuptake blockers showed no significant change,[16,19,52,53] an increase,[9,20,54,55] or in the case of fluoxetine, a decrease[50] in CSF levels of HVA. A decrease in CSF levels of HVA after short-term treatment may be evident only with fluoxetine because it seems to cause the greatest proportional decrease in CSF levels of 5-HIAA, which has been positively correlated with changes in CSF levels of HVA in this study and several others using a variety of antidepressants.[18,19,20,50,54,56] The decrease in HVA levels in our long-term study of clomipramine had not been observed in several short-term clomipramine treatment studies and suggests that the HVA response to serotonin-reuptake blockade with clomipramine may continue to change for at least several months.

The functional significance of the observed changes in CSF levels of monoamine metabolites is not at all clear. Recent studies indicate that CSF levels of 5-HIAA and HVA do not directly or independently reflect serotonin and dopamine turnover, respectively.[14,57-60] Because monoamine oxidase is located intracellularly, monoamines released into the synapse must undergo reuptake to be metabolized. Thus, although decreased central monoamine turnover should be reflected in decreased CSF metabolite levels, it is also possible that during treatment with a monoamine-reuptake blocker, decreased metabolite levels could be found in association with increased activity of monoamine systems. Consistent correlation of baseline 5-HIAA and HVA levels in CSF[33,56] and positive correlation of changes in CSF levels of 5-HIAA and HVA in this study and others[18-20,50,54,56] is expected in light of the well-documented functional interrelationships between these two monoamine systems.[16,56]

Our finding of an increase in the CSF HVA–5-HIAA ratio after clomipramine treatment is also compatible with prior reports that serotonin-reuptake blockers are distinguished from other antidepressants by producing proportionally greater reductions in CSF levels of 5-HIAA than in CSF levels of HVA or MHPG, thus causing an increase

in the HVA–5-HIAA and MHPG–5-HIAA ratios.*

The two patients who were taking L-tryptophan as well as clomipramine at the time of the posttreatment lumbar puncture had two of the smallest decreases in CSF levels of 5-HIAA with treatment. Changes in other CSF levels of monoamine metabolites and peptides in the patients receiving L-tryptophan augmentation did not seem to differ from those seen in the group as a whole.

It is important to note that although we did not directly assess the effect of sample storage time on neuropeptide and monoamine metabolite measurements, six of the seven observed neurochemical changes with treatment were reductions in the posttreatment values compared with pretreatment values. Because the posttreatment samples had been stored for shorter periods of time, this could only have reduced the likelihood of finding the observed changes.

It remains to be determined whether the CSF neuropeptide and monoamine changes found in this group of 17 clomipramine responders are a proximate cause of symptom relief, result from the symptomatic improvement, or occur independently of such improvement. Neurochemical changes in the one patient in our study who was studied 8 months after discontinuing treatment with clomipramine were consistent with the changes found in the rest of the group still receiving clomipramine. The parallel changes noted after treatment of nonpathological states, ie, animal studies[14,46,47] and studies conducted in normal volunteers,[40,63] suggest that these central neuropeptide and monoamine changes actually result from drug treatment and are not secondary to the amelioration of pathological symptoms. The study in depressed patients by Banki et al[43] suggests that central peptide changes may determine the response to treatment because they found reductions in CSF levels of CRH in sustained responders to antidepressant treatment only. On the other hand, changes in CSF levels of monoamine metabolites did not correspond to the clinical response in a large study of the treatment of depression with amitriptyline and imipramine,[17] which is consistent with the findings of the clomipramine study described herein.

Further support for a role of CSF neuropeptide and/or monoamine changes in symptom reduction would come from evidence that the time course of maximal neurochemical changes corresponds to the time of maximal symptom reduction. Such studies have not yet been performed in clinical populations. In rats, reduction in hypothalamic CRH mRNA[64] and changes in monoamine receptor function[65,66] are seen only after several weeks of treatment with antidepressants. This several-week latency in the development of neuropeptide and monoamine receptor changes following antidepressant treatment raises the possibility that drug-induced changes in neuropeptides and monoamines may persist for several weeks after withdrawal of antidepressant treatment. The current standard drug-free period prior to biological studies of patient populations is based on the time needed for the elimination of circulating levels of medication. However, this 4- to 5-week period may be inadequate to return to a baseline neurochemical state. The fact that none of our patients had been treated previously with clomipramine or a serotonin-selective reuptake blocker and only five had been treated with antidepressants within the 3 months preceding the study may have enhanced our ability to detect these neurochemical changes in the CSF.

*References 16, 17, 20, 21, 49, 50, 58, 61, 62.

Accepted for publication August 1, 1994.

We acknowledge the assistance of Candace Davis in the performance of somatostatin assays and Wilma Davis in manuscript preparation.

Reprint requests to NIMH/LCS, Bldg 10, Room 3D-41, 10 Center Dr, MSC 1256, Bethesda, MD 20892-1264 (Dr Altemus).

REFERENCES

1. Altemus M, Pigott T, Kalogeras KT, Demitrack M, Dubbert B, Murphy DL, Gold PW. Abnormalities in the regulation of vasopressin and corticotropin releasing factor secretion in obsessive-compulsive disorder. *Arch Gen Psychiatry.* 1992; 49:9-20.
2. Altemus M, Pigott T, L'Heureux F, Davis CL, Rubinow DR, Murphy DL, Gold PW. CSF somatostatin in obsessive-compulsive disorder. *Am J Psychiatry.* 1993; 150:460-464.
3. Swedo SE, Leonard HL, Kruesi MJP, Rettew DC, Listwak SJ, Berrettini W, Stipetic M, Hamburger S, Gold PW, Potter WZ, Rapoport JL. Cerebrospinal fluid neurochemistry in children and adolescents with obsessive-compulsive disorder. *Arch Gen Psychiatry.* 1992;49:29-36.
4. Bohus B, Kovács GL, DeWeid D. Oxytocin, vasopressin and memory: opposite effects on consolidation and retrieval processes. *Brain Res.* 1978;157:414-417.
5. Sahgal A. A critique of the vasopressin-memory hypothesis. *Psychopharmacology.* 1984;83:215-228.
6. Koob GF. Behavioral responses to stress. In: Brown MR, Koob GR, Rivier C, eds. *Stress: Neurobiology and Neuroendocrinology.* New York, NY: Marcel Dekker Inc; 1991:255-271.
7. Havlicek V, Rezek M, Freisen H. Somatostatin and thyrotropin-releasing hormone: central effects on sleep and motor systems. *Pharmacol Biochem Behav.* 1976;4:445-451.
8. Vecsei L, Winderlov E. Effects of intracerebroventricularly administered somatostatin on passive avoidance, shuttle-box and openfield activity in rats. *Neuropeptides.* 1988;12:237-242.
9. Thoren P, Asberg M, Bertelsson L, Mellstrom B, Sjoqvist F, Traskman L. Clomipramine treatment of obsessive-compulsive disorder, II: biochemical aspects. *Arch Gen Psychiatry.* 1980;37:1289-1294.
10. Calogero AE, Bagdy G, Szemeredi K, Tartaglia ME, Gold PW, Chrousos GP. Mechanisms of serotonin receptor agonist-induced activation of the hypothalamic-pituitary-adrenal axis in the rat. *Endocrinology.* 1990;126:1888-1894.
11. Calogero AE, Gallucci WT, Chrousos GP, Gold PW. Catecholamine effects upon rat hypothalamic corticotropin releasing hormone secretion in vitro. *J Clin Invest.* 1988;82:839-846.
12. Pergola PE, Alper RH. Vasopressin and autonomic mechanisms mediate cardiovascular actions of central serotonin. *Am J Physiol.* 1991;260:R1188-R1193.
13. Kakigi T, Maeda K. Effect of serotonergic agents on regional concentrations of somatostatin and neuropeptide Y-like immunoreactivities in rat brain. *Brain Res.* 1992;599:49-50.
14. Altemus M, Cizza G, Gold PW. Chronic fluoxetine treatment reduces hypothalamic vasopressin secretion in vitro. *Brain Res.* 1992;593:311-313.
15. Saydoff JA, Rittenhouse PA, van de Kar LD, Brownfield MS. Enhanced serotonergic neurotransmission stimulates oxytocin secretion in conscious male rats. *J Pharmacol Exp Ther.* 1991;257:95-99.
16. Risby ED, Hsiao JK, Sunderland T, Agren H, Rudorfer MV, Potter WZ. The effects of antidepressants on the cerebrospinal fluid homovanillic acid/5-hydroxyindoleacetic acid ratio. *Clin Pharmacol Ther.* 1987;42:547-554.
17. Bowden CL, Koslow SH, Hanin I, Maas JW, Davis JM, Robins E. Effects of amitriptyline and imipramine on brain amine neurotransmitter metabolites in cerebrospinal fluid. *Clin Pharmacol Ther.* 1985;37:316-324.
18. Bertilsson L, Asberg M, Thoren P. Differential effect of clorimipramine and

nortriptyline on cerebrospinal fluid metabolites of serotonin and noradrenaline in depression. *Eur J Clin Pharmacol.* 1974;7:365-367.
19. Martensson B, Wagner A, Beck O, Brodin K, Montero D, Asberg M. Effects of clomipramine treatment on cerebrospinal fluid monoamine metabolites and platelet 3-H-imipramine binding and serotonin uptake and concentration in major depressive disorder. *Acta Psychiatr Scand.* 1991;83:125-133.
20. Bjerkenstedt L, Edman G, Flyckt L, Hagenfeldt L, Sedvall G, Wiesel FA. Clinical and biochemical effects of citalopram, a selective 5-HT reuptake inhibitor: a dose-response study in depressed patients. *Psychopharmacology.* 1985;87: 253-259.
21. Potter WZ, Scheinin M, Golden RN, Rudorfer MV, Cowdry RW, Calil HM, Ross RJ, Linnoila M. Selective antidepressants and cerebrospinal fluid. *Arch Gen Psychiatry.* 1985;42:1171-1177.
22. Leonard HL, Swedo SE, Rapoport JL, Koby E, LeNane M, Cheslow D, Hamburger S. Treatment of obsessive-compulsive disorder with clomipramine and desipramine in children and adolescents: a double-blind crossover comparison. *Arch Gen Psychiatry.* 1989;46:1088-1092.
23. American Psychiatric Association. *Diagnostic and Statistical Manual of Mental Disorders, Third Edition.* Washington, DC: American Psychiatric Association; 1980.
24. Welner Z, Reich W, Herjanic B, Jung KG, Amado H. Reliability, validity and parent-child agreement studies of the Diagnostic Interview for Children and Adolescents (DICA). *J Am Acad Child Adolesc Psychiatry.* 1987;26:649-653.
25. Patel YC, Reichlin S. Somatostatin. In: Jaffe BM, Beheman HR, eds. *Methods of Hormone Radioimmunoassay.* Orlando, Fla: Academic Press Inc; 1979.
26. Roy A, Pickar DS, Paul S, Doran AR, Chrousos GP, Gold PW. CSF corticotropin releasing hormone in depressed patients and normal control subjects. *Am J Psychiatry.* 1987;44:641-645.
27. Demitrack MA, Lesem MD, Listwak SJ, Brandt HA, Jimerson DC, Gold PW. CSF oxytocin in anorexia nervosa and bulimia nervosa: clinical and pathophysiologic considerations. *Am J Psychiatry.* 1990;147:882-886.
28. Seppala T, Scheinin M, Capone A, Linnoila M. Liquid chromatographic assay for CSF catecholamines using electrochemical detection. *Acta Pharmacol Toxicol.* 1984;55:81-97.
29. Berg CZ, Whitaker A, Davies M, Flament MF, Rapoport JL. The survey form of the Leyton Obsessional Inventory–Child Version. *J Am Acad Child Adolesc Psychiatry.* 1988;27:759-763.
30. Flament M, Rapoport JL, Berg C, Sceery W, Kilts C, Mellstrom B, Linnoila M. Clomipramine treatment of childhood obsessive-compulsive disorder. *Arch Gen Psychiatry.* 1985;42:977-983.
31. Hamilton M. Development of a rating scale for primary depressive illness. *Br J Soc Clin Psychol.* 1967;6:278-296.
32. Murphy DL, Pickar D, Alterman IS. Methods for the quantitative assessment of depressive and manic behavior. In: Burdock EI, Sudilovsky A, Gershon S, eds. *Quantitative Techniques for the Evaluation of the Behavior of Psychiatric Patients.* New York, NY. Marcel Dekker Inc; 1982:355-392.
33. Riddle MA, Anderson GM, McIntosh S, Harcherik DF, Shaywitz BA, Cohen DJ. Cerebrospinal fluid monoamine precursor and metabolite levels in children treated for leukemia: age and sex effects and individual variability. *Biol Psychiatry.* 1986;21:69-83.
34. Seifert WE, Foxx JF, Butler IJ. Age effect on dopamine and serotonin metabolite levels in cerebrospinal fluid. *Ann Neurol.* 1980;8:38-42.
35. Leckman JF, Cohen DJ, Shaywitz BA, Caparulo BK, Heninger GR, Bowers MB. CSF monoamine metabolites in child and adult psychiatric patients. *Arch Gen Psychiatry.* 1980;37:677-681.
36. Young SN, Gauthier S, Anderson GM, Purdy WC. Tryptophan, 5-hydroxyindoleacetic acid and indoleacetic acid in human cerebrospinal fluid: interrelationships and the influence of age, sex, epilepsy and anticonvulsant drugs. *J Neurol Neurosurg Psychiatry.* 1980;43:438-445.
37. DeBellis MD, Gold PW, Geracioti TD, Listwak SJ, Kling MA. Association of fluoxetine treatment with reductions in CSF concentrations of corticotropin-releasing hormone and arginine vasopressin in patients with major depression. *Am J Psychiatry.* 1993;150:656-657.
38. Kruesi MJP, Swedo S, Leonard H, Rubinow DR, Rapoport JL. CSF somatostatin in childhood psychiatric disorders: a preliminary investigation. *Psychiatry Res.* 1990;33:277-284.
39. Herkenham M. Mismatches between neurotransmitter and receptor localization in brain: observations and implications. *Neuroscience.* 1987;23:1-38.
40. Heuser I, Bissette G, Gotthardt U, Schmider J, Lammers CH, Dettling M, Deuschle M, Schweiger U, Nemeroff CB, Holsboer F. Effects of amitryiptyline upon HPA-system regulation. *Biol Psychiatry.* 1993;33:72A. Abstract.
41. Nemeroff CB, Bissette G, Akil H, Fink M. Neuropeptide concentrations in the cerebrospinal fluid of depressed patients treated with electroconvulsive therapy: corticotrophin-releasing factor, β-endorphin and somatostatin. *Br J Psychiatry.* 1991;158:59-63.
42. Rubinow DR, Gold PW, Post RM, Ballenger JC, Cowdry RW. Somatostatin in patients with affective illness and in normal volunteers. In: Post RM, Ballenger JC, eds. *Neurobiology of Mood Disorders.* Baltimore, Md. Williams & Wilkins; 1984:369-387.
43. Banki CM, Karmacsi L, Bissette G, Nemeroff CB. CSF corticotropin-releasing hormone and somatostatin in major depression: response to antidepressant treatment and relapse. *Eur Neuropsychopharmacol.* 1992;2:107-113.
44. Kling AS, Metter EJ, Riegge WH. Comparison of PET measurement of local brain glucose metabolism and CAT measurement of brain atrophy in chronic schizophrenia and depression. *Am J Psychiatry.* 1986;143:175-180.
45. Rudorfer MV, Risby ED, Osman OT, Gold PW, Potter WZ. Hypothalamic-pituitary-adrenal axis and monoamine transmitter activity in depression: a pilot study of central and peripheral effects of electroconvulsive therapy. *Biol Psychiatry.* 1991;29:253-264.
46. Brady LS, Gold PW, Herkenham M, Lynn AB, Whitfield HJJ. The antidepressants fluoxetine, idazoxan and phenelzine alter corticotropin-releasing hormone and tyrosine hydroxylase mRNA levels in rat brain: therapeutic implications. *Brain Res.* 1992;572:117-125.
47. Kakigi T, Tanimoto K, Maeda K. The effect of various antidepressants on the concentration of somatostatin in the rat brain. *Jpn J Psychiatry Neurol.* 1990; 44:145.
48. Papeschi R, McClure DJ. Homovanillic and a 5-hydroxyindoleacetic acid in cerebrospinal fluid of depressed patients. *Arch Gen Psychiatry.* 1971;25:354-358.
49. Asberg M, Ringerger V-A, Sjoqvist F, Thoren P, Traskman L, Tuck JR. Monoamine metabolites in cerebrospinal fluid and serotonin uptake inhibition during treatment with chlorimipramine. *Clin Pharmacol Ther.* 1977;21:201-207.
50. Martensson B, Nyberg S, Toresson G, Brodin E, Bertilsson L. Fluoxetine treatment of depression. *Acta Psychiatr Scand.* 1989;79:586-596.
51. Post RM, Goodwin FK. Effects of amitriptyline and imipramine on amine metabolites in the CSF of depressed patients. *Arch Gen Psychiatry.* 1974;30:234-239.
52. Greenhill LL, Stanley M, Setterberg S, Elzohairy B, Shaffer D. Biological studies in suicidal adolescents: stability of CSF measures. Presented at the 38th Annual Meeting of the American Academy of Child and Adolescent Psychiatry; October 1991; San Francisco, Calif.
53. DeBellis MD, Gold PW, Geracioti TD, Altemus M, Kling MA. Effects of fluoxetine treatment on CSF monoamine metabolites in patients with major depression. *Biol Psychiatry.* 1993;33:636-641.
54. Traskman L, Asberg M, Bertilsson L. Plasma levels of clomipramine and its demethyl metabolite during treatment of depression. *Clin Pharmacol Ther.* 1979; 26:600-610.
55. Asberg-Wistedt A, Alvariza M, Bertilsson L, Malmgren R, Wachtmeister H. Alaproclate a novel antidepressant? a biochemical and clinical comparison with zimelidin. *Acta Psychiatr Scand.* 1985;71:256-278.
56. Hsaio JK, Agren H, Bartko JJ, Rudorfer MV, Linnoila M, Potter WZ. Monoamine neurotransmitter interactions and the prediction of antidepressant response. *Arch Gen Psychiatry.* 1987;44:1078-1083.
57. Trulson ME. Dietary tryptophan does not alter the function of brain serotonin neurons. *Life Sci.* 1985;37:1067-1072.
58. Murphy DL. Peripheral indices of central serotonin function in humans. *Ann N Y Acad Sci.* 1990;600:282-296.
59. Commissiong JW. Monoamine metabolites: their relationship and lack of relationship to monoaminergic neuronal activity. *Biochem Pharmacol.* 1985;34: 1127-1131.
60. Kopin KG. Catecholamine metabolism: basic aspects and clinical significance. *Pharmacol Rev.* 1985;37:333-364.
61. Major LF, Lake CR, Lipper S, Lerner P, Murphy DL. The central noradrenergic system and affective response to MAO inhibitors. *Prog Neuropsychopharmacol Biol Psychiatry.* 1979;3:535-542.
62. Bertilsson L, Asberg M. Amine metabolites in the cerebrospinal fluid as a measure of central neurotransmitter function: methodological aspects. *Adv Biochem Psychopharmacol.* 1984;39:27-34.
63. Veith RC, Lewis N, Langohr JI. Effect of desipramine on cerebrospinal fluid concentrations of corticotropin-releasing factor in humans. *Psychiatry Res.* 1993; 46:1-8.
64. Brady LS, Whitfield HJ, Fox RJ, Gold PW, Herkenham M. Long-term antidepressant administration alters corticotropin-releasing hormone, tyrosine hydroxylase, and mineralocorticoid receptor gene expression in rat brain. *J Clin Invest.* 1991;87:831-837.
65. Charney DS, Menkes DB, Heninger GR. Receptor sensitivity and the mechanism of action of antidepressant treatment: implications for the etiology and therapy of depression. *Arch Gen Psychiatry.* 1981;38:1160-1180.
66. Surge MF. Chronic antidepressant therapy and associated changes in central monoaminergic receptor functioning. *Pharmacol Ther.* 1983;21:1-33.

ORIGINAL ARTICLE

Neuropsychological Impairments in Deficit vs Nondeficit Forms of Schizophrenia

Robert W. Buchanan, MD; Milton E. Strauss, PhD; Brian Kirkpatrick, MD; Constanze Holstein, MS; Alan Breier, MD; William T. Carpenter, Jr, MD

Background: Previous studies have suggested that functional impairments of the frontal and parietal lobes are related to the deficit symptoms of schizophrenia. The purpose of the current study was to examine whether neuropsychological measures of frontal and parietal lobe function differentiated deficit from nondeficit patients. Neuropsychological measures of temporal lobe function were used as contrast measures.

Methods: The performance of 18 deficit and 21 nondeficit schizophrenic patients was examined on neuropsychological measures of executive, visuospatial, and memory functions, selected on the basis of their association with lesions of either the frontal, parietal, or temporal lobes. The results from the schizophrenic subgroups were compared with the results on the same measures obtained from 30 normal controls.

Results: Deficit patients performed more poorly than nondeficit patients on two frontal lobe measures, the Stroop Color-Word Interference and Trails Making B tests, and one parietal lobe measure, the Mooney Faces Closure Test. There were no differences in performance on the temporal lobe measures between the two groups. Both groups performed more poorly on the tests than the normal controls.

Conclusion: The results suggest that deficit patients may have greater performance impairments on neuropsychological measures associated with frontal and parietal neuropsychological abnormalities.

(Arch Gen Psychiatry. 1994;51:804-811)

THE VALIDITY of using primary, enduring negative or deficit symptoms to define subgroups of schizophrenia has been examined in a number of studies.[1-6] These studies have demonstrated the temporal stability and long-term predictive validity of the deficit-nondeficit distinction[6] and shown deficit patients to have poorer premorbid adjustment,[1] increased social and physical anhedonia,[2] a differential pattern of associated psychopathological features,[5] and a diminished response to methylphenidate hydrochloride (D. Mayerhoff, MD, S. Alvir, MD, J. Lieberman, MD; unpublished data, 1991). Deficit patients have also been shown to be more neurologically impaired, especially with respect to neurological signs sensitive to parietal lobe function[1]; exhibit increased volitional saccadic latency,[3] an eye-tracking measure sensitive to frontal and/or parietal lobe impairment[7]; and have reduced glucose utilization as assessed with positron emission tomography in the frontal and parietal cortices and thalamus.[4]

The neurological signs, eye-tracking, and results of positron emission tomography studies have been consistent in their implication of the frontal and parietal lobes in the neuroanatomical substrate of deficit symptoms. The possible involvement of the frontal and parietal lobes in the neural substrate underlying the production of deficit symptoms is further supported by the results of multiple functional imaging studies that have found a relationship between nega-

From the Department of Psychiatry, Maryland Psychiatric Research Center, University of Maryland School of Medicine, Baltimore (Drs Buchanan, Kirkpatrick, and Carpenter and Ms Holstein); the Department of Psychology, Case Western Reserve University, Cleveland, Ohio (Dr Strauss); and the Experimental Therapeutics Branch, National Institute of Mental Health, Rockville, Md (Dr Breier).

See Methods on next page

METHODS

SUBJECTS

Thirty-nine patients meeting *DSM-III-R*[24] criteria for schizophrenia were selected from the Maryland Psychiatric Research Center Outpatient Clinic, Baltimore, for entry into the study. All available deficit patients (N=18) were entered into the study. The nondeficit patients (N=21) were selected from the clinic population on the basis of their similarity to the deficit patients on the following demographic variables: age, race, and sex. Diagnoses were made using a best estimate diagnostic approach that used all available information from direct assessment, family informants, and past medical records. Patients with an organic brain disorder, mental retardation, a history of severe head trauma, or a history of drug abuse/dependence were excluded from the study.

The 30 normal controls were selected from the general population through neighborhood newspaper notices and flyers. The controls did not have a past or current *DSM-III-R* Axis I or II disorder, as determined by results of the Structured Clinical Interview for *DSM-III-R*–Patient Version,[25] or a history of organic brain disorder, mental retardation, or severe head trauma.

The patients and normal controls gave informed consent prior to participating in the study. The normal controls were reimbursed for their participation in the study.

CLINICAL ASSESSMENTS

The patients were categorized into deficit and nondeficit subgroups on the basis of the consensus diagnosis of two of us (R.W.B. and B.K.), using the Schedule for the Deficit Syndrome (SDS), a semistructured interview of documented reliability in this population.[26] The SDS provides specific criteria for assessing the presence of negative symptoms, the duration of the symptoms, and whether the symptoms are primary or secondary. Patients were interviewed while they were between episodes, during periods of clinical stability. Additional information was obtained from clinicians with long-standing contact with the patients and from family members. The Brief Psychiatric Rating Scale (BPRS) Thought Disorder Factor was used to measure positive symptoms. Anticholinergic doses were expressed in benztropine equivalents, and mean neuroleptic doses for each group were determined using the conversion system developed by Schooler.[27]

NEUROPSYCHOLOGICAL ASSESSMENTS

The neuropsychological test battery is presented in **Table 1**.[28-38] The tests are measures of executive, visuospatial, and memory functions and were selected on the basis of their association with lesions of either the frontal, parietal, or temporal lobes.[20,38-41] Although performance on the tests selected for this study is adversely affected by lesions of the stated brain regions, neuropsychological test performance is dependent on the functional integrity of multiple brain structures, and performance on these tests may be affected by lesions of other brain regions.[38,42] Therefore, to increase the likelihood of detecting functional disturbances in a specific cortical brain region or system of which it is a part, multiple tests are used to provide a comprehensive assessment of functions associated with each of the cortical brain regions.

The neuropsychological tests were administered according to standardized testing procedures, with minimal reinforcement and extraneous interaction to maximize the similarity in testing situations for each subject. The test battery was administered to the schizophrenic patients while they were clinically stable; patients had been judged to be stable for a median of 18.0 weeks (range, 1 to 121 weeks). All patients were receiving neuroleptics at the time of testing. The test battery was administered to the normal controls on completion of their diagnostic evaluation. The tests were administered in a fixed rather than random order to ensure that more difficult tasks did not occur consecutively, and short tasks were interspersed between longer ones.[38] Frequent breaks were allowed, and, if necessary, the tests were administered over two test sessions. The total time for the administration of the test battery was 3 hours. The subject's attentiveness, effort, and motivation for each of the tests was assessed and coded as adequate or inadequate by the examiner. The assessment of the adequacy of the subjects' performances on the tests was based on the subjects' behavior and comments during the testing session and indicates the examiner's judgment about the degree to which the subjects' performances reflect their abilities. Test scores for which performance was characterized by inadequate attention, effort, and motivation, as determined by the examiner prior to analyses and blind to the study hypotheses and SDS categorizations, were excluded from the analyses. Four subjects had test scores excluded: two deficit patients (from Trails Making B and Benton Judgment of Lines tests) and two nondeficit patients (Wisconsin Card Sorting Test [WCST] and Benton Judgment of Lines Test).

STATISTICAL ANALYSES

The variables used to assess test performance are presented in Table 1. The distribution of each variable was examined to determine if it was normally distributed. The only variables that were not normally distributed were the total times required to complete Trails Making A and B tests. Log transformation was used to normalize these scores.

Derived scores were developed for the Trails Making and Stroop Color-Word Interference tests to have measures specifically focused on the executive (frontal) function construct we wished to measure.[38] For the Trails Making tests, the measure of interest is the influence of set maintenance and set shift requirements

Continued on next page

(Trails Making B Test) independent of general psychomotor efficiency and sequential responding (Trails Making A Test). To evaluate impairments in set functioning, we measured the difference between each subject's actual Trails Making B score and the Trails Making B score estimated by the regression of the log-transformed Trails Making A time on log-transformed Trails Making B time. The regression equation was computed using the data from the normal controls. Accordingly, the mean discrepancy score for the normal control group was zero. The higher the average discrepancy score was for the two schizophrenic subgroups, the slower the Trails Making B time was than expected from the correlation of Trails Making A and B times in normal controls. A similar approach was used to estimate the residual score for the Stroop Color-Word Interference Test measure. The residual score was the difference between the observed Color-Word score and the score predicted by the Color-Word score with Color score regression in normal controls.

The following modification was made in the procedure used to assess performance on the Benton Judgment of Lines Test. This test is usually scored by counting the number of correctly identified line pairs. To measure the magnitude of errors in judgment, as well as their frequency, we calculated the number of positions by which the subject misidentified the correct location of the lines. This score can range from 0 to 355. Weighted raw scores were used for the individual Wechsler Memory Scale–Revised subscales.[43] Scores on the Figural Memory and Visual Pairs subscale were summed, on the basis of the similarity of the memory function assessed by both scales, to maximize the similarity in the number of variables used to assess frontal, parietal, and temporal lobe function. The standard measures were used on each of the remaining tests.

Multivariate analysis of variance (MANOVA) was performed to compare neuropsychological test performance among deficit patients, nondeficit patients, and normal controls. All subjects with complete data sets were included in the MANOVA. Analyses of variance (ANOVAs) were performed to assess group differences on the individual neuropsychological tests. All subjects with valid scores for a particular test were included in the ANOVAs. The significance level was set at $\alpha=.05$.

The ANOVAs were performed to determine if deficit and nondeficit patients differed on medication (ie, anticholinergic and neuroleptic dosages) and clinical variables (ie, level of psychotic symptoms and duration of illness) that could potentially confound deficit-nondeficit comparisons on neuropsychological test performance.[44-47] When differences in control variables were observed, analyses of covariance (ANCOVAs) were performed to assess the effect of each variable on group differences in neuropsychological test performance.

Differences in intelligence or general ability may also be associated with differences in group performance on neuropsychological measures. Therefore, the Wechsler Adult Intelligence Scale–Revised (WAIS-R) Vocabulary and Picture Completion subscale scores were used to estimate General Ability (WAIS-R General Ability).[35] These two measures were selected because they are the two WAIS-R verbal and performance measures, respectively, with the highest correlation with general ability.[38] An ANOVA was performed to assess if deficit and nondeficit patients differed in general ability, and, if differences were significant, ANCOVAs were performed to assess the effect of group differences in intelligence on deficit-nondeficit differences in neuropsychological test performance. The summed age-corrected Vocabulary and Picture Completion subscale scaled scores from the WAIS-R were used as the covariate.

Prior to conducting any ANCOVA analysis, the relationship between the dependent and control variables was assessed in each schizophrenic subgroup to determine if the assumption of homogeneity of regression was met.[48]

tive symptoms and decreased glucose utilization[8,9] or decreased regional cerebral blood flow (rCBF)[10,11] in the frontal lobes and between negative symptoms and decreased rCBF in the inferior parietal cortex.[10] The frontal and parietal cortices have extensive reciprocal interconnections[12,13] and extensive connections with the thalamus, the other brain region implicated in the study of glucose utilization.[14,15] The frontal and parietal cortices are also connected through their involvement in the basal ganglia-thalamocortical circuits described by Alexander[16] and Alexander and Crutcher.[17] Each of these parallel segregated circuits is hypothesized to subserve a discrete range of functions. We have hypothesized the involvement of the dorsolateral prefrontal circuit in the production of deficit symptoms, as it is composed of the brain regions, ie, the dorsolateral prefrontal and inferior parietal cortices and the thalamus, implicated in the pathophysiological features of the deficit syndrome.[1,3,4]

In the present study, the functional integrity of the frontal, parietal, and temporal lobes was assessed in deficit and nondeficit patients with neuropsychological measures selected on the basis of their sensitivity to lesions of these areas. To provide a framework for interpreting the deficit-nondeficit comparisons, the results from the two schizophrenic subgroups were compared with those obtained from normal controls. On the basis of our hypothesis of dorsolateral prefrontal circuit involvement in the production of deficit symptoms, the deficit patients were hypothesized to perform more poorly on frontal and parietal measures than the nondeficit patients. The neuropsychological measures sensitive to temporal lobe lesions were used as control tasks. The two groups were

Table 1. Neuropsychological Test Battery

Test	Variable
Frontal function tests	
Wisconsin Card Sorting	Percent of perseverative errors
Controlled Oral Word Association	Total number of words produced
Stroop Color-Word Interference	Total number of color-word items correctly completed*
Trails Making B	Total number of seconds*
Parietal function tests	
Mooney Faces Closure	Total number of faces correctly identified
Benton Judgment of Lines	Total number of positions by which lines were misidentified
Wechsler Adult Intelligence Scale–Revised Block Design	Total number of points, age-corrected
Temporal function measures	
Wechsler Memory Scale–Revised	
Logical Memory subscale	Total number of items correctly repeated
Figural Memory and Visual Pairs subscale	Total number of designs correctly identified and total number of correct color-figure associations
Verbal Pairs subscale	Total number of correct word associations
Visual Reproduction subscale	Total number of accuracy criteria met in drawing designs

*See the "Methods" section of the text for a more detailed description of scoring procedures.

Table 2. Demographic and Clinical Characteristics

Characteristic	Patients: Deficit (N=18)	Patients: Nondeficit (N=21)	Normal Controls (N=30)
Mean (±SD) age, y	35.3±6.8	32.3±5.6	34.2±7.4
Sex, No. of M/F	15/3	17/4	20/10
Race, No. of black/white/other	6/12/0	4/17/0	4/25/1
Handedness, No. of R/L	16/2	19/2	26/4
Mean (±SD) No. of years of education	11.4±1.7	12.7±2.7	14.2±2.5
Mean (±SD) socioeconomic status*			
Patient	4.6±0.6	3.8±1.1	3.1±0.7
Head of household	3.4±0.9	3.0±1.1	3.1±1.2
Mean (±SD) age at onset, y	20.1±6.0	19.8±4.8	...
Mean (±SD) duration of illness, y	15.3±6.4	12.4±5.6	...
Brief Psychiatric Rating Scale-Factor 1	5.1±3.0	8.1±3.3	...
Mean (±SD) neuroleptic dosage†	3.1±1.1	3.4±0.9	...
Mean (±SD) anticholinergic dosage, mg	3.7±2.3	4.0±2.5	...

*Determined by the Hollingshead-Redlich rating of one to five, in which 1 is the highest and 5 the lowest. Socioeconomic status could not be determined for one deficit patient (N=17) and was not available for three heads of households (N=15) of deficit patients.

†Based on a scale of zero to four, in which 0 indicates no drug; 1, low dosage; and 4, high dosage.

hypothesized not to differ in their performance on these tasks, because temporal lobe abnormalities have been implicated in the production of positive symptoms,[18] and both patient groups were characterized by the presence of these symptoms. However, both schizophrenic groups were expected to perform less well on these measures than the normal controls.[19-21] Two design features distinguished the current study from previous studies of the neuropsychology of negative symptoms. First, the differentiation of deficit symptoms from other types of negative symptoms restricts the scope of investigation to those negative symptoms that were most likely to represent intrinsic trait features of the schizophrenic illness.[22] Second, subjects were prospectively selected on the basis of their exhibition of the psychopathological features of interest, ie, deficit symptoms, and their similarity in demographic and clinical variables. These features optimized the ability to interpret study results in the context of deficit symptoms.[23]

RESULTS

The demographic and clinical characteristics of the study sample are presented in **Table 2**. There were no significant differences between the two schizophrenic subgroups and normal controls in age, sex, or race distribution or handedness. Deficit patients, compared with nondeficit patients, had significantly lower socioeconomic status (SES) (F=8.12; *df*=1,36; *P*<.01). However, there was no significant difference between the deficit and nondeficit patients with respect to head of household SES in the family of origin (F=1.64; *df*=1,34; *P*=.21). The deficit and nondeficit patients had similar numbers of years of education. The normal controls had significantly more years of education and higher SES than both the deficit and nondeficit patients, but there were no significant differences between head of household SES among the normal controls and the schizophrenic subgroups.

Anticholinergic and neuroleptic dosages, length of illness, and age at onset were similar between the two schizophrenic subgroups. The deficit patients had less severe psychotic symptoms than the nondeficit patients at the time of the neuropsychological testing (F=8.88; *df*=1,37; *P*<.01). The test for homogeneity of regression revealed a significant group by BPRS-Factor 1 interaction for multiple neuropsychological measures. The failure to meet the assumption of homogeneity of regression for all the neuropsychological measures precluded the ANCOVA analyses.

The overall MANOVA for the neuropsychological

Table 3. Mean (±SD) Neuropsychological Test Scores

Test	Patients: Deficit (N=18)	Patients: Nondeficit (N=21)	Normal Controls (N=30)
Frontal function tests			
Wisconsin Card Sorting	0.31±0.18*	0.24±0.17†‡	0.14±0.10
Verbal Fluency	29.7±11.8*	36.3±11.9‡	44.3±11.4
Stroop Color-Word Interference	9.6±7.1*§	4.3±8.1	0.0±10.4
Trails Making B	0.17±0.18*§‖	0.04±0.17	0.00±0.12
Parietal function tests			
Mooney Faces Closure	18.4±1.5*§	20.0±2.2	20.5±2.3
Benton Judgment of Lines	15.2±15.6*‖	7.8±6.8†‡	5.2±3.6
Wechsler Adult Intelligence Scale–Revised Block Design	8.7±3.0*	9.5±3.5‡	11.9±2.6
Temporal function subscales¶			
Logical Memory	27.8±16.3*	37.0±18.5‡	57.5±13.0
Figural Memory and Visual Pairs	7.1±3.2*	8.8±2.9‡	11.5±2.0
Verbal Pairs	15.3±5.2*	18.0±4.7‡	20.4±2.7
Visual Reproduction	27.8±7.1*	29.0±9.4‡	36.6±3.8
Other measures			
Wechsler Adult Intelligence Scale–Revised General Ability	13.6±4.0	18.0±5.1	...

*$P<.05$, for deficit patients vs normal controls.
†Scores of one nondeficit patient were excluded.
‡$P<.05$, for nondeficit patients vs normal controls.
§$P<.05$, for deficit vs nondeficit patients.
‖Scores of one deficit patient were excluded.
¶Subscales are from the Wechsler Memory Scale–Revised.

test performance demonstrated a significant group by test interaction (n=65; F=3.07; *df*=22,104; $P<.0001$). The result indicates that the pattern of deficit, nondeficit, and normal control group differences varied across the tests. Univariate tests were performed to assess specific group differences for each test.

Deficit vs Nondeficit

The mean±SD scores for the deficit and nondeficit patients are presented in **Table 3**. The deficit patients performed significantly more poorly on two of the four executive/frontal measures—the Stroop Color-Word Interference (F=4.69; *df*=1,37; *P*=.04) and the Trails Making B tests (F=5.92; *df*=1,36; *P*=.02)—and on one of the three visuospatial/parietal measures—the Mooney Faces Closure Test (F=7.14; *df*=1,37; *P*=.01). There were no significant differences between the two schizophrenic subgroups on any of the memory/temporal measures.

The deficit patients, compared with the nondeficit patients, had significantly lower WAIS-R General Ability scores (F=8.35; *df*=1,36; $P<.01$). Because the regressions between the WAIS-R General Ability scores and neuropsychological test performance in both groups did not differ, the General Ability measure was used as a covariate to determine its influence on the group differences on the neuropsychological test measures. The general pattern of deficit-nondeficit group differences did not change, but the magnitudes of the differences were reduced. The differences on the Stroop Color-Word Interference (F=3.03; *df*=1,35; *P*=.09) and Mooney Faces Closure tests (F=3.80; *df*=1,35; *P*=.06) were reduced to trend levels, and the differences on the Trails Making B Test (F=0.83; *df*=1,34; *P*=.36) were no longer significant.

Schizophrenic Subgroups vs Normal Controls

The mean±SD scores for the normal controls are presented in Table 3. The deficit patients performed significantly worse than the normal controls on all the neuropsychological measures. The same pattern appears with the nondeficit patients, except that there were no significant differences between nondeficit patients and normal controls on the three tests (ie, Stroop Color-Word Interference, Trails Making B, and Mooney Faces Closure) that significantly differentiated deficit from nondeficit patients.

COMMENT

The overall MANOVA demonstrated a significant interaction between group and neuropsychological test, indicating that there were nonuniform group performance differences across the tests. The follow-up univariate analyses revealed that deficit and nondeficit patients differed in performances on selected frontal and parietal measures. Deficit patients performed significantly more poorly on two of the four frontal tests, the Stroop Color-Word Interference and Trails Making B tests, and on one of three parietal tests, the Mooney Faces Closure Test. There were no significant performance differences between the two schizophrenic subgroups on the other frontal or parietal measures. The deficit patients performed significantly more poorly than the normal controls on all the frontal and parietal lobe measures. The differences between the nondeficit patients and normal controls were not as numerous; the two groups did not differ on the three frontal and parietal measures, ie, the Stroop Color-Word Interference, Trails Making B, and Mooney Faces Closure tests, that significantly differentiated the deficit from the nondeficit patients. The results are consistent with the a priori hypothesis that deficit patients, compared with nondeficit patients, are characterized by impairments in frontal and parietal lobe functions. The similarity between the two groups on multiple clinical and demographic variables enhances the likelihood that the observed deficit-nondeficit neuropsychological test performance differences are due to deficit symptoms. The correlation of test performance with the results of either structural or functional imaging mea-

sures of the frontal and parietal lobes are required to confirm the involvement of these brain regions in the impaired test performance.[49]

THE ASSOCIATION of frontal lobe functional impairment and deficit symptoms is consistent with the findings of previous neuropsychological studies of negative symptoms. Most,[50-54] but not all,[55-57] studies have demonstrated a relationship between negative symptoms and impaired performance on neuropsychological tests sensitive to frontal lobe dysfunction. Examination of the studies that used some of the same frontal measures used in the current study reveals a fairly consistent pattern of results. In the current study, we failed to find a unique relationship between the WCST or Verbal Fluency Test performance and deficit symptoms, ie, deficit and nondeficit patients both performed poorly on the tasks. In three studies that have examined the concurrent relationship between WCST performance and negative symptoms, one study found WCST perseverative errors to be significantly correlated with both positive and negative symptoms,[50] and two studies were unable to document a significant relationship between WCST perseverative errors and negative symptoms.[56,57] Similarly, Liddle and Morris[56] found Verbal Fluency performance to be associated with both negative symptoms and thought disorder, and Morrison-Stewart et al[57] were unable to demonstrate a relationship between Verbal Fluency Test performance and negative symptoms. In contrast, Stolar et al[54] observed Verbal Fluency Test performance to be significantly and inversely related to alogia and affective flattening and not related to positive symptoms. The contrast with the findings of the current study may be related to their emphasis on alogia in defining their negative symptom construct. Only Breier et al[53] have found a unique relationship between WCST performance and negative symptoms. They also found Verbal Fluency Test performance to be uniquely related to negative symptoms. In that study, the reported relationships were between index neuropsychological test performance and follow-up negative symptom ratings. Finally, Liddle and Morris[56] did not find an association between negative symptoms and measures of performance on the Stroop Color-Word Interference and Trails Making B tests, similar measures to those used in the current study. In summary, the majority of studies, despite major methodological differences, are consistent in their failure to find a unique relationship between WCST and Verbal Fluency Test performance and negative symptoms. There are less data with respect to the performance on the Stroop Color-Word Interference and Trails Making B tests, but only the current study was designed to specifically isolate primary and enduring negative symptoms for study.

There have been relatively few studies examining the relationship between neuropsychological measures of parietal lobe function and negative symptoms, although Green and Walker[58] did find performance on the Purdue Pegboard and Block Design tests related to negative symptoms. In addition, Liddle et al[10] reported a relationship between decreased rCBF in the inferior parietal cortex and negative symptoms.

There were no significant deficit-nondeficit differences on any of the temporal lobe/memory measures. Both schizophrenic subgroups performed, as predicted, less well than the normal controls on the temporal lobe tasks. The observation of impaired memory function in the two schizophrenic subgroups is consistent with previous studies documenting memory impairments in schizophrenic patients.[20,21,55] Moreover, the shared impairments in memory function support hypotheses of temporal lobe involvement in the production of psychotic symptoms,[4,59-61] as both groups were characterized by the presence of psychotic symptoms.

There are several methodological issues that require comment. First, although the deficit and nondeficit patients were similar on multiple clinical and demographic variables, the nondeficit patients did have a significantly higher level of psychotic symptoms at the time of neuropsychological testing than the deficit patients. The failure to meet the assumption of homogeneity of regression precluded the use of BPRS-Factor 1 as a covariate to statistically assess the effect of the level of psychotic symptoms on deficit-nondeficit differences on neuropsychological test performance. It is unlikely that differences in the level of psychotic symptoms underlie the deficit-nondeficit differences on the Stroop Color-Word Interference, Trails Making B, and Mooney Faces Closure tests, as psychotic symptoms would be more likely to interfere with test performance. However, the possibility exists that the higher level of psychotic symptoms in the nondeficit patients differentially interfered with their performance on the neuropsychological test measures, leading to the failure to find deficit-nondeficit performance differences on the other neuropsychological test measures. The selection of deficit and nondeficit patients with comparable levels of psychotic symptoms is required to examine this possibility.

Second, the addition of the intelligence/general ability measure as a covariate altered the magnitude of deficit-nondeficit group differences on the Stroop Color-Word Interference, Mooney Faces Closure, and Trails Making B tests. An examination of the ω^2 value, an estimation of the effect size due to the experimental manipulation (ie, the deficit-nondeficit categorization[62]), suggests that the deficit-nondeficit group differences on the Stroop Color-Word Interference and Mooney Faces Closure tests, although reduced to a trend level, are nontrivial and remain potentially meaningful. The effect sizes for the three tests, prior to covariance adjustment for intelligence/general abil-

ity, were .14 for the Stroop Color-Word Interference Test; .09 for the Mooney Faces Closure Test; and .12 for the Trails Making B Test. After the covariance adjustment for intelligence/general ability, the effect sizes for the Stroop Color-Word Interference and Mooney Faces Closure tests were .09 and .05, respectively. The effect size for the Trails Making B Test was zero. Parenthetically, the effect sizes for the three temporal lobe measures that were greater than zero prior to covariance adjustment for intelligence, ie, Logical Memory, Verbal Pairs, and Figural Memory and Visual Pairs subscales, equaled zero after covariance adjustment for intelligence. By way of comparison, the ω^2 value for the effect of cigarette smoking on heart disease in the Framingham study was .01.[63] This was, of course, statistically significant because of the large sample size in that epidemiological study, whereas the power in the present study was much less because of the small sample sizes, and so our findings are suggestive rather than conclusive.

Understanding the role of intelligence/general ability in deficit-nondeficit performance differences is an important issue in interpreting the present study results. When this study was designed, intelligence/general ability was construed as a "nuisance" variable that required control, ie, the intelligence/general ability measure was to control for group performance differences unrelated to the deficit/nondeficit categorization. This may have been an incorrect perspective. A number of investigations have reported significant relationships between intelligence and negative symptoms.[50,54,64,65] In addition, intelligence in schizophrenic patients has also been related to other features that differentiate deficit and nondeficit patients, specifically neurological signs and poor premorbid adjustment.[66-68] Further, SES has also been shown to be correlated with intelligence, and, in the current study, deficit patients had a lower SES than nondeficit patients. Thus, it is not clear that intelligence/general ability should be conceptualized as a nuisance variable. The complex interaction between intelligence/general ability and the deficit syndrome suggests that it may not be possible to disentangle the effects of intelligence from more specific impairments on standardized neuropsychological tests using statistical means.

Third, the possibility exists that the deficit-nondeficit differences on the selected frontal and parietal measures are due to the differential discriminating power of the neuropsychological measures and not specific behavioral abnormalities.[69] Alternatively, discriminating power differences could also account for the failure of all of the frontal and parietal measures to differentiate deficit from nondeficit patients. In the future, it may be necessary to develop psychometrically matched tasks designed to tap specific neuropsychological functions of research interest to effectively deal with the problem of differential deficit in studies concerned with the identification of neurocognitive functional differences within schizophrenic subgroups.[69]

In conclusion, the results of the current study provide tentative support for the hypothesis that deficit symptoms are associated with frontal and parietal neuropsychological impairments. If the results are confirmed, important questions arise concerning how these impairments are related to the production of deficit symptoms. Future studies will attempt to elucidate the specific cognitive impairments occurring in deficit patients and combine theoretically based, rather than clinically derived, behavioral measures with structural and functional imaging measures to examine more precisely the involvement of the frontal and parietal cortices and other components of the dorsolateral prefrontal basal ganglia-thalamocortical circuit in the production of deficit symptoms.

Accepted for publication June 23, 1994.

Supported by grants MH40279, MH45074, MH48225, and MH00925 from the National Institute of Mental Health, Rockville, Md, and by the National Alliance for Research in Schizophrenia and Depression, Chicago, Ill, (Drs Buchanan and Kirkpatrick).

Reprint requests to Psychiatric Research Center, PO Box 21247, Baltimore, MD 21228 (Dr Buchanan).

REFERENCES

1. Buchanan RW, Kirkpatrick B, Heinrichs DW, Carpenter WT. Clinical correlates of the deficit syndrome of schizophrenia. *Am J Psychiatry.* 1990;147:290-294.
2. Kirkpatrick B, Buchanan RW. Anhedonia and the deficit syndrome of schizophrenia. *Psychiatry Res.* 1989;31:25-30.
3. Thaker G, Kirkpatrick B, Buchanan RW, Ellsberry R, Lahti A, Tamminga CA. Oculomotor abnormalities and their clinical correlates in schizophrenia. *Psychopharmacol Bull.* 1989;25:491-498.
4. Tamminga CA, Thaker GK, Buchanan R, Kirkpatrick B, Alphs LD, Chase TN, Carpenter WT. Limbic system abnormalities identified in schizophrenia using positron emission tomography with fluorodeoxyglucose and neocortical alterations with deficit syndrome. *Arch Gen Psychiatry.* 1992;49:522-530.
5. Gur RE, Mozley PD, Resnick SM, Levick S, Erwin R, Saykin AJ, Gur RC. Relations among clinical scales in schizophrenia. *Am J Psychiatry.* 1991;148: 472-478.
6. Fenton WS, McGlashan TH. Testing systems for assessment of negative symptoms in schizophrenia. *Arch Gen Psychiatry.* 1992;49:179-184.
7. Pierrot-Deseilligny CH, Rivaud S, Gaymard G, Agid Y. Cortical control of reflexive visually-guided saccades. *Brain.* 1991;114:1473-1485.
8. Volkow ND, Wolf AP, Van Gelder P, Brodie JD, Overall JE, Cancro R, Gomez-Mont F. Phenomenological correlates of metabolic activity in 18 patients with chronic schizophrenia. *Am J Psychiatry.* 1987;144:151-158.
9. Wolkin A, Sanfilipo M, Wolf AP, Angrist B, Brodie JD, Rotrosen J. Negative symptoms and hypofrontality in chronic schizophrenia. *Arch Gen Psychiatry.* 1992;49:959-965.
10. Liddle PF, Friston KJ, Frith CD, Hirsch SR, Jones T, Frackowiak RSJ. Patterns of cerebral blood flow in schizophrenia. *Br J Psychiatry.* 1992;160:179-186.
11. Andreasen NC, Rezai K, Alliger R, Swayze VW III, Flaum M, Kirchner P, Cohen G, O'Leary DS. Hypofrontality in neuroleptic-naive patients and in patients with chronic schizophrenia: assessment with Xenon 133 single-photon emission computed tomography and the Tower of London. *Arch Gen Psychiatry.* 1992; 49:943-958.
12. Cavada C, Goldman-Rakic PS. Posterial parietal cortex in Rhesus monkey, I: parcellation of areas based on distinctive limbic and sensory corticocortical connections. *J Comp Neurol.* 1989;287:393-421.
13. Cavada C, Goldman-Rakic PS. Posterior parietal cortex in Rhesus monkey, II: evidence for segregated corticocortical networks linking sensory and limbic areas with the frontal lobe. *J Comp Neurol.* 1989;287:422-445.

14. Mesulam M-M. *Principles of Behavioral Neurology.* Philadelphia, Pa: FA Davis Co Publishers; 1985.
15. Fuster JM. *The Prefrontal Cortex.* New York, NY: Raven Press; 1989.
16. Alexander GE. Parallel organization of functionally segregated circuits linking basal ganglia and cortex. *Annu Rev Neurosci.* 1986;9:357-381.
17. Alexander GE, Crutcher MD. Functional architecture of basal ganglia circuits: neural substrates of parallel processing. *Trends Neurosci.* 1990;13:266-270.
18. Buchanan RW, Carpenter WT. Domains of psychopathology: concept and validity. *J Nerv Ment Dis.* 1994;182:193-204.
19. Kolb B, Whishaw IQ. Performance of schizophrenic patients on tests sensitive to left or right frontal, temporal, or parietal function in neurological patients. *J Nerv Ment Dis.* 1983;171:435-443.
20. Gruzelier J, Seymour K, Wilson L, Jolley A, Hirsch S. Impairments on neuropsychologic tests of temporohippocampal and frontohippocampal functions and word fluency in remitting schizophrenia and affective disorders. *Arch Gen Psychiatry.* 1988;45:623-629.
21. Saykin AJ, Gur RC, Gur RE, Mozley D, Mozley LH, Resnick SM, Kester DB, Stafiniak P. Neuropsychological function in schizophrenia: selective impairment in memory and learning. *Arch Gen Psychiatry.* 1991;48:618-624.
22. Carpenter WT Jr, Heinrichs DW, Wagman AMI. Deficit and nondeficit forms of schizophrenia: the concept. *Am J Psychiatry.* 1988;145:578-583.
23. Carpenter WT Jr, Buchanan RW, Kirkpatrick B, Tamminga C, Wood F. Strong inference, theory testing, and the neuroanatomy of schizophrenia. *Arch Gen Psychiatry.* 1993;50:825-831.
24. American Psychiatric Association, Committee on Nomenclature and Statistics. *Diagnostic and Statistical Manual of Mental Disorders, Revised Third Edition.* Washington, DC: American Psychiatric Association; 1987.
25. Spitzer RL, Williams JBW, Gibbon M, First MB. *Structured Clinical Interview for DSM-III-R–Patient Version (SCID-P, 5/1/89).* New York, NY: Biometrics Research Dept, New York State Psychiatric Institute; 1989.
26. Kirkpatrick B, Buchanan RW, McKenney PD, Alphs LD, Carpenter WT Jr. The Schedule for the Deficit Syndrome: an instrument for research in schizophrenia. *Psychiatry Res.* 1989;30:119-123.
27. Schooler N. Antipsychotic medications in schizophrenia: their effect in acute and maintenance treatment. In: Cromwell RL, ed. *Schizophrenia: Origins, Processes, Treatment, and Outcome.* New York, NY: Oxford University Press; 1993.
28. Heaton RK. *Wisconsin Card Sorting Test, Manual.* Odessa, Fla: Psychological Assessment Resources; 1981.
29. Taylor LB. Psychological assessment of neurosurgical patients. In: Rasmussen T, Marino R, eds. *Functional Neurosurgery.* New York, NY: Raven Press; 1979:165-180.
30. Milner B. Some effects of frontal lobectomy in man. In: Warren JM, Akert K, eds. *The Frontal Granular Cortex and Behavior.* New York, NY: McGraw-Hill International Book Co; 1964:313-334.
31. Golden CJ. *Stroop Color and Word Test: A Manual for Clinical and Experimental Uses.* Chicago, Ill: Stoelting Co; 1978.
32. Reitan RM, Wolfson D. *The Halstead-Reitan Neuropsychological Test Battery: Theory and Clinical Interpretation.* Tucson, Ariz: Neuropsychology Press; 1985.
33. Mooney CM. Age in the development of closure ability in children. *Can J Psychol.* 1957;11:219-226.
34. Benton AL, Hannay HJ, Varney NR. Visual perception of line direction in patients with unilateral disease. *Neurology.* 1975;25:907-910.
35. Wechsler D. *Wechsler Adult Intelligence Scale–Revised, Manual.* Cleveland, Ohio: The Psychological Corp; 1981.
36. Wechsler D. A standardized memory scale for clinical use. *J Psychol.* 1945; 19:87-95.
37. Russell EW. A multiple scoring method for assessment of complex memory functions. *J Consult Clin Psychol.* 1975;43:800-809.
38. Lezak MD. *Neuropsychological Assessment.* 2nd ed. New York, NY: Oxford University Press; 1983.
39. Perrett E. The left frontal lobe of man and the suppression of habitual responses in verbal categorical behaviour. *Neuropsychologia.* 1974;12:323-330.
40. Fried I, Mateer C, Ojemann G, Wohns R, Fedio P. Organization of visuospatial functions in human cortex. *Brain.* 1982;105:349-371.
41. Goldberg TE, Kelsoe JR, Weinberger DR, Pliskin NH, Kirwin PD, Berman KF. Performance of schizophrenic patients on putative neuropsychological tests of frontal lobe function. *Int J Neurosci.* 1988;42:51-58.
42. Anderson SW, Damasio H, Jones RD, Tranel D. Wisconsin Card Sorting Test performance as a measure of frontal lobe damage. *J Clin Exp Neuropsychol.* 1991;13:909-922.
43. Wechsler D. *WMS-R, Wechsler Memory Scale—Revised Manual.* New York, NY: The Psychological Corporation, Harcourt Brace Jovanovich, Inc; 1987.
44. Perlick D, Stastny P, Katz I, Mayer M, Mattis S. Memory deficits and anticholinergic levels in chronic schizophrenia. *Am J Psychol.* 1986;143:230-232.
45. Strauss ME, Reynolds KA, Jayaram G, Tune LE. Effects of anticholinergic medication on memory in schizophrenia. *Schizophr Res.* In press.
46. Medalia A, Gold J, Merriam A. The effects of neuroleptics on neuropsychological test results of schizophrenics. *Arch Clin Neuropsychol.* 1988;3:249-271.
47. Cassens G, Inglis AK, Appelbaum PS, Gutheil TG. Neuroleptics: effects on neuropsychological function in chronic schizophrenic patients. *Schizophr Bull.* 1990; 16:477-499.
48. Stevens J. *Applied Multivariate Statistics for the Social Sciences.* Hillsdale, NJ: Lawrence Erlbaum Associates; 1986.
49. Goldstein G. Comprehensive neuropsychological test batteries and research in schizophrenia. In: Steinhauer SR, Gruzelier JH, Zubin Z, eds. *Handbook of Schizophrenia: Neuropsychology, Psychophysiology and Information Processing.* New York, NY: Elsevier Science Publishers; 1991;5:525-551.
50. Braff DL, Heaton R, Kuck J, Cullum M, Moranville J, Grant I, Zisook S. The generalized pattern of neuropsychological deficits in outpatients with chronic schizophrenia with heterogeneous Wisconsin Card Sorting Test results. *Arch Gen Psychiatry.* 1991;48:891-898.
51. Guy JD, Liaboe GP, Wallace CJ. Premorbid adjustment in adult male schizophrenics, as related to process vs reactive, chronic vs acute, age of onset, and neurologically impaired vs non-impaired. *J Clin Psychol.* 1986;42:62-67.
52. Kemali D, Maj M, Galderisi S, Monteleone P, Mucci A. Conditional associative learning in drug-free schizophrenic patients. *Neuropsychobiology.* 1987;17: 30-34.
53. Breier A, Schreiber JL, Dyer J, Pickar D. National Institute of Mental Health longitudinal study of chronic schizophrenia: prognosis and predictors of outcome. *Arch Gen Psychiatry.* 1990;48:239-246.
54. Stolar N, Berenbaum H, Banich MT, Barch D. Neuropsychological correlates of alogia and affective flattening in schizophrenia. *Biol Psychiatry.* 1994;35:164-172.
55. Goldberg TE, Ragland JD, Fuller-Torrey E, Gold JM, Bigelow LB, Weinberger DR. Neuropsychological assessment of monozygotic twins discordant for schizophrenia. *Arch Gen Psychiatry.* 1990;47:1066-1072.
56. Liddle PF, Morris DL. Schizophrenic syndromes and frontal lobe performance. *Br J Psychiatry.* 1991;158:340-345.
57. Morrison-Stewart SL, Williamson PC, Corning WC, Kutcher SP, Snow WG, Merskey H. Frontal and non-frontal lobe neuropsychological test performance and clinical symptomatology in schizophrenia. *Psychol Med.* 1992;22:353-359.
58. Green M, Walker E. Neuropsychological performance and positive and negative symptoms in schizophrenia. *J Abnorm Psychol.* 1985;94:460-469.
59. Weinberger DR. Implications of normal brain development for the pathogenesis of schizophrenia. *Arch Gen Psychiatry.* 1987;44:660-669.
60. Barta PE, Pearlson GD, Powers RE, Richards SS, Tune LE. Auditory hallucinations and smaller superior temporal gyral volume in schizophrenia. *Am J Psychiatry.* 1990;147:1457-1462.
61. Cleghorn JM, Franco S, Szechtman B, Kaplan RD, Szechtman H, Brown GM, Nahmias C, Garnett ES. Toward a brain map of auditory hallucinations. *Am J Psychiatry.* 1992;149:1062-1069.
62. Keppel G. *Design and Analysis: A Researcher's Handbook.* Englewood Cliffs, NJ: Prentice-Hall International Inc; 1973.
63. Rosenthal R, Rosenow RL. *Essentials of Behavioural Research: Methods and Data Analysis.* New York, NY: McGraw Hill International Book Co; 1991.
64. Crow TJ. The two-syndrome concept: origins and current status. *Schizophr Bull.* 1985;11:471-486.
65. Addington J, Addington D, Maticka-Tyndale E. Cognitive functioning and positive and negative symptoms in schizophrenia. *Schizophr Res.* 1991;5:123-134.
66. Mosher LR, Pollin W, Stabenau JR. Identical twins discordant for schizophrenia. *Arch Gen Psychiatry.* 1971;24:422-430.
67. Manschreck TC, Ames D. Neurologic features and psychopathology. *Biol Psychiatry.* 1948;19:703-719.
68. Garmezy N. Process and reactive schizophrenia: some conceptions and issues. In: Katz MM, Cole JO, Barton WE, eds. *The Role and Methodology of Classification in Psychiatry and Psychopathology.* Washington, DC: US Government Printing Office; 1968. US Dept of Health, Education, and Welfare publication 1584.
69. Chapman LJ, Chapman JP. The measurement of differential deficits. *J Psychiatr Res.* 1978;14:303-311.

Autonomic Abnormalities in Schizophrenia

State or Trait Indicators?

Michael E. Dawson, PhD; Keith H. Nuechterlein, PhD; Anne M. Schell, PhD; Michael Gitlin, MD; Joseph Ventura, MA

Background: Tonic electrodermal measures have been widely used to index autonomic abnormalities in schizophrenia, whereas phasic electrodermal nonresponsiveness has been frequently used to index attentional orienting abnormalities. The primary objective of the present study was to assess whether these electrodermal abnormalities are episode indicators or vulnerability indicators.

Methods: Twenty patients with a recent first episode of schizophrenia were tested during symptomatically remitted states and psychotic states. Twenty demographically matched normal controls were tested at two comparable intervals. Testing for stability of abnormalities across remitted and psychotic states allowed us to determine whether tonic and phasic electrodermal measures qualify as episode indicators or vulnerability indicators.

Results: Tonic electrodermal activity was abnormally elevated only during the psychotic state, which indicates that it is an episode indicator in schizophrenia. Phasic hyporesponsiveness relative to levels of general activation was present in both the remitted and the psychotic states, most strikingly during the psychotic state, and the proportion of patients who were electrodermally nonresponsive tended to be abnormally high during the remission test.

Conclusion: Tonic electrodermal hyperarousal appears to be a state-sensitive episode indicator, whereas phasic electrodermal hyporesponsiveness to innocuous stimuli relative to activation level appears to be a mediating vulnerability factor.

(Arch Gen Psychiatry. 1994;51:813-824)

SCHIZOPHRENIA IS a disorder that is characterized by impairments in attention and information processing and by dysfunctions in autonomic nervous system activation. Electrodermal activity has been used frequently to index abnormalities in both of these realms.[1-8] Electrodermal activity is a peripheral measure of electrical conductivity of the skin and is widely employed in the study of both normal and pathological populations because it indexes sympathetic nervous system activity and is sensitive to psychological processes. Electrodermal activity is distinctive from other autonomic measures in that it is mediated by sympathetic processes rather than by a combination of sympathetic and parasympathetic processes. It is common to distinguish between relatively long-lasting tonic electrodermal activity and more transient phasic electrodermal activity. *Tonic* electrodermal measures such as skin conductance level and frequency of nonspecific skin conductance responses have been used to index general sympathetic nervous system arousal and activation, whereas stimulus-elicited *phasic* skin conductance responses have been used to examine attention allocation, orienting, and information processing. Recent books[9,10] and chapters of books[11,12] provide detailed presentations of the physiological and psychological significance of electrodermal measures.

Two prominent electrodermal abnormalities have been identified in schizophrenia. One abnormality is the reduced frequency of phasic skin conductance orienting responses (SCORs), particularly to

From the Department of Psychology, the University of Southern California (Dr Dawson); the Department of Psychiatry and Biobehavioral Sciences, the University of California–Los Angeles (Drs Nuechterlein and Gitlin and Mr Ventura); and the Department of Psychology, Occidental College (Dr Schell), Los Angeles.

See Subjects and Methods on next page

SUBJECTS AND METHODS

SUBJECTS

A total of 20 schizophrenic patients and 20 matched normal controls served as subjects. Demographics and other characteristics of the schizophrenic patients and the normal subjects are provided in **Table 1**. All of the patients received a diagnosis of schizophrenia by Research Diagnostic Criteria.[25] Patients with schizoaffective disorders were not included in the present sample, although they were included in an earlier preliminary summary of the present study.[13] The normal control subjects were matched to the patients on an individual basis in terms of age (±2 years), sex, ethnicity, and educational level (±2 years). Other inclusionary and exclusionary criteria for patient and control selection are given in Nuechterlein et al.[26]

OVERALL DESIGN

The patients and controls were selected from participants in a larger longitudinal follow-through study of the early phase of schizophrenia.[26] This project involved the repeated assessments of schizophrenic patients whose first psychotic symptoms began not longer than 2 years before project entry. Patients were treated at the Aftercare Program at the University of California–Los Angeles, using a common starting dosage of 12.5 mg of injectable fluphenazine decanoate (Prolixin) every 2 weeks as soon as their clinical state stabilized. Dosage was decreased if intolerable side effects occurred and increased as clinically indicated if significant symptoms recurred. After at least 1 year of neuroleptic treatment, patients who had sufficient clinical stability were invited to enter into a 24-week drug-placebo crossover study, followed by an open drug-withdrawal phase. A battery of information-processing, psychophysiological, and other measures was administered on prespecified occasions throughout the entire longitudinal protocol. The test occasions included the intake point, a clinically stabilized point on the injectable medication (about 3 months after hospital discharge), a point of symptomatic remission, and a point at which psychotic symptoms returned, if one occurred. Matched normal controls were administered the same battery of tests at intervals that were matched to those of individual schizophrenic patients. Informed consent was obtained from each patient and normal control prior to participation. Subjects signed written consent forms and also were provided additional information orally to enhance their understanding of the research project.

The electrodermal data reported here were collected on two test occasions, one while the schizophrenic patients were in a state of symptomatic remission and the other while the patients were in a psychotic state. The vast majority of the test occasions (33 [83%] of 40 tests) occurred during the initial phase of antipsychotic medication treatment at the Aftercare Program; the remaining tests occurred during the subsequent drug crossover and withdrawal phase. Test occasions were selected for instances in which dosages of fluphenazine decanoate were at identical or nearly identical levels (mean dosage was 12.22 mg on each test occasion). Also, when clinically possible, antiparkinsonian medications with anticholinergic effects (most commonly benztropine mesylate [Cogentin]) were not taken for at least 24 hours before each electrodermal test. This was possible for all tests in this sample except four psychotic-state tests. At the remission test, four patients had not taken antiparkinsonian medications for 24 hours and 16 had not taken such medication for 48 hours or longer; at the psychotic-state test, four patients were taking antiparkinsonian medications, seven had not taken them for 24 hours, and nine had not taken them for 48 hours or longer. Any anticholinergic effect of antiparkinsonian medications would lower electrodermal activity,[27] which, in the present design, would only serve to offset the hypothesized increase in electrodermal activity during psychotic episodes.

For most of the patients (17 [85%] of 20), the remission test occurred before the psychotic test. The median interval between the two tests was approximately 8 months. Any effects of habituation that are associated with this order of testing would work against the hypothesized greater electrodermal activity during the psychotic state. Moreover, the matched controls had a similar test order and interval between their test occasions.

IDENTIFICATION OF CLINICAL STATES

The Brief Psychiatric Rating Scale (BPRS)[28] was used to define the remitted and the psychotic states. Remission was defined as having all ratings on the standard 18 BPRS items[29] at 3 or less on a scale scored from 1 to 7 for a period of at least 1 month. Ratings of 3 or less correspond to the nonpathological range according to the BPRS anchor points.[30,31] A psychotic testing state was defined as having one or more of the three BPRS psychotic items (unusual thought content, hallucinations, or conceptual disorganization) rated at least a 4 on the day of testing.

ELECTRODERMAL TESTS

Each electrodermal test session began with the attachment of recording electrodes and was followed by a 5-minute rest period and three successive auditory stimulation phases. Each of the three auditory phases was separated by approximately 3 minutes, during which time the instructions were given about the next phase and 1 minute of silence followed before the first stimulus of the next phase was presented.

The first auditory stimulation phase measured SCORs to mild nonsignal tones in a standard orienting and habituation paradigm. Fifteen moderate-intensity tones were binaurally presented through headphones, with the subjects instructed to simply sit quietly with their eyes open. The tones were 1.0 second in duration, 78 dB (sound pressure level, C weighting) in intensity, with controlled rise times and fall times of 25 milliseconds. These auditory stimulus values were selected to replicate the conditions under which SCOR orient-

ing and habituation abnormalities have been found previously.[1,21] The first 12 tones were 1000 Hz and the last three tones were 1200 Hz; only the data from the first 12 tones are reported herein. The intertone intervals varied between 30, 40, and 50 seconds in block-randomized order.

The second auditory stimulation phase measured SCORs to task-significant tones. It consisted of 12 monaurally presented tones that alternated regularly between the left ear and the right ear. The tone characteristics were the same as those used during the preceding phase, except that the tone frequency was 500 Hz. The tones used during the second phase were given task significance by instructing the subjects to move their eyes to a black dot on the wall approximately 30° to the left when the tone was presented to the left ear and to a similar dot approximately 30° to the right when the tone was presented to the right ear.

The third auditory stimulation phase measured skin conductance responses to aversive loud noises, a condition that reportedly elicits exceptionally vigorous electrodermal responses in the offspring of schizophrenic patients.[32] This phase consisted of a series of 12 bursts of loud white noise presented binaurally, each 1.0 second in duration and 98 dB in intensity with fast rise times and fall times.

EQUIPMENT

Electrodermal measures were recorded using standard methods.[11] Skin conductance was recorded using silver–silver chloride electrodes (SensorMedics, Anaheim, Calif) that were filled with isotonic electrode paste and attached with adhesive collars (1 cm in diameter) to the volar surface of the distal phalanges of the index and second fingers of each hand. The electrode paste consisted of a neutral cream (Unibase, Warner Chilcott Laboratories, Morris Plains, NJ) containing sodium chloride (0.05 mol/L). A constant 0.5 V was applied across each pair of electrodes from a skin conductance coupler (9844, SensorMedics). A polygraph (Dynograph Recorder, SensorMedics) was used to obtain rectilinear tracings of skin conductance on paper moving at a chart speed of 10 mm/s.

Auditory stimuli (tones and white noises) were delivered from a stereo tape recorder through stereophonic headphones (TDH 49, Grason-Stadler, Concord, Mass). During the initial taping of the auditory stimuli, the tones originated from an oscillator (Hewlett-Packard, Palo Alto, Calif), and the white noises originated from a noise generator (829C, Grason-Stadler).

TONIC AND PHASIC ELECTRODERMAL MEASURES

Although electrodermal activity was recorded from both hands simultaneously, for the sake of simplicity, only data from the right hand are reported here. Three tonic and three phasic electrodermal measures were analyzed. The three tonic electrodermal measures were the number of nonspecific skin conductance responses per minute, the skin conductance level, and the slope of the change in the skin conductance level over time within a test session. Nonspecific skin conductance responses were defined as responses of at least 0.05 microsiemen that occurred during the rest phase or during the intertone intervals of the stimulation phases, were averaged across the entire test session, and were expressed as the number per minute. Skin conductance level was defined as the mean of the logarithm of the skin conductance readings that were taken each minute during the rest phase and at tone onset during each auditory stimulation phase. The slope of the changes in the skin conductance level was defined as the regression of the logarithm of the skin conductance level on trial number during the loud noise auditory stimulation phase.

The three phasic measures of electrodermal responsiveness that were obtained during the auditory stimulation phases were the proportion of subjects who were identified as SCOR nonresponders to innocuous tones, the number of trials before habituation of the SCOR occurred (habituation was defined as three consecutive trials without a SCOR), and the number of stimulus-elicited SCORs. To score stimulus-elicited SCORs, one must select the minimum amplitude of change in skin conductance that may be considered a response as well as a latency window following each stimulus during which a skin conductance response is considered to be an orienting response elicited by the stimulus. In the present study, the minimum amplitude was 0.05 microsiemen, and the placement of the latency window was individually adjusted for each subject by examining the minimum response latency to the bursts of loud noise. If the minimum latency was less than 2 seconds, then the latency window was set at 1.0 to 3.0 seconds. If the minimum latency was greater than 2 seconds, then the latency window was set at 2.0 to 4.0 seconds. Thus, the latency window was 2 seconds in duration for all subjects, with the beginning and ending points individually adjusted.

A SCOR nonresponder was defined in two ways: in the standard way,[1] as one who did not exhibit a response to any of the first three mild innocuous tones, and in the original and more strict sense,[21] as one who did not give a SCOR to all 12 innocuous tones.

STATISTICAL ANALYSES

For each electrodermal measure, a 2 (diagnosis: schizophrenia vs normal)×2 (schizophrenic state: remitted vs psychotic test occasion) repeated measures analysis of variance (ANOVA) was carried out. The normal subjects, of course, were not in states of remission and psychosis but rather were tested at intervals that were matched to those between the remitted and psychotic test occasions of the patients. The diagnosis variable was treated as a repeated measure variable because each schizophrenic patient was matched with a normal control subject of the same sex, ethnicity, approximate age, and approximate educational level. If an ANOVA showed either a significant main effect of diagnosis or a significant diagnosis-by-state interaction, repeated-measures *t* tests were computed to compare the two groups at the remitted and the psychotic states to evaluate the tripartite distinction that is summarized in **Figure 1**.

Table 1. Characteristics of Schizophrenic and Normal Comparison Samples

Characteristic	Schizophrenic Patients, Mean (SD)	Normal Subjects, Mean (SD)
Sample size, No.	20	20
Age, y	22.8 (3.5)	23.7 (3.3)
Education, y	12.6 (1.6)	13.2 (1.6)
Sex, No.		
M	16	16
F	4	4

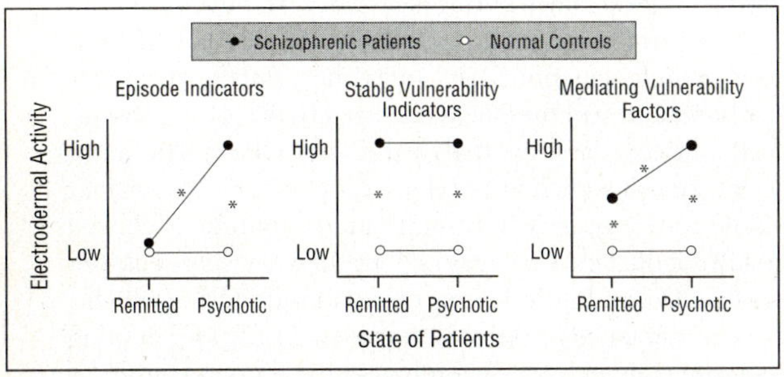

Figure 1. *Distinctive characteristics of episode indicators (left), stable vulnerability indicators (center), and mediating vulnerability factors (right) when patients and controls are tested during the remitted and psychotic states of the patients. Asterisks indicate significant differences. Adapted from Nuechterlein and Dawson.[24]*

mild innocuous tones. Typically, between 40% and 50% of schizophrenic patients do not exhibit SCORs to novel mild innocuous tones (nonresponders) compared with approximately a 10% rate of nonresponders frequently reported in normal subjects.[1,3,5,6] The majority of the patients who do respond (responders) also exhibit reduced autonomic phasic responsiveness in that their SCORs generally habituate quickly.[1,5] The second electrodermal abnormality is that schizophrenic patients who are SCOR responders exhibit abnormally high tonic autonomic activity, as indicated by a raised skin conductance level, an elevated frequency of nonspecific skin conductance responses, and an abnormally slow rate of decrease in skin conductance level across time within a session.[3,5] Thus, it appears that some schizophrenic patients exhibit phasic electrodermal (SCOR) hyporeactivity to innocuous stimuli, whereas others exhibit tonic electrodermal hyperactivity.[3,5,13]

Although electrodermal abnormalities have been hypothesized to be related to vulnerability to schizophrenia,[2,3,5,14] the issue of whether the abnormalities represent vulnerability-linked traits or symptom-linked states has received little direct empirical testing. Bernstein[15] has reviewed several indirect lines of evidence suggesting that SCOR nonresponsiveness in particular is a traitlike vulnerability indicator in schizophrenia. Among the lines of evidence cited by Bernstein for the hypothesized vulnerability status of SCOR nonresponsiveness are findings of larger than normal proportions of SCOR nonresponders among first-degree relatives of SCOR nonresponder schizophrenic probands[16] and among remitted schizophrenics.[17] Furthermore, at least three studies have found that the proportion of SCOR nonresponders remains stable when the same patients are tested when symptoms are mild and when symptoms are severe.[18-20]

However, seemingly inconsistent with the notion of electrodermal activity as a stable vulnerability indicator is the finding in basic research with normal subjects that electrodermal measures are exquisitely sensitive to changes in psychological states. For example, the anticipation and the performance of practically any task will increase both the skin conductance level and the frequency of nonspecific skin conductance responses, as well as increase the frequency of SCORs and delay their habituation to discrete stimuli.[11]

Changes in phasic and tonic electrodermal activity have been reported to vary with changes in psychological and behavioral states in schizophrenic patients as well, further questioning the hypothesis that such activity is a stable index of vulnerability to schizophrenia. For example, in the initial identification of phasic SCOR responders and nonresponders among schizophrenic patients, Gruzelier and Venables[21(p285)] noted that "repeated testing with some noninstitutionalized schizophrenics has shown that nonresponding is a temporary phase accompanying periods of inactive behavior." Gruzelier and Venables[21] also reported changes in tonic electrodermal data that were recorded on 3 successive days from a young catatonic schizophrenic patient. On the first 2 days, the patient exhibited euphoric mood and restless behavior accompanied by high skin conductance levels; then on the third day, there was a marked change to a state of dulled affect and inert posture, accompanied by a low skin conductance level.

In summary, electrodermal measures reportedly exhibit characteristics of either state-sensitive episode indicators or trait-sensitive vulnerability indicators or both. Thus, electrodermal measures may not fit neatly into a dichotomous distinction between episode indicators and vulnerability indicators.[22,23] Considerations such as these prompted the proposal of a tripartite distinction between episode indicators, stable vulnerability indicators, and mediating vulnerability factors.[3,24]

The tripartite distinction is illustrated in Figure 1. The differences between episode indicators, stable vulnerability indicators, and mediating vulnerability factors are shown in the different patterns of abnormalities during remitted and psychotic states. As shown in the left panel of Figure 1, episode indicators do not differ from normal at remission, differ from normal during psychotic episodes, and are significantly more severely abnormal during the psychotic state than during the remitted state.

As can be seen in the center panel of Figure 1, stable vulnerability indicators differ from normal at remission, differ from normal during psychotic episodes, and are not more severely abnormal during the psychotic state than during the remitted state.

Finally, as shown in the right panel of Figure 1, mediating vulnerability factors differ from normal at remission, differ from normal during psychotic episodes, and are significantly more severely abnormal during the psychotic state than during the remitted state.

We report herein electrodermal measures obtained during clinically remitted and psychotic states in patients with recent-onset schizophrenia who were receiving equivalent medications during both states and in matched normal controls who were tested at comparable time intervals. The inclusion of these matched normal controls is a unique feature of the present design compared with other studies that have tested schizophrenic patients in different symptomatic states. This group by state design allows us to evaluate the criteria outlined above to determine whether electrodermal phasic and tonic measures qualify as episode indicators, stable vulnerability indicators, or mediating vulnerability factors in schizophrenia. It was previously proposed that electrodermal anomalies may be mediating vulnerability factors in schizophrenia.[3] The present study tests that hypothesis.

RESULTS

SYMPTOM STATUS DURING REMITTED AND PSYCHOTIC TESTS

The BPRS was administered on each test occasion to document the clinical state of the patients on the day of each test. **Table 2** shows the mean scores for the three BPRS psychotic items, the five BPRS factors, and the total 18-item BPRS on the day of the remission test and on the day of the psychotic test. As can be seen, symptom ratings were consistently higher on the day of the psychotic test than on the day of the remission test. This subgroup of patients showed particularly low ratings at the remission test point, with scores being near the lowest possible anchor point. When the differences in symptom ratings on the two test occasions were expressed as effect sizes,[33] the differences varied between moderate and strong effects for all items and for all factors except activation. The increases in thought disturbance and total BPRS scores on the day of the psychotic test were particularly strong effects. Thus, the BPRS data indicate that symptom levels were substantially higher during the psychotic test occasion than during the remission test occasion.

Table 2. Mean Scores of Brief Psychiatric Rating Scale (BPRS) at Remission and Psychotic-State Test Points*

BPRS Measure	Remission Test	Psychotic Test	Effect Size
Psychotic items			
Unusual thought content	1.00 (0.00)	4.21 (1.81)	1.77†
Hallucinations	1.10 (0.45)	3.05 (2.37)	0.85†
Conceptual disorganization	1.00 (0.00)	1.65 (1.27)	0.51‡
Factors			
Thought disturbance	1.02 (0.11)	2.82 (0.87)	2.05†
Anxiety/depression	1.22 (0.32)	2.21 (1.05)	1.02†
Anergia	1.42 (0.35)	2.09 (1.02)	0.60‡
Hostility	1.10 (0.22)	1.80 (0.70)	0.89†
Activation	1.20 (0.31)	1.48 (0.58)	0.40§
Total scores (18 items)	21.60 (2.58)	38.35 (9.99)	1.67†

*Values in parentheses are SDs.
†Strong effect size.
‡Moderate effect size.
§Weak effect size.*

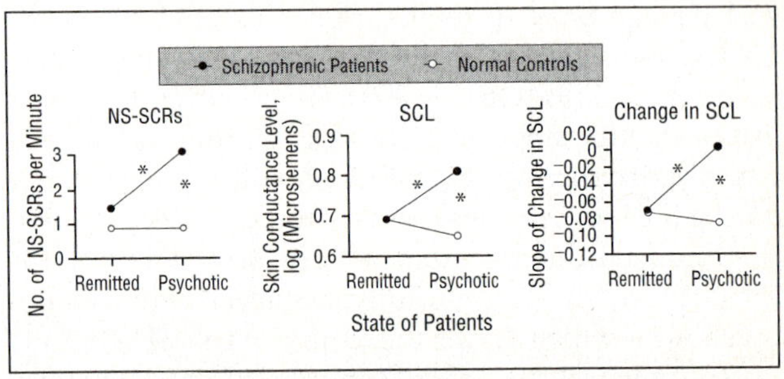

Figure 2. *Results of three tonic electrodermal measures (nonspecific skin conductance responses [NS-SCRs], skin conductance level [SCL], and slope of change in SCL) that were obtained from schizophrenic patients and normal controls when tested during the remitted and psychotic states of the patients. Asterisks indicate significant differences.*

TONIC ELECTRODERMAL ACTIVITY

Figure 2 summarizes the results for the three tonic electrodermal measures for schizophrenic patients during the remitted and the psychotic states and for normal controls at matched intervals. The findings will be described by reference to the criteria that were described earlier and depicted in Figure 1 for distinguishing between episodes indicators, stable vulnerability indicators, and mediating vulnerability factors.

First, for the number of nonspecific skin conductance responses, a diagnosis by state ANOVA revealed a significant diagnosis main effect ($F[1,19]=9.47$; $P<.01$), a significant state main effect ($F[1,19]=5.30$, $P<.04$), and a significant diagnosis-by-state interaction ($F[1,19]=6.23$, $P<.03$). Simple effects tests confirmed that the frequency of nonspecific responses for schizophrenic patients did not differ from normal during clinical remission, was significantly higher than normal at the psychotic test point ($t[19]=3.98$; $P<.01$), and was significantly higher during the psychotic period than during the remitted period ($t[19]=2.43$; $P<.03$), whereas this measure did not change significantly for the controls across the two test occasions. Thus, an elevated number of non-

specific skin conductance responses satisfies all three criteria for an episode indicator.

Second, for the logarithm of the skin conductance level seen in the center panel of Figure 2, a diagnosis-by-state ANOVA revealed a highly significant diagnosis-by-state interaction ($F[1,19]=8.59$; $P<.01$). Simple effects tests confirmed that the skin conductance level of the schizophrenic patients did not differ from normal during the remission test, was significantly higher than normal during the psychotic test ($t[19]=2.61$; $P<.02$), and was significantly higher during the symptomatic test than during the remission test ($t[19]=2.66$; $P<.02$), whereas the normal controls did not show a significant change across test sessions. Thus, elevated skin conductance level also satisfies all three criteria for an episode indicator.

Third, for the slope of the change in skin conductance level across trials of the loud-noise phase, the data from two schizophrenic patients were missing because of their refusal to continue testing during this phase. The data of the remaining 18 patients are summarized in the right panel of Figure 2. A diagnosis-by-state ANOVA revealed a significant diagnosis main effect ($F[1,17]=4.98$; $P<.04$) and a highly significant diagnosis-by-state interaction ($F[1,17]=11.46$; $P<.005$). Simple effects tests confirmed that the slope of the change in skin conductance of the schizophrenic patients did not differ from normal during the remission test, was significantly less negative than normal during the psychotic test ($t[18]=4.43$; $P<.001$), and was significantly less negative during the psychotic test than during the remission test ($t[18]=3.11$; $P<.01$), whereas the normal controls did not change significantly across test sessions. Thus, a reduced slope of decrease in skin conductance level across trials also satisfies all three criteria for an episode indicator.

The nature of the significant effects for the slope of the change in skin conductance level over trials is clarified by examination of **Figure 3**. This figure shows the logarithm of skin conductance level for the schizophrenic patients and the matched normal controls at the onset of each of the 12 loud noises during the remitted state and during the psychotic state. As can be seen, during the remission test, the skin conductance level of the patients is only slightly and nonsignificantly above normal and declines at a similar rate across trials for the patients and controls. During the psychotic state, in contrast, the skin conductance level for the patients is significantly higher than normal and shows a significantly reduced downward slope across trials.

In sum, the tonic electrodermal measures indicate that schizophrenic patients during psychotic periods are in a state of abnormally high sympathetic activation that is slow to adapt over time within a test session. These abnormalities, however, do not exist when the same patients are in symptomatic remission. Thus, tonic electrodermal hyperactivity is an episode indicator rather than an indicator of the vulnerability to schizophrenia in the present sample of patients with recent-onset schizophrenia.

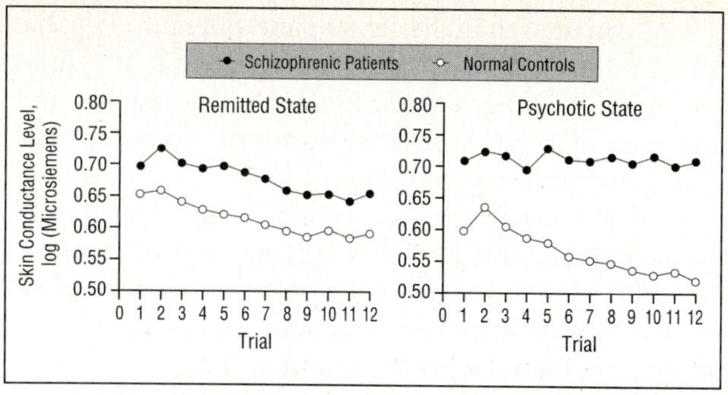

Figure 3. *Mean logarithm of the skin conductance level during 12 loud-noise trials presented to schizophrenic patients and normal controls during the remitted and psychotic states of the patients.*

We also analyzed the three tonic electrodermal measures that were obtained solely during the initial rest phase of each test session to determine whether this simple procedure would yield the same results as did the analyses of the tonic measures described above. The number of nonspecific skin conductance responses and the skin conductance level measured during the rest phase satisfied all of the criteria described above for an episode indicator. That is, the ANOVAs revealed significant diagnosis-by-state interactions, and the *t* tests demonstrated that patients did not differ from normal during the remission test, did differ from normal during the symptomatic phase, and did exhibit a significant increase across the two test occasions. The decline in skin conductance level over time measured during rest, however, showed a less consistent pattern. The decline in skin conductance level over time for the patients did not differ from normal during the remission test occasion and did differ from normal during the psychotic test occasion; however, the difference for the patients across the two test occasions was not significant. When considered in its entirety, these data indicate that tonic electrodermal episode indicators generally can be detected by recording these measures during a simple nonstimulation rest period.

PHASIC SKIN CONDUCTANCE RESPONDING

Proportion of SCOR Nonresponders

Each patient was classified as either a responder or a nonresponder based on the standard criterion of whether any of the first three presentations of the innocuous tone elicited a SCOR, as well as by the strict criterion of whether any of the 12 innocuous tones elicited a SCOR. The results obtained with the two criteria are summarized in **Figure 4**. One control subject was missing phasic SCOR data for the innocuous tones at the psychotic-state test, and therefore, analyses of the nonresponder data during the psychotic test are based on 19 pairs of subjects rather than 20 pairs.

With the standard three-trial criterion applied to the patients, there were 15 nonresponders (75%) during the remission test and eight nonresponders (42%) during the

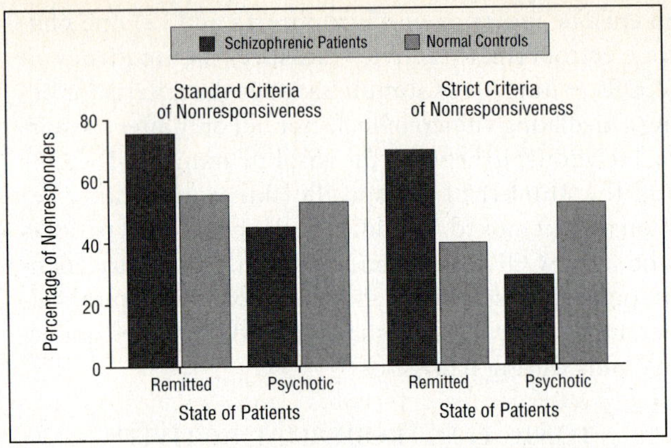

Figure 4. *Percentage of SCOR (skin conductance orienting response) nonresponders according to the standard and the strict criteria of nonresponsiveness in schizophrenic patients and normal controls tested during the remitted and psychotic states of patients.*

psychotic test. By contrast, among the controls there were 11 nonresponders (55%) during the equivalent of the remission test and 10 nonresponders (53%) during the equivalent of the psychotic test. With the strict 12-trial criterion, among the patients, there were 14 nonresponders (70%) during the remission test and only six nonresponders (32%) during the psychotic test, whereas among the controls, there were eight nonresponders (40%) during the equivalent of the remission test and 10 nonresponders (53%) during the equivalent of the psychotic test. The reason for the different results with the different criteria is that some patients who did not respond to the first three tones (and hence were classified as nonresponders by the standard criterion) nevertheless responded to later tones (and hence were classified as responders by the strict criterion).

With the strict criterion, the proportion of patients who were nonresponders was marginally greater than the proportion of controls who were nonresponders during the remission test (McNemar test; $\chi^2[1]=3.00$; $P<.09$), was not significantly different from the proportion of controls who were nonresponders during the psychotic test, and was significantly greater during the remission test than during the psychotic test (McNemar test; $\chi^2[1]=8.00$; $P<.005$), with eight of the 14 schizophrenic patients who were nonresponders during remission becoming responders when in the psychotic state.

This pattern of results was not anticipated in our tripartite distinction. That is, we did not anticipate the possibility that patients would differ from normal when in remission but not when in a psychotic state. This unexpected pattern of results indicates that SCOR nonresponsiveness might be a vulnerability indicator when scored in this way but one that is abnormal only during remission and that normalizes during the psychotic episode.[34(p484)] Similar analyses were performed on the proportion of nonresponders defined by the standard definition and, although effects were in the same direction, the level of statistical significance was not as high. This pattern of results suggests that the strict criterion of nonresponsiveness is somewhat more sensitive to group and state differences than is the standard criterion of SCOR nonresponsiveness.

Number of SCORs and Trials Before Habituation

Figure 5 shows the mean number of SCORs elicited during the three auditory phases from patients during the remitted- and psychotic-state tests and from the normal controls during the matched tests. As can be seen, the frequency of SCORs tends to increase among patients from the remitted to the psychotic states during the innocuous tone and task-significant tone phases. However, a series of ANOVAs and *t* tests did not reveal critical significant effects for the raw number of SCORs. That is, the schizophrenic patients and normal controls did not differ significantly during any of the auditory phases at either the remitted- or the psychotic-state test point, and there were no significant changes across remitted- and psychotic-state test points among schizophrenic patients. Thus, the absolute number of SCORs does not qualify as either an episode indicator, stable vulnerability indicator, or a mediating vulnerability factor in the present sample. Similar analyses that were performed on the number of trials before habituation occurred revealed the same lack of significant effects.

Observed vs Predicted SCORs

The tendency for specific SCORs to increase from the remitted test to the psychotic test and for the number of SCOR nonresponders to decrease must be interpreted within the context of a significantly increased number of nonspecific skin conductance responses. The frequency of nonspecific responses is, as was already pointed out, a measure of nonspecific arousal and activation, and as arousal increases, orienting to specific stimuli in the environment ordinarily increases as well. Thus, the number of SCORs and the number of nonspecific responses are usually positively correlated,[35,36] which was also true in the present samples of patients and normal controls during both the remission and psychotic-state test occasions (all Pearson *r*'s were significantly positive, ranging from .61 to .87). To take these correlations into account in interpreting the tendency for the number of SCORs to be higher during the psychotic-state test occasion, we computed regression equations based on the normal control group data so that the number of SCORs to innocuous tones could be predicted, given the number of nonspecific responses for each subject. A difference score was then computed by subtracting the predicted frequency of SCORs from the observed frequency of SCORs for each normal and schizophrenic subject. Thus, the resulting score represents the degree to which subjects were electrodermally responsive to innocuous

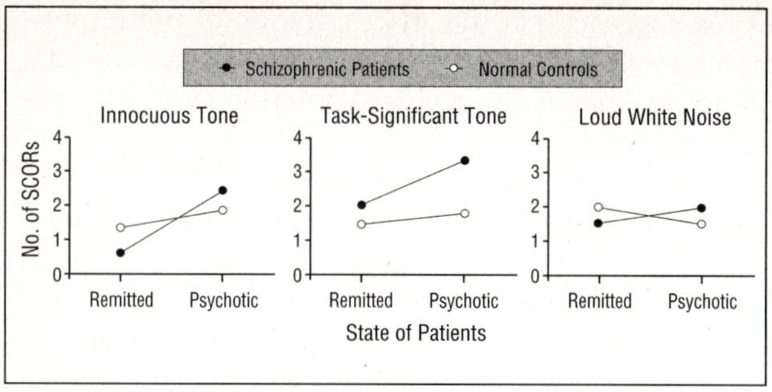

Figure 5. *Mean number of skin conductance orienting responses (SCORs)to innocuous tones, task-significant tones, and loud white noises in schizophrenic patients and normal controls tested during the remitted and psychotic states of the patients.*

tones after the normal relationship between SCORs and nonspecific responses was taken into account. For each schizophrenic subject, this score is the difference between actual responsiveness and the responsiveness that a normal control would be predicted to have at that arousal level. Negative scores indicate hyporesponsiveness, whereas positive scores indicate hyperresponsiveness.

The mean SCOR observed-predicted difference scores for patients and controls during the two test occasions are shown in **Figure 6**. As can be seen, patients had fewer SCORs than predicted based on their frequency of nonspecific responses during both remitted- and psychotic-state tests, with the psychotic-state test showing the most striking score. A diagnosis-by-state ANOVA confirmed a significant diagnosis main effect ($F[1,18]=12.94$; $P<.003$) as well as a significant diagnosis-by-state interaction effect ($F[1,18]=4.76$; $P<.05$). Simple effects tests revealed that the mean observed-predicted difference score of the schizophrenic patients was significantly greater in magnitude than that of the normal controls during the remitted-state test ($t[19]=3.13$; $P<.01$), was significantly greater than that of the normal controls during the psychotic-state test ($t[18]=3.26$; $P<.01$), and was significantly greater at the psychotic-state test point than at the remitted-state test point ($t[19]=2.76$; $P<.05$). These results indicate that, although the absolute number of SCORs tended to increase from the remitted test point to the psychotic test point, they did not increase as much as expected based on the increased number of nonspecific responses. Thus, the frequency of SCORs to innocuous stimuli in the present sample of schizophrenic patients is actually less than that which would normally be predicted based on the frequency of nonspecific responses, and in fact, the observed-predicted difference score satisfies all three criteria for a mediating vulnerability factor.

COMMENT

The two principal findings of the present longitudinal study are as follows: (1) tonic electrodermal activation measures clearly and consistently satisfy the criteria for an episode indicator in schizophrenia and (2) one phasic electrodermal reactivity measure, the frequency of SCORs to innocuous stimuli, satisfies the criteria for being a mediating vulnerability factor but only after the normal relationship between the absolute number of SCORs and the number of nonspecific skin conductance responses is removed. In addition, the number of patients who were SCOR nonresponders according to a strict definition of nonresponsiveness appears to be an atypical vulnerability indicator that shows a tendency to be abnormal only during remission.

TONIC ELECTRODERMAL ACTIVITY

The finding that tonic electrodermal activation becomes abnormally high during a psychotic state has both theoretical and applied implications. Theoretically, this finding may help shed light on the processes underlying psychotic breakdown. These electrodermal findings suggest that schizophrenic psychotic states are accompanied by elevated sympathetic nervous system activation. These findings are consistent with reports that plasma 3-methoxy-4-hydroxyphenylglycol values are elevated in high-psychosis phases compared with low-psychosis phases in drug-free chronic schizophrenic patients[37] and are lower when psychotic symptoms are reduced by drug treatment.[38] However, significant increases in autonomic activity can occur without corresponding changes in symptoms.[39] Thus, although elevated autonomic activation occurs during the psychotic episode, it is certainly not an infallible indicator of the psychotic state.

A major unanswered theoretical question concerns the functional role of sympathetic activation in the return of psychotic symptoms. Is it merely a secondary consequence of the symptoms (eg, reflecting anxiety and turmoil associated with the presence of psychotic symptoms or with attempts to cope with the intrusive symptoms), or does it play a causal mediating role in the chain of events leading to a psychotic episode? We hypothesize that sympathetic arousal plays an active mediating role in the psychotic decompensation process or at least indexes the processes that play such a role. A heuristic vulnerability-stress model has been proposed that explicitly incorporates this notion.[24,26,40,41] In this model, autonomic hyperactivation is a transient intermediate state that is elicited in part by stressful environmental stimuli and that precedes psychotic episodes and contributes to the return of schizophrenic symptoms in vulnerable individuals. Preliminary supportive evidence for this notion was found in that some patients exhibit increased electrodermal activation in the week or two before a psychotic exacerbation,[13] which is clearly contrary to the hypothesis that the elevated electrodermal activation is a secondary reaction to the presence of psychotic symptoms.

Other behavioral evidence that elevated sympathetic activation may occur early in the formation of posi-

tive psychotic symptoms and is not merely a secondary consequence of the symptoms is that commonly reported prodromal symptoms include nervousness, tension, anxiety, and "trouble sleeping."[42-47] Biochemical evidence consistent with this view is that the administration of methylphenidate, a sympathetic nervous system stimulant, increases positive symptoms in many schizophrenic patients.[48-50] Thus, we view a psychotic episode as an event resulting from underlying processes that are frequently characterized by heightened autonomic activation.

In addition to the theoretical implications, identifying measures that are state sensitive can potentially serve many useful purposes. A noninvasive, nonverbal, involuntary measure that changes during the psychotic state and returns to normal at other times can be used to index the onset, duration, and offset of an episode.[22,34] Such an index may be valuable in comparing the efficacy of different treatments for resolving schizophrenic episodes. Furthermore, if some episode indicators are sensitive to the early prodromal stages occurring just before an episode, as preliminary evidence suggests that tonic electrodermal hyperactivation may be,[13] then these indicators might be useful in predicting the impending return of psychotic symptoms. If reliable precursors of psychotic symptoms can be established, effective early intervention becomes more feasible.

PHASIC ELECTRODERMAL ACTIVITY

The present phasic electrodermal data suggest that one derived variable, reduced number of SCORs to innocuous tones corrected for the frequency of nonspecific responses, may be a mediating vulnerability factor. Another phasic variable, the proportion of SCOR nonresponders using a strict definition of nonresponsiveness, tends to appear as an atypical vulnerability indicator that is abnormal only in the remitted state. This atypical pattern of apparent normalization during the psychotic phase, however, may be due to the overall increased level of activation during the psychotic phase. That is, the expected frequency of SCORs is less than normal during both the remitted and the psychotic phases, especially during the psychotic phase, based on the frequency of nonspecific conductance responses. In a similar vein, other investigators[51,52] computed the ratio of elicited responses to nonspecific responses and found that schizophrenic patients show fewer elicited responses per number of nonspecific responses than do normal controls. Overall, these findings suggest that increased autonomic arousal indexed by tonic electrodermal activity may be the principal change during the psychotic phase and that any increase in SCORs is a secondary by-product of the increased tonic activity.

Schizophrenic patients appear abnormally hyporesponsive to innocuous stimuli during symptomatic re-

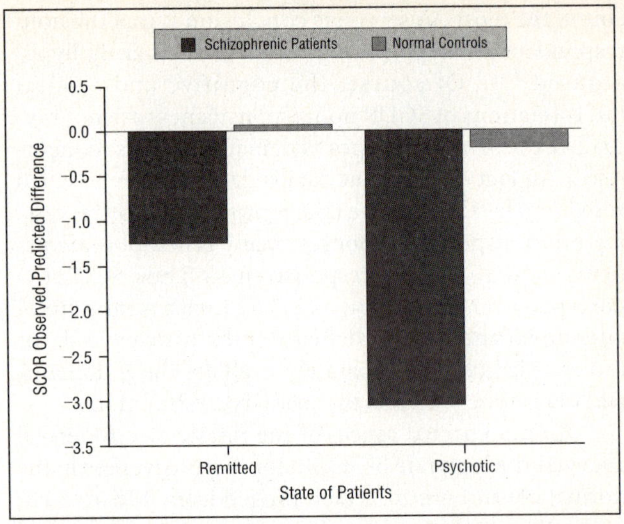

Figure 6. *Mean observed-predicted difference scores for the frequency of skin conductance orienting response (SCOR) in schizophrenic patients and normal controls tested during the remitted and psychotic states of the patients.*

mission, whether one measures the proportion of SCOR nonresponders with the strict criterion or one computes the predicted frequency of SCORs based on the frequency of nonspecific responses. What is the psychological significance of the SCOR hyporesponsiveness and/or nonresponsiveness during remission? This abnormality can be interpreted in terms of deficits in cognitive processes and/or arousal processes. From the cognitive perspective, the SCOR is associated with attentional responses to environmental stimuli.[53-57] According to this theoretical viewpoint, SCOR hyporesponsiveness indexes a deficit in active attention and processing of environmental stimuli. That is, at least some schizophrenic patients have attenuated processing of incoming environmental information or might actively gate-out such information. The presence of abnormal SCOR hyporesponsiveness to innocuous tones during clinical remission indicates that a subtle cognitive deficit is present even when clinical symptoms are absent. Thus, SCOR hyporesponsiveness and nonresponsiveness may index an attentional deficit that is related to an enduring vulnerability to schizophrenic symptoms, which is consistent with other performance-based measures of attention and information processing.[58]

The SCOR hyporesponsiveness and/or nonresponsiveness also can be interpreted from the theoretical perspective of physiological arousal. According to one possible version of this view, SCOR hyporesponsiveness reflects general physiological hypoarousal. Consistent with this view, SCOR nonresponders have been found to have lower tonic electrodermal activity,[19,21] cardiovascular activity,[59] serum cortisol levels,[60] and brain glucose activity[61] than do responders. However, when the nonresponders are compared with normal controls and when the possible effects of medications are taken into ac-

count, the most conservative conclusion is that the nonresponders are hyporeactive and not necessarily hypoaroused.[3,5,13] Of course, the cognitive and arousal interpretations of SCOR nonresponsiveness are not mutually exclusive. Both types of deficits may exist concurrently. In fact, the present data suggest that, even when activation level effects are taken into account by regressing out nonspecific responses, many schizophrenic patients show SCOR hyporesponsiveness. Thus, SCOR hyporesponsiveness may be associated with a mixture of attentional and arousal deficits, and a primary task for future research is to separately evaluate these domains and determine which is the primary dysfunction.

An unexpected aspect of the phasic electrodermal data was the high rate of SCOR nonresponsiveness in the normal control group, which ranged from 40% to 55%, depending on the test occasion and the criterion of nonresponsiveness (Figure 4). As indicated earlier, one traditionally expects a nonresponsiveness rate of approximately 10% among normal controls. However, higher than expected rates of nonresponsiveness have been reported in several recent studies.[13,62,63] It has been noted that higher than expected rates of nonresponsiveness are found particularly among normal controls who are demographically matched to schizophrenic patients,[13,62] such as those in the present study. However, there also have been reports of high rates of SCOR nonresponsiveness even among normal college students that have been hypothesized to be due to a low intensity of the SCOR-eliciting innocuous tone (A. Raine, PhD; T. Lencz, MA; A. Scerbo, PhD; D. Benishay, MA, unpublished data, 1993). Although we, too, have suggested that absolute tone intensity is important,[13] we also believe that the ratio of tone intensity to background noise intensity may be critical. The background noise in the present study was moderately high (approximately 68 dB) relative to the innocuous tone intensity of 78 dB, which may have contributed to the present high rate of SCOR nonresponsiveness. The important point is that the patient-control differences in SCOR may depend on the type of normal control selected, as well as on the physical characteristics of the environmental stimuli used to elicit phasic SCOR responsiveness.

PREVIOUS REPEATED-TESTING ELECTRODERMAL STUDIES

As noted earlier, three prior studies[18-20] measured electrodermal activity in both relatively symptomatic and relatively remitted states within the same schizophrenic patients. All three of these studies reported that both tonic and phasic electrodermal activity were generally stable across symptomatic states. However, all three of the studies tested hospitalized patients who did not appear to be as completely remitted as our outpatients with recent-onset schizophrenia. Our remission point in these analyses involved very low symptom ratings at or near the lowest possible BPRS ratings. Also, all three previous studies tested patients while the use of neuroleptic agents was discontinued for a week or more, at least during the symptomatic phase. Patients participating in the present study, in contrast, were tested with low-to-moderate dosages of a single neuroleptic agent on both test occasions. The discontinuation of the use of medication in the previous studies may have increased electrodermal activity, whereas our moderate levels of antipsychotic medication may have reduced electrodermal activity. Finally, unlike the present study, none of the three previous studies included tests of matched normal subjects at intervals matched to the remitted and psychotic tests of the patients. Clearly, more research is needed to clarify the generality of the present findings across different patient populations, different neuroleptic states, and different symptom levels and configurations during the psychotic state. Moreover, further research is needed with other diagnostic groups to determine whether the phasic and tonic electrodermal anomalies are specific to schizophrenia.

THE PRESENT findings indicate that tonic electrodermal activity is abnormally high in schizophrenic outpatients during symptomatic periods only and, therefore, is an episode indicator. Absolute phasic nonresponsiveness, on the other hand, appears to be a possible atypical vulnerability indicator that tends to be abnormal during nonpsychotic periods. Phasic hyporesponsiveness to innocuous external stimuli relative to levels of electrodermal activation was present in both remitted and psychotic states and was significantly greater in the psychotic state. Thus, phasic SCOR hyporesponsiveness appears to be a mediating vulnerability factor that may be related to attentional deficits.

The state sensitivity of the tonic electrodermal measures casts new light on the theoretical importance of these measures and their dysfunctions in schizophrenia. Specifically, tonic electrodermal measures may be more useful than previously thought in understanding the nature of the process by which psychotic symptoms return and in obtaining objective early warning signs of that process. Phasic electrodermal measures, on the other hand, appear to be more complicated but may prove to be useful in understanding the processes that occur during nonpsychotic periods and that are possibly related to the vulnerability to schizophrenia. The measurement of phasic skin conductance responses after correcting for nonspecific response frequency is a new and promising measure that warrants additional consideration in this context. Finally, given the importance of the symptomatic state

as a determiner of electrodermal activity, we strongly recommend that future research fully document and report the patients' clinical state at the time of testing with electrodermal and other autonomic measures.

Accepted for publication June 13, 1994.

This research was supported by research grant RO1 MH37705 (Dr Nuechterlein), Research Scientist Development Award 1 KO2 MH01086 (Dr Dawson), and Mental Health Clinical Research Center grant MH30911 (Robert P. Liberman, MD) from the National Institute of Mental Health, Bethesda, Md.

We wish to acknowledge the contributions of the staff of the University of California–Los Angeles Aftercare Program, Craig Childress, MA, and Rhonda Daily for their careful laboratory testing, and Rosemary Collier, MS; Sally Friedlob, MSW, OTR; Debbie Gioia-Hasick, MSW; David Lukoff, PhD; Sandy Rappe, MSW; Margie Stratton, MS; and Joseph Tietz, PhD, for serving as caring case managers who completed repeated administrations of the Brief Psychiatric Rating Scale. We also thank an anonymous reviewer for suggesting that the frequency of nonspecific skin conductance responses be taken into account in reporting frequency of skin conductance orienting responses. Finally, we thank the patients for their participation and generous cooperation throughout this project.

Reprint requests to Department of Psychology, SGM 501, University of Southern California, Los Angeles, CA 90089-1061 (Dr Dawson).

REFERENCES

1. Bernstein AS, Frith CD, Gruzelier JH, Patterson T, Straube E, Venables PH, Zahn TP. An analysis of the skin conductance orienting response in samples of American, British and German schizophrenics. *Biol Psychol.* 1982;14:155-211.
2. Bernstein AS. Orienting response research in schizophrenia: where we have come and where we might go. *Schizophr Bull.* 1987;13:623-641.
3. Dawson ME, Nuechterlein KH. Psychophysiological dysfunctions in the developmental course of schizophrenic disorders. *Schizophr Bull.* 1984;10:204-232.
4. Holzman PS. Recent studies of psychophysiology in schizophrenia. *Schizophr Bull.* 1987;13:49-75.
5. Öhman A. Electrodermal activity and vulnerability to schizophrenia: a review. *Biol Psychol.* 1981;12:87-145.
6. Spohn HE, Patterson T. Recent studies of psychophysiology in schizophrenia. *Schizophr Bull.* 1979;5:581-611.
7. Zahn TP. Psychophysiological approaches to psychopathology. In: Coles MGH, Donchin E, Porges SW, eds. *Psychophysiology: Systems, Processes, and Applications.* New York, NY: Guilford Press; 1986:508-610.
8. Zahn TP, Frith CD, Steinhauer SR. Autonomic functioning in schizophrenia: electrodermal activity, heart rate, pupillography. In: Steinhauer S, Gruzelier J, Zubin J, eds. *Handbook of Schizophrenia: Neuropsychology, Psychophysiology, and Information Processing.* Amsterdam, the Netherlands: Elsevier Science Publishers; 1991;5:185-224.
9. Boucsein W. *Electrodermal Activity.* New York, NY: Plenum Press; 1992.
10. Roy JC, Boucsein W, Fowles DC, Gruzelier JH. *Progress in Electrodermal Research.* New York, NY: Plenum Press; 1993.
11. Dawson ME, Schell AM, Filion DL. The electrodermal system. In: Cacioppo JT, Tassinary LG, eds. *Principles of Psychophysiology.* Cambridge, England: Cambridge University Press; 1990:295-324.
12. Fowles DC. The eccrine system and electrodermal activity. In: Coles MGH, Donchin E, Porges SW, eds. *Psychophysiology: Systems, Processes, and Applications.* New York, NY: Guilford Press; 1986:51-96.
13. Dawson ME, Nuechterlein KH, Schell AM. Electrodermal anomalies in recent-onset schizophrenia: relationships to symptoms and prognosis. *Schizophr Bull.* 1992;18:295-311.
14. Cannon TD, Mednick SA, Parnas J. Antecedents of predominantly negative- and predominantly positive-symptom schizophrenia in a high-risk population. *Arch Gen Psychiatry.* 1990;47:622-632.
15. Bernstein AS. The orienting response as an index of attentional dysfunction in schizophrenia. In: Campbell BA, Hayne H, Richardson R, eds. *Attention and Information Processing in Infants and Adults: Perspectives From Human and Animal Research.* Hillsdale, NJ: Lawrence Erlbaum Associates Inc; 1992:297-323.
16. Ficken J, Iacono WG. Electrodermal deviations in first-episode psychiatric patients and their relations. *Psychophysiology.* 1990;27(suppl):S30.
17. Iacono WG. Bilateral electrodermal habituation-dishabituation and resting EEG in remitted schizophrenics. *J Nerv Ment Dis.* 1982;170:91-101.
18. Olbrich R. The contributions of psychophysiology to vulnerability models. In: Häfner H, Gattaz WF, eds. *Search for the Causes of Schizophrenia.* Berlin, Germany: Springer-Verlag; 1991;2:192-204.
19. Spohn HE, Coyne L, Wilson JK, Hayes K. Skin-conductance orienting response in chronic schizophrenics: the role of neuroleptics. *J Abnorm Psychol.* 1989;98:478-486.
20. Zahn TP, Carpenter WT, McGlashan TH. Autonomic nervous system activity in acute schizophrenia, II: relationship to short-term prognosis and clinical state. *Arch Gen Psychiatry.* 1981;38:260-266.
21. Gruzelier JH, Venables PH. Skin conductance orienting activity in a heterogeneous sample of schizophrenics: possible evidence of limbic dysfunction. *J Nerv Ment Dis.* 1972;155:277-287.
22. Zubin J, Spring B. Vulnerability: a new view of schizophrenia. *J Abnorm Psychol.* 1977;86:103-126.
23. Cromwell RL, Spaulding W. How schizophrenics handle information. In: Fann WF, Karacan I, Pokorny AD, Williams RL, eds. *Phenomenology and Treatment of Schizophrenia.* Jamaica, NY: Spectrum Publishers; 1978:127-162.
24. Nuechterlein KH, Dawson ME. A heuristic vulnerability/stress model of schizophrenic episodes. *Schizophr Bull.* 1984;10:300-312.
25. Spitzer RL, Endicott J, Robins E. Research Diagnostic Criteria: rationale and reliability. *Arch Gen Psychiatry.* 1978;35:773-782.
26. Nuechterlein KH, Dawson ME, Gitlin M, Ventura J, Goldstein MJ, Snyder KS, Yee CM, Mintz J. Developmental Processes in Schizophrenic Disorders: longitudinal studies of vulnerability and stress. *Schizophr Bull.* 1992;18:387-425.
27. Schnur DB. Effects of neuroleptics on electrodermal activity in schizophrenic patients: a review. *Psychopharmacology.* 1990;102:429-437.
28. Overall JE, Gorham DR. The brief psychiatric rating scale. *Psychol Rep.* 1962;10:799-812.
29. Overall JE, Klett CJ. *Applied Multivariate Analysis.* New York, NY: McGraw-Hill International Book Co; 1972.
30. Ventura J, Lukoff D, Nuechterlein KH, Liberman RL, Green MF, Shaner A. Brief Psychiatric Rating Scale (BPRS), Expanded Version (4.0): scales, anchor points and administration manual. *Int J Methods Psychiatr Res.* 1993;3:227-243.
31. Lukoff D, Nuechterlein KH, Ventura J. Manual for expanded Brief Psychiatric Rating Scale (BPRS). *Schizophr Bull.* 1986;12:594-602.
32. Mednick SA, Schulsinger F. Some premorbid characteristics related to breakdown in children with schizophrenic mothers. In: Rosenthal D, Kety SS, eds. *Transmission of Schizophrenia.* New York, NY: Pergamon Press Inc; 1968:267-291.
33. Cohen J. *Statistical Power Analysis for the Behavioral Sciences.* 2nd ed. Hillsdale, NJ: Lawrence Erlbaum Associates Inc; 1988.
34. Zubin J, Steinhauer S. How to break the logjam in schizophrenia: a look beyond genetics. *J Nerv Ment Dis.* 1981;169:477-492.
35. Crider A. Electrodermal response lability-stability: individual difference correlates. In: Roy JC, Boucsein W, Fowles DC, Gruzelier JH, eds. *Progress in Electrodermal Research.* New York, NY: Plenum Publishing Corp; 1993:173-186.
36. Schell AM, Dawson ME, Filion DL. Psychophysiological correlates of electrodermal lability. *Psychophysiology.* 1988;25:619-632.
37. Ko GN, Jimerson DC, Wyatt RJ, Bigelow LB. Plasma 3-methoxy-4-hydroxyphenylglycol changes associated with clinical state and schizophrenic subtype. *Arch Gen Psychiatry.* 1988;45:842-846.
38. Mazure CM, Nelson JC, Jatlow PI, Bowers MB. Plasma free homovanillic acid (HVA) as a predictor of clinical response in acute psychosis. *Biol Psychiatry.* 1991;30:475-482.

39. Hommer D, Zahn T, Pickar D, van Kammen D. Prazosin, a specific alpha 1–noradrenergic receptor antagonist, has no effect on symptoms but increases autonomic arousal in schizophrenic patients. *Psychiatry Res.* 1984;11:193-204.
40. Dawson ME, Neuchterlein KH. The role of autonomic dysfunctions within a vulnerability/stress model of schizophrenic disorders. In: Magusson D, Ohman A, eds. *Psychopathology: An Interactional Perspective.* New York, NY: Academic Press Inc; 1987:41-57.
41. Dawson ME, Nuechterlein KH, Liberman RP. Relapse in schizophrenic disorders: possible contributing factors and implications for behavior therapy. In: Rosenbaum M, Franks CM, Jaffe Y, eds. *Perspectives on Behavior Therapy in the Eighties.* New York, NY: Springer-Verlag; 1983:265-286.
42. Birchwood M, Smith J, Macmillan F, Hogg B, Prasad R, Harvey L, Bering S. Predicting relapse in schizophrenia: the development and implementation of an early signs monitoring system using patients and families as observers in preliminary investigation. *Psychol Med.* 1989;19:649-656.
43. Docherty JP, Van Kammen DP, Siris SG, Marder SR. Stages of onset of schizophrenic psychosis. *Am J Psychiatry.* 1978;135:420-426.
44. Herz MI, Melville C. Relapse in schizophrenia. *Am J Psychiatry.* 1980;137:801-805.
45. Heinrichs DW, Carpenter WT. Prospective study of prodromal symptoms in schizophrenic relapse. *Am J Psychiatry.* 1985;142:371-373.
46. Marder S, Wirshing W, Van Putten T, Mintz J, McKenzie J, Johnston-Cronk K. Fluphenazine vs placebo supplementation for prodromal signs of relapse in schizophrenia. *Arch Gen Psychiatry.* 1994;51:280-287.
47. Subotnik KL, Nuechterlein KH. Prodromal signs and symptoms of schizophrenic relapse. *J Abnorm Psychol.* 1988;97:405-412.
48. Janowsky DS, El-Yousef MK, Davis JM, Sekerke HJ. Provocation of schizophrenic symptoms by intravenous administration of methylphenidate. *Arch Gen Psychiatry.* 1973;28:185-191.
49. Lieberman JA, Kane JM, Sarantakos S, Gadaleta D, Woerner M, Alvir J, Ramos-Lorenzi J. Prediction of relapse in schizophrenia. *Arch Gen Psychiatry.* 1987; 44:597-603.
50. Sharma RP, Javaid JI, Pandey GN, Janicak PG, Davis JM. Behavioral and biochemical effects of methylphenidate in schizophrenic and nonschizophrenic patients. *Biol Psychiatry.* 1991;30:459-466.
51. Zahn TP, Carpenter WT, McGlashan TH. Autonomic nervous system activity in acute schizophrenia, I: method and comparison with normal controls. *Arch Gen Psychiatry.* 1981;38:251-259.
52. Öhman A, Nordby H, D'Elia G. Orienting in schizophrenia: habituation to auditory stimuli of constant and varying intensity in patients high and low in skin conductance responsivity. *Psychophysiology.* 1989;26:48-61.
53. Sokolov EN. *Perception and the Conditioned Reflex.* New York, NY: Macmillan Publishing Co Inc; 1963.
54. Kahneman D. *Attention and Effort.* Englewood Cliffs, NJ: Prentice-Hall International Inc; 1973.
55. Öhman A. Orienting and attention: preferred preattentive processing of potentially phobic stimuli. In: Campbell BA, Hayne H, Richardson R, eds. *Attention and Information Processing in Infants and Adults: Perspectives From Human and Animal Research.* Hillsdale, NJ: Lawrence Erlbaum Associates Inc; 1992: 263-295.
56. Dawson ME, Filion DL, Schell AM. Is elicitation of the autonomic orienting response associated with allocation of processing resources? *Psychophysiology.* 1989;26:560-572.
57. Siddle DAT, Spinks JA. Orienting, habituation, and the allocation of processing resources. In: Campbell BA, Hayne H, Richardson R, eds. *Attention and Information Processing in Infants and Adults: Perspectives From Human and Animal Research.* Hillsdale, NJ: Lawrence Erlbaum Associates Inc; 1992:227-262.
58. Nuechterlein KH, Dawson ME. Information processing and attentional functioning in the developmental course of schizophrenic disorders. *Schizophr Bull.* 1984;10:160-203.
59. Gruzelier JH. The cardiac responses of schizophrenics to orienting, signal and non-signal tones. *Biol Psychology.* 1975;3:143-155.
60. Gruzelier JH, Hammond NV. The effect of chlorpromazine upon psychophysiological, endocrine and information processing measures in schizophrenia. *J Psychiatr Res.* 1978;14:167-182.
61. Hazlett EA, Dawson ME, Buchsbaum MS, Nuechterlein KH. Reduced regional brain glucose metabolism assessed by PET in electrodermal nonresponder schizophrenics: a pilot study. *J Abnorm Psychol.* 1993;102:39-46.
62. Iacono WG, Ficken JW, Beiser M. Electrodermal nonresponding in first-episode psychosis as a function of stimulus significance. In: Roy JC, Boucsein W, Fowles DC, Gruzelier JH, eds. *Electrodermal Activity: From Physiology to Psychology.* New York, NY: Plenum Publishing Corp; 1993:239-256.
63. Levinson DF. Skin conductance orienting response in unmedicated RDC schizophrenic, schizoaffective, depressed, and control subjects. *Biol Psychiatry.* 1991; 30:663-683.

Keep your professional career on the right track . . .

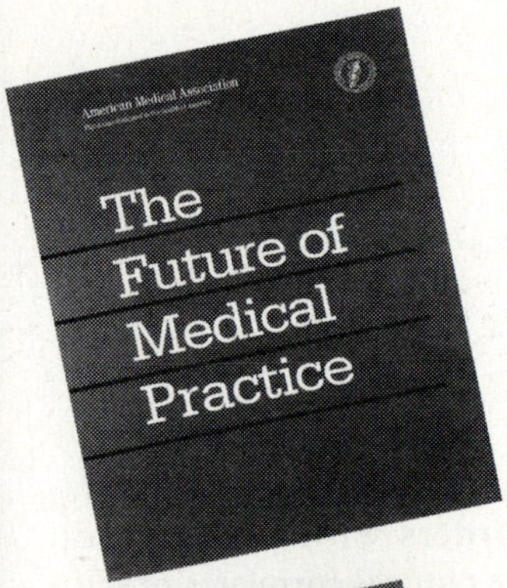

The Future of Medical Practice

This major new study from the AMA Council on Long Range Planning and Development analyzes 33 potential trends that are likely to occur during the next 10 to 15 years. Provides solid, reliable information about the future of medicine to use to develop effective strategies for dealing with the fast-changing health care system. An indispensable guide to ensuring the future success of any medical practice.

ISBN 0-89970-479-4. 108 pages, softbound. Publication date: August 1994. Order #: OP211594NT. AMA member price: $35.00. Nonmember price: $49.00.

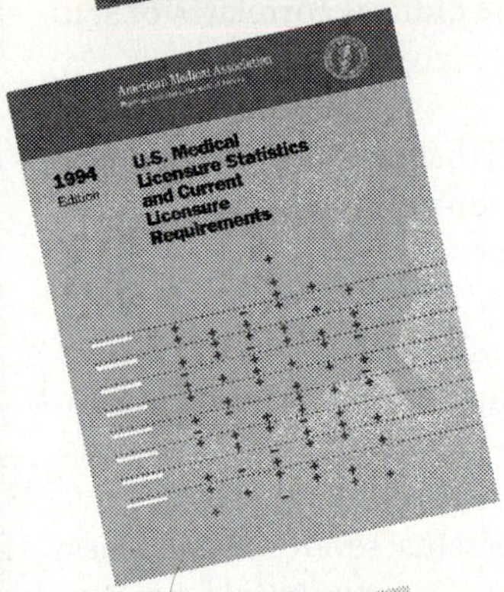

US Medical Licensure Statistics and Current Licensure Requirements, 1994 Edition

Whether you're starting a new practice or moving an established one, this new edition will save you time and aggravation. It's the only reference that gives statistics and licensure information for every state in the US in a single source.
• All state board licensing policies as of January 1994. • New US Medical Licensing Examination information. • National Board and ECFMG requirements. • Reciprocity and endorsement policies. • Fees, renewal intervals, and CME requirements. • Current guidance for Department of Defense licensure. • Immigration overview of international medical graduates

The most up-to-date, practical guide for students, residents, graduates of foreign medical schools, and physicians contemplating a move.

ISBN 0-89970-544-8. 85 pages, 30 tables, softbound. Publication date: 1994; annual. Order #: OP399094NT. AMA member price: $50.00. Nonmember price: $75.00.

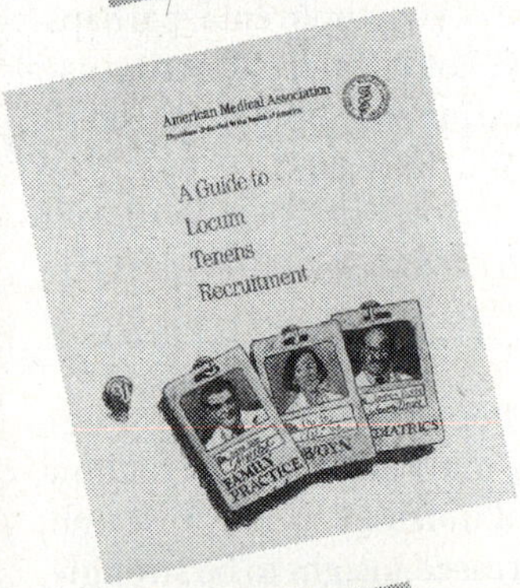

Guide to Locum Tenens Recruitment

Recruiting locum tenens physicians? This resource describes how to create and manage an effective recruitment program for physicians who will take temporary assignments in a practice. Includes how to find qualified candidates, design a compensation package, and write an employment contract as well as details on practice and professional liability.

ISBN 0-89970-415-8. 14 pages, softbound. Publication date: 1992. Order #: OP392292NT. AMA member price: $20.00. Nonmember price: $25.00.

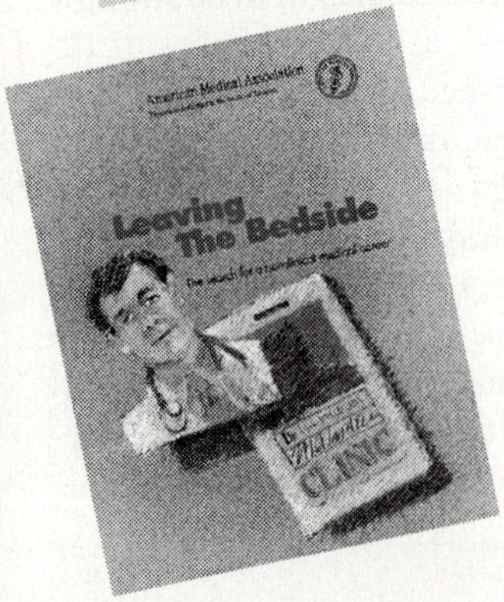

Leaving the Bedside: The Search for a Non-clinical Medical Career

Physicians in the process of considering a career change need information about themselves and their options in order to make informed decisions. *Leaving the Bedside* offers physicians guidance in assessing professional and personal strengths, developing self-marketing strategies, and identifying and evaluating career options for the future.

ISBN 0-89970-464-6. 120 pages, softbound. Publication date: 1993. Order #: OP392092NT. AMA member price: $24.95. Nonmember price: $29.95.

To order, call toll free 800 621-8335

American Medical Association
Physicians dedicated to the health of America

ORIGINAL ARTICLE

Awareness of Illness in Schizophrenia and Schizoaffective and Mood Disorders

Xavier F. Amador, PhD; Michael Flaum, MD; Nancy C. Andreasen, MD, PhD; David H. Strauss, MD; Scott A. Yale, MSW; Scott C. Clark, MD; Jack M. Gorman, MD

Background: The literature on insight, or self-awareness, in schizophrenia suggests that this cognitive dimension may be of nosological value. Poor insight has descriptive validity at the phenomenological and neuropsychological levels of schizophrenia and has prognostic validity in terms of the prediction of the course of illness. The lack of empirical data on the diagnostic specificity of poor insight to schizophrenia and the previous use of insight measures with questionable reliability and validity have limited this interpretation.

Methods: In the present study, we assessed insight into multiple aspects of mental disorder using a measure with demonstrated reliability and validity. A sample of 412 patients with psychotic and mood disorders coming from geographically diverse regions of the United States and one international site was studied. The main aims were to determine the prevalence of self-awareness deficits in patients in whom schizophrenia was diagnosed, to examine the relative severity of self-awareness deficits associated with schizophrenia compared with that of schizoaffective and mood disorders with and without psychosis, and to evaluate the clinical correlates of self-awareness in patients with schizophrenia.

Results: The results indicated that poor insight is a prevalent feature of schizophrenia. A variety of self-awareness deficits are more severe and pervasive in patients with schizophrenia than in patients with schizoaffective or major depressive disorders with or without psychosis and are associated with poorer psychosocial functioning.

Conclusions: The results suggest that severe self-awareness deficits are a prevalent feature of schizophrenia, perhaps stemming from the neuropsychological dysfunction associated with the disorder, and are more common in schizophrenia than in other psychotic disorders.

(Arch Gen Psychiatry. 1994;51:826-836)

From the Department of Clinical Psychobiology, Schizophrenia Research Unit, New York State Psychiatric Institute (Drs Amador, Strauss, Clark, and Gorman and Mr Yale), the Department of Psychiatry, College of Physicians and Surgeons, Columbia University (Drs Amador, Strauss, Clark, and Gorman and Mr Yale), and New York University Graduate School of Arts and Sciences (Dr Amador), New York, NY; and the Mental Health Clinical Research Center, the University of Iowa Hospitals and Clinics, and the Department of Psychiatry, the University of Iowa College of Medicine, Iowa City (Drs Flaum and Andreasen).

SEVERAL INVESTIGATORS[1-3] have proposed that schizophrenia is best conceptualized as a disorder that encompasses multiple aspects of psychopathology. In this context, the literature on poor insight into illness in schizophrenia suggests that this deficit may have nosological value. Poor insight appears to have descriptive validity at the phenomenological and neuropsychological levels of schizophrenia. For example, based on cluster analytic analyses of the signs and symptoms of schizophrenia, poor insight had descriptive validity as a symptom on which patients could be subtyped.[4,5] The results of a more recent study[6] indicated that the severity of poor insight was strongly correlated with the degree of neuropsychological dysfunction of the frontal lobes. Poor insight also has prognostic validity in terms of the prediction of the course of illness. Previous research has found decreased insight to be strongly correlated with a poorer course of illness, impoverished psychosocial functioning, and noncompliance with treatment.[7-13]

Nonetheless, it has been difficult to generalize from the results of previous studies because the majority did not use measures of insight with proven reliability and validity.[11] In addition, until re-

See Patients and Methods on next page

PATIENTS AND METHODS

SAMPLE

Patients were recruited from eight sites: Columbia University and the New York State Psychiatric Institute, New York City; Long Island Jewish Medical Center, Hillside (NY) Hospital; McLean Hospital, Harvard University, Belmont, Mass; the Medical College of Virginia, Richmond; the University of Arkansas, Fayetteville; the Clinical Research Center, the University of Iowa, Iowa City; the University of Nuevo Leon, Monterey, Mexico; and Yale Psychiatric Institute, Yale University, New Haven, Conn. All patients gave informed consent to participate in the study. **Table 1** presents descriptive data on the sample.

PROCEDURES

Disorders of all patients were diagnosed by *DSM-III-R* criteria. The diagnoses given by the raters were confirmed using the symptom ratings to ensure that the categorization of psychosis in mood disorders was particularly rigorous and stringent. Final diagnoses of mood disorder were derived from the symptom data collected by the interviewers using computer-programmed algorithms based on *DSM-III-R* criteria. All necessary symptom severity and duration data were available to make these diagnoses. Patients with major depressive disorder who were also psychotic (PMDD) were arbitrarily defined as those individuals scoring at least a 3 (moderate) or higher on the Scale to Assess Positive Symptoms' hallucination and/or delusion item(s) while also meeting the *DSM-III-R* criteria for a major depressive syndrome. Consequently, a small number of the patients in whom major depressive disorder without psychosis (MDD) was ultimately diagnosed actually were rated as having questionable or mild hallucinations and/or delusions. Nonetheless, the algorithmically derived diagnoses were generally in agreement with the rater diagnoses (bipolar [BP] disorder, 100% agreement; MDD, 92% agreement; and PMDD, 77% agreement). The main difference was that fewer patients with PMDD were identified by the computer owing to the more stringent criteria.

The moderate to severe cutoff scores were chosen so that the psychotic mood disorder group would be limited to those patients with unambiguous symptoms of psychosis of a severity equal to that of the patients with schizophrenia (SZ). In fact, a one-way analysis of variance contrasting the patients with SZ, schizoaffective (SA) disorder, BP disorder, and PMDD revealed no significant differences in the severity of delusions among groups ($F=1.5$, $df=3$, $P=.20$). Although the BP group had less severe hallucinations, the SZ, SA, and PMDD groups did not differ from each other in the severity of hallucinations ($F=2.8$, $df=2$, $P=.44$).

For the current study, measures included the field trial instrument developed for the Schizophrenia and Psychotic Disorders Field Trial[17] and an abbreviated version of the SUMD (**Figure 1**). The field trial instrument consisted of several scales adapted from the Comprehensive Assessment of Symptoms and History,[18] eg, the Scale to Assess Positive Symptoms, the Scale to Assess Negative Symptoms, the Global Assessment Scale,[19] and depressive and manic syndrome scales. A shortened version of the SUMD was used because of interview time constraints. Scores for each of the nine items (**Table 2**) ranged from 1 to 3, with higher scores indicating poorer awareness. This version was nearly identical to that reported on recently[12] with the exception that several symptom items, the retrospective awareness scales, and all of the attributional scales were omitted. The omission of symptom items made the calculation of the awareness subscale total, as described by Amador et al,[12] impossible. Consequently, each item was examined separately.

At least one of the following positive or negative symptoms had to be currently present to at least a mild degree for a subject to be included in the study: delusions, hallucinations, disorganized speech, flat affect, poverty of speech, or passive, apathetic social withdrawal. Sampling pools were

Continued on next page

cently, most assessments of insight reported in the literature were not standardized and were deficient in evaluating the multidimensional nature of this phenomenon.[11,12,14,15] Amador et al[12] argued that poor insight is best viewed as a symptom (or sign) comprising multiple components, not unlike affective flattening, and developed a rating scale based on this notion. The Scale to Assess Unawareness of Mental Disorder (SUMD) samples discrete and global aspects of insight across a variety of manifestations of illness. Data that indicate that the SUMD has convergent and criterion validities and can be used reliably with minimal training have been reported.[12]

In the present study, we assessed insight into, or awareness of, multiple dimensions of mental disorder. In addition to evaluating patients' general awareness of having a mental disorder, we also assessed their awareness of the efficacy of pharmacotherapy, the social consequences of mental disorder, and six common symptoms of schizophrenia. For the purposes of this discussion, the term insight will be used interchangeably with awareness. *Awareness* refers to the recognition of particular causal relationships, eg, recognition that having a mental disorder has contributed to one's long-standing unemployment or that taking medications has been associated with decreased hospitalizations. In addition, awareness can refer to the recognition of aberrant aspects of one's appearance or functioning (ie, symptoms of the mental disorder). In this study, our assessment of a patient's awareness of the signs and symptoms of the mental disorder focused solely on whether the subject recognized the essential features of the particular sign or symptom that he or she had, eg, that he or she had dis-

identified at each site and included both inpatient and outpatient facilities. Information was obtained from subject interviews, current and past medical records, and informant interviews. Although diagnoses were made by several criteria, only *DSM-III-R* diagnoses are reported here.

A training session was conducted on the field trial instrument for the coordinators at each site, and they, in turn, supervised the raters at their respective sites. No formal training on the administration of the SUMD was provided other than the directions given on the scale itself. Interviewers ranged from master's level clinicians to senior psychiatrists, and all had substantial experience working with and evaluating patients with psychotic disorders. Between four and eight raters participated at each site. It is noteworthy that of the 412 patients interviewed, 190 (46%) were simultaneously assessed by two raters and another 188 (46%) were rated in a test-retest condition (no more than 48 hours apart). Consequently, extensive reliability data were generated for all of the psychopathological assessments, diagnoses, and insight ratings. Data from only the primary interviewer were used in all analyses other than those involving the examination of rater reliabilities. A more detailed description of the assessment procedure and rater characteristics will be given elsewhere.[17]

RELIABILITY OF DIAGNOSTIC, SYMPTOM, AND AWARENESS RATINGS

Diagnosis and Symptoms

Interrater and test-retest intraclass correlation coefficients (ICCs) (*r*) were calculated using the formula in Fleiss.[20] Rater agreement on *DSM-III-R* diagnoses were in the good to excellent range, as reflected by κ's for overall diagnosis of 0.74 and 0.64 for interrater and test-retest reliability, respectively, and 0.77 and 0.74, respectively, for the diagnosis of SZ. Similarly, interrater and test-retest reliability on the psychopathological ratings from the Field Trial Instrument ranged from adequate to excellent. A more detailed description of the reliability of the diagnoses and symptom ratings will be reported elsewhere.[17]

Awareness Ratings

The one previous report of the reliability of the SUMD was based on ratings made at two SZ research centers.[12] In the present study, a large proportion of the sample and many of the raters came from hospitals and clinics that were not actively involved in clinical research. In addition, the raters did not receive formal training on the SUMD. Nonetheless, the SUMD ratings were made reliably. The interrater ICC was .95 and test-retest ICC was .62 for the first item, the general insight measure, ie, awareness of mental disorder. The other insight items all had excellent interrater ICCs (between .76 to .99; median, .89) and fair to good test-retest ICCs (.36 to .80; median, .51). Mean±SD ratings from the nine items of the SUMD ranged from 0.82±1.03 to 1.85±1.18. Item 6, awareness of thought disorder, had the greatest variability with an SD of 1.35, whereas item 1, awareness of mental disorder, had the lowest (SD=0.90).

STATISTICAL ANALYSES

Pearson's correlation coefficients were used to assess hypothesized relationships between insight scores and psychopathological and demographic variables.

Because all but the first item on the SUMD are not necessarily relevant for each subject, multivariate analyses such as a factor analysis or an analysis of variance (ANOVA) were not possible. For example, of the total sample of 221 patients with SZ, only 151 were rated on the awareness of hallucinations item (ie, awareness of this symptom was assessed only in those patients with moderate to severe hallucinations). Meanwhile, the sample size for awareness of anhedonia was 129. Consequently, to examine differences between groups on the SUMD, we used two-tailed independent *t* tests with and without Bonferroni corrections for multiple comparisons.

organized speech, false perceptions, or impoverished speech. A more detailed discussion of the assessment of the multiple dimensions of insight appears elsewhere.[12]

Herein, we assessed awareness of illness in a sample of 412 patients with psychotic disorders from geographically diverse regions of the United States and one international site. To our knowledge, this is the first study to evaluate many of the component dimensions of awareness of illness (eg, awareness of signs and/or symptoms and effects of medication) using an instrument with demonstrated reliability and validity and the first to contrast different diagnostic groups on this cognitive capacity. This study was conducted in collaboration with the work group impaneled by the American Psychiatric Association, Washington, DC, for the purpose of revising the diagnostic criteria for schizophrenia and related disorders in the *DSM-III-R*.[16] The main objectives of this aspect of the field trial study were to determine the prevalence of various aspects of poor insight in patients in whom schizophrenia was diagnosed, to examine the extent of poor insight in patients with schizophrenia relative to that in patients with schizoaffective or mood disorders with and without psychosis, and to evaluate the clinical correlates of insight in patients with schizophrenia.

RESULTS

THE PREVALENCE OF POOR INSIGHT IN PATIENTS WITH SCHIZOPHRENIA

As can be seen in **Figure 2**, 57.4% of the patients with SZ showed a moderate to severe lack of awareness of hav-

Table 1. Descriptive Characteristics of the Sample*

Disorder	No. of Patients	Age, y†	Age at Onset, y†	Education, y†	GAS Score†	Sex, M/F	Married, %
SZ	221	34.4±11.2	22.0±7.0	12.0±3.0	34.5±10.0	146/75	7.7
SA disorder	49	33.6±12.1	20.1±6.5	13.0±3.0	37.6±12.6	27/22	12.2
BP disorder	40	32.4±12.5	26.2±12.0	14.1±3.1	37.3±10.9	29/11	32.5
PMDD	24	30.1±14.6	25.0±14.1	13.0±3.3	41.6±15.6	11/13	16.7
Nonpsychotic MDD	14	35.4±12.7	25.0±11.0	13.8±3.0	39.8±13.3	8/6	21.4

**GAS indicates Global Assessment Scale; SZ, schizophrenia; SA, schizoaffective; BP, bipolar; MDD, major depressive disorder; PMDD, psychotic MDD.*
†Values are expressed as mean±SD.

DIRECTIONS:

For each symptom item on the Unawareness Scale, it must first be ascertained that the subject has had the symptom during the time period being rated. Using the ratings you made earlier to determine this. Symptom ratings of 3 or higher are required. Circle the relevant items, then inquire as to the patient's awareness of it.

In order to evidence some awareness, the subject does not have to give precise attributions for symptoms. For example, "I hear voices because of the implant the researchers put in my brain" would constitute a "Somewhat Aware/Unaware" response.

In the current episode column, rate the highest level of awareness during the current exacerbation.

RATING KEY:

unk: UNKNOWN
There is inadequate information to assess.
0: NOT APPLICABLE
Item is not relevant.
1: AWARE
Subject clearly believes that he or she has a mental disorder.
2: SOMEWHAT AWARE/UNAWARE
Subject is unsure about whether he or she has a mental disorder but can entertain the idea.
3: SEVERELY UNAWARE
Subject believes he or she does not have a mental disorder.

Figure 1. *Scale to Assess Unawareness of Mental Disorder (SUMD), short form.*

ing a mental disorder (SUMD item 1). In addition, 31.5% had severe unawareness (ie, a score of 3) of the social consequences of mental disorder and 21.7% were rated as having severe unawareness of the efficacy of medication. **Figure 3** shows the percentage of patients with SZ with a severe unawareness of the signs and symptoms of mental disorder. Proportions of the sample that were unaware ranged from 27.8% to 57.6%, depending on the particular sign or symptom.

COMPARISON OF DIAGNOSTIC GROUPS

Table 3 shows the mean SUMD scores of the five diagnostic groups. Differences between the SZ group and each of the other diagnostic groups were tested independently using two-tailed *t* tests with correction for multiple comparisons.

As can be seen in Table 3, relative to the patients with SZ, the patients with SA disorder were more aware of having a mental disorder (t=2.24, df=264, P=.02) and of having four of the six symptoms that were evaluated.

Table 2. Scale to Assess Unawareness of Mental Disorder (Abridged)

1. **Awareness of mental disorder:** In the most general terms, does the subject believe that he or she has a mental disorder?
2. **Awareness of the consequences of mental disorder:** What is the subject's belief regarding the reason(s) he or she has been unemployed, evicted, hospitalized, etc?
3. **Awareness of the effects of medication:** Does the subject believe that medications have diminished the severity of his or her symptoms (if applicable)?
4. **Awareness of hallucinatory experiences:** Does the subject believe that he or she experiences hallucinations as such? Rate his or her ability to interpret this experience as primarily hallucinatory.
5. **Awareness of delusions:** Does the subject believe that he or she experiences delusions as such, that is, as internally produced erroneous beliefs? Rate his or her awareness of the implausibility of the belief if applicable.
6. **Awareness of thought disorder:** Does the subject believe that his or her communications are disorganized?
7. **Awareness of flat or blunt affect:** Rate the subject's awareness of his or her affect as communicated by his or her expressions, voice, gestures, etc. Do not rate his or her evaluation of his or her mood.
8. **Awareness of anhedonia:** Is the subject aware that his or her behavior reflects an apparent decrease in experiencing pleasure while participating in activities normally associated with such feelings?
9. **Awareness of asociality:** Is the subject aware that he or she shows no interest in social relationships?

Specifically, patients with SA disorder were significantly more aware of hallucinations (t=2.31, df=186, P=.02), delusions (t=3.10, df=228, P=.002), anhedonia (t=2.30, df=156, P=.03), and asociality (t=3.10, df=193, P=.003) than were patients with SZ.

Of the 40 patients in whom BP disorder was diagnosed, 37 (93%) met *DSM-III-R* criteria for current manic episode. This severely manic BP group scored as poorly as the SZ group on the majority of the items. The one exception to this pattern was the awareness of delusion item: patients with BP disorder were significantly more aware of currently having delusions (t=2.2, df=224, P=.02) than were patients with SZ. However, only the awareness of delusion and thought disorder items had large

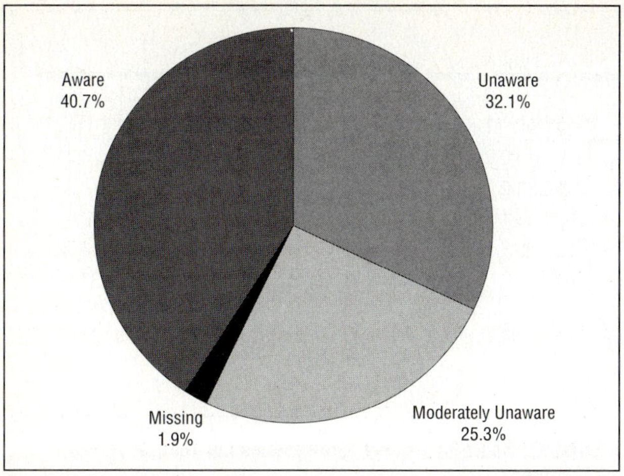

Figure 2. *Percentage of patients with schizophrenia with unawareness of mental disorder. N=221.*

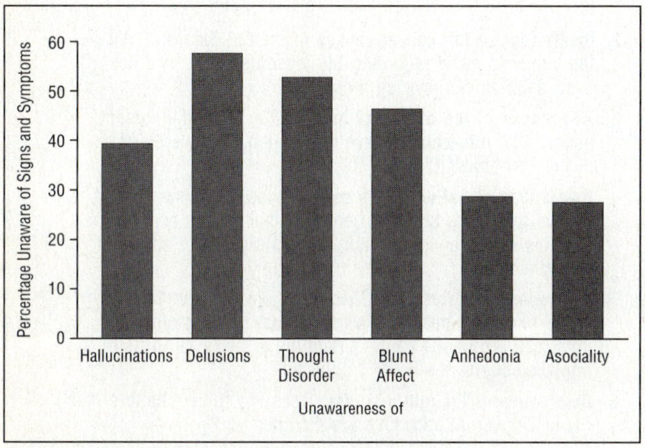

Figure 3. *Percentage of patients with schizophrenia with severe unawareness of signs and symptoms of mental disorder. Sample sizes ranged from n=129 (patients with anhedonia) to n=191 (patients with delusions) because only patients with a symptom rating of moderate to severe intensity were rated for awareness.*

enough numbers to provide an adequate statistical power to detect differences.

Patients with PMDD were also generally more aware than were the patients with SZ despite having clear-cut psychosis of equal severity. Specifically, patients with PMDD were significantly more aware of having a mental disorder (t=2.02, df=239, P=.04), of the social consequences of the mental disorder (t=2.7, df=233, P=.007), and of delusions (t=3.14, df=212, P=.002) and tended to be more aware of anhedonia (t=1.75, df=143, P=.08). It is noteworthy that the symptom items with nonsignificant results all had very small sample sizes resulting in a low statistical power to detect differences.

Finally, relative to the SZ group, the nonpsychotic MDD group was found to be significantly more aware of having a mental disorder (t=3.31, df=229, P=.001) and of the social consequences of having a mental disorder (t=2.53, df=225, P=.01). They also showed significantly better awareness of all three negative symptoms evaluated (flat affect, t=2.2, df=141, P=.03; anhedonia, t=2.7, df=139, P=.008; and asociality, t=2.2, df=176, P=.03). The number of patients with MDD and positive symptoms (ie, of questionable to mild severity) was too small to yield a sufficient power to detect any differences in awareness of positive symptoms.

Table 4 shows the proportion of patients in each diagnostic group with severe unawareness. As can be seen, statistically significant diagnostic group differences in the incidence of severe unawareness were found on the awareness of mental disorder, the awareness of delusion, and the awareness of anhedonia items. Diagnostic groups also tended to differ on the awareness of asociality item. Although not always statistically significant, the highest incidence of severe unawareness was observed in the SZ sample. The SZ group exhibited the highest incidence of severe unawareness relative to the other groups on the awareness of mental disorder, social consequences, medication efficacy, delusion, and asociality items. The BP sample showed the highest incidence of severe unawareness on the awareness of hallucination, flat affect, and anhedonia items. The high percentages on the awareness of negative symptom items in the BP group were attributable to a few patients because the sample sizes were very small (n=6 and n=9). Meanwhile, both the SA and SZ groups had nearly identical proportions with severe unawareness of thought disorder (54.5% and 53.1%, respectively).

To determine whether group differences on the insight measure were due to differences in overall level of functioning, we compared groups on the Global Assessment Scale (GAS) and also repeated the insight analyses using GAS scores as a covariate. A one-way ANOVA comparing the five diagnostic groups on current GAS scores revealed that the SZ group ($\bar{x}$=34.5; SD=10.0) did not differ significantly from the SA ($\bar{x}$=37.6; SD=12.6), MDD ($\bar{x}$=39.8; SD=13.3), or BP ($\bar{x}$=37.3; SD=10.9) groups. Only the patients with PMDD ($\bar{x}$=41.6; SD=15.6), (F=3.3, df=4, P=.01) had a significantly higher level of functioning. Next, we conducted a one-way ANOVA comparing the five diagnostic groups on the SUMD using the current GAS score as a covariate, and we found a main effect for diagnosis on general awareness of mental disorder (F=26.1, df=4, P=.02), awareness of hallucinations (F=3.0, df=3, P=.03), awareness of delusion (F=6.6, df=3, P=.0001), and awareness of asociality (F=3.2, df=4, P=.01). Post hoc analyses comparing each group with the SZ sample using GAS scores as a covariate revealed that the SZ group still had poorer awareness on many of the insight items than did the patients with SA disorder, PMDD, and nonpsychotic MDD but did not differ from the patients with BP disorder. Specifically, relative to the SA group, patients with SZ had less awareness of hallucinations (F=3.5, df=1, P=.01), delusions (F=13.6, df=1, P=.0001), anhedonia (F=3.3, df=1, P=.06), and asociality (F=8.0, df=1, P=.006).

Table 3. Average Awareness Scores on the SUMD for Each Diagnostic Group*

Awareness of:	SZ	SA Disorder	BP Disorder	PMDD	Nonpsychotic MDD
Mental disorder†	1.9±.85 (217)	1.6±.80 (49)‡	1.7±.82 (40)	1.5±.80 (24)‡	1.1±.54 (14)§
Consequences	1.9±.90 (213)	1.7±.90 (48)	1.7±.81 (40)	1.4±.72 (22)§	1.3±.61 (14)‡
Medication efficacy	1.7±.81 (173)	1.6±.80 (48)	1.6±.71 (39)	1.5±.74 (22)	1.4±.77 (14)
Hallucinations†	2.1±.85 (151)	1.7±.83 (31)‡	2.2±.90 (15)	1.8±1.0 (17)	1.0±.00 (2)
Delusions†	2.4±.80 (191)	2.0±.90 (39)§	2.0±.80 (35)‡	1.8±.90 (23)§	2.0±1.0 (7)
Thought disorder	2.3±.81 (119)	2.3±.90 (22)	2.3±.80 (27)	1.9±.84 (8)	1.7±.60 (3)
Flat affect	2.2±.90 (133)	2.0±.84 (25)	2.3±.90 (9)	2.1±.83 (11)	1.6±.70 (10)‡
Anhedonia	1.8±.90 (129)	1.4±.70 (29)‡	2.0±.90 (6)	1.4±.62 (16)‖	1.1±.30 (12)§
Asociality†	1.8±.84 (169)	1.3±.70 (26)§	1.9±.83 (8)	1.5±.71 (17)	1.2±.44 (9)‡

*Scale to Assess Unawareness of Mental Disorder (SUMD) scores range from 1 to 3, with higher scores indicating increased unawareness. In addition to a one-way analysis of variance (ANOVA) using Global Assessment Scale (GAS) scores as a covariate, each of the nonschizophrenia groups was independently compared with the schizophrenia (SZ) group using t tests. All comparisons were two-tailed. Values are expressed as mean±SD (No.). SA indicates schizoaffective; BP, bipolar; MDD, major depressive disorder; and PMDD, psychotic MDD.
†One-way ANOVA, using current GAS score as a covariate. Main effect for diagnostic group (P ranged from .0001 to .03).
‡P<.04.
§P<.008. Significant after Bonferonni correction: P of .05÷9=.006.
‖P<.09.

Relative to the PMDD group, patients with SZ tended to have less awareness of mental disorder (F=3.5, *df*=1, *P*=.06), less awareness of the consequences of mental disorder (F=3.0, *df*=1, *P*=.08), and significantly less awareness of hallucinations (F=4.0, *df*=1, *P*=.04) and delusions (F=7.7, *df*=1, *P*=.006). Compared with the patients with MDD, patients with SZ had less awareness of mental disorder (F=7.6, *df*=1, *P*=.006) and less awareness of the consequences of mental disorder (F=3.8, *df*=1, *P*=.05). The only differences between the MDD and SZ groups that were not confirmed with this analysis were the ones involving awareness of negative symptoms.

CLINICAL CORRELATES AMONG PATIENTS WITH SZ

We examined the relations between global positive symptoms from the Scale to Assess Positive Symptoms and the nine insight scores for the SZ group. Modest correlations were obtained for the relations between delusions and several dimensions of unawareness. Specifically, an increase in the severity of delusions was modestly correlated with less awareness of mental disorder, the social consequences of mental disorder, the efficacy of medication, hallucinations, and delusions (*r* ranged from .14 to .23, all *P* values <.04). Delusions were additionally categorized with respect to whether they were bizarre. Of the 198 patients with SZ with current delusions, those with bizarre delusions (n=120) differed from those with nonbizarre delusions (n=72) only on the awareness of hallucination item (*t*=2.4, *df*=143, *P*=.01, n=145 for this comparison). This result was in the direction of poorer awareness of hallucinations being associated with bizarre delusions. Among patients who did not have SZ, no significant differences between those with (n=43) and those without (n=63) bizarre delusions were found on any SUMD item.

Increased formal thought disorder was also modestly correlated with less awareness of mental disorder, the social consequences of mental disorder, hallucinations, delusions, anhedonia, and asociality (*r* ranged from .18 to .24, all *P* values <.03). Similarly, disorganized behavior was modestly correlated with less awareness of mental disorder, the social consequences of mental disorder, the efficacy of medication, hallucinations, delusions, and anhedonia (*r* ranged from .15 to .30, all *P* values <.04).

Generally, negative symptoms from the Scale to Assess Negative Symptoms were not significantly correlated with any SUMD score, with the exception of social isolation. Increased social isolation was modestly correlated with less awareness of mental disorder, the social consequences of mental disorder, the efficacy of medication, delusions, and anhedonia (*r* ranged from .16 to .20, all *P* values <.03).

To examine the relations between mood symptoms and insight, we divided the SZ group into patients who did and did not meet the *DSM-III-R* criteria for hypomania, mania, and major depressive syndrome. No significant differences were found between hypomanic and nonhypomanic patients or between manic and nonmanic patients on any of the SUMD items. On the other hand, patients with SZ who also met the criteria for a major depressive syndrome were significantly more aware of current thought disorder (*t*=2.1, *df*=124, *P*=.03), blunt affect (*t*=2.8, *df*=126, *P*<.006), and anhedonia (*t*=3.2, *df*=125, *P*=.002) and tended to be more aware of asociality (*t*=1.8, *df*=161, *P*=.08).

Average SUMD sores did not differ between schizophrenics with a chronic course and those with a subchronic course as categorized by *DSM-III-R* criteria. In

Table 4. Proportion of Patients in Each Diagnostic Group With Severe Unawareness Scores on the SUMD*

	Mental Disorder	Social Consequences	Medication Efficacy	Hallucination	Delusion	Thought Disorder	Flat or Blunt Affect	Anhedonia	Asociality
SZ, % (No.)	32.7 (71/217)	31.5 (67/213)	21.7 (43/198)	39.5 (62/157)	57.6 (110/191)	53.1 (69/130)	46.6 (62/133)	28.7 (37/129)	27.8 (47/169)
SA disorder, % (No.)	18.4 (9/49)	25 (12/48)	16.7 (8/48)	22.6 (7/31)	33.3 (13/39)	54.5 (12/22)	36.0 (9/25)	10.3 (3/29)	11.5 (3/26)
BP disorder, % (No.)	22.5 (9/40)	22.5 (9/40)	12.8 (5/39)	46.7 (7/15)	34.3 (12/35)	44.4 (12/27)	55.6 (5/9)	33.3 (2/6)	25.0 (2/8)
PMDD, % (No.)	16.7 (4/24)	13.6 (3/22)	13.6 (3/22)	35.3 (6/17)	30.4 (7/23)	25.0 (2/8)	36.4 (4/11)	6.3 (1/16)	11.8 (2/17)
Nonpsychotic MDD, % (No.)	7.1 (1/14)	7.1 (1/14)	14.3 (2/14)	0 (0/2)	42.9 (3/7)	0 (0/3)	10 (1/10)	0 (0/12)	0 (0/9)
χ^2†	9.8	7.3	2.7	4.9	15.7	6.0	6.4	11.6	7.8
P	.04	.11	.60	.28	.003	.19	.16	.02	.09

*SUMD indicates Scale to Assess Unawareness of Mental Disorder; SZ, schizophrenia; SA, schizoaffective; BP, bipolar; MDD, major depressive disorder; and PMDD, psychotic MDD.
†All df=4.

addition, the number and duration of hospitalizations were not significantly correlated with any SUMD score.

On the other hand, as can be seen in **Table 5**, the level of functioning at the time of the interview, as measured by the GAS, was negatively correlated with all but one of the SUMD items in the direction of less awareness being modestly associated with poorer functioning. Functioning during the previous year was also assessed. The GAS scores for the previous year were negatively correlated with all nine of the SUMD scores in the direction of poorer functioning being associated with less awareness. The GAS ratings for the previous 5 years were generally not significantly correlated with any current awareness score. The exceptions to this pattern were the awareness of blunt affect and social isolation scores. Gender, age, and level of education were not significantly correlated with any SUMD score.

COMMENT

The results indicate that poor insight is a prevalent feature of SZ and that severe unawareness is more common in patients with SZ than in those with SA disorder or MDD with or without psychosis. The other diagnostic groups studied, most notably the BP sample, also exhibited a relatively high incidence of unawareness. However, very small sample sizes on several of the SUMD items where high percentages of unawareness were found in the BP group limit the interpretation of these data. Regardless, the SZ group generally had poorer average awareness scores and a higher incidence of severe unawareness than did the other groups. In patients with SZ, less awareness of various aspects of mental disorder was associated with poorer psychosocial functioning.

PREVALENCE OF POOR AWARENESS IN SCHIZOPHRENIA

Over half of the patients with SZ (57%) had moderate to severe unawareness of having a mental disorder. This finding is in agreement with the results from the International Pilot Study of Schizophrenia report and the Classification of Chronic Hospitalized Schizophrenics study, which both indicate that a majority of patients with SZ appear to be unaware of having a mental disorder.[4,8] Both of these investigations studied very large samples coming from multiple settings around the world. However, a major limitation of these studies was their reliance on a measure of insight that was dichotomous and conceptually narrow. Patients were judged as having poor insight if they "denied being ill" and as having good insight if they did not. In the present study, we used a measure of insight that was more complex, allowing the assessment of multiple aspects of insight. Between 27% and 57% of the patients with SZ were severely unaware of specific signs and symptoms, ie, hallucinations, delusions, thought disorder, blunt affect, anhedonia, and asociality. These results suggest that patients with SZ have multiple deficits in self-awareness and that this unawareness can be modality specific, ie, one can have poor awareness of thought disorder but recognize that he or she suffers from false perceptions.

The finding that patients with SZ had pervasive deficits in awareness of signs and symptoms has important implications for psychoeducation interventions. One goal of most psychoeducation programs is to educate patients about the warning signs of acute exacerbations of illness. Early symptom detection relies not only on knowledge about symptoms but also on self-awareness or recognition that the symptom is occurring. To our knowl-

edge, the prevalence of unawareness of signs and symptoms has not been reported previously in the literature. In the sample with SZ studied here, a large proportion of patients appeared completely unaware of various signs and symptoms. These results suggest that psychoeducation programs should also address the remediation of self-awareness deficits in addition to educating patients about the nature of symptoms more generally.

DIAGNOSTIC GROUP DIFFERENCES IN UNAWARENESS

Although the data presented herein do not demonstrate that self-awareness deficits are specific to SZ, they nonetheless indicate that severe deficits in awareness of illness are more common in this disorder. To our knowledge, the finding that self-awareness deficits were more severe in patients in whom SZ was diagnosed than in those in whom SA disorder or mood disorder was diagnosed has not been reported previously in the literature.[11] However, Carpenter et al[21(p1275)] did report that "poor insight" was one of 12 signs and symptoms that were "especially discriminating between SZ and other psychiatric disorders." A relevant difference between this earlier study and the one reported herein is that Carpenter and his colleagues used a single dichotomous item to measure insight so that the degree and type of unawareness were not assessed. The strengths and limitations of this approach vs the SUMD method are discussed elsewhere.[11,12] In the present study, patients with SZ had significantly poorer awareness of having a mental disorder, hallucinations, delusions, anhedonia, and social isolation than did the patients with SA disorder. Furthermore, patients with MDD with or without psychosis were also more aware of many aspects of illness than were the patients with SZ. The only exceptions to this pattern were on those items with small sample sizes. In the context of inadequate statistical power, negative results from the comparisons of patients with MDD with schizophrenics are inconclusive. In short, these results suggest that some aspects of disordered self-awareness may be characteristic of SZ rather than of psychosis more generally.

The finding that psychosocial functioning was correlated with degree of insight in the SZ group raises the question of whether group differences on awareness were due to differences in the overall severity of illness. However, except for the patients with PMDD, the diagnostic groups had similarly poor psychosocial functioning as reflected in their GAS scores. More importantly, when GAS scores were used as a covariate, the patients with SZ still had significantly worse insight than all groups except the patients with BP disorder.

The BP group had significantly better awareness of delusions than did the SZ group. In all other respects, however, these two groups did not appear to differ. It would be premature, however, to conclude that the BP sample had equally poor insight as that of the SZ group because awareness of only three positive symptoms was evaluated and the BP sample sizes were very small for the three negative symptoms (for all samples, $n \leq 9$). Because patients with BP disorder were severely ill when interviewed, we do not have data on whether the observed unawareness persists during periods of remission. It may be that unawareness is state related in patients with BP disorder, whereas it is trait related in patients with SZ. In the present study, patients with SZ in remission did not differ from those in acute exacerbation on any insight item. Furthermore, longitudinal studies of insight in patients with SZ suggest that unawareness is stable in this group.[9] Future comparisons of patients with SZ and patients with BP disorder should longitudinally assess a broader range of awareness dimensions to more directly examine the trait vs state question and to better characterize the phenomenologic aspects of self-awareness in these groups.

It is noteworthy that the one SUMD item that most consistently distinguished the patients with SZ from the other psychotic patients regardless of the statistical analysis employed was the one that assessed awareness of delusion. This difference was not due to differences in the severity of delusion because the groups were equivalent in the severity of their delusions (see sample description in the "Patients and Methods" section). Rather, these results reflect group differences in awareness of delusion. Previously, the importance of evaluating multiple aspects of delusional beliefs (eg, awareness of illogicality, implausibility, or falseness of the belief) when assessing insight into delusion was emphasized.[12,15] One interpretation of the data reported herein is that patients with SZ are less aware of various violations of reality testing that are manifested in their thinking. In other words,

Table 5. Correlations Between Awareness and Global Assessment Scale (GAS) Scores in the Schizophrenia Sample

	Correlation		
Awareness of:	Current GAS	Past Year GAS	Past 5 Years' GAS
Mental disorder	−.26 (P<.0001)	−.16 (P=.01)	−.03
Consequences	−.28 (P<.0001)	−.17 (P=.01)	−.09
Medication efficacy	−.23 (P<.001)	−.18 (P=.01)	−.08
Hallucinations	−.13	−.16 (P=.05)	−.12
Delusions	−.29 (P<.0001)	−.15 (P=.04)	−.10
Thought disorder	−.32 (P<.0001)	−.25 (P=.004)	−.16
Flat affect	−.25 (P=.004)	−.22 (P=.01)	−.17 (P=.04)
Anhedonia	−.28 (P=.001)	−.26 (P=.003)	−.15
Asociality	−.26 (P=.001)	−.25 (P=.001)	−.15 (P=.05)

although they were equivalent to the other psychotic patients in the severity of their delusions (ie, effect on behavior and preoccupation), patients with SZ were less aware of the faultiness of their logic and the implausibility of their beliefs.

NOT SURPRISINGLY, the rate of bizarre delusions was significantly higher in the patients with SZ than in the other psychotic patients studied. One could argue that the group differences in awareness found could be explained in part on the basis of bizarre delusions. However, the presence of bizarre delusions was not generally associated with poorer awareness on eight of the nine SUMD items. Nonetheless, the patients with SZ and bizarre delusions were significantly less aware of having hallucinations than were patients with SZ without bizarre delusions. Extreme illogicality and implausibility are defining features of bizarre delusional beliefs. It may be the case that bizarre delusions and particular deficits in self-awareness (ie, awareness of false perceptions) are caused in part by similar breakdowns in reality testing. We have considered two deficits. First, unawareness of illness and bizarre delusions may result from a deficit in the capacity to recognize the extent to which one's experience of one's self and circumstances differs from the views communicated by others. Alternatively, in patients who can recognize the illogicality of a belief or perception (ie, a bizarre delusion or perception that someone is speaking to them despite the fact that they are alone), the psychological mechanism implicated involves an increased tolerance for illogicality in one's thinking. An individual with either psychological deficit could be expected to be little influenced by the views held by family, friends, and mental health professionals when describing a bizarre delusion and when explaining why they do not think the voices they hear are false perceptions.

The results of this study are consistent with our contention that many self-awareness deficits in SZ are manifestations of the neuropsychological deficits associated with the disorder.[11] Unlike the other diagnostic groups studied, patients with SZ evidenced pervasive unawareness across all of the insight dimensions assessed. Previously, it was suggested that frontal lobe dysfunction may be implicated in the self-awareness deficits observed in patients with SZ.[11] We have preliminary data that support this view, and one independent investigation[6] has also found significant correlations between SUMD scores and performance on neuropsychological tests that are sensitive to frontal lobe dysfunction. Specifically, Young and colleagues[6] administered the SUMD, the Wisconsin Card Sorting Test (WCST), a test of verbal fluency, and Trails A and B to a sample of 31 patients with chronic SZ diagnosed according to *DSM-III-R* criteria. The percentage of perseverative responses on the WCST were found to significantly correlate with the SUMD total awareness of symptoms score (r=.49, P<.01) and the total attributions for symptoms score (r=.42, P<.05). Similar correlations were found between the number of categories completed on the WCST and the SUMD total awareness of symptoms score (r=.59, P<.001) and the total attributions for symptoms score (r=.50, P<.01).

Young and colleagues[6] also dichotoimized the sample with respect to "high" vs "low" awareness and performed a discriminant function analysis to determine which variables most significantly differentiated the high vs low awareness groups. The variables examined were inpatient vs outpatient status, IQ, number of WCST categories completed, percentage of perseverative responses, and average symptom severity (using a seven-point Likert scale developed by Young et al[6]). A linear combination of perseverative responses on the WCST and average symptom severity correctly categorized 83.9% of the patients in the high and low awareness groups. The other variables made no statistically significant contribution to the discrimination.

Another research group found that unlike poor-insight SZ patients with normal frontal functioning, poor-insight SZ patients with neuropsychological dysfunction of the frontal lobes did not show improvement in insight following psychosocial treatment.[22] It is noteworthy that two of the studies mentioned did not find significant correlations between the level of awareness and measures of overall cognitive functioning (ie, full scale, verbal, or performance IQ), and the study by Young et al[6] did not find that IQ contributed significantly to the discrimination of patients with high vs low awareness. These data suggest that generalized cognitive impairment did not account for the degree of unawareness observed. The hypothesis that neuropsychological dysfunction of the frontal lobes underlies self-awareness deficits in SZ was not tested in the present study. However, the fact that the patients with SZ studied herein had significantly poorer awareness than did patients with SA disorder or psychotic depressive disorder is consistent with our suggestion that severe self-awareness deficits may be a unique feature of SZ rather than of psychosis and that they stem from the neuropsychological dysfunction that is commonly associated with the disorder.

CLINICAL CORRELATES OF UNAWARENESS IN SCHIZOPHRENIA

In general, the level of awareness was unrelated to symptom severity. Noteworthy exceptions to this pattern include the finding that an increase in the severity

of delusions, thought disorder, and disorganized behavior were modestly correlated with less awareness of mental disorder, of the social consequences of mental disorder, and of several positive symptoms. Negative symptoms were not significantly correlated with any SUMD score, with the exception of social isolation. Because the social isolation rating used in this analysis did not distinguish between primary and secondary negative symptoms, it is possible that a proportion of the variance on this item can be accounted for by positive symptoms. The associations between symptoms and insight were small; consequently, it would be premature to suggest that patients with SZ and an increase in delusions, thought disorder, social isolation, and disorganized behavior are more likely to have poor insight. Nonetheless, these data suggest such a relationship, and replications should be attempted. Another possibility is that rater bias may have accounted for these correlations. In other words, the interviewers may have been predisposed to view poor insight and increased positive symptoms as covarying with one another. Longitudinal studies that assess insight and symptoms during acute exacerbations and during remission would provide more direct information about the relationship between these two psychopathological dimensions.

Recently, two of us (X.F.A. and S.A.Y.) completed a follow-up evaluation of patients with SZ at the Maryland Psychiatric Research Center, Baltimore, Md, in collaboration with William T. Carpenter, Jr, MD, and Brian Kirkpatrick, MD, MSPH. These patients previously had been characterized with respect to the deficit syndrome. Current deficit syndrome status was assessed, and awareness of illness was evaluated with the SUMD. Patients with SZ and the deficit syndrome had significantly poorer SUMD scores than did nondeficit schizophrenics (X.F.A., S.A.Y., W. T. Carpenter, Jr, MD, and B. Kirkpatrick, MD, MSPH, unpublished data, 1994). The associations found between unawareness and primary negative symptoms were much stronger than the associations between positive and negative symptoms and unawareness that are reported herein. These data suggest that poor awareness may be associated with primary negative symptoms in SZ. If subsequent studies confirm these results, it could be argued that particular aspects of unawareness (eg, emotional indifference or anosodiaphoria) reflect in part a decrement in the ability to experience emotion.

With regard to insight and mood, at least in patients with SZ, the results do not support Van Putten et al's[13] contention that manic mood states and grandiosity are inversely related to insight. We found no significant differences between hypomanic and nonhypomanic patients with SZ or between manic and nonmanic patients with SZ on any insight item. Interestingly, however, patients with SZ who met the criteria for a major depressive syndrome were significantly more aware of current thought disorder and anhedonia and tended to be more aware of asociality. The relationship between awareness of anhedonia and increased depression may be somewhat tautological. Regardless, these data can be interpreted as suggesting that patients who are aware of significant thought disorder and social isolation may also be more likely to be depressed.

In the study reported herein, schizophrenic patients with poorer insight were more likely to have poorer psychosocial functioning during the present episode and the previous year. This finding is consistent with previous reports.[7,23-25] Whether schizophrenic patients with poor awareness function less well because of a neuropsychological deficit, decreased cooperation with regard to treatment, or other factors was not evaluated in the present study. Future work in this area could address this question by evaluating the relations between insight, treatment adherence, neuropsychological deficit, and psychosocial functioning. Nonetheless, the data reported herein suggest that there is both descriptive and prognostic value in characterizing awareness of illness in SZ. These data also suggest that the relationship between psychosocial functioning and awareness of illness should be studied in other disorders in addition to SZ.

Accepted for publication July 5, 1994.

Supported in part by grants from the National Alliance for Research in Schizophrenia and Affective Disorders, Chicago, Ill, and the Scottish Rite Schizophrenia Research Program, Lexington, Mass; and grants TO1 MH19627 and MH47200, a National Institute of Mental Health Faculty Scholar Award, and Mental Health Clinical Research Center Grant MH43271 from the National Institutes of Mental Health, Bethesda, Md.

Patients at the New York site also were recruited from the St Lukes/Roosevelt Hospital Center and the Washington Heights Community Service at the New York State Psychiatric Institute, New York, NY.

We wish to thank Ewald Horwath, MD; Chrysoula Kasapis, MA; and David Klahr, MD, for assisting in patient recruitment; Jean Endicott, PhD; Richard S. E. Keefe, PhD; and William T. Carpenter, Jr, MD, for commenting on earlier drafts of this article; Gary Tyrrell, MA, for data management of the entire field trial; Stephan Arndt, PhD, for statistical consultation; the DSM-IV *Work Group on Schizophrenia; and the* DSM-IV *Field Trial Site Coordinators (H. Stefan Bracha, MD; William Edell, PhD; Jeffrey Lieberman, MD; Ananda Pandurangi, MD; Delbert Robinson, MD;*

Patrick McGorry, MBBS; Alfonso Ontiveros, MD, MSc; and Mauricio Tohen, MD.

Reprint requests to Department of Clinical Psychobiology, Unit 2, New York State Psychiatric Institute, 722 W 168th St, New York, NY 10032 (Dr Amador).

REFERENCES

1. Andreasen NC, Carpenter WT Jr. Diagnosis and classification of schizophrenia. *Schizophr Bull.* 1993;19:199-214.
2. Carpenter WT Jr, Kirkpatrick B. The heterogeneity of the long-term course of schizophrenia. *Schizophr Bull.* 1988;14:645-651.
3. Carpenter WT Jr, Heinrichs DW, Wagman AMI. Deficit and nondeficit forms of schizophrenia: the concept. *Am J Psychiatry.* 1988;145:578-583.
4. World Health Organization. *Report of the International Pilot Study of Schizophrenia.* Geneva, Switzerland: World Health Organization Press; 1973.
5. Carpenter WT Jr, Bartko JJ, Carpenter CL, and Strauss JS. Another view of schizophrenia subtypes. *Arch Gen Psychiatry.* 1976;33:508-516.
6. Young DA, Davila R, Scher H. Unawareness of illness and neuropsychological performance in chronic schizophrenia. *Schizophr Res.* 1993;10:117-124.
7. McGlashan TH, Carpenter WT Jr. Does attitude toward psychosis relate to outcome? *Am J Psychiatry.* 1981;138:797-801.
8. Wilson WH, Ban TA, Guy W. Flexible system criteria in chronic schizophrenia. *Compr Psychiatry.* 1986;27:259-265.
9. McEvoy JP, Freter S, Everett G, Geller JL, Appelbaum P, Apperson LJ, Roth L. Insight and the clinical outcome of schizophrenics. *J Nerv Ment Dis.* 1989; 177:48-51.
10. McEvoy JP, Apperson LJ, Appelbaum PS, Ortlip P, Brecosky J, Hammill K. Insight in schizophrenia: its relationship to acute psychopathology. *J Nerv Ment Dis.* 1989;177:43-47.
11. Amador XF, Strauss DH, Yale SA, Gorman JM. Awareness of illness in schizophrenia. *Schizophr Bull.* 1991;17:113-132.
12. Amador XF, Strauss DH, Yale S, Gorman JM, Endicott J. The assessment of insight in psychosis. *Am J Psychiatry.* 1993;150:873-879.
13. Van Putten T, Crumpton E, Yale C. Drug refusal in schizophrenia and the wish to be crazy. *Arch Gen Psychiatry.* 1976;33:1443-1446.
14. David AS. On insight and psychosis: discussion paper. *J R Soc Med.* 1990; 83:325-329.
15. Amador XF, Strauss DH. Poor insight in schizophrenia. *Psychiatr Q.* 1993;64: 305-318.
16. American Psychiatric Association. *Diagnostic and Statistical Manual of Mental Disorders, Revised Third Edition.* Washington, DC: American Psychiatric Association; 1987.
17. Flaum M, Amador XF, Bracha HS, Edell W, Gorman J, Kendler K, Lieberman J, McGlashan T, McGorry P, Ontiveros A, Pandurangi A, Robinson D, Tohen M. *DSM-IV* Field Trial for Schizophrenia and Related Psychotic Disorders. *Am J Psychiatry.* In press.
18. Andreasen NC, Flaum M, Arndt S. The Comprehensive Assessment of Symptoms and History (CASH): an instrument for assessing diagnosis and psychopathology. *Arch Gen Psychiatry.* 1992;49:615-623.
19. Endicott J, Spitzer RL, Fleiss JL, Cohen J. The Global Assessment Scale: a procedure for measuring overall severity of Psychiatric disturbance. *Arch Gen Psychiatry.* 1976;33:766-771.
20. Fleiss JL. *The Design and Analysis of Clinical Experiments.* New York, NY: John Wiley & Sons; 1986.
21. Carpenter WT Jr, Strauss JS, Bartko JJ. Flexible system for the diagnosis of schizophrenia: report from the WHO international pilot study of schizophrenia. *Science.* 1973;182:1275-1277.
22. Lysaker P, Bell M. Impaired insight in schizophrenia: advances from psychosocial treatment research. In: Amador XF, David A, eds. *Insight and Psychosis.* Oxford, England: Oxford University Press. In press.
23. Lin IF, Spiga R, Fortsch W. Insight and adherence to medication in chronic schizophrenics. *J Clin Psychiatry.* 1979;40:430-432.
24. Bartko G, Herczog I, Zador G. Clinical symptomatology and drug compliance in schizophrenic patients. *Acta Psychiatr Scand.* 1988;77:74-76.
25. Heinrichs DW, Cohen BP, Carpenter WT Jr. Early insight and the management of schizophrenic decompensation. *J Nerv Ment Dis.* 1985;173:133-138.

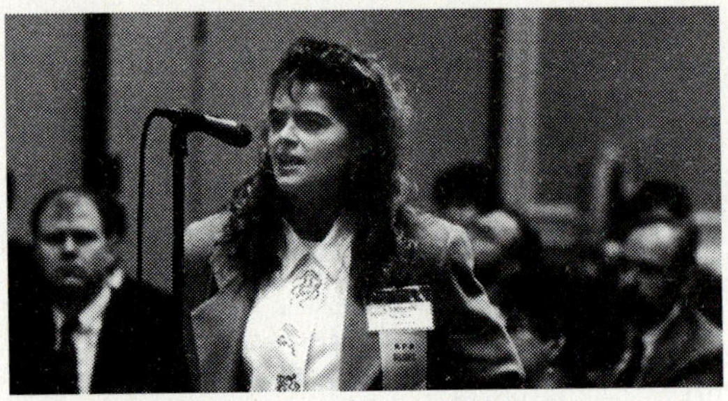

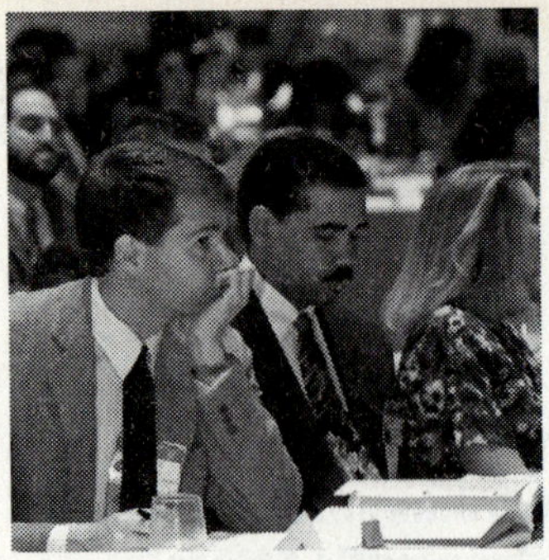

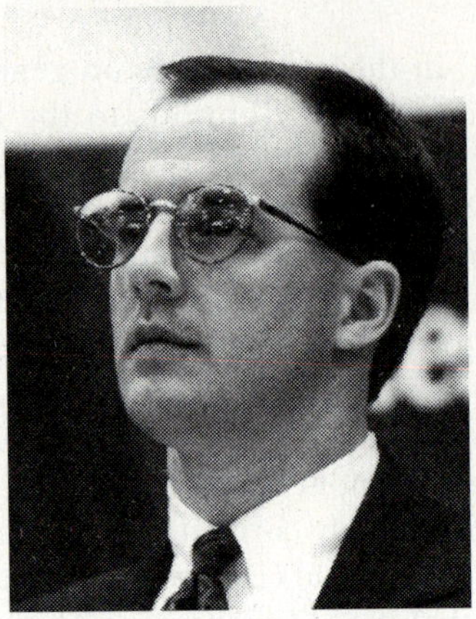

Genetic and Environmental Influences of Twins in Posttraumatic Stress

True et al,[1] in their twin study on genetic and environmental contributions to the liability for posttraumatic stress symptoms in Vietnam veterans, use a bivariate model to postulate significant genetic influences on symptom liability and state that there is no evidence that shared environment contributes to the development of posttraumatic stress symptoms.

This model is erroneous, however, since it is based on the assumption that noncombat environmental influences are not more highly correlated in monozygotic (MZ) twins than in dizygotic (DZ) twins. The authors' own data indicate that the MZ twins have a higher concordance for combat exposure than do DZ twins (0.34 vs 0.17). To assume that their environments previous to this are somehow no more concordant seems obviously false.

In addition, the fact that MZ twins are so much more alike in appearance, tend to play together, and have other childhood similarities, seems to guarantee that their environments will be more concordant. Studies of concordance rates for schizophrenia demonstrate the importance of this similarity of environment. Dizygotic twins, no more genetically alike than nontwin siblings, have higher concordance rates for schizophrenia than do siblings.[2,3] Similarly, same-sex DZ twins have higher concordance rates for schizophrenia than do different-sex DZ twins.[2,4,5] Considering these data, it seems justified to make the assumption that environmental influences are no more concordant for MZ twins than for DZ twins. It is, therefore, unjustified to conclude, as the authors do, that environmental factors do not contribute to susceptibility for posttraumatic stress disorder symptoms.

Unfortunately, our psychiatric literature is replete with such reductionist assumptions that obscure the importance of gene-environment interactions. Such reductionism limits our ability to understand our patients and limits our treatment options.

Scott Lurie, MD
Pleas Geyer, MD
Carolinas Medical Center
501 Billingsley Rd
Charlotte, NC 28211

1. True WR, Rice J, Eisen SA, Heath AC, Goldeberg J, Lyons MJ, Nowac J. A twin study of genetic and environmental contributions to liability for posttraumatic stress symptoms. *Arch Gen Psychiatry.* 1993;50:257-264.
2. Slater E. *Psychotic and Neurotic Illnesses in Twins.* London, England: Her Majesty's Stationery Office; 1953. Special Report Series 278.
3. Fischer M. Genetic and environmental factors in schizophrenia: a study of schizophrenic twins and their families. *Acta Psychiatr Scand.* 1973;238(suppl):9-142.
4. Rosanoff AJ, Handy LM, Plesset IR, Brush S. The etiology of so-called schizophrenic psychoses with special reference to their occurrence in twins. *Am J Psychiatry.* 1934;91:247-286.
5. Kallmann FJ. The genetic theory of schizophrenia: an analysis of 691 schizophrenic twin index families. *Am J Psychiatry.* 1946;103:309-322.

In reply

Lurie and Geyer question our finding that shared environment did not contribute to susceptibility to posttraumatic stress disorder symptoms in our study of 2224 MZ and 1818 DZ male veteran twins.[1] They base their argument on the validity of the equal environments assumption of twin studies, which is that MZ and DZ twins do not differ in exposure to etiologically relevant environmental influences.

Although, as stated in the article, we did not have data in our study to test directly this assumption, the issue has received considerable critical attention in the twin literature, most recently in Kendler's[2] comprehensive review of the role of twin studies of psychiatric illness and in a review of genetic approaches to personality by Eaves et al.[3] The issue is that if the phenotypic similarity of MZ twins is actually attributed to shared environments that are more uniform, then genetic contributions will be overestimated. Evidence has been presented that MZ twins may be more often treated alike,[4] but the argument turns on whether these similarities actually affect mature phenotypes, such as posttraumatic stress symptoms.

This point has been vigorously addressed in the literature.[2] Kendler reviews approaches that have been used for assessing the equal environments assumption to determine if observed childhood similarities of MZ environment produce increased similarities in later measured phenotypes. Most pertinent to the phenotype considered here is evidence that MZ twins who experienced more similar environments "imposed" on them by parents and "elicited" by their own behavior was unrelated to later behavioral similarity in neuroticism, anxiety, and depression.[5] Similarly, although MZ twins may have been dressed alike or shared the same room, there is little evidence that such similarities influence a wide range of twin phenotypic correlations, including pertinent psychiatric disorders and a number of other common behavior manifestations.[2] If there

is little evidence that these shared environments affect common phenotypes, we believe that it is unlikely that there would be mechanisms whereby they would affect such a severe disorder as posttraumatic stress disorder.

Further, the concordance data for combat exposure (0.34 for MZ twins and 0.17 for DZ twins) are not pertinent to the equal environments assumption because we specifically chose the analysis strategy of the bivariate model to address the issue of environmental and genetic contributions to both exposure to and sequelae of combat. A genetic analysis of these data on combat exposure has been conducted.[6]

Finally, Lurie and Geyer cite older data on genetics of schizophrenia to assert the importance of environmental influences. This literature has been considerably amplified in recent years with research designs using identical twins reared apart and adoption studies that directly addressed questions of environmental and genetic contributions to schizophrenia. These studies have been reviewed[7,8] *and do not support the assertion that twin correlations in schizophrenia are caused by shared environmental influences.*

William R. True, PhD, MPH
St Louis University School of Public Health
St Louis, MO 63108
John Rice, PhD
Andrew C. Heath, DPhil
Washington School of Medicine
St Louis, Mo

1. True WR, Rice J, Eisen SA, Heath AC, Goldberg J, Lyons MJ, Nowak J. A twin study of genetic and environmental contributions to liability for posttraumatic stress symptoms. *Arch Gen Psychiatry.* 1993;50:257-264.
2. Kendler KS. Twin studies of psychiatric illness. *Arch Gen Psychiatry.* 1993; 50:905-915.
3. Eaves LJ, Eysenck HJ, Martin NG. *Genes, Culture and Personality: An Empirical Approach.* London, England: Academic Press Ltd; 1989.
4. Loehlin JC, Nichols RC. *Heredity, Environment and Personality: A Study of 850 Sets of Twins.* Austin: University of Texas Press; 1976.
5. Morris-Yates A, Andrews G, Howie P, Henderson S. Twins: a test of the equal environments assumption. *Acta Psychiatr Scand.* 1990;81:322-326.
6. Lyons MJ, Goldberg J, Eisen SA, True W, Meyer J, Tsuang MT, Henderson W. Do genes influence exposure to trauma? a twin study of combat. *Am J Med Genet (Neuropsychiatr Genet).* 1993;48:22-27.
7. Gottesman II, Shields J. *Schizophrenia: The Epigenetic Puzzle.* Cambridge, England: Cambridge University Press; 1982.
8. Kendler KS. Overview: a current perspective on twin studies of schizophrenia. *Am J Psychiatry.* 1983;140:1413-1425.

Theme Issues on Cancer and Health Promotion and Disease Prevention

The *Journal of the American Medical Association* is planning to publish a theme issue on cancer in February 1995 and another theme issue on health promotion and disease prevention in April 1995. The *Archives of General Psychiatry* will also consider papers on these topics for its concurrent issues.

The purpose of these theme issues is to expose *JAMA*'s and the *ARCHIVES*' broad readerships to the latest high-quality research and critical thinking in these areas.

Original research contributions, special communications, and review articles dealing with any aspect of the above issues will be considered. All submissions will be subject to *JAMA*'s or the *ARCHIVES*' rigorous review process.

Professional Opportunities

Archives of General Psychiatry is an exceptional journal that provides physicians with the latest medical and technological information in the psychiatric field. It is an excellent source for recruiting, reaching over 30,220 psychiatrists each month.

All advertising orders must be submitted in writing by mail or fax. Although the American Medical Association believes the classified advertisements in these pages to be from reputable sources, the Association does not assume liability concerning them. Acceptance of advertising is restricted to physician recruitment opportunities, practices for sale, medical office space for sale or rent, and medical equipment for sale.

You can mail your ad materials to *Archives of General Psychiatry* Classifieds, 515 N State St, Chicago, IL 60610 or fax to 312-464-5909.

Confidential box numbers are available to advertisers for an additional $20.00 per issue. All confidential box replies must be in writing and must cite the box number in the ad, example: Box XXXX, c/o *Archives of General Psychiatry,* 515 N State St, Chicago, IL 60610.

All cancellations/changes must be received at least 25 days prior to the issue date by phone, mail, or fax to the *Archives of General Psychiatry* Classified office.

For information on rates, deadlines, and policies for *Archives of General Psychiatry* Classifieds, contact your classified service representative at 800-AMA-2260 or 312-464-2475/2490/2491/4485.

Psychiatry

CORRECTIONAL/ACADEMIC PSYCHIATRIST, CHICAGO, ILlinois: The Isaac Ray Center and Cermak Health Services, both nationally recognized forensic mental health teams, seek full-time, flexible-schedule BC/BE psychiatrist to provide clinical, clinical supervision, and academic services in the psychiatric facilities of the Cook County Jail. Be an integral part of a unique new partnership of academics and public policy. You will be an employee of the Isaac Ray Center with a faculty position at Rush Medical College. Salary $100K+ with generous benefit package. Participate in training of residents, fellows, and psychology graduate students in an active, innovative training setting. The positions do not involve or require specialized forensic evaluations for court/testimony. Openings are available after 9/1/94. Eligibility for Illinois medical license required. Send CV with inquiry to Mark R. McClung, MD; Vice President, Educational Services; Isaac Ray Center; 1725 West Harrison Street; Suite 110; Chicago, IL 60612.

Nationwide
PSYCHIATRY
&
NEUROLOGY
Positions
We know how busy you are.
Let us do the mundane busy work.
1 (800) 428-4406
Physician Search Associates

STAFF PSYCHIATRIST FOR NEVADA COUNTY MENTAL Health, a comprehensive mental health program. Board-certified, public service–oriented psychiatrist who believes in the importance of community mental health services and enjoys working as part of a multidisciplinary treatment team. Beautiful, mountainous, rural area, one hour from Lake Tahoe and Sacramento. Contract position; county provides malpractice insurance. Contact Diane Chenoweth, Mental Health Director, 916-265-1437, or fax 916-265-7065, or write 10433 Willow Valley Road, Nevada City, CA 95959, and indicate preference—inpatient, outpatient, or both.

UNIVERSITY OF WISCONSIN–MADISON: THE DEPARTMENT of Psychiatry is seeking a Psychiatrist (MD) for an academically oriented, tenure-track position. Responsibilities include: development and supervision of a newly-created, integrated psychiatric/medical clinic devoted to training psychiatric and medical residents to work together in providing coordinated care for the broad range of psychiatric problems occurring in primary care settings; providing outpatient psychiatric care in VA and UW settings; training medical students & psychiatric residents in clinical and didactic settings; developing own area of research or collaborating with other ongoing research projects in psychiatry & medicine. Send CV and cover letter to Dr Dean Krahn, D6/248-2475, Dept of Psychiatry, University of WI Medical School, 600 Highland Ave, Madison, WI 53792. The University of WI is an Equal Opportunity/Affirmative Action Employer.

Fellowships

Postdoctoral Fellowships in Drug Abuse Treatment Research

The NIH/National Institute on Drug Abuse, and the DHHS/PHS/FDA/Center for Drug Evaluation and Research are sponsoring three-year postdoctoral fellowships. This program will train physicians for careers in drug abuse treatment research, and the design, conduct, and interpretation of clinical trials to develop new medications for treatment of drug abuse. The fellowship includes clinical, research management, and drug regulatory training.

Fellowships begin in July. Physicians must be United States citizens, or plan citizenship within one year, and be board eligible upon entering the program. Stipends begin at around $40,000 per year.

Application deadline is January 15, 1995. **For further information, contact Fellowships Coordinator, Mail Code HFD-6, Parklawn 9B-04, 5600 Fishers Lane, Rockville, MD 20857.**

Locum Tenens Wanted

HKA LOCUM TENENS is looking for quality general psychiatry physicians to do Locum Tenens. We have opportunities coast-to-coast. We furnish Occurrence Malpractice Insurance (no tail necessary). Please call **HKA LOCUM TENENS at (800)226-6347, Extension AM7.1.**

Chiefs/Department Heads/Directors

CHIEF, PSYCHIATRY SERVICE VACANCY. A SENIOR, ACAdemically-oriented, board-certified psychiatrist is sought for the position of Chief, Psychiatry Service, VA Medical Center, Long Beach, CA. The Medical Center is a tertiary care medical center and is an integral part of the College of Medicine, University of California at Irvine. Candidates should have a strong background in clinical psychiatry, a significant record of research accomplishments, and possess demonstrated teaching and management skills. The successful candidate will qualify for academic appointment at the associate or full professor level. US citizenship is required. The Department of Veterans Affairs is an Equal Opportunity Employer. A letter of application along with a CV should be sent to Evelyne Mindes, MD (11A), Long Beach VA Medical Center, 5901 E 7th St, Long Beach, CA 90822.

CHAIR OF PSYCHIATRY, CERMAK MENTAL HEALTH SERvices, Cook County Jail, Chicago, and Vice President for Correctional Services, Isaac Ray Center, Inc: The Isaac Ray Center, the nation's largest private, not-for-profit forensic mental health services corporation, was recently awarded a three-year $4.1 million contract by the Cook County Board of Commissioners to provide psychiatric and psychological leadership and services for Cook County Jail, which has one of the largest correctional mental health programs in the country. Applications for the Chair of Psychiatry are being sought from board-certified psychiatrists with strong clinical, administrative, and academic qualifications to lead this pioneering effort in restructuring of Cook County's "Cermak Mental Health Services" into a premier service system combining the resources of both the public and private sectors. Included in the restructured program will be training experiences for senior psychiatric residents and postdoctoral forensic fellows from several universities in the Chicago area. The successful applicant will also be a Vice President of the Isaac Ray Center and a member of its management committee. The applicant must be eligible for a senior academic appointment in the Department of Psychiatry at Rush Medical College. Salary is negotiable based on qualifications, experience, and seniority. An Illinois medical license is required. Applicant must be available to begin on or before January 1, 1995. Isaac Ray Center is an EO/AA employer. Please address a letter of inquiry with a current CV to James L. Cavanaugh, Jr, MD, Professor of Psychiatry, Rush Medical College, and Chairman of the Board, Isaac Ray Center, 1725 West Harrison Street, #110, Chicago, IL 60612. Fax 312 829-1476.

UNIVERSITY OF WISCONSIN–MADISON: THE DEPARTMENT of Psychiatry is seeking a board-certified/eligible Child and Adolescent Psychiatrist to fill the position of the Director of the Pediatric Consultation-Liaison Service. This is a full-time faculty position, and applicants should possess excellent clinical, teaching, and administrative skills. It is envisioned that patient care and teaching will occur in both inpatient and outpatient settings. Opportunities for research exist and such scholarly activities are strongly encouraged. Faculty rank and salary are dependent upon experience and qualifications. Send CV and cover letter to Dr William Swift, Director, Division of Child and Adolescent Psychiatry, Dept of Psychiatry, University of WI Medical School, 600 Highland Ave, Madison, WI 53792. The University of WI is an Equal Opportunity/Affirmative Action Employer.

Academic/Faculty

BUFFALO, NEW YORK: THE BUFFALO VA MEDICAL CENTER has two excellent opportunities for academically-oriented physicians. Current positions include Director, Division of Substance Abuse and Director, Division of Anxiety and Affective Disorders, both of which incorporate inpatient and ambulatory programs. Protected time for research is provided, as is access to both a PET Center and excellent laboratory facilities in a new research building. The VA Medical Center is affiliated with the Department of Psychiatry, SUNY at Buffalo which, under new leadership, is developing clinical research programs in schizophrenia, substance abuse, posttraumatic stress disorder, as well as other targeted areas of interest. Board eligibility or certification in psychiatry is required and academic appointment will be at the Assistant or Associate Professor level depending on experience. The Buffalo/Niagara Falls region is culturally and scenically rich, providing for an exceptionally high quality of life. Please send CV to Human Resources Management Office, VA Medical Center, 3495 Bailey Avenue, Buffalo, NY 14215. Equal Opportunity Employer. Applicants are subject to random drug testing.

For more **Professional Opportunities** please refer to the **Classified** sections in ***JAMA*** and ***AMNews***.

Diagnostic Interview for Genetic Studies

Rationale, Unique Features, and Training

John I. Nurnberger, Jr, MD, PhD; Mary C. Blehar, PhD; Charles A. Kaufmann, MD; Carolyn York-Cooler; Sylvia G. Simpson, MD; Jill Harkavy-Friedman, PhD; Joanne B. Severe, MS; Dolores Malaspina, MD; Theodore Reich, MD; and collaborators from the NIMH Genetics Initiative

This article reports on the development and reliability of the Diagnostic Interview for Genetic Studies (DIGS), a clinical interview especially constructed for the assessment of major mood and psychotic disorders and their spectrum conditions. The DIGS, which was developed and piloted as a collaborative effort of investigators from sites in the National Institute of Mental Health (NIMH) Genetics Initiative, has the following additional features: (1) polydiagnostic capacity; (2) a detailed assessment of the course of the illness, chronology of psychotic and mood syndromes, and comorbidity; (3) additional phenomenologic assessments of symptoms; and (4) algorithmic scoring capability. The DIGS is designed to be employed by interviewers who exercise significant clinical judgment and who summarize information in narrative form as well as in ratings. A two-phase test-retest (within-site, between-site) reliability study was carried out for *DSM-III-R* criteria–based major depression, bipolar disorder, schizophrenia, and schizoaffective disorder. Reliabilities using algorithms were excellent (0.73 to 0.95), except for schizoaffective disorder, for which disagreement on estimates of duration of mood syndromes relative to psychosis reduced reliability. A final best-estimate process using medical records and information from relatives as well as algorithmic diagnoses is expected to be more reliable in making these distinctions. The DIGS should be useful as part of archival data gathering for genetic studies of major affective disorders, schizophrenia, and related conditions.

(Arch Gen Psychiatry. 1994;51:849-859)

RATIONALE

Recent inconsistent and nonreplicated findings in psychiatric genetics may stem in part from differences in phenotypic assessment. The definition of spectrum disorders for major mood disorders and schizophrenia (SZ) is still problematic, especially as one moves toward the milder, less incapacitating variants. Substance use increases the uncertainty about diagnosis and complicates genetic studies. Quantitative rather than categorical phenotypes may be helpful in analysis if in fact multiple susceptibility traits rather than a disease gene predispose one to a major psychiatric disorder.

Based on such considerations, collaborators from the National Institute of Mental Health (NIMH) Genetics Initiative developed the Diagnostic Interview for Genetic Studies (DIGS). The DIGS is designed to be used in combination with the Family Instrument for Genetic Studies (to be described separately) and medical record information as part of a final best-estimate diagnostic procedure.[1-3]

From the Departments of Psychiatry at Indiana University Medical Center, Indianapolis (Dr Nurnberger and Ms York-Cooler), Columbia University, New York, NY (Drs Kaufmann, Harkavy-Friedman, and Malaspina), The Johns Hopkins University, Baltimore, Md (Dr Simpson), and Washington University, St Louis, Mo (Dr Reich); and the National Institute of Mental Health (NIMH) Division of Clinical and Treatment Research, Rockville, Md (Dr Blehar and Ms Severe). A list of the NIMH Genetics Initiative Collaborators appears at the end.

DIAGNOSTIC CAPACITY

Diagnosis in Multiple-Criterion Systems

The polydiagnostic approach involves recording clinical information accurately

Table 1. Diagnoses and Corresponding Criteria Systems Covered by the Diagnostic Interview for Genetic Studies*

Diagnosis	*DSM-III-R*	*DSM-III*	*DSM-IV* Compatible	Modified RDC	OPCRIT 3.0†	RDC	Feighner et al[17]	*ICD-10*
Major depressive disorder	X	X	X	X	X	X		
Mania	X	X	X	X	X	X		
Hypomania	X		X			X		
Dysthymia	X							
Hyperthymic personality				X				
Depressive personality				X				
Schizophrenia	X	X	X	X	X	X	X	X
Delusional disorder	X							
Schizoaffective disorder	X		X	X		X		
Psychotic disorder not otherwise specified	X							
Schizotypal personality disorder	X		X					
Schizoid personality disorder	X							
Paranoid personality disorder	X							
Schizophreniform disorder	X							
Brief reactive psychosis	X							
Obsessive-compulsive disorder	X			X		X		
Agoraphobia	X		X	X		X		
Social phobia	X		X	X		X		
Simple phobia	X		X	X		X		
Panic disorder	X		X	X		X		
Anorexia nervosa	X							
Bulimia nervosa	X							
Pathological gambling	X							
Antisocial personality disorder	X							
Somatization disorder	X		X					
Alcohol dependence	X							
Alcohol abuse	X							
Alcoholism (definite)							X	
Alcoholism (probable)							X	
Drug dependence	X							
Drug abuse	X							

**RDC indicates Research Diagnostic Criteria;* ICD-10, International Classification of Diseases, 10th Revision.
†*OPCRIT 3.0 indicates Operational Criteria Checklist, version 3.0 of McGuffin and Farmer.*[15]

and in sufficient detail to allow differing definitions of an illness to be applied.[4,5] **Table 1** lists the diagnoses and corresponding criterion systems covered by the DIGS. This feature was incorporated for several reasons. First, it creates the broadest possible dataset for investigators in psychiatric genetics. Because the etiologic and pathophysiologic characteristics of bipolar (BP) disorder and SZ are unknown, valid definitions for these diagnoses are ambiguous.

See also page 863

Second, it ensures maximum comparability with other data sets. The BP and SZ centers initially plan to categorize subjects using *DSM-III-R* criteria.[6] It is clearly advantageous, however, for our work to be compatible with *DSM-IV*,[7] and the working criteria for *DSM-IV* were consulted with this in mind. No significant changes in the DIGS will be required to make *DSM-IV* diagnoses of the disorders noted other than the addition of one or two questions. A new version of the DIGS will be issued soon after *DSM-IV* appears in its final form. In addition, we wish to be able to compare rates of illness found in relatives of probands in our research with rates reported in family studies that used different criterion systems, eg, the NIMH Collaborative Depression Study,[8] the family study data of Gershon et al,[3,9] the St Louis Family Study,[10] the Iowa-500 studies,[11] and the Epidemiologic Catchment Area Study.[12]

The European Science Foundation is currently sponsoring a multicenter genetic study of BP disorder and SZ. These investigators are using either the Schedule for Affective Disorders and Schizophrenia (SADS)[13] or the Present State Exam,[14] but all have agreed to use the Operational Criteria (OPCRIT) Checklist[15] (which draws from 11 operational definitions of the major psychoses)[6,16-20] as the final common pathway for diagnosis. To attain comparability between the NIMH and European Science Foundation efforts, we included additional items necessary to complete the OPCRIT checklist in the DIGS.

Diagnosis-Independent Ratings

The DIGS provides more details regarding the phenomenology of mood disorders and SZ than many other available instruments. To an extent, this is an inevitable consequence of its polydiagnostic aspect since each diagnostic system requires some items not found in other systems. In the DIGS, other items have been included expressly for gathering phenomenologic information not required by any other current diagnostic scheme. Among other uses, phenomenologic detail may permit the construction of quantitative phenotypes or recon-

figuration of information gathered into new biologically based categories. For example, questions regarding mixed states of mania and depression, rapid cycling, suicidality, and comorbidity are included, as well as a time line to help specify the course of illness (as in Roy-Byrne et al[21]). In the psychosis section of the DIGS, experiences of depersonalization, derealization, and disorientation are assessed. The course of psychotic illness is characterized graphically, and positive and negative symptoms are rated using the Scale for the Assessment of Negative Symptoms[22] and the Scale for the Assessment of Positive Symptoms.[23]

Diagnoses Included in the DIGS

For both BP disorder and SZ, the genetic phenotype appears to be broader than the core diagnosis.[24] Comorbidity in a proband further complicates family studies of a given spectrum. Additional conditions have been demonstrated to aggregate in family studies, but considerable uncertainty over boundaries remains.

For our genetic study of BP illness, bipolar I (BPI) and schizoaffective (SA) disorder (bipolar type [SA/BP]) were chosen as the core disorders. The spectrum conditions were designated as bipolar II (BPII) (recurrent major depression and hypomania), recurrent major depression, and cyclothymia.[25] For cyclothymia, we used the Modified Research Diagnostic Criteria[3,26] category of cyclothymic personality (a combination of depressive personality and hyperthymic personality) because this appeared to aggregate in previous family studies.[10,24] In addition, investigators agreed on the clinical significance of *DSM-III-R* dysthymia and included a section with criteria for this diagnosis. A section on suicidal behavior has also been included in the DIGS.

Chronic SZ and SA disorder, depressed type, were considered core phenotype diagnoses for SZ because they appear to cluster in the same families in many but not in all studies.[27,28] The psychosis section was also designed to permit the diagnosis of delusional disorder,[29] brief reactive psychosis, schizophreniform disorder, and psychotic disorder not otherwise specified (all of which may or may not be part of the schizophrenic spectrum).

Regarding the personality disorders, the evidence for inclusion of schizotypal personality disorder in the SZ spectrum was considered strong, and the evidence for including schizoid and paranoid personality disorders was considered mixed.[30] A modified form of the Structured Interview for Schizotypy[31] was included for use by investigators specifically interested in the familial spectrum of SZ. A shorter operationalized version of the *DSM-III-R* criteria for schizotypal personality disorder was created for other investigators.

It should be noted that the use of spectrum diagnoses may be advantageous for linkage analysis under some, but not all, models. A narrow definition of the phenotype may be beneficial in some cases of oligogenic inheritance because the probability of replication is increased in a second sample of reasonable size.[32] A narrow phenotype may also reduce false-positive attributions of affected status, which are more damaging to linkage studies than false negatives.[33]

INTERVIEW ASPECTS OF DIGS

Development

Items previously tested in other research interviews were incorporated into the DIGS. These instruments include the SADS,[13] Structured Clinical Interview for *DSM-III-R*,[34,35] Diagnostic Interview Schedule,[36] and Comprehensive Assessment of Symptoms and History.[37,38] Concurrent development of a research interview for the Collaborative Study on the Genetics of Alcoholism, the Semi-Structured Assessment for Genetic Studies of Alcoholism,[39] permitted the inclusion of comparable items in the affective disorders and substance abuse sections.

The DIGS evolved from multiple drafts that were field tested by researchers at the participating centers. Each group conducted field trials with psychiatric inpatients, outpatients, and controls (more than 70 patients at seven sites). Frequent collaborator meetings were held to discuss modifications to the drafts.

A comprehensive DIGS training manual was written to accompany the interview.[40] It covers general topics such as background information, administrative procedures, and coding conventions and provides numerous examples of probing and coding various subject responses. The manual addresses numerous complex or potentially confusing situations that may arise during the course of interviewing (eg, managing information about organic precipitants in the major depression section).

Format of the Interview

Because of the semistructured nature of the DIGS, clinical judgment is often required to code responses properly. The interviewer is directed to probe for further information and note examples of behavior that support the codes. Standard probe questions and criterion-based definitions are provided. If there is clear evidence that a symptom is present, it should be scored and a marginal note made even if the subject denies that symptom.

Sections of the DIGS typically begin with one or two closed-end questions that invite a yes or no response. A denial of symptoms in these screening questions permits one to skip the remainder of the section. If the subject responds positively to the initial screening questions, comprehensive symptom-based information is obtained. A series of questions systematically covers the diagnostic criteria for the various systems (integrated for ease of flow and efficiency). "Skip-outs" are used only if no symptoms are reported so that clinical descriptive information is not lost. Organic factors; age of onset; and recency, severity, frequency, and duration of symptoms/syndromes are assessed.

The time required to conduct the interview may vary considerably, from 30 minutes for an unaffected subject to 4 hours for a patient with complex symptoms. The median time required is 2½ hours

for symptomatic individuals. Following the interview, 30 to 40 minutes of the interviewer's time may be required to review the information and write a narrative. More than 1300 DIGS interviews have been performed successfully in affected families by the collaborating centers as of October 1993.

SECTIONS OF THE DIGS

Introduction

A modified Mini-Mental State examination[41] is included to permit early termination of the interview with subjects of diminished cognitive capacity. In the demographics section, in addition to standard information, subjects are asked about adoption status and country of birth. Ethnic background is detailed to permit comparisons of allele frequencies or disorder rates among subpopulations in genetic studies. The medical history screens for developmental factors and medical disorders that are known to be associated with psychiatric syndromes including neurological disorders, head injuries, hormonal disturbances, vitamin deficiencies, and birth and developmental abnormalities. Cigarette smoking history is quantified. Female subjects are asked about the association of psychiatric disturbances with pregnancy, childbirth, and menopause and the association of mood disturbance with the premenstrual and menstrual periods.

Somatization

This section is placed following medical history to enhance interview flow. Subjects are asked about problems with body pains in 10 physical systems. If four body pains are scored as medically unexplained, the interviewer proceeds to cover neurological, gastrointestinal, sexual, and other complaints. The interviewer is also alerted to consider panic disorder instead of somatization if the symptom complex is appropriate for this.

Overview

This section begins by recording the subject's age at the first psychiatric treatment, any psychotropic agents used, the formal psychiatric assessment, and the number of hospitalizations. The remainder is an open-ended history of the subject's psychopathologic episodes and treatment. A course of illness table is provided for interviewers to summarize the information.

A time line (**Figure**) is provided to chart the chronologic interaction of affective, psychotic, and other key symptoms over the lifetime course of illness. The interviewer will refer back to this framework to anchor information gathered in the specific diagnostic sections, and it is particularly useful in making differential diagnoses of mood, schizophrenic, and SA syndromes.

Mood Disorders

The major depression section assesses symptoms for both the current and most severe episode (it is recommended that the two episodes be assessed in series rather than in parallel). If delusions and/or hallucinations have occurred during the episode, descriptive information is obtained to classify symptoms as mood congruent or incongruent. The presence of psychotic symptoms prior to and beyond the resolution of affective symptoms is also assessed (to distinguish *DSM-III-R* SA disorder). To permit diagnosis using Modified Research Diagnostic Criteria,[3,26] multiple impairment items are included, and the interviewer must further rate whether the subject was impaired or incapacitated in the major life role. Possible specific precipitants of affective syndromes[42] are considered and an attempt is made to establish the existence of at least one "clean" episode without such a specific precipitant. A symptom checklist is used for reviewing a second episode to establish recurrent major depression. The age of onset and the number of episodes are also recorded.

The mania/hypomania section assesses a current and most severe episode, the presence and quality of any psychotic features, the presence of psychosis prior to and beyond resolution of affective symptoms, impairment/incapacitation, organic factors,[43] and treatment-seeking behavior. Screening questions include a brief summary of prominent symptoms for those who do not recognize or admit to mood changes and probes to separate brief situational mood changes from clinical mania. Mixed affective states and rapid cycling are assessed. The total number of episodes, age of onset, and recency are recorded. For the subjects who skip out of the mania section, a second series of questions deliberately designed to assess hypomania is included. Dysthymia is assessed in a separate section.

The cyclothymic personality section is adapted from the modified SADS of Gershon and coworkers,[3,26] as a combination of two subsections that assess modified Research Diagnostic Criteria depressive personality and hyperthymic personality. This is similar to cyclothymia as described by Akiskal et al.[44]

Substance Use Disorders

The DIGS offers a comprehensive assessment of the consumption of both alcohol and other drugs, abuse, and dependence. These sections are similar to those in the Semi-Structured Assessment for Genetic Studies of Alcoholism.[39] Two optional tables at the beginning of the alcohol section permit the interested researcher to record the number of drinks consumed each day of the week prior to the interview and the time it took to consume the alcoholic beverage.

A screen is built into the alcohol section to enable a skip-out if the subject reports any of the follow-

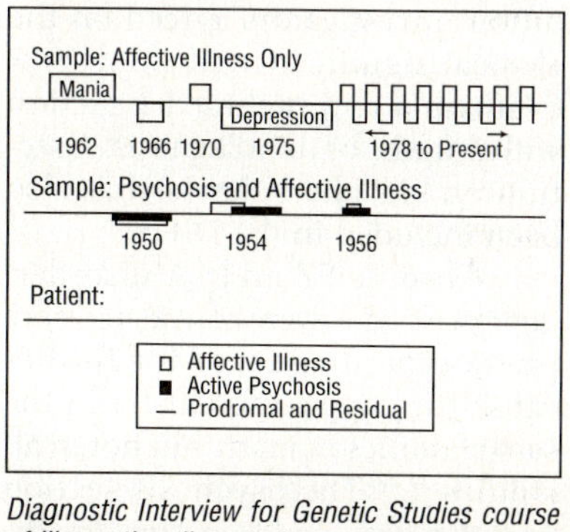

Diagnostic Interview for Genetic Studies course of illness time line used to summarize the history of psychopathologic symptoms.

ing: never had a drink of alcohol, never drank regularly (defined as at least once a week for 6 months or more), never became drunk (operationalized as slurred speech, unsteady gait), or never drank more than three alcoholic beverages in a 24-hour period. The final screening questions are those of the CAGE questionnaire.[45,46]

The marijuana section has been separated from the general drug section because of the high specific prevalence of its use. In the general drug abuse section, subjects are shown a list of commonly abused drugs (using vernacular terms) in the following categories: cocaine, stimulants, sedatives, hypnotics, tranquilizers, opiates, PCP (phencyclidine hydrochloride), hallucinogens, solvents, combination drugs, and a miscellaneous category. All drug users are asked about intravenous drug use.

Alcohol and other drug withdrawal syndromes are assessed by asking about individual symptoms associated with each substance, the co-occurrence of withdrawal symptoms, and whether the subject used the substance to ameliorate the discomfort of withdrawal symptoms. Medical and psychological consequences of substance abuse are evaluated. The clustering of symptoms is assessed for alcohol and drug abuse or dependence by rating the persistence of specific cognitive, behavioral, and physiologic symptoms for at least 1 month. Treatment, age of onset, and the recency and the date of last use of each substance are recorded.

Psychosis

The psychosis section offers a detailed assessment of psychotic symptoms as well as items to distinguish specific psychotic syndromes. Standard probes are used throughout the section to verify that the positive responses are in fact indicative of psychosis.

After positive response to probe questions, the subject is initially asked about 25 different types of delusions and hallucinations. Judgments are also made regarding formal thought disorder, bizarre behavior, catatonic motor behavior, avolition or apathy, flat and/or inappropriate affect, depersonalization, and derealization (after questions or observations).

Individual symptoms are recorded on a lifetime basis as well as anchored to the current or most recent episode. An array is used to specify whether symptoms occurred during depression, mania, substance use, a medical illness,[47-49] or in the absence of these conditions. The onset of the first symptoms or episode is explored and the number of episodes is recorded (chronic psychosis, including prodromal and residual periods, is considered to be one extended period of illness). Prodromal and residual symptoms are evaluated separately.

For SZ studies, the DIGS includes the modified Structured Interview for Schizotypy[31] to assess schizotypal, schizoid, and paranoid personality disorders in relatives. These sections are not used if psychosis was reported previously. A briefer schizotypal personality features section is also included for use in studies of affective disorder.

Comorbidity

Given the possibility that substance abuse can mimic mood and psychotic syndromes[42,43,48,49] and the extensive comorbidity noted in epidemiologic samples,[25] a distinct comorbidity assessment was incorporated into the DIGS. The crux of this section is to establish the temporal relationship between major affective disorder, psychosis, and substance abuse. One attempts to characterize the pattern of comorbidity by evaluating whether one disorder typically or always occurs first, if the disorders always co-occur, if one disorder persists in the absence of the other, and the duration of the persistence.

Suicidal Behavior

A separate section for the assessment of suicidal behavior characterizes the most serious suicide attempt in terms of intent, lethality, and the symptomatic context in which it occurred, eg, during an episode of mood disorder, psychosis, or substance abuse.

Anxiety Disorders

The major anxiety disorders were included because they are common familial conditions with an overlap in symptom profile and perhaps genetic vulnerability factors with affective illnesses.[50-52] Generalized anxiety disorder was excluded because of a lack of compelling family data. The temporal relationship to other major psychiatric disorders is noted, and subjects are asked to describe the specific content of their phobic or obsessive symptoms. Obsessive-compulsive disorder, panic disorder, agoraphobia, social phobia, and simple phobia are assessed.

Eating Disorders

Because some but not all[53-55] family studies have indicated a familial relationship between affective and eating disorders, sections on anorexia and bulimia were included in the DIGS. The anorexia section includes a table to determine whether the subject meets the *DSM-III-R* body weight criterion for anorexia (15% below the expected body weight). The table entries are made according to gender, height, and body frame size. Those who continue are assessed for a distortion of body image and presence of an intense fear of gaining weight despite being underweight. Possible organic contributors are ruled out. Symptoms, age of onset, and recency of first and last regularly occurring binges are recorded in the bulimia section.

Sociopathy

Antisocial personality disorder was included as a disorder from a different genetic spectrum[56] that should generally be excluded from studies of affective illness and SZ. Questions are taken strictly from *DSM-III-R* criteria for this section. The interviewer is directed not to include behavior that is solely related to abuse of alcohol or other drugs.

CLINICAL RATINGS AND SUMMARY OF SECTIONS

At the conclusion of the individual diagnostic sections the interviewer completes a series of assessment

scales based on information and observations obtained during the interview, including the Global Assessment Scale,[57] the Scale for the Assessment of Negative Symptoms,[22] and the Scale for the Assessment of Positive Symptoms.[23] The ratings are based on the month prior to the interviews.

Interviewers rate their assessment of the reliability of information obtained in each major diagnostic category as either good, fair, or unreliable. A brief narrative is then written to provide extra detail beyond the ratings, including the outline of psychiatric disorders, crucial and/or uncertain points, difficulties in conducting the interview, conflicting data, and reliability of the data.

SELECTING TEST ADMINISTRATORS

The most suitable personnel to administer the DIGS are mental health professionals with clinical experience and knowledge of the multiple diagnostic criteria systems. The interviewer must have a basic understanding of psychiatric disorders and be able to make clinical judgments about manifest psychopathologic symptoms. Interviewers employed by the BP and SZ centers for the NIMH Genetics Initiative have varied professional backgrounds that include psychiatry, psychology, psychiatric nursing, and psychiatric social work.

TRAINING METHODS

Three multicenter interviewer training sessions were held at The Johns Hopkins University, Baltimore, Md; Indiana University Medical Center, Indianapolis; and Washington University, St Louis, Mo. The training included demonstration interviews by senior clinicians to illustrate specific diagnostic distinctions; ultimately, each trainee administered a DIGS to a patient under the observation of a group of interviewers and a clinician. Three videotaped patient interviews were circulated among the centers for supplemental training.

RELIABILITY

As part of overall interview development, we conducted a two-phase reliability study that had three major goals: (1) to determine the reliability of four diagnoses critical in initial phases of the genetic research, (2) to determine the feasibility of automated scoring of the DIGS using external diagnostic algorithms, and (3) to assess the comparability of diagnostic reliability among collaborating sites.

Subjects in the NIMH collaborative genetic studies will ultimately receive best-estimate diagnoses using procedures similar to those described in previous studies.[1-3] Before that stage, however, core DIGS diagnoses in a minimum set of first-degree relatives must be identified and will determine whether further interviewing of other family members is initiated. For this reason, we sought to ensure that study interviewers had extensive experience with these diagnoses rather than less intensive experience with a wider variety of diagnoses.

We based our primary reliability analyses on the algorithmic diagnosis made from items scored in the instrument, even if this diagnosis disagreed with the interviewer's clinical impression. Interviewers were blinded to all corollary information. In adopting these procedures, we sought to test the adequacy of the DIGS as an information-gathering instrument and as an assessment of the role of algorithms in diagnostic procedures.

Because our plans to combine data from different sites depend on the uniform implementation of a study protocol, including diagnostic evaluations, we sought to determine the success of our efforts at providing DIGS interviewers with comparable training in the second phase of our study.

The study design called for test-retest reliability assessment in two phases. Six weeks of independent interviewing at each of six sites (phase 1) was followed by 2 weeks of cross-site interviewing at three sites (phase 2). In phase 1, 60% of subjects were reinterviewed within 7 days, 90% between 4 and 10 days after the initial interview. In phase 2, 100% of subjects were reinterviewed in a 4- to 10-day interval.

Nineteen interviewers participated in phase 1 (between two and four per site). Fourteen interviewers (two from each site) also participated in phase 2 assessments. All but one of the interviewers had prior clinical interviewing experience using semistructured instruments such as the SADS.[13]

SUBJECT SELECTION CRITERIA

We attempted to enter equal numbers of clinical subjects who met *DSM-III-R* criteria for primary lifetime diagnoses of SZ, SA disorder, BP disorder, and major depression into the study at each site for both phases. Site study coordinators obtained referrals from a variety of sources, and referrals were based on lifetime *DSM-III-R* clinical or research diagnoses. At the Washington University site, all of the subjects had clinical diagnoses made by psychiatrists working at the Barnes Hospital Psychiatry Clinic in St Louis, Mo; and at the Johns Hopkins site, by psychiatrists at The Johns Hopkins Outpatient Clinic. At the Columbia University, New York, NY, site, subject referrals were based primarily on clinical diagnoses made by psychiatrists at the New York State Psychiatric Institute in New York City, although eight of 58 subjects had previously received research diagnoses. At the Harvard University, Boston, Mass, site, all but two of the subjects were referred by treating clinicians at the Brockton (Mass) Veterans Affairs Medical Center, based on research diagnoses. At Indiana University, 23 of 43 subjects had research diagnoses, and the remaining subjects were recruited from clinics at four university-affiliated hospitals. Only four of 150 clinical subjects seen in phase 1 were inpatients, and in phase 2, all were outpatients.

In addition to the four clinical groups, a fifth nonpatient group was added to the design to make the overall diagnostic process closer to a naturalistic situation in which well family members are assessed. These subjects were not interviewed beforehand and were recruited primarily by word of mouth from among employees working at the research

Table 2. Demographics by Entry Diagnosis (Between Site and Within Site Combined)

	Major Depression	Bipolar I Disorder	Schizophrenia	Schizoaffective Disorder	No Diagnosis
Mean age, y	41.8	46.5	36.6	37.0	42.7
% Female	60	56	29	40	64
% White	76	79	50	72	83
% Never married	29	29	88	63	26
Mean years of school	15.3	14.3	12.3	13.5	14.7

sites. At the Columbia University site, however, subjects were well family members from other genetic studies or previous normal control subjects in biological studies. **Table 2** summarizes the demographic characteristics of the patient and nonpatient groups.

Over all sites, 72% of the sample was white, 10% was black, and 18% was either of Hispanic origin or mixed origin including Alaskan or American Indian. The schizophrenic group had a lower mean age, fewer years of schooling, and a higher proportion of nonwhite subjects.

DESIGN PHASES

Phase 1: Within-Site Design

In phase 1, each of the six sites was asked to obtain 30 subjects (six in each of the four referral diagnostic groups and in the nonpatient group); 179 pairs were actually obtained. During this phase, interviewers completed a summary at the end of the DIGS; they did not consistently state one *DSM-III-R* diagnosis as their diagnostic first choice based on their clinical impressions but instead listed alternatives or provided descriptive details. In phase 2, interviewers were asked to make a clear diagnostic first choice. In both phases, subjects within each of the five groups were assigned randomly and blindly to interviewers, and each interviewer saw a variety of diagnostic types.

Phase 2: Between-Site Design

In this phase, Washington University (36 subjects), Columbia University (24 subjects), and Indiana University (24 subjects) hosted simultaneous 2-week reliability studies to which interviewers traveled from their home sites. Eighty-one subjects completed both interviews.

In week 1, one interviewer from each of seven sites traveled to a host site to interview 12 subjects (one to two per day over a 7- to 32-day period). Every interviewer was assigned at least two subjects from each of the five groups. In week 2, seven other interviewers (one from that of each site) repeated this schedule, but at a host site different from that of the other home site interviewer. Of the 12 subjects seen by an interviewer in the first week, six each were interviewed by two interviewers in the second week. Because in the genetic studies data from three SZ sites will be pooled as will data from four BP sites in the intersite reliability study design, an attempt was made to pair at least one of the two participating interviewers from a site with an interviewer from a similar collaborating site. Five of six possible pairings of the four collaborating BP sites were made, and all three collaborating SZ site pairings were made. In this phase, interviewers reviewed their own DIGS following an interview, and this was followed by a second review for completeness (eg, items filled in) by host site coordinators.

DATA MANAGEMENT

DSM-III-R algorithms for the four diagnoses were applied to DIGS items by five scorers different from the interviewers and blinded to the referral diagnosis. Scorer edits were done in cases of interviewer data entry error. For instance, the *DSM-III-R* SZ criterion D includes prodromal, active, and residual phases in calculations of total duration of disorder. In phase 1, however, some interviewers entered duration of a brief recent exacerbation of psychosis in the DIGS item used to score the criterion, despite noting elsewhere a long-standing psychosis. Such an item was edited before algorithms were applied. Before phase 2, this item and a few others were clarified by changing wording slightly or by adding additional instructions. As a result, DIGS editing was minimal in phase 2.

DATA ANALYTIC APPROACH

For reliability analyses, we disregarded referral diagnosis and used actual algorithmic agreement. We also observed hierarchical diagnostic rules and did not double-count subjects with more than one diagnosis. Diagnostic agreement was strictly defined: a diagnosis of BPI vs recurrent major depression or BPII was coded as a disagreement; although in the latter case, two interviews might differ only in whether impairment was rated during the manic episode. In the genetic study, BPI but not recurrent major depression or BPII is used to identify a proband, and a false-positive BPI diagnosis might invalidate the ascertainment of an entire family. Diagnoses of BPI vs SA and SZ vs SA were defined as disagreement in all but one analysis (see below). In the NIMH Genetics Initiative, the distinction between the two subtypes of SA disorder, depressed (SA/D) and bipolar (SA/BP), is an important one. Schizoaffective disorder/bipolar depression is defined as a core spectrum diagnosis closely related to BPI, and SA/D is defined as a core spectrum diagnosis closely related to SZ. In this scheme, a diagnostic confusion of BPI and SA/BP or of SZ and SA/D would not invalidate a family's ascertainment, but a confusion of SA/BP and SA/D would. To see how interviewers performed at this practically important level of reli-

Table 3. Reliability by Diagnostic Category Within Phase (All Sites Combined) and Between Phase (All Host Sites Combined)

Entry Diagnosis vs All Others	Phase 1 (Within Site) Algorithmic Diagnosis, κ (95% CI*) (n=179)	Phase 2 (Between Site) Diagnosis, κ (95% CI) (n=81)	
		Algorithmic	Clinical
Major depression	0.84 (0.70-0.98	0.94 (0.72-1.0)	0.86 (0.64-1.0)
Bipolar disorder	0.78 (0.64-0.92)	0.96 (0.74-1.0)	0.85 (0.63-1.0)
Schizoaffective disorder	0.39 (0.25-0.53)	0.31 (0.11-0.51)	0.45 (0.23-0.67)
Schizophrenia	0.73 (0.59-0.87)	0.75 (0.53-0.97)	0.90 (0.68-1.0)
No target diagnosis/other	0.87 (0.73-1.0)	0.86 (0.64-1.0)	0.96 (0.74-1.0)
Overall	0.78 (0.70-0.86)	0.85 (0.73-0.97)	0.84 (0.72-0.96)

**CI indicates confidence interval.*

ability, subjects with a diagnosis of SA were subtyped based on affective symptoms in one analysis. Reliability coefficients were calculated defining agreement as BPI-BPI and BPI-SA/BP interview pairs; or alternatively, SZ-SZ and SZ-SA/D interview pairs.

For each phase, data were analyzed using the same general strategy. In phase 1, 5×5 tables were constructed for each of the six sites representing the four major target diagnoses plus "other" (ie, no target diagnosis) at interview 1 vs interview 2. This approach yielded an overall kappa (κ) per site. Data from the sites were then combined and 2×2 κ's computed for each category vs all others. In phase 2, using the same analytic strategy, overall κ's were computed for each host site. Then, combining across host sites, separate 2×2 κ's were computed for each target diagnosis plus "no target diagnosis" vs all others. In phase 2, κ's were also calculated in the same manner for interviewer clinical diagnoses.

Referral diagnosis was compared with DIGS algorithmic diagnosis as another indication of consensual diagnostic validity as follows: No. of pairs of DIGS diagnoses that agreed with a given referral diagnosis/total No. of subjects with that referral diagnosis.

The following *DSM-III-R* syndromal criteria were also examined: major depressive episode A criterion, manic episode A and B criteria, and SZ A criterion. This approach disregarded hierarchical diagnostic rules so that a subject could receive multiple syndromal criterion scores. A criterion was defined as present if both interviewers scored it. In one analysis, the reliability of syndromal criteria was examined for the entire sample. In a second analysis, groups of subjects entered with the different referral diagnoses were compared on syndrome criterion scores.

Because phase 1 goals included those of training as well as the establishment of baseline reliability, phase 2 findings are considered to represent a more rigorous test of DIGS reliability. Phase 1 findings, however, are consistent with phase 2 results, and where applicable, are summarized along with them.

RESULTS

In phase 1, overall κ's ranged from 0.66 to 0.86 at the six sites (agreement of 0.70 or above is defined as excellent; 0.50 to 0.70 as fair; and less than 0.50 as poor). Differences among the sites were not significant (χ^2=3.24, *df*=4). In phase 2, κ's ranged from 0.81 to 0.88 at the three host sites, also not significantly different (χ^2=0.172, *df*=2).

Because there were no significant site differences in overall agreement in either phase of the reliability study, data were combined within each phase for analysis of individual diagnoses. Findings are summarized in **Table 3**.

For all target diagnoses except SA, κ's obtained for algorithmic and interviewer clinical diagnoses were in the excellent range, 0.73 to 0.96. In phase 2, where they were consistently available, interviewer clinical diagnoses yielded slightly higher κ's than did algorithms for the psychotic disorders. For both affective disorder target diagnoses, algorithm κ's exceeded those for clinical diagnoses. Algorithmic diagnosis was unsatisfactory for SA and phase 2 clinical diagnosis was only slightly better. A notable source of unreliability stemmed from differences in rating of the SA C criterion, which requires mood syndromes to be "not brief" relative to psychotic syndromes. (It should be noted that we have arbitrarily defined brief as 30% of total time with psychosis. Thus, 12 weeks of depression in the course of 3 years of psychosis would be brief, but 12 months would not be brief.) When SA was subtyped according to affective subtype and paired with either BPI or SZ depending on that subtype, reliability improved substantially for SA (0.67 for clinical diagnosis, phase 2).

From **Table 4** it can be seen that agreement of algorithmic with referral diagnosis of recurrent major depression was high in both phases of the study. Likewise, algorithmic diagnosis agreed well with referral diagnosis of BPI. When a disagreement occurred, algorithmic diagnosis was most often BPII, the interview failing to provide evidence of impairment necessary to make the lifetime diagnosis of BPI.

For SZ, the agreement between algorithmic and referral diagnoses was 76% in phase 2 but only 47% in phase 1. In some cases, no algorithmic diagnosis was made from either DIGS interview (and hence interviewers agreed) because subjects either denied symptoms or failed to provide information on other aspects of their psychosis necessary for the algorithm. However, clinical summaries indicated that interviewers had a clear impression of SZ.

Of 48 interview pairs with referral subjects with SA, only two resulted in an SA algorithmic diagnosis in both interviews and hence met

Table 4. Agreement Between Referral Diagnosis and Diagnostic Interview for Genetic Studies (DIGS) Algorithmic Diagnosis

	No. of Agreements/Total No. of Subjects (% Agreement)*		
Diagnosis	Phase 1 (Within Site)	Phase 2 (Between Site)	Within and Between Sites Combined
Depression	31/36 (86)	14/17 (82)	45/53 (85)
Bipolar disorder	28/38 (74)	14/17 (82)	42/55 (76)
Schizophrenia	16/34 (47)	13/17 (76)	29/51 (57)
Schizoaffective disorder	2/34 (6)	0/14 (0)	2/48 (4)

Number of agreements is based on agreement between both raters' DIGS algorithmic diagnosis and the referral diagnosis; total number of subjects is the number of subjects entered with each diagnosis.

our definition of agreement. For only 12 of the 48 subjects was the algorithmic diagnosis of SA made by even one interviewer. In these cases as well, it is of note that the second diagnosis was more often of SZ and less frequently of an affective disorder with mood incongruent psychotic symptoms. When algorithmic assessments agreed on another diagnosis, agreement was most frequently on SZ.

For the entire sample, agreement on algorithmic criteria defining specific syndrome patterns was high: *DSM-III-R* major depressive episode criterion A, 87%, κ=0.78; manic episode criteria A and B, 71%, κ=0.72; and SZ criterion A, 74%, κ=0.77.

For subjects referred with a diagnosis of SA, the diagnostically requisite *DSM-III-R* SZ A criterion was more reliably agreed on than the DIGS diagnosis of the full disorder. The SA and SZ referral groups did not differ significantly on the presence of this criterion (63% vs 73%). As expected, the SA group had more depressive symptoms (major depressive episode criterion A) (71% vs 49%; χ^2=4.89, *df*=1, *P*<.05) and more manic symptoms (manic episode criteria A and B) (50% vs 16%; χ^2=13.31, *df*=1, *P*<.001).

COMMENT

It is our hope that the DIGS will be of particular use to investigators doing comprehensive psychiatric family genetic studies. It has a detailed focus on SZ, affective disorders, and substance abuse and is expected to be useful in any study of these conditions, their spectrum manifestations, or their interaction.

The DIGS will be useful for those investigators interested in comparing data with previous studies using criterion systems other than *DSM-III-R*. This may be particularly important for biologic marker studies in which populations may be compared over many years.

The instrument will play a special role for individual investigators or groups with a long history of using an older instrument. To enable a transition from the criteria systems of Feighner et al[17] or Research Diagnostic Criteria to *DSM-III-R* or *DSM-IV*, the investigator may use the DIGS in a new sample and observe the relationship between results in the same sample diagnosed using different criteria. It will not be necessary to use two installments on the same sample.

The DIGS increases the potential for developing quantitative phenotypes in addition to categorical phenotypes. A numerical rating of symptoms can be derived, leading to a judgment of severity. This has important implications for lifetime diagnoses. The data of Rice et al[58,59] showed the stability of lifetime affective diagnoses to be directly proportional to the number of symptoms present.

The DIGS is not designed for routine clinical use. It cannot easily be used by lay interviewers or with cognitively disorganized subjects. It should be a useful addition, however, to most biologic, phenomenologic, or prospective clinical research programs. It is designed to be employed by trained personnel using significant clinical judgment and summarizing information in narrative form as well as in ratings for algorithmic diagnosis, present symptom state, and representation of life course.

The results of the reliability study indicate generally satisfactory performance of the DIGS in characterizing the types of clinically and diagnostically complex subjects who must be identified at the outset of ascertainment in the genetic study, and algorithms appear to be a feasible way of abstracting interview information. Phase 2 results indicate that cross-site training procedures were successful in yielding a group of clinical interviewers who would apply a skilled and uniform approach to this ascertainment.

An automated system for DIGS data entry and editing is currently under development and will flag many potential errors as well as internal inconsistencies. However, we would not advocate a strictly automated approach to final diagnosis. Certain information may be gleaned more accurately from records. Medical interpretation is required to determine whether alcohol or other drugs or another organic factor is a precipitant for a psychiatric syndrome, and a clinician's interpretation is important in judging the relative severity of psychopathologic symptoms described or denied by the subject.

It must be noted that diagnoses such as BPII and schizotypal personality, which are likely to be found in family members of BP or SZ subjects, were not included in this initial assessment. A reliability assessment of these diagnoses will be conducted using relatives of probands identified in the course of the genetic studies.

In using algorithms to measure agreement, we anticipated that reliabilities might be lower than those from other studies,[16,45,60,61] which were based on broader sources of information and used primarily inpatient samples. However, as seen in **Table 5**, this proved generally not to be the case.

Clinical reliabilities from our study, computed in phase 2, may be considered most directly compa-

Table 5. Test-Retest Reliability Comparisons*

Diagnosis	SCID (n=390)	CASH (n=30)	SADS (n=36)	SADS (RDC) (n=60)	DIGS (n=81) Algorithmic	DIGS (n=81) Clinical
Biopolar disorder	.84	.90	.49	.77	.96	.86
Major depression	.64	.65	.46	.71	.94	.85
Schizophrenia	.65	.72	.71	.73	.75	.90
Schizoaffective disorder	.63	.52	.27	.70	.31	.45

All diagnoses lifetime, based on DSM-III-R criteria except where indicated. SCID indicates Structured Clinical Interview for DSM-III-R; CASH, Comprehensive Assessment of Symptoms and History; SADS, Schedule for Affective Disorders and Schizophrenia; RDC, Research Diagnostic Criteria; and DIGS, Diagnostic Interview for Genetic Studies.

rable to the results of other studies. For the psychotic disorders of SA and SZ, clinical diagnoses based on the DIGS yielded better reliabilities than strict algorithm scoring. For the mood disorders, however, the algorithmic approach appears superior to clinical diagnosis. This suggests that algorithm scoring may have an advantage in precision if the informant is able to respond accurately to key interview questions.

Our reliability coefficients for SA are much lower than for the other diagnoses. This may be owing to the small number of subjects actually diagnosed with the disorder. However, it seems as likely that the *DSM-III-R* SA C criterion (duration of all episodes of a mood syndrome not brief relative to total duration of psychotic disturbance) may be difficult to assess reliably, as was noted in our study and in one other recent reliability assessment.[61] Experienced clinicians rating identical case records for the European Science Foundation psychiatric genetics effort also had special difficulty in making reliable ratings for relative duration of mood and psychotic syndromes (Anne Farmer, MD, oral communication, 1992). These judgments are quite difficult under the best of circumstances but are probably best made by combining all available sources of information in a best-estimate process, as noted previously. Studies on the reliability of the best-estimate process are projected as part of the NIMH Genetics Initiative.

Accepted for publication June 24, 1994.

Development of the DIGS instrument and training manual was supported by the NIMH Diagnostic Centers for Psychiatric Linkage Studies (extramural grant Nos. U01 MH46276, 46289, 46318, 46274, 46282, 46280); the Clinical Neurogenetics Branch, Intramural Research Program, NIMH; and the Division of Clinical and Treatment Research, NIMH.

Other participants in the NIMH Genetics Initiative who helped in the development of the DIGS include Sandra Barton, Deborah Brookshire, Christopher Cottrell, Katharina Crombie, Caroline Drain, David Goldfinger, Robin Green, Diane Kazuba, Dawn Lawrence, Aimee Mayeda, MD, Francis McMahon, MD, Martin McElhiney, Catharine Monaco, Beth O'Dell, H. Matthew Quitkin, Diane Raasch, RN, Leela Rau, MD, Carrie Smiley, RN, Scott Yale, and Ruth Yarrington.

The authors thank Jean Endicott, PhD, Kenneth Kendler, MD, Philip Lavori, PhD, and Lee Robins, PhD, for critical review of the instrument and John Bartko, PhD, and Michael Borenstein, PhD, for their consultation on the design and statistical analysis of the reliability study.

Reprint requests to Institute of Psychiatric Research, Department of Psychiatry, Indiana University School of Medicine, 791 Union Dr, Indianapolis, IN 46202-4887 (Dr Nurnberger).

NIMH Genetics Initiative Collaborators

Department of Psychiatry, Indiana University Medical Center, Indianapolis: Marvin Miller, MD; Elizabeth S. Bowman, MD. **Department of Psychiatry, The Johns Hopkins University, Baltimore, Md:** J. Raymond DePaulo, MD. **Department of Psychiatry, Washington University, St Louis, Mo:** C. Robert Cloninger; Gordon Robinson, MD; Steven Moldin, PhD. **NIMH Intramural Research Program, Rockville, Md:** Elliot S. Gershon, MD; M. Elizabeth Maxwell, MSW; Juliet J. Guroff, MSW; Darrell Kirch, MD. **NIMH Division of Clinical and Treatment Research:** Debra Wynne, MSW; Kate Berg, PhD. **Brockton/West Roxbury (Mass) Veterans Affairs Medical Center/Harvard Schools of Medicine and Public Health:** Ming T. Tsuang, MD, PhD, DSc; Stephen V. Faraone, PhD; John R. Pepple, PhD. **SRA Technologies Incorporated, Falls Church, Va:** A. Louise Ritz, MBA.

REFERENCES

1. Leckman JF, Sholomskas D, Thompson WD, Belanger A, Weissman MM. Best estimate of lifetime psychiatric diagnosis: a methodological study. *Arch Gen Psychiatry.* 1982;39:879-883.
2. Weissman MM, Merikangas KR, John K, Wickramaratne P, Prusoff BA, Kidd KK. Family genetic studies of psychiatric disorders: developing technologies. *Arch Gen Psychiatry.* 1986;43:1104-1116.
3. Gershon ES, Hamovit J, Guroff JJ, Dibble E, Leckman JF, Sceery W, Targum SD, Nurnberger JI, Goldin LR, Bunney WE. A family study of schizoaffective, bipolar I, bipolar II, unipolar, and normal control probands. *Arch Gen Psychiatry.* 1982;39:1157-1167.
4. Kendell RE. The choice of diagnostic criteria for biological research. *Arch Gen Psychiatry.* 1982;39:1334-1339.
5. Berner P, Gabriel E, Katschnig H, Keiffer W, Kohler K. *Diagnostic Criteria for Schizophrenia and Affective Psychoses.* Washington, DC: World Psychiatric Association, American Psychiatric Press Inc; 1983.
6. American Psychiatric Association. *Diagnostic and Statistical Manual of Mental Disorders, Revised Third Edition.* Washington, DC: American Psychiatric Association; 1987.
7. American Psychiatric Association. *Diagnostic and Statistical Manual of Mental Disorders, Fourth Edition.* Washington, DC: American Psychiatric Association; 1994.
8. Andreason NC, Scheftner W, Reich T, Hirschfeld RM, Endicott J, Keller MB. The validation of the concept of endogenous depression: a fam-

ily study approach. *Arch Gen Psychiatry.* 1986; 43:246-351.

9. Gershon ES, Hamovit JH, Guroff JJ, Nurnberger JI. Birth-cohort changes in manic and depressive disorders in relatives of bipolar and schizoaffective patients. *Arch Gen Psychiatry.* 1987; 44:314-319.
10. Reich T, Clayton PJ, Winokur G. Family history studies, V: the genetics of mania. *Am J Psychiatry.* 1969;125:1358.
11. Tsuang MT, Winokur G, Crowe RR. Morbidity risks of schizophrenia and affective disorders among first-degree relatives of patients with schizophrenia, mania, depression, and surgical conditions. *Br J Psychiatry.* 1980;137:497-504.
12. Regier DA, Myers JK, Kramer M, Robins LN, Blazer DG, Hough RL, Eaton WW, Locke BZ. The NIMH Epidemiologic Catchment Area program: historical context, major objectives, and study population characteristics. *Arch Gen Psychiatry.* 1984; 41:934-941.
13. Endicott J, Spitzer RL. A diagnostic interview: the Schedule for Affective Disorders and Schizophrenia. *Arch Gen Psychiatry.* 1978;35:837-844.
14. Wing JK, Birley JLT, Cooper JE, Graham P, Isaacs AD. Reliability of a procedure for measuring and classifying 'present psychiatric state.' *Br J Psychiatry.* 1967;113:499-515.
15. McGuffin P, Farmer AE. *Operational Criteria (OPCRIT) Checklist.* Version 3.0. Cardiff: University of Wales; 1990.
16. Spitzer RL, Endicott J, Robins E. Research diagnostic criteria. *Arch Gen Psychiatry.* 1978;35: 773-782.
17. Feighner JP, Robin SE, Guze SB, Woodruff RA, Winokur G, Munoz R. Diagnostic criteria for use in psychiatric research. *Arch Gen Psychiatry.* 1972; 26:57-63.
18. American Psychiatric Association, Committee on Nomenclature and Statistics. *Diagnostic and Statistical Manual of Mental Disorders, Third Edition.* Washington, DC: American Psychiatric Association; 1980.
19. Schneider K; Hamilton M, trans. *Clinical Psychopathology.* New York, NY: Grune & Stratton Inc; 1959.
20. Farmer AE, McGuffin P, Gottesmall IL. Searching for a split in schizophrenia: a twin study perspective. *Psychiatry Res.* 1984;13:109-118.
21. Roy-Byrne P, Post RM, Uhde TW, Porcu T, Davis D. The longitudinal course of recurrent affective illness: life chart data from research patients at the NIMH. *Acta Psychiatr Scand Suppl.* 1985; 317:1-34.
22. Andreasen NC. *The Scale for the Assessment of Negative Symptoms (SANS).* Iowa City: University of Iowa; 1983.
23. Andreasen NC. *The Scale for the Assessment of Positive Symptoms (SAPS).* Iowa City: University of Iowa; 1984.
24. Gershon ES, Mark A, Cohen N, Belizon N, Baron M, Knobe KE. Transmitted factors in the morbid risk of affective disorders: a controlled study. *J Psychiatr Res.* 1975;12:283-299.
25. Nurnberger JI, Gershon ES. Genetics. In: Paykel ES, ed. *Handbook of Affective Disorders.* 2nd ed. Edinburgh, Scotland: Churchill Livingstone; 1992: 131-148.
26. Mazure C, Gershon ES. Blindness and reliability in lifetime psychiatric diagnosis. *Arch Gen Psychiatry.* 1979;36:521-525.
27. Guze SB, Cloninger CR, Martin RM, Clayton PJ. A follow-up and family study of schizophrenia. *Arch Gen Psychiatry.* 1983;40:1273-1276.
28. Gershon ES, DeLisi LE, Hamovit J, Nurnberger JI Jr, Maxwell ME, Schreiber J, Dauphinais D, Dingman CW II, Guroff JJ. A controlled family study of chronic psychoses. *Arch Gen Psychiatry.* 1988;45:328-336.
29. Kendler KS, Gruenberg AM, Tsuang MT. Psychiatric illness in first-degree relatives of schizophrenic and surgical control patients. *Arch Gen Psychiatry.* 1985;42:770-779.
30. Tsuang MT, Gilbertson MV, Faraone SV. Genetic transmission of negative and positive symptoms in the biological relatives of schizophrenics. In: Marneros A, Tsuang MT, Andreasen NC, eds. *Negative Versus Positive Schizophrenia.* New York, NY: Springer-Verlag; 1991.
31. Kendler KS, Lieberman JA, Walsh D. The Structured Interview for Schizotypy (SIS): a preliminary report. *Schizophr Bull.* 1989;15:559-571.
32. Suarez BK. Problems of replicating linkage claims in psychiatry. Presented at the Annual Meeting of the American Psychopathological Association; March 5-7, 1992; New York, NY.
33. Lander E. Mapping complex genetic traits in humans. In: Davies K, ed. *Genome Analysis.* Oxford, England: IRL Press; 1988.
34. Spitzer RL, Williams JB, Gibbon M, First MB. *Structured Clinical Interview for* DSM-III-R, *Patient Edition.* New York: Biometrics Research Department, New York State Psychiatric Institute; 1989.
35. Andreasen NC, Flaum M, Arndt S. The Comprehensive Assessment of Symptoms and History (CASH): an instrument for assessing diagnosis and psychopathology. *Arch Gen Psychiatry.* 1992; 49:615-623.
36. Robins LN, Helzer JE, Croughon J, Ratcliff KS. National Institute of Mental Health Diagnostic Interview Schedule: its history, characteristics, and validity. *Arch Gen Psychiatry.* 1981;38:381-389.
37. Andreasen NC. *Comprehensive Assessment of Symptoms and History.* Iowa City: University of Iowa; 1987.
38. Spitzer RL, Williams JBW, Gibbon M, First MB. The Structured Clinical Interview for *DSM-III-R* (SCID). *Arch Gen Psychiatry.* 1992;49:624-629.
39. Bucholz K, Cadoret R, Cloninger CR, Dinwiddie S, Hesselbrock V, Nurnberger JI Jr, Reich T, Schmidt I, Schuckit M. Semi-Structured Assessment for the Genetics of Alcoholism (SSAGA). *J Stud Alcohol.* 1993:149-158.
40. National Institute of Mental Health. *Molecular Genetics Initiative: Diagnostic Interview for Genetic Studies, Training Manual.* Bethesda, Md: National Institute of Mental Health; May 13, 1992.
41. Cockrell JR, Folstein MF. Mini-Mental State examination (MMSE). *Psychopharmacol Bull.* 1988; 24:689-692.
42. Wood KA, Harris MJ, Morreale A, Rizos AL. Drug-induced psychosis and depression in the elderly. *Psychiatr Clin North Am.* 1984;11:167-193.
43. Krauthammer C, Klerman GL. Secondary mania: manic syndromes associated with antecedent physical illness or drugs. *Arch Gen Psychiatry.* 1978;35:1333-1339.
44. Akiskal HS, Kheni MK, Scott-Strauss A. Cyclothymic temperamental disorders. *Psychiatr Clin North Am.* 1979;2:527-554.
45. Mayfield D, McLeod G, Hall P. Alcoholism screening instrument. *Am J Psychiatry.* 1974;131:1121-1123.
46. Bush B, Shaw S, Cleary P, Delbanco TL, Aronson MD. Screening for alcohol abuse using the CAGE questionnaire. *Am J Med.* 1987;82:231-235.
47. Propping P. Genetic disorders presenting as schizophrenia: Karl Bonhoeffer's early view of the psychoses in the light of medical genetics. *Hum Genet.* 1983;65:1-10.
48. Davison K, Bagley CR. Schizophrenia-like psychoses associated with organic disorders of the central nervous system: a review of the literature. In: Herrington RH, ed. *Current Problems in Neuropsychiatry, Schizophrenia, Epilepsy, the Temporal Lobe. Br J Psychiatry.* 1969;4:113-184. Special publication.
49. Cummings JL. Organic psychoses: delusional disorders and secondary mania. *Psychiatr Clin North Am.* 1986;9:292-311.
50. Coryell W, Endicott J, Andreasen NC, Keller MB, Clayton PJ, Hirschfeld RMA, Scheftner WA, Winokur G. Depression and panic attacks: the significance of overlap as reflected in follow-up and family study data. *Am J Psychiatry.* 1988; 145:293-300.
51. Leckman JF, Weissman MM, Merikangas KR, Pauls DL, Prusoff BA. Panic disorder and major depression: increased risk of depression, alcoholism, panic and phobic disorders in families of depressed probands with panic disorder. *Arch Gen Psychiatry.* 1983;40:1055-1060.
52. Fyer AJ, Mannuzza S, Gallops MS, Martin LY, Aaronson C, Gorman J, Liebowitz MR, Klein DF. Familial transmission of simple phobias and fears. *Arch Gen Psychiatry.* 1990;47:252-256.
53. Gershon ES, Hamovit JR, Schreiber JL, Dibble ED, Kaye W, Nurnberger JI Jr, Andersen A, Ebert M. Anorexia nervosa and major affective disorders associated in families: a preliminary report. In: Guze SB, Earls FJ, Barrett JE, eds. *Child Psychopathology and Development.* New York, NY: Raven Press Ltd; 1983:279-286.
54. Kassett JA, Gershon ES, Maxwell ME, Guroff JJ, Kazuba DM, Smith AL, Brandt HA, Jimerson DC. Psychiatric disorders in the first-degree relatives of probands with bulimia nervosa. *Am J Psychiatry.* 1989;146:1468-1471.
55. Levy AB, Dixon KN, Stern SL. How are depression and bulimia related? *Am J Psychiatry.* 1989; 146:162-169.
56. Cloninger CR, Reich T, Guze SB. The multifactorial model of disease transmission, III: familial relationship between sociopathy and hysteria (Briquet's syndrome). *Br J Psychiatry.* 1975; 127:23-32.
57. Endicott J, Spitzer RL, Fleiss JL, Cohen J. The Global Assessment Scale: a procedure for measuring overall severity of psychiatric disturbance. *Arch Gen Psychiatry.* 1976;33:766-771.
58. Rice J, Endicott J, Knesevich MA. The estimation of diagnostic sensitivity using stability data: an application to major depressive disorder. *J Psychiatr Res.* 1987;21:337-345.
59. Rice J, Reich T, Andreasen NC, Endicott J, Van Eerdeweigh M, Fishman R, Hirschfeld RMA, Klerman GL. The familial transmission of bipolar illness. *Arch Gen Psychiatry.* 1987;44:441-447.
60. LeBoyer M, Maier W, Teherani M, Lichtermann D, D'Amato T, Franke P, Lepine J, Minges J, McGuffin P. The reliability of the SADS-LA in a family study setting. *Eur Arch Psychiatry Clin Neurosci.* 1991;241:165-169.
61. Williams JBW, Gibbon M, First MB, Spitzer RL, Davies M, Borus J, Howes MJ, Kane J, Poper HG, Rousaville B, Wittchen H. The Structured Clinical Interview for *DSM-III-R* (SCID), II: multisite test-retest reliability. *Arch Gen Psychiatry.* 1992; 49:630-636.

UNITED STATES POSTAL SERVICE™

Statement of Ownership, Management, and Circulat
(Required by 39 U.S.C.

1. Publication Title: Archives of General Psychiatry
2. Publication No.: 0 2 9 - 6 4 0
3. Filing Date: 9-30-94
4. Issue Frequency: Monthly
5. No. of Issues Published Annually: 12
6. Annual Subscription Price: $90.00
7. Complete Mailing Address of Known Office of Publication *(Street, City, County, State, and ZIP+4) (Not Printer)*: 515 N. State Street, Chicago, Cook, IL 60610
8. Complete Mailing Address of Headquarters or General Business Office of Publisher *(Not Printer)*: 515 N. State Street, Chicago, Cook, IL 60610
9. Full Names and Complete Mailing Addresses of Publisher, Editor, and Managing Editor *(Do Not Leave Blank)*

Publisher *(Name and Complete Mailing Address)*: American Medical Association, 515 N. State Street, Chicago, IL 60610

Editor *(Name and Complete Mailing Address)*: Jack D. Barchas, M.D., 515 N. State Street, Chicago, IL 60610

Managing Editor *(Name and Complete Mailing Address)*: None

10. Owner *(If owned by a corporation, its name and address must be stated and also immediately thereafter the names and addresses of stockholders ow or holding 1 percent or more of the total amount of stock. If not owned by a corporation, the names and addresses of the individual owners must be gi owned by a partnership or other unincorporated firm, its name and address as well as that of each individual must be given. If the publication is publis by a nonprofit organization, its name and address must be stated.) (Do Not Leave Blank.)*

Full Name	Complete Mailing Address
American Medical Association	515 N. State Street, Chicago, IL 60610

11. Known Bondholders, Mortgagees, and Other Security Holders Owning or Holding 1 Percent or More of Total Amount of Bonds, Mortgages, or Other Securities. If none, check here. ☒ None

Full Name	Complete Mailing Address
None	

12. For completion by nonprofit organizations authorized to mail at special rates. The purpose, function, and nonprofit status of this organization and the e status for federal income tax purposes: *(Check one)*
☒ Has Not Changed During Preceding 12 Months
☐ Has Changed During Preceding 12 Months
(If changed, publisher must submit explanation of change with this statement)

PS Form **3526**, October 1994 *(See Instructions on Reverse)*

13. Publication Name: Archives of General Psychiatry
14. Issue Date for Circulation Data Below: 9/94

15. Extent and Nature of Circulation	Average No. Copies Each Issue During Preceding 12 Months	Actual No. Copies of Single Is Published Nearest to Filing D
a. Total No. Copies *(Net Press Run)*	10/93-9/94 31,220	31,273
b. Paid and/or Requested Circulation (1) Sales Through Dealers and Carriers, Street Vendors, and Counter Sales *(Not Mailed)*	575	575
(2) Paid or Requested Mail Subscriptions *(Include Advertisers' Proof Copies/Exchange Copies)*	28,131	27,851
c. Total Paid and/or Requested Circulation *(Sum of 15b(1) and 15b(2))*	28,706	28,426
d. Free Distribution by Mail *(Samples, Complimentary, and Other Free)*	0	0
e. Free Distribution Outside the Mail *(Carriers or Other Means)*	0	0
f. Total Free Distribution *(Sum of 15d and 15e)*	0	0
g. Total Distribution *(Sum of 15c and 15f)*	28,706	28,426
h. Copies Not Distributed (1) Office Use, Leftovers, Spoiled	2,514	2,847
(2) Return from News Agents	0	0
i. Total *(Sum of 15g, 15h(1), and 15h(2))*	31,220	31,273
Percent Paid and/or Requested Circulation *(15c / 15g x 100)*	100%	100%

16. This Statement of Ownership will be printed in the 11/94 issue of this publication. ☐ Check box if not required to publish.
17. Signature and Title of Editor, Publisher, Business Manager, or Owner: V.P. - Publishing Date: October 11, 1994

I certify that all information furnished on this form is true and complete. I understand that anyone who furnishes false or misleading information on this form who omits material or information requested on the form may be subject to criminal sanctions *(including fines and imprisonment)* and/or civil sanctions *(including multiple damages and civil penalties).*

Instructions to Publishers

1. Complete and file one copy of this form with your postmaster on or before October 1, annually. Keep a copy of the completed form for your records.
2. Include in items 10 and 11, in cases where the stockholder or security holder is a trustee, the name of the person or corporation for wh the trustee is acting. Also include the names and addresses of individuals who are stockholders who own or hold 1 percent or more of total amount of bonds, mortgages, or other securities of the publishing corporation. In item 11, if none, check box. Use blank sheets if more space is required.
3. Be sure to furnish all information called for in item 15, regarding circulation. Free circulation must be shown in items 15d, e, and f.
4. If the publication had second-class authorization as a general or requester publication, this Statement of Ownership, Management, and Circulation must be published; it must be printed in any issue in October or the first printed issue after October, if the publication is not published during October.
5. In item 16, indicate date of the issue in which this Statement of Ownership will be printed.
6. Item 17 must be signed.

Failure to file or publish a statement of ownership may lead to suspension of second-class authorization.

PS Form **3526**, October 1994 *(Reverse)*

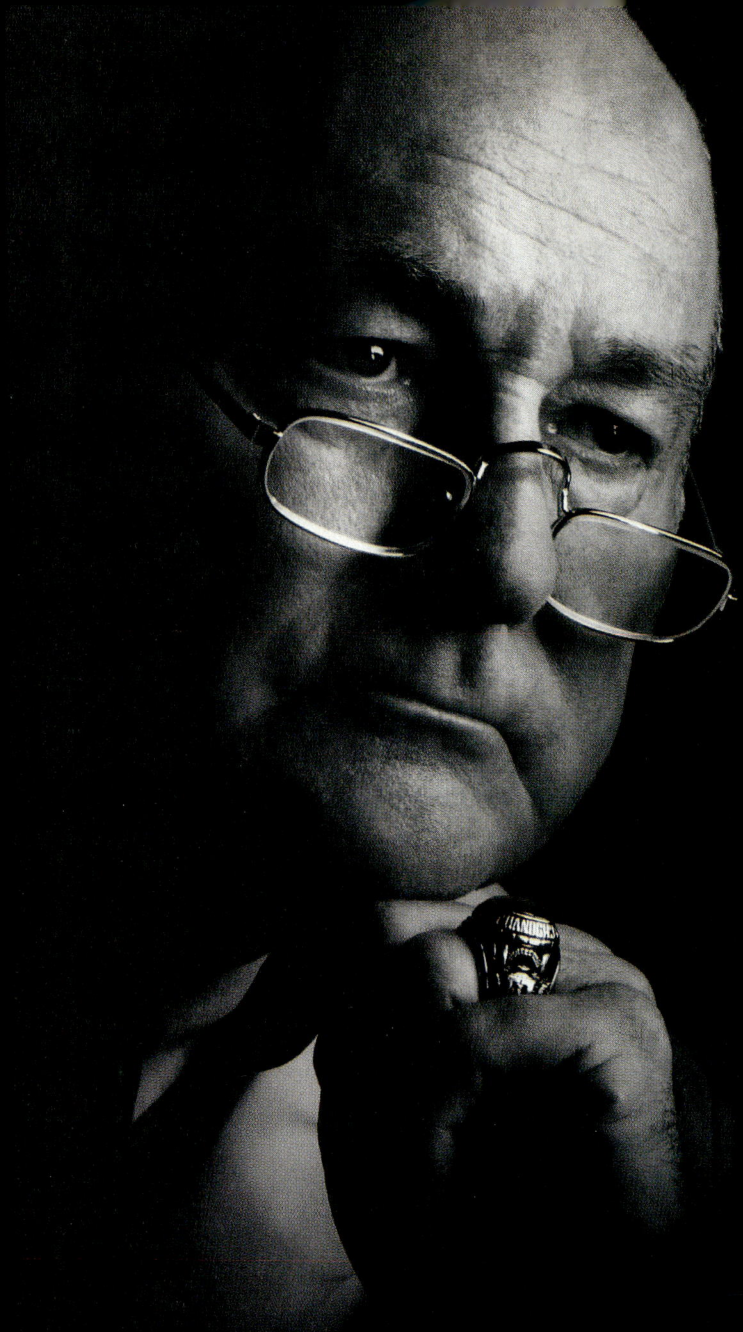

LITHOBID®

(Lithium Carbonate, USP)
Slow-Release Tablets, 300 mg

There Is No Substitute For Confidence

BRIEF SUMMARY:

The following is a brief summary only. Before prescribing, see complete prescribing information in LITHOBID® Slow-Release Tablets product labeling.

WARNING

Lithium toxicity is closely related to serum lithium levels, and can occur at doses close to therapeutic levels. Facilities for prompt and accurate serum lithium determinations should be available before initiating therapy. (See DOSAGE AND ADMINISTRATION in Full Prescribing Information.)

INDICATIONS:

Lithium is indicated in the treatment of manic episodes of manic-depressive illness. Maintenance therapy prevents or diminishes the intensity of subsequent episodes in those manic-depressive patients with a history of mania.

Typical symptoms: of mania include pressure of speech, motor hyperactivity, reduced need for sleep, flight of ideas, grandiosity, elation, poor judgment, aggressiveness, and possibly hostility. When given to a patient experiencing a manic episode, lithium may produce a normalization of symptomatology within 1 to 3 weeks.

WARNINGS:

Lithium should generally not be given to patients with significant renal or cardiovascular disease, severe debilitation, dehydration, sodium depletion, and to patients receiving diuretics, or angiotensin converting enzyme (ACE) inhibitors, since the risk of lithium toxicity is very high in such patients. If the psychiatric indication is life threatening, and if such a patient fails to respond to other measures, lithium treatment may be undertaken with extreme caution, including daily serum lithium determinations and adjustment to the usually low doses ordinarily tolerated by these individuals. In such instances, hospitalization is a necessity.

Chronic lithium therapy may be associated with diminution of renal concentrating ability, occasionally presenting as nephrogenic diabetes insipidus, with polyuria and polydipsia. Such patients should be carefully managed to avoid dehydration with resulting lithium retention and toxicity. This condition is usually reversible when lithium is discontinued.

Morphologic changes with glomerular and interstitial fibrosis and nephron atrophy have been reported in patients on chronic lithium therapy. Morphologic changes have also been seen in manic-depressive patients never exposed to lithium. The relationship between renal function and morphologic changes and their association with lithium therapy have not been established.

Kidney function should be assessed prior to and during lithium therapy. Routine urinalysis and other tests may be used to evaluate tubular function (e.g., urine specific gravity or osmolality following a period of water deprivation, or 24-hour urine volume) and glomerular function (e.g., serum creatinine or creatinine clearance). During lithium therapy, progressive or sudden changes in renal function, even within the normal range, indicate the need for reevaluation of treatment.

An encephalopathic syndrome (characterized by weakness, lethargy, fever, tremulousness and confusion, extrapyramidal symptoms, leukocytosis, elevated serum enzymes, BUN and FBS) has occurred in a few patients treated with lithium plus a neuroleptic, most notably haloperidol. In some instances, the syndrome was followed by irreversible brain damage. Because of possible causal relationship between these events and the concomitant administration of lithium and neuroleptic drugs, patients receiving such combined therapy or patients with organic brain syndrome or other CNS impairment should be monitored closely for early evidence of neurologic toxicity and treatment discontinued promptly if such signs appear. This encephalopathic syndrome may be similar to or the same as Neuroleptic Malignant Syndrome (NMS).

Lithium toxicity is closely related to serum lithium concentrations and can occur at doses close to the therapeutic concentrations. (See DOSAGE AND ADMINISTRATION in Full Prescribing Information.)

Outpatients and their families should be warned that the patient must discontinue lithium therapy and contact his physician if such clinical signs of lithium toxicity as diarrhea, vomiting, tremor, mild ataxia, drowsiness, or muscular weakness occur.

Lithium may prolong the effects of neuromuscular blocking agents. Therefore, neuromuscular blocking agents should be given with caution to patients receiving lithium.

Usage in Pregnancy: Adverse effects on nidation in rats, embryo viability in mice, and metabolism in vitro of rat testis and human spermatozoa have been attributed to lithium, as have teratogenicity in submammalian species and cleft palate in mice.

In humans, lithium may cause fetal harm when administered to a pregnant woman. Data from lithium birth registries suggest an increase in cardiac and other anomalies, especially Ebstein's anomaly. If this drug is used in women of childbearing potential, or during pregnancy, or if a patient becomes pregnant while taking this drug, the patient should be apprised by their physician of the potential hazard to the fetus.

Usage in Nursing Mothers: Lithium is excreted in human milk. Nursing should not be undertaken during lithium therapy except in rare and unusual circumstances where, in the view of the physician, the potential benefits to the mother outweigh possible hazard to the child. Signs and symptoms of lithium toxicity such as hypertonia, hypothermia, cyanosis and ECG changes have been reported in some infants.

Usage in Children: Since the safety and effectiveness of lithium in children under 12 years of age has not been established, its use in such patients is not recommended at this time.

There has been a report of transient syndrome of acute dystonia and hyperreflexia occurring in a 15 kg child who ingested 300 mg of lithium carbonate.

PRECAUTIONS:

The ability to tolerate lithium is greater during the acute manic phase and decreases when manic symptoms subside. (See DOSAGE AND ADMINISTRATION in Full Prescribing Information.)

The distribution space of lithium approximates that of total body water. Lithium is primarily excreted in urine with insignificant excretion in feces. Renal excretion of lithium is proportional to its plasma concentration. The elimination half-life of lithium is approximately 24 hours. Lithium decreases sodium reabsorption by the renal tubules which could lead to sodium depletion. Therefore, it is essential for the patient to maintain a normal diet, including salt, and an adequate fluid intake (2500-3500 mL) at least during the initial stabilization period. Decreased tolerance to lithium has been reported to ensue from protracted sweating or diarrhea and, if such occur, supplemental fluid and salt should be administered under careful medical supervision and lithium intake reduced or suspended until the condition is resolved.

In addition to sweating and diarrhea, concomitant infection with elevated temperatures may also necessitate a temporary reduction or cessation of medication.

Previously existing thyroid disorders do not necessarily constitute a contraindication to lithium treatment. Where hypothyroidism preexists, careful monitoring of thyroid function during lithium stabilization and maintenance allows for correction of changing thyroid parameters and/or adjustment of lithium doses, if any. If hypothyroidism occurs during lithium stabilization and maintenance, supplemental thyroid treatment may be used.

In general, the concomitant use of diuretics or angiotensin converting enzyme (ACE) inhibitors with lithium carbonate should be avoided. In those cases where concomitant use is necessary, extreme caution is advised since sodium loss from these drugs may reduce the renal clearance of lithium resulting in increased serum lithium concentrations with the risk of lithium toxicity. When such combinations are used, the lithium dosage may need to be decreased, and more frequent monitoring of lithium serum concentrations is recommended. (See WARNINGS for additional caution information.)

Concomitant administration of carbamazepine and lithium may increase the risk of neurotoxic side effects.

The following drugs can lower serum lithium concentrations by increasing urinary lithium excretion: acetazolamide, urea, xanthine preparations and alkalinizing agents such as sodium bicarbonate.

Concomitant extended use of iodide preparations, especially potassium iodide, with lithium may produce hypothyroidism. Indomethacin and piroxicam have been reported to significantly increase steady state serum lithium concentrations. In some cases lithium toxicity has resulted from such interactions. There is also some evidence that other nonsteroidal, anti-inflammatory agents may have a similar effect. When such combinations are used, increased serum lithium concentrations monitoring is recommended.

Concurrent use of calcium channel blocking agents with lithium may increase the risk of neurotoxicity in the form of ataxia, tremors, nausea, vomiting, diarrhea and/or tinnitus. Concurrent use of metronidazole with lithium may provoke lithium toxicity due to reduced renal clearance. Patients receiving such combined therapy should be monitored closely.

Concurrent use of fluoxetine with lithium has resulted in both increased and decreased serum lithium concentrations. Patients receiving such combined therapy should be monitored closely.

Lithium may impair mental and/or physical abilities. Patients should be cautioned about activities requiring alertness (e.g., operating vehicles or machinery).

Usage in Pregnancy: Pregnancy Category D (see WARNINGS).

Usage in Nursing Mothers: Because of the potential for serious adverse reactions in nursing infants from lithium, a decision should be made whether to discontinue nursing or to discontinue the drug, taking into account the importance of the drug to the mother (see WARNINGS).

Usage in Children: Safety and effectiveness in children below the age of 12 have not been established (see WARNINGS).

Usage in the Elderly: Elderly patients often require lower lithium dosages to achieve therapeutic serum concentrations. They may also exhibit adverse reactions at serum concentrations ordinarily tolerated by younger patients. Additionally, patients with renal impairment may also require lower lithium doses (see WARNINGS).

ADVERSE REACTIONS:

The occurrence and severity of adverse reactions are generally directly related to serum lithium concentrations and to individual patient sensitivity to lithium. They generally occur more frequently and with greater severity at higher concentrations.

Adverse reactions may be encountered at serum lithium concentrations below 1.5 mEq/L. Mild to moderate adverse reactions may occur at concentrations from 1.5-2.5 mEq/L, and moderate to severe reactions may be seen at concentrations from 2.0 mEq/L and above.

Fine hand tremor, polyuria and mild thirst may occur during initial therapy for the acute manic phase, and may persist throughout treatment. Transient and mild nausea and general discomfort may also appear during the first few days of lithium administration.

These side effects usually subside with continued treatment or with a temporary reduction or cessation of dosage. If persistent, a cessation of lithium therapy may be required. Diarrhea, vomiting, drowsiness, muscular weakness and lack of coordination may be early signs of lithium intoxication, and can occur at lithium concentrations below 2.0 mEq/L. At higher concentrations giddiness, ataxia, blurred vision, tinnitus and a large output of dilute urine may be seen. Serum lithium concentrations above 3.0 mEq/L may produce a complex clinical picture involving multiple organs and organ systems. Serum lithium concentrations should not be permitted to exceed 2.0 mEq/L during the acute treatment phase.

The following reactions have been reported and appear to be related to serum lithium concentrations, including concentrations within the therapeutic range:

Central Nervous System: tremor, muscle hyperirritability (fasiculations, twitching, clonic movements of whole limbs), hypertonicity, ataxia, choreoathetotic movements, hyperactive deep tendon reflex, extrapyramidal symptoms including acute dystonia, cogwheel rigidity, blackout spells, epileptiform seizures, slurred speech, dizziness, vertigo, downbeat nystagmus, incontinence of urine or feces, somnolence, psychomotor retardation, restlessness, confusion, stupor, coma, tongue movements, tics, tinnitus, hallucinations, poor memory, slowed intellectual functioning, startle response, worsening of organic brain syndromes. Cases of Pseudotumor Cerebri (increased intracranial pressure and papilledema) have been reported with lithium use. If undetected, this condition may result in enlargement of the blind spot, constriction of visual fields and eventual blindness due to optic atrophy. Lithium should be discontinued, if clinically possible, if this syndrome occurs. **Cardiovascular:** cardiac arrhythmia, hypotension, peripheral circulatory collapse, bradycardia, sinus node dysfunction with severe bradycardia (which may result in syncope); **Gastrointestinal:** anorexia, nausea, vomiting, diarrhea, gastritis, salivary gland swelling, abdominal pain, excessive salivation, flatulence, indigestion; **Genitourinary:** glycosuria, decreased creatinine clearance, albuminuria, oliguria, and symptoms of nephrogenic diabetes insipidus including polyuria, thirst and polydipsia; **Dermatologic:** drying and thinning of hair, alopecia, anesthesia of skin, acne, chronic folliculitis, xerosis cutis, psoriasis or its exacerbation, generalized pruritus with or without rash, cutaneous ulcers, angioedema; **Autonomic Nervous System:** blurred vision, dry mouth, impotence/sexual dysfunction; **Thyroid Abnormalities:** euthyroid goiter and/or hypothyroidism (including myxedema) accompanied by lower T_3 and T_4. ^{131}Iodine uptake may be elevated (see PRECAUTIONS). Paradoxically, rare cases of hyperthyroidism have been reported. **EEG Changes:** diffuse slowing, widening of frequency spectrum, potentiation and disorganization of background rhythm. **EKG Changes:** reversible flattening, isoelectricity or inversion of T-waves. **Miscellaneous:** Fatigue, lethargy, transient scotomata, exophthalmos, dehydration, weight loss, leucocytosis, headache, transient hyperglycemia, hypercalcemia, hyperparathyroidism, albuminuria, excessive weight gain, edematous swelling of ankles or wrists, metallic taste, dysgeusia/taste distortion, salty taste, thirst, swollen lips, tightness in chest, swollen and/or painful joints, fever, polyarthralgia, and dental caries.

Some reports of nephrogenic diabetes insipidus, hyperparathyroidism and hypothyroidism which persist after lithium discontinuation have been received.

A few reports have been received of the development of painful discoloration of fingers and toes and coldness of the extremities within one day of starting lithium treatment. The mechanism through which these symptoms (resembling Raynaud's Syndrome) developed is not known. Recovery followed discontinuance.

OVERDOSAGE:

The toxic concentrations for lithium (≥1.5 mEq/L) are close to the therapeutic concentrations (0.6-1.2 mEq/L). It is therefore important that patients and their families be cautioned to watch for early toxic symptoms and to discontinue the drug and inform the physician should they occur. (Toxic symptoms are listed in detail under ADVERSE REACTIONS.)

Treatment: No specific antidote for lithium poisoning is known. Treatment is supportive. Early symptoms of lithium toxicity can usually be treated by reduction or cessation of dosage of the drug and resumption of the treatment at a lower dose after 24 to 48 hours. In severe cases of lithium poisoning, the first and foremost goal of treatment consists of elimination of this ion from the patient.

Treatment is essentially the same as that used in barbiturate poisoning: 1) gastric lavage, 2) correction of fluid and electrolyte imbalance and 3) regulation of kidney functioning. Urea, mannitol, and aminophylline all produce significant increases in lithium excretion. Hemodialysis is an effective and rapid means of removing the ion from the severely toxic patient. However, patient recovery may be slow.

Infection prophylaxis, regular chest X-rays, and preservation of adequate respiration are essential.

SOLVAY PHARMACEUTICALS
Marietta, GA 30062

20E0803 Rev 7/94

REFERENCES:

1. Data on file, Solvay Pharmaceuticals. 2. Kirkwood CK, Wilson SK, Hayes PE, et al. Single-dose bioavailability of two extended-release lithium carbonate products. *Am J Hosp Pharm.* February 1994;51:486-489. 3. Cooper TB, Simpson GM, Lee JH, Bergner P-EE. Evaluation of slow-release lithium carbonate formulation. *Am J Psychiatry.* August 1978;135(8):917-922. 4. Grof P, MacCrimmon D, Saxena B, et al. Bioavailability and side effects of different lithium carbonate products. *Neuropsychobiology.* 1976;2:313-323. 5. Shaw DM, Hewland R, Johnson AL, et al. Comparison of serum levels of two sustained-release preparations of lithium carbonate. *Curr Med Res Opin.* 1974;2:90-94.

SOLVAY PHARMACEUTICALS
901 Sawyer Road
Marietta, Georgia 30062

S&R0296 October 1994

COMMENT

The Diagnostic Interview for Genetic Studies

THE GOOD news is that we are probably at the brink of a revolution in our understanding of the genetics of the major psychiatric disorders. The bad news is that the steps we must take in getting there will not always be pretty or easy. We must recognize that this research enterprise is inherently a bootstrapping operation that will have to make the best of a useful but imperfect diagnostic system. Under optimal conditions, genetic studies are aimed at disorders with clear-cut diagnostic markers. Unfortunately, our classification of mental disorders is based on the definition of their descriptive characteristics and is largely uninformed by an understanding of underlying pathogenesis. For the most part, we lack diagnostic tests with sufficient sensitivity and specificity to be of much use in clinical practice or research investigations. What this means is that genetic studies of the psychiatric disorders must sort out the noise introduced by the limited level of accuracy provided by our diagnostic system. We will have to make the best of the cards we can play at this stage of our knowledge and be thankful that at least we can diagnose more or less reliably even if we are not always confident about validity. We must hope that an interactive back-and-forth process between our limited current methods and emerging new findings will gradually allow the diagnostic system to inform and be informed by advances in our understanding.

The Diagnostic Interview for Genetic Studies (DIGS) reported by Nurnberger et al[1] in this issue of the ARCHIVES will help a great deal in this bootstrapping operation. It offers many advantages over other available methods of diagnostic assessment. The DIGS is especially comprehensive and includes questions that are derived not only from the most important current diagnostic methods but also from earlier methods. Such comprehensiveness has two virtues. First, it increases the likelihood that possibly important items will not be overlooked. There is no reason to believe that any of the available diagnostic systems has any monopoly on diagnostic validity, and the more data gathered the more likely we are to find important relationships. Second, the DIGS provides an opportunity for comparability across data sets, which is crucial if we are to get as much leverage as possible from the information that has been, and is being, gathered using different systems.

A second advantage of the DIGS is that it can be scored quantitatively (by symptom dimension score) as well as qualitatively (by categorical syndromal diagnosis). This is important because our descriptive syndromal system has great limitations in dealing with the frequently encountered boundary cases that do not fall neatly within a given category (eg, schizoaffective disorder) or that may possibly represent an incomplete spectrum penetrance of what in more severe and characteristic form would be the classic presentation of the disorder (eg, schizotypal personality disorder). Boundary cases cannot be discarded in genetic studies because the information they offer may be crucial in understanding patterns of transmission. Unfortunately, however, boundary cases also provide great potential noise in genetic studies because we have no way to be certain on descriptive grounds alone what sorts best with what. This is illustrated by the sad state of the diagnosis of schizoaffective disorder. One possible way out of the quagmire caused by the fuzzy-set nature of categorical psychiatric diagnosis is to assess and analyze psychopathology by dimensions as well as by categories. Dimensional systems save information, are more accurate in labeling boundary cases, and avoid the need for a priori assumptions concerning spectrum relationships.

See also page 849

A third advantage of the DIGS is its careful attention to the substance-induced forms of psychopathology. This is especially important because substances (both drugs of abuse and prescribed medication) are increasingly implicated as a cause of psychopathological symptoms. Whenever a substance etiology is ignored and the condition is incorrectly considered to be primary, misleading information is introduced into the genetic modeling because of the elevated rates of false positives.

The DIGS is also to be commended for its emphasis on clinical observation and judgment. The items written as criteria in the various diagnostic systems do not generally diagnose themselves. Patient self-report is fallible and likely to be subject to either the false-positive overinterpretation of the clinical significance of some symptoms or the false-negative denial of others. While clinical

judgment also is of course fallible, it does remove some noise from the system and increases the likelihood of accurate descriptive diagnosis. The additional provision of an algorithmic scoring system increases the convenience of using the DIGS and also reduces the risk of clinician halo effects in sorting symptoms into categories. It also will be useful to compare results derived from clinician vs algorithmic diagnosis.

Finally, it is reassuring that the DIGS has undergone a careful process of reliability testing. Most important, and unfortunately unusual, was the fairly extensive cross-site rater reliability study reported in the article.[1] Many studies test only the within-site reliabilities, which are much easier to achieve and maintain owing to the development of local cultures and common diagnostic habits. It is much more difficult to maintain reliability among raters who do not work together every day. The DIGS is off to an excellent start in achieving acceptable cross-site reliability. It will be particularly useful to determine whether the cross-site reliability remains high over time or whether there is drift as the study progresses and particularly as the initial raters are replaced.

In summary, then, the DIGS is an important and welcome methodological step forward that will greatly facilitate studies on the genetics of psychiatric disorders. It provides a thorough and well-tested assessment and communication tool for descriptive diagnosis that is compatible with a number of different diagnostic instruments. The DIGS represents the state of our current descriptive diagnostic art that desperately needs to be informed by a more basic understanding of pathogenesis. The limitations of the DIGS are the limitations of our current diagnostic accuracy. The diagnostic system is imperfectly reliable, and especially so when it most counts in the diagnosis of boundary cases (eg, schizoaffective disorder). Even if it were perfectly reliable, however, any descriptive system without proven validity and accurate diagnostic markers would remain extremely problematic. In nature, different underlying causes frequently have similar phenotypes. This also will almost certainly be the case for psychiatric disorders. There is no reason to expect a single genetic answer for each descriptive category, given that each of the categories is likely to be a final common pathway for a heterogeneous array of different causes. Currently, we have no way to classify except by descriptive similarity. This is indeed a primitive, but necessary, means. Progress will come from using the hypotheses that are represented in the diagnostic system to learn more about the causes of disorders. This will lead us to more refined hypotheses embodied in more specifically defined diagnostic categories that will facilitate even clearer answers and so forth. We must, however, be patient and cautious in interpreting early findings.

Allen Frances, MD
Department of Psychiatry
Duke University Medical Center
Box 3950
Durham, NC 27710

Accepted for publication August 22, 1994.

REFERENCE

1. Nurnberger JI Jr, Blehar MC, Kaufmann CA, York-Cooler C, Simpson SG, Harkavy-Friedman J, Severe JB, Malaspina D, Reich T, the NIMH Genetics Initiative. Diagnostic Interview for Genetic Studies: rationale, development, training, and reliability. *Arch Gen Psychiatry.* 1994;51:849-859.

Correction

Error in Reported Data. In the article "A Multicenter Investigation of Fixed-Dose Fluoxetine in the Treatment of Obsessive-compulsive Disorder" published in the July 1994 issue of the ARCHIVES (1994;51:559-567), an error appears in the "Results" section on page 563. Under the "Safety" heading in the right-hand column, six lines from the top, the numbers in parentheses should read "(3.45%, 3/87)."

ORIGINAL ARTICLE

Serotonin and the Neurobiology of Depression

Effects of Tryptophan Depletion in Drug-Free Depressed Patients

Pedro L. Delgado, MD; Lawrence H. Price, MD; Helen L. Miller, MD; Ronald M. Salomon, MD; George K. Aghajanian, MD; George R. Heninger, MD; Dennis S. Charney, MD

Objective: To investigate the effects of tryptophan depletion in untreated depressed patients. Rapid dietary depletion of the precursor of serotonin synthesis, tryptophan, causes a transient return of depression in 67% of patients who have had a therapeutic antidepressant response.

Method: Forty-three untreated depressed patients underwent tryptophan depletion in a double-blind, placebo-controlled cross-over study. After testing, they received open sequential antidepressant treatment.

Results: Mood did not change when tryptophan was depleted but did change on the day after the depletion test. Relative to the control test, 37% of the patients had 10-point or greater *decrease* in Hamilton Depression Rating Scale (Ham-D) score, while 23% had a 10-point or greater *increase* in Ham-D score on the day after the tryptophan depletion test. Change in mood was correlated to treatment response after testing. Patients whose condition worsened proved to be highly refractory to treatment while those who showed improvment were more likely to respond.

Conclusions: That tryptophan depletion did not rapidly worsen depression argues that serotonin function is not linearly related to the level of depression and if reduced serotonin function does cause depression, then it is either as predisposing factor or due to a postsynaptic deficit in the utilization of serotonin.

(Arch Gen Psychiatry. 1994;51:865-874)

THE NEUROBIOLOGY of depression remains poorly understood. Recent focus has been on a dysfunction within the serotonin (5-HT) system leading to a decreased level of 5-HT neurotransmission.[1,2] The original 5-HT hypothesis of depression[3-5] proposes decreased presynaptic function in 5-HT neurons similar to reduced dopamine function in Parkinson's disease. Failure to identify decreased brain levels of 5-HT shifted attention to postsynaptic dysfunction, suggesting that postsynaptic neurons were not able to respond to normal 5-HT levels.[6] A model for this hypothesis might be insulin-resistant diabetes.

Investigations of brain 5-HT function in drug-free depressed patients do not consistently support one particular hypothesis of the pathophysiology of depression.[7,8] Findings of lower plasma tryptophan (TRP) levels,[9,10] reduced cerebrospinal fluid 5-hydroxyindoleacetic acid levels,[11,12] and decreased platelet 5-HT uptake[13,14] support presynaptic 5-HT dysfunction. Less conclusive data could support either a presynaptic or postsynaptic dysfunction. These data include increased 5-HT_2 receptors in the brains of suicide victims[15-18]; the blunted prolactin responses to TRP infusion,[19-22] fenfluramine hydrochloride,[23,24] and clomipramine hydrochloride administration[25]; and the preliminary reports of a blunted hypothermic response to the 5-HT_{1A} partial agonist ipsapirone hydrochloride.[26,27]

The presynaptic dysfunction hypotheses would generally predict that decreasing brain 5-HT content should worsen depression in depressed patients. The postsynaptic dysfunction hypotheses would tend to predict that decreasing 5-HT function would have less of an effect on mood because postsynaptic cells might be less responsive to 5-HT anyway.

We attempted to assess the 5-HT hypothesis of depression and antidepressant action directly by using rapid TRP depletion to transiently decrease the central ner-

See Subjects and Methods on next page

From the Department of Psychiatry, Yale University School of Medicine, New Haven, Conn (Drs Delgado, Price, Miller, Salomon, Aghajanian, Heninger, and Charney); the Department of Veterans Affairs Medical Center, Psychiatry Service 116A1, West Haven, Conn (Drs Delgado, Miller, Salomon, and Charney); and the Connecticut Mental Health Center, New Haven (Drs Price, Aghajanian, and Heninger). Dr Delgado is now with the Department of Psychiatry, University of Arizona College of Medicine, Tucson.

SUBJECTS AND METHODS

SUBJECTS

Fifty drug-free depressed patients (31 inpatient, 19 outpatient; 26 female, 24 male; aged 23 to 69 years) gave written informed consent to participate in a research study of the behavioral effects of TRP depletion. A summary of some of the findings contained herein have been presented in abstract form and published in a preliminary report.[40] Fifteen of the 50 patients in the present sample were again tested after having had therapeutic responses to antidepressant treatment. The findings in these 15 patients have been published previously.[39]

Complete medical and neurologic evaluations revealed each patient to be free of medical or neurologic illness. Patients with a history of substantial substance abuse were excluded from the study. Admission criteria included a diagnosis of major depressive episode[41] and a minimum score of 21 on the 25-item modified Hamilton Depression Rating Scale (Ham-D).[42] Diagnoses were made on admission to the study by consensus of the authors using *DSM-III-R* criteria.[41] Diagnoses were based on direct interview with use of the Yale Depression Inventory[42] and review of medical records.

Demographic and clinical information regarding previous antidepressant treatment and response were obtained by two of us (P.L.D. and L.H.P.) during a clinical interview on admission to the study. The number of unsuccessful antidepressant trials before admission was determined by consensus of the authors based on patient report, review of medical records, and direct contact with previous clinicians. A previously unsuccessful antidepressant trial was defined as follows: (1) failure to return to the premorbid level of functioning, (2) insufficient improvement to permit discharge from the short-term treatment setting, *or* (3) need for a major medication change within 4 weeks of discharge from acute treatment *and* at least 4 weeks of treatment with either a therapeutic blood level[43] or an adequate dose (≥300 mg/d of imipramine hydrochloride or its equivalent) of an antidepressant. To count only true previous antidepressant treatment failures, previous antidepressant trials in which an adequate dose was not achieved or in which there was less than a 4-week treatment period at an adequate dose were not counted.

Information regarding specific antidepressant treatments used and responses after TRP depletion testing were obtained from our treatment records by a research assistant who was blinded to the results of the TRP depletion testing. The number of antidepressant trials that failed during the treatment phase in the research program and the status of the patient at the time of discharge (treatment responders, partial responders, and nonresponders) were based on the criteria specified below for treatment response. For this purpose, the mean of the last two Ham-D ratings for a patient compared with baseline scores while drug free (before TRP depletion testing) was used.

Before a patient is discharged from our research program as a treatment nonresponder, he or she is usually offered trials of at least one tricyclic antidepressant drug, a selective 5-HT reuptake inhibitor, a monoamine oxidase inhibitor, and lithium augmentation of one or all of the previous antidepressant drugs. Electroconvulsive therapy is available but not routinely used. Weekly ratings of mood are obtained during sequential antidepressant treatment.

As in previous studies by our group,[39,44] treatment responders were defined as meeting criteria of (1) sufficient improvement in global functioning, by consensus of patient, treating staff, and family, to warrant discharge from the short-term treatment setting, and (2) a 50% or greater improvement on the Ham-D, with a total score of 17 or lower following at least 4 weeks of antidepressant treatment with either a therapeutic blood level[43] or an adequate dose (≥300 mg/d of imipramine hydrochloride or its equivalent) of an antidepressant drug. Partial responders were defined as having met criterion 1 but not criterion 2. All other subjects were nonresponders.

Seven patients did not complete the testing phase of the protocol and were therefore dropped from the study. These included three men and four women, all of whom were inpatients. Two of these patients were unable to tolerate the procedure, and the remaining five completed the procedure but could not be rated on at least one of the rating days before or after the testing.

PROCEDURE

The experiment was conducted in a double-blind, placebo-controlled, balanced cross-over fashion. The TRP depletion test consisted of a 24-hour, 160-mg/d TRP diet (day 1) with blue placebo capsules taken three times daily, followed the next morning by a TRP-free, 15–amino acid drink (day 2). Control testing consisted of a 24-hour, 160-mg/d TRP diet supplemented with blue capsules containing 500 mg of L-TRP taken three times daily, followed the next morning by a 16–amino acid drink containing 2.3 g of L-TRP. Testing occurred after a minimum of 2 weeks drug free. All patients were rated again between 11 AM and 1 PM on the day after the TRP depletion or control test (day after testing). The depletion procedure was as follows: patients received 500 mg of L-TRP orally on the evening of day 2 and 500 mg of L-TRP orally three times a day on the day after testing (after both the control and TRP depletion tests).

The low-TRP diet[39] (diet available on request) consisted of food chosen in consultation with the research dietitians of Yale–New Haven (Conn) Hospital to provide an adequate protein (48 g/d) and energy intake (10 500 J/d) but containing the minimum possible amount of TRP (160 mg/d). Inpatients ate the low-TRP diet food at their regular meal times (8 AM, noon, and 5 PM) and outpatients were allowed to take the diet food home with them. Patients were

vous system 5-HT content in drug-free and antidepressant-treated patients. The TRP depletion paradigm is based on preclinical literature suggesting that dietary depletion of the precursor of 5-HT, TRP, specifically reduces brain 5-HT function.[28-32] Ingestion of TRP-free amino acid mixtures in vervet monkeys decreases plasma TRP and cerebrospinal fluid TRP and 5-hydroxyindoleacetic acid levels, with no change in cerbrospinal fluid tyrosine, homovanillic acid, or methoxy-4-hydroxyphenylethylene glycol levels.[31] Ingestion of TRP-free amino acid mixtures in laboratory animals leads to extremely rapid changes in both plasma TRP and brain 5-HT levels, with maximal reductions of brain 5-HT levels occurring within 2 hours of ingestion of the TRP-free mixture.[31,32]

instructed to eat all of the food and were allowed to drink water, apple juice, coffee without milk or cream, and carbonated soft drinks.

The amino acid drink was composed of 15 amino acids with or without 2.3 g of L-TRP, as described by Young et al.[37] Because of the unpleasant taste of methionine, cysteine, and arginine, these amino acids were encapsulated, and patients took the capsules 15 minutes before drinking the remaining amino acids dissolved in water (300 mL) at room temperature and flavored with chocolate syrup. Patients drank the solution quickly through a straw. Patients returned to unrestricted dietary intake immediately following the completion of test day 2 (at 4 to 5 PM).

Patients were rated and plasma for free and total TRP levels was obtained at 9 AM before starting the diet (test day 1), 15 minutes before, and 5 and 7 hours after the drink (test day 2). Ratings were obtained again between 11 AM and 1 PM the day after each amino acid drink (the day after testing). Ratings were obtained by one of the investigators or by a trained nurse-clinician. Raters had established reliability on the rating instruments used (interrater reliability for Ham-D ranged from 88% to 95%) and were blinded to the sequence of placebo or active TRP supplementation. Whenever possible, ratings were obtained by the same rater throughout the testing.

On the day of each amino acid drink, patients were kept in a specialized procedure room. They were allowed to drink water and fruit juice but could not eat food for the 7-hour assessment period. Patients were allowed to go to the bathroom freely, but interaction with others was kept to a minimum. They were encouraged to try to read as they wished or to listen to the radio but were not allowed to watch television.

Behavioral rating scales consisted of the Ham-D, the Hamilton Anxiety Rating Scale (Ham-A),[45] and the Symptom Checklist.[46]

BIOCHEMICAL METHODS

Total plasma TRP concentration was assayed by high-performance liquid chromatography with flourometric detection.[47] Free plasma TRP concentration was assayed by obtaining the ultrafiltrate of plasma through a commercially available anisotropic, hydrophilic ultrafiltration membrane system (Amicon Co, Beverly, Mass) centrifuged (1000g) at room temperature and subjecting the ultrafiltrate to the high-performance liquid chromatography with fluorometric detection method.

DATA ANALYSIS

Change in plasma free and total TRP concentrations were assessed by analysis of variance (ANOVA) with repeated measures. This allowed an assessment of the main effects of test dose (control vs TRP depletion) and time (changes over the time points sampled). The interaction of test dose × time indicates the effect of the TRP depletion in the sample as a whole. Significant interactions revealed by ANOVA were further examined with paired *t* tests to determine when significant effects occurred and the magnitude of the changes.

Change in behavioral ratings (Ham-D, Ham-A, and Symptom Checklist) were also assessed by ANOVA with repeated measures (test dose, time, and test dose×time interaction). As with the plasma TRP analyses, when significant test dose×time interactions were observed, paired *t* tests were used to determine the time course and magnitude of the changes.

Change in depressive symptoms on the Ham-D was further assessed by categorization of the data in an attempt to define clinically meaningful changes in depression. The categories constructed were based on our clinical experience using the Ham-D. Change in depressive symptoms was categorized as much better (≥10-point decrease in total Ham-D score), better (5- to 9-point decrease), no change (0- to 4-point change), worse (5- to 9-point increase), or much worse (≥10-point increase in Ham-D score). The changes in Ham-D score were assessed across two points: *during* the TRP depletion (420-minute time point, day 2 score minus baseline score, day 2) and on *the day after* the depletion (day after rating minus the 420-minute time point rating, day 2). Because plasma TRP levels reach their minimum value 5 to 7 hours after the amino acid drink and then return toward baseline with refeeding and TRP supplementation, behavioral changes that occurred after testing were defined as those occurring between the 420–time point on day 2 and the next day rating. To control for nonspecific effects of the procedure, the change in Ham-D score during the control test was subtracted from the change in Ham-D score during the TRP depletion test at the two time points described above. Normality of these data was assessed using the Shapiro-Wilks test.[48]

The relationship of behavioral change during the TRP depletion testing to ultimate antidepressant treatment response was assessed by the interaction of treatment response grouping (responders, partial responders, and nonresponders) with test dose and time on an ANOVA with repeated measures. When significant group × dose × time interactions were encountered, the dose × time interactions for each group were calculated. Then, *t* tests were used to assess the time course and magnitude of changes in behavioral ratings.

Pearson's correlation coefficients were calculated to evaluate the relationship between plasma TRP levels and behavioral changes. Results were considered significant when $P \leq .05$. Trends are also reported when $P \leq .10$. All tests were two tailed. For data analysis and graphic presentation, we used SAS,[49] BMDP,[50] Statview 512+,[51] Super Anova,[52] and Cricket Graph[53] computer programs.

In healthy humans, TRP-free or low-TRP diets cause a reduction of plasma TRP levels.[33-36] Rapid plasma TRP depletion (by 70% to 80% within 5 hours following the TRP-free amino acid load) causes decreased concentration and an increased reporting of negative mood states in healthy male subjects.[37,38] While low-TRP diets reduce plasma TRP levels by restricting dietary intake of TRP, a TRP-free amino acid mixture rapidly depletes plasma TRP levels by inducing hepatic protein synthesis, using up plasma TRP stores in the anabolic process.[39]

A combination of a 24-hour, 160-mg/d, low-TRP diet followed the next day by a 15–amino acid, TRP-free drink administered in a double-blind, placebo-controlled, cross-

over fashion to antidepressant-treated depressed patients led to a transient depressive relapse in 67% of these patients.[39] Patients successfully treated with the selective norepinephrine reuptake inhibitor, desipramine hydrochloride, were less likely to relapse (only 20% relapse rate). Patients successfully treated with a selective 5-HT reuptake inhibitor or monoamine oxidase inhibitor were more likely to relapse (90% relapse rate).[39,40]

Herein, we describe the effects of rapid TRP depletion in drug-free depressed patients. We hypothesized that if decreased 5-HT function caused depressive symptoms, then rapid TRP depletion would lead to a transient worsening of mood in drug-free depressed patients. We further predicted that those patients whose condition worsened during the TRP depletion test might have a specific dysfunction of the 5-HT system and might therefore be more likely to have a therapeutic response to antidepressant drugs that directly increased 5-HT function.

RESULTS

CLINICAL CHARACTERISTICS

The present study group comprised a heterogeneous group of patients. Antidepressant treatment before admission included zero to seven treatment failures. The number of unsuccessful treatment trials following testing was also variable. These patients underwent a mean of 3.3 antidepressant trials after TRP depletion testing (range, 0 to 12). After participating in the testing phase and undergoing sequential antidepressant treatment, 10 patients were discharged as antidepressant nonresponders, 12 as partial responders, and 20 as antidepressant responders; one patient was discharged after an inadequate trial. As expected, treatment nonresponders were more likely to have had a larger number of failed adequate antidepressant trials during the treatment phase (mean±SD, 4.4±3.1) than antidepressant responders (2.5±1.5). Treatment nonresponders (five of 10) and partial responders (five of 12) were more likely to have been concomitantly diagnosed on admission as having a *DSM-III-R* personality disorder than were antidepressant responders (one of 20) (Fisher's Exact Test, P=.018).

EFFECT OF TESTING ON PLASMA FREE AND TOTAL TRP LEVELS

A 1-day low-TRP diet (160 mg/d of TRP) followed the next morning by a TRP-free amino acid drink led to a profound depletion of plasma total and free TRP within 5 hours following ingestion of the amino acid drink. A TRP-supplemented diet (1660 mg/d of TRP) followed by a TRP-supplemented (2.3 g of TRP) amino acid drink caused modest elevations of plasma free and total TRP levels. Baseline total and free TRP values were not significantly different between the TRP depletion (total TRP level, 55.4±14.5 μmol/L; free TRP level, 8.7±3.4 μmol/L) and control tests (total TRP level, 54.9±14.5 μmol/L; free TRP level, 8.7±2.4 μmol/L). An ANOVA of changes in free TRP level during TRP depletion and control testing revealed significant effects of test dose (F=60.69; df=1,29; P<.0001) and time (F=6.03; df=2,58; P<.005). The interaction of test dose × time for change in free TRP level was also highly significant (F=43.83; df=2,58; P<.0001). An ANOVA of changes in total TRP levels also revealed significant effects of test dose (F=167.33; df=1,31; P<.0001), a trend toward significance for time (F=2.80; df=2,62; P<.07), and a significant interaction of test dose × time (F=141.94; df=2,62; P<.0001).

The low-TRP diet itself caused nonsignificant decreases in fasting morning plasma total (7% mean decrease) and free (5% mean decrease) TRP levels. The TRP-free amino acid drink was responsible for most of the decrease in plasma free and total TRP levels, with peak effects (83% decrease) occurring 5 hours after ingestion of the amino acid drink.

EFFECTS OF TRP DEPLETION ON DEPRESSED MOOD

In general, little change in mood was observed *during* the time when TRP was being rapidly depleted. However, clinically meaningful changes in mood (as reflected by the Ham-D score) were observed on *the day after* testing, when TRP was being repleted. A placebo-subtracted (depletion minus control) frequency histogram of the change in Ham-D score *during* TRP depletion testing (available on request) shows that there was minimal change in Ham-D score on the day the amino acid drink was ingested (day 2). These data are normally distributed, with the median Ham-D change score near 0, as would be expected of a procedure having little or no behavioral effect.

Figure 1 depicts a placebo-subtracted frequency histogram of the change in Ham-D score on *the day after* TRP depletion testing. In contrast to the minimal change in Ham-D score during the time when TRP was being depleted, a marked change in Ham-D score was observed on the day after the TRP depletion testing relative to the control test. These data are not normally distributed (Shapiro-Wilks test, P=.02): this histogram is bimodal, with some patients becoming more depressed and others becoming less depressed.

The extremes of this bimodal pattern consisted of 16 patients (37%) who experienced a transient improvement of mood (≥10-point decrease in Ham-D score; mean score, 17±8) and 10 (23%) who experienced a transient worsening of mood (≥10-point increase in Ham-D score; mean score, 36±8) on return to normal food intake *the day after* the TRP depletion test. Individual change scores for the Ham-D ranged from a 20-point decrease to a 25-point increase.

RELATIONSHIP TO TREATMENT RESPONSE

Nine of the 10 patients who were discharged as treatment nonresponders were classified into the "worse" or "much worse" category for change in Ham-D score on the day after TRP depletion testing relative to control. Only five of 20 treatment responders were worse or much worse (Fisher's Exact Test, P=.029). While none of the treatment nonresponders were categorized as "better" or "much better" on the day after TRP depletion, 13 of 20

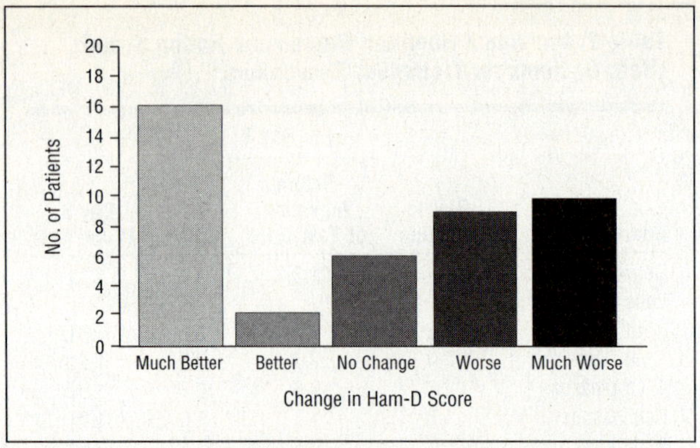

Figure 1. *Relative change in Hamilton Depression Rating Scale[42] (Ham-D) score on the day after tryptophan depletion testing, ie, the change in Ham-D score from the 420-minute time point on day 2 to day 3 during the tryptophan depleting test minus the same measurement on the control test. The Ham-D score change categories are much better (≥10-point decrease in total Ham-D score), better (5- to 9-point decrease), no change (0- to 4-point change), worse (5- to 9-point increase), or much worse (≥10-point increase).*

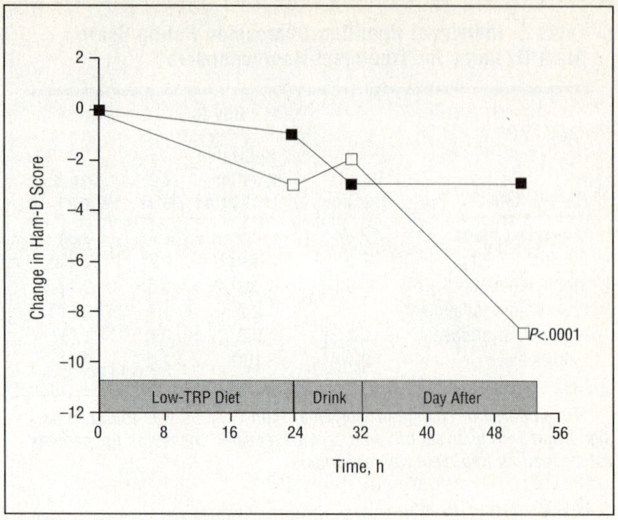

Figure 2. *Total Hamilton Depression Rating Scale[42] (Ham-D) score for treatment responders throughout control testing (solid squares) and tryptophan (TRP) depletion testing (open squares) (P<.0001).*

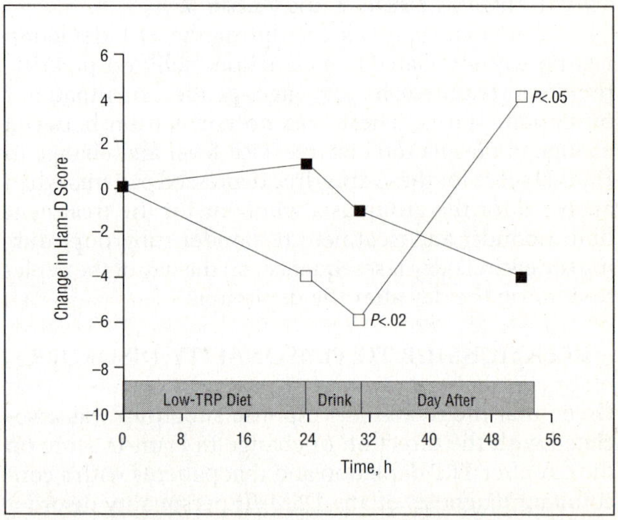

Figure 3. *Total Hamilton Depression Rating Scale[42] (Ham-D) score for treatment nonresponders throughout control testing (solid squares) and tryptophan (TRP) depletion testing (open squares) (P<.05).*

of the treatment responders were better or much better (Fisher's Exact Test, *P*=.0006). Partial responders were evenly distributed into worse and much worse categories (four of 12), "no change" (three of 12), and better or much better (five of 12).

In further examining these data, we assessed the interaction of eventual treatment response grouping (antidepressant responders, partial responders, and nonresponders) with test dose and time using ANOVA with repeated measures. This revealed a highly significant test dose × time × group interaction (F=4.54; *df*=6,117; *P*=.0004), supporting the observation that the pattern of change in mood with TRP depletion testing was related to the ultimate antidepressant treatment response category.

Separate ANOVA tests for each treatment response subgroup revealed significant test dose × time interactions for the treatment nonresponder (F=8.47; *df*=3,27; *P*=.0004) and responder (F=2.95; *df*=3,57; *P*=.04) subgroups. There was no significant test dose × time interaction (F=0.77; *df*=3,33; *P*=.52) for the partial responder subgroup. Further analysis to identify the direction and magnitude of change in total Ham-D score during control and depletion tests was not performed for the partial responder subgroup.

The pattern of changes in mood throughout the TRP depletion test differed considerably between the antidepressant nonresponder and responder subgroups. Relative to baseline, treatment responders showed improvement on the day after the TRP depletion test while the condition of treatment nonresponders worsened. In contrast, both subgroups showed gradual mild improvement in depressive symptoms throughout the control test. **Figure 2** and **Figure 3**, which depict the total Ham-D scores during the 3-day test sequence for the treatment responder and nonresponder subgroups, respectively, also show when significant changes in total Ham-D score from baseline occurred.

We subsequently assessed the change in each individual item of the Ham-D during and after TRP depletion and control testing for the treatment nonresponder and responder subgroups. For the treatment nonresponders, there was a trend for significant test dose × time interaction for "depressed mood" (F=9.33; *df*=3,27; *P*=.0002), "suicidal thinking" (F=8.51; *df*=3,27; *P*=.0004), "motor retardation" (F=5.56; *df*=3,27; *P*=.004), "worthlessness/failure" (F=2.75; *df*=3,27; *P*=.06), "retardation of speech" (F=2.45; *df*=3,27; *P*=.09), and "helplessness" (F=2.39; *df*=3,27; *P*=.09).

For treatment responders, there were trends or significant dose × time interactions for depressed mood (F=3.53; *df*=3,54; *P*=.02), "loss of energy" (F=3.57; *df*=3,54; *P*=.02), "loss of interest" (F=3.06; *df*=3,54; *P*=.04), "loss of pleasure" (F=2.92; *df*=3,54; *P*=.04), helplessness (F=7.41; *df*=3,54; *P*=.0003), and "agitation" (F=2.17; *df*=3,54; *P*=.10). Post hoc *t* tests identifying the magnitude and time course of the changes in these items dur-

Table 1. Individual Hamilton Depression Rating Scale[34] (Ham-D) Items for Treatment Nonresponders*

Ham-D Item	Day 1: Baseline	Day 2: Before Ingestion of Test Drink	Day 2: 7 h After	Day 3: 11 AM-1 PM
Depressed mood	2.3	2.5	2.7†	2.8‡
Suicidal thinking	2.0	1.0‡	1.2†	2.7†
Motor retardation	0.9	0.8	0.5	2.1‡
Worthlessness/failure	2.2	2.2	1.9	2.6†
Retardation of speech	0.8	0.8	0.6	1.8‡
Helplessness	2.1	1.9	2.0	2.3

*Time course of change in individual Ham-D items was found to be significant with analysis of variance with repeated measures for patients categorized as treatment nonresponders.
†P<.03.
‡P<.01.

Table 2. Individual Hamilton Depression Rating Scale[34] (Ham-D) Items for Treatment Responders*

Ham-D Item	Day 1: Baseline	Day 2: Before Ingestion of Test Drink	Day 2: 7 h After	Day 3: 11 AM-1 PM
Depressed mood	2.4	2.3	2.4	1.8†
Loss				
Of energy	2.2	2.3	2.6	1.5‡
Of interest	2.4	2.4	2.6	1.7‡
Of pleasure	2.7	2.6	2.7	1.9‡
Helplessness	1.8	1.7	1.9	1.0‡
Agitation	0.7	0.5	1.1	0.6†

*Time course of change in individual Ham-D items was found to be significant with analysis of variance with repeated measures for patients categorized as treatment responders.
†P<.03.
‡P<.01.

ing the TRP depletion test for the treatment nonresponder and treatment responder subgroups, respectively, are presented in **Table 1** and **Table 2**.

Change in Ham-D score during the TRP depletion testing was not related to melancholic subtype, polarity, previous treatment history, age, gender, or inpatient/outpatient status. There was no correlation between change in plasma total or free TRP level and change in Ham-D score for these drug-free depressed patients when analyzed for the group as a whole or for the treatment nonresponder and treatment responder subgroups during the entire 3-day test sequence, on the day of the depletion, or on the day after the depletion.

RELATIONSHIP TO PERSONALITY DISORDER

Given that the treatment response subgroup was associated with the direction of change in Ham-D score on the day after TRP depletion and that patients with a concomitant diagnosis of any *DSM-III* personality disorder were more likely to have been treatment nonresponders, we further evaluated the relationship of personality disorder in this regard. Seven of the 11 patients who were diagnosed as having a personality disorder were classified into the worse (n=4) or much worse (n=3) category for change in Ham-D score on the day after TRP depletion testing relative to control. By comparison, 12 of 32 patients without personality disorder were categorized as worse (n=5) or much worse (n=7) (Fisher's Exact Test, *P*=.09).

OTHER BEHAVIORAL EFFECTS OF TESTING

In contrast to depression scores, anxiety (based on Ham-A scores) was not significantly affected by the TRP depletion test relative to the control test. There were no significant test dose × time interactions. There was a significant main effect of time for total Ham-A score (F=9.36; *df*=3,105; *P*=.0001), suggesting nonspecific changes. Post hoc *t* tests revealed that this was accounted for by a gradual reduction of anxiety during both the TRP depletion and the control tests.

Side effects of the control and TRP depletion amino acid drinks were minimal, making it difficult to distinguish between them. Of the 15 items on the Symptom Checklist, only "nausea" was found to differentiate between the two test days. The test dose × time interaction for nausea was highly significant (F=8.35; *df*=1,40; *P*=.006). Post hoc *t* tests revealed the difference in reporting of nausea between the two conditions to be accounted for primarily by an increase in reporting on the TRP depletion test (*t*=−4.67, *P*=.0001), with no significant change on the control test. There were no interactions for any of the items on the Symptom Checklist when treatment response was used as a grouping variable.

Significant main effects of time with no test dose × time interaction were noted for several Symptom Checklist items. This suggests that these symptoms were nonspecific side effects of both the TRP depletion and the control amino acid drinks. There was a significant increase in the reporting of "faintness" (F=5.71; *df*=1,40; *P*=.02), a trend for an increased reporting of "increased appetite" (F=3.13; *df*=1,40; *P*=.09), and a decreased reporting of "frequent urination" (F=13.45; *df*=1,40; *P*=.0007), "ringing in the ears" (F=6.07; *df*=1,40; *P*=.02), "tremors" (F=5.90; *df*=1,40; *P*=.02), "skin rash" (F=6.27; *df*=1,40; *P*=.02), "decreased appetite" (F=5.89; *df*=1,40; *P*=.02), and "stiffness in muscles" (F=4.99; *df*=1,40; *P*=.03).

EFFECTS OF SEQUENCE OF TESTING

Twenty-two patients received the TRP depletion test first and the control test second, while 21 patients received the control test first followed by the TRP depletion test. There were no significant interactions between test dose × time × sequence of testing for all patients (F=0.12; *df*=3,123; *P*=.95) or for any of the three treatment response subgroups separately.

Long-lasting effects from the TRP depletion test appeared to occur in three patients. Two of these three patients experienced hypomania following the TRP depletion testing. One continued to experience hypomanic symptoms for 10 days after the TRP depletion test, then gradually became depressed again. Another became hy-

pomanic for 2 days and then continued to have significantly reduced depression scores, with no further hypomania for another 8 days. The third patient showed marked improvement and did not require further treatment after 4 weeks of follow-up subsequent to testing.

RELATIONSHIP TO SPECIFIC ANTIDEPRESSANT DRUGS

Forty-one of the patients received at least one adequate trial of a tricyclic antidepressant drug alone, 25 patients received at least one trial of either a monoamine oxidase inhibitor or a 5-HT reuptake inhibitor, and 33 patients received at least one trial of the combination of lithium with another antidepressant drug. Based on current response criteria, three patients responded to a tricyclic antidepressant therapy alone, while two had partial responses and 36 were nonresponders. Six patients responded to a monoamine oxidase inhibitor or a 5-HT reuptake inhibitor, while three were partial responders and 16 were nonresponders. Six patients responded to a lithium augmentation of an antidepressant drug therapy, while five patients had partial responses and 22 were nonresponders.

When test dose × time × treatment response (responders, partial responders, and nonresponders) interactions were assessed for each of these groupings, no significant interactions were seen. There was a trend for significance for patients who received a trial of lithium in combination with another antidepressant medication ($F=1.84$; $df=6,90$; $P=.10$).

COMMENT

Depressed mood in drug-free depressed patients did not worsen while plasma TRP was being depleted. This contrasts sharply with the dramatic and rapid return of depression in patients tested following therapeutic antidepressant treatment.[39] Fifteen of the 43 patients subsequently received TRP depletion after successful antidepressant treatment.[39] While none of these patients became more depressed during the drug-free depletion tests, nine of 15 had a relapse of depression[39] when tested after a successful antidepressant treatment. The neurobiologic response to TRP depletion may be dramatically different when the test is administered to the same patient after successful antidepressant treatment than when drug free. If rapid TRP depletion can so quickly disrupt the therapeutic effects of antidepressant medications in depression, then why does it not worsen depression in drug-free depressed patients? Equally important, why do some drug-free depressed patients become less depressed and some become more depressed on *the day after* the TRP depletion test?

An important unresolved question is whether the behavioral effects seen during plasma TRP depletion reflect decreases in 5-HT neurotransmission. No direct measures of 5-HT content of neurotransmission are available, and any association of the behavioral effects of TRP depletion with 5-HT function are implicit, requiring further study. It is possible that the behavioral changes observed with TRP depletion are not related to the changes in 5-HT function. However, much evidence shows that TRP depletion lowers not only 5-HT content but also 5-HT function. Preclinical studies have convincingly shown that brain TRP and 5-HT levels are dependent on plasma levels of TRP.[28-32] Tryptophan-free diets and TRP-free amino acid drinks rapidly reduce brain TRP and 5-HT levels and alter behaviors such as pain sensitivity and aggression that are dependent on 5-HT.[54-60] Our TRP depletion test led to an 83% decrease in plasma free and total TRP levels within 5 hours after ingestion of the drink (similar to the 87% to 90% decrease seen in our prior study[39]). In rats, this degree of plasma TRP depletion leads to a 60% to 70% decrease in brain 5-HT level,[31,32] and the decrease in brain 5-HT level correlated best with the pool of free plasma TRP.[32]

IF A SIMILAR RELATIONSHIP exists in humans, then the drug-free patients should have had similar decreases in brain 5-HT content, as did the antidepressant-treated patients in our prior study. No data are available regarding the effects of plasma TRP depletion on brain 5-HT function in animals with and without antidepressant drugs. Indeed, antidepressant drugs increase plasma and brain TRP levels,[61,62] and this might oppose the effects of the TRP depletion. It is possible that antidepressant drugs somehow increase the impact of lowering 5-HT level on 5-HT function, perhaps owing to the adaptive changes induced by antidepressant drugs.[63]

The effects of antidepressant drugs on other neurotransmitter systems may also be a factor. Most antidepressant drugs have long-lasting effects on the noradrenergic and dopaminergic systems. Therefore, it may be that a critical balance among neurotransmitter systems is disturbed in a different manner when 5-HT level is reduced in a patient taking an antidepressant drug compared with the drug-free state.

It is also possible that 5-HT function is already diminished in drug-free depressed patients; hence, lowering it further does not exacerbate depression. However, there should have been some worsening in those patients with mild depression, and this was not observed. In Parkinson's disease, where dopamine function is directly involved in movement, lowering dopaminergic function further will rapidly exacerbate symptoms, especially in those with severe illness.

BIMODAL CHANGES OF MOOD ON THE DAY AFTER TRP DEPLETION

There were robust changes of mood in some patients on the day after the depletion test. At that time, these patients had returned to unrestricted food intake and received oral TRP supplementation. As described above, the changes of mood showed a bimodal response, with 37% of patients becoming much less depressed and 23% becoming much more depressed. This change occurred *after* the experimental procedure and did not correlate with the magnitude of TRP depletion, complicating its interpretation.

Serotonin function may have been transiently enhanced in some patients because of the rapid TRP depletion and repletion. The prolactin and corticosterone responses to 5-hydroxytryptamine are enhanced after a 14-day TRP-free diet in rats,[60] and the prolactin response to TRP infusion in healthy humans is enhanced the day after a 10-day low-TRP diet compared with the prediet response.[36] These studies suggest that TRP restriction may lead to supersensitivity within the 5-HT system analogous to that seen on neuronal denervation. Such a supersensitivity could be related to increases in TRP transport across the blood-brain barrier, increased neuronal uptake of TRP, increased activity of TRP hydroxylase, increased release of 5-HT, or increased postsynaptic receptor or neuronal sensitivity.

ANOTHER POSSIBILITY is that rapid TRP depletion may have an effect that is similar to that of sleep deprivation, either by changing sleep rhythms or by blocking the nighttime melatonin surge. This is possible because melatonin is synthesized from 5-HT and might be influenced by TRP depletion. Also, TRP depletion followed by rapid repletion could be causing alterations in the activity of other neurotransmitter systems or neuronal processes due to the metabolic perturbation.

More difficult to understand is the small subset of patients who became transiently more depressed on the day after the TRP depletion. These patients could have had longer-lasting decreases in 5-HT function and therefore more pronounced negative effects. This could have been due to different rates of TRP or 5-HT repletion to differences in dietary intake after the test or differences in 5-HT repletion because of differences dietary intake after the test or difference in the rate of 5-HT synthesis. Because we lack direct measures of brain 5-HT content or control over dietary intake on the day after testing, we cannot assess the functional state of the 5-HT system.

RELATIONSHIP TO TREATMENT RESPONSE AND PERSONALITY DISORDER

The direction of change in Ham-D score on the day after TRP depletion was correlated with eventual treatment response. This finding should be interpreted with caution, as this was an open clinical trial. Furthermore, while the patients considered refractory to treatment were in fact highly refractory, responders were also relatively refractory. Treatment responders were receiving combination treatments, and a trial of a tricyclic antidepressant alone had failed in most. These factors limit interpretations and warrant future prospective studies.

The fact that treatment responders more often showed improvement the day after TRP depletion compared with nonresponders is consistent with the hypothesis that enhancement of 5-HT neurotransmission is involved in antidepressant action.[63] If there is a transient enhancement (or overshoot) of 5-HT function on the day after TRP depletion, then patients who show improvement on that day may be the ones most likely to show improvement with a treatment that potently enhances 5-HT function (such as lithium combined with an antidepressant drug).

Patients whose condition worsens the day after TRP depletion may be the ones with a primary dysfunction of the 5-HT system. Perhaps a serotonergic antidepressant drug may not be effective if that system is abnormal. These patients may have an impaired ability to restore "baseline" levels of function within an impaired 5-HT system. Therefore, the effects of transient TRP depletion may be more pronounced or more prolonged in these patients. The "normal" response to TRP depletion and TRP repletion may be the development of a transient state of enhanced 5-HT function. A transient improvement of depressive symptoms on the day after TRP depletion may reflect the beneficial effects on depression of enhanced 5-HT function in patients with a "normal" 5-HT system.

There was a trend for condition of patients with personality disorder to worsen on the day after TRP depletion. This is a provocative but highly preliminary finding. The diagnosis of personality disorder was not made on the basis of a structured interview, and we do not know whether the finding is owing to the presence of personality disorder per se or to the fact that most of these patients were antidepressant nonresponders.

RELEVANCE TO THE NEUROBIOLOGY OF DEPRESSION AND FUTURE DIRECTIONS

If TRP depletion alters 5-HT function in humans in a similar manner as in laboratory animals, our data support a major role for the 5-HT system in the pathophysiology of depression. However, this role is clearly more complex than originally proposed. If presynaptic 5-HT dysfunction is present in some depressed patients, it may only predispose to the state of depression, rather than directly regulate the level of depression.

Depression may also result from postsynaptic 5-HT dysfunction. Brain cells receiving a 5-HT input may not be able to utilize this input in depression, possibly owing to an abnormality at the level of the 5-HT receptor, G-protein coupling, or second or third messenger systems or in gene transcription. If an inability to utilize 5-HT were present, then the sudden raising of the 5-HT level would not immediately alleviate depression and the rapid lowering of the 5-HT level would not make depression worse. In this model, antidepressant drugs would be working by causing a time-dependent alteration in the ability of postsynaptic neurons to utilize 5-HT. Once that process had occurred, then lowering the 5-HT level would again disrupt neurotransmission, explaining why drug-free patients are not affected while antidepressant-treated patients are affected.

It is also possible that brain 5-HT function might only be involved in the therapeutic response to some antidepressant drugs but not in the pathophysiology of depression. Antidepressant drugs may not be correcting the underlying deficit in affective states but simply compensating for it. Many treatments in medicine simply restore normal function by reestablishing a critical homeostatic balance rather than directly cor-

recting the underlying condition. This is true for cardiac arrhythmias, hypertension, heart failure, colitis, diarrhea, headache, autoimmune disorders, and many other conditions.

The rapid improvement of mood in some drug-free depressed patients the day after the TRP depletion suggests that depletion followed by repletion may cause neurochemical alterations that transiently improve depression, possibly by enhancing 5-HT function. The worsening of depression the day after TRP depletion may reflect an increased vulnerability to depression and a decreased ability to respond to antidepressant drugs. Both replication and within-subject test-retest data will be important for further tests of these notions.

Future studies will begin to explore the relationships between neurotransmitter systems. The role of the 5-HT system in the modulation of neuropeptides, as well as in the modulation of the catecholeamines, needs to be further understood. The functional status of the 5-HT system on the day after the TRP depletion test will be studied with cerebrospinal fluid measurements and brain imaging. If we could understand how TRP depletion followed by TRP repletion can so quickly improve depressive symptoms in some patients, then more rapidly acting antidepressant medications with similar actions might be developed.

Accepted for publication August 1, 1994.

This work was supported by grants MH 25642, MH 36229, MH 00579, and MH 30929 from the National Institutes of Mental Health, Rockville, Md; by the Department of Veterans Affairs (Merit Review Grant, "Behavioral Effects of Acute Tryptophan Depletion"); and the state of Connecticut.

Presented in part in abstract form at the 141st Annual Meeting of the American Psychiatric Association, Montreal, Quebec, May 11, 1988; the New York Academy of Sciences Symposium "Neuropharmacology of Serotonin," New York, NY, July 15, 1989; the 19th Annual Meeting of the Society for Neuroscience, New Orleans, La, November 27, 1989; the annual meeting of the American College Neuropsychopharmacology, Maui, Hawaii, December 13, 1989; and the 143rd Annual Meeting of the American Psychiatric Association, New York, NY, May 16, 1990.

Amino acids were obtained from Ajinomoto USA Inc, New York, NY.

The study could not have been accomplished without expert assistance from Kathy Colonese, Lisa Roach, Linda Grisgrabber, RN, and Barbara Aiken, RN. Statistical consultation and analyses were performed by Pedro Mendia, PhD.

Reprint request to the Department of Psychiatry, University of Arizona College of Medicine, 1501 N Campbell Ave, Tucson, AZ 85724 (Dr Delgado).

REFERENCES

1. Heninger GR, Charney DS. Mechanism of action of antidepressant treatments: implications for the etiology and treatment of depressive disorders. In: Meltzer HY, ed. *Psychopharmacology: The Third Generation of Progress.* New York, NY: Raven Press; 1987:535-544.
2. Meltzer HY, Lowy MT. The serotonin hypothesis of depression. In: Meltzer HY, ed. *Psychopharmacology: The Third Generation of Progress.* New York, NY: Raven Press; 1987:513-526.
3. Coppen A. The biochemistry of affective disorders. *Br J Psychiatry.* 1967;113: 1237-1264.
4. Lapin IP, Oxenkrug GF. Intensification of the central serotonergic processes as a possible determinant of the thymoleptic effect. *Lancet.* 1969;1:132-136.
5. Murphy DL, Cambell I, Costa JL. Current status of the indoleamine hypothesis of the affective disorders. In: Lipton MA, DiMascio A, Killam KF, eds. *Psychopharmacology: A Generation of Progress.* New York, NY: Raven Press; 1978: 1235-1247.
6. Charney DS, Menekes DB, Heninger GR. Receptor sensitivity and the mechanism of action of antidepressant treatment. *Arch Gen Psychiatry.* 1981;38: 1160-1180.
7. Delgado PL, Charney DS. Neuroendocrine challenge studies in affective disorders. In: Horton RW, Katona C, eds. *Biological Aspects of Affective Disorders.* Orlando, Fla: Academic Press Inc; 1991:146-190.
8. Delgado PL, Charney DS. Neurochemistry of affective disorders. In: Paykel ES, ed. *Handbook of Affective Disorders.* 2nd ed. New York, NY: Churchill Livingstone Inc; 1992:219-253.
9. Coppen A, Eccleston EG, Peet M. Total and free tryptophan concentration in the plasma of depressed patients. *Lancet.* 1973;2:60-63.
10. Cowen PJ, Parry-Billings M, Newsholme EA. Decreased plasma tryptophan levels in major depression. *J Affect Disord.* 1989;16:27-31.
11. Åsberg M, Schalling D, Traskman-Bendz L, Wagner A. Psychobiology of suicide, impulsivity, and related phenomena. In: Meltzer HY, ed. *Psychopharmacology: The Third Generation of Progress.* New York, NY: Raven Press; 1987: 655-668.
12. Roy A, Virkkunen M, Linnoila M. Serotonin in suicide, violence, and alcoholism. In: Coccaro EF, Murphy DL, eds. *Serotonin in Major Psychiatric Disorders.* Washington, DC: American Psychiatric Press; 1990:187-208.
13. Pare CMB, Trenchard A, Turner P. 5-Hydroxytryptamine in depression. *Adv Biochem Psychopharmacol.* 1974;11:275-279.
14. Healy D, Leonard BE. Monoamine transport in depression: kinetics and dynamics. *J Affect Disord.* 1987;12:91-103.
15. Stanley M, Mann JJ. Increased serotonin-2 binding sites in frontal cortex of suicide victims. *Lancet.* 1983;1:214-216.
16. Yates M, Leake A, Candy JM, Fairbairn AF, McKeith IG, Ferrier IN. 5-HT-2 receptor changes in major depression. *Biol Psychiatry.* 1990;27:489-496.
17. Arora RC, Meltzer HY. Serotonergic measures in the brains of suicide victims: 5-HT_2 binding sites in the frontal cortex of suicide victims and control subjects. *Am J Psychiatry.* 1989;146:730-736.
18. Arango V, Ernsberger P, Marzuk PM, et al. Autoradiographic demonstration of increased serotonin 5-HT_2 and β-adrenergic receptor binding sites in the brain of suicide victims. *Arch Gen Psychiatry.* 1990;47:1038-1047.
19. Heninger GR, Charney DS, Sternberg DE. Serotonergic function in depression: prolactin response to intravenous tryptophan in depressed patients and healthy subjects. *Arch Gen Psychiatry.* 1984;41:398-402.
20. Cowen PJ, Charig EM. Neuroendocrine responses to tryptophan in major depression. *Arch Gen Psychiatry.* 1987;44:958-966.
21. Deakin JFW, Pennell I, Upadhyaya AJ, Lofthouse R. A neuroendocrine study of 5HT function in depression: evidence for biological mechanisms of endogenous and psychosocial causation. *Psychopharmacology.* 1990;101:85-92.
22. Price LH, Charney DS, Delgado PL, Heninger GR. Serotonin function and depression: neuroendocrine and mood responses to intravenous L-tryptophan in *DSM-III-R* depressive subtypes and healthy controls. *Am J Psychiatry.* 1991; 148:1518-1525.
23. Siever LJ, Murphy DL, Slater S, de la Vega E, Lipper S. Plasma prolactin changes following fenfluramine in depressed patients compared to controls: an evaluation of central serotonergic responsivity in depression. *Life Sci.* 1984;34: 1029-1039.
24. Mitchell P, Smythe G. Hormonal responses to fenfluramine in depressed and control subjects. *J Affect Disord.* 1990;19:43-51.
25. Golden RN, Hsiao JK, Lane E, et al. Abnormal neuroendocrine responsivity to acute IV clomipramine challenge in depressed patients. *Psychiatry Res.* 1990; 31:39-47.
26. Lesch KP, Mayer S, Disselkamp-Tietze J, Hoh A, Schoelnhammer G, Schulte HM. Subsensitivity of the 5-hydroxytryptamine $_{1A}$ (5-HT_{1A}) receptor medicated hypothermic response to ipsapirone in unipolar depression. *Life Sci.* 1990;46: 1271-1277.
27. Lesch KP, Disselkamp-Tietze J, Schmidtke A. 5-HT1a receptor function in depression: effect of chronic amitriptyline treatment. *J Neural Transm.* 1990;80: 157-161.
28. Fernstrom JD. Effects of the diet on brain neurotransmitters. *Metabolism.* 1977; 26:207-223.

29. Curzon G. Relationships between plasma, CSF and brain tryptophan. *J Neural Transm.* 1979;15(suppl):93-105.
30. Curzon G. Influence of plasma tryptophan on brain 5HT synthesis and serotonergic activity. In: Haber B, Gabay S, eds. *Serotonin: Current Aspects of Neurochemistry and Function.* New York, NY: Plenum Press; 1981:207-219.
31. Young SN, Ervin FR, Pihl RO, Finn P. Biochemical aspects of tryptophan depletion in primates. *Psychopharmacology.* 1989;98:508-511.
32. Moja EA, Cipollo P, Castoldi D, Tofanetti O. Dose-response decrease in plasma tryptophan and in brain tryptophan and serotonin after tryptophan-free amino acid mixtures in rats. *Life Sci.* 1989;44:971-976.
33. Rose WC, Haines WJ, Warner DT. The amino acid requirements of man. *J Biol Chem.* 1954;206:421-430.
34. Young VR, Hussein MA, Murray E, Scrimshaw NS. Tryptophan intake, spacing of meals, and diurnal fluctuations of plasma tryptophan in men. *Am J Clin Nutr.* 1969;22:1563-1567.
35. Young VR, Hussein MA, Murray E, Scrimshaw NS. Plasma tryptophan response curve and its relation to tryptophan requirements in young adult men. *J Nutr.* 1971;101:45-60.
36. Delgado PL, Charney DS, Price LH, Landis H, Heninger GR. Neuroendocrine and behavioral effects of dietary tryptophan restriction in healthy subjects. *Life Sci.* 1989;45:2323-2332.
37. Young SN, Smith SE, Pihl R, Ervin FR. Tryptophan depletion causes a rapid lowering of mood in normal males. *Psychopharmacology.* 1985;87:173-177.
38. Smith SE, Pihl RO, Young SW, Ervin FR. A test of possible cognitive and environmental influences on the mood lowering effect of tryptophan depletion in normal males. *Psychopharmacology.* 1987;91:451-457.
39. Delgado PL, Charney DS, Price LH, Aghajanian GK, Landis H, Heninger GR. Serotonin function and the mechanism of antidepressant action: reversal of antidepressant induced remission by rapid depletion of plasma tryptophan. *Arch Gen Psychiatry.* 1990;47:411-418.
40. Delgado PL, Price LH, Miller HL, Salomon RM, Licinio J, Krystal JH, Heninger GR, Charney DS. Rapid serotonin depletion as a provocative challenge test for patients with major depression: relevance to antidepressant action and the neurobiology of depression. *Psychopharmacol Bull.* 1991;27:321-330.
41. American Psychiatric Association. *Diagnostic and Statistical Manual of Mental Disorders, Revised Third Edition.* Washington, DC: American Psychiatric Association; 1987.
42. Mazure CM, Nelson JC, Price LH. Reliability and validity of the symptoms of major depressive illness. *Arch Gen Psychiatry.* 1986;43:451-456.
43. Task Force on the Use of Laboratory Tests in Psychiatry. Tricyclic antidepressants: blood level measurements and clinical outcome: an APA Task Force report. *Am J Psychiatry.* 1985;142:155-162.
44. Delgado PL, Price LH, Charney DS, Heninger GR. Efficacy of fluvoxamine in treatment-refractory depression. *J Affect Disord.* 1988;15:55-60.
45. Hamilton M. The assessment of anxiety states by rating. *Br J Med Psychol.* 1959;32:51-53.
46. Woods SW, Charney DS, Goodman WK, Heninger GR. Carbon dioxide–induced anxiety. *Arch Gen Psychiatry.* 1988;45:43-52.
47. Anderson GM, Young JG, Cohen DJ, Schlicht KR, Patel N. Liquid-chromatographic determination of serotonin and tryptophan in whole blood and plasma. *Clin Chem.* 1981;27:775-776.
48. Conover WJ. *Practical Nonparametric Statistics.* 2nd ed. New York, NY: John Wiley & Sons Inc; 1980.
49. *SAS User's Guide: Statistics, 1982 Edition.* Cary, NC: SAS Institute Inc; 1982.
50. Dixon WJ, Brown MB, Engelman L, Frane JW, Hill MA, Jennvick RI, Toporek JD. *BMDP Statistical Software.* Berkley, Calif: University of California Press; 1983.
51. BrainPower, Inc. *Statview 512+.* 1986. 24009 Ventura Blvd, Calabasas, CA 91302.
52. *Super ANOVA User's Guide.* 1989. Abacus Concepts, Inc, 1984 Bonita Ave, Berkley, CA 94704.
53. Cricket Software. *Cricket Graph Users Guide.* 1986. 40 Valley Stream Parkway, Malvern, PA 19355.
54. Lytle LD, Messing RB, Fisher L, Phebus L. Effects of long-term corn consumption on brain serotonin and the response to electric shock. *Science.* 1975;190:692-694.
55. Messing RB, Fisher LA, Phebus L, Lytle LD. Interaction of diet and drugs in the regulation of brain 5-hydroxyindoles and the response to painful electric shock. *Life Sci.* 1976;18:707-714.
56. Walters JK, Davis M, Sheard MH. Tryptophan-free diet: effects on the acoustic startle reflex in rats. *Psychopharmacology.* 1979;62:103-109.
57. Gibbons JL, Barr GA, Bridger WH, Leibowitz SF. Manipulations of dietary tryptophan: effects on mouse killing and brain serotonin in the rat. *Brain Res.* 1979;169:139-153.
58. Vergnes M, Kempf E. Tryptophan deprivation: effects on mouse-killing and reactivity in the rat. *Psychopharmacol Aggression Soc Behav.* 1981;14:19-23.
59. Moja EA, Mendelson WB, Stoff DM, Gillin JC, Wyatt RJ. Reduction of REM sleep by a tryptophan-free amino acid diet. *Life Sci.* 1979;24:1467-1470.
60. Clemens JA, Bennett DR, Fuller RW. The effect of a tryptophan-free diet on prolactin and corticosterone release by serotonergic stimuli. *Horm Metab Res.* 1980;12:35-38.
61. Badawy AA-B. Minireview: the functions and regulation of tryptophan pyrrolase. *Life Sci.* 1977;21:755-768.
62. Badawy AA-B, Evans M. Inhibition of rat liver tryptophan pyrrolase activity and elevation of brain tryptophan concentration by acute administration of small doses of antidepressants. *Br J Pharmacol.* 1982;77:59-67.
63. Blier P, de Montigny, Chaput Y. A role for the serotonin system in the mechanism of action of antidepressant treatments: preclinical evidence. *J Clin Psychiatry.* 1990;51(suppl):14-20.

Dose-Response Studies With Protirelin

James C. Garbutt, MD; James P. Mayo, MD; Karley Y. Little, MD; Gregory M. Gillette, MD; George A. Mason, PhD; Bess Dew, RN; Arthur J. Prange, Jr, MD

Background: A reduced thyrotropin (TSH) response to thyrotropin-releasing hormone (protirelin [TRH]) has been found consistently in a portion of patients with major depression. One hypothesis to explain this observation is that pituitary TRH receptors are downregulated in major depression. One prediction stemming from this hypothesis is that prolactin (PRL) as well as TSH responses to TRH should be attenuated. To adequately test the pattern of protirelin-induced TSH and PRL responses with a protirelin dose-response design is necessary.

Methods: Four doses of protirelin (25, 100, 500, and 800 μg) were infused in an ascending schedule at intervals of 3 to 7 days in patients with major depression and in control subjects. Seven women and six men with major depression were compared with age- and gender-matched controls (five women and seven men). The TSH and PRL responses were measured at regular intervals following each dose of protirelin.

Results: No significant group differences in baseline levels of thyroid hormones or cortisol were present. Depressed men exhibited significant reductions in both TSH and PRL responses to protirelin across all doses compared with control men. Depressed women exhibited significant reductions in TSH responses but not in PRL responses compared with control women.

Conclusions: The findings that men with major depression exhibit reductions in both protirelin-induced TSH and PRL responses support the hypothesis that TRH receptors are downregulated in depression. The findings in women are less clear and may represent the greater variance in the protirelin-induced PRL responses found in women.

(Arch Gen Psychiatry. 1994;51:875-883)

A REDUCED thyrotropin (TSH) response to protirelin (thyrotropin-releasing hormone [TRH]) was first reported in depressed patients in 1972 by Prange et al[1] and Kastin et al.[2] Since these initial reports, many groups have replicated the finding, and a reduced TSH response to protirelin is presently one of the best documented biological markers in major depression. Loosen and Prange[3] and Loosen[4] have thoroughly reviewed the clinical studies concerning the diagnostic, prognostic, and biological aspects of this marker. In brief, they note that: (1) 25% to 30% of patients with major depression have a reduced TSH response to protirelin (maximal change from baseline TSH [ΔmaxTSH] <5 mU/L using a TSH radioimmunoassay) compared with about 5% of psychiatrically healthy controls; (2) standard subtypes or severity of depression do not predict a reduced TSH response; (3) patients with certain other psychiatric disorders, notably alcoholism, have rates of a reduced TSH response similar to that found in major depression; and (4) the underlying biological reason for the fault is unknown. Although an association between diagnostic subtypes of depression and a reduced TSH response has not been found, there have been reports that panic attacks,[5,6] suicidal intent and lethality,[7,8] and agitation[8,9] are related to a low TSH response in depressed patients.

Many factors can produce a low TSH response to protirelin: elevated levels of thyroid hormones,[10] cortisol,[11] somatostatin,[12] or dopamine[13]; calcium channel blockade[14]; and reduced energy intake.[15] In an attempt to understand the reduced TSH response to protirelin in depression, several of these factors have been investigated. Some reports suggest that an in-

From the Department of Psychiatry (Drs Garbutt, Mayo, Little, Mason, and Prange) and the Brain and Development Research Center (Drs Mason and Prange), University of North Carolina at Chapel Hill; the Clinical Research Unit (Drs Garbutt, Mayo, Little, and Prange and Ms Dew), Dorothea Dix Hospital, Raleigh, NC; and the Department of Psychiatry, University of Arkansas, Little Rock (Dr Gillette).

See Subjects and Methods on next page

SUBJECTS AND METHODS

SUBJECTS

Seven women and six men with a Research Diagnostic Criteria[42] diagnosis of major depression participated in the study. All depressed subjects were studied as inpatients and were selected from consecutive admissions to the Clinical Research Unit at Dorothea Dix Hospital if they met the following criteria: (1) Research Diagnostic Criteria diagnosis of major depression; (2) no evidence of significant medical problems as determined from physical examination and laboratory testing (complete blood cell count, serum chemistry determinations, thyroid panel and TSH determination, serologic tests, urinalysis, and electrocardiogram); and (3) no diagnoses of alcoholism or substance dependence. A minimal level of depressive symptoms was not required, given evidence that this is not a predictor of TSH response.[3]

At the time of testing, the subjects had been free of antidepressant and benzodiazepine use for at least 2 weeks, with three exceptions: one woman completed a course of doxepin hydrochloride therapy 10 days prior to the study; one woman received a dose of diazepam 5 days prior to the study; and one woman received a dose of alprazolam 6 days prior to the study. Four weeks prior to the study, one woman had received phenelzine sulfate but no other subjects had recently received a monoamine oxidase inhibitor. No subjects had received lithium carbonate, carbamazepine, or depot neuroleptics within 8 weeks prior to the study. During the study, the subjects remained free of psychotropic drug use with the exception of two men who each received two doses of temazepam. It has been shown that clinically relevant doses of benzodiazepines do not alter the pituitary response to protirelin in humans.[43]

Five women and seven men were studied as control subjects. The control subjects were recruited from responses to advertisements and through word of mouth. They were studied on an "outpatient" basis. They were screened with a detailed psychiatric interview and a medical evaluation. To be eligible for participation, control subjects were required to have no evidence of current or past psychiatric problems, including alcoholism or substance abuse. Of the control women, none had a first- or second-degree relative with a history of alcoholism or substance abuse. None of the control men had a first-degree relative with a history of mental illness or alcoholism, although one man had an alcoholic uncle. Control subjects were in good medical health and were not receiving medication for either medical or psychiatric reasons.

The mean (±SD) age of the depressed women was 39±11 years (range, 24 to 56 years) and of the control women, 39±6 years (range, 29 to 46 years) ($t[10]=-0.15$, $P=.89$); the mean (±SD) age of the depressed men was 42±8 years (range, 33 to 53 years) and of the control men, 41±9 years (range, 30 to 51 years) ($t[11]=.12$, $P=.90$). The mean (±SD) body surface area of the depressed women was 1.85±0.28 m^2 compared with 1.64±0.10 m^2 for the control women ($t[10]=1.58$, $P=.14$) and was 1.96±0.07 m^2 for the depressed men compared with 1.94±0.11 m^2 for the control men ($t[11]=0.46$, $P=.65$). Five depressed women were premenopausal and two were postmenopausal. All five control women were premenopausal. Older, postmenopausal women do not exhibit different TSH or PRL responses to protirelin from those of premenopausal women.[25,44] Premenopausal women were studied at different phases of their menstrual cycle. Findings from two studies are relevant to this point: no effects of menstrual cycle hormonal changes on the TSH and PRL responses to protirelin were found by one group of investigators[45] using a within-subjects design; another group[46] found a greater TSH response in the postovulatory period using an across-subjects design.

Prior to entering the study, all of the subjects gave informed consent to participate in a protocol that had been approved by the Committee for the Protection of the Rights of Human Subjects, School of Medicine, University of North Carolina at Chapel Hill.

DIAGNOSTIC AND RATING METHODS

For depressed subjects, consensus diagnoses were made at a diagnostic conference using information from psychiatric interviews, social history, and information from the Schedule for Affective Disorders and Schizophrenia.[47] All six men met criteria for recurrent unipolar major depression and two also met criteria for endogenous depression. Three women met criteria for recurrent major depression, two of whom had endogenous subtype. An additional three women met criteria for major depression (single episode) and one met criteria for bipolar depression. The Schedule for Affective Disorders and Schizophrenia was completed on all patients by a psychiatric social worker trained in its administration. For the control subjects, psychiatric screening was completed through the use of a detailed psychiatric interview.

The Hamilton Depression Rating Scale (HDRS),[48] items 1 through 17, was completed on all subjects at baseline and on each study day by a psychiatrist (J.P.M., K.Y.L., or

crease in thyroid hormone levels may be partly responsible for a low TSH response in depression,[16,17] but this has not been uniformly found (see references 3 and 4 for review). Clearly, the reduced TSH response to protirelin in depressed patients is not secondary to overt hyperthyroidism, although it may be caused sometimes by transient hyperthyroxinemia or even by increases in thyroid hormone levels within normal physiological boundaries. Given that many depressed patients exhibit hypercortisolemia,[18] excess cortisol could be responsible for the reduced TSH response. However, a clear dissociation between measures of hypercortisolemia and TSH response has been found.[19,20] Similarly, evidence argues against an important involvement of dopamine[21] or starvation.[22] The possible roles of somatostatin and calcium channel dysfunction have not been well investigated.

One leading hypothesis that has been advanced to explain the reduced TSH response in depression is that pituitary TRH receptors are downregulated secondary to TRH hypersecretion from the hypothalamus. This hypothesis was initially formulated from studies in animals[23] and derives support from a series of basic and clinical studies.

Protirelin is known to release prolactin (PRL) and TSH from the pituitary gland[24,25] through TRH receptors located on the cell membranes of lactotrophs and thyrotrophs. In vitro, protirelin administration produces re-

G.M.G.). Interrater reliability for those administering the HDRS as determined by Spearman's correlation was greater than 0.8 for all relevant pairs of raters.

PROTOCOL DESIGN

The purpose of this study was to test the TSH and PRL responses to protirelin in depressed patients across a full spectrum of protirelin doses. Accordingly, four doses of protirelin were selected (25, 100, 500, and 800 μg) that spanned the range from submaximal to supramaximal for both TSH and PRL responses.[24,25] Each subject received each dose of protirelin, administered by intravenous injection, in an ascending dose design with intervals of 3 to 7 days between injections. The mean intertest intervals between injection days 1 and 2, 2 and 3, and 3 and 4 for depressed women vs control women were 3.4 vs 3.4, 3.3 vs 3.6, and 4.5 vs 4.0 days, respectively. For depressed men vs control men, the intertest intervals were 3.0 vs 3.6, 3.3 vs 3.7, and 3.8 vs 4.6 days, respectively. These differences were not statistically significant for either gender.

The ascending dose design was chosen over a random or balanced design to minimize the possibility of an effect of one protirelin test on a subsequent test. Haigler et al[49] reported that daily testing with a 500-μg dose of protirelin led to a reduced TSH response after 2 to 3 days, whereas no reduction was found with an every-other-day schedule. Winokur et al[50] reported reductions in TSH response when 500 μg of protirelin was given at weekly intervals for 3 to 4 weeks. Therefore, an ascending dose design with a 3-to 5-day interval was used. This design produces TSH and PRL responses that are comparable to those found with a random-dose schedule.[24,25,51]

On each protirelin test day, after the subject had fasted overnight, an intravenous catheter was inserted into an antecubital vein at 8:30 AM and kept patent by the slow infusion of normal saline solution. At 9 AM, protirelin was injected intravenously over 1 minute. Blood samples for hormone measures were drawn 15 minutes before, just prior to, and 15, 30, 45, 60, 120, and 180 minutes after the protirelin injection. The blood was allowed to clot at 40°C, and then the serum was separated and stored at −20°C until it was assayed in duplicate. Preprotirelin injection measures included TSH, PRL, thyroxine (T_4), triiodothyronine (T_3), T_3 uptake, cortisol, estradiol, progesterone, and testosterone. The free T_4 index was calculated from T_4 and T_3 uptake values. Measurements of TSH and PRL were then taken at all time points following protirelin injection.

Baseline hormone values represent the mean of the two preinjection measures. Changes in TSH and PRL responses (ΔmaxTSH, ΔmaxPRL) after protirelin injection are calculated as the maximal TSH or PRL values minus baseline values and represent the variable used for the TSH and PRL analyses.

ASSAY METHODS

All hormones were assayed with commercial radioimmunoassay kits. The hormone, the manufacturer of the kit used, and the respective sensitivities and intra-assay and interassay coefficients of variation of each kit, respectively, are as follows: TSH, Hybritech Inc, 0.3 mU/L, 6% and 9% at 2.4 mU/L, 3% and 3% at 25 mU/L; PRL, Serono Laboratories Inc, Braintree, Mass, 0.5 μg/L, 3.8% and 6.1%; T_4, Becton-Dickinson Immunodiagnostics, Orangeburg, NY, 8 nmol/L, 5.5% and 7.0%; T_3, 0.077 nmol/L, 6.0% and 7.0%, T_3 uptake, Ames Co, Elkhart, Ind, 4.6% and 7.3%; cortisol, Becton-Dickinson Immunodiagnostics, 1 nmol/L, 5% and 5%; testosterone, Serono Laboratories Inc, 0.1 nmol/L, 5.3% and 8.8%; estradiol, Serono Laboratories Inc, 5 pmol/L, 8.1% and 10.1%; and progesterone, Serono Laboratories Inc, 0.318 nmol/L, 4.5% and 8.9%.

STATISTICAL ANALYSIS

Because of the well-documented differences in the PRL response to protirelin between men and women,[25] results for men and women were analyzed separately. A separate analysis of TSH and PRL responses was also completed on the subgroup of premenopausal women.

Baseline measures that were taken prior to each infusion trial were assessed for diagnostic group differences and carryover effects using repeated measures analysis of variance. Probability values were derived using Wilks' λ statistics.

For analysis of TSH and PRL responses, the independent variables were group (depressed vs control), trial (25, 100, 500, 800 μg of protirelin), and group×trial interaction. Analysis of variance was the statistical method employed, with Tukey's Honestly Significant Difference Test applied in examining differences among levels for actors with more than two levels in those cases where a test for the main effect proved significant. In analyses where both ΔmaxTSH and ΔmaxPRL served as response variables, multivariate analysis of variance (MANOVA) was used. Test statistics reported by MANOVA were associated with computed values of Wilks' λ.

ductions in TRH binding sites in cell cultures of both thyrotrophs[26] and lactotrophs.[27] Repetitive administration of protirelin in humans does tend to reduce both the TSH[28-30] and the PRL response[28,31] to protirelin, though the latter has not been uniformly found.[30] Therefore, parallel reductions in the protirelin-induced responses of TSH and PRL in depressed patients would provide supportive evidence for the TRH-receptor downregulation hypothesis.

Clinical evidence in support of the downregulation hypothesis comes from two areas: cerebrospinal fluid (CSF) and neuroendocrine studies. Two groups of investigators[32,33] have found that depressed patients have an elevation in TRH levels in CSF, although a direct association between protirelin-induced TSH response and CSF TRH was not found in either of these studies. Second, reductions have been found in the protirelin-induced PRL response as well as in the TSH response in depressed patients,[34-37] although not by all groups.[38,39] Several studies have found concordance between the TSH and the PRL responses to protirelin in depression,[36-40] yet again, not all studies are confirmatory.[38,41]

One problem in interpreting the TSH and PRL responses to protirelin in humans is that TSH and PRL exhibit different dose-response characteristics.[24,25] When compared with the TSH response, the PRL response is more robust at a low dose, 6.25 μg, and reaches a maximum re-

Table 1. Baseline Hormone Values Across Protirelin Infusions for Depressed and Control Women*

Hormone	Protirelin Dose, μg: 25	100	500	800	MANOVA *P*: Trial	Group×Trial
TSH, mU/L						
Depressed	1.3±0.5	1.6±0.8	1.5±0.6	1.8±0.9	.42	.56
Control	1.8±0.7	1.5±0.6	1.4±0.7	1.9±0.7		
PRL, %μg/L						
Depressed	8.4±6.0	8.4±4.8	7.5±5.0	11.0±10.2	.56	.86
Control	9.1±2.2	9.2±2.0	9.1±1.8	10.0±2.3		
T_4, nmol/L (μg/dL)						
Depressed	77±17 (5.9±1.3)	65±13 (5.0±1.0)	74±23 (5.7±1.8)	65±19 (5.1±1.5)	.11	.52
Control	81±10 (6.3±0.8)	81±15 (6.3±1.2)	82±13 (6.4±1.0)	73±7 (5.7±0.5)		
T_3, nmol/L						
Depressed	1.1±0.5	0.8±0.3	0.9±0.4	1.0±0.4	.08	.79
Control	1.4±0.2	1.2±0.1	1.2±0.2	1.1±0.2		
T_3 uptake, %						
Depressed	0.52±0.01	0.51±0.01	0.51±0.02	0.49±0.03	.13	.77
Control	0.50±0.05	0.48±0.05	0.49±0.04	0.48±0.04		
FTI, nmol/L						
Depressed	81±13	73±13	79±19	70±16	.08	.72
Control	85±17	83±21	85±16	74±9		
Cortisol, nmol/L						
Depressed	440±190	470±150	440±140	490±190	.83	.62
Control	350±200	300±140	320±180	330±200		
Estradiol, pmol/L (pg/mL)						
Depressed	660±450 (180±123)	590±390 (161±106)	660±70 (180±19)	940±450 (256±123)	<.03	<.07
Control	750±560 (204±152)	530±670 (144±182)	780±650 (212±177)	310±330 (84±90)		
Progesterone, nmol/L						
Depressed	16±4	8±4	4±4	8±8	.06	.10
Control	20±2	22±16	20±10	4±2		

**Data are expressed as mean±SD. MANOVA indicates multivariate analysis of variance; TSH, thyrotropin; PRL, prolactin; T_4, thyroxine; T_3, triiodothyronine; and FTI, free T_4 index.*

sponse at 100 μg, compared with 400 μg for the TSH response.[24,25] Therefore, to adequately characterize the TSH and PRL responses to protirelin, it is necessary to employ a range of protirelin doses that elicit submaximal to supramaximal responses for both hormones. This strategy allows for both the interpretation of the TSH and PRL responses within subjects and for the assessment of whether supramaximal stimulation with protirelin can overcome blunted TSH and/or PRL responses resulting from reduced TRH-receptor affinity. Thus, the purpose of the present study was to determine the dose-response patterns of TSH and PRL in patients with major depression and, by doing so, to obtain further information on the TRH-receptor downregulation hypothesis.

RESULTS

Prior to the first infusion, depressed women had significantly higher HDRS scores (mean±SD) than control women, 24.7±10.9 vs 2.2±1.9, respectively ($F[1,10]=20.47$, $P=.001$), and depressed men had higher HDRS scores than did control men, 17.8±7.3 vs 0.9±0.9, respectively ($F[1,11]=37.42$, $P=.0001$). By the fourth infusion, HDRS scores were 15.3±10.9 for depressed men, a nonsignificant decline from the first infusion ($F[3,9]=1.78$, $P=.22$). For depressed women, HDRS scores were 19.2±10.6 at the fourth infusion, a slight but significant decline from the first infusion ($F[3,8]=5.39$, $P=.025$). The HDRS scores did not change for the control subjects.

Baseline measures of each hormone were tested for the effects of group, trial, and group×trial interaction. **Table 1** presents the means±SDs of baseline hormone values for female subjects. **Table 2** presents baseline hormone data for male subjects. For the female subjects, no statistically significant group differences were found in any of the hormones measured at baseline at any of the four trials, including differences in estrogen and progesterone. A trial effect was detected for estradiol, indicating that estradiol values changed over the course of the study in keeping with expected estrogen fluctuations in premenopausal women. Among men, depressed subjects exhibited lower baseline TSH levels than controls on the first trial (univariate $F[1,11]=8.60$, $P=.014$), but not at any other trial. Because of the lack of any consistent differences in baseline hormone values across groups, these values were not used in any analyses of covariance.

Analyses of TSH and PRL responses to protirelin revealed significant group effects for both genders and a trial effect for men for TSH (**Table 3**). The findings for trial effects for men indicate that the different dosages of protirelin used produced different TSH responses, as has been shown previously.[24] The findings for group effects revealed that depressed women had lower ΔmaxTSH responses to protirelin than control women and that depressed men had lower ΔmaxTSH and ΔmaxPRL responses than did control men. None of the subjects had evidence for an enhanced TSH response (>25 mU/L) at the 500-μg protirelin dose. **Figure 1** and **Figure 2** show the

Table 2. Baseline Hormone Values Across Protirelin Infusions for Depressed and Control Men*

Hormone	Protirelin Dose, μg: 25	100	500	800	MANOVA P: Trial	Group×Trial
TSH, mU/L						
Depressed	1.3±0.3	1.6±0.4	1.3±0.5	1.5±0.5	.27	.31
Control	2.2±0.7	2.3±0.7	1.9±0.5	2.0±0.6		
PRL, μg/L						
Depressed	5.1±3.4	5.3±3.2	4.9±2.3	5.1±3.6	<.04	.51
Control	5.8±2.1	6.1±1.3	5.2±1.4	5.2±1.5		
T_4, nmol/L (μg/dL)						
Depressed	88±13 (6.8±1.0)	90±19 (7.0±1.5)	95±35 (7.4±2.7)	85±24 (6.6±1.9)	.53	.44
Control	79±16 (6.1±1.2)	68±18 (5.3±1.4)	59±16 (4.5±1.2)	61±17 (4.7±1.3)		
T_3, nmol/L						
Depressed	1.3±0.6	1.2±0.4	1.6±0.7	1.6±0.9	.86	.26
Control	1.2±0.6	1.1±0.4	1.0±0.3	1.0±0.3		
T_3 uptake, %						
Depressed	0.52±0.03	0.52±0.05	0.50±0.04	0.50±0.05	.23	.29
Control	0.52±0.05	0.50±0.06	0.52±0.05	0.54±0.04		
FTI, nmol/L						
Depressed	88±15	92±18	86±29	82±27	.41	.56
Control	79±15	69±18	61±16	63±18		
Cortisol, nmol/L						
Depressed	330±70	330±50	380±90	330±40	.66	.52
Control	390±120	370±60	360±110	320±60		
Testosterone, nmol/L (ng/mL)						
Depressed	22.0±5.5 (6.3±1.6)	24.0±5.0 (6.9±1.4)	23.5±6.5 (6.8±1.9)	23.5±8.0 (6.8±2.3)	.43	.85
Control	20.5±4.2 (5.9±1.2)	21.1±3.8 (6.1±1.1)	20.5±4.5 (5.9±1.3)	22.2±3.0 (6.4±0.9)		

**Data are expressed as mean±SD. See Table 1 for explanation of abbreviations.*

Table 3. Thyrotropin and Prolactin Responses to Protirelin in Depressed and Control Men and Women*

Sex	Response	Predictor	F Ratio	df	P	Tukey's Honestly Significant Difference Test
F	ΔmaxTSH	Group	15.13	1, 40	.0004	NL>MD
		Dose	2.13	3, 40	.11	
		Group×dose	0.23	3, 40	.87	
F	ΔmaxPRL	Group	0.00	1, 39	.95	
		Dose	0.45	3, 39	.72	
		Group×dose	0.92	3, 39	.44	
M	ΔmaxTSH	Group	12.04	1, 44	.001	NL>MD
		Dose	6.92	3, 44	.0006	800, 500, and 100 μg>25 μg
		Group×dose	0.26	3, 44	.87	
M	ΔmaxPRL	Group	4.81	1, 44	.03	NL>MD
		Dose	0.94	3, 44	.43	
		Group×dose	0.26	3, 44	.85	

**ΔmaxTSH indicates maximal change from baseline thyrotropin; ΔmaxPRL, maximal change from baseline prolactin; NL, normal controls; and MD, patients with major depression.*

ΔmaxTSH and ΔmaxPRL values for depressed and control women across all four protirelin infusions. **Figure 3** and **Figure 4** show the ΔmaxTSH and ΔmaxPRL values for depressed and control men across all four protirelin infusions. The analysis for premenopausal women revealed similar findings: a significant group effect for ΔmaxTSH ($F[1,32]=11.38$, $P=.002$) but no group effect for ΔmaxPRL ($F[1,32]=0.23$, $P=.63$).

To examine the relationship between TSH and PRL responses to protirelin within subjects, Pearson correlations were calculated on ΔmaxTSH and ΔmaxPRL at each dose of protirelin by gender, combining depressed and control subjects. For women, the correlations at the four ascending protirelin doses were .16 (25 μg), −.32 (100 μg), −.57 (500 μg), and −.17 (800 μg) and for men the values were .29, .50, .35, and .57, respectively. None of these correlations were significant. A relationship between TSH and PRL response within gender and diagnostic category was tested for. These results are shown in **Table 4** and indicate positive correlations between TSH and PRL responses for depressed men across the range of protirelin doses that reaches significance at the 25-μg protirelin dose.

COMMENT

The results of this study indicate that depressed men and women have a reduced TSH response to protirelin compared with age- and gender-matched controls across a

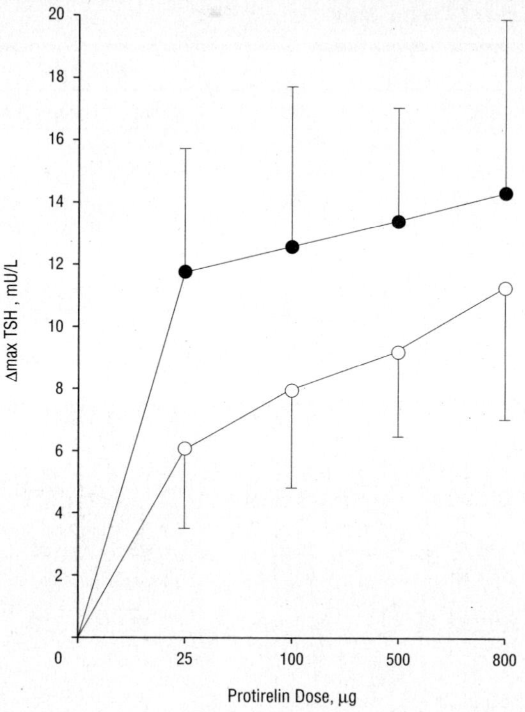

Figure 1. *Maximal change from baseline thyrotropin (ΔmaxTSH) values, expressed as mean±SD, for depressed (open circles) and control (solid circles) women at each of the four protirelin infusions. Group effect by analysis of variance, F=15.13,* P*=.0004.*

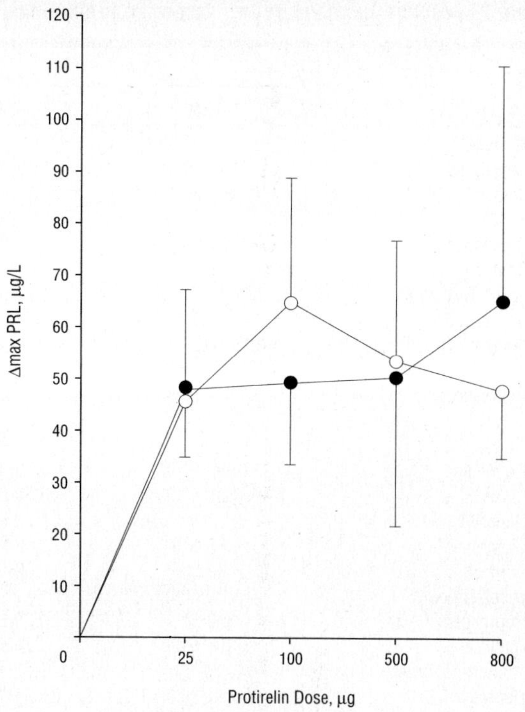

Figure 2. *Maximal change from baseline prolactin (ΔmaxPRL) values, expressed as mean±SD, for depressed (open circles) and control (solid circles) women at each of the four protirelin infusions. Group effect by analysis of variance, F=0.0,* P*=.95.*

range of protirelin doses. Furthermore, depressed men have a reduced protirelin-induced PRL response compared with control men. These findings confirm the well-documented reduction in protirelin-induced TSH release in depression[3,4] and offer new insights into possible underlying pathophysiological mechanisms.

First, the use of the dose-response design with supramaximal as well as submaximal doses allows for the conclusion that increasing the dose of protirelin does not normalize either the TSH or the PRL response to protirelin in depression. This observation suggests that if the fault is at the level of the TRH receptor, then it is a decrease in receptor number rather than in affinity that is responsible for low TSH and PRL responses to protirelin in depression. One possible cause for this would be TRH hypersecretion from the hypothalamus.

Two main lines of evidence support the concept of TRH hypersecretion in depression: the findings of elevated CSF TRH[32,33] and the findings presented herein and elsewhere[35,36,38,40] of parallel reductions in protirelin-induced TSH and PRL response. The CSF findings provide direct evidence for higher central nervous system levels of TRH in depression but do not address whether the elevation is secondary to increased synaptic release or decreased inactivation, the neuroanatomical source of the TRH, or the functional significance of the elevation. With regard to the last point, it is of interest that no relationship between CSF-TRH and TSH response to protirelin was reported in either of the CSF studies in depression.[32,33]

In contrast to the CSF data, the neuroendocrine data, on balance, provide support for the hypothesis of TRH hypersecretion from the hypothalamus. Repetitive administration of protirelin to humans clearly reduces TSH response to protirelin,[28-30] even in the absence of release of thyroid hormones,[29] and in some studies has been found to reduce PRL response.[28,31] In the case of PRL release in humans, the protirelin-induced desensitization has been shown to be specific to TRH-mediated release. For example, pimozide, a dopamine blocker, produces a robust PRL release following long-term protirelin administration, whereas the PRL response to protirelin is markedly reduced.[31] Radioligand binding data also reveal that continuous exposure to protirelin reduces the number of TRH receptors in cell culture models of both thyrotroph and lactotroph cells without altering the affinity of the TRH receptor.[26,27]

One part of the present data appears to contradict the downregulation hypothesis: if TRH receptors are downregulated in depressed women, why were there no reductions in PRL responses as well as in TSH responses? First, it should be noted that reductions in PRL responses in depressed women in fact have been reported in many[36,37,39,40] but not all studies.[38,41] Consistent with the sex differences in protirelin-induced pituitary response found in the present study, a sex difference has been reported in normal subjects. Mongioi et al[31] found reduced TSH and PRL responses in men following continuous protirelin infusion; Frey and Haug[30] found that prolonged protirelin administration in women reduced TSH but not PRL responses. Another point to consider is that women have a much greater variance in their PRL responses to protirelin than do men.[25] Therefore, detect-

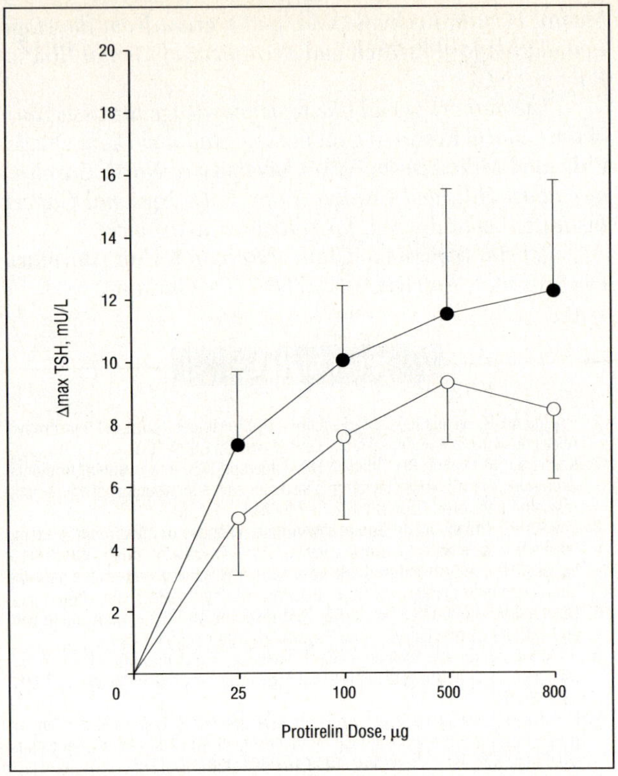

Figure 3. *Maximal change from baseline thyrotropin (ΔmaxTSH) values, expressed as mean±SD, for depressed (open circles) and control (solid circles) men at each of the four protirelin infusions. Group effect by analysis of variance, F=12.04, P=.001.*

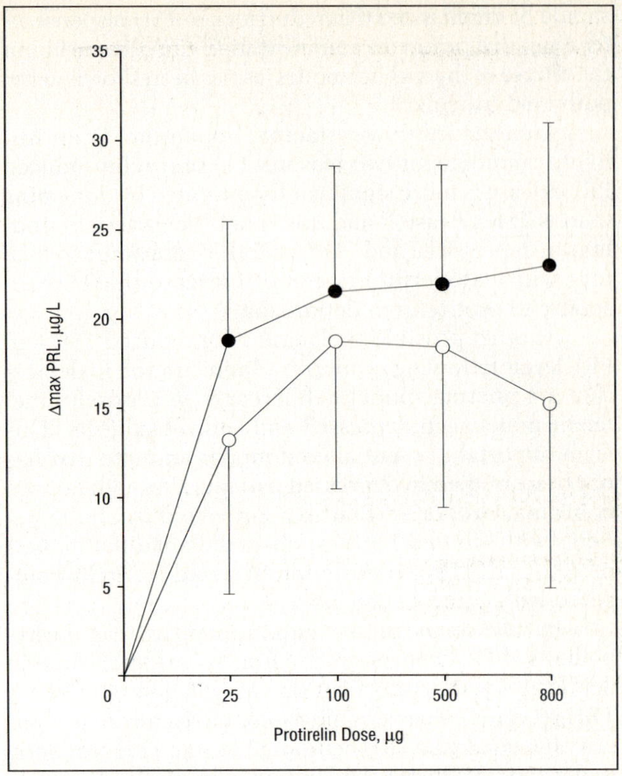

Figure 4. *Maximal change from baseline prolactin (ΔmaxPRL) values, expressed as mean±SD, for depressed (open circles) and control (solid circles) men at each of the four protirelin infusions. Group effect by analysis of variance, F=4.81, P=.03.*

ing differences in PRL response between groups of women requires more statistical power than for groups of men.

Another aspect of the present data needs consideration in the context of the downregulation hypothesis: the lack of a significant relationship between the protirelin-induced TSH and PRL responses in women. Women's greater variance in PRL response may help explain this. For depressed men, there were consistent positive correlations between the TSH and PRL responses across all of the protirelin infusion doses that reached statistical significance for the 25-μg dose. This finding does support the downregulation hypothesis in depression, at least in men.

Of course, other factors must be considered to explain the present TSH and PRL response results. As noted earlier, evidence has accumulated to suggest that thyroid hormones are involved in the reduced TSH response to protirelin in depression.[16,17] It is well known that thyroid hormones inhibit the TSH response to protirelin more than they inhibit the PRL response.[52,53] Therefore, activation of the thyroid gland would lead to reductions in TSH response but only weakly affect PRL response. This could explain the more robust decrements in ΔmaxTSH compared with ΔmaxPRL in the depressed men and help to explain why ΔmaxTSH was reduced in depressed women in the presence of no change in ΔmaxPRL. In fact, Rabello et al[28] reported greater reductions in protirelin-induced TSH response compared with PRL response after repetitive protirelin administration in humans and linked this to the release of thyroid hormones. However, given the relative insensitivity of the protirelin-induced PRL response to the inhibitory effects of thyroid hormones,[52,53] the present find-

Table 4. Pearson Correlations Between ΔmaxTSH and ΔmaxPRL in Depressed and Control Men and Women at Four Doses of Protirelin*

Protirelin Dose, μg	Women: Depressed	Women: Control	Men: Depressed	Men: Control
25	.79†	−.20	.84†	−.41
100	−.25	−.08	.67	.26
500	−.62	−.68	.51	.24
800	−.38	−.30	.69	.33

*ΔmaxTSH indicates maximal change from baseline thyrotropin; ΔmaxPRL, maximal change from baseline prolactin.
†P<.05.

ing of low PRL responses in depressed men suggests that a mechanism separate from the release of thyroid hormones is operative. Based on our results, one could postulate a two-factor model in depression whereby TRH overdrive produces both pituitary TRH-receptor downregulation and activation of the thyroid gland. Alternatively, stimulation of the thyroid gland may occur independent of TRH and TSH release, eg, via direct sympathetic innervation of the gland.[54] Given the evidence of increased plasma levels of norepinephrine in depression,[55] this could provide another mechanism for the release of thyroid hormone and the subsequent inhibition of TSH. In fact, Maes et al[17] found a significant relationship between increased urinary norepinephrine output, increased thyroid hormone levels, and decreased baseline TSH levels in depression. However, it

should be emphasized that reductions in TSH response after repetitive protirelin administration can occur without the release of thyroid hormones, as has been shown in hypothyroid patients.[29]

Another inhibitory factor, dopamine, is an unlikely candidate for two reasons: (1) protirelin-induced PRL release is more significantly inhibited by dopamine than is TSH release,[56] and this is not the pattern of findings in depression; and (2) blockade of dopamine receptors with haloperidol does not increase the TSH response to protirelin in depression.[21]

Another possible explanation for reduced TSH and PRL levels following protirelin administration in depression are pharmacokinetic differences in protirelin metabolism between depressed and control subjects. This is an important potential confounder and one that has not been studied in depressed patients although Loosen et al[57] have reported that two euthyroid alcoholic patients with blunted TSH responses did not differ in their metabolism of exogenously administered protirelin compared with control subjects.

In balance, the present data are supportive of the hypothesis of TRH hypersecretion from the hypothalamus in depression with subsequent downregulation of pituitary TRH receptors. The pathophysiological factors that could drive hypothalamic TRH neurons to secrete TRH are poorly understood. Reductions in thyroid hormone levels can increase TRH synthesis in the hypothalamic paraventricular nucleus in the rat,[58] but reductions in thyroid hormone levels are not linked to a reduced TSH response in depressed patients.[3,4] Central catecholaminergic, presumably noradrenergic, neurons synapse directly on hypothalamic TRH neurons in rodents.[59] Given the strong evidence for a central noradrenergic dysfunction in depression,[60] a primary dysfunction in this system could affect hypothalamic TRH neurons. Such hypothesized changes in TRH neurons could be part of a homeostatic response to neurobiological processes associated with depression.[61] Indeed, there is evidence that activation of brain TRH and the thyroid axis may improve outcome in depression.[62-65]

In summary, the results of our present study when combined with findings of prior neuroendocrine and behavioral studies in animals and humans continue to support the hypothesis that some forms of depression are associated with an increased drive in brain TRH neurons. Direct tests of this hypothesis will require the development of new imaging technology or postmortem examination in patients with histories of depression and in controls to examine TRH precursor levels and receptors in the hypothalamus and other brain regions. Postmortem audioradiographic studies of pituitary TRH receptors would be useful to document whether pituitary TRH receptors are, in fact, reduced in depression. Elucidation of the relationship of the changes in the hypothalamic-pituitary-thyioid axis in depression to other brain TRH systems and to the phenomenology and course of depressive illnesses will clarify the pathophysiology of depression and perhaps lead to new treatment strategies.

Accepted for publication August 1, 1994.

This work was completed with the assistance of grants MH33127 and M1122536 from the National Institute of Mental Health, Rockville, Md, and a grant from the Hope Foundation for Research and Treatment of Mental Illness, Raleigh, NC.

The authors would like to acknowledge the assistance of the Clinical Research Unit nursing staff and Dana Quade, PhD, and Mike Senger, MA, University of North Carolina at Chapel Hill, and Carolyn Frey, PhD, National Cancer Institute, Bethesda, Md, for statistical assistance.

Reprint requests to Clinical Research Unit, Dorothea Dix Hospital, Raleigh, NC 27603 (Dr Garbutt).

REFERENCES

1. Prange AJ Jr, Wilson IC, Lara PP, Alltop LB, Breese OR. Effects of thyrotropin-releasing hormone in depression. *Lancet.* 1972;11:999-1002.
2. Kastin AJ, Ehrensing RH, Schalch DS, Anderson MS. Improvement in mental depression with decreased thyrotropin response after administration of thyrotropin-releasing hormone. *Lancet.* 1972;11:740-742.
3. Loosen PT, Prange AJ Jr. Serum thyrotropin response to thyrotropin-releasing hormone in psychiatric patients: a review. *Am J Psychiatry.* 1982;139:405-416.
4. Loosen PT. The TRH-induced TSH response in psychiatric patients: a possible neuroendocrine marker. *Psychoneuroendocrinology.* 1985;10:237-260.
5. Gillette GM, Garbutt JC, Quade DE. TSH response to TRH in depression with and without panic attacks. *Am J Psychiatry.* 1989;146:743-748.
6. Stein MB, Uhde TW. Endocrine, cardiovascular, and behavioral effects of intravenous protirelin in patients with panic disorder. *Arch Gen Psychiatry.* 1991; 48:148-156.
7. Linkowski P, Van Wettere JP, Kerkhofs M, Brauman H, Mendlewicz J. Thyrotropin response to thyreostimulin in affectively ill women: relationship to suicidal behavior. *Br J Psychiatry.* 1983;143:401-405.
8. Corrigan MHC, Gillette GM, Quade D, Garbutt JC. Panic, suicide, and agitation. *Biol Psychiatry.* 1992;31:984-982.
9. Calloway SP, Dolan RI, Fonagy VFA, De Souza VF, Wakeling A. Endocrine changes and clinical profiles in depression, II. *Psychol Med.* 1984;14:759-765.
10. Larsen PR. Thyroid-pituitary interaction: feedback regulation of thyrotropin secretion by thyroid hormones. *N Engl J Med.* 1982;306:23-32.
11. Wilber JF, Utiger RD. The effect of glucocorticoids on the thyrotropin secretion. *J Clin Invest.* 1969;48:2096-2103.
12. De Rosa G, Corsello SM, Della Cassa S, De Rosa E, Raimondo S. Effect of somatostatin on the pituitary-thyroid axis. *Ann Endocrinol (Paris).* 1983;44:355-360.
13. Rojdmark S. Influence of central dopaminergic activity on thyrotropin responsiveness to thyrotropin-releasing hormone in normal and thyrotoxic subjects. *Horm Metab Res.* 1986;18:407-410.
14. Barbarino A, De Marinis L. Calcium antagonists and hormone release, II. *J Clin Endocrinol Metab.* 1980;51:749-753.
15. Vinik AI, Kalk WJ, McLaren H, Hendricks S, Pimstone BL. Fasting blunts the TSH response to synthetic thyrotropin-releasing hormone (TRH). *J Clin Endocrinol Metab.* 1975;40:509-513.
16. Unden F, Ljunggren JG, Kjellman BF, Beck-Friis J, Wetterberg L. Twenty-four-hour serum levels of T_4 and T_3 in relation to decreased TSH serum levels and decreased TSH response to TRH in affective disorders. *Acta Psychiatr Scand.* 1986;73:358-365.
17. Maes M, Vandewoude M, Maes L, Schotte C, Cosyns P. A revised interpretation of the TRH test results in female depressed patients, part 1 responses. *J Affect Dis.* 1989;16:203-213.
18. Sachar EJ, Hellman L, Roffarg HP, Halpern FS, Fukushima DK, Gallagher TF. Disrupted 24-hour patterns of cortisol secretion in psychiatric depression. *Arch Gen Psychiatry.* 1973;28:19-24.
19. Kirkegaard C, Carroll BJ. Dissociation of TSH and adrenocortical disturbances in endogenous depression. *Psychiatry Res.* 1980;3:253-264.
20. Kupfer DJ, Jarrett DB, Frank E. Relationship among selected neuroendocrine and sleep measures in patients with recurrent depression. *Biol Psychiatry.* 1984; 19:1525-1536.
21. Loosen PT, Garbutt JC, Tipermas A. The TRH test during dopamine receptor blockade in depressed patients. *Psychoneuroendocrinology.* 1986;11:327-336.
22. Baumgartner A, Graf KJ, Kurten I, Meinhold H. The hypothalamic-pituitary axis in psychiatric patients and healthy subjects, I. *Psychiatry Res.* 1988;24:271-332.
23. Nemeroff CB, Bissette U, Martin JB, Brazeau P, Vale Y, Kizer JS, Prange AJ Jr. Effect of chronic treatment with thyrotropin-releasing hormone (TRH) or an analog of TRH (linear β-alanine TRH) on the hypothalamic-pituitary-thyroid axis. *Neuroendocrinology.* 1980;30:193-199.
24. Snyder PJ, Utiger RD. Response to thyrotropin-releasing hormone (TRH) in normal man. *J Clin Endocrinol.* 1972;34:380-385.
25. Jacobs LS, Snyder PJ, Utiger RD, Daughaday WH. Prolactin response to thyrotropin-releasing hormone in normal subjects. *J Clin Endocrinol Metab.* 1973; 36:1069-1073.
26. Gershengorn MC. Bihormonal regulation of the thyrotropin-releasing hormone receptor in mouse pituitary thyrotropic tumour cells in culture. *J Clin Invest.*

1978;62:937-943.
27. Hinkle PM, Tashjian AH Jr. Thyrotropin-releasing hormone regulates the number of its own receptors in the GH3 strain of pituitary cells in culture. *Biochem.* 1975;14:3845-3851.
28. Rabello MM, Snyder PJ, Utiger RD. Effects on the pituitary-thyroid axis and prolactin secretion of single and repetitive oral doses of thyrotropin-releasing hormone (TRH). *J Clin Endocrinol Metab.* 1974;39:571-578.
29. Staub JJ, Girard J, Mueller-Brand J, Noelpp B, Werner-Zodrow I, Baur U, Heitz P, Gemsenjaeger E. Blunting of TSH response after repeated oral administration of TRH in normal and hypothyroid subjects. *J Clin Endocrinol Metab.* 1978; 46:260-266.
30. Frey HMM, Haug E. Effect of prolonged oral administration of TRH on plasma levels of thyrotropin and prolactin in normal individuals and in patients with primary hypothyroidism. *Acta Endocrinol.* 1977;85:744-752.
31. Mongioi A, Aliffi A, Vicari E, Coniglione F, Scapagnini U, D'Agata R. Down-regulation of prolactin secretion in men during continuous thyrotropin-releasing hormone infusion. *J Clin Endocrinol Metab.* 1983;56:904-907.
32. Kirkegaard C, Faber J, Hummer L, Rogowski P. Increased levels of TRH in cerebrospinal fluid from patients with endogenous depression. *Psychoneuroendocrinology.* 1979;4:227-235.
33. Banki CM, Bissette G, Arato M, Nemeroff CB. Elevation of immunoreactive CSF TRH in depressed patients. *Am J Psychiatry.* 1988;145:1526-1531.
34. Linkowski P, Brauman H, Mendlewicz J. Prolactin secretion in women with unipolar and bipolar depression. *Psychiatry Res.* 1980;3:265-271.
35. Winokur A, Amsterdam J, Oler J, Mendels J, Snyder PJ, Caroff SN, Brunswick DJ. Multiple hormonal responses to protirelin (TRH) in depressed patients. *Arch Gen Psychiatry.* 1983;40:525-531.
36. Witschy JK, Schlesser MA, Fulton CL, Orsulak PJ, Giles DE, Fairchild C, Crowley G, Rush J. TRH-induced prolactin release is blunted in females with endogenous unipolar major depression. *Psychiatry Res.* 1984;12:321-331.
37. Garbutt JC, Loosen PT, Blacharsh J, Prange AJ Jr. The prolactin response to thyrotropin-releasing hormone in depressed patients and normal subjects. *Psychoneuroendocrinology.* 1986;11:213-219.
38. Unden F, Ljunggren JG, Kjelhnan BF, Beck-Friis J, Wetterberg L. Unaltered 24-h serum PRL levels and PRL response to TRH in contrast to decreased 24-h serum TSH levels and TSH response to TRH in major depressive disorder. *Acta Psychiatr Scand.* 1987;75:131-138.
39. Kirkegaard C, Eskildsen PC, Bjorum N. Parallel changes of the responses of thyrotropin, growth hormone, and prolactin to thyrotropin-releasing hormone in endogenous depression. *Psychoneuroendocrinology.* 1981;6:253-259.
40. Targum SD, Sullivan AC, Byrnes SM. Compensatory pituitary-thyroid mechanisms in major depressive disorder. *Psychiatry Res.* 1982;6:85-96.
41. Maes M, Vandewoude M, Maes L, Schotte C, Cosyns P. A revised interpretation of the TRH test results in female depressed patients, II: prolactin responses. *J Affect Dis.* 1989;16:215-221.
42. Spitzer RL, Endicott J, Robins E. Research Diagnostic Criteria: rationale and reliability. *Arch Gen Psychiatry.* 1978;35:773-782.
43. Wainer JA, Garbutt JC, Gillette GM, Mason GA, Quade D. Failure of chlordiazepoxide to antagonize the thyrotropin or prolactin response to thyrotropin-releasing hormone in humans. *Neuroendocrinology Lett.* 1991;13:431-436.
44. Snyder PJ, Utiger RD. Thyrotropin response to thyrotropin-releasing hormone in normal females over forty. *J Clin Endocrinol Metab.* 1972;34:1096-1098.
45. Sawin CT, Hershman JM, Boyd AE III, Longcope C, Bacharach P. The relationship of changes in serum estradiol and progesterone during the menstrual cycle to the thyrotropin and prolactin responses to thyrotropin-releasing hormone. *J Clin Endocrinol Metab.* 1978;47:1296-1302.
46. Sanchez-Frances F, Cacicedo G, Martin-Zurro A, Del Ray FE. Influence of the sex phase of the menstrual cycle on thyrotropin (TSH) response to thyrotropin-releasing hormone (TRH). *J Clin Endocrinol Metab.* 1973;37:736-740.
47. Endicott J, Spitzer RL. A diagnostic interview: The Schedule for Affective Disorders and Schizophrenia. *Arch Gen Psychiatry.* 1978;35:837-844.
48. Hamilton M. A rating scale for depression. *J Neurol Neurosurg Psychiatry.* 1960;23:56-62.
49. Haigler ED, Pittman JA Jr, Heishman JM, Baugh CM. Direct evaluation of pituitary thyrotropin reserve utilizing synthetic thyrotropin-releasing hormone. *J Clin Endocrinol Metab.* 1971;33:573-581.
50. Winokur A, Caroff SN, Amsterdam JD, Maislin G. Administration of thyrotropin-releasing hormone at weekly intervals results in a diminished thyrotropin response. *Biol Psychiatry.* 1984;19:695-702.
51. Garbutt JC, Mayo JP, Gillette GM, Little KY, Hicks RE, Mason GA, Prange AJ Jr. Dose-response studies with thyrotropin-releasing hormone (TRH) in abstinent male alcoholics. *J Stud Alcohol.* 1991;52:275-280.
52. Snyder PJ, Jacobs LS, Utiger RD, Daughaday WH. Thyroid hormone inhibition of the prolactin response to thyrotropin-releasing hormone. *J Clin Invest.* 1973; 52:2324-2329.
53. Carlson HE, Sawin CT, Krugman LG, Meyer NC, Hershman JM. Effect of thyroid hormones on the prolactin response to thyrotropin-releasing hormone in normal persons and euthyroid goitrous patients. *J Clin Endocrinol Metab.* 1978; 47:275-279.
54. Melander A, Westgren U, Ericson L, Sundler F. Influence of the sympathetic nervous system on the secretion and metabolism of thyroid hormone. *Endocrinology.* 1976;101:1228-1237.
55. Lake CR, Pickar D, Ziegler MG, Lipper S, Slater S, Murphy DL. High plasma norepinephrine levels in patients with major affective disorders. *Am J Psychiatry.* 1982;139:1315-1318.
56. Besses GS, Burrow GN, Spaulding SW, Donabedian RK. Dopamine infusion acutely inhibits the TSH and prolactin response to TRH. *J Clin Endocrinol Metab.* 1975;41:985-987.
57. Loosen PT, Youngblood W, Dew B. Plasma levels of exogenous TRH in normal subjects and two patients with TSH blunting. *Psychopharmacol Bull.* 1983; 19:325-327.
58. Segerson TP, Kauer J, Wolfe HC, Mobtaker H, Wu P, Jackson I, Lechan RM. Thyroid hormone regulates TRH biosynthesis in the paraventricular nucleus of the rat hypothalamus. *Science.* 1987;238:78-80.
59. Shioda S, Nakai Y, Sato A, Sunayama S, Shimoda Y. Electromicroscopic cytochemistry of the catecholaminergic innervation of TRH neurons in the rat hypothalamus. *Cell Tissue Res.* 1986;245:247-252.
60. Siever LJ. Role of noradrenergic mechanisms in the etiology of affective disorders. In: Meltzer HY, ed. *Psychopharmacology: The Third Generation of Progress.* New York, NY: Raven Press; 1987:493-504.
61. Post RM, Weiss SRB. Endogenous biochemical abnormalities in affective illness: therapeutic versus pathogenic. *Biol Psychiatry.* 1992;32:469-484.
62. Kirkegaard C. The thyrotropin response to thyrotropin-releasing hormone in endogenous depression. *Psychoneuroendocrinology.* 1981;6:189-212.
63. Whybrow PC, Prange AJ Jr. A hypothesis of thyroid-catecholamine receptor interaction: its relevance to affective illness. *Arch Gen Psychiatry.* 1981;38:106-113.
64. Metcalf G. Regulatory peptides as a source of new drugs. *Brain Res Rev.* 1982; 4:389-408.
65. Prange AJ Jr, Loosen PT, Wilson IC, Lipton MA. The therapeutic use of hormones of the thyroid axis in depression. In: Post RM, Ballenger JC, eds. *Neurobiology of Mood Disorders.* Baltimore, Md: Williams & Wilkins; 1984:311-322.

Conversions From Système International (SI) Units to Traditional Units (Modified From *The SI Manual in Health Care*)

System	Component	SI Reference Interval*	SI Unit	Conversion Factor (Divide by)	Traditional Reference Interval*	Traditional Unit
Serum	Cortisol					
	8 AM	110-520	nmol/L	27.59	4-19	μg/dL
	4 PM	50-410	nmol/L	27.59	2-15	μg/dL
	Midnight	<140	nmol/L	27.59	<5	μg/dL

**These reference values are not intended to be definitive since each laboratory determines its own values. They are provided for illustration only.*

ORIGINAL ARTICLE

Regional Cerebral Blood Flow in Mood Disorders, III

Treatment and Clinical Response

Mitchell S. Nobler, MD; Harold A. Sackeim, PhD; Isak Prohovnik, PhD; James R. Moeller, PhD; Sukdeb Mukherjee, MD; David B. Schnur, MD; Joan Prudic, MD; D. P. Devanand, MD

Background: Global and regional deficits in cerebral blood flow and glucose metabolism have been reported in major depression, but there is limited information on the effects of somatic treatment and clinical recovery on these abnormalities.

Methods: We assessed cortical blood flow with the xenon 133 technique in depressed patients prior to a course of electroconvulsive therapy (ECT), 30 minutes before and 50 minutes after a single treatment, and during the week following ECT. Acute (preictal and postictal) effects of a single treatment also were studied in manic patients.

Results: In the depressed and manic groups, larger blood flow reductions in the acute period, both globally and in particular patterns of brain regions, were associated with a superior clinical outcome following the treatment course. In depressed patients, similar patterns were observed for the blood flow changes over a full treatment course. Blood flow reductions in anterior cortical regions were strongly associated with a positive clinical response in both depression and mania.

Conclusions: The findings indicated that cerebral blood flow abnormalities in major depression were not reversed by successful treatment with ECT. Rather, particularly in responders, ECT resulted in additional perfusion reductions. The therapeutic properties of ECT are related to reduced functional brain activity in specific neural regions.

(Arch Gen Psychiatry. 1994;51:884-897)

SEVERAL STUDIES have found that patients experiencing episodes of major depression have abnormal patterns of cerebral blood flow (CBF) and cerebral metabolic rate (CMR) for glucose.[1] In comparison with normal controls, globally reduced CBF or CMR,[2-12] as well as specific topographic abnormalities,[2-4,8,13-22] has been reported. Most commonly, the topographic disturbances have also reflected CBF or CMR deficits, with widely distributed spatial patterns. Some investigators[2-3,9,13-17,19,22] have emphasized cortical reductions in frontal regions, and reduced CBF and CMR have also been observed in the basal ganglia.[2,13,16,18,22] In contrast, the more limited information on manic patients is inconsistent, with reports of normal, decreased, or increased CBF and CMR during episodes of illness.[2,6,23,24]

It is not known whether these abnormalities reverse with the resolution of affective episodes or whether they reflect persistent deficits. A related issue is the impact of somatic treatments on the baseline CBF and CMR abnormalities. Preclinical research has demonstrated marked effects of antidepressant medications and electroconvulsive shock on cerebral capillary permeability, CBF, and CMR in rodents and primates.[25-28] However, information is lacking at the clinical level, with a few reports indicating that antidepressant medications reverse baseline abnormalities,[2,3] have no effect,[20] or reverse some abnormalities while not affecting others.[8,18,29] It is difficult to draw conclusions from this work because sample sizes have been small and treatment regimens and follow-up intervals often were not standardized. A few reports have indicated that CBF and CMR decrease shortly after electroconvulsive therapy (ECT),[23,30-35] but there are virtually no studies of relations with clinical outcome or of long-term ECT effects.[36]

From the Departments of Biological Psychiatry (Drs Nobler, Sackeim, Moeller, Prudic, and Devanand) and Brain Imaging (Dr Prohovnik), the New York State Psychiatric Institute; the Departments of Psychiatry (Drs Nobler, Sackeim, Prohovnik, Moeller, Prudic, Devanand), Neurology (Dr Prohovnik), and Radiology (Dr Prohovnik), the College of Physicians and Surgeons, Columbia University; and the Department of Psychiatry, Mount Sinai School of Medicine (Dr Schnur), New York, NY; and the Departments of Psychiatry and Neurology, Medical College of Georgia, Augusta (Dr Mukherjee).

See Patients and Methods on next page

PATIENTS AND METHODS

PATIENTS

Depressed patients met the Research Diagnostic Criteria[41] for major depressive disorder, endogenous subtype, and had scores of at least 18 on the Hamilton Rating Scale for Depression (HRSD) (24-item).[42] Patients were excluded if they had a history of schizophrenia, schizoaffective disorder, other functional psychosis, rapid-cycling bipolar disorder, neurological illness or insult (including stroke or transient ischemic attack), substance abuse within the past year or any history of substance dependence, ECT within the previous 6 months, or any significant current medical condition. Sixty-eight depressed patients participated in one or both of the substudies reported herein. The 10 manic patients who participated met the Research Diagnostic Criteria for definite bipolar disorder, manic episode, on the basis of the Schedule for Affective Disorders and Schizophrenia.[43] They had scores of at least 30 on the Modified Mania Scale[44] at study entry. The same exclusion criteria were applied to this sample as to the depressed sample. In addition, prior to ECT, all of the manic patients did not respond to at least one pharmacological trial that involved at least 2 weeks of lithium carbonate, with blood levels between 1.0 and 1.5 mEq/L, or 2 weeks of neuroleptic treatment at dosages equivalent to at least 1500 mg of chlorpromazine hydrochloride per day. **Table 1** presents demographic and clinical features of the patient samples.

TREATMENT AND CLINICAL EVALUATION PROCEDURES

Methods of ECT administration were identical in the depressed and the manic groups, except where noted.[44-47] With the exception of lorazepam administration (up to 3 mg/d, as needed), depressed patients underwent a minimum 5-day psychotropic medication washout prior to the first rCBF assessment and the start of ECT. The 68 depressed patients averaged 18.5±7.7 days (mean±SD) (30-day upper limit) of washout prior to ECT and 1.2±1.0 mg (mean±SD) of lorazepam per day in the 48 hours prior to the first ECT. Manic patients underwent a 4- to 7-day washout of all psychotropic medications prior to ECT, with the exception of amobarbital sodium (up to 500 mg/d, intramuscularly, as needed). Other than these exceptions, both groups were maintained free of psychotropic medications until the completion of assessments during the week following ECT. Electroconvulsive therapy was administered with a constant-current, bidirectional, brief-pulse stimulus device (MECTA Corporation, Lake Oswego, Ore). Medications during the time of ECT were restricted to atropine sulfate (0.4 mg, intravenously), methohexital sodium (0.75 mg/kg), and succinylcholine chloride (0.5 mg/kg), with dosage adjustment after the first treatment. Patients were oxygenated (100% oxygen) from the administration of the anesthetic until the resumption of spontaneous respiration. Motor and electroencephalographic (EEG) seizure manifestations were monitored to ensure adequate duration.[45-47] The d'Elia placement was used for unilateral ECT.

The depressed patients participated in consecutive research protocols. In one study,[45] patients were randomly assigned to right unilateral or bilateral ECT, with stimulus intensity maintained just above seizure threshold (low dose). In the subsequent studies,[46] patients were randomized to either right unilateral or bilateral ECT, but with electrical dosage either just above seizure threshold (low dose) or substantially in excess of the initial seizure threshold (high dose, 150% or 450% above threshold). The number of ECT treatments and the clinical response were determined by a blind evaluation team. Patients received at least eight treatments before being classified as nonresponders. Patients who showed substantial clinical benefit received ECT until they were asymptomatic or had plateaued over at least two treatments. Relative to pre-ECT baseline, responders had at least a 60% reduction in HRSD scores at assessment the day following the final treatment, had a maximal post-ECT HRSD score of 16, and maintained these gains at least 1 week following ECT. A relatively high HRSD cutoff of 16 was used so as not to prejudge the issue of whether maximal response to ECT in patients with "double depression" involved a relatively asymptomatic state or a return to a dysthymic baseline.[48] However, only five of the 35 patients who were classified as ECT responders had HRSD scores of 10 or greater 1 week following ECT.

The manic patients were randomly assigned to left unilateral, right unilateral, or bilateral ECT, with the electrical dose 150% above the initial seizure threshold in all cases.[47] Nonresponders received a minimum of 10 treatments. Responders could not meet the Research Diagnostic Criteria for either mania or hypomania at least 1 week following the end of ECT.

rCBF MEASUREMENT

The rCBF procedures have been described previously.[37] Assessments were made under resting, supine conditions in a quiet, darkened room, with blinders placed over the patients' eyes. The measurements were made using a commercial device (Novo Cerebrograph 32c, Novo Diagnostics Systems, Copenhagen, Denmark), establishing head positioning by orienting a helmet that housed 32 scintillation detectors (16 per hemisphere) in relation to light markers that were aligned to the canthomeatal line. Extensive quality control procedures were used as documented elsewhere.[49] End-tidal P_{CO_2} was continuously monitored during the 11-minute measurement period. Clearance curves were analyzed with a six-unknown model, which provides greater sensitivity under low flow conditions and more accurate artifact removal, as well as with the traditional four-unknown model.[50,51] The major dependent variable was the six-unknown model initial slope index.[52]

rCBF ASSESSMENT INTERVALS

Depressed patients could undergo resting rCBF measurements on four occasions: pretreatment baseline (pre-ECT), 30 minutes before a specific ECT treatment (preictal), 50 minutes following that treatment (postictal), and during the week following the ECT course (post-ECT) (**Table 2**). To maximize sample sizes, separate analyses examined acute (preictal vs postictal) and short-term (pre-ECT vs post-ECT) effects. In both data sets, the sub-

Continued on next page

groups defined by electrode placement and response status were equivalent in age, sex distribution, pre-ECT HRSD scores, P_{CO_2} during each measurement, and number of ECT treatments. Data on manic patients are presented only for the acute interval because too few measurements at other time points met quality standards.

Depression

Acute ECT Effects. Fifty-four depressed patients contributed preictal and postictal rCBF measurements, which were almost always conducted at the sixth treatment (mean±SD, 6.2±1.1 treatments). Response rates tended to be superior with bilateral ECT (65.4%) relative to right unilateral ECT (39.3%) (χ^2=3.68, *P*=.06). As seen in Table 2, HRSD assessment at the time of the rCBF measurements indicated that patients ultimately classified as ECT responders had already achieved greater symptomatic reduction compared with nonresponders (*t*=4.68, *P*<.0001).

Short-term Effects. Cerebral blood flow measurements were available at pretreatment and during the week following the ECT course for 50 patients, who averaged 15.0±9.0 days (mean±SD) of psychotropic medication washout prior to the baseline rCBF measurement. Thirty-six of these 50 patients participated in the substudy on acute effects. The post-ECT measurement occurred 4.6±2.8 days (mean±SD) (range, 2 to 10 days) following the last treatment. Response rates were superior with bilateral ECT (76.0%) compared with right unilateral ECT (32.0%) (χ^2=9.74, *P*<.002).

Acute ECT Effects for Mania

Ten manic patients (Table 1) had rCBF measurements 30 minutes before and 50 minutes following their fifth ECT treatment. Three patients were treated with left unilateral ECT (one responder), four patients received right unilateral ECT (two responders), and three patients received bilateral ECT (three responders). One week following ECT, responders (n=6) had a mean±SD Modified Mania Scale score of 7.3±4.1 compared with a score of 34.0±12.4 in nonresponders (n=4).

STATISTICAL ANALYSES

The results are reported as the mean±SD. The same analytic strategy was applied to all data sets, each of which involved a patient sample (depressed or manic) that was studied at two time points (ie, preictal vs postictal). In the total sample, we used paired *t* tests to determine whether P_{CO_2} and global CBF values changed over time. Analyses of covariance (ANCOVAs) were then applied to the changes in global values (preictal CBF minus postictal CBF or pre-ECT CBF minus post-ECT CBF), using the change in P_{CO_2} as a covariate and electrode placement and response status as between-subject factors.

To examine topographic effects, we used both a conventional multivariate strategy and SSM.[38] For the conventional approach, we computed ratio scores for the CBF values at each of the 32 brain regions: (postictal [or post-ECT] CBF values/preictal [or pre-ECT] CBF values) ×100. A multivariate analysis of variance (MANOVA) was conducted on these ratios, with electrode placement and response status as between-subject factors and hemisphere (two levels) and brain region (16 levels) as repeated measures. The significance of multivariate effects was assessed with the F test associated with Wilks' λ. Significant multivariate interactions were followed by the performance of analyses of variance (ANOVAs) (electrode placement by response status) on the ratio scores at each brain region.

The mathematical properties of SSM, its statistical assumptions, and the computational procedures have been described elsewhere.[38-40] All SSM variables were derived blind to subject and time-point information. The method involves a principal components factor analysis conducted on the portion of rCBF values that is dependent on the subject, the brain region, and the time point. The SSM yields an estimate of a global scaling factor (GSF). This variable quantifies individual differences in global values, removing the contributions of topographic effects. The SSM also produces a set of principal component factors that characterize the covariance relations among brain regions. The weights of each brain region on a factor describe the topographic structure. The loading of a subject on that factor quantifies the extent to which the topographic pattern was manifested by the subject (pattern scores). The number of factors retained was determined by applying the scree test, and we limited each analysis to a maximum of three topographic patterns. Paired *t* tests determined whether the total sample changed in GSF and the pattern scores. Analyses of covariance were then conducted on the post-ECT SSM variables, with electrode placement and response status as between-subject factors and the pre-ECT scores as the covariate.

In a previous study,[37,38] it was found that at baseline, depressed patients had a topographic disturbance that was characterized by bilateral CBF reductions in selective frontal, central, superior temporal, and anterior parietal regions. To track changes in this pattern over the course of treatment, we also computed scores for each depressed subject at each time point on this depression profile. Thirty-two of the 68 depressed patients in the current study had participated in the earlier study. The term "depression profile" is used descriptively, without implying that this CBF abnormality will show sufficient sensitivity and specificity to be of diagnostic utility or that the abnormality is independent of treatment history. However, previous work has suggested that manifestation of this abnormality in the absence of other topographic disturbances distinguishes patients with major depression from those with Alzheimer's disease.[38]

The analyses focused on the CBF changes associated with clinical response and electrode placement, and they were collapsed across electrical dosage conditions because cell sizes were too small to examine the contributions of all three factors. All ANCOVAs using baseline CBF variables (pre-ECT or preictal) as covariates were preceded by ANCOVAs (global values) or ANOVAs (pattern scores) on these baseline values, using response status and electrode placement as between-subject factors. The absence of significant between-group effects in these analyses justified the use of the baseline values as covariates.

Table 1. Demographic and Clinical Features for the Total Depressed and Manic Samples*

Variable	Depressed Patients (n=68) Mean	SD	Manic Patients (n=10) Mean	SD
Age, y	56.8	14.1	36.0	12.5
Sex, % female	61.8	...	60.0	...
Education, y	13.4	3.2	11.6	3.9
Bipolar disorder, %	33.8	...	100	...
Psychosis, %	35.3	...	50.0	...
Pretreatment HRSD score	31.3	7.5	NA	...
Pretreatment MMS score	NA	...	50.9	13.7
Age at onset, y	38.9	18.0	20.6	5.9
Duration of illness, y	17.7	14.0	15.4	11.6
Duration of episode, wk†	42.5	33.2	17.0	8.4
Previous affective episodes, No.‡	4.2	3.4	NA	...
Previous psychiatric hospitalizations, No.‡	2.6	2.7	NA	...

*NA indicates not available; HRSD, Hamilton Rating Scale for Depression; and MMS, Modified Mania Scale.
†Maximum of 104 weeks applied.
‡Maximum of 10 applied.

Previously, a sample of medication-free, elderly depressed patients were studied with the xenon 133 (^{133}Xe) regional CBF (rCBF) technique and were compared with matched normal controls.[37,38] The depressed group had a marked deficit in global cortical CBF, averaging approximately 12% to 14% below control values. In applying a statistical method that reveals abnormal regional patterns by isolating covariance patterns (Scaled Subprofile Model [SSM]),[38-40] it was found that depressed patients also had CBF reductions in a specific cortical pattern, involving selective frontal, central, superior temporal, and anterior parietal regions. Herein, we report on the effects of ECT and clinical response on rCBF in depressed and manic patients.

RESULTS

MAJOR DEPRESSION

Acute Effects

Global Effects. Among the 54 depressed patients (acute effects sample), P_{CO_2} values were higher 50 minutes following the treatment (38.6±5.1 mm Hg) compared with a half hour before the treatment (37.3±4.7 mm Hg) (t=3.84, P<.0005). Despite increased P_{CO_2}, there was a significant decrease in global CBF (average value across the 32 brain regions; preictal, 44.8±7.2; postictal, 43.1±7.2) (t=2.07, P<.05) and in GSF, the SSM measure of region-independent global blood flow (preictal, 44.9±6.7; postictal, 42.8±6.81) (t=2.86, P<.01). The change in P_{CO_2} correlated positively with both the change in global CBF (r=.51, P<.0001) and the change in GSF (r=.47, P<.0005), which suggests that the reductions in global CBF and GSF underestimated the change in cerebral metabolism.

Table 2. Characteristics of the Subsamples of Depressed Patients*

Variable	Acute Effects Sample	Short-term Sample
rCBF measurements	Preictal vs postictal	Pre-ECT vs post-ECT
Gender	21 M, 33 F	19 M, 31 F
Mean±SD age, y	58.2±14.3	55.6±14.7
ECT modality,† No. of patients		
Right unilateral	18, low dose 10, high dose	12, low dose 13, high dose
Bilateral	15, low dose 11, high dose	15, low dose 10, high dose
ECT treatments, mean±SD No.	9.5±2.4	9.4±2.2
Mean±SD pre-ECT washout, d	19.0±7.7	18.4±7.7
Mean±SD seizure duration per treatment, s		
Motor	46.4±13.5	46.8±13.3
EEG	58.8±17.3	59.7±16.2
Mean±SD lorazepam dosage, mg/d‡	0.9±0.9	1.1±1.0
Responders, No.	28	27
Pre-ECT HRSD score, mean±SD	31.0±7.6	32.3±6.9
HRSD score at sixth ECT, mean±SD	12.3±8.2	13.5±9.1
Post-ECT HRSD score, mean±SD	3.5±2.3	4.8±3.1
1-wk post-ECT HRSD score, mean±SD	5.5±4.3	5.6±3.7
Nonresponders, No.	26	23
Pre-ECT HRSD score, mean±SD	30.6±7.9	31.7±8.5
HRSD score at sixth ECT, mean±SD	23.8±9.9	22.7±9.6
Post-ECT HRSD score, mean±SD	24.3±9.1	19.7±10.2
1-wk post-ECT HRSD score, mean±SD	25.4±7.9	22.7±6.9

*Preictal measurements were conducted 30 minutes prior to a treatment and postictal measurements were conducted 50 minutes following that treatment. Pre-electroconvulsive therapy (ECT) measurements were performed following psychotropic medication washout and prior to the start of ECT. Post-ECT measurements were made between 2 and 10 days following the end of ECT. rCBF indicates regional cerebral blood flow; EEG, electroencephalographic; and HRSD, Hamilton Rating Scale for Depression.
†Low-dose treatment involved a stimulus intensity just above seizure threshold. For bilateral ECT, high-dose treatment involved a stimulus intensity 150% above threshold. High-dose unilateral ECT involved a stimulus intensity 150% or 450% above seizure threshold.
‡Average daily dose of lorazepam during the ECT course.

Clinical outcome following the ECT course was associated with the extent of global CBF reduction. The ANCOVA conducted on the change in global CBF yielded a main effect of response status (F=4.56, P<.05). Adjusting for P_{CO_2}, ECT responders averaged a 6.3%±12.1% decrease in global CBF, whereas nonresponders averaged a 1.1%±12.4% increase (unadjusted means, −6.0%±12.3% vs 0.3%±14.6%). Other than the covariate term, no effects were significant in the ANCOVA on the change in GSF. Simultaneous regression analyses were also conducted using the change in P_{CO_2} and the changes in either global CBF or GSF to predict the percentage change in HRSD scores (1-week post-ECT values relative to pre-ECT baseline values). Greater reductions in both global CBF (P<.005) and GSF (P=.02) during the

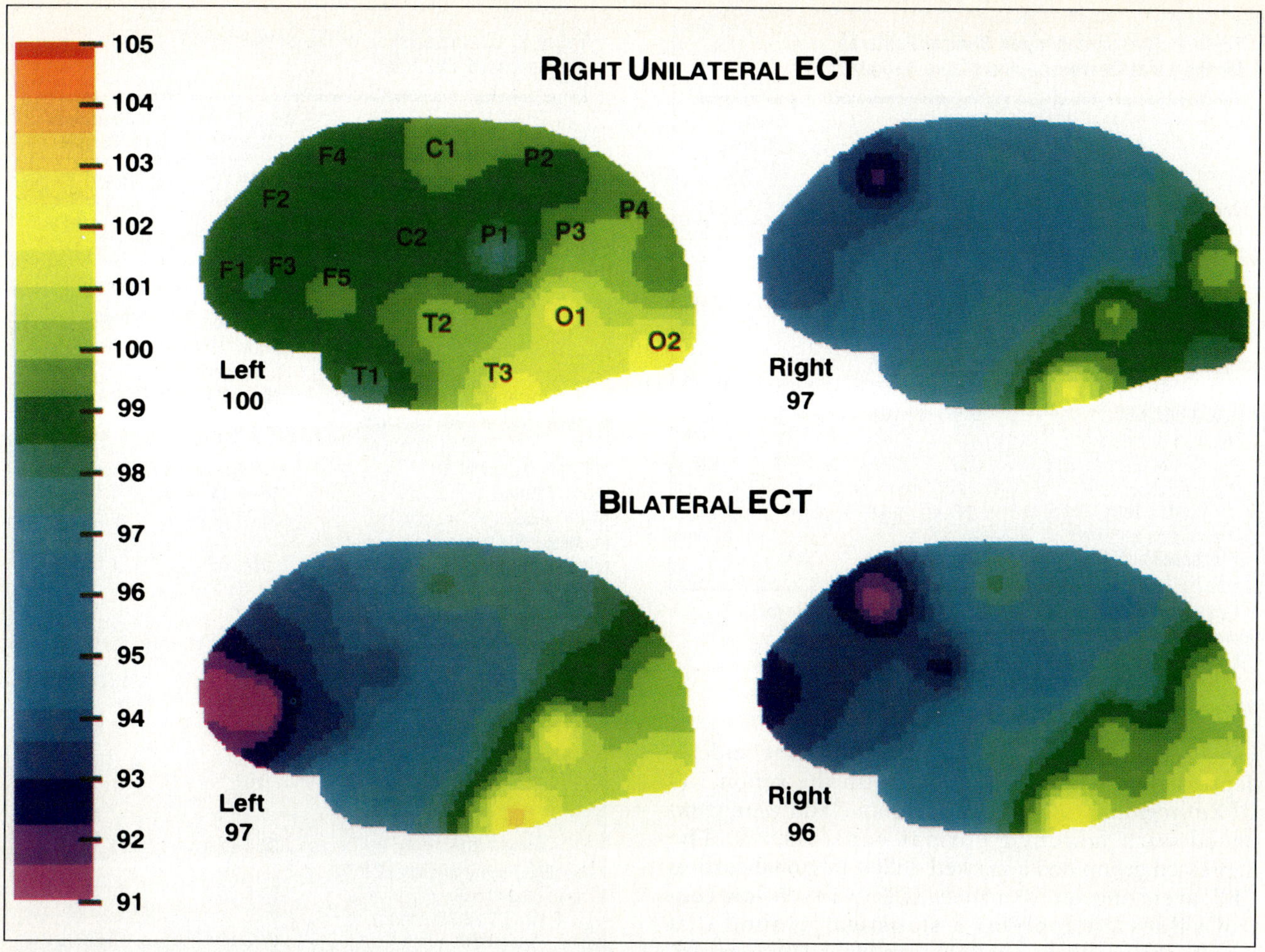

Figure 1. *Mean changes in regional cerebral blood flow (rCBF) as a function of electrode placement in depressed patients during the acute period following a single electroconvulsive therapy (ECT) treatment. Changes in the left and right hemispheres are presented separately for patients who were treated with right unilateral ECT (n=28) or bilateral ECT (n=26). Relative positions of the rCBF detectors are labeled on the representation of the left hemisphere of patients treated with right unilateral ECT. Cerebral blood flow (CBF) values at 32 brain regions were expressed as ratios of the values obtained 50 minutes after a treatment relative to those obtained 30 minutes before the treatment ([posttreatment values/pretreatment values] × 100). Values of 100 indicate no change following the treatment compared with before the treatment. The ratio scores were color coded so that purple and blue correspond to postictal CBF reductions, whereas orange and red correspond to postictal CBF increases. The brain shapes are displayed in a 185 × 112-pixel matrix. Pixels were interpolated from all 16 detectors in each hemisphere, with each detector value multiplied by an inverse square factor equal to $2^{18}/r^2$, with r being the distance in pixels to the center of each detector. All pixels within a radius of 5 pixels from the center of each detector were set to the value of that detector.*

acute period were associated with greater clinical improvement following the treatment course.

Topographic Effects. **Figure 1** depicts the CBF changes during the acute period for each cortical region as a function of electrode placement (right unilateral ECT vs bilateral ECT). **Figure 2** presents these changes as a function of response status. The MANOVA produced main effects of response status (F=4.91, *P*=.03), hemisphere (F=13.97, *P*=.0005), and brain region (F=5.24, *P*<.0001), with significant interactions between electrode placement and hemisphere (F=8.83, *P*<.005) and between response status and brain region (F=2.86, *P*<.005). The main effect of response status was due to greater global CBF reductions in responders (Figure 2). The electrode placements differed in lateralized effects. Right unilateral ECT resulted in reductions that were restricted to the right hemisphere, with no change in the left hemisphere (−3.7%±10.5% vs −0.7%±11.4%). In contrast, bilateral ECT resulted in symmetric CBF reductions (right hemisphere, −3.8%±15.9%; left hemisphere, −3.5%±17.1%) (Figure 1). The CBF reductions were topographically distributed, with the greatest changes in the anterior cortex (Figures 1 and 2). This accounted for the main effect of region and the response-by-region interaction. The follow-up ANOVAs produced significant main effects of response status (*P*<.05) at 11 regions (right hemisphere: F_1, F_2, F_3, F_5, and T_1; left hemisphere: F_1, F_2, F_4, F_5, T_2, and P_1) (Figure 1 illustrates the detector locations). In contrast, none of the effects that involved electrode placement were significant. These analyses of ratio scores indicated that right unilateral and bilateral ECT differed in hemispheric effects. Furthermore, independent of electrode placement, ECT responders had greater postictal CBF reductions than did nonresponders, particularly in anterior cortical regions.

The three topographic patterns revealed by SSM are depicted in **Figure 3**. The first pattern described a bilateral anterior-posterior gradient that involved the complete frontal cortex (F_1 through F_5) and the anterior tem-

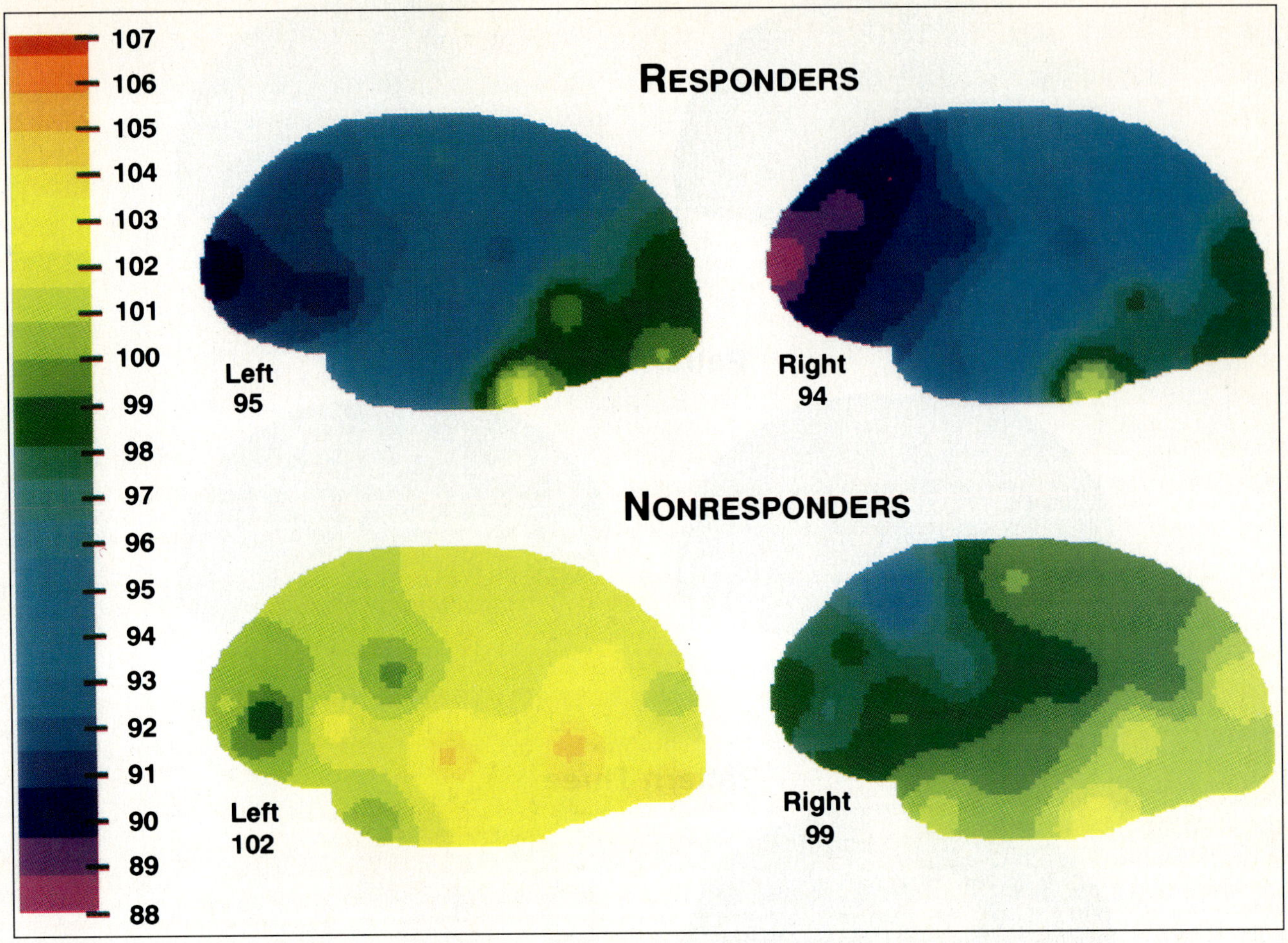

Figure 2. *Mean changes in regional cerebral blood flow as a function of clinical outcome following the treatment course in depressed patients during the acute period following a single electroconvulsive therapy (ECT) treatment (n=28 for ECT responders and n=26 for ECT nonresponders). See Figure 1 for color coding and the interpolation algorithm.*

poral cortex (T_1). Across the sample, there was marked CBF reduction in this pattern following ECT (t=6.77, P<.0001). The second pattern involved a bilateral distribution of relatively high CBF in anterior temporal regions (T_1), coupled with relatively low CBF in selective frontal (F_2 and F_3), central (C_2), and anterior parietal (P_1 and P_2) regions. Cerebral blood flow in this network was unchanged following ECT. The third pattern reflected lateralized effects that involved 10 right-sided regions (F_1, F_2, F_3, F_4, F_5, C_1, C_2, T_2, P_2, and O_2) but also included central (C_2) and superior temporal (T_2) regions in the left hemisphere. Across the sample, scores on this pattern changed following ECT in the direction of reduced CBF in the critical regions (t=2.05, P<.05).

Figure 4 presents the change in scores on each of these three patterns for the subgroups defined by electrode placement and response status. The ANCOVAs revealed a significant main effect of response status for the first pattern (F=7.35, P=.01) and a main effect of electrode placement for the third pattern (F=10.78, P<.002). Other than the contribution of the covariates, no other effects were significant. Responders to either unilateral or bilateral ECT showed more prominent changes in the first pattern than did nonresponders. Positive clinical outcome following the ECT course was associated with greater CBF reduction in this grouping of frontal and anterior temporal regions. The main effect of electrode placement for the third pattern was due to both responders and nonresponders to unilateral ECT manifesting a pattern of asymmetries that was not observed with bilateral ECT. A regression analysis that predicted the percentage change in HRSD scores on the basis of change in GSF, the three patterns, and P_{CO_2} was also conducted. The change in GSF (P<.05) and in the first pattern (P=.01) predicted the magnitude of clinical improvement. These effects found with SSM were fully consistent with the findings obtained using traditional multivariate statistics. Each approach indicated that superior clinical outcome was associated with larger CBF reductions, both globally and in a pattern of anterior cortical regions.

At both preictal and postictal measurements, patients were scored for manifestation of the depression profile identified in previous research.[37] Depression profile scores changed markedly from the preictal to postictal time point (t=7.76, P<.0001). Immediately following ECT, 49 (90.7%) of the 54 patients showed deepening of this topographic abnormality (sign test, P<.0001). An ANCOVA (electrode placement by response status) on the postictal scores, using the preictal score as a covariate, yielded a main effect of response status (F=9.38,

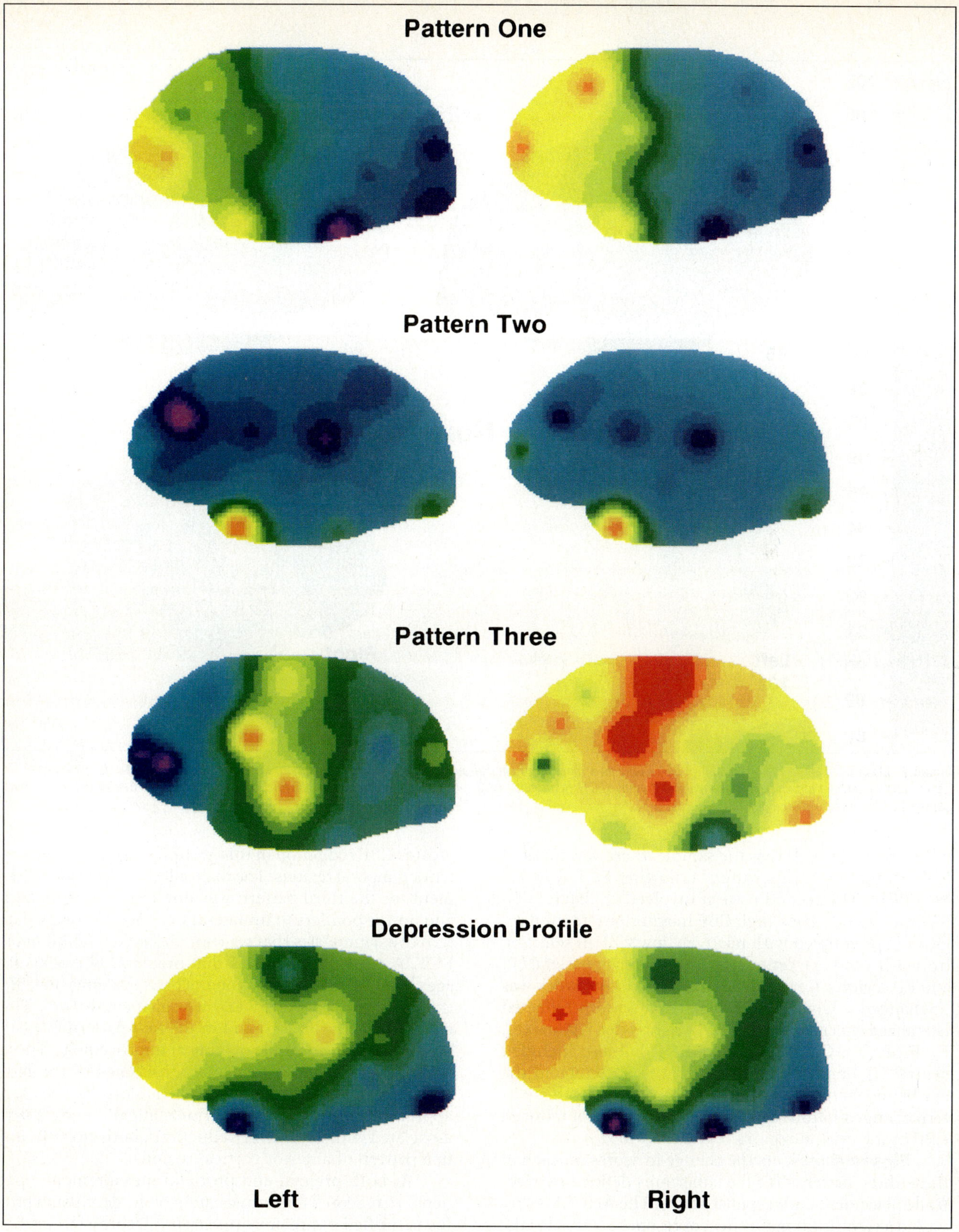

Figure 3. *Three topographic patterns that emerged in the Scaled Subprofile Model (SSM) analysis of acute electroconvulsive therapy (ECT) effects and the original topographic pattern linked to major depression. The color scales denote the weight of brain regions on each pattern. See Figure 1 for the interpolation algorithm. Pattern One corresponded to an anterior-posterior gradient, with high cerebral blood flow (CBF) in bilateral frontal and anterior temporal regions and low CBF in posterior regions. Electroconvulsive therapy resulted in reduced scores on this pattern because of CBF reductions in the critical anterior regions. This effect was most pronounced in treatment responders. Pattern Two corresponded to a pattern of low CBF in selective frontal, central, and anterior parietal regions, with higher CBF in anterior temporal regions. Pattern Three reflected a pattern of asymmetry, involving 10 right-sided regions and two left-sided regions. Right unilateral ECT resulted in an asymmetric pattern of CBF reductions in these critical regions. High region weights on the Depression Profile (orange and red) denote the topographic deficit that was previously linked to major depression.[37] This abnormal pattern was further deepened in the acute period following ECT, particularly in treatment responders.*

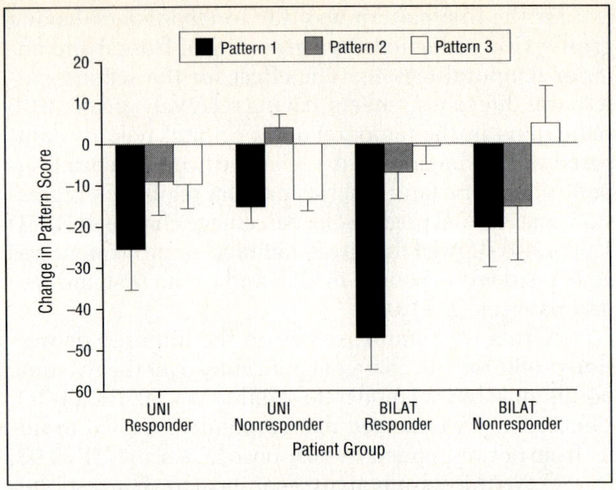

Figure 4. *Mean changes in manifestation of three topographic patterns during the acute period following an electroconvulsive therapy (ECT) treatment as a function of both electrode placement (UNI [right unilateral ECT] vs BILAT [bilateral ECT]) and clinical outcome following the treatment course (responder vs nonresponder). Error bars indicate SEM.*

$P<.005$). Depression profile scores of responders changed more than those of nonresponders. Postictal depression profile scores were also strongly associated with the percentage change in HRSD scores over the treatment course ($r=.48$, $P=.0002$). These analyses indicated that the abnormality, which was previously identified in an overlapping sample as characteristic of major depression, intensified in virtually all patients in the acute period following ECT. Patients who manifested the greatest clinical improvement at the completion of ECT showed the greatest deepening of this topographic deficit.

Prediction of Outcome. To explore whether the observed effects were sufficiently robust to be useful in the prediction of ECT response, a predictive discriminant function analysis was performed that classified patients as responders or nonresponders following ECT on the basis of changes in global CBF during the acute period, the first SSM topographic pattern (anterior-posterior gradient), the imposed SSM depression profile, and PCO_2. Overall classification accuracy was strong (likelihood ratio, $\chi^2=16.18$; $P<.0001$). Of the 28 ECT responders, 19 (68%) were correctly classified, whereas 22 (85%) of 26 ECT nonresponders were correctly classified. This latter aspect was particularly critical because presumably the greatest clinical need pertains to the identification of potential nonresponders. The logistic regression associated with this classification analysis indicated that the changes in the SSM scores for the anterior-posterior topography and for the depression profile were most contributory, without any relation observed with a change in PCO_2.

Medication and Seizure Effects. Analyses of variance were conducted, contrasting the groups defined by electrode placement and clinical response in the number of days of psychotropic medication washout until the CBF measurements and methohexital dose, succinylcholine dose, and motor and EEG measurements of seizure duration at the ECT treatment. There were no significant differences between the groups. Correlations were computed between these variables and the acute-period change in global CBF values and the scores on the topographic patterns revealed by SSM. Higher methohexital dosage tended to be associated with a smaller postictal reduction in global CBF ($r=-.24$, $P<.1$). The duration of motor manifestations of seizure was associated with the changes in global CBF ($r=.42$, $P=.002$), the first SSM topographic pattern ($r=.27$, $P=.05$), and the imposed depression profile ($r=.46$, $P=.001$). These effects were mirrored in the EEG duration measurement and indicated that longer seizures were associated with larger global CBF reductions and with larger CBF decreases in the regions defined by the two topographic patterns. Therefore, similar CBF changes during the acute period were independently associated with positive clinical outcome and longer seizure duration.

During the 48 hours preceding the rCBF measurements, the average daily dose of lorazepam was greater in patients who were later classified as ECT nonresponders (1.3±1.1 mg/d) compared with responders (0.4±0.5 mg/d) ($F=17.0$, $P<.0001$). Nonresponders were more symptomatic and required administration of the anxiolytic agent for anxiety and insomnia (Table 2). However, correlational analyses did not yield any significant relations between lorazepam dosage and global or topographic CBF changes. The findings reported above also were unchanged when lorazepam dosage was included as a covariate in multivariate and univariate ANCOVAs. As a further check, all analyses were repeated, restricting the sample to patients who had averaged 1 mg of lorazepam or less per day in the 48 hours prior to measurement. In this restricted sample, the 26 responders and 13 nonresponders were equivalent in average lorazepam dosage (0.3±0.4 vs 0.4±0.5 mg/d, respectively), yet the differences in the change in global CBF, the first SSM pattern (anterior-posterior gradient), and the imposed depression profile all remained significant.

Effects of the ECT Course

Global CBF Effects. There was no change in PCO_2 among the 50 patients studied at pretreatment baseline and during the week following treatment. There also was no change in global CBF (pre-ECT measurement, 45.8±8.2; post-ECT measurement, 45.4±8.5) or GSF (pre-ECT measurement, 45.4±7.8; post-ECT measurement, 45.5±8.2). Global flow values showed moderate stability, with a test-retest correlation of .65 for global CBF and .61 for GSF (P's$<.0001$). The ANCOVA on the change in global CBF yielded a trend for a main effect of response status ($F=3.06$, $P=.09$). This effect was significant in the analysis of GSF ($F=5.91$, $P<.02$). At the post-ECT measurement, global CBF was reduced by 5.2%±14.6% in responders and increased by 6.9%±17.7% in nonresponders. The ECT responders averaged a 6.0%±13.1% decrease in GSF, whereas nonresponders had a 9.3%±16.8% increase. The within-group change in global CBF was significant among responders ($t=2.20$, $P<.05$), whereas the GSF changes were significant for both responders ($t=2.56$, $P<.02$) and nonresponders ($t=2.44$, $P<.02$). These effects were confirmed with re-

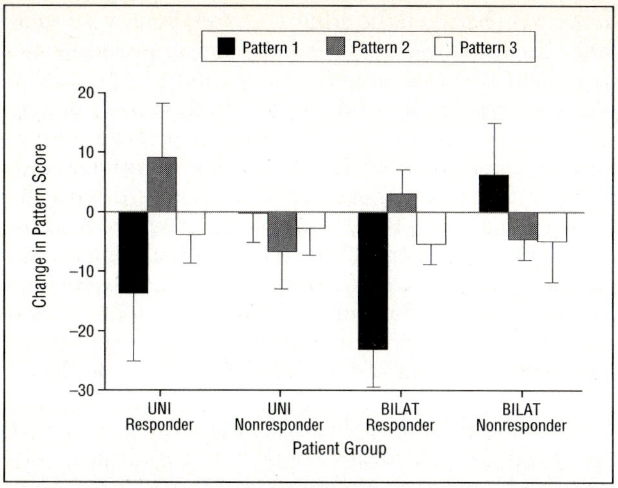

Figure 5. *Mean changes in the manifestation of three topographic patterns over the complete treatment course as a function of both electrode placement (UNI [right unilateral electroconvulsive therapy] vs BILAT [bilateral electroconvulsive therapy]) and clinical outcome following the treatment course (responder vs nonresponder). Error bars indicate SEM.*

gression analyses. The greater the reduction in global CBF ($P<.05$) or GSF ($P<.02$), the greater the percentage change in HRSD scores.

Topographic Effects. The MANOVA conducted on the 32 ratio scores (post-ECT CBF/pre-ECT CBF) yielded a trend for a main effect of response status (F=3.57, P=.06), an interaction between response status and brain region (F=2.73, $P<.01$), and an interaction between electrode placement, hemisphere, and brain region (F=2.50, P=.02). The main effect reflected the greater global CBF reduction in responders than in nonresponders. The interactions indicated that clinical response and electrode placement were associated with changes in topography. Follow-up ANOVAs on the ratio scores yielded significant main effects of response status (P's<.05) at 10 locations (right hemisphere: F_4, T_1, T_2, P_3, P_4, and O_2; left hemisphere: F_3, F_4, F_5, and T_1), all in the direction of lower values in responders. The ANOVAs did not produce a significant effect involving electrode placement.

The first pattern in the SSM analysis was similar to the first pattern in the analysis of acute effects, whereas the second pattern was very similar to the depression profile reported in previous work[37] but had greater emphasis on preserved CBF in anterior temporal regions (T_1). The third pattern was dominated by a right prefrontal region (F_1), with smaller contributions from the left hemisphere's superior and posterior temporal regions (T_2 and T_3). The total sample showed a significant change in the first pattern (t=2.44, $P<.02$) and tended to change in the third pattern (t=1.80, P=.08). In both cases, these changes reflected CBF reductions in the regions defining these patterns. The ANCOVAs conducted on the post-ECT pattern scores produced a significant main effect of response status for the first pattern (F=4.95, $P<.05$) and a trend for the second pattern (F=2.94, P=.09). There were no effects of electrode placement in any of the analyses. As seen in **Figure 5**, compared with nonresponders, ECT responders showed a greater change in the first and second patterns. As in the analysis of acute effects, the effect for the first pattern was due to responders' having greater CBF reductions in a grouping of frontal and anterior temporal regions. The effect for the second pattern was due to responders' having relatively greater CBF reductions in the temporal and occipital regions compared with reductions in the selective frontal, central, superior temporal, and anterior parietal regions. A regression analysis that predicts the percentage change in HRSD scores also showed that greater clinical improvement was associated with changes in GSF and in the first and second patterns (P's<.05).

Across the sample, scores on the imposed depression profile did not change significantly over the two time points and showed moderate stability (r=.50, $P<.0001$). The ANCOVA indicated that responders tended to differ from nonresponders in their post-ECT scores (F=2.93, P=.09). Within-group analyses indicated that responders tended to decrease in their magnitude of abnormality following ECT relative to pretreatment (t=1.79, P=.09), whereas nonresponders were unchanged. Change in manifesting this profile was not associated with change in HRSD scores. In addition, the trend for improved scores on the depression profile among responders was not due to enhanced CBF in the regions that were previously found to be characterized by CBF deficits. Rather, at the post-ECT measurement, responders had a less differentiated topography because of CBF reductions in the anterior temporal and occipital regions, areas originally identified as preserved in major depression.

Medication and Seizure Effects. Analyses of variance contrasted the groups in the number of days of psychotropic washout until the pre-ECT CBF measurement, the interval between the last ECT and the post-ECT CBF measurement, and methohexital dose, succinylcholine dose, and motor and EEG measurements of seizure duration, each averaged across all treatments. There were no significant effects. Correlational analyses indicated that none of these measures or the number of ECT treatments was associated with the change in global CBF or in scores on any of the SSM patterns.

An ANOVA indicated that the average daily lorazepam dose was greater in nonresponders than in responders when averaged over the treatment course (1.5±1.1 mg/d vs 0.7±0.7, respectively) and during the 48 hours preceding the post-ECT CBF measurement (1.2±1.2 mg/d vs 0.3±0.5 mg/d, respectively) (P's<.005). However, there were no associations between lorazepam dosage and the changes in CBF values, and inclusion of lorazepam dosage as a covariate term in the major analyses yielded no change in the findings. In addition, we repeated the major analyses, restricting the sample to patients who received an average daily dose of 1 mg of lorazepam or less throughout the ECT course and in the 48 hours preceding the final CBF measurement. These subgroups of 23 responders and 10 nonresponders were virtually identical in average lorazepam dosage (eg, during ECT: responders, 0.5±0.4 mg/d; nonresponders, 0.4±0.3 mg/d), but responders still manifested significantly greater reductions in global CBF, GSF, and change in scores for the first SSM topographic pattern (anterior-posterior gradient).

MANIA: ACUTE EFFECTS

Among the 10 manic patients, PCO_2 values were unchanged 50 minutes following the treatment (41.1±4.1 mm Hg) compared with a half hour before the treatment (40.7±4.6 mm Hg). There was a large reduction in global CBF (preictal CBF, 59.3±7.5; postictal CBF, 51.8±8.2) (t=3.83, P<.005) but no change in GSF (preictal GSF, 56.5±5.5; postictal GSF, 54.0±7.8). The lack of change in GSF indicated that a large proportion of the global CBF reduction was due to changes in topography. Separate ANCOVAs were conducted on the changes in global CBF and GSF with either response status or electrode placement as a between-subjects factor. None of the effects of electrode placement was significant. Responders had larger global CBF decreases (−18.0%±9.2%) than did nonresponders (−4.0%±5.2%) (F=5.70, P<.05), with no difference for GSF.

A repeated measures ANOVA was conducted on the ratio scores at the 32 regions with response status as a between-subjects factor and with hemisphere (two levels) and region (16 levels) as repeated measures. There were main effects of response status (F=7.58, P<.02) and of region (F=3.95, P<.002) and an interaction between response status and region (F=2.33, P<.05). Follow-up t tests indicated that responders had significantly lower ratio scores (P's<.05) than did nonresponders at four right hemisphere regions (F_1, F_3, T_1, and P_1) and 11 left hemisphere regions (F_1, F_3, F_4, F_5, C_1, T_1, T_2, P_1, P_2, P_3, and O_1).

The first pattern that emerged in the SSM analysis described the characteristic anterior-posterior gradient, with heavy weighting of anterior frontal regions. The second pattern was unique to the manic sample and was defined by relatively high CBF in bilateral anterior temporal regions (T_1) and left hemisphere prefrontal regions (F_1 and F_3) and low CBF in bilateral central regions (C_1 and C_2). The third pattern expressed hemispheric asymmetry, with CBF higher in all left hemisphere regions than in all right hemisphere regions. The total sample changed significantly in expression of the first and second patterns (P's<.05). The change in the first pattern reflected decreased CBF in bilateral frontal regions at the postictal assessment. The change in the second pattern reflected bilateral decreases in central regions. In ANCOVAs on the postictal pattern scores, there was a significant effect of response status for the first pattern (F=5.21, P<.05). Responders evidenced greater bilateral frontal reductions than did nonresponders. These analyses were repeated, substituting electrode placement for response status. There was a trend for a main effect of electrode placement for the third pattern (F=4.60, P<.06). Post hoc comparisons indicated that patients undergoing left and right unilateral ECT differed in their scores on this laterality pattern, with right unilateral ECT associated with greater CBF reductions in the right hemisphere and left unilateral ECT associated with greater CBF reductions in the left hemisphere.

COMMENT

The majority of functional imaging studies in major depression have found pretreatment deficits in global and/or topographic CBF and CMR.[2-23] Nonetheless, the most striking finding in this study was that depressed patients who responded to ECT had further CBF reductions. Relative to baseline, ECT responders had reduced global CBF in the acute period following a single treatment and during the week following the treatment course. In addition, all the topographic changes that distinguished responders from nonresponders were due to greater regional CBF reductions in the patients who improved. In a small group of manic patients, ECT responders also showed greater global and topographic reductions during the acute period than did nonresponders.

The largest CBF changes were observed in the acute-effects studies. In the manic sample, responders averaged an 18% global CBF decrease following a single treatment. Among depressed patients, CBF decreases in the acute period were most marked in a set of frontal and anterior temporal regions, averaging approximately 12% among responders. At the intervals studied herein, the short-acting barbiturates used for anesthesia did not appear to alter CBF. Silfverskiöld[36] found no CBF changes 1 to 2 hours following sham ECT, ie, administration of anesthetic medications alone, but observed the characteristic global reduction with real ECT. In our study, ECT electrode placement was associated with distinct CBF regional patterns only at the acute time point. Bilateral ECT resulted in symmetric CBF reductions, whereas in both depression and mania, unilateral ECT produced decreases restricted mainly to the hemisphere ipsilateral to stimulation (Figure 1). Longer seizure duration was associated with more marked CBF reductions at the acute time point, but seizure duration was not related to CBF changes across the treatment course or to clinical outcome.

The acute-effects studies were conducted at the fifth treatment in manic patients and typically at the sixth treatment in depressed patients. In both samples, ECT responders had greater global and topographic CBF decreases during the acute period than did nonresponders. Indeed, the postictal CBF reductions, especially in an anterior-posterior gradient and in the depression profile, were predictive of eventual ECT outcome, with high accuracy in forecasting nonresponse. Therefore, functional imaging studies may have clinical utility in predicting clinical response to ECT if it is found that this power to predict outcome applies to acute-effects studies conducted at early treatments. In contrast, it could be argued that the differences in acute changes between responders and nonresponders at the sixth treatment were due to the responder group's being already partially remitted. This suggests that the larger reductions in the acute period observed in responders, rather than being predictive of the change in clinical state, were a result of an already improved clinical state. However, arguing against this possibility are preliminary reports that the magnitude of the global CBF reduction in the acute period is greatest at early treatments and attenuates at later treatments.[31,53] Nonetheless, future studies should examine differences between responders and nonresponders at early treatments to more directly test these competing hypotheses.

During the week following ECT, we observed some of the same, albeit less profound, general effects on CBF

as were observed in the acute-effects analyses. Global CBF was significantly reduced in responders compared with baseline, whereas it tended to increase in nonresponders. In all three data sets examined in this study, the first topographic pattern corresponded to an anterior-posterior gradient, reflecting higher CBF in selective frontal and anterior temporal regions and lower CBF in posterior regions. The patients who responded to ECT showed reduced manifestation of this pattern because of CBF decreases in selective frontal and anterior temporal regions. In the depressed sample, this induction of hypofrontality was more marked in responders than in nonresponders at both the postictal time point and several days following the end of ECT. Similarly, the induction of hypofrontality in the acute period was greater in manic responders than in nonresponders. In both patient samples, this CBF reduction in anterior cortical regions was the topographic change most consistently related to superior clinical outcome. This phenomenon is of particular interest because the most common cortical deficit reported at pretreatment in major depression has been reduced CBF or CMR in frontal regions.[2,3,7,13-15,17,20]

In the acute period following ECT, abnormal scores on the imposed depression profile were intensified in virtually all depressed patients. This effect was particularly marked among ECT responders. In contrast, following the treatment course, ECT responders showed nonsignificant improvement in depression profile scores. This seeming improvement was not due to increased CBF in regions manifesting abnormalities at baseline. Rather, after treatment, responders had further CBF reductions in these selective frontal, central, superior temporal, and anterior parietal regions, but the magnitude of these reductions was less than in the anterior temporal and occipital regions that had been notably preserved at baseline. Therefore, in this study, there was no evidence that pretreatment deficits in major depression reversed with clinical response to ECT. Rather, short-term clinical response was associated with further global and topographic CBF reductions.

Our findings that ECT produces CBF reductions in the acute and short-term periods are in agreement with other studies. In schizophrenic patients, using the nitrous oxide method, Kety et al[54] observed 35% reductions in global CBF 15 minutes following ECT. Postictal reductions in CMR for glucose have also been observed with positron emission tomography[25] and in CBF using the ^{133}Xe-inhalation[31,53] and hexamethylpropyleneamine oxime (HM-PAO) single-photon emission computed tomography[34] techniques. Rosenberg et al,[32] using single-photon emission computed tomography, and Volkow et al,[35] employing positron emission tomography, found decreased CBF and CMR, respectively, 24 hours following ECT. These findings were consistent with the marked postictal decreases in CBF and CMR in animals following induced seizures[25,55] and interictally in epileptic patients following some types of spontaneous seizures.[56,57] This study is the first to contrast the CBF profiles of a large group of ECT responders and nonresponders and suggests that the magnitude of the CBF reductions in the acute and short-term periods is related to the antidepressant effects of ECT.

LIMITATIONS OF THE STUDY

Several limitations of the study should be considered. This research used forms of ECT that varied in electrode placement and stimulus dosage. Our analyses focused on the CBF changes associated with clinical response and electrode placement and ignored dosage effects. This strategy was adopted because of the limited size of subgroups. Elsewhere, it has been documented that higher-intensity stimulation enhances the efficacy of right unilateral ECT, raising the possibility that the clinical outcome findings were confounded by dosage effects.[46] Three facts argue against this possibility. First, all of the findings that distinguished depressed responders and nonresponders applied equally to groups treated with right unilateral or bilateral ECT. It was also shown that higher-intensity stimulation does not enhance the efficacy of bilateral ECT.[46] Second, we reanalyzed the data on acute effects in major depression, restricting the sample to patients treated with low electrical intensity (data not shown). All major effects were maintained. Third, similar acute effects were observed in the manic and depressed samples. The manic patients all received high-dosage stimulation.

Another limitation concerns possible order effects. In some studies,[58,59] normal controls have had higher global CBF at first measurement than at second and subsequent measurements. Thus, the findings of decreased global CBF in ECT responders might be viewed as an adaptation to the measurement conditions. This possibility is also unlikely. First, in the acute-effects studies, the preictal measurement was used as the baseline. In both the depressed and manic samples, all patients had participated in at least one measurement prior to the preictal assessment, which rules out first measurement effects. Second, the major findings pertained to differences between ECT responders and nonresponders. Both groups were evaluated at equivalent time points. Third, in a group of 11 patients, we obtained serial CBF measurements at pretreatment baseline, following an unsuccessful ECT course, and after response to a crossover course of high-dosage bilateral ECT (data not shown). Compared with pretreatment, global CBF was slightly increased following the unsuccessful treatment course but was significantly reduced following the successful crossover treatment. Therefore, the findings relating CBF reductions to superior clinical outcome did not appear to be contingent on first measurement effects.

Perhaps the most important limitation concerns the use of the ^{133}Xe-inhalation lateral probe technique. This method provides absolute CBF quantification, is particularly sensitive to cortical phenomena, and because it assesses CBF in perfused tissue only, is less subject to partial volume artifacts than are tomographic approaches. However, the method has limited spatial resolution, and its inability to observe subcortical effects is a major drawback. We found that in addition to topographic effects, clinical response was associated with global cortical CBF reductions. The global changes may have reflected decreased excitatory or increased inhibitory input from subcortical nuclei, with widespread cortical projection. In addition, CBF is typically assessed in psychiatric disor-

ders as an indirect measure of cerebral metabolism and neuronal activity. In the normal brain, CBF and glucose metabolism are tightly coupled on a local basis.[60,61] Particularly with respect to acute effects, it is conceivable that ECT results in a decoupling of CBF and glucose metabolism, given that increases in CBF outstrip increases in metabolic rate during seizures[55,62] and that there is transient postictal disruption of the blood-brain barrier.[63,64] For these reasons, direct measurement of the effects of ECT on regional glucose metabolism with positron emission tomography would be valuable.

rCBF ABNORMALITIES IN MAJOR DEPRESSION

This study highlights a theoretical paradox. A number of studies[2-22] have reported that compared with controls, untreated depressed patients have global and regional CBF and CMR deficits. Comparison with matched normal controls has also shown marked deficits in the depressed patients studied herein.[37,38] Yet, in this study, effective treatment with ECT resulted in further global and topographic reductions. Before the possible resolutions of this paradox can be considered more than speculation, we may have to await a better understanding of the pathophysiology of major depression and of the mechanisms of action of antidepressant treatments. Nonetheless, we offer our perspective.

Our findings are compatible with the theory that the anticonvulsant properties of ECT are related to its antidepressant and antimanic properties.[65,66] Electroconvulsive therapy is a powerful anticonvulsant. In animals and humans, there is a progressive increase in seizure threshold with repeated electrical induction of seizures.[45,67] Seizure duration also displays a progressive decrease over the ECT course.[68] Traditionally, the defining characteristics of compounds with anticonvulsant activity have been the ability to increase seizure threshold and/or reduce seizure manifestations.[69] Electroconvulsive therapy also results in decreased neurometabolic activity and cerebral circulation,[23,25,30-35] as well as enhanced EEG slow-wave activity. In animals, electroconvulsive shock can prevent the development of kindled seizures or block seizure expression in already kindled animals.[66,70] There are also limited clinical data that suggest that ECT may be useful in reducing the frequency of spontaneous seizures in some cases of intractable seizure disorder.[65,71-73] The anticonvulsant theory posits that ECT triggers an endogenous process that terminates the generalized seizure and results in enhanced postictal inhibition of functional activity. Systems that involve γ-aminobutyric acid,[74,75] endogenous opioids,[76] adenosine,[77] and/or endogenous monoamine oxidase inhibition[78] have been implicated in these anticonvulsant effects.

Some studies have suggested that the magnitude of the increase in seizure threshold during ECT is associated with clinical outcome. In both depressed[68,79,80] and manic[81] samples, larger increases in seizure threshold have correlated with superior clinical response. Similarly, the findings in this study suggest that larger CBF reductions, globally and in a pattern of frontal and anterior temporal regions, are associated with positive clinical outcome in both major depression and mania. As Post et al[66] have pointed out, the fact that ECT is effective in both depression and mania lends credence to the anticonvulsant hypothesis. This spectrum is not shared by traditional antidepressant medications but may be observed with some anticonvulsant agents.[82] In short, the findings of this study are compatible with the view that enhanced inhibition, both transcortically and specifically in an anterior cortical pattern, is linked to the efficacy of ECT.

The baseline rCBF abnormalities in the depressed sample did not reverse at either time point. Although complicated by medication status, preliminary 2-month follow-up data on 17 patients (data not shown) indicated that global CBF remained significantly reduced relative to baseline, despite sustained euthymia. At 2-month follow-up, patients showed strong stability in their baseline topographic deficit. Therefore, our findings suggest that in the relatively elderly and severely depressed sample studied herein, the pretreatment global and topographic CBF deficits are persistent abnormalities.

In accounting for the persistence of baseline abnormalities in the depressed sample, one possibility is that, despite the relatively long medication washout, the baseline deficits reflect long-term effects of prior treatment. In this respect, the changes associated with response to ECT accentuate the persistent effects of previous antidepressant therapies. Another possibility is that the baseline deficits reflect secondary compensatory changes, in effect, the response of the brain to the state of major depression. According to this view, ECT results in an accentuation of these compensatory alterations. However, a third possibility suggests that the CBF deficits in elderly depressed patients are a trait characteristic. There is growing evidence that such samples have a high prevalence of subcortical gray and white matter magnetic resonance imaging signal abnormalities, which is suggestive of an ischemic cerebrovascular disease process.[1,83-85] It is possible that the persistent CBF deficits that we observed are linked to such a cerebrovascular disease process and are related to the fixed structural abnormalities. Similar magnetic resonance imaging hyperintensities in other populations consistently have been associated with perfusion deficits,[86-90] and research that examines the covariation between the extent and the location of structural and functional brain abnormalities in major depression is needed.

Critically, the findings of this study, linking clinical response with CBF reductions, also suggest that there are state-related abnormalities. Depressive episodes may be associated with enhanced functional activity in one or more neural systems.[18] However, particularly in pretreatment cross-sectional comparisons, the presence of marked trait CBF deficits would obscure the identification of such smaller state-dependent regional increases in functional activity. Effective antidepressant treatments such as ECT may produce clinical remission by reducing functional activity in these putatively disinhibited systems, without influencing the background of persistent functional deficit. If this view is correct, it may prove useful in understanding why treatments such as ECT are remarkably powerful in suppressing the symptomatic expression of episodes but have little impact on the underlying disease process.

Accepted for publication August 17, 1994.

This study was supported in part by grants MH35636, MH44779, and MH47739 from the National Institute of Mental Health and grant AG05433 from the National Institute of Aging, Bethesda, Md; an Established Investigator Award (Dr Sackeim) and a Young Investigator Award (Dr Nobler) from the National Alliance for Research in Schizophrenia and Depression, Chicago, Ill; and the Jean and Louis Dreyfus Foundation, and the Dana Foundation, New York, NY.

We thank Claire D. Metz, PhD, for designing the rCBF display software.

Reprint requests to Department of Biological Psychiatry, Unit 72, New York State Psychiatric Institute, 722 W 168th St, New York, NY 10032 (Dr Nobler).

REFERENCES

1. Sackeim HA, Prohovnik I. Studies of brain imaging in mood disorders. In: Mann JJ, Kupfer D, eds. *The Biology of Depressive Disorders: Part A: A Systems Perspective.* New York, NY: Plenum Publishing Corp; 1993:205-258.
2. Baxter LR Jr, Phelps M, Maziotta J, Schwartz J, Gerner R, Selin C, Sumida R. Cerebral metabolic rates for glucose in mood disorders. *Arch Gen Psychiatry.* 1985;42:441-447.
3. Baxter LR Jr, Schwartz JM, Phelps ME, Mazziotta JC, Guze BH, Selin CE, Gerner RH, Sumida RM. Reduction of prefrontal cortex glucose metabolism common to three types of depression. *Arch Gen Psychiatry.* 1989;46:243-250.
4. Devous MS. Imaging brain function by single-photon emission computer tomography. In: Andreasen N, ed. *Brain Imaging: Applications in Psychiatry.* Washington, DC: American Psychiatric Press; 1989:147-234.
5. Kanaya T, Yonekawa M. Regional cerebral blood flow in depression. *Jpn J Psychiatry Neurol.* 1990;44:571-576.
6. Kishimoto H, Takazu O, Ohno S, Yamaguchi T, Fujita H, Kuwahara H, Ishii T, Matsushita M, Yokoi S, Iio M. 11C-glucose metabolism in manic and depressed patients. *Psychiatry Res.* 1987;22:81-88.
7. Kumar A, Newburg A, Alavi A, Berlin J, Smith R, Reivich M. Regional cerebral glucose metabolism in late-life depression and Alzheimer disease: a preliminary positron emission tomography study. *Proc Natl Acad Sci U S A.* 1993; 90:7019-7023.
8. Martinot JL, Hardy P, Feline A, Huret JD, Mazoyer B, Attar-Levy D, Pappata S, Syrota A. Left prefrontal glucose hypometabolism in the depressed state: a confirmation. *Am J Psychiatry.* 1990;147:1313-1317.
9. Mathew R, Meyer J, Francis D, Semchuk K, Mortel K, Claghorn J. Cerebral blood flow in depression. *Am J Psychiatry.* 1980;137:1449-1450.
10. O'Connell RA, Van Heertum RL, Billick SB, Holt AR, Gonzalez A, Notardonato H, Luck D, King LN. Single photon emission computed tomography (SPECT) with $^{[123]}$ IMP in the differential diagnosis of psychiatric disorders. *J Neuropsychiatry Clin Neurosci.* 1989;1:145-153.
11. Schlegel S, Aldenhoff JB, Eissner D, Linder P, Nickel O. Regional cerebral blood flow in depression: associations with psychopathology. *J Affect Disord.* 1989; 17:211-218.
12. Warren L, Butler R, Katholi C, McFarland C, Crews E, Halsey J Jr. Focal changes in cerebral blood flow produced by monetary incentive during a mental mathematics task in normal and depressed subjects. *Brain Cogn.* 1984;3:71-85.
13. Austin MP, Dougall N, Ross M, Murray C, O'Carroll RE, Moffoot A, Ebmeier KP, Goodwin GM. Single photon emission tomography with ^{99m}Tc-exametazime in major depression and the pattern of brain activity underlying the psychotic/neurotic continuum. *J Affect Disord.* 1992;26:31-43.
14. Bench CJ, Friston KJ, Brown RG, Frackowiak RSJ, Dolan RJ. Regional cerebral blood flow in depression measured by positron emission tomography: the relationship with clinical dimensions. *Psychol Med.* 1993;23:579-590.
15. Buchsbaum MS, DeLisi L, Holcomb H, Cappelletti J, King A, Johnson J, Hazlett E, Dowling-Zimmerman S, Post R, Morihisa J, Carpenter W, Cohen R, Pickar D, Weinberger D, Margolin R, Kessler R. Anteroposterior gradients in cerebral glucose use in schizophrenia and affective disorders. *Arch Gen Psychiatry.* 1984; 41:1159-1166.
16. Buchsbaum MS, Wu J, DeLisi LE, Holcomb H, Kessler R, Johnson J, King AC, Hazlett E, Langston K, Post RM. Frontal cortex and basal ganglia metabolic rates assessed by positron emission tomography with [18F]2-deoxyglucose in affective illness. *J Affect Disord.* 1986;10:137-152.
17. Cohen RM, Semple WE, Gross M, Nordahl TE, King AC, Pickar D, Post RM. Evidence for common alterations in cerebral glucose metabolism in major affective disorders and schizophrenia. *Neuropsychopharmacology.* 1989;2:241-254.
18. Drevets WC, Raichle ME. Neuroanatomical circuits in depression: implications for treatment mechanisms. *Psychopharmacol Bull.* 1992;28:261-274.
19. Hagman JO, Buchsbaum MS, Wu JC, Rao SJ, Reynolds CA, Blinder BJ. Comparison of regional brain metabolism in bulimia nervosa and affective disorder assessed with positron emission tomography. *J Affect Disord.* 1990;19:153-162.
20. Hurwitz TA, Clark C, Murphy E, Klonoff H, Martin WR, Pate BD. Regional cerebral glucose metabolism in major depressive disorder. *Can J Psychiatry.* 1990; 35:684-688.
21. Mayberg HS, Starkstein SE, Sadzot B, Preziosi T, Andrezejewski PL, Dannals RF, Wagner HN Jr, Robinson RG. Selective hypometabolism in the inferior frontal lobe in depressed patients with Parkinson's disease. *Ann Neurol.* 1990; 28:57-64.
22. Post RM, DeLisi LE, Holcomb HH, Uhde TW, Cohen R, Buchsbaum MS. Glucose utilization in the temporal cortex of affectively ill patients: positron emission tomography. *Biol Psychiatry.* 1987;22:545-553.
23. Silfverskiöld P, Risberg J. Regional cerebral blood flow in depression and mania. *Arch Gen Psychiatry.* 1989;46:253-259.
24. Migliorelli R, Starkstein SE, Teson A, de Quiros G, Vazquez S, Leiguarda R, Robinson RG. SPECT findings in patients with primary mania. *J Neuropsychiatry Clin Neurosci.* 1993;5:379-383.
25. Ackermann RF, Engel J Jr, Baxter L. Positron emission tomography and autoradiographic studies of glucose utilization following electroconvulsive seizures in humans and rats. *Ann N Y Acad Sci.* 1986;462:263-269.
26. Caldecott-Hazard S, Mazziotta J, Phelps M. Cerebral correlates of depressed behavior in rats, visualized using 14C-2-deoxyglucose autoradiography. *J Neurosci.* 1988;8:1951-1961.
27. Gerber JC III, Choki J, Brunswick DJ, Reivich M, Frazer A. The effect of antidepressant drugs on regional cerebral glucose utilization in the rat. *Brain Res.* 1983;269:319-325.
28. Preskorn SH, Raichle ME, Hartman BK. Antidepressants alter cerebrovascular permeability and metabolic rate in primates. *Science.* 1982;217:250-252.
29. Goodwin GM, Austin MP, Dougall N, Ross M, Murray C, O'Carroll RE, Moffoot A, Prentice N, Ebmeier KP. State changes in brain activity shown by the uptake of ^{99m}Tc-exametazime with single photon emission tomography in major depression before and after treatment. *J Affect Disord.* 1993;29:243-253.
30. Guze BH, Baxter LR Jr, Schwartz JM, Szuba MP, Liston EH. Electroconvulsive therapy and brain glucose metabolism. *Convulsive Ther.* 1991;7:15-19.
31. Prohovnik I, Sackeim H, Decina P, Malitz S. Acute reductions of regional cerebral blood flow following electroconvulsive therapy: interactions with modality and time. *Ann N Y Acad Sci.* 1986;462:249-262.
32. Rosenberg R, Vostrup S, Andersen A, Bolwig T. Effect of ECT on cerebral blood flow in melancholia assessed with SPECT. *Convulsive Ther.* 1988;4:62-73.
33. Sackeim HA, Prohovnik I, Apter S, Lucas L, Decina P, Mukherjee S, Prudic J, Malitz S. Regional cerebral blood flow in affective disorders: relations to phenomenology and effects of treatment. In: Takahashi R, Flor-Henry P, Gruzelier J, Niwa S-I, eds. *Cerebral Dynamics, Laterality and Psychopathology.* New York, NY: Elsevier Science Publishing; 1987:477-492.
34. Scott AIF, Dougall N, Ross M, O'Carroll RE, Riddle W, Ebmeier KP, Goodwin GM. Short-term effects of electroconvulsive treatment on the uptake of ^{99m}Tc-exametazime into brain in major depression shown with single photon emission tomography. *J Affect Disord.* 1994;30:27-34.
35. Volkow ND, Bellar S, Mullani N, Jould L, Dewey S. Effects of electroconvulsive therapy on brain glucose metabolism: a preliminary study. *Convulsive Ther.* 1988;4:199-205.
36. Silfverskiöld P. *Depression and Mania: Clinical and Neurophysiological Aspects and Effects of ECT.* Lund, Sweden: University of Lund; 1987.
37. Sackeim HA, Prohovnik I, Moeller JR, Brown RP, Apter S, Prudic J, Devanand DP, Mukherjee S. Regional cerebral blood flow in mood disorders, I: comparison of major depressives and normal controls at rest. *Arch Gen Psychiatry.* 1990;47:60-70.
38. Sackeim HA, Prohovnik I, Moeller JR, Mayeux R, Stern Y, Devanand DP. Regional cerebral blood flow in mood disorders, II: comparison of major depression and Alzheimer's disease. *J Nucl Med.* 1993;34:1090-1101.
39. Moeller J, Strother S, Sidtis J, Rottenberg D. Scaled subprofile model: a statistical approach to the analysis of functional patterns in positron emission tomographic data. *J Cereb Blood Flow Metab.* 1987;7:649-658.
40. Moeller JR, Strother SC. A regional covariance approach to the analysis of functional patterns in positron emission tomographic data. *J Cereb Blood Flow Metab.* 1991;11:A121-A135.
41. Spitzer R, Endicott J, Robins E. *Research Diagnostic Criteria for a Selected Group of Functional Disorders.* New York, NY: Biometrics Research Division,

New York State Psychiatric Institute; 1977.
42. Hamilton M. Development of a rating scale for primary depressive illness. *Br J Soc Clin Psychol.* 1967;6:278-296.
43. Endicott J, Spitzer R. A diagnostic interview: the Schedule for Affective Disorders and Schizophrenia. *Arch Gen Psychiatry.* 1978;35:837-844.
44. Blackburn IM, London JB, Ashworth CM. A new scale for measuring mania. *Psychol Med.* 1977;7:454-458.
45. Sackeim H, Decina P, Prohovnik I, Malitz S. Seizure threshold in electroconvulsive therapy: Effects of sex, age, electrode placement, and number of treatments. *Arch Gen Psychiatry.* 1987;44:355-360.
46. Sackeim HA, Prudic J, Devanand DP, Kiersky JE, Fitzsimons L, Moody BJ, McElhiney MC, Coleman EA, Settembrino JM. Effects of stimulus intensity and electrode placement on the efficacy and cognitive effects of electroconvulsive therapy. *N Engl J Med.* 1993;328:839-846.
47. Mukherjee S, Sackeim HA, Lee C. Unilateral ECT in the treatment of manic episodes. *Convulsive Ther.* 1988;4(suppl):74-80.
48. Prudic J, Sackeim HA, Devanand DP, Kiersky JE. The efficacy of ECT in double depression. *Depression.* 1993;1:38-44.
49. Prohovnik I. Data quality, integrity, and interpretation. In: Knezevic S, Maximilian V, Mubrin Z, Prohovnik I, Wade J, eds. *Handbook of Regional Cerebral Blood Flow.* Hillsdale, NJ: Lawrence Erlbaum Associates Inc; 1988:51-78.
50. Prohovnik I, Knudsen E, Risberg J. Accuracy of models and algorithms for determination of fast-compartment flow by non-invasive 133-Xe clearance. In: Magistretti P, ed. *Functional Radionuclide Imaging of the Brain.* New York, NY: Raven Press; 1983:87-115.
51. Obrist W, Wilkinson W, Wang H, Harel D. The noninvasive 133-Xe method: influence of the input function on computed rCBF values. In: Knezevic S, Maximilian V, Mubrin Z, Prohovnik I, Wade J, eds. *Handbook of Regional Cerebral Blood Flow.* Hillsdale, NJ: Lawrence Erlbaum Associates Inc; 1988:37-50.
52. Prohovnik I, Knudsen E, Risberg J. Theoretical evaluation and simulation test of the initial slope index for noninvasive rCBF. In: Hartmann A, Hoyer S, eds. *Cerebral Blood Flow and Metabolism Measurement.* Berlin, Germany: Springer-Verlag; 1985:56-60.
53. Silfverskiöld P, Gustafson L, Risberg J, Rosén I. Acute and late effects of electroconvulsive therapy: clinical outcome, regional cerebral blood flow, and electroencephalogram. *Ann N Y Acad Sci.* 1986;462:236-248.
54. Kety SS, Woodford RB, Harmel MH, Freyhan FA, Appel KE, Schmidt CF. Cerebral blood flow and metabolism in schizophrenia. *Am J Psychiatry.* 1948;104:765-770.
55. Ingvar M. Cerebral blood flow and metabolic rate during seizures: relationship to epileptic brain damage. *Ann N Y Acad Sci.* 1986;462:194-206.
56. Engel J Jr. New concepts of the epileptic focus. In: Wiesser HG, Speckman EJ, Engel J Jr, eds. *The Epileptic Focus.* London, England: John Libbey; 1987:83-94.
57. Theodore WH, Newmark ME, Sato S, De LaPaz R, DiChiro G, Brooks R, Patronas N, Kessler RM, Manning R, Margolin R, Channing M, Porter RJ. ^{18}F-fluorodeoxyglucose positron emission tomography in refractory complex partial seizures. *Ann Neurol.* 1984;14:429-437.
58. Risberg J, Maximilian VA, Prohovnik I. Changes of cortical activity patterns during habituation to a reasoning test: a study with the 133-Xe technique for measuring regional cerebral blood flow. *Neuropsychologia.* 1977;15:793-798.
59. Warach S, Gur RC, Gur RE, Skolnick B, Obrist W, Reivich M. The reproducibility of the 133-Xe inhalation method technique in resting studies: task order and sex-related effects in healthy young adults. *J Cereb Blood Flow Metab.* 1987;7:702-708.
60. Baron JC, Lebrun-Grandie P, Collard P, Crouzel C, Mestelan GT, Bousser MG. Noninvasive measurement of blood flow, oxygen consumption and glucose utilization in the same brain regions in man by positron emission tomography. *J Nucl Med.* 1982;23:391-399.
61. McCulloch, J. The physiology and regulation of cerebral blood flow. In: Knezevic S, Maximilian V, Mubrin Z, Prohovnik I, Wade J, eds. *Handbook of Regional Cerebral Blood Flow.* Hillsdale, NJ: Lawrence Erlbaum Associates Inc; 1988:1-24.
62. Posner JB, Plum F, Van Poznak A. Cerebral metabolism during electrically induced seizures in man. *Arch Neurol.* 1969;20:388-395.
63. Bolwig TG, Hertz MM, Paulson OB, Spotoft H, Rafaelsen OJ. The permeability of the blood-brain barrier during electrically induced seizures in man. *Eur J Clin Invest.* 1977;7:87-93.
64. Preskorn SH, Irwin GH, Simpson S, Friesen D, Rinne J, Jerkovich G. Medical therapies for mood disorders alter the blood-brain barrier. *Science.* 1981;213:469-471.
65. Sackeim HA, Decina P, Prohovnik I, Malitz S, Resor SR. Anticonvulsant and antidepressant properties of electroconvulsive therapy: a proposed mechanism of action. *Biol Psychiatry.* 1983;18:1301-1310.
66. Post RM, Putnam F, Uhde TW, Weiss SR. Electroconvulsive therapy as an anticonvulsant: implications for its mechanism of action in affective illness. *Ann N Y Acad Sci.* 1986;462:376-388.
67. Green A, Nutt D, Cowen P. Increased seizure threshold following convulsion. In: Sandler M, ed. *Psychopharmacology of Anticonvulsants.* Oxford, England: Oxford University Press; 1982:16-26.
68. Sackeim HA, Decina P, Portnoy S, Neeley P, Malitz S. Studies of dosage, seizure threshold, and seizure duration in ECT. *Biol Psychiatry.* 1987;22:249-268.
69. Swinyard EA, Woodhead JH. Experimental detection, quantification, and evaluation of anticonvulsants. In: Woodbury DM, Penry JK, Pippenger CE, eds. *Antiepileptic Drugs.* New York, NY: Raven Press; 1982:111-126.
70. Babington RG, Wedeking PW. Blockade of tardive seizures in rats by electroconvulsive shock. *Brain Res.* 1975;88:141-144.
71. Caplan G. Electrical convulsion therapy in treatment of epilepsy. *J Ment Sci.* 1946;92:784-793.
72. Schnur DB, Mukherjee S, Silver J, Degreef G, Lee C. Electroconvulsive therapy in the treatment of episodic aggressive dyscontrol in psychotic patients. *Convulsive Ther.* 1989;5:353-361.
73. Viparelli U, Viparelli G. ECT and grand mal epilepsy. *Convulsive Ther.* 1992;8:39-42.
74. Green A, Nutt D. Psychopharmacology of repeated seizures: possible relevance to the mechanisms of action of electroconvulsive therapy. In: Iversen L, Iversen S, Snyder S, eds. *Handbook of Psychopharmacology.* New York, NY: Plenum Press; 1987;19:375-419.
75. Lloyd KG, Morselli PL, Bartholini G. GABA and affective disorders. *Med Biol.* 1987;65:159-165.
76. Tortella FC, Long JB. Characterization of opioid peptide-like anticonvulsant activity in rat cerebrospinal fluid. *Brain Res.* 1988;456:139-146.
77. Gleiter CH, Deckert J, Nutt DJ, Marangos PJ. Electroconvulsive shock (ECS) and the adenosine neuromodulatory system: effect of single and repeated ECS on the adenosine A1 and A2 receptors, adenylate cyclase, and the adenosine uptake site. *J Neurochem.* 1989;52:641-646.
78. Bhattacharya SK, Banerjee PK, Glover V, Sandler M. Augmentation of rat brain endogenous monoamine oxidase inhibitory activity (tribulin) by electroconvulsive shock. *Neurosci Lett.* 1991;125:65-68.
79. Roemer RA, Dubin WR, Jaffe R, Lipschutz L, Sharon D. An efficacy study of single- versus double-seizure induction with ECT in major depression. *J Clin Psychiatry.* 1990;51:473-478.
80. Yatham LN, Barry S, Dinan TG, Webb M. Which patients will respond to ECT? *Br J Psychiatry.* 1989;879-880.
81. Mukherjee S. Mechanisms of the antimanic effect of electroconvulsive therapy. *Convulsive Ther.* 1989;5:227-243.
82. Kahn D. Carbamazepine and other antiepileptic drugs in refractory depression. In: Roose SP, Glassman AH, eds. *Treatment Strategies for Refractory Depression.* Washington, DC: American Psychiatric Press; 1990:77-107.
83. Coffey CE, Figiel GS, Djang WT, Weiner RD. Subcortical hyperintensity on magnetic resonance imaging: a comparison of normal and depressed elderly subjects. *Am J Psychiatry.* 1990;147:187-189.
84. Coffey CE, Wilkinson WE, Weiner RD, Parashos IA, Djang WT, Webb MC, Figiel GS, Spritzer CE. Quantitative cerebral anatomy in depression: a controlled magnetic resonance imaging study. *Arch Gen Psychiatry.* 1993;50:7-16.
85. Zubenko GS, Sullivan P, Nelson JP, Belle SH, Huff FJ, Wolf GL. Brain imaging abnormalities in mental disorders of late life. *Arch Neurol.* 1990;47:1107-1111.
86. Fazekas F, Niederkorn K, Schmidt R, Offenbacher H, Horner S, Bertha G, Lechner H. White matter signal abnormalities in normal individuals: correlation with carotid ultrasonography, cerebral blood flow measurements, and cerebrovascular risk factors. *Stroke.* 1988;19:1285-1288.
87. Herholz K, Heindel W, Rackl A, Neubauer I, Steinbrich W, Pietrzyk U, Erasmi-Körber H, Heiss W. Regional cerebral blood flow in patients with leuko-araiosis and atherosclerotic carotid artery disease. *Arch Neurol.* 1990;47:392-396.
88. Kobari M, Meyer JS, Ichijo M. Leuko-araiosis, cerebral atrophy, and cerebral perfusion in normal aging. *Arch Neurol.* 1990;47:161-168.
89. Kawamura J, Meyer JS, Terayama Y, Weathers S. Leukoaraiosis correlates with cerebral hypoperfusion in vascular dementia. *Stroke.* 1991;22:609-614.
90. DeReuck J, Decoo D, Strijckmans K, Lemahieu I. Does the severity of leukoaraiosis contribute to senile dementia? a comparative computerized and positron emission tomographic study. *Eur Neurol.* 1992;32:199-205.

ORIGINAL ARTICLE

Specificity of Ethanollike Effects Elicited by Serotonergic and Noradrenergic Mechanisms

John H. Krystal, MD; Elizabeth Webb; Ned Cooney, PhD; Henry R. Kranzler, MD; Dennis S. Charney, MD

Background: This study evaluated the specificity of the ethanollike effects of the serotonergic receptor partial agonist *m*-chlorophenylpiperazine hydrochloride (MCPP) relative to the α_2-adrenergic receptor antagonist yohimbine hydrochloride and the placebo in recently detoxified alcoholics. It also examined the relationship between ethanollike discriminative properties and the induction of craving in these patients. Both MCPP and yohimbine are anxiogenic in humans; thus, this study evaluated the role of anxiogenic and ethanollike effects in the elicitation of craving.

Methods: Twenty-two male inpatients who met *DSM-III-R* criteria for alcohol dependence and who had not consumed alcohol for 12 to 26 days prior to the study completed 3 days of testing that involved the intravenous infusion of MCPP (0.1 mg/kg), yohimbine hydrochloride (0.4 mg/kg), or a saline solution over 2 weeks under double-blind conditions. Ethanollike subjective effects were assessed using the Sensation Scale and visual analog scales to measure the degree of similarity to the effects of ethanol, cocaine, and marijuana. Five components of craving for alcohol were assessed using visual analog scales. The effects of the drugs on mood were assessed using visual analog scales. Plasma levels of cortisol, prolactin, and 3-methoxy-4-hydroxyphenylethyleneglycol were also measured during the test days.

Results: *m*-Chlorophenylpiperazine and yohimbine produced significant increases compared with placebo in Sensation Scale scores and the visual analog scale score for nervousness. However, the effects of MCPP were rated as more similar to those of ethanol, cocaine, and marijuana than were those of either yohimbine or placebo. Also, MCPP but not yohimbine or placebo significantly increased craving for alcohol. Yohimbine and MCPP increased plasma prolactin and cortisol levels relative to placebo, whereas only yohimbine increased plasma 3-methoxy-4-hydroxyphenylethyleneglycol levels.

Conclusions: *m*-Chlorophenylpiperazine produced ethanollike effects and alcohol craving in recently detoxified alcoholics. Yohimbine increased Sensation Scale scores but was not recognized as ethanollike by patients. Although both drugs produced comparable levels of nervousness, yohimbine did not increase craving for alcohol. These data further implicate serotonergic systems in the discriminative properties of ethanol and may indicate a serotonergic contribution to craving. Noradrenergic systems contributed to the discriminative properties of ethanol but not to those features of ethanol response that were salient to craving in this population.

(Arch Gen Psychiatry. 1994;51:898-911)

From the Department of Psychiatry, the Veterans Affairs–Yale Alcoholism Research Center, Veterans Affairs Medical Center, Yale University School of Medicine, West Haven, Conn (Drs Krystal, Cooney, Kranzler, and Charney and Ms Webb), and the Department of Psychiatry, the University of Connecticut School of Medicine, Farmington (Dr Kranzler).

SEROTONERGIC AND noradrenergic systems have been implicated in the discriminative properties of alcohol and the propensity to consume alcohol. However, the relative or differential contributions of noradrenergic and serotonergic systems to the discriminative properties of ethanol in humans has yet to be formally assessed. In rats, the effects of the serotonin (5-HT) partial agonist 1-(*m*-trifluoromethyl) piperazine were recognized as similar to those of ethanol,[1] whereas *m*-chlorophenylpiperazine hydrochloride (MCPP) showed discriminative stimulus properties that were similar to those of ethanol dosages lower than 2.0 g/kg.[2] Recently, some detoxified alcoholics reported experiencing a "high" and a craving for alcohol following the administration of the 5-HT partial agonists MCPP[3] and MK-212.[4] Although these studies suggest that the stimulation of 5-HT receptors produces sensations that are associated with ethanol intoxication, the degree of similarity to the effects of ethanol was not formally assessed. Also, the reported propensity of MCPP to increase irritability[5] or to stimulate anxiety[6] could have accounted for the alcohol craving pro-

See Patients and Methods on next page

PATIENTS AND METHODS

PATIENTS

Twenty-two male inpatients (mean±SEM age, 39.3±1.7 years; mean±SEM weight, 73.7±2.3 kg) who met *DSM-III-R* criteria for alcohol dependence[41] determined by the Structured Clinical Interview for *DSM-III-R*[42] participated in testing. The demographic characteristics of this patient sample are summarized in the **Table**. Patients began drinking at a mean±SEM age of 13.7±0.8 years, regular drinking at 16.2±0.5 years, regular drinking to intoxication at 20.5±1.6 years, and their heaviest level of drinking at 24.6±1.9 years. Patients had a mean±SEM 15.6±1.8-year history of alcoholism. They underwent a mean±SEM of 7.9±3.6 inpatient alcohol detoxifications (range, 1 to 66). Thirteen (59%) of the 22 patients had a first-degree relative with a history of alcoholism. Nine (69%) of the 13 patients had fathers with a history of alcoholism, six (46%) of the 13 patients had brothers with a history of alcoholism, and the mother of one (8%) of the 13 patients had a history of alcoholism.

The mean±SEM score for the patients on the Socialization Scale of the California Psychological Inventory, a validated measure of the degree of sociopathy in alcoholics,[43,44] was 20.9±1.2 (range, 12 to 31). Patients estimated that their mean±SEM daily consumption of alcohol in the month prior to detoxification was the equivalent of 171±21 mL of absolute alcohol per day. The mean±SEM Michigan Alcoholism Screening Test score[45] was 38.6±2.2. All of the patients in this study met the criteria of von Knorring et al[46] for type 2 alcoholism. All but one of the patients met the more stringent early alcoholism onset criteria of 20 years that was suggested by Lamparski et al.[47] Patients were medically stable at the time of entry into the study based on medical history, physical examination, and routine laboratory testing. Patients were admitted to the study if their liver function tests were less than 1.5 times the maximum normal range at our clinical laboratory.

Patients were excluded if they met the criteria for another substance use disorder other than nicotine dependence in the year prior to testing. Subjects were also excluded if they met the criteria for another Axis I diagnosis on the Structured Clinical Interview for *DSM-III-R* during a period that was free of alcohol consumption. Because posttraumatic stress disorder may influence the response to yohimbine and MCPP,[48,49] one patient was excluded because of a score greater than 108 on the Mississippi Scale for posttraumatic stress disorder,[50] despite the fact that the patient did not meet *DSM-III-R* criteria for posttraumatic stress disorder. The absence of other current substance abuse was supported by negative results of urine toxicologic screens prior to testing.

Patients were inpatients at the Substance Abuse Treatment Research Unit of the West Haven (Conn) Veterans Affairs Medical Center. They participated in testing an average of 23.3±1.7 days (mean±SEM) (range, 12 to 26 days) after consuming their last alcoholic beverage. Nine of the 22 patients underwent benzodiazepine-assisted alcohol detoxification (oxazepam, n=7; chlordiazepoxide hydrochloride, n=2) prior to participating in this study. The mean±SEM period between the administration of the last benzodiazepine dose and the first pharmacologic test day was 12.6±2.4 days (range, 5 to 25 days). On their first test day, nine patients received placebo, six patients received yohimbine, and seven patients received MCPP.

TESTING PROCEDURES

After obtaining informed consent for human investigation, each patient completed 3 test days separated by 48 to 96 hours in a randomized order under double-blind conditions. On each test day, subjects received two 10-minute infusions. On the saline solution test day, both infusions consisted of 0.9% saline solution. On the MCPP test day, both infusions contained MCPP (0.05 mg/kg for a total of 0.1 mg/kg over 20 minutes). On the yohimbine test day, one infusion contained yohimbine hydrochloride (0.4 mg/kg administered over 10 minutes), and the other infusion consisted of saline solution infused over 10 minutes. Thus, the MCPP and yohimbine doses and rates of infusion were identical to those of previously reported studies in healthy subjects[6,51] and in patients with panic disorder,[6,51] posttraumatic stress disorder,[48,49] obsessive-compulsive disorder,[52] and schizophrenia.[53] For each test session, participants fasted overnight and remained in the fasting state during the test session. They presented for testing at approximately 8:30 AM, and an intravenous line was placed at that time. Blood for the determination of the norepinephrine metabolite 3-methoxy-4-hydroxyphenylethyleneglycol (MHPG) and for the determination of hormone levels was sampled via the intravenous line at 30 and 15 minutes prior to the infusion, immediately following the 20-minute infusion, and at 20, 40, 100, and 160 minutes following the termination of the infusion.

Ratings were performed to characterize subjective responses to MCPP and yohimbine. Patients completed visual analog scales for feelings of anger, anxiety, high, ner-

Continued on next page

duced by this drug in alcoholics. The clinical significance of serotonergic contributions to the discriminative properties of alcohol was further questioned by a study that suggested that reductions in 5-HT synthesis via tryptophan depletion did not decrease the effects of ethanol in healthy subjects.[7]

Central noradrenergic systems also may mediate or modulate the discriminative properties of alcohol. Noradrenergic systems were activated by ethanol administration in rats,[8-10] which is consistent with preclinical evidence that noradrenergic systems contributed to the rewarding properties of ethanol.[11] Ethanol inhibited some noradrenergic neurons via a mechanism blocked by the α_2-adrenergic receptor antagonist yohimbine hydrochloride.[12] Ethanol also attenuated stress-induced noradrenergic activation,[13] which is consistent with its anxiolytic effects. In rats, α_2-adrenergic receptor antagonists reduced the effects of ethanol on exploratory behavior[14] and ataxia[15] without affecting the effects of ethanol on locomotor behavior.[14]

In healthy humans, short-term ethanol administration increased norepinephrine turnover.[16,17] Yohimbine produced ethanollike sensations and increased aspects of the behavioral effects of ethanol but did not enhance ethanol-induced euphoria.[17] Inhibition of cat-

vousness, and sadness.[51,54] Briefly, anxiety was defined as "a mental awareness of worry," whereas nervousness was defined as "a physical feeling of jitteriness, tension, heart throbbing, breathlessness, or other similar symptoms." These scales consisted of 100-mm lines (0 indicated none; 100, maximum possible) marked proportionately to the perceived intensity of the experience.

Patients completed two indexes of alcohollike subjective effects: the Sensation Scale,[55] a 31-item scale with items that assess responses that are associated with alcohol administration on a 10-point scale, and a self-rated visual analog scale for measuring the similarity to alcohol (0 indicated not at all similar; 100, identical). The similarity of the effects of the tested drugs to those produced by cocaine and marijuana was also assessed using a self-rated visual analog scale in subjects with histories of exposure to these drugs (cocaine, n=14; marijuana, n=18). The Sensation Scale and the visual analog scales were intended to assess different aspects of alcohollike subjective effects. The Sensation Scale is a validated measure that assesses a broad range of alcohollike responses, particularly physical effects, without prioritizing particular responses.[55] The visual analog scales measuring the similarity of effects to the subjective effects of drugs of abuse were intended to identify the degree of similarity of the effects of the tested drugs to the subjective effects associated with alcohol that were most important to the patient group.

Craving for ethanol was assessed using five self-rated visual analog scales that evaluated the five key components of drug craving identified by Tiffany and colleagues[56,57]: "I would like to drink alcohol," "I intend to drink alcohol in the near future," "Alcohol will make me feel better," "Alcohol would get rid of any discomfort I am feeling," and "I feel I can control my drinking of alcohol." Visual analog scales, assessment of alcohollike effects, craving, and vital signs were assessed at 30 and 15 minutes prior to the infusion, immediately following the termination of the infusion, and at 20, 40, 100, 160, and 220 minutes following the termination of the infusion.

BIOCHEMICAL METHODS

Radioimmunoassay kits were used to determine plasma levels of prolactin (GammaCoat Prolactin, Clinical Assays Inc, Stillwater, Minn) (intra-assay and interassay coefficients of variance were 3% and 7%, respectively) and cortisol (GammaCoat Cortisol, Clinical Assays Inc) (intra-assay and interassay coefficients of variance were 3% and 5%, respectively). Plasma free levels of MHPG[58] were measured by gas chromatography and mass spectrometry using deuterated internal standards. Samples were assayed in duplicate, and the reported values are the means of these two measures. The intra- and interassay coefficients of variance were 6% and 11% for MHPG.

DATA ANALYSIS

Subjective responses initially were evaluated using repeated measures analysis of variance (ANOVA) with the within-subjects factors of drug (placebo, MCPP, and yohimbine) and time. These ANOVAs were tested for lack of sphericity, and Huynh-Feldt adjustments were made when appropriate. Huynh-Feldt adjustments to *df* are noted in the text by the subscript HF. Post hoc repeated measures ANOVAs were then performed separately, comparing the responses following MCPP administration with those following placebo administration and the responses following yohimbine administration with those following placebo administration.

Baseline values were compared between test days using paired *t* tests with Bonferroni's correction made to decrease the impact of multiple comparisons. To evaluate the change from baseline on each test day, Dunnett's *t* test was used to control for multiple comparisons with baseline.[59] Changes in responses following the administration of MCPP or yohimbine compared with the responses following the administration of placebo were adjusted for placebo–test-day responses by comparing the change from baseline with each time point for the active drug and placebo using Dunnett's *t* tests.

To examine the relationship between sociopathy and selected outcome variables, partial correlations were calculated between California Psychological Inventory socialization scale scores and peak scores on selected outcome measures. This procedure permitted the assessment of the relationship between California Psychological Inventory scores and peak responses, covarying for baseline values.[60] Spearman correlation matrixes were created to examine the relationship between the five peak-MCPP–induced visual analog scales measuring craving (5×5 correlation matrix) and to examine the correlations of peak increases in anxiety, high, similarity to ethanol, and scores on the five craving scales on the MCPP test day (3×5 matrix). Bonferroni's corrections were employed to adjust the level of significance for the multiple comparisons involved in these correlation matrixes. Data were analyzed using the Statistical Package for the Social Sciences (SPSS Inc, Chicago, Ill).

echolamine synthesis with α-methyl-*p*-tyrosine decreased ethanol-induced elation and talkativeness but not the reported degree of intoxication.[18] Consistent with these reports, catecholamine release that was evoked by dextroamphetamine sulfate did not enhance ethanol intoxication.[19] These studies suggest that the noradrenergic contributions to the short-term subjective effects of alcohol may be limited to selected aspects of ethanol intoxication. Thus, the nature of ethanollike discriminative properties of noradrenergic activating drugs such as yohimbine in alcoholics needs further characterization.

Serotonergic systems have been consistently implicated in the propensity to self-administer alcohol. Preclinical studies[20-22] suggested that alcohol-preferring rat strains differ in several indexes of serotonergic regulation from non–alcohol-preferring rat strains. Drugs that modulate 5-HT function also differentially reduced alcohol consumption relative to food consumption in rats.[23] Researchers noted that some pharmacologic reductions in alcohol consumption could be indirect consequences of generalized suppression of consummatory behavior[23] or aversive properties of the drugs that were studied.[24] In humans, tryptophan depletion did not affect alcohol consumption rates in in-

Characteristics of Alcoholic Patients*

Patient No./ Age, y	Age at Onset of Heavy Drinking, y	No. of Detoxifications	Family History of Alcoholism	No. of Drinks per Drinking Day†	No. of Drinking Days per Month†	Peak Change in Desire to Drink on MCPP Test Day
1/30	17	1	−	20	30	24.0
2/32	18	4	+	32	30	7.5
3/41	21	0	+	48	30	0
4/50	20	3	+	12	30	0
5/35	14	7	−	24	30	0
6/21	18	0	+	10	12	0
7/46	34	0	−	34	30	0
8/31	30	0	+	24	30	0
9/40	21	5	−	13	30	16.0
10/44	40	6	+	7	30	2.5
11/41	38	0	+	24	30	13.0
12/43	21	0	−	10	12	0
13/44	17	65	+	12	30	75.0
14/38	23	0	+	14	30	100.0
15/49	27	50	−	24	30	0
16/29	27	1	−	16	30	13.0
17/29	22	0	−	22	30	7.5
18/54	50	0	+	12	30	0
19/34	17	20	+	24	30	0
20/39	20	3	+	27	30	81.0
21/47	25	8	+	18	30	16.0
22/47	22	1	−	12	30	0

**MCPP indicates* m*-chlorophenylpiperazine hydrochloride; plus sign, family history of alcoholism; and minus sign, no family history of alcoholism.*
†Applies to the month prior to detoxification.

dividuals without an identified risk for alcoholism.[25] However, deficits in 5-HT synthesis, turnover, or receptor function have been described in chronic alcoholism.[3,4,26-30] Pharmacotherapies for alcoholism based on modulating 5-HT function, such as the 5-HT reuptake inhibitors,[31] showed promise in initial trials.[23,31,32]

The role of noradrenergic systems in alcohol self-administration is less clear. Alcohol-preferring rat strains do not differ from non–alcohol-preferring strains in their brain norepinephrine turnover rates[20] or the number or affinity of brain noradrenergic receptors.[33] Depletion of norepinephrine both increased[34] and decreased[35] ethanol self-administration in rats. Both α_2-adrenergic receptor agonists[36] and α_2-adrenergic receptor antagonists[37] reduced alcohol consumption in rats. Noradrenergic-based pharmacotherapies for alcoholism have received relatively little attention. Heterocyclic norepinephrine-reuptake blockers have been studied in alcoholics primarily as treatment for comorbid depression.[38] Also, the α_2-adrenergic receptor agonist clonidine hydrochloride suppresses aspects of the alcohol withdrawal syndrome.[39,40]

The current study evaluated whether the 5-HT partial agonist MCPP or the α_2-adrenergic receptor antagonist yohimbine produced ethanollike effects or craving for alcohol in recently detoxified alcoholics. In doing so, this study provided an initial examination of the magnitude and the specificity of the contributions of serotonergic and noradrenergic systems to alcohollike subjective effects in recently detoxified alcoholics. The comparison of the effects of two anxiogenic drugs in alcoholic patients also permitted the evaluation of the relationship between drug-induced mood states and the craving for alcohol.

RESULTS

EVIDENCE OF ETHANOLLIKE EFFECTS

Data analysis revealed that both MCPP and yohimbine produced a high and ethanollike sensations in recently detoxified alcoholic patients. Results are presented in **Figure 1**.

Self-reported High

Analysis of data from the visual analog scale assessing the high effect with repeated measures ANOVA revealed significant effects of time (F_{HF}[2.5,52.3]=4.9, *P*=.007) and of the drug-by-time interaction (F_{HF}[4.9,103.5]=4.3, *P*=.001) but not of the drug. Post hoc repeated measures ANOVAs revealed that both MCPP (drug-by-time interaction, F_{HF}[2.3,47.6]=6.9, *P*=.002) and yohimbine (drug-by-time interaction, F_{HF}[3.8,80.5]=2.9, *P*=.03) had euphorigenic effects relative to placebo. There was a nonsignificant trend for MCPP to be more euphorigenic than was yohimbine (drug-by-time interaction, F_{HF}[2.8,58.6]=2.7, *P*=.06). Baseline scores did not differ between test days. The placebo did not produce a significant change from baseline on the visual analog scale for high. Yohimbine did not significantly increase scores from baseline. However adjusting for the nonsignificant placebo–test-day decrease, yohimbine increased scores (*t*[3,252]=3.8, *P*<.05) at the 20-minute time point. *m*-Chlorophenylpiperazine significantly increased scores from baseline at the 20-minute (*t*[7,252]=5.1, *P*<.01) and 40-minute (*t*[7,252]=3.2, *P*<.05) time points, and these effects remained significant after adjusting for placebo–test-day responses.

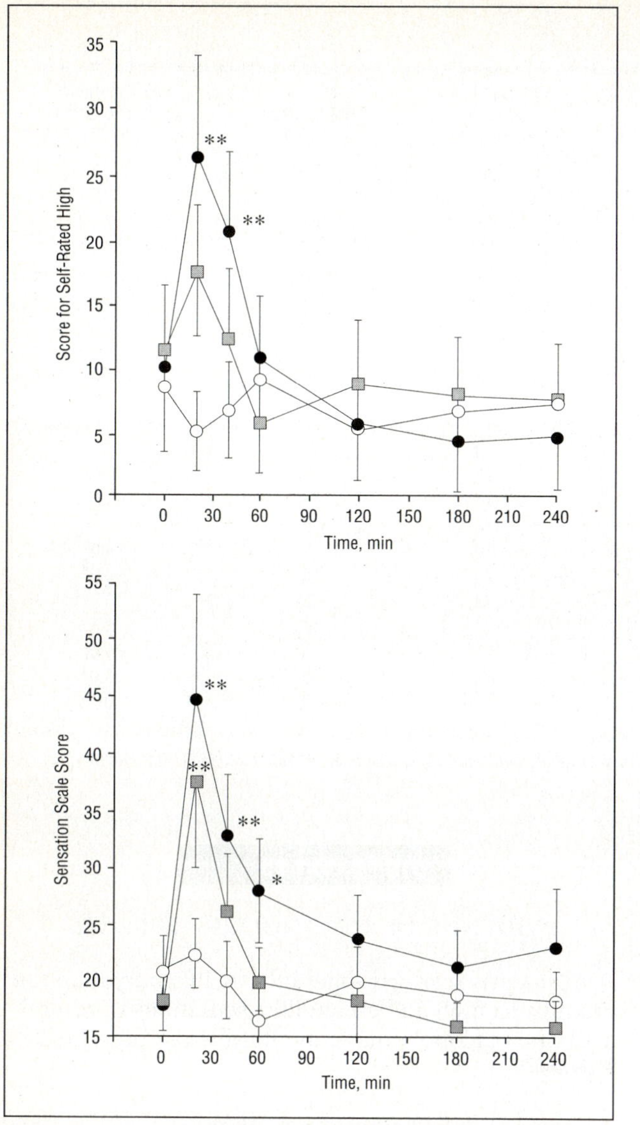

Figure 1. *Effects of placebo (open circles),* m*-chlorophenylpiperazine hydrochloride (solid circles), and yohimbine hydrochloride (shaded squares) on self-rated high (top) and Sensation Scale scores (bottom) in recently detoxified alcoholic patients (n=22). Values are expressed as mean±SEM. Increases from baseline were evaluated using Dunnett's* t *test. Single asterisk indicates* $P<.05$*; double asterisks,* $P<.01$*. See "Patients and Methods" and "Results" sections for explanation of all other statistics.*

Sensation Scale

The repeated measures ANOVA that was performed on Sensation Scale scores revealed significant effects of drug ($F[2.42]=4.4$, $P=.02$), time ($F_{HF}[1.8,37.7]=13.6$, $P=.0001$), and the drug-by-time interaction ($F_{HF}[4.0,84.5]=3.7$, $P=.008$). Both MCPP (drug-by-time interaction, $F_{HF}[2.3,48.6]=6.0$, $P=.003$) and yohimbine (drug-by-time interaction, $F_{HF}[2.1,43.3]=5.5$, $P=.007$) significantly increased Sensation Scale scores relative to placebo, although the effects of MCPP and yohimbine did not differ significantly. There were no statistically significant differences in baseline scores between the test days. On the placebo test day, Sensation Scale scores did not significantly increase from baseline at any time point. Yohimbine significantly increased scores from baseline at the 20-minute time point ($t[7,252]=5.8$, $P<.01$), and this effect remained significant when adjusting for placebo–test-day responses. *m*-Chlorophenylpiperazine significantly increased scores from baseline at 20 ($t[7,252]=8.0$, $P<.01$), 40 ($t[7,252]=4.41$, $P<.01$), and 60 ($t[7,252]=2.9$, $P<.05$) minutes following the initiation of drug infusion. Adjusting for placebo–test-day responses did not affect the level of significance of the effects of MCPP.

SPECIFICITY OF ETHANOLLIKE EFFECTS

As presented in **Figure 2**, the effects of MCPP were judged to be more similar than was yohimbine or placebo to the effects of ethanol, marijuana, and cocaine.

Ethanol

Repeated measures ANOVA of visual analog scale data evaluating the degree of similarity between the effects of the tested drugs and those of ethanol revealed significant effects of drug ($F[2,40]=3.9$, $P=.03$), time ($F_{HF}[2.2,44.3]=16.86$, $P=.0001$), and the drug-by-time interaction ($F_{HF}[4.3,86.2]=3.2$, $P=.01$). Post hoc repeated measures ANOVAs revealed that MCPP was more ethanollike than were placebo (drug-by-time interaction, $F_{HF}[1.9,37.2]=5.3$, $P=.01$) and yohimbine (drug-by-time interaction, $F_{HF}[3.0,61.9]=2.9$, $P=.04$). Yohimbine did not significantly affect scores on this visual analog scale. There were no significant differences in baseline scores between the test days. On the placebo test day, scores did not increase significantly from baseline. On the yohimbine test day, scores increased relative to baseline at the 20-minute time point ($t[7,240]=3.5$, $P=.05$). However, adjusting for the placebo–test-day increase at this time point, the effect of yohimbine was no longer significant. The effects of MCPP were judged to be significantly ethanollike relative to baseline ($P<.01$) at 20 and 40 minutes following the initiation of MCPP infusion. This effect remained significant ($P<.01$) after adjusting for placebo–test-day changes.

Marijuana

The similarity between the effects of the tested drugs and those of marijuana was assessed in patients with reported histories of marijuana use (n=18). Repeated measures ANOVA of data that evaluated the degree of similarity between the effects of the tested drugs and those of marijuana revealed a nonsignificant trend for a drug effect ($F_{HF}[1.6,26.4]=2.5$, $P=.1$) and significant effects of time ($F_{HF}[2.1,35.6]=3.9$, $P=.03$) and the drug-by-time interaction ($F_{HF}[3.9,66.7]=2.7$, $P=.04$). Both MCPP (drug-by-time interaction, $F_{HF}[2.9,49.1]=0.03$)and yohimbine (drug-by-time interaction, $F_{HF}[3.1,52.6]=0.04$)were judged to be more similar to marijuana than was the placebo, although the effects of MCPP and yohimbine did not differ significantly. There were no significant differences in baseline scores between the test days. Scores did not significantly increase from baseline on the placebo or yohimbine test days. The effects of MCPP were judged to be marijuanalike relative to baseline at 20 ($t[7,204]=5.0$, $P<.01$), 40 ($t[7,204]=4.4$, $P<.01$), and 60 ($t[7,204]=2.7$, $P<.05$) minutes following the initiation of MCPP infusion. These effects remained significant ($P<.05$) after adjusting for placebo–test-day responses.

Cocaine

Similarity between the effects of the tested drugs and those of cocaine was assessed in patients with reported histories of cocaine use (n=14). Repeated measures ANOVA of data that evaluated the degree of similarity between the effects of the tested drugs and those of cocaine revealed nonsignificant trends for drug ($F_{HF}[1.1,14.0]=3.1$, $P=.1$) and the drug-by-time interaction ($F_{HF}[2.2,28.3]=2.3$, $P=.1$) and a significant time effect ($F_{HF}[1.8,23.7]=4.9$, $P=.02$). Post hoc repeated measures ANOVAs revealed that both MCPP (drug-by-time interaction, $F_{HF}[1.7,21.8]=3.2$, $P=.07$) and yohimbine (drug-by-time interaction, $F_{HF}[1.3,16.4]=2.4$, $P=.1$) nonsignificantly elicited cocainelike effects when compared with placebo. However, MCPP and yohimbine did not significantly differ in this capacity. There were no significant differences in baseline scores between the test days. Patients did not significantly increase scores from baseline on the placebo or yohimbine test days. The effects of MCPP were judged to be significantly cocainelike relative to baseline ($P<.01$) at 20, 40, and 60 minutes following the initiation of MCPP infusion. This effect remained significant ($P<.01$) after adjusting for placebo–test-day changes.

INDUCTION OF CRAVING

As presented in **Figure 3**, MCPP but not yohimbine or placebo elicited a desire to drink alcohol in these recently detoxified patients. Repeated measures ANOVA revealed nonsignificant trends for the effects of drug ($F[2,42]=2.5$, $P=.1$), time ($F_{HF}[2.6,54.5]=1.9$, $P=.1$), and drug-by-time interaction ($F_{HF}[4.3,89.6]=2.3$, $P=.06$). Post hoc repeated measures ANOVAs found that relative to placebo, MCPP (drug-by-time interaction, $F_{HF}[2.5,51.4]=2.9$, $P=.05$) but not yohimbine increased the desire to drink alcohol. There were also nonsignificant trends for MCPP to elicit a greater desire to drink alcohol than did yohimbine (drug, $F[1,21]=4.1$, $P=.06$; time, $F_{HF}[2.5,51.7]=2.7$, $P=.07$; drug-by-time interaction, $F_{HF}[2.2,46.6]=2.7$, $P=.07$). There were no statistically significant differences in baseline scores between test days. Neither placebo nor yohimbine significantly increased the desire to drink alcohol from baseline. After adjusting for placebo–test-day effects, yohimbine reduced the desire to drink alcohol ($P<.05$) at the 40-, 60-, 120-, and 180-minute time points. *m*-Chlorophenylpiperazine increased this urge at 20 ($t[7,252]=4.6$, $P<.01$) and 40 ($t[7,252]=3.3$, $P<.05$) minutes following the initiation of drug infusion; these effects remained significant ($P<.05$) after adjusting for placebo–test–day responses. After adjusting for baseline craving levels on the MCPP test day in a stepwise multiple regression, neither the age of onset of regular drinking (partial $r=-.25$), regular drinking to intoxication (partial $r=-.14$), or heaviest drinking (partial $r=-.22$) correlated significantly with the peak levels of desire to consume alcohol following MCPP infusion. Also, patients with a family history of alcoholism did not differ significantly from patients without a family history of alcoholism on the peak MCPP-induced increase in desire to drink alcohol or any of the other visual analog scales of craving.

m-Chlorophenylpiperazine but not yohimbine increased the patients' feeling that drinking would make them feel better. The ANOVA revealed significant drug

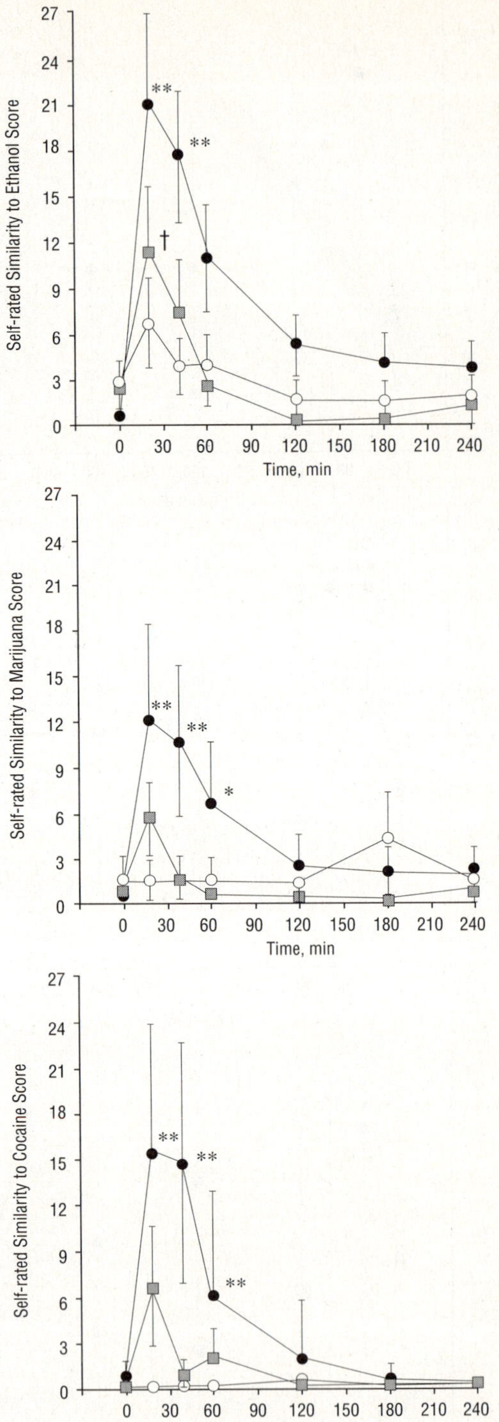

Figure 2. *Similarity of the effects of placebo (open circles), m-chlorophenylpiperazine hydrochloride (solid circles), and yohimbine hydrochloride (shaded squares) to ethanol (top, n=21), marijuana (center, n=18), and cocaine (bottom, n=14). Values are expressed as mean±SEM. Scores were based on a scale from 0 to 100. Increases from baseline were evaluated using Dunnett's* t *test. Single asterisk indicates* $P<.05$*; double asterisks,* $P<.01$*; and dagger,* $P<.05$ *on the yohimbine–test-day but nonsignificant after adjusting for placebo–test-day response (all other significant increases from baseline retained their level of significance after adjusting for placebo–test-day responses). See "Patients and Methods" and "Results" sections for explanation of all other statistics.*

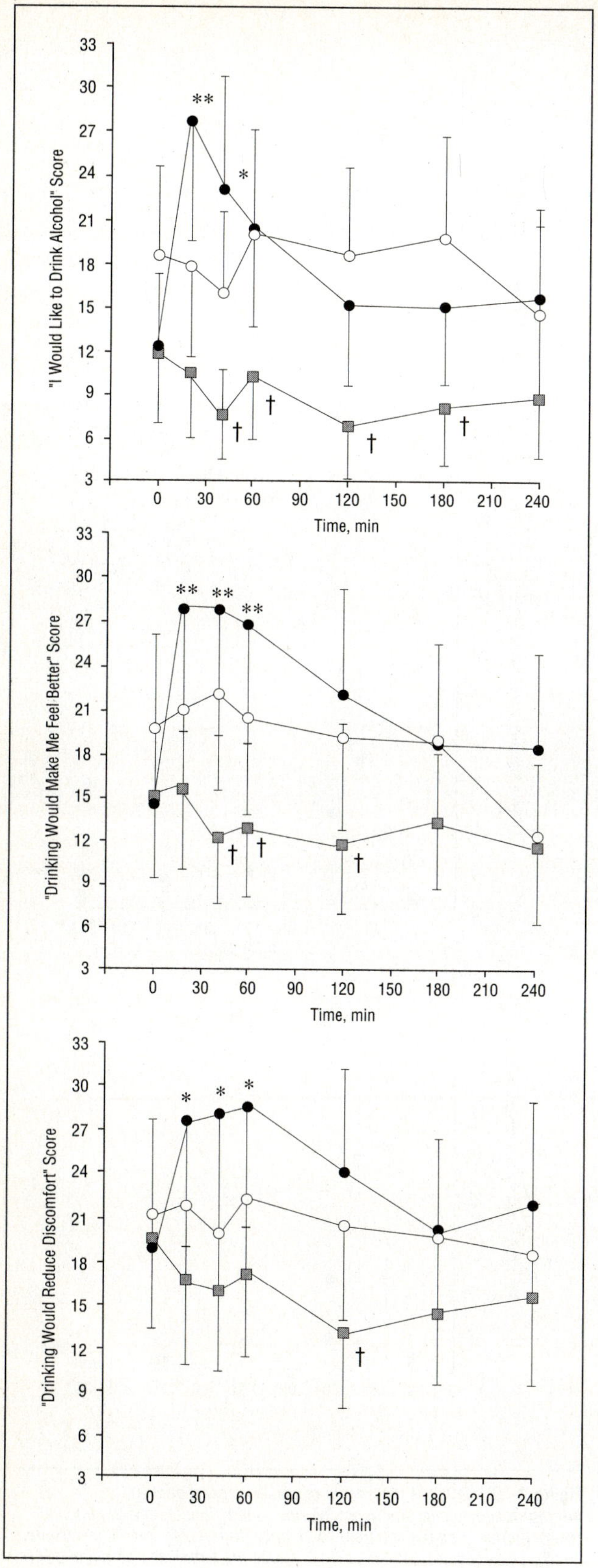

Figure 3. *Effects of placebo (open circles),* m*-chlorophenylpiperazine hydrochloride (solid circles), and yohimbine hydrochloride (shaded squares) on dimensions of craving for alcohol (n=22). Values are expressed as mean±SEM. Scores were based on a scale from 0 to 100. Increases from baseline were evaluated using Dunnett's* t *test. Single asterisk indicates* $P<.05$*; double asterisks,* $P<.01$*; and dagger,* $P<.05$ *after nonsignificant decreases from baseline were reexamined, adjusting for the placebo–test-day effects using Dunnett's* t *test. See "Patients and Methods" and "Results" sections for explanation of all other statistics. There were no statistically significant effects in the two dimensions of craving that were not depicted: intention to drink and loss of control over drinking.*

($F[2,42]=3.2$, $P=.05$) and time ($F_{HF}[3.0,62.3]=3.1$, $P=.03$) effects and a nonsignificant trend for a drug-by-time interaction ($F_{HF}[4.3,89.6]=2.3$, $P=.06$). Post hoc repeated measures ANOVAs found that relative to placebo, MCPP (time, $F[2.6,53.8]=4.2$, $P=.01$) but not yohimbine significantly increased the feeling that alcohol would enhance their behavioral state. *m*-Chlorophenylpiperazine also increased this sense relative to yohimbine (drug, $F[1,21]=5.2$, $P=.03$; time, $F_{HF}[2.7,56.8]=2.4$, $P=0.09$; drug-by-time interaction, $F_{HF}[2.7,57.1]=3.2$, $P=.03$). There were no significant differences in baseline values between test days. Neither placebo nor yohimbine significantly increased from baseline the impression that alcohol would lead to feeling better. However, adjusting for placebo–test-day responses, yohimbine significantly decreased scores from baseline ($P<.05$) at 40, 80, and 120 minutes following the initiation of drug infusion. *m*-Chlorophenylpiperazine increased scores from baseline ($P<.01$) at 20, 40, and 60 minutes following the initiation of drug infusion. The effects at the 20- and 60-minute time points reached the level of nonsignificant trends ($P<.1$) after adjusting for placebo–test-day responses.

m-Chlorophenylpiperazine but not yohimbine generated the feeling that alcohol would reduce discomfort. Repeated measures ANOVA revealed a nonsignificant trend for a drug-related effect ($F[2,42]=2.4$, $P=.1$) on this aspect of craving. Although post hoc ANOVAs did not reveal yohimbine effects, there was a nonsignificant trend for a time effect in the MCPP-placebo comparison ($F_{HF}[3.1,65.0]=2.1$, $P=.1$). Also, relative to yohimbine, MCPP increased the impression that alcohol would reduce discomfort (drug, $F[1,21]=4.9$, $P=.04$). Neither placebo nor yohimbine significantly increased from baseline the impression that alcohol would lead to feeling better. However, adjusting for placebo–test-day responses, yohimbine significantly ($t[3,252]=2.2$, $P<.05$) decreased scores from baseline 120 minutes following the initiation of drug infusion. *m*-Chlorophenylpiperazine increased scores from baseline ($P<.05$) at 20, 40, and 60 minutes following the initiation of drug infusion. After adjusting for placebo–test-day responses, only the increase at the 40-minute time point retained significance ($t[3,252]=2.5$, $P<.05$).

Repeated measures ANOVA did not reveal significant test-day effects for the intention to drink ethanol (drug-by-time interaction, $F[12,252]=0.9$, $P=.6$) or the sense of loss of control over drinking (drug-by-time interaction, $F[12,252]=0.7$, $P=.7$).

The five craving subscales showed a high degree of intercorrelation that remained significant after adjusting for multiple comparisons using Bonferroni's correction. On the MCPP test day, the peak increase in the desire to drink was significantly correlated with the peak increase in the intention to drink ($r=.80$, $P<.05$), the peak increase in the sense that alcohol would lead to feeling better ($r=.83$, $P<.05$), and the peak increase in the perception that alcohol would reduce discomfort ($r=.86$,

P<.05). The peak increase in the intention to drink alcohol on the MCPP test day was also correlated with the sense that alcohol would lead to feeling better (*r*=.69, *P*<.05) and with the peak increase in the impression that alcohol would reduce discomfort (*r*=.72, *P*<.05). The effects of MCPP on the sense that alcohol would lead to feeling better and the impression that alcohol would reduce discomfort were highly correlated (*r*=.94, *P*<.05). The effects of MCPP on feelings of control over drinking did not correlate significantly with any other visual analog scale assessing craving.

SELF-RATED VISUAL ANALOG SCALES OF MOOD STATES

The assessments of mood responses to pharmacologic testing are presented in **Figure 4**.

Anger

m-Chlorophenylpiperazine appeared to produce sustained feelings of anger that persisted or increased as both nervousness and high declined. Yohimbine had little effect on anger. Repeated measures ANOVAs performed on the visual analog scale for anger revealed a nonsignificant trend for a drug effect (F_{HF}[1.1,23.8]=3.1, *P*=.09) but no drug-by-time interaction (F_{HF}[2.8,59.2]=1.5, *P*=.2). Post hoc repeated measures ANOVAs revealed that MCPP significantly increased anger relative to yohimbine (drug, F[1,21]=4.2, *P*=.05) but not to placebo (drug, F[1,21]=2.3, *P*=.2). There were no significant differences in baseline anger scores between test days and no significant increases from baseline on the placebo and yohimbine test days. *m*-Chlorophenylpiperazine increased anger from baseline at 20 (*t*[7,252]=2.7, *P*<.05) and 60 (*t*[7,252]=3.8, *P*<.01) minutes following the initiation of drug infusion. Both increases remained significant after adjusting for placebo–test-day responses. A stepwise regression did not suggest any significant relationship between scores on the Socialization Scale of the California Psychological Inventory and baseline levels of anger (partial *r*=−.25) or peak anger levels (partial *r*=−.14) on the MCPP test day.

Anxiety and Nervousness

As shown in Figure 3, both MCPP and yohimbine increased nervousness, whereas MCPP appeared more potent than yohimbine in stimulating anxiety. The repeated measures ANOVA performed on nervousness revealed significant effects of time (F_{HF}[3.2,67.4]=8.6, *P*=.0001) and the drug-by-time interaction (F_{HF}[5.7,118.7]=2.8, *P*=.02). Post hoc repeated measures ANOVAs revealed significant drug-by-time interactions for the comparisons of both MCPP (F_{HF}[4.3,90.5]=4.3, *P*=.002) and yohimbine (F_{HF}[2.6,57.6]=3.5, *P*=.02) with placebo. However, the effects of MCPP and yohimbine did not differ significantly (F_{HF}[2.8,58.1]=1.1, *P*=.4). There were no significant differences in the baseline values between test days. The placebo did not significantly alter self-ratings of nervousness. *m*-Chlorophenylpiperazine increased nervousness from baseline (*P*<.05) at both 20 and 40 minutes

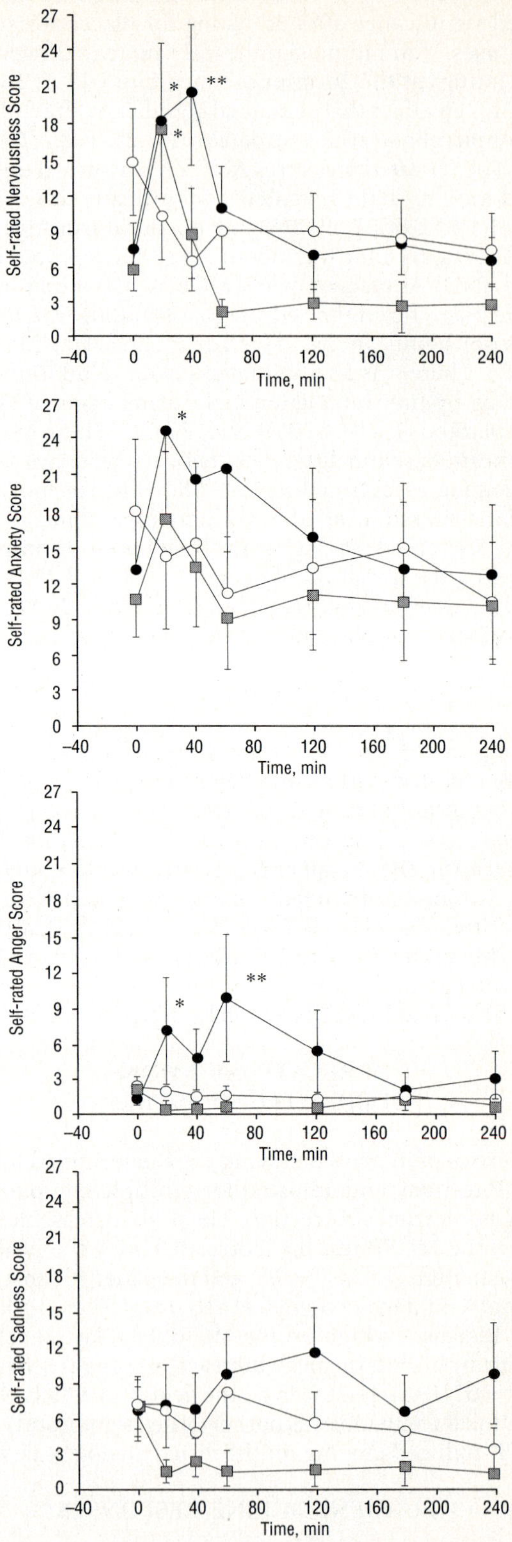

Figure 4. *Effects of placebo (open circles),* m-*chlorophenylpiperazine hydrochloride (solid circles), and yohimbine hydrochloride (shaded squares) on self-rated visual analog scales of mood states (n=22). Figures represent data from visual analog scales for nervousness, anxiety, anger, and sadness. Values are expressed as mean±SEM. Scores were based on a scale from 0 to 100. Increases from baseline were evaluated using Dunnett's* t *test. Single asterisk indicates* P<.05; *double asterisks,* P<.01. *See "Patients and Methods" and "Results" sections for definitions for the visual analog scales and explanation of all other statistical analyses.*

following the start of drug infusion, an effect that retained significance after adjusting for placebo–test-day responses. Yohimbine significantly increased nervousness ratings at the 20-minute time point ($t[7,252]=3.4$, $P<.01$), an effect that remained significant after adjusting for placebo–test-day responses ($t[3,252]=2.2$, $P=.05$).

The repeated measures ANOVA performed on self-rated anxiety data revealed a significant time effect ($F_{HF}[4.1,85.3]=2.7$, $P=.04$) but no significant drug effect or drug-by-time interaction. Post hoc repeated measures ANOVAs that compared MCPP with yohimbine revealed a significant time effect ($F_{HF}[3.8,80.6]=2.9$, $P=.03$) and a nonsignificant trend for a drug effect ($F[1,21]=3.5$, $P=.08$). There was also a nonsignificant trend found for the drug-by-time interaction in the comparison of MCPP with placebo ($F_{HF}[9.4,98.4]=2.0$, $P=.09$). There were no significant baseline differences between test days or significant increases from baseline following placebo or yohimbine infusion. *m*-Chlorophenylpiperazine significantly increased anxiety from baseline at 20 minutes following the initiation of drug infusion ($t[7,252]=3.0$, $P<.05$), an effect that remained significant ($P<.05$) after adjusting for placebo–test-day responses.

Sadness

The repeated measures ANOVA that evaluated sadness scores revealed significant effects of drug ($F[2,42]=4.0$, $P=.03$) but not of time or the drug-by-time interaction. Post hoc repeated measures ANOVAs revealed that MCPP produced no significant effects relative to placebo. However, yohimbine reduced sadness compared with placebo (drug, $F[1,21]=5.0$, $P=.04$; time, $F_{HF}[4.9,102.8]=3.6$, $P=.005$) and MCPP (drug, $F[1,21]=6.5$, $P=.02$; drug-by-time interaction, $F_{HF}[3.7,77.9]=1.9$, $P=.1$). There were no significant baseline differences between test days.

CORRELATIONS AMONG SUBJECTIVE MEASURES

Correlates of increased craving were determined for the MCPP test day and adjusted for multiple comparisons using Bonferroni's correction. The peak increase in anxiety on the MCPP test day correlated with the peak increase in high ($r=.51$, $P=.04$) and the patients' sense that alcohol would make them feel better ($r=.54$, $P=.04$). The peak increase in high on the MCPP test day correlated significantly with the peak increase in similarity to alcohol ($r=.62$, $P<.04$). However, the degree to which MCPP was similar to ethanol was not correlated significantly with MCPP-induced craving on the visual analog scales.

NEUROENDOCRINE RESPONSES

Prolactin

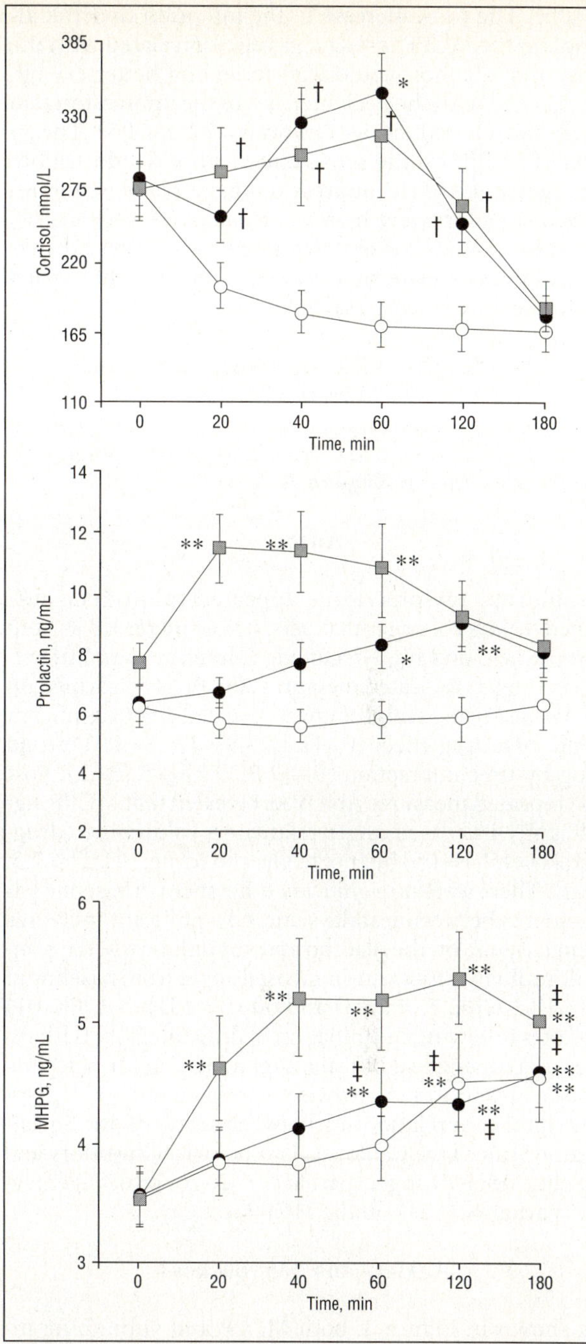

Figure 5. *Effects of placebo (open circles),* m*-chlorophenylpiperazine hydrochloride (solid circles), and yohimbine hydrochloride (shaded squares) on levels of cortisol, prolactin, and 3-methoxy-4-hydroxyphenylethyleneglycol (MHPG) in recently detoxified alcoholic patients (n=22). Values are expressed as mean±SEM. Increases from baseline were evaluated using Dunnett's* t *test. Single asterisk indicates* P<.05*; double asterisks,* P<.01*; dagger,* P<.05 *after nonsignificant increases from baseline were reexamined adjusting for the placebo–test-day effects using Dunnett's* t *test (after adjusting for placebo–test-day responses, all significant increases from baseline retained their significance); and double dagger,* P<.05 *but no longer significant after adjusting for placebo–test-day effects.*

As indicated in **Figure 5**, both MCPP and yohimbine produced small increases in prolactin levels (drug, $F_{HF}[1.2,25.8]=9.4$, $P=.003$; time, $F_{HF}[2.9,61.0]=5.1$, $P=.003$; drug-by-time interaction, $F_{HF}[3.5,74.1]=8.1$, $P=.0001$). Although, relative to placebo, both MCPP (drug-by-time interaction, $F_{HF}[2.7,55.9]=8.1$, $P=.0003$) and yohimbine (drug-by-time interaction, $F_{HF}[2.3,48.0]=9.4$, $P=.0002$) increased prolactin levels, yohimbine produced greater increases than did MCPP (drug-by-time interaction, $F_{HF}[2.5,52.6]=7.0$, $P=.0009$). There were no significant differences in basal levels of prolactin between test days. There

were no statistically significant changes in prolactin level from baseline on the placebo test day. Prolactin levels increased from baseline on the MCPP test day at 60 ($t[7,210]=3.0, P<.02$) and 120 ($t[7,210]=4.3, P<.01$) minutes following the initiation of drug infusion. Adjusting for placebo–test-day responses, MCPP produced significant increases ($P<.01$) beginning 40 minutes following the initiation of drug infusion and persisting throughout the assessment period. Yohimbine increased prolactin ($P<.01$) at the 20-, 40-, and 60-minute time points. After adjusting for placebo–test-day responses, yohimbine significantly increased prolactin levels ($P<.01$) at all postinfusion time points.

Cortisol

Both MCPP and yohimbine increased cortisol levels (Figure 5). Repeated measures ANOVA found significant effects of drug ($F_{HF}[1.7,34.8]=10.4$, $P=.0006$), time ($F_{HF}[2.9,60.2]=17.5$, $P=.0001$), and the drug-by-time interaction ($F_{HF}[3.4,70.4]=7.1$, $P=.0002$). Post hoc repeated measures ANOVAs revealed that relative to placebo, MCPP and yohimbine produced comparable increases in cortisol levels as indicated by the drug-by-time interaction effects (MCPP vs placebo, $F_{HF}[2.5,52.9]=19.1$, $P=.0001$; yohimbine vs placebo, $F_{HF}[2.7,55.8]=8.7$, $P=.0001$; MCPP vs yohimbine, $F_{HF}[1.9,39.2]=1.1$, $P=.4$). There were no significant differences in baseline values between test days. On the placebo test day, there was a significant decrease in cortisol levels ($P<.01$) at all postinfusion time points. On the MCPP test day, cortisol levels were increased from baseline 60 minutes after initiating the infusion ($t[6,210]=3.1$, $P<.05$) and were significantly decreased relative to baseline at the 180-minute time point ($t[6,210]=5.3$, $P<.01$). After adjusting for the placebo–test-day decreases, MCPP produced significant increases in cortisol levels ($P<.05$) at all postinfusion time points except the 180-minute time point. Yohimbine did not produce a significant increase in cortisol levels from baseline but eliminated a significant test-day decline in cortisol levels from baseline at all but the 180-minute time point. Adjusting for placebo–test-day effects, yohimbine significantly increased cortisol levels ($P<.05$) at all but the 180-minute time point.

3-Methoxy-4-hydroxyphenylethyleneglycol

Figure 5 illustrates the finding that relative to both MCPP and placebo, yohimbine increased plasma MHPG levels. The repeated measures ANOVA revealed significant effects of drug ($F_{HF}[1.6,33.1]=8.0$, $P=.003$), time ($F_{HF}[2.2,46.3]=18.7$, $P=.0001$), and the drug-by-time interaction ($F_{HF}[3.4,70.6]=3.1$, $P=.03$). Post hoc repeated measures ANOVAs indicated that relative to placebo, yohimbine (drug-by-time interaction, $F_{HF}[2.3,47.3]=4.0$, $P=.02$) but not MCPP ($F_{HF}[3.6,75.5]=1.9$, $P=.12$) increased plasma MHPG levels. Relative to MCPP, yohimbine also increased MHPG levels (drug, $F[1,21]=8.2$, $P=.009$; drug-by-time interaction, $F_{HF}[2.2,46.6]=2.6$, $P=.08$). There were no significant baseline differences between test days. Plasma MHPG levels increased relative to baseline during the placebo test day, reaching significance ($P<.01$) at the 120- and 180-minute time points. *m*-Chlorophenylpiperazine produced significant increases in plasma MHPG levels from baseline ($P<.05$) at the 40-, 80-, 120-, and 180-minute time points. However, none of the MCPP–test-day effects retained statistical significance after adjusting for placebo–test-day changes. Yohimbine significantly increased plasma MHPG levels at all postinfusion time points ($P<.01$). After adjusting for placebo–test-day increases in plasma MHPG levels, these increases retained significance ($P<.05$) at all time points except 180 minutes after starting the infusion.

For the MCPP test day, partial correlations that controlled for baseline levels were calculated between the peak levels of prolactin, cortisol, and MHPG and the peak levels of high, similarity to alcohol, and the desire to drink alcohol. No significant correlations emerged in this analysis.

PHYSIOLOGIC RESPONSES

Yohimbine produced the greatest increases in systolic and diastolic blood pressures relative to MCPP and placebo. Repeated measures ANOVA for systolic blood pressure data revealed significant effects of drug ($n=21$; $F[2,40]=19.6$, $P=.0001$), time ($F_{HF}[3.3,64.9]=6.2$, $P=.0007$), and the drug-by-time interaction ($F_{HF}[5.3,105.1]=2.5$, $P=.03$). Post hoc repeated measures ANOVAs indicated that yohimbine significantly increased systolic blood pressure relative to placebo (drug-by-time interaction, $F_{HF}[2.6,51.1]=3.9$, $P=.02$), although none of the other comparisons reached significance. Baseline values (mean±SEM) did not differ significantly between the test days (baseline placebo, 111.9±2.4 mm Hg; baseline MCPP, 109.2±1.8 mm Hg; baseline yohimbine, 111.4±1.7 mm Hg). Systolic blood pressure (mean±SEM) peaked at 40 minutes following the initiation of the infusion (placebo, 112.4±2.5 mm Hg; MCPP, 117.7±3.0 mm Hg; yohimbine, 130.6±3.4 mm Hg). Neither MCPP nor placebo significantly increased systolic blood pressure relative to baseline, although the MCPP-induced increase at 180 minutes following the initiation of the infusion was greater than the placebo-induced increase (mean±SEM) (placebo, 105.0±2.6; MCPP, 113.1±3.1 mm Hg). At all but the 240-minute time point, yohimbine significantly increased systolic blood pressure relative to baseline ($P<.05$) and the change from baseline was significantly greater ($P<.01$) than that produced by placebo.

Repeated measures ANOVA for diastolic blood pressure data revealed significant effects of drug ($n=21$; $F[2,40]=6.7$, $P=.003$), time ($F_{HF}[4.3,85.4]=2.8$, $P=.03$), and the drug-by-time interaction ($F_{HF}[6.1,121.4]=2.4$, $P=.03$). Post hoc repeated measures ANOVAs found that MCPP (drug-by-time interaction, $F_{HF}[5.1,107.0]=4.2$, $P=.002$) produced significantly greater increases than did placebo, there was a nonsignificant trend for yohimbine to increase diastolic blood pressure relative to placebo ($F_{HF}[3.1,62.8]=2.3$, $P=.09$), and MCPP and yohimbine test days did not differ significantly. Baseline values (mean±SEM) did not differ significantly between the test days (baseline placebo, 68.6±1.7 mm Hg; baseline MCPP, 66.7±1.5 mm Hg; baseline yohimbine, 68.1±1.7 mm Hg). Systolic blood pressure (mean±SEM) peaked at 20 minutes following the initiation of the infusion for placebo and yohimbine and 40 minutes following drug infusion for MCPP (20 minutes after infusion of placebo, 69.3±1.8

mm Hg; 40 minutes after infusion of MCPP, 72.0±2.3 mm Hg; 20 minutes after infusion of yohimbine, 74.4±2.6 mm Hg). Diastolic blood pressure did not increase significantly from baseline on the placebo test day. On the MCPP test day, diastolic blood pressure increased significantly ($P<.05$) from baseline at the 20-, 40-, and 60-minute time points. Adjusting for placebo–test-day changes, MCPP significantly increased diastolic blood pressure ($P<.05$) at 20, 40, 120, and 180 minutes following the initiation of drug infusion. Yohimbine significantly increased diastolic blood pressure from baseline ($P<.05$) at all but the 240-minute time point. After adjusting for placebo–test-day responses, yohimbine increased diastolic blood pressure ($P<.01$) at all postinfusion time points.

Repeated measures ANOVA for pulse rate did not indicate significant drug (n=21; $F[2,40]=1.1$, $P=.3$) or drug-by-time interaction ($F_{HF}[7.6,152.4]=1.2$, $P=.3$) effects. Also, none of the post hoc repeated measures ANOVAs showed significant drug-by-time interaction effects.

COMMENT

The principal finding of this study was that some of the ethanollike effects of the 5-HT partial agonist MCPP showed pharmacologic specificity in recently detoxified alcoholics, ie, they were not produced by placebo or by the α_2-adrenergic receptor antagonist yohimbine. Both drugs increased blood pressure and produced nervousness, ethanollike physical sensations, and euphoria. However, MCPP produced a greater degree of anxiety and anger. Also, the effects of MCPP were rated more similar to those of ethanol than were those of either yohimbine or placebo. In addition, MCPP but not yohimbine or placebo elicited three of the five components of craving identified by Tiffany and colleagues.[56,57] The elicitation of ethanollike responses and cravings in alcoholics by MCPP replicates earlier findings reported for the 5-HT partial agonists MCPP[3] and MK-212.[4] Both MCPP and yohimbine increased prolactin and cortisol levels. However, relative to placebo, yohimbine produced greater increases in prolactin levels than did MCPP. Also, relative to both MCPP and placebo, yohimbine increased plasma MHPG levels. None of the neuroendocrine measures significantly correlated with self-ratings of high or craving for alcohol. Yohimbine produced the greatest increases in systolic blood pressure, whereas yohimbine and MCPP comparably increased diastolic blood pressure. Neither drug significantly affected pulse rate.

These data further implicate 5-HT systems in the discriminative properties and craving for alcohol in recently detoxified alcoholics. *m*-Chlorophenylpiperazine interacts with the 5-HT transporter[61] and several 5-HT receptor subtypes, including, in descending affinity, the 5-HT_3, 5-HT_{2C}, 5$HT_{2A/B}$, 5-HT_7, 5-HT_{1A}, and 5-HT_{1D} receptors.[62-66] *m*-Chlorophenylpiperazine is a partial agonist of 5-HT_1 receptor subtypes,[65,67] a partial agonist or antagonist of the 5-HT_2 receptor,[68-70] and an antagonist of 5-HT_3 receptors.[71,72] Although its highest affinity is for 5-HT receptors, it has a lower but significant affinity at noradrenergic receptors and low affinity for dopamine receptors.[63] The ethanollike effects of MCPP could arise from MCPP actions at a 5-HT receptor subtype or from an indirect modulation of dopamine function by actions at these receptors.[73] Hormonal responsivity to MCPP has been used as a probe of 5-HT receptor function in humans,[74,75] yet neither prolactin nor cortisol responses to MCPP correlated significantly with the degree to which MCPP increased self-rated high, alcohollike sensations, or craving for alcohol. The absence of a correlation between hormonal and behavioral measures raises questions concerning the mechanisms underlying the behavioral effects of MCPP in the current study. However, previous studies with MCPP in healthy subjects and anxious patients found significant correlations between cortisol responses and anxiety but not other behaviors.[6] Also, there is evidence that hormonal responses to MCPP and other 5-HT direct and indirect agonists may be blunted in alcoholic patients relative to healthy subjects,[3,4,26,76] perhaps altering the relationships between hormonal measures and the behavioral measures most directly relevant to alcoholism.

m-Chlorophenylpiperazine produced ethanollike effects as assessed by the Sensation Scale that were similar in magnitude to short-term ethanol intoxication in healthy subjects in a previous study.[17] *m*-Chlorophenylpiperazine also produced a high that was recognized by alcoholics as moderately ethanollike. In patients who had used other drugs, the effects of MCPP were recognized as similar to cocaine and, to a lesser extent, marijuana. This finding raises the possibility that 5-HT systems contribute to important subjective effects of several drugs of abuse. These effects could be direct effects of serotonergic stimulation or indirect consequences of serotonergic modulation of dopamine function.[71,77] Given the lack of specificity of MCPP in its similarity to several drugs of abuse, one might more accurately label its ethanollike responses "abused substance–like." Future studies should evaluate whether MCPP differentially stimulates craving for alcohol relative to other abused substances in alcoholic patients.

m-Chlorophenylpiperazine but not yohimbine increased three highly intercorrelated aspects of craving relative to preinfusion levels on MCPP test days and relative to placebo infusions. The craving subscale scores that were increased by MCPP included the desire to drink alcohol, the sense that alcohol would reduce discomfort, and the impression that alcohol consumption would result in feeling better. Under the test conditions, MCPP did not increase self-reports of the intention to drink alcohol or the sense of loss of control over drinking. Several cognitive processes could have contributed to the elicitation of craving by MCPP. *m*-Chlorophenylpiperazine served as an ethanollike cue. Cues associated with alcohol consumption,[78,79] including a priming dose of alcohol,[80,81] stimulate craving for alcohol in alcoholics.[82]

The capacity of MCPP to generate dysphoric affects probably contributed to its capacity to stimulate craving for alcohol. Whereas MCPP and yohimbine produced nervousness, MCPP more potently stimulated dysphoric affective states, including anger and anxiety. The negative mood states may have independently provoked craving[83] or may have increased the capacity of the ethanollike properties of MCPP to produce an increase in craving.[84] Both of these possibilities are consistent with

the significant correlations between MCPP-induced anxiety and the increase in the feeling that drinking alcohol would lead to feeling better. Neither MCPP nor yohimbine appeared to have a direct effect on consummatory processes as suggested by self-reports of the intention to drink alcohol or the sense of loss of control over alcohol consumption. However, contextual factors, particularly the fact that patients were studied during inpatient substance abuse treatment, may have affected the patients willingness to report intentions to consume alcohol or capacity to accurately assess or report feelings of loss of control over alcohol consumption. Consistent with these concerns, the visual analog scale that assessed control over alcohol consumption did not correlate highly with the other visual analog scales that measured craving.

THE MCPP RESPONSES that were observed in the current study may have been influenced by the subtype of the alcoholic patients who formed the patient sample. All of the patients in the current study met von Knorring et al's[46] criteria for type 2 alcoholism based on their early onset and significant detrimental social consequences of drinking. An increasing body of literature suggests that serotonergic dysregulation is more prominent in type 2 alcoholics relative to type 1 alcoholics and healthy subjects.[85,86] The current findings also replicate a report from Benkelfat et al[3] that suggested that the ethanollike properties of MCPP are more prominent in type 2 alcoholics than in type 1 alcoholics or healthy subjects. This group also reported blunted hormonal responses to MCPP in type 2 alcoholics relative to type 1 alcoholics and healthy subjects. Both Cloninger[87] and von Knorring et al[46] suggested that type 2 alcoholics are prone to violence during intoxication. The current study found that MCPP produced small but consistent increases in anger in patients. *m*-Chlorophenylpiperazine–induced anger has been reported in patients with generalized anxiety disorder[88] but not in healthy subjects or patients in whom panic disorder or major depression was diagnosed.[89] Patients with antisocial personality disorder, a component of type 2 alcoholism in the Cloninger schema,[87] also exhibit increased irritability following MCPP administration.[3] Ongoing evaluation of serotonergic contributions to anger and aggression in alcoholic patients appears warranted.

These data question the clinical importance of noradrenergic contributions to the discriminative properties of ethanol. Yohimbine produced a high that was not similar to alcohol or other drugs of abuse, and it did not stimulate craving. This finding suggests that yohimbine increased the dimensions of the Sensation Scale scores that were unrelated to the key discriminative properties of ethanol in the patient group. In healthy subjects, neither yohimbine nor idazoxan elicited euphoria.[54] The coadministration of yohimbine (given intravenously) and ethanol in healthy subjects enhanced ethanol-induced increases in Sensation Scale scores but not in euphoria.[17] Both yohimbine and ethanol increase noradrenergic turnover and produced nervousness or restlessness in healthy subjects[17,54,90-92]; thus, yohimbine-induced increases in Sensation Scale scores may reflect this common property. The capacity of yohimbine to induce nervousness or anxiety has been attributed to increased noradrenergic neuronal activity that results from the blockade of presynaptic α_2-adrenergic receptors.[93,94] Other effects of yohimbine may be mediated by postsynaptic α_2-adrenergic receptor antagonism,[95] dopamine$_2$ antagonism,[96] and blockade of 5-HT$_{1D}$ receptors.[97] However, the behavioral effects of yohimbine in humans are similar to those of the more selective α_2-adrenergic receptor antagonist idazoxan.[54] Also, the current study found that relative to both placebo and MCPP, yohimbine increased plasma MHPG levels, which is consistent with increased norepinephrine turnover.

The fact that yohimbine did not generate ethanollike interoceptive cues or elicit ethanol craving questions a direct involvement of the noradrenergic systems in generating a craving for alcohol. However, the current data do not rule out noradrenergic modulation of reactivity to alcohol-related cues in alcoholics, perhaps by affecting levels of arousal or anxiety. This hypothesis is consistent with evidence that cerebrospinal fluid levels of the noradrenaline metabolite MHPG but not the 5-HT metabolite 5-hydroxyindoleacetic acid predict the magnitude of craving elicited in alcoholics on exposure to an ethanol cue.[98] Future studies should directly examine the effects of noradrenergic and serotonergic drugs in modulating alcohol cue reactivity in alcoholics.

In the current study, the inability to evaluate multiple doses and administration strategies for the agents under investigation limits the interpretation of the relative contributions to craving of serotonergic and noradrenergic systems. The doses and durations of administration for each agent were selected on the basis of previous studies conducted at this institution.[6,48,49,51-53] However, the rewarding properties of drugs of abuse are affected by pharmacokinetic factors.[99] It is possible that the ethanollike effects of MCPP and yohimbine are dependent on dose and method of drug administration. It is also possible that both the central and the peripheral effects of these drugs contributed to the responses observed in the current studies. Future studies will be needed to characterize pharmacokinetic contributions to the findings of this study.

The current results suggest that MCPP has ethanollike properties in type 2 alcoholics and that these properties show pharmacologic specificity and clinical relevance. Future investigation is required to determine whether MCPP responses predict the outcome of psychosocial and pharmacologic therapies for alcoholism. If so, then the pharmacologic capacity to block the ethanollike effects of MCPP in alcoholics might serve to identify pharmacotherapeutic agents with therapeutic potential for type 2 alcoholics. Antagonists of the 5-HT$_2$ receptor block MCPP-induced anxiety and hormonal responses in healthy subjects[100] and patient groups,[101,102] making them suitable initial candidate drugs for this purpose. Investigation of the interactions of 5-HT$_7$ antagonists with MCPP in humans would also be of interest in light of the relatively high affinity of both MCPP and ritanserin for this receptor.[66] Given the rapidly progressive clinical course of this alcoholic subtype,[103] the clinical implications of this approach are potentially substantial.

Accepted for publication August 1, 1994.

This research was supported by the Department of Veterans Affairs, Washington, DC, through funding of the Veterans Affairs–Yale Alcoholism Research Center, West Haven. Additional funding came from grant MH-30929 from the National Institute of Mental Health and grant K20-AA00143 from the National Institute on Alcohol Abuse and Alcoholism, Bethesda, Md.

We wish to acknowledge the critical contributions to this research made by the clinical and research staffs of the Biostudies Unit and Substance Abuse Treatment Unit of the West Haven Veterans Affairs Medical Center. We also thank Pedro Mendia, MS, for statistical consultation.

Reprints not available.

REFERENCES

1. Signs SA, Schechter MD. The role of dopamine and serotonin receptors in the mediation of the ethanol interoceptive cue. *Pharmacol Biochem Behav.* 1988;30:55-64.
2. Grant KA, Colombo G, Gatto GJ. Characterization of 5-HT_1 receptor agonists and the mediation of ethanolmimetic discriminative stimulus effects. *Alcohol Clin Exp Res.* 1993;17:334. Abstract.
3. Benkelfat C, Murphy DL, Hill JL, George DT, Nutt D, Linnoila M. Ethanollike properties of the serotonergic partial agonist m-chlorophenylpiperazine in chronic alcoholic patients. *Arch Gen Psychiatry.* 1991;48:383.
4. Lee MA, Meltzer HY. Neuroendocrine responses to serotonergic agents in alcoholics. *Biol Psychiatry.* 1991;30:1017-1030.
5. Moss HB, Yao JK, Panzak GL. Serotonergic responsivity and behavioral dimensions in antisocial personality disorder with substance abuse. *Biol Psychiatry.* 1990;28:325-328.
6. Charney DS, Woods SW, Goodman WK, Heninger GR. Serotonin function in anxiety, II: effects of the serotonin agonist MCPP in panic disorder patients and healthy subjects. *Psychopharmacology.* 1987;92:14-24.
7. Zacchia C, Pihl RO, Young S, Ervin F. The influence of altered tryptophan availability on ethanol intoxication in normal men. *J Stud Alcohol.* 1987;48:535-540.
8. Corrodi H, Fuxe K, Hockfelt T. The effect of ethanol on the activity of the catecholamine neurons in the rat brain. *J Pharm Pharmacol.* 1966;18:821-823.
9. Poherecky LA, Jaffe LS. Noradrenergic involvement in the acute effects of ethanol. *Res Commun Chem Pathol Pharmacol.* 1975;12:433-447.
10. Karoum F, Wyatt RJ, Majchrowicz E. Brain concentrations of biogenic-amine metabolites in acutely treated and ethanol dependent rats. *Br J Pharmacol.* 1976;56:403-411.
11. Amit Z, Brown ZW. Actions of drugs of abuse on brain reward systems: a reconsideration with specific attention to alcohol. *Pharmacol Biochem Behav.* 1982;17:233-238.
12. Verbanck P, Seutin V, Massotte L, Dresse A. Yohimbine can induce ethanol tolerance in an in vitro preparation of rat locus coeruleus. *Alcohol Clin Exp Res.* 1991;15:1036-1039.
13. Shiirao I, Tsuda A, Ida Y, Tsujimaru S, Satoh H, Oguchi M, Tanaka M, Inanaga K. Effect of acute ethanol administration on noradrenaline metabolism in brain regions in stressed and non-stressed rats. *Pharmacol Biochem Behav.* 1988;30:769-773.
14. Durcan MJ, Lister RG, Linnoila M. Behavioral effects of alpha 2 adrenoceptor antagonists and their interactions with ethanol in tests of locomotion, exploration and anxiety in mice. *Psychopharmacology.* 1989;97:189-193.
15. Lister RG, Durcan MJ, Nutt DJ, Linnoila M. Attenuation of ethanol intoxication by alpha adrenoceptor antagonists. *Life Sci.* 1989;44:111-119.
16. Borg S, Kvande H, Sedvall G. Central norepinephrine metabolism during alcohol intoxication in addicts and healthy volunteers. *Science.* 1981;213:1135-1137.
17. McDougle CJ, Krystal JH, Price LH, Heninger GR, Charney DS. Noradrenergic response to acute ethanol administration in healthy human subjects: comparison with intravenous yohimbine. *Psychopharmacology.* In press.
18. Ahlenius S, Carlsson A, Engel J, Svensson T, Sodersten P. Antagonism by alpha methyltyrosine of the ethanol-induced stimulation and euphoria in man. *Clin Pharmacol Ther.* 1973;14:586-591.
19. Perez-Reyes M, White WR, McDonald SA, Hicks RE. Interaction between ethanol and dextroamphetamine: effects on psychomotor performance. *Alcohol Clin Exp Res.* 1992;16:75-81.
20. Murphy JM, McBride WJ, Lumeng L, Li T-K. Contents of monoamines in forebrain regions of alcohol-preferring (P) and -nonpreferring (NP) lines of rats. *Pharmacol Biochem Behav.* 1987;26:389-392.
21. Wong DT, Threlkeld PG, Lumeng L, Li T-K. Higher density of serotonin-1A receptors in the hippocampus and cerebral cortex of alcohol-preferring P rats. *Life Sci.* 1990;46:231-235.
22. Korpi ER, Paivarinta P, Abi-Dargham A, Honkanen A, Laruelle M, Tuominen K, Hiilakivi LA. Binding of serotonergic ligands to brain membranes of alcohol-preferring AA and alcohol-avoiding ANA rats. *Alcohol.* 1992;9:369-374.
23. Sellers EM, Higgins GA, Sobell MB. 5-HT and alcohol abuse. *Trends Pharmacol Sci.* 1992;13:69-75.
24. Holman RB, Hoyland V, Shillito EE. The failure of p-chlorophenylalanine to affect voluntary alcohol consumption in rats. *Br J Pharmacol.* 1975;53:299-304.
25. Pihl RO, Young SN, Ervin FR, Plotnick S. Influence of tryptophan availability on selection of alcohol and water by men. *J Stud Alcohol.* 1987;48:260-264.
26. Coccaro EF, Siever LJ, Klar HM, Maurer G, Cochrane K, Cooper TB, Mohs RC, Davis KL. Serotonergic studies in patients with affective and personality disorders: correlates with suicidal and impulsive aggressive behavior. *Arch Gen Psychiatry.* 1989;46:587-599.
27. Friedman MJ, Krstulovic AM, Severinghaus JM, Brown SJ. Altered conversion of tryptophan to kynurenine in newly abstinent alcoholics. *Biol Psychiatry.* 1988;23:89-93.
28. Olsen RE, Gursey D, Vester J. Evidence for a defect in tryptophan metabolism in chronic alcoholism. *N Engl J Med.* 1960;263:1169-1174.
29. Ballenger JC, Goodwin FK, Major LF, Brown GL. Alcohol and central serotonin metabolism in man. *Arch Gen Psychiatry.* 1979;36:224-227.
30. Thomson SM Jr, McMillen BA. Test for decreased serotonin/tryptophan metabolite ratios in abstinent alcoholics. *Alcohol.* 1987;4:1-5.
31. Naranjo CA, Sellers EM, Lawrin MO. Modulation of ethanol intake by serotonin uptake inhibitors. *J Clin Psychiatry.* 1986;47(suppl 4):16-22.
32. Kranzler HR, Meyer RE. An open trial of buspirone in alcoholics. *J Clin Psychopharmacol.* 1989;9:379-380.
33. Wong DR, Lumeng L, Threlkeld PG, Reid LR, Li T-K. Serotonergic and adrenergic receptors in alcohol-preferring and non-preferring rats. *J Neural Transm.* 1988;71:207-218.
34. Kiianmaa K, Fuxe K, Jonsson G, Ahtee L. Evidence for involvement of central NA neurons in alcohol intake: increased alcohol consumption after degeneration of the NA pathway to the cortex cerebri. *Neurosci Lett.* 1975;1:41-45.
35. Mason ST, Corcoran ME, Fibiger HC. Noradrenaline and ethanol intake in the rat. *Neurosci Lett.* 1979;12:137-142.
36. Hubbell CL, Delconte JD, Amendola CA, Nichols ML, Reid LD. Adrenergic drugs and rats' intake of alcoholic beverage. *Soc Neurosci Abstracts.* 1991;16:1422. Abstract 565.6.
37. Opitz K. The effect of clonidine and related substances on voluntary ethanol consumption in rats. *Drug Alcohol Depend.* 1990;25:43-48.
38. Meyer RE. Prospects for a rational pharmacotherapy of alcoholism. *J Clin Psychiatry.* 1989;50:403-412.
39. Bjorkquist SE. Clonidine in alcohol withdrawal. *Acta Psychol Scand.* 1975;52:256-263.
40. Baumgartner GR, Rowen RC. Clonidine vs chlordiazepoxide in the management of acute alcohol withdrawal syndrome. *Arch Intern Med.* 1987;147:1223-1226.
41. American Psychiatric Association. *Diagnostic and Statistical Manual of Mental Disorders, Revised Third Edition.* Washington, DC: American Psychiatric Association; 1987.
42. Spitzer RI, Williams JBW, Gibbgon M, First MB. The Structured Clinical Interview for *DSM-III-R*, I: history, rationale, and description. *Arch Gen Psychiatry.* 1992;49:624-629.
43. Gough HG, ed. *CPI Administrator's Guide.* Palo Alto, Calif: Consulting Psychologists Inventory Press Inc; 1987.
44. Cooney NL, Kadden RM, Litt MD. A comparison of methods for assessing sociopathy in male and female alcoholics. *J Stud Alcohol.* 1990;51:42-48.
45. Selzer ML. The Michigan Alcoholism Screening Test: the quest for a new diagnostic instrument. *Am J Psychiatry.* 1971;127:1653-1658.
46. von Knorring AL, Bohman M, von Knorring L, Oreland L. Platelet MAO activity as a biological marker in subgroups of alcoholism. *Acta Psychiatr Scand.* 1985;72:51-58.
47. Lamparski DM, Roy A, Nutt DJ, Linnoila M. The criteria of Cloninger et al and von Knorring et al for subgrouping alcoholics: a comparison in a clinical population. *Acta Psychiatr Scand.* 1991;84:497-502.
48. Southwick SM, Krystal JH, Morgan CA, Johnson D, Nagy LM, Nicolau A, Heninger GR, Charney DS. Abnormal noradrenergic function in posttraumatic stress disorder. *Arch Gen Psychiatry.* 1993;50:266-274.
49. Southwick SM, Krystal JH, Morgan A, Nagy LM, Dan E, Johnson D, Bremner D, Charney DS. Yohimbine and *m*-chlorophenylpiperazine in PTSD. In: 1991 New Research Program and Abstracts, American Psychiatric Association, 144th Annual Meeting; May 11-16, 1991; New Orleans, La. Abstract NR348.
50. Keane TM, Caddell JM, Taylor KL. Mississippi scale for combat-related posttraumatic stress disorder: three studies in reliability and validity. *J Consult Clin Psychol.* 1988;56:85-90.
51. Charney DS, Woods SW, Krystal JH, Nagy LM, Heninger GR. Noradrenergic neuronal dysregulation in panic disorder: the effects of intravenous yohimbine and clonidine in panic disorder patients. *Acta Psychiatr Scand.* 1992;86:273-282.
52. Charney DS, Goodman WK, Price LH, Woods SW, Rasmussen SA, Heninger GR. Serotonin function in obsessive-compulsive disorder: a comparison of the effects of tryptophan and *m*-chlorophenylpiperazine in patients and healthy subjects. *Arch Gen Psychiatry.* 1988;45:177-185.
53. Krystal JH, Seibyl JP, Price LH, Woods SW, Heninger GR, Aghajanian GK, Charney DS. *m*-Chlorophenylpiperazine effects in neuroleptic-free schizophrenic patients: evidence implicating serotonergic systems in the positive

symptoms of schizophrenia. *Arch Gen Psychiatry.* 1993;50:624-635.
54. Krystal JH, McDougle CJ, Woods SW, Price LH, Heninger GR, Charney DS. Dose response relationship for oral idazoxan effects in healthy human subjects: comparison with oral yohimbine. *Psychopharmacology.* 1992;108:313-319.
55. Maisto SA, Conners GJ, Tucker JA, McCollam JB, Addesso VJ. Validation of the sensation scale: a measure of subjective physiological responses to alcohol. *Behav Res Ther.* 1980;18:37-43.
56. Tiffany ST, Drobes DJ. Development and validation of a questionnaire on smoking urges. *Br J Addict.* 1991;86:1467-1476.
57. Tiffany ST, Singleton E, Haertzen C, Henningfield JE. The development of a cocaine craving questionnaire. *Drug Alcohol Depend.* In press.
58. Maas JW, Hattox SE, Landis DH, Roth RH. The determination of a brain arteriovenous difference for 3-methoxy-4-hydroxyphenylethylene glycol (MHPG). *Brain Res.* 1976;118:167-173.
59. Winer BJ. *Statistical Principles in Experimental Design.* 2nd ed. New York, NY: McGraw-Hill International Book Co; 1971.
60. American Psychiatric Association Commission on Psychotherapies. *Psychotherapy Research: Methodological and Efficacy Issues.* Washington, DC: American Psychiatric Press; 1982.
61. Wolf WA, Kuhn DM. The 5-HT transporter is an additional site of action for the 5-HT agonists RU 24969 and TFMPP. *Neurochem Int.* 1991;19:39-44.
62. Hoyer D. Functional correlates of serotonin 5-HT_1 recognition sites. *J Recept Res.* 1988;8:59-81.
63. Hamik A, Peroutka SJ. 1-(*m*-chlorophenyl)piperazine interactions with neurotransmitter receptors in the human brain. *Biol Psychiatry.* 1989;25:569-575.
64. Glennon RA, Ismaiel AE-KM, McCarthy BG, Peroutka SJ. Binding of arylpiperazines to 5-HT_3 serotonin receptors: results of a structure-affinity study. *Eur J Pharmacol.* 1989;168:387-392.
65. Schoeffter P, Hoyer D. Interaction of arylpiperazines with 5-HT_{1A}, 5-HT_{1B}, 5-HT_{1C} and 5-HT_{1D} receptors: do discriminatory 5-HT_{1B} receptor ligands exist? *Arch Pharmacol.* 1989;339:675-683.
66. Shen Y, Monsma FJ Jr, Metcalf MA, Jose PA, Hamblin MW, Sibley DR. Molecular cloning and expression of a 5-hydroxytryptamine$_7$ receptor subtype. *J Biol Chem.* 1993;268:18200-18204.
67. Sheldon PW, Aghajanian GK. Excitatory responses to serotonin (5-HT) in neurons of the rat piriform cortex: evidence for mediation by 5-HT_{1C} receptors in pyramidal cells and 5-HT_2 receptors in interneurons. *Synapse.* 1991;9:208-218.
68. Conn PJ, Sanders-Bush E. Relative efficacies of piperazines at the phosphoinositide hydrolysis-linked serotonergic (5-HT_2 and 5-HT_{1C}) receptors. *J Pharmacol Exp Ther.* 1987;2142:552-557.
69. Sheldon PW, Aghajanian GK. Serotonin (5-HT) induces IPSP's in pyramidal layer cells of rat piriform cortex: evidence for the involvement of a 5-HT_2 activated interneuron. *Brain Res.* 1990;506:62-69.
70. Carver JG, Grahame-Smith DG, Johnson ES, Madgwick Z. The effects of 5-HT and *m*-chlorophenylpiperazine (m-CPP) on the efflux of [^{3}H]-5-HT from human perfused platelets. *Br J Clin Pharmacology.* 1993;35:473-478.
71. Ireland SJ, Tyers MB. Pharmacological characterization of 5-hydroxytryptamine-induced depolarization of the rabbit isolated vagus nerve. *Br J Pharmacol.* 1987;90:229.
72. Robertson DW, Bloomquist W, Wong DT, Cohen ML. MCPP but not TFMPP is an antagonist at cardiac 5-HT_3 receptors. *Life Sci.* 1992;50:599-605.
73. Benloucif S, Galloway MP. Facilitation of dopamine release in vivo by serotonin agonists: studies with microdialysis. *Eur J Pharmacol.* 1991;200:1-8.
74. Siever LJ, Kahn RS, Lawlor BA, Trestman RL, Lawrence TL, Coccaro EF. Critical issues in defining the role of serotonin in psychiatric disorders. *Pharmacol Rev.* 1991;43:509-525.
75. Murphy DL, Lesch KP, Aulakh CS, Pigott TA. Serotonin-selective arylpiperazines with neuroendocrine, behavioral, temperature, and cardiovascular effects in humans. *Pharmacol Rev.* 1991;43:528-552.
76. Krystal JH, Webb E, Kranzler H, Cooney N, Heninger GR, Charney DS. Yohimbine and MCPP effects in alcoholics and healthy subjects. *Alcohol Clin Exp Res.* 1992;16:234.
77. Di Chiara G, Imperato A. Drugs abused by humans preferentially increase synaptic dopamine concentrations in the mesolimbic system of freely moving rats. *Proc Natl Acad Sci U S A.* 1988;85:5274-5278.
78. Pomerleau OF, Fertig J, Baker L, Cooney N. Reactivity to alcohol cues in alcoholics and non-alcoholics: implications for a stimulus control analysis of drinking. *Addict Behav.* 1983;8:1-10.
79. Rohsenow DJ, Niaura RS, Childress AR, Abrams DB, Monti PM. Cue reactivity in addictive behaviors: theoretical and treatment implications. *Int J Addict.* 1991;25:957-993.
80. Engle KB, Williams TK. Effect of an ounce of vodka on alcoholics desire for alcohol. *Q J Stud Alcohol.* 1972;33:1099-1105.
81. Ludwig AM, Wikler A, Stark L. The first drink: psychobiological aspects of craving. *Arch Gen Psychiatry.* 1974;30:539-547.
82. Hodgson R, Rankin H, Stockwell T. Alcohol dependence and the priming effect. *Behav Res Ther.* 1979;17:379-387.
83. Childress AR, Ehrman R, McLellan AT, Natale M, O'Brien CP. Mood states can elicit drug craving and conditioned withdrawal in opiate abuse patients. *NIDA Res Monogr.* 1986;76:137-144.
84. Litt MD, Cooney NL, Kadden RM, Gaupp L. Reactivity to alcohol cues and induced moods in alcoholics. *Addict Behav.* 1990;15:137-146.
85. Buydens-Branchey L, Branchey MH, Noumair D, Lieber CS. Age of alcoholism onset, II: relationship to susceptibility to serotonin precursor availability. *Arch Gen Psychiatry.* 1989;46:231-236.
86. Roy A, Virkkunen M, Linnoila M. Reduced central serotonin turnover in a subgroup of alcoholics? *Prog Neuropsychopharmacol Biol Psychiatry.* 1987; 11:173-177.
87. Cloninger CR. Neurogenetic adaptive mechanisms in alcoholism. *Science.* 1987; 236:410-416.
88. Germaine M, Goddard AW, Woods SW, Charney DS, Heninger GR. Anger and anxiety responses to *m*-chlorophenylpiperazine in generalized anxiety disorder. *Biol Psychiatry.* 1992;32:457-461.
89. Wetzler S, Kahn RS, Asnis GM, Korn M, van Praag HM. Serotonin receptor sensitivity and aggression. *Psychiatry Res.* 1991;37:271-279.
90. Holmberg G, Gershon S. Autonomic and psychic effects of yohimbine hydrochloride. *Psychopharmacologia (Berl).* 1961;2:93-106.
91. Ingram CG. Some pharmacologic actions of yohimbine and chlorpromazine in man. *Clin Pharmacol Ther.* 1962;3:345-352.
92. Charney DS, Heninger GR, Sternberg DE. Assessment of α_2 autoreceptor function in humans: effects of oral yohimbine. *Life Sci.* 1982;30:2033-2041.
93. Charney DS, Woods SW, Price LH, Goodman WK, Glazer WM, Heninger GR. Noradrenergic dysregulation in panic disorder. In: Ballenger JC, ed. *Neurobiology of Panic Disorder.* New York, NY: Alan R Liss Inc; 1990:91-105.
94. Redmond DE Jr. New and old evidence for the involvement of a brain norepinephrine system in anxiety. In: Fann WE, ed. *The Phenomenology and Treatment of Anxiety.* New York, NY: Plenum Publishing Corp; 1979:153-203.
95. Goldberg MR, Robinson D. Yohimbine: a pharmacological probe for study of the α_2 adrenoreceptor. *Pharmacol Rev.* 1983;35:143-180.
96. van Oene JC, de Vries JB, Horn AS. The effectiveness of yohimbine in blocking rat central dopamine autoreceptors in vivo. *Naunyn Schmiedebergs Arch Pharmacol.* 1984;327:304-311.
97. Peroutka SJ, Switzer JA, Hamik A. Identification of 5-hydroxytryptamine$_{1D}$ binding sites in human brain membranes. *Synapse.* 1989;3:61-66.
98. Petrakis I, Webb E, Abi-Dargham A, Cooney N, Charney DS, Krystal JH. Serotonin contributions to cue-induced craving in alcoholics. *Alcohol Clin Exp Res.* 1993;17:335. Abstract.
99. Schuster CR, Balster RL. The discriminative stimulus properties of drugs. *Adv Behav Pharmacol.* 1977;1:85-138.
100. Seibyl JP, Krystal JH, Price LH, Woods SW, D'Amico C, Heninger GR, Charney DS. Effects of ritanserin on the behavioral, neuroendocrine and cardiovascular responses to *m*-chlorophenylpiperazine in healthy human subjects. *Psychiatry Res.* 1991;38:227-236.
101. Krystal JH, Seibyl JP, Karper L, Erdos J, Wong ML, Heninger GR, Charney DS. Clozapine versus haloperidol blockade of M-CPP in schizophrenia. In: 1992 New Research Program and Abstracts, American Psychiatric Association, 145th Annual Meeting; May 2-7, 1992; Washington, DC. Abstract NR428.
102. Krystal JH, Seibyl JP, Karper L, Wong ML, Erdos J, Heninger GR, Charney DS. Ritanserin blockade of M-CPP effects in schizophrenia. In: 1992 New Research Program and Abstracts, American Psychiatric Association, 145th Annual Meeting; May 2-7, 1992; Washington, DC. Abstract NR429.
103. Babor TF, Hofmann M, DelBoca FK, Hesselbrock V, Meyer RE, Dolinsky ZS, Rounsaville B. Types of alcoholics, I: evidence for an empirically derived typology based on indicators of vulnerability and severity. *Arch Gen Psychiatry.* 1992;49:599-608.

Conversions From Système International (SI) Units to Traditional Units (Modified From *The SI Manual in Health Care*)

System	Component	SI Reference Interval*	SI Unit	Conversion Factor (Divide by)	Traditional Reference Interval*	Traditional Unit
Serum	Cortisol					
	8 AM	110-520	nmol/L	27.59	4-19	μg/dL
	4 PM	50-410	nmol/L	27.59	2-15	μg/dL
	Midnight	<140	nmol/L	27.59	<5	μg/dL

**These reference values are not intended to be definitive since each laboratory determines its own values. They are provided for illustration only.*

ORIGINAL ARTICLE

Allelic Variation in the D_4 Dopamine Receptor (DRD4) Gene Does Not Predict Response to Clozapine

Peter A. Rao, MD; David Pickar, MD; Pablo V. Gejman, MD; Anca Ram, MD; Elliot S. Gershon, MD; Joel Gelernter, MD

Objective: To test the hypothesis that interindividual differences in response to clozapine therapy might be attributable to the D_4 dopamine receptor (DRD4) alleles they carry. Different alleles of the D_4 dopamine receptor, coded by the DRD4 gene, differ in the affinity with which they bind the atypical antipsychotic drug clozapine in vitro. This may have physiologic implications. Clinical response to clozapine therapy varies among patients. The observation that, in vitro, clozapine binds the protein products of different DRD4 alleles with differing affinity characteristics suggested this hypothesis.

Method: The region of the DRD4 gene that encodes the putative third cytoplasmic loop of the D_4 receptor contains a 48–base pair sequence repeated a variable number of times. With use of polymerase chain reaction amplification, we assessed this variable number of tandem repeats polymorphism in a series of schizophrenic and schizoaffective subjects who had been treated with clozapine, and related genotype with treatment response, to test the hypothesis that DRD4 alleles lead to varying response to clozapine.

Results: Allelic variation at the DRD4 locus does not predict clinical response to clozapine relative to either fluphenazine hydrochloride or placebo in subjects with treatment-refractory schizophrenia or schizoaffective disorder.

Conclusions: DRD4 alleles do not predict therapeutic response to clozapine in schizophrenic and schizoaffective patients. There are implications from these data for the pathophysiology of schizophrenia and the mechanism of clozapine's therapeutic effect are discussed.

(Arch Gen Psychiatry. 1994;51:912-917)

From the Department of Psychiatry, West Haven (Conn) Veterans Affairs Medical Center (Drs Rao and Gelernter); the Department of Psychiatry, Division of Molecular Psychiatry, Yale University School of Medicine, New Haven, Conn (Drs Rao and Gelernter); the Experimental Therapeutics Branch, National Institute of Mental Health, Bethesda, Md (Dr Pickar); and the Clinical Neurogenetics Branch, National Institute of Mental Health, Bethesda, Md (Drs Gejman, Ram, and Gershon). Dr Rao is now at the Department of Psychiatry, Columbia University, New York, NY.

SCHIZOPHRENIA IS a disease of high morbidity that affects 1% of the population worldwide.[1] The mainstay of treatment for the past 40 years has been the antipsychotic medications, drugs characterized experimentally by their ability to induce catalepsy in animal models and pharmacologically by their ability to bind to dopamine receptors with high affinity.[2] The D_2 dopamine receptor is believed to be the primary target of antipsychotic medications.[2] However, the four other known dopamine receptors may also play a role. The D_1 dopamine receptor is present in the brain in greatest number[3] and is functionally linked to the D_2 receptor in animal models of motor function.[4] In recent years, molecular biologists have identified and characterized other dopamine receptors (D_3,[5] D_4,[6] and D_5[7] dopamine receptors) that were previously not known. The dopamine receptors belong to a family of G protein–coupled receptors that contain seven putative transmembrane regions.[8] The role these receptors play in the therapeutic actions of antipsychotic medications is unknown.

Many schizophrenic patients do not respond to the "typical" antipsychotic drugs. The dibenzodiazepine clozapine shows increased efficacy in schizophrenia. It is the prototype "atypical" antipsychotic drug because of its inability to cause catalepsy in animal models and extrapyramidal side effects or increased serum prolactin levels in humans.[9] In a study of patients with treatment-refractory schizophrenia, clozapine was shown to be effective in improving symptomatology for 30% of patients, while only 4% showed improvement with chlorpromazine hydrochloride.[10]

It would be very useful to know why clozapine is more effective than other antipsychotic drugs. Initial speculation about the mechanism of clozapine's superior therapeutic effects focused on several possibilities, including its higher affinity for the D_2 and serotonin S_2 (5-HT2) recep-

See Subjects and Methods on next page

SUBJECTS AND METHODS

Subjects were recruited from individuals referred to the Experimental Therapeutics Branch of the National Institute of Mental Health. Subjects accepted into the study met *DSM-III-R*[24] criteria for schizophrenia or schizoaffective disorder and met criteria established by the Clozapine Compassionate Use Protocol (Sandoz 71): (1) drug intolerance, as reflected by marked tardive dyskinesia or extrapyramidal symptoms, or (2) a history of treatment-refractoriness, defined as a lack of satisfactory clinical response to at least two different antipsychotic drugs given in adequate doses and for adequate periods.[22] A total of 41 subjects met criteria and participated in a cross-over, double-blind study of clozapine efficacy vs that of fluphenazine and placebo, the design for which has been described in detail elsewhere.[22] Subjects (all of whom had been treated with typical antipsychotic drugs for at least 3 months before entry into the study) started treatment with fluphenazine, the dose of which was adjusted based on clinical response, for a minimum of 4 weeks (average, 6 weeks). Subsequently, subjects were switched to placebo for a minimum of 2.5 weeks (average, 5 weeks), after which they underwent a two-part clozapine treatment phase, the first being a trial of clozapine at a "moderate" dose for a minimum of 3 weeks (average, 7 weeks) and the second being a trial of clozapine at an "optimized" dose for an average of 15 weeks. Subjects were assessed at weekly intervals during the trial with the modified Brief Psychiatric Rating Scale[25] 18-item inventory and the Bunney-Hamburg Scale for Psychosis.[26] Responsivity was determined with use of a priori criteria modified from those of Kane et al[10]: responsivity to clozapine relative to that to placebo and clozapine relative to that to fluphenazine was defined as (1) a 20% or more decrease in Brief Psychiatric Rating Scale score *and* (2) a Brief Psychiatric Rating Scale score less than 36 or Bunney-Hamburg Global Psychosis Rating of less than 6 (mild psychosis).[22]

Control subjects were derived from two cohorts. The first consisted of 27 subjects recruited for research at either the West Haven (Conn) Veterans Affairs Medical Center or the Department of Psychiatry, University of Connecticut, Farmington, 17 of whom were judged to have no psychiatric illness and no family history of psychiatric illness based on a psychiatric interview and 10 of whom were psychiatrically unassessed, genotyped by us. The second consisted of 115 white subjects studied and genotyped by Sommer et al.[27]

From each subject, DNA was extracted from blood by standard procedures. Polymerase chain reaction amplification of genomic DNA within the DRD4 third intracytoplasmic loop was performed with the use of oligonucleotide primers and conditions described by Lichter et al.[23] The PCR primers were D4-3 (5'-*GCG ACT ACG TGG TCT ACT CG*-3') and D4-42 (5'-*AGG ACC CTC ATG GCC TTG*-3').[23] Polymerase chain reaction amplification was performed in 25-μL volume reactions with the following components: 50 ng of genomic DNA; 10 mmol/L of TRIS hydrochloride; 50 mmol/L of potassium chloride; 1 mmol/L of magnesium chloride; 10% dimethyl sulfoxide; 200 μmol/L each of dATP, dTTP, and dCTP; 100 μmol/L each of dGTP and 7-deaza-dGTP; 0.5 μmol/L each of primers D4-3 and D4-42; and 0.05 U/μL of Taq DNA polymerase (Amplitaq, Perkin Elmer Cetus, Norwalk, Conn). Genomic DNA was heated to 99°C for 1 minute before the addition of 25 μL of a cocktail composed of the other reaction components just described. Subsequently, samples were heated to 95°C for 5 minutes, after which amplification was effected on a PCR cycler (GeneAmp PCR System 9600, Perkin Elmer Cetus) with 40 temperature cycles, each consisting of 20 seconds at 95°C, 20 seconds at 54°C, and 40 seconds at 72°C. The PCR products were then separated by electrophoresis in a modified agarose gel composed of 0.7% agarose (SeaKem LE, FMC Bioproducts, Rockland, Me) and 0.75% Synergel (Diversified Biotech, obtained from Research Products International, Mount Prospect, Ill) and stained with ethidium bromide, and visualized by UV transillumination. Alleles were assigned by comparison with a 100-base pair DNA ladder marker. Allele assignments were made blindly with respect to clozapine response.

Depending on the expected number of observations in cells for an allele, χ^2 statistic (wherever possible) or Fisher's Exact Test was used sequentially to test the null hypothesis that the distribution of each allele (relative to that of the sum of all other allele types) between groups is no different from chance distribution.

tors relative to other neuroreceptors[11] and its differential effect on electrophysiologic functioning of A10 vs A9 dopaminergic neurons.[12,13] The cloning of the D_4 dopamine receptor (DRD4)[6] raised other possibilities because clozapine binds to the D_4 receptor with an affinity 10 times greater than to the D_2 receptor,[6] differentiating it from the typical antipsychotic drugs; thus, clozapine might exert its primary antipsychotic effect at the level of the D_4 receptor. The D_4 receptor might have a specific role in the development of schizophrenia given its high density (compared with the D_2 and D_3 dopamine receptors) in the frontal cortex and amygdala,[6] areas believed to be involved in the pathophysiology of schizophrenia. In addition, it has been argued that the density of D_4 receptors is elevated in postmortem schizophrenic brains based on the differential binding of tritiated nemonapride and tritiated raclopride to D_2, D_3, and D_4 receptors.[14]

A variable number of tandem repeats (VNTR) polymorphism was identified in the putative third cytoplasmic loop of the D_4 receptor.[15] (We had previously used this polymorphism, detected as a restriction fragment length polymorphism, to map DRD4 to the distal short arm of chromosome 11[16] [**Figure 1**].) The third cytoplasmic loop, located between the fifth and sixth transmembrane regions, is believed to be a binding site (along with transmembrane region two) for G proteins in this family of receptors.[8,18,19] DRD4 alleles corresponding to the VNTR polymorphism variants have been shown to differ by up to a factor of four in their dissociation constant for inhibition of tritiated spiperone binding by clozapine when tested in sodium chloride–free conditions in vitro.[15] These differences in binding affinity characteristics for clozapine found in vitro may have physiologic significance in vivo and suggest that there may be differences in binding affinity of clozapine in vivo between the protein products of different DRD4 alleles. (The criti-

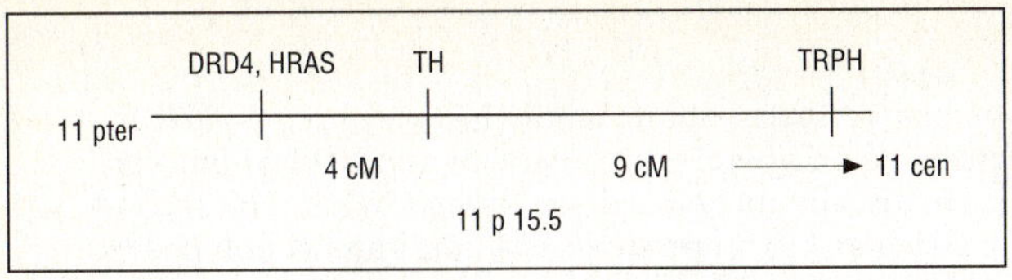

Figure 1. *Genetic map of distal chromosome 11p including D_4 dopamine receptor (DRD4).*[16,17] *HRAS indicates Harvey* ras *oncogene; TH, tyrosine hydroxylase; TRPH, tryptophan hydroxylase; cM, centimorgan, and cen, centromere.*

cal recognition sites for ligands in this receptor family are located in the transmembrane regions.[20])

It has previously been demonstrated[21] that DRD4 is not linked to schizophrenia and, at least in the informative families studied, a mutation in DRD4 therefore cannot in itself account for susceptibility to schizophrenia. However, clozapine still might have its primary effect on the D_4 receptor, and differences among individuals in response to clozapine might be attributable to the DRD4 alleles they carry.[15] If differential response to clozapine were in fact attributable to DRD4 alleles, there might be an overrepresentation of lower-affinity alleles in nonresponders; lack of treatment response might then be due to the inability to increase the clozapine dose above a threshold for toxicity (generally 900 mg/d) to compensate for differences in the dissociation constant of clozapine for the protein products of different alleles. These hypotheses, ie, that clozapine's actions at the level of the D_4 receptor might determine not only its overall antipsychotic efficacy but also its differential effectiveness over typical antipsychotic drugs in the treatment-resistant population, are a natural consequence of the finding of a seeming selectivity of clozapine for the D_4 dopamine receptor in general and of differential clozapine binding to the protein products of different DRD4 alleles in particular. We tested these hypotheses in a group of subjects with treatment-refractory schizophrenia and schizoaffective disorder who participated in a three-phase cross-over study of clozapine responsivity conducted at the National Institute of Mental Health, Bethesda, Md.[22] The polymerase chain reaction (PCR) was used to amplify the DRD4 VNTR region.[23] Allele frequencies were compared in schizophrenic and control subjects and in responders and nonresponders to clozapine treatment.

RESULTS

Allele frequencies were compared in the three groups of control subjects (**Table 1** and **Figure 2**). There was no statistically significant difference in frequency for any allele compared with normal and no diagnosis control groups. Comparison of a composite of these two control groups with the control group of Sommer et al[27] revealed no statistically significant difference in allele frequencies. Subsequently, all analyses were conducted with use of a composite control group made up of pooled data from these three groups.

Of the original 41 subjects, 34 were white; of these, 29 completed the clinical protocol. Allele frequencies may only be compared between patients of similar racial background because of the wide variation in allele frequencies often seen between different racial groups,[23,28,29] so all subsequent analyses were performed only on white subjects.

Table 1. D_4 Allele Frequencies in Three Control Groups*

	Normal Subjects		No Diagnosis		
D_4 Allele	All (n=17)	White (n=13)	All Subjects (n=10)	White Subjects (n=7)	Subjects of Sommer et al[27] (White Subjects) (n=115)
2	0.1 (4)	0.2 (4)	0.2 (3)	0.2 (3)	0.10 (24)
3	0 (0)	0 (0)	0 (0)	0 (0)	0.065 (15)
4	0.65 (22)	0.62 (16)	0.65 (13)	0.6 (8)	0.574 (132)
5	0 (0)	0 (0)	0 (0)	0 (0)	0.004 (1)
6	0.03 (1)	0.04 (1)	0 (0)	0 (0)	0.009 (2)
7	0.2 (7)	0.2 (5)	0.2 (4)	0.2 (3)	0.23 (54)
8	0 (0)	0 (0)	0 (0)	0 (0)	0.009 (2)

**Allele frequencies of the D_4 variable number of tandem repeats polymorphism. Numbers in parentheses are raw allele counts. Control groups are (1) normal subjects; (2) unselected (no diagnosis) subjects; and (3) subjects of Sommer et al.*[27] *Depending on the expected number of observations in cells for an allele, either the χ^2 statistic (wherever possible) or Fisher's Exact Test was used sequentially to test the null hypothesis that the distribution of each allele (relative to that of the sum of all other allele types) between groups (affected vs controls) is no different from chance distribution. Normal vs no diagnosis subjects (white only): alleles 2, 3, 5, 6, 7, and 8: Fisher's Exact Test, all alleles not significant at $P \geq .471$; allele 4: $\chi^2=0.004$, df=1, not significant $P=.950$. Normal and no diagnosis subjects (combined) vs subjects of Sommer et al*[27] *(white only): alleles 2, 3, 5, 6, and 8: Fisher's Exact Test, all alleles not significant at $P>.0841$; alleles 4 and 7: $\chi^2<0.0779$, df=1, both alleles not significant at $P>.780$.*

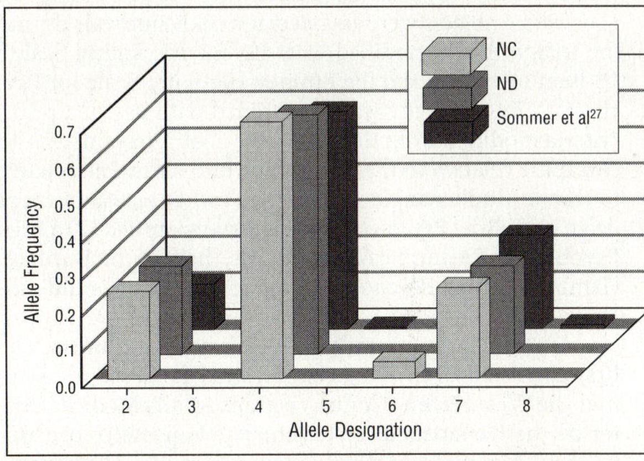

Figure 2. *Allele frequencies at D_4 dopamine receptor in three control groups: NC indicates normal control (normal by psychiatric evaluation); ND, no diagnosis (no psychiatric evaluation done); and Sommer et al,*[27] *controls (Table 1).*

The DRD4 allele frequencies were compared between subjects receiving clozapine (both schizophrenic [n=28] and schizoaffective [n=6]) from whom DRD4 data were available and the composite control group (**Table 2** and **Figure 3**). As shown in Table 2, χ^2 statistic and Fisher's Exact Tests of differences in allele frequency for each allele between subjects receiving clozapine and control groups revealed no statistically significant differences for any allele. Data analysis employing only schizophrenic subjects receiving clozapine similarly showed no statistically significant difference compared with the control group (Table 2).

Subjects who completed the clinical protocol and for whom DRD4 data were available (schizophrenic, n=25; schizoaffective, n=4; total, N=29) were categorized by responsivity to clozapine relative to other treatments: group 1, those who responded to clozapine over both fluphenazine and placebo; group 2, those who responded to cloza-

Table 2. D_4 Allele Frequencies in Schizophrenic, Schizoaffective, and Pooled Control Subjects*

D_4 Allele	All Subjects Receiving Clozapine (Schizophrenic and Schizoaffective d/o) (n=34)	Subjects Receiving Clozapine (Schizophrenic Only) (n=28)	Control Subjects, Pooled Data (n=135)
2	0.07 (5) χ^2=0.61, *df*=1, *P*=.44	0.05 (30 χ^2=1.3, *df*=1, *P*=.26†	0.11 (31)
3	0.07 (5) χ^2=0.075, *df*=1, *P*=.78	0.09 (5) FET, *P*=.25	0.056 (15)
4	0.56 (38) χ^2=0.021, *df*=1, *P*=.88	0.55 (31) χ^2=0.034, *df*=1, *P*=.85	0.578 (156)
5	0 (0) FET, *P*=.80	0 (0) FET, *P*=.83	0.004 (1)
6	0 (0) FET, *P*=.51	0 (0) FET, *P*=.57	0.01 (3)
7	0.29 (20) χ^2=0.90, *df*=1, *P*=.34	0.30 (17) χ^2=1.0, *df*=1, *P*=.32	0.23 (62)
8	0 (0) FET, *P*=.64	0 (0) FET, *P*=.69	0.007 (2)

**Allele frequencies of the D_4 variable number of random repeats polymorphism. Numbers in parentheses are raw allele counts. All subjects were white.* P *values result from statistical comparison of subjects receiving clozapine (with either schizophrenia and schizoaffective disorder [column 2] or schizophrenia only [column 3]) with control subjects (pooled data from Table 1 [column 4]). Depending on the expected number of observations in cells for an allele, either the χ^2 statistic (wherever possible) or Fisher's Exact Test (FET) was used sequentially to test the null hypothesis that the distribution of each allele (relative to that of the sum of all other allele types) between groups (affected vs controls) is no different from chance distribution.*

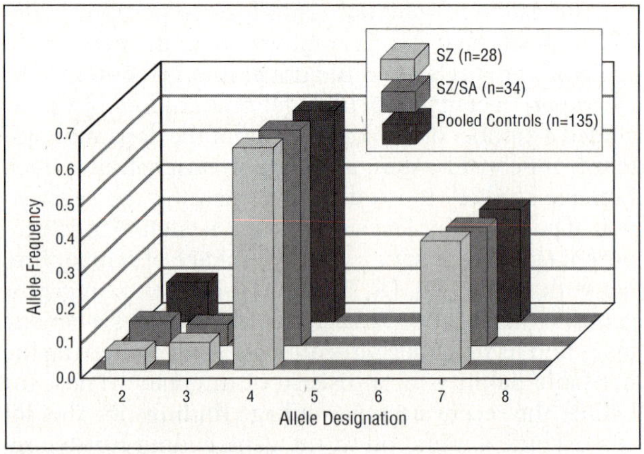

Figure 3. *Allele frequencies at D_4 dopamine receptor in schizophrenic subjects alone (SZ), schizophrenic subjects and schizoaffective subjects (SZ/SA), and pooled white control subjects (Table 2).*

pine over placebo but who did not show greater improvement while receiving clozapine compared with fluphenazine; and group 3, those who did not respond to clozapine over placebo (**Table 3** and **Figure 4**). The χ^2 statistic and Fisher's Exact Tests for allelic differences across groups revealed no statistically significant difference between group 1 and a composite of groups 2 and 3 (ie, between responders and nonresponders, respectively, to clozapine relative to fluphenazine and/or placebo; Table 3) and between group 3 and a composite of groups 1 and 2 (ie, between [typical and atypical] drug nonresponders and responders, respectively, relative to placebo; Table 3). Analysis of the data including only subjects with schizophrenia similarly showed no statistically significant difference (data not shown).

COMMENT

Thirty percent to 50% of patients with treatment-refractory schizophrenia respond to clozapine. The description of the D4 receptor (DRD4) and its high binding affinity (relative to the D_2 receptor) for clozapine raised the possibility that this might be an important site for the pathophysiology of schizophrenia and for the therapeutic action of clozapine. Furthermore, the report that a VNTR polymorphism in the third cytoplasmic loop is associated with differences in binding affinity characteristics to clozapine suggested that this variation might have a role in the determination of responsivity to clozapine in patients with treatment-refractory schizophrenia. Our study shows that allele frequencies at DRD4 are not significantly different between schizophrenic and schizoaffective individuals and controls. (This replicates previous findings by both Sommer and colleagues,[27] who studied European whites, and Nanko and colleagues,[30] who studied a Japanese population, that there is no DRD4 allelic difference between schizophrenic and control subjects. In addition, these findings were replicated by us in a separate study in which we found no differences in allelic variation at DRD4 between unrelated schizophrenic, schizoaffective, and control subjects [unpublished data, January 1993].) We have also provided evidence that DRD4 alleles are not associated with response to clozapine relative to either fluphenazine or placebo. This result makes it less likely that differential response to clozapine among patients with treatment-refractory disease is attributable to variation in their DRD4 genes. Had this hypothesis been correct, one might have expected an overrepresentation of "lower-affinity" alleles among the nonresponders to clozapine; lack of treatment response would then have been due to limitations in the maximum dose of clozapine allowable or to a phenotypic difference other than receptor binding affinity associated with or linked to these alleles. Our results (overall allele frequencies in schizophrenics and controls as well as the comparison between clozapine responders and nonresponders), together with the prior linkage results,[21] suggest (but do not prove) that the pharmacologic data that hinted at a special role for DRD4 in schizophrenia[14,31] may not actually have direct clinical relevance. Although it would be very difficult to test clinically, it still may be that responders to clozapine who carry the "higher-affinity" alleles require a lower dose of clozapine than people who carry "lower-affinity" alleles. If this could be demonstrated, it would suggest strongly (contrary to the present results) that DRD4 is in fact a major site of action for clozapine in vivo. Another possibility is that the in vitro differences in clozapine affinity for the protein products of different DRD4 alleles may not result in any in vivo binding affinity differences between them.

These conclusions need to be viewed with several methodologic limitations in mind. It is possible that we committed a type II error (ie, that we incorrectly accepted the null hypothesis of no association or prediction) because of our small sample sizes. Confirmation of these findings would

Table 3. D_4 Allele Frequency in Schizophrenic and Schizoaffective Subjects According to Clozapine Responsivity*

D_4 Allele	Group 1 (n=13)	Group 2 (n=6)	Group 3 (n=10)
2	0.08 (2) FET, *P*=.60†	0.08 (1)	0.1 (2) FET, *P*=.57‡
3	0.08 (2) FET, *P*=.61†	0.08 (1)	0.05 (1) FET, *P*=.57‡
4	0.58 (15) χ^2=0.0068, *df*=1, *P*=.93†	0.5 (6)	0.55 (11) χ^2=0.067, *df*=1, *P*=.80‡
7	0.3 (7) χ^2=0.0049, *df*=1, *P*=.94†	0.3 (4)	0.3 (6) χ^2=0.048, *df*=1, *P*=.83‡

Allele frequencies of the D_4 variable number of tandem repeats polymorphism. Numbers in parentheses are raw allele counts. Schizophrenics were categorized by clozapine responsivity relative to other treatments: group 1, those who responded to clozapine over both fluphenazine and placebo; group 2, those who responded to clozapine over placebo but who did not show a greater improvement while receiving clozapine compared with fluphenazine; and group 3, those who did not respond to clozapine over placebo.

†Statistical comparison of group 1 with combined groups 2 and 3.

‡Statistical comparison of combined groups 1 and 2 with group 3. Depending on the expected number of observations in cells for an allele, either the χ^2 statistic (wherever possible) or Fisher's Exact Test (FET) was used sequentially to test the null hypothesis that the distribution of each allele (relative to that of the sum of all other allele types) between groups is no different from chance distribution.

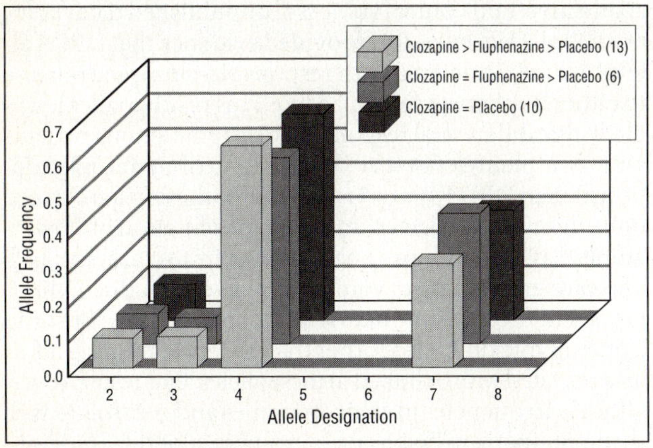

Figure 4. *Allele frequencies at D_4 dopamine receptor by response to clozapine compared fluphenazine and placebo in schizophrenic and schizoaffective subjects (Table 3).*

require replication in future studies with larger sample sizes. A second source for a type II error (only in the comparison between diagnostic groups, not by medication response) might be our control population, which, while controlling for race, did not control for ethnicity.[29] While there is no current evidence that DRD4 allele frequencies differ among white ethnic groups relative to the known differences between different racial groups,[23] the genotyping of more individuals from different ethnic backgrounds might reveal otherwise, thus potentially affecting our results. Ideally, although studies of this sort should be controlled for ethnicity as well as race, in an ethnically diverse country, such as the United States, this is generally difficult. Such matching for ethnicity is most likely important where the rate of illness varies by ethnicity (and therefore either the ill or well group might draw preferentially from a certain ethnic group); that is not thought to be the case for schizophrenia[1] nor is it known to be the case for treatment response *within* populations with schizophrenia, the phenotype of most concern to us herein.

Other sites of allelic variation have been identified recently within the DRD4 gene.[32] Although the alleles we studied would be likely to be in linkage disequilibrium (ie, not to have undergone a recombinant event) with other genetic systems at this locus (because they are within the gene themselves), this would not *necessarily* be the case. This possibility could be examined by a mutation detection strategy.[33]

Subjects with schizoaffective disorder were included in our study because this disorder is likely to belong to the schizophrenia spectrum, based on findings of family, twin, and adoption studies.[34] Our finding that analyses with the use of either the composite schizophrenia-schizoaffective group or the schizophrenia only group gave the same statistical results is consistent with this hypothesis.

Generally, it may be difficult to identify disease associations with VNTR polymorphisms (when used as markers) because of their high mutation rate. Because of this high mutation rate, VNTRs may rapidly lose linkage disequilibrium with disease-causing mutations. However, for this VNTR, it is the VNTR polymorphism itself that is hypothesized to be related to the phenotype (in this case, treatment response). In population-based studies such as this one, the mutation rate therefore does not pose increased risk of error; if a subject has received an allele that is the result of a new mutation, his or her phenotype should correspond to that (new) allele, and the new allele is what is assessed directly.

The dopamine hypothesis, a major theory regarding the cause of schizophrenia for the past three decades, posits that the pathophysiologic disturbance in schizophrenia relates to the dopaminergic system.[4,35,36] However, recent molecular genetic studies have excluded a number of the components of the dopamine system from consideration as common susceptibility loci. Linkage studies (ie, studies that examine the segregation of polymorphic loci vis-à-vis disease status) in schizophrenia pedigrees have excluded linkage of schizophrenia with the D_1, D_2, D_3, D_4, and D_5 dopamine receptor genes.[21,37] A negative linkage finding excludes a genetic locus and its neighboring sequences from conferring the heritable liability for a disease of interest.[38] Thus, for DRD4, the recent negative linkage findings for this locus exclude a mutation in the gene coding for this receptor from being an inherited cause of schizophrenia in the families studied. These linkage studies do not address variation in drug response, however; clozapine responsivity in affected individuals was not studied.

The prior exclusion of genetic linkage between DRD4 and schizophrenia is of only limited relevance to our present study. Association studies can provide information about both known genetic polymorphisms and new mutations that may increase liability for a disorder but can also identify attributes of a subtype within that diagnostic entity.[33] Thus, a negative linkage study does not exclude the possibility of a positive association finding of the disease with that locus. Although a mutation at DRD4 has been excluded from being causative for schizophre-

nia based on linkage studies (in the families studied), a mutation at this locus might have been associated with treatment-refractory schizophrenia or differential responsivity to a drug such as clozapine.

Although clozapine responsivity has not been found to be associated with allelic variation at DRD4, the D_4 receptor may still be the primary site for the therapeutic actions of clozapine (or typical antipsychotic drugs for that matter). Other possibilities include the D_1, D_2, 5-HT_2, serotonin S_3, M_1 muscarinic cholinergic, α_1-adrenergic, and α_2-adrenergic receptors[9,39]; serotonin S_6[40] receptors; and serotonin S_7[41] receptors, all of which are candidate genes for study of differential responsivity to clozapine therapy. Furthermore, differential responsivity to clozapine therapy may reflect heterogeneity in the pathophysiology of schizophrenia, the nature of which has yet to be determined.

Accepted for publication August 1, 1994.

This work was supported in part by funds from the US Department of Veterans Affairs (USDVA) (USDVA National Center for Schizophrenia Research, USDVA National Center for PTSD Research, the VA-Yale Alcoholism Research Center, the VA Medical Research Program [Merit Review grant to Dr Gelernter], and the USDVA Research Training Fellowship in Psychiatry [Dr Rao]), the Mental Health Clinical Research Center at Yale University School of Medicine, New Haven, Conn (National Institute of Mental Health grant MH30929), and National Institute of Mental Health Scientist Development Award-Clinicians grant MH00931 to Dr Gelernter.

Neil Risch, PhD, provided advice about statistical analyses and made helpful comments concerning the manuscript. We thank Henry Kranzler, MD, for providing access to assessed normal controls. We thank Ariel Deutsch, PhD, Robert Innis, MD, PhD, and Eric J. Nestler, MD, PhD, for helpful discussions during the writing of the manuscript. Laura A. Green, MS, provided technical assistance.

Reprint requests to Psychiatry 116A2, West Haven Veterans Affairs Medical Center, 950 Campbell Ave, West Haven, CT 06516 (Dr Gelernter).

REFERENCES

1. Karno M and Norquist GS. Schizophrenia: epidemiology. In: Kaplan HI, Sadock BJ, eds. *Comprehensive Textbook of Psychiatry.* 5th ed. Baltimore, Md: Williams & Wilkins; 1989:699-705.
2. Creese I, Burt DR, Snyder SH. Dopamine receptor binding predicts clinical and pharmacological potencies of antischizophrenic drugs. *Science.* 1976;192:481-483.
3. Rao PA, Molinoff P, Joyce JN. Ontogeny of dopamine D_1 and D_2 receptor subtypes in rat basal ganglia: a quantitative autoradiographic study. *Dev Brain Res.* 1991:60:161-177.
4. Seeman P. Dopamine receptors and the dopamine hypothesis of schizophrenia. *Synapse.* 1987;1:133-152.
5. Sokoloff P, Giros B, Martres M-P, Bouthenet M-L, Schwartz J-C. Molecular cloning and characterization of a novel dopamine receptor (D_3) as a target for neuroleptics. *Nature.* 1990;347:146-151.
6. Van Tol HHM, Bunzow JR, Guan H-C, et al. Cloning of the gene for a human dopamine D_4 receptor with high affinity for the antipsychotic clozapine. *Nature.* 1991;350:610-614.
7. Sunahara RK, Guan H-C, O'Dowd BF, et al. Cloning of the gene for a human dopamine D5 receptor with higher affinity for dopamine than D1. *Nature.* 1991; 350:614-619.
8. O'Dowd BF, Hnatowich M, Lefkowitz RL. Adrenergic and related G protein coupled receptors, structure and function. In: Dulbecco R, ed. *Encyclopedia of Human Biology.* Orlando, Fla: Academic Press Inc; 1991;1:81-92.
9. Deutch AY, Moghaddam B, Innis RB, et al. Mechanisms of action of atypical antipsychotics drugs: implications for novel therapeutic strategies for schizophrenia. *Schizophrenia Res.* 1991;4:121-156.
10. Kane J, Honigfeld G, Singer J, Meltzer H, and the Clozaril Collaborative Study Group. Clozapine for the treatment-resistant schizophrenic. *Arch Gen Psychiatry.* 1988;45:789-796.
11. Meltzer HY, Matsubara S, Lee J-C. Classification of typical and atypical antipsychotic drugs on the basis of dopamine D-1, D-2 and serotonin-2 pKi values. *J Pharmacol Exp Ther.* 1989;251:238-246.
12. Chiodo LA, Bunney BS. Typical and atypical neuroleptics: differential effects of chronic administration on the activity of A9 and A10 midbrain dopaminergic neurons. *J Neurosci.* 1983;3:1607-1619.
13. Bunney BS. Effects of acute and chronic neuroleptic treatment on the activity of midbrain dopamine neurons. *Ann N Y Acad Sci.* 1988;537:77-85.
14. Seeman P, Guan H-C, Van Tol HHM. Dopamine D4 receptors elevated in schizophrenia. *Nature.* 1993;365:441-445.
15. Van Tol HHM, Caren MW, Guan H-C, et al. Multiple dopamine D_4 receptor variants in the human population. *Nature.* 1992;358:149-152.
16. Gelernter J, Kennedy J, van Tol HHM, Civelli O, Kidd KK. The D_4 dopamine receptor (DRD4) maps to distal 11p close to HRAS. *Genomics.* 1992;13:208-210.
17. Nielsen DA, Dean M, Goldman D. Genetic mapping of the human tryptophan hydroxylase gene on chromosome 11, using an intronic conformational polymorphism. *Am J Hum Genet.* 1992;51:1366-1371.
18. Strader CD, Dixon RA, Cheung AH, Candelore MR, Blake AD, Sigal IS. Mutations that uncouple the β-adrenergic receptor from Gs and increase agonist affinity. *J Biol Chem.* 1987;262:16439-16443.
19. Kobilka BK, Kobilka TS, Daniel K, Regan JW, Caron MG, Lefkowitz RJ. Chimeric α2- and β2-adrenergic receptors: delineation of domains involved in effector coupling and ligand binding specificity. *Science.* 1988;240:1310-1316.
20. Mansour A, Meng F, Meador-Woodruff JH, Taylor LP, Civelli O, Akil H. Site-directed mutagenesis of the human dopamine D_2 receptor. *Eur J Pharmacol.* 1992;227:205-214.
21. Coon H, Byerley W, Holik J, et al. Linkage analysis of schizophrenia with five dopamine receptor genes in nine pedigrees. *Am J Hum Genet.* 1993;52:327-334.
22. Pickar D, Owen RR, Litman RE, Konicki PE, Gutierrez R, Rapaport MH. Clinical and biologic response to clozapine in patients with schizophrenia. *Arch Gen Psychiatry.* 1992;49:345-353.
23. Lichter JB, Barr CL, Kennedy JL, Van Tol HHM, Kidd KK, Livak KJ. A hypervariable segment in the human dopamine receptor D_4 (DRD4) gene. *Hum Mol Genet.* 1993;2:767-773.
24. American Psychiatric Association, Committee on Nomenclature and Statistics. *Diagnostic and Statistical Manual of Mental Disorders, Revised Third Edition.* Washington, DC: American Psychiatric Association; 1987.
25. Overall JE, Gorham DR. The Brief Psychiatric Rating Scale. *Psychol Rep.* 1962; 10:799-812.
26. Bunney WE Jr, Hamburg DA. Methods for reliable longitudinal observation of behavior. *Arch Gen Psychiatry.* 1963;9:280-294.
27. Sommer SS, Lind TJ, Heston LL, Sobell JL. Dopamine D4 receptor variants in unrelated schizophrenic cases and controls. *Am J Med Genet.* 1993;48:90-93.
28. Gelernter J, O'Malley S, Risch N, et al. No association between an allele at the D_2 dopamine receptor gene (DRD2) and alcoholism. *JAMA.* 1991;266:1801-1807.
29. Gelernter J, Goldman D, Risch N. The A1 allele at the D_2 dopamine receptor gene and alcoholism: a reappraisal. *JAMA.* 1993;269:1673-1677.
30. Nanko S, Hattori M, Ikeda K, Sasaki T, Kazamatsuri H, Kuwata S. Dopamine D4 receptor polymorphism and schizophrenia. *Lancet.* 1993;341:689-690.
31. Seeman P. Dopamine receptor sequences: therapeutic levels of neuroleptics occupy D_2 receptors, clozapine occupies D_4. *Neuropsychopharmacology.* 1992; 7:261-284.
32. Catalano M, Nobile M, Novelli E, Nothen MM, Smeraldi E. Distribution of a novel mutation in the 1st exon of the human dopamine D_4 receptor gene in psychotic patients. *Biol Psychiatry.* 1993;34:459-464.
33. Gejman PV, Gelernter J. Mutational analysis of candidate genes in psychiatric disorders. *Am J Med Genet.* 1993;48:184-191.
34. Kendler KS. The genetics of schizophrenia and related disorders: a review. In: Dunner DL, Gershon ES, Barrett JE. *Relatives at Risk for Mental Disorder.* New York, NY: Raven Press; 1988.
35. Van Rossum JM. The significance of dopamine-receptor blockade for the action of neuroleptic drugs. In: Brill H, Cole JO, Deniker P, Hippius H, Bradley PB, eds. *Proceedings of the Fifth International Congress of the Collegium Internationale Neuropsychopharmacologicum.* Amsterdam, the Netherlands: Excerpta Medica Foundation; 1967:321-329.
36. Losonczy MF, Davidson M, Davis KL. The dopamine hypothesis of schizophrenia. In: Meltzer HY, ed. *Psychopharmacology: The Third Generation of Progress.* New York, NY: Raven Press; 1987:715-726.
37. Moises HW, Gelernter J, Giuffra LA, et al. No linkage between D_2-dopamine receptor gene region and schizophrenia. *Arch Gen Psychiatry.* 1991;48:643-647.
38. Gelernter J, Kidd KK. The current status of linkage studies in schizophrenia. In: McHugh P, McKusick VA, eds. *Brain and Behavior.* New York, NY: Raven Press; 1990:137-152.
39. Tandon R and Kane JM. Neuropharmacologic basis for clozapine's unique profile. *Arch Gen Psychiatry.* 1993;50:158-159.
40. Monsma FJ, Shen Y, Ward RP, Hamblin MW, Sibley DR. Cloning and expression of a novel serotonin receptor with high affinity for tricyclic psychotropic drugs. *Mol Pharmacol.* 1993;43:320-327.
41. Shen Y, Monsma FJ, Metcalf MA, Jose PA, Hamblin MW, Sibley DR. Molecular cloning and expression of a 5-hydroxytrypamine$_7$ serotonin receptor subtype. *J Biol Chem.* 1993;268:18200-18204.

ORIGINAL ARTICLE

Hypochondriasis and Panic Disorder

Boundary and Overlap

Arthur J. Barsky, MD; Maria C. Barnett, MPH; Paul D. Cleary, PhD

Background: To determine the nosological and phenomenological overlap and boundaries between panic disorder and hypochondriasis, we compared the symptoms, disability, comorbidity, and medical care of primary care patients with each diagnosis.

Methods: Patients with *DSM-III-R* panic disorder were recruited by screening consecutive primary care clinic attenders and then administering a structured diagnostic interview for panic disorder. Patients also completed self-report questionnaires, and their primary care physicians completed questionnaires about them. They were then compared with patients with *DSM-III-R* hypochondriasis from the same setting who had been studied previously.

Results: One thousand six hundred thirty-four patients were screened; 135 (71.0% of the 190 eligible patients) completed the research battery; 100 met lifetime panic disorder criteria. Twenty-five of these had comorbid hypochondriasis. Those without comorbid hypochondriasis (n=75) were then compared with patients with hypochondriasis without comorbid panic disorder (n=51). Patients with panic disorder were less hypochondriacal ($P<.001$), somatized less ($P<.05$), were less disabled ($P<.001$), were more satisfied with their medical care ($P<.001$), and were rated by their physicians as less help rejecting ($P<.05$) and less demanding ($P<.01$). Major depression was more prevalent in the group with panic disorder (66.7% vs 45.1%; $P<.05$), as were phobias (76.0% vs 37.3%; $P<.001$), but somatization disorder symptoms ($P<.0001$) and generalized anxiety disorder were less prevalent (74.5% vs 16.0%; $P<.001$) in panic disorder than was hypochondriasis.

Conclusions: While hypochondriasis and panic disorder co-occur to some extent in a primary care population, the overlap is by no means complete. These patients are phenomenologically and functionally differentiable and distinct and are viewed differently by their primary care physicians.

(Arch Gen Psychiatry. 1994;51:918-925)

From the Departments of Psychiatry (Dr Barsky) and Health Care Policy (Dr Cleary), Harvard Medical School, the Division of Psychiatry, Brigham and Women's Hospital (Dr Barsky), and the Psychiatry Service, Massachusetts General Hospital (Ms Barnett), Boston, Mass.

THE NOSOLOGICAL boundaries between hypochondriasis and the anxiety disorders remain largely uncharted. It is unclear whether the key features of hypochondriasis, such as a cognitive schema about disease, visceral sensitivity, and prominent sick-role behavior, are unique to it or whether they are nonspecific features of many psychiatric disorders, including anxiety disorders. Fundamentally, we do not know whether hypochondriasis is better understood as a somatoform or an anxiety disorder, that is, whether it is a disorder of bodily perception and cognitive misinterpretation (ie, a way of perceiving and thinking about illness) or fundamentally a disorder of excessive alarm and anxiety in which the fear of disease is only one of several fears. There has been debate about whether to place hypochondriasis within the anxiety or somatoform disorder sections of the *DSM-IV*,[1] but adequate empirical data to resolve this question are lacking. The debate has major clinical implications since pharmacotherapy, cognitive and behavioral treatment, and better techniques of reassurance and explanation all require a clearer understanding of the fundamental nature of hypochondriasis.

It is therefore important to determine how much hypochondriasis shares with the anxiety disorders (particularly panic disorder, obsessive-compulsive disorder, disease phobia, and generalized anxiety disorder) and how distinct and differentiable it is from them. There are four reasons why the boundaries with panic dis-

See Methods on next page

METHODS

SUBJECTS AND SETTING

The study was conducted in the general medicine clinic of the Massachusetts General Hospital, Boston. The clinic serves 29 000 patients who make over 50 000 visits annually. It is staffed by 36 attending physicians and 65 house officers, all of whom provide primary, rather than specialty, medical care. All patients of primary care physicians were eligible. The exclusion criteria were illiteracy, inability to speak English, and major sensory or communication deficits.

DESIGN AND PROCEDURE

Consecutive clinic attenders on randomly selected days completed a self-report panic disorder screening questionnaire (discussed below). A cutoff score was chosen to maximize sensitivity at the expense of specificity; we were willing to accept a relatively large number of false-positive diagnoses to minimize the number of false-negative ones. Those patients with a score exceeding the predetermined cutoff were telephoned at home and asked whether the somatic symptoms they had endorsed on the screening questionnaire had a known medical basis. If not, they were then asked to return to the hospital to undergo the research battery. This included a structured diagnostic interview for *DSM-III-R*[28] panic disorder, and these interview-positive patients constitute the sample with panic disorder. All instruments were administered by research assistants with masters' degrees. After the research interview, each patient's medical record was audited blindly by one of us (A.J.B.) to assess medical morbidity. In addition, the patient's primary physician completed a 10-item questionnaire about the patient. Subjects received $40 for participating.

The data gathered from these patients are compared in the "Results" section of the text with data obtained from hypochondriacal patients in a previous study conducted in the same setting, using similar methods, and described elsewhere.[5,27,29,30] Consecutive attenders in the general medicine clinic underwent screening with a questionnaire and then completed a structured diagnostic interview to obtain a sample of patients meeting *DSM-III-R* criteria for hypochondriasis. A random sample of the remaining nonhypochondriacal patients in the clinic served as the comparison group.

VARIABLES AND THEIR MEASUREMENTS

Psychiatric Variables

The 15-item Screener for Panic Disorder, developed by Rost et al,[31] was used. This questionnaire was developed by expert panel consensus for use in medical settings with medically ill respondents. It has high sensitivity and acceptable specificity and has been validated against the Anxiety Disorders Interview Schedule.[31] It employs a yes-no response format and asks about the occurrence in the preceding 6 months of the diagnostic symptoms embedded in the *DSM-III-R* definition of panic disorder.

The clinical diagnosis of panic disorder was made with the Diagnostic Interview Schedule, Version 3R (DIS-3R).[32] This highly structured interview generates criterion-standard psychiatric diagnoses in conformity with *DSM-III-R* nosology. It has been widely used in medical outpatient settings as well as community samples. The panic disorder section of the DIS-3R was modified slightly, as discussed by Katon et al,[14,33] to obviate the tendency of patients with panic disorder encountered in medical settings to somatize, thereby minimizing their cognitive and affective symptoms.

Hypochondriasis that met *DSM-III-R* criteria was diagnosed with the Structured Diagnostic Interview for Hypochondriasis, developed in previous work.[34] This interview is based on operationalized *DSM-III-R* criteria and follows the format of the Structured Clinical Interview for *DSM-III-R*.[35] There are four probe questions, followed by eight questions covering the *DSM-III-R* diagnostic criteria. Based on the patient's responses, the interviewer judges whether each of the diagnostic criteria is met. The Structured Diagnostic Interview for Hypochondriasis has good interrater reliability and convergent and predictive validity.[34]

Hypochondriacal symptoms were assessed with the Whiteley Index and the Somatic Symptom Inventory. The Whiteley Index[36] consists of 14 hypochondriacal attitudes and concerns. Responses are scored on a five-point ordinal scale. It yields three factors on principal components

Continued on next page

order in particular are of interest. Epidemiologically and phenomenologically, the co-occurrence and overlap of these two disorders appear to be high. Nosologically, the debate over placing hypochondriasis in the anxiety disorder section of *DSM-IV* calls into question the fundamental nature of hypochondriasis as either a somatoform or an anxiety disorder. In terms of pathogenesis, recent thinking suggests that the two disorders may share a similar pathogenic mechanism (the cognitive misinterpretation of benign bodily sensations, which results in excessive alarm). Clinically, both are commonly encountered in general medical practice and frequently confused with each other.

Hypochondriasis and panic disorder overlap phenomenologically. Hypochondriacs are fearful, anxious, and have an increased prevalence of comorbid anxiety disorder[2-7]; conversely, patients with panic disorder have prominent hypochondriacal features and somatize intensely both during and between panic attacks.[8-13] They also fear medical disease,[9,14,15] and diagnosable hypochondriasis develops.[9,14] These hypochondriacal features have been reported to decline with successful treatment of the panic disorder.[9,10,16]

Recent cognitive research suggests similarities in the pathogenesis of the two conditions. It has been found that amplification of benign bodily sensation occurs prominently in hypochondriacal patients.[17-21] A similar pathogenic mechanism has been proposed for the panic attack, which has been characterized as an acutely hypochondriacal state in which the patient misattributes the sensations of benign physiological arousal to serious medical disease, "catastrophizes" them, and mistakes them for a

analysis: disease fear, disease conviction, and bodily preoccupation. Its internal consistency, test-retest reliability, and discriminant and convergent validity have been established.[36-39] Hypochondriacal somatic complaints were assessed with a 26-item Somatic Symptom Inventory composed of items drawn from the Minnesota Multiple Personality Inventory Hypochondriasis and Hopkins Symptom Check List Somatization subscales.[40,41] Responses are scored on an ordinal scale from 1 to 5. The test-retest and intrascale reliability of this instrument have been demonstrated.[42,43] In previous work in this setting, the Whiteley Index and Somatic Symptom Inventory were highly intercorrelated (r=.52; P=.0001) and together identified medical outpatients with a syndrome consistent with *DSM-III* hypochondriasis.[44]

Role Performance

Disability was assessed with the Functional Status Questionnaire (FSQ), a valid and reliable self-report instrument developed for use in ambulatory medical populations.[45] We employed the 31 items that constitute four of its six subscales: Basic Activities, Intermediate Activities, Social Activities, and Work Performance. The FSQ is scored by computer, which provides numerical ratings from 1 to 100 (100 indicates maximal functional ability).

Medical Morbidity

Aggregate medical morbidity was assessed with an audit of the patient's medical record. All recorded medical diagnoses were abstracted and rated for seriousness using explicit, preestablished criteria. A weighted score was calculated for aggregate morbidity. Two rating systems were employed. The first was based on our own criteria for seriousness of illness. This method has been employed in previous work and was found to have satisfactory interrater reliability and to correlate significantly with physician ratings of morbidity.[29] The second was the Duke Severity of Illness Scale.[46] The former method reflected total morbidity over the entire period under review, while the latter emphasized the patient's current medical status at the time of the review.

In addition to the record audit, each patient's primary care physician rated the patient's current, aggregate, medical morbidity and future medical prognosis, using a five-point ordinal scale.

The Medical Care Process

Each primary care physician also completed an eight-item questionnaire about the patient, employing a five-point ordinal response format. Three items with face validity asked the physician to note the degree to which he or she considered the patient to be hypochondriacal, anxious, and depressed. Four additional items asked: (1) "How effective are you in treating this patient's symptoms?" (2) "How demanding, dependent, and clinging do you find this patient?" (3) "How much does this patient thwart your attempts to help?" and (4) "How emotionally taxing and frustrating do you find this patient?"

The patient's satisfaction with medical care was measured with three items taken from the FSQ. The intrascale reliability of these three items in a previous study was .76 (Cronbach's α).[27]

Patients were asked about all use of medical care in the preceding 12 months, including scheduled physician visits, walk-in and emergency department visits, the number of days hospitalized, and outpatient mental health visits.

Statistical Methods

To compare the average value of continuous variables between two groups, we used t tests. To compare categorical variables, we used the χ^2 test. In two-by-two tables in which expected cell sizes were less than five, we used Fisher's Exact Test. To compare groups while controlling for potentially confounding variables, we used general linear models that were estimated using ordinary least squares. We used the characteristic of interest (eg, disease fear score) as the dependent variable and included the potentially confounding variables (eg, age and race) and group membership (eg, the sample with or without comorbid hypochondriasis) as covariates. Because measures of physician visits were highly skewed, we analyzed both the actual number of visits and the natural log of the number of visits. We added 0.01 to each measure of visits prior to calculating the natural log to allow calculation of a value when there were no visits.

grave medical emergency.[22-25] Panic anxiety is also accompanied by bodily hypervigilance and an attentional bias toward threatening and danger-related information,[10,11,16,26] cognitive characteristics that have also been reported in hypochondriasis.[17-21]

Finally, these two disorders overlap clinically. They often have similar presentations and present primary care physicians with similar clinical difficulties and dilemmas. Both are major causes of somatization in ambulatory medical populations and sources of excessive use of medical care, and tend to obscure other comorbid psychiatric disorders from the primary care physician's view.[14,27] Panic disorder itself is also underdiagnosed and undertreated in general medical practice.[14]

In this article, we compare the phenomenological features, disability, medical morbidity, use of medical care, and primary care physician impressions of medical outpatients with panic disorder and hypochondriasis.

RESULTS

A total of 1634 consecutive attenders on randomly selected days completed the panic disorder screening questionnaire over a 7-month period. Of the 248 patients (15.1%) who exceeded the cutoff score, three patients (1.2%) could not be reached; 58 (23.4%) met exclusion criteria, failed to meet inclusion criteria, or clearly had medical causes for their panic symptoms on the screening questionnaire; and 52 (21.0%) refused to be interviewed. One hundred thirty-five patients (71.0% of the 190 patients eligible) returned to the hospital to undergo the research battery. One hun-

Table 1. Sociodemographic Descriptors of Study Groups

	Patient Groups*		Comparison Group Without Hypochondriasis or Panic Disorder (n=96)	P†	P‡
	"Pure" Panic Disorder (n=75)	"Pure" Hypochondriasis (n=51)			
Mean (±SD) age, y	44.1 (12.9)	57.1 (15.6)	58.8 (14.8)	<.0001	<.0001
% Male	42.7	25.5	28.1	.07	.07
Mean (±SD) social class§	3.2 (1.1)	3.3 (1.1)	3.0 (1.1)	.59	.27
Marital status, % of subjects					
Single	28.0	17.6	13.5	.26	.03
Married	36.0	51.0	62.5	.14	.001
Widowed	6.7	15.7	11.5	.18	.01
Divorced or separated	29.3	15.7	12.5	.12	.01
Race, % of subjects					
White	97.3	80.4	94.8	.002	.34
Other	2.7	19.6	5.2	.009	.66

*"Pure" panic disorder and "pure" hypochondriasis are described in the "Results" section of the text.
†Based on comparisons between the groups of patients with pure panic disorder and pure hypochondriasis.
‡Based on comparisons between the group of patients with pure panic disorder and the comparison group.
§Measured on a scale of 1 to 5, where 1 is highest and 5, lowest.

dred patients (74.1%) in this group received a diagnosis of lifetime *DSM-III-R* panic disorder using the DIS-3R. Ninety-four of these patients had current (within the last 6 months) panic disorder. In 74, panic disorder was present within the last month.

The sociodemographic characteristics of the sample with panic disorder without comorbid hypochondriasis are presented in **Table 1**, where they are compared with those of the two other groups who were studied in this setting and previously described[5,27,29,30]: 60 patients meeting *DSM-III-R* criteria for hypochondriasis and 96 randomly selected nonhypochondriacal medical outpatients. In the following analyses, we have removed from the hypochondriacal group those patients who had comorbid panic disorder (n=9). Table 1 reveals that patients with panic disorder were significantly younger than hypochondriacal patients and significantly more likely to be white. When compared with the sample from the medical clinic, the sample with panic disorder was younger and less likely to be married.

Twenty-five percent of the subjects with panic disorder met criteria for current (within the last 6 months) hypochondriasis. Conversely, in our previous study of patients with *DSM-III-R* hypochondriasis, the prevalence of current panic disorder was 13.3%; lifetime panic disorder was found in 15.0%; and 1-month panic disorder was present in 10.0%. On a statistical basis alone, panic and hypochondriasis would be expected to co-occur in approximately 3.8% of all patients in this setting. The overlap found is significantly higher than that expected by chance.

Do patients with panic disorder, with and without comorbid hypochondriasis, differ in their clinical characteristics? **Figure 1** indicates that, as expected, those with comorbid hypochondriasis have significantly more severe hypochondriacal symptoms (disease fear, disease conviction, and bodily preoccupation) and more severe somatization. They also have a consistent pattern of greater disability (**Figure 2**). Primary care physicians distinguish between their patients with panic disorder with and without comorbid hypochondriasis (**Figure 3**). Those with hypochondriasis are considered to be significantly more hypochondriacal, anxious, depressed, demanding, and frustrating to treat. From the patients' viewpoint, those with both disorders are significantly more dissatisfied with their medical care than those with panic disorder alone. Finally, in terms of their use of medical care (**Figure 4**), those with comorbid hypochondriasis make significantly more emergency department visits. Analyses using the natural log of use yielded comparable results. All of these analyses were repeated after adjusting statistically for group differences in age and the proportion of nonwhite subjects, and all results were entirely comparable.

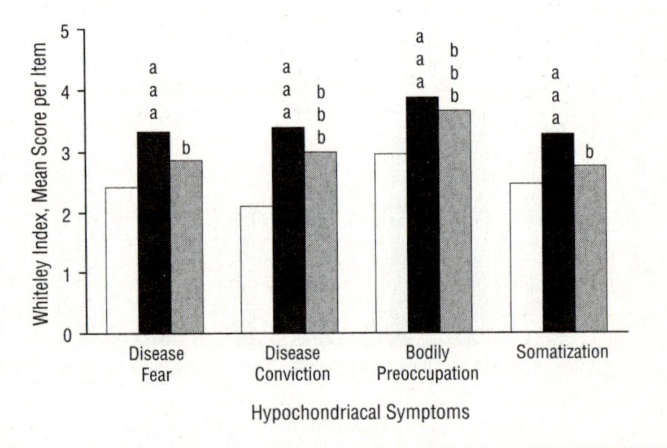

Figure 1. *Hypochondriacal symptoms. Open bars indicate patients with "pure" panic disorder (n=75); solid bars, patients with panic disorder with hypochondriasis (n=25); shaded bars, patients with "pure" hypochondriasis (n=51); a, comparison between patients with panic disorder with and without comorbid hypochondriasis; b, comparison between patients with pure panic disorder and hypochondriacal patients; one symbol,* P<*.05; and three symbols,* P<*.001. Pure panic disorder and pure hypochondriasis are described in the "Results" section of the text.*

Next, we compared "pure" panic disorder (seen in the 75 patients with panic disorder without comorbid hypochondriasis) with "pure" hypochondriasis (seen in the

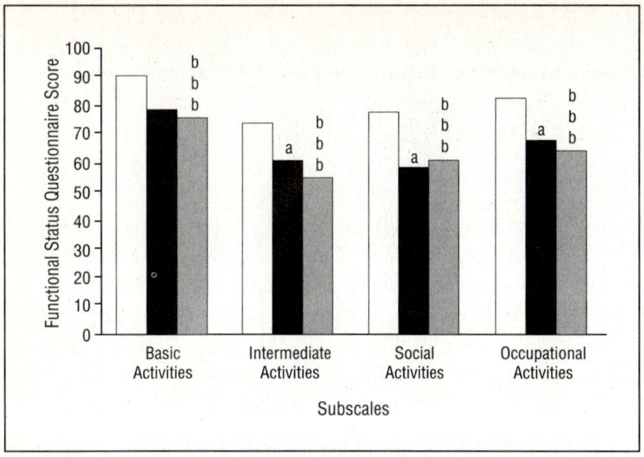

Figure 2. *Functional status and role impairment. Open bars indicate patients with "pure" panic disorder (n=75); solid bars, patients with panic disorder with hypochondriasis (n=25); shaded bars, patients with "pure" hypochondriasis (n=51); a, comparison between patients with panic disorder with and without comorbid hypochondriasis; b, comparison between patients with pure panic disorder and hypochondriacal patients; one symbol,* P<.05*; and three symbols,* P<.001*. Pure panic disorder and pure hypochondriasis are described in the "Results" section of the text.*

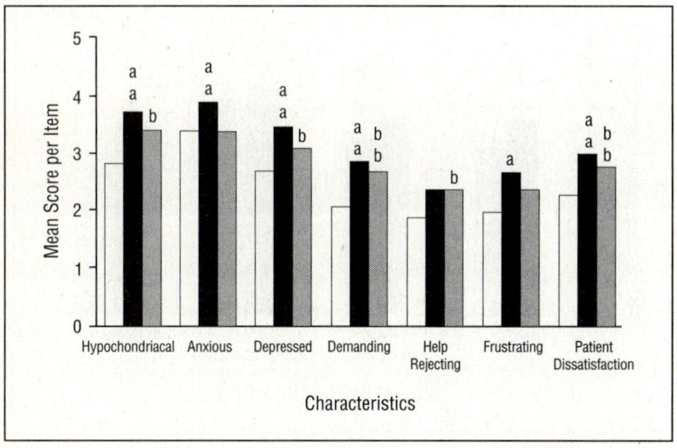

Figure 3. *Physician and patients ratings of the patient care process. All characteristics except dissatisfaction are derived from physician ratings of patients; dissatisfaction was rated by patients. Open bars indicate patients with "pure" panic disorder (n=75); solid bars, patients with panic disorder with hypochondriasis (n=25); shaded bars, patients with "pure" hypochondriasis (n=51); a, comparison between patients with panic disorder with and without comorbid hypochondriasis; b, comparison between patients with pure panic disorder and hypochondriacal patients; one symbol,* P<.05*; and two symbols,* P<.01*. Pure panic disorder and pure hypochondriasis are described in the "Results" section of the text.*

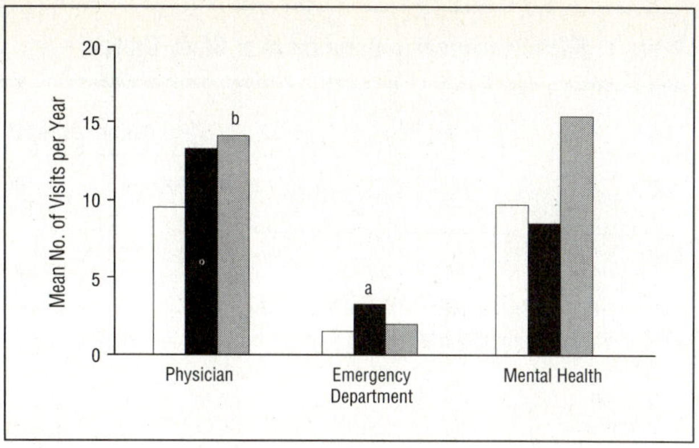

Figure 4. *Use of medical care. Open bars indicate patients with "pure" panic disorder (n=75); solid bars, patients with panic disorder with hypochondriasis (n=25); shaded bars, patients with "pure" hypochondriasis (n=51); a, comparison between patients with panic disorder with and without comorbid hypochondriasis; and b, comparison between patients with pure panic disorder and hypochondriacal patients. For all comparisons,* P<.05*. Pure panic disorder and pure hypochondriasis are described in the "Results" section of the text.*

Table 2. Aggregate Medical Morbidity

	Patient Groups		
	Panic Disorder Without Comorbid Hypochondriasis (n=75)	Hypochondriasis Without Comorbid Panic Disorder (n=51)	*P*
Mean (±SD) physician-rated morbidity*	2.5 (1.0)	2.5 (1.0)	.88
Mean (±SD) physician-rated prognosis*	2.8 (1.3)	2.6 (1.2)	.32
Mean No. of major medical diagnoses (%)	0.2 (0.05)	0.8 (1.2)	.005
Mean No. of moderate medical diagnoses (%)	1.2 (1.5)	3.1 (2.3)	.0001
Mean No. of minor medical diagnoses (%)	1.9 (1.3)	2.7 (1.6)	.03

**Ratings are based on a scale of 1 to 5.*

51 hypochondriacal patients from the previous study without comorbid lifetime panic disorder). These data also appear in Figures 1 through 4. Hypochondriacal patients have significantly more disease fear, disease conviction, bodily preoccupation, and somatization than patients with panic disorder. They report significantly more disability and impairment of role performance and more dissatisfaction with their medical care. Primary care physicians consider their hypochondriacal patients to be significantly more hypochondriacal and more depressed, but not more anxious, than their patients with panic disorder. They also rate the hypochondriacs as more demanding and help rejecting (the difference in physician frustration does not attain significance). Hypochondriacal patients make significantly more physician visits per year, but not more emergency department visits or significantly more mental health visits. All these analyses were repeated after statistically adjusting for group differences in age and the proportion of nonwhite subjects, and all results were comparable.

The medical morbidity data (**Table 2**) present an inconsistent picture. While physician-rated aggregate medical morbidity does not differ, the medical record audit indicates that hypochondriacal patients have significantly more major, moderate, and minor medical diagnoses.

We also compared the pattern of psychiatric comorbidity in hypochondriacal patients and patients with panic disorder. **Figure 5** presents prevalence rates for selected DIS Axis I diagnoses in both samples. When all hypochondriacs and all patients with panic disorder are compared, the sample with panic disorder has a significantly higher prevalence of major depression, phobias,

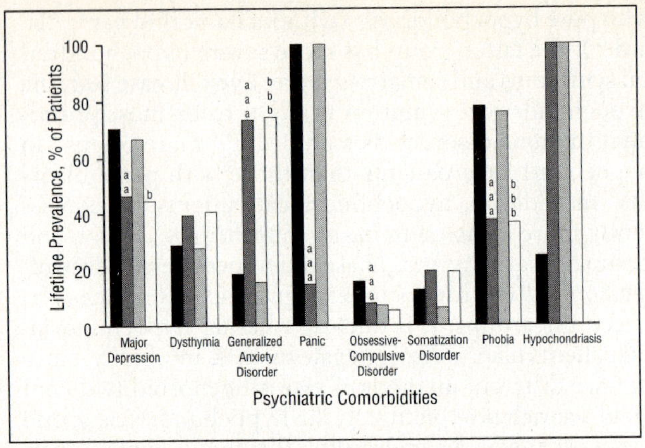

Figure 5. *Axis I lifetime psychiatric comorbidity in samples with panic disorder and hypochondriasis. Solid bars indicate all patients with panic disorder (n=100); darker shaded bars, all hypochondriacal patients (n=60); lighter shaded bars, patients with "pure" panic disorder (n=75); open bars, patients with pure hypochondriasis (n=51); a, comparison between all patients with panic disorder and all hypochondriacal patients; b, comparison between patients with pure panic disorder and patients with "pure" hypochondriasis; one symbol,* P<.05; *two symbols,* P<.01; *and three symbols,* P<.001. *Pure panic disorder and pure hypochondriasis are described in the "Results" section of the text.*

and obsessive-compulsive disorder and a significantly lower prevalence of generalized anxiety disorder. Figure 5 also compares the nonoverlapping groups with pure panic disorder and pure hypochondriasis and reveals the same pattern: the patients with panic disorder have more depression and phobias and less generalized anxiety disorder. The overlap of these two disorders with somatization disorder is of particular interest. When all patients with panic disorder are compared with all hypochondriacal patients, the rates of somatization disorder, 13.0% and 20.0%, respectively, do not differ significantly. However, the mean number of somatization disorder symptoms is significantly higher in the hypochondriacal group (9.4 [±4.1] vs 6.8 [±4.6]; *P*=.0004). The same pattern is seen when groups with pure panic disorder and pure hypochondriasis are compared: although the prevalence of full-blown somatization disorder does not differ significantly, the mean number of somatization disorder symptoms is significantly higher in the hypochondriacal group (9.4 [±4.3] vs 5.7 [±3.9]; *P*<.0001).

When the sample with panic disorder is compared with the random sample of patients from the general medicine clinic of our institution, as expected, the sample with panic disorder is significantly more hypochondriacal, somatizes more, is more disabled, and is considered more difficult to treat.

COMMENT

LIMITATIONS OF THE PRESENT STUDY

Several caveats are in order before interpreting these results. First, the generalizability of these findings is limited by the characteristics of our setting—a large, urban, academic teaching hospital. Furthermore, the patients with panic disorder encountered in medical settings may be a biased subsample of all patients with the disorder; they are likely, for example, to have a high degree of somatization and be especially concerned about their medical health. Second, some of the differences between pure panic disorder and pure hypochondriasis may partly result from the definitions of these two disorders. The group with pure panic disorder omits those patients who would be most similar to the hypochondriacal sample, namely, the ones with comorbid hypochondriasis. Third, the sensitivity of the screening instrument has not been established. We estimate it to be high, however, since a low cutoff was deliberately chosen to maximize sensitivity at the expense of specificity. While 14.1% of the clinic population exceeded the cutoff, only slightly more than half of them received a diagnosis of panic disorder. We did not, however, determine the rate of false-negative diagnoses in those below the cutoff. That underdiagnosis was minimal is suggested by the relatively high estimated prevalence of panic disorder that emerges from these data—8.4%. (Comparable studies in medical outpatient settings have reported panic disorder prevalence rates in the vicinity of 2% to 6%.[8,11,47,48]) Fourth, the eligibility criteria for the samples with hypochondriasis and panic disorder differed slightly. Patients were included in the hypochondriasis study only if they had had at least one prior visit to their primary care physician and had been followed up at our hospital for at least 2 years. In addition, only patients of staff physicians were eligible. In contrast, all clinic attenders were eligible for the panic disorder study. However, based on other analyses of these two groups, we do not think that these differences in eligibility introduced very profound or systematic differences between the samples. Finally, the hypochondriacal sample received the DIS Version 3A, which yields *DSM-III* diagnoses, while the sample with panic disorder was given DIS-3R, which yields *DSM-III-R* diagnoses.

EPIDEMIOLOGICAL AND NOSOLOGICAL BOUNDARIES

Our findings suggest that some overlap exists between panic disorder and hypochondriasis in an ambulatory medical population, but that it is by no means complete. Far more patients have each of these disorders separately than concurrently. One quarter of patients with panic disorder have comorbid, current hypochondriasis, while 13.3% of hypochondriacal patients have comorbid, current panic disorder. Although the estimates of comorbidity in previous reports tend to be somewhat higher than ours, *DSM-III*[49] and *DSM-III-R*[28] diagnostic criteria for hypochondriasis have not been employed in previous studies. Buglass et al,[50] for instance, reported that more than half of patients with panic disorder had persistent fears and worries about health when not acutely anxious. Starcevic et al[51] found that 50% of patients with panic disorder scored in the clinically hypochondriacal range on a hypochondriasis self-report questionnaire (the Illness Attitude Scale). Sheehan et al[10] reported that 68% of patients with panic disorder believed that something was seriously wrong with their bodies. Conversely, Warwick and Salkovskis[52] site their own unpublished finding that 59% of hypochondriacal patients met *DSM-III* criteria for panic disorder. These studies, however, vary

in their sampling frames, diagnostic criteria, use of validated and reliable instruments, and appropriate comparison groups. In particular, hypochondriasis is defined in these studies as a symptom score and is assessed with self-report inventories. The present study, in contrast, defines hypochondriasis more stringently as a disorder that meets the *DSM-III-R* diagnostic criteria and assesses it with a structured diagnostic interview.

The pattern of Axis I comorbidity differs in these two conditions. Hypochondriasis is accompanied less often by major depression, phobias, and obsessive-compulsive disorder and more often by generalized anxiety disorder than panic disorder. Hypochondriasis appears to have a greater overlap with somatization disorder than panic disorder, but the prevalence of somatization disorder in the sample with panic disorder was still relatively high (13.0%). The relevant literature on psychiatric comorbidity is limited. One study[51] comparing patients with panic disorder with and without comorbid hypochondriasis reported that the former have more agoraphobia and isolated phobias but not more Axis II disorder caseness or more severe depressive, obsessive-compulsive, and anger symptoms. These authors also noted that hypochondriacal patients were most interested in an explanation and understanding of their conditions, as opposed to simple symptom palliation.[51] The literature seems to suggest that panic disorder may overlap more with somatization disorder than hypochondriasis. In one study, 40% of female psychiatric outpatients with somatization disorder had panic disorder[53]; in another, 71% of patients with panic disorder met diagnostic criteria for somatization disorder.[54] By contrast, we found somatization disorder in 13% of patients with panic disorder and hypochondriasis in 25% of them.

We estimate the prevalence of current *DSM-III-R* panic disorder to be 8.5% in this primary care setting. This assumes that the prevalence of panic disorder among eligible patients who were not studied is the same as the prevalence determined in those who were interviewed. The prevalence of *DSM-III-R* hypochondriasis in this same setting was estimated at between 4.2% and 6.3%.[30]

DESCRIPTIVE AND PHENOMENOLOGICAL OVERLAP

Our results suggest that patients with panic disorder with and without comorbid hypochondriasis differ significantly in a number of respects. Hypochondriacal patients with comorbid panic disorder somatize more, report more basic, social, and occupational role impairment, and visit emergency departments more frequently. Their physicians also distinguish between these two groups of patients with panic disorder, viewing those with comorbid hypochondriasis as more hypochondriacal, more anxious, more depressed, more demanding, and more frustrating to treat. The patients themselves seem to concur in that those with hypochondriasis are more dissatisfied with their medical care. These differences persist even after controlling statistically for sociodemographic differences between the two groups.

When patients with pure panic disorder (those without comorbid hypochondriasis) are compared with those with pure hypochondriasis (without comorbid panic disorder), the latter group has more severe hypochondriacal symptoms and somatizes more. Even disease fear, the hypochondriacal symptom thought to be most prominent in panic disorder, is significantly more intense in hypochondriacal patients than those with panic disorder. In addition, hypochondriacal patients are consistently more disabled in basic, intermediate, social, and occupational activities. These differences persist even after controlling for sociodemographic differences between the groups. It is unclear whether hypochondriacal patients have more aggregate medical morbidity, since the two different methods of assessing morbidity do not yield a conclusive picture. If the hypochondriacal group has more medical comorbidity, this might explain their greater disability. There is some prior research that bears on these findings but little that directly compares hypochondriacal patients with patients with panic disorder. Thus Fava et al[16] and Otto et al[15] report that patients with panic disorder score high on scales assessing fears and catastrophic thoughts associated with the somatic symptoms of anxiety, but disease conviction and disease beliefs are relatively less elevated in patients with panic disorder compared with nonanxious controls. Kellner et al[55] found higher levels of disease fear, disease conviction, and attention to bodily sensation in patients with panic disorder than in other anxious psychiatric patients. Noyes et al[9] found that the severity of hypochondriacal attitudes and beliefs in patients with panic disorder approached those found in hypochondriacal psychiatric inpatients. Elevated somatization has been reported in panic disorder by Noyes et al,[9] Sheehan et al,[10] and Fava et al.[16]

Finally, primary care physicians distinguish between the two disorders: patients with panic disorder are judged by their physicians to be less hypochondriacal, less depressed (although they actually have a higher prevalence of major depression), less demanding, and less help rejecting. The two groups are perceived to be equally anxious. In keeping with these results, the hypochondriacal group is more dissatisfied with their medical care. Hypochondriacs have been thought to establish a distinctive physician-patient relationship characterized by a peculiarly frustrating combination of demanding neediness on the one hand and a help-rejecting refractoriness to treatment on the other hand.[27] The physician ratings in our study were entirely compatible with this clinical impression. In terms of use of medical care, a consistent but largely nonsignificant trend is evident in which hypochondriacal patients use more medical care than patients with panic disorder.

CONCLUSIONS

These findings suggest that although some diagnostic overlap exists between hypochondriasis and panic disorder, the two conditions are distinct and have discriminant validity. They occur separately far more often than together in the same individual, and they appear to be phenomenologically and functionally differentiable and distinguishable. The most central features of hypochondriasis are significantly more prominent in hypochondriacal patients than in patients with panic disorder, and

their primary care physicians distinguish these two groups of patients. However, this study is far from definitive. Further investigation is in order, since the discriminant validity of the somatoform disorders and their boundaries with affective and anxiety disorders remains unclear.

Accepted for publication July 1, 1994.

Supported by research grant MH-40487 from the National Institute of Mental Health, Rockville, Md.

Reprint requests to Psychiatry Division, Brigham and Women's Hospital, 75 Francis St, Boston, MA 02115 (Dr Barsky).

REFERENCES

1. American Psychiatric Association. *Diagnostic and Statistical Manual of Mental Disorders, Fourth Edition.* Washington, DC: American Psychiatric Association; 1994.
2. Kenyon FE. Hypochondriasis: a clinical study. *Br J Psychiatry.* 1964;110:478-488.
3. Kellner R, Abbott P, Winslow WW, Pathak D. Anxiety, depression, and somatization in *DSM-III* hypochondriasis. *Psychosomatics.* 1989;30:57-64.
4. Bianchi GN. Patterns of hypochondriasis: a principal components analysis. *Br J Psychiatry.* 1973;122:541-548.
5. Barsky AJ, Wyshak G, Klerman GL. Psychiatric comorbidity in *DSM-III-R* hypochondriasis. *Arch Gen Psychiatry.* 1992;49:101-108.
6. Kellner R, Slocumb JC, Wiggins RJ. The relationship of hypochondriacal fears and beliefs to anxiety and depression. *Psychiatr Med.* 1987;4:15-24.
7. Fava GA, Grandi S, Saviotti FM, Conti S. Hypochondriasis with panic attacks. *Psychosomatics.* 1990;31:351-353.
8. Katon W. Panic disorder: epidemiology, diagnosis and treatment. *J Clin Psychiatry.* 1986;47:21-27.
9. Noyes R, Reich J, Clancy J, O'Gorman TW. Reduction in hypochondriasis with treatment of panic disorder. *Br J Psychiatry.* 1986;149:631-635.
10. Sheehan DV, Ballenger J, Jacobson G. Treatment of endogenous anxiety with phobic, hysterical and hypochondriacal symptoms. *Arch Gen Psychiatry.* 1980; 37:51-59.
11. Katon W. Panic disorder and somatization: a review of 55 cases. *Am J Med.* 1984;77:101-106.
12. Katon W, Vitaliano PP, Russo J, Jones M, Anderson K. Panic disorder: epidemiology in primary care. *J Fam Pract.* 1986;23:233-239.
13. Lader MH, Marks IM. *Clinical Anxiety.* New York, NY: Grune & Stratton; 1971.
14. Katon W. *Panic Disorder in the Medical Setting.* Washington, DC: American Psychiatric Press Inc; 1991.
15. Otto M, Pollack MH, Sachs GS, Rosenbaum JF. Hypochondriacal concerns, anxiety sensitivity, and panic disorder. *J Anxiety Disord.* 1992;6:93-104.
16. Fava GA, Kellner R, Zielezny M, Grandi S. Hypochondriacal fears and beliefs in agoraphobia. *J Affect Disord.* 1988;14:239-244.
17. Simon GE. Somatization and psychiatric disorders. In: Kirmayer LJ, Robbins JM, eds. *Current Concepts of Somatization: Research and Clinical Perspectives.* Washington, DC: American Psychiatric Press Inc; 1991:37-62.
18. Robbins JM, Kirmayer LJ. Cognitive and social factors in somatization. In: Kirmayer LJ, Robbins JM, eds. *Current Concepts of Somatization: Research and Clinical Perspectives.* Washington, DC: American Psychiatric Association; 1991: 107-142.
19. Barsky AJ, Wyshak G. Hypochondriasis and somatosensory amplification. *Br J Psychiatry.* 1990;157:404-409.
20. Barsky AJ, Wyshak G, Klerman GL. The Somatosensory Amplification Scale and its relationship to hypochondriasis. *J Psychiatr Res.* 1990;24:323-334.
21. Barsky AJ. Amplification, somatization, and the somatoform disorders. *Psychosomatics.* 1992;33:28-34.
22. Clark DM, Salkovskis PM, Gelder M, Koehler C, Martin M, Anastasiades P, Hackman A, Middleton H, Jeavons A. Tests of a cognitive theory of panic. In: Hand I, Wittchen HU, eds. *Panic and Phobias.* 2nd ed. New York, NY: Springer-Verlag NY Inc; 1988:149-158.
23. Clark DM. A cognitive approach to panic. *Behav Res Ther.* 1986;24:461-470.
24. Beck AT, Emery G, Greenberg RC. *Anxiety Disorders and Phobias: A Cognitive Perspective.* New York, NY: BasicBooks Inc Publishers; 1985.
25. Hibbert GA. Ideational components of anxiety: their origin and content. *Br J Psychiatry.* 1984;144:618-624.
26. Sheehan DV, Sheehan KH. The classification of phobic disorders. *Int J Psychiatry Med.* 1982;12:243-266.
27. Barsky AJ, Wyshak G, Latham KS, Klerman GL. Hypochondriacal patients, their physicians, and their medical care. *J Gen Intern Med.* 1991;6:413-419.
28. American Psychiatric Association. *Diagnostic and Statistical Manual of Mental Disorders, Revised Third Edition.* Washington, DC: American Psychiatric Association; 1987.
29. Barsky AJ, Wyshak G, Latham KS, Klerman GL. The relationship between hypochondriasis and medical illness. *Arch Intern Med.* 1991;151:84-88.
30. Barsky AJ, Wyshak G, Klerman GL, Latham KS. The prevalence of hypochondriasis in medical outpatients. *Soc Psychiatry Psychiatr Epidemiol.* 1990;25: 89-94.
31. Rost K, Smith GR, Hollenberg J. *Mental Health Outcomes, Module Development and Testing: Validation of the Panic Outcomes Module.* Kalamazoo, Mich: The Upjohn Co; 1994.
32. Robins LN, Helzer JE, Croughan J, Ratcliff KS. National Institute of Mental Health Diagnostic Interview Schedule: its history, characteristics, and validity. *Arch Gen Psychiatry.* 1981;38:381-389.
33. Katon W, Vitaliano PP, Russo J, Jones M, Anderson K. Panic disorder: spectrum of severity and somatization. *J Nerv Ment Dis.* 1987;175:12-19.
34. Barsky AJ, Cleary PD, Wyshak G, Spitzer RL, Williams JBW, Klerman GL. A structured diagnostic interview for hypochondriasis. *J Nerv Ment Dis.* 1992; 180:20-27.
35. Spitzer RJL, Williams JBW. *Structured Clinical Interview for* DSM-III *(SCID).* New York, NY: New York State Psychiatric Institute, Biometric Research; 1984.
36. Pilowsky I. Dimensions of hypochondriasis. *Br J Psychiatry.* 1967;113:89-93.
37. Pilowsky I. A general classification of abnormal illness behaviors. *Br J Med Psychol.* 1978;51:131-137.
38. Pilowsky I, Murrell TGC, Gordon A. The development of a screening method for abnormal illness behavior. *J Psychosom Res.* 1979;23:203-207.
39. Beaber RJ, Rodney WM. Underdiagnosis of hypochondriasis in family practice. *Psychosomatics.* 1984;24:39-45.
40. Derogatis LR, Lipman RS, Covi L, Rickels K, Uhlenhuth EH. The Hopkins Symptom Checklist (HSCL): a self-report symptom inventory. *Behav Sci.* 1974;19: 1-15.
41. Lipman RS, Covi L, Shapiro AK. The Hopkins Symptom Checklist (HSCL): factors derived from the HSCL-90. *Psychopharmacol Bull.* 1977;13:43-45.
42. Barsky AJ, Wyshak G, Klerman GL. Transient hypochondriasis. *Arch Gen Psychiatry.* 1990;47:746-752.
43. Weinstein MC, Berwick DM, Goldman PA, Murphy JM, Barsky AJ. A comparison of three psychiatric screening tests using Receiver Operation Characteristic (ROC) analysis. *Med Care.* 1989;27:593-607.
44. Barsky AJ, Wyshak G, Klerman GL. Hypochondriasis: an evaluation of the *DSM-III* criteria in medical outpatients. *Arch Gen Psychiatry.* 1986;43:493-500.
45. Jette AM, Davies AR, Cleary PD, Calkins DR, Rubenstein LV, Fink A, Kosecoff J, Young RT. The Functional Status Questionnaire: reliability and validity when used in primary care. *J Gen Intern Med.* 1986;1:143-149.
46. Parkerson GR, Michener JL, Wu LR, Finch JN, Muhlbaier LH, Macgruder-Habib K, Kertesz JW, Clapp-Channing N, Morrow DS, Chen ALT, Jokerst E. Associations among family support, family stress, and personal functional health status. *J Clin Epidemiol.* 1989;42:217-229.
47. Schulberg HC, Saul M, McClelland M, Ganguli M, Christy W, Frank R. Assessing depression in primary medical and psychiatric practices. *Arch Gen Psychiatry.* 1985;42:1164-1170.
48. Von Korff M, Shapiro S, Burke JD, Teitlebaum M, Skinner EA, German P, Turner RW, Klein L, Burns B. Anxiety and depression in a primary care clinic. *Arch Gen Psychiatry.* 1987;44:152-156.
49. American Psychiatric Association. *Diagnostic and Statistical Manual of Mental Disorders, Third Edition.* Washington, DC: American Psychiatric Association; 1980.
50. Buglass D, Clarke J, Henderson AS, Kreitman N, Presley AS. A study of agoraphobic housewives. *Psychol Med.* 1977;7:73-86.
51. Starcevic V, Dellner R, Uhlenhuth EH, Pathak D. Panic disorder and hypochondriacal fears and beliefs. *J Affect Disord.* 1992;24:73-85.
52. Warwick HMC, Salkovskis PM. Hypochondriasis. *Behav Res Ther.* 1990;28: 105-117.
53. Liskow B, Othmer E, Penich EC. Is Briquet's Syndrome a heterogeneous disorder? *Am J Psychiatry.* 1986;143:626-629.
54. Sheehan DV, Sheehan KH. The classification of anxiety and hysterical states, I: historical review and empirical delineation. *J Clin Psychopharmacol.* 1982; 1:235-244.
55. Kellner R, Abbott P, Winslow WW, Pathak D. Fears, beliefs and attitudes in *DSM-III* hypochondriasis. *J Nerv Ment Dis.* 1987;175:20-25.

The Effect of Diagnostic Hierarchy in Genetic Epidemiological Studies of Psychiatric Disorders

In a recent article in the ARCHIVES, Weissman et al[1] reported the rates of late-onset major depression (MD) (onset after 30 years of age) in relatives of subjects with panic disorder only, with panic disorder and MD, with early-onset MD (onset before 30 years of age), and never mentally ill. By the definition of their diagnostic hierarchy, an individual with early-onset MD cannot have a diagnosis of late-onset MD. However, to compute the risk for late-onset MD, Weissman et al divided the number of relatives with late-onset MD by the total number of relative-years at risk in each group, including relatives with early-onset MD. One may argue that subjects with early-onset MD should not be considered at risk for late-onset MD, since the diagnostic hierarchy used precludes making a diagnosis of late-onset MD in such subjects.[2] Therefore, the situation of subjects with early-onset MD is analogous to that of individuals in epidemiological studies who died or did not reach the period at risk and who are considered "censored," ie, those who are not included among individuals at risk.[3] Then, including individuals with early-onset MD with relatives at risk for late-onset MD would cause an underestimation of the true risk for late-onset MD. Moreover, because of differences in the rates of early-onset MD according to the proband's diagnosis, the extent of this underestimation would vary among groups of relatives and could bias a comparison of the risk of late-onset MD according to the proband's diagnosis.

To examine the impact of hierarchy effects on the results reported by Weissman and colleagues, we approximated corrected risk estimates for late-onset MD in relatives according to the proband's diagnosis using the following simple formula:

Corrected Risk = Age-Adjusted Reported Risk for Late-Onset MD/(1 − Reported Proportion of Relatives With Early-Onset MD, Not Adjusted for Age).

This formula is only an approximation because it assumes that the age of relatives with early-onset MD is comparable to that of relatives without early-onset MD. The **Table** reports the uncorrected (reported in Table 4 of the article by Weissman et al) and the corrected risk estimates in relatives according to the proband's diagnosis. Our table shows that the risk in relatives was underestimated for all four groups, but to a larger extent for relatives of early-onset MD probands. We examined the impact of this underestimation on the patterns of familial aggregation by computing the odds ratio for late-onset MD in relatives of early-onset MD probands vs relatives of subjects who were not mentally ill, using the uncorrected vs the corrected rates. The uncorrected odds ratio was 1.73 and the corrected odds ratio was 2.17. Because we did not have the number of person-years at risk, we could not perform statistical testing. However, because the comparison reported by Weissman et al was close to statistical significance, it is quite likely that it would have become significant with the use of the rates of late-onset MD corrected for hierarchy effects, then potentially changing their conclusion about the familial relationship between early-onset and late-onset MD.

Age-Adjusted Risk for Late-Onset Major Depression in Relatives

Proband's Diagnosis	Risk for Late-Onset Major Depression, %: Uncorrected for Hierarchy Effects	Corrected for Hierarchy Effects
Panic disorder only	20.2	21.7
Panic disorder + major depression	14.4	15.9
Early-onset major depression	16.3	20.6
Never mentally ill	10.1	10.7

In the article by Weissman and colleagues, the correction for hierarchy effects resulted in small yet potentially significant effects on hypothesis testing; however, in other instances, this effect could be much more significant. For example, let us hypothesize that early-onset alcoholism develops in 50% of monozygotic (MZ) cotwins and 20% of dizygotic (DZ) twins of alcoholic subjects. Therefore, 50% of MZ and 80% of DZ cotwins would be at risk for late-onset alcoholism. Then, let us hypothesize that among the cotwins at risk for late-onset alcoholism that late-onset alcoholism develops in 25% of the MZ and 10% of the DZ cotwins. These rates are therefore corrected for hierarchy effects, since relatives with early-onset alcoholism were excluded from the group of individuals at risk for late-onset alcoholism. The corrected odds ratio for late-onset alcoholism in MZ vs DZ cotwins of alcoholic subjects would then be 3.00, thereby strongly supporting genetic transmission. Conversely, the uncorrected risk for late-onset alcoholism would be 12.5% in MZ, and 8% in DZ cotwins, and the uncorrected odds ratio would be 1.64, providing much weaker evidence for genetic transmission.

In conclusion, our intent was not to repeat a comprehensive review of the factors that influence the effect of diagnostic hierarchy on the prevalence of a disorder,[2] but rather to illustrate how this effect can be relevant for genetic epidemiological studies of psychiatric disorders. Therefore, we hope that this letter will serve to raise this issue for general consideration by investigators in this field.

Marc-André Roy, MD
Centre de Recherche
Université Laval Robert-Giffard
2601 de la Canardière
Beauport, Quebec
Canada G1J 2G3
Kenneth S. Kendler, MD
Richmond, Va

1. Weissman MM, Wickramaratne P, Adams PB, Lish JD, Horwath E, Charney D, Woods SW, Leeman E, Frosch E. The relationship between panic disorder and

major depression: a new family study. *Arch Gen Psychiatry*. 1993;50:767-780.
2. Kendler KS. The impact of diagnostic hierarchies on prevalence estimates for psychiatric disorders. *Compr Psychiatry*. 1988;29:218-227.
3. Hennekens CH, Buring JE, eds. *Epidemiology in Medicine*. Boston, Mass: Little Brown & Co; 1987.

In reply

We welcome this opportunity to further clarify the concepts underlying the method that was used in our article[1] to compute the risks for late-onset MD. There appears to be some confusion regarding our definition of late-onset MD. In this article[1] as well as in our previous publications on this topic,[2,3] we have defined late-onset MD as cases in which the first onset of MD occurs after age 30 years. In other words, the event of interest is that an individual remains free of MD until age 30, and then his or her first episode of MD develops after age 30. The rationale for this definition is that we are hypothesizing that individuals who have a first onset of MD after age 30 have a different form of the disorder from individuals who have a first onset of MD before age 30. Any recurrent episode of MD occurring before or after this age is not considered to be relevant. With these definitions, early-onset and late-onset MD are considered to be mutually exclusive disorders, not because we have imposed a diagnostic hierarchy, but rather because an individual cannot have a first onset of MD both before and after age 30 years.

Using our definition, the risk of late-onset MD developing in an individual is the risk that an individual remains free of MD until age 30 and then has MD develop after age 30. This risk can be shown (using standard probability theory) to be equal to the number of individuals with the first onset of MD after age 30 divided by the total number of individuals (with and without MD).

It appears to us that what Roy and Kendler are attempting to estimate is the risk of having an episode of MD after age 30, regardless of whether it is the first episode of MD. This risk is not of relevance to the hypothesis that we are postulating in our article,[1] although we certainly agree that this may be of relevance in other situations.

Priya Wickramaratne, PhD
Myrna M. Weissman, PhD
College of Physicians and Surgeons
Columbia University
722 W 168th St
New York, NY 10032

1. Weissman MM, Wickramaratne PJ, Adams PB, Lish JD, Horwath E, Charney D, Woods SW, Leeman E, Frosch E. The relationship between panic disorder and major depression: a new family study. *Arch Gen Psychiatry*. 1993;50:767-780.
2. Weissman MM, Wickramaratne PJ, Merikangas KR, Leckman JF, Prusoff BA, Caruso KA, Kidd KK, Gammon GD. Onset of major depression in early adulthood: increased familial loading and specificity. *Arch Gen Psychiatry*. 1984;41:1136-1143.
3. Wickramaratne PJ, Prusoff BA, Merikangas KR, Weissman MM. The use of survival time models with nonproportional hazard functions to investigate age of onset in family studies. *J Chronic Dis*. 1986;39:389-397.

Brain Atrophy or Dystrophy in Schizophrenia: When Did It Happen?

Breier et al,[1] reporting on a quantitative magnetic resonance imaging investigation of 44 neuroleptic-treated schizophrenic patients and 29 healthy volunteers, found a decrease in volume of left and right amygdala-hippocampal complex and a smaller volume of right and left prefrontal white matter in the schizophrenic group. These findings support and extend similar results by others from previous imaging and quantitative postmortem studies.[2-6]

This study[1] also measured total cerebral and cerebrospinal fluid volume based on an outline of the dura on serial magnetic resonance imaging slices, excluding the brain stem and cerebellum. There was no significant difference between the schizophrenic cohort and controls in this measure of total cerebral volume, which may be considered to be equivalent to the measurement of head circumference. Many investigators consider that a reduction in the volume of the medial temporal lobe and other structures in schizophrenia represents a "neurodevelopmental disorder," ie, a smaller volume in these brain structures is present from birth or even before birth. If this is the case, total head size, which reflects brain growth and development, should be smaller in these schizophrenic subjects, yet this study[1] and others[7,8] indicate it is not, which suggests that the reported differences in volume of areas of frontal and temporal lobes occurred after the attainment of adult head size.

An even more precise evaluation of the cranial-cerebral size relationship could be obtained by measurement of subdivisions of the cranial vault. In the days before cerebral imaging, when clinicians were required to diagnose temporal lobe atrophy or dystrophy from plain skull roentgenograms, a smaller temporal lobe fossa and elevation of the sphenoid ridge were used to detect prenatal or early-life atrophy or the lack of normal development of medial temporal lobe structures. This strategy was often used to corroborate other evidence in determining the side of a temporal lobe epileptic focus. Measurement of the volume of the temporal lobe fossae can also be accomplished from magnetic resonance imaging and should correlate with the volume of the medial temporal lobe structures and be smaller than that of matched controls if the reported dystrophy or atrophy occurred prenatally or in early life. Measurement of the temporal lobe fossae volume could thus give more decisive information about the timing of the presumed dystrophic or atrophic process in individuals with smaller mesial temporal lobe volumes.

Janice R. Stevens, MD
Departments of Neurology and Psychiatry
Oregon Health Sciences University
3181 SW Sam Jackson Park Rd
Portland, OR 97201

1. Breier A, Buchanan RW, Elkashef A, Munson RC, Kirkpatrick B, Gellad F. Brain morphology and schizophrenia: a magnetic resonance imaging study of limbic, prefrontal cortex, and caudate structures. *Arch Gen Psychiatry*. 1992;49:921-926.
2. Bogerts B, Meertz E, Schonfeldt-Bausch R. Basal ganglia and limbic system pathology in schizophrenia. *Arch Gen Psychiatry*. 1985;42:784-791.
3. Shelton RC, Karson CN, Doran AR, Pickar D, Bigelow LB, Weinberger DR. Cerebral structural pathology in schizophrenia: evidence for a selective prefrontal cortical defect. *Am J Psychiatry*. 1988;145:154-163.
4. Bogerts B, Ashtari M, Degreef G, Alvir JMJ, Bilder RM, Lieberman JA. Reduced temporal limbic structure volumes on magnetic resonance images in first episode schizophrenia. *Psychiatry Res*. 1990;35:1-13.
5. Suddath RL, Christison GW, Torrey EF, Casanova MF, Weinberger DR. Anatomical abnormalities in the brains of monozygotic twins discordant for schizophrenia. *N Engl J Med*. 1990;322:789-794.
6. DeLisi LE, Hoff AL, Schwartz JE, Shields GW, Halthore SN, Gupta SM, Henn FA, Anand AK. Brain morphology in first-episode schizophrenic-like psychotic patients: a quantitative magnetic resonance imaging study. *Biol Psychiatry*. 1991;29:159-175.
7. Andreasen NC, Ehrhardt JC, Swayze VW, Alliger RJ, Yuh WTC, Cohen G, Ziebell S. Magnetic resonance imaging of the brain in schizophrenia. *Arch Gen Psychiatry*. 1990;47:35-46.
8. Grove WM, Lebow BS, Medus C. Head size in relation to schizophrenia and schizotypy. *Schizophr Bull*. 1991;17:157-161.

Professional Opportunities

Archives of General Psychiatry is an exceptional journal that provides physicians with the latest medical and technological information in the psychiatric field. It is an excellent source for recruiting, reaching over 30,220 psychiatrists each month.

All advertising orders must be submitted in writing by mail or fax. Although the American Medical Association believes the classified advertisements in these pages to be from reputable sources, the Association does not assume liability concerning them. Acceptance of advertising is restricted to physician recruitment opportunities, practices for sale, medical office space for sale or rent, and medical equipment for sale.

For information on rates, deadlines, and policies for *Archives of General Psychiatry* Classifieds, contact your classified service representative at 800-AMA-2260 or 312-464-2475/2490/2491/4485.

Psychiatry

CLINICAL PSYCHIATRIST: ENTHUSIASTIC TEAM PLAYER needed for new 18-bed inpatient unit. Must be available for January relocation. Salary plus benefits for 37.5 hr work week. Call 1:4. Affordable, beautiful living 30 miles from Albany, 2.5 hrs from NYC. Theatre, music, antiques, skiing, all in the immediate area. Confidential replies to Christine Ross, RN, 1-800-776-5776 or fax CV to 314-863-1327.

Psychiatry

Nationwide

PSYCHIATRY

&

NEUROLOGY

Positions

We know how busy you are.
Let us do the mundane busy work.

1 (800) 428-4406

Physician Search Associates

Locum Tenens Wanted

HKA LOCUM TENENS is looking for quality general psychiatry physicians to do Locum Tenens. We have opportunities coast-to-coast. We furnish Occurrence Malpractice Insurance (no tail necessary). Please call **HKA LOCUM TENENS at (800)226-6347, Extension AM7.1.**

Fellowships

Postdoctoral Fellowships in Drug Abuse Treatment Research

The NIH/National Institute on Drug Abuse, and the DHHS/PHS/FDA/Center for Drug Evaluation and Research are sponsoring three-year postdoctoral fellowships. This program will train physicians for careers in drug abuse treatment research, and the design, conduct, and interpretation of clinical trials to develop new medications for treatment of drug abuse. The fellowship includes clinical, research management, and drug regulatory training.

Fellowships begin in July. Physicians must be United States citizens, or plan citizenship within one year, and be board eligible upon entering the program. Stipends begin at around $40,000 per year.

Application deadline is January 15, 1995. For further information, contact Fellowships Coordinator, Mail Code HFD-6, Parklawn 9B-04, 5600 Fishers Lane, Rockville, MD 20857.

Call 800-AMA-2260
for rate and deadline information.

CORRECTIONAL/ACADEMIC PSYCHIATRIST, CHICAGO, ILLINOIS: THE ISAAC RAY CENTER and Cermak Health Services, both nationally recognized forensic mental health teams, seek full-time, flexible-schedule BC/BE psychiatrist to provide clinical, clinical supervision, and academic services in the psychiatric facilities of the Cook County Jail. Be an integral part of a unique new partnership of academics and public policy. You will be an employee of the Isaac Ray Center with a faculty position at Rush Medical College. Salary $100K+ with generous benefit package. Participate in training of residents, fellows, and psychology graduate students in an active, innovative training setting. The positions do not involve or require specialized forensic evaluations for court/testimony. Openings are available after 9/1/94. Eligibility for Illinois medical license required. Send CV with inquiry to Mark R. McClung, MD; Vice President, Educational Services; Isaac Ray Center; 1725 West Harrison Street; Suite 110; Chicago, IL 60612.

Chiefs/Department Heads/Directors

CHAIR OF PSYCHIATRY, CERMAK MENTAL HEALTH SERVICES, COOK COUNTY JAIL, CHIcago, and Vice President for Correctional Services, Isaac Ray Center, Inc: The Isaac Ray Center, the nation's largest private, not-for-profit forensic mental health services corporation, was recently awarded a three-year $4.1 million contract by the Cook County Board of Commissioners to provide psychiatric and psychological leadership and services for Cook County Jail, which has one of the largest correctional mental health programs in the country. Applications for the Chair of Psychiatry are being sought from board-certified psychiatrists with strong clinical, administrative, and academic qualifications to lead this pioneering effort in restructuring of Cook County's "Cermak Mental Health Services" into a premier service system combining the resources of both the public and private sectors. Included in the restructured program will be training experiences for senior psychiatric residents and postdoctoral forensic fellows from several universities in the Chicago area. The successful applicant will also be a Vice President of the Isaac Ray Center and a member of its management committee. The applicant must be eligible for a senior academic appointment in the Department of Psychiatry at Rush Medical College. Salary is negotiable based on qualifications, experience, and seniority. An Illinois medical license is required. Applicant must be available to begin on or before January 1, 1995. Isaac Ray Center is an EO/AA employer. Please address a letter of inquiry with a current CV to James L. Cavanaugh, Jr, MD, Professor of Psychiatry, Rush Medical College, and Chairman of the Board, Isaac Ray Center, 1725 West Harrison Street, #110, Chicago, IL 60612. Fax312-829-1476.

THE DEPARTMENT OF PSYCHIATRY AT THE UNIVERSITY OF NORTH CAROLINA AT CHAPEL Hill is seeking a new Director for the UNC Mental Health Clinical Research Center (UNC MHCRC), as the founding Director, Dr Arthur J. Prange, Jr, plans to step down in order to return to full-time research and teaching. The UNC MHCRC is funded from federal, state, and private sources. Its personnel have primary appointments in any of several departments of the UNC School of Medicine, School of Public Health, School of Pharmacy, and at the Dorothea Dix Hospital in Raleigh, where a sixteen-bed research unit and support facilities occupy their own building. The UNC MHCRC also enjoys a close working relationship with the UNC General Clinical Research Center (GCRC). Applicants must be board-certified psychiatrists with considerable experience in research and research administration. Two essential qualities are a proven ability to obtain independent research funding and the ability to foster research in a collaborative environment. Academic rank and salary are dependent on qualifications, but it is expected that the successful candidate will qualify for appointment as tenured Professor or Associate Professor. Application deadline is January 1, 1995. Applicants should submit a letter of application and curriculum vitae to Robert Golden, MD, Professor and Chair, Department of Psychiatry, Campus Box #7160, University of North Carolina, Chapel Hill, NC 27599-7160. The University of North Carolina is an equal opportunity/affirmative action employer. Women and minority applicants are encouraged to apply.

Multiple Specialties/Group Practice

Your next job is on the line.

1·800·233·9330

Finally you have direct access to career opportunities across the country. The new **Practice Opportunity Line** offers an easy, no pressure, confidential way to conduct a thorough job search on your own, 24 hours a day. All you have to do is call, follow the prompts and research the openings. Then send a voice mail mini-CV to the opportunities you wish to pursue. It's the newest, fastest and simplest way to get the job you want.

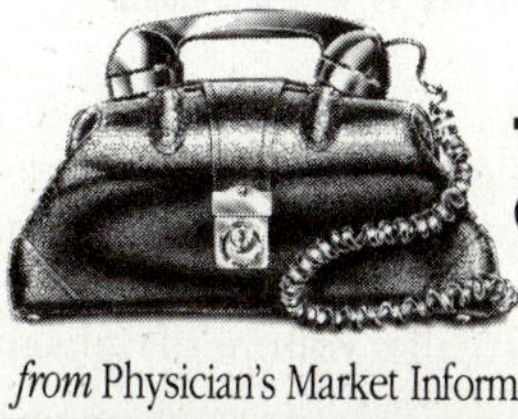

The Practice Opportunity Line

We're on call for you.

from Physician's Market Information Center **1·800·423·1229**

REVIEWERS FOR 1994

The constituency of the ARCHIVES comprises a "university" of often interchangeable writers and readers, students, knowledgeable practitioners, and scholars of medicine and the sciences underlying the field of psychiatry. The editors are deeply grateful for the generous assistance in editorial critique and review of the many colleagues listed below. The donation of their special expertise is a necessary contribution on which intellectual standards in the field heavily depend.

Amir Abduljalli
Ralph H. Abraham
Richard Abrams
Robert F. Ackermann
Lawrence E. Adler
George Aghajanian
W. Stewart Agras
Tim Ahles
Salman Akhtar
Huda Akil
Hagop S. Akiskal
Marilyn Albert
A. Alderman
Georgios Alexopoulos
Albert John Allen
Margaret Altemus
Lori Altshuler
Jose Alvir
Farooq Amin
Jay Amsterdam
S. M. Anderson
Gavin Andrews
Carol Aneshensel
Burton Angrist
James C. Anthony
Paul Appelbaum
Victoria Arango
Robert Asarnow
Marie Asberg
Boris Astrachan
Thomas Babor
Lee Baer
Peggy Baker
Samuel Ball
James C. Ballenger
David Barlow
Miron Baron
Herbert Barry III
Arthur Barsky
John J. Bartko
George Bartzokis
Ellen Bassuk
Lance Bauer
Mark Bauer
Andrew Baum
Lewis Baxter
Aaron T. Beck
Mace Beckson
Henri Begleiter
Allan Beigel
Alan S. Bellack
Ruth Benca
Elisa Benedek
Francine Benes
Chawki Benkelfat
Neal Benowitz
Sarah Berga
Cathy Berkman
Karen Faith Berman
Wade Berrettini
Joseph Biederman
Robert Bilder
Eric Bing
Hector Bird
Boris Birmaher
Bruce Black
Donald Black
Deborah Blacker
Jack Blaine
R. Clifford Blair
Jack Blanchard
Dan G. Blazer
Kenneth Blum
Hans Boeltzer
William Bondareff
Kyle Boone
Michael Borenstein
David Bornstein
Gilbert Botvin
David Braff
Alan Breier
David Brent
Naomi Breslau
Timothy D. Brewerton
Darla Broberg
Ian Brockington
Evelyn Bromet
Judith Brook
George W. Brown
Joan Heller Brown
Tim Brown
Gerard E. Bruder
Robert W. Buchanan
Kathy Bucholz
Monte Buchsbaum
Jennifer S. Buchwald
Benjamin S. Bunney
William E. Bunney
Jack D. Burke
Margit Burmeister
Audrey Burnam
Barbara Burns
Nelson Butters
Daniel Buysse
Robert Byck
Matthew Byerley
William Byne
Alexander Bystritsky
Jean lud Cadet
Remi Cadoret
Eric Caine
Avraham Calev
Enoch Calloway
Oliver Cameron
Anthony Campagnoni
Scott Campbell
Dennis Cantwell
Greg Carey
Gabrielle Carlson
Dorit Carmelli
William Carpenter
Bernard J. Carroll
Rosland Cartwright
Manuel Casanova
B. J. Casey
Daniel E. Casey
Regina Casper
Ned Cassem
F. Xavier Castellanos
Verne Caviness
Phillip B. Chappell
Dennis S. Charney
Michael Chase
Ching-Piao Chien
Howard Chilcoat
C. Chiles
Diane Chugani
Harry Chugani
Roland D. Ciaranello
David Clark
Duncan Clark
John Clark
John Clarkin
Paula Clayton
Bretle Clemente
Pat Coble
Emil Coccaro
C. Edward Coffey
Donald Cohen
Howard L. Cohen
Jonathan Cohen
Robert Cohen
David E. Comings
Margaret Compton
Robert Conley
P. Michael Conneally
John Constantino
Brian L. Cook
Edwin H. Cook
Richard Coppola
Jody Corey-Bloom
Jack Cornelius
William Coryell
Jane Costello
Guylan Cote
Rex Cowdry
David Cox
Thomas Craig
Paul Crits-Christoph
Tim Crow
Raymond Crowe
Thomas Crowley
John Csernansky
Joe Cubells
Jeffrey Cummings
Charles Czeisler
Antonio R. Damasio
Jonathan Davidson
Lucy Davidson
Michael Davidson
Richard Davidson
John M. Davis
Kenneth Davis
Michael Davis
Michael E. Dawson
Claude De Montigny
Lynn DeLisi
Raymond Deicken
Pedro Delgado
William C. Dement
Steven Demeter
Mark A. Demitrack
Michael Devlin
Eric Devor
Mary Amanda Dew
Victoria DiSclafani
Park Elliot Dietz
Herbert Dietze
Steven Dilsaver
Joel E. Dimsdale
Jeri Doane
John Docherty
Nancy Docherty
Ed Domino

Wayne C. Drevets
Connie C. Duncan
W. C. Duncan
David Dunner
Renee Dupont
Mary Durham
Maurice Dysken
Felton Earls
Charmane Eastman
Craig Edelbrock
Robert H. Edwards
Cindy L. Ehlers
Burr Eichelman
Glenn Elliott
Jean Endicott
Joseph T. English
Susan Essock
Christopher Evans
Dwight Evans
Christopher Fairburn
Ted Fallon
Stephen Faraone
Mary Farmer
Kym Faull
Jan Fawcett
Fawzy I. Fawzy
George Fein
Irwin R. Feinberg
Wayne S. Fenton
John Fernstrom
Steven Ferris
Gary Figiel
Max Fink
Marion Fischman
Barbara Fish
Baruch Fishman
Michael Flaum
Kirsten Fleming
Edna B. Foa
Laura Fochtmann
Marshal F. Folstein
Susan Folstein
Judith Ford
David Foulkes
Allen Frances
Andrew Francis
Ellen Frank
Richard Frank
Robert Freedman
Arnold J. Friedhoff
C. D. Frith
Paul Fudala
Ray Fuller
Joaquin M. Fuster
Abby Fyer
Barbara Jones Galaty
Mary Ganguli
Rohan Ganguli
Jesus Garcia-Sevilla
William Gardner
George Gardos
Paul Garfinkel
David M. Garner
Tom Garrick
M. Garvey
Constantine Gatsonis
Frank Gawin
Mike Gazzaniga
Alan Gelenberg
Joel Gelernter
Linda George
Elliot Gershon
Sam Gershon
Mark Geyer
Robert D. Gibbons
Jay Giedd
Donna Giles
T. Conrad Gilliam
J. Christian Gillin
Michael Gitlin
Rachel Gittleman
Stanton Glantz
Ronald Glaser
William Glazer
Shirley Glynn
James Gold
Phillip W. Gold
Richard Goldberg
Terry E. Goldberg
Lynn Goldin
Jacqueline M. Golding
Howard Goldman
Patricia Goldman-Rakic
Michael Goldstein
Rise Goldstein
Junius Gonzales
Daniel Goodman
Wayne Goodman
Donald Goodwin
David Gorelick
Jack Gorman
Ian Gotlib
Irving Gottesman
Igor Grant
John Greden
Michael Green
Richard Green
David Greenberg
David Greenblatt
David Greenfeld
Joel Greenhouse
Steven Greenwald
Tom Greider
John H. Greist
E. Griez
Roland Griffiths
Christina Grillon
Ruth Gross-Isseroff
Luis Guiffra
John G. Gunderson
Sanjay Gupta
Raquel Gur
Ruben Gur
Thomas Gutheil
Donald Guthrie
Barry Guze
Samuel Guze
Harry E. Gwirtsman
Laszlo Gyulai
Gretchen Haas
Romaine Hain
Uriel Halbreich
Eric Halgren
Katherine Halmi
Susan Hamburger
Constance Hammen
Leonard Handlesman
John Hanley
Sydney Hans
William Hargreaves
Martin Harrow
Beth Hart
Roger Haskett
Richard Hauger
Peter Hauri
James Haustad
Heidi Heard
Robert Heaton
Don Hedecker
Larry Hedges
Richard G. Heimberg
John E. Helzer
Robert Henden
Hugh Hendrie
George Heninger
Jack E. Henningfield
Kevin Hensen
Mary Herman
Victor Hesselbrock
J. D. Higley
Shirley Hill
Ann Hinsberger
Robert Hirschfeld
Robert Hitzemann
Kimberly Hoagwood
Susan Hodge
Sheilagh Hodgins
Ann Hoff
Ralph Hoffman
Gerald E. Hogarty
Ann Hohmann
Jimmie C. Holland
Eric Hollander
Philip Holzman
Ewald Horwath
Robert Howland
John Hsiao
James Hudson
John Hughes
Stephen Hurt
Steven Hyman
William G. Iacono
Stanley Imber
Loring Ingraham
Thomas R. Insel
Michael Irwin
Rolf Jacob
Barry L. Jacobs
Jerome H. Jaffe
David M. Janowsky
Lissy Jarvik
Murray Jarvik
Donald Jasinski
Daniel C. Javitt
Michael Jenike
J. Richard Jennings
Terry Jernigan
Dilip Jeste
Tong Joh
Chris-Ellen Johansen
Robin Johnson
Reese Jones
Lewis L. Judd
Charles Kaelber
Bruce Kagan
Tatsu Kakuma
Denise Kandel
John Kane
Gurneet Kanwal
Bert Kaplan
Marvin Karno
Craig Karson
Javad H. Kashani
Roger Kathol
Wayne Katon
Ira Katz
C. Kaufman
Joan Kaufman
Walter Kaye
Samuel Keith
Martin Keller
Steven Keller
Margaret Kemeny
Kenneth Kendler
Cille Kennedy
Ronald Kessler
Seymour Kety
Kenneth Kidd
Joel Killen
Bryan King
Raymond King
Darrell Kirch
Brian Kirkpatrick
Herbert D. Kleber
Joel Kleinman
Thomas Knauss
James Knowles
James H. Kocsis
Sharon Koele
Robert Kohn
Alexander Kopelowicz
Lorrin Koran
Conan Kornetsky
Thomas Kosten
Maria Kovacs
Beatrice Kovasznay
Mark Kowaleski
Helena Kraemer
Dean Krahn
Rachel Kramer
Henry Richard Kranzler
Mary Jane Kreek
Marcus Kruesi
Lauren Krupp
John Krystal
Michael J. Kuhar
Walter Kukull
Samuel Kuperman
Andrew Kurtiz
Michelle La Buda
David La Porte
Asenath LaRue
Malcolm Lader
Ben Lahey
H. Richard Lamb
Douglas Langbehn
Philip Lavori
William B. Lawson
James Leckman
Marguerite Lederberg
Julian Leff
Tony Lehman

Ellen Leibenluft
Robert Lenox
Andrew Leon
Henrietta L. Leonard
Ira M. Lesser
Andrew Leuchter
Bennett Leventhal
Seymour Levine
Deborah Levy
Norman Levy
Richard Lewine
Collins Lewis
Alfred Lewy
T. K. Li
Robert Liberman
Jeffrey A. Lieberman
Morton Lieberman
Michael Liebowitz
Kelvin Lim
Keh-Ming Lin
Marsha Linehan
Walter Ling
Paul Linkowski
Markku Linnoila
Jennifer Lish
Robert Litman
Edythe London
Armand Loranger
Lester Luborsky
Elliot D. Luby
Daniel Luchins
Suniya Luthar
R. Bruce Lydiard
David Lykken
Jeffrey Lyness
Michael Lyons
James Maas
Paul MacLean
James MacMurray
Michael Maes
Kathyrn Magruder
Nigel Maidment
Anil Malhotra
Arnold Mandell
J. John Mann
William Manning
Salvatore Mannuzza
Joseph Marcus
Stephen Marder
John Markowitz
Isaac Marks
Laura Marsh
B. D. Marshall
Ronald Martin
Mauri Marttunen
Jack Maser
Brian Masterson
Aleksander Mathe
Roy J. Mathew
Susan Mathews
Jeff Mattes
Steven Matthysse
Matig Mavissakalian
Carolyn Mazure
John Mazziotta
Una McCann
Robert W. McCarley
James T. McCracken
Bruce S. McEwen
Thomas P. McGlashan
Peter McGuffin
Michael McGuire
Paul McHugh
James McKay
William McKinney
A. Thomas McLellan
James Meader-Woodruff
Sarnoff Mednick
Deb Medoff
Paul E. Meehl
Nancy Mello
Herbert Y. Meltzer
Robert Mendelson
Wallace Mendelson
Chantal Merette
Kathleen Merikangas
Ernst Meyer
James L. Meyerhoff
Barnett Meyers
Alexander Miller
Andrew Miller
Del Miller
Eric N. Miller
Frank C. Miller
Robert B. Millman
Jim Mintz
Steven Mirin
A. Mirsky
James E. Mitchell
Phillip Mitchell
Steven O. Moldin
Margaret Moline
John Monahan
Donna Moreau
Hal Morgenstern
Eve K. Moscicki
Laura Mufson
Declan Murphy
Dennis Murphy
George Murphy
Jane Murphy
Robin M. Murray
Bengt Muthen
James L. Myerhoff
Lisa M. Najavits
William E. Narrow
Henry A. Nasrallah
Mike Neale
Craig Nelson
Charles Nemeroff
Eric Nestler
Paul Nestor
Rosalind Neuman
John Newcomer
Thomas Newton
David Nichols
David A. Nielsen
Ernest Noble
Eric Nofzinger
Peggy Nopoulos
Thomas Nordahl
Carol North
Russell Noyes
Keith Nuechterlein
Ned Nunes
John I. Nurnberger
David Nutt
Charles O'Brien
M. O'Hara
Stephanie O'Malley
David R. Offord
John Oldham
Mark Olfson
Richard Olsen
T. F. Oltmanns
J. Ormel
Martin Orne
Jurg Ott
Michael Otto
David Page
German Palafox
Jose Pardo
William M. Pardrige
Barbara Parry
Oscar Parsons
Michelle Pato
Thomas L. Patterson
David Pauls
Eugene Paykel
Godfrey D. Pearlson
John C. Pecknold
Roger Peele
Deborah Perlick
Jay Pettegrew
Cynthia Pfeffer
Adolf Pfefferbaum
Bruce Pfohl
Michael E. Phelps
R. Philibert
David Phillips
Katherine Phillips
David Pickar
Roy Pickens
Teresa Pigott
Paul Pilkonis
Nancy Pilott
Harold Pincus
Andrew Pitts
Joseph Piven
Michael Pogue-Geile
Russell Poland
John Polich
Simka Pollock
Vickie Pollock
John Pomeroy
Nancy Poole
Michael Popkin
Michael Posner
Robert Post
Steve Potkin
Arthur Prange
Lawrence H. Price
Jim W. Prichard
Robert Pynoos
Donald Quinlan
Frederic Quitkin
Peter Rabins
Judith Rabkin
Richard Rada
Marcus E. Raichle
Michael J. Raleigh
Mark H. Rapaport
Allen Raskin
Murray Raskind
Scott Rauch
Rebecca Rausch
Darrel Regier
Theodore Reich
Eric Reiman
Barry Reisberg
Alan Reiss
David Reiss
Ronald A. Remick
Richard Rende
Susan Resnick
Charles Reynolds
Howard Rhoades
John P. Rice
Charles Rich
John Richters
Karl Rickels
Craig Risch
Neil Risch
Marjorie Robertson
Lee Robins
Donald Robinson
William Rogers
Barbara Rohland
John Rohrbough
Steven Roose
Jed Rose
Robert Rose
Jerrold Rosenbaum
Norman E. Rosenthal
Elliot Ross
Loren Roth
Sir Martin Roth
Walton Roth
Bruce Rounsaville
Alec Roy
Marc-Andre Roy
Peter Roy-Byrne
Lalofaye Royne
John Rubenstein
Eugene Rubin
Robert Rubin
David Rubinow
Matthew V. Rudorfer
David Rumelhart
Judith Rumsey
Agnes Rupp
A. John Rush
Michael Rutter
Neal D. Ryan
Harold Sackheim
Michael H. Sacks
Bruce Sales
R. M. Saloman
Jacqueline Samsan
Paul Satz
Cary R. Savage
Andrew Saykin
L. Scahill
Alan F. Schatzburg
Richard Scheffler
Arnold Scheibel
Mark Schmidt
Franklin Schneier
Nina Schooler
Marc Schuckit
Leslie Schuh
H. Charles Schulberg

S. Charles Schulz
Charles R. Schuster
Edward Schwiezer
Mark Sedler
Goran Sedvall
Phillip Seeman
Jerome Segal
J. P. Seigel
Edward M. Sellers
Edward C. Senay
Michael Sernyak
Sally Severino
Richard I. Shader
David Shaffer
Mohammed Shafii
Charles Shagass
Andrew Shaner
David Shapiro
Theodore Shapiro
Steven S. Sharfstein
Katherine M. Shear
David V. Sheehan
Martha Shenton
David Shern
Richard Shiffrin
James Shore
Patrick E. Shrout
Marc Shuckit
Ben Siegel
Carol Siegel
Larry Siever
Soren Sigvordsson
Peter Silberfarb
David Silbersweig
Jeremy Silverman
James Simmons
Roberta Simmons
Peter Simon
George Simpson
J. Sines
Andrew E. Skodol
Sue Smadley
Gary Small
Joyce Small
Gerard P. Smith
Richard G. Smith
Robert C. Smith
Louis Sokoloff
Paul H. Soloff
David Solomon
Susan Solomon
Barbara Sommer
Susan Sorenson
James E. Spar
M. Anne Spence
David Spiegel
Robert L. Spitzer
Herbert Spohn
Stephen M. Stahl
Michael Stanley
Daniel Stein
Leonard Stein
Marvin Stein
Murray B. Stein
Stuart Steinhauer
Donald Steinwachs
Emily Stern
Yaakov Stern
Janice R. Stevens
Maxine Stitzer
David Stoff
Julie C. Stout
Robert Stout
Rick Strassman
John Strauss
Michael Strober
Albert J. Stunkard
Kenneth Subotnik
Edith Sullivan
Mark Sullivan
Trey Sunderland
Andrew Suollolund
Ezra Susser
Dragan Svrakic
Susan Swedo
John Sweeney
Robert Sweet
Neil Swerdlow
Martin Szuba
Carol Tamminga
Radiv Tandon
Peter E. Tanguay
Kenneth Tardiff
Alvin Tarlov
C. B. Taylor
Lawrence Tecott
Auke Tellegen
Linda Teri
Leonore Terr
Joseph Terwilliger
Gunvant Thaker
Leon Thal
Allen Tien
Pekka Tienani
Gary Tischler
Allan J. Tobin
Richard Todd
Mauricio Tohen
E. Fuller Torrey
Daniel Tranel
Ming T. Tsuang
Gary Tucker
Thomas Uhde
George R. Uhl
E. H. Uhlenhuth
Richard Ulrich
Robert Utiger
Heiddes Valdimarsdottir
George Valliant
Wilfred Van Gorp
Ronald Van Heertum
Daniel Van Kammen
Herman Van Praag
Bessel Van der Kolk
Herbert Vaughan
Richard Veith
Joseph Ventura
Milton Viederman
Benedetto Vitiello
Gerald Vogel
Michael Vogel
George Vogler
Ecford Voit
Jan Volavka
Nora Volkow
Michael R. Von Korff
Mark Von Zastrow
John L. Waddington
Daniel Wagner
Dale Walker
B. Timothy Walsh
Royce W. Waltrip II
Virginia Warner
Meredith Warshaw
Christine Waternaux
Rafiq Waziri
William Weddington
Tom Wehr
Daniel Weinberger
Richard Weiner
Herbert Weingartner
Roger D. Weiss
Michael Welch
Kenneth Wells
Paul H. Wender
Robert Wesner
Joseph Westermeyer
Lennart Wetterberg
Richard Wetzel
Nancy Wexler
Patricia Whitaker-Azmita
Kerrin White
Peter Whybrow
Priya Wickramaratne
Thomas A. Widiger
Jeff Wilkins
Janet B. W. Williams
R. B. Williams
P. C. Williamson
Joe P. Windham
Andrew Winokur
Anna Wirz-Justice
Thomas Wise
Sandra Witelson
Margaret G. Woerner
Peter Wolff
Susan Wolk
Adam Wolkin
Owen Wolkowitz
Dean F. Wong
Chris Wood
Catherine Woodman
Scott Woods
George Woody
G. Fred Wooten
Margaret Worner
Richard Jed Wyatt
Lyman Wynne
Joe Yamamoto
William R. Yates
Elizabeth Young
Arthur Yuwiler
Theodore Zahn
Alan Zametkin
Vincent Zarcone
Mark Zimmerman
Robert Zipursky
Athanasios Zis
Cheryl Zlotnick
George Zubenko
Deborah Zurin

ORIGINAL ARTICLE

Backward Masking in Schizophrenia and Mania

I. Specifying a Mechanism

Michael Foster Green, PhD; Keith H. Nuechterlein, PhD; Jim Mintz, PhD

Background: Backward masking is a neuropsychological procedure that involves the earliest phases of visual processing. Compared with normal controls, the performance of schizophrenic patients is more disrupted by a visual mask. Masking procedures used previously with schizophrenic patients have combined two separate masking mechanisms (interruption and integration), which prevent interpretation of the nature of the abnormality. The current study systematically limited the masking mechanism to interruption to specify the underlying mechanisms. Manic patients were included to examine diagnostic specificity.

Methods: Sixty-three schizophrenic inpatients, 31 manic inpatients, and 48 normal controls received three versions of the backward masking procedure. One version used a high-energy mask that combines both integration and interruption mechanisms. Another procedure used a low-energy mask that works mainly through interruption. A final condition altered the features of the mask so that masking was almost entirely through interruption.

Results: Schizophrenic patients showed performance deficits across masking conditions, even in procedures that were largely limited to masking by interruption. The masking performance of the patients did not appear to fit a simple generalized deficit. Manic patients performed significantly worse than normal controls and comparably with the schizophrenic patients.

Conclusions: Schizophrenic patients have abnormalities at least with interruptive mechanisms. The results suggest that deficits on masking procedures are not entirely specific to schizophrenia because comparable masking deficits were found in manic inpatients with chronic disease. The current study addresses the neuropsychological mechanisms of the masking deficit. The next step will be to investigate the contributions of two distinct neuroanatomical visual pathways to the masking abnormality in schizophrenia.

(Arch Gen Psychiatry. 1994;51:939-944)

BACKWARD MASKING is a neuropsychological process that involves the earliest phases of visual information processing. In backward masking, two very brief visual stimuli are presented in rapid succession. Typically, the subject's task is to identify the first, or *target* stimulus. The *mask* (ie, the second stimulus) makes the task more difficult, even though it is presented after the target is no longer present: hence the name "backward masking." Masking effects occur for normal as well as psychiatrically disordered people, but schizophrenic patients have consistently been found to exhibit deficits in backward masking tasks, meaning that the mask interferes even more with the visual processing of the target for schizophrenic patients than for normal individuals.[1-6]

Although the existence of schizophrenic performance deficits on backward masking procedures has been known for some 20 years,[1] the diagnostic specificity and underlying mechanisms have not been extensively studied. There is some evidence that masking performance deficits may be traitlike characteristics of schizophrenic patients. They have been found in schizophrenic patients during periods of relative symptom remission.[7] They are probably not an artifact of neuroleptics, which may actually improve visual processing among schizophrenic patients. In one study, at least, schizophrenic patients who were receiving neuroleptics showed less performance deficit than patients receiving no medication, despite the fact that the patients receiving medication were more symptomatic.[6] These perceptual processing deficits may

From the Department of Psychiatry and Biobehavioral Sciences, University of California–Los Angeles (Drs Green, Nuechterlein, and Mintz), and the Veterans Affairs Medical Center, West Los Angeles, Calif (Drs Green and Mintz).

See Methods on next page

METHODS

SUBJECTS

Schizophrenic (N=63; 21 female) and manic (N=31; 15 female) subjects were recruited from the inpatient units of Camarillo (Calif) State Hospital. All patients received diagnoses according to *DSM-III-R* criteria, based on an expanded version of the Present State Examination[19] that was supplemented with items from the Schedule for Affective Disorders and Schizophrenia[20] and Structured Clinical Interview for *DSM-III-R*–Patient Version.[21] Interviewers were trained to a sensitivity of at least 0.85 and a specificity of at least 0.90 for key psychotic and affective symptoms by the Diagnosis and Psychopathology Unit of the University of California–Los Angeles Clinical Research Center for the Study of Schizophrenia (principal investigator, Robert P. Liberman, MD). Potential subjects were excluded if they had a history of drug or alcohol dependence, an identifiable neurological disorder, any signs of mental retardation, or were over 55 years of age. For the schizophrenic and manic patients, mean (±SD) ages were 33.2±6.2 years and 37.7±9.2 years, respectively; mean years of education, 11.7±2.0 and 13.3±2.3, respectively; and mean number of years since first hospitalization, 14.0±6.3 and 14.5±7.5, respectively.

The normal controls (N=48; 27 female) were drawn from the Psychiatric Technician Training Program at Camarillo State Hospital. Normal controls were given the expanded Present State Examination and sections of the Structured Clinical Interview for *DSM-III-R*[22] that probed for schizotypal, paranoid, and borderline personality disorder. The exclusion criteria were the same for the normal controls as for the patients, with the additional provision that normal controls were excluded if they met criteria for any of these personality disorders or had a first-degree relative with a history of a psychotic disorder. Mean (±SD) age for normal controls was 33.5 years ±10.1, and mean years of education was 13.8±1.8.

The groups were unmatched for gender, with the schizophrenic group having relatively more men. The manic group differed from the other two groups in age, and the schizophrenic group differed from the other two groups in education. As a result of these demographic differences, the primary analyses for the current study (repeated measure analyses of variance [ANOVAs]), were also conducted as repeated measure analyses of covariance in which age, education, and gender served as covariates. The results were essentially the same with the covariates. For the current study, we present the data from the ANOVAs.

TESTING PROCEDURES

The subjects underwent testing on a three-channel Gerbrands projection tachistoscope (model #G1176, Gerbrands, Arlington, Mass). The projectors used flat-field lenses with a focal length of 102 mm. Subjects sat 1 meter away from a rear-projection screen and were presented with one of four target letters (S, C, O, or Q), which could appear at any one of four locations that were 2.2° of visual angle away from fixation (top, right, bottom, or left). The target letters subtended 0.3° of visual angle. The lens-to-screen distance was 95 cm. Luminance was determined with a Gossen Luna Pro light meter (Gossen, Woodside, NY) that was held 1 meter from the screen at eye level. Ambient light (with a light diffuser) was approximately 350 lux, and the luminance of both target and mask stimuli (without light diffuser) was approximately 2300 lux. A fixation point was presented for 400 milliseconds, and it ended 200 milliseconds prior to the target presentation.

even be a marker of vulnerability to schizophrenia, having been found in individuals whom some would consider to be in the "schizophrenia spectrum" based on their symptoms, a Minnesota Multiphasic Personality Profile, or scores on a psychosis-proneness scale.[8-12]

The diagnostic specificity of backward masking deficits is not clear, however, as they have been found in other diagnostic groups. Furthermore, in at least some clinical populations, the severity of masking deficits may covary with clinical state. Depressed and manic (described as mainly hypomanic) patients did not differ from normal controls in one study that used a traditional backward masking protocol,[2] but in another study of actively psychotic schizoaffective and bipolar patients, the same authors did find backward masking deficits.[4] In our own prior work,[3] a sample of bipolar patients performed more poorly than normal controls, but the difference was not statistically significant. The patients in these studies differed in symptom severity, which raises questions concerning the role of clinical state in masking performance, at least for patients with affective disorders.

Two fundamental mechanisms underlie the backward masking effect.[13] *Integration* occurs when the visual representations (called the *icons*[14]) initiated by the mask and target fuse because of the close temporal and spatial proximity of the stimuli. The result is a confusing, composite image, rather like a double-exposed photograph. Integration is strongest when the mask has high energy or intensity and overlaps the target spatially and when the interval between the target and mask (termed the *interstimulus interval* [ISI]) is shortest. Visual processing performance under masking by integration is thus an exponential function of time, being most impaired when the mask and target are presented simultaneously and steadily rising to a plateau as the ISI increases.

A second, distinct masking process is called masking by *interruption*. In this type of masking, fusion of icons does not occur. Rather, the visual processes triggered by the onset of the masking stimulus interrupt and disrupt later-stage processing of the target. Masking by interruption is a bell-shaped function of the ISI. In normal individuals, disruption of visual performance is negligible at the shortest ISIs (eg, below 20 milliseconds). It initially increases as the ISI is lengthened, reaching a maximum somewhere between 20 and 70 milliseconds, and then decreases again. Masking by interruption is most clearly seen when the energy of the mask is weak relative to that of the target or when the mask is presented around the target rather than over it. In those cases, the effects of integration on visual processing are minimized or elimi-

In all but the last substudy reported herein, the mask consisted of four groups of overlapping *X*'s, one at each of the four possible target locations. As noted below, our initial attempt to minimize masking by integration by reducing mask energy was not completely successful. As a result, we attempted to eliminate residual integration effects in our final substudy by changing the mask to overlapping circles. A forced-choice procedure was used throughout testing to reduce any differences in the response criterion. To ensure that subjects remained aware of all possible targets, the four target letters were displayed on a card in front of the subjects throughout testing.

During practice, the target was presented without the mask at a duration of 10 milliseconds. Subjects were required to identify the target on at least eight of 10 trials, which was generally easy for them. Next, subjects practiced with both target and mask at an ISI of 100 milliseconds, which we assumed was sufficiently long for target identification in all groups (our subsequent results challenge that assumption). Subjects were required to correctly identify four of five targets at this ISI before proceeding with the test. If the subjects could not identify the target during practice at the criterion level, the duration of the target was increased by 4-millisecond increments until subjects met the criterion. For those who required adjustment (23 schizophrenic patients, six manic patients, and one normal control), the duration of the mask was adjusted in the experimental conditions to maintain a constant target-mask ratio across subjects.

In the studies reported herein, both high- and low-energy masks were used. The energy of a brief stimulus is defined as the luminance multiplied by the duration. In the current studies, which used a projection tachistoscope, the duration could be altered. The duration of the high-energy mask was set at twice that of the target (eg, 20 milliseconds for a 10-millisecond target), and the duration of the low-energy mask at one half that of the target (eg, 5 milliseconds for a 10-millisecond target). The conditions were administered in a counterbalanced order across subjects. The ISIs were 5, 10, 20, 40, 70, and 100 milliseconds, with 12 target presentations at each ISI. Both the targets and the ISIs were presented in a block-randomized fashion.

STATISTICAL ANALYSES

Data were initially analyzed using a repeated measures ANOVA design, with one between-groups factor (diagnosis) and one within-groups factor (ISI). We used conventional repeated measures analysis (with Greenhouse-Geisser correction for the within-groups effects). The repeated measures ANOVA also reports univariate ANOVA results at each ISI. Interactions of significant diagnosis by ISI were followed by simple F tests at each ISI. Separate ANOVAs using only a subset of ISIs were performed when they would clarify the results of overall ANOVA models. When the results of univariate F tests were significant, pairwise group contrasts were evaluated with simple *t* tests. When the results of univariate ANOVAs did not reach statistical significance, Tukey pairwise contrasts were examined to control for type I error. The timing of recovery from masking was analyzed by coding the first ISI at which performance improved and comparing groups using survival models and univariate ANOVA (with square root transformation). Results of both analytic methods were comparable, and only the former are reported here. To simplify presentation of results, we employ the subscripts N, S, and M to reference normal, schizophrenic, and manic subjects, respectively, for paired comparisons. Thus, an F ratio contrasting normal and schizophrenic samples would be written as F_{NS}. When all three samples are included in a comparison, no subscript is used.

nated, because the composite icon formed by integration is no longer confusing.

With very few exceptions,[15,16] the research on backward masking in schizophrenia to date has used high-energy masks that spatially overlap the target. In this masking procedure, both integration and interruption occur simultaneously, and masking by interruption can be obscured by strong integration. In addition, some studies have used ISIs that completely miss the "window" in which interruption occurs. As a result, the relative role of these two masking mechanisms in the backward masking deficit observed in schizophrenia is not clear.[17,18] In the case of masking through integration, a deficit could be owing to difficulty in deciphering a complex icon. If masking is through interruption, the deficits could be owing to slow information transfer or fragile visual icon formation. Similarly, it is not known whether the masking deficits observed in various diagnostic groups are based on the same mechanisms.

The current study represents an attempt to systematically explore the backward masking performance deficit in schizophrenia and determine its diagnostic specificity, using methods that allow us to more precisely specify the underlying mechanisms involved. In a series of related studies, we manipulated characteristics of the mask to more fully explore both the integration and interruption mechanisms. In addition, we included a sample of manic patients to determine the specificity of the findings to schizophrenia.

RESULTS

HIGH-ENERGY MASK

All of the ANOVA effects were significant (for diagnosis, F=25.37, *df*=2,139, *P*<.0001; for ISI, F=429.58, *df*=5,695, *P*<.0001; for interaction of diagnosis by ISI, F=6.29, *df*=10,695, *P*<.0001). The results are displayed in **Figure 1**. Relative to normal subjects, schizophrenic and manic patients clearly showed masking performance deficits; differences between the patient samples were not significant (F_{NS}=8.56, *df*=5,695, *P*<.0001; F_{NM}=8.92, *df*=5,695, *P*<.0001; F_{SM}=1.39, *df*=5,695, *P*=.22).

At the shortest ISI (5 milliseconds), all three groups performed at chance levels (mean levels ranged from 3.1 to 3.2, all nonsignificantly different from random guessing; *P*=.25 to .66). As the ISI increased, performance improved in all groups, but more rapidly among normal subjects than patients (log-rank χ^2=6.46, *df*=2, *P*=.04; χ^2_{NS}=5.15, *df*=1, *P*=.02; χ^2_{NM}=4.40, *df*=1, *P*=.04; χ^2_{SM}=.38,

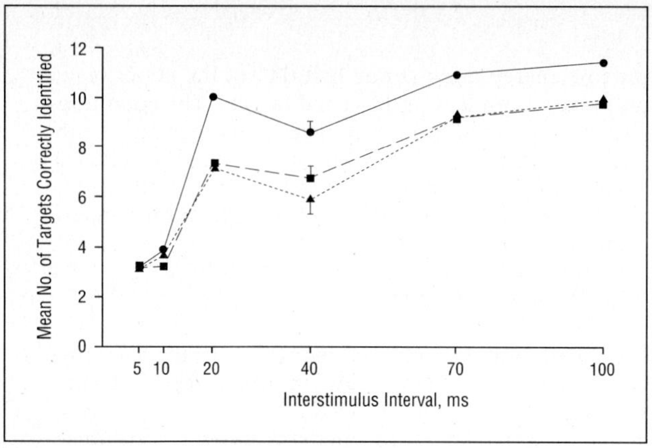

Figure 1. *Results of masking by integration and interruption with a high-energy mask. Squares indicate the performance of schizophrenic patients; triangles, manic patients; and circles, normal controls. Mean SE bars are shown at the 40-millisecond interstimulus interval.*

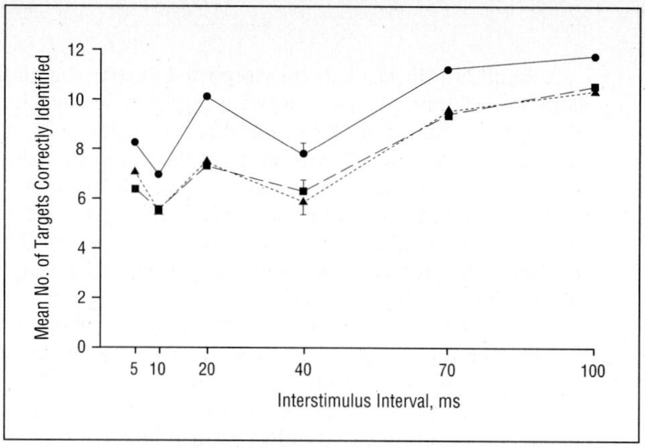

Figure 2. *Results of masking primarily by interruption with a low-energy mask. Squares indicate the performance of schizophrenic patients; triangles, manic patients; and circles, normal controls. Mean SE bars are shown at the 40-millisecond interstimulus interval.*

df=1, *P*=.54). The patient groups also improved less overall. At all ISIs of 20 milliseconds or more, normal controls performed significantly better (F_{NS}=42.72, *df*=1,130, *P*<.0001; F_{NM}=35.55, *df*=1,139, *P*<.0001; all univariate ANOVA contrasts between normal controls and both patient groups at ISIs of 20 milliseconds or more were significant at *P*≤.01).

In short, visual recognition of letters showed susceptibility to high-energy masking for longer intervals in the schizophrenic and manic subjects than normal controls. These results thus confirm the existence of deficits associated with high-energy masking in schizophrenic patients. Further, they indicate that these deficits are not specific to schizophrenic subjects; manic patients also showed a deficit in this condition. It must be recalled, however, that one limitation of the high-energy masking procedure is that it causes both strong integration and interruption effects. For example, the strong suppression of performance at the shorter ISIs is largely due to masking by integration, and the dip in performance in all groups at 40 milliseconds is mainly the result of weak masking by interruption.[23] Both mechanisms are presumed to operate to some degree throughout. For this reason, the results obtained with the high-energy mask do not permit unambiguous interpretation of the masking mechanism underlying the diagnostic differences.

LOW-ENERGY MASK

In this condition, the main effects of diagnosis (F=21.21, *df*=2,139, *P*<.0001) and ISI (F=142.31, *df*=5,695, *P*<.0001) were significant, but the interaction of diagnosis by ISI was not significant (F=1.58, *df*=10,695, *P*<.12). Pairwise diagnostic group contrasts showed a consistent pattern (**Figure 2**). Normal controls performed significantly better than both the schizophrenic and manic patients at every ISI (for main effect, F_{NS}=37.02, *df*=1,139, *P*<.0001; F_{NM}=24.21, *df*=1,139, *P*<.0001; all pairwise contrasts were significant). The patient groups did not differ significantly from each other at any ISI (F_{MS}<1, nonsignificant).

Thus, both patient groups showed similar masking deficits in a low-energy masking procedure that we had hoped would limit the masking mechanism to interruption. However, inspection of the results (Figure 2) suggested that we were not entirely successful in eliminating all masking effects of integration. Instead of a simple, U-shaped function that would be consistent with interruption alone, we saw two dips (at 10 and 40 milliseconds). Both of these drops were statistically significant in all three groups (*P*<.01).

The dip at 40 milliseconds, which also was seen to a lesser extent in the high-energy masking condition, was owing to the interruption mechanism. However, we believe that the dip at 10 milliseconds was owing to the fact that integration was weakened but not eliminated, and it therefore represented the combined effects of strong interruption and attenuated integration.[23]

FURTHER ISOLATION OF MASKING BY INTERRUPTION

We reasoned that masking by integration may have continued to be a factor despite weakening the energy of the mask, because the perceptual features of the mask and target were very different (rounded vs straight-line). If so, a purer U-shaped function would result if we used a mask and target with similar features. This manipulation should largely eliminate masking by integration while maintaining or even increasing masking through interruption.[24] The intention of this manipulation was thus to obtain a purer example of masking by interruption.

To test this hypothesis, we recruited a subsample of 10 schizophrenic patients and 10 normal controls from the larger samples described above. The new mask was constructed of adjacent circles that covered all possible target locations. The target-mask ratio was set to 2:1, similar to the conditions with a low-energy mask. We were primarily interested in mapping the early part of the masking function, where the dips were observed in Figure 2. Hence, the ISIs were set at simultaneous onset, contiguous presentation, and 10, 20, 30, 40, 50, and 60 milliseconds. Ten target stimuli were presented for each ISI.

The results from this procedure are shown in **Figure 3**. The normal controls show a masking curve

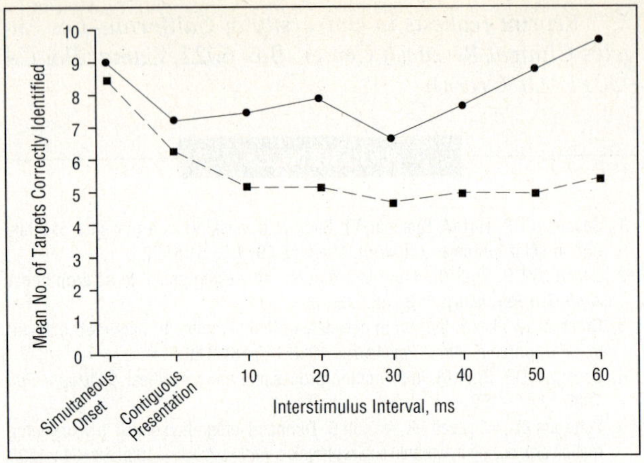

Figure 3. *Results of further isolation of interruption with a low-energy mask consisting of circles. Squares indicate the performance of schizophrenic patients; circles, normal controls.*

that is much closer to a classical U-shaped function. The patients show the descending but not the ascending portion of the U-shaped function. We would expect to see the ascending part of the curve for the patients if we sampled longer ISIs. The effects of group ($F=10.54$, $df=1,18$, $P<.005$) and ISI ($F=5.79$, $df=7,126$, $P<.001$) were significant. In addition, the interaction of group by ISI was significant ($F=2.76$, $df=7,126$, $P<.05$), indicating that the groups were comparable at the initial ISIs and then diverged from each other.

Slopes on the descending portion (at or below the 40-millisecond ISI) of the function were steeper for the schizophrenic patients than for normal controls (mean slope, -0.08 ± 0.07 vs -0.04 ± 0.09, respectively) but not significantly different ($t=1.32$, $df=18$, $P=.20$). However, recovery was much slower. The mean slope after a 40-millisecond ISI was 0.02 (±0.05) for schizophrenic subjects vs 0.10 (±0.07) for normal controls ($t=2.94$, $df=18$, $P=.0088$). The results from this manipulation indicate that schizophrenic patients show deficits on a relatively pure interruption task in which integration has been largely eliminated, and their visual recognition remains susceptible to masking by interruption for longer intervals than that of normal controls.

COMMENT

In the current series of studies, schizophrenic patients showed visual masking performance deficits, even when the mechanism involved was largely limited to masking by interruption. To our knowledge, there is one unpublished study (cited by Schuck and Lee[15]) but no published studies that have shown this effect. By using a mask with features similar to the target, we obtained a U-shaped masking function that we believe indicates relatively pure masking by interruption. In this masking condition, patients showed a markedly longer period during which visual masking occurred, compared with normal controls. We conclude that schizophrenic patients have abnormalities involving at least interruptive mechanisms, and the deficits observed on masking procedures cannot be explained solely in terms of difficulty deciphering composite stimuli (integration processes).

Several of our results suggest that schizophrenic patients may manifest deficits on masking procedures for far longer periods than we had previously supposed. The performance of schizophrenic patients remained impaired and showed slow recovery even at relatively long ISIs. Michaels and Turvey[23] have suggested that a deflection of attention from the target to the subsequent mask is likely to be involved in slow recovery of performance at long ISIs. Thus, in addition to difficulties associated with interruption, schizophrenic patients may be unusually susceptible to such attentional disruption by the mask at relatively long ISIs.

Our methods did not completely rule out the existence of a generalized sensory input deficit as a contributing factor, but the tendency for the performance of schizophrenic patients to converge with that of normal controls at the shortest and longest ISIs, taken together with the pronounced lack of parallelism displayed in Figure 3, argues against an obvious generalized deficit. A number of previous studies have come to the same conclusion.[7-12,25]

With regard to the question of diagnostic specificity, the visual processing of manic patients was comparable to or perhaps even slightly worse than that of the schizophrenic patients across all of the masking conditions. The results thus suggest that backward masking deficits are not entirely specific to schizophrenia, and comparable masking deficits are found in hospitalized manic inpatients with chronic disease.

Although the manic patients were hospitalized at the time of testing, they were not as symptomatic as the schizophrenic patients, based on the Brief Psychiatric Rating Scale.[26] The groups differed significantly on several Brief Psychiatric Rating Scale symptom clusters,[27] including the Thinking Disturbance Factor score (7.6 vs 10.9, $t=3.94$, $P<.0002$), the Withdrawal-Retardation Factor score (4.2 vs 7.6, $t=5.99$, $P<.0001$), and the score from a depressive factor that included depressed mood, guilt, and suicidality (3.9 vs 5.3, $t=3.15$, $P<.005$) for manic vs schizophrenic patients, respectively. To the extent that masking deficits are associated with psychiatric symptoms, we might have expected the manic patients to perform better than schizophrenic patients, but they clearly did not. It should be emphasized that these manic patients had a fairly chronic and severe illness, so the generalizability of these findings to a healthier sample of bipolar patients is open to question.

There is some debate in the field as to the relative importance of *stimulus onset asynchrony,* which refers to the time lapse between the onset of the target and that of the mask, vs the ISI, which refers to the lapse between the offset of the target and onset of the mask.[13] Most previous studies of backward masking have controlled only the latter. In the typical experimental procedure called *critical stimulus duration,*[2,11] the target duration is set individually for each subject at a threshold level. The timing of the mask is then set relative to the offset of the target. This procedure has the advantage of approximately equating subjects in terms of sensory input factors, so that remaining deficits can be attributed more unambiguously to the effects of the mask. However, there is a disadvantage to the critical stimulus duration pro-

cedure for studies of interruption, such as the current one. When the duration of the target differs from subject to subject, the time lapse between the onsets of the target and mask (ie, the stimulus onset asynchrony) also varies. This effect may make a critical difference when the mechanism of interest is interruption.[14]

Our initial intention was to use a constant target duration for all subjects by setting it at a level that would be sufficiently long for everyone to identify the target and hold both the stimulus onset asynchrony and the ISI constant across subjects. We were not entirely successful, because more subjects than expected required adjustments to their target durations. This is a limitation of the current procedures. Another potential limitation is that patients who underwent retesting in the subsequent analyses might have benefited from repeated exposure to the masking procedure. Although a practice effect cannot be ruled out, it seems unlikely to account for the pattern of results that was observed in Figure 3.

The current findings help us to interpret the nature of the visual masking performance in major mental illness and suggest some methodological refinements and directions. We believe that our findings are the first to demonstrate that masking by interruption is at least one of the mechanisms responsible for deficits in early visual processing in schizophrenic subjects. Furthermore, our data provide no evidence that these deficits are specific to schizophrenia, as comparable performance deficits were found among manic subjects in each condition evaluated. Susceptibility to masking by interruption occurs over a longer interval after stimulus presentation than we originally suspected. Even in masking conditions designed to markedly attenuate or eliminate the effects of masking by integration, masking deficits persisted at ISIs of at least 100 milliseconds, suggesting that additional disruption due to deflection of attention from the target to the mask is probably involved. At the physiological level, masking through interruption involves a complex interaction of transient and sustained visual channels in which the transient channels of the mask inhibit (interrupt) the sustained channels of the target.[24,28] The relative contributions of these visual channels to the backward masking deficit will be considered in a following article.

Accepted for publication July 8, 1994.

Funding for this project came from grant MH-43292 of the National Institute of Mental Health, Rockville, Md (Dr Green).

The authors thank Maryam Aslani, David Chavez, Cynthia Christenson, Donna Gaier, Daniel Gutkind, Robert Kern, PhD, David King, PhD, Susan G. Hellman, Sharon Mitchell, MA, Chad Nelson, Julie Van Sickle, MA, and Jennifer Smith for their help in subject recruitment and data collection. Bruno Breitmeyer, PhD, consulted on the design of this project and the interpretation of the results. The statistical analyses were conducted by Sun Hwang, MS, MPH, of the Methodology and Statistical Support Unit of the University of California–Los Angeles Clinical Research Center for the Study of Schizophrenia. The patients were recruited through the excellent cooperation of the staff and administration of Camarillo State Hospital.

Reprint requests to University of California–Los Angeles Clinical Research Center, Box 6022, Camarillo, CA 93011 (Dr Green).

REFERENCES

1. Saccuzzo DP, Hirt M, Spenser TJ. Backward masking as a measure of attention in schizophrenia. *J Abnorm Psychol.* 1974;83:512-522.
2. Saccuzzo DP, Braff DL. Early information processing deficit in schizophrenia. *Arch Gen Psychiatry.* 1981;38:175-179.
3. Green M, Walker E. Symptom correlates of vulnerability to backward masking in schizophrenia. *Am J Psychiatry.* 1986;143:181-186.
4. Saccuzzo DP, Braff DL. Information-processing abnormalities. *Schizophr Bull.* 1986;12:447-459.
5. Schwartz BD, Winstead DK, Adinoff B. Temporal integration deficit in visual information processing by chronic schizophrenics. *Biol Psychiatry.* 1983;18:1311-1320.
6. Braff DL, Saccuzzo DP. Effect of antipsychotic medication on speed of information processing in schizophrenic patients. *Am J Psychiatry.* 1982;139:1117-1130.
7. Miller S, Saccuzzo D, Braff D. Information processing deficits in remitted schizophrenics. *J Abnorm Psychol.* 1979;88:446-449.
8. Steronko RJ, Woods DJ. Impairment in early stages of visual information processing in nonpsychotic schizotypic individuals. *J Abnorm Psychol.* 1978;87:481-490.
9. Braff DL. Impaired speed of information processing in nonmedicated schizotypal patients. *Schizophr Bull.* 1981;7:499-508.
10. Balogh DW, Merritt RD. Susceptibility to type A backward pattern masking among hypothetically psychosis-prone college students. *J Abnorm Psychol.* 1985;94:377-383.
11. Saccuzzo DP, Schubert DL. Backward masking as a measure of slow processing in schizophrenia spectrum disorders. *J Abnorm Psychol.* 1981;90:305-312.
12. Merritt RD, Balogh DW. The use of a backward masking paradigm to assess information-processing deficits among schizotypics: a re-evaluation of Steronko and Woods. *J Nerv Ment Dis.* 1984;172:216-224.
13. Turvey MT. On peripheral and central processes in vision: inferences from an information-processing analysis of masking with patterned stimuli. *Psychol Rev.* 1973;80:1-52.
14. Neisser U. *Cognitive Psychology.* New York, NY: Appleton-Century-Crofts; 1967.
15. Schuck JR, Lee RG. Backward masking, information processing, and schizophrenia. *Schizophr Bull.* 1989;15:491-500.
16. Merritt RD, Balogh DW, Leventhal DB. Use of a metacontrast and a paracontrast procedure to assess the visual information processing of hypothetically schizotypic college students. *J Abnorm Psychol.* 1986;95:74-80.
17. Nuechterlein KH, Dawson ME. Information processing and attentional functioning in the developmental course of schizophrenic disorders. *Schizophr Bull.* 1984;10:160-203.
18. Braff DL, Saccuzzo DP, Geyer MA. Information processing dysfunctions in schizophrenia: studies of visual backward masking, sensorimotor gating, and habituation. In: Steinhauer SR, Gruzelier JH, Zubin J, eds. *Handbook of Schizophrenia: Neuropsychology, Psychophysiology, and Information Processing.* Amsterdam, the Netherlands: Elsevier Science Publishers; 1991;5:303-334.
19. Wing JK, Cooper JE, Sartorius N. *The Measurement and Classification of Psychiatric Symptoms.* New York, NY: Cambridge University Press; 1974.
20. Endicott J, Spitzer RL. A diagnostic interview: the Schedule for Affective Disorders and Schizophrenia. *Arch Gen Psychiatry.* 1978;35:837-844.
21. Spitzer RL, Williams JBW, Gibbon M, First MB. *Structured Clinical Interview for DSM-III-R–Patient Edition (SCID-P, Version 1.0).* Washington, DC: American Psychiatric Press; 1990.
22. Spitzer RL, Williams JBW, Gibbon M, First MB. *Structured Clinical Interview for DSM-III-R–Personality Disorders (SCID-II, Version 1.0).* Washington, DC: American Psychiatric Press; 1990.
23. Michaels CF, Turvey MT. Central sources of visual masking: indexing structures supporting seeing at a single, brief glance. *Psychol Res.* 1979;41:1-61.
24. Breitmeyer BG. *Visual Masking: An Integrative Approach.* New York, NY: Oxford University Press; 1984.
25. Brody D, Saccuzzo DP, Braff DL. Information processing for masked and unmasked stimuli in schizophrenia and old age. *J Abnorm Psychol.* 1980;89:617-622.
26. Lukoff D, Nuechterlein KH, Ventura J. Appendix A: manual for the expanded Brief Psychiatric Rating Scale (BPRS). *Schizophr Bull.* 1986;12:594-602.
27. Overall JE, Hollister LE, Pichot P. Major psychiatric disorders: a four-dimensional model. *Arch Gen Psychiatry.* 1967;16:146-161.
28. Breitmeyer BG, Ganz L. Implications of sustained and transient channels for theories of visual pattern masking, saccadic suppression, and information processing. *Psychol Rev.* 1976;83:1-36.

Backward Masking in Schizophrenia and Mania

II. Specifying the Visual Channels

Michael Foster Green, PhD; Keith H. Nuechterlein, PhD; Jim Mintz, PhD

Background: The backward masking procedures that have been used in psychopathology research have confounded two types of masking mechanisms (integration and interruption) and two types of visual channels (transient and sustained). In an earlier study, we attempted to limit the masking mechanism to interruption. The current study limited the role of sustained (parvocellular) visual channels to masking performance.

Methods: Masking procedures were altered in the following two ways to reduce reliance on sustained visual channels: (1) the spatial frequency was lowered by blurring the target and (2) a location task was used instead of an identification task. Manic patients were included to examine the specificity of deficits on these tasks to schizophrenia and to test the hypothesis that mania is associated with abnormalities on visuospatial tasks.

Results: Schizophrenic patients differed significantly from normal controls on both masking conditions. Manic patients also showed deficits relative to normal controls. Manic patients showed a significantly different masking function from that of schizophrenic patients on the location condition.

Conclusions: Schizophrenic deficits within masking paradigms may involve abnormalities in transient, as opposed to sustained, visual channels. Masking performance deficits were also found in manic patients, but the underlying processes are probably different. A reformulation is offered concerning the nature of early visual processing deficits in schizophrenia.

(Arch Gen Psychiatry. 1994;51:945-951)

BACKWARD MASKING procedures used with schizophrenic patients have typically confounded two types of masking mechanisms (integration and interruption) and two types of visual channels (transient and sustained).[1-3] As a result, it is difficult to understand the nature of the deficit that patients show on these procedures. Our initial study[4] attempted to limit the masking mechanisms to interruption. The current study addresses the contribution of two types of visual channels (transient and sustained) to masking performance.

At the physiological level, masking involves the interaction of two types of visual pathways: transient (also called magnocellular) and sustained (parvocellular).[5,6] These visual channels differ in their anatomical distributions and psychophysiological characteristics. The transient cells show a short response latency and are sensitive to low spatial frequency (eg, coarse features of a stimulus). They convey information about the onset, offset, and location of a stimulus. The sustained cells have a relatively long response latency and are sensitive to high spatial frequency (eg, the fine details of a stimulus). These pathways conduct a more detailed analysis of objects and are important for identification of stimuli. The characteristics of the visual channels are summarized in the **Table**.

Breitmeyer and Ganz[5] and Breitmeyer[6] proposed a comprehensive model to explain masking in terms of these visual channels. According to their model, the target first initiates activity in the transient channels (needed to locate the stimulus), followed by activity in the sustained channels (needed to identify the stimulus). Backward masking by interruption occurs because the transient channels of the mask (presented after the target) interrupt the sustained channel activity of the target. Masking by integration occurs

From the Department of Psychiatry and Biobehavioral Sciences, University of California–Los Angeles (Drs Green, Nuechterlein, and Mintz), and the Veterans Affairs Medical Center, West Los Angeles, Calif (Drs Green and Mintz).

See Methods on next page

METHODS

SUBJECTS

The present study used 62 (20 female) schizophrenic patients, 31 (14 female) bipolar manic patients, and 48 (27 female) normal controls. These patient samples overlapped but were not identical to the samples in our previous article.[4] The specific inclusionary and exclusionary criteria are listed in our initial article.[4] The mean (±SD) ages were 33.5±6.2 years, 37.2±9.0 years, and 33.5±10.1 years and mean education was 11.8 ±2.0 years, 13.3±2.4 years, and 13.8±1.8 years for the schizophrenic patients, manic patients, and normal controls, respectively. The mean number of years since first hospitalization was 14.1±6.4 for the schizophrenic patients and 14.0±7.1 for the manic patients.

The schizophrenic group had relatively more male subjects than the other groups. The manic group was older than the other two groups, and the schizophrenic group had less education than the other two groups. To determine whether these demographic differences influenced the results, analyses of covariance were conducted (for each condition) in which age, education, and gender served as covariates. The results were essentially the same with or without the inclusion of the covariates.

The Gerbrands tachistoscopic equipment (Gerbrands, Arlington, Mass) and the stimuli were the same as described in the initial study[4]: one of four possible targets (O, S, Q, and C) appeared at one of four possible target locations (up, down, left, and right), and the mask consisted of overlapping *X*'s. Two masking conditions were used, and the order was counterbalanced across subjects.

CONDITIONS

Reducing Reliance on Sustained Visual Channels

In this condition, we reduced reliance on sustained channels by using an identification task in which the target was blurred to eliminate high spatial frequency information. The target was blurred to a standardized degree by changing the lens-to-screen distance from 95 to 107.5 cm (which defocuses the stimuli) and then refocusing the mask but not the target. As a by-product of blurring, the visual discrimination became more difficult. Based on pilot data, we selected parameters that yielded a test of approximately the same difficulty level as the masking condition, with the low-energy mask of our initial study.[4] The duration of the target was doubled (eg, 20 milliseconds for a target duration of 10 milliseconds), and the duration of the mask was set to one fourth the duration of the target (eg, 5 milliseconds for a 20-millisecond target). Twelve targets were presented at each of six interstimulus intervals (ISIs) of 5, 10, 20, 40, 70, and 100 milliseconds.

Further Restriction of Sustained Channels

For this condition, subjects stated the location of a clearly focused target (up, down, left, and right) but did not need to identify it. To reduce any confusion, a response card was placed in front of the subject, which displayed the four possible responses in their respective spatial locations. This task relies heavily on transient channels. Because locating is generally easier than identifying a target, we made the task more difficult by setting the target-mask ratio at 1:1 (eg, 10 milliseconds for both the target and mask). The transient channels have a shorter latency than sustained channels, so the sampling of ISIs was compressed and included 5, 10, 15, 20, 30, and 50 milliseconds (12 targets at each ISI).

when the activity from the visual channels becomes combined. Typically, this type of masking involves the sustained activity of the mask integrating with the sustained activity of the target.

Figure 1, based on the model of Breitmeyer and Ganz,[5] illustrates these concepts. The spatial frequency (eg, amount of fine detail) of a target and the type of task (location vs identification) will influence which channels are needed for the visual analysis. Specifically, identification of a target with fine detail (high spatial frequency) relies heavily on the sustained channels, while the visual analysis of a low spatial frequency (blurry) target relies primarily on transient channels and relatively little on the sustained channels. Likewise, if task requirements are changed so that subjects are asked to locate but not identify a target, only the transient channels are needed. To our knowledge, masking research in schizophrenia has exclusively involved identification tasks, which require detailed scrutiny through the use of the sustained channels.

Abnormalities of transient and/or sustained channels could underlie the masking deficit in schizophrenia, but opinions have differed on this matter.[7,8] Schuck and Lee[7] noted that schizophrenic patients appear to have deficits on backward but not forward masking,[3] which is consistent with abnormal transient activity, because forward masking uses mainly sustained channels. In contrast, a study of visible persistence by Schwartz and Winstead[9] reported that paranoid schizophrenic patients showed deficits with a stimulus of high but not low spatial frequency. The finding was consistent with an abnormality of the sustained visual channels because of their sensitivity to higher spatial frequency.

In the present study, two manipulations were used to investigate the contribution of the transient and sustained visual channels to masking performance in schizophrenia. First, we lowered the spatial frequency of the target (by blurring) to reduce reliance on sustained visual channels and hence increase reliance on the transient channels. Second, we used a location task (as opposed to an identification task) to further restrict processing by sustained channels. If the deficit that patients show on masking procedures is due to abnormalities in the sustained channels, these manipulations should reduce the degree of the deficit.

Manic patients were included, not merely to test the specificity to schizophrenia among psychotic disorders, but also to address an additional research question. Bipolar patients in a depressed phase have been described as performing poorly relative to other affective groups

Properties of Visual Channels

Properties	Type of Channel: Transient*	Sustained†
Anatomical distributions		
Retinal origin	Type A ganglion cells	Type B ganglion cells
Projections to lateral geniculate	Magnocellular layers	Parvocellular layers
Projections to visual cortex	Layer 4C alpha, then layer 4B alpha	Layer 4C beta, then layers 2 and 3 beta
Psychophysiological characteristics		
Receptive field	Large	Small
Response	Onset and offset	Maintained
Latency	Short	Long
Spatial frequency	Low	High

*Transient channels are used to convey information about the onset, offset, and location of stimuli.
†Sustained channels are used to convey information about fine details of stimuli.

on left hemifield (right hemisphere) tachistoscopic visuospatial tasks.[10,11] Such a finding is consistent with the theory that bipolar mood disorder is associated with a right hemisphere abnormality. The right hemisphere appears to be especially suited for identifying stimuli of low spatial frequency[12] and locating objects.[13-15] For reasons that are not yet understood, the same conditions that increase reliance on transient channels also increase reliance on right hemisphere processing. If mania is associated with a right hemisphere abnormality, we would expect the performance of manic patients to be particularly affected by these manipulations.

RESULTS

For each masking condition, a multivariate analysis of variance was conducted for the three groups (normal controls, schizophrenic patients, and manic patients) and six ISIs. The masking conditions were usually counterbalanced across subjects. The blurred condition was given priority and was occasionally administered first when patients were not considered to be fully cooperative. Four manic patients completed the blurred identification condition but not the location condition. Pairwise contrasts were conducted for each ISI (each patient group was compared with normal controls and then each other), with the criterion for significance set at the .05 level.

IDENTIFICATION OF BLURRED TARGET

The results from the blurred target identification condition are displayed in **Figure 2**. The effects of group ($F=3.36$, $df=12,266$, $P<.0001$) and ISI ($F=108.39$, $df=5,134$, $P<.0001$) were significant. The overall interaction of group by ISI was significant ($F=2.01$, $df=10,268$, $P=.03$). This interaction was due to a significant interaction between normal controls and schizophrenic patients ($F=3.42$, $df=5,134$, $P<.01$). The interaction of group by ISI was not significant between the normal controls and the manic patients or between two patients groups.

The pairwise contrasts revealed significant differences between normal controls and schizophrenic patients at each ISI except the second (10 millisecond) and the fourth (40 millisecond) ones. Normal controls and manic patients differed at each ISI except the second one. The manic patients tended to perform worse than schizophrenic patients ($P=.08$) at the 40-millisecond ISI. Inspection of the data (Figure 2) as well as pairwise comparisons reveal that the group interaction of normal controls by schizophrenic patients was largely due to a convergence of the groups at the 10-millisecond ISI.

LOCATION OF TARGET

The results from the location condition are shown in **Figure 3**. The effects of group ($F=40.36$, $df=2,134$, $P<.0001$) and ISI ($F=92.80$, $df=5,130$, $P<.0001$) were significant. The overall interaction of group by ISI ($F=3.12$, $df=10,260$, $P<.0009$) was significant. The simple interaction was significant for the normal controls vs the manic patients ($F=3.42$, $df=5,130$, $P<.006$) but not for the normal controls vs the schizophrenic patients. Importantly, the interaction was significant when the schizophrenic patients were compared with the manic patients ($F=5.71$, $df=5,130$, $P<.0001$).

The normal controls correctly located more targets than the schizophrenic and manic patients at every ISI. In addition, the manic patients performed significantly worse ($P<.0001$) than the schizophrenic patients at the fifth ISI (30 milliseconds) and tended to perform worse at the fourth ISI (20 milliseconds). Inspection of the data and pairwise contrasts suggests that the significant interactions come from the separation of the two patient groups after the 15-millisecond ISI, with the manic patients showing a pronounced dip at the 30-millisecond ISI.

COMMENT

COMPARISON OF NORMAL CONTROLS AND SCHIZOPHRENIC PATIENTS

Schizophrenic patients both identified blurred targets and located clearly focused targets significantly more poorly than normal controls across ISIs in the present study. Hence, restricting the role of sustained visual channels (consequently increasing reliance on transient channels) did not eliminate the performance deficit on the masking procedures.

The conditions of the present study also did not re-

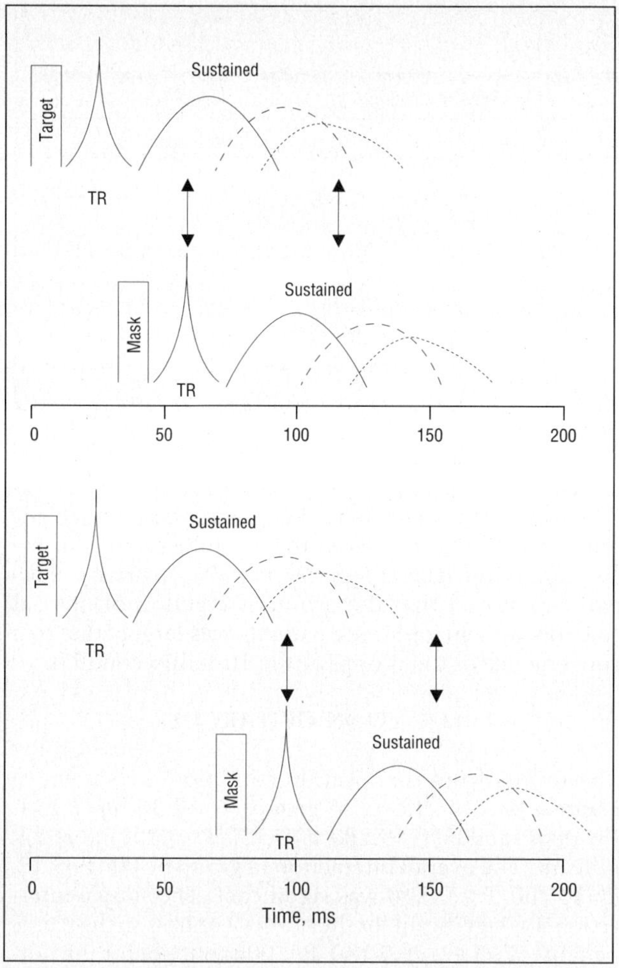

Figure 1. *Proposed interactions of sustained and transient channels. The figures show backward masking at two different interstimulus intervals. The transient channel activity is shown by the spike labeled TR, and the sustained channel activity is shown by three curves that represent increasing spatial frequency. The interactions of the visual channels are represented by the vertical arrows. Solid curves indicate lowest spatial frequency; dashed curves, increasing spatial frequency; and dotted curves, highest spatial frequency. Adapted from Breitmeyer and Ganz.*[5]

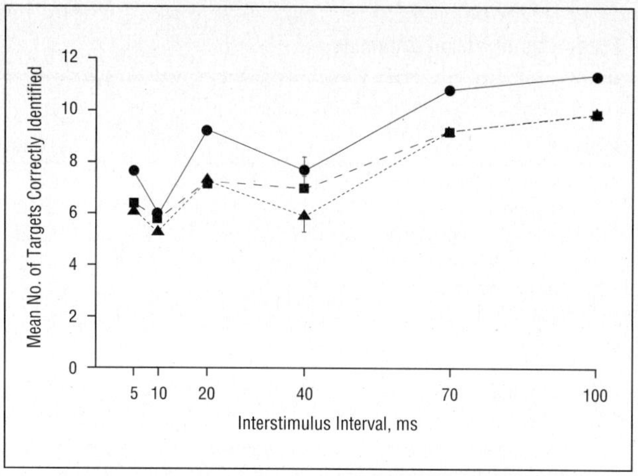

Figure 2. *Results of identification task with a blurred target. Squares indicate the performance of schizophrenic patients; triangles, manic patients; and circles, normal controls. Mean SE bars are shown at the 40-millisecond interstimulus interval.*

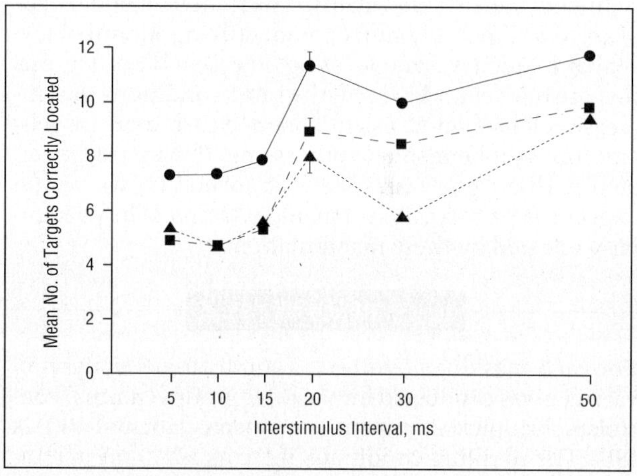

Figure 3. *Results of location task with a clear target. Squares indicate the performance of schizophrenic patients; triangles, manic patients; and circles, normal controls. Mean SE bars are shown at the 20-millisecond interstimulus interval.*

duce the performance deficit when compared with conditions from our initial study, which relied heavily on sustained channels. The mean effect size across ISIs between schizophrenic patients and normal controls in the low-energy masking condition of our initial study[4] was 1.17. By comparison, the mean effect sizes in the current study are somewhat smaller for the blurred identification condition (0.75) but larger for the location condition (1.46). The location task provided a stronger test of the role of transient channels because sustained channels are not required for this task. Thus, when the task conditions rely heavily on transient channels stimulated by the target, the magnitude of the masking effect in schizophrenia appears to be at least as large as the effect when both transient and sustained channels are needed for target processing. Given these results, the deficit on masking procedures might be mediated by abnormalities of the transient channels.

An assumption of the current study was that experimental manipulations that decrease reliance on the sustained channels of normal subjects have the same effects on schizophrenic patients. Although not directly tested, this assumption seems reasonable because the characteristics of the transient and sustained visual channels (Table) derive from basic single-cell response characteristics, and these differences exist across species.[6]

COMPARISON OF MANIC AND SCHIZOPHRENIC PATIENTS

The manic patients appeared to be somewhat more affected by the manipulations of the current study than the schizophrenic patients. This pattern occurred despite the fact that the manic patients were less symptomatic on the Thinking Disturbance and Withdrawal-Retardation clusters of the Brief Psychiatric Rating Scale, as shown in our initial article.[4] The results argue against the notion that poor performance under visual masking conditions is specific to schizophrenia among the psychotic disorders. Such a finding is perhaps not surprising, given the strong similarities in cross-sectional symptoms between severe bipolar disorder and schizophrenia.[16] The similarities be-

tween these two disorders in terms of phenomenological features, information processing, and biological markers have prompted some investigators to consider a unitary view of psychoses in which schizophrenia and bipolar disorders fall along a single dimension.[17,18]

Although our results are somewhat consistent with a unitary view in that both groups show poor performance, the significant interaction of diagnostic group by ISI for the location condition suggests that the groups performed poorly for different reasons. The masking functions appear to diverge when the manic patients show a pronounced dip at the 30-millisecond ISI. Perhaps the manic patients are especially sensitive to a relatively late masking effect with a task that would normally rely on transient channel activity.

As mentioned earlier, the manipulations that increased reliance on transient channels also increased reliance on processes associated with the right cerebral hemisphere, such as sensitivity to low spatial frequencies[12] and locating objects in space.[13-15] The performance of the manic patients in the current study is consistent with that seen in previous studies, which indicated that bipolar patients have a right hemisphere deficit compared with unipolar depressed patients and normal controls.[10,11] These results, which clearly need replication, suggest that visual processing in mania might be particularly susceptible to disruption under conditions that emphasize transient channel activity and/or right hemisphere processing. The findings also suggest a time course by implicating the interruptive component of the masking function (ISI of approximately 30-milliseconds). Future studies may wish to present stimuli to the right or left of midline to allow clear assessment of hemifield effects and more directly test the question of right hemisphere involvement with manic patients. In addition, it would also be informative for subsequent studies to sample more ISIs from the middle region (ISIs of 30 to 60 milliseconds) of the masking function so that the critical aspects of the masking function could be better mapped.

REFORMULATION OF BACKWARD MASKING IN SCHIZOPHRENIA

Based on the results of these experiments as well as the work of Breitmeyer and Ganz[5] and Braff et al,[19] we can refine our view of the nature of the schizophrenic performance deficit on visual masking procedures. This discussion will focus on schizophrenia, which has received the lion's share of the research. It may be too early to develop a formulation for masking performance in mania.

Our results indicate that visual masking performance deficits in schizophrenia probably involve abnormalities in the interruption of target processing. Specifically, what process is being interrupted? The traditional explanations for the masking deficit in schizophrenia have assumed that the problems begin after the icon of the target is clear and well formed. However, this assumption is inconsistent with the model of Breitmeyer and Ganz[5] presented in Figure 1, in which the icon is not formed instantaneously. Instead, the icon is formed in waves of neural activity that provide information of progressively higher spatial frequency. According to this model, the icon is "not a static representation but rather an ongoing, dynamic process,"[5(p226)] and it is this dynamic neural process that is interrupted by masking.

METHODOLOGICAL differences among studies of icon integrity in schizophrenia have been associated with differing results. For example, using a temporal integration technique, Knight et al[20] and Spaulding et al[21] found that icon storage and decay are intact in schizophrenia. Temporal integration involves the presentation of two separate stimuli separated by a brief ISI. Neither stimulus is interpretable by itself, but the two become a meaningful stimulus (picture or number) when they are integrated. In contrast with the temporal integration studies, Schwartz and Winstead[8] reported slower rates of visual decay in schizophrenic patients using a two-pulse temporal resolution task. In this task, two stimuli are presented with varying ISIs, and subjects decide whether they saw one or two stimuli. Both of these methods provide direct indices of visual persistence or icon *decay*, but they are not well suited for assessing the processes involved with the icon *formation*. The finding that schizophrenic patients show normal temporal integration[20,21] suggests that schizophrenic patients have normal visual persistence (ie, normal integration of sustained channel activity from successive stimuli), but it does not address the question of interruption. Likewise, the finding of slow icon decay rates with the temporal resolution task[8] does not address interruptive processes either, because interference with processing of a target stimulus was not assessed.

A plausible alternative is that icon formation in schizophrenic patients is especially susceptible to disruption, either because the process of icon formation of the target is fragile, or the effects of the mask are unusually disruptive. The latter explanation fits well with the growing literature on sensory gating abnormalities in schizophrenia.[19] Specifically, backward masking might be viewed as a special condition of the general phenomenon of sensory gating deficits in schizophrenia. In sensory gating experiments, schizophrenic patients usually fail to gate normally (ie, fail to attenuate) the second of two stimuli that are closely linked in time. One example of a sensory gating procedure is the startle-blink paradigm, in which electromyogram amplitude is measured to a blink-eliciting stimulus such as a loud tone. When the blink-eliciting stimulus is preceded by a prepulse, the amplitude of the blink is normally reduced. However, schizophrenic patients fail to attenuate the response to the second stimulus.[22] Interestingly, normal attenuation of the second stimulus is largest when the interval between the prepulse and blink-eliciting stimuli is around 60 to 120 milliseconds, an interval that is quite comparable to the time course of visual masking effects. Within the context of sensory gating, the backward masking deficits could be seen as a failure to attenuate the disruptive effects of the mask. At a physiological level, prepulse inhibition has been explained in terms of fast and slow neurons,[23] which is comparable to the explanation by Breit-

meyer and Ganz[5] of masking in terms of transient sustained visual channels.[19] The possibility that masking is a type of sensory gating abnormality could be tested by examining the degree of association between performance on backward masking and other sensory gating procedures.

IF THE BACKWARD masking deficit reflects a failure to attenuate the physiological events associated with the mask, we can predict that any alteration that increases the transient activity of the mask (and increases its ability to interrupt target processing) should increase the magnitude of the masking performance deficit. Although such data do not exist for schizophrenic patients, a relevant study was conducted in which undergraduates, who were considered schizotypal based on their responses to psychosis proneness scales, were compared with a control group.[24] Subjects received two backward masking procedures: one with a low spatial frequency mask and one with a high spatial frequency mask. The hypothesis was that the psychometrically defined schizotypal subjects would be especially susceptible to a mask of low spatial frequency, because it would increase transient channel activity. In fact, group differences were found for the low but not the high spatial frequency mask. The authors speculated that these presumed schizotypal subjects had overly active transient channels that were enhanced by the low spatial frequency mask.

The goal of the current study was to separate the effects of transient from sustained channels in visual masking. The next step will be to better characterize the nature of the abnormalities of the transient channels. At this point, it appears that suggestions of overly active transient channels[7,24] have merit. If we reconsider Figure 3 in our initial study,[4] the masking function of the patients in that relatively small subsample shows a more noticeable dip than that of the normal controls. Such a steep descending slope and slow ascending slope is consistent with overly active transient channels. Overly active transient channel response to the mask would be highly disruptive to the sustained channel response to the target and yield a more pronounced dip in the masking function.

Final interpretation of the source of the masking abnormality must await specialized masking procedures, such as forward and backward procedures with stimuli that rely on processing by transient channels. The hypothesis that transient activity is abnormally strong in schizophrenia leads to a specific and rather paradoxical prediction: under certain *forward* masking conditions, schizophrenic patients should have performance that is at least as good, and perhaps superior, to that of normal controls. In forward masking, the overly active transient activity of the target should be less susceptible to interruption by the sustained channels of the mask. We can predict a performance advantage in forward masking tasks that rely on transient channel activity (such as location tasks) and should occur as the ISIs approach 0 milliseconds (where the sustained channels of the mask would normally be disruptive to processing by the transient channel activity of the target).

CONCLUSIONS

In our initial study,[4] we addressed one limitation of the literature on early visual processing in schizophrenic patients. These studies have depended heavily on visual masking studies but have not separated masking by interruption and integration. We found substantial deficits under masking conditions that limited the mechanism to interruption. The current article addresses another limitation of this literature: the techniques have not allowed for the separation of transient and sustained visual channels. We reduced the role of sustained visual channels by lowering the spatial frequency of the target and also by using a location task. Schizophrenic patients continued to show deficits of comparable or greater magnitude under these conditions, suggesting that the relatively poor masking performance of schizophrenic patients may involve abnormalities in transient channels.

Our data indicate that masking performance deficits also occur with manic patients and are not specific to schizophrenia among the major psychotic disorders. We speculate that manic patients perform poorly on masking tasks for different reasons, possibly involving interruptive mechanisms when the processing of the target relies heavily on transient channels and/or right hemisphere processes.

Based on the results of the current experiments and theoretical contexts provided by Breitmeyer and Ganz,[5] Breitmeyer,[6] and Braff et al,[19] we propose the following hypotheses to serve as points of departure for future studies of visual masking in schizophrenia: (1) the schizophrenic deficit in masking paradigms involves some interruptive (not simply integrative) component; (2) the interruption affects icon formation (as opposed to posticonic processes); (3) backward masking procedures can be considered a special condition of a more general sensory gating deficit; (4) the deficits that patients show in these procedures may be explained by abnormalities in transient, not sustained, visual channels; and (5) the abnormality in transient channels may stem from overactive responses of the pathways.

Accepted for publication July 8, 1994.

Funding for this project came from grant MH-43292 of the National Institute of Mental Health, Rockville, Md (Dr Green).

The authors thank Maryam Aslani, David Chavez, Cynthia Christenson, Donna Gaier, Daniel Gutkind, Robert Kern, PhD, David King, PhD, Susan G. Hellman, Sharon Mitchell, MA, Chad Nelson, Julie Van Sickle, MA, and Jennifer Smith for their help in subject recruitment and data collection. Bruno Breitmeyer, PhD, provided valuable consultation on the design of this project and the interpretation of the results. The statistical analyses were conducted by Sun Hwang, MS, MPH, of the Methodology and Statistical Support Unit of the University of California–Los Angeles Clinical Research Center for the Study of Schizophrenia. The patients were recruited through the excellent cooperation of the staff and administration of Camarillo (Calif) State Hospital.

Reprint requests to University of California–Los Angeles Clinical Research Center, Box 6022, Camarillo, CA 93011 (Dr Green).

REFERENCES

1. Braff DL. Impaired speed of information processing in nonmedicated schizotypal patients. *Schizophr Bull.* 1981;7:499-508.
2. Green M, Walker E. Symptom correlates of vulnerability to backward masking in schizophrenia. *Am J Psychiatry.* 1986;143:181-186.
3. Saccuzzo DP, Braff DL. Early information processing deficit in schizophrenia. *Arch Gen Psychiatry.* 1981;38:175-179.
4. Green MF, Nuechterlein KH, Mintz J. Backward masking in schizophrenia and mania, I: specifying a mechanism. *Arch Gen Psychiatry.* 1994;51:939-944.
5. Breitmeyer BG, Ganz L. Implications of sustained and transient channels for theories of visual pattern masking, saccadic suppression, and information processing. *Psychol Rev.* 1976;83:1-36.
6. Breitmeyer BG. *Visual Masking: An Integrative Approach.* New York, NY: Oxford University Press; 1984.
7. Schuck JR, Lee RG. Backward masking, information processing, and schizophrenia. *Schizophr Bull.* 1989;15:491-500.
8. Schwartz BD, Winstead DK. Visual processing deficits in acute and chronic schizophrenics. *Biol Psychiatry.* 1982;17:1377-1387.
9. Schwartz BD, Winstead DK. Visible persistence in paranoid schizophrenics. *Biol Psychiatry.* 1988;23:3-12.
10. Bruder GE, Stewart JW, Towey JP, Friedman D, Tanke CE, Volgmaier MM, Leite P, Cohen P, Quitkin FM. Abnormal cerebral laterality in bipolar depression: convergence of behavioral and brain event–related potential findings. *Biol Psychiatry.* 1992;32:33-47.
11. Bruder GE, Quitkin FM, Stewart JW, Martin C, Volgmaier MM, Harrison WM. Cerebral laterality and depression: differences in perceptual asymmetry among diagnostic subtypes. *J Abnorm Psychology.* 1989;98:177-186.
12. Sergent J. The cerebral balance of power: confrontation or cooperation? *J Exp Psychol Hum Percept Perform.* 1982;8:253-272.
13. Hannay HJ, Varney NR, Benton AL. Visual localization in patients with unilateral brain disease. *J Neurol Neurosurg Psychiatry.* 1976;39:307-313.
14. Kimura D. Spatial localization in the left and right visual fields. *Can J Psychol.* 1969;23:445-458.
15. Kosslyn SM, Koenig O, Barrett A, Cave CB, Tang J, Gabrieli JDE. Evidence for two types of spatial representations: hemispheric specialization for categorical and coordinate relations. *J Exp Psychol Hum Percept Perform.* 1989;15:723-735.
16. Carlson GA, Goodwin FK. The stages of mania: a longitudinal analysis of the manic episode. *Arch Gen Psychiatry.* 1973;28:221-228.
17. Meltzer HY. Schizoaffective disorder: is the news of its nonexistence premature? *Schizophr Bull.* 1984;10:11-13.
18. Crow TJ. The continuum of psychosis and its implication for the structure of the gene. *Br J Psychiatry.* 1986;149:419-429.
19. Braff DL, Saccuzzo DP, Geyer MA. Information processing dysfunctions in schizophrenia: studies of visual backward masking, sensorimotor gating, and habituation. In: Steinhauer SR, Gruzelier JH, Zubin J, eds. *Handbook of Schizophrenia: Neuropsychology, Psychophysiology, and Information Processing.* Amsterdam, the Netherlands: Elsevier Science Publishing; 1991;5:303-334.
20. Knight R, Sherer M, Putchat C, Carter G. A picture integration task for measuring iconic memory in schizophrenics. *J Abnorm Psychol.* 1978;87:314-321.
21. Spaulding W, Rosenzweig L, Huntzinger R, Cromwell RL, Briggs D, Hayes T. Visual pattern integration in psychiatric patients. *J Abnorm Psychol.* 1980;89:635-643.
22. Braff DL, Grillon C, Geyer MA. Gating and habituation of the startle reflex in schizophrenic patients. *Arch Gen Psychiatry.* 1992;49:206-215.
23. Graham FK. The more or less startling effects of weak prestimuli. *Psychophysiology.* 1975;12:238-248.
24. Merritt RD, Balogh DW. Backward masking spatial frequency effects among hypothetically schizotypal individuals. *Schizophr Bull.* 1989;15:573-583.

Parsing Cognition

The Power of Psychology Paradigms

THE EARLIEST systematic descriptions of psychotic disorders noted that attention is disturbed in these conditions. Kraepelin,[1(p6)] for example, wrote that in schizophrenia, there is "a certain unsteadiness of attention" and it is quite difficult for these patients to "keep their attention fixed for any length of time." Kraepelin explained these variations in attention (*aufmerksamkeit* in German is less ambiguous than *attention* in English) as manifestations of impaired volition, even a kind of inattention, as it were, and therefore an epiphenomenon of the disorder. Recent explorations of schizophrenic psychopathology, however, strongly suggest that attentional dysfunctions are primary manifestations of the disease process in schizophrenia (as Bleuler[2] believed), and that the earliest as well as the later phases of attention are disordered, as exemplified in the studies by Green et al.[3,4]

The term "phases of attention" requires clarification. Until the middle of the 19th century, scientists believed that impulses were transmitted through the central nervous system at speeds that approached the speed of light. Hermann von Helmholtz, in the 1860s, was among the first to demonstrate that the journey of an impulse from the periphery to the brain took about 20 milliseconds. That discovery marked the beginning of what can be called the serial model of mental processing, which proposes that there is a series of successive stages between the appearance of a physical stimulus and the organism's response to it. Each stage that makes up the sequence takes a finite and measurable period of time. The model further assumes that these stages can be regarded as subsystems that have specialized functions for processing information. That there can be simultaneous, parallel processing of information from several input sources does not invalidate the assumption that serial processing also occurs.

Many cognitive scientists have studied this serial aspect of information processing, which informs our understanding of psychopathology in a "top down" manner, just as the biochemistry of the central nervous system informs us about psychopathology in a "bottom up" manner. The seminal work on mental chronometry by Posner[5] contains an extended discussion of the area, and readers are urged to peruse that work.

See also pages 939 and 945

Imagine that a small flying object appears suddenly in the periphery of one's visual field. Several events follow. First, the sensory system becomes activated, informing the organism that some event is occurring. This stage may be thought of as a reflexive organismic alerting response that prepares one to act with regard to the stimulus. It is induced primarily by the stimulus (although a state of preparedness or expectation can have an effect on the magnitude of the activation), and it can therefore be called an exogenous event. Next, attention is turned toward the disturbance, which may be accomplished by turning the eyes toward the external event, although eye movements are not always necessary, since attention can be engaged without them. This action makes possible the detection of the stimulus. Detection is then followed by identification or recognition of what the disturbance is—a mosquito! The detection and recognition stages are considered primarily endogenous, inasmuch as they make contact with the person's stored experiences, explicit and implicit. This modularization of information processing parallels the modularization of the brain itself.

The exact sequence and timing of these stages tend to vary with the particular sensory modality that is involved, but a roughly similar sequence of stages occurs in all sensory activity. It is therefore possible to trace the time course of information processing in the central nervous system by manipulating the time that a person has available to interact with a stimulus at any particular phase. This view implies that at one and the same time, information processing is a physiological and psychological activity that is detectable by experiments in both domains.

If all that is disordered in schizophrenic information processing is attention, and these patients are distracted (Kraepelin's *aufmerksamkeit*), then the issue is trivial. Patients who suffer from

almost any disease are distracted, preoccupied, and inattentive. However, if there is more to the claim of attentional dysfunction in schizophrenia, we are obliged to determine what aspects of this attentional process are impaired. Attention, then, becomes not necessarily an explanation of schizophrenic defect, but an arena for discovering which finer psychological processes are malfunctioning.

THE STAGE MODEL of information processing presents a rich scheme for reducing a global concept to manageable units of analysis, and that is the procedure adopted by Green et al[3,4] in their studies of backward masking in schizophrenia. The technique of backward masking controls the time that a person has available for processing a stimulus. Recall the example given above of the mosquito coming into view. Each phase of the processing sequence (activation, orientation, detection, and identification) takes time. The temporal epochs consume only fractions of a second, yet, as mentioned, any part of the sequence can be rather precisely measured. Since the entire sequence does not happen instantaneously, an experimenter can interrupt the sequence at any phase to test the status of the stimulus-generated event.

In the typical backward masking paradigm, the question asked is, "How long does it take for the processing of a stimulus to move from one phase to another?" The experimenter presents a stimulus, the letter *Q* for example, for a brief instant but long enough to be identified and recognized for what it is (the recognition threshold). After having determined what that recognition threshold is (it may be as short as 10 milliseconds), the experimenter presents Q again, but shortly after presents another letter, this time a *P*. At a particular interval that separates the presentation of the two stimuli, the first letter, Q, is not consciously seen. It is as if the letter had not been flashed at all. The second stimulus, the *P*, masked the Q, and one acceptable interpretation is that the second stimulus interrupted the processing of the information about the *Q* before it had reached the detection and identification stages. By manipulating the time interval during which the mask is effective, one can discover how long it takes for the first stimulus to progress to the recognition phase.

Almost a decade ago, Braff and Sacuzzo[6] reported that a backward visual mask had a greater effect on information processing of schizophrenic patients than on that of normal subjects. In schizophrenic patients, a mask presented as long as 500 milliseconds after the first stimulus was effective in interrupting processing, whereas in normal subjects, the mask ceased to be effective after about 100 milliseconds. It thus appeared that the identification of a stimulus is slower in schizophrenic patients than in normal subjects. That result required further probing and experimental manipulation to discover the process that produces the persistence of the masking effect in schizophrenic patients. Is the information processing stuck at the phase of orientation? Is the formation of the final percept interrupted prior to detection and recognition, and thus obliterated by the mask? Does the initial representation persist in a prerecognition stage for a longer than usual amount of time and therefore suffer the fate of interruption by the mask? Slowed recognition would reflect higher neural events; increased visual persistence of a representation would indicate problems at an early phase of the sequence. Either of these possibilities or both may be correct. Any of these explanations will move us further toward identifying the nature of the anomaly. This is the task that Green and colleagues[3,4] set for themselves, although they addressed other parts of the processing sequence.

In their first study, Green et al[3] tested whether the backward masking deficits in schizophrenic patients occur because the visual representations of the target stimulus and mask fuse with each other (integrate) or because the mask interrupts the information processing of the target just prior to the recognition stage. They manipulated the temporal proximity between target and mask and their relative intensities. Fusing of the target and mask is strongest when the mask overlaps the target spatially and when the time between target and mask is shortest. Interruption, they state, occurs at a slightly later stage of processing of the target and can be seen when the mask is relatively weak with respect to the target or when it does not spatially overlap the target. While they were not entirely successful in understanding the role of integration, they were able to show that interrupting the processing of the icon is a crucial factor in the backward masking deficit of schizophrenic patients because patients continue to show deficits when fusion of the target and mask does not occur. They also found that hospitalized patients with chronic mania showed similar interruption abnormalities.

In their second study, they focused on the earlier detection stages of information processing.[4] They accomplished this by requiring subjects simply to identify the presence and location of blurred targets (blurred by the experimenters to impede recognition) but not to recognize the targets. The authors presumed that this task taps transient rather than sustained visual channels. The former, sometimes referred to as magnocellular, are responsive to low spatial frequencies (or coarse features of a stimulus) and show a short response latency; the latter, sometimes referred to as parvocellular, are responsive to high spatial frequencies (or the finer details of a stimulus) and have longer response latencies. Schizophrenic patients were poorer than normal subjects in locating targets and identifying the blurred images, indicating that a performance deficit is present even at the early stages of processing. The patients with chronic mania, too, showed a deficit on this task. The evidence thus suggests that transient visual channels are disordered in schizophrenic patients, even when sus-

tained channels are not normally required. A similar but not identical pattern occurs in chronic mania. The experiments are, however, not yet decisive, and more refined work is necessary to understand the pathological process.

These studies are examples of a program of experimental "reductivism" that is required for discovering the essence of abnormalities in major behavioral disorders. The procedure is not a simple-minded reductionism that denies the reality of psychological events by rushing to translate them into physical events and thereby consider the psychological events as nothing but the physical ones. That is a vain and misguided exercise. The experimental reductivism described herein is an attempt to discover the smallest number of elements or units that make up a behavior and can explain how the more complex behaviors work. Such experimental reductivism sparks progress. The discovery by Watson and Crick of the double helix structure of DNA represents a triumph of such reductivism. In that case, the reductivist assertion is that living organisms from the simplest to the most complex can be explained as the outcome of a simple inherited design coded as four bases arranged as triads. Although they are a necessary cause of the organism, they must not be mistaken for the organism, any more than the function of attention should be mistaken for neural firing in a specific brain area.

My colleagues Levy[7] and Matthysse[8] have independently written about this method, which they have described as a parsing effort that dissects behavior into smaller but essential chunks whose lawfulness and interrelations can then be understood more clearly. Physicists use the term "coarse graining" to describe a similar method that searches for essential details of a process. They focus on increasingly simpler entities and then stop when the reductive process no longer yields useful information. In psychopathology, too, we can reach a level at which the successive parsing has reached its limit and the phenomenon of interest disappears, just as in the progressive enlargement of a photograph one reaches a point where only the grain but not the object becomes the image. This process of coarse graining of attention in schizophrenia informs us that the earliest exogenous as well as the later endogenous phases of attention are impaired. Cognitive psychological explorations will surely pursue the reductive or parsing process to discover the locus of the failures in the attentional system, which Kraepelin[1] and Bleuler[2] had earlier discussed. In this process, psychiatry relies on psychology as one of its basic sciences, and the articles by Green and colleagues[3,4] provide an instructive example of this reductive effort.

Philip S. Holzman, PhD
Laboratory of Psychology
McLean Hospital
115 Mill St
Belmont, Mass

Accepted for publication October 19, 1994.

Reprint requests to Dr Holzman.

REFERENCES

1. Kraepelin E; Barclay RM, trans. *Dementia Praecox and Paraphrenia.* Edinburgh, Scotland: S and S Livingstone; 1919.
2. Bleuler E; Zinkin H, trans. *Dementia Praecox or the Group of Schizophrenias.* New York, NY: International Universities Press;1911.
3. Green MF, Nuechterlein KH, Mintz J. Backward masking in schizophrenia and mania, I: specifying a mechanism. *Arch Gen Psychiatry.* 1994; 51:939-944.
4. Green MF, Nuechterlein KH, Mintz J. Backward masking in schizophrenia and mania, II: specifying the visual channels. *Arch Gen Psychiatry.* 1994;51:945-951.
5. Posner MI. *Chronometric Explorations of Mind.* Hillsdale, NJ: Lawrence Erlbaum & Associates; 1978.
6. Braff DS, Sacuzzo DP. The time course of information-processing deficits in schizophrenia. *Am J Psychiatry.* 1985;142:170-174.
7. Levy DL. Location, location, location: the pathway from behavior to brain locus in schizophrenia. In: Matthysse SW, Levy DL, Benes F, Kagan J, eds. *Psychopathology: The Evolving Science of Mental Disorder.* New York, NY: Cambridge University Press. In press.
8. Matthysse SW. *Drosophila* eye and the genetics of schizophrenia. In: Matthysse SW, Levy DL, Benes F, Kagan J, eds. *Psychopathology: The Evolving Science of Mental Disorder.* New York, NY: Cambridge University Press. In press.

ORIGINAL ARTICLE

Developmental Brain Abnormalities in the Offspring of Schizophrenic Mothers

II. Structural Brain Characteristics of Schizophrenia and Schizotypal Personality Disorder

Tyrone D. Cannon, PhD; Sarnoff A. Mednick, PhD, DrMed; Josef Parnas, MD; Fini Schulsinger, MD; Johannes Praestholm, MD; Aage Vestergaard, MD

Background: We examined differences in ventricular and sulcal cerebrospinal fluid-to-brain ratios as a function of lifetime psychiatric diagnosis in the offspring of schizophrenic mothers (high-risk sample) and in the offspring of normal parents (low-risk sample).

Methods: We used a cohort analytic study of 17 high-risk individuals with schizophrenia, 31 high-risk individuals with schizotypal personality disorder, 33 high-risk individuals with nonschizophrenia-spectrum psychiatric disorders, 45 high-risk individuals with no disorders, 31 low-risk individuals with psychiatric disorders of all types, and 46 low-risk individuals with no disorders, evaluated initially in 1962 when they were a mean age of 15 years, and reexamined from 1986 through 1989 with psychiatric interviews and computed tomographic scans of the brain.

Results: High-risk individuals with schizophrenia and schizotypal personality disorder evidenced an equivalent degree of cortical sulcal enlargement, and both groups evidenced significantly greater sulcal enlargement than did high-risk individuals with nonschizophrenia-spectrum disorders and no disorders and low-risk individuals with psychiatric disorders and no disorders. High-risk individuals with schizophrenia evidenced significantly greater ventricular enlargement than did high-risk and low-risk subjects with other disorders and no disorders, including those with schizotypal personality disorder. These differences were independent of age, gender, history of substance dependence, and history of organic brain syndromes and head injuries.

Conclusions: Among the offspring of schizophrenic parents, cortical abnormalities are expressed equally across the range of syndromes in the schizophrenia spectrum. Subcortical abnormalities (ie, ventricular enlargement) are more pronounced in the more severe syndrome (ie, schizophrenia).

(Arch Gen Psychiatry. 1994;51:955-962)

In the first report[1] of this series, we examined the contributions of genetic and perinatal factors to regional brain abnormalities in the offspring of schizophrenic and normal parents. Genetic risk for schizophrenia was found to be related to increased cerebrospinal fluid (CSF)–brain ratios in the sulcal regions of the cerebral cortex. That is, individuals with two affected parents evidenced greater cortical sulcal enlargement than did individuals with one affected parent, who in turn evidenced greater cortical sulcal enlargement than did individuals with no affected parents. In addition, genetic risk for schizophrenia and complications at delivery were found to interact in the prediction of the subcortical (ie, ventricular) CSF-brain ratio. The increase in the ventricular-brain ratio associated with delivery complications was greater among individuals with two affected parents compared with individuals with one affected parent, and greater among individuals with one affected parent compared with individuals with no affected parents. These effects were significant after controlling for age, gender, history of substance abuse, and history of organic brain syndromes and head injuries.

Together with the results of our earlier pilot study,[2,3] the findings just summarized support the hypothesis that cortical and subcortical brain abnormalities in schizophrenia result from the independent and interacting influences of genetic risk for schizophrenia and perinatal complications. The finding that the brain abnormalities were related to genetic and perinatal factors after controlling for ma-

From the Departments of Psychology and Psychiatry, University of Pennsylvania, Philadelphia (Dr Cannon); the Social Science Research Institute, University of Southern California, Los Angeles (Dr Mednick); and the Institute of Preventive Medicine, Copenhagen Health Services, Kommunehospitalet (Drs Parnas and Schulsiner), and Departments of Psychiatry (Drs Parnas and Schulsinger) and Diagnostic Radiology (Drs Praestholm and Vestergaard), Hvidovre Hospital, Copenhagen, Denmark.

See Subjects and Methods on next page

SUBJECTS AND METHODS

SUBJECTS

To identify early markers of schizophrenia, in 1962, Mednick and Schulsinger[14] initiated a prospective, longitudinal study of 207 HR children (offspring of severely schizophrenic mothers) and 104 matched LR controls. In 1962, the children were a mean age of 15.1 years (age range, 10 to 19 years), and none qualified for a psychiatric diagnosis. There have been two major diagnostic follow-ups since 1962. The first reevaluation[15] was conducted from 1972 through 1974 when the subjects were a mean age of 25 years. The second reevaluation[4] was conducted from 1986 through 1989 when the subjects were a mean age of 39 years and nearly through the risk period for developing schizophrenia. Included in this later follow-up was an assessment of structural brain abnormalities by computed tomographic (CT) scans. In addition to these major assessment waves, in 1980, we conducted a pilot CT examination on 34 HR subjects.[2,3]

PSYCHIATRIC DIAGNOSES

The 1972 through 1974 diagnostic assessment used two structured psychiatric interviews (Present State Examination[16] and Current and Past Psychopathology Scales[17]) and a set of additional items focusing on subschizophrenic characteristics.[15] The psychopathological data from this assessment have been converted into diagnoses according to *DSM-III-R*[18] criteria, as described in detail by Parnas et al.[4] The 1986 through 1989 diagnostic assessment consisted of three structured psychiatric interviews (Schedule for Affective Disorders and Schizophrenia-Lifetime version,[19] Present State Examination, and Personality Disorders Examination).[20] The interviewing psychiatrist assigned diagnoses using *DSM-III-R* criteria. At each assessment, the interviewing psychiatrist also prepared a detailed (four- to five-page) written summary of psychiatric, medical, social, educational, and occupational functioning for each subject. The written case summaries from each assessment were stripped of identifying and diagnostic information and were blindly reviewed by a team of noninterviewing investigators (T.D.C., S.A.M., and J.P.), who then assigned an independent set of *DSM-III-R* diagnoses for each case summary at each assessment. Comparison of the independently assigned diagnoses with the diagnoses assigned by the original interviewers indicated a high degree of diagnostic reliability (ie, mean κ coefficient of agreement, 0.95).[4] Although this procedure does not permit assessment of diagnostic reliability based on independent evaluations of the actual clinical interviews, the case summaries included detailed descriptions of psychiatric symptoms reported by the subject and observed by the interviewer during the interviews. The results of our reliability procedure are thus likely to be equivalent to one in which blind reviews of videotaped interviews are performed. It is important to note that in either procedure, the information used to assign independent diagnoses depends on the psychiatric symptoms elicited during the interviews by the interviewing psychiatrist.

For the purpose of this report, each subject was assigned a primary lifetime diagnosis representing his or her most severe Axis I or II diagnosis at either assessment wave. Since our hypotheses focus on spectrum disorders, SPD was considered primary to all disorders other than schizophrenia. If a subject had a diagnosis available for only one assessment, this diagnosis was used as the lifetime diagnosis. See the report by Parnas et al[4] for a comparison of morbid risks for schizophrenia and other diagnostic outcomes in the HR and LR samples.

CT SCAN PROCEDURES AND MEASUREMENTS

A total of 126 HR and 77 LR subjects underwent CT scanning as part of the 1986 through 1989 assessment. The lifetime *DSM-III-R* diagnoses of the HR subjects who were given a scan is as follows (the number of LR subjects are enclosed in parentheses): 17 with schizophrenia (n=1), 31 with SPD (n=4), 33 with nonspectrum psychiatric disorders (n=26), and 45 with no disorders (n=46). Subjects who were given a scan were representative of the original sample with respect to age, gender, risk status, lifetime psychiatric diagnosis, and history of perinatal complications.[1]

Scans were performed on a CT scanner (Somaton DRG, Siemens, Iselin, NJ) at Hvidovre Hospital in Copenhagen,

jor secondary contributors suggests that the abnormalities are at least in part neurodevelopmental in origin and may play a role in the cause of the disorder.

The purpose of this article is to report on differences in regional brain abnormalities as a function of lifetime diagnostic outcome in the offspring of schizophrenic and normal parents. The major advantage of the high-risk (HR) design in this context is that the subjects manifest the full range of disorders that are genetically linked to schizophrenia. It is thus possible to address the issue of how various brain abnormalities are expressed among the different clinical syndromes in the schizophrenia spectrum and to examine specificity of abnormalities to spectrum conditions in individuals with a schizophrenic parent. We can also assess specificity of schizophrenia-spectrum–related patterns of brain abnormalities with respect to demographically matched low-risk (LR) controls (some of whom have psychiatric disorders).

In view of the substantial body of evidence indicating a genetic relationship between schizophrenia and schizotypal personality disorder (SPD),[4-11] one would expect to find a similar distribution of the brain abnormalities that are related to genetic liability to schizophrenia among individuals with these conditions. Thus, we predicted that among the offspring of schizophrenic parents, those who develop schizophrenia and SPD will evidence an equivalent degree of cortical sulcal enlargement, and that both groups will evidence greater cortical sulcal enlargement than HR individuals with nonspectrum psychiatric disorders and no disorders, and LR individuals with psychiatric disorders and no disorders. In addition, in view of the finding that the HR individuals who developed schizophrenia suffered significantly more de-

Denmark. An average of 13 slices were taken parallel to the supraorbitomeatal line, each with a thickness of 8 mm and no overlap. Images were processed on a 256×256 matrix.

A semiautomated computer algorithm was used to obtain volumetric, area, and linear measurements of the CSF spaces in the regions of the ventricles and cortical sulci (both overall and for the frontal interhemispheric fissure and the right and left sylvian fissures separately), which were then expressed as percentages of (total or hemispheric) brain volume, area, and width, respectively. All measurements were then standardized to the same metric (ie, mean=5, SD=1). For the primary analyses (see below), we used the same standardized measures of ventricular-brain ratio and sulcal-brain ratio that were used in the first report in this series (where each measure represents the average of the standardized measures available for that region). Separate measures of the ventricular, sulcal, and brain components of these ratios were available only for the area and linear measurements. Unfortunately, the component measurements of the volumetric ratios were not saved independently in the scoring algorithm. Measurements of cerebellar CSF were also obtained but were not used in this report because we detected no association of abnormalities in this region with genetic risk for schizophrenia or perinatal complications. Intrarater and interrater reliabilities were adequate for all of the measurements (ie, intraclass correlations ranged from .73 to .99). A more detailed description of the CT scan assessment can be found in the report by Cannon et al.[1]

STATISTICAL ANALYSES

To test our hypotheses concerning differences in regional brain abnormalities by lifetime *DSM-III-R* diagnostic outcomes, we conducted a repeated-measures analysis of variance and covariance (ANCOVA), where brain region (ie, ventricular vs sulcal CSF-brain ratio) served as a within-subject variable. Preliminary analyses demonstrated no significant differences between the five LR subjects with spectrum disorders and the 26 LR subjects with nonspectrum psychiatric disorders (the mean of the former group was not higher than the mean of the latter group on any of the CT variables); these individuals were therefore collapsed into a single category of LR subjects with psychiatric disorders. The diagnosis variable contrasted the following six groups: (1) HR subjects with schizophrenia (n=17), (2) HR subjects with SPD (n=31), (3) HR subjects with nonspectrum psychiatric disorders (n=33), (4) HR subjects with no disorders (n=45), (5) LR subjects with psychiatric disorders (n=31), and (6) LR subjects with no disorders (n=46). In addition to testing the overall diagnosis effect, single *df* contrasts were performed comparing HR subjects with schizophrenia with the remaining subjects and comparing HR subjects with schizophrenia spectrum disorders (ie, schizophrenia and SPD combined) with the remaining subjects. Selectivity of the hypothesized diagnostic differences according to brain region was examined by comparing the strength of the relevant diagnostic contrast between the two brain regions (ie, CONTRAST option of the REPEATED statement[21]). Age (as a continuous variable), gender, history of substance dependence, and history of organic brain syndromes and head injuries were also modeled to determine whether any diagnostic differences were independent of these factors. In addition, since gender and history of substance dependence might be expected to have differential effects on brain morphological characteristics among different diagnostic classes (see the article by Flaum et al[22]), we examined the two-way interactions between diagnosis, gender, and history of substance dependence. The three-way interaction term (diagnosis by gender by history of substance dependence) was not modeled since some of the cell sizes were prohibitively low to provide a meaningful test (ie, included only one subject).

The analyses used type III (regression) sums of squares, which tests the significance of each effect controlling for all of the other effects in the model simultaneously. This approach is more conservative than the traditional type I (hierarchical) sums of squares, since the results are not unstable with respect to different ways of ordering the independent variables. Where significant effects were obtained, secondary analyses were conducted to determine if the effects pertained exclusively (or more strongly) to the CSF or brain components of each measure or to a particular cortical lobe or cerebral hemisphere.

The above analyses were repeated, excluding the subjects who had undergone scanning as part of our 1980 pilot study.[2,3] This provided a test of the independence of the findings.

livery complications than did those with other outcomes,[12,13] one would expect to find a dissimilar distribution of the brain abnormalities linked to delivery complications among individuals with schizophrenia compared with those with other diagnoses. Thus, we predicted that HR individuals with schizophrenia will evidence a greater degree of ventricular enlargement than HR individuals with SPD, nonspectrum psychiatric disorders, and no disorders, and LR individuals with psychiatric disorders and no disorders.

RESULTS

SAMPLE CHARACTERISTICS

Table 1 provides a breakdown of the major demographic characteristics of the sample. There were no differences in age, gender, or parental socioeconomic status among the six diagnostic subgroups. The prevalence of history of substance dependence was equivalent among subjects with psychiatric disorders of any type. More than 90% of the substance disorders in this sample pertained to alcohol. The remainder pertained to cannabis and opiates. A larger percentage of HR subjects with schizophrenia and LR subjects with psychiatric disorders had histories of organic brain syndromes and head injuries compared with the other groups.

DIAGNOSTIC COMPARISONS

Ventricular and Sulcal CSF-Brain Ratios

Table 2 gives the results of the repeated-measures ANCOVA examining ventricular and sulcal CSF-brain ra-

Table 1. Demographic Characteristics of the Six Diagnostic Subgroups*

	High-Risk Group				Low-Risk Group	
	Schizophrenia	SPD	Nonspectrum Disorders	No Disorders	Psychiatric Disorders	No Disorders
No. of subjects	17	31	33	45	31	46
Female, No. (%)†	6 (35.3)	9 (29.0)	14 (41.4)	26 (57.7)	14 (45.2)	20 (43.5)
Substance dependence, No. (%)‡	5 (29.4)	4 (12.9)	5 (14.7)	0 (0)	7 (22.6)	0 (0)
Organic brain syndrome or head injury, No. (%)§	4 (23.5)	4 (12.9)	3 (8.8)	1 (2.2)	5 (16.1)	0 (0)
Mean (SD) age, y‖	37.9 (3.4)	38.9 (3.5)	38.9 (3.4)	38.7 (2.9)	38.2 (3.2)	38.8 (3.1)
Mean (SD) parental socioeconomic status¶	2.0 (1.8)	2.0 (2.0)	1.9 (1.9)	2.2 (1.8)	2.0 (2.1)	2.2 (1.9)

*SPD indicates schizotypal personality disorder. Mean parental socioeconomic status is based on a scale of 0 (low) to 6 (high).
†$\chi^2[5]=6.9$, $P=.23$.
‡$\chi^2[3]=2.6$, $P=.45$.
§$\chi^2[5]=14.8$, $P<.01$.
‖$F[5,197]=0.5$, $P=.77$.
¶$F[5,197]=0.1$, $P=.98$.

tios as a function of age, history of organic brain syndromes and head injuries, gender, history of substance dependence, and lifetime psychiatric diagnosis. There was a significant overall main effect of diagnosis, and significant overall contrasts between HR subjects with schizophrenia vs the other diagnostic categories and between HR subjects with spectrum disorders vs the other diagnostic categories. The region by diagnosis interaction term was not significant. There was, however, a significant interaction between region and the contrast comparing HR subjects with spectrum disorders with the remaining subjects, such that sulcal enlargement was more strongly associated with spectrum disorder outcome than was ventricular enlargement.

The mean (±SEM) standardized ventricular and sulcal CSF-brain ratios of the six diagnostic subgroups are shown in **Figure 1**. High-risk subjects with schizophrenia had significantly higher ventricular-brain ratios than did HR subjects with SPD, HR subjects with nonspectrum psychiatric disorders, HR subjects with no disorders, LR subjects with psychiatric disorders, and LR subjects with no disorders (who did not differ significantly from each other). High-risk subjects with schizophrenia and SPD did not differ from each other on the sulcal measure, and both groups had significantly higher scores on this measure than did HR subjects with nonspectrum psychiatric disorders, HR subjects with no disorders, LR subjects with psychiatric disorders, and LR subjects with no disorders (who did not differ significantly from each other).

While the main effects of history of substance dependence and the other secondary contributors were not significant, there was a trend for history of substance dependence to interact with diagnosis independently of brain region (*P*<.06). When this interaction term was decomposed by comparing subjects with and without substance dependence on overall CSF-brain ratio (ie, average of ventricular and sulcal CSF-brain ratios) within each diagnostic class, the history of substance dependence effect was significant only among the HR subjects with schizophrenia. As shown in **Figure 2**, substance dependence is associated with a significant increase in overall CSF-brain ratio among HR subjects with schizophrenia but not among the remaining subjects. Figure 2 also shows that HR subjects with schizophrenia who did not have a history of substance dependence had larger overall CSF-brain ratios than did subjects with other diagnostic outcomes, regardless of substance dependence status. This difference was significant only in comparison with subjects with other outcomes who did not have a history of substance dependence.

Ventricular, Sulcal, and Brain Components

Secondary analyses were conducted to determine if the diagnostic differences noted above pertained exclusively (or more strongly) to the CSF or brain components of each ratio. In an ANCOVA, identical to the one just described but this time using the ventricular and sulcal CSF area measures uncorrected for brain area, all effects were the same as in the analysis of the measures expressed as ratios to brain. **Figure 3** shows the mean (±SEM) standardized ventricular, sulcal, and brain area measures of the six diagnostic subgroups. The diagnostic differences on the ventricular and sulcal CSF measures uncorrected for brain area follow the same pattern as those observed on the corresponding ratio measures. In contrast, HR subjects with schizophrenia and SPD did not differ from each other or from any of the other diagnostic subgroups in terms of brain area (the contrast between HR subjects with schizophrenia and HR subjects with no disorders approached significance; *P*<.08). Low-risk subjects with no disorders had a significantly larger mean brain area than did HR subjects with nonspectrum psychiatric disorders, HR subjects with no disorders, and LR subjects with psychiatric disorders.

Regional Cortical and Hemispheric Differences

Secondary analyses were also conducted on the temporal and frontal fissure measures and on the right and left hemisphere measures of the cortical sulci, temporal fissures, and lateral ventricles. In the former case, lobe served as a repeated-measures variable, and in the latter cases,

Table 2. Results of Repeated-Measures Analysis of Variance and Covariance on Ventricular and Sulcal CSF-Brain Ratios*

	Total Sample (n=203)			Replication Sample (n=178)		
Source	df	MS	F	df	MS	F
Factor						
Age	1	0.58	0.63	1	1.69	1.97
Organic brain syndrome or head injury	1	0.23	0.25	1	0.11	0.13
Gender	1	2.15	2.34	1	0.06	0.06
Substance dependence	1	0.71	0.77	1	1.62	1.89
Diagnosis	5	3.17	3.44†	5	1.73	2.02‡
Gender × substance dependence	1	0.11	0.12	1	0.95	1.10
Gender × diagnosis	5	0.10	0.11	5	0.57	0.66
Substance dependence × diagnosis	3	2.34	2.54§	3	2.19	2.56§
Error	184	0.92	...	159	0.86	...
Diagnostic contrast: schizophrenia	1	13.20	14.35‖	1	6.14	7.14†
Diagnostic contrast: spectrum	1	17.96	19.52‖	1	7.35	8.55†
Region	1	0.48	1.33	1	0.44	1.25
Region × age	1	0.66	1.83	1	0.78	2.22
Region × organic brain syndrome/head injury	1	0.01	0.02	1	0.05	0.13
Region × gender	1	0.00	0.00	1	0.03	0.08
Region × substance dependence	1	0.46	1.25	1	0.78	2.23
Region × diagnosis	5	0.41	1.14	5	0.42	1.19
Region × gender × substance dependence	1	0.11	0.30	1	0.06	0.16
Region × gender × diagnosis	5	0.13	0.36	5	0.14	0.40
Region × substance dependence × diagnosis	3	0.16	0.44	3	0.47	1.34
Error	184	0.36	...	159	0.35	...
Region × diagnostic contrast: schizophrenia	1	0.11	0.31	1	0.88	2.51
Region × diagnostic contrast: spectrum	1	1.53	4.25¶	1	2.73	7.80†

**CSF indicates cerebrospinal fluid; MS, mean square; diagnostic contrast: schizophrenia, the contrast testing for the difference between subjects with schizophrenia vs all other subjects (combined); and diagnostic contrast: spectrum, the contrast testing for the difference between subjects with schizophrenia and spectrum personality disorders (combined) vs all other subjects (combined).*

†$P<.01$.
‡$P<.08$.
§$P<.06$.
‖$P<.001$.
¶$P<.05$.

hemisphere served as a repeated-measures variable. These analyses did not produce interactions involving lobe or hemisphere and recapitulated the results reported above with respect to the corresponding measurements collapsed across lobe and hemisphere.

Treatment and Illness Variables

Among the 17 HR subjects with schizophrenia diagnoses, there were no significant correlations between any of the CT measures (ie, ventricular CSF-brain ratio, sulcal CSF-brain ratio, ventricular area, sulcal area, and brain area) and age at onset, duration of illness, or duration of neuroleptic treatment (all ρ values=−0.38 to 0.01, all *P* values>.10). There were also no significant correlations between any of the CT measures and severity of positive and negative symptoms in the 1972 through 1974 or 1986 through 1989 assessments (all ρ values=−0.41 to 0.40, all *P* values>.10). (The description of the positive and negative symptom scales is found in the article by Cannon and Mednick.[23])

Replication Analyses

As mentioned previously, 34 HR subjects were given CT scans in our 1980 pilot study.[2,3] The 1980 psychiatric diagnoses of these 34 subjects were as follows: 10 with schizophrenia, 10 with SPD, and 14 with no disorders. Twenty-five of these 34 subjects were also given CT scans in the 1986 through 1989 assessment and were used in the present report. (Only 19 of the 25 overlapping subjects had all of the relevant birth information available for the previous report in this series[1]; thus, only 19 subjects were excluded for the replication portion of that report.) The 1980 psychiatric diagnoses of these 25 subjects were as follows: eight with schizophrenia, eight with SPD, and nine with no disorders.

The above analyses were repeated, excluding these 25 subjects. The results are shown in the right-hand section of Table 2. The overall main effect of diagnosis was reduced to a trend (*P*<.06), but the overall contrasts comparing HR subjects with schizophrenia with the other diagnostic subgroups and comparing HR subjects with spectrum disorders with the other subgroups remained significant. In addition, the interaction between region and the contrast comparing subjects with spectrum disorders with the other subgroups remained significant, confirming that spectrum disorder outcome is more strongly related to sulcal enlargement than to ventricular enlargement.

COMMENT

Adult offspring of schizophrenic parents were found to express different patterns of neuroanatomical

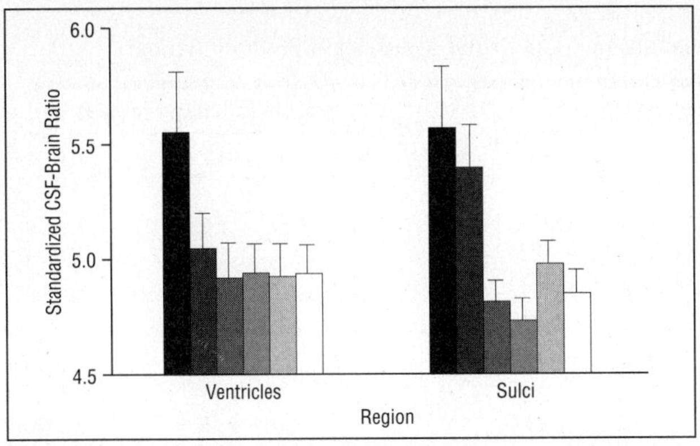

Figure 1. *Mean (±SEM) standardized ventricular and sulcal cerebrospinal fluid (CSF)–brain ratios by lifetime* DSM-III-R[18] *diagnosis. The groups compared, from right to left, are: high-risk subjects with schizophrenia, high-risk subjects with schizotypal personality disorder, high-risk subjects with nonspectrum psychiatric disorders, high-risk subjects with no disorders, low-risk subjects with psychiatric disorders, and low-risk subjects with no disorders. Pairwise* t *tests indicated that the schizophrenic group was significantly different from each of the other five groups on the ventricular measure and that the schizophrenic and schizotypal personality disorder groups did not differ from each other and were significantly different from the other four groups on the sulcal measure.*

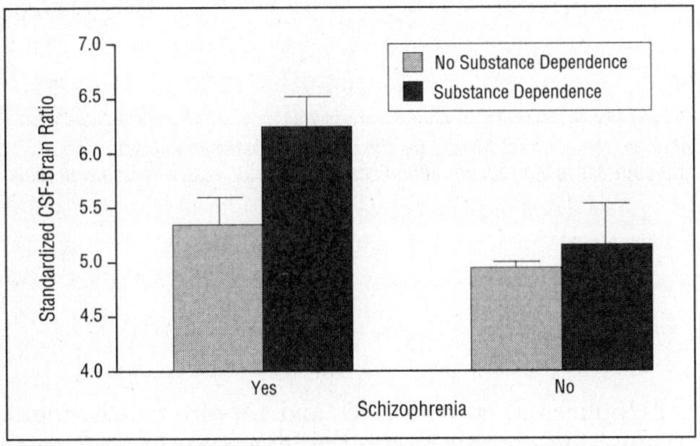

Figure 2. *Mean (±SEM) standardized overall cerebrospinal fluid (CSF)–brain ratios (ie, average of ventricular and sulcal CSF-brain ratios) by schizophrenia diagnosis and substance dependence status. A history of substance dependence was associated with a significant increase in overall CSF-brain ratio among the schizophrenic subjects, but not among the remaining subjects. Schizophrenic subjects without histories of substance dependence had significantly larger overall CSF-brain ratios than did the nonschizophrenic subjects without histories of substance dependence.*

abnormality on CT scans, depending on their diagnostic outcome as follows: (1) those with diagnoses of schizophrenia and SPD evidenced significantly greater sulcal enlargement than did those with nonspectrum psychiatric disorders and no disorders, and matched LR offspring with psychiatric disorders and no disorders; and (2) those with schizophrenia evidenced significantly greater ventricular enlargement than did those with SPD, nonspectrum pychiatric disorders, and no disorders, and LR offspring with psychiatric disorders and no disorders. These effects were evident with and without correction for brain size and persisted after controlling for the effects of age, gender, history of substance dependence, and history of organic brain syndromes or head injuries. Together, these results suggest that while cortical abnormalities are expressed equally across the range of syndromes in

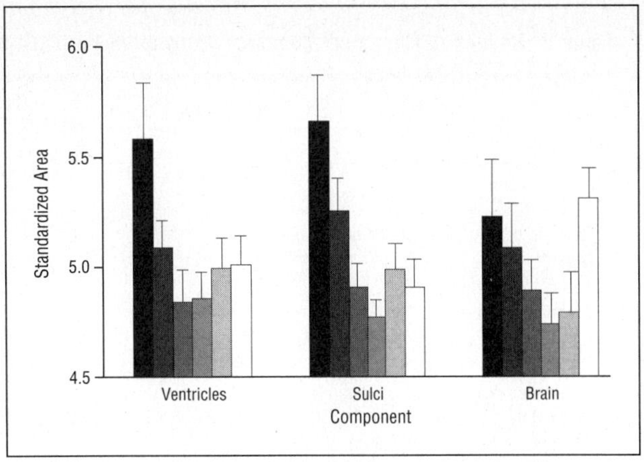

Figure 3. *Mean (±SEM) standardized ventricular cerebrospinal fluid (CSF), sulcal CSF, and brain areas (at the cella media level) by lifetime* DSM-III-R[18] *diagnosis. The groups compared are as described in Figure 1. Pairwise* t *tests indicated that the schizophrenic group was significantly different from each of the other five groups on the ventricular measure, that the schizophrenic and schizotypal personality disorder groups did not differ from each other and were significantly different from the other four groups on the sulcal measure, and that the low-risk subjects with no disorders were significantly different from the high-risk subjects with nonspectrum disorders and no disorders and from the low-risk subjects with psychiatric disorders on the brain area measure.*

the schizophrenia spectrum, subcortical abnormalities (ie, ventricular enlargement) are more pronounced in the more severe syndrome (ie, *DSM-III-R* schizophrenia).

These findings are consistent with a previously proposed diathesis-stress model of schizophrenia-spectrum disorders.[2,13,23] According to this model, schizophrenia and SPD are unified by a common genetic diathesis, one expression of which is cellular migratory failure and other signs of dysgenesis in various regions of the cerebral cortex. Among individuals with this genetic diathesis, those who experience severe delivery complications develop subcortical abnormalities in addition to the genetically mediated cortical abnormalities; the subcortical abnormalities then contribute to the development of overt schizophrenia.

The two reports in this series further substantiate this model by demonstrating that (1) cortical abnormalities increase in severity with increasing level of genetic risk for schizophrenia and are expressed equally among individuals with diagnoses of schizophrenia and SPD, and (2) ventricular enlargement is predicted primarily by the interaction of genetic risk for schizophrenia and perinatal complications and is expressed more severely among individuals with diagnoses of schizophrenia compared with those with SPD. The findings thus support the status of cortical and subcortical structural abnormalities as markers of basic pathophysiologic influences in the schizophrenia spectrum. Further work is needed to investigate whether the brain abnormalities are themselves pathophysiologic mechanisms (ie, with cortical abnormalities underlying behavioral characteristics common to the schizophrenia spectrum and subcortical abnormalities underlying behavioral characteristics specific to schizophrenia). See the study by Mirsky et al[24] for preliminary evidence consistent with this hypothesis.

The finding that sulcal prominence and ventricular enlargement are equally sensitive as indicators of schizophrenia is contrary to the conclusion of a quantitative review[25] that noted that the effect size associated with sulcal prominence in imaging studies of schizophrenia is smaller than that associated with ventricular enlargement. However, most of the studies included in the review used width measurements of the broadest visible sulci. The method of measurement is known to influence the sensitivity of structural brain indexes as illness markers, with volumetric measures superior to area measures, and area measures superior to linear measures.[26] All three approaches to quantitation of the ventricular and sulcal CSF spaces were used in the present study. It is also important to note that in more recent studies with magnetic resonance imaging (which has greater contrast and spatial resolution than CT), increased sulcal CSF volume[27] and reduced cortical tissue volume, particularly in the left temporal lobe,[28-33] have been consistently reported. That the diagnostic differences in this study were not specific with respect to cortical lobe or cerebral hemisphere may reflect the lower contrast and spatial resolution of CT compared with magnetic resonance imaging studies.

THE DIAGNOSTIC differences in this study were independent of several secondary contributors to brain abnormalities (ie, age, gender, history of substance dependence, history of organic brain syndromes or head injuries). In addition, there were no significant correlations between the brain abnormalities and several indexes of treatment and chronicity within the schizophrenic group. There was, however, a significant interaction between history of substance dependence (primarily alcohol in this sample) and diagnosis, such that substance dependence was associated with significantly larger overall CSF-brain ratios among HR subjects with schizophrenia, but not among any of the other diagnostic subgroups. The meaning of this effect is not entirely clear. It is possible that prolonged exposure to alcohol (and possibly other substances) interacts with factors that predispose to schizophrenia and thereby magnifies the extent of brain abnormalities in these subjects. It is also possible that the schizophrenic patients with histories of substance dependence were more severely affected with the illness, in which case history of substance dependence may not play a direct role but may merely mark a proportion of the schizophrenic population with a more severe form of the disease. In any case, it is important to emphasize that schizophrenic patients without histories of substance dependence still had larger overall CSF-brain ratios than did nonschizophrenic subjects, regardless of substance dependence status, although this effect was significant only in comparison to the nonschizophrenic subjects without a history of substance dependence. This result indicates that some portion of the structural brain abnormalities in schizophrenia is independent of the effects of substance dependence.

In the present study, the offspring of schizophrenic parents who developed SPD had significantly greater sulcal enlargement than did those with nonspectrum outcomes, but did not differ from nonspectrum HR subjects (and LR subjects) in terms of ventricular enlargement. In our earlier pilot study[2] using a subsample of this cohort, subjects with SPD had smaller (but not significantly so) mean ventricle-brain ratios than did HR subjects with no mental illness, and did not differ from nonmentally ill subjects in terms of cortical sulcal prominence. Discrepancies between the present findings and those of the pilot study are most likely owing to an increase in sample size and statistical power (ie, the group sizes are three to five times greater) and the use of a superior method of quantitation in the present study.

Two other studies have examined structural abnormalities in individuals with SPD or schizotypal traits who were recruited from community or psychiatric samples. Raine et al[34] found an association between schizotypal traits and reduced frontal lobe volume on magnetic resonance imaging scan in a college population. This effect would appear to be consistent with the present findings in implicating cortical abnormalities in SPD. In a preliminary study using a sample of clinic patients meeting *DSM-III-R* criteria for SPD, Rotter et al[35] found significantly larger lateral ventricular and frontal horn areas in patients with SPD compared with normal controls. This result is contrary to the findings of the present study in which the offspring of schizophrenic parents who developed SPD did not differ from normal HR or LR subjects in terms of ventricular enlargement, a discrepancy that may be accounted for by differences in the nature of the study populations (ie, clinic patients with SPD vs the offspring of schizophrenic parents with SPD). Unfortunately, the study by Rotter et al[35] did not attempt to examine sulcal abnormalities in the schizotypal sample.

In summary, HR subjects who developed schizophrenia and SPD were found to show a similar degree of cortical sulcal prominence, with both groups showing significantly greater sulcal prominence than HR and LR subjects with other disorders and no disorders; in contrast, ventricular enlargement was more pronounced in HR subjects who developed schizophrenia compared with those with SPD and with HR and LR subjects with other disorders and no disorders.

Accepted for publication August 24, 1994.

This research was supported by grant R29 MH 48207 (Dr Cannon), grant R01 37692 and Research Scientist Award 1 K05 MH 00619 (Dr Mednick), and grant R01 MH 41469 (Dr Parnas) from the National Institute of Mental Health, Bethesda, Md.

Reprint requests to Department of Psychology, University of Pennsylvania, 3815 Walnut St, Philadelphia, PA 19104-6196 (Dr Cannon).

REFERENCES

1. Cannon TD, Mednick SA, Parnas J, Schulsinger F, Praestholm J, Vestergaard A. Developmental brain abnormalities in the offspring of schizophrenic mothers, I: contributions of genetic and perinatal factors. *Arch Gen Psychiatry.* 1993; 50:551-564.
2. Cannon TD, Mednick SA, Parnas J. Genetic and perinatal determinants of structural brain deficits in schizophrenia. *Arch Gen Psychiatry.* 1989;46:883-889.

3. Schulsinger F, Parnas J, Petersen ET, Schulsinger H, Teasdale TW, Mednick SA, Moller L, Silverton L. Cerebral ventricular size in the offspring of schizophrenic mothers. *Arch Gen Psychiatry.* 1984;41:602-606.
4. Parnas J, Cannon TD, Jacobsen B, Schulsinger H, Schulsinger F, Mednick SA. Lifetime *DSM-III-R* diagnostic outcomes in the offspring of schizophrenic mothers: results from the Copenhagen high-risk study. *Arch Gen Psychiatry.* 1993; 50:707-714.
5. Kety SS. The significance of genetic factors in the etiology of schizophrenia: results from the national study of adoptees in Denmark. *J Psychiatr Res.* 1987; 4:423-429.
6. Farmer AE, McGuffin P, Gottesman II. Twin concordance for *DSM-III* schizophrenia. *Arch Gen Psychiatry.* 1987;44:634-641.
7. Kendler KS, Gruenberg AM, Strauss JS. An independent analysis of the Copenhagen sample of the Danish Adoption Study of schizophrenia, II: the relationship between schizotypal personality disorder and schizophrenia. *Arch Gen Psychiatry.* 1981;38:982-984.
8. Baron M, Gruen R, Asnis L, Kane J. Familial relatedness of schizophrenia and schizotypal states. *Am J Psychiatry.* 1983;140:1437-1442.
9. Siever LJ, Silverman JM, Horvath TB, Klar H, Coccaro E, Keefe RSE, Pinkham L, Rinaldi P, Mohs RC, Davis KL. Increased morbid risk for schizophrenia-related disorders in relatives of schizotypal personality disordered patients. *Arch Gen Psychiatry.* 1990;47:634-640.
10. Thaker G, Adami H, Moran M, Lahti A, Cassady S. Psychiatric illnesses in families of subjects with schizophrenia-spectrum personality disorders: high morbidity risks for unspecified functional psychoses and schizophrenia. *Am J Psychiatry.* 1993;150:66-71.
11. Kendler KS, McGuire M, Gruenberg AM, O'Hare A, Spellman M, Walsh D. The Roscommon Family Study, III: schizophrenia-related personality disorders in relatives. *Arch Gen Psychiatry.* 1993;50:781-788.
12. Parnas J, Schulsinger F, Teasdale TW, Schulsinger H, Feldman PM, Mednick SA. Perinatal complications and clinical outcome within the schizophrenia spectrum. *Br J Psychiatry.* 1982;140:416-420.
13. Cannon TD, Mednick SA, Parnas J. Antecedents of predominantly negative- and predominantly positive-symptom schizophrenia in a high-risk population. *Arch Gen Psychiatry.* 1990;47:622-632.
14. Mednick SA, Schulsinger F. A longitudinal study of children with a high risk for schizophrenia: a preliminary report. In: Vandenberg S, ed. *Methods and Goals in Human Behavior Genetics.* Orlando, Fla: Academic Press Inc; 1965:255-296.
15. Schulsinger H. A ten-year follow-up of children of schizophrenic mothers: clinical assessment. *Acta Psychiatr Scand.* 1976;53:371-386.
16. Wing JK, Cooper JE, Sartorious N. *The Measurement and Classification of Psychiatric Symptoms.* London, England: Cambridge University Press; 1974.
17. Endicott J, Spitzer R. Current and past psychopathology scales (CAPPS). *Arch Gen Psychiatry.* 1972;27:678-687.
18. American Psychiatric Association. *Diagnostic and Statistical Manual of Mental Disorders, Revised Third Edition.* Washington, DC: American Psychiatric Association; 1987.
19. Spitzer RL, Endicott J. *Schedule for Affective Disorders and Schizophrenia—Lifetime Version.* New York: New York Psychiatric Institute; 1978.
20. Loranger AW, Sussman VL, Oldham JM, Russakoff LM. *Personality Disorder Examination: A Structured Interview for Making Diagnosis of DSM-III-R Personality Disorders.* White Plains, NY: Cornell Medical College; 1985.
21. *SAS/STAT User's Guide.* Cary, NC: SAS Institute; 1988.
22. Flaum M, Arndt S, Andreasen NC. The role of gender in studies of ventricle enlargement in schizophrenia: a predominantly male effect. *Am J Psychiatry.* 1990;147:1327-1332.
23. Cannon TD, Mednick SA. The schizophrenia high-risk project in Copenhagen: three decades of progress. *Acta Psychiatr Scand.* 1993;370:33-47.
24. Mirsky AF, Lochhead SJ, Jones BP, Kugelmass S, Walsh D, Kendler KS. On familial factors in the attentional deficit in schizophrenia: a review and report of two new subject samples. *J Psychiatr Res.* 1992;26:383-403.
25. Raz S, Raz N. Structural brain abnormalities in the major psychoses: a quantitative review of the evidence from computerized imaging. *Psychol Bull.* 1990; 108:93-108.
26. Raz S, Raz N, Weinberger DR, Boronow J, Pickar D, Bigler ED, Turkheimer E. Morphological brain abnormalities in schizophrenia determined by computed tomography: a problem of measurement? *Psychiatry Res.* 1987;22:91-98.
27. Gur RE, Mozley PD, Resnick SM, Shtasel D, Kohn M, Zimmerman R, Herman G, Atlas S, Grossman R, Erwin R, Gur RC. Magnetic resonance imaging in schizophrenia, I: volumetric analysis of brain and cerebrospinal fluid. *Arch Gen Psychiatry.* 1991;48:407-412.
28. DeLisi LE, Hoff AL, Schwartz JE, Shields GW, Halthore SN, Gupta SM, Henn FA, Anand AK. Brain morphology in first-episode schizophrenic-like psychotic patients: a quantitative magnetic resonance imaging study. *Biol Psychiatry.* 1991; 29:159-175.
29. Dauphinais ID, DeLisi LE, Crow TJ, Alexandropoulos K, Colter N, Tuma I, Gershon E. Reduction in temporal lobe size in siblings with schizophrenia: a magnetic resonance imaging study. *Psychiatry Res.* 1990;35:137-147.
30. Johnstone EC, Owens DG, Crow TJ, Frith CD, Alexandropolis K, Bydder G, Colter N. Temporal lobe structure as determined by nuclear magnetic resonance in schizophrenia and bipolar affective disorder. *J Neurol Neurosurg Psychiatry.* 1989;52:736-741.
31. Rossi A, Stratta P, D'Albenzio L, Tartaro A, Schiazza G, di Michele V, Bolino F, Casacchia M. Reduced temporal lobe areas in schizophrenia: preliminary evidences from a controlled multiplanar magnetic resonance imaging study. *Biol Psychiatry.* 1990;27:61-68.
32. Rossi A, Stratta P, di Michele V, Gallucci M, Splendiani A, de Cataldo S, Casacchia M. Temporal lobe structure by magnetic resonance in bipolar affective disorders and schizophrenia. *J Affect Disord.* 1991;21:19-22.
33. Suddath RL, Casanova MF, Goldberg TE, Daniel DG, Kelsoe JR Jr, Weinberger DR. Temporal lobe pathology in schizophrenia: a quantitative magnetic resonance imaging study. *Am J Psychiatry.* 1989;146:464-472.
34. Raine A, Sheard C, Reynolds GP, Lencz T. Pre-frontal structural and functional deficits associated with individual differences in schizotypal personality. *Schizophr Res.* 1992;7:237-247.
35. Rotter M, Kalus O, Losonczy M, Guo L, Trestman RL, Coccaro E, Davidson M, Davis KL, Siever LJ. Lateral ventricle enlargement in schizotypal personality disorder. *Biol Psychiatry.* 1991;29(addendum issue):43a-185a.

Clinical Characteristics and Predisposing Factors in Acute Drug-Induced Akathisia

Perminder Sachdev, MD, PhD, FRANZCP, Jane Kruk, BSc(Hons)

Background: As subtypes of drug-induced akathisia have become accepted and attempts have been made at establishing diagnostic criteria, a prospective study of the clinical features and predisposing factors of acute akathisia is a significant deficiency in the literature.

Methods: One hundred consecutive inpatients with nonorganic psychotic disorders, not receiving neuroleptics or other drugs and free of akathisia and related disorders at admission, were assessed for psychiatric status and movement disorders at baseline and daily for 2 weeks, with detailed examinations on days 7 and 14. Multiple operational criteria for akathisia were used. The following risk factors were examined: age, sex, current neuroleptic dose, rate of increment of dose, drug type, duration of illness, past use of neuroleptics, extrapyramidal side effects score, Zung Depression Scale score, Spielberger State Anxiety Inventory score, psychosis score, and smoking.

Results: Using a global rating, mild akathisia developed in 41% and moderate-to-severe akathisia in 21%. The symptoms that best discriminated akathisia from nonakathisia were shifting weight from foot to foot or walking on the spot, inability to keep legs still, feelings of inner restlessness, and shifting of body position in the chair. The subjective and objective symptoms loaded on separate factors. Akathisia ratings had low correlations with the anxiety and Zung scores. Receiver operating characteristic analysis suggested a cutoff score of 4 on our 10-item Akathisia Scale as optimal for the diagnosis of akathisia, with a stricter criterion of scores of 2 or more on both the subjective and objective items being more suitable for research diagnosis. The most significant predisposing factors were the extrapyramidal side effects score and current neuroleptic dose and its rate of increment, with lesser contributions from serum iron status and medication type. Predictability was, however, modest.

Conclusion: Acute akathisia is a common syndrome with well-defined clinical features. Its occurrence can be predicted with only modest accuracy.

(Arch Gen Psychiatry. 1994;51:963-974)

From the Neuropsychiatric Institute, The Prince Henry Hospital, Matraville, New South Wales (Dr Sachdev), and the School of Psychiatry, University of New South Wales, Sydney (Dr Sachdev and Ms Kruk), Australia.

AKATHISIA (from Greek, literally, "not to sit") is a common and extremely distressing side effect of neuroleptics and some other drugs.[1,2] While its clinical importance in psychiatric patients was recognized in the 1950s and 1960s,[3,4] it was relatively ignored by researchers until the 1980s, when the first detailed clinical descriptions of the disorder were published.[1,5-8] Most investigators emphasized two components of akathisia: a subjective or psychological component and an objective or movement component, with disagreement on the relative importance of these two aspects.[1,2,9-12] Many issues with regard to the diagnosis of akathisia remain unresolved. There is no general agreement regarding which clinical features are specific to the disorder. Clinical judgment is called on to decide if the patient's movements are manifestations of akathisia, anxious restlessness, dyskinesia, or some other abnormality and whether the distress the patient reports is akathisia or anxiety, depression, agitation, or an exacerbation of psychosis or has some other psychiatric cause. Further, a number of subtypes of akathisia have been identified,[1,2] which include acute (AA), chronic, tardive, and withdrawal akathisia and pseudoakathisia. Akathisialike syndromes not related to drugs are also well recognized, and these include the restless legs syndrome (RLS)[13,14] and akathisia related to Parkinson's disease[15] or other brain disorders.[16]

See Methods on next page

METHODS

SELECTION OF SAMPLE

The sample consisted of consecutive patients (N=100) admitted to the psychiatric inpatient units of two teaching hospitals affiliated with the University of New South Wales, Sydney, Australia, who met the following inclusion criteria: (1) presence of a nonorganic psychotic illness, making the patient eligible for treatment with neuroleptics; (2) freedom from dopamine antagonists for a minimum of 2 weeks (6 weeks if a depot preparation had been used) prior to the day of admission; (3) freedom from acetylcholine (ACh) or β-adrenergic (βA) antagonists for 2 weeks prior to admission; (4) freedom from nonneuroleptics known to sometimes cause or modify akathisia, eg, lithium carbonate, heterocyclic antidepressants, calcium channel antagonists, and serotonin reuptake inhibitors[2]; (5) absence of akathisia on day 1 on clinical assessment and a baseline global akathisia rating of 0; (6) no current replacement iron therapy; (7) no history of sympathomimetic use (including nonprescription forms) in the previous 2 weeks by patient report and a urine screen negative for amphetamines, cocaine, and phencyclidine; (8) no history of RLS, Parkinson's disease, peripheral neuropathy, diabetes mellitus, or peripheral vascular disease; and (9) likeliness to stay in the hospital or be otherwise available for assessment for a minimum of 2 weeks.

INITIAL ASSESSMENT (BASELINE OR DAY 1)

Potential subjects were examined within 48 hours of admission, and if inclusion criteria were met, they underwent a detailed assessment prior to the initiation of neuroleptic therapy (except the nine patients in whom an emergency neuroleptic was used prior to baseline assessment). The assessment consisted of (1) a 16-item akathisia rating scale (Long Scale)[18] adapted and modified from Braude et al,[5] later modified to a 10-item Akathisia Scale[18] (**Table 1**); (2) a global akathisia rating scale; (3) a 10-item questionnaire specially constructed to elicit the patients' descriptions of akathisia, consisting of 10 items (sample items: Do you think you are restless? [yes or no]; If yes, where does this restlessness come from? [mind or whole body or legs]; Do you have a feeling of discomfort in your arms or legs? [arms or legs or neither]); (4) the Abnormal Involuntary Movement Scale (AIMS),[19] with the sum of the first four items yielding the Oral-Buccal-Lingual-Facial score; items five through seven, the Limb-Truncal (LT) score; and the sum of items one through seven, the AIMS score; (5) the Simpson and Angus Scale for Extrapyramidal Side Effects (EPSE),[20] with the sum of 10 items yielding the EPSE score; (6) Zung Depression Scale,[21] the sum of the items yielding the Zung score; (7) Spielberger's State Anxiety Inventory,[22] the sum of the items yielding the anxiety score; and (8) the Brief Psychiatric Rating Scale (BPRS),[23] the scores on some individual items being used, and a psychosis score obtained by summing the following six items: Conceptual Disorganization, Mannerisms and Posturing, Suspiciousness, Hallucinatory Behavior, Bizarre Behavior, and Unusual Thought Content. The Anxiety and Motor Hyperactivity items of the BPRS were also rated. A morning blood sample was obtained for hemoglobin, serum iron, and transferrin levels in the first half of the sample. A urinary screen for drugs was performed on admission.

MEDICATION

The actual treatment decisions were made by individual psychiatrists responsible for the care of different patients. Both units, however, cooperated in the study by attempting to (1) not initiate neuroleptic treatment, as far as was clinically possible, until after the baseline assessment and (2) not use ACh and βA antagonists routinely, introducing them only after consultation with the research team. Patients in whom acute dystonia developed and who were treated with regular ACh antagonists and manic patients treated with lithium in the first 2 weeks were excluded. The choices of the neuroleptic, initial dose, and rate of increment of the dose were clinical decisions not involving the research team. If a subject was noted by us to have moderate-to-severe akathisia and the clinical team was unaware of it, this was communicated to the appropriate nurse or psychiatrist, but no instructions regarding management were given.

ASSESSMENT IN FIRST WEEK (DAYS 2 TO 6)

Each subject underwent assessment daily in the morning, and the current medication and its major side effects were noted. The global akathisia rating was performed, and if it was 1 or more, the Long Scale for akathisia was administered. A diagnosis of akathisia agreed on by both investigators (P.S. and J.K.) allowed the subject to proceed to day 7 assessment. The subjects were interviewed before the ratings so that there was no intense physical activity for at least 15 minutes (usually longer) before the ratings.

The most well-recognized subtype is that of AA, which is related to the recent introduction or dose increase of neuroleptic therapy or a change to a high-potency drug.[2] There is only one published study that has examined the clinical features of AA in some detail.[5] This was a naturalistic study, the methods of which did not necessarily exclude subjects who had akathisia or tardive dyskinesia (TD) at baseline. Relatively little is known of factors, other than those related to drugs, that predispose to AA. Age and gender do not seem to be important,[2,5] and the relevance of previous neuroleptic exposure and past extrapyramidal symptoms has not been investigated. Whether poor iron status is a risk factor has found only inconsistent support in the literature.[17]

In this study, we report the investigation of a series of patients admitted for the treatment of an acute psychotic illness with neuroleptics, who had been free of neuroleptics for at least 2 weeks (6 weeks in the case of depot preparations) prior to their admission and were free of akathisia and related syndromes at the time of initial assessment. These subjects underwent assessment daily for 2 weeks, with detailed assessments at the end of weeks 1 and 2. Treatment with antiakathisia medication or neuroleptic dose reduction was undertaken only after a thorough evalu-

DAY 7 ASSESSMENT

On day 7, following admission or earlier if akathisia developed (global score, ≥3), the subjects underwent the same detailed assessment as on day 1 except for the laboratory tests. These assessments were performed in the morning or early afternoon. The global akathisia, Long Scale, and AIMS rating procedures were videotaped for later review and reliability assessment. The mode of intervention in those in whom akathisia developed was again a clinical decision and involved one of the following: a reduction in neuroleptic dose, a change from high- to low-potency neuroleptics, or treatment with an ACh (benztropine mesylate) or βA antagonist (propranolol hydrochloride).

ASSESSMENT IN SECOND WEEK (DAYS 8 TO 14)

Assessments on days 8 to 13 were similar to those in the first week, and in the second week subjects (n=91) proceeded to a day 14 assessment similar to that on day 7.

Follow-up after day 14 was incomplete and not systematic.

AKATHISIA SCALES

The following rating scales were used for the assessment of akathisia.

The Long Scale consisted of 16 items drawn from the questionnaire by Braude et al[5] and listed in Table 1. From this, a shorter 10-item Akathisia Scale[18] was derived. Acceptable reliability and validity of this scale have been documented elsewhere.[18] Each item was rated on a scale from 0 to 3. The subjective items were rated as absent, mild, moderate, or severe on the basis of the patient's response to specific questions. The objective items were rated on the basis of both intensity and severity. There was a categorical shift from 0 to 1, denoting absence or presence, and the rating of 1, 2, or 3 was then made regarding severity. A standardized procedure was followed for the examinations, with subjects examined in the sitting, standing, and lying positions and two distracting procedures (counting backward from 30 and finger tapping for 15 seconds) were used. The subjects were also observed as they listened to a recorded passage for 2 minutes. The objective ratings were performed first. Observations outside the period of the rating were noted but not used in the ratings. The 10-item Akathisia Scale was used for most of the analyses. The sum of the three subjective items gave the sum subjective score; the sum of the seven objective items, the sum objective score; and the sum of all 10 items, the total akathisia score.

A global akathisia rating scale was included, based on an abbreviated version of the Long Scale examination described above, on a scale of 0 to 3 (absent, mild, moderate, or severe), using the overall clinical judgment of the investigators and incorporating reports of the nursing staff. A description of these ratings is as follows: 0 indicates both subjective and objective symptoms questionable; 1, mild restlessness, wish to move, or inability to stay still subjectively, with mild limb movements and shifting body position on observation (can sit, stand, or lie for 10 minutes); 2, moderate feelings of restlessness and distress, with moderate movements suggestive of akathisia (unable to sit, stand, or lie for more than 5 minutes); and 3, marked distress, compulsion to move, preoccupation with symptoms or restlessness, or aggravation of psychosis, with almost constant leg and/or arm movements, rocking or pacing (cannot sit, stand, or lie still more than 1 minute). A rating of 1 or more represented definite akathisia as judged clinically. For the day 7 and 14 assessments, global ratings were performed separately in the sitting, standing, and lying positions. The proportion of observation time during which akathisia was present was rated on days 7 and 14 on the following scale: 0 indicates none; 1, a quarter; 2, a quarter to half; 3, more than half; and 4, continuously.

ANALYSIS OF DATA

The sociodemographic and clinical features were initially examined qualitatively. The psychiatric and drug-related variables were quantified. The profile of scores on the different items of the Long Scale and the 10-item Akathisia Scale was examined for days 7 and 14. To determine the factor structure of the akathisia ratings, they were subjected to a principal components analysis using the SPSS-PC+ statistical package.[24] Both strict and loose criteria were used for the diagnosis of akathisia at days 7 and 14 (**Table 2**). The relationship of all akathisia scores with drug dose was examined. The akathisia scores were correlated with the Zung, anxiety, and EPSE scores. Subjects were divided into akathisic and nonakathisic groups using different criteria and contrasted on the important variables known or suggested to be associated with the development of akathisia. Further, a logistic regression analysis was performed for the same variables to determine variables that best predicted the development of akathisia on days 7 or 14.

ation. The major potential predisposing factors were systematically studied.

RESULTS

DESCRIPTION OF THE SAMPLE (N=100)

The subjects (45 men; 55 women) had a mean (±SD) age of 34.4±10.8 years. Sixty-six were receiving Social Security benefits, 12 were housewives, eight were students, and the remaining 14 were currently employed. Sixteen had received tertiary education. Sixty-eight were never married, 12 were currently married, and 20 had been married previously. Their psychiatric diagnoses, using *DSM-III-R* criteria,[25] were schizophrenic disorder (n=75), manic bipolar disorder (n=4), delusional disorder (n=8), brief reactive psychosis (n=4), and other psychotic disorders (n=9). The current episode of illness for which they had been admitted was less than 1 week in duration in 20 and less than 1 month in 63. The majority (67%) were smokers, with 14 smoking more than 25 cigarettes per day. Only four reportedly consumed more than 10 g of alcohol per day. Ninety-one subjects underwent assessment on day 14; five were discharged early in the second week and refused daily outpatient follow-up, and four were

Table 1. Subjects With a Positive Rating on the Different Items of the Long Scale*

Item (Description)	% of Subjects Day 1 (N=100)	Day 7 (N=100)	Day 14 (n=91)	Days 7 and 14, Order of Symptom Frequency
Subjective item 1 (distressing sensations in the limbs)	3	21	31.9	5
Subjective item 2 (feeling of inner restlessness)†	18	52	53.8	1
Subjective item 3 (inability to remain still, standing, and/or sitting)†	9	32	36.6	3
Subjective item 4 (inability to keep legs still)†	6	25	25.3	6
Sitting item 1 (inability to remain seated)†	6	14	9.9	13
Sitting item 2 (semipurposeful or purposeless normal leg and/or feet movements)†	12	35	45.1	2
Sitting item 3 (inability to keep toes still)	1	21	25.3	9
Sitting item 4 (shifting of body position in chair)†	13	27	29.7	4
Sitting item 5 (semipurposeful hand and/or arm movements)†	4	16	17.6	10
Standing item 1 (shifting weight from foot to foot and/or walking on one spot)†	6	26	20.9	8
Standing item 2 (other purposeless [normal] foot movements)†	4	25	25.3	6
Standing item 3 (inability to remain standing on one spot [walked or paced])†	8	13	12.1	12
Lying item 1 (coarse tremor of legs and/or feet)	0	5	3.4	16
Lying item 2 (myoclonic jerks of the feet)	1	8	8.0	15
Lying item 3 (semipurposeful or purposeless leg and/or feet movements)	2	19	12.5	11
Lying item 4 (inability to remain lying down)	4	11	12.5	14

**Adapted from Braude et al.[5] Positive indicates a rating of 1 or higher. Rating is explained the "Akathisia Scales" subsection of the "Methods" section of the text. No subject received a clinical diagnosis of akathisia on day 1.*

†Indicates items from which our shorter 10-item Akathisia Scale was adapted.

withdrawn to participate in a drug study because of the development of significant akathisia.

MEDICATION HISTORY

The majority (83%) had both a history of psychiatric disorder and of receiving neuroleptics in the past. The mean (±SD) age at commencement of any psychiatric treatment was 22.0±12.6 years, and the mean duration of neuroleptic use was 19.3 months. They had been treated with a mean (±SD) of 2.4±1.9 different neuroleptics in the past, and the average proportions of time for receiving and not receiving neuroleptics since commencement had been 55% and 45%, respectively.

All subjects started receiving medication on day 1, with a mean (±SD) dose of 413±233 mg of chlorpromazine equivalents (CPZE), using the neuroleptic equivalence data published by Davis.[26] The mean (±SD) days 7 and 14 doses were 541±393 and 589±377 mg of CPZE, and the mean maximum dose in the first 2 weeks was 595±672 mg of CPZE. On day 1, 36 received low-potency (chlorpromazine hydrochloride or thioridazine hydrochloride), and 55 high-potency (haloperidol, trifluoperazine hydrochloride, pimozide, or fluphenazine hydrochloride) neuroleptics, and nine received both.

BASELINE ASSESSMENT

No subject had TD at baseline. The mean (±SD) psychosis score was 15.9±5.4, and the mean (±SD) Zung and anxiety scores were 44.5±7.6 and 45.0±9.9, respectively. The subjects had a mean (±SD) score of 1.3±0.9 (possible range, 1 to 5) on the Motor Hyperactivity item of the BPRS. Even though all these subjects were judged as not akathisic and they had been free of neuroleptics for at least 2 weeks, they rated positively on some Long Scale items. Subjectively, 18 had feelings of inner restlessness; nine, an inability to remain still; six, an inability to keep their legs still; and four, distressing sensations in their limbs. Objectively, semipurposeful leg movements were observed to a mild degree in 12 and mild shifting of body position in the chair in 13. Six subjects tended to pace and had difficulty sitting in the chair for 5 minutes. In the standing position, movements were less, with only four subjects demonstrating restless leg movements and six tending to shift their weight to a mild degree. The movements were even less obvious in the lying position. The mean baseline sum subjective score was 0.47 and sum objective score was 0.59. The six subjects who had a baseline sum subjective score of 2 or more were all acutely disturbed, with a mean psychosis score of 17.5, and showed marked motor agitation. However, the overall correlations of the akathisia total scores with the anxiety, Zung, and BPRS Motor Hyperactivity item scores were low and nonsignificant.

To determine whether the subjects who had positive ratings on one or more items of the 10-item Akathisia Scale at baseline had a greater propensity to receive a diagnosis of akathisia on day 7 or 14, we examined their scores separately. Of the 18 subjects who had baseline ratings of 1 or greater on subjective item 2 of the scale, nine had global akathisia ratings of 1 or greater on day 7 or 14 (nonsignificant difference from overall incidence). Of the six subjects with sum subjective scores of 2 or greater at baseline, three had global akathisia ratings of 1 or greater on day 7 or 14. The incidence of aka-

Table 2. Akathisia Diagnosis Using Different Criteria

Criterion No. (Description)	No. of Patients With Akathisia: Day 7 (N=100)	Day 14 (n=91)	Total (N=100)	Comment*
1 (global score, ≥1)†	32	31	40	Reference standard
2 (global score, ≥2)†	15	18	21	Moderate-to-severe akathisia
3 (total score, ≥4)‡	31	33	41	Acceptable cutoff on ROC analysis
4 (total score, ≥5)‡	25	27	32	Appropriate cutoff on ROC analysis
5 (sum subjective score, ≥2; sum objective score ≥2)§	23	26	31	Strict subjective and objective criterion, suitable for research
6 (sum subjective score, ≥1; sum objective score, ≥1)§	39	48	55	Loose criterion, likely to result in overdiagnosis
7 (total score, ≥2)‡	53	58	61	Very loose criterion, will certainly result in overdiagnosis

*ROC indicates receiver operating characteristic.

†Global score (range, 0 to 3) is a global akathisia rating based on an abbreviated version of the Long Scale described in the "Akathisia Scales" subsection of the "Methods" section of the text.

‡Total score is obtained from the sum of subjective and objective items on our 10-item Akathisia Scale. Items are described in Table 1.

§Sum subjective score is obtained from the sum of the three subjective items on our 10-item Akathisia Scale; sum objective score, from the seven objective items.

thisia in those with positive baseline ratings on the restlessness item on the scale was, therefore, not significantly different from the incidence in those with a rating of 0. The sum subjective scores at baseline had a low overall correlation with the sum subjective scores on day 7 (r=.03) or 14 (r=.02). The sum objective scores at baseline had a slightly higher, but nonsignificant, correlation with sum objective scores on day 7 (r=.20) or 14 (r=.29).

RELIABILITY OF AKATHISIA RATINGS

The reliability of the akathisia ratings was examined in the following manner. The two investigators (P.S. and J.K.) subsequently rated one in three videotapes for day 7 or 14 assessments. The ratings correlated highly (P<.01) on all items of the scale, with κ coefficients from 0.40 to 0.75, and the global rating with a κ value of 0.65. A new group of 50 patients treated with neuroleptics were administered the short version of the rating scale. The interrater validity for two raters was again high (κ range, 0.42 to 0.81 on various items). Twenty-five videotaped assessments were rated by two independent psychiatrists and one of us (P.S.), and a good concordance between the raters on the global ratings was achieved (κ=0.67).

INCIDENCE OF AKATHISIA

Akathisia developed in three subjects on the first day and another subject on the second day. From day 3 until day 6, the rate increased rapidly. When the akathisic and nonakathisic subjects, using criterion 3 (Table 2) on day 7, were compared on their daily global akathisia scores using Student's t test, there was a consistent difference in the scores from day 5 onward. The increment in dose had occurred sharply on day 1 (to a mean [±SD] dose of 416±393 mg of CPZE), and more slowly subsequently. The mean (±SD) dose on day 7 was 541±393 and on day 14 was 589±377 mg of CPZE. This suggested a delay of 5 to 6 days between an increase in the dose of the neuroleptics and the greatest likelihood of receiving a diagnosis of akathisia. During the second week, the population with akathisia was, however, not static, with some patients improving and akathisia developing in others for the first time.

The incidence of akathisia depends on the criteria used for diagnosis. Both strict and loose criteria were applied to our data, and these are presented in Table 2. We had realized, from our examination of the baseline data, that patients rated positively on many of the items of the Akathisia Scale even when they did not receive a clinical diagnosis of akathisia. We therefore decided on the clinical global score as our reference standard for diagnosis (criterion 1). By this criterion (ie, global rating of 1 or more), 32 patients had akathisia on day 7 and 31 (34%) of 91 patients on day 14. Of the 68 subjects not akathisic on day 7, akathisia developed in eight during the second week, thereby giving a 2-week incidence of 40% for akathisia. However, the majority of patients had only a mild disorder, which did not appear to be clinically significant and was often not noted by the treating team. A stricter standard was therefore agreed on as the need to intervene because of akathisia (ie, reduction in dose, change in type of neuroleptic, or introduction of antiakathisia medication). To us, this was akin to the diagnosis of moderate-to-severe akathisia (global rating of 2 or 3) (criterion 2). By this more strict criterion, 15 subjects had akathisia on day 7 and 18 (19.8%) on day 14. Of the 85 patients not akathisic on day 7 according to the criterion, akathisia developed in six during the second week, giving an overall incidence of 21% in the first 2 weeks.

EVALUATION OF DIAGNOSTIC CRITERIA

We examined the performance of the diagnostic criteria presented above using receiver operating characteristic (ROC) analysis. The ROC curves were constructed using criteria 1 and 2 for the classification of akathisia or nonakathisia on days 7 and 14 and the dif-

ferent scores on the sum of the items of the 10-item Akathisia Scale as the individual points. The curves for day 7 are presented in the **Figure** (top left and right) and suggest that a cutoff total sum score of 4 or 5 yielded the optimal balance of sensitivity and specificity for the diagnosis of akathisia. The different criteria presented in Table 2 were also examined for their sensitivity and specificity, again using criteria 1 and 2 for the classification of akathisia or nonakathisia. The day 7 results are presented in the Figure (bottom left and right) and suggest that criteria 3 and 4 yielded similar probabilities of true- or false-positive diagnoses. This again suggested a total sum of 4 or more as being optimal. Criterion 5 (sum subjective and sum objective scores of 2 or more) led to greater specificity but with reduced sensitivity and may arguably be an appropriate criterion for research diagnoses. The day 14 results were similar to those for day 7. The data, therefore, suggested that, if one used the rating scale, criterion 3 was appropriate for clinical diagnosis and criterion 5 for a more strict research diagnosis.

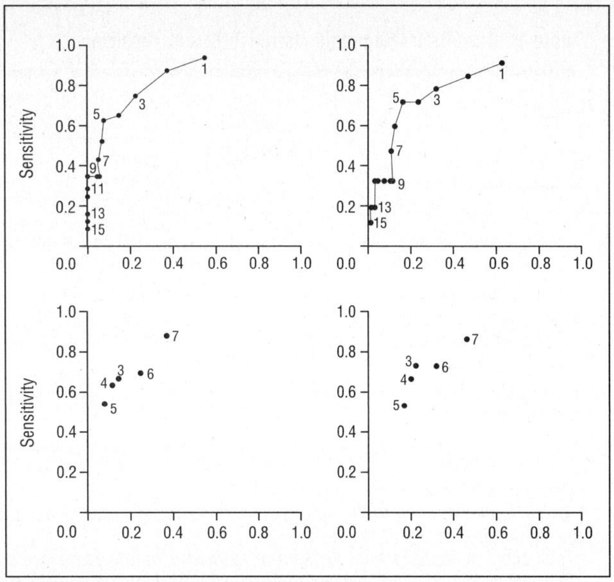

Receiver operating characteristic (ROC) curves for total 10-item Akathisia Scale scores from 1 to 15 (top left and top right) and criteria 3 to 7 (bottom left and bottom right) on day 7. Subjects were arranged into akathisic or nonakathisic groups according to criterion 1 or 2. The ROC curves represent the relationship between sensitivity (true-positive rate) and 1 minus specificity (false-positive rate) of the different proposed criteria in relation to criterion 1 (top left and bottom left) or 2 (top right and bottom right). Criteria are listed in Table 2.

SYMPTOM PROFILE OF AKATHISIA

Patients used adjectives and descriptors like "restless," "nervous," "fidgety," "unable to keep still," "nervy," "compelled to move," "on the go," "like jumping out of my skin," "uncomfortable," "legs want to keep moving," "unable to sit or stand in one place," "like ants crawling in my legs," "like pins and needles in my legs," etc, to describe their akathisia. Nearly all subjects judged to be akathisic (n=40) described themselves as being restless on direct query, with a few (n=5) exceptions. On further inquiry, six (15%) said that this restlessness stemmed from the mind, 12 (30%) said that it was in the body and mind, and 22 (55%) said that it was in the body, primarily the legs. Tension was described by 21 (52.5%), which was in the mind or body for about a quarter each and in both the mind and body in the rest. Twenty-one (52.5%) described discomfort in the arms or legs, and five (12.5%) described a feeling of pins and needles. Four (10%) had abdominal discomfort, and 10 (25%) had difficulty in sleeping because of the restlessness.

The majority of the patients had some relief of symptoms in the lying position; 16 (40%) said that they felt worst when standing and 24 (60%) when they were sitting. The ratings on the Long Scale in the three positions were consistent with this. As Table 1 demonstrates, the ratings on the lying items were positive in fewer subjects, and they also tended to be less intense. The global ratings in the different positions again supported the finding that akathisia was least prominent in the lying position, with the mean global ratings for all subjects on day 7 being 0.41, 0.32, and 0.23 and on day 14 being 0.47, 0.34, and 0.21 in the sitting, standing, and lying positions, respectively. All subjects who had positive ratings on the lying items also rated similar or greater severity on the other items. While some subjects reported a worsening of akathisia if they were asked to stand in one spot for a prolonged period, akathisia was not necessarily worse in the standing compared with the sitting position. The movements were not constant and were usually apparent for only a proportion of the observation period.

Table 1 gives the percentage of subjects who rated positively on the various rating scale items. The most common symptom was the subjective report of restlessness. However, this was present in 18% of all subjects at initial assessment, even though they were not judged to have akathisia. Inability to keep legs or feet still as assessed objectively was also frequent. Inability to remain still (subjectively) and tendency to shift body position in the chair were the next most common features. The ratings on the 10-item Akathisia Scale were subjected to a factor analysis. A two-factor solution was obtained for both day 7 and 14 ratings. As an examination of the factor coefficients suggests (**Table 3**), the subjective items had a high loading on factor 2, for which only one objective item loaded highly. A varimax rotation of the matrix suggested the first factor as the objective factor and the second as the subjective factor. Oblique rotations produced similar factor solutions, with the correlations between the factors being .45 for both day 7 and 14 ratings. The relative factorial separation supported the decision to separately rate the subjective and objective features of akathisia, but for a diagnosis of akathisia we insisted on the presence of both features.

To determine which symptoms best characterized akathisia, we first compared akathisic (n=32 for day 7) with nonakathisic (n=68 for day 7) subjects on the rating scores on different items of the Long Scale (**Table 4**). The scores were significantly different (analysis of variance [ANOVA], $P<.01$) on all items. We then performed a discriminant function analysis on the scale items,

Table 3. Factor Analysis of Our 10-Item Akathisia Scale on Day 7 and Day 14*

	Day 7 (N=100)			Day 14 (n=91)		
	Mean Score (SD)	Rotated Factors		Mean Score (SD)	Rotated Factors	
Items		1	2		1	2
Subjective item 2	0.59 (0.8)	.14	.81	0.71 (0.8)	.20	.77
Subjective item 3	0.41 (0.7)	.06	.86	0.33 (0.6)	.13	.80
Subjective item 4	0.26 (0.5)	.30	.71	0.30 (0.5)	.26	.67
Sitting item 1	0.19 (0.5)	.45	.63	0.11 (0.3)	.55	.30
Sitting item 2	0.43 (0.73)	.57	.59	0.56 (0.7)	.65	.50
Sitting item 4	0.33 (0.68)	.76	.31	0.37 (0.6)	.64	.37
Sitting item 5	0.19 (0.5)	.85	.05	0.19 (0.4)	.61	.43
Standing item 1	0.39 (0.7)	.78	.46	0.29 (0.6)	.70	.40
Standing item 2	0.34 (0.6)	.85	.20	0.27 (0.5)	.70	.16
Standing item 3	0.16 (0.4)	.77	.20	0.14 (0.4)	.84	−.05

**The factor loadings on varimax analysis rotated factor matrices. Items are described in Table 1.*

using criteria 1 and 3 to classify subjects into akathisic or nonakathisic groups to determine the most discriminating items. While different items emerged as most discriminating using different criteria, the items that were most consistently discriminating were standing item 1 (shifting of weight from foot to foot or walking on the spot), subjective item 4 (inability to keep legs still, subjectively), subjective item 2 (feelings of inner restlessness), and sitting item 4 (shifting of body position in the chair).

Patients reported that the characteristic movements of akathisia described above were voluntary and in response to the subjective distress. The movements were suppressible for at least short periods of time in all subjects. The subjects who had observable movement disorder without reported distress also were able to suppress the movements with focused attention.

SUBJECTIVE OR OBJECTIVE AKATHISIA OR BOTH?

While we considered both subjective and objective features for the global ratings, and the presence of both was necessary for a definitive diagnosis, there were patients with subjective symptoms who did not manifest any motor restlessness and others with characteristic motor abnormalities without any subjective complaints. The correlations between the sum subjective and sum objective scores on days 7 and 14 were .57 and .60 ($P<.001$), respectively, suggesting a moderate correspondence between the two. On day 7, seven subjects had sum subjective scores of 2 or more, with ratings of 0 on all objective items. Over the next week, five received a diagnosis of akathisia (three mild and two moderate in severity), with both features being present. All five were treated with benztropine, and two had a positive response. Four subjects had day 7 sum objective ratings greater than 2, with 0 on all subjective items; three of these later received a diagnosis of akathisia, with two responding to benztropine. One patient, receiving a large dose of haloperidol, had very characteristic akathisic movements (sum objective score, 12) but did not report any subjective distress. This patient was also acutely psychotic, hostile, and uncooperative, and as his psychotic symptoms improved, his subjective distress due to akathisia came to the fore.

AKATHISIA, ANXIETY, DEPRESSION, HYPERACTIVITY, AND PSYCHOSIS

We determined the Spearman's correlation coefficients between subjective and objective akathisia scores and anxiety scores, Zung scores, and BPRS Anxiety and Motor Hyperactivity item scores. The sum objective scores were significantly correlated with the Motor Hyperactivity item scores on day 7 ($r=.26$, $P<.01$) but not on day 14 ($r=.18$), suggesting that akathisic movements may also sometimes receive a rating on this BPRS item. More importantly, the akathisia ratings did not have significant correlations with the BPRS Anxiety item ratings, suggesting that it was possible to distinguish the subjective experience of akathisia from that of anxiety. The sum subjective score had correlations of .17 and .11 with the anxiety score and .05 and −.05 with the BPRS Anxiety item rating on days 7 and 14, respectively. The correlations of sum objective scores with the BPRS Anxiety item ratings were similarly low (−.04 to .09). The subjective rating had a significant correlation with self-rated depression[21] on day 7 ($r=.20$, $P<.05$) but not on day 14 ($r=.04$), suggesting a weak relationship. When akathisic subjects, as defined by criterion 1, 2, or 3, were compared with nonakathisic patients using ANOVA, the two groups did not differ significantly on the measures of anxiety, depression, or psychosis.

AKATHISIA AND OTHER DRUG-INDUCED MOVEMENT DISORDERS

The objective akathisia score had a significant correlation with the EPSE score on days 7 ($r=.25$, $P<.05$) and 14 ($r=.40$, $P<.001$). The same was true for the total akathisia scores ($r=.30$ and .30, $P<.01$). The correlations were

Table 4. Akathisic and Nonakathisic Subjects With Positive Rating on the Items of the Long Scale on Day 7*

Items	% of Subjects: Akathisic (n=32)	% of Subjects: Nonakathisic (n=68)
Subjective item 1	43.7	10.3
Subjective item 2	86.2	35.3
Subjective item 3	59.4	19.1
Subjective item 4	56.2	10.3
Sitting item 1	37.2	2.9
Sitting item 2	65.6	20.6
Sitting item 3	43.7	10.3
Sitting item 4	58.1	14.7
Sitting item 5	31.2	8.8
Standing item 1	65.6	7.4
Standing item 2	53.1	11.8
Standing item 3	31.2	4.4
Lying item 1	18.1	0
Lying item 2	19.4	2.9
Lying item 3	45.2	7.4
Lying item 4	25.8	4.4

**Items are described in Table 2. Positive indicates a rating of 1 or higher. Ratings are described in the "Akathisia Scales" subsection of the "Methods" section of the text.*

significant ($P<.01$ or .05) for both elbow rigidity and tremor (correlation with global scores: day 7, .26 and .44, respectively; day 14, .31 and .33, respectively). Akathisic patients were significantly more likely to have tremor of the hands (χ^2 *df* 1; day 7, $P<.001$; day 14, $P<.05$). The correlation between tremor and elbow rigidity was also high (day 7, $r=.53$, $P<.001$). While no subject met diagnostic criteria for TD, a number received positive scores on some items, in particular those pertaining to limb and truncal movements. The LT dyskinesia scores had a positive correlation with the sum objective scores (day 7, $r=.29$, $P<.01$; day 14, $r=.23$, $P<.05$), which were interpreted to reflect the difficulty in distinguishing some akathisic movements from dyskinetic ones when they involved the limbs, in particular the lower limbs. A few subjects had myoclonic jerks. Of the eight subjects in whom severe akathisia developed, five had myoclonic jerks of the legs or toes that were clearly involuntary. These jerks were present only in the severe cases and were distressing; a few jerks persisted in sleep.

INFLUENCE OF DISTRACTING MANEUVERS

The videotapes of the days 7 and 14 assessments of the akathisic patients were reviewed to investigate the influence of the distracting maneuvers on akathisic movements. Of the 40 subjects so studied, 26 (65%) demonstrated a reduction of their movements, with the rest not showing any perceptible change. In no subject were the movements exacerbated by these.

RISK FACTORS AND PREDICTORS OF AKATHISIA

We performed a logistic regression analysis to determine the variables that best predicted the development of akathisia in our sample. This method was selected over discriminant function analysis because the assumption of multivariate normality of the independent variables that the latter requires was not fulfilled by our data. The groups were defined separately by two sets of criteria, criteria 1 (our reference standard) and 3 (criterion supported by ROC analysis) and the analysis performed for days 7 and 14 using presence or absence of akathisia as the dependent variable. The independent variables entered into the analysis were based on evidence from the literature, theoretical considerations, and a preliminary examination of the data. These were age, sex, current neuroleptic (CPZE) dose, rate of increment of dose in the last week (milligrams of CPZE per day), drug type used (low-, high-, or mixed-potency), duration of illness, past use of neuroleptics (present or absent), EPSE score, Zung score, anxiety score, psychosis score, and smoking (number of cigarettes per day). For the subgroup (n=50) in whom serum iron and ferritin levels were also available, these were also entered into a separate analysis. The method used for the logistic regression was that of forward stepwise selection. Some subjects (**Table 5** indicates the number in each analysis) were excluded because of one or more missing variables. To start with, the model contained only the constant. At each step, the variable with the smallest significance level for the score statistic was added to the model, provided it was less than the chosen cutoff ($P=.15$). The criterion used to determine the variables to be removed from the model was the likelihood-ratio test[27] at the cutoff significance level of $P<.2$. The day 7 data yielded the most satisfactory results, partly because by day 14 intervention had occurred in a number of cases. The variables that emerged to be significant on the analysis that included all cases were the EPSE score, the current neuroleptic dose, and the rate of increment of dose, producing a nearly 80% correct classification. When the subset with the iron data was analyzed (n=42 because of missing data), the EPSE score was again entered on step 1. The additional significant variables were drug type and serum iron levels. All five variables produced an overall correct classification of 93%. Two additional variables tended toward significance: duration of illness ($P=.05$) and history of neuroleptic use ($P=.12$). The results of the logistic regression are presented in Table 5. Correlations were determined between global akathisia ratings on days 7 and 14 and the neuroleptic doses. The correlation between day 7 ratings and dose was .3 ($P<.01$) and between day 14 ratings and dose was .27 ($P<.01$). Day 14 akathisia ratings had significant correlations with dose from day 5 onward. We also examined the role of psychiatric diagnosis by comparing the proportions of subjects with schizophrenia (n=75) and nonschizophrenic disorders (n=25) in whom akathisia developed, using the χ^2 test. The difference was not significant.

The final model that deals with the contributions of the examined variables toward the development of AA is presented in **Table 6**. The effect size (ES) index[28] for each variable is presented. For continuous variables, this

Table 5. Results of a Logistic Regression Analysis*

No. of Subjects	Variables†	Regression Coefficient	SE	Adjusted Odds Ratio	P	% of Subjects Correctly Classified: Overall	% of Subjects Correctly Classified: With Akathisia
			Entire Sample				
	Day 7						
97	EPSE score	0.302	0.18	1.652	.01	76.3	37.5
	Rate of dose increment	0.001	0.00	1.001	.09		
	Age	0.337	0.23	1.034	.15		
	Day 14						
87	EPSE score	0.209	0.09	1.232	.02	77.0	42.9
	Current CPZE dose	0.003	0.00	1.003	.04		
	Rate of dose increment	−0.002	0.00	0.998	.14		
			Half Sample				
	Day 7						
42	EPSE score	1.602	0.67	4.963	.02	88.1	76.57
	Medication type	−4.581	2.07	0.010	.03		
	Serum iron level	−0.472	0.22	0.624	.03		
	Duration of illness	0.250	0.13	1.285	.05		
	Day 14						
37	EPSE score	0.341	0.18	1.410	.05	75.7	62.5
	Current CPZE dose	0.002	0.00	1.002	.09		
	Serum iron level	−0.157	0.10	0.855	.13		

*Analysis used presence or absence of akathisia as the dependent variable and 12 independent variables (described in the "Risk Factors and Predictors of Akathisia" subsection of the "Results" section of the text) in a stepwise procedure. P=.15 inclusion; P=.20 for removal.

†ESPE score indicates score on the Simpson and Angus[20] Scale for Extrapyramidal Side Effects; CPZE, chlorpromazine equivalents. Only variables significant at the .15 level are presented.

was the product-moment correlation coefficient (r) between the variable and global akathisia rating on day 7. For discrete variables (sex, medication type, previous exposure to neuroleptics, and smoking), the ES index was calculated as suggested by Cohen,[28(p216-217)] using the χ^2 test (w). The magnitude of ES was determined using conventional definitions[28]: small for 0.10, medium for 0.30, and large for 0.50. No variable had a large ES. Four variables (EPSE score, rate of dose increment, current neuroleptic dose, and serum iron levels) had a medium ES. These effect sizes are "unadjusted" in the sense that they do not represent effects over and above the other variables in the model.

COMMENT

We have presented a prospective study of the clinical characteristics of AA and the potential factors that predict its development. The study used strict inclusion criteria such that subjects who already had akathisia or RLS at the time of initiation of neuroleptic therapy were excluded. The clinical description, therefore, is of the acute syndrome without contamination with related syndromes. The study confirms and extends what is already known about AA.

Acute akathisia has a range of manifestations that characterize it as both a mental and motor disorder. The subjective features are described variously by the patients, but usually reflect an inner feeling of restlessness that seems to stem most commonly from the legs and can be unrelenting. Subjective restlessness cannot be considered diagnostic of the disorder, however, as it is often reported by psychiatric patients not being treated with neuroleptics and without other features of akathisia. When this report is combined with the complaint of an inability to keep legs still, akathisia is more likely to be present. These findings are consistent with previous reports of AA.[5,7] An urge to move was a common symptom, but an inability to sit (the literal meaning of akathisia) was not so. A small proportion of akathisic patients reported symptoms in the upper limbs or abdomen, and a few reported paresthesia in the extremities, again consistent with the published literature.[5] Patients improved in the lying position, but only a proportion felt worse in the standing position, unlike previous reports.[5,7] The factorial separation of subjective and objective items is of interest, although it is difficult to rule out the possibility of this being a method-related artifact. However, it supports the decision to rate these features separately. In most patients, there is a moderately high correspondence between the subjective and objective features, but some may present with subjective or objective features alone. Many clinicians believe that subjective features precede the development of motor abnormality in most patients. While this may be true in some cases, our data suggest that these are a minority, and both subjective and objective features develop concomitantly in most patients. Further, the full syndrome does not develop in all patients who present with the typical subjective or objective features. We, therefore, recommend a definitive diagnosis of akathisia only when both features are present, especially if the diagnosis is being made for research purposes. At the same time, the clinical implications of a false-negative diagnosis of akathisia may be serious, and a high index of suspicion is necessary.

Table 6. Effect Size Indices (Unadjusted) for the Variables Examined as Putative Risk Factors for Acute Akathisia*

Variables†	Effect Size Index‡	Comment
Medium effect size		
EPSE score, *r*	.40	...
Rate of increment of dose (mg of CPZE per day), *r*	.40	...
Current neuroleptic dose (mg of CPZE), *r*	.37	...
Serum iron level, *r*	−.35	First half of sample examined only
Small effect size		
Medication type, *w*	0.28	High-potency drugs more likely to cause akathisia
Anxiety score, *r*	.25	Spielberger's State Anxiety Inventory was used
Previous exposure to neuroleptics, *w*	0.23	Past exposure had a negative effect on akathisia
Psychosis score, *r*	.16	...
Age, *r*	.15	...
Sex, *w*	0.133	Slightly more akathisia in women
Smoking, *w*	0.11	Slightly more akathisia in smokers
Zung score, *r*	.10	...
Duration of illness, *r*	−.08	...

*Day 7 data were utilized for all calculations.

†EPSE score indicates score on the Simpson and Angus[20] Scale for Extrapyramidal Side Effects; CPZE, chlorpromazine equivalents.

‡The value of Pearson's correlation (r) for continuous variables and the χ^2 test for proportions effect size index (w) for categorical variables (as suggested by Cohen[28]) are presented.

The motor disorder of akathisia is again varied in its manifestation, but the most characteristic symptom is the inability to maintain posture, either sitting or standing. This again is in agreement with some previous reports judging the inability to maintain a particular posture as indicative of severe akathisia.[29,30] That myoclonic jerks of the legs and toes may occur in severe akathisia, as seen in our subjects, has been previously described.[31] Myoclonic jerks have also been described as part of Ekbom syndrome.[32] Acute akathisia has a strong association with parkinsonian symptoms like tremor and rigidity, but dyskinetic movements suggestive of TD are not seen. We do not consider tremor to be a feature of akathisia, however. While the tremor ratings had a significant correlation with the akathisia ratings, their correlation with rigidity was much higher and consistent on different examinations. Distracting maneuvers resulted in reduction of akathisia movements, which is in contrast with dyskinetic movements that are often exacerbated or brought out by such tasks. A similar observation has previously been made by other investigators.[33] This information is of potential utility in distinguishing akathisia from dyskinetic movements, especially if it can be shown that the movement disorder of tardive akathisia behaves similarly to AA in this respect.

The movements were recognized as voluntary by most subjects and could be suppressed for varying periods of time. They were, nevertheless, in response to an irresistible urge and were, therefore, not intentional. A parallel can be drawn with motor tics, which are also experienced by patients as being in response to an irresistible urge to move and can be voluntarily suppressed temporarily.[34] In spite of this, tics are generally recognized as being involuntary.[25] One difference between tics and akathisic movements is that tics are stereotyped and nonpurposive, whereas akathisic movements are complex and semipurposeful in most patients. Myoclonic jerks, when they do form part of akathisia, are clearly involuntary. A report of unilateral akathisia in a patient with acquired immunodeficiency syndrome and a toxoplasmosis subthalamic abscess[35] suggests that the nonstereotyped nature of the movement disorder in akathisia does not argue against its involuntary nature.

Our investigation supports earlier reports that akathisia is very common. We report an incidence of 40% in the first 2 weeks after the initiation of neuroleptic therapy in patients not being treated with any potentially antiakathisic medication. Using more conservative criteria, the rate is at least 21% according to our data. Previous studies have reported variable rates for AA. Freyhan[35] reported a prevalence of 14.4% in patients receiving one of four phenothiazines. In a large survey of drug-induced extrapyramidal reactions, Ayd[4] reported a rate of 21.2%. Braude et al,[5] who included mild cases, reported a rate of 25% in all patients admitted to a psychiatric unit who required antipsychotic medication. Higher rates were reported by Van Putten[9]—45% in a sample of 110 patients at some time during the course of treatment with antipsychotic drugs. The variability in the rates may be explained by different definitions used, nature of concomitant medication, acute or chronic administration of neuroleptics, use of high- or low-potency drugs, and different drug regimens used. We argue that the rigor of our investigation, the strict definitions, and the minimal amount of concomitant medication used make it likely that it reflects the true incidence of the disorder. One limitation of the study was that most patients were not followed up systematically after the first 2 weeks. Our figures therefore may be an underestimate but are unlikely to be far away from the real figures. In the study by Braude et al,[5] the disorder developed in 85% of the patients within a week of starting the medication therapy and nearly all by the second week. Akathisia developed in 90% of the patients receiving depot fluphenazine seen by Ayd[4] within 4 days of the injection.

We should point out some further limitations of our data. Even though we had initially intended to do so, we were unable to control the type and dose of neuroleptic because of clinical constraints. We were also unable to monitor plasma levels of the drugs to account for pharmacokinetic factors that may have affected the results. Since subjects were interviewed on multiple occasions, it is possible that they were sensitized to the anticipated side effects and consequently overreported them. Against this suggestion is the fact that the relative ratings on the subjective and objective features did not change from day 7 to 14. We were also aware of the possibility of an upward drift in the investigator's ratings. To guard against

this, one of us (P.S.) met periodically with the research assistant to compare their ratings, and videotapes of examinations by one were rated by the other independently.

EVEN THOUGH we have described in some detail the clinical features of AA, a clinical diagnosis of akathisia is often uncertain. We have demonstrated that the ratings on the akathisia scale do not correlate highly with the BPRS Anxiety or Motor Hyperactivity item ratings, and do so only modestly with self-rated depression. The low correlation between akathisia and anxiety is of interest and suggests that subjects, when closely questioned, are able to separate the subjective restlessness and urge to move of akathisia from feelings of anxiety that were often present concomitantly. In spite of this, clinical experience suggests that mild akathisia can be difficult to diagnose, especially in an acutely psychotic patient who does not provide a clear account of the subjective experience. A high index of suspicion is therefore necessary in the setting in which AA is most likely to occur, ie, in patients who have recently started neuroleptic therapy or in whom the dose of the drug was significantly increased or the drug changed to a high-potency one. Inclusion of cases with both subjective and objective features is likely to reduce the false-positive rates. Sometimes multiple examinations of the patient at different times of the day, as well as observations by nurses, may be of assistance. If the diagnosis is still uncertain, a reduction in dose or a switch to a low-potency drug may help confirm it. Alternately, a trial of an ACh or βA antagonist drug may be attempted, although the results of such a trial may not necessarily aid the diagnosis, as these drugs are not specific to akathisia and not all patients with akathisia respond to them.

Akathisia can be predicted in an individual patient with only modest accuracy. The most significant predictor that emerged in our study was the presence of parkinsonian side effects, in particular tremor and rigidity. In other words, akathisia was more likely to develop in patients in whom marked extrapyramidal symptoms developed. This may reflect a common vulnerability to extrapyramidal symptoms and should not be considered to suggest that parkinsonian symptoms in themselves produced the restlessness of akathisia. That parkinsonian symptoms and akathisia may share some pathophysiological mechanisms is also suggested by the fact that akathisia may be a feature of postencephalitic or idiopathic parkinsonism.[15] The possibility was also considered that the predictive value of the EPSE score for akathisia indicated a lack of complete neuroleptic washout and receptor readaptation. Against this was the absence of a significant correlation between length of washout and the presence of akathisia on day 7 or 14 ($r=-.1$ for both). Our study did not examine the time course of development of extrapyramidal symptoms. Therefore, the question of whether extrapyramidal symptoms precede akathisia and can therefore be used to predict it cannot be answered from our data. Previous studies[4,35-37] that examined the development of drug-induced parkinsonism reported its time course to be similar to that of akathisia or somewhat delayed. This would suggest that the EPSE score may not be useful in predicting akathisia in clinical practice. Certain drug-related factors were important predictors, in particular the current dose, the type of drug (high-potency drugs being more likely), and the rate of increment of the dose. These findings are consistent with earlier reports.[4,38,39] There was also a suggestion that past exposure to neuroleptics and a long history of psychiatric illness tended to reduce the likelihood of akathisia developing. Another factor that made akathisia more likely was a low serum iron level. When the serum iron and transferrin status of akathisic and nonakathisic subjects were compared, however, the differences were nonsignificant, thus suggesting that the contribution of poor iron status was small.[40] Age and gender did not emerge to be significant predictors, and this is again consistent with the published literature.[1,5,38] It must be emphasized, however, that our subjects were mostly young, and the effect of age may be more apparent in the older age group. Similarly, gender may interact with age, so that its effect may also be more apparent later in life. Future studies should, therefore, include elderly subjects to address this question. Even when all significant variables were entered into the equation, a major portion of the likelihood of the development of akathisia remained unexplained. We refer to this as individual vulnerability, thus acknowledging our ignorance.

In conclusion, our report describes a prospective study of AA, giving its incidence, detailing its clinical features, and examining various criteria for its diagnosis. It suggests factors that may predict its development in an individual patient in whom neuroleptic therapy is being initiated. The study reasserts the clinical importance of this common and distressing side effect of psychotropic medication.

Accepted for publication July 21, 1994.

Supported by a grant from the National Health and Medical Research Council of Australia, Canberra, Australian Capital Territory.

Celia Loneragan assisted with data collection and Doreen Hanlon with manuscript preparation. We are grateful to Gordon Parker, MD, PhD, Anthony Kuk, PhD, Dusan Hadzi-Pavlovic, MPsychol, all the psychiatrists who permitted us to investigate their patients (in particular, the unit directors, Charles Doutney, FRANZCP, and Kay Wilhelm, MD, FRANZCP), the Medical Illustration Unit of the University of New South Wales, and Eastpath Laboratories, Sydney.

Reprints not available.

REFERENCES

1. Barnes TRE, Braude WM. Akathisia variants and tardive dyskinesia. *Arch Gen Psychiatry.* 1985;42:874-878.
2. Sachdev P, Loneragan C. The present status of akathisia. *J Nerv Ment Dis.* 1991;179:381-391.
3. Steck H. Le syndrome extrapyramidal et d'encephalique au cours des traitements au largactil et au serpasil. *Ann Med Psychol (Paris).* 1954;112:737-

743.
4. Ayd FJ. A survey of drug-induced extrapyramidal reactions. *JAMA.* 1961;175:1054-1060.
5. Braude W, Barnes TRE, Gore SM. Clinical characeristics of akathisia: a systematic investigation of acute psychiatric inpatient admissions. *Br J Psychiatry.* 1983;143:139-150.
6. Gibb WRG, Lees AJ. The clinical phenomenon of akathisia. *J Neurol Neurosurg Psychiatry.* 1986;49:861-866.
7. Burke RE, Kang UJ, Fahn S. Tardive akathisia: motor phenomena and treatment. *Neurology.* 1987;37(suppl 1):124-125.
8. Burke RE, Kang UJ, Jankovic J, Miller LG, Fahn S. Tardive akathisia: an analysis of clinical features and response to open therapeutic trials. *Mov Disord.* 1989;4:157-175.
9. Van Putten T. The many faces of akathisia. *Compr Psychiatry.* 1975;16:43-47.
10. Akathisia and antipsychotic drugs. *Lancet.* 1986;2:1131-1132. Editorial.
11. Stahl SM. Akathisia and tardive dyskinesia. *Arch Gen Psychiatry.* 1985;42:915-917.
12. Lang AE. Other hyperkinetic and paroxysmal movements. *Curr Opin Neurol Neurosurg.* 1989;2:334-342.
13. Ekbom KA. Restless legs syndrome. *Neurology.* 1960;10:868-873.
14. Gibb WRG, Lees AJ. The restless legs syndrome. *Postgrad Med J.* 1986;62:329-333.
15. Lang AE, Johnson K. Akathisia in idiopathic Parkinson's disease. *Neurology.* 1987;37:477-481.
16. Carrazana E, Rossitch E Jr, Martinez J. Unilateral 'akathisia' in a patient with AIDS and a toxoplasmosis subthalamic abscess. *Neurology.* 1989;39:449-450.
17. Sachdev P. The neuropsychiatry of brain iron. *J Neuropsychiatry Clin Neurosci.* 1993;5:18-29.
18. Sachdev PS. A rating scale for drug-induced akathisia: development, reliability and validity. *Biol Psychiatry.* 1994;35:263-271.
19. National Institute of Mental Health. Abnormal Involuntary Movement Scale. In: Guy W, ed. *Early Clinical Drug Evaluation Unit Assessment Manual.* Rockville, Md: US Dept of Health and Human Services; 1976:534-537.
20. Simpson G, Angus JWS. A rating scale for extrapyramidal side effects. *Acta Psychiatr Scand.* 1970;212:11-19.
21. Zung WWK. A self-rating depression scale. *Arch Gen Psychiatry.* 1965;12:63-70.
22. Spielberger CD, Gorsuch RL, Lushene RE. *State-Trait Anxiety Inventory.* Tallahassee, Fla: Florida State University; 1967.
23. Lukoff D, Nuechterlein KH, Ventura J. Brief Psychiatric Rating Scale. *Schizophr Bull.* 1986;12:594-601.
24. SPSS Inc. *Statistical Package for Social Sciences, PC+.* Chicago, Ill: SPSS Inc; 1988.
25. American Psychiatric Association. *Diagnostic and Statistical Manual of Mental Disorders, Revised Third Edition.* Washington, DC: American Psychiatric Association; 1987.
26. Davis JM. Comparative doses and costs of antipsychotic medication. *Arch Gen Psychiatry.* 1976;33:858-861.
27. Hosmer D, Lemeshow S. *Applied Logistic Regression.* New York, NY: John Wiley & Sons Inc; 1989.
28. Cohen J. *Statistical Power Analysis for the Behavioral Sciences.* Hillsdale, NJ: Erlbaum Associates; 1988.
29. Raskin D. Akathisia: a side effect to be remembered. *Am J Psychiatry.* 1972;129:345-347.
30. Sovner R, DiMascio A. Extrapyramidal syndromes and other neurological side effects of psychotropic drugs. In: Lipton MA, DiMascio A, Killam KF, eds. *Psychopharmacology: A Generation of Progress.* New York, NY: Raven Press; 1978:1021-1032.
31. Braude W, Charles IP, Barnes TRE. Coarse, jerky foot tremor: tremographic investigation of an objective sign of akathisia. *Psychopharmacology.* 1984;82:95-101.
32. Boghen D, Peyronnard JM. Myoclonus in familial restless legs syndrome. *Arch Neurol.* 1976;33:368-370.
33. Fleischhacker WW, Miller CH, Barnes C, Bergman K, Perovich R, Alvir JMJ, Leiberman JA, Kane JM. The effect of activation procedures on neuroleptic-induced akathisia. *Br J Psychiatry.* 1993;163:781-784.
34. Kurlan R, Lichter D, Hewitt D. Sensory tics in Tourette's syndrome. *Neurology.* 1989;39:731-734.
35. Freyhan FA. Therapeutic implications of different effects of new phenothiazine compounds. *Am J Psychiatry.* 1959;115:577-585.
36. Medinar C, Kramen MD, Kurland AA. Biperiden in the treatment of phenothiazine-induced extrapyramidal reactions. *JAMA.* 1982;182:1127-1128.
37. Levinson DF, Simpson GF, Singh H, Yadalam K, Jain A, Stephanos MJ, Silver P. Fluphenazine dose, clinical response, and extrapyramidal symptoms during acute treatment. *Arch Gen Psychiatry.* 1990;47:761-768.
38. Braude W, Barnes TRE. Late-onset akathisia: an indicant of covert dyskinesia: two case reports. *Am J Psychiatry.* 1982;140:611-612.
39. Van Putten T, May PRA, Marder SR. Akathisia with haloperidol and thiothixene. *Arch Gen Psychiatry.* 1984;41:1036-1039.
40. Sachdev P, Loneragan C. Acute drug-induced akathisia is not associated with low serum iron status. *Psychopharmacology.* 1991;103:138-139.

The Boundary of Social Phobia

Exploring the Threshold

Jonathan R. T. Davidson, MD; Dana C. Hughes, RN, PhD; Linda K. George, PhD; Dan G. Blazer, MD, PhD

Background: Individuals with subthreshold social phobia (SSP) in the community are characterized relative to nonphobic, healthy controls (C), and diagnosed social phobics (SP).

Methods: Data from 1488 subjects from the Duke University Epidemiological Catchment Area Study were examined. Bivariate and multivariate methods were used to compare the SSP, SP, and C groups on 10 sets of variables.

Results: Compared with C respondents, SSP respondents were more likely to be female and unmarried and to report less income and education. The SSP respondents were also more likely to report work attendance problems, poor grades in school, symptoms of conduct disturbance, impaired subjective social support, lack of self-confidence, lack of a close friend, use of psychotropic drugs in past year, and a greater number of life changes, chronic medical problems, and mental health visits within the past 6 months. In a multivariate logistic regression model with group membership as the dependent variable, compared with C respondents, SSP respondents were more likely to be female, to have less education, and to report more indicators of poor school performance and symptoms of adolescent conduct disturbance. In contrast, in a similar but separate multivariate model, compared with SP respondents, SSP respondents met the criteria for fewer *DSM-III* psychiatric disorders and were less likely to report impaired instrumental support.

Conclusion: Social phobia adversely affects over 10% of the population. Previous epidemiologic catchment area–based prevalence estimates have probably been unrealistically low.

(Arch Gen Psychiatry. 1994;51:975-983)

SOCIAL ANXIETY is a relatively common phenomenon, although in the National Institute of Mental Health Epidemiological Catchment Area (ECA) Project[1] social phobia affected less than 4% of the population, with lifetime prevalence ranging from 1.8% to 3.8% across the four ECAs examined. More recent surveys suggest a much higher prevalence of social phobia, based on the adoption of different interview assessments from that used in the ECA Study.[2,3]

In the Piedmont region of North Carolina, one of the four ECAs examined by the National Institute of Mental Health, 10.5% of the participating adults reported the presence of at least one of the three listed social phobic/public situations (ie, fear of eating in public, speaking in front of small groups, or speaking to strangers), but only 3.8% fulfilled the Diagnostic Interview Schedule (DIS)/*DSM-III* diagnostic threshold criteria for social phobia.[4] Thus, an additional 6.7% of the population reported one of the listed social phobic symptoms. However, they denied that these symptoms substantially interfered with their activities or led to their seeking medical assistance.

Community and clinical studies have shown that social phobics carry a heavy burden, in that this disorder develops early in life and has a low spontaneous recovery rate.[1,4,5] In comparison with controls, social phobics report higher rates of childhood and adolescent disturbances, greater impairment on social support and quality-of-life measures, more suicide attempts, more physical and mental health problems, and increased utilization of health services.[1,4] Is it possible that individuals who report one or more symptoms of social phobia but without significant avoid-

From the Anxiety and Traumatic Stress Program (Dr Davidson), the Departments of Psychiatry (Drs Davidson, George, and Blazer), Medicine (Dr Hughes), and Sociology (Dr George), the School of Nursing (Dr Hughes), and the Office of Medical Education (Dr Blazer), Duke University Medical Center, Durham, NC.

See Methods on next page

ance are equally burdened? Broadhead and colleagues[6] reported that "minor" depressives, defined as subjects who reported some depressive symptoms but an insufficient number to meet *DSM-III* criteria for the diagnosis of major depression, reported a substantial level of morbidity and could benefit from treatment. In this study, we question whether subjects who have at least one of the three listed social phobic symptoms but fail to meet the DIS/*DSM-III* diagnostic criteria for social phobia are troubled enough to warrant diagnosis and treatment. That is, are subthreshold social phobics (SSPs) more similar to social phobics or to healthy controls?

We examine the characteristics of participants in the North Carolina ECA Study who reported SSP symptoms. The SSP respondents are compared with respondents in each of two groups: (1) nonphobic, nonpsychiatric controls (Cs) without any lifetime *DSM-III* diagnosis or phobic symptoms and (2) diagnosed *DSM-III* social phobics (SPs).

Subjects in the three groups are compared on the following sets of variables, which have been identified as correlates of social phobia by previous investigators or clinicians examining this disorder[1-3,5,7]: demographics, familial characteristics, impaired school performance, conduct disturbance in adolescence, social support, self-confidence, stressful life events, health status measures, health-seeking behaviors, and psychiatric comorbidity. The question of major interest is whether SSP subjects more closely resemble C or SP subjects.

METHODS

The ECA program has been described elsewhere.[8-11] The Duke University site comprised a five-county catchment area in the Piedmont region of North Carolina. Using a multistage sampling procedure, 3921 households were screened to yield 3015 respondents and an elderly oversample of 906. One year later, 2993 (76%) of these respondents were reinterviewed. Subjects (N=1488) examined in this study are those wave I respondents who participated in both surveys and who, at the first interview, reported symptoms of social phobia above (n=123) or below (n=248) the *DSM-III* diagnostic threshold and those who did not report a phobic symptom or meet the criteria for any DIS/*DSM-III* diagnosis (n=1117). Most data examined in this study were taken from the initial interview. However, data that allowed us to make a *DSM-III* diagnosis of generalized anxiety disorder (GAD) and posttraumatic stress disorder (PTSD) were taken from the wave II interview. Prevalence rates of these two disorders were adjusted for their occurrence prior to the baseline interview.

Subjects participated in a 2-hour interview that included the structured DIS, developed for use by lay interviewers in epidemiological studies.[12] Questions were asked about demographic characteristics, symptoms associated with a variety of mental disorders, a family history of alcohol abuse and/or mental disorders, a history of childhood behavior problems, the presence of several chronic illnesses, the use of health services within the past year, and at the Duke site, items concerned with social support and stressful life events experienced during the past year.

Subjects were asked if they tried to avoid the following situations because of unreasonable fear: (1) eating in public, (2) speaking in front of a small group, and (3) speaking to strangers. A positive diagnosis was given if the respondent endorsed at least one of the questions and gave an affirmative answer to the question of whether "having to avoid the situation interfered with your life or activities a lot." Subthreshold social phobia was defined as phobic avoidance of public speaking and/or meeting strangers or eating in public not associated with significant functional interference.

VARIABLES ASSESSED

Ten sets of variables that have been associated with the onset or course of social phobia were examined to assess whether SSP respondents were more similar to SP or C individuals[1,5,7]:

1. *Demographic characteristics:* urban residence, gender, race, marital status, employment status, income, age, and level of education.
2. *Familial characteristics:* family history of psychiatric disorder or alcohol abuse, parental abuse, early separation or divorce of parents, and parental poverty.
3. *Impaired school performance:* poor grades, repetition of grades, expulsion from school, and repeatedly playing hooky.
4. *Conduct disturbance in adolescence:* trouble with misbehavior, fighting, runaway behavior, stealing, and juvenile arrest.
5. *Social support measures:* subjective support, interaction, network size, instrumental support, and the presence of at least one close friend, as assessed by the Duke Social Support Index.[13] Subjective social support, a summative scale of 10 items, is concerned with feeling understood, feeling useful, being listened to, having a role in family, being able to count on family/friends in times of trouble, and being satisfied with relationships. Instrumental support, a summative scale of 13 items, is concerned with the types of help received from family/friends, such as helping out when sick, running errands, fixing things around the house, and giving advice. Social interaction includes the number of contacts via telephone, in person, or in meetings the subject had within the past week, and social network refers to the number of household members and other family members who are living within one hour's travel, and time spent talking with others at work/school. The social support scales were arbitrarily dichotomized into impaired vs nonimpaired following examination of the psychometric properties of each scale completed by more than 2700 of the community-based respondents participating in both ECA surveys with complete data on the social support items (D.C.H., D.G.B., and C. Hybels, MPH, unpublished technical report, April 1990). Approximately 15% (weighted data) of the wave I respondents were considered impaired on each of the four support scales. The Cronbach α reliability coefficient for subjective social support at wave I was .79, the mean score was 26.1 (high-positive) (SD, 2.7). Respondents who scored 23 or less were considered impaired. The mean score for instrumental support was 10.3 (SD, 2.5). Respondents who scored less than 18 were considered impaired. The mean score for social interaction was 6.3 (SD, 2.7). Sub-

jects who scored less than 4 were considered impaired. The mean score for social network was 5.0 (SD, 3.1). Respondents who scored less than 3 were considered impaired. Reliability coefficients were not computed for the instrumental, interaction, and network scales because the items that made up each of these scales were not considered to have a common cause.

6. *Self confidence,* as determined by whether or not the subject feels capable of dealing with problems on his or her own.

7. *Stressful life events in the past year:* total number and number of negative events.

8. *Health status:* number of chronic medical disorders, number of days sick in the past 90 days, and lifetime number of alcohol symptoms.

9. *Health-seeking behaviors:* number of medical visits in previous 6 months and number of mental health visits in previous year; and *medication use:* use of hypnotic, tranquilizer, and antidepressant medications in the past year.

10. *Psychiatric comorbidity:* number of lifetime DIS/*DSM-III* diagnoses and incidence of suicidal thoughts and attempts.

METHODS OF ANALYSIS

The three groups were compared with one another on all the above characteristics utilizing parametric and nonparametric bivariate and multivariate procedures. To minimize the chance of type II errors with the multiple comparisons made, the Bonferroni correction was used to calculate the level of probability considered statistically significant. For the bivariate analyses, only those variables with $P \leq .0001$ were considered statistically significant. However, variables significant at $P \leq .01$ are also shown in the tables, as they represent a trend we believe merits attention.

We used χ^2 analysis to determine the presence of associations among and between the three groups for each of the categorical variables. Fisher's Exact Test was used when cell tables were sparse and χ^2 analysis was unreliable.

An analysis of variance procedure was used to compare mean scores of the continuous variables with a normal distribution across the three groups, and the *t* test was used to compare means across pairs of groups (SSP vs SP, SSP vs C, and SP vs C). The Kruskal-Wallis Test was used for comparisons of the continuous variables with a nonnormal distribution across all three groups, and the Mann-Whitney *U* test was used for paired comparisons. All bivariate analyses were repeated comparing means across the three groups and the pairs of groups after excluding cases of lifetime comorbid psychiatric disorder, except for simple phobia. These analyses were repeated excluding respondents with simple phobia. Results of these analyses (available on request from the authors) are not reported, because the diminished size of the SP group reduced our confidence in the results.

In some instances, the percentage difference between the SP and SSP groups was greater than that between the SSP and C groups. For example, 2.9% more SSP than C respondents reported a psychiatric illness in the family, compared with 5.8% more SP than SSP respondents. Nevertheless, the χ^2 value did not reach the threshold for statistical significance. This may have been a result of there being insufficient power to detect a "true" difference because of the small size of the SSP and SP groups relative to the C group. To determine whether the sample size influenced our ability to find "true" differences between the two diagnostic groups, one additional test was performed on all variables in which the difference between the SSP and SP groups was the same as or greater than the difference between the SSP and C groups. We calculated the sample size that would be required of each group to determine whether the observed difference was a "true" difference at $P=.0001$ and a power of .80. We reasoned that if the sample size required for each group was equal to or less than that of the control group (n=1117), the larger number of respondents in the SSP and SP groups would have resulted in the group differences being statistically significant. If the sample size required for each of the social phobic groups was greater than that of the control group, the observed difference between the SSP and SP groups could have happened by chance.

Multivariate modeling with group membership (SSP vs C, SP vs C, SP vs SSP) as the dependent variable was conducted using a logistic regression procedure. Categorical and continuous variables examined in the bivariate analyses that demonstrated an association with either the SSP or SP group were the independent variables included in each model. These variables were selected to determine whether the statistically significant bivariate associations held when other variables associated with group membership were statistically controlled.

RESULTS

Altogether, there were 1488 subjects in the analyses. The rates of SSP (n=248) and SP (n=123) were 6.7% and 3.8%, respectively, yielding a lifetime prevalence of social phobia of 10.5% in the total population.

DEMOGRAPHICS

Bivariate group comparisons on the demographic characteristics are presented in **Table 1**. Comparisons that remained significant after subjects with psychiatric comorbidity were excluded are shown in brackets. Statistically significant overall differences among the three diagnostic groups were found for sex, marital status, work behaviors, personal income, and years of education. In the paired comparisons, SSP subjects were more likely than C subjects to be female, to be unmarried, and to report repeated lateness/absences from work, lower income, and fewer years of education. There was a trend for SSP respondents to report a lower rate of employment. When comorbid SP subjects were deleted from the sample and the analyses were repeated, SSP respondents were more likely to be female and to report less income and fewer years of education.

Similar differences were observed between the SP and C groups with respect to marital status, work behaviors, personal income, and years of education. These

Table 1. Comparisons of Demographic Characteristics Among Nonpsychiatric Controls (C), Subthreshold Social Phobics (SSP), and Social Phobics (SP)

	C (n=1117)	SSP (n=248)*	SP (n=123)*	χ^2 or F Value†‡ Overall	C vs SSP	C vs SP
Urban residence, %	46.9	49.2	52.0	NS	NS	NS
Male, %	46.6	26.2	31.7	40.6§ [34.7§]	34.6§ [30.9§]	10.0‖
White, %	72.6	64.9	68.3	NS	NS	NS
Married, %	60.1	46.8	41.5	26.6§ [8.5‖]	14.7§ [8.0‖]	15.8§
Employed, %	61.0	49.6	52.0	12.9‖	10.8¶	NS
Repeated lateness/absence, %#	2.6	9.4	15.9	52.6§	24.1§ [7.4‖]	48.3§
Personal income quartile, %**						
1	13.8	27.5	29.3	NS	NS	NS
2	29.9	38.5	41.5	92.8§ [36.6§]	62.3§ [33.0§]	41.5§
3	32.0	28.3	23.6	NS	NS	NS
4	24.2	5.7	5.7	NS	NS	NS
Age, y††	49.4±19.3	49.5±19.7	46.3±19.2	NS	NS	NS
Education, y††‡‡	12.1±3.4	10.6±3.5	10.4±3.3	31.2§ [10.9§]	42.5§ [20.2§]	28.0§

Noncomorbid groups: SSP (n=135) and SP (n=36).
†*Values in brackets are significant after eliminating comorbidity. NS indicates not significant.*
‡*For SSP vs SP, no values were significant.*
§*P<.0001.*
‖*P<.01.*
¶*P<.001.*
#*Data were missing for 74 cases.*
***Data were missing for four cases.*
††*Values are mean±SD.*
‡‡*Data were missing for two cases.*

differences disappeared when subjects with identified psychiatric comorbidity were removed from the sample.

No differences were found between respondents in the SSP and SP groups.

FAMILIAL, SCHOOL PERFORMANCE, AND CONDUCT DISTURBANCE VARIABLES

Group comparisons on familial, school performance, and conduct disturbance characteristics with and without psychiatric comorbidity are presented in **Table 2**. Significant overall differences were found with respect to early parental separation or divorce. There was a trend for differences on familial psychiatric history, familial alcohol abuse, and parental poverty. Respondents in the SSP and SP groups showed greater disturbance than respondents in the C group. Statistically significant overall differences were found with respect to three school performance measures: poor grades, repeating grades, and expulsion from school. There was a trend for group differences on the variable, "played hooky repeatedly." Significant overall differences were also found with regard to three of the five conduct disturbance variables examined: frequently in trouble for misbehaving, in trouble for fighting, and runaway behavior. There was a trend for group differences for repeated theft. A greater percentage of SSP and SP respondents than C respondents reported these behaviors.

In the paired group comparisons, SSP subjects were significantly more disturbed than C subjects with respect to parental poverty, poor grades, frequently in trouble for misbehavior, and runaway behavior. Compared with C respondents, SP respondents were more likely to report the following: early parental separation/divorce, poor grades, had to repeat school grade, expelled from school, frequently in trouble for misbehavior, in trouble for fighting, and runaway behavior.

If the SSP and SP groups had been considerably larger, with increased power (.80) to detect "true" differences between the groups, it is likely that SSP and SP respondents would have differed from one another with respect to early parental separation/divorce, having to repeat a school grade, and repeated stealing.

After subjects with psychiatric comorbidity other than simple phobia were eliminated, overall significant differences between groups in the paired comparison were found with respect to poor grades. Compared with C respondents, SSP respondents were more likely to report poor grades. No significant differences were found in the noncomorbid SP-vs-C or SSP-vs-SP comparisons.

SOCIAL SUPPORT MEASURES AND LACK OF CONFIDENCE

Group comparisons on social support measures and lack of confidence with and without psychiatric comorbidity are presented in **Table 3**. Overall differences were noted with respect to greater impairment of SSP and SP subjects in subjective support, instrumental support, presence of close friends, and lack of confidence in handling problems alone. There was a trend for more SSP and SP respondents than C respondents to be impaired on social interaction.

In the paired comparisons, SSP respondents differed from C respondents on impaired subjective support, lack of a close friend, and lack of confidence in handling problems. More SP than C respondents reported

Table 2. Comparisons of Familial, Childhood, School, and Conduct Characteristics Among Nonpsychiatric Controls (C), Subthreshold Social Phobics (SSP), and Social Phobics (SP)

	C (n=1117), %	SSP (n=248), %*	SP (n=123), %*	χ^2 Value† Overall	C vs SSP	C vs SP	SSP vs SP
Familial‡							
Familial psychiatric disorder	7.6	10.5	16.3	9.8§ [10.3§]	NS	9.0§ [10.1§]	NS
Familial alcohol abuse	11.8	17.3	20.6	9.4§	NS	6.3§	NS
Parental abuse	3.0	3.5	5.1	NS	NS	NS	NS
Early parental separation/divorce	6.4	8.5	16.5	16.4‖	NS	16.4‖	¶
Parental poverty	42.9	54.8	53.9	12.4§ [9.0§]	9.6§	NS	NS
School Performance#							
Poor grades	4.1	11.1	16.1	37.6‖ [15.5‖]	18.9‖ [12.9‖]	30.3‖	NS
Had to repeat grades	21.6	30.3	41.3	27.7‖	8.4§ [7.1§]	23.4‖	**
Expelled from school	6.6	11.4	15.6	16.2‖	6.8§	12.9‖	NS
Played hooky repeatedly	17.0	22.4	27.9	11.1§	NS	8.8§	NS
Conduct Disturbance‡							
Frequently in trouble for misbehavior	4.1	10.5	13.0	27.0‖	16.6‖	18.4‖	NS
In trouble for fighting	8.0	13.9	18.8	19.9‖	8.5§	15.7‖	NS
Runaway from home	1.2	4.9	9.8	40.6‖	15.3‖	41.4‖	NS
Repeatedly stole	7.2	9.7	16.3	12.3§	NS	12.0††	‡‡
Arrested as juvenile	1.5	2.4	4.1	NS	NS	NS	NS

*Noncomorbid groups: SSP (n=135) and SP (n=36).
†Values in brackets are significant after eliminating comorbidity. NS indicates not significant.
‡The number of subjects with data varied from 1469 to 1487.
§P<.01.
‖P<.0001.
¶If the sample size were 735 or greater in each group, the observed difference would represent a "true" difference.
#The number of subjects with data varied from 1396 to 1479.
**If the sample size were 804 or greater in each group, the observed difference would represent a "true" difference.
††P<.001.
‡‡If the sample size were 1107 or greater in each group, the observed difference would represent a "true" difference.

Table 3. Comparisons of Social Support Measures, Lack of Confidence, and Recent Life Events Among Nonpsychiatric Controls (C), Subthreshold Social Phobics (SSP), and Social Phobics (SP)

	C (n=1117)	SSP (n=248)*	SP (n=123)*	χ^2 or z Value† Overall	C vs SSP	C vs SP	SSP vs SP
Social Support‡							
Impaired subjective support, %	7.0	17.4	31.1	78.9§	26.3§	73.6§	‖
Impaired social interaction, %	11.0	18.4	18.8	14.2¶	10.3¶	6.6#	NS
Impaired network size, %	24.6	17.7	21.5	NS	NS	NS	NS
Impaired instrumental support, %	9.7	15.8	23.5	23.9§ [14.7¶]	7.42#	21.0§ [13.9§]	NS
Presence of at least one close friend, %	95.9	89.0	86.8	28.8§ [15.2§]	18.6§ [15.2§]	18.9§	NS
No confidence in handling problems, %	4.6	13.6	24.6	72.9§ [10.7#]	27.0§ [8.5#]	68.7§	**
Recent Life Changes (Past Year)‡							
No. of life events	0.88±1.14	1.46±1.38	1.52±1.64	64.0§ [17.5¶]	7.11§ [4.1§]	4.7§	NS
No. of negative events	0.26±0.58	0.53±0.88	0.66±0.88	60.8§ [11.7¶]	5.51§ [3.1§]	6.6§	NS

*Noncomorbid groups: SSP (n=123) and SP (n=36).
†Values in brackets are significant after eliminating comorbidity. NS indicates not significant.
‡The number of subjects with data varied from 1430 to 1480.
§P<.0001.
‖If the sample size were 418 or greater in each group, the observed difference would represent a "true" difference.
¶P<.001.
#P<.01.
**If the sample size were 138 or greater in each group, the observed difference would represent a "true" difference.

impaired subjective and instrumental support, lack of at least one close friend, and lack of confidence. If the SSP and SP groups had been considerably larger, with increased power to detect "true" differences between the groups, it is likely that fewer SSP than SP respondents would have been impaired on subjective social support and confidence in handling problems.

When subjects with psychiatric comorbidity were eliminated from the sample, overall differences were found on only one social support variable, presence of at least one close friend. Compared with C respondents, SSP respondents were less likely to report having a close friend. No significant differences were found between SSP and SP respondents.

Table 4. Comparison of Health Status, Health-Seeking Behaviors, and Medication Use Among Nonpsychiatric Controls (C), Subthreshold Social Phobics (SSP), and Social Phobics (SP)

	C (n=1117)	SSP (n=248)*	SP (n=123)*	χ^2 or z Value† Overall	C vs SSP	C vs SP	SSP vs SP
Health Status							
No. of chronic medical disorders‡	0.87±1.14	1.27±1.38	1.27±1.38	24.9§ [11.1‖]	4.2§ [3.3¶]	3.3¶	NS
No. of days sick in past 90 d‡	3.13±13.72	4.38±14.37	6.92±18.62	35.0§	3.9§	5.1§	NS
Lifetime No. of alcohol symptoms‡	0.18±0.58	0.94±2.62	1.28±3.40	26.2§	4.1§	3.8§	NS
Health-Seeking Behaviors							
No. of medical visits in past 6 mo‡	1.69±4.10	2.05±4.25	3.12±5.34	12.0‖	NS	3.4¶	#
No. of mental health visits in past 6 mo‡	0.23±1.93	1.06±4.82	4.08±15.97	70.7§ [27.3¶]	4.6§	8.3§ [5.2§]	**
Medication Use in Past Year							
Hypnotic medication, %	7.8	15.7	22.8	36.0§	15.3§ [6.1‖]	29.5§	NS
Tranquilizers, %	6.6	16.2	23.6	51.4§ [10.3‖]	24.2§ [9.7‖]	41.8§	NS
Antidepressants, %	1.2	4.9	10.6	45.7§	15.3§	47.7§	††

*Noncomorbid groups: SSP (n=135) and SP (n=36).
†Values in brackets are significant after eliminating comorbidity. NS indicates not significant.
‡Values are mean±SD.
§$P<.0001$.
‖$P<.01$.
¶$P<.001$.
#If the sample size were 653 or greater in each group, the observed difference would represent a "true" difference.
**If the sample size were 387 or greater in each group, the observed difference would represent a "true" difference.
††If the sample size were 945 or greater in each group, the observed difference would represent a "true" difference.

RECENT LIFE CHANGES

Group comparisons on recent life changes with and without psychiatric comorbidity are also presented in Table 3. An overall significant difference was found in both the total number of life events in the past year and the total number of negative life events, with the SSP and SP groups both differing from the C group. When comorbid cases were excluded, trends toward significant group differences were still found in the overall comparisons and in the SSP-vs-C comparisons. No significant differences were found in the SSP-vs-SP comparisons.

HEALTH STATUS AND HEALTH-SEEKING BEHAVIORS

Group comparisons on health status are presented in **Table 4**. Statistically significant overall differences were found on the following health status measures: number of chronic medical disorders, number of days sick in last 90 days, and lifetime number of alcohol symptoms (all greater in the SSP and SP groups). In the paired comparisons, differences were found in all three health status variables for the SSP vs C respondents and in days sick and alcohol symptoms for the SP vs C respondents. Respondents in the SSP vs SP groups reported greater impairment than respondents in the C group. No significant differences were found on health status variables in the SSP-vs-SP comparisons.

When comorbid cases were eliminated and the above analyses repeated, no statistically significant differences were found between the groups. However, a trend was observed for SSP vs C respondents to report more chronic illnesses.

Comparisons of health-seeking behaviors and psychotropic drug use are also presented in Table 4. Overall differences among the three groups were found for number of mental health visits in the past year and use of hypnotic, tranquilizer, and antidepressant medication over the past year, all of which were greater in the SSP and SP groups than in the C group. In the SSP-vs-C and SP-vs-C comparisons, there were significant differences in the number of mental health visits and the use of all three categories of psychotropic medications. Compared with C respondents, SSP and SP respondents reported more visits and were more likely to report use of hypnotic, tranquilizer, and antidepressant medications. If the sample of respondents in the SSP and SP groups had been considerably larger, with sufficient power to detect "true" differences between groups, the two groups would have differed in number of medical and mental health visits and use of antidepressant medications during the past year, with the SSP group demonstrating less impairment.

When subjects with comorbidity were eliminated from the sample and the analyses repeated, the abovementioned statistically significant overall group differences were eliminated. However, a trend was observed for number of mental health visits, with SP respondents reporting more visits than SSP and C respondents. A trend was also observed for more noncomorbid SSP than C respondents to report use of hypnotic and tranquilizer medications during the past year.

COMORBIDITY

Lifetime comorbidities of psychiatric illness and of suicidal thoughts and behavior were compared between the SSP and SP groups (**Table 5**). Significant increases were noted in the SP group with respect to the total number

Table 5. Comparison of Subthreshold Social Phobics (SSP) and Social Phobics (SP) on Lifetime Prevalence Rates of DIS/*DSM-III* Mental Disorders and Suicidality*

	SSP (n=248)	SP (n=123)	χ^2 or *z* Value	*P*†	Base Rate in Population (n=3801)‡
No. of *DSM-III* disorders§	1.06±1.46	2.51±2.46	6.26‖	.0001	...
Affective disorders, %					
Major depression	5.2	13.8	8.14	.004	3.9
Bipolar disorder	0.4	0.8	0.26	NS	0.2
Alcohol/substance use disorders, %					
Alcohol abuse/dependence	10.5	12.2	0.23	NS	8.7
Drug abuse/dependence	0.4	3.2	5.01	NS	1.1
Anxiety disorder, %					
Panic disorder	2.8	9.8	8.14	.004	1.6
Agoraphobia	9.7	47.1	67.1	.0001	7.8
Simple phobia	24.2	63.4	54.1	.0001	17.4
Posttraumatic stress disorder	1.0	3.0	1.68	NS	0.9
Generalized anxiety disorder	10.5	20.4	5.44	NS	8.8
Obsessive-compulsive disorder	4.4	17.1	16.7	.0001	3.3
Others, %					
Somatization disorder	1.6	4.9	3.34	NS	0.4
Schizophrenia/schizophreniform disorder	1.6	9.8	13.1	.0001	1.6
Suicidality, %					
Thought about suicide	11.3	30.1	20.0	.0001	9.3
Attempted suicide	1.6	9.8	13.2	.0001	1.5

**DIS indicates Diagnostic Interview Schedule.*
†NS indicates not significant.
‡Rates are weighted percentages and are included for reference purposes only.
§Values are mean±SD.
‖z score.

of DIS/*DSM-III* disorders as well as the specific diagnoses of major depression, four of the six anxiety disorders (panic disorder, agoraphobia, simple phobia, and obsessive-compulsive disorder), and schizophrenia/schizophreniform disorder. In addition, a greater percentage of SP subjects reported thoughts about and attempts at suicide.

MULTIVARIATE ANALYSES

Although several variables differentiated the SSP and SP respondents from the C respondents, we questioned whether these associations would hold up in a multivariate analysis if SSP-vs-C, SP-vs-C, or SSP-vs-SP group membership was regressed on these variables in three separate multivariate logistic regression analyses. Sixteen independent variables were placed in each regression model: sex, marital status, age, highest grade, number of school performance problems (range, 0-4), number of conduct disturbance problems (range, 0-4), parental poverty, four measures of impaired social support (lack of close friend, subjective support, social interaction, and instrumental support), lack of self-confidence, number of negative life events, number of chronic illnesses (range, 0-8), number of mental health visits, and use of psychotropic medications. One additional independent variable (number of *DSM-III* psychiatric disorders) was placed in the SSP-vs-SP regression model. This variable was not included in the other two models given that the C subjects were selected because they did not have an identified *DSM-III* disorder.

When SSP-vs-C group membership was regressed on the above 16 variables, four were statistically significant at $P \leq .01$: being female, having fewer years of formal education, having a greater number of school performance problems, and having a greater number of adolescent conduct disturbance symptoms (overall model: χ^2=160.5, 16 *df*, *P*=.0001). These same four variables were statistically significant at $P \leq .01$ when SP-vs-C group membership was regressed on the same set of variables (overall model: χ^2=219.27, 16 *df*, *P*=.0001). In addition, impaired instrumental support, lack of self-confidence, and a greater number of mental health visits were statistically significant predictors of SP group membership. In contrast, when SSP-vs-SP group membership was regressed on the 16 variables identified above and the number of *DSM-III* disorders, only two variables were statistically significant: impaired instrumental support and total number of *DSM-III* disorders (overall model: χ^2=48.97, 17 *df*, *P*=.0001). On both variables, SSP subjects were less impaired.

COMMENT

Subthreshold forms of social phobia have not been well studied in the past. Thus, it is difficult to know whether SSP individuals more closely resemble SP individuals or C individuals, many of whom may be presumed to exhibit some degree of social anxiety as a normal trait. In the present study we examined the differences among these three groups.

Many statistically significant overall differences were found, nearly all of which were accounted for by the SSP-vs-C and SP-vs-C comparisons. Only a few differences

were observed between SSP and SP respondents after adjustments were made for the smaller size of these two groups. Some of these differences were expected on the basis of sample definition (eg, more clinic visits and greater comorbidity). Considering both the number and pattern of observed differences among the SSP, SP, and C groups, we conclude that the condition we have labeled subthreshold social phobia is closely related to social phobia.

ONE OF THE important findings of this report lies in the socioeconomic disadvantages and impaired quality of life as well as increased treatment seeking of SSP individuals. In this regard, our findings are similar to those of Broadhead and colleagues' study of depression[6]; the groups showed substantial morbidity among subthreshold or so-called "minor" social phobia and depression, respectively. In reality, minor forms of psychiatric disorders should be taken seriously both in their own right and because they often serve as precursors to more serious events and disorders. There remains some doubt as to the real prevalence of clinically meaningful social phobia; a recent study by Stein and colleagues[2] noted that the prevalence of social phobia ranged from 1.9% to 18.7% depending on where the case threshold was set and also depending on the degree to which interviewers probed for feared situations. Stein and colleagues examined psychosocial interference, distress, and the presence of "pure" public speaking separately as criteria. Our results as well as those of recent studies[2,3] add to the growing evidence that over 10% of the population experiences social phobia to an extent that produces a significant clinical and socioeconomic impact.

Despite initially denying the screen question (ie, denying interference), SSP respondents were impaired or disadvantaged in many ways. It is possible that they denied interference from their social phobia on first questioning because they were insufficiently aware of the effects of their fear, because of lifelong adaptation to a phobic lifestyle, because of stigma, or for some other reason. We believe, on the basis of our results, that the DIS/*DSM-III* algorithm for social phobia was too restrictive and that previously reported rates based on the ECA[1,4,14] underestimate substantially the true prevalence and burden of social phobia.

Many of the SSP-vs-C differences remained significant when lifetime comorbidity was excluded. Among the demographic variables, SSP subjects were more likely to be female, to be earning a lower income, and to be less educated. In contrast to a previous report[11] that found increased risk of phobias among nonwhites, we found no difference between blacks and whites. However, in the original report,[11] the increased prevalence of phobias among blacks was restricted to agoraphobia and simple phobia.

The SSP group was also more impaired than the C group on subjective social support and lack of close friends. The latter variable remained significant in the noncomorbid groups. There was also a trend for the SSP-vs-C respondents to report impairment on social interaction and instrumental support. Given that SSP respondents also indicated less confidence in their ability to handle problems on their own, their failure to obtain adequate instrumental support from others puts them at a major disadvantage in terms of coping. The importance of this association takes on added significance with our finding that SSP subjects also reported higher numbers of total and negative life events during the preceding year and that hypnotic or minor tranquilizer (ie, benzodiazepines and barbiturates) medications had been prescribed for 16% of the SSP respondents during the previous year, even though they did not suffer from any major DIS psychiatric disorder. Reduced instrumental support, low self-confidence, more negative life events, and increased use of prescription psychotropic medications represent an unfortunate tetrad of characteristics among noncomorbid SSP individuals that, to our knowledge, has not previously received attention.

The increased use of prescribed anxiolytic and hypnotic medications in one out of six individuals in a 1-year period was surprising and calls for further consideration. The rate of tranquilizer use (14.0%) remained high among SSP subjects even after adjusting for comorbidity, although it did diminish somewhat in noncomorbid SP subjects, to 11.1%. Antidepressant use dropped considerably in both the SSP and SP noncomorbid groups, to 1.4% and 0, respectively. Our database did not explain the reasons for or the source of such treatment, but the SSP group made more visits for medical problems during the prior 6 months (mean, 2.05 visits) than they made for mental health problems during the previous year (mean, 1.06 visits), which suggests that a primary care physician or possibly a nonpsychiatric specialist prescribed medication. It is doubtful whether the prescribing physician recognized the presence of social phobic symptoms, since fully diagnosed SP subjects were not recognized as such when they presented for treatment to their physician because of psychological problems.[4] We stress the need for greater physician awareness of social phobia at all levels of severity, coupled with early and vigorous treatment. We also speculate from our data that increased levels of stress can give rise either to psychosomatic problems or to adjustment-related difficulties in subclinical SP individuals, and these may often be the reason for treatment seeking. We urge better elicitation of the presenting complaints of such individuals.

Subthreshold phobia was not associated with disturbed familial measures, except the possibility of greater parental poverty. However, higher rates of poor school performance were noted for SSP respondents, even for the noncomorbid SSP respondents, indicating a possible early manifestation of phobic anxiety. The increased frequency of early conduct disorder disappeared after comorbid conditions were excluded.

Logistic regression analyses revealed the importance of sociodemographic and developmental factors with respect to the characterization of SSP and SP. The increased risk of school performance and adolescent be-

havior problems in both groups may reflect what has been referred to elsewhere[15] as social-emotional learning disability. Women were more likely to be in the SSP and SP groups than the C group.

In a previous report using the ECA database,[16] we observed a relationship between chronic posttraumatic stress disorder and social phobia, which suggested the existence of a subtype of traumatically induced social phobia. The results here do not suggest this to be an important issue for the SSP group, which did not demonstrate an increased risk of posttraumatic stress disorder or of early parental abuse or early sexual trauma.

We should acknowledge some limitations of our study. While the DIS algorithm for social phobia shows acceptable validity relative to an independent psychiatric clinical diagnosis,[17] some problems may still exist.[18] By asking about only three feared situations, the DIS likely resulted in an underestimate of the prevalence of social phobia, since studies that asked about more situations yielded higher rates.[2,3] Moreover, the psychometric properties of the DIS algorithm for subthreshold social phobia have not been established. A second limitation arises from the use of *DSM-III* criteria, which are not identical to those of *DSM-III-R*. If anything, the *DSM-III* criteria are more restrictive and do not encompass the severe forms of generalized social phobia. Moreover, the DIS does not address fear of embarrassment or humiliation, both of which are central to social phobia. The DIS requires avoidance, whereas the *DSM-IV* requires avoidance or endurance with distress.

Our findings (1) suggest that the community prevalence and burden of social phobia are larger than has been realized, (2) reveal increased use of health services and tranquilizers by noncomorbid SSP individuals; (3) show that subthreshold social phobia in many respects closely resembles social phobia diagnosed according to DIS/*DSM-III* criteria; (4) suggest that clinicians should not limit treatment to patients with obvious impairment; and (5) suggest that researchers should be as willing to study cases below the diagnostic threshold as cases that meet the standard diagnostic criteria.

Accepted for publication August 17, 1994.

This study was supported by grant UO1MH35386 from the US Public Health Service to Drs Blazer and George.

Reprint requests to Box 3812, Duke University Medical Center, Durham, NC 27710 (Dr Davidson).

REFERENCES

1. Schneier FR, Johnson J, Hornig CD, Liebowitz MR, Weissman MM. Social phobia: comorbidity and morbidity in an epidemiological sample. *Arch Gen Psychiatry.* 1992;49:282-291.
2. Stein MB, Walker JR, Forde DR. Setting diagnostic thresholds for social phobia: considerations from a community study of social anxiety. *Am J Psychiatry.* 1994;152:408-412.
3. Kessler RC, McGonagle KA, Zhao S, Nelson CB, Hughes M, Eshleman S, Wittchen H-U, Kendler KS. Lifetime and 12-month prevalence of *DSM-III-R* psychiatric disorders in the United States: results from the National Comorbidity Survey. *Arch Gen Psychiatry.* 1994;51:8-19.
4. Davidson JRT, Hughes DC, George LK, Blazer DG. The epidemiology of social phobia: findings from the Duke Epidemiological Catchment Area Study. *Psychol Med.* 1993;23:709-718.
5. Amies PL, Gelder MG, Shaw PM. Social phobia: a comparative clinical study. *Psychiatry.* 1983;142:174-179.
6. Broadhead WE, Blazer DG, George LK, Tse CK. Depression, disability days, and days lost from work in a prospective epidemiological survey. *JAMA.* 1990; 264:2524-2528.
7. Solyom L, Ledwidge B, Solyom C. Delineating social phobia. *Br J Psychiatry.* 1986;149:464-470.
8. Eaton WW, Kessler LG. *Epidemiological Field Methods in Psychiatry: The NIMH Epidemiological Catchment Area Program.* Orlando, Fla: Academic Press Inc; 1985.
9. Blazer DG, George LK, Landerman R, Pennybacker M, Melville ML, Woodbury M, Manton KG, Jordan K, Locke B. Psychiatric disorders. *Arch Gen Psychiatry.* 1985;42:651-656.
10. Kessler LG, Folsom R, Royall R, Forsythe A, McEvoy L, Holzer CE, Rae DS, Woodbury M. Parameter and variance estimation. In: Eaton WW, Kessler LG, eds. *Epidemiological Field Methods in Psychiatry: The NIMH Epidemiologic Catchment Area Program.* Orlando, Fla: Academic Press Inc; 1985:327-348.
11. Eaton WW, Dryman A, Weissman MM. Panic and phobia. In: Robins LN, Regier DA, eds. *Psychiatric Disorders in America: The Epidemiological Catchment Area Study.* New York, NY: Free Press; 1991:155-179.
12. Robins LN, Helzer JE, Croughlan JL, Williams JBW, Spitzer RL. *NIMH Diagnostic Interview Schedule–Version III.* Rockville, Md: National Institute of Mental Health; 1981. Publication PHS ADM-T-42-3.
13. George LK, Blazer DG, Hughes DC, Fowler N. Social support and outcome of major depression. *Br J Psychiatry.* 1989;154:478-485.
14. Myers JK, Weissman MM, Tischler GL, Holzer CE, Leaf PJ, Orvaschal H, Anthony JC, Boyd JH, Burke JD, Kramer M, Stoltzman R. Six month prevalence of psychiatric disorders in three communities: 1980-1982. *Arch Gen Psychiatry.* 1984;41:959-967.
15. Voeller KSS. Social-emotional learning disabilities. *Psychiatr Ann.* 1991;21: 735-741.
16. Davidson JRT, Hughes DC, Blazer DG, George LK. Posttraumatic stress disorder in the community: an epidemiological study. *Psychol Med.* 1991;21:713-721.
17. Helzer JE, Robins LN, McEvoy LT, Spitznagel EL, Stollizman RK, Farmer A, Brockington IF. A comparison of clinical and Diagnostic Interview Schedule diagnosis. *Arch Gen Psychiatry.* 1985;42:657-664.
18. Anthony JC, Folstein M, Romanowski AJ, von Korff MR, Nestodt GR, Chahol R, Merchant A, Brown CH, Shapiro S, Kramer M, Gruemberg EM. Comparison of the lay Diagnostic Interview Schedule and a standardized psychiatric diagnosis. *Arch Gen Psychiatry.* 1985;42:667-675.

Birth Complications Combined With Early Maternal Rejection at Age 1 Year Predispose to Violent Crime at Age 18 Years

Adrian Raine, DPhil; Patricia Brennan, PhD; Sarnoff A. Mednick, PhD

Background: This study tests the biosocial interaction hypothesis that birth complications when combined with early maternal rejection of the infant predispose to adult violent crime.

Methods: This hypothesis was tested using a cohort of 4269 consecutive live male births on whom measures of birth complications (age 0), early maternal rejection (age 1 year), and violent crime (age 18 years) were collected.

Results: A significant interaction ($P<.0001$) between birth complications and early maternal rejection indicated that those who suffered both birth complications and early child rejection were most likely to become violent offenders in adulthood. While only 4.5% of the subjects had both risk factors, this small group accounted for 18% of all violent crimes. The effect was specific to violence and was not observed for nonviolent criminal offending.

Conclusions: To our knowledge, this is the first study to show that birth complications in combination with early child rejection predispose to violent crime. The findings illustrate the critical importance of integrating biological with social measures to fully understand how violence develops and also suggest that prenatal, perinatal, and early postnatal health care interventions could significantly reduce violence.

(Arch Gen Psychiatry. 1994;51:984-988)

THE RECENT report on understanding and preventing violence from the National Research Council suggests that birth complications may predispose to violence,[1(pp364-365)] but empirical support for this link is currently very limited. While several studies have indicated that perinatal factors are linked to later antisocial and criminal behavior,[2-7] not all studies have confirmed this relationship.[8]

There are four limitations to these important but initial studies that may help explain conflicting findings. First, samples tend not to have been representative of the general population. Second, it is unclear whether the effect is specific to violence or can be observed for nonviolent crime or repeated criminal offending; most previous research has found it difficult to isolate specific correlates of violent crime as opposed to correlates of criminal behavior in general.[1(p359)] Third, and most important, previous studies have not considered the possibility that birth complications may additionally require a negative early psychosocial environment to result in the specific outcome of violent behavior in adulthood. Research on school performance, for example, has indicated that the combination of birth complications and a negative family environment is associated with poor school performance.[9] While the interaction between biological and environmental variables is commonly believed to be important in explaining violent behavior,[1,3,10,11] there is surprisingly little hard empirical evidence to support such a view.[1(p102)] Fourth, previous studies have not assessed the potential importance of early child rejection in predisposing to violence. Maternal rejection of the infant and disruption to the mother-infant bond, in conjunction with a biological predisposition to violence, could prove critical in disrupting interpersonal development and predis-

See Methods on next page

From the Department of Psychology, University of Southern California–Los Angeles (Drs Raine, Brennan, and Mednick), and the Institute of Preventive Medicine, Copenhagen Health Services, Copenhagen, Denmark (Dr Mednick).

METHODS

SUBJECTS

Male subjects (N=4269) were drawn from a total cohort of 9125 consecutive births of males and females that took place in the maternity department of the State University Hospital (Rigshospitalet) in Copenhagen, Denmark, between September 1959 and December 1961. All live deliveries of over 20 weeks' gestation were included. Informed consent for human investigation was obtained from the parents. Further details of the birth cohort used in this study have been reported elsewhere.[12] Only data from males were analyzed because the very low rates of criminal violence in females (0.3%) precluded meaningful statistical analyses.

BIRTH COMPLICATIONS

Birth complications and conditions were recorded at the time of delivery by an obstetrician assisted by a midwife. This study uses a frequency birth complications score developed through the collaboration of American and Danish obstetricians and pediatric neurologists.[13,14] Examples of delivery complications on this scale include forceps extraction, breech delivery, umbilical cord prolapse, preeclampsia, and long birth duration. For analysis purposes, the subjects were divided into two groups: those with no delivery complications and those with one or more complications.

EARLY CHILD REJECTION AND SOCIAL CIRCUMSTANCE MEASURES

Demographic, family, and psychosocial variables were collected during pregnancy and when the child was 1 year old. Variables collected during pregnancy relevant to our analyses include whether the pregnancy was wanted or unwanted, the mother's attempts to abort the fetus, and the mother's age. Year 1 follow-up interview variables included home conditions, marital status, and placement of infant for care into a full-time public institution for more than 4 months of the first year. The socioeconomic status of the family (based on educational and occupational levels) was obtained at 1 year from the Danish Central Persons' Register.

A factor analysis using principal component analysis followed by a varimax rotation produced two factors with eigenvalues greater than 1. The two factors were defined as follows (factor loadings in parentheses): factor 1, "poor social circumstances": unmarried mother (.71); low socioeconomic status (.67); poor home conditions (.65); young maternal age (.64); unwanted pregnancy (.59); and factor 2, "early child rejection": public institutional care of infant (.68); attempt to abort fetus (.65); unwanted pregnancy (.44).

Having an unwanted pregnancy was the only measure common to both factors, but this variable was associated with two different psychosocial patterns. In factor 2, this lack of planning was coupled with a more "rejecting" pattern of behavior as indicated by the fact that the mother had attempted to abort her pregnancy, followed after birth by the child being sent to an institution for at least 4 months in the first year. Conversely, in factor 1, the unwanted pregnancy was not linked to these variables but instead was linked to poor family and social circumstances, including low social class, paternal absence, poor home conditions, and young maternal age. Consequently, factor 1 was tentatively labeled "poor social circumstances" while factor 2 was labeled "early child rejection."

Data were complete on all variables in this study with the exception that socioeconomic status information was missing for 653 subjects. In the results reported below, the data were analyzed in two ways: (1) using the reduced sample of 3616 and (2) using the entire sample of 4269. In analyses of the entire sample, the early maternal rejection factor was recomputed with the loading of social class (which did not load significantly on this factor) omitted.

VIOLENT CRIMINAL OFFENDING

Criminal status was assessed when the offspring were aged 17 to 19 years by a search of the Danish National Criminal Register in which all police contacts and court decisions involving Danish citizens are recorded. This is viewed as one of the most comprehensive and accurate registers in the Western world.[15] The definition of violence used by the National Academy of Sciences Panel on the Understanding and Control of Violence ("behaviors by individuals that intentionally threaten, attempt, or inflict physical harm on others") was used.[1] Consequently, violent crime was defined by the following offenses: murder, attempted murder, assault (including domestic assault), rape, armed robbery, illegal possession of a weapon, and threats of violence. Nonviolent crime was defined as theft, breaking and entering, fraud, forgery, blackmail, embezzlement, vandalism, prostitution, pimping, and narcotic offenses. One hundred forty-five subjects were classified as violent criminals (3.4%), 540 as nonviolent criminals (12.6%), and 3584 as noncriminals (84.0%). The total criminality rate of 16% in this Danish sample is similar to the rate of 17% found by Raine et al[16] for a community sample of English males.

posing to more callous, violent interpersonal behavior in later life.

The study reported herein attempts to overcome some problems associated with previous studies to better test the biosocial interaction hypothesis that birth complications interact with negative early psychosocial environment in predisposing to adult violent offending. In particular, the possibility that early child rejection may be a specific and important aspect of a negative psychosocial environment in predisposing to violence was tested. Specificity to violent as opposed to nonviolent crime was also assessed.

RESULTS

VIOLENT OFFENDERS VS NONCRIMINALS

A logistic regression analysis indicated a highly significant interaction between delivery complications and early child rejection in predicting violence (χ^2 [df=1, N=3175]=10.4, P<.002) and indicated that those who experienced both birth complications and early child rejection were most likely to become violent. To exemplify this relationship diagrammatically, rates of

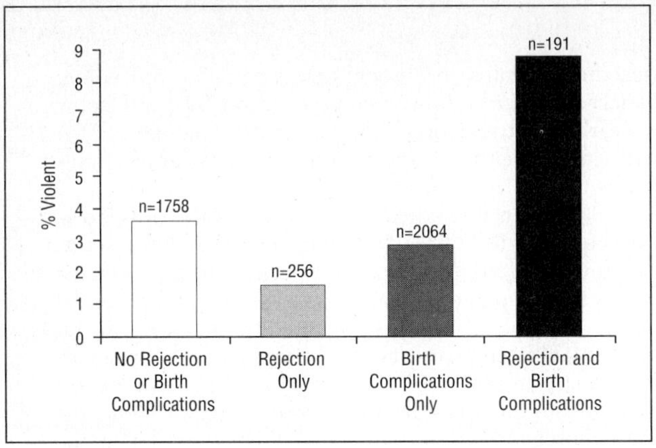

Illustration of the significant interaction (P<.0001) observed between birth complications and early maternal rejection at age 1 year in predicting outcome for criminal violence at age 18 years.

violence were calculated for those subjects who had both risk factors, ie, birth complications and severe maternal rejection (defined by mothers' negative attitude to pregnancy and either attempted abortion or institutionalization). Rates of violence for this group were compared with three other comparison groups: (1) those with neither risk factor, (2) those with severe maternal rejection only, and (3) those with birth complications only. Results of these analyses are shown in the **Figure**. Using this more severe criterion of maternal rejection, the interaction was again significant (χ^2 [df=1, N=3175]=14.4, $P<.0001$).

The interaction was specific to early maternal rejection in that no such interaction was observed between poor social circumstances and birth complications ($P>.66$). As has been observed in previous research,[1] a main effect was observed for poor social circumstances (χ^2 [df=1, N=3175]=40.6, $P<.00001$). No main effects were observed for birth complications ($P>.90$) or early child rejection ($P>.62$).

VIOLENT OFFENDERS VS NONVIOLENT CRIMINALS

The above interaction is specific to violent offending and is not found for nonviolent crime. A significant interaction between birth complications and early child rejection was observed when violent criminals were compared with nonviolent criminals in a logistic regression analysis (χ^2 [df=1, N=557]=6.3, $P<.02$). The interaction indicated that those who experienced both high birth complications and early child rejection were most likely to become violent criminals, ie, of offenders who had both risk factors, 47.2% became violent compared with 19.7% of offenders who had neither risk factor or only one.

In this comparison of violent with nonviolent criminals, the interaction effect is again specific to maternal rejection. No interaction effect was observed for poor social circumstances and birth complications ($P>.80$). In addition, main effects were not found for early child rejection ($P>.39$), poor social circumstances ($P>.08$), or birth complications ($P>.23$).

POTENTIAL CONFOUNDERS

Reduced Sample Size Due to Missing Data

The effect of the interaction of birth complications and early maternal rejection was reanalyzed for the total sample of 4269 by recomputing scores on the early maternal rejection factor as described above. The interaction between birth complications and early child rejection was again significant when comparing violent criminals with noncriminals (χ^2 [df=1, N=3729]=12.3, $P<.0005$) and when comparing violent criminals with nonviolent criminals (χ^2 [df=1, N=685]=7.2, $P<.007$).

Controlling for Recidivism

The interaction between birth complications and early child rejection in predisposing to violence cannot be accounted for by the fact that violent offenders commit more crime in general than nonviolent criminals. When violent offenders were compared with nonviolent offenders, the interaction between birth complications and early child rejection in predisposing to violent crime remained significant and in the predicted direction when the total number of crimes was entered as a covariate (χ^2 [df=1, N=557]=6.56, $P<.01$). Furthermore, when violent offenders were matched on total number of crimes committed with an equal number of nonviolent offenders, the interaction remained significant and in the predicted direction (χ^2 [df=1, N=332]=4.2, $P<.05$). These results indicate that the biosocial interaction applies to all violent offenders whether they commit repeated offenses or not.

COMMENT

To our knowledge, this is the first study to provide evidence from a large birth cohort to show that birth complications in combination with a negative psychosocial environment (specifically early child rejection) are associated with violent crime in early adulthood. In contrast, the very few previous biosocial studies have neither shown specificity for violence nor highlighted the specific importance of early child rejection.[9,14] The interaction between biological and social predispositions appears to be critically important in understanding violent offending[17,18] because possession of only one risk factor (ie, birth complications alone or early child rejection alone) was not associated with increased rates of violence. This interaction effect was found to be specific to violent crime and not crime in general, whereas most previous biological research has not obtained specificity for violent crime per se.[1(p359)]

The fact that birth complications combined with child rejection but not the more general factor of poor social circumstances in predisposing to violence helps establish a more specific biosocial pathway toward violent crime. Poor social circumstances such as low social class and poor home conditions have been found to be general, weak correlates of violent and nonviolent crime, whereas there is some evidence that variables related to child rejection such as child neglect, lack of maternal warmth, and separation from parents may be more spe-

cific predispositions toward violent crime in particular.[19-21] Disruption to the mother-infant bonding processes due to institutionalization has been associated with affectionless psychopathic criminal behavior.[22,23] Poor early bonding may therefore lead to more callous, affectionless, unempathic interpersonal relationships that in turn may increase the likelihood of violent interpersonal behavior, particularly when combined with a preexisiting biological predisposition to violence.

It is not known precisely how birth complications predispose to violence, but it is possible that such complications result in brain dysfunction and associated neurological and neuropsychological deficits that in turn directly and indirectly predispose to violence.[3,24-26] For example, birth complications could lead to cognitive deficits that in turn lead to school failure, occupational failure, and ultimately violence. Similarly, birth complications may contribute to neuropsychiatric deficits and lack of self-control, resulting in explosive, impulsive aggression.[7] The effects of any such brain dysfunction may in turn be exacerbated by a negative early psychosocial environment.[3,9]

While prospective longitudinal studies can help tease out causality by establishing temporal ordering of variables, they cannot establish causality per se, and several causal pathways are feasible other than the one described above. Specifically, it is possible that a third factor underlies the link between birth complications/parental rejection and violence. For example, it is conceivable that there are genetic predispositions to birth complications, negative parenting, and violence and that genetic factors underlie the observed relationships.

It could be argued that birth complications and maternal rejection are not independent events. Specifically, children with birth complications might be more likely to be rejected by their mothers. This scenario seems unlikely, however, for two reasons. First, two of the three variables making up the construct of early child rejection precede birth in time (unwanted pregnancy, attempts to abort fetus) rather than postdating birth complications. Second, birth complications and early child rejection were not positively correlated in this sample ($\tau = -.029$), indicating that these constructs reflect processes that are largely independent.

We would caution against the overgeneralization of our findings to other populations at this stage and emphasize the need for replication of our findings in the United States. Denmark is a relatively homogeneous society and future studies are needed to confirm this biosocial interaction in countries such as the United States with its higher rates of violent crime. Such homogeneity in Denmark may, however, reduce the amount of variance in violence and attenuate our findings; as such, it is anticipated that similar findings to those observed in Denmark might be expected in a future replication study in the United States. We also would caution that these findings do not demonstrate causal links between birth complications/early child rejection and later violence, although the prospective, longitudinal nature of the study helps to provide some support for such an interpretation. Furthermore, it is recognized that birth complications and early child rejection are only two of many risk factors for violence, which also include learning deficits,[27] parental criminality,[28] low serotonin levels,[29] parental absence,[21,30] neuropsychological deficits,[24,31,32] poor parental supervision,[33,34] child abuse,[20,32] low arousal,[16] poor affective relationships,[35,36] and parental criminality.[37]

Results of this study raise two important questions with respect to efforts to reduce rates of violence that focus on biological and psychosocial risk factors. The first question concerns whether interventions aimed at providing better antenatal health care to underserved populations could have an effect in reducing rates of violence. The recent National Research Council report on understanding and preventing violence recommended that serious consideration be given to conducting such interventions to reduce perinatal complications,[1(pp383-384)] although this recommendation was based on limited empirical data. In the present study, we found that although only 4.5% of population had both birth complications and early child rejection, this small group accounted for 18% of all violent crimes perpetrated by the entire sample of 4269. Assuming early interventions could successfully reduce birth complications and the link between birth complications and violence is causal, these findings suggest that such interventions could conceivably reduce violence in the next generation by as much as 18%. The current findings lend some support for the consideration of initial perinatal intervention research studies to test whether the link between birth complications/early child rejection and violence is causal.

The second question concerns whether changing the psychosocial environment can help reduce violence in society. Very little is known regarding what factors protect a biologically predisposed individual from becoming violent. The finding that birth complications do not predispose to violence when combined with a nonrejecting early home environment (Figure) is of potential importance because it suggests that a good psychosocial home environment can protect against the otherwise negative effects of birth complications. This is consistent with previous findings that good parental care and the opportunity to bond with a caregiver in the first year of life can reduce the deleterious cognitive and behavioral effects of birth complications.[2,9] Psychosocial interventions aimed at increasing caregiving skills to parents may conceivably help suppress this biological predisposition to later adult violence.

Accepted for publication August 2, 1994.

This research was conducted with the support of Research Scientist Development Award K02MH01114-01 (Dr Raine) and Research Scientist Award 5 K05MH00619-08 (Dr Mednick) from the National Institute of Mental Health, Rockville, Md, and a grant from the Harry Frank Guggenheim Foundation (Dr Brennan).

Presented at the Annual Meeting of the American Association for the Advancement of Science, San Francisco, Calif, February 23, 1994.

Reprint requests to Department of Psychology, S.G.M. Building, University of Southern California–Los Angeles, Los Angeles, CA 90089-1061 (Dr Raine).

REFERENCES

1. Reiss AJ, Roth JA, eds. *Understanding and Preventing Violence.* Washington, DC: National Academy Press; 1993.
2. Werner EE, Smith RS. *Overcoming the Odds: High Risk Children From Birth to Adulthood.* Ithaca, NY: Cornell University Press; 1992.
3. Raine A. *The Psychopathology of Crime: Criminal Behavior as a Clinical Disorder.* San Diego, Calif: Academic Press; 1993.
4. Brennan P, Mednick SA, Kandel E. Congenital determinants of violent and property offending. In: Pepler DJ, Rubin KH, eds. *The Development and Treatment of Childhood Aggression.* Hillsdale, NJ: Lawrence Erlbaum Associates; 1993:81-92.
5. Kandel E, Mednick SA. Perinatal complications predict violent offending. *Criminology.* 1991;29:519-529.
6. Litt SM. *Perinatal Complications and Criminality.* Ann Arbor: University of Michigan; 1971. Doctoral dissertation.
7. Mungas D. An empirical analysis of specific syndromes of violent behavior. *J Nerv Ment Dis.* 1983;171:354-361.
8. Denno DJ. *Biology, Crime and Violence: New Evidence.* Cambridge, England: Cambridge University Press; 1989.
9. Drillien CM. *The Growth and Development of the Prematurely Born Infant.* Baltimore, Md: Williams & Williams; 1964.
10. Mednick SA, Christiansen KO. *Biosocial Bases of Criminal Behavior.* New York, NY: Gardner; 1977.
11. Raine A, Mednick SA. Biosocial longitudinal research into antisocial behavior. *Rev Epidemiol Sante Publique.* 1989;37:515-524.
12. Zachau Christiansen B, Ross EM. *Babies: Human Development During the First Year.* London, England: Wiley & Sons; 1975.
13. Mednick SA, Mura E, Schulsinger F, Mednick B. Perinatal conditions and infant development in the children of schizophrenic parents. *Soc Biol.* 1971;18:5103-5113.
14. Baker RL, Mednick BR. *Influences on Human Development: A Longitudinal Analysis.* Boston, Mass: Kluwer; 1984.
15. Wolfgang ME. Foreword. In: Mednick SA, Christiansen KO, eds. *Biosocial Bases of Criminal Behavior.* New York, NY: Gardner; 1977:v-vi.
16. Raine A, Venables PH, Williams M. Relationships between CNS and ANS measures of arousal at age 15 and criminality at age 24. *Arch Gen Psychiatry.* 1990;47:1003-1007.
17. Eichelman B. Neurochemical and psychopharmacological aspects of aggressive behavior. *Ann Rev Med.* 1970;41:149-158.
18. Widom CS. Does violence beget violence? a critical examination of the literature. *Psychol Bull.* 1991;109:130.
19. Farrington DP. Childhood aggression and adult violence: early precursors and later life outcomes. In: Pepler DJ, Rubin KH, eds. *The Development and Treatment of Childhood Aggression.* Hillsdale, NJ: Lawrence Erlbaum Associates; 1991:5-29.
20. Widom CS. The cycle of violence. *Science.* 1989;244:160-166.
21. McCord JM. A longitudinal view of the relationship between paternal absence and crime. In: Gunn J, Farrington DP, eds. *Abnormal Offenders, Delinquency, and the Criminal Justice System.* Chichester, England: Wiley & Sons; 1982: 113-127.
22. Bowlby J. *Forty-four Juvenile Thieves: Their Characters and Home Life.* London, England: Baillere Tindall & Cox; 1946.
23. Rutter M. *Maternal Deprivation Reassessed.* 2nd ed. Harmondsworth, England: Penguin; 1982.
24. Moffitt TE. The neuropsychology of juvenile delinquency: a critical review. In: Tonry M, Morris N, eds. *Crime and Justice: A Review of the Literature.* Chicago, Ill: University of Chicago Press; 1990.
25. Moffitt TE, Henry B. Neuropsychological studies of juvenile delinquency and juvenile violence. In: Milner JS, ed. *Neuropsychology of Aggression.* Boston, Mass: Kluwer; 1991:131-146.
26. Lewis DO, Pincus JH, Bard B, Richardson E, Prichep LS, Feldman M, Yeager C. Neuropsychiatric, psycho-educational, and family characteristics of 14 juveniles condemned to death in the United States. *Am J Psychiatry.* 1988;145: 584-589.
27. Wilson JQ, Herrnstein RJ. *Crime and Human Nature.* New York, NY: Simon & Schuster; 1985.
28. Loeber R, Dishion T. Early predictors of male delinquency: a review. *Psychol Bull.* 1983;94:68-99.
29. Linnoila VMI, Virkkunen M. Aggression, suicidality, and serotonin. *J Clin Psychiatry.* 1992;53:46-51.
30. Ellis L. The victimful-victimless crime distinction, and seven universal demographic correlates of victimful criminal behavior. *Pers Individual Differ.* 1988; 9:525-548.
31. Ellis L. Left and mixed handedness and criminality: explorations for a probable relationship. In: Coran S, ed. *Left Handedness: Behavioral Implications and Anomalies.* Amsterdam, the Netherlands: Elsevier Science Publishers; 1990.
32. Lewis DO. From abuse to violence: psychophysiological consequences of maltreatment. *J Am Acad Child Adolesc Psychiatry.* 1992;31:383-391.
33. Loeber R. Development and risk factors of juvenile antisocial behavior and delinquency. *Clin Psychol Rev.* 1990;10:1-41.
34. Loeber R, Stouthamer-Loeber M. Family factors as correlates and predictors of juvenile conduct problems and delinquency. In: Tonry M, Morris N, eds. *Crime and Justice.* Chicago, Ill: Chicago University Press; 1986;7:29-149.
35. McCord J. Long-term perspectives on parental absence. In: Robins LN, Rutter M, eds. *Straight and Devious Pathways From Childhood to Adulthood.* Cambridge, England: Cambridge University Press; 1990:116-134.
36. Farrington DP, Hawkins JD. Predicting participation, early onset, and later persistence in officially recorded offending. *Criminal Behav Ment Health.* 1991; 1:1-33.
37. Farrington DP. Early predictors of adolescent aggression and adult violence. *Violence Victims.* 1989;4:79-100.

ORIGINAL ARTICLE

One-Year Follow-up of Psychotherapy and Pharmacotherapy for Cocaine Dependence

Delayed Emergence of Psychotherapy Effects

Kathleen M. Carroll, PhD; Bruce J. Rounsaville, MD; Charla Nich, MS; Lynn T. Gordon, RN, MPA; Philip W. Wirtz, PhD; Frank Gawin, MD

Background: Neither the durability of brief ambulatory treatments for cocaine dependence nor the relative ability of psychotherapy vs pharmacotherapy to effect lasting change has been evaluated in well-controlled randomized trials.

Methods: We conducted a 1-year naturalistic follow-up of 121 ambulatory cocaine abusers who underwent psychotherapy (cognitive-behavioral relapse prevention or clinical management) and pharmacotherapy (desipramine hydrochloride or placebo) in a 2×2 design. Subjects were interviewed 1, 3, 6, or 12 months after the termination of a 12-week course of outpatient treatment. Eighty percent (n=97) of the subjects who were randomized to treatment were followed up at least once.

Results: First, the effects of study treatments appeared durable over the follow-up; as for the full sample, measures of cocaine use indicated either improvement or no change over posttreatment levels. Second, abstinence during treatment was strongly associated with less cocaine use during follow-up. Third, random effects regression models indicated significant psychotherapy-by-time effects, suggesting a delayed improved response during follow-up for patients who received cognitive-behavioral relapse prevention compared with supportive clinical management.

Conclusions: Our findings suggest a delayed emergence of the effects of cognitive-behavioral relapse prevention, which may reflect the subjects' implementation of the generalizable coping skills conveyed through that treatment. Moreover, these data underline the importance of conducting follow-up studies of substance abusers and other groups because delayed effects may occur after the cessation of short-term treatments.

(Arch Gen Psychiatry. 1994;51:989-997)

AN IMPORTANT question regarding recently developed pharmacologic and psychotherapeutic treatments for cocaine dependence is whether these typically brief therapies can effect a sustained improvement in substance use and psychosocial functioning. A related issue concerns the relative ability of psychotherapy and pharmacotherapy to effect lasting change, given differences in their hypothesized mechanisms of action and time to effect.[1,2] Previous follow-ups from clinical trials of psychotherapy, including studies of opiate addicts,[3] have pointed to the durability of psychotherapy effects with such consistency that some investigators have called for more selective use of costly follow-up studies.[4] However, the durability of well-defined psychotherapeutic treatments for cocaine abuse has heretofore not been evaluated systematically; thus, the value of follow-up studies in this area is unknown.

Regarding the durability of pharmacotherapy effects, a 6-month follow-up of a previous investigation by Kosten et al[5] suggested better outcomes for patients treated with desipramine hydrochloride than for those treated with placebo through a 6-month follow-up, although this finding has not been replicated by other groups.[6] Moreover, in the study by Gawin et al,[7] all subjects received interpersonal psychotherapy in combination with desipramine; thus, the effectiveness of desipramine without intensive psychotherapy in sustaining improvement has not been evaluated.

The present study reports follow-up data from a study of psychotherapy and pharmacotherapy, alone and in combination, as treatment for 121 ambulatory co-

From the Division of Substance Abuse, the Department of Psychiatry, Yale University School of Medicine (Drs Carroll and Rounsaville and Ms Nich), and the APT Foundation (Ms Gordon), New Haven, Conn; the Departments of Psychology and Management Science, George Washington University, Washington, DC (Dr Wirtz); and the Laboratory for the Study of Addiction, the University of California–Los Angeles (Dr Gawin).

See Subjects and Methods on next page

caine abusers.[8] Subjects were randomly assigned to one of four conditions that were offered over a 12-week abstinence-initiation trial: (1) relapse prevention (a cognitive-behavioral treatment)[9] plus desipramine, (2) clinical management (a psychotherapy control condition),[10] plus desipramine, (3) relapse prevention plus placebo, and (4) clinical management plus placebo in a 2×2 factorial design. At posttreatment, all groups reported a sig-

SUBJECTS AND METHODS

Because the study protocol has been described in detail,[8] subjects, treatments, design, and procedures are summarized briefly below.

SUBJECTS

Subjects were recruited from individuals seeking treatment at the Substance Abuse Treatment Unit of the Connecticut Mental Health Center, New Haven, or from respondents to newspaper advertisements or public service announcements. Subjects were included who met current *DSM-III-R*[11] criteria for cocaine dependence and who had used at least 12 g of cocaine during the past 3 months. Individuals were excluded who (1) were currently physically dependent on opiates, barbiturates, or alcohol or whose principal drug of dependence was not cocaine, (2) met current *DSM-III-R* criteria for an Axis I disorder other than depressive or anxiety disorders, met lifetime criteria for schizophrenia or mania, or expressed significant current suicidal or homicidal ideation and presented substantial risk, (3) had a current medical condition that would contraindicate ambulatory tricyclic antidepressant therapy, (4) had been treated for substance use during the previous 2 months or were currently involved in psychotherapy or pharmacotherapy for any other psychiatric disorder, or (5) had conditions of probation or parole that required reports of drug use to officers of the court.

One hundred twenty-one individuals were determined to be eligible for the study, provided informed consent, were randomized, and began treatment. Of these, 110 (91%) received 2 or more weeks of study treatment, and 49 (40%) completed treatment and were fully compliant with medications; the mean number of sessions completed for all subjects was 7.2 (SD, 3.6). As described in greater detail in a previous report,[8] there were no statistically significant differences by treatment group for any baseline demographic, substance use, or psychosocial functioning variable. In the original sample, 27% of the subjects were women, 54% were African American or Hispanic, 71% were single or divorced, and 52% were working full- or part-time. Thirty-four percent had some college education, 42% were high school graduates, and 24% did not complete high school. The mean age of the sample was 28.8 years (SD, 5.8). Subjects reported using an average of 4.4 g (SD, 3.3) of cocaine per week for an average of 4.2 years. Sixty-two percent reported predominantly freebase use of cocaine, 29% were intranasal users, and 9% were intravenous users. Thirty percent had some previous exposure to treatment.

THERAPISTS

There were 11 doctoral-level therapists (seven psychiatrists and four psychologists) who saw an average of 11 patients (range, one to 23). Therapists selected were experienced in and committed to the type of treatment they conducted in the trial, averaging 4.4 years of postdoctoral experience. All therapists received extensive training that included a 2-day didactic seminar and successful completion of at least one closely supervised training case. To promote adherence to manual guidelines and prevent drift through the main phase of the study, therapists in each condition met weekly with study investigators to discuss case material and review session videotapes.

TREATMENTS

Each of the study treatments was manual-guided and was delivered to patients in weekly individual sessions that were offered over 12 weeks. All training and main phase sessions were videotaped for supervision and process assessment. Evaluation of 103 session videotapes by raters who were blind to treatment condition using an adaptation of the Collaborative Study Psychotherapy Rating Scale[12,13] indicated that the treatments were discriminable.[8]

DESIPRAMINE

Subjects received an average of 200 mg of desipramine hydrochloride per day (or four placebo pills) to a maximum dosage of 300 mg/d. Initial target plasma level ranges were 300 to 750 nmol/L. Dosage adjustments were made by nonblind study psychiatrists in response to serum blood levels and reported side effects and were yoked to dose changes for subjects who received placebo to maintain a medication double blind.

COGNITIVE-BEHAVIORAL COPING SKILLS TRAINING

The cognitive-behavioral treatment was based on techniques described by Marlatt and Gordon,[14] which were adapted for use with cocaine users.[9] The goal of this treatment was abstinence from cocaine and other substances through the identification of high-risk situations for relapse and the implementation of more effective coping strategies. Specific techniques included fostering the resolution to stop cocaine use through exploring positive and negative consequences of continued use, self-monitoring to identify high-risk situations for relapse, and the development of strategies for coping with and avoiding cocaine craving and high-risk situations.

CLINICAL MANAGEMENT

Clinical management was adapted from the guidelines developed for the National Institute of Mental Health Collaborative Study on the Treatment of Depression by Fawcett and colleagues.[10] The provision of clinical management was intended (1) to provide nonspecific elements of a psychotherapeutic relationship, including a supportive physician-patient relationship, education, empathy, and the instillation of hope, without providing active ingredients that are specific to relapse prevention; (2) to provide medication management and the opportunity to monitor patients' clinical status during treatment; and (3) to provide a convincing therapeutic rationale and foster greater retention in the protocol and compliance with medication.

FOLLOW-UP PROCEDURES

We attempted to follow up all 121 subjects who were randomized to treatment, regardless of whether they completed the treatment phase of the protocol. Subjects who did complete treatment were given a debriefing session after their posttreatment assessment in which their medication type was revealed. Administration of desipramine was tapered off over a 2-week period.

Follow-up was naturalistic; thus, we did not seek to control subjects' treatment involvement after they completed their study treatment. Although exposure to nonstudy treatments during the follow-up period could confound the interpretation of long-term effects of study treatments, cocaine dependence is a chronically relapsing disorder, and we believed it would be unethical as well as unfeasible to discourage patients from seeking treatment during follow-up. Therefore, subjects who requested further treatment or who continued cocaine abuse were referred to the Substance Abuse Treatment Unit outpatient cocaine clinic, where the modal form of treatment was weekly supportive group therapy.

OUTCOME AND FOLLOW-UP ASSESSMENT

Patients were assessed before treatment, weekly during treatment, after treatment, and at follow-up interviews conducted 1, 3, 6, and 12 months after termination by an independent clinical evaluator who was blind to both psychotherapy and pharmacotherapy condition. The effectiveness of blinding procedures have been described in detail in a previous report.[15] Rater training included an initial 2-day didactic training in the Addiction Severity Index (ASI) and other instruments, followed by frequent recalibration meetings. Patients were paid $25 for each follow-up interview.

Patient self-reports were verified through urine toxicology screens, which were obtained at each follow-up. Of 168 urine samples collected, 70% were consistent with patient self-report (sensitivity, 0.75; specificity, 0.56). Of the 51 discrepant urinalysis reports, 21 results (12% of the total) were negative for cocaine, although the patient reported recent cocaine use, and 30 results (18%) were positive for cocaine in cases in which the patient had denied use. Because urinalysis data would reflect only very recent cocaine use, in the follow-up, urine screen results were used as a check on the validity of self-reports rather than as outcome measures (there were no significant differences between treatments on rates of urine samples that tested positive for cocaine at any follow-up). However, in cases of discrepancy between self-reports and urine reports, subjects were reclassified as nonabstinent in analyses of rates of continuous abstinence.

The ASI[16] was administered at each follow-up as a secondary measure to assess multidimensional aspects of outcome (psychosocial functioning). We supplemented the drug abuse section of the ASI to calculate separate composite scores for cocaine vs other drug use, resulting in eight, rather than seven, domains (medical, employment/support, legal, cocaine, alcohol, other drug, family/social, and psychological). Composite scores vary from 0 to 1, with higher scores indicating a greater need for treatment. In addition, we added several questions that assessed the quantity and frequency of cocaine and other drug use, the duration of consecutive periods of abstinence, and the level and type of treatment involvement in the month prior to each interview.

Our two primary outcome variables for the analyses of treatment effects were a frequency measure (days of cocaine use in the past 30 days) and a composite measure that tapped frequency, intensity, and the problems associated with cocaine use (the ASI cocaine composite score). Correlations between these two measures at baseline and posttreatment were only moderate (posttreatment Pearson's $r=.42$, $P<.001$), which suggests that these variables tapped related but somewhat different aspects of cocaine use. Secondary outcome variables included the remaining ASI composite scores, which assessed psychosocial functioning. We selected point-prevalence variables over measures of continuous abstinence (in which the treatment of patients who relapse briefly and then recover is permanently classified as relapsed) because point-prevalence data have the advantages of offering both a better reflection of the dynamic nature of periods of abstinence and cocaine use when few subjects can be expected to be continuously abstinent throughout the follow-up period and a greater opportunity to validate the subjects' self-reports through biochemical measures such as urinalysis.[17]

DATA ANALYSES

The principal analysis for the effects of study treatments across time was a random effects regression model (D. Hedeker, PhD, unpublished software and manual, 1993) for the two primary outcome variables. Time was represented in logarithmic form to account for nonsynchronous intervals between follow-up evaluations (1, 3, 6, and 12 months). Random-effects regression models have several advantages in follow-up data from clinical trials, including this one, in which subjects are unlikely to attend follow-up evaluations precisely at the desired fixed points, not all subjects attend all follow-up evaluations, and intervals between follow-up occasions are not constant.[18] By treating time as a random effect, an individual's behavior is modeled as a function of an individual growth trajectory, and by treating time as a fixed effect, the individual change trajectories are modeled by treatment group. Thus, random effects regression models permit a more flexible approach for studying change over time.[18,19] Furthermore, in contrast to repeated measures analyses of variance, which usually involve the exclusion of subjects with missing data or imputing values for missing data points, random effects regression models allow the use of all available data. The MIXREG program (D. Hedeker, PhD, unpublished software and manual, 1993) was used for these analyses. Analysis of variance, χ^2 tests, and log-linear regression were used to analyze representativeness of the follow-up sample and level of treatment involvement during follow-up by treatment group.

nificant decrease in cocaine use and improvement in several domains of psychosocial functioning over the 12-week course of treatment. However, significant main effects for medication or psychotherapy were not found for treatment retention, reduction in cocaine use, or other outcomes. Exploratory analyses suggested that subjects with more severe cocaine use at baseline had better outcomes when treated with relapse prevention than with

clinical management, whereas clinical management was associated with better outcomes for less severe cocaine abusers. Desipramine significantly reduced cocaine use compared with the placebo through 6 but not 12 weeks of treatment and appeared to be most effective for less severe cocaine use.

However, those results reflect immediate posttreatment outcomes only and leave unanswered many questions relating to patients' sustained improvement after the completion of study treatments. Based on data from a 1-year follow-up from that investigation, we will address the following research questions:

1. How durable are the gains made during short-term outpatient treatment for cocaine dependence? That is, are treatment gains sustained or does cocaine use rebound from posttreatment levels? This is a particularly important issue for desipramine, where rebound effects after the cessation of desipramine treatment have been reported in cocaine-abusing methadone-maintained opioid addicts.[6] A related question concerns the relationship between cocaine use during treatment and long-term outcome. For example, are individuals who become abstinent during treatment more likely to remain abstinent than individuals with poorer initial outcome?

2. Do psychotherapy and pharmacotherapy differ in their ability to effect enduring change? Regarding the effects of psychotherapy, we hypothesized that relapse prevention, through fostering the development of coping strategies that are generalizable to several problem areas, would be associated with more enduring changes in more areas of functioning than would supportive clinical management. Regarding pharmacotherapy effects, data from the study by Gawin et al[7] indicated a desipramine effect both at posttreatment[7] and at follow-up.[5] However, in the present study, we had not seen posttreatment main effects for desipramine; thus, the emergence of effects after the cessation of desipramine treatment was considered unlikely.

RESULTS

FOLLOW-UP SAMPLE

Ninety-seven (80%) of the 121 individuals who began treatment had at least one face-to-face follow-up interview. An additional two subjects completed telephone interviews only. Of the 22 subjects who were never interviewed, eight did not respond to contacts for interview, four repeatedly did not keep interview appointments, eight moved without leaving a forwarding address, one was in prison and refused to be interviewed, and one had died several months after leaving the study.

While 80% of the subjects were interviewed at least once, most subjects did not attend all four follow-ups. Of the 97 subjects in the follow-up sample, 64 (66%) were interviewed at least twice, 49 (50%) were interviewed three or more times, and 24 (25%) were interviewed at all four time points. Across time, 56 subjects had a 1-month follow-up, 65 had a 3-month follow-up, 57 had a 6-month follow-up, and 59 had a 12-month follow-up. As shown in **Table 1**, there were no statistically significant differences by treatment group for the number of subjects followed up at least once, the number of follow-ups (all groups had a comparable number of follow-up data points), and the timing of follow-ups (all groups had comparable rates of follow-up at each time point).

Across treatment conditions, subjects who completed treatment were more likely to be reached for follow-up than were subjects who dropped out (96% vs 72%, χ^2=10.75, $P<.001$). Similarly, there was a strong correspondence between the level of exposure to study treatment and the number of follow-ups, with subjects with better retention in study treatment overrepresented in the follow-up data. For example, the 22 subjects who were never followed up averaged 4 weeks of treatment, whereas subjects who were followed up four times averaged 10 weeks of treatment (F=11.2, $P<.001$). However, subjects who achieved significant abstinence during treatment (eg, 3 or more consecutive weeks) were no more likely to be followed up than were subjects who did not (89% vs 84%, P=.48).

To evaluate whether there were systematic differences between subjects who were and were not reached for follow-up or the number of follow-up interviews completed by group, by baseline demographic (age, education, gender, race, marital status, occupational status, and socioeconomic status), and by clinical characteristics (ASI composite scores, quantity and frequency of cocaine use, route of administration, treatment history, and Axis I and II psychiatric disorders), we conducted a series of χ^2 tests, two- and three-factor analyses of variance (eg, number of follow-ups by treatment group by characteristic), and log-linear regressions (predicting baseline characteristics based on the number of follow-up interviews completed and treatment group). In addition to the close relationship between retention in treatment and number of follow-ups that was reported above, significant differences were found only for occupational status, where subjects who were employed at baseline were more likely to be reached for follow-up (90% of the employed vs 75% of the unemployed subjects were reached, χ^2=4.12, P=.04). Baseline characteristics of the follow-up sample by treatment group are presented in Table 1.

HOW DURABLE ARE GAINS MADE DURING SHORT-TERM OUTPATIENT TREATMENT FOR COCAINE DEPENDENCE?

As a group, subjects' cocaine outcomes either improved or did not change with respect to posttreatment levels. That is, the random regression model indicated significant effects for time for the ASI cocaine composite score, indicating that most patients reported continuing improvement in cocaine-related problems through the course of the follow-up (estimate, −0.063; SE=0.026; z=2.41; P=.01). As shown in **Table 2**, no effect for time was seen for the frequency of cocaine use, indicating that no significant change in the reported frequency of cocaine use from posttreatment levels occurred for the sample as a whole. Significant differences across time for secondary outcomes (ASI composite scores) were also not seen, suggesting that continuing improvement from posttreatment levels was confined to cocaine use and not seen for psychosocial outcomes. This may, however, reflect ceiling effects because both pretreatment and posttreatment scores for most ASI domains were comparatively

Table 1. Baseline Characteristics of Follow-up Sample and Rates of Subjects Reached for Follow-up by Treatment Group (n=97)

	Treatment Group*				
	CM and DMI (n=24)	RP and DMI (n=27)	CM and PLA (n=21)	RP and PLA (n=25)	Total
Demographics, No. (%)					
Female	7 (29.2)	8 (29.6)	10 (47.6)	4 (16.0)	**29** (29.9)
White	12 (50.0)	16 (59.3)	9 (42.9)	11 (44.0)	**48** (49.5)
Single or divorced	16 (66.7)	17 (63.0)	17 (81.0)	21 (84.0)	**71** (73.2)
Unemployed	9 (37.5)	13 (48.1)	12 (57.1)	8 (32.0)	**42** (43.3)
Completed high school	17 (70.8)	17 (63.3)	15 (71.4)	14 (56.0)	**63** (64.9)
Age, mean (SD)	28.9 (5.1)	29.6 (6.7)	28.4 (6.1)	27.7 (4.1)	28.7 (5.6)
Baseline cocaine use, mean (SD)					
ASI cocaine composite score†	.68 (.18)	.72 (.17)	.70 (.19)	.62 (.16)	.68 (0.19)
No. of days used/past 30 d	13.7 (9.1)	17.1 (7.9)	15.6 (6.8)	12.2 (7.3)	14.7 (8.0)
Grams used per week	4.0 (2.6)	6.2 (5.6)	5.1 (5.6)	3.8 (2.8)	4.8 (4.4)
Treatment involvement, No. (%)					
Completed treatment‡	11 (45.8)	15 (55.6)	10 (47.6)	11 (44.0)	**47** (48.5)
No. of treatment sessions, mean (SD)	6.5 (3.5)	7.9 (4.2)	7.3 (3.7)	7.4 (3.9)	7.3 (3.8)
Follow-up involvement					
No. of follow-ups completed, mean (SD)	2.5 (1.2)	2.4 (1.2)	2.7 (1.0)	2.2 (1.2)	2.4 (1.2)
Attended 1-mo follow-up, No. (%)	14 (58.3)	18 (66.7)	12 (57.1)	12 (48.0)	**56** (57.7)
Attended 3-mo follow-up, No. (%)	16 (66.7)	16 (59.3)	14 (66.7)	19 (76.0)	**65** (67.0)
Attended 6-mo follow-up, No. (%)	15 (62.5)	15 (55.6)	16 (76.2)	11 (44.0)	**57** (58.8)
Attended 12-mo follow-up, No. (%)	14 (58.3)	15 (55.6)	14 (66.7)	14 (56.0)	**57** (58.8)
Attended 0 follow-ups, No.§	3	6	7	8	**24**
Attended 1 follow-up, No.	9	9	4	10	**32**
Attended 2 follow-ups, No.	1	7	3	5	**16**
Attended 3 follow-ups, No.	8	3	10	4	**25**
Attended 4 follow-ups, No.	6	8	4	6	**24**

**CM indicates clinical management; DMI, desipramine hydrochloride; RP, relapse prevention; and PLA, placebo.*

†From the Addiction Severity Index (ASI) interview. Composite scores range from 0 to 1; higher scores indicate higher severity. Cocaine composite score modeled on calculation for alcohol composite score.

‡Indicates patients who attended all 12 sessions and were compliant with study medication.

§Indicates the 24 subjects who did not attend any follow-up interviews and are not included in the follow-up sample (n=97).

low, and therefore little additional improvement in these measures was possible.

To evaluate potential desipramine rebound effects, which have been reported after the cessation of desipramine treatment in methadone-maintained opioid addicts who also abuse cocaine,[6] we evaluated the number of subjects by treatment group whose cocaine use at follow-up equaled or exceeded either their pretreatment or posttreatment levels. These data suggest a rebound effect was less rather than more likely for the desipramine-treated subjects: at the two early follow-ups, desipramine-treated subjects were less likely than were placebo-treated subjects to have a cocaine composite score that exceeded their posttreatment scores (at 1 month, rates for placebo-treated subjects were 58% and for desipramine-treated subjects were 31%, χ^2=4.1, *P*=.04; at 3 months, rates were 21% vs 15%, respectively, *P*=.56). A similar pattern was seen for the comparison with pretreatment data. Similarly, the rates of continuous abstinence were 38% for desipramine-treated subjects and 36% for placebo-treated subjects at the 1-month follow-up (*P*=.89).

WHAT IS THE RELATIONSHIP BETWEEN COCAINE USE DURING TREATMENT AND FOLLOW-UP?

As shown in **Figure 1**, results from the random regression model revealed that subjects who accrued 4 or more weeks of consecutive abstinence at the end of treatment had significantly better outcomes during follow-up than did subjects who did not attain a stable period of abstinence during treatment (estimate, −0.291; SE=0.058; *z*=4.96; *P*<.001).

This pattern of results was consistent across outcome variables, including ASI cocaine composite scores and frequency of cocaine use in the 30 days prior to the follow-up interview. These findings closely paralleled results from the study of Kosten et al,[5] which suggested that abstinence initiation during treatment is an important indicator of longer-term prognosis.

DO PSYCHOTHERAPY AND PHARMACOTHERAPY DIFFER IN THEIR ABILITY TO EFFECT ENDURING CHANGE?

Twenty-seven subjects (28%) reported continuous abstinence at all follow-ups, and although χ^2 analyses indicated trends favoring relapse prevention, no significant effects for treatment type were seen. As noted above, however, analyses using dichotomous variables such as continuous abstinence are limited in that they do not reflect the dynamic nature of periods of relapse and abstinence in cocaine abusers and they do not differentiate infrequent, low-intensity use from continuous, heavy use—limitations that can be addressed by random regression models.

Results from the random effects regression analy-

Table 2. Random Regression Analyses: Effects of Time and Treatment From Posttreatment to 12-Month Follow-up for Primary Outcome Measures (n=97)

	Parameter Estimate	SE	z	P
ASI cocaine composite*				
Fixed effects				
Intercept (end-point value)	0.447	0.051	8.83	.001
Time (improvement rate)†	−0.062	0.026	−2.49	.02
Psychotherapy‡	0.038	0.047	0.80	.42
Medication§	−0.042	0.047	−0.88	.38
Psychotherapy by time	−0.061	0.026	−2.39	.02
Medication by time	0.008	0.026	0.30	.76
Psychotherapy by medication	−0.051	0.047	−1.07	.28
Psychotherapy by medication by time	0.030	0.025	1.17	.24
Random effects (variance)				
Intercept‖	0.030	0.010	2.87	.001
Slope¶	0.005	0.003	1.46	.07
Covariance#	−0.004	0.004	−0.92	.35
Days of cocaine use in past 30 days				
Fixed effects				
Intercept (end-point value)	6.14	1.36	4.50	.001
Time (improvement rate)	0.12	0.69	0.17	.86
Psychotherapy	0.92	1.26	0.72	.46
Medication	−0.32	1.27	−0.25	.80
Psychotherapy by time	−1.43	0.68	−2.11	.03
Medication by time	−0.51	0.68	−0.75	.45
Psychotherapy by medication	−1.46	1.27	−1.14	.25
Psychotherapy by medication by time	0.12	0.68	0.18	.85
Random effects (variance)				
Intercept	26.18	5.88	4.44	.001
Slope	3.53	1.67	2.12	.02
Covariance	3.68	2.54	−1.44	.15

*ASI indicates Addiction Severity Index.
†Log (months+1) from posttreatment to month 12.
‡Relapse prevention vs clinical management.
§Desipramine hydrochloride vs placebo.
‖Variance of β_0.
¶Variance of β_1.
#Relationship of β and α.

ses are shown in Table 2 and **Figure 2**. For the ASI cocaine composite scores, these analyses indicate a significant time-by-psychotherapy interaction (estimate, 0.061; SE=0.02; z=2.38; P=.01), which suggests emergent effects of relapse prevention over clinical management across time. For frequency of cocaine use in the past 30 days, the emergent relapse prevention effect was also seen (estimate, 1.43; SE=0.677; z=2.11; P=.03). The data are illustrated in Figure 2, which plots regression estimates across time by treatment group, psychotherapy condition, and medication condition.

Moreover, this pattern of findings was consistent across outcome variables when covarying for retention in the active treatment phase and level of baseline cocaine use. Although covarying for these variables did not change either the significance or the direction of the emergent effect for cognitive-behavioral treatment, it should be noted that both of the covariates were significant (P<.001). This suggests that retention in treatment was associated with less cocaine use during follow-up, and more severe cocaine use before treatment was associated with more cocaine use during follow-up.

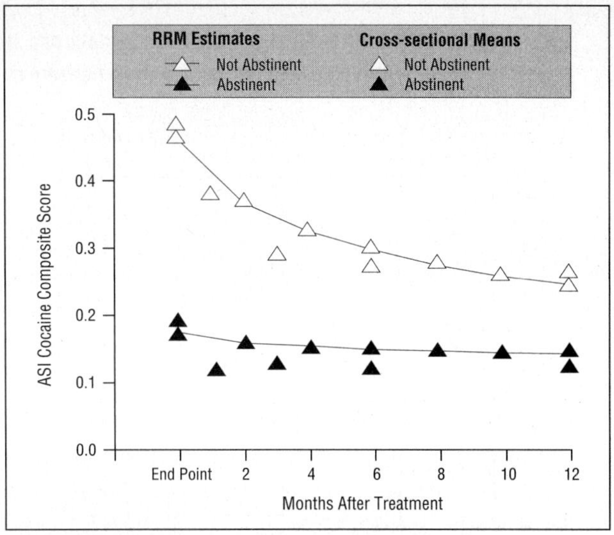

Figure 1. *Cocaine use during follow-up: comparison of subjects who were abstinent during treatment (n=15) with subjects who did not attain 1 month or more of abstinence (n=82). Plots are the results of random regression and cross-sectional analyses. ASI indicates Addiction Severity Index; RRM, random regression model.*

The data presented above suggest that the effects of relapse prevention emerged over time but do not address when these effects emerged. To explore this issue, we repeated the random regression model with four variables representing time and interactions with time (rather than a single term for time). These analyses indicated that significant effects of relapse prevention were not present at the 1- and 3-month points but did emerge by the 6-month follow-up and were the most apparent at the 12-month follow-up.

Regarding secondary outcomes, the random regression model did not converge for three variables (employment and legal and family functioning), which indicates that change in these variables over time was not well represented by a linear model. The random regression model did converge for medical, alcohol, noncocaine drug use, and psychological functioning, but there were no significant effects for treatment group or treatment by time. There was a significant effect for time for the alcohol composite score, which indicates that across groups, subjects reported decreasing their alcohol use from posttreatment through the end of follow-up.

TREATMENT INVOLVEMENT DURING FOLLOW-UP

Thirty-nine subjects reported participating in some form of treatment during follow-up. Fifteen received outpatient individual or group psychotherapy at the Substance Abuse Treatment Unit cocaine clinic, nine received pharmacotherapy (either desipramine or methylphenidate), four participated in family therapy, three entered inpatient treatment, two entered residential treatment, and 19 attended self-help groups. The number of subjects involved in any form of treatment was highest at the 1-month follow-up (mean, 2.4 d/mo) and dropped off sharply at subsequent follow-ups (3-month follow-up, 1.1 d/mo; 6-month follow-up, 1.0 d/mo; and 12-month follow-up, 1.1 d/mo). There were no statisti-

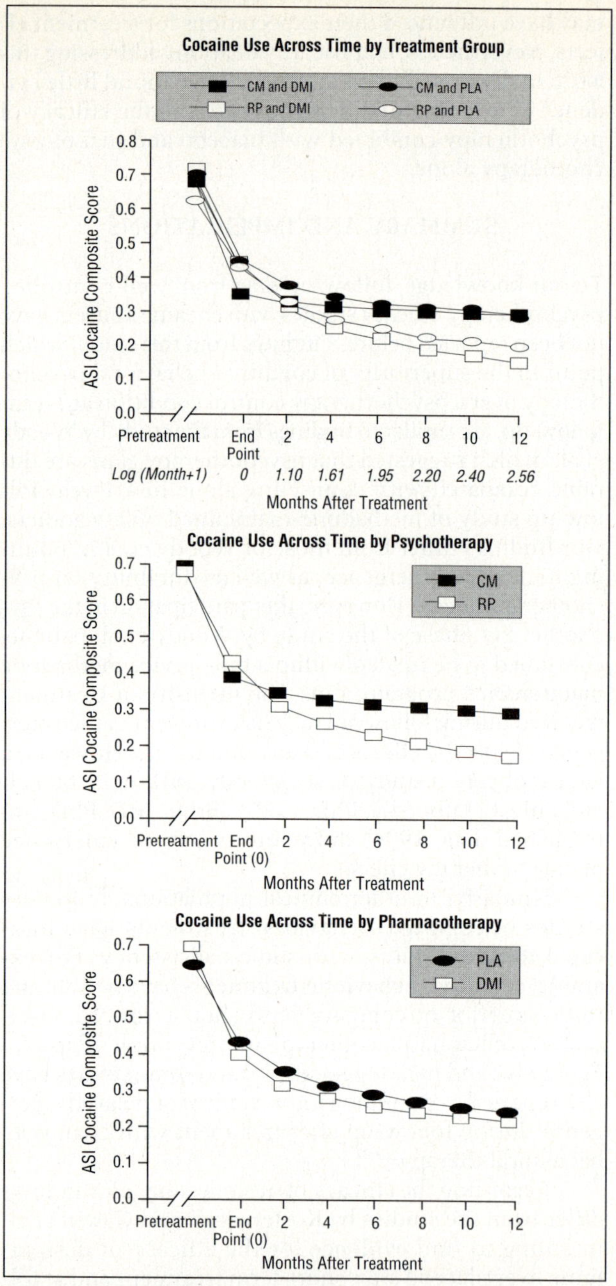

Figure 2. *Cocaine use across time by treatment group, psychotherapy, and pharmacotherapy condition (n=97). Plots are of random regression analyses. ASI indicates Addiction Severity Index; CM, clinical management; RP, relapse prevention; DMI, desipramine hydrochloride; and PLA, placebo.*

cally significant differences by treatment group for involvement or type of treatment received during follow-up. Although type of study treatment was not associated with differential treatment seeking during follow-up, subjects who received any formal treatment during follow-up were significantly more likely to have completed treatment (41% vs 68%, χ^2=6.4, *P*=.01) and to have lower (eg, less severe) end-point ASI cocaine composite scores (0.51 vs 0.39, F=5.74, *P*=.02). Otherwise, there were no significant differences between subjects who sought further formal treatment during the follow-up year and those who did not.

To evaluate the impact of nonstudy treatment received during follow-up on cocaine use during follow-up, we added days of formal treatment received during follow-up as a time-varying covariate to the random regression model described above. The covariate was significant, which indicates that treatment exposure during follow-up was associated with better outcome (estimate, −0.006; SE=0.002; *z*=2.84; *P*<.001). However, adding this covariate to the model did not affect the significance or the direction of the psychotherapy-by-time interaction described above, which suggests that the emergent effect of cognitive-behavioral relapse prevention treatment occurred even in the presence of some exposure to other treatments during follow-up.

COMMENT

This 1-year naturalistic follow-up of psychotherapy and pharmacotherapy for cocaine dependence suggested the following: First, overall, subjects' cocaine use decreased or remained stable with respect to posttreatment levels. Rebound effects after the cessation of desipramine treatment were not seen. Second, across time, there was consistent evidence of delayed emergence of effects for cognitive-behavioral psychotherapy over a psychotherapy control condition for cocaine outcomes. No study treatment was associated with greater involvement with formal treatment seeking or self-help during follow-up, and the pattern of results presented herein was not affected by controlling for such exposures.

DELAYED EMERGENCE OF TREATMENT EFFECTS

These findings raise the question of why there were no main effects of psychotherapy or pharmacotherapy condition at treatment termination but there were significant treatment-by-time effects for relapse prevention psychotherapy at follow-up. Because the emergence of psychotherapy effects at follow-up did not appear to be related to nonstudy treatment received during follow-up, we hypothesize that these effects may be due to the delayed emergence of the specific effects of cognitive-behavioral relapse prevention treatment. That is, during the active phase of treatment, all subjects received a variety of nonspecific interventions that included weekly urine monitoring, frequent assessment of cocaine use and other symptoms, support and encouragement from therapists and research staff, and expectations for medication and other treatment effects. These nonspecific interventions may have been powerfully therapeutic and overwhelmed treatment-specific effects. However, the cessation of these nonspecific interventions at termination may have provided the conditions under which the more durable and specific effects of treatment had an opportunity to emerge. That is, cognitive-behavioral coping skills treatment is intended to impart generalizable coping skills that can be implemented long after patients leave treatment, whereas supportive clinical management may be effective during short-term treatment but may have provided patients with fewer enduring resources on which they could draw after treatment termination.

LIMITATIONS

This study is unique among treatment efficacy research with cocaine abusers as it reports comparatively extended outcomes for both psychotherapeutic and pharmacotherapeutic treatments with appropriate controls for each form of treatment, 80% of all subjects randomized to treatment were reached for at least one follow-up, data were collected from face-to-face interviews with a clinical evaluator who was blind to the subjects' study treatment condition, subjects' self-reports were validated through urine toxicology screens, and standardized instruments were used to assess multidimensional aspects of outcome.

A limitation of this study is incomplete data at some time points; that is, not all subjects were reached for all follow-ups. However, the random regression model used herein addresses, to a large extent, the statistical problems usually associated with missing follow-up data.[18,19] Furthermore, although we evaluated our follow-up data carefully for sources of bias (eg, differential contribution to the dataset by treatment group and other characteristics) and found no significant effects other than those reported and controlled for herein, it is possible that other, undetected sources of bias exist. Also, given the strong relationship between the subjects' retention in treatment and representation in the follow-up data, it is possible that poorer-functioning cocaine abusers who dropped out of treatment early were underrepresented in the follow-up data. However, because (1) there were no treatment differences in retention in the main phase of the study and controlling for level of treatment exposure did not affect the emergent effects of relapse prevention, (2) relapse prevention was associated with better retention of subjects with high-severity cocaine use, and (3) all treatment groups appeared comparably represented in the follow-up data, it is unlikely that this issue would create a bias in favor of the emergent psychotherapy effects reported herein.

Another limitation of this and any naturalistic follow-up study is uncontrolled exposure to treatments during the follow-up that might be different from subjects' study treatment. In this study, although a significant minority of subjects participated in some treatment during follow-up, such exposures were typically abbreviated, were not systematically associated with any study treatment, and appeared to have a positive but minimal influence on extended outcomes. Most important, our findings of the delayed emergence of treatment effects were not altered when controlling for exposure to other treatments.

It should also be noted that the analyses presented in this report are exploratory as our primary hypotheses concerned only the short-term outcomes, and confirmation of these findings through replication with other samples is needed. Conclusions about the durability of treatment effects for the sample as a whole must be tempered with the recognition that an untreated control group was not included in this study and that little is now known about the natural course of cocaine dependence in untreated samples. Finally, all subjects who received psychotherapy also received active or inert medication that may have influenced their expectations for treatment effects. Nevertheless, empirical evaluations addressing this issue in depressed populations[20,21] have found little evidence of meaningful differences between the efficacy of psychotherapy combined with placebo and that of psychotherapy alone.

SUMMARY AND IMPLICATIONS

To our knowledge, follow-up data from well-controlled psychotherapy efficacy studies with cocaine abusers have not been reported before. Findings from this study, which point to the superiority of cognitive-behavioral psychotherapy over a psychotherapy control condition at 1-year follow-up, are similar to findings from the study by Woody et al,[3] which suggested that psychotherapy gains are durable compared with counseling alone in a 1-year follow-up study of methadone-maintained opiate addicts. Our findings differ from those of Woody et al in pointing to delayed emergence, as well as durability, of psychotherapy effects. However, after participation in the psychotherapy phase of the study by Woody et al, patients continued to be treated within a full-service methadone maintenance program; thus, the intensity of treatment received during follow-up may have prevented the emergence of specific effects of study treatments. However, a later replication study (G. E. Woody, MD, A. T. McLellan, PhD, L. Luborsky, PhD, C. P. O'Brien, MD, PhD, unpublished data, 1994) did point to delayed emergence of psychotherapy effects.

Similarly, in other clinical populations, follow-up studies of cognitive-behavioral treatments have indicated their durability with some consistency. For example, cognitive-behavioral treatments have been found to be superior or comparable to short-term or continued tricyclic pharmacotherapy in preventing relapse of depressive and panic episodes,[22-24] and some studies have also reported a continuing improvement or delayed emergence during follow-up after treatment with cognitive-behavioral therapy.[25-27]

Regarding the efficacy of desipramine, our findings differ from the studies by Kosten et al[5] and Gawin et al[7] in failing to find evidence for the efficacy of desipramine over placebo after short-term treatment and at follow-up. They are consistent, however, with findings from other groups that have suggested that the effects of desipramine treatment are modest and most apparent in the initial phases of treatment. Our data underscore the importance of providing a potent psychosocial treatment to cocaine users and that desipramine should be conceived only as an adjunctive treatment for use in some populations and settings. Furthermore, both this follow-up study and that of Kosten et al[5] have not found evidence of rebound effects after desipramine treatment in independent samples of primary cocaine abusers. This runs counter to reports of rebound effects following the cessation of desipramine treatment for methadone-maintained patients who also abuse cocaine.[6] Differences across these studies may be due to differences in the subject populations (primary cocaine addicts vs opiate addicts), as well as the type and intensity of treatment received during follow-up (patients in the study by

Arndt et al[6] continued full-service methadone maintenance after the cessation of desipramine treatment).

Finally, our findings underscore the importance of conducting follow-ups in clinical trials of cocaine abusers and other clinical groups. Psychotherapy researchers have argued that outcomes at follow-up frequently do not differ from those seen at posttreatment.[4] Therefore, the expense of conducting follow-ups may not be justified, given that little new information is usually obtained from them. However, our findings suggest that differential treatment effects may emerge only after the cessation of short-term treatment. Follow-ups from clinical trials evaluating psychotherapeutic treatments should be done more frequently than they have been, both to confirm the findings of the present study and to evaluate the potentially emergent and enduring benefits of other types of treatment.

Accepted for publication September 5, 1994.

Support was provided by grants RO1-DA04299, R18-DA06963, and K05-DA00089 from the National Institute on Drug Abuse, Rockville, Md.

We gratefully acknowledge Michael Barrios, PhD; Lisa Fenton, PsyD; Andrew Grunebaum, PhD; Daniel Keller, PhD; Robert Malison, MD; Ismene Petrakis, MD; Glen Pickett, MD; Merrill Rotter, MD; Marlene Steinberg, MD; and Robert Sbriglio, MD, who made many contributions to the success of this project through their work as therapists. Roseann Bisighini, MS; Tami Frankforter; and Julia Kasl assisted in the data collection and analyses. We also wish to acknowledge the helpful consultation of Donald Hedeker, PhD, in the application of the MIXREG software.

Reprint requests to Yale University School of Medicine, 34 Park St/SAC 208, New Haven, CT 06519 (Dr Carroll).

REFERENCES

1. Elkin I, Pilkonis PA, Docherty JP, Sotsky SM. Conceptual and methodological issues in comparative studies of psychotherapy and pharmacotherapy, I: active ingredients and mechanisms of change. *Am J Psychiatry.* 1988;145:909-917.
2. Elkin I, Pilkonis PA, Docherty JP, Sotsky SM. Conceptual and methodological issues in comparative studies of psychotherapy and pharmacotherapy, II: nature and timing of treatment effects. *Am J Psychiatry.* 1988;145:1070-1076.
3. Woody GE, McLellan AT, Luborsky L, O'Brien CP. Twelve-month follow-up of psychotherapy for opiate dependence. *Am J Psychiatry.* 1987;144:590-596.
4. Nicholson RA, Berman JS. Is follow-up necessary in evaluating psychotherapy? *Psychol Bull.* 1983;93:61-78.
5. Kosten TR, Gawin FH, Kosten TA, Morgan C, Rounsaville BJ, Schottenfeld R, Kleber HD. Six-month follow-up of short-term pharmacotherapy for cocaine dependence. *Am J Addict.* 1992;1:40-49.
6. Arndt IO, Dorozynsky L, Woody GE, McLellan AT, O'Brien CP. Desipramine treatment of cocaine dependence in methadone-maintained patients. *Arch Gen Psychiatry.* 1992;49:888-893.
7. Gawin FH, Kleber HD, Byck R, Rounsaville BJ, Kosten TR, Jatlow PI, Morgan CB. Desipramine facilitation of initial cocaine abstinence. *Arch Gen Psychiatry.* 1989;46:117-121.
8. Carroll KM, Rounsaville BJ, Gordon LT, Nich C, Jatlow P, Bisighini RM, Gawin FH. Psychotherapy and pharmacotherapy for ambulatory cocaine abusers. *Arch Gen Psychiatry.* 1994;51:177-187.
9. Carroll KM, Rounsaville BJ, Keller DS. Relapse prevention strategies in the treatment of cocaine abuse. *Am J Drug Alcohol Abuse.* 1991;17:249-265.
10. Fawcett J, Epstein P, Fiester SJ, Elkin I, Autry JH. Clinical management—imipramine/placebo administration manual: NIMH Treatment of Depression Collaborative Research Program. *Psychopharmacol Bull.* 1987;23:309-324.
11. American Psychiatric Association. *Diagnostic and Statistical Manual of Mental Disorders, Revised Third Edition.* Washington, DC: American Psychiatric Association; 1987.
12. Hill CE, O'Grady KE, Elkin I. Applying the Collaborative Study Psychotherapy Rating Scale to rate therapist adherence in cognitive-behavior therapy, interpersonal therapy, and clinical management. *J Consult Clin Psychol.* 1992;60:73-79.
13. Hollon SD, Waskow IE, Evans M, Lowery HA. Systems for rating therapies for depression. Presented at the 91st Annual Convention of the American Psychiatry Association; May 1984; Los Angeles, Calif.
14. Marlatt GA, Gordon JR, eds. *Relapse Prevention: Maintenance Strategies in the Treatment of Addictive Behaviors.* New York, NY: Guilford Press; 1985.
15. Carroll KM, Rounsaville BJ, Nich C. Blind man's bluff? the effectiveness and significance of psychotherapy and pharmacotherapy blinding procedures in a randomized clinical trial. *J Consult Clin Psychol.* 1994;62:276-280.
16. McLellan AT, Luborsky L, Woody GE, O'Brien CP. An improved diagnostic evaluation instrument for substance abuse patients: the Addiction Severity Index. *J Nerv Mental Dis.* 1980;168:26-33.
17. Velicer WF, Prochaska JO, Rossi JS, Snow MG. Assessing outcome in smoking cessation studies. *Psychol Bull.* 1992;111:23-41.
18. Gibbons RD, Hedeker D, Elkin I, Waternaux C, Kraemer HC, Greenhouse JB, Shea MT, Imber SD, Sotksy SM, Watkins JT. Some conceptual and statistical issues in analyses of longitudinal psychiatric data: application to the NIMH Treatment of Depression Collaborative Research Program dataset. *Arch Gen Psychiatry.* 1993;50:739-750.
19. Bryk AS, Raudenbush SW. Application of hierarchical linear models to assessing change. *Psychol Bull.* 1987;101:147-158.
20. Frank E, Kupfer DJ. Does a placebo tablet affect psychotherapeutic treatment outcome? results from the Pittsburgh Study of Maintenance Therapies in Recurrent Depression. *Psychother Res.* 1992;2:102-111.
21. Klerman GL, DiMascio A, Weissman M, Prusoff B, Paykel ES. Treatment of depression by drugs and psychotherapy. *Am J Psychiatry.* 1974;131:186-190.
22. Hollon SD, Beck AT. Cognitive and cognitive-behavioral therapies. In: Garfied SL, Bergin AE, eds. *Handbook of Psychotherapy and Behavior Change: An Empirical Analysis.* 4th ed. New York, NY: John Wiley & Sons Inc; 1994.
23. Shea MT, Elkin I, Imber SD, Sotsky SM, Watkins JT, Collins JF, Pilkonis PA, Beckham E, Glass DR, Dolan RT, Parloff MB. Course of depressive symptoms over follow-up: findings from the National Institute of Mental Health Treatment of Depression Collaborative Research Program. *Arch Gen Psychiatry.* 1992;49:782-787.
24. Margraf J, Barlow DH, Clark DM, Telch MJ. Psychological treatment of panic: work in progress on outcome. *Behav Res Ther.* 1993;31:1-8.
25. Beutler LE, Scogin F, Kirkish P, Schretlen D, Corbishley A, Hamblin D, Meredith K, Potter R, Bamford CR, Levenson AI. Group cognitive therapy and alprazolam in the treatment of depression in older adults. *J Consult Clin Psychol.* 1987;55:550-556.
26. O'Farrell TJ, Choquette KA, Cutter HS, Brown ED, McCorte WF. Behavioral marital therapy with and without additional relapse prevention sessions for alcoholics and their wives. *J Stud Alcohol.* 1993;54:652-666.
27. Goldstein MG, Niaura R, Follick MJ, Abrams DB. Effects of behavioral skills training and schedule of nicotine gum administration on smoking cessation. *Am J Psychiatry.* 1989;146:56-60.

Conversions From Système International (SI) Units to Traditional Units (Modified From *The SI Manual in Health Care*)

System	Component	SI Reference Interval*	SI Unit	Conversion Factor (Divide by)	Traditional Reference Interval*	Traditional Unit
Plasma	Desipramine, therapeutic	170-700	nmol/L	3.754	50-200	ng/mL

**These reference values are not intended to be definitive since each laboratory determines its own values. They are provided for illustration only.*

Some Issues for the New Director of NIMH

DAN FREEDMAN'S last editorial in the ARCHIVES[1] dealt with funding issues for the National Institute of Mental Health (NIMH). Now, 18 months later, it is with a certain trepidation that we follow so eminent a spokesperson for psychiatry with our first editorial, trying to pick up where he left off. We are compelled to take up the subject of NIMH again, because interviews with candidates for the directorship of the Institute are ongoing.

The change in leadership at NIMH comes at an auspicious time, with the transition of the Institute back under the direct aegis of the National Institutes of Health (NIH) and changes in the organization of health care taking place throughout the marketplace, at the level of the individual states as well as through potential federal legislation. The choice of the director will have a profound effect on our field: setting research priorities and financing them, shaping the careers of scientists, providing funding for cash-strapped medical school departments, and influencing the clinical practice of psychiatry. The new director will have several daunting challenges; only a few of the research issues are highlighted here.

INCREASING FUNDING FOR RESEARCH

The new director will need to seek creative ways both to ensure the continued level of funding available for research and, ideally, obtain additional funds. After a period of substantive gain, in recent years the annual budget of NIMH has increased at a rate that barely keeps pace with inflation.[2,3] In some review cycles, very few proposals are funded, even though many are of high quality. The average percentile score of projects that eventually receive funding has fallen dramatically. However, in a period of fiscal belt-tightening by the federal government, an increased budget will not be achieved easily.

The new director will have to articulate clearly the importance of basic science, clinical, and epidemiological research in mental health to a divided legislature, a somewhat cynical public, and perhaps even a skeptical NIH. This role is particularly crucial as NIMH becomes a component of an agency that has its own financial problems. Mental disorders once given special attention, if only because of stigmatization, are now lumped together to compete for funding with other equally deserving public health problems such as cancer, heart disease, acquired immunodeficiency syndrome, and diabetes. The director will have to convince his constituency not only by word but by deed that money allocated will be well spent and will get results. At the same time, the director must acknowledge the inevitable blind alleys of any worthy scientific endeavor. Money spent that does not produce results may well be worth the risk taking required to advance science.

The search for new funding comes at a particularly defining moment for clinical research. With money from clinical practices drying up, academic institutions will no longer be able to underwrite the research activities of young faculty members. In many settings, changes in reimbursement from third-party payers, including the federal government, as well as shortened lengths of stay, have reduced the opportunities for inpatient-based research. The allotment of time and space for outpatient-based research is costly and difficult. The new director must ensure that clinical research is not imperiled so as to threaten the advance of clinical practice. The issues of funding for clinical research and careers in clinical investigation cross all areas of biomedical research—as considered in a recent Institute of Medicine study chaired by William Kelley[4]—and the director must take a leadership role in addressing them for the mental health community.

The scarcity of money available to academic institutions makes the research money received by them seem even more precious. This may allow the director new opportunities to explore creative partnerships with universities. However, this should also make the new director wary of academic administrators who are simply not committed to research and eye research dollars as a way to plug their own deficits.

Indeed, the new director may have to devise creative ways to enhance NIMH funding by interacting more directly with voluntary organizations, private philanthropy, foundations, and perhaps even companies. This will prove tricky for all parties involved, all of whom have their own missions and agendas and may expect, therefore, to be full-fledged captains. However, these organizations, which are usually too small to finance large research proposals, have been crucial in providing seed money for many young investigators to acquire pilot data or for more experienced ones to sail in uncharted waters. The growth of an organization such as the National Alliance for Research in Schizophrenia and Depression (NARSAD), with its inspired leadership, has been one of the great success stories of the past decade.

SETTING RESEARCH PRIORITIES

The new director will clearly be instrumental in setting the research agenda for the next decade. However, that agenda cannot, with the limited funding available, be a limitless one. Priorities will have to be set for the goals that are sought, the topics that are covered, and even the research tools that are used. Priorities have to be established at a time when the outcome of the health care debate is far from over, and supervisionary skill is required to know how the landscape will look in 10 years. An Institute of Medicine study chaired by Floyd Bloom[5] deals with this topic and provides a framework for considering the issues as they arise for all components of NIH. It emphasizes the importance of maintaining a variety of research support mechanisms and the necessity of supporting the development of young investigators and providing for the ongoing needs for equipment and facilities, regardless of the financial climate. The history of science repeatedly demonstrates that our discipline will advance only if there is a deep commitment to research in the field's fundamental biological and psychosocial underpinnings as well as in specific disorders.

A major challenge within the goal-setting process continues to be the tension between basic science and technology. Projects that will yield findings only in the long term must be balanced with those that will provide more immediate results. Likewise, projects that generate new hypotheses not directly relevant to clinical practice must be balanced with those that document the efficacy of existing or new treatments.

The research topics that are funded will have to be examined, but so will the ways in which we construe topics as "research areas." It is tempting to fund research only for diseases that affect many people or that are severe (ideally, both), but the director will have to ensure that disorders that meet neither criteria or behaviors that are not technically disorders get a fair shot at research dollars. Perhaps we will have a shift from categorical thinking about research areas to a more dimensional one that allows cross-fertilization of ideas, including the ways in which biological and psychosocial processes interact. The challenge of redefining the research domains to give a greater coherence and unity of purpose will necessitate radical thinking about how scientific review committees are structured and staffed.

The new director will also feel the pull of new research tools. The exciting advances in molecular genetics and brain imaging allow us to solve some research problems and generate new ones never before conceptualized. However, the director must ensure that these important and glamorous tools exclusively do not set the research agenda. The importance of psychosocial research, which is more abstruse, must not be lost. The NIMH director will have to assert what we know: psychosocial research is of enormous value for understanding mental disorders, and psychosocial treatments are effective in reducing health care costs of many medical and psychiatric illnesses and of direct importance for primary care. Finally, an appropriate priority must be assigned to prevention and services research, one which takes into account prevailing social pressures but is not dictated by them.

ANOTHER AREA to which the new director will urgently need to attend is child psychiatry. An Institute of Medicine study chaired by James Leckman and Glen Elliott[6] noted the disparity between the importance of studying disorders that affect children and adolescents and the available funding. The needs in child psychiatry cry out for more research in many areas. As a start, the organization of the NIMH-sponsored study of the epidemiology of childhood disorders may need to be reconsidered, with the inclusion of more centers in the program.

The setting of research priorities—the goals, topics, and tools—will of course have major ramifications for how money is disbursed and to whom. Should NIMH underwrite a larger cottage industry of research, or will it resort to a more centralized approach, concentrating its money in centers that have a critical mass of researchers? The importance of research conducted by individual researchers is clear. It is also apparent that outstanding investigator-initiated research has been accomplished using large-program projects and centers.

Without priorities, money cannot be raised. How and where the research portfolio should be broadened or deepened will be one of the most important decisions for the new director.

WORKING WITHIN THE NIH SYSTEM

The new director of NIMH will face all the promises and perils of working within the organizational structure of NIH. The Institute may learn new things from its sister organizations, who may also have much to learn from it. Indeed, extraordinary opportunities for collaboration are now presented by the recent appointments of Zach Hall as director of the National Institute of Neurological Disorders and Alan Leshner as director of the National Institute on Drug Abuse. Similar situations exist with regard to the Alcoholism Institute and other programs at NIH. However, it will take great diplomacy to prevent precious time from being wasted on turf battles, budget skirmishes, and power struggles.

The new director will also inherit a vast intramural program. Among the major NIH institutes, NIMH allocates one of the highest percentages of its overall budget to intramural research. The intramural program has a number of outstanding scholars and a tradition of great accomplishments. At the same time, consideration must be given to the appropriate size of the program. There is severe crunch of space and resources. Among the issues to be considered are the number of intramural laboratories and their size and role, the areas of research represented, the appropriate development of programs, the need for new facilities,

the protection of clinical research, and the relocation of some intramural laboratories extramurally, which might benefit the field as a whole.

BOOSTING MORALE

The new director must not forget that he or she is dealing with people, not just budgets and programs. The new director must seek to preserve the integrity of the scientific process and must be deeply concerned about the ethical conduct of research. In addition, we all feel discouraged to see promising young investigators wracked by anxiety over finding ways to finance their ideas and then persistently disheartened by lack of funding. Middle- and senior-level investigators either share that panic or experience the pain of the long-distance runner. The new director must keep open the pipeline of bright, enthusiastic young investigators guided by refreshed, stimulating senior mentors.

Disentangling all of these challenges and somehow creatively reintegrating them into a coherent goal will probably be, in itself, the hardest challenge faced by the director. An outstanding committee has been appointed for the review and selection process. The word on the street is that an equally superb group of individuals are candidates. As the highest public health official in the nation in the field of mental health, with a constituency of federal legislators, intramural and extramural scientists, clinicians, educators, university administrators, and the public, the new director will be expected to be many different things to many different people. He or she will have to be the consummate advocate, politician, salesman, campaigner, cheerleader, coach, accountant, teacher, scientist, student, and visionary—and not necessarily in that order. The excellent example set by previous directors gives us hope that such a person can be found and will accept the position.

Jack D. Barchas, MD
Peter M. Marzuk, MD

REFERENCES

1. Freedman DX. Black days for research: the NIH Admissions Tax. *Arch Gen Psychiatry.* 1993;50:513-516.
2. Barchas JD, Elliott GR, Berger PA, Barchas PR, Solomon F. The ultimate stigma: inadequate funding for research on mental illness and addictive disorders. *Am J Psychiatry.* 1985;142:838-839.
3. Research on mental illness and addictive disorders: progress and prospects. *Am J Psychiatry.* 1985;142(suppl):1-41.
4. Kelley WN, Randolph MA. *Careers in Clinical Research: Obstacles and Opportunities.* Washington, DC: National Academy Press; 1994.
5. *Funding Health Sciences Research: A Strategy to Restore Balance.* Washington, DC: Institute of Medicine, National Academy Press; 1990.
6. *Research on Children and Adolescents With Mental, Behavioral, and Developmental Disorders: Mobilizing a National Initiative.* Washington, DC: Institute of Medicine, National Academy Press; 1989.

Clinical Action of Remoxipride

Expectations for new neuroleptics with improved antipsychotic action have been high since the demonstration of differential antipsychotic efficacy with clozapine.[1] The exact mechanism of clozapine's unique antipsychotic action is unknown, so directions for new drug development have been speculative. Remoxipride hydrochloride is a substituted benzamide of the sulpiride family; it has highly selective dopamine D_2 antagonist activity and in vivo selectivity for limbic D_2 receptors.[2] Although this neuroleptic is not now in active development in the United States for toxicity reasons, its known clinical actions and preclinical properties can provide information for future drug development. Remoxipride has already been shown to produce significantly fewer motor side effects than the standard neuroleptic, haloperidol.[3] Herein, we report preliminary data suggesting that remoxipride, like clozapine, has unique antipsychotic activity in neuroleptic-resistant schizophrenic individuals.

Sixteen *DSM-III-R*[4] schizophrenic subjects were characterized as neuroleptic resistant, according to previous criteria.[1] After a prospective negative trial of a traditional neuroleptic, they underwent testing in a 6-week, double-blind, drug-drug, parallel groups study, comparing the antipsychotic action of remoxipride with that of haloperidol. The two study groups were matched on critical clinical parameters, including age, sex, length of illness, hospital stay, and prestudy Brief Psychiatric Rating Scale (BPRS) score (mean [±SD] baseline BPRS score, 50±9 for the haloperidol group vs 48±7 for the remoxipride group). After a 1- to 2-week neuroleptic washout, study medication was administered blindly and adjusted within a fixed range over 2 weeks to the optimal clinical dose; the dose remained fixed during the last 4 weeks of study. The mean treatment dose of remoxipride hydrochloride was 413±69 mg (range, 300 to 450 mg) and of haloperidol was 25±4.6 mg (range, 20 to 30 mg). Clinical state was rated weekly using the BPRS and Clinical Global Inventory weekly throughout the trial.

Subjects were considered "improvers" if their total BPRS score fell by 20% compared with the prestudy optimal treatment evaluation score and if at least moderate improvement occurred, as judged by their treating clinician. One haloperidol-treated patient who experienced no improvement was dropped from the study for administrative reasons without being included in the data analysis. Using these criteria, three (38%) of eight remoxipride-treated subjects were improvers, whereas zero (0%) of seven of the haloperidol group responded (**Table**). This magnitude of antipsychotic response in the neuroleptic-resistant patients is comparable to the 30% rate of response previously reported for clozapine.[1]

The remoxipride group had significantly lower BPRS scores at optimal dose treatment than haloperidol-treated patients (40±9 for the remoxipride group vs 49±7 for the haloperidol group; *P*=.046). The mean improvement in positive symptoms was also numerically greater for the remoxipride group (18% for the remoxipride group vs 2% for the haloperidol group), but the difference was not significant. No group differences were seen in negative symptoms, as measured by the BPRS Anergia score. Two of the seven haloperidol-treated patients received benztropine mesylate for emergent pseudoparkinsonism, whereas no remoxipride-treated patients required the drug.

These data suggest that remoxipride may have differential efficacy in neuroleptic-resistant schizophrenic patients. Subsequent study of this drug is not currently possible because of its association with aplastic anemia, albeit at a low incidence. Although the patient numbers in this study are low and replication presumably cannot be done, these results encourage an interest in remoxipride's clozapinelike preclinical characteristics for effective atypical antipsychotic action in patients not responsive to traditional neuroleptics. The low affinity of this drug for striatal D_2 receptors and its differential in vivo affinity for the limbic striatal areas might be important characteristics in this regard.[2]

Response to Study Drugs*

Drug	No Response	Response
Haloperidol	7	0
Remoxipride hydrochloride	5	3

**For comparisons between drugs, P<.07, (χ^2 test).*

Robert Conley, MD
Carol A. Tamminga, MD
James An Nguyen, MD
Maryland Psychiatric Research Center
PO Box 21247
Baltimore, MD 21228

1. Kane J, Honigfeld G, Singer J, Meltzer H, the Clozaril Collaborative Study Group. *Arch Gen Psychiatry*. 1988;45:789-796.
2. Kohler C, Hall H, Mangnusson O, Lewander T, Gustafsson K. *Acta Psychiatr Scand Suppl*. 1990;102:27-36.
3. Lewander T, Westerbergh SE, Morrison D. *Acta Psychiatr Scand Suppl*. 1990; 102:92-98.
4. American Psychiatric Association. *Diagnostic and Statistical Manual of Mental Disorders, Revised Third Edition*. Washington, DC: American Psychiatric Association; 1987.

All Prepaid Health Care Systems Are Not Equal

The article by Rogers et al[1] concerning the different outcomes of adults with depression as a function of their means of payment raises many questions in trying to account for the discrepancy seen in psychiatrists' patients receiving fee-for-service (FFS) or prepaid (PP) care.

The major question that needs answering to evaluate this study is how the mental health program was managed compared with the FFS program. Were case managers evaluating the treatment along with the caregivers? Were any limitations placed on the caregivers, especially the psychiatrists, as to what they could or could not do? Were there limitations as to the number of visits or length of time per visit? Unless one knows the differences between the programs, the difference in outcomes is meaningless.

Since those with no insurance were included in the FFS group, how much did their presence lower the median income? In general, was this group of a higher socioeconomic status than the PP group? If so, the FFS group also might be a more psychiatrically sophisticated population and more likely to comply with instructions, continue taking medication, and stay in treatment. I wonder if those whose depression was improving would get a better job and therefore change from a PP plan to an FFS plan, whereas the opposite would be true for those doing poorly. This might account for the differences in limitations in role/physical functioning associated with changing payment plans.

Another factor that was not considered was whether the primary care physicians in the PP system of care were "gatekeepers" in that the patients required their referral to the psychiatrist, or were the primary care physicians given an incentive NOT to refer patients to specialists. If either of these factors was present, it would be expected that the more depressed, harder to treat patients (including those who were less compliant with medication management) would be the ones referred to a psychiatrist, while the primary care physician would treat the less difficult patients himself or herself. One assumes that the FFS patients had open access to a psychiatrist, so they would be able to obtain psychiatric care for symptoms perceived as problematic (no matter how mild) by the patient himself or herself, not by another physician.

The type of medication used is another consideration. Were the PP group more likely to be prescribed generic antidepressant medications compared with the FFS group? Many times, patients doing well using a brand-name product start doing poorly when they are changed to a generic product. This is another factor of cost containment that needs to be examined.

Just because a health care provision system is PP does not necessarily mean that poor care is given. Regardless of the form of reimbursement, if there is a commitment to quality, with well-trained, skilled physicians (primary care physicians and psychiatrists), access to care with a minimal time for entry into the system, plus a continuum of care (hospital, day treatment, halfway houses, ancillary caregivers, etc) so that patients can be cared for in the least restrictive environment, then the patients will receive the best care available.

Abby L. Wasserman, MD
United Behavioral Systems
12125 Woodcrest Executive Dr
Suite 320
St Louis, MO 63141

Reprint requests to Dr Wasserman.

1. Rogers WH, Wells KB, Meredith LS, Sturm R, Burnam MA. Outcomes for adult outpatients with depression under prepaid or fee-for-service financing. *Arch Gen Psychiatry*. 1993;50:517-525.

In reply

Wasserman commented that it is meaningless to analyze differences in outcomes without studying differences in other aspects of delivery systems. We agree that it is important to understand differences across systems of care in programs, management structures, and process of care, but this does not make outcome comparisons meaningless. A central feature of PP care is that it is provided in different settings and under different incentives than FFS care, ie, there are likely to be many programmatic and management differences. Yet, it is not clear whether entirely different systems of care are associated with different patient outcomes, and this is the subject of the analysis by Rogers et al (1993).[1]

However, because we found significant outcome differences among patients of psychiatrists, it now becomes worthwhile to focus on unraveling the mystery of the "black box" of the different systems of care—especially within psychiatry. Some of that can be done in the Medical Outcomes Study and is the subject of ongoing research[2,3]; some of that will require other studies specifically designed for that purpose. For example, we mentioned[1] that, over time, there were outcome differences in switches in type of insurance and in continuation of antidepressant medication by initial type of payment among patients of psychiatrists. The latter especially is suggestive of a clinically important difference in treatment style, since there is very strong support in the literature for the efficacy of antidepressant medications in major depression. Interestingly, in the Medical Outcomes Study, the PP patients perceived themselves as having similar or more generous benefits for mental health care than the FFS patients (even excluding the uninsured).[1]

Wasserman wondered whether income differences by type of payment (especially the inclusion of the uninsured in the FFS group) could explain outcome differences by type of payment. Our conclusions were not sensitive to the exclusion of the uninsured from the FFS group and the analysis adjusted for patient demographic characteristics, including income. Wasserman's argument that depressed patients whose condition were deteriorating would switch from FFS to PP care, while patients whose conditions were improving would do the opposite, is inconsistent with the

data reported in the study by Rogers et al[1] and with plan enrollment procedures. Specifically, psychiatric patients switching out of PP and into FFS care were more likely to be deteriorating in physical and role functioning than were those switching from FFS and into PP care (but the absolute numbers in these categories are small in this study). Furthermore, patients whose job functioning is deteriorating would not, as Wasserman suggests, be more likely to switch to PP care because PP care is more tied than is FFS care to being employed. Wasserman is right to suggest, however, that more work is needed on the dynamics of insurance switching and its relationship to health among depressed patients, and we address this in the article by Sturm et al.[2]

Wasserman also raises the issue of differences in use of antidepressant medication by type of payment. In a recent article,[3] we show that FFS patients of psychiatrists initially have a similar level of use of antidepressant medications as PP patients. Furthermore, the percentage of those medicated who use a subtherapeutic dosage is similar by type of payment. However, PP depressed patients are twice as likely to use minor tranquilizers (despite similar levels of comorbid anxiety disorder) as FFS depressed patients across specialty sectors and within psychiatry specifically. Because of sedating effects of minor tranquilizers but uncertain efficacy in depression, this difference in use by type of payment, combined with the difference by payment in exposure to antidepressant medications over time described in the study by Rogers et al,[1] could have contributed to outcome differences by type of payment in psychiatry. With a nonexperimental design, of course, we cannot be sure of the cause.

Kenneth B. Wells, MD, MPH
Roland Sturm, PhD
RAND Corp
1700 Main St
Santa Monica, CA 90407-2138

1. Rogers WH, Wells KB, Meredith LS, Sturm R, Burnam MA. Outcomes for adult outpatients with depression under prepaid or fee-for-service financing. *Arch Gen Psychiatry.* 1993;50:517-525.
2. Sturm R, McGlynn EA, Meredith LS, Wells KB, Manning WG, Rogers WH. Switches between prepaid and fee-for-service health systems among depressed outpatients: results from the Medical Outcomes Study. *Med Care.* 1994; 32:917-929.
3. Wells KB, Katon W, Rogers B, Camp P. Use of minor tranquilizers and antidepressant medications by depressed outpatients: results from the Medical Outcomes Study. *Am J Psychiatry.* 1994;151:694-700.

Serotonin$_{2A}$ Receptors in Schizophrenia: Relation to Suicide

Laruelle et al[1] reported no difference in B_{max} (maximum number of ligand-binding sites) for serotonin$_{2A}$ (5-HT_{2A}) receptors in the frontal cortex of six schizophrenic patients and six schizoaffective patients compared with 13 normal controls, using tritiated ketanserin as a ligand. There was a trend for B_{max} to be decreased in both patient groups compared with nine nonpsychotic suicide victims. The psychotic patients included seven suicides and five nonsuicides. According to the abstract in their article, the B_{max} of the five chronic psychotics who died of natural causes was less than that of the controls, the psychotics dying of suicide, and the nonpsychotic suicide victims. However, no statistical analysis to support this potentially important difference between schizophrenic or schizoaffective patients who suicided and those who did not was provided.

The authors should have cited our data,[2] published in 1991, of a significant decrease in B_{max} of 5-HT_{2A} receptors in the frontal cortex of 11 schizophrenic patients compared with 11 normal controls, using tritiated spiperone as a ligand. All the patients in that study died of natural causes. The B_{max} values we reported were very similar to those of Laruelle et al.[1]

Joyce et al[3] failed to find any difference in B_{max} of 5-HT_2 receptors in the frontal cortex of schizophrenics using tritiated lysergic acid diethylamide (LSD) as a ligand and autoradiography. This may have been due to combining data from four suicide victims and six schizophrenic patients who died of natural causes. The discrepancy between the study of Joyce et al[3] and our study[2] may be owing to the use of tritiated LSD as the ligand, since tritiated LSD labels multiple 5-HT receptor subtypes, as well as their combining data from suicides and nonsuicides. Mita et al[4] previously reported data similar to ours, using tritiated ketanserin as a ligand. They, too, studied only schizophrenic patients who died of natural causes. Thus, there are now, to my knowledge, three studies that suggest that schizophrenic patients who died of natural causes have decreased 5-HT_{2A} receptors in the frontal cortex. Future studies must clearly report data from patients with schizophrenia who die of natural causes and suicide.

Herbert Y. Meltzer, MD
Case Western Reserve University
School of Medicine
2074 Abbington Rd
Cleveland, OH 44106

1. Laruelle M, Abi-Dargham A, Casanova MF, Toti R, Weinberger DR, Kleinman JE. Selective abnormalities of prefrontal serotonergic receptors in schizophrenia. *Arch Gen Psychiatry.* 1993;50:810-818.
2. Arora RC, Meltzer HY. Serotonin$_2$ (5-HT_2) receptor binding in the frontal cortex of schizophrenic patients. *J Neural Transm.* 1991;85:19-29.
3. Joyce JN, Shane A, Lexow N, Winokur A, Casanova MF, Kleinman JE. Serotonin uptake sites and serotonin receptors are altered in the limbic system of schizophrenia. *Neuropsychopharmacology.* 1993;8:315-335.
4. Mita T, Hanada S, Nishono N, Kuno T, Nikai H, Yamadori T, Mizoi Y, Tanaka C. Decreased serotonin S_2 and increased dopamine D_2 receptors in chronic schizophrenics. *Biol Psychiatry.* 1986;21:1407-1414.

In reply

The density of 5-HT_2 receptors in the frontal cortex of patients with schizophrenia has been reported to be decreased in three studies[1-3] and unchanged in four studies.[4-7] Obviously, this discrepancy could be due to several factors, such as differences in ligands (iodine 125–labeled LSD vs tritiated ketanserin vs tritiated spiperone), differences in prior medication exposure, or differences in the clinical and demographic characteristics of the patients.

In our study, the patients with schizophrenia who died of natural causes had frontal 5-HT_2 receptor B_{max} values (mean±SEM; n=7, 76±16 fmol/mg of protein) significantly lower than controls (n=13, 164±14 fmol/mg of pro-

tein), schizophrenic patients who committed suicide (n=5, 162±25 fmol/mg of protein), and nonschizophrenic suicide victims (n=9, 205±22 fmol/mg of protein). The overall difference among groups was significant (analysis of covariance, P=.006) and the post hoc comparison revealed that the group of patients with schizophrenia who died of natural causes had a significantly lower B_{max} than the three other groups (Duncan New Multiple Range Test, P<.01). Furthermore, this factor could not be attributed to a medication effect.

As pointed out by Meltzer, it is interesting to note that the studies of Mita et al[2] and Arora and Meltzer[3] that reported decreased levels of $5\text{-}HT_2$ receptors in the frontal cortex included only patients dying of natural causes. The incidence of suicide in the schizophrenic population studied by Bennett et al,[1] Whitaker et al,[4] and Reynolds et al[7] was not reported. The group of schizophrenic patients studied by Joyce et al[6] included both suicides and nonsuicides.

Thus, available data are consistent with the hypothesis that decreased $5\text{-}HT_2$ density is observed only in a subgroup of schizophrenic patients characterized by the absence of suicide. However, this observation needs replication and its significance remains to be elucidated. As discussed in our article, it is conceivable that the decrease in $5\text{-}HT_2$ density is secondary to a loss of cortical GABAergic interneurons[8] and may be associated with prominent negative symptoms and a lower incidence of suicide.

We hope that these issues will be addressed in further postmortem or in vivo studies.

We apologize for overlooking the study of Arora and Meltzer in the reference list and appreciate Meltzer's comments.

Marc Laruelle, MD
Anissa Abi-Dargham, MD
Department of Psychiatry
Yale School of Medicine
West Haven Veterans Affairs Medical Center
950 Campbell Ave
West Haven, CT 06511
Manuel F. Casanova, MD
Augusta, Ga
Daniel R. Weinberger, MD
Joel E. Kleinman, MD, PhD
Washington, DC

1. Bennett JP, Enna SJ, Bylund DB, Gillin JC, Wyatt RJ, Snyder SH. Neurotransmitter receptors in frontal cortex of schizophrenics. *Arch Gen Psychiatry*. 1979; 36:927-934.
2. Mita T, Hanada S, Nishino N, Kuno T, Nakai H, Yamadori T, Mizoi Y, Tanaka C. Decreased serotonin S2 and increased dopamine D2 receptors in chronic schizophrenics. *Biol Psychiatry*. 1986;21:1407-1414.
3. Arora RC, Meltzer H. Serotonin ($5\text{-}HT_2$) receptor binding in the frontal cortex of schizophrenic patients. *J Neural Transm*. 1991;815:19-29.
4. Whitaker PM, Crow TJ, Ferrier IN. Tritiated LSD binding in frontal cortex schizophrenia. *Arch Gen Psychiatry*. 1981;38:278-280.
5. Laruelle M, Abi-Dargham A, Casanova MF, Toti R, Weinberger DR, Kleinman JE. Selective abnormalities of prefrontal serotonergic receptors in schizophrenia: a postmortem study. *Arch Gen Psychiatry*. 1993;50:810-818.
6. Joyce JN, Shane A, Lexow N, Winokur A, Casanova MF, Kleinman JE. Serotonin uptake sites and serotonin receptors are altered in the limbic system of schizophrenics. *Neuropsychopharmacology*. 1993;8:315-336.
7. Reynolds GP, Rossor MN, Ivesen LL. Preliminary studies of human cortical $5\text{-}HT_2$ receptors and their involvement in schizophrenia and neuroleptic drug action. *J Neural Transm*. 1984;18(suppl):273-277.
8. Sheldon P, Aghajanian GK. Excitatory responses to serotonin (5-HT) in neurons of the rat piriform cortex: evidence for mediation by $5\text{-}HT_2$ receptors in pyramidal cells and $5\text{-}HT_{1C}$ receptors in interneurons. *Synapse*. 1991;9:208-218.

Effects of Alterations in Plasma Tryptophan Levels on Aggressive Feelings

We read with interest the recent correspondence with regard to the dangers of amino acid supplements, given the effect of tryptophan-free amino acid mixtures in lowering mood.[1] We have been using the technique of rapid enhancement or depletion of plasma tryptophan levels to investigate the control of aggression. Recent work[2] has suggested that impulsivity rather than aggression, per se, may be affected by central serotonin function. Thus, in depressed patients, reduced serotonin activity is associated with suicide,[3] and in violent offenders, with measures of aggression and hostility[2]; the changes in impulsivity are manifested by the underlying traits. Previous studies that measured provoked aggression[4] and subjective hostility[5] after tryptophan depletion have not measured preexisting aggressive traits, which may have accounted for their failure to find an effect.

We looked at 24 male subjects who were selected because they had high levels of trait aggression based a score of greater than 40 of 75 on the Buss-Durkee hostility inventory. Subjects drank either a standard 100-g tryptophan-free mixture of 15 amino acids (T−)[4,5] or the same mixture with the addition of 10.3 g of tryptophan (T+) in a double-blind design. *P* values are given for two-tailed *t* tests. The mean total plasma tryptophan level decreased from 57.2 to 12.0 μmol/L in the T− group and increased from 59.4 to 656 μmol/L in the T+ group (*P*<.001). Subjects completed an aggression rating scale and a mood rating scale at baseline and at 5 hours after ingestion of the mixture. Both of these measures involved completing visual analog scales and were scored out of 100. In addition, there were three factors derivable from the mood rating scale: anxiety, well-being, and sedation.

After subtracting baseline scores, the T− group rated themselves significantly higher than did the T+ group on the variables angry (30 percentage points difference; *P*=.009), aggressive (29 percentage points difference; *P*=.01), annoyed (29 percentage points difference; *P*=.04), quarrelsome (29 percentage points difference; *P*=.01), and hostile (20 percentage points difference; *P*=.01). The changes were of approximately equal magnitude in opposite directions in the two groups. The overall change in mean score for all 13 items on the aggression rating scale also showed a significant difference (*P*=.04). One item on the mood rating scale was significant: discontent, which increased with T− and decreased with T+ (20 percentage points difference; *P*=.04). Of the three factors, one showed a trend to significance: well-being increased with T+ and decreased with T− (11 percentage points difference; *P*=.06).

We believe that these results show a clear effect of both tryptophan depletion and enhancement on aggression in subjects who have preexisting aggressive traits. The concerns that amino acid supplements that lack tryp-

tophan could inadvertently cause tryptophan depletion and, subsequently, serious adverse mood changes in those who are prone to depression are well founded. We believe that these concerns may apply equally to those who are prone to aggression.

Anthony J. Cleare, MBBS
Alyson J. Bond, PhD
Institute of Psychiatry
De Crespigny Park
Denmark Hill
London, England SE5 8AF

1. Norden M. Risk of tryptophan depletion following amino acid supplementation. *Arch Gen Psychiatry*. 1993;50:1000.
2. Virkkunen M, Rawlings R, Tokola R, Poland RE, Guidotti A, Nemeroff C, Bissette G, Kalogeras K, Karonen SL, Linnoila M. CSF biochemistries, glucose metabolism, and diurnal activity rhythms in alcoholics, violent offenders, fire setters, and healthy volunteers. *Arch Gen Psychiatry*. 1994;51:20-27.
3. Stanley M, Stanley B. Postmortem evidence for serotonin's role in suicide. *J Clin Psychiatry*. 1990;51(suppl 4):22-28.
4. Smith SE, Pihl RO, Young SN, Ervin FR. Elevation and reduction of plasma tryptophan and their effects on aggression and perceptual sensitivity in normal males. *Aggressive Behav*. 1986;12:393-407.
5. Young SN, Smith S, Pihl RO, Ervin FR. Tryptophan depletion causes a rapid lowering of mood in normal males. *Psychopharmacology*. 1985;87:173-177.

IN MEMORIAM

Mary Catherine Neidigh Freedman
August 2, 1921 - October 21, 1994

It is with great sadness that we must inform our readership of the death of Mary Freedman of chronic obstructive lung disease at her home in Los Angeles, Calif. An accomplished artist and a woman of great depth and dignity, Mrs Freedman was known and loved by many in the ARCHIVES collegium of contributors and reviewers. At the time of his death in June 1993, Daniel X. Freedman, this journal's editor for over two decades, and Mary had been married for 47 years.

She will be fondly remembered and deeply missed.

ARCHIVES
OF
GENERAL PSYCHIATRY

Index to

Volume 51

January through December 1994

AUTHOR INDEX TO VOLUME 51

In this index in alphabetical order are listed names of authors of all articles and letters. Full citation is given under first author only; reference is made from joint authors. Names which begin with a prefix are entered under the prefix. The month is given as a two-letter notation in parentheses.

A

Abi-Dargham A see Laruelle M
Adams PB see Goldstein RB
Aghajanian GK see Delgado PL
Akil H see Young EA
Akiskal HS see Coryell W; Kovacs M
Allgulander C: Suicide and mortality patterns in anxiety neurosis and depressive neurosis, 708 (Se)
Alpert NM see Rauch SL
Altemus M, Swedo SE, Leonard HL, Richer D, Rubinow DR, Potter WZ, Rapoport JL: Changes in cerebrospinal fluid neurochemistry during treatment of obsessive-compulsive disorder with clomipramine, 794 (Oc)
Alterman AI see Volpicelli JR
Alvarez E see Artigas F
Alvir J see Koreen AR
Amador XF, Flaum M, Andreasen NC, Strauss DH, Yale SA, Clark SC, Gorman JM: Awareness of illness in schizophrenia and schizoaffective and mood disorders, 826 (Oc)
Amin F see Koreen AR
An Nguyen J see Conley R
Anderson B see Frank E
Anderson GM see Leckman JF
Andrade C, Rao NSK: Naltrexone and alcohol dependence: some methodological issues (letter) 335 (Ap)
Andreasen N see Wang ZW
Andreasen NC see Amador XF
Andreoli A see Loranger AW
Annable L see Bradwejn J
Armstrong HE see Linehan MM
Artigas F, Perez V, Alvarez E: Pindolol induces a rapid improvement of depressed patients treated with serotonin reuptake inhibitors (letter) 248 (Mr)
Ashleigh EA see Veith RC

B

Babor TF see Kranzler HR
Badger GJ see Higgins ST
Baer L, Rauch SL, Jenike MA, Cassem NH, Ballantine HT, Manzo PA, Martuza RL: Cingulotomy in a case of concomitant obsessive-compulsive disorder and Tourette's syndrome (letter) 73 (Ja)
Baer L see Breiter HC; Rauch SL
Baldessarini RJ see Popli AP
Ballantine HT see Baer L
Barchas JD, Marzuk PM: Some issues for the new director of NIMH, 998 (De)
Barkley C see Paykel ES
Barnes GJ, Jones Q: Maintenance therapy in depression (letter) 503 (Je)
Barnes RF see Veith RC
Barnett MC see Barsky AJ
Barr LC, Goodman WK, McDougle CJ, Delgado PL, Heninger GR, Charney DS, Price LH: Tryptophan depletion in patients with obsessive-compulsive disorder who respond to serotonin reuptake inhibitors, 309 (Ap)
Barr LC see Leckman JF
Barsky AJ, Barnett MC, Cleary PD: Hypochondriasis and panic disorder: boundary and overlap, 918 (No)
Bass N see DeLisi LE
Beardsall L see Paykel ES
Benes FM, Turtle M, Khan Y, Farol P: Myelination of a key relay zone in the hippocampal formation occurs in the human brain during childhood, adolescence, and adulthood, 477 (Je)
Benkelfat C, Ellenbogen MA, Dean P, Palmour RM, Young SN: Mood-lowering effect of tryptophan depletion: enhanced susceptibility in young men at genetic risk for major affective disorders, 687 (Se)
Berger D, Suematsu H, Ono Y: Theories of sexual orientation: a reappraisal (letter) 432 (My)
Berger P see Loranger AW
Bermanzohn PC see Siris SG
Bickel WK see Higgins ST
Bing EG see Maj M
Bird HR: Correction and amplification (letter) 429 (My)
Bisighini RM see Carroll KM
Bissette G see Marangell LB; Virkkunen M
Black DW see Wang ZW
Black JE see McDougle CJ
Blake D see Mason J
Blaney NT see Goodkin K
Blazer DG see Davidson JRT
Blehar MC see Nurnberger JI Jr
Boccio A see DeLisi LE
Bohn MJ see Kranzler HR
Bond AJ see Cleare AJ
Boone KB see Lesser IM
Bowers MB Jr see Krystal JH
Bradwejn J, Koszycki D, Couëtoux du Tertre A, van Megen H, den Boer J, Westenberg H, Annable L: Panicogenic effects of cholecystokinin-tetrapeptide are antagonized by L-365,260, a central cholecystokinin receptor antagonist, in patients with panic disorder, 486 (Je)
Braff D see Heaton R
Braff DL see Swerdlow NR
Brasseur M see Linkowski P
Brayne C see Paykel ES
Breier A see Buchanan RW
Breiter HC, Filipek PA, Kennedy DN, Baer L, Pitcher DA, Olivares MJ, Renshaw PF, Caviness VS Jr, Jenike MA: Retrocallosal white matter abnormalities in patients with obsessive-compulsive disorder (letter) 663 (Au)
Breiter HCR see Rauch SL
Bremner D see Mason J
Bremner JD see Krystal JH
Brennan P see Hollister JM; Raine A
Brown GW, Harris TO, Hepworth C: Life events and endogenous depression: puzzle reexamined, 525 (Jy)
Brown J see Kranzler HR
Bryois C, Ferrero F: Mania induced by citalopram (letter) 664 (Au)
Buchanan RW see Carpenter WT Jr
Buchanan RW, Strauss ME, Kirkpatrick B, Holstein C, Breier A, Carpenter WT Jr: Neuropsychological impairments in deficit vs nondeficit forms of schizophrenia, 804 (Oc)
Buchheim P see Loranger AW
Budney AJ see Higgins ST
Buesching DP see Fifer SK
Burleson JA see Kranzler HR
Butters N see Gillin JC
Byne W, Parsons B: Theories of sexual orientation: a reappraisal (letter) 432 (My)

C

Calil HM see Maj M
Cannon TD, Mednick SA, Parnas J, Schulsinger F, Praestholm J, Vestergaard A: Developmental brain abnormalities in the offspring of schizophrenic mothers: II. structural brain characteristics of schizophrenia and schizotypal personality disorder, 955 (De)
Cannon TD, Zorrilla LE, Shtasel D, Gur RE, Gur RC, Marco EJ, Moberg P, Price RA: Neuropsychological functioning in siblings discordant for schizophrenia and healthy volunteers, 651 (Au)
Cannon TD see Hollister JM
Carpenter WT Jr, Buchanan RW, Kirkpatrick B, Tamminga C, Wood F: Neural circuits in schizophrenia (letter) 516 (Jy)
Carpenter WT Jr see Buchanan RW
Carroll KM, Rounsaville BJ, Gordon LT, Nich C, Jatlow P, Bisighini RM, Gawin FH: Psychotherapy and pharmacotherapy for ambulatory cocaine abusers, 177 (Mr)
Carroll KM, Rounsaville BJ, Nich C, Gordon LT, Wirtz PW, Gawin F: One-year follow-up of psychotherapy and pharmacotherapy for cocaine dependence: delayed emergence of psychotherapy effects, 989 (De)
Casanova MF see Laruelle M
Cassem NH see Baer L
Castillo S see Veith RC
Cavallini MC see Macciardi F
Caviness VS Jr see Breiter HC
Chakos M see Koreen AR
Channabasavanna SM see Loranger AW
Chappell PB see Leckman JF
Charney D see Goldstein RB; Mason J
Charney DS see Barr LC; Delgado PL; Krystal JH
Clark DC, Fawcett J: Relation of parenthood to suicide (letter) 160 (Fe)
Clark SC see Amador XF
Cleare AJ, Bond AJ: Effects of alterations in plasma tryptophan levels on aggressive feelings (letter) 1004 (De)
Cleary PD see Barsky AJ
Cloitre M see Shear MK
Coccaro EF, Silverman JM, Klar HM, Horvath TB, Siever LJ: Familial correlates of reduced central serotonergic system function in patients with personality disorders, 318 (Ap)
Cohen DJ see Leckman JF
Cohen RM see Sunderland T
Coid B see Loranger AW
Cole JO see Popli AP
Conley R, Tamminga CA, An Nguyen J: Clinical action of remoxipride (letter) 1001 (De)
Cooney N see Krystal JH
Cooper T see Koreen AR
Copinschi G see Linkowski P
Coryell W, Akiskal HS, Leon AC, Winokur G, Maser JD, Mueller TI, Keller MB, National Institute of Mental Health Collaborative Program on the Psychobiology of Depression—Clinical Studies: Time course of nonchronic major depressive disorder: uniformity across episodes and samples, 405 (My)
Couëtoux du Tertre A see Bradwejn J
Crowe RR see Wang ZW

D

Dahl A see Loranger AW
Davidson JRT, Hughes DC, George LK, Blazer DG: Boundary of social phobia: exploring the threshold, 975 (De)
Davis KL see Silverman JM
Dawson ME, Nuechterlein KH, Schell AM, Gitlin M, Ventura J: Autonomic abnormalities in schizophrenia: state or trait indicators? 813 (Oc)
Dean P see Benkelfat C
Del Boca FK see Kranzler HR
Delaney R see Krystal JH
Delgado PL, Price LH, Miller HL, Salomon RM, Aghajanian GK, Heninger GR, Charney DS: Serotonin

and the neurobiology of depression: effects of tryptophan depletion, 865 (No)
Delgado PL see Barr LC
D'Elia L see Maj M
DeLisi LE, Bass N, Boccio A, Shields G, Morganti C, Vita A: Age of onset in familial schizophrenia (letter) 334 (Ap)
Demodena A see Gillin JC
den Boer J see Bradwejn J
Devanand DP see Nobler MS
Dew B see Garbutt JC
Diekstra RFW see Loranger AW
Dingemans PM see Linszen DH
Dobkin PL see Tremblay RE
Dohrenwend BP see Skodol AE
Dominguez RA see Tollefson GD
Donham R see Higgins ST

E

Eaton WW see Wittchen H-U
Ellenbogen MA see Benkelfat C
Escriba PV, Sastre M, Garcia-Sevilla JA: Increased density of guanine nucleotide-binding proteins in the postmortem brains of heroin addicts, 494 (Je)
Eshleman S see Kessler RC

F

Faber B see Kety SS
Farol P see Benes FM
Fawcett J see Clark DC
Fenton WS, Wyatt RJ, McGlashan TH: Risk factors for spontaneous dyskinesia in schizophrenia, 643 (Au)
Ferguson B see Loranger AW
Ferrero F see Bryois C
Fiero PL see Leibenluft E
Fifer SK, Mathias SD, Patrick DL, Mazonson PD, Lubeck DP, Buesching DP: Untreated anxiety among adult primary care patients in a health maintenance organization, 740 (Se)
Filipek PA see Breiter HC
Fischman AJ see Rauch SL
Flaum M see Amador XF
Fletcher MA see Goodkin K
Foeg FE see Higgins ST
Frances A: Diagnostic Interview for Genetic Studies, 863 (No)
Frank E, Anderson B, Reynolds CF III, Ritenour A, Kupfer DJ: Life events and the research diagnostic criteria endogenous subtype: confirmation of the distinction using the Bedford College methods, 519 (Jy)
Frank E, Kupfer DJ: Maintenance therapy in depression (letter) 504 (Je)
Freeman GK see Krystal JH

G

Garbutt JC, Mayo JP, Little KY, Gillette GM, Mason GA, Dew B, Prange AJ Jr: Dose-response studies with protirelin, 875 (No)
Garcia-Sevilla JA see Escriba PV
Gatsonis C see Kovacs M
Gawin F see Carroll KM
Gawin FH see Carroll KM
Gehlhaar E see Paykel ES
Gejman PV see Rao PA
Gelernter J see Rao PA
Genduso LA see Tollefson GD
George LK see Davidson JRT
George MS see Marangell LB
Gershon ES see Rao PA
Geyer MA see Swerdlow NR
Geyer P see Lurie S
Gill C see Paykel ES
Gillette GM see Garbutt JC
Gillin JC, Smith TL, Irwin M, Butters N, Demodena A, Schuckit M: Increased pressure for rapid eye movement sleep at time of hospital admission predicts relapse in nondepressed patients with primary alcoholism at 3-month follow-up, 189 (Mr)
Girling DM see Paykel ES
Gitlin M see Dawson ME
Gold JM, Hermann BP, Randolph C, Wyler AR, Goldberg TE, Weinberger DR: Schizophrenia and temporal lobe epilepsy: a neuropsychological analysis, 265 (Ap)
Goldberg TE see Gold JM
Goldman D see Nielsen DA
Goldstein RB, Weissman MM, Adams PB, Horwath E, Lish JD, Charney D, Woods SW, Sobin C, Wickramaratne PJ: Psychiatric disorders in relatives of probands with panic disorder and/or major depression, 383 (My)
Goodkin K, Mulder CL, Blaney NT, Ironson G, Kumar M, Fletcher MA: Psychoneuroimmunology and human immunodeficiency virus type 1 infection revisited (letter) 246 (Mr)
Goodman W see Tollefson GD
Goodman WK see Barr LC; Leckman JF; McDougle CJ
Gordon LT see Carroll KM
Gorman JM see Amador XF
Green MF, Nuechterlein KH, Mintz J:
Backward masking in schizophrenia and mania: I. specifying a mechanism, 939 (De)
Backward masking in schizophrenia and mania: II. specifying the visual channels, 945 (De)
Gruenberg AM see Kendler KS
Grunhaus L see Young EA
Guidotti A see Virkkunen M
Gur RC see Cannon TD; Saykin AJ
Gur RE see Cannon TD; Saykin AJ
Gusman F see Mason J

H

Halter JB see Veith RC
Harkavy-Friedman J see Nurnberger JI Jr
Harris MJ see Heaton R
Harris TO see Brown GW
Haskett RF see Young EA
Heard HL see Linehan MM
Heath AC see True WR
Heaton R, Paulsen JS, McAdams LA, Kuck J, Zisook S, Braff D, Harris MJ, Jeste DV: Neuropsychological deficits in schizophrenics: relationship to age, chronicity, and dementia, 469 (Je)
Heninger GR see Barr LC; Delgado PL; Krystal JH; McDougle CJ
Hepworth C see Brown GW
Hermann BP see Gold JM
Hietala J, Syvälahti E, Vuorio K, Någren K, Lehikoinen P, Ruotsalainen U, Räkköläinen V, Lehtinen V, Wegelius U: Striatal D_2 dopamine receptor characteristics in neuroleptic-naive schizophrenic patients studied with positron emission tomography, 116 (Fe)
Higgins ST, Budney AJ, Bickel WK, Foerg FE, Donham R, Badger GJ: Incentives improve outcome in outpatient behavioral treatment of cocaine dependence, 568 (Jy)
Higley JD, Mehlman PT, Taub D, Suomi SJ, Higley SB, Vickers JM, Linnoila M: Are stress hormones and serotonin related to aggression in primates? (letter) 73 (Ja)
Higley SB see Higley JD
Hodgins S: Violence in the severely mentally ill (letter) 71 (Ja)
Hollister JM, Mednick SA, Brennan P, Cannon TD: Impaired autonomic nervous system habituation in those at genetic risk for schizophrenia, 552 (Jy)
Holstein C see Buchanan RW
Holzman PS: Parsing cognition: the power of psychology paradigms, 952 (De)
Hong WW see Pickar D
Horrobin DF see Peet M
Horvath TB see Coccaro EF
Horwath E see Goldstein RB
Høyer G, Lund E: Relation of parenthood to suicide (letter) 160 (Fe)
Hsiao JK see Pickar D
Hubain P see Linkowski P
Huggins T see Marangell LB
Hughes DC see Davidson JRT
Hughes M see Kessler RC
Huppert FA see Paykel ES

I

Ingraham LJ see Kety SS
Ironson G see Goodkin K
Irwin M see Gillin JC

J

Jacobsberg LB see Loranger AW
Jacobsen B see Kety SS
Janssen R see Maj M
Jansson L see Kety SS
Jatlow P see Carroll KM
Jenike MA see Baer L; Breiter HC; Rauch SL; Tollefson GD
Jeste DV see Heaton R
Johnson D see Mason J
Johnston-Cronk K see Marder SR
Jones P: Schizophrenia after prenatal exposure to the Dutch Hunger Winter of 1944-1945 (letter) 333 (Ap)
Jones Q see Barnes GJ

K

Kallio E see Virkkunen M
Kalogeras K see Virkkunen M
Karonen S-L see Virkkunen M
Karper LP see Krystal JH
Katz DL see Pope HG Jr
Kaufmann CA see Nurnberger JI Jr
Keller MB see Coryell W
Kellner R see Strassman RJ
Kendler KS, Gruenberg AM, Kinney DK: Independent diagnoses of adoptees and relatives as defined by *DSM-III* in the provincial and national samples of the Danish Adoption Study of Schizophrenia, 456 (Je)
Kendler KS see Kessler RC; Roy M-A; Walsh D
Kennedy DN see Breiter HC
Kennedy JL see Macciardi F
Kerkhofs M see Linkowski P
Kessler RC, McGonagle KA, Zhao S, Nelson CB, Hughes M, Eshleman S, Wittchen H-U, Kendler KS: Lifetime and 12-month prevalence of *DSM-III-R* psychiatric disorders in the United States: results from the National Comorbidity Survey, 8 (Ja)
Kessler RC see Wittchen H-U
Kester DB see Saykin AJ
Kety SS, Wender PH, Jacobsen B, Ingraham LJ, Jansson L, Faber B, Kinney DK: Mental illness in the biological and adoptive relatives of schizophrenic adoptees: replication of the Copenhagen Study in the rest of Denmark, 442 (Je)
Khan Y see Benes FM
Kinney DK see Kendler KS; Kety SS
Kirkpatrick B see Buchanan RW; Carpenter WT Jr
Klar HM see Coccaro EF
Klein DF: Klein's suffocation theory of panic (letter) 506 (Je)
Kleinman JE see Laruelle M
Koran LM see Tollefson GD
Koreen AR, Lieberman J, Alvir J, Mayerhoff D, Loebel A, Chakos M, Amin F, Cooper T: Plasma homovanillic acid levels in first-episode schizophrenia: psychopathology and treatment response, 132 (Fe)
Korner P see Kranzler HR
Kosten TR see McDougle CJ
Koszycki D see Bradwejn J
Kovacs M, Akiskal HS, Gatsonis C, Parrone PL: Childhood-onset dysthymic disorder: clinical features and prospective naturalistic outcome, 365 (My)
Kovacs M, Gatsonis C, Pollock M, Parrone PL: Controlled prospective study of *DSM-III* adjustment disorder in childhood: short-term prognosis and long-term predictive validity, 535 (Jy)
Kranzler HR, Burleson JA, Del Boca FK, Babor TF, Korner P, Brown J, Bohn MJ: Buspirone treatment of anxious alcoholics: placebo-controlled trial, 720 (Se)
Kranzler HR see Krystal JH
Kruk J see Sachdev P
Krystal JH, Karper LP, Seibyl JP, Freeman GK, Delaney R, Bremner JD, Heninger GR, Bowers MB Jr, Charney DS: Subanesthetic effects of the noncompetitive NMDA antagonist, ketamine, in humans: psychotomimetic, perceptual, cognitive, and neuroendocrine responses, 199 (Mr)
Krystal JH, Southwick SM, Charney DS: Alcohol dependence may be the missing link between posttraumatic stress disorder and panic (letter) 430 (My)
Krystal JH, Webb E, Cooney N, Kranzler HR, Charney DS: Specificity of ethanollike effects elicited by serotonergic and noradrenergic mechanisms, 898 (No)
Kuck J see Heaton R
Kumar M see Goodkin K
Kupfer DJ see Frank E

L

Laruelle M, Abi-Dargham A, Casanova MF, Weinberger DR, Kleinman JE: Serotonin $_{2a}$ receptors in schizophrenia: relation to suicide (letter) 1003 (De)
Laugharne JDE see Peet M
Lawlor BA see Sunderland T
Lebell M see Marder SR
Leckman JF, Goodman WK, North WG, Chappell PB, Price LH, Pauls DL, Anderson GM, Riddle MA, McSwiggan-Hardin M, McDougle CJ, Barr LC, Cohen DJ: Elevated cerebrospinal fluid levels of oxytocin in obsessive-compulsive disorder: comparison with Tourette's syndrome and healthy controls, 782 (Oc)
Leckman JF see McDougle CJ
Leclercq R see Linkowski P
Lee NC see McDougle CJ
Lee S: Diagnostic Interview Schedule and anorexia nervosa in Hong Kong (letter) 251 (Mr)
Lehikoinen P see Hietala J
Lehtinen V see Hietala J
Leibenluft E, Fiero PL, Rubinow DR: Effects of the menstrual cycle on dependent variables in mood disorder research, 761 (Oc)
Lenior ME see Linszen DH
Leon AC see Coryell W; Shear MK
Leonard HL see Altemus M
Lesser IM, Mena I, Boone KB, Miller BL, Mehringer CM, Wohl M: Reduction of cerebral blood flow in older depressed patients, 677 (Se)
Levav I see Skodol AE
Lewis N see Veith RC
L'Hermite-Balériaux M see Linkowski P
Li G see Silverman JM
Liberman RP see Marder SR
Lieberman J see Koreen AR
Lin SP see Susser E
Linares OA see Veith RC
Linehan MM, Heard HL, Armstrong HE: Naturalistic follow-up of a behavioral treatment for chronically parasuicidal borderline patients, 50:971 (De); correction, 51: 422 (My)
Linkowski P, Kerkhofs M, Van Onderbergen A, Hubain P, Copinschi G, L'Hermite-Balériaux M, Leclercq R,

Brasseur M, Mendlewicz J, Van Cauter E: 24-hour profiles of cortisol, prolactin, and growth hormone secretion in mania, 616 (Au)
Linnoila M see Higley JD; Nielsen DA; Virkkunen M
Linszen DH, Dingemans PM, Lenior ME: Cannabis abuse and the course of recent-onset schizophrenic disorders, 273 (Ap)
Lish JD see Goldstein RB
Litman RE see Pickar D
Little KY see Garbutt JC
Loebel A see Koreen AR
Loranger AW, Sartorius N, Andreoli A, Berger P, Buchheim P, Channabasavanna SM, Coid B, Dahl A, Diekstra RFW, Ferguson B, Jacobsberg LB, Mombour W, Pull C, Ono Y, Regier DA: International Personality Disorder Examination: The World Health Organization/Alcohol, Drug Abuse, and Mental Health Administration International Pilot Study of Personality Disorders, 215 (Mr)
Luabeya M'A-K see Maj M
Lubeck DP see Fifer SK
Lubin H see Mason J
Lund E see Høyer G
Lundberg GD see Springer MD
Lurie S, Geyer P: Genetic and environmental influences of twins in posttraumatic stress (letter) 838 (Oc)

M

Macciardi F, Petronis A, Van Tol HHM, Marino C, Cavallini MC, Smeraldi E, Kennedy JL: Analysis of the D_4 dopamine receptor gene variant in an Italian schizophrenia kindred, 288 (Ap)
Maj M, Janssen R, Starace F, Zaudig M, Satz P, Sughondhabirom B, Luabeya M'A-K, Riedel R, Ndetei D, Calil HM, Bing EG, St Louis M, Sartorius N: WHO Neuropsychiatric AIDS Study, Cross-sectional Phase I: study design and psychiatric findings, 39 (Ja)
Maj M, Satz P, Janssen R, Zaudig M, Starace F, D'Elia L, Sughondhabirom B, Mussa M, Naber D, Ndetei D, Schulte G, Sartorius N: WHO Neuropsychiatric AIDS Study, Cross-sectional Phase II: neuropsychological and neurological findings, 51 (Ja)
Malaspina D see Nurnberger JI Jr
Malison RT see McDougle CJ
Manzo PA see Baer L
Marangell LB, George MS, Bissette G, Pazzaglia P, Huggins T, Post RM: Carbamazepine increases cerebrospinal fluid thyrotropin-releasing hormone levels in affectively ill patients, 625 (Au)
Marco EJ see Cannon TD
Marder SR, Wirshing WC, Van Putten T, Mintz J, McKenzie J, Johnston-Cronk K, Lebell M, Liberman RP: Fluphenazine vs placebo supplementation for prodromal signs of relapse in schizophrenia, 280 (Ap)
Marino C see Macciardi F
Markowitz JC see Weissman MM
Martuza RL see Baer L
Marzuk PM see Barchas JD
Maser JD see Coryell W; Shear MK
Mason GA see Garbutt JC
Mason J, Southwick S, Yehuda R, Wang S, Riney S, Bremner D, Johnson D, Lubin H, Blake D, Zhou G, Gusman F, Charney D: Elevation of serum free triiodothyronine, total triiodothyronine, thyroxine-binding globulin, and total thyroxine levels in combat-related posttraumatic stress disorder, 629 (Au)
Mason SE see Siris SG
Mathias SD see Fifer SK
Mayerhoff D see Koreen AR
Mayo JP see Garbutt JC
Mazonson PD see Fifer SK
McAdams LA see Heaton R
McCarley RW, Shenton ME, O'Donnell BF, Nestor PG: Neural circuits in schizophrenia (letter) 515 (Jy)
McConaghy N: Biologic theories of sexual orientation (letter) 431 (My)
McDougle CJ, Black JE, Malison RT, Zimmermann RC, Kosten TR, Heninger GR, Price LH: Noradrenergic dysregulation during discontinuation of cocaine use in addicts, 713 (Se)
McDougle CJ, Goodman WK, Leckman JF, Lee NC, Heninger GR, Price LH: Haloperidol addition in fluvoxamine-refractory obsessive-compulsive disorder: a double-blind, placebo-controlled study in patients with and without tics, 302 (Ap)
McDougle CJ see Barr LC; Leckman JF
McGlashan TH see Fenton WS
McGonagle KA see Kessler RC
McKenzie J see Marder SR
McSwiggan-Hardin M see Leckman JF
Mednick SA see Cannon TD; Hollister JM; Raine A
Mehlman PT see Higley JD
Mehringer CM see Lesser IM
Mellow AM see Sunderland T
Meltzer HY: Serotonin $_{2a}$ receptors in schizophrenia: relation to suicide (letter) 1003 (De)
Mena I see Lesser IM
Mendlewicz J see Linkowski P
Miller BL see Lesser IM
Miller HL see Delgado PL
Mintz J see Green MF; Marder SR
Moberg P see Cannon TD
Moeller JR see Nobler MS
Mohs RC see Silverman JM
Molchan S see Sunderland T
Mombour W see Loranger AW
Morganti C see DeLisi LE
Mozley LH see Saykin AJ
Mueller EA see Sunderland T
Mueller TI see Coryell W
Mukherjee S see Nobler MS
Mulder CL see Goodkin K
Murburg MM see Veith RC
Murphy DL see Sunderland T
Mussa M see Maj M

N

Naber D see Maj M
Någren K see Hietala J
National Institute of Mental Health Collaborative Program on the Psychobiology of Depression—Clinical Studies see Coryell W
Ndetei D see Maj M
Nelson CB see Kessler RC
Nemeroff C see Virkkunen M
Nestor PG see McCarley RW
Newhouse PA see Sunderland T
Nich C see Carroll KM
Nielsen DA, Goldman D, Virkkunen M, Tokola R, Rawlings R, Linnoila M: Suicidality and 5-hydroxyindoleacetic acid concentration associated with a tryptophan hydroxylase polymorphism, 34 (Ja)
NIMH Genetics Initiative see Nurnberger JI Jr
Nobler MS, Sackeim HA: Lithium prophylaxis in American patients with unipolar disorder (letter) 502 (Je)
Nobler MS, Sackeim HA, Prohovnik I, Moeller JR, Mukherjee S, Schnur DB, Prudic J, Devanand DP: Regional cerebral blood flow in mood disorders, III: treatment and clinical response, 884 (No)
North WG see Leckman JF
Nuechterlein KH see Dawson ME; Green MF
Nurnberger JI Jr, Blehar MC, Kaufmann CA, York-Cooler C, Simpson SG, Harkavy-Friedman J, Severe JB, Malaspina D, Reich T, NIMH Genetics Initiative: Diagnostic Interview for Genetic Studies: rationale, unique features, and training, 849 (No)

O

O'Brien CP see Volpicelli JR
O'Connor D see Paykel ES
O'Donnell BF see McCarley RW
Olivares MJ see Breiter HC
Ono Y see Berger D; Loranger AW

P

Palmour RM see Benkelfat C
Pande A see Young EA
Parnas J see Cannon TD
Parrone PL see Kovacs M
Parsons B see Byne W
Pascualy M see Veith RC
Patrick DL see Fifer SK
Pauls DL see Leckman JF
Paulsen JS see Heaton R
Paykel ES, Brayne C, Huppert FA, Gill C, Barkley C, Gehlhaar E, Beardsall L, Girling DM, Pollitt P, O'Connor D: Incidence of dementia in a population older than 75 years in the United Kingdom, 325 (Ap)
Pazzaglia P see Marangell LB
Peet M, Laugharne JDE, Horrobin DF, Reynolds GP: Arachidonic acid: a common link in the biology of schizophrenia? (letter) 665 (Au)
Perez V see Artigas F
Perry S, Rabkin J: Psychoneuroimmunology and human immunodeficiency virus type 1 infection revisited (letter) 247 (Mr)
Peskind ER see Veith RC
Petronis A see Macciardi F
Pickar D, Litman RE, Hong WW, Su TP, Weissman EM, Hsiao JK, Potter WZ: Clinical response to clozapine in patients with schizophrenia (letter) 159 (Fe)
Pickar D see Rao PA
Pihl RO see Tremblay RE
Pilkonis PA see Shear MK
Pitcher DA see Breiter HC
Poland RE see Virkkunen M
Pollitt P see Paykel ES
Pollock M see Kovacs M
Pope HG Jr, Katz DL: Psychiatric and medical effects of anabolic-androgenic steroid use: a controlled study of 160 athletes, 375 (My)
Popli AP, Baldessarini RJ, Cole JO: Interactions of serotonin reuptake inhibitors with tricyclic antidepressants (letter) 666 (Au)
Post RM see Marangell LB
Potter WZ see Altemus M; Pickar D
Potvin JH see Tollefson GD
Praestholm J see Cannon TD
Prange AJ Jr see Garbutt JC
Price LH see Barr LC; Delgado PL; Leckman JF; McDougle CJ
Price RA see Cannon TD
Prohovnik I see Nobler MS
Prudic J see Nobler MS
Pull C see Loranger AW

Q

Qualls CR see Strassman RJ

R

Rabkin J see Perry S
Rachman S see Taylor S
Raine A, Brennan P, Mednick SA: Birth complications combined with early maternal rejection at age 1 year predispose to violent crime at age 18 years, 984 (De)
Räkköläinen V see Hietala J
Ram A see Rao PA
Rampey AH Jr see Tollefson GD
Randolph C see Gold JM
Rao NSK see Andrade C
Rao PA, Pickar D, Gejman PV, Ram A, Gershon ES, Gelernter J: Allelic variation in the D_4 dopamine receptor (DRD4) gene does not predict response to clozapine, 912 (No)
Rapoport JL see Altemus M
Raskind MA see Veith RC
Rauch SL, Jenike MA, Alpert NM, Baer L, Breiter HCR, Savage CR, Fischman AJ: Regional cerebral blood flow measured during symptom provocation in obsessive-compulsive disorder using oxygen 15—labeled carbon dioxide and positron emission tomography, 62 (Ja)
Rauch SL see Baer L
Rawlings R see Nielsen DA; Virkkunen M
Regier DA see Loranger AW
Reich T see Nurnberger JI Jr
Renshaw PF see Breiter HC
Reus VI: Are stress hormones and serotonin related to aggression in primates? (letter) 72 (Ja)
Reynolds CF III see Frank E
Reynolds GP see Peet M
Rice J see True WR
Richer D see Altemus M
Riddle MA see Leckman JF
Riedel R see Maj M
Riney S see Mason J
Ritenour A see Frank E
Rounsaville BJ see Carroll KM
Roy M-A, Kendler KS: Effect of diagnostic hierarchy in genetic epidemiological studies of psychiatric disorders (letter) 926 (No)
Rubinow DR see Altemus M; Leibenluft E
Ruotsalainen U see Hietala J
Rush AJ see Tollefson GD

S

Sachdev P, Kruk J: Clinical characteristics and predisposing factors in acute drug-induced akathisia, 963 (De)
Sackeim HA see Nobler MS
Salomon RM see Delgado PL
Sartorius N see Loranger AW; Maj M
Sastre M see Escriba PV
Satz P see Maj M
Savage CR see Rauch SL
Saykin AJ, Shtasel DL, Gur RE, Kester DB, Mozley LH, Stafiniak P, Gur RC: Neuropsychological deficits in neuroleptic naive patients with first-episode schizophrenia, 124 (Fe)
Schell AM see Dawson ME
Schmeidler J see Silverman JM
Schnur DB see Nobler MS
Schou M: Lithium prophylaxis in American patients with unipolar disorder (letter) 502 (Je)
Schuckit M see Gillin JC
Schulsinger F see Cannon TD
Schulte G see Maj M
Schwartz S see Skodol AE
Seibyl JP see Krystal JH
Severe JB see Nurnberger JI Jr
Shear MK, Maser JD: Standardized assessment for panic disorder research: conference report, 346 (My)
Shear MK, Pilkonis PA, Cloitre M, Leon AC: Cognitive behavioral treatment compared with nonprescriptive treatment of panic disorder, 395 (My)
Shear MK see Tollefson GD
Shenton ME see McCarley RW
Shields G see DeLisi LE
Shrout PE see Skodol AE
Shtasel D see Cannon TD
Shtasel DL see Saykin AJ
Shuwall MA see Siris SG
Siever LJ see Coccaro EF
Silverman JM, Li G, Zaccario ML, Smith CJ, Schmeidler J, Mohs RC, Davis KL: Patterns of risk in first-degree relatives of patients with Alzheimer's disease, 577 (Jy)
Silverman JM see Coccaro EF

Simpson SG see Nurnberger JI Jr
Siris SG, Bermanzohn PC, Mason SE, Shuwall MA: Maintenance imipramine therapy for secondary depression in schizophrenia: a controlled trial, 109 (Fe)
Skodol AE, Schwartz S, Dohrenwend BP, Levav I, Shrout PE: Minor depression in a cohort of young adults in Israel, 542 (Jy)
Smeraldi E see Macciardi F
Smith CJ see Silverman JM
Smith RC: Lower-dose therapy with traditional neuroleptics in chronically hospitalized schizophrenic patients (letter) 427 (My)
Smith TL see Gillin JC
Sobin C see Goldstein RB
Southwick S see Mason J
Southwick SM see Krystal JH
Springer MD, Lundberg GD: Third editor of the ARCHIVES—Jack D Barchas, MD, 173 (Mr)
St Louis M see Maj M
Stafiniak P see Saykin AJ
Starace F see Maj M
Stevens JR: Brain atrophy or dystrophy in schizophrenia: when did it happen? (letter) 927 (No)
Strassman RJ, Qualls CR: Dose-response study of N,N-dimethyltryptamine in humans: I. neuroendocrine, autonomic, and cardiovascular effects, 85 (Fe)
Strassman RJ, Qualls CR, Uhlenhuth EH, Kellner R: Dose-response study of N,N-dimethyltryptamine in humans: II. subjective effects and preliminary results of a new rating scale, 98 (Fe)
Strauss DH see Amador XF
Strauss ME see Buchanan RW
Sturm R see Wells KB
Su TP see Pickar D
Suematsu H see Berger D
Sughondhabirom B see Maj M
Sunderland T, Cohen RM, Molchan S, Lawlor BA, Mellow AM, Newhouse PA, Tariot PN, Mueller EA, Murphy DL: High-dose selegiline in treatment-resistant older depressive patients, 607 (Au)
Suomi SJ see Higley JD
Susser E, Lin SP: Schizophrenia after prenatal exposure to the Dutch Hunger Winter of 1944-1945 (letter) 333 (Ap)
Susser E, Wanderling J: Epidemiology of nonaffective acute remitting psychosis vs schizophrenia: sex and sociocultural setting, 294 (Ap)
Swedo SE see Altemus M
Swerdlow NR, Braff DL, Taaid N, Geyer MA: Assessing the validity of an animal model of deficient sensorimotor gating in schizophrenic patients, 139 (Fe)
Syvälahti E see Hietala J

T

Taaid N see Swerdlow NR
Tamminga C see Carpenter WT Jr
Tamminga CA see Conley R
Tariot PN see Sunderland T
Taub D see Higley JD
Taylor S, Rachman S: Klein's suffocation theory of panic (letter) 505 (Je)
Tokola R see Nielsen DA; Virkkunen M
Tollefson GD, Rampey AH Jr, Potvin JH, Jenike MA, Rush AJ, Dominguez RA, Koran LM, Shear MK, Goodman W, Genduso LA:
Multicenter investigation of fixed-dose fluoxetine in the treatment of obsessive-compulsive disorder, 559 (Jy); correction, 864 (No)
Torrey EF: Prevalence of schizophrenia in Ireland (letter) 513 (Jy)
Tremblay RE, Pihl RO, Vitaro F, Dobkin PL: Predicting early onset of male antisocial behavior from preschool behavior, 732 (Se)
True WR, Rice J, Heath AC: Genetic and environmental influences of twins in posttraumatic stress (letter) 838 (Oc)
Turtle M see Benes FM

U

Uhlenhuth EH see Strassman RJ

V

Van Cauter E see Linkowski P
van Megen H see Bradwejn J
Van Onderbergen A see Linkowski P
Van Putten T see Marder SR
Van Tol HHM see Macciardi F
Veith RC, Lewis N, Linares OA, Barnes RF, Raskind MA, Villacres EC, Murburg MM, Ashleigh EA, Castillo S, Peskind ER, Pascualy M, Halter JB: Sympathetic nervous system activity in major depression: basal and desipramine-induced alterations in plasma norepinephrine kinetics, 411 (My)
Ventura J see Dawson ME
Vestergaard A see Cannon TD
Vickers JM see Higley JD
Villacres EC see Veith RC
Virkkunen M, Kallio E, Rawlings R, Tokola R, Poland RE, Guidotti A, Nemeroff C, Bissette G, Kalogeras K, Karonen S-L, Linnoila M: Personality profiles and state aggressiveness in Finnish alcoholic, violent offenders, fire setters, and healthy volunteers, 28 (Ja)
Virkkunen M, Rawlings R, Tokola R, Poland RE, Guidotti A, Nemeroff C, Bissette G, Kalogeras K, Karonen S-L, Linnoila M: CSF biochemistries, glucose metabolism, and diurnal activity rhythms in alcoholic, violent offenders, fire setters, and healthy volunteers, 20 (Ja)
Virkkunen M see Nielsen DA
Vita A see DeLisi LE
Vitaro F see Tremblay RE
Volpicelli JR, Alterman AI, O'Brien CP: Naltrexone and alcohol dependence: some methodological issues (letter) 335 (Ap)
Vuorio K see Hietala J

W

Walsh D, Kendler KS: Prevalence of schizophrenia in Ireland (letter) 513 (Jy)
Wanderling J see Susser E
Wang S see Mason J
Wang ZW, Black DW, Andreasen N, Crowe RR: No evidence of a schizophrenia locus in a second pseudoautosomal region (letter) 427 (My)
Wasserman AL: All prepaid health care systems are not equal (letter) 1002 (De)
Watson SJ see Young EA
Webb E see Krystal JH
Wegelius U see Hietala J
Weiler MA: Violence in the severely mentally ill (letter) 71 (Ja)
Weinberg VM see Young EA
Weinberger DR see Gold JM; Laruelle M
Weissman EM see Pickar D
Weissman MM, Markowitz JC: Interpersonal psychotherapy: current status, 599 (Au)
Weissman MM see Goldstein RB; Wickramaratne P
Wells KB, Sturm R: All prepaid health care systems are not equal (letter) 1002 (De)
Wender PH see Kety SS
Westenberg H see Bradwejn J
Wickramaratne P, Weissman MM: Effect of diagnostic hierarchy in genetic epidemiological studies of psychiatric disorders (letter) 927 (No)
Wickramaratne PJ see Goldstein RB
Winokur G see Coryell W
Wirshing WC see Marder SR
Wirtz PW see Carroll KM
Wiseman EJ: Alcohol dependence may be the missing link between posttraumatic stress disorder and panic (letter) 429 (My)
Wittchen H-U see Kessler RC
Wittchen H-U, Zhao S, Kessler RC, Eaton WW: *DSM-III-R* generalized anxiety disorder in the National Comorbidity Survey, 355 (My)
Wohl M see Lesser IM
Wood F see Carpenter WT Jr
Woods SW see Goldstein RB
Wright S: Familial obsessive-compulsive disorder presenting as pathological jealousy successfully treated with fluoxetine (letter) 430 (My)
Wyatt RJ see Fenton WS
Wyler AR see Gold JM

Y

Yale SA see Amador XF
Yehuda R see Mason J
York-Cooler C see Nurnberger JI Jr
Young EA, Haskett RF, Grunhaus L, Pande A, Weinberg VM, Watson SJ, Akil H: Increased evening activation of the hypothalamic-pituitary-adrenal axis in depressed patients, 701 (Se)
Young SN see Benkelfat C

Z

Zaccario ML see Silverman JM
Zaudig M see Maj M
Zhao S see Kessler RC; Wittchen H-U
Zhou G see Mason J
Zimmerman M: Diagnosing personality disorders: a review of issues and research methods, 225 (Mr)
Zimmermann RC see McDougle CJ
Zisook S see Heaton R
Zorrilla LE see Cannon TD

SUBJECT INDEX TO VOLUME 51

The following index is an alphabetical list of significant subjects presented in this volume. The month is given as a two-letter notation in parentheses.

A

Abnormalities
Developmental brain abnormalities in the offspring of schizophrenic mothers: II. structural brain characteristics of schizophrenia and schizotypal personality disorder [Cannon] 955 (De)

Acquired Immunodeficiency Syndrome
WHO Neuropsychiatric AIDS Study, Cross-sectional Phase I: study design and psychiatric findings [Maj] 39 (Ja)
WHO Neuropsychiatric AIDS Study, Cross-sectional Phase II: neuropsychological and neurological findings [Maj] 51 (Ja)

Activities of Daily Living
WHO Neuropsychiatric AIDS Study, Cross-sectional Phase II: neuropsychological and neurological findings [Maj] 51 (Ja)

Adjustment Disorders
Controlled prospective study of *DSM-III* adjustment disorder in childhood: short-term prognosis and long-term predictive validity [Kovacs] 535 (Jy)
Correction and amplification (letter) [Bird] 429 (My)

Adolescence
Myelination of a key relay zone in the hippocampal formation occurs in the human brain during childhood, adolescence, and adulthood [Benes] 477 (Je)

Adolescent Behavior
Birth complications combined with early maternal rejection at age 1 year predispose to violent crime at age 18 years [Raine] 984 (De)

Adolescent Psychiatry
Controlled prospective study of *DSM-III* adjustment disorder in childhood: short-term prognosis and long-term predictive validity [Kovacs] 535 (Jy)

Adoption
Independent diagnoses of adoptees and relatives as defined by *DSM-III* in the provincial and national samples of the Danish Adoption Study of Schizophrenia [Kendler] 456 (Je)
Mental illness in the biological and adoptive relatives of schizophrenic adoptees: replication of the Copenhagen Study in the rest of Denmark [Kety] 442 (Je)

Adrenergic Alpha Receptors see Receptors, Adrenergic, Alpha

Adult
Minor depression in a cohort of young adults in Israel [Skodol] 542 (Jy)
Myelination of a key relay zone in the hippocampal formation occurs in the human brain during childhood, adolescence, and adulthood [Benes] 477 (Je)

Affect
Psychiatric and medical effects of anabolic-androgenic steroid use: a controlled study of 160 athletes [Pope] 375 (My)
Serotonin and the neurobiology of depression: effects of tryptophan depletion [Delgado] 865 (No)
Affective Disorders
Awareness of illness in schizophrenia and schizoaffective and mood disorders [Amador] 826 (Oc)
Carbamazepine increases cerebrospinal fluid thyrotropin-releasing hormone levels in affectively ill patients [Marangell] 625 (Au)
Childhood-onset dysthymic disorder: clinical features and prospective naturalistic outcome [Kovacs] 365 (My)
Diagnostic Interview for Genetic Studies: rationale, unique features, and training [Nurnberger] 849 (No)
Effects of the menstrual cycle on dependent variables in mood disorder research [Leibenluft] 761 (Oc)
Lifetime and 12-month prevalence of *DSM-III-R* psychiatric disorders in the United States: results from the National Comorbidity Survey [Kessler] 8 (Ja)
Mood-lowering effect of tryptophan depletion: enhanced susceptibility in young men at genetic risk for major affective disorders [Benkelfat] 687 (Se)
Plasma homovanillic acid levels in first-episode schizophrenia: psychopathology and treatment response [Koreen] 132 (Fe)
Regional cerebral blood flow in mood disorders, III: treatment and clinical response [Nobler] 884 (No)
Time course of nonchronic major depressive disorder: uniformity across episodes and samples [Coryell] 405 (My)
Tryptophan depletion in patients with obsessive-compulsive disorder who respond to serotonin reuptake inhibitors [Barr] 309 (Ap)
Affective Disorders, Psychotic
Autonomic abnormalities in schizophrenia: state or trait indicators? [Dawson] 813 (Oc)
Awareness of illness in schizophrenia and schizoaffective and mood disorders [Amador] 826 (Oc)
DSM-III-R generalized anxiety disorder in the National Comorbidity Survey [Wittchen] 355 (My)
Interpersonal psychotherapy: current status [Weissman] 599 (Au)
Age Factors
High-dose selegiline in treatment-resistant older depressive patients [Sunderland] 607 (Au)
Neuropsychological deficits in schizophrenics: relationship to age, chronicity, and dementia [Heaton] 469 (Je)
Age of Onset
Age of onset in familial schizophrenia (letter) [DeLisi] 334 (Ap)
Effect of diagnostic hierarchy in genetic epidemiological studies of psychiatric disorders (letter) [Roy] 926 (reply) [Wickramaratne] 927 (No)
Aged
Incidence of dementia in a population older than 75 years in the United Kingdom [Paykel] 325 (Ap)
Reduction of cerebral blood flow in older depressed patients [Lesser] 677 (Se)
Aged, 80 and Over
Incidence of dementia in a population older than 75 years in the United Kingdom [Paykel] 325 (Ap)
Aggression
Are stress hormones and serotonin related to aggression in primates? (letter) [Reus] 72 (reply) [Higley] 73 (Ja)
CSF biochemistries, glucose metabolism, and diurnal activity rhythms in alcoholic, violent offenders, fire setters, and healthy volunteers [Virkkunen] 20 (Ja)
Effects of alterations in plasma tryptophan levels on aggressive feelings (letter) [Cleare] 1004 (De)
Personality profiles and state aggressiveness in Finnish alcoholic, violent offenders, fire setters, and healthy volunteers [Virkkunen] 28 (Ja)
Psychiatric and medical effects of anabolic-androgenic steroid use: a controlled study of 160 athletes [Pope] 375 (My)
Agoraphobia
Cognitive behavioral treatment compared with nonprescriptive treatment of panic disorder [Shear] 395 (My)
Psychiatric disorders in relatives of probands with panic disorder and/or major depression [Goldstein] 383 (My)
AIDS see Acquired Immunodeficiency Syndrome
AIDS Seropositivity see HIV Seropositivity
Akathisia, Drug-Induced
Clinical characteristics and predisposing factors in acute drug-induced akathisia [Sachdev] 963 (De)
Alcohol Abuse see Alcoholism
Alcohol, Drug Abuse, and Mental Health Administration (U.S.) see United States Alcohol, Drug Abuse, and Mental Health Administration
Alcohol, Ethyl
Specificity of ethanollike effects elicited by serotonergic and noradrenergic mechanisms [Krystal] 898 (No)
Alcoholism
Alcohol dependence may be the missing link between post-traumatic stress disorder and panic (letter) [Wiseman] 429 (reply) [Krystal] 430 (My)
Buspirone treatment of anxious alcoholics: placebo-controlled trial [Kranzler] 720 (Se)
CSF biochemistries, glucose metabolism, and diurnal activity rhythms in alcoholic, violent offenders, fire setters, and healthy volunteers [Virkkunen] 20 (Ja)
Familial correlates of reduced central serotonergic system function in patients with personality disorders [Coccaro] 318 (Ap)
Increased pressure for rapid eye movement sleep at time of hospital admission predicts relapse in nondepressed patients with primary alcoholism at 3-month follow-up [Gillin] 189 (Mr)
Naltrexone and alcohol dependence: some methodological issues (letter) [Andrade] (reply) [Volpicelli] 335 (Ap)
One-year follow-up of psychotherapy and pharmacotherapy for cocaine dependence: delayed emergence of psychotherapy effects [Carroll] 989 (De)
Personality profiles and state aggressiveness in Finnish alcoholic, violent offenders, fire setters, and healthy volunteers [Virkkunen] 28 (Ja)
Specificity of ethanollike effects elicited by serotonergic and noradrenergic mechanisms [Krystal] 898 (No)
Suicidality and 5-hydroxyindoleacetic acid concentration associated with a tryptophan hydroxylase polymorphism [Nielsen] 34 (Ja)
Alleles
Allelic variation in the D_4 dopamine receptor (DRD4) gene does not predict response to clozapine [Rao] 912 (No)
Alzheimer's Disease
Patterns of risk in first-degree relatives of patients with Alzheimer's disease [Silverman] 577 (Jy)
Amenorrhea
Diagnostic Interview Schedule and anorexia nervosa in Hong Kong (letter) [Lee] 251 (Mr)
Amino Acids
Effects of alterations in plasma tryptophan levels on aggressive feelings (letter) [Cleare] 1004 (De)
Anabolic Steroids
Psychiatric and medical effects of anabolic-androgenic steroid use: a controlled study of 160 athletes [Pope] 375 (My)
Androgens
Psychiatric and medical effects of anabolic-androgenic steroid use: a controlled study of 160 athletes [Pope] 375 (My)
Anesthetics, Dissociative
Subanesthetic effects of the noncompetitive NMDA antagonist, ketamine, in humans: psychotomimetic, perceptual, cognitive, and neuroendocrine responses [Krystal] 199 (Mr)
Animals, Laboratory
Assessing the validity of an animal model of deficient sensorimotor gating in schizophrenic patients [Swerdlow] 139 (Fe)
Anorexia Nervosa
Diagnostic Interview Schedule and anorexia nervosa in Hong Kong (letter) [Lee] 251 (Mr)
Anticholinergic Agents see Parasympatholytics
Anticonvulsants
Carbamazepine increases cerebrospinal fluid thyrotropin-releasing hormone levels in affectively ill patients [Marangell] 625 (Au)
Antidepressant Drugs
All prepaid health care systems are not equal (letter) [Wasserman] (reply) [Wells] 1002 (De)
Pindolol induces a rapid improvement of depressed patients treated with serotonin reuptake inhibitors (letter) [Artigas] 248 (Mr)
Serotonin and the neurobiology of depression: effects of tryptophan depletion [Delgado] 865 (No)
24-hour profiles of cortisol, prolactin, and growth hormone secretion in mania [Linkowski] 616 (Au)
Antidepressants see Antidepressive Agents
Antidepressive Agents
Assessing the validity of an animal model of deficient sensorimotor gating in schizophrenic patients [Swerdlow] 139 (Fe)
Lithium prophylaxis in American patients with unipolar disorder (letter) [Schou] (reply) [Nobler] 502 (Je)
Mood-lowering effect of tryptophan depletion: enhanced susceptibility in young men at genetic risk for major affective disorders [Benkelfat] 687 (Se)
Time course of nonchronic major depressive disorder: uniformity across episodes and samples [Coryell] 405 (My)
Antidepressive Agents, Tricyclic
Interactions of serotonin reuptake inhibitors with tricyclic antidepressants (letter) [Popli] 666 (Au)
Antipsychotic Agents see Tranquilizing Agents, Major
Antisocial Personality Disorder
Lifetime and 12-month prevalence of *DSM-III-R* psychiatric disorders in the United States: results from the National Comorbidity Survey [Kessler] 8 (Ja)
Predicting early onset of male antisocial behavior from preschool behavior [Tremblay] 732 (Se)
Psychiatric disorders in relatives of probands with panic disorder and/or major depression [Goldstein] 383 (My)
Anxiety
Buspirone treatment of anxious alcoholics: placebo-controlled trial [Kranzler] 720 (Se)
Cognitive behavioral treatment compared with nonprescriptive treatment of panic disorder [Shear] 395 (My)
Controlled prospective study of *DSM-III* adjustment disorder in childhood: short-term prognosis and long-term predictive validity [Kovacs] 535 (Jy)
Dose-response study of N,N-dimethyltryptamine in humans: II. subjective effects and preliminary results of a new rating scale [Strassman] 98 (Fe)
Naltrexone and alcohol dependence: some methodological issues pgnum335 (reply) [Volpicelli] 335 (Ap)
Standardized assessment for panic disorder research: conference report [Shear] 346 (My)
Anxiety Disorders
Cannabis abuse and the course of recent-onset schizophrenic disorders [Linszen] 273 (Ap)
Childhood-onset dysthymic disorder: clinical features and prospective naturalistic outcome [Kovacs] 365 (My)
Correction and amplification (letter) [Bird] 429 (My)
DSM-III-R generalized anxiety disorder in the National Comorbidity Survey [Wittchen] 355 (My)
Haloperidol addition in fluvoxamine-refractory obsessive-compulsive disorder: a double-blind, placebo-controlled study in patients with and without tics [McDougle] 302 (Ap)
Hypochondriasis and panic disorder: boundary and overlap [Barsky] 918 (No)
Lifetime and 12-month prevalence of *DSM-III-R* psychiatric disorders in the United States: results from the National Comorbidity Survey [Kessler] 8 (Ja)
Mental illness in the biological and adoptive relatives of schizophrenic adoptees: replication of the Copenhagen Study in the rest of Denmark [Kety] 442 (Je)
Naltrexone and alcohol dependence: some methodological issues (letter) [Andrade] 335 (Ap)
Suicide and mortality patterns in anxiety neurosis and depressive neurosis [Allgulander] 708 (Se)
Untreated anxiety among adult primary care patients in a health maintenance organization [Fifer] 740 (Se)
Anxiety Neuroses see Anxiety Disorders
Anxiolytic Agents see Tranquilizing Agents, Minor
Apomorphine
Assessing the validity of an animal model of deficient sensorimotor gating in schizophrenic patients [Swerdlow] 139 (Fe)
Arachidonic Acid
Arachidonic acid: a common link in the biology of schizophrenia? (letter) [Peet] 665 (Au)
ARCHIVES OF GENERAL PSYCHIATRY
Reviewers for 1994, 933 (De)
Third editor of the ARCHIVES—Jack D Barchas, MD [Springer] 173 (Mr)
Arginine Vasopressin see Argipressin
Argipressin
Elevated cerebrospinal fluid levels of oxytocin in obsessive-compulsive disorder: comparison with Tourette's syndrome and healthy controls [Leckman] 782 (Oc)
Asphyxia
Klein's suffocation theory of panic (letter) [Taylor] 505 (Je)
Athletics see Sports
Atrophy
Brain atrophy or dystrophy in schizophrenia: when did it happen? (letter) [Stevens] 927 (No)
Attention
Autonomic abnormalities in schizophrenia: state or trait indicators? [Dawson] 813 (Oc)
Neuropsychological deficits in neuroleptic naive patients with first-episode schizophrenia [Saykin] 124 (Fe)
Parsing cognition: the power of psychology paradigms [Holzman] 952 (De)
Schizophrenia and temporal lobe epilepsy: a neuropsychological analysis [Gold] 265 (Ap)
Autonomic Nervous System
Autonomic abnormalities in schizophrenia: state or trait indicators? [Dawson] 813 (Oc)
Impaired autonomic nervous system habituation in those at genetic risk for schizophrenia [Hollister] 552 (Jy)

B

Barchas, Jack D
Third editor of the ARCHIVES—Jack D Barchas, MD [Springer] 173 (Mr)
Basal Ganglia
Retrocallosal white matter abnormalities in patients with obsessive-compulsive disorder (letter) [Breiter] 663 (Au)
Behavior
Incentives improve outcome in outpatient behavioral treatment of cocaine dependence [Higgins] 568 (Jy)
Behavior Therapy
Cognitive behavioral treatment compared with nonprescriptive treatment of panic disorder [Shear] 395 (My)
Behavioral Interventions
Psychoneuroimmunology and human immunodeficiency virus type 1 infection revisited (letter) [Goodkin] 246 (reply) [Perry] 247 (Mr)
Behavioral Medicine
Naturalistic follow-up of a behavioral treatment for chronically parasuicidal borderline patients [Linehan], 50:971 (De); **correction,51:422 (My)**
Regional cerebral blood flow measured during symptom provocation in obsessive-compulsive disorder using oxy-

gen 15—labeled carbon dioxide and positron emission tomography [Rauch] 62 (Ja)
Benzodiazepines
Lower-dose therapy with traditional neuroleptics in chronically hospitalized schizophrenic patients (letter) [Smith] 427 (My)
Benztropine
Maintenance imipramine therapy for secondary depression in schizophrenia: a controlled trial [Siris] 109 (Fe)
Biological Markers
Life events and the research diagnostic criteria endogenous subtype: confirmation of the distinction using the Bedford College methods [Frank] 519 (Jy)
Biological Psychiatry
Assessing the validity of an animal model of deficient sensorimotor gating in schizophrenic patients [Swerdlow] 139 (Fe)
Bipolar Disorder
Childhood-onset dysthymic disorder: clinical features and prospective naturalistic outcome [Kovacs] 365 (My)
Diagnostic Interview for Genetic Studies: rationale, unique features, and training [Nurnberger] 849 (No)
High-dose selegiline in treatment-resistant older depressive patients [Sunderland] 607 (Au)
Mental illness in the biological and adoptive relatives of schizophrenic adoptees: replication of the Copenhagen Study in the rest of Denmark [Kety] 442 (Je)
Blood Chemical Analysis
Effects of alterations in plasma tryptophan levels on aggressive feelings (letter) [Cleare] 1004 (De)
Blood Glucose
Regional cerebral blood flow in mood disorders, III: treatment and clinical response [Nobler] 884 (No)
Bonding (Psychology) see Object Attachment
Brain
Brain atrophy or dystrophy in schizophrenia: when did it happen? (letter) [Stevens] 927 (No)
Developmental brain abnormalities in the offspring of schizophrenic mothers: II. structural brain characteristics of schizophrenia and schizotypal personality disorder [Cannon] 955 (De)
Increased density of guanine nucleotide-binding proteins in the postmortem brains of heroin addicts [Escriba] 494 (Je)
Myelination of a key relay zone in the hippocampal formation occurs in the human brain during childhood, adolescence, and adulthood [Benes] 477 (Je)
Buspirone
Buspirone treatment of anxious alcoholics: placebo-controlled trial [Kranzler] 720 (Se)

C

Cannabis
Specificity of ethanollike effects elicited by serotonergic and noradrenergic mechanisms [Krystal] 898 (No)
Carbamazepine
Carbamazepine increases cerebrospinal fluid thyrotropin-releasing hormone levels in affectively ill patients [Marangell] 625 (Au)
Catecholamines
Mania induced by citalopram (letter) [Bryois] 664 (Au)
Sympathetic nervous system activity in major depression: basal and desipramine-induced alterations in plasma norepinephrine kinetics [Veith] 411 (My)
CCK-4 see Tetragastrin
Cerebral Cortex
Developmental brain abnormalities in the offspring of schizophrenic mothers: II. structural brain characteristics of schizophrenia and schizotypal personality disorder [Cannon] 955 (De)
Regional cerebral blood flow in mood disorders, III: treatment and clinical response [Nobler] 884 (No)
Cerebral Ischemia
Reduction of cerebral blood flow in older depressed patients [Lesser] 677 (Se)
Cerebral Ventricles
Developmental brain abnormalities in the offspring of schizophrenic mothers: II. structural brain characteristics of schizophrenia and schizotypal personality disorder [Cannon] 955 (De)
Cerebrospinal Fluid
Are stress hormones and serotonin related to aggression in primates? (letter) [Reus] 72 (reply) [Higley] 73 (Ja)
Carbamazepine increases cerebrospinal fluid thyrotropin-releasing hormone levels in affectively ill patients [Marangell] 625 (Au)
Changes in cerebrospinal fluid neurochemistry during treatment of obsessive-compulsive disorder with clomipramine [Altemus] 794 (Oc)
CSF biochemistries, glucose metabolism, and diurnal activity rhythms in alcoholic, violent offenders, fire setters, and healthy volunteers [Virkkunen] 20 (Ja)
Elevated cerebrospinal fluid levels of oxytocin in obsessive-compulsive disorder: comparison with Tourette's syndrome and healthy controls [Leckman] 782 (Oc)
Personality profiles and state aggressiveness in Finnish alcoholic, violent offenders, fire setters, and healthy volunteers [Virkkunen] 28 (Ja)
Suicidality and 5-hydroxyindoleacetic acid concentration associated with a tryptophan hydroxylase polymorphism [Nielsen] 34 (Ja)
Cerebrum see Brain
Child Behavior Disorders
Boundary of social phobia: exploring the threshold [Davidson] 975 (De)
Controlled prospective study of *DSM-III* adjustment disorder in childhood: short-term prognosis and long-term predictive validity [Kovacs] 535 (Jy)
Predicting early onset of male antisocial behavior from preschool behavior [Tremblay] 732 (Se)
Child Custody
Relation of parenthood to suicide (letter) [Clark] 160 (reply) [Høyer] 160 (Fe)
Child, Preschool
Predicting early onset of male antisocial behavior from preschool behavior [Tremblay] 732 (Se)
Child Psychiatry
Some issues for the new director of NIMH [Barchas] 998 (De)
Childhood
Myelination of a key relay zone in the hippocampal formation occurs in the human brain during childhood, adolescence, and adulthood [Benes] 477 (Je)
Chlorophenylpiperazine Hydrochloride
Specificity of ethanollike effects elicited by serotonergic and noradrenergic mechanisms [Krystal] 898 (No)
Cholecystokinin
Panicogenic effects of cholecystokinin-tetrapeptide are antagonized by L-365,260, a central cholecystokinin receptor antagonist, in patients with panic disorder [Bradwejn] 486 (Je)
Cholecystokinin-Tetrapeptide see Tetragastrin
Circadian Rhythm
CSF biochemistries, glucose metabolism, and diurnal activity rhythms in alcoholic, violent offenders, fire setters, and healthy volunteers [Virkkunen] 20 (Ja)
Citalopram
Mania induced by citalopram (letter) [Bryois] 664 (Au)
Classification
Diagnosing personality disorders: a review of issues and research methods [Zimmerman] 225 (Mr)
Clinical Trials
Multicenter investigation of fixed-dose fluoxetine in the treatment of obsessive-compulsive disorder [Tollefson] 559 (Jy); correction, 864 (No)
Clomipramine
Changes in cerebrospinal fluid neurochemistry during treatment of obsessive-compulsive disorder with clomipramine [Altemus] 794 (Oc)
Clozapine
Allelic variation in the D_4 dopamine receptor (DRD4) gene does not predict response to clozapine [Rao] 912 (No)
Assessing the validity of an animal model of deficient sensorimotor gating in schizophrenic patients [Swerdlow] 139 (Fe)
Clinical response to clozapine in patients with schizophrenia (letter) [Pickar] 159 (Fe)
Cocaine
Incentives improve outcome in outpatient behavioral treatment of cocaine dependence [Higgins] 568 (Jy)
Noradrenergic dysregulation during discontinuation of cocaine use in addicts [McDougle] 713 (Se)
One-year follow-up of psychotherapy and pharmacotherapy for cocaine dependence: delayed emergence of psychotherapy effects [Carroll] 989 (De)
Psychotherapy and pharmacotherapy for ambulatory cocaine abusers [Carroll] 177 (Mr)
Specificity of ethanollike effects elicited by serotonergic and noradrenergic mechanisms [Krystal] 898 (No)
Cognition
Parsing cognition: the power of psychology paradigms [Holzman] 952 (De)
Cognition Disorders
Neuropsychological deficits in schizophrenics: relationship to age, chronicity, and dementia [Heaton] 469 (Je)
Schizophrenia and temporal lobe epilepsy: a neuropsychological analysis [Gold] 265 (Ap)
Cognitive Therapy
Klein's suffocation theory of panic (letter) [Taylor] 505 (reply) [Klein] 506 (Je)
Naturalistic follow-up of a behavioral treatment for chronically parasuicidal borderline patients [Linehan], 50:971 (De); correction,51:422 (My)
Comorbidity
Controlled prospective study of *DSM-III* adjustment disorder in childhood: short-term prognosis and long-term predictive validity [Kovacs] 535 (Jy)
Hypochondriasis and panic disorder: boundary and overlap [Barsky] 918 (No)
Lifetime and 12-month prevalence of *DSM-III-R* psychiatric disorders in the United States: results from the National Comorbidity Survey [Kessler] 8 (Ja)
Compulsive Personality Disorder
Regional cerebral blood flow measured during symptom provocation in obsessive-compulsive disorder using oxygen 15—labeled carbon dioxide and positron emission tomography [Rauch] 62 (Ja)
Conduct Disorders, Child see Child Behavior Disorders
Corpus Callosum
Retrocallosal white matter abnormalities in patients with obsessive-compulsive disorder (letter) [Breiter] 663 (Au)
Corpus Luteum
Effects of the menstrual cycle on dependent variables in mood disorder research [Leibenluft] 761 (Oc)
CORRECTIONS
Correction and amplification (letter) [Bird] 429 (My)
Multicenter investigation of fixed-dose fluoxetine in the treatment of obsessive-compulsive disorder, 559 (Jy); correction, 864 [Tollefson] 864 (No)
Naturalistic follow-up of a behavioral treatment for chronically parasuicidal borderline patients [Linehan], 50:971 (De); correction,51:422 (My)
Corticotropin-Releasing Hormone
Increased evening activation of the hypothalamic-pituitary-adrenal axis in depressed patients [Young] 701 (Se)
Cortisol see Hydrocortisone
Crime
Birth complications combined with early maternal rejection at age 1 year predispose to violent crime at age 18 years [Raine] 984 (De)
Violence in the severely mentally ill (letter) [Weiler] (reply) [Hodgins] 71 (Ja)
Custody, Child see Child Custody

D

Data Collection
Correction and amplification (letter) [Bird] 429 (My)
Diagnostic Interview for Genetic Studies: rationale, unique features, and training [Nurnberger] 849 (No)
Data Interpretation, Statistical
Effect of diagnostic hierarchy in genetic epidemiological studies of psychiatric disorders (letter) [Roy] 926 (reply) [Wickramaratne] 927 (No)
Delivery
Birth complications combined with early maternal rejection at age 1 year predispose to violent crime at age 18 years [Raine] 984 (De)
Developmental brain abnormalities in the offspring of schizophrenic mothers: II. structural brain characteristics of schizophrenia and schizotypal personality disorder [Cannon] 955 (De)
delta(9)-THC see Tetrahydrocannabinol
Delusions
Neural circuits in schizophrenia (letter) [McCarley] 515 (reply) [Carpenter] 516 (Jy)
Dementia
Incidence of dementia in a population older than 75 years in the United Kingdom [Paykel] 325 (Ap)
Neuropsychological deficits in schizophrenics: relationship to age, chronicity, and dementia [Heaton] 469 (Je)
Patterns of risk in first-degree relatives of patients with Alzheimer's disease [Silverman] 577 (Jy)
Denmark
Independent diagnoses of adoptees and relatives as defined by *DSM-III* in the provincial and national samples of the Danish Adoption Study of Schizophrenia [Kendler] 456 (Je)
Mental illness in the biological and adoptive relatives of schizophrenic adoptees: replication of the Copenhagen Study in the rest of Denmark [Kety] 442 (Je)
Depression
DSM-III-R generalized anxiety disorder in the National Comorbidity Survey [Wittchen] 355 (My)
Depression, Bipolar see Bipolar Disorder
Depression, Endogenous see Depressive Disorder
Depressive Disorder
All prepaid health care systems are not equal (letter) [Wasserman] (reply) [Wells] 1002 (De)
Childhood-onset dysthymic disorder: clinical features and prospective naturalistic outcome [Kovacs] 365 (My)
Controlled prospective study of *DSM-III* adjustment disorder in childhood: short-term prognosis and long-term predictive validity [Kovacs] 535 (Jy)
Diagnostic Interview for Genetic Studies: rationale, unique features, and training [Nurnberger] 849 (No)
Dose-response studies with protirelin [Garbutt] 875 (No)
Effect of diagnostic hierarchy in genetic epidemiological studies of psychiatric disorders (letter) [Roy] 926 (reply) [Wickramaratne] 927 (No)
Haloperidol addition in fluvoxamine-refractory obsessive-compulsive disorder: a double-blind, placebo-controlled study in patients with and without tics [McDougle] 302 (Ap)
High-dose selegiline in treatment-resistant older depressive patients [Sunderland] 607 (Au)
Hypochondriasis and panic disorder: boundary and overlap [Barsky] 918 (No)
Increased evening activation of the hypothalamic-pituitary-adrenal axis in depressed patients [Young] 701 (Se)
Interpersonal psychotherapy: current status [Weissman] 599 (Au)
Life events and endogenous depression: puzzle reexamined [Brown] 525 (Jy)
Life events and the research diagnostic criteria endogenous subtype: confirmation of the distinction using the Bedford College methods [Frank] 519 (Jy)

Lifetime and 12-month prevalence of *DSM-III-R* psychiatric disorders in the United States: results from the National Comorbidity Survey [Kessler] 8 (Ja)
Lithium prophylaxis in American patients with unipolar disorder (letter) [Schou] (reply) [Nobler] 502 (Je)
Maintenance imipramine therapy for secondary depression in schizophrenia: a controlled trial [Siris] 109 (Fe)
Maintenance therapy in depression (letter) [Barnes] 503 (reply) [Frank] 504 (Je)
Mania induced by citalopram (letter) [Bryois] 664 (Au)
Mental illness in the biological and adoptive relatives of schizophrenic adoptees: replication of the Copenhagen Study in the rest of Denmark [Kety] 442 (Je)
Minor depression in a cohort of young adults in Israel [Skodol] 542 (Jy)
Mood-lowering effect of tryptophan depletion: enhanced susceptibility in young men at genetic risk for major affective disorders [Benkelfat] 687 (Se)
Pindolol induces a rapid improvement of depressed patients treated with serotonin reuptake inhibitors (letter) [Artigas] 248 (Mr)
Psychiatric disorders in relatives of probands with panic disorder and/or major depression [Goldstein] 383 (My)
Reduction of cerebral blood flow in older depressed patients [Lesser] 677 (Se)
Regional cerebral blood flow in mood disorders, III: treatment and clinical response [Nobler] 884 (No)
Serotonin and the neurobiology of depression: effects of tryptophan depletion [Delgado] 865 (No)
Suicide and mortality patterns in anxiety neurosis and depressive neurosis [Allgulander] 708 (Se)
Sympathetic nervous system activity in major depression: basal and desipramine-induced alterations in plasma norepinephrine kinetics [Veith] 411 (My)
Time course of nonchronic major depressive disorder: uniformity across episodes and samples [Coryell] 405 (My)
Tryptophan depletion in patients with obsessive-compulsive disorder who respond to serotonin reuptake inhibitors [Barr] 309 (Ap)
Untreated anxiety among adult primary care patients in a health maintenance organization [Fifer] 740 (Se)
WHO Neuropsychiatric AIDS Study, Cross-sectional Phase I: study design and psychiatric findings [Maj] 39 (Ja)

Desipramine
Interactions of serotonin reuptake inhibitors with tricyclic antidepressants (letter) [Popli] 666 (Au)
One-year follow-up of psychotherapy and pharmacotherapy for cocaine dependence: delayed emergence of psychotherapy effects [Carroll] 989 (De)
Psychotherapy and pharmacotherapy for ambulatory cocaine abusers [Carroll] 177 (Mr)
Sympathetic nervous system activity in major depression: basal and desipramine-induced alterations in plasma norepinephrine kinetics [Veith] 411 (My)

Dexamethasone
Increased evening activation of the hypothalamic-pituitary-adrenal axis in depressed patients [Young] 701 (Se)

Diagnosis
Clinical characteristics and predisposing factors in acute drug-induced akathisia [Sachdev] 963 (De)
Correction and amplification (letter) [Bird] 429 (My)
Effect of diagnostic hierarchy in genetic epidemiological studies of psychiatric disorders (letter) [Roy] 926 (reply) [Wickramaratne] 927 (No)
International Personality Disorder Examination: The World Health Organization/Alcohol, Drug Abuse, and Mental Health Administration International Pilot Study of Personality Disorders [Loranger] 215 (Mr)

Diagnostic Interview for Genetic Studies
Diagnostic Interview for Genetic Studies [Frances] 863 (No)
Diagnostic Interview for Genetic Studies: rationale, unique features, and training [Nurnberger] 849 (No)

Diet Therapy
Tryptophan depletion in patients with obsessive-compulsive disorder who respond to serotonin reuptake inhibitors [Barr] 309 (Ap)

N,N-Dimethyltryptamine
Dose-response study of N,N-dimethyltryptamine in humans: I. neuroendocrine, autonomic, and cardiovascular effects [Strassman] 85 (Fe)
Dose-response study of N,N-dimethyltryptamine in humans: II. subjective effects and preliminary results of a new rating scale [Strassman] 98 (Fe)

Disabled
Hypochondriasis and panic disorder: boundary and overlap [Barsky] 918 (No)

Dissociation see Dissociative Disorders

Dissociative Disorders
Dose-response study of N,N-dimethyltryptamine in humans: II. subjective effects and preliminary results of a new rating scale [Strassman] 98 (Fe)
Subanesthetic effects of the noncompetitive NMDA antagonist, ketamine, in humans: psychotomimetic, perceptual, cognitive, and neuroendocrine responses [Krystal] 199 (Mr)

Diurnal Rhythm see Circadian Rhythm

Dopamine
Plasma homovanillic acid levels in first-episode schizophrenia: psychopathology and treatment response [Koreen] 132 (Fe)

Dopamine Agonists see Dopaminergic Agents

Dopamine D2 Receptors see Receptors, Dopamine D2

Dopamine Receptors see Receptors, Dopamine

Dopaminergic Agents
Assessing the validity of an animal model of deficient sensorimotor gating in schizophrenic patients [Swerdlow] 139 (Fe)

Dose-Response Relationship, Drug
Dose-response studies with protirelin [Garbutt] 875 (No)
Dose-response study of N,N-dimethyltryptamine in humans: II. subjective effects and preliminary results of a new rating scale [Strassman] 98 (Fe)

Drug Abuse see Substance Abuse

Drug Addiction see Substance Dependence

Drug Dependence see Substance Dependence

Drug Therapy
All prepaid health care systems are not equal (letter) [Wasserman] (reply) [Wells] 1002 (De)
Incentives improve outcome in outpatient behavioral treatment of cocaine dependence [Higgins] 568 (Jy)
One-year follow-up of psychotherapy and pharmacotherapy for cocaine dependence: delayed emergence of psychotherapy effects [Carroll] 989 (De)
Psychotherapy and pharmacotherapy for ambulatory cocaine abusers [Carroll] 177 (Mr)

Drug Treatment Centers
Increased pressure for rapid eye movement sleep at time of hospital admission predicts relapse in nondepressed patients with primary alcoholism at 3-month follow-up [Gillin] 189 (Mr)

DSM-III-R
DSM-III-R generalized anxiety disorder in the National Comorbidity Survey [Wittchen] 355 (My)
Prevalence of schizophrenia in Ireland (letter) [Torrey] (reply) [Walsh] 513 (Jy)
Standardized assessment for panic disorder research: conference report [Shear] 346 (My)

Dyskinesia see Movement Disorders

Dysthymic Disorder see Depressive Disorder

E

Eating Disorders
Diagnostic Interview Schedule and anorexia nervosa in Hong Kong (letter) [Lee] 251 (Mr)

Electroconvulsive Therapy
Lithium prophylaxis in American patients with unipolar disorder (letter) [Schou] (reply) [Nobler] 502 (Je)
Regional cerebral blood flow in mood disorders, III: treatment and clinical response [Nobler] 884 (No)

Environment
Genetic and environmental influences of twins in posttraumatic stress (letter) [Lurie] (reply) [True] 838 (Oc)

Epidemiologic Methods
Correction and amplification (letter) [Bird] 429 (My)

Epidemiology
Effect of diagnostic hierarchy in genetic epidemiological studies of psychiatric disorders (letter) [Roy] 926 (reply) [Wickramaratne] 927 (No)
Epidemiology of nonaffective acute remitting psychosis vs schizophrenia: sex and sociocultural setting [Susser] 294 (Ap)

Epilepsy, Temporal Lobe
Schizophrenia and temporal lobe epilepsy: a neuropsychological analysis [Gold] 265 (Ap)

Estrogens
Effects of the menstrual cycle on dependent variables in mood disorder research [Leibenluft] 761 (Oc)

Ethanol see Alcohol, Ethyl

Euphoria
Dose-response study of N,N-dimethyltryptamine in humans: II. subjective effects and preliminary results of a new rating scale [Strassman] 98 (Fe)

F

Family
Patterns of risk in first-degree relatives of patients with Alzheimer's disease [Silverman] 577 (Jy)

Fee for Service, Medical see Fees, Medical

Fees, Medical
All prepaid health care systems are not equal (letter) [Wasserman] (reply) [Wells] 1002 (De)

Fenfluramine
Familial correlates of reduced central serotonergic system function in patients with personality disorders [Coccaro] 318 (Ap)

Finland
Personality profiles and state aggressiveness in Finnish alcoholic, violent offenders, fire setters, and healthy volunteers [Virkkunen] 28 (Ja)

Firesetting Behavior
CSF biochemistries, glucose metabolism, and diurnal activity rhythms in alcoholic, violent offenders, fire setters, and healthy volunteers [Virkkunen] 20 (Ja)
Personality profiles and state aggressiveness in Finnish alcoholic, violent offenders, fire setters, and healthy volunteers [Virkkunen] 28 (Ja)

5-HT2 Receptors see Receptors, Serotonin

Fluorescent in Situ Hybridization see In Situ Hybridization, Fluorescence

Fluoxetine
Cingulotomy in a case of concomitant obsessive-compulsive disorder and Tourette's syndrome (letter) [Baer] 73 (Ja)
Familial obsessive-compulsive disorder presenting as pathological jealousy successfully treated with fluoxetine (letter) [Wright] 430 (My)
Multicenter investigation of fixed-dose fluoxetine in the treatment of obsessive-compulsive disorder [Tollefson] 559 (Jy); correction, 864 (No)

Fluphenazine
Fluphenazine vs placebo supplementation for prodromal signs of relapse in schizophrenia [Marder] 280 (Ap)
Maintenance imipramine therapy for secondary depression in schizophrenia: a controlled trial [Siris] 109 (Fe)

Fluvoxamine
Haloperidol addition in fluvoxamine-refractory obsessive-compulsive disorder: a double-blind, placebo-controlled study in patients with and without tics [McDougle] 302 (Ap)

Follow-Up Studies
Increased pressure for rapid eye movement sleep at time of hospital admission predicts relapse in nondepressed patients with primary alcoholism at 3-month follow-up [Gillin] 189 (Mr)

Freedman, Mary Catherine Neidigh (1921-1994)
Mary Catherine Neidigh Freedman (August 2, 1921 - October 21, 1994) 1005 (De)

Frontal Lobe
Cingulotomy in a case of concomitant obsessive-compulsive disorder and Tourette's syndrome (letter) [Baer] 73 (Ja)
Neuropsychological impairments in deficit vs nondeficit forms of schizophrenia [Buchanan] 804 (Oc)

Fumarates
Dose-response study of N,N-dimethyltryptamine in humans: I. neuroendocrine, autonomic, and cardiovascular effects [Strassman] 85 (Fe)

G

Gender see Sex

Genes
Allelic variation in the D_4 dopamine receptor (DRD4) gene does not predict response to clozapine [Rao] 912 (No)

Genetics
Genetic and environmental influences of twins in posttraumatic stress (letter) [Lurie] (reply) [True] 838 (Oc)
Impaired autonomic nervous system habituation in those at genetic risk for schizophrenia [Hollister] 552 (Jy)
Mental illness in the biological and adoptive relatives of schizophrenic adoptees: replication of the Copenhagen Study in the rest of Denmark [Kety] 442 (Je)
Mood-lowering effect of tryptophan depletion: enhanced susceptibility in young men at genetic risk for major affective disorders [Benkelfat] 687 (Se)
Neuropsychological functioning in siblings discordant for schizophrenia and healthy volunteers [Cannon] 651 (Au)
Patterns of risk in first-degree relatives of patients with Alzheimer's disease [Silverman] 577 (Jy)
Prevalence of schizophrenia in Ireland (letter) [Torrey] (reply) [Walsh] 513 (Jy)

Genetics, Medical
Developmental brain abnormalities in the offspring of schizophrenic mothers: II. structural brain characteristics of schizophrenia and schizotypal personality disorder [Cannon] 955 (De)
Diagnostic Interview for Genetic Studies [Frances] 863 (No)
Diagnostic Interview for Genetic Studies: rationale, unique features, and training [Nurnberger] 849 (No)
Effect of diagnostic hierarchy in genetic epidemiological studies of psychiatric disorders (letter) [Roy] 926 (reply) [Wickramaratne] 927 (No)
Independent diagnoses of adoptees and relatives as defined by *DSM-III* in the provincial and national samples of the Danish Adoption Study of Schizophrenia [Kendler] 456 (Je)

Glucose Tolerance Test
CSF biochemistries, glucose metabolism, and diurnal activity rhythms in alcoholic, violent offenders, fire setters, and healthy volunteers [Virkkunen] 20 (Ja)
Personality profiles and state aggressiveness in Finnish alcoholic, violent offenders, fire setters, and healthy volunteers [Virkkunen] 28 (Ja)

Glutamates
Arachidonic acid: a common link in the biology of schizophrenia? (letter) [Peet] 665 (Au)

Gonadal Dysgenesis
Neuropsychological functioning in siblings discordant for schizophrenia and healthy volunteers [Cannon] 651 (Au)

Great Britain
Incidence of dementia in a population older than 75 years in the United Kingdom [Paykel] 325 (Ap)

Growth Hormone-Releasing Hormone see Somatotropin-Releasing Hormone

Guanine Nucleotides
Increased density of guanine nucleotide-binding proteins in the postmortem brains of heroin addicts [Escriba] 494 (Je)

H

Habituation (Psychophysiology)
Impaired autonomic nervous system habituation in those at genetic risk for schizophrenia [Hollister] 552 (Jy)
Hall, Zach
Some issues for the new director of NIMH [Barchas] 998 (De)
Hallucinations
Neural circuits in schizophrenia (letter) [McCarley] 515 (reply) [Carpenter] 516 (Jy)
Hallucinogens
Dose-response study of N,N-dimethyltryptamine in humans: I. neuroendocrine, autonomic, and cardiovascular effects [Strassman] 85 (Fe)
Dose-response study of N,N-dimethyltryptamine in humans: II. subjective effects and preliminary results of a new rating scale [Strassman] 98 (Fe)
Haloperidol
Assessing the validity of an animal model of deficient sensorimotor gating in schizophrenic patients [Swerdlow] 139 (Fe)
Haloperidol addition in fluvoxamine-refractory obsessive-compulsive disorder: a double-blind, placebo-controlled study in patients with and without tics [McDougle] 302 (Ap)
Health Maintenance Organizations
Untreated anxiety among adult primary care patients in a health maintenance organization [Fifer] 740 (Se)
Hereditary Diseases
Age of onset in familial schizophrenia (letter) [DeLisi] 334 (Ap)
Independent diagnoses of adoptees and relatives as defined by *DSM-III* in the provincial and national samples of the Danish Adoption Study of Schizophrenia [Kendler] 456 (Je)
Heroin Dependence
Increased density of guanine nucleotide-binding proteins in the postmortem brains of heroin addicts [Escriba] 494 (Je)
Heterosexuality see Sex Behavior
Hippocampus
Myelination of a key relay zone in the hippocampal formation occurs in the human brain during childhood, adolescence, and adulthood [Benes] 477 (Je)
Histrionic Personality Disorder
Predicting early onset of male antisocial behavior from preschool behavior [Tremblay] 732 (Se)
HIV
WHO Neuropsychiatric AIDS Study, Cross-sectional Phase I: study design and psychiatric findings [Maj] 39 (Ja)
WHO Neuropsychiatric AIDS Study, Cross-sectional Phase II: neuropsychological and neurological findings [Maj] 51 (Ja)
HIV Seropositivity
WHO Neuropsychiatric AIDS Study, Cross-sectional Phase I: study design and psychiatric findings [Maj] 39 (Ja)
HIV-1
Psychoneuroimmunology and human immunodeficiency virus type 1 infection revisited (letter) [Goodkin] 246 (reply) [Perry] 247 (Mr)
WHO Neuropsychiatric AIDS Study, Cross-sectional Phase I: study design and psychiatric findings [Maj] 39 (Ja)
WHO Neuropsychiatric AIDS Study, Cross-sectional Phase II: neuropsychological and neurological findings [Maj] 51 (Ja)
Homosexuality
Biologic theories of sexual orientation (letter) [McConaghy] 431 (reply) [Byne] 432 (My)
Theories of sexual orientation: a reappraisal (letter) [Berger] (reply) [Byne] 432 (My)
Homovanillic Acid
Plasma homovanillic acid levels in first-episode schizophrenia: psychopathology and treatment response [Koreen] 132 (Fe)
Hong Kong
Diagnostic Interview Schedule and anorexia nervosa in Hong Kong (letter) [Lee] 251 (Mr)
Hormones
24-hour profiles of cortisol, prolactin, and growth hormone secretion in mania [Linkowski] 616 (Au)
5-HT see Serotonin
Human Immunodeficiency Virus Type 1 see HIV-1
Human Immunodeficiency Viruses see HIV
Hunger
Schizophrenia after prenatal exposure to the Dutch Hunger Winter of 1944-1945 (letter) [Jones] (reply) [Susser] 333 (Ap)
Hydrocortisone
Are stress hormones and serotonin related to aggression in primates? (letter) [Reus] 72 (reply) [Higley] 73 (Ja)
24-hour profiles of cortisol, prolactin, and growth hormone secretion in mania [Linkowski] 616 (Au)
Hydroxyindoleacetic Acid
Are stress hormones and serotonin related to aggression in primates? (letter) [Reus] 72 (reply) [Higley] 73 (Ja)
CSF biochemistries, glucose metabolism, and diurnal activity rhythms in alcoholic, violent offenders, fire setters, and healthy volunteers [Virkkunen] 20 (Ja)
Personality profiles and state aggressiveness in Finnish alcoholic, violent offenders, fire setters, and healthy volunteers [Virkkunen] 28 (Ja)
Suicidality and 5-hydroxyindoleacetic acid concentration associated with a tryptophan hydroxylase polymorphism [Nielsen] 34 (Ja)
Hyperthyroidism
Elevation of serum free triiodothyronine, total triiodothyronine, thyroxine-binding globulin, and total thyroxine levels in combat-related posttraumatic stress disorder [Mason] 629 (Au)
Hypochondriasis
Hypochondriasis and panic disorder: boundary and overlap [Barsky] 918 (No)
Hypothalamo-Hypophyseal System
Increased evening activation of the hypothalamic-pituitary-adrenal axis in depressed patients [Young] 701 (Se)

I

Imipramine
Maintenance imipramine therapy for secondary depression in schizophrenia: a controlled trial [Siris] 109 (Fe)
Maintenance therapy in depression (letter) [Barnes] 503 (reply) [Frank] 504 (Je)
Impulsive Behavior
CSF biochemistries, glucose metabolism, and diurnal activity rhythms in alcoholic, violent offenders, fire setters, and healthy volunteers [Virkkunen] 20 (Ja)
Personality profiles and state aggressiveness in Finnish alcoholic, violent offenders, fire setters, and healthy volunteers [Virkkunen] 28 (Ja)
Suicidality and 5-hydroxyindoleacetic acid concentration associated with a tryptophan hydroxylase polymorphism [Nielsen] 34 (Ja)
In Situ Hybridization, Fluorescence
Analysis of the D_4 dopamine receptor gene variant in an Italian schizophrenia kindred [Macciardi] 288 (Ap)
Incidence
Incidence of dementia in a population older than 75 years in the United Kingdom [Paykel] 325 (Ap)
Information Processing, Human see Mental Processes
Injections, Intravenous
Dose-response study of N,N-dimethyltryptamine in humans: II. subjective effects and preliminary results of a new rating scale [Strassman] 98 (Fe)
Insurance Benefits
All prepaid health care systems are not equal (letter) [Wasserman] (reply) [Wells] 1002 (De)
Interview, Psychological
Diagnostic Interview for Genetic Studies [Frances] 863 (No)
Diagnostic Interview for Genetic Studies: rationale, unique features, and training [Nurnberger] 849 (No)
International Personality Disorder Examination: The World Health Organization/Alcohol, Drug Abuse, and Mental Health Administration International Pilot Study of Personality Disorders [Loranger] 215 (Mr)
Interviews
Diagnosing personality disorders: a review of issues and research methods [Zimmerman] 225 (Mr)
Lifetime and 12-month prevalence of *DSM-III-R* psychiatric disorders in the United States: results from the National Comorbidity Survey [Kessler] 8 (Ja)
Ireland
Prevalence of schizophrenia in Ireland (letter) [Torrey] (reply) [Walsh] 513 (Jy)
Irritable Mood
Psychiatric and medical effects of anabolic-androgenic steroid use: a controlled study of 160 athletes [Pope] 375 (My)
Israel
Minor depression in a cohort of young adults in Israel [Skodol] 542 (Jy)

J

Jealousy
Familial obsessive-compulsive disorder presenting as pathological jealousy successfully treated with fluoxetine (letter) [Wright] 430 (My)
Juvenile Delinquency
Predicting early onset of male antisocial behavior from preschool behavior [Tremblay] 732 (Se)

K

Ketamine
Subanesthetic effects of the noncompetitive NMDA antagonist, ketamine, in humans: psychotomimetic, perceptual, cognitive, and neuroendocrine responses [Krystal] 199 (Mr)
Kinetics
Sympathetic nervous system activity in major depression: basal and desipramine-induced alterations in plasma norepinephrine kinetics [Veith] 411 (My)

L

Language
Neuropsychological deficits in neuroleptic naive patients with first-episode schizophrenia [Saykin] 124 (Fe)
Schizophrenia and temporal lobe epilepsy: a neuropsychological analysis [Gold] 265 (Ap)
Leshner, Alan
Some issues for the new director of NIMH [Barchas] 998 (De)
Life Change Events
Boundary of social phobia: exploring the threshold [Davidson] 975 (De)
Life events and endogenous depression: puzzle reexamined [Brown] 525 (Jy)
Linkage (Genetics)
Analysis of the D_4 dopamine receptor gene variant in an Italian schizophrenia kindred [Macciardi] 288 (Ap)
Familial correlates of reduced central serotonergic system function in patients with personality disorders [Coccaro] 318 (Ap)
No evidence of a schizophrenia locus in a second pseudo-autosomal region (letter) [Wang] 427 (My)
Lithium
Lithium prophylaxis in American patients with unipolar disorder (letter) [Schou] (reply) [Nobler] 502 (Je)
Luteal Phase
Effects of the menstrual cycle on dependent variables in mood disorder research [Leibenluft] 761 (Oc)
Lysergic Acid Diethylamide
Dose-response study of N,N-dimethyltryptamine in humans: I. neuroendocrine, autonomic, and cardiovascular effects [Strassman] 85 (Fe)

M

Magnetic Resonance Imaging
Brain atrophy or dystrophy in schizophrenia: when did it happen? (letter) [Stevens] 927 (No)
Neural circuits in schizophrenia (letter) [McCarley] 515 (reply) [Carpenter] 516 (Jy)
Regional cerebral blood flow measured during symptom provocation in obsessive-compulsive disorder using oxygen 15—labeled carbon dioxide and positron emission tomography [Rauch] 62 (Ja)
Mania see Manic Disorder
Manic Disorder
Backward masking in schizophrenia and mania: I. specifying a mechanism [Green] 939 (De)
Backward masking in schizophrenia and mania: II. specifying the visual channels [Green] 945 (De)
Mania induced by citalopram (letter) [Bryois] 664 (Au)
Regional cerebral blood flow in mood disorders, III: treatment and clinical response [Nobler] 884 (No)
24-hour profiles of cortisol, prolactin, and growth hormone secretion in mania [Linkowski] 616 (Au)
Marijuana Abuse
Cannabis abuse and the course of recent-onset schizophrenic disorders [Linszen] 273 (Ap)
Marijuana see Cannabis
m-Chlorophenylpiperazine Hydrochloride
Specificity of ethanollike effects elicited by serotonergic and noradrenergic mechanisms [Krystal] 898 (No)
Medical Record Linkage
Suicide and mortality patterns in anxiety neurosis and depressive neurosis [Allgulander] 708 (Se)
Melancholia see Depressive Disorder
Memory
Neural circuits in schizophrenia (letter) [McCarley] 515 (reply) [Carpenter] 516 (Jy)
Memory Disorders
Neuropsychological deficits in schizophrenics: relationship to age, chronicity, and dementia [Heaton] 469 (Je)
Menstrual Cycle, Luteal Phase see Luteal Phase
Mental Disorders
Awareness of illness in schizophrenia and schizoaffective and mood disorders [Amador] 826 (Oc)
Diagnostic Interview for Genetic Studies [Frances] 863 (No)
Violence in the severely mentally ill (letter) [Weiler] (reply) [Hodgins] 71 (Ja)
WHO Neuropsychiatric AIDS Study, Cross-sectional Phase I: study design and psychiatric findings [Maj] 39 (Ja)
Mental Health Services
All prepaid health care systems are not equal (letter) [Wasserman] (reply) [Wells] 1002 (De)
Mental Processes
Autonomic abnormalities in schizophrenia: state or trait indicators? [Dawson] 813 (Oc)
Parsing cognition: the power of psychology paradigms [Holzman] 952 (De)
Metabolic Diseases
Neuropsychological functioning in siblings discordant for schizophrenia and healthy volunteers [Cannon] 651 (Au)
Methoxyhydroxyphenylglycol
Noradrenergic dysregulation during discontinuation of cocaine use in addicts [McDougle] 713 (Se)
N-Methylaspartate
Subanesthetic effects of the noncompetitive NMDA antagonist, ketamine, in humans: psychotomimetic, percep-

tual, cognitive, and neuroendocrine responses [Krystal] 199 (Mr)
Metyrapone
Increased evening activation of the hypothalamic-pituitary-adrenal axis in depressed patients [Young] 701 (Se)
Monoamine Oxidase
High-dose selegiline in treatment-resistant older depressive patients [Sunderland] 607 (Au)
Mood Disorders, Non-Psychotic see Affective Disorders
Mood Disorders, Psychotic see Affective Disorders, Psychotic
Mood see Affect
Mortality
Suicide and mortality patterns in anxiety neurosis and depressive neurosis [Allgulander] 708 (Se)
Mother-Child Relations
Birth complications combined with early maternal rejection at age 1 year predispose to violent crime at age 18 years [Raine] 984 (De)
Mothers
Developmental brain abnormalities in the offspring of schizophrenic mothers: II. structural brain characteristics of schizophrenia and schizotypal personality disorder [Cannon] 955 (De)
Motor Skills
Neuropsychological deficits in neuroleptic naive patients with first-episode schizophrenia [Saykin] 124 (Fe)
Movement Disorders
Risk factors for spontaneous dyskinesia in schizophrenia [Fenton] 643 (Au)
Myelin Sheath
Myelination of a key relay zone in the hippocampal formation occurs in the human brain during childhood, adolescence, and adulthood [Benes] 477 (Je)

N

Naltrexone
Naltrexone and alcohol dependence: some methodological issues (letter) [Andrade] (reply) [Volpicelli] 335 (Ap)
National Institute of Mental Health (US)
Some issues for the new director of NIMH [Barchas] 998 (De)
National Institutes of Health (US)
Some issues for the new director of NIMH [Barchas] 998 (De)
Netherlands
Schizophrenia after prenatal exposure to the Dutch Hunger Winter of 1944-1945 (letter) [Jones] (reply) [Susser] 333 (Ap)
Neural Conduction
Neural circuits in schizophrenia (letter) [McCarley] 515 (reply) [Carpenter] 516 (Jy)
Neuroanatomy
Regional cerebral blood flow measured during symptom provocation in obsessive-compulsive disorder using oxygen 15—labeled carbon dioxide and positron emission tomography [Rauch] 62 (Ja)
Neurochemistry
Changes in cerebrospinal fluid neurochemistry during treatment of obsessive-compulsive disorder with clomipramine [Altemus] 794 (Oc)
Neuroleptics see Tranquilizing Agents, Major
Neurology
WHO Neuropsychiatric AIDS Study, Cross-sectional Phase I: study design and psychiatric findings [Maj] 39 (Ja)
WHO Neuropsychiatric AIDS Study, Cross-sectional Phase II: neuropsychological and neurological findings [Maj] 51 (Ja)
Neuropsychological Tests
Neuropsychological deficits in neuroleptic naive patients with first-episode schizophrenia [Saykin] 124 (Fe)
Schizophrenia and temporal lobe epilepsy: a neuropsychological analysis [Gold] 265 (Ap)
Neuropsychology
WHO Neuropsychiatric AIDS Study, Cross-sectional Phase I: study design and psychiatric findings [Maj] 39 (Ja)
WHO Neuropsychiatric AIDS Study, Cross-sectional Phase II: neuropsychological and neurological findings [Maj] 51 (Ja)
Neuroregulators
Arachidonic acid: a common link in the biology of schizophrenia? (letter) [Peet] 665 (Au)
Life events and the research diagnostic criteria endogenous subtype: confirmation of the distinction using the Bedford College methods [Frank] 519 (Jy)
Neurosis, Depressive see Depressive Disorder
Neurotransmitters see Neuroregulators
N-Methyl-D-aspartate see N-Methylaspartate
Noradrenaline see Norepinephrine
Norepinephrine
Are stress hormones and serotonin related to aggression in primates? (letter) [Reus] 72 (reply) [Higley] 73 (Ja)
Specificity of ethanollike effects elicited by serotonergic and noradrenergic mechanisms [Krystal] 898 (No)
Sympathetic nervous system activity in major depression: basal and desipramine-induced alterations in plasma norepinephrine kinetics [Veith] 411 (My)

O

Obituary
Mary Catherine Neidigh Freedman (August 2, 1921 - October 21, 1994) 1005 (De)
Object Attachment
Birth complications combined with early maternal rejection at age 1 year predispose to violent crime at age 18 years [Raine] 984 (De)
Obsessive-Compulsive Disorder
Changes in cerebrospinal fluid neurochemistry during treatment of obsessive-compulsive disorder with clomipramine [Altemus] 794 (Oc)
Cingulotomy in a case of concomitant obsessive-compulsive disorder and Tourette's syndrome (letter) [Baer] 73 (Ja)
Elevated cerebrospinal fluid levels of oxytocin in obsessive-compulsive disorder: comparison with Tourette's syndrome and healthy controls [Leckman] 782 (Oc)
Familial obsessive-compulsive disorder presenting as pathological jealousy successfully treated with fluoxetine (letter) [Wright] 430 (My)
Haloperidol addition in fluvoxamine-refractory obsessive-compulsive disorder: a double-blind, placebo-controlled study in patients with and without tics [McDougle] 302 (Ap)
Hypochondriasis and panic disorder: boundary and overlap [Barsky] 918 (No)
Multicenter investigation of fixed-dose fluoxetine in the treatment of obsessive-compulsive disorder [Tollefson], 559 (Jy); correction, 864 (No)
Regional cerebral blood flow measured during symptom provocation in obsessive-compulsive disorder using oxygen 15—labeled carbon dioxide and positron emission tomography [Rauch] 62 (Ja)
Retrocallosal white matter abnormalities in patients with obsessive-compulsive disorder (letter) [Breiter] 663 (Au)
Tryptophan depletion in patients with obsessive-compulsive disorder who respond to serotonin reuptake inhibitors [Barr] 309 (Ap)
Odds Ratio
Effect of diagnostic hierarchy in genetic epidemiological studies of psychiatric disorders (letter) [Roy] 926 (reply) [Wickramaratne] 927 (No)
Opioid Receptors see Receptors, Endorphin
Orientation
Biologic theories of sexual orientation (letter) [McConaghy] 431 (reply) [Byne] 432 (My)
Ovulation
Effects of the menstrual cycle on dependent variables in mood disorder research [Leibenluft] 761 (Oc)
Oxytocin
Elevated cerebrospinal fluid levels of oxytocin in obsessive-compulsive disorder: comparison with Tourette's syndrome and healthy controls [Leckman] 782 (Oc)

P

Panic
Alcohol dependence may be the missing link between posttraumatic stress disorder and panic (letter) [Wiseman] 429 (reply) [Krystal] 430 (My)
Panic Attacks see Panic Disorder
Panic Disorder
Cognitive behavioral treatment compared with nonprescriptive treatment of panic disorder [Shear] 395 (My)
DSM-III-R generalized anxiety disorder in the National Comorbidity Survey [Wittchen] 355 (My)
Hypochondriasis and panic disorder: boundary and overlap [Barsky] 918 (No)
Klein's suffocation theory of panic (letter) [Taylor] 505 (reply) [Klein] 506 (Je)
Noradrenergic dysregulation during discontinuation of cocaine use in addicts [McDougle] 713 (Se)
Panicogenic effects of cholecystokinin-tetrapeptide are antagonized by L-365,260, a central cholecystokinin receptor antagonist, in patients with panic disorder [Bradwejn] 486 (Je)
Psychiatric disorders in relatives of probands with panic disorder and/or major depression [Goldstein] 383 (My)
Standardized assessment for panic disorder research: conference report [Shear] 346 (My)
Paranoid Disorders
Diagnosing personality disorders: a review of issues and research methods [Zimmerman] 225 (Mr)
Paranoid Personality Disorder
Independent diagnoses of adoptees and relatives as defined by *DSM-III* in the provincial and national samples of the Danish Adoption Study of Schizophrenia [Kendler] 456 (Je)
Parasympatholytics
Neuropsychological deficits in neuroleptic naive patients with first-episode schizophrenia [Saykin] 124 (Fe)
Parent-Child Relations
Relation of parenthood to suicide (letter) [Clark] 160 (reply) [Høyer] 160 (Fe)
Parietal Lobe
Neuropsychological impairments in deficit vs nondeficit forms of schizophrenia [Buchanan] 804 (Oc)
Paroxetine
Interactions of serotonin reuptake inhibitors with tricyclic antidepressants (letter) [Popli] 666 (Au)
Patient Admission
Increased pressure for rapid eye movement sleep at time of hospital admission predicts relapse in nondepressed patients with primary alcoholism at 3-month follow-up [Gillin] 189 (Mr)
Patient Satisfaction
Hypochondriasis and panic disorder: boundary and overlap [Barsky] 918 (No)
Perceptual Masking
Backward masking in schizophrenia and mania: I. specifying a mechanism [Green] 939 (De)
Backward masking in schizophrenia and mania: II. specifying the visual channels [Green] 945 (De)
Parsing cognition: the power of psychology paradigms [Holzman] 952 (De)
Periodicals
Third editor of the ARCHIVES—Jack D Barchas, MD [Springer] 173 (Mr)
Personality
Predicting early onset of male antisocial behavior from preschool behavior [Tremblay] 732 (Se)
Personality Disorder, Antisocial see Antisocial Personality Disorder
Personality Disorder, Schizotypal see Schizotypal Personality Disorder
Personality Disorders
Developmental brain abnormalities in the offspring of schizophrenic mothers: II. structural brain characteristics of schizophrenia and schizotypal personality disorder [Cannon] 955 (De)
Diagnosing personality disorders: a review of issues and research methods [Zimmerman] 225 (Mr)
Familial correlates of reduced central serotonergic system function in patients with personality disorders [Coccaro] 318 (Ap)
International Personality Disorder Examination: The World Health Organization/Alcohol, Drug Abuse, and Mental Health Administration International Pilot Study of Personality Disorders [Loranger] 215 (Mr)
Serotonin and the neurobiology of depression: effects of tryptophan depletion [Delgado] 865 (No)
Personality Inventory
Personality profiles and state aggressiveness in Finnish alcoholic, violent offenders, fire setters, and healthy volunteers [Virkkunen] 28 (Ja)
Pharmacotherapy see Drug Therapy
Phenethylamines
Dose-response study of N,N-dimethyltryptamine in humans: I. neuroendocrine, autonomic, and cardiovascular effects [Strassman] 85 (Fe)
Phobia, Social see Phobic Disorders
Phobias see Phobic Disorders
Phobic Disorders
Boundary of social phobia: exploring the threshold [Davidson] 975 (De)
Hypochondriasis and panic disorder: boundary and overlap [Barsky] 918 (No)
Psychiatric disorders in relatives of probands with panic disorder and/or major depression [Goldstein] 383 (My)
Standardized assessment for panic disorder research: conference report [Shear] 346 (My)
Pindolol
Pindolol induces a rapid improvement of depressed patients treated with serotonin reuptake inhibitors (letter) [Artigas] 248 (Mr)
Pituitary-Adrenal System
Increased evening activation of the hypothalamic-pituitary-adrenal axis in depressed patients [Young] 701 (Se)
Placebo Effect
Buspirone treatment of anxious alcoholics: placebo-controlled trial [Kranzler] 720 (Se)
Plasma
Plasma homovanillic acid levels in first-episode schizophrenia: psychopathology and treatment response [Koreen] 132 (Fe)
Polymerase Chain Reaction
Analysis of the D_4 dopamine receptor gene variant in an Italian schizophrenia kindred [Macciardi] 288 (Ap)
No evidence of a schizophrenia locus in a second pseudoautosomal region (letter) [Wang] 427 (My)
Polymorphism (Genetics)
Analysis of the D_4 dopamine receptor gene variant in an Italian schizophrenia kindred [Macciardi] 288 (Ap)
Suicidality and 5-hydroxyindoleacetic acid concentration associated with a tryptophan hydroxylase polymorphism [Nielsen] 34 (Ja)
Positron-Emission Tomography see Tomography, Emission-Computed
Post-Traumatic Stress Disorders see Stress Disorders, Post-Traumatic
Predictive Value of Tests
Controlled prospective study of *DSM-III* adjustment disorder in childhood: short-term prognosis and long-term predictive validity [Kovacs] 535 (Jy)
Fluphenazine vs placebo supplementation for prodromal signs of relapse in schizophrenia [Marder] 280 (Ap)

Prenatal Exposure Delayed Effects
Schizophrenia after prenatal exposure to the Dutch Hunger Winter of 1944-1945 (letter) [Jones] (reply) [Susser] 333 (Ap)
Prepaid Health Plans
All prepaid health care systems are not equal (letter) [Wasserman] (reply) [Wells] 1002 (De)
Prevalence
Incidence of dementia in a population older than 75 years in the United Kingdom [Paykel] 325 (Ap)
Lifetime and 12-month prevalence of *DSM-III-R* psychiatric disorders in the United States: results from the National Comorbidity Survey [Kessler] 8 (Ja)
Primary Health Care
All prepaid health care systems are not equal (letter) [Wasserman] (reply) [Wells] 1002 (De)
Untreated anxiety among adult primary care patients in a health maintenance organization [Fifer] 740 (Se)
Primates
Are stress hormones and serotonin related to aggression in primates? (letter) [Reus] 72 (reply) [Higley] 73 (Ja)
Probability
Correction and amplification (letter) [Bird] 429 (My)
Progesterone
Effects of the menstrual cycle on dependent variables in mood disorder research [Leibenluft] 761 (Oc)
Prolactin
Dose-response studies with protirelin [Garbutt] 875 (No)
Familial correlates of reduced central serotonergic system function in patients with personality disorders [Coccaro] 318 (Ap)
24-hour profiles of cortisol, prolactin, and growth hormone secretion in mania [Linkowski] 616 (Au)
Protirelin
Carbamazepine increases cerebrospinal fluid thyrotropin-releasing hormone levels in affectively ill patients [Marangell] 625 (Au)
Dose-response studies with protirelin [Garbutt] 875 (No)
Psilocybine
Dose-response study of N,N-dimethyltryptamine in humans: I. neuroendocrine, autonomic, and cardiovascular effects [Strassman] 85 (Fe)
Psychiatric Status Rating Scales
Serotonin and the neurobiology of depression: effects of tryptophan depletion [Delgado] 865 (No)
Psychiatry
Third editor of the ARCHIVES—Jack D Barchas, MD [Springer] 173 (Mr)
WHO Neuropsychiatric AIDS Study, Cross-sectional Phase I: study design and psychiatric findings [Maj] 39 (Ja)
Psychiatry, Biological see Biological Psychiatry
Psychomotor Performance
Assessing the validity of an animal model of deficient sensorimotor gating in schizophrenic patients [Swerdlow] 139 (Fe)
Psychoneuroimmunology
Psychoneuroimmunology and human immunodeficiency virus type 1 infection revisited (letter) [Goodkin] 246 (reply) [Perry] 247 (Mr)
Psychopathology
Awareness of illness in schizophrenia and schizoaffective and mood disorders [Amador] 826 (Oc)
Plasma homovanillic acid levels in first-episode schizophrenia: psychopathology and treatment response [Koreen] 132 (Fe)
Psychoses, Alcoholic
Naltrexone and alcohol dependence: some methodological issues (letter) [Andrade] (reply) [Volpicelli] 335 (Ap)
Psychoses see Psychotic Disorders
Psychoses, Substance-Induced
Subanesthetic effects of the noncompetitive NMDA antagonist, ketamine, in humans: psychotomimetic, perceptual, cognitive, and neuroendocrine responses [Krystal] 199 (Mr)
Psychosocial Deprivation
Birth complications combined with early maternal rejection at age 1 year predispose to violent crime at age 18 years [Raine] 984 (De)
Psychotherapy
Buspirone treatment of anxious alcoholics: placebo-controlled trial [Kranzler] 720 (Se)
Interpersonal psychotherapy: current status [Weissman] 599 (Au)
One-year follow-up of psychotherapy and pharmacotherapy for cocaine dependence: delayed emergence of psychotherapy effects [Carroll] 989 (De)
Psychotherapy and pharmacotherapy for ambulatory cocaine abusers [Carroll] 177 (Mr)
Psychotic Disorders
Age of onset in familial schizophrenia (letter) [DeLisi] 334 (Ap)
Allelic variation in the D_4 dopamine receptor (DRD4) gene does not predict response to clozapine [Rao] 912 (No)
Awareness of illness in schizophrenia and schizoaffective and mood disorders [Amador] 826 (Oc)
Cannabis abuse and the course of recent-onset schizophrenic disorders [Linszen] 273 (Ap)
Clinical characteristics and predisposing factors in acute drug-induced akathisia [Sachdev] 963 (De)
Diagnostic Interview for Genetic Studies: rationale, unique features, and training [Nurnberger] 849 (No)
Epidemiology of nonaffective acute remitting psychosis vs schizophrenia: sex and sociocultural setting [Susser] 294 (Ap)
Independent diagnoses of adoptees and relatives as defined by *DSM-III* in the provincial and national samples of the Danish Adoption Study of Schizophrenia [Kendler] 456 (Je)
Lower-dose therapy with traditional neuroleptics in chronically hospitalized schizophrenic patients (letter) [Smith] 427 (My)
Parsing cognition: the power of psychology paradigms [Holzman] 952 (De)
Puerto Rico
Correction and amplification (letter) [Bird] 429 (My)

R

Raclopride
Striatal D_2 dopamine receptor characteristics in neuroleptic-naive schizophrenic patients studied with positron emission tomography [Hietala] 116 (Fe)
Radioisotopes
Striatal D_2 dopamine receptor characteristics in neuroleptic-naive schizophrenic patients studied with positron emission tomography [Hietala] 116 (Fe)
Randomized Controlled Trials
Fluphenazine vs placebo supplementation for prodromal signs of relapse in schizophrenia [Marder] 280 (Ap)
Subanesthetic effects of the noncompetitive NMDA antagonist, ketamine, in humans: psychotomimetic, perceptual, cognitive, and neuroendocrine responses [Krystal] 199 (Mr)
Rapid Eye Movements see Sleep, REM
Receptors, Adrenergic, Alpha
Sympathetic nervous system activity in major depression: basal and desipramine-induced alterations in plasma norepinephrine kinetics [Veith] 411 (My)
Receptors, Dopamine
Allelic variation in the D_4 dopamine receptor (DRD4) gene does not predict response to clozapine [Rao] 912 (No)
Analysis of the D_4 dopamine receptor gene variant in an Italian schizophrenia kindred [Macciardi] 288 (Ap)
Arachidonic acid: a common link in the biology of schizophrenia? (letter) [Peet] 665 (Au)
Neuropsychological deficits in neuroleptic naive patients with first-episode schizophrenia [Saykin] 124 (Fe)
Receptors, Dopamine D2
Striatal D_2 dopamine receptor characteristics in neuroleptic-naive schizophrenic patients studied with positron emission tomography [Hietala] 116 (Fe)
Receptors, Endorphin
Increased density of guanine nucleotide-binding proteins in the postmortem brains of heroin addicts [Escriba] 494 (Je)
Receptors, Serotonin
Dose-response study of N,N-dimethyltryptamine in humans: I. neuroendocrine, autonomic, and cardiovascular effects [Strassman] 85 (Fe)
Serotonin $_{2a}$ receptors in schizophrenia: relation to suicide (letter) [Meltzer] (reply) [Laruelle] 1003 (De)
Receptors, Thyrotropin-Releasing Hormone
Dose-response studies with protirelin [Garbutt] 875 (No)
Record Linkage, Medical see Medical Record Linkage
Recurrence
Fluphenazine vs placebo supplementation for prodromal signs of relapse in schizophrenia [Marder] 280 (Ap)
Increased pressure for rapid eye movement sleep at time of hospital admission predicts relapse in nondepressed patients with primary alcoholism at 3-month follow-up [Gillin] 189 (Mr)
Naltrexone and alcohol dependence: some methodological issues (letter) [Andrade] (reply) [Volpicelli] 335 (Ap)
Psychotherapy and pharmacotherapy for ambulatory cocaine abusers [Carroll] 177 (Mr)
Regional Blood Flow
Reduction of cerebral blood flow in older depressed patients [Lesser] 677 (Se)
Regional cerebral blood flow in mood disorders, III: treatment and clinical response [Nobler] 884 (No)
Rejection (Psychology)
Birth complications combined with early maternal rejection at age 1 year predispose to violent crime at age 18 years [Raine] 984 (De)
Relapse see Recurrence
Reliability and Validity see Reproducibility of Results
Remoxipride
Clinical action of remoxipride (letter) [Conley] 1001 (De)
Reproducibility of Results
Diagnosing personality disorders: a review of issues and research methods [Zimmerman] 225 (Mr)
Diagnostic Interview for Genetic Studies [Frances] 863 (No)
Diagnostic Interview for Genetic Studies: rationale, unique features, and training [Nurnberger] 849 (No)
Research
Diagnosing personality disorders: a review of issues and research methods [Zimmerman] 225 (Mr)
Standardized assessment for panic disorder research: conference report [Shear] 346 (My)
Research Support
Some issues for the new director of NIMH [Barchas] 998 (De)
Reviewers
Reviewers for 1994, 933 (De)
Risk
Patterns of risk in first-degree relatives of patients with Alzheimer's disease [Silverman] 577 (Jy)
Risk Factors
Risk factors for spontaneous dyskinesia in schizophrenia [Fenton] 643 (Au)
Schizophrenia after prenatal exposure to the Dutch Hunger Winter of 1944-1945 (letter) [Jones] (reply) [Susser] 333 (Ap)
Risk Ratio see Odds Ratio

S

Schizoaffective Disorder see Psychotic Disorders
Schizophrenia
Age of onset in familial schizophrenia (letter) [DeLisi] 334 (Ap)
Allelic variation in the D_4 dopamine receptor (DRD4) gene does not predict response to clozapine [Rao] 912 (No)
Analysis of the D_4 dopamine receptor gene variant in an Italian schizophrenia kindred [Macciardi] 288 (Ap)
Arachidonic acid: a common link in the biology of schizophrenia? (letter) [Peet] 665 (Au)
Assessing the validity of an animal model of deficient sensorimotor gating in schizophrenic patients [Swerdlow] 139 (Fe)
Autonomic abnormalities in schizophrenia: state or trait indicators? [Dawson] 813 (Oc)
Awareness of illness in schizophrenia and schizoaffective and mood disorders [Amador] 826 (Oc)
Backward masking in schizophrenia and mania: I. specifying a mechanism [Green] 939 (De)
Backward masking in schizophrenia and mania: II. specifying the visual channels [Green] 945 (De)
Brain atrophy or dystrophy in schizophrenia: when did it happen? (letter) [Stevens] 927 (No)
Cannabis abuse and the course of recent-onset schizophrenic disorders [Linszen] 273 (Ap)
Clinical action of remoxipride (letter) [Conley] 1001 (De)
Clinical response to clozapine in patients with schizophrenia (letter) [Pickar] 159 (Fe)
Developmental brain abnormalities in the offspring of schizophrenic mothers: II. structural brain characteristics of schizophrenia and schizotypal personality disorder [Cannon] 955 (De)
Diagnostic Interview for Genetic Studies: rationale, unique features, and training [Nurnberger] 849 (No)
Epidemiology of nonaffective acute remitting psychosis vs schizophrenia: sex and sociocultural setting [Susser] 294 (Ap)
Fluphenazine vs placebo supplementation for prodromal signs of relapse in schizophrenia [Marder] 280 (Ap)
Genetic and environmental influences of twins in posttraumatic stress (letter) [Lurie] (reply) [True] 838 (Oc)
Impaired autonomic nervous system habituation in those at genetic risk for schizophrenia [Hollister] 552 (Jy)
Independent diagnoses of adoptees and relatives as defined by *DSM-III* in the provincial and national samples of the Danish Adoption Study of Schizophrenia [Kendler] 456 (Je)
Lower-dose therapy with traditional neuroleptics in chronically hospitalized schizophrenic patients (letter) [Smith] 427 (My)
Maintenance imipramine therapy for secondary depression in schizophrenia: a controlled trial [Siris] 109 (Fe)
Mental illness in the biological and adoptive relatives of schizophrenic adoptees: replication of the Copenhagen Study in the rest of Denmark [Kety] 442 (Je)
Neural circuits in schizophrenia (letter) [McCarley] 515 (reply) [Carpenter] 516 (Jy)
Neuropsychological deficits in neuroleptic naive patients with first-episode schizophrenia [Saykin] 124 (Fe)
Neuropsychological functioning in siblings discordant for schizophrenia and healthy volunteers [Cannon] 651 (Au)
Neuropsychological impairments in deficit vs nondeficit forms of schizophrenia [Buchanan] 804 (Oc)
No evidence of a schizophrenia locus in a second pseudo-autosomal region (letter) [Wang] 427 (My)
Parsing cognition: the power of psychology paradigms [Holzman] 952 (De)
Plasma homovanillic acid levels in first-episode schizophrenia: psychopathology and treatment response [Koreen] 132 (Fe)
Prevalence of schizophrenia in Ireland (letter) [Torrey] (reply) [Walsh] 513 (Jy)
Risk factors for spontaneous dyskinesia in schizophrenia [Fenton] 643 (Au)
Schizophrenia after prenatal exposure to the Dutch Hunger Winter of 1944-1945 (letter) [Jones] (reply) [Susser] 333 (Ap)
Schizophrenia and temporal lobe epilepsy: a neuropsychological analysis [Gold] 265 (Ap)
Serotonin $_{2a}$ receptors in schizophrenia: relation to suicide (letter) [Meltzer] (reply) [Laruelle] 1003 (De)

Striatal D_2 dopamine receptor characteristics in neuroleptic-naive schizophrenic patients studied with positron emission tomography [Hietala] 116 (Fe)
Subanesthetic effects of the noncompetitive NMDA antagonist, ketamine, in humans: psychotomimetic, perceptual, cognitive, and neuroendocrine responses [Krystal] 199 (Mr)
Schizophrenia, Disorganized
Neuropsychological deficits in schizophrenics: relationship to age, chronicity, and dementia [Heaton] 469 (Je)
Schizophrenic Disorders see Schizophrenia
Schizotypal Personality Disorder
Developmental brain abnormalities in the offspring of schizophrenic mothers: II. structural brain characteristics of schizophrenia and schizotypal personality disorder [Cannon] 955 (De)
Independent diagnoses of adoptees and relatives as defined by *DSM-III* in the provincial and national samples of the Danish Adoption Study of Schizophrenia [Kendler] 456 (Je)
Science
Some issues for the new director of NIMH [Barchas] 998 (De)
Selegiline
High-dose selegiline in treatment-resistant older depressive patients [Sunderland] 607 (Au)
Semantics
Schizophrenia and temporal lobe epilepsy: a neuropsychological analysis [Gold] 265 (Ap)
Sensitivity and Specificity
Fluphenazine vs placebo supplementation for prodromal signs of relapse in schizophrenia [Marder] 280 (Ap)
Sensory Motor Performance see Psychomotor Performance
Serotonin
Are stress hormones and serotonin related to aggression in primates? (letter) [Reus] 72 (reply) [Higley] 73 (Ja)
CSF biochemistries, glucose metabolism, and diurnal activity rhythms in alcoholic, violent offenders, fire setters, and healthy volunteers [Virkkunen] 20 (Ja)
Effects of alterations in plasma tryptophan levels on aggressive feelings (letter) [Cleare] 1004 (De)
Familial correlates of reduced central serotonergic system function in patients with personality disorders [Coccaro] 318 (Ap)
Interactions of serotonin reuptake inhibitors with tricyclic antidepressants (letter) [Popli] 666 (Au)
Mania induced by citalopram (letter) [Bryois] 664 (Au)
Mood-lowering effect of tryptophan depletion: enhanced susceptibility in young men at genetic risk for major affective disorders [Benkelfat] 687 (Se)
Multicenter investigation of fixed-dose fluoxetine in the treatment of obsessive-compulsive disorder [Tollefson] 559 (Jy); correction, 864 (No)
Personality profiles and state aggressiveness in Finnish alcoholic, violent offenders, fire setters, and healthy volunteers [Virkkunen] 28 (Ja)
Serotonin and the neurobiology of depression: effects of tryptophan depletion [Delgado] 865 (No)
Specificity of ethanollike effects elicited by serotonergic and noradrenergic mechanisms [Krystal] 898 (No)
Serotonin Agonists
Dose-response study of N,N-dimethyltryptamine in humans: I. neuroendocrine, autonomic, and cardiovascular effects [Strassman] 85 (Fe)
Specificity of ethanollike effects elicited by serotonergic and noradrenergic mechanisms [Krystal] 898 (No)
Serotonin Receptor Agonists see Serotonin Agonists
Serotonin Receptors see Receptors, Serotonin
Serotonin Reuptake Inhibitors see Serotonin Uptake Inhibitors
Serotonin Uptake Inhibitors
Haloperidol addition in fluvoxamine-refractory obsessive-compulsive disorder: a double-blind, placebo-controlled study in patients with and without tics [McDougle] 302 (Ap)
Interactions of serotonin reuptake inhibitors with tricyclic antidepressants (letter) [Popli] 666 (Au)
Pindolol induces a rapid improvement of depressed patients treated with serotonin reuptake inhibitors (letter) [Artigas] 248 (Mr)
Tryptophan depletion in patients with obsessive-compulsive disorder who respond to serotonin reuptake inhibitors [Barr] 309 (Ap)
Sex
Epidemiology of nonaffective acute remitting psychosis vs schizophrenia: sex and sociocultural setting [Susser] 294 (Ap)
Schizophrenia after prenatal exposure to the Dutch Hunger Winter of 1944-1945 pgnum333 (reply) [Susser] 333 (Ap)
Sex Behavior
Biologic theories of sexual orientation (letter) [McConaghy] 431 (reply) [Byne] 432 (My)
Theories of sexual orientation: a reappraisal (letter) [Berger] (reply) [Byne] 432 (My)
Sex Factors
Epidemiology of nonaffective acute remitting psychosis vs schizophrenia: sex and sociocultural setting [Susser] 294 (Ap)
Schizophrenia after prenatal exposure to the Dutch Hunger Winter of 1944-1945 (letter) [Jones] 333 (Ap)
Sibling Relations
Neuropsychological functioning in siblings discordant for schizophrenia and healthy volunteers [Cannon] 651 (Au)
Single-Photon Emission-Computed Tomography see Tomography, Emission-Computed, Single-Photon
Sleep Disorders
Increased pressure for rapid eye movement sleep at time of hospital admission predicts relapse in nondepressed patients with primary alcoholism at 3-month follow-up [Gillin] 189 (Mr)
Sleep, REM
Increased pressure for rapid eye movement sleep at time of hospital admission predicts relapse in nondepressed patients with primary alcoholism at 3-month follow-up [Gillin] 189 (Mr)
Socioeconomic Factors
Boundary of social phobia: exploring the threshold [Davidson] 975 (De)
Somatization Disorder see Somatoform Disorders
Somatoform Disorders
Hypochondriasis and panic disorder: boundary and overlap [Barsky] 918 (No)
Somatotropin-Releasing Hormone
24-hour profiles of cortisol, prolactin, and growth hormone secretion in mania [Linkowski] 616 (Au)
Space Perception
Backward masking in schizophrenia and mania: II. specifying the visual channels [Green] 945 (De)
Sports
Psychiatric and medical effects of anabolic-androgenic steroid use: a controlled study of 160 athletes [Pope] 375 (My)
Street Drugs
Cannabis abuse and the course of recent-onset schizophrenic disorders [Linszen] 273 (Ap)
Stress
Cognitive behavioral treatment compared with nonprescriptive treatment of panic disorder [Shear] 395 (My)
Life events and endogenous depression: puzzle reexamined [Brown] 525 (Jy)
Stress Disorders, Post-Traumatic
Alcohol dependence may be the missing link between posttraumatic stress disorder and panic (letter) [Wiseman] 429 (reply) [Krystal] 430 (My)
Elevation of serum free triiodothyronine, total triiodothyronine, thyroxine-binding globulin, and total thyroxine levels in combat-related posttraumatic stress disorder [Mason] 629 (Au)
Genetic and environmental influences of twins in posttraumatic stress (letter) [Lurie] (reply) [True] 838 (Oc)
Substance Abuse
Cingulotomy in a case of concomitant obsessive-compulsive disorder and Tourette's syndrome (letter) [Baer] 73 (Ja)
Diagnostic Interview for Genetic Studies [Frances] 863 (No)
Increased density of guanine nucleotide-binding proteins in the postmortem brains of heroin addicts [Escriba] 494 (Je)
Psychiatric disorders in relatives of probands with panic disorder and/or major depression [Goldstein] 383 (My)
Psychotherapy and pharmacotherapy for ambulatory cocaine abusers [Carroll] 177 (Mr)
Violence in the severely mentally ill (letter) [Weiler] (reply) [Hodgins] 71 (Ja)
Substance Dependence
Incentives improve outcome in outpatient behavioral treatment of cocaine dependence [Higgins] 568 (Jy)
Noradrenergic dysregulation during discontinuation of cocaine use in addicts [McDougle] 713 (Se)
One-year follow-up of psychotherapy and pharmacotherapy for cocaine dependence: delayed emergence of psychotherapy effects [Carroll] 989 (De)
Violence in the severely mentally ill (letter) [Weiler] (reply) [Hodgins] 71 (Ja)
Substance Use Disorders
Lifetime and 12-month prevalence of *DSM-III-R* psychiatric disorders in the United States: results from the National Comorbidity Survey [Kessler] 8 (Ja)
Suffocation see Asphyxia
Suicide
Maintenance imipramine therapy for secondary depression in schizophrenia: a controlled trial [Siris] 109 (Fe)
Naturalistic follow-up of a behavioral treatment for chronically parasuicidal borderline patients [Linehan], 50:971 (De); correction,51:422 (My)
Relation of parenthood to suicide (letter) [Clark] 160 (reply) [Høyer] 160 (Fe)
Serotonin $_{2A}$ receptors in schizophrenia: relation to suicide (letter) [Meltzer] (reply) [Laruelle] 1003 (De)
Suicide and mortality patterns in anxiety neurosis and depressive neurosis [Allgulander] 708 (Se)
Suicide, Attempted
Suicidality and 5-hydroxyindoleacetic acid concentration associated with a tryptophan hydroxylase polymorphism [Nielsen] 34 (Ja)
Sweden
Suicide and mortality patterns in anxiety neurosis and depressive neurosis [Allgulander] 708 (Se)
Sympathetic Nervous System
Sympathetic nervous system activity in major depression: basal and desipramine-induced alterations in plasma norepinephrine kinetics [Veith] 411 (My)

T

Technology
Some issues for the new director of NIMH [Barchas] 998 (De)
Temporal Lobe
Brain atrophy or dystrophy in schizophrenia: when did it happen? (letter) [Stevens] 927 (No)
Neuropsychological impairments in deficit vs nondeficit forms of schizophrenia [Buchanan] 804 (Oc)
Testosterone
CSF biochemistries, glucose metabolism, and diurnal activity rhythms in alcoholic, violent offenders, fire setters, and healthy volunteers [Virkkunen] 20 (Ja)
Personality profiles and state aggressiveness in Finnish alcoholic, violent offenders, fire setters, and healthy volunteers [Virkkunen] 28 (Ja)
Tetragastrin
Panicogenic effects of cholecystokinin-tetrapeptide are antagonized by L-365,260, a central cholecystokinin receptor antagonist, in patients with panic disorder [Bradwejn] 486 (Je)
Tetrahydrocannabinol
Cannabis abuse and the course of recent-onset schizophrenic disorders [Linszen] 273 (Ap)
Thyrotropin
Dose-response studies with protirelin [Garbutt] 875 (No)
Thyrotropin Releasing Hormone Receptors see Receptors, Thyrotropin-Releasing Hormone
Thyrotropin-Releasing Hormone see Protirelin
Thyroxine-Binding Globulin see Thyroxine-Binding Proteins
Thyroxine-Binding Proteins
Elevation of serum free triiodothyronine, total triiodothyronine, thyroxine-binding globulin, and total thyroxine levels in combat-related posttraumatic stress disorder [Mason] 629 (Au)
Tic
Cingulotomy in a case of concomitant obsessive-compulsive disorder and Tourette's syndrome (letter) [Baer] 73 (Ja)
Haloperidol addition in fluvoxamine-refractory obsessive-compulsive disorder: a double-blind, placebo-controlled study in patients with and without tics [McDougle] 302 (Ap)
Time
Increased evening activation of the hypothalamic-pituitary-adrenal axis in depressed patients [Young] 701 (Se)
Time course of nonchronic major depressive disorder: uniformity across episodes and samples [Coryell] 405 (My)
Time Factors
One-year follow-up of psychotherapy and pharmacotherapy for cocaine dependence: delayed emergence of psychotherapy effects [Carroll] 989 (De)
Tomography, Emission-Computed
Neural circuits in schizophrenia (letter) [McCarley] 515 (reply) [Carpenter] 516 (Jy)
Neuropsychological impairments in deficit vs nondeficit forms of schizophrenia [Buchanan] 804 (Oc)
Regional cerebral blood flow measured during symptom provocation in obsessive-compulsive disorder using oxygen 15—labeled carbon dioxide and positron emission tomography [Rauch] 62 (Ja)
Retrocallosal white matter abnormalities in patients with obsessive-compulsive disorder (letter) [Breiter] 663 (Au)
Tomography, Emission-Computed, Single-Photon
Reduction of cerebral blood flow in older depressed patients [Lesser] 677 (Se)
Regional cerebral blood flow measured during symptom provocation in obsessive-compulsive disorder using oxygen 15—labeled carbon dioxide and positron emission tomography [Rauch] 62 (Ja)
Tourette Syndrome
Cingulotomy in a case of concomitant obsessive-compulsive disorder and Tourette's syndrome (letter) [Baer] 73 (Ja)
Elevated cerebrospinal fluid levels of oxytocin in obsessive-compulsive disorder: comparison with Tourette's syndrome and healthy controls [Leckman] 782 (Oc)
Tranquilizing Agents, Major
Assessing the validity of an animal model of deficient sensorimotor gating in schizophrenic patients [Swerdlow] 139 (Fe)
Autonomic abnormalities in schizophrenia: state or trait indicators? [Dawson] 813 (Oc)
Clinical action of remoxipride (letter) [Conley] 1001 (De)
Clinical characteristics and predisposing factors in acute drug-induced akathisia [Sachdev] 963 (De)
Clinical response to clozapine in patients with schizophrenia (letter) [Pickar] 159 (Fe)
Haloperidol addition in fluvoxamine-refractory obsessive-compulsive disorder: a double-blind, placebo-controlled study in patients with and without tics [McDougle] 302 (Ap)

Lower-dose therapy with traditional neuroleptics in chronically hospitalized schizophrenic patients (letter) [Smith] 427 (My)
Maintenance imipramine therapy for secondary depression in schizophrenia: a controlled trial [Siris] 109 (Fe)
Neuropsychological deficits in neuroleptic naive patients with first-episode schizophrenia [Saykin] 124 (Fe)
Plasma homovanillic acid levels in first-episode schizophrenia: psychopathology and treatment response [Koreen] 132 (Fe)
Risk factors for spontaneous dyskinesia in schizophrenia [Fenton] 643 (Au)

Tranquilizing Agents, Minor
Assessing the validity of an animal model of deficient sensorimotor gating in schizophrenic patients [Swerdlow] 139 (Fe)

Treatment Outcome
Naturalistic follow-up of a behavioral treatment for chronically parasuicidal borderline patients [Linehan], 50:971 (De); correction,51:422 (My)
Psychotherapy and pharmacotherapy for ambulatory cocaine abusers [Carroll] 177 (Mr)

Treatment Refusal
Reduction of cerebral blood flow in older depressed patients [Lesser] 677 (Se)

Tricyclic Antidepressive Agents see Antidepressive Agents, Tricyclic

Triiodothyronine
Elevation of serum free triiodothyronine, total triiodothyronine, thyroxine-binding globulin, and total thyroxine levels in combat-related posttraumatic stress disorder [Mason] 629 (Au)

Tryptophan
Effects of alterations in plasma tryptophan levels on aggressive feelings (letter) [Cleare] 1004 (De)
Mood-lowering effect of tryptophan depletion: enhanced susceptibility in young men at genetic risk for major affective disorders [Benkelfat] 687 (Se)
Serotonin and the neurobiology of depression: effects of tryptophan depletion [Delgado] 865 (No)
Tryptophan depletion in patients with obsessive-compulsive disorder who respond to serotonin reuptake inhibitors [Barr] 309 (Ap)

Tryptophan Hydroxylase
Suicidality and 5-hydroxyindoleacetic acid concentration associated with a tryptophan hydroxylase polymorphism [Nielsen] 34 (Ja)

Twins
Genetic and environmental influences of twins in posttraumatic stress (letter) [Lurie] (reply) [True] 838 (Oc)

U

Unipolar Depression see Depressive Disorder

United States Alcohol, Drug Abuse, and Mental Health Administration
International Personality Disorder Examination: The World Health Organization/Alcohol, Drug Abuse, and Mental Health Administration International Pilot Study of Personality Disorders [Loranger] 215 (Mr)

V

Variation (Genetics)
Allelic variation in the D_4 dopamine receptor (DRD4) gene does not predict response to clozapine [Rao] 912 (No)

Veterans
Increased pressure for rapid eye movement sleep at time of hospital admission predicts relapse in nondepressed patients with primary alcoholism at 3-month follow-up [Gillin] 189 (Mr)

Violence
Birth complications combined with early maternal rejection at age 1 year predispose to violent crime at age 18 years [Raine] 984 (De)
CSF biochemistries, glucose metabolism, and diurnal activity rhythms in alcoholic, violent offenders, fire setters, and healthy volunteers [Virkkunen] 20 (Ja)
Personality profiles and state aggressiveness in Finnish alcoholic, violent offenders, fire setters, and healthy volunteers [Virkkunen] 28 (Ja)
Suicidality and 5-hydroxyindoleacetic acid concentration associated with a tryptophan hydroxylase polymorphism [Nielsen] 34 (Ja)
Violence in the severely mentally ill (letter) [Weiler] (reply) [Hodgins] 71 (Ja)

Visual Pathways
Backward masking in schizophrenia and mania: II. specifying the visual channels [Green] 945 (De)

Visual Perception
Backward masking in schizophrenia and mania: I. specifying a mechanism [Green] 939 (De)
Backward masking in schizophrenia and mania: II. specifying the visual channels [Green] 945 (De)
Parsing cognition: the power of psychology paradigms [Holzman] 952 (De)

Volition
Dose-response study of N,N-dimethyltryptamine in humans: II. subjective effects and preliminary results of a new rating scale [Strassman] 98 (Fe)

W

World Health Organization
International Personality Disorder Examination: The World Health Organization/Alcohol, Drug Abuse, and Mental Health Administration International Pilot Study of Personality Disorders [Loranger] 215 (Mr)
WHO Neuropsychiatric AIDS Study, Cross-sectional Phase I: study design and psychiatric findings [Maj] 39 (Ja)

X

X Chromosome
No evidence of a schizophrenia locus in a second pseudoautosomal region (letter) [Wang] 427 (My)

Y

Y Chromosome
No evidence of a schizophrenia locus in a second pseudoautosomal region (letter) [Wang] 427 (My)

Yohimbine
Noradrenergic dysregulation during discontinuation of cocaine use in addicts [McDougle] 713 (Se)
Specificity of ethanollike effects elicited by serotonergic and noradrenergic mechanisms [Krystal] 898 (No)

Professional Opportunities

Archives of General Psychiatry is an exceptional journal that provides physicians with the latest medical and technological information in the psychiatric field. It is an excellent source for recruiting, reaching over 30,220 psychiatrists each month.

All advertising orders must be submitted in writing by mail or fax. Although the American Medical Association believes the classified advertisements in these pages to be from reputable sources, the Association does not assume liability concerning them. Acceptance of advertising is restricted to physician recruitment opportunities, practices for sale, medical office space for sale or rent, and medical equipment for sale.

You can mail your ad materials to *Archives of General Psychiatry* Classifieds, 515 N State St, Chicago, IL 60610 or fax to 312-464-5909.

Confidential box numbers are available to advertisers for an additional $20.00 per issue. All confidential box replies must be in writing and must cite the box number in the ad, example: Box XXXX, c/o *Archives of General Psychiatry,* 515 N State St, Chicago, IL 60610.

All cancellations/changes must be received at least 25 days prior to the issue date by phone, mail, or fax to the *Archives of General Psychiatry* Classified office.

For information on rates, deadlines, and policies for *Archives of General Psychiatry* Classifieds, contact your classified service representative at 800-AMA-2260 or 312-464-2475/2490/2491/4485.

Psychiatry

CORRECTIONAL/ACADEMIC PSYCHIATRIST, CHICAGO, Illinois: The Isaac Ray Center and Cermak Health Services, both nationally recognized forensic mental health teams, seek full-time, flexible-schedule BC/BE psychiatrist to provide clinical, clinical supervision, and academic services in the psychiatric facilities of the Cook County Jail. Be an integral part of a unique new partnership of academics and public policy. You will be an employee of the Isaac Ray Center with a faculty position at Rush Medical College. Salary $100K+ with generous benefit package. Participate in training of residents, fellows, and psychology graduate students in an active, innovative training setting. The positions do not involve or require specialized forensic evaluations for court/testimony. Openings are available after 9/1/94. Eligibility for Illinois medical license required. Send CV with inquiry to Mark R. McClung, MD; Vice President, Educational Services; Isaac Ray Center; 1725 West Harrison Street; Suite 110; Chicago, IL 60612.

For more **Professional Opportunities** please refer to the **Classified** sections in ***JAMA*** and ***AMNews***.

Nationwide

PSYCHIATRY & NEUROLOGY

Positions

We know how busy you are. Let us do the mundane busy work.

1 (800) 428-4406

Physician Search Associates

PENNSYLVANIA (LEBANON) — PSYCHIATRIST, Board Certified or Board Eligible, needed for 2 full-time positions at the Department of Veterans Affairs Medical Center, Lebanon, Pennsylvania, to start approximately July 1, 1995. Starting salary $90,000 to $112,000 based on experience and training. The Lebanon VA Medical Center is affiliated with the Medical College of Penn State University. Positions are in general psychiatry and geriatric psychiatry. Position holds potential for faculty appointment and/or research. The Lebanon VA Medical Center is located in the heart of the Pennsylvania Dutch country close to Hershey (Chocolatetown, USA). Excellent housing and schools within easy reach of Philadelphia, New York City, and Baltimore. Low crime, low cost, clean, quiet area — a great place to raise a family. Excellent work hours and fringe benefits. **Contact Raymer A. Kent, Human Resources Management Service (05), VA Medical Center, Lebanon, PA 17042, 717-272-6621, extension 4273.**

EQUAL OPPORTUNITY EMPLOYER.

Locum Tenens Wanted

HKA LOCUM TENENS is looking for quality general psychiatry physicians to do Locum Tenens. We have opportunities coast-to-coast. We furnish Occurrence Malpractice Insurance (no tail necessary). Please call **HKA LOCUM TENENS at (800)226-6347, Extension AM7.1.**

Chiefs/Department Heads/Directors

THE DEPARTMENT OF PSYCHIATRY AT THE UNIVERSITY of North Carolina at Chapel Hill is seeking a new Director for the UNC Mental Health Clinical Research Center (UNC MHCRC), as the founding Director, Dr Arthur J. Prange, Jr, plans to step down in order to return to full-time research and teaching. The UNC MHCRC is funded from federal, state, and private sources. Its personnel have primary appointments in any of several departments of the UNC School of Medicine, School of Public Health, School of Pharmacy, and at the Dorothea Dix Hospital in Raleigh, where a sixteen-bed research unit and support facilities occupy their own building. The UNC MHCRC also enjoys a close working relationship with the UNC General Clinical Research Center (GCRC). Applicants must be board-certified psychiatrists with considerable experience in research and research administration. Two essential qualities are a proven ability to obtain independent research funding and the ability to foster research in a collaborative environment. Academic rank and salary are dependent on qualifications, but it is expected that the successful candidate will qualify for appointment as tenured Professor or Associate Professor. Application deadline is January 1, 1995. Applicants should submit a letter of application and curriculum vitae to Robert Golden, MD, Professor and Chair, Department of Psychiatry, Campus Box #7160, University of North Carolina, Chapel Hill, NC 27599-7160. The University of North Carolina is an equal opportunity/affirmative action employer. Women and minority applicants are encouraged to apply.

THE SCHOOL OF MEDICINE OF THE STATE UNIVERSITY OF New York at Stony Brook announces a search for a Chairperson of its Department of Psychiatry and Behavioral Science. The Medical Center at Stony Brook is the only comprehensive university medical center on Long Island. It is an integral part of the Health Sciences Center on the campus of The State University of New York at Stony Brook located approximately 50 miles from New York City. SUNY Stony Brook is a comprehensive research university with over 17,000 students and more than 100 degree-granting programs. The Department has educational responsibilities in each of the four years of the undergraduate curriculum. There are fully-accredited residency programs in adult and child psychiatry and a variety of continuing education offerings. The department enjoys a strong and growing network of academic and clinical affiliates, including 283 beds at VAMC Northport. The successful candidate will be selected on the basis of his or her academic and research accomplishments, educational goals, clinical skills, and administrative and managerial abilities. The individual must hold the MD degree, be qualified for a senior faculty appointment, have specialty board certification in psychiatry, and be eligible to practice in New York State. The State University of New York is an Equal Opportunity Employer and qualified minority candidates are particularly solicited. Applications will be accepted until February 15, 1995. Interested persons are asked to submit a CV and 2-3 page personal statement to the Chairman of the Search Committee, Richard N. Fine, MD, Professor and Chairman of Pediatrics, c/o Office of the Dean, School of Medicine, University at Stony Brook, Stony Brook, NY 11794-8430.

CHAIR OF PSYCHIATRY, CERMAK MENTAL HEALTH SERvices, Cook County Jail, Chicago, and Vice President for Correctional Services, Isaac Ray Center, Inc: The Isaac Ray Center, the nation's largest private, not-for-profit forensic mental health services corporation, was recently awarded a three-year $4.1 million contract by the Cook County Board of Commissioners to provide psychiatric and psychological leadership and services for Cook County Jail, which has one of the largest correctional mental health programs in the country. Applications for the Chair of Psychiatry are being sought from board-certified psychiatrists with strong clinical, administrative, and academic qualifications to lead this pioneering effort in restructuring of Cook County's "Cermak Mental Health Services" into a premier service system combining the resources of both the public and private sectors. Included in the restructured program will be training experiences for senior psychiatric residents and postdoctoral forensic fellows from several universities in the Chicago area. The successful applicant will also be a Vice President of the Isaac Ray Center and a member of its management committee. The applicant must be eligible for a senior academic appointment in the Department of Psychiatry at Rush Medical College. Salary is negotiable based on qualifications, experience, and seniority. An Illinois medical license is required. Applicant must be available to begin on or before January 1, 1995. Isaac Ray Center is an EO/AA employer. Please address a letter of inquiry with a current CV to James L. Cavanaugh, Jr, MD, Professor of Psychiatry, Rush Medical College, and Chairman of the Board, Isaac Ray Center, 1725 West Harrison Street, #110, Chicago, IL 60612. Fax 312-829-1476.

Academic/Faculty

THE DEPARTMENT OF PSYCHIATRY OF THE UNIVERSITY of Rochester School of Medicine and Dentistry is recruiting junior faculty–level psychiatrists, with strong interests in research and teaching, together with a dedication to clinical care. We are developing academic programs in the following areas: the Comprehensive Psychiatric Emergency Program; the Inpatient Service of Strong Memorial Hospital; neuropsychiatry in the Program in Geriatrics and Neuropsychiatry; our innovative, outpatient Long-Term Care Program; geropsychiatry on our unique, University-affiliated, 30-bed community psychogeriatric intermediate care unit, based at the Rochester Psychiatric Center. Mentoring and research support are available, and faculty are expected to develop productive academic careers. Interested applicants should send a CV to Mary Lou Meyers, MD, Department of Psychiatry, University of Rochester Medical Center, 300 Crittenden Boulevard, Rochester, NY 14642-8409. The University of Rochester is an equal opportunity/affirmative action employer. Applications from women and minority groups are encouraged. A license to practice in New York State will be required.